PLASTIC SURGERY

Editor

JOSEPH G. McCARTHY, M.D.

Lawrence D. Bell Professor of Plastic Surgery and
Director of the Institute of Reconstructive Plastic Surgery
New York University Medical Center
New York, New York

Editors, Hand Surgery Volumes

JAMES W. MAY, JR., M.D.

Director of Plastic Surgery and Hand Surgery Service
Massachusetts General Hospital
Associate Clinical Professor of Surgery
Harvard Medical School
Boston, Massachusetts

J. WILLIAM LITTLER, M.D.

Past Professor of Clinical Surgery
College of Physicians and Surgeons
Columbia University, New York
Senior Attending Surgeon
The St. Luke's–Roosevelt Hospital Center
New York, New York

PLASTIC SURGERY

VOLUME 2

THE FACE

Part 1

W.B. SAUNDERS COMPANY

A Division of Harcourt Brace & Company

Philadelphia ▪ London ▪ Toronto
Montreal ▪ Sydney ▪ Tokyo

W. B. SAUNDERS COMPANY
A Division of
Harcourt Brace & Company

The Curtis Center
Independence Square West
Philadelphia, PA 19106

Library of Congress Cataloging-in-Publication Data

Plastic surgery.
Contents: v. 1. General principles—v. 2–3.
The face—v. 4. Cleft lip & palate and craniofacial anomalies—[etc.]
1. Surgery, Plastic. I. McCarthy, Joseph G., 1938–
[DNLM: 1. Surgery, Plastic. WO 600 P7122]

RD118.P536 1990 617′.95 87–9809

ISBN 0–7216–1514–7 (set)

Editor: W. B. Saunders Staff
Designer: W. B. Saunders Staff
Production Manager: Frank Polizzano
Manuscript Editor: David Harvey
Illustration Coordinator: Lisa Lambert
Indexer: Kathleen Garcia
Cover Designer: Ellen Bodner

Volume 1 0–7216–2542–8
Volume 2 0–7216–2543–6
Volume 3 0–7216–2544–4
Volume 4 0–7216–2545–2
Volume 5 0–7216–2546–0
Volume 6 0–7216–2547–9
Volume 7 0–7216–2548–7
Volume 8 0–7216–2549–5
Plastic Surgery 8 Volume Set 0–7216–1514–7

Printed in the United States of America.

Last digit is the print number: 9 8 7 6 5 4 3

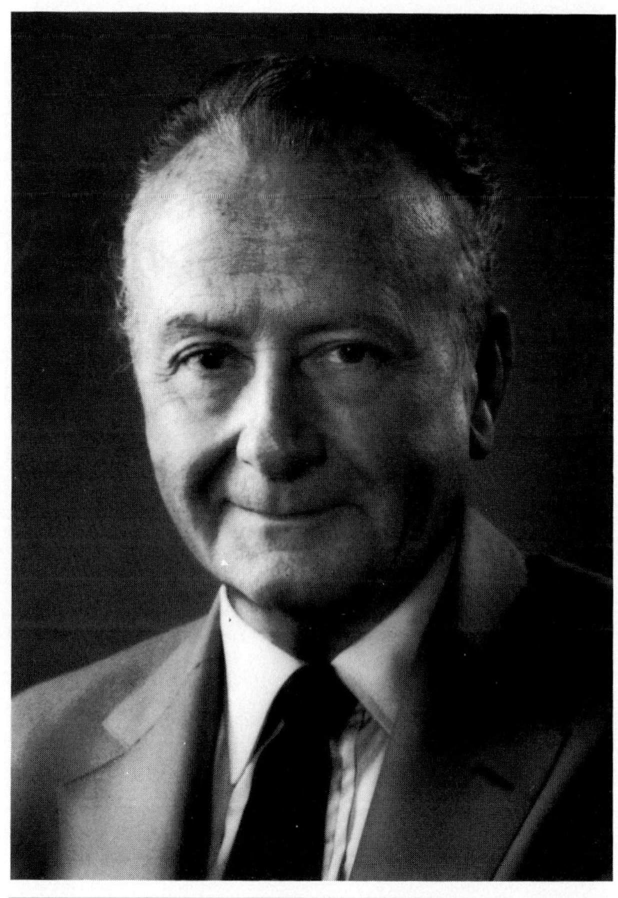

John Marquis Converse

(1909–1981)

This book is dedicated to John Marquis Converse. His enthusiasm for plastic surgery was unrivaled and his contributions to the field were legendary. Through his many writings he not only educated and inspired the plastic surgeon in the era after World War II, but also helped to define modern plastic surgery. This book is a testimony to his professional accomplishments.

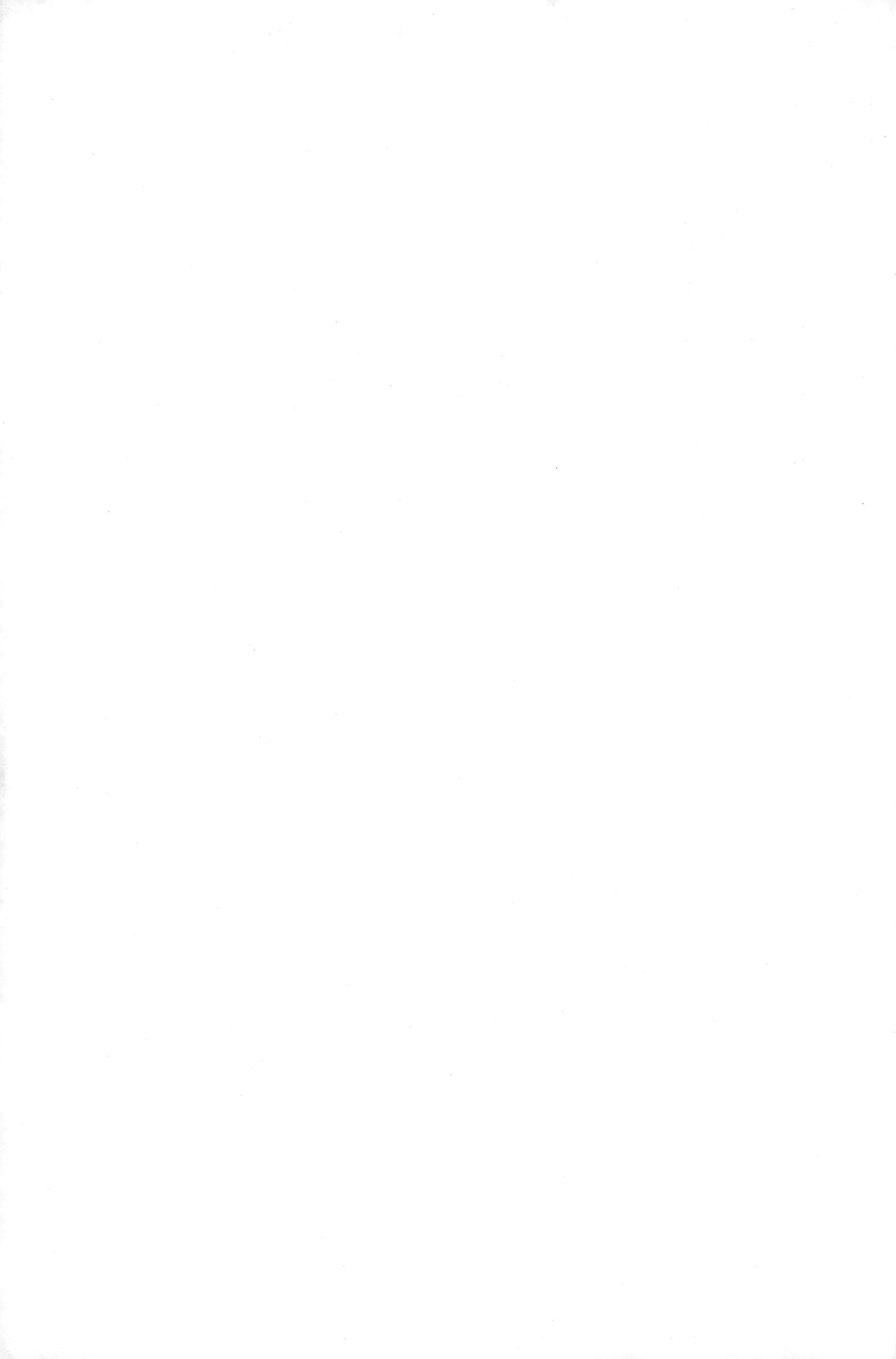

Contributors

PETER J. COCCARO, D.D.S.
Formerly Associate Professor of Orthodontics, New York University School of Dentistry, and Research Professor of Clinical Surgery (Orthodontics), New York University School of Medicine, New York, New York.

STEPHEN R. COLEN, M.D., D.D.S.
Assistant Professor of Surgery (Plastic Surgery), New York University School of Medicine; Attending Surgeon, University Hospital, Bellevue Hospital Center, Manhattan Eye, Ear & Throat Hospital, and New York Eye & Ear Infirmary, New York, New York.

CRAIG R. DUFRESNE, M.D.
Assistant Professor of Plastic Surgery, Johns Hopkins University School of Medicine; Director, The Facial Rehabilitation Center and Cleft Lip and Palate Clinic, Johns Hopkins Hospital and Children's Hospital; Chief of Plastic Surgery Service, Loch Raven Veterans Administration Medical Center; Attending Physician in Plastic Surgery, The Maryland Institute of Emergency Medical Services Systems, Baltimore, Maryland.

BARRY H. GRAYSON, D.D.S.
Associate Professor of Clinical Surgery (Orthodontics), New York University School of Medicine; Associate Professor of Clinical Orthodontics, New York University School of Dentistry, New York, New York.

GLENN W. JELKS, M.D.
Associate Professor of Surgery (Plastic Surgery), New York University School of Medicine; Attending Surgeon, University Hospital, Bellevue Hospital, Manhattan Eye, Ear & Throat Hospital, Manhattan Veterans Administration Hospital, and New York Eye & Ear Infirmary, New York, New York.

HENRY K. KAWAMOTO, JR., M.D., D.D.S.
Associate Clinical Professor, UCLA Division of Plastic Surgery, Los Angeles, California.

PAUL N. MANSON, M.D.
Professor of Plastic Surgery, Johns Hopkins University School of Medicine; Director of Plastic Surgery, The Maryland Institute of Emergency Medical Services Systems; Attending Surgeon, Johns Hopkins Hospital, University Hospital, Children's Hospital and Center for Reconstructive Surgery, and Francis Scott Key Medical Center, Baltimore, Maryland.

DANIEL MARCHAC, M.D.
Professor, Collège de Médecine des Hôpitaux de Paris; Director, Center for Cranio-facial Anomalies, Hôpital Necker-Enfants-Malades, Paris, France.

JOSEPH G. McCARTHY, M.D.
Lawrence D. Bell Professor of Plastic Surgery, New York University School of Medicine; Director, Institute of Reconstructive Plastic Surgery, New York University Medical Center; Attending Surgeon, University Hospital, Bellevue Hospital, Manhattan Eye, Ear and Throat Hospital, and Veterans Administration Hospital, New York, New York.

BYRON C. SMITH, M.D.
Consultant in Ophthalmic Plastic Surgery, Manhattan Eye, Ear & Throat Hospital and New York Eye & Ear Infirmary; Attending Surgeon, Mount Sinai Medical Center, New York, New York.

AUGUSTUS J. VALAURI, D.D.S.
Professor of Surgery (Maxillofacial Prosthetics), New York University School of Medicine; Clinical Professor of Removable Prosthodontics and Occlusion, New York University School of Dentistry;

Chief of the Maxillofacial Prosthetics Service, Institute of Reconstructive Plastic Surgery, New York University Medical Center, New York, New York.

CHARLES P. VALLIS, M.D.
Clinical Instructor in Plastic Surgery, Harvard Medical School; Clinical Instructor in Plastic Surgery and Dermatology, Tufts University School of Medicine; Attending Surgeon, Atlanticare Center, Boston, Massachusetts.

DONALD WOOD-SMITH, M.D., F.R.C.S.E.
Professor of Surgery (Plastic Surgery), New York University School of Medicine; Chairman, Department of Plastic Surgery, New York Eye & Ear Infirmary; Attending Surgeon (Plastic Surgery), Bellevue Medical Center; Attending Surgeon, New York University Hospital, New York Veterans Administration Hospital, and Manhattan Eye, Ear & Throat Hospital, New York, New York.

BARRY M. ZIDE, D.M.D., M.D.
Assistant Professor of Surgery (Plastic Surgery), New York University Medical Center; Attending Surgeon, Bellevue Hospital Center, Manhattan Veterans Administration Hospital, and Manhattan Eye, Ear & Throat Hospital, New York, New York.

Preface

Where does a book begin? Initially, I think of a warm September afternoon in a hotel in Madrid when I first organized an outline of the chapters while waiting for an international surgery meeting to begin. However, a scientific book is only an extension of earlier publications. This text is descended from *Reconstructive Plastic Surgery*, edited in 1964 by my predecessor John Marquis Converse, and reedited in 1977. I had been Assistant Editor of the latter. Many of the ideas and principles, if not the exact words, that were integral to the teaching and writing of Dr. Converse live on in the present volumes. *Reconstructive Plastic Surgery* in turn was derived from his earlier collaboration with V. H. Kazanjian, *The Surgical Treament of Facial Injuries*, published in 1949, 1959, and 1974.

Earlier textbooks by Nélaton and Ombrédanne (1904), Davis (1919), Gillies (1920), and Fomon (1939) had played a germinal role in the development of modern plastic surgery. However, even these books represented only a continuum of publications extending back over the centuries to Tagliacozzi and Sushruta. Indeed, there are also the many surgeons who never published but who by their teachings contributed greatly to the body of knowledge that is represented in the present publication. Their concepts, too, have found their way into the plastic surgery literature for the edification of another generation of students.

My own career has been greatly influenced by my teachers, and their spirit has remained an integral part of my personal and professional life. This heritage of the plastic surgeon–teacher represents the spirit of this book.

The title defines the subject—*Plastic Surgery*. Adjectives such as *reconstructive* or *esthetic* are misleading and redundant and represent artificial divisions of this surgical specialty. The parents of the infant undergoing cleft lip repair are more interested in the *esthetic* aspects of the procedure, which traditionally has been regarded as *reconstructive*. The contemporary face lift, long perceived as an *esthetic* operation, represents a surgical reconstruction of the multiple layers of the soft tissues of the face. Plastic surgery, a term first popularized by Zeis in 1838, is preferred.

With the deliberate exception of parts of Chapters 1 and 35, originally written by Dr. Converse and revised through subsequent editions of various books, few paragraphs in these volumes remain unchanged from the 1977 edition. Many of the authors, however, have used material from the previous editions. Line drawings prepared for these editions by Daisy Stillwell have been reproduced again where appropriate. With the death of Ms. Stillwell, I was fortunate to recruit yet another outstanding medical artist, Craig Luce, to draw hundreds of new illustrations to reflect the continuing developments in this specialty.

The purpose of this book is to define the specialty of plastic surgery. To accomplish this goal, contributions have been sought from the acknowledged leaders of this discipline in all of its ramifications. The clinical applications of plastic surgery, practiced over the whole of the human anatomy, range from skin grafting to the management of uncommon craniofacial clefts, to replantation of the lower extremity. Its practice varies from uncomplicated procedures to sophisticated multistage reconstructions that ally the plastic surgeon with other specialists. The chapters that follow vary in the same way from the short and direct to the lengthy and complex. More than any other, this type of surgery strives for the restoration or improvement of form as well as the restoration of function. The teaching of plastic surgery thus lends itself to illustration. The contributors to this book have been encouraged to use drawings and photographs liberally as an enhancement of the principles and techniques described in the text. Special attention has been given to the sizing and placement of more than 5000 illustrations submitted in accordance with this plan. The contributors and publisher have also made every effort to acknowledge and cite the work of other authors. In a text of this magnitude any omission, while understandable, is regrettable.

In Volume 1 will be found discussions of the essential principles basic to all plastic surgery: wound healing, circulation of the skin, microneurovascular repairs, skin expansion, and grafting of tendons, nerves, and bone, as well as their associated methods of repair. This is the largest of the volumes and testifies to the broadening scope of the field. Much of what is now fundamental to the training of a plastic surgeon was only imagined a generation ago.

After the discussion of general principles in Volume 1, the organization of the text is by anatomic regions. Volumes 2 and 3 are devoted to the face; here, as throughout the book, each chapter draws upon the expertise of acknowledged master surgeons particularly experienced in the subjects on which they have written.

Clefts of the lip and palate as well as severe craniofacial anomalies make up Volume 4. In addition to plastic surgery, these chapters incorporate contributions from the allied fields of embryology, craniofacial growth and development, orthodontics, prosthodontics, speech pathology, and neurosurgery.

Volume 5 covers tumors of the skin and head and neck and Volume 6 the trunk, lower extremity, and genitourinary system. Of particular note, the text details recent advances in reconstruction that involve newly developed flaps of ingenious design and considerable sophistication.

The application of plastic surgical principles and techniques of the upper extremity are discussed in Volumes 7 and 8 under the editorship of Drs. James W. May, Jr., and J. William Littler. The latter, one of the most esteemed and influential hand surgeons of the modern era, edited the upper extremity section in 1964 and 1977. He has been joined in this edition by Dr. May, who is qualified in both hand surgery and microsurgical reconstruction. Both, who are my personal friends, brought their usual enthusiasm, experience, and equanimity to bear on this project. Because surgery of the upper extremity is practiced so extensively, ample space has been afforded for the comprehensive description of the reconstructive procedures specifically designed for the restoration of injured parts. Much of the current progress in plastic surgery of the upper extremity has been made possible by the gradual perfection of microvascular techniques, and these newer developments have been incorporated into the text.

Continuing change, the hallmark of all medical and surgical practice, dictates the need for a reference book such as this and makes its accomplishment a challenging task for everyone involved. With the writing of these words the lengthy process of revising, updating, and improving is ended. The book is committed to the press with the promise that it is both complete and current, in the belief that readers will find it an invaluable resource, and with the hope that it makes a contribution to the body of plastic surgery knowledge and to the education of tomorrow's plastic surgeon.

JOSEPH G. MCCARTHY, M.D.

Acknowledgments

The authors or contributors, all with heavy clinical responsibilities and demands, have contributed greatly and are responsible for this text. In addition to outlining their personal views, they have conducted exhaustive literature searches and have organized their illustrative material. They represent the heart and soul of the book.

I wish also to acknowledge my fellow faculty members at the Institute of Reconstructive Plastic Surgery, since their work and concepts, as well as their encouragement, have been so important in the development of this text: Sherrell J. Aston, Donald L. Ballantyne, Robert W. Beasley, Phillip R. Casson, David T.W. Chiu, Peter J. Coccaro, Stephen R. Colen, Court B. Cutting, Barry H. Grayson, V. Michael Hogan, Glenn W. Jelks, Frances C. Macgregor, Thomas D. Rees, Blair O. Rogers, William W. Shaw, John W. Siebert, Charles H. M. Thorne, Augustus J. Valauri, Donald Wood-Smith, and Barry M. Zide. Dr. Frank Cole Spencer, George David Stewart Professor of Surgery and Chairman of the Department of Surgery at the New York University Medical Center, has always championed the goals of the Institute and has especially encouraged development in the newer areas of craniofacial surgery and microsurgery.

I should also pay tribute to Ms. Karen Singer, who did so much of the bibliographic study, and Wayne Pearson and Harry Weissfisch, who provided photographic support. I must also acknowledge my associates at the Institute, Robert E. Bochat, Linda Gerson, Donna O'Brien, Caren Crane, Marilyn Deaton, Margy Maroutsis, Marjorie Huggins, and others for acts of kindness and support during the years of preparation of this book.

Mr. Albert Meier, Senior Editor at Saunders, had a major share in the organization and editing of this book. A friend and colleague since 1974 when we began the Second Edition, I have benefited immensely from his advice and counsel. He has also shown an unusual sense of understanding throughout this project. Special thanks are also due to David Harvey, Frank Polizzano, and Richard Zorab of the W. B. Saunders Company for their support.

I am also grateful to the residents and fellows at the Institute of Reconstructive Plastic Surgery, whose boundless enthusiasm is ever encouraging and who have given generously of their time to proofread manuscripts and galleys: Christopher Attinger, Constance Barone, Richard Bartlett, P. Craig Hobar, William Hoffman, Armen Kasabian, Gregory LaTrenta, George Peck, Rosa Razaboni, Gregory Ruff, John Siebert, R. Kendrick Slate, Henry Spinelli, Michael Stevens, Charles Thorne, and Douglas Wagner.

Special thanks are also due to my colleagues and friends at the National Foundation for Facial Reconstruction, whose support and encouragement have provided a unique environment at the Institute that is conducive to writing and research.

Finally, I want to thank my family, Karlan, Cara, and Stephen, for their love and understanding during the demanding years of this project, especially those times spent at a desk when I may have appeared distracted or lost in thought. They remain my main support and life focus.

I also want to thank my friends, especially Charles and Heather Garbaccio, who had the ability to offer those special moments of lightheartedness, good cheer, and camaraderie.

JGM

Contents

Volume 2

The Face (Part 1)

27

Facial Injuries 867
Paul N. Manson

28

Pediatric Facial Trauma 1142
Craig R. Dufresne • Paul N. Manson

29

Surgery of the Jaws 1188
Joseph G. McCarthy • Henry K. Kawamoto
Barry H. Grayson • Stephen R. Colen
Peter J. Coccaro • Donald Wood-Smith

30

The Temporomandibular Joint 1475
Barry M. Zide

31

Hair Replacement Surgery 1514
Charles P. Vallis

32

Deformities of the Forehead, Scalp, and Cranial Vault 1538
Daniel Marchac

33

The Orbit and Zygoma 1574
Joseph G. McCarthy • Glenn W. Jelks
Augustus J. Valauri • Donald Wood-Smith
Byron C. Smith

34

Reconstruction of the Eyelids and Associated Structures 1671
Glenn W. Jelks • Byron C. Smith

Index i

27

Paul N. Manson

Facial Injuries*

INITIAL ASSESSMENT
- Timing of Facial Injury Treatment
- Evaluation of the Multiply Injured Patient
- Head Injuries
- Cervical Spine Injuries
- Emergency Treatment
- Clinical Examination

ROENTGENOGRAPHIC DIAGNOSIS

TREATMENT OF SOFT TISSUE WOUNDS
- Tetanus Prophylaxis
- Delayed Primary Wound Closure
- Cleaning of the Wound
- Photography
- Preoperative Considerations
- Anesthesia
- Debridement and Care

FRACTURES OF THE CRANIOFACIAL SKELETON
- Dentition
- Fractures of the Mandible
- Fractures of the Nasal Bones and Cartilages
- Fractures of the Zygoma
- Fractures of the Maxilla
- Complex (Panfacial) Fractures
- Orbital and Nasoethmoido-orbital Fractures
- Fractures of Frontobasilar Region

GUNSHOT WOUNDS OF THE FACE

POST-TRAUMATIC FACIAL PAIN

Few injuries are as challenging as those of the face. Physicians have a dual responsibility: repair of the esthetic defect (restore the preinjury appearance) and restoration of function. A unique aspect of facial injuries is that the restoration of appearance may be the chief indication for treatment. In other cases, injuries might require surgery solely to restore function.

Although there are few facial emergencies, the literature has underemphasized the advantages of prompt definitive reconstruction of facial injuries and the contribution of early treatment to superior esthetic and functional results. Economic, sociologic, and psychologic factors operating in a competitive society make it imperative that an aggressive, expedient, and well-planned program be outlined, executed, and maintained in order to return the patient to an active, productive life as soon as possible with minimal esthetic and functional disability. A facial injury victim often sustains multiple injuries to other organ systems (Fig. 27–1). Thus, early definitive care of the maxillofacial injury must be accomplished safely at the same time that other (perhaps life-threatening) conditions are being evaluated and treated. After the life threatening injuries have been managed, the patient's principal concerns frequently involve residual facial deformity.

The incidence of facial injuries is high because the face is exposed and because there is little protective covering. Two-thirds of patients admitted to the Maryland Institute for Emergency Medical Services Systems (MIEMSS), an area-wide trauma center receiving injury victims from the state of Maryland, have injuries of the head and face. The causes of facial injuries in the United States

*Portions of this chapter are revised from sections of Chapters 24 and 25 in the predecessor of this book, Converse, J.M. (Ed.): *Reconstructive Plastic Surgery* (2nd ed., 1977), which was prepared by R.O. Dingman, J.M. Converse, B. Smith, and D. Wood Smith.

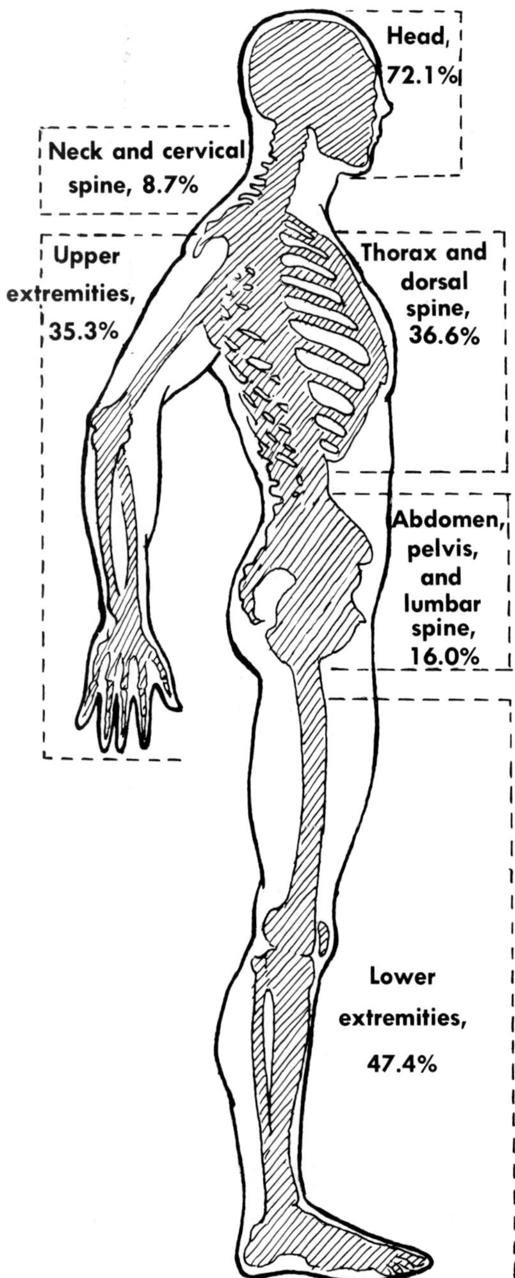

Figure 27–1. Motor vehicle accidents can result in multiple injuries. Two-thirds of the victims suffer injuries to the head and facial area. Other anatomic areas also are often involved. (From Patterns of Disease, a publication of Parke, Davis & Co.)

include motor vehicle accidents, assaults and altercations, animal bites, bicycle accidents, home and industrial accidents, and athletic injuries (Rowe and Killey, 1968; Dingman and Natvig, 1964; Kazanjian and Converse, 1974). The automobile is frequently responsible for the most devastating facial injuries. In automobile accidents, injuries to the head, face, and cervical spine occur in over 75 per cent of all victims. There are over 50,000 traffic fatalities each year in the U.S. In addition to the number killed, 40 patients require hospitalization for every person who is fatally injured. Thus, over 4,000,000 people are injured in automobile accidents in the U.S. each year and many have a facial injury.

Statistics on the number of facial injuries due to various etiologic factors are not significant: there is a wide variation in different samples because of social, economic, and geographic factors. Whereas smaller emergency rooms may see a greater proportion of injuries due to altercations, falls, and home and athletic accidents, the major trauma centers treat a patient group in whom the etiologic factor is either a motor vehicle accident or a ballistic injury. Alcohol abuse is frequently a contributing factor. The concepts advanced in this chapter were developed at MIEMSS. The proportion of severe (as opposed to minor or moderate) injuries is high. The concepts, however, can be modified appropriately for general use in the treatment of lesser degrees of facial trauma.

There have been a number of advances in the construction of automobiles and the regulation of traffic that relate to protection from injury. The use of restraints, the introduction of padded dashboards, the multilaminated windshield, and improvements in the design of rear-view mirrors and steering wheels have reduced the severity of injuries. The introduction of the 55 mph speed limit resulted in a decreased incidence of major (Le Fort and panfacial) fractures. Other factors, such as check points, stiffer penalties for "drunk driving," and the increased economic burden of more expensive motor fuels have contributed to the decrease in facial injuries from motor vehicle accidents. At MIEMSS fewer facial ballistic injuries have been observed and, in those currently seen, less destructive weapons have been involved. Unfortunately, the popularity of the motorcycle is still a major factor in the etiology of major facial trauma.

INITIAL ASSESSMENT

The management of facial fractures has undergone significant changes within the last ten years.

1. The injuries are now diagnosed with a high degree of radiologic accuracy through

the routine use of computed tomographic (CT) scanning. The scans visualize both soft tissue and bone with unexcelled clarity. Relationships previously not discernible from plain films are clearly apparent.

2. The advent of regional trauma centers has provided improved diagnostic and supportive care for multiply injured patients. A system of invasive diagnosis and continuous monitoring of all organ systems allows patients with facial injuries to be operated on at an early time with safety.

3. The application of craniofacial techniques of exposure (Jones, Whitaker, and Murtagh, 1977; Wolfe, 1982) has improved the ability to restore the preinjury facial appearance.

4. The techniques (Gruss, 1985; Gruss and associates, 1985b; Manson and associates, 1985, 1986b, 1988) of extended open reduction of facial fractures and replacement of missing or unusable bone with grafts as a primary procedure, and the use of multiple interfragment wire or plate and screw fixation have improved the functional and esthetic results of facial fracture treatment.

Timing of Facial Injury Treatment

Timing is especially important in the optimal management of facial injuries. It is axiomatic that soft tissue and bone injuries in the facial area be managed as soon as is consistent with the patient's general condition (Mektubjian, 1982). Time and time again, it has been the author's impression that early, skillful management decreases the possibility of permanent facial disfigurement and limits serious functional disturbances. Although facial soft tissue and bone injuries are rarely acute surgical emergencies (as far as closure of the wounds or reduction of fractures is concerned), there are few patients whose injuries cannot be definitively managed within a short time after admission. Some exceptions to acute treatment include patients who have ongoing significant blood loss (such as pelvic fractures), whose intracranial pressure exceeds 25 torr, or whose pulmonary ventilation pressures are rapidly increasing.

Table 27–1. Glasgow Coma Scale (GCS)

I. Best Verbal Response	
None	1
Incomprehensible sound	2
Inappropriate words	3
Confused	4
Oriented	5
II. Eyes Open	
None	1
To pain	2
To speech	3
Spontaneously	4
III. Best Motor Response	
None	1
Abnormal extension	2

Evaluation of the Multiply Injured Patient

Patients with dramatic facial injuries are often rapidly (and inappropriately) assigned to a subspecialty service. It is important, therefore, that subspecialists consider first whether the patient has been adequately evaluated for the presence of multiple injuries (see Fig. 27–1) (Schultz, 1967; Gwyn and associates, 1971; Christian, 1976). This includes provision for control of the airway, control of external bleeding, insertion of intravenous lines, and insertion of a Foley catheter. The usual protocol for systems evaluation at MIEMSS includes examination for head injuries (Glasgow Coma Scale) (Table 27–1), upright chest and cervical spine radiographs, peritoneal lavage, and radiographs of the pelvis and appropriate extremities. Diagnostic failures occur in 12 per cent of motor vehicle accident victims and 23 per cent of motorcycle victims in some series (Chan, Ainscow, and Sikorski, 1980). Frequent errors include clinical misjudgments, failure to follow routine systems protocols, false interpretation of obtained examinations, and inadequate radiographs. In multiply injured or comatose patients, all organ systems must be evaluated by protocol and continuously monitored throughout the initial resuscitation and operative treatment.

While the protocol systems examinations are in progress, the face may be examined. Facial wounds may be cleansed and protected with a sterile dressing, or the margins of the wound may be tacked together with a few well-placed sutures. These measures limit further contamination. Bleeding facial lacerations are usually controlled with direct pressure. Blind probing or clamping with hemostats without direct visualization is contraindicated, to avoid injury to delicate structures such as branches of the facial nerve. It should be noted that branches of the facial nerve are frequently located adjacent to arterial branches.

Head Injuries

Cerebral injury includes that due to mechanical damage to neurons and that resulting from secondary ischemia and edema (Gurdjian and Webster, 1958). Ischemia is aggravated by the presence of mass lesions, brain swelling, and increased intracranial pressure, which lead (in a progressive cycle) to intracranial hypertension, increased pressure, and progressive ischemia. Patients with head injuries should be evaluated by a clinical examination that classifies the severity of injury according to the Glasgow Coma Scale (Table 27–1). This scale relates the patient's level of consciousness, eye opening response, and ability to speak and move extremities to the prognosis. A CT scan identifies mass lesions, cerebral contusion, shift of the midline, extradural or intradural hematoma, skull fractures, and intracranial air. Patients with head injuries have a less favorable prognosis with increasing age, decreasing Glasgow Coma score, decreasing systemic blood pressure, and abnormal posturing. Additional factors correlating with prognosis include spontaneous and reflex eye movements and pupil reactivity to light. Accompanying spinal injuries, pulmonary injuries, and shock worsen the prognosis. Children have a more favorable prognosis than do adults.

The presence of coma should not contraindicate the treatment of a maxillofacial injury (Teasdale and Jennett, 1974; Becker and associates, 1977). Neurosurgical studies have shown that patients in coma that has lasted more than one week to one month have a hopeful prognosis in terms of returning to a functional role in society. In one study, one-fourth of patients in coma whose duration exceeded one week died, one-fourth were disabled, and one-half returned to useful work (McDonald, 1980). Thus, the presence of coma should never be used as an excuse to defer treatment of the facial injury. This practice relegates the esthetic and functional result that might be achieved by treatment to a substandard level. Head injury patients who survive especially need the benefit of the improved esthetic and functional results obtainable by early treatment. Safe anesthesia is achieved with intracranial pressure monitoring (Fig. 27–2).

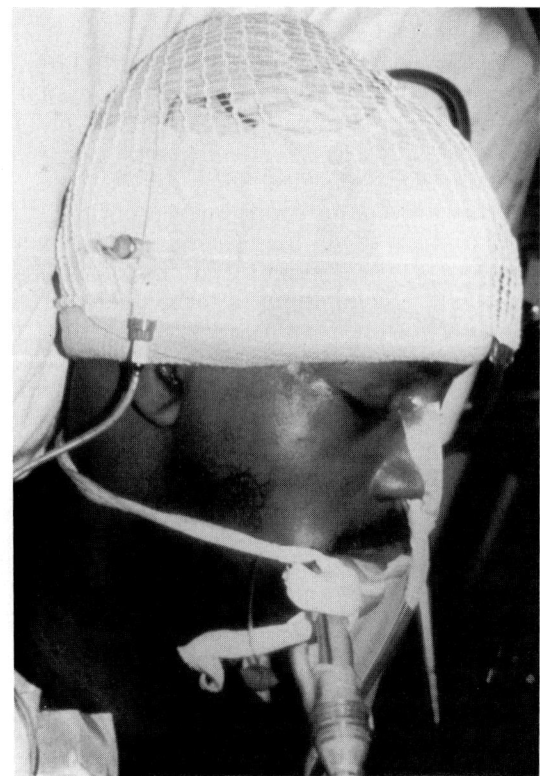

Figure 27–2. Intracranial pressure is monitored continuously in patients with head injuries.

Despite the progress that has occurred in the treatment of major head injuries, one should not assume that minor head injuries do not have significant permanent sequelae. Even in patients in whom the duration of coma was less than 20 minutes, 80 per cent demonstrate some late symptoms such as headaches, memory difficulty, and problems with interpersonal relationships. Decreased attention span and concentration and judgment problems reflect some degree of organic brain damage. The patients, who frequently relate problems in work, school, and home, can benefit from intervention by a head injury rehabilitation center program or from proper guidance.

Cervical Spine Injuries

Injuries to the cervical spine often accompany those of the head and face. A significant cervical cord injury exists in one out of 300 accident victims, or one out of 14 occupants who are ejected from their cars (Babcock, 1976; Bucholz and associates, 1979; Huelke,

O'Day, and Mendelsohn, 1981). All patients (especially those who are unconscious) should be considered to have a spinal injury until it is proved otherwise. Patients who fail to move their extremities on command or sternal pressure, who have penetrating trauma to the neck, who complain of pain in the neck, or who describe disturbances in sensation or motor function must be assumed to have a cervical injury. The association of facial and cervical injuries has been documented in a large study in which 10 per cent of those with facial fractures had a cervical spine injury, and 18 per cent of those with cervical spine injuries had a maxillofacial injury (Gwyn and associates, 1971; Lewis and associates, 1985). The study also documented an association between fractures of the mandible and those of the upper cervical spine. Upper facial injuries were associated with cervical hyperextension injuries at all levels. Careful reviews of cervical injuries indicated that the most commonly missed lesions involved the base of the skull—C1/C2 and C6/C7. These areas are notoriously more difficult to visualize on radiographs and the failure to adequately demonstrate these areas allows the fractures to be missed. CT scans are more accurate than plain radiographs and may require less patient neck movement. Both cerebral and cervical spine injuries may occur secondary to whiplash without head contact or skull or facial fracture. The diagnostic principle to be emphasized is that if one is unable to visualize the whole cervical spine radiographically and confirm that the patient is asymptomatic, he must be treated as if he has a cervical fracture, by proper immobilization and limited movement of the head.

Anterior cervical cord compression produces a syndrome of motor paralysis and loss of pain and temperature sense below the level of the lesion, with preservation of dorsal column sensation (pain, touch, and vibration). *Posterior cord compression* affects dorsal column sensation. Acute central cord compression results in greater motor impairment of the upper limbs than of the lower, and is usually due to central hemorrhage and bruising. Many cervical cord injuries are incomplete and thus can be aggravated by improper diagnosis and treatment. There is evidence that the cycle of ischemia and vasoconstriction, mentioned in the cycle of cerebral injury progression, can also occur and aggravate the cervical cord lesion.

The treatment of maxillofacial injuries should be organized in several phases:

1. Emergency measures.
2. Early treatment.
3. Delayed treatment.

Emergency Treatment

There are three life-threatening facial emergencies:

1. Respiratory obstruction.
2. Hemorrhage.
3. Aspiration.

RESPIRATORY OBSTRUCTION

Establishment and control of the airway is a primary and important consideration in the clinical management of the acutely injured patient. Asphyxia is an ever-present threat in patients with injuries to the lower jaw, combined facial injuries, or laryngeal trauma. The mouth must be cleared of broken teeth, fractured dentures, foreign bodies, and clots that might be causing obstruction. Traction on the mandible or tongue pulls these structures away from the pharynx and allows removal or retrieval of objects displaced into that location (Fig. 27–3). In fractures of the mandible that are unstable, the jaw may be displaced posteriorly with the tongue falling against the posterior wall of the pharynx, obstructing respiration (Fig. 27–3). In these cases, it helps to place the patient in a prone or sitting position with the head down and forward if he can be turned or moved into that location without aggravating other injuries. Anterior traction on the tongue with a towel clip, suture, forceps, or fingers may avert asphyxia in patients who cannot be turned so that the tongue would be displaced forward by gravity.

Respiratory obstruction is most likely to occur with combined fractures of the maxilla, mandible, and nose, or in patients with massive hemorrhage or soft tissue swelling. Patients especially prone to difficulty are those with stupor or coma resulting from head injury. Consideration should be given to immediate intubation in these cases. Patients with laryngeal or tracheal injuries and significant facial burns benefit from intubation.

Respiratory obstruction may result in rapid demise. Only a short time exists between the onset of significant symptoms of respiratory

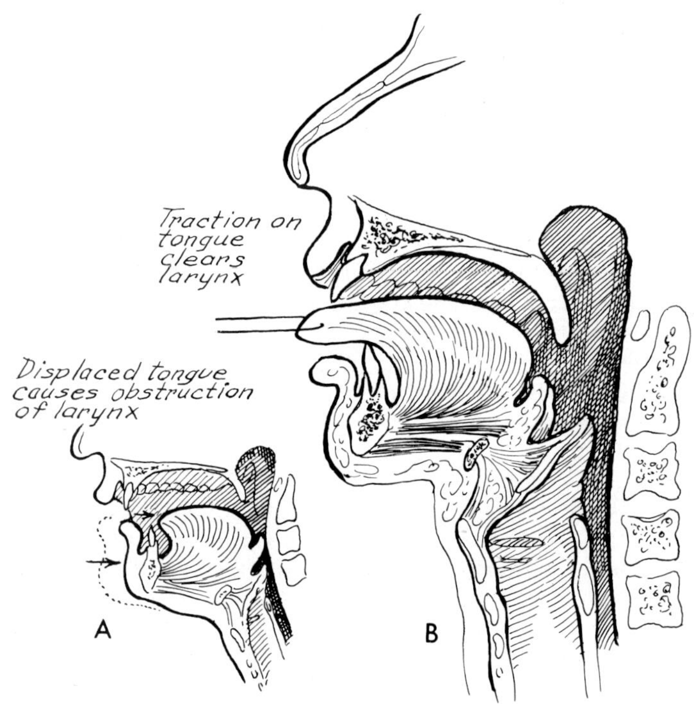

Figure 27–3. When the mandible is unsupported because of bilateral fractures (the body or subcondylar), respiratory obstruction can be produced by the mandible falling backward, allowing the tongue to lie against the posterior pharyngeal wall *(A)*. Holding the tongue or the anterior portion of the mandible forward with traction *(B)* clears the obstruction. If the patient can be turned to the prone position, the action of gravity displaces the tongue structures anteriorly.

obstruction (e.g., stridor, hoarseness, retraction, drooling, inability to swallow, restlessness, air hunger, cyanosis, tracheal tug, or retraction of supraclavicular, intercostal, or epigastreal areas) and total inability to breathe. An alert clinician anticipates an advancing respiratory obstruction and performs a prophylactic intubation before a crash or chaotic emergency intubation or tracheostomy becomes necessary. In extremely urgent cases, when oral or nasal intubation is not feasible, a cricothyroidotomy or coniotomy is the preferred treatment, incising transversely through the skin and cricothyroid ligament (conic ligament) between the thyroid and cricoid cartilages (Fig. 27–4). Cricothyroidotomy is the preferred emergency surgical treatment of airway obstruction. After the procedure, the coniotomy should be closed after conversion to tracheotomy; the latter avoids the damage that occurs when a coniotomy is used for long-standing intubation.

An emergency (low) tracheotomy may be performed in the following manner. The trachea is grasped between the fingers and the thumb. An incision is made through the skin in the midline between the thyroid cartilage and the sternal notch, and deepened into the trachea (vertically); the tracheal incision should be below the second tracheal ring. A cannula, catheter, or endotracheal tube or tracheostomy tube is inserted to keep the opening patent.

Elective Tracheotomy

Early tracheotomy is an advantage in patients with panfacial fractures and in those with head or chest injuries when they are

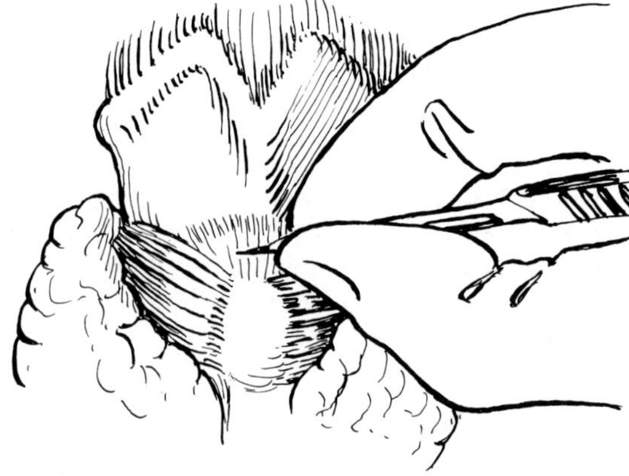

Figure 27–4. Coniotomy. The cricothyroid membrane, following a skin incision, is incised transversely. The direction of the cricothyroid membrane fibers favors opening of the wound to provide an airway, especially with the head extended. The knife should be grasped firmly to prevent the inadvertent entrance of the knife into the esophagus and development of an acute tracheoesophageal fistula.

unlikely to be awake or be able to manage the airway within a brief period (one week). The tracheotomy facilitates placing the patient in intermaxillary fixation and clears the oral or nasal area of obstructing tubes. Patients in whom the floor of the mouth, tongue, and hypopharynx are becoming increasingly edematous, and who require intermaxillary fixation, should also be considered for tracheotomy. Patients who have an adequate airway but are maintaining it only by sheer effort will be more comfortable (and the surgeon will be more secure) if an airway is established by intubation or tracheotomy. The tracheotomy provides a route by which a general anesthetic may be administered and one that does not interfere with the reduction of fractures in the facial area.

Indications for Tracheotomy. These include:

1. Unrelieved obstruction of the airway in the region of the larynx or the hypopharynx.
2. The probability that edema might result in serious decrease in size of the airway above the larynx.
3. Intracranial or chest injury with difficulty in maintaining adequate ventilation by normal reflex activity or endotracheal intubation.
4. Chest or high spinal cord injuries with loss of normal cough reflexes to clear the bronchial tree of fluids, blood, or secretions.
5. The possibility of prolonged postoperative airway problems.
6. The need for intermaxillary fixation in comatose patients or those with chest injuries.
7. Panfacial fractures.
8. Severe facial burns.
9. Concern about a difficult reintubation.

Techniques of Tracheotomy. The *coniotomy* procedure is useful in extreme emergencies when time is of the essence. Coniotomy is performed by making an incision (or passing a large-bore needle or two) through the cricothyroid membranes (conus elasticus). Although not recommended as a routine procedure, coniotomy may be employed as a lifesaving measure (see Fig. 27–4). The cricothyroid membrane lies superficially and the overlying tissues are relatively avascular except for the anterior jugular veins that are close to the operative incision.

When there is sufficient time to carry out an elective procedure, or when a semiurgent situation exists under satisfactory conditions, the low tracheotomy is the operation of choice. The *low tracheotomy* is made below the thyroid isthmus. The opening is generally in the second and third, or preferably in the third and fourth, tracheal rings.

The patient should be placed in the dorsal recumbent position (Fig. 27–5). The shoulders should be elevated by a sheet and the head extended if this position is permitted by the absence of cervical injury (Fig. 27–5). The neck is extended (if there are no cervical fractures) as much as feasible in order to bring the trachea into the best relationship for exposure and incision. Positioning is especially important when the neck is short or thick, or when the patient has heavy neck musculature.

Tracheotomy may be performed relatively easily, under a local anesthetic or with a general anesthetic when an endotracheal tube is in place. If a local anesthetic is to be used, the skin is infiltrated, as well as the deep structures down to the tracheal level. When the trachea is entered, the endotracheal tube is retracted to the superior level of the tracheal opening, and the tracheostomy tube can be immediately inserted and the inner trochar removed. The endotracheal tube is still in place in the event of emergency. The anesthetic connections can be applied to the tracheotomy cannula and the general anesthetic continued if indicated.

The *elective tracheotomy* operation (Fig. 27–6) is performed through a 4 cm transverse incision approximately 2 to 3 cm above the suprasternal notch (Fig. 27–6*A*). The incision is planned to be directly over the tracheal opening. The incision line should fall exactly within skin creases. Hypertrophy of the scar has been noticed in the exact area of an incision that has strayed from the relaxed lines of skin tension (Rubin, 1948). Location

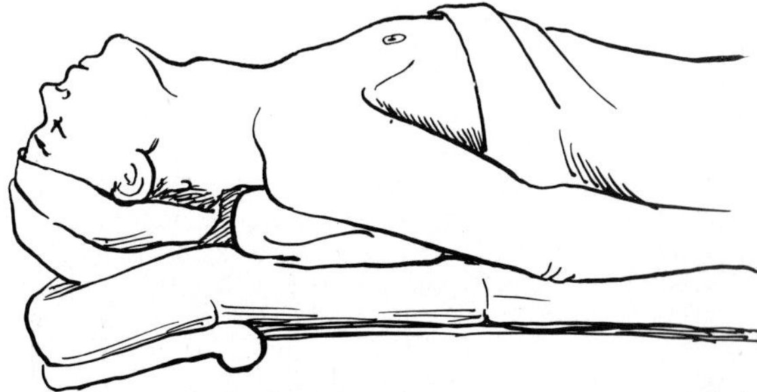

Figure 27–5. The tracheotomy is most easily performed with the patient in the dorsal recumbent position, the head and shoulders being placed on a roll to extend the neck.

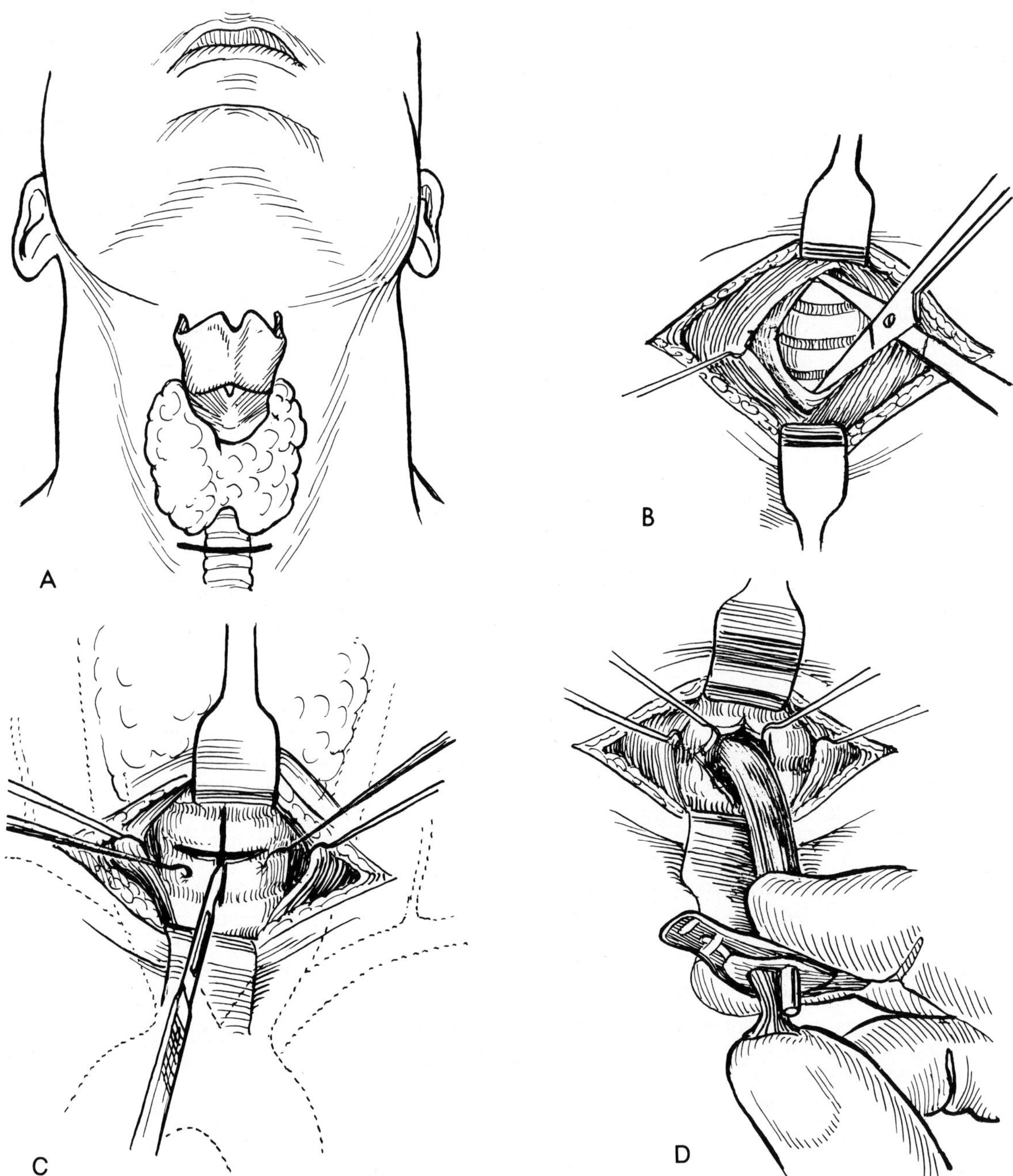

Figure 27–6. Exposure of the trachea for tracheotomy. *A,* A 5 cm incision approximately 2 fingerbreadths above the sternal notch provides excellent exposure and a scar that is in the relaxed lines of skin tension. The incision is deepened through the superficial fascia of the neck to expose the strap muscles. *B,* Dissection is performed separating the strap muscles in the midline by dividing the fascia. Blunt dissection with scissors exposes the trachea. *C,* The trachea is stabilized by hooks to prevent rotation. A cruciate or longitudinal incision is made. *D,* Retraction of the edges of the incision of the trachea allows the insertion of an appropriately sized and pretested cuffed tracheostomy tube.

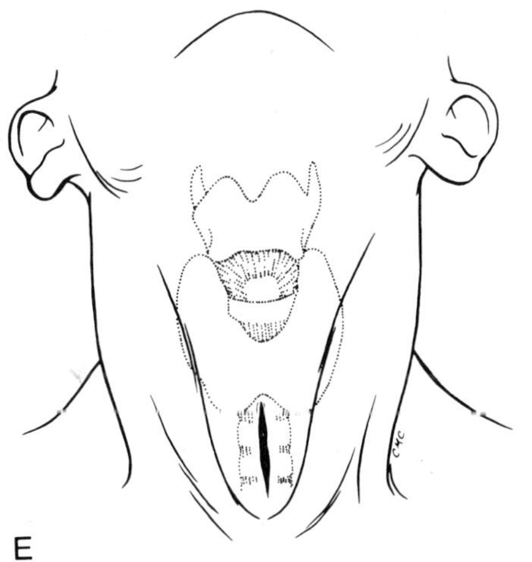

E

Figure 27–6 *Continued E,* The tracheal opening is made through the third and fourth tracheal rings, and the incision is separated for the insertion of the tube.

of the skin incision directly over the tracheal opening avoids irritation of the skin, dislodgement of the tube, or tension on the skin.

The incision should be made through the skin and subcutaneous tissue to the level of the superficial fascia of the neck. Small bleeding vessels should be clamped and electrocoagulated. Larger veins, such as the anterior jugular, if transected, should be ligated with silk sutures. An incision is made vertically in the fascia between the strap muscles exactly in the midline of the neck (Fig. 27–6*B*). The isthmus of the thyroid should be located after separation of the strap muscles of the neck. If it cannot be conveniently retracted, the isthmus should be incised in a vertical direction after ligation with suture ligatures. The deep fascia overlying the trachea is apparent and the glistening cartilages are easily identified. Both the lower portion of the larynx and the cricoid cartilage below the larynx should be palpated. A sharp hook is then placed in each side of the trachea and the trachea is raised into a position for incision. The anesthesiologist, if present, should be warned before an incision is made in the trachea. The balloon on the cuff of an endotracheal tube should be deflated at this time. Rotation of the trachea before the incision is made should be avoided. The tracheal incision was formerly made in a cruciate manner (Fig. 27–6*C*) between the third and fourth tracheal rings. It is the author's preference to make this in a vertical manner (Fig. 27–6*E*), spreading the edges and inserting the endotracheal tube. No cartilage is removed.

Some surgeons prefer to place a suture in the sides of the tracheal incision and to bring these sutures out through the skin. The purpose of this precaution is to allow easy and direct retraction of the trachea if inadvertent decannulation occurs. These sutures can be trimmed in the early postoperative period.

After the tracheal incision has been made, a tracheostomy tube of adequate diameter and length, with the trochar in place, which has been previously tested for cuff integrity, is inserted into the trachea under direct vision (Fig. 27–6*D*). Tracheostomy tubes have been inadvertently placed in the fascial spaces of the neck and alongside or in front of the trachea. If the tracheostomy tube is too long, it may irritate the carina or ventilate only one lung by intubation of one of the main stem bronchi. If the tube is too firm or curved too acutely, it can erode the surface of the trachea and cause necrosis of the tracheal wall, resulting in a fistula. The esophagus or a major blood vessel may be involved. Soft, low pressure (cuff) tracheostomy tubes are preferred. Semiflexible silicone material seems to cause less irritation and the tubes are less likely to result in complications than are metal tubes. After the tracheostomy tube has been inserted, the edges of the skin incision are closed with several interrupted sutures and the tube may be secured to the cervical skin both by means of sutures and by a tie through the edges of the cuff on the tracheostomy tube. These two measures prevent dislodgement. Fabric tape is tied around the neck at the close of the procedure. The fixation must be sufficiently secure so that the tube cannot be dislodged from the trachea when the patient coughs or moves the neck. Blood and secretions are carefully aspirated from the trachea through the tube periodically.

After insertion of the tracheostomy tube, the wound should not be allowed to close too tightly, otherwise trapped air may pass along the fascial spaces of the face and neck, resulting in troublesome subcutaneous emphysema. The wound is sutured loosely, leaving it funnel shaped outwardly so that the air cannot be trapped in the subcutaneous tissue and fascial spaces.

Postoperative care of tracheostomy patients requires diligence. It is distressing to see patients who have retained secretions with tracheostomy tubes partially plugged by mucus and crust, and an infected tracheotomy wound with macerated skin surrounding it, or patients unable to make their wants known or to communicate. All these conditions can be avoided by proper care.

The tracheostomy tube should be aspirated frequently with a sterile disposable catheter, using a glove. The nature of tracheal secretions should be monitored and appropriate cultures taken if indicated. The tracheotomy wound itself should be cleansed with hydrogen peroxide on cotton-tipped applicators, and a lubricating antibiotic ointment may be applied as necessary. The wound may be protected with a gauze dressing to keep it dry and clean until healing has occurred. Since a tracheotomized patient is unable to speak, a pad of paper and a pencil at the bedside are helpful in maintaining communication and providing a sense of security. Oxygen should be humidified and delivered through a cuff or tent over the tracheostomy stoma. The humidification is necessary to prevent excessive drying of the respiratory mucosa. Humidification moistens the gases passing into the bronchi and facilitates the removal of secretions that would otherwise become dry and inspissated. Particular attention should be paid to the task of intermittently deflating the balloon of the cuff of the tracheostomy tube. If the tube has more than one balloon, they should be inflated alternately. Such care prevents continuous mucosal pressure and the development of tracheal necrosis, erosion, and fistula.

Complications of Tracheotomy. As with all seemingly simple operative procedures, complications (Meade, 1961; Cambell, 1962) may follow, but these are mostly avoidable.

Operative Complications. These may include:

1. Severe hemorrhage from vessels of the neck, which may be difficult to control if exposure, lighting, and assistants are inadequate. If too low an exposure is attempted, the large vessels in the chest may be damaged. Hemorrhage from the innominate artery or thyroid arteries may occur from inappropriate dissection.

2. Inadvertent damage to the larynx or cricoid cartilage from inappropriately placed incisions.

3. Cutting through the back wall of the trachea, producing a tracheoesophageal fistula. Inadequate exposure is the cause of this complication, which most often occurs in children.

4. Pneumothorax from damage to the apex of the pleura or one or both lungs.

Postoperative Complications. These may include:

1. Secondary hemorrhage from vessels within the immediate operative dissection or from erosion of the tracheostomy tube through the trachea and into a large vessel, such as the innominate artery.

2. Subcutaneous emphysema from air leaking into the fascial spaces of the neck.

3. Dislodgement of the tracheostomy tube. After dislodgement, the tube is frequently reinserted hurriedly, often in a region outside the trachea.

4. Infection of the wound.

5. Erosion of the trachea with tracheomalacia and stenosis.

6. Tracheoesophageal fistula.

7. Aerophagia, which may result in distressing abdominal distention, gastrointestinal atony, paralytic ileus, and death.

8. Recurrent respiratory obstruction from blood, mucus, and purulent materials in the tube.

9. Ulcerative tracheobronchitis.

10. Retained tracheobronchial secretions with lung abscess.

Late Complications. These may include:

1. Unsightly scar formation.

2. Adherence of the scar to the trachea (routine following decannulation of a tracheostomy that has been present for some time).

3. Injury to the trachea or tracheal cartilage with tracheomalacia, tracheal atresia, or stenosis. Collapse of the trachea may occur from inadequate support, or the tracheal opening may be narrowed by scarring or granulation tissue. A bronchoscopy is necessary to establish this diagnosis.

4. Persistent tracheocutaneous fistula after long-standing tracheostomy.

CONTROL OF SEVERE HEMORRHAGE IN FACIAL WOUNDS

Lacerations and crush injuries of the facial region may result in significant hemorrhage that may be life threatening. Methods of control include local pressure, dressings, the application of fine clamps, ligation, or packing. Hemostatic materials and nasal tamponade to pack the nasal cavity and sinuses may be required (Fig. 27–7). Such packs may be gradually removed over a two to three day period or may be removed as soon as the patient's general condition improves and the hemorrhage has abated. Approximation of wound edges with a few sutures or reduction of the fracture often diminishes hemorrhage. Careful final suturing can be accomplished later when adequate exposure and time permit a precise repair. Secondary bleeding is occasionally observed in facial injuries but usually responds to the methods described for acute bleeding. Since hemorrhage may be rapid and exsanguinating, evaluation of the effective circulating blood volume with replacement therapy is indicated if blood loss has been significant. It is not uncommon for patients to swallow several hundred milliliters of blood from severe nasal, oral, or pharyngeal bleeding. Alternatively, significant quantities of blood can be aspirated into the pulmonary tracheobronchial system. Patients seem to be swallowing frequently and epigastric distention may be noted; significant hemorrhage may be disguised and unrecognized because of the persistent swallowing of blood.

There are three techniques for control of closed hemorrhage from the nasopharyngeal region, which is usually due to lacerations of arteries or veins in fractured sinus cavities of the face. The internal maxillary artery is commonly the source of bleeding.

Anteroposterior Nasal Packing (Fig. 27–7). Efficient anteroposterior nasal packing can be achieved with two 30 to 50 ml balloon Foley catheters. One is inserted through each nostril, inflated in the pharynx, and pulled to occlude the posterior nasopharyngeal opening on each side. This maneuver provides a posterior obturator. Several packs of oxytetracycline (Terramycin) ointment–soaked Vaseline gauze are carefully packed into the recesses of each nasal cavity. Care must be taken to avoid entering the orbit or anterior cranial fossa in cases of severe comminuted fractures. The packing provides compression, which can be supplemented by tying or securing the ends of the Foley catheters over the columella. Necrosis of the columella must be avoided by intermittently relaxing this pressure (Fig. 27–7*C*). A period of several hours of pressure is usually sufficient to stop the bleeding. The columella pressure can then be relaxed; the packing is removed after 24 to 48 hours. If a cerebrospinal fluid leak is present, most surgeons prefer that the packing be removed as early as possible in order to limit the possibility of an infection ascending into the meningeal area.

External Compression Dressing. This dressing (with a Barton circumferential bandage) may reduce bleeding. In practice, this dressing is rarely necessary.

Selective Arterial Ligation. Selective arterial ligation or embolization (done under radiographic control) is reserved for those few patients who continue to hemorrhage despite the above measures, including reduction of the maxillary fracture and placement of the intermaxillary fixation. Frequently, the placement of the maxilla in intermaxillary fixation limits the hemorrhage. Selective arterial ligation may include the internal maxillary or ethmoidal arteries. In severe cases, the bilateral external carotid and superficial temporal arteries are ligated.

Massive uncontrolled hemorrhage secondary to closed maxillofacial trauma occasionally occurs, and one must be prepared to administer multiple transfusions and to monitor the state of the coagulation factors hourly, correcting any abnormalities. Coagulation factor abnormalities are frequently observed in patients with combined cerebral and maxillofacial injuries on an almost immediate basis.

ASPIRATION

Pulmonary aspiration of oral secretions, gastric contents, or blood frequently accompanies maxillofacial trauma, especially if there is a concomitant cerebral injury. Noisy respirations, low arterial oxygen content, and a decrease in compliance are rapidly seen. A chest radiograph usually shows an infiltrate. Appropriate cleansing by aspiration of the tracheobronchial tree is indicated. Tracheal lavage and steroids are advocated by some but probably are not more effective than aspiration and positive pressure ventilation.

Planning of Treatment

Because of the complexity of the face, a team approach to the management of severe facial injuries has become popular in many centers in which specialists in various disciplines compete for cases. Plastic surgeons, otolaryngologists, oral surgeons, ophthalmologists, neurosurgeons, general surgeons, and critical care specialists constitute the team. It is preferable, however, for a single individual with broad training to be primarily responsible for the facial injury and to coordinate consultations and operative activities of

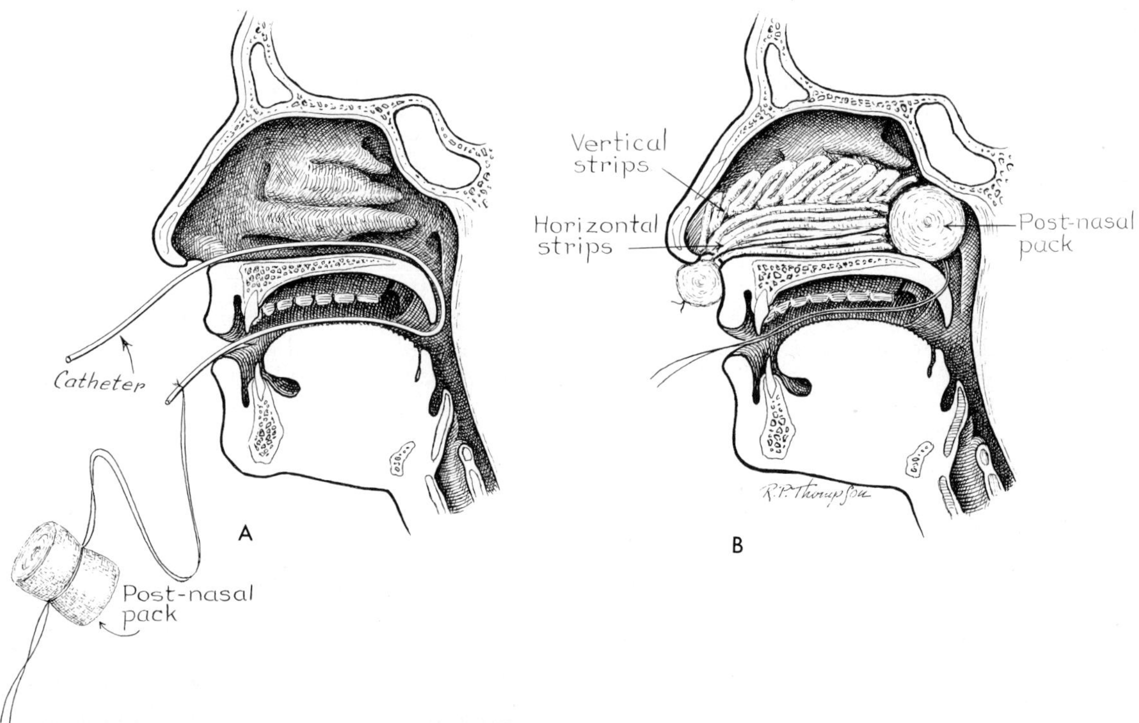

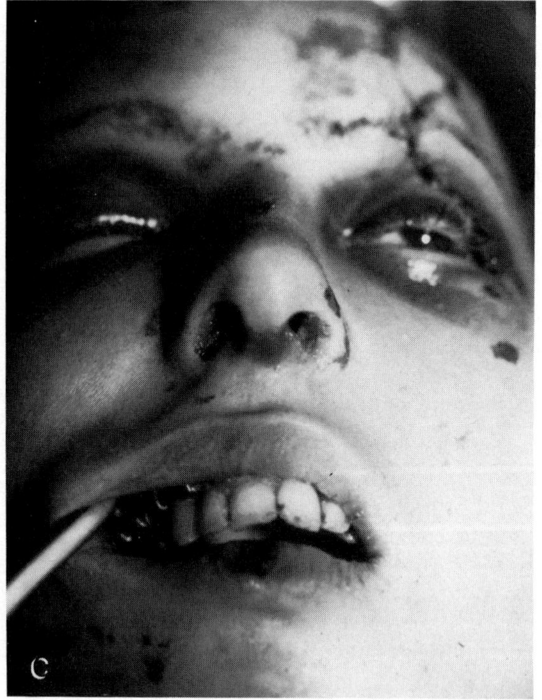

Figure 27–7. Technique of anteroposterior nasal packing for the arrest of severe nasopharyngeal bleeding. *A,* The nasal pack is guided into the nasal pharynx by a suture attached to a Foley catheter. Alternatively, a Foley catheter can be inflated in the posterior pharynx. *B,* With either a Foley catheter or a posterior nasal pack in place, the nasal cavity is packed with strips of antibiotic impregnated gauze. The entire cavity of the nose should be thoroughly packed, creating a light pressure. If the bleeding persists, the anterior pack should be removed and the recesses of the nasal cavity carefully repacked. In severe fractures, one should take care not to enter the anterior cranial fossa floor or the orbit. *C,* Excessive pressure on the columella from tying the rubber catheters may produce columella necrosis. The nasal pack can be removed 24 to 48 hours after the bleeding has been controlled. The columella pressure should be released within a matter of hours.

the team members. When all the information and suggestions are available, the surgeon-in-charge should make the final decisions regarding treatment and ensure that the plan is executed with skill and expediency.

Clinical Examination

A careful history and clinical examination form the basis for the diagnosis of most facial injuries. A thorough examination is indicated, even if the patient has only minor superficial wounds or abrasions. An abrasion, a contusion, or a laceration may be the most apparent symptom of an underlying fracture or abnormality. A facial laceration may be the only sign of a penetrating injury that has entered the eye, nose, ear, or cranial cavity. Facial lacerations may often be repaired during the treatment of injuries in other parts of the body without the need for an additional operative session. Treatment of facial lacerations should not be deferred. Superficial lacerations or abrasions may leave disfiguring scars despite their inconsequential appearance if not adequately managed. Careful cleansing of all wounds, debridement when necessary, and meticulous closure minimize conspicuous permanent deformity (Fig. 27–8).

Facial injuries should be considered in three categories: (1) soft tissue injuries, (2) wounds involving soft tissue associated with fractures of the bone, and (3) facial fractures without soft tissue wounds.

Soft tissue injuries may be clean and sharp lacerations, ragged lacerations, contusions, abrasions, avulsions (with or without missing tissue), puncture wounds, ballistic injuries such as gunshot and shotgun wounds, and thermal injuries (burns).

Bone injuries should be suggested by overlying soft tissue injuries, such as contusions and abrasions. Ecchymoses or edema over a bony prominence should prompt an evaluation to rule out fracture. Subconjunctival hemorrhage with ecchymosis and edema in the region of the orbit and a palpebral hematoma (Fig. 27–9) suggest a fracture of the nose, zygoma, orbit and nasoethmoidal or frontal bone region (Fig. 27–10). Ecchymotic and contused intraoral tissues over the surface of the mandible suggest a fracture of the lower jaw (Fig. 27–11).

Fractures of the facial bones may be diagnosed on the basis of malocclusion of the teeth (Fig. 27–12) or open bite deformity due to displacement of the upper or lower jaw. A fracture of the mandibular condyle (Fig. 27–13), for instance, may produce pain, deviation with motion, and inability to occlude the upper and lower jaw properly. Pain with movement of the jaw (trismus) may be caused by a fracture of the zygoma or upper or lower jaw. Unequal globe levels and double vision indicate zygomatic, orbital, or maxillary fractures. A thorough palpation of all areas of the facial bones should be performed.

An orderly examination of the facial structures should be accomplished, progressing from either superior to inferior or inferior to

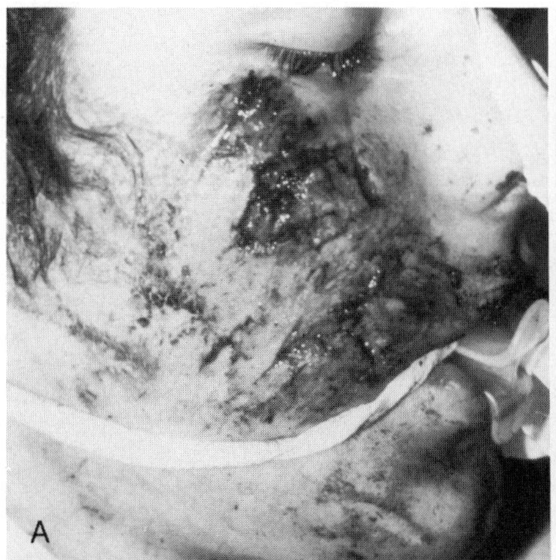

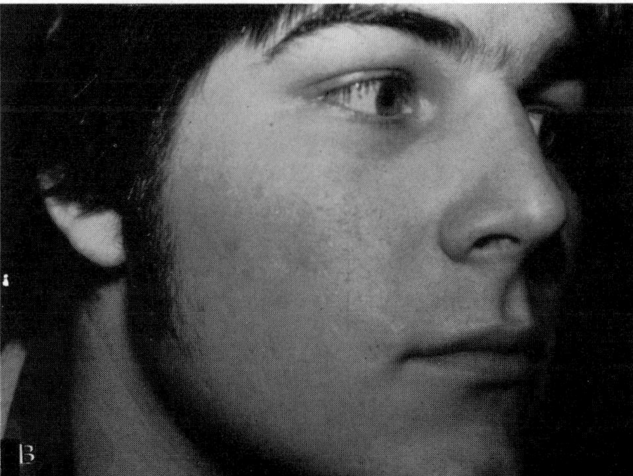

Figure 27–8. *A*, Abrasive laceration. *B*, Result obtained following thorough removal of all foreign material and careful suturing of each small laceration.

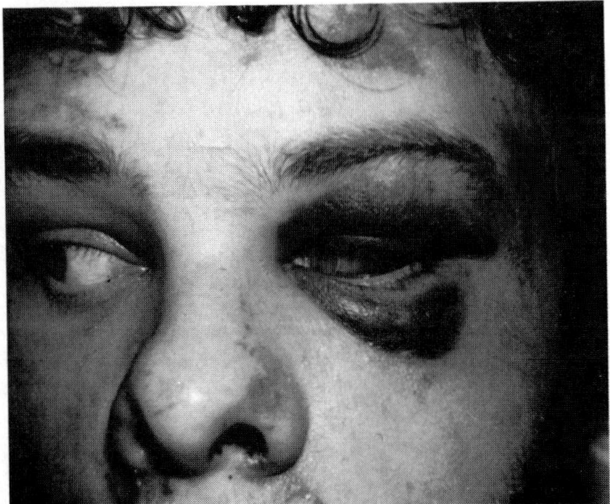

Figure 27–9. The combination of a periorbital hematoma and a subconjunctival hematoma indicates the possibility of a fracture of the orbit.

superior. Symptoms and signs produced by facial injuries include pain or localized tenderness, crepitation from areas of underlying bone fracture, hypoesthesia in the distribution of a specific nerve, paralysis in the distribution of a specific nerve, malocclusion, visual disturbance, facial asymmetry, deformity, obstructed respiration, lacerations, bleeding, and contusions.

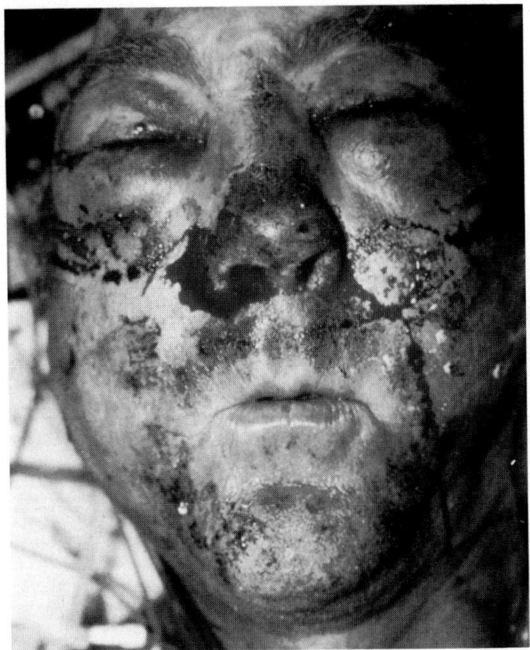

Figure 27–10. Bilateral palpebral hematoma and facial swelling are present in this patient with a significant Le Fort fracture.

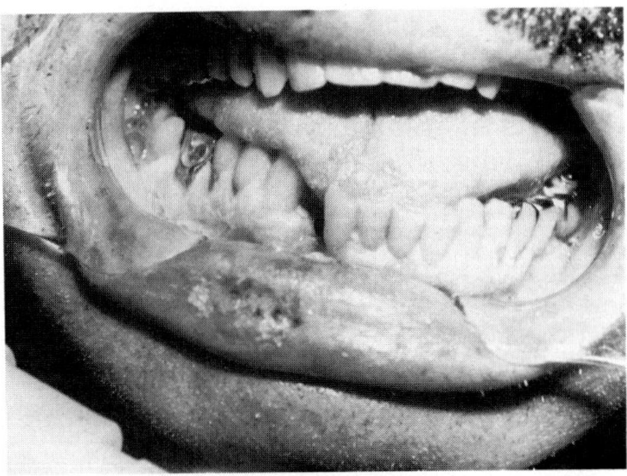

Figure 27–11. Intraoral examination demonstrating a parasymphyseal fracture and oral laceration.

The clinical examination should begin with evaluation for symmetry and deformity. The clinical examination should begin with inspection of the face, comparing one side with the other. Palpation of all bony surfaces follows in an orderly manner. The orbital rims, superior (Fig. 27–14*A*) and inferior (Fig. 27–14*B*); the nose (Fig. 27–15); the brows; the zygomatic arches (Fig. 27–16); the malar eminence; and the border of the mandible should be evaluated. A thorough inspection of the intraoral area (Fig. 27–17) should be made to detect lacerations or abnormalities of the dentition. Palpation of the dental arches follows the inspection, noting mobility. The maxillary and mandibular dental arches are carefully visualized and palpated to detect bone irregularity, bruise, hematoma, swelling, movement (Fig. 27–18), tenderness, or

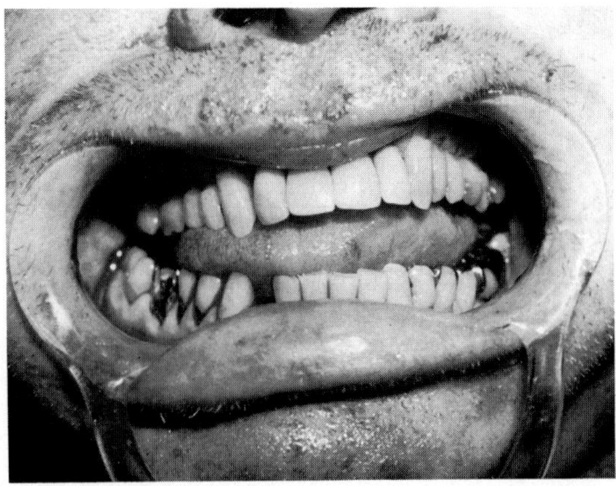

Figure 27–12. Intraoral examination demonstrates fractures of the mandible and maxilla, with widening of both dental arches, malocclusion, and open bite.

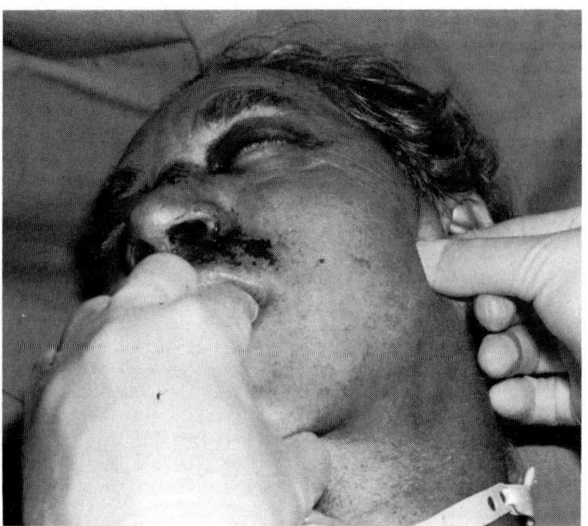

Figure 27–13. The mandible is grasped with one hand, and the condyle area is bimanually palpated with one finger in the ear canal and one finger over the condyle. Abnormal movement or crepitation indicates a condylar fracture.

crepitus. Evaluation of the sensory and motor nerve function in the facial area is performed. The presence of hypoesthesia or anesthesia in the distribution of the supraorbital, infraorbital, and mental nerve should suggest a fracture somewhere along the path of these sensory nerves.

Extraocular movements (cranial nerves III, IV, and VI) and the muscles of facial expression (cranial nerve VII) must be examined in the conscious cooperative patient. Pupillary size and symmetry, globe turgor, globe excursion, eyelid excursion, double vision, and visual loss are noted (Barton and Berry, 1982). A funduscopic examination should be performed. The presence of a hyphema or visual disturbance (field defect, visual loss, double vision, decreased vision, or absent vision) should be noted and appropriate consultation requested. A penetrating ocular injury or globe rupture should be suspected with any injury to the eye or periorbital area. The presence of a periorbital hematoma with the eye swollen shut should not deter the clinician from examining the globe. Indeed, some have suggested that the globe examination be performed with a determination inversely proportional to the difficulty. It should be emphasized, however, that care must be exercised to avoid extrusion of globe contents through a globe laceration. It is only by means of a thorough examination that globe ruptures and penetrating globe injuries are not missed.

The excursion and deviation of the jaws with motion, the presence of pain upon opening the jaw, the relationship of the teeth, the symmetry of the dental arches, and the ability to bring the teeth into a maximal intercuspal relationship are important clues to the diagnosis of fractures involving the dentition. A finger in the ear canal can detect condylar movement (see Fig. 27–13). The presence of a fractured or missing tooth (Fig. 27–19) should imply the possibility of more significant maxillary or mandibular injury, which must be confirmed by further examination for mobility (Fig. 27–20) and appropriate radiographs. Fractures of the mandible may be detected by pulling forward on the jaw

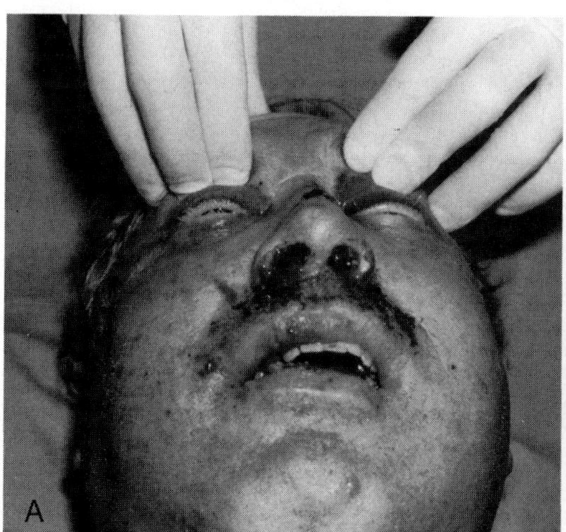

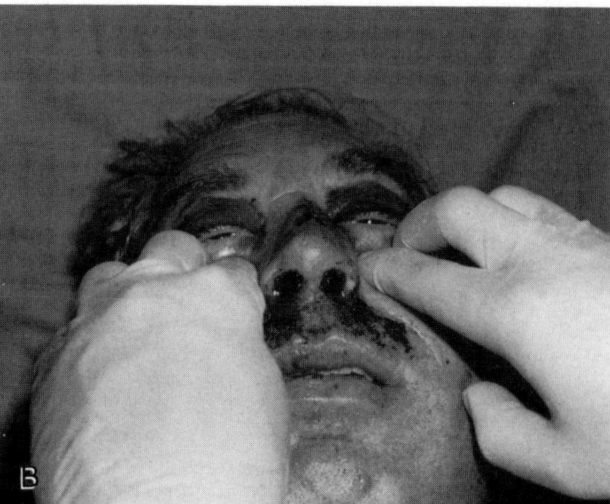

Figure 27–14. Palpation of the orbital rims. *A,* The superior rims. *B,* The inferior rims.

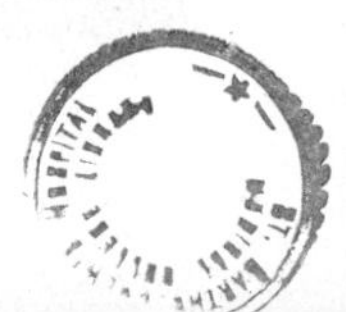

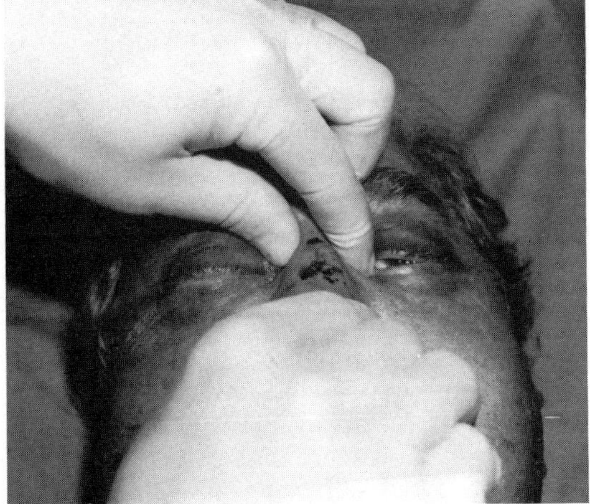

Figure 27–15. The nasoethmoid region should be palpated for fractures of the nose and the finger should also be placed deeply over the medial orbital rims to detect mobility, which is indicative of a nasoethmoidal fracture.

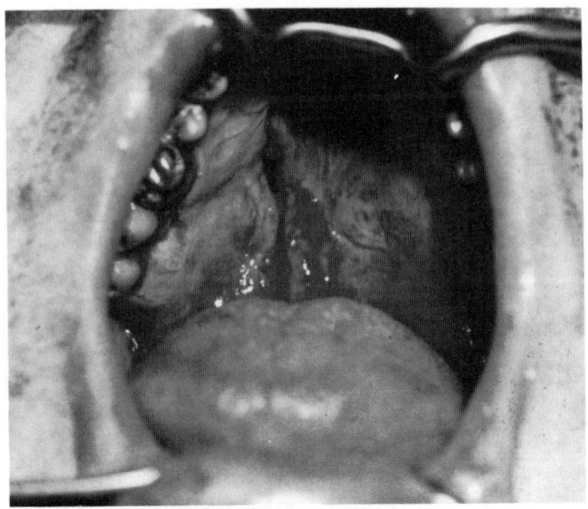

Figure 27–17. Examination of the roof of the mouth discloses a sagittal fracture of the palate, accompanied by a mucosal laceration of the palatal mucoperiosteum.

(see Fig. 27–13), or by applying up and down manual pressure on the anterior portion of the mandible, having supported the angle. Instability, crepitus, and pain may be noted when this maneuver is performed. Edema and hemorrhage may mask facial asymmetry. Bleeding accompanying facial fractures may disguise a cerebrospinal fluid leak. Bleeding or fluid draining from the ear canal may indicate a laceration in the ear canal, a condylar dislocation, or a middle cranial fossa fracture. Bleeding from the nose may indicate nasal or septal injuries, Le Fort, zygomatic, or orbital fractures, or fractures of the anterior cranial fossa. Mobility of the middle third of the facial skeleton indicates a fracture of the Le Fort type. Basilar skull fractures or cribriform plate fractures should be suspected when cerebrospinal fluid leak or bleeding from the ears is present. Central nervous system injury is implied by paralysis of one or more of the cranial nerves, unconsciousness, depressed sensorium, unequal size of the pupils, paralysis of one or more of the extremities, abnormal neurologic reflexes, convulsions, delirium, or irrational behavior.

ROENTGENOGRAPHIC DIAGNOSIS

Patients with serious or multiple injuries should not be sent without monitoring or

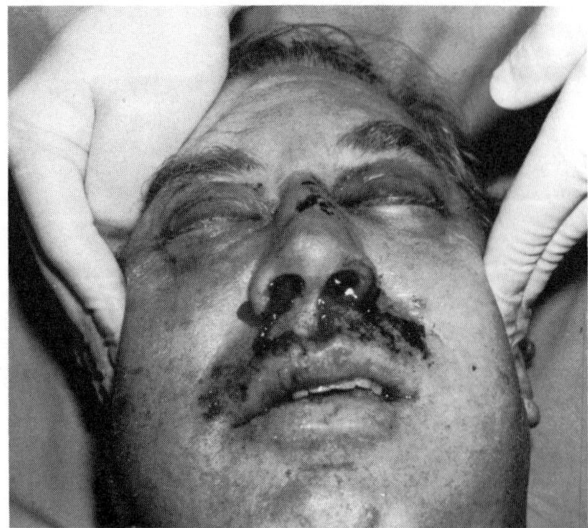

Figure 27–16. The zygomatic arches are palpated.

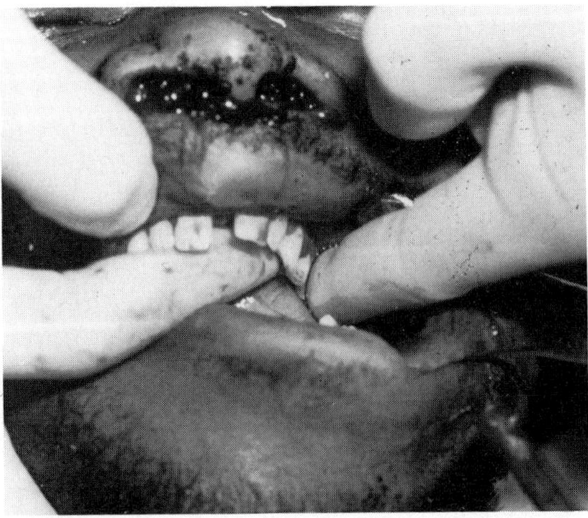

Figure 27–18. Lateral mobility of the entire dental arch should be assessed for both the upper and lower jaw. A fracture of the maxillary tuberosity area is common in more extensive midfacial injuries.

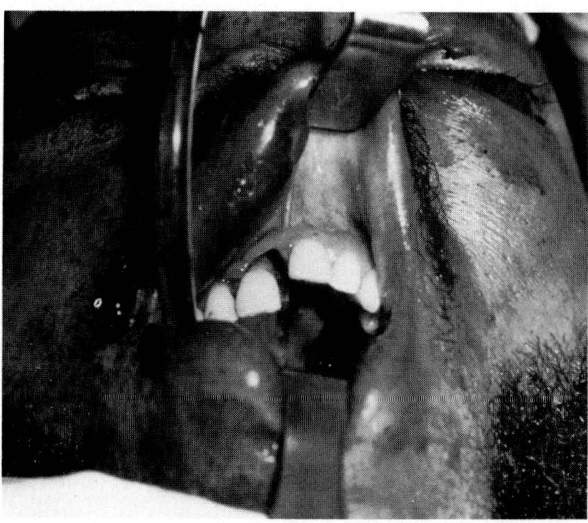

Figure 27–19. A split palate (sagittal fracture of the maxilla) is often accompanied by a laceration in the upper buccal sulcus adjacent to the frenulum.

support personnel for extensive radiographic evaluation of facial injuries. Simple bedside radiographs combined with a thorough clinical examination can provide much of the information necessary for emergency diagnosis and treatment.

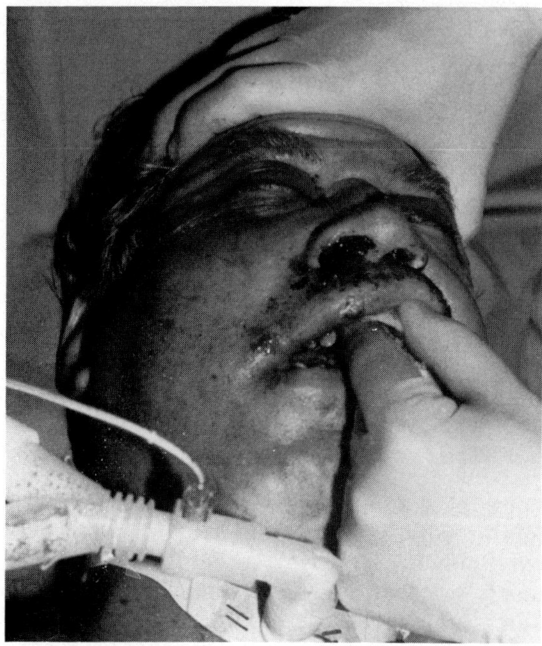

Figure 27–20. With the head securely grasped, the midface is assessed for movement. One must be careful not to allow the head to move so as to avoid the false impression of maxillary mobility. Loose dentures or bridgework should not be confused with mobility of the maxilla. Higher Le Fort fractures demonstrate, as a rule, less mobility if they exist as a single piece fracture than do lower Le Fort fractures. More comminuted fractures demonstrate extreme mobility.

Roentgenographic evaluation is indispensable in the evaluation of a patient with head and face injuries. However, it does not under any circumstances replace the clinical examination, which is the most sensitive indication of facial injury (Fig. 27–21*A*). A complete radiographic evaluation of the cranial and facial bone structure should be obtained when clinical symptoms are present. Previously plain films, stereoscopic views, and tomograms were the important roentgenographic evaluations, but they have largely been completely replaced in most modern units by a craniofacial CT scan. Even though the clinical evaluation may demonstrate obvious fracture and suggest a standard type of management, a thorough roentgenographic examination should be made. It may be quite obvious that a patient has a fracture through the premolar region of the mandible on one side with mild malocclusion. It would be reasonable to apply intermaxillary fixation and to bring the teeth into occlusion. One might miss, however, the documentation of the contralateral subcondylar area or of the zygomatic arch. Even though the plan of treatment would be the same, the presence of a condylar fracture should be known to the surgeon and to the patient. Because of the high incidence of litigation arising from injuries, it is of prime importance to have a thorough documentation of all bone injuries even if treatment is not required.

It should be emphasized that roentgenographic examination is only one of the means of establishing the diagnosis of a fracture. The roentgenogram, however, provides absolute evidence of the bone injury. The appearance of a fracture on plain radiographs or CT scan may require clinical interpretation (Fig. 27–21*B*). The extent and amount of displacement of the fragments, for instance, may be difficult to determine by roentgenographic study alone. In many views, the fracture is partially or totally obscured in plain films by overlying or superimposed bone structures of the face, skull, or spine. The clinical picture in most cases may be more serious than suspected from cursory evaluation of the roentgenographic anatomy alone.

Plain Facial Films

The most valuable and the most often employed views of the face are the facial bone

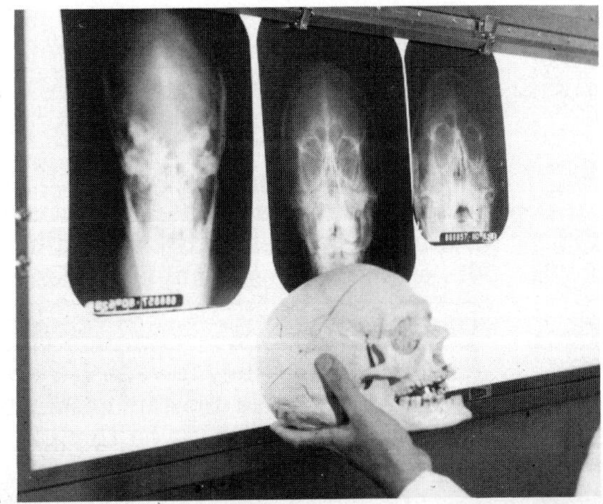

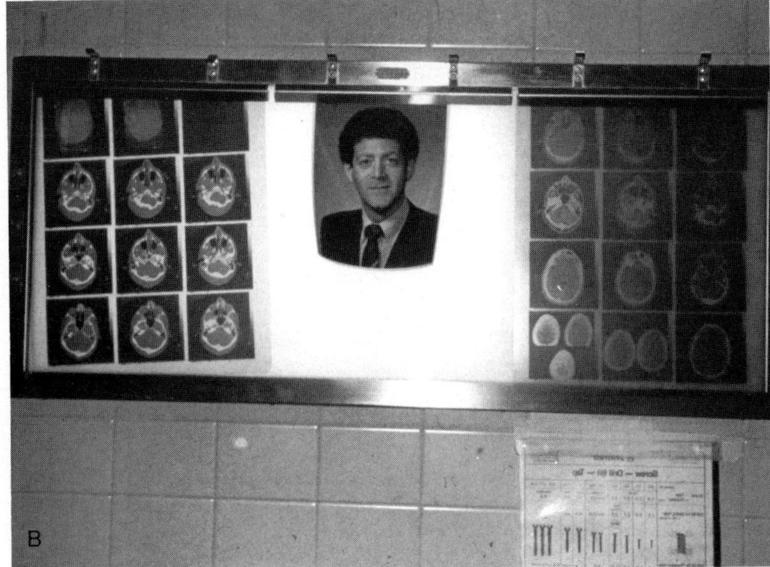

Figure 27–21. *A,* Examination of a skull is helpful in the interpretation of plain facial bone roentgenograms or computed tomographic (CT) examinations. *B,* Preinjury photographs are as important as the CT scan as a guide to reconstructing the patient's former appearance.

series, which includes the Caldwell, submentovertex, Waters, Towne, and lateral skull views (Ayella, 1978). Anteroposterior and lateral oblique views of the mandible are also obtained. Specialized views of the mandible, such as the panoramic roentgenogram and occlusal or apical views of the teeth, may disclose detailed anatomy. Specialized roentgenograms, such as cephalometric examination, may be necessary and soft tissue may be included with profile views. The middle and upper facial structures are most accurately evaluated with a detailed CT examination. The evaluation of the frontal bone, sinuses, orbit, and midface may require both axial and coronal CT for the most accurate documentation.

ROENTGENOGRAPHIC POSITIONS FOR STANDARD FACIAL FILMS

Waters Position. The posteroanterior projection is employed for an oblique anterior view of the upper facial bones; the orbits, malar bones, and zygomatic arches are also well shown. This view is helpful in the diagnosis of fractures of the maxilla, maxillary sinuses, orbital floor, infraorbital rim, zygomatic bone, and zygomatic arches. To a lesser extent, the view documents the nasal bones, nasal process of the maxilla, and supraorbital rim (Fig. 27–22).

Caldwell Position. The posteroanterior projection is primarily used to demonstrate the frontal sinuses, frontal bone, anterior ethmoidal cells, and zygomaticofrontal su-

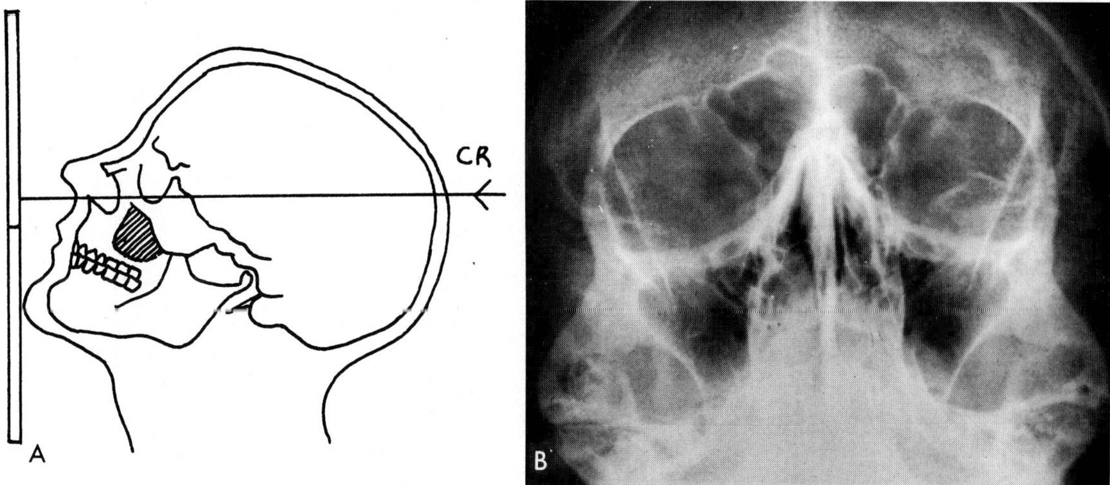

Figure 27–22. Waters position. Posteroanterior view for visualization of the maxillary sinuses, maxilla, orbits, and zygomatic arches. This projection may also be helpful in demonstrating fractures of the nasal bones and nasal processes of the maxilla. In this view, the petrous ridges are projected just below the floors of the maxillary sinuses. *A,* Position of the patient in relation to the film and the central ray. *B,* Waters view showing fractures of the middle third of the face. (The drawings in Figures 27–22 to 27–44 are reproduced from Kazanjian and Converse.)

ture. The orbital margin, the lateral walls of the maxillary sinuses, the petrous ridges, and the mandibular rami are also demonstrated in this projection (Fig. 27–23).

Fronto-Occipital Projection. This view is used when injuries prevent examination of the facial bones with the patient in a prone or seated position. The projection gives a satisfactory view of the orbits and the lesser and greater wings of the sphenoid, frontal bone, frontal and ethmoidal sinuses, nasal septum, floor of the nose, hard palate, mandible, and upper and lower dental arches (Fig. 27–24).

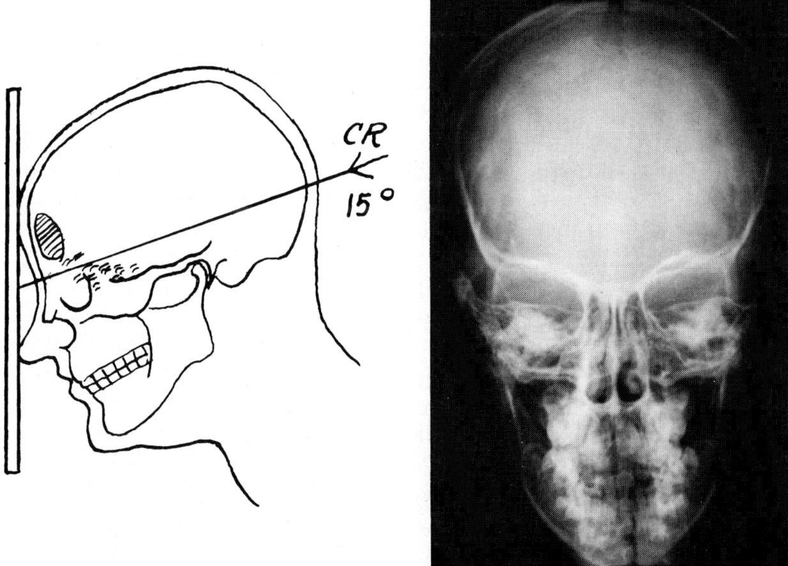

Figure 27–23. Caldwell position. Posteroanterior view of the skull. This position is used to study fractures of the frontal bone, orbital margins, zygomaticofrontal sutures, and lateral walls of the maxillary sinuses. The paranasal sinuses are shown in this projection. The petrous ridges are shown at a level between the lower and middle thirds of the orbits.

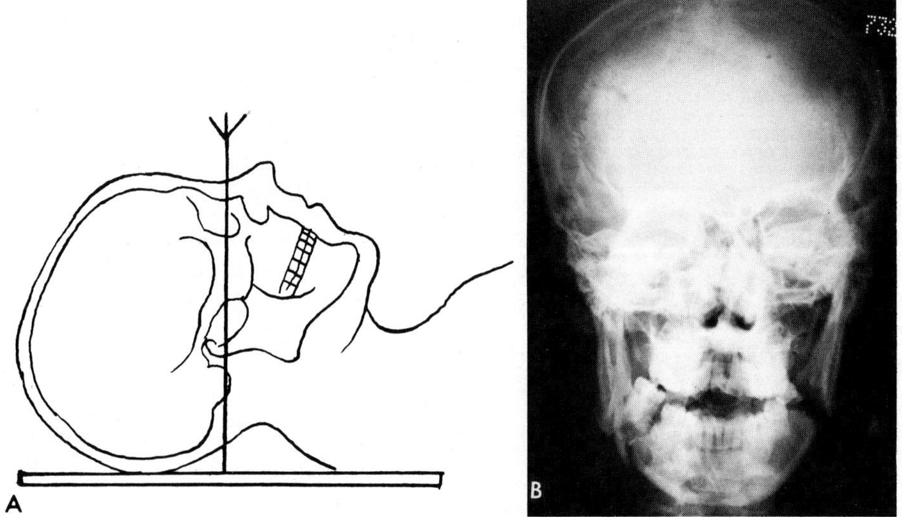

Figure 27–24. The fronto-occipital anteroposterior projection. When injuries prevent positioning of the patient in the prone or seated posteroanterior position, this position or the reverse Waters projection may be used. *A*, The examination is made with the patient in the dorsal recumbent position. *B*, Lateral mandibular fractures are demonstrated with the fronto-occipital anteroposterior projection.

Reverse Waters Position. The mento-occipital position is also used to demonstrate the facial bones when the patient cannot be placed in the prone position. This projection is used to demonstrate fractures of the orbits, maxillary sinuses, zygomatic bone, and zygomatic arches. The increased patient-to-film distance magnifies the upper facial structures, but otherwise the film is similar to that obtained with the Waters position (Fig. 27–25).

Optic Foramen—Oblique Orbital Position. This view is best demonstrated by stereoscopic projections and shows the optic foramen in its relationship to the posterior ethmoidal and sphenoidal sinuses. It also demonstrates the lateral wall of the frontal sinus, the vertical plate of the frontal bone, and the roof and lateral wall of the dependent orbit. Under a bright spotlight, the lateral wall of the opposite orbit may be clearly defined (Fig. 27–26).

Semiaxial (Superoinferior) Projection (Titterington Position). The zygomatic arches, facial bones, and orbits are well shown in this projection (Fig. 27–27).

Lateroanterior Projection (Fuchs Position). This projection gives an oblique view of the zygomatic arch projected free of superimposed structures. The lateral wall of the maxillary sinus is also well shown in this view (Fig. 27–28).

Lateral and Profile View of Face. Stereoscopic projections may be made with this view because of the complexity of the superimposed shadows of the face. This projection demonstrates the lateral profile of the facial bones and soft tissues of the face. The study is important in the evaluation of maxillary-mandibular relationships and fractures of the vertical plate of the frontal bone (Fig. 27–29).

Nasal Bones, Lateral Views. This projection gives a detailed view of the nasal bones of the side nearest the film and of the soft structures of the nose. Both sides should be examined radiographically. One view with this projection should be made with intensifying screens to show the frontal sinuses. Fractures of the nasal bones, the anterior nasal spine, and the frontal processes of the maxilla are demonstrated in this view (Fig. 27–30*A*).

Nasal Bones, Axial Projection. The axial superoinferior view of the nasal bones is used to demonstrate medial or lateral displacement of the bony fragments that are not shown on lateral views. The thin nasal bones do not have sufficient body to cast a shadow through the superimposed frontal bone of the anterior maxillary structures. This view demonstrates only those positions of the nasal bones that project beyond a line anterior to the glabella and upper incisor teeth. The view

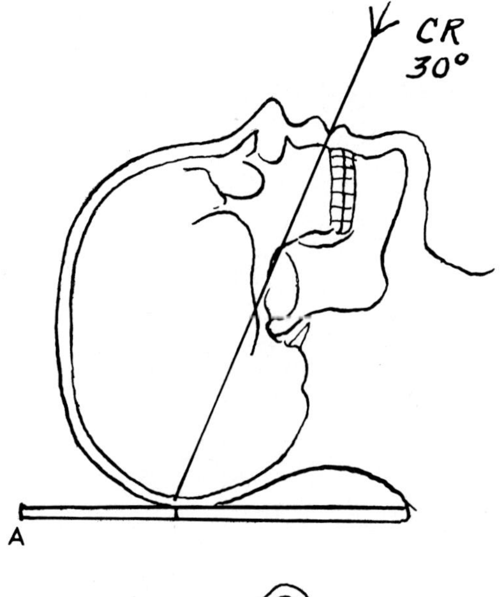

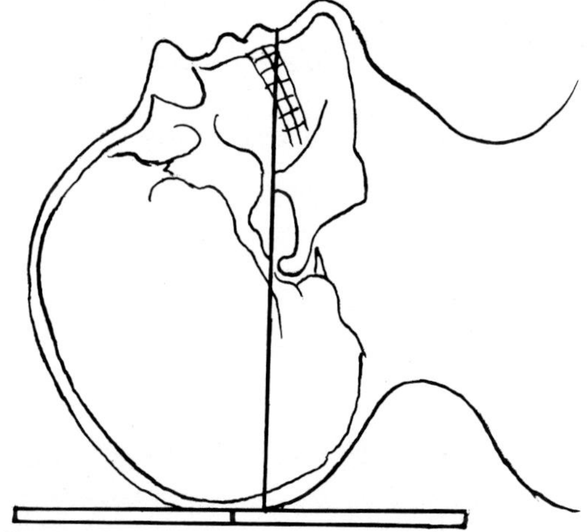

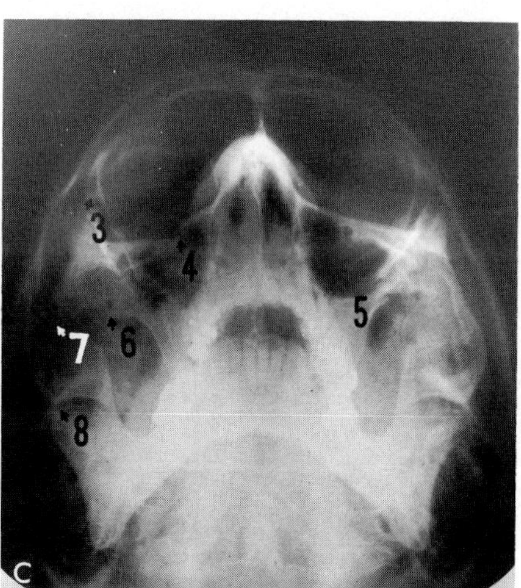

Figure 27–25. The reverse Waters position. *A, B,* The mento-occipital position or reverse Waters projection is a view of the facial bones similar to Waters view except for the greater magnification of the facial bones due to the increased distance between the face and the film. *C,* Fractures of the orbits, maxillary sinuses, zygomatic bones, and arches are identified.

is not helpful in children or adults who have short nasal bones, a concave face, or protruding maxillary teeth (Fig. 27–30*B*).

Superoinferior Occlusal Views of Hard Palate. Fractures of the hard palate may be demonstrated by occlusal views with superoinferior projections, the x-ray tube being focused and positioned to demonstrate the angle of interest.

Superoinferior Central Occlusal View of Hard Palate. This view demonstrates the palatine process of the maxilla and the horizontal plates of the palatine bones in the entire dental arch (Fig. 27–31).

Superoinferior Anterior Occlusal View of Hard Palate. This projection gives a view of the anterior part of the hard palate, the alveolar process, and the upper incisor teeth in greater bone detail than the central occlusal view because the obliquely focused central ray does not penetrate any superimposed structures (Fig. 27–32).

Oblique Superoinferior Posterior Occlusal View of Hard Palate. This projection gives an oblique occlusal view of the posterior part of the hard palate (unilateral) and the alveolar process and all the teeth of the upper quadrant of the maxilla. Fractures of the teeth or alveolar process may also be demonstrated (Fig. 27–33).

Submentovertex and Verticosubmental Positions for Base of Skull. These views give an axial projection of the mandible; the coronoid and condyloid process of the mandib-

Text continued on page 893

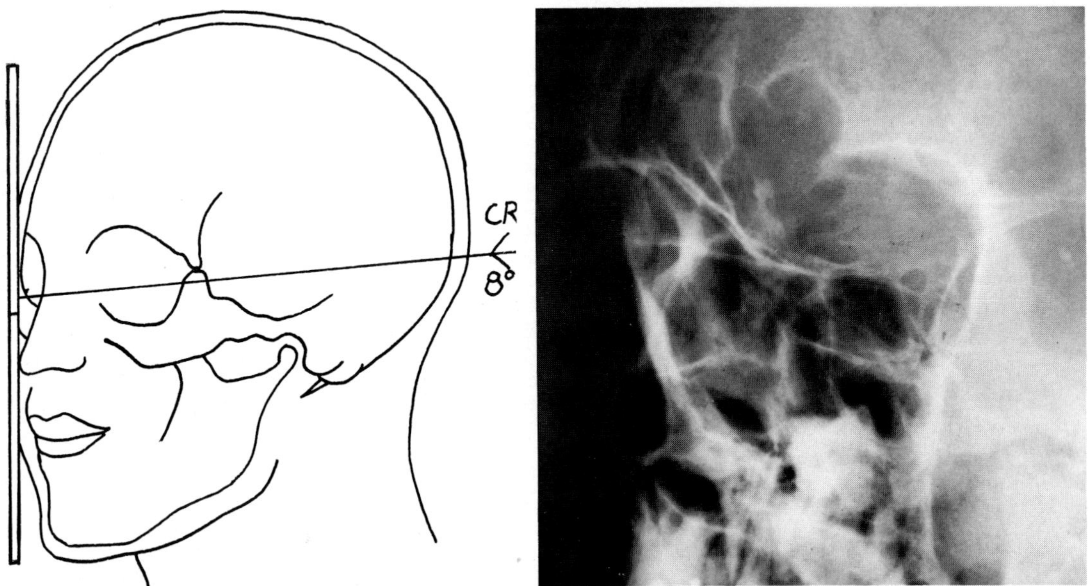

Figure 27–26. Optic foramen—oblique orbital position. The oblique posteroanterior view of the facial bones shows the optic foramen and the lower inferior quadrant of the orbit in relation to the posterior ethmoid and sphenoid sinuses.

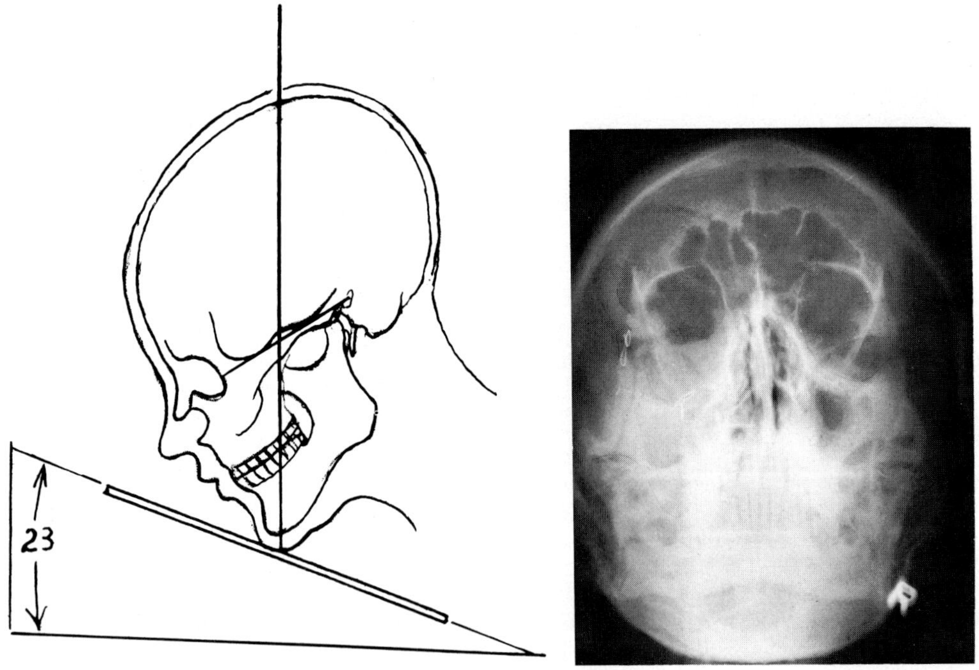

Figure 27–27. The semiaxial position known as the Titterington position. The projection is helpful in the study of fractures of the zygomatic arches, lateral walls of the maxilla, orbital floors, and orbital margins. The maxillary, ethmoid, and frontal sinuses, and the inferior border of the mandible are well shown in this projection.

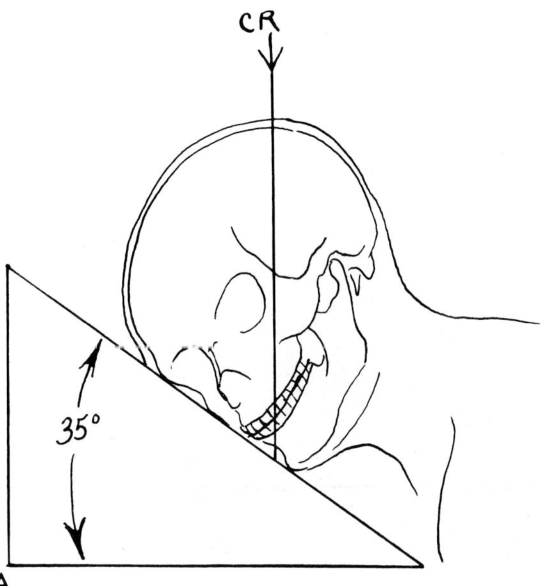

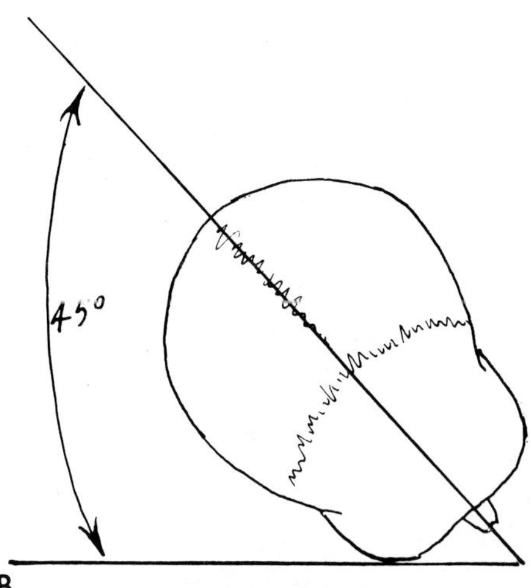

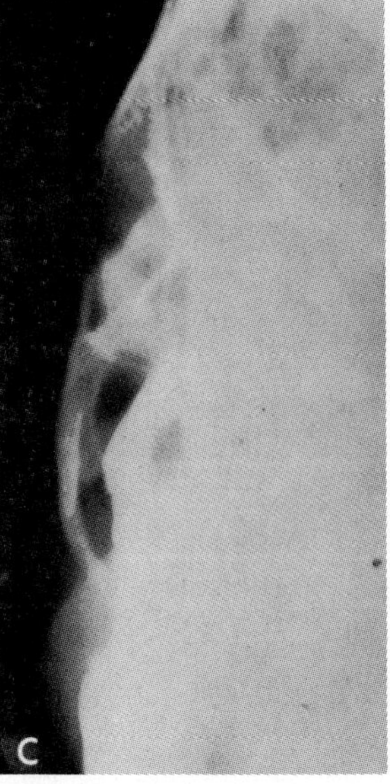

Figure 27–28. *A, B,* The lateroanterior projection is an excellent view of the zygomatic arch projected free of superimposed structures. Fractures of the lateral wall of the maxillary sinus may also be studied in this view. *C,* Fractures of the zygomatic arch are demonstrated by the lateroanterior projection.

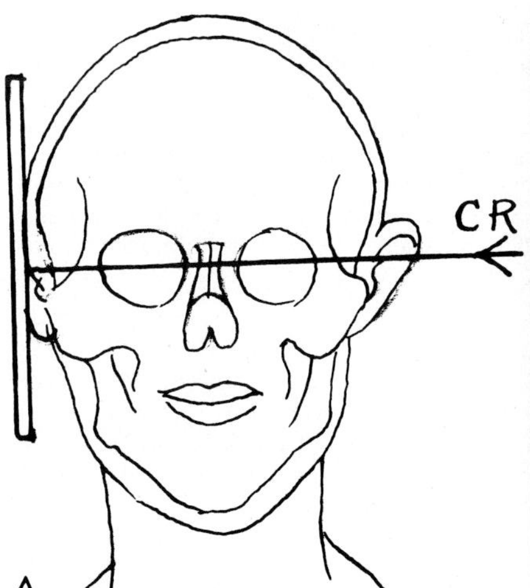

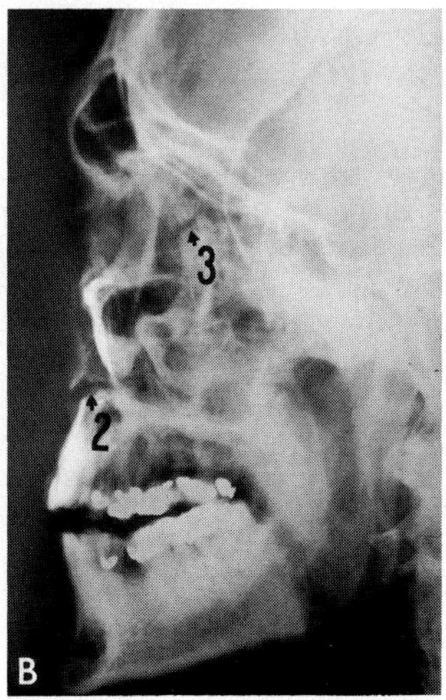

Figure 27–29. Lateral and profile view of the face. The view is helpful in the study of fractures of the frontal sinuses, lateral walls of the orbit, maxilla, and mandible. *A,* Position of part to film. *B,* Lateral profile view of the face demonstrating fractures of the zygomaticofrontal suture *(3)* and the maxilla at the level of the floor of the nose *(2).*

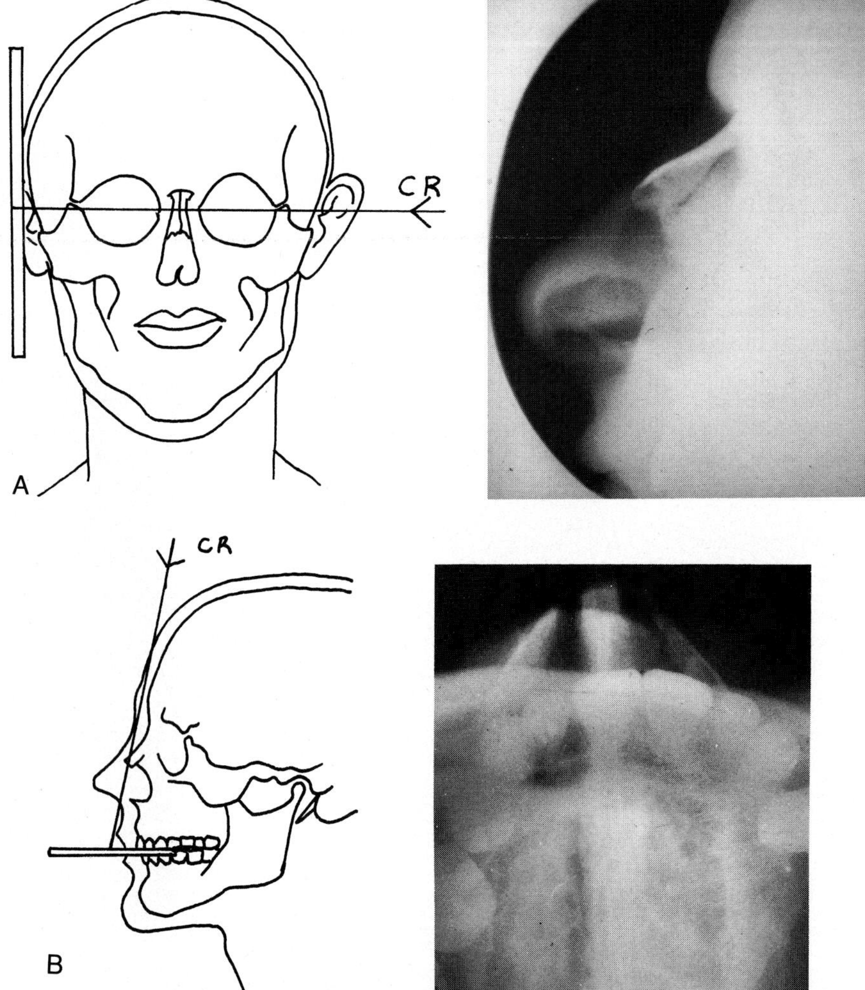

Figure 27–30. *A,* Nasal bones, lateral view. This projection provides a detailed view of the nasal bone nearest the side of the film. Views from both sides are helpful in the study of fractures of the nasal bones, anterior nasal spine, and nasal processes of the maxilla. *B,* The axial view of the nasal bones may reveal fractures with medial or lateral displacement that are not demonstrated on lateral views. Only those portions of the nasal bones that project anteriorly to the line between the glabella and the upper incisor teeth can be demonstrated in this projection. This view is not helpful in the examination of children or adults who have relatively smaller or depressed nasal bones and projecting upper teeth or forehead.

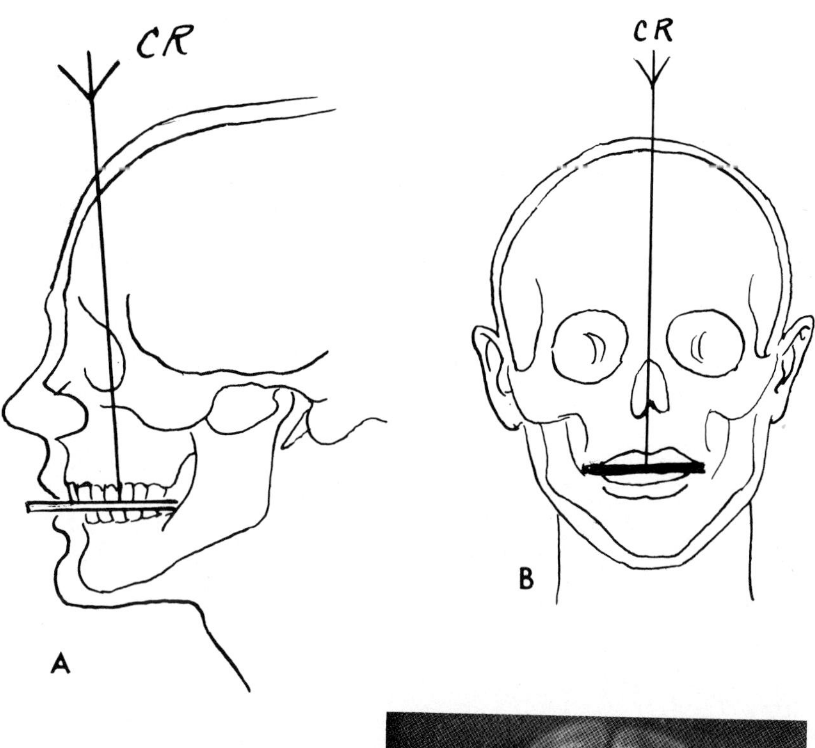

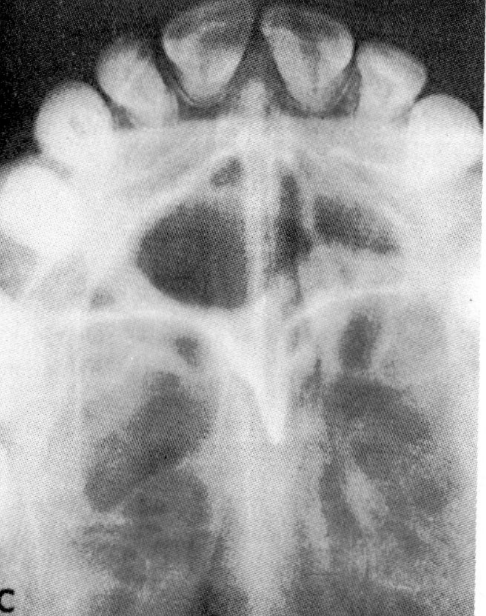

Figure 27–31. Superoinferior central occlusal view of the hard palate. The view helps to demonstrate fractures of the alveolar process or hard palate. Cysts and bone malformations or defects of the upper dental arch may be shown by this view. *A* and *B* demonstrate the path of the central ray. *C* is a radiographic example.

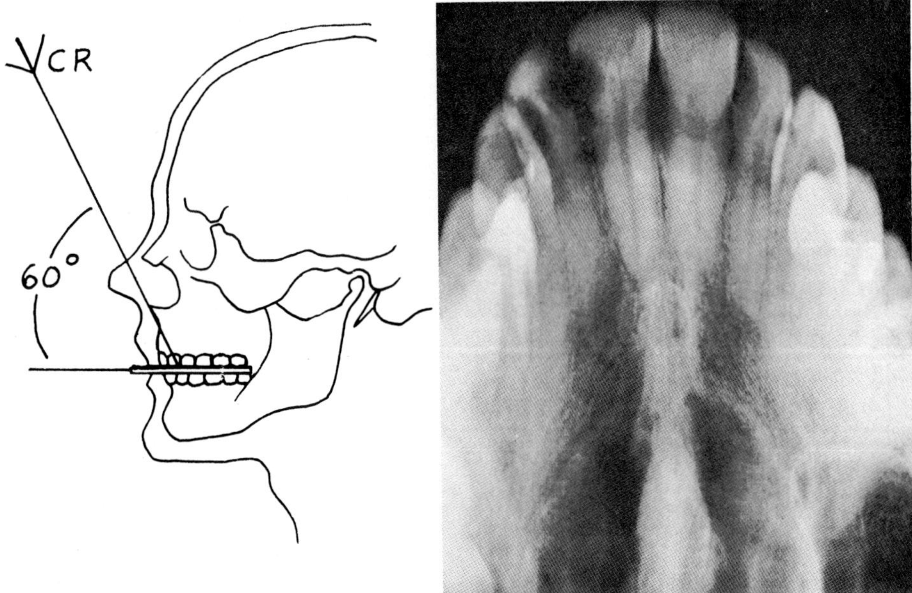

Figure 27–32. Superoinferior anterior occlusal view of the hard palate. This view gives details of the maxillary anterior teeth, the alveolar processes, and the anterior portion of the hard palate. The incisive canal is well demonstrated by this view.

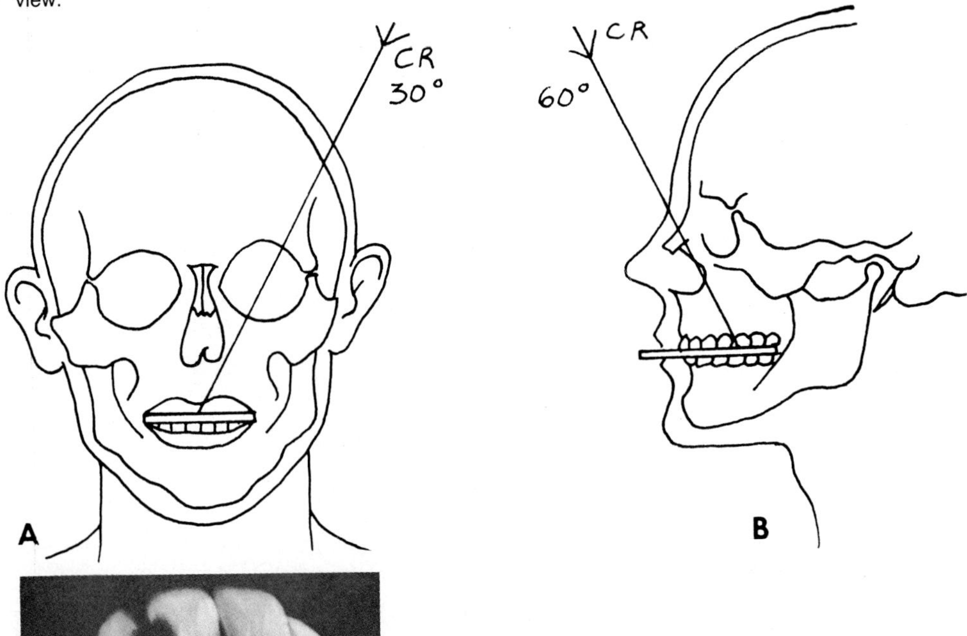

C

Figure 27–33. The oblique superoinferior posterior occlusal view of the hard palate. This projection gives an oblique occlusal view of the posterior part of the hard palate on one side. *A, B,* Path of the central ray. *C,* The alveolar process in the teeth and the upper quadrant of the maxilla are demonstrated in detail. Fractures of the alveolar process or teeth may be demonstrated by this view.

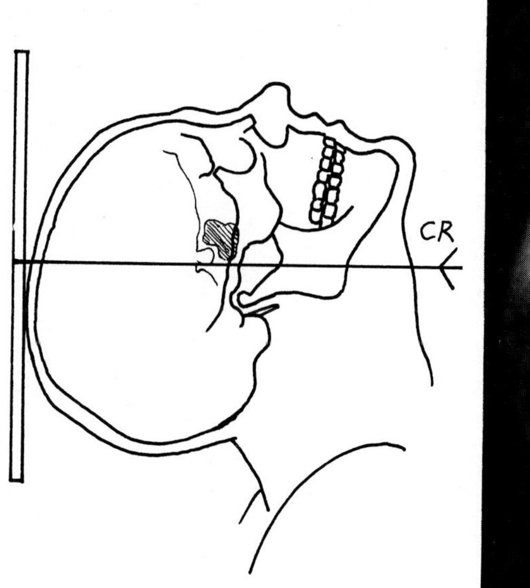

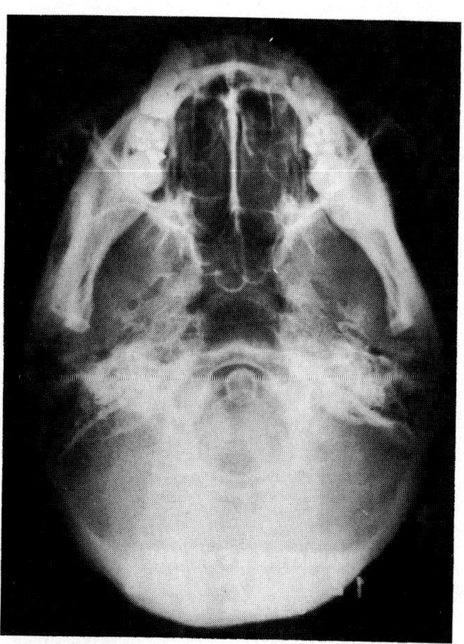

Figure 27–34. The verticosubmental projection of the base of the skull gives an axial projection of the mandible, including the coronoid and condyloid processes of the rami; the zygomatic arches; the base of the skull and its foramina; the petrous pyramids; the sphenoid, posterior ethmoid, and maxillary sinuses; and the nasal septum.

ular rami; the zygomatic arches; the base of the skull and its foramina; the petrous pyramid; the sphenoidal, posterior ethmoid, and maxillary sinuses; and the bony septum (Fig. 27–34).

Occlusal Inferosuperior Views of Mandible. Medial or lateral bone displacement in anterior mandibular fractures is well shown by occlusal inferosuperior views of the mandible. This view affords bone detail of the entire lower dental arch, mandibular body, symphysis, lower alveolar process, and teeth.

Occlusal Inferosuperior Projection. This projection is used to demonstrate mesial or lateral displacement of fragments in fractures of the anterior portion of the mandible (Fig. 27–35).

Oblique Inferosuperior Projection. This projection gives an oblique occlusal view of the anterior mandibular area showing the symphysis, alveolar process, and incisor teeth. The bone detail is excellent and a fracture of the symphysis region, alveolar process, or teeth can be well demonstrated (Fig. 27–36).

Oblique Superoinferior Submental Projection of Mandibular Symphysis. This view gives an oblique anteroposterior

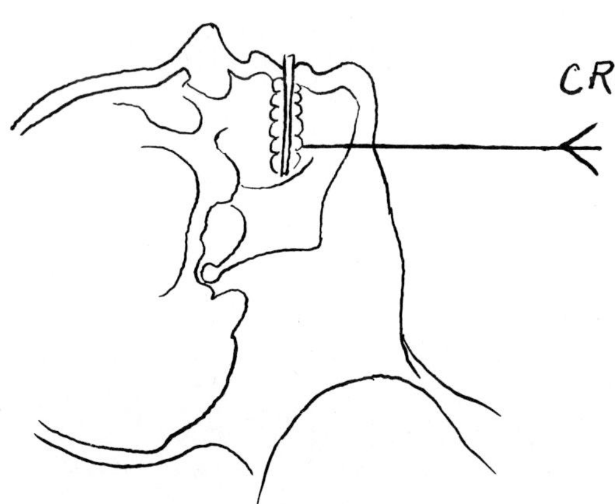

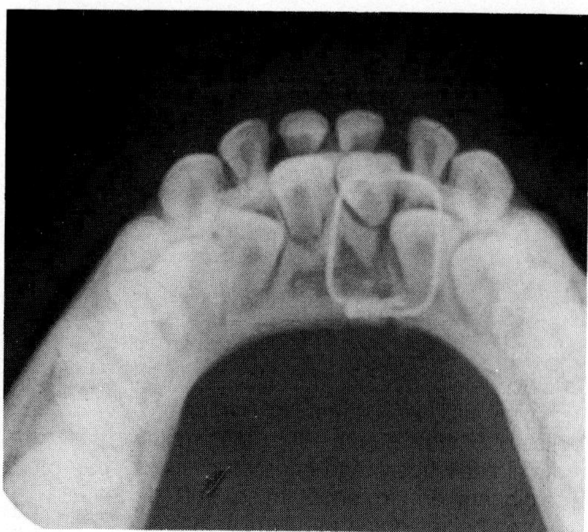

Figure 27–35. Inferosuperior occlusal projection of the mandible. The symphyseal area is well demonstrated. A fracture has been wired in the parasymphyseal area.

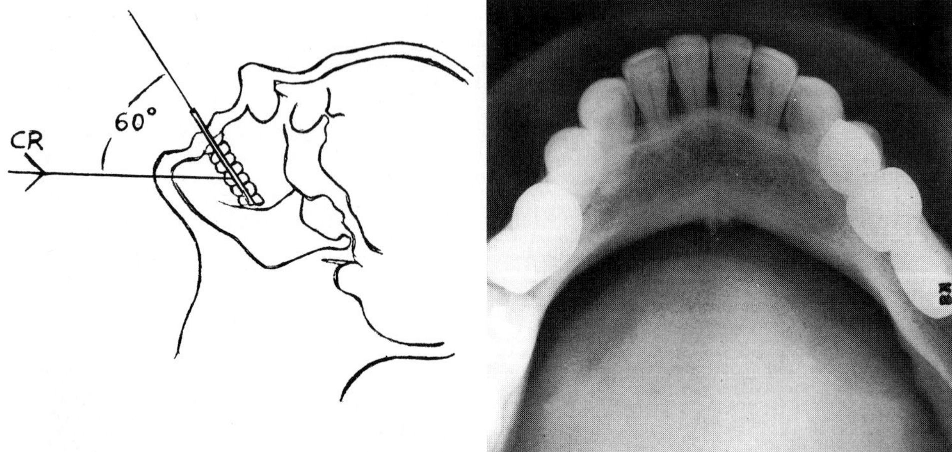

Figure 27–36. Oblique inferosuperior projection. This projection shows the mental symphysis, the incisor and canine teeth, and the alveolar process with excellent bone detail.

projection of the mandibular symphysis (Fig. 27–37).

Oblique Lateral Views of Mandible. These positions are used to demonstrate fractures of the mandibular ramus, body of the mandible, and symphysis region.

Body of Mandible. This projection provides a lateral view of the mandible posterior to the cuspid tooth and includes a portion of the ramus of the mandible (Fig. 27–38).

Ramus of Mandible. This posteriorly directed oblique lateral view shows fractures of the ramus, mandibular condyle, condylar and condyloid processes, and posterior body of the mandible (Fig. 27–39).

Symphysis of Mandible. The anteriorly directed oblique lateral projection of the symphysis of the mandible demonstrates fractures of the mandibular symphysis, mental foramen region, and body of the mandible (Fig. 27–40).

Posteroanterior View of Mandible. Medial and lateral displacement of fractured segments of the mandible may be demonstrated by this view. It demonstrates the symphysis, body and rami of the mandible, condyloid and coronoid processes, and temporomandibular joints (Fig. 27–41).

Temporomandibular Joints

Oblique Anteroposterior, Fronto-occipital View of Temporomandibular Joints. This projection provides an oblique posterior view of the condyloid processes of the mandible and mandibular fossa, temporal bones, petrous bones, internal auditory canals, occipital bone, posterior cranial fossa, and for-

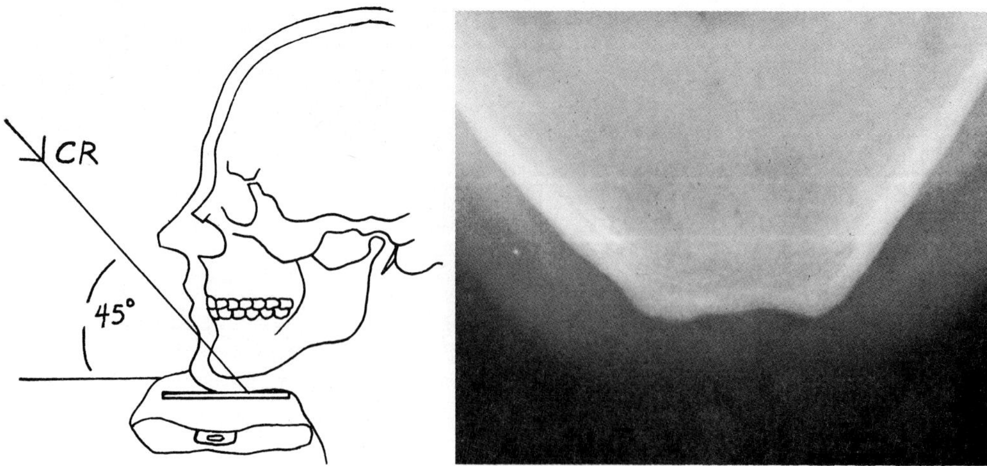

Figure 27–37. Oblique superoinferior submental projection of the mental symphysis.

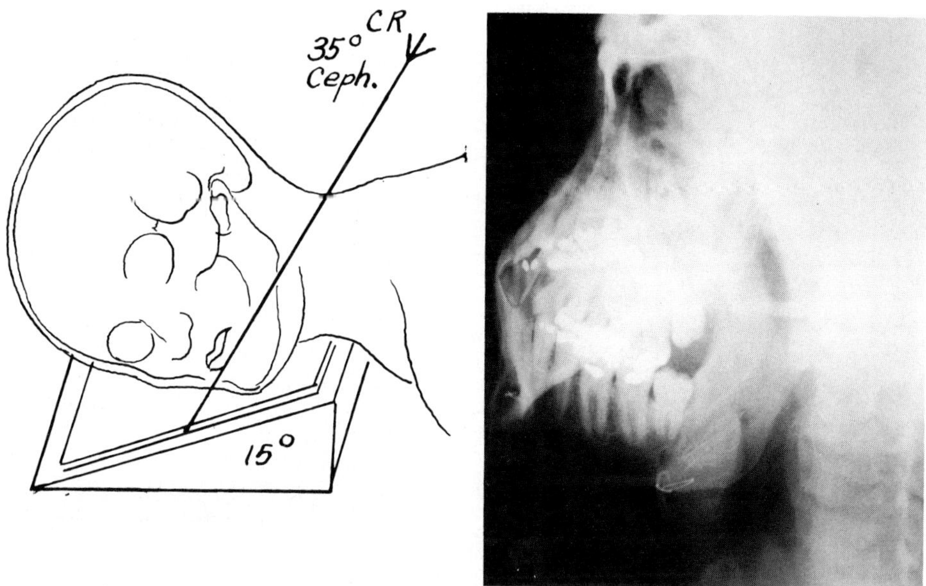

Figure 27–38. The body of the mandible. The angle and most of the mandibular ramus are demonstrated in this projection.

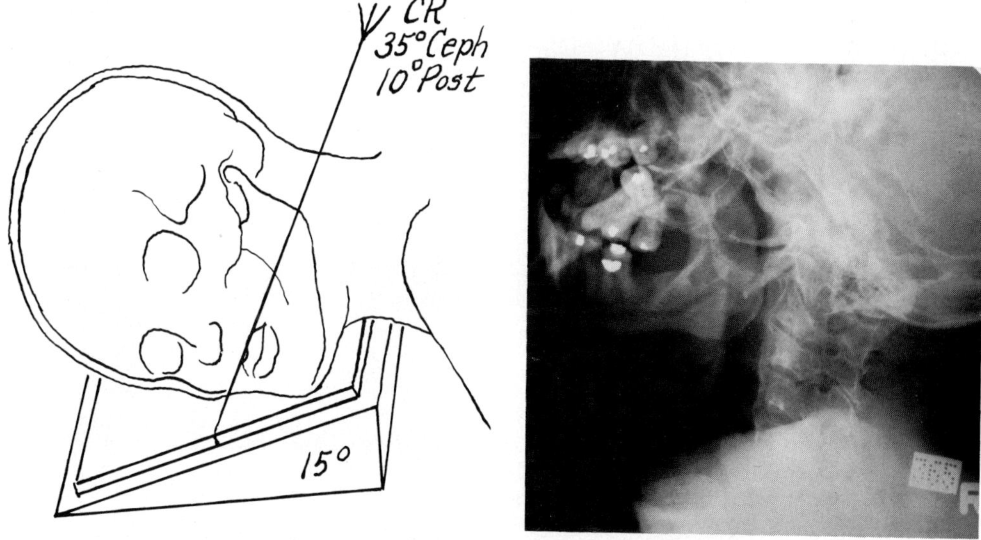

Figure 27–39. The ramus of the mandible, in a posteriorly directed oblique lateral view.

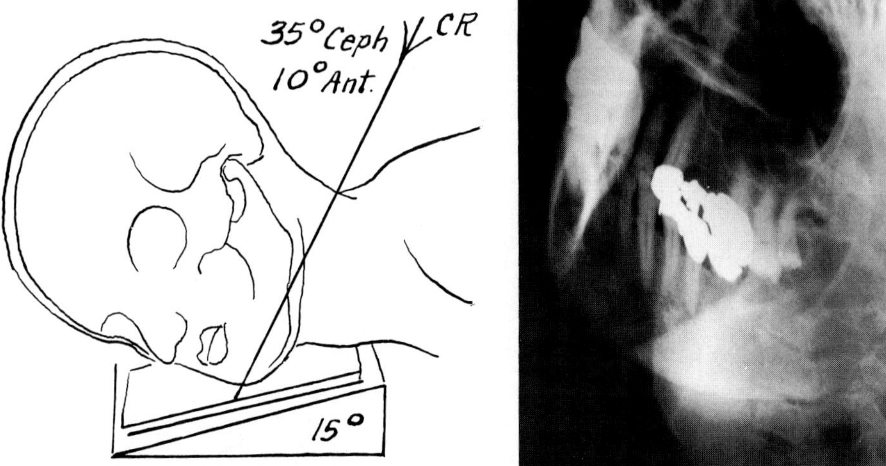

Figure 27–40. The symphysis of the mandible is shown by an anteriorly directed oblique lateral view. The regions of the mental foramen and the body of the mandible are also shown in detail.

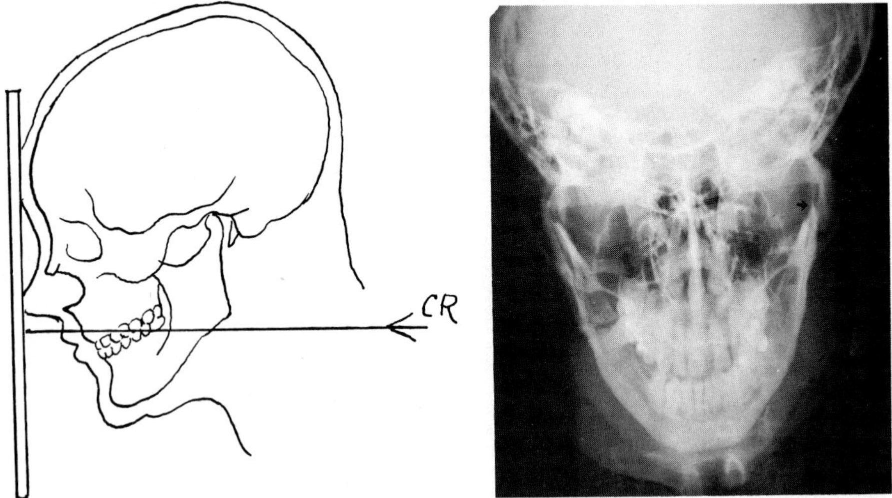

Figure 27–41. Posteroanterior view of the mandible. This view demonstrates the symphysis, the body and the rami of the mandible, including the coronoid and condyloid processes, and the articular surfaces of the temporomandibular joints. Angle and bilateral subcondylar fractures are demonstrated on the radiographs.

amen magnum. Fractures in the region of the temporomandibular joints with displacement medially or laterally can be detected in these views (Fig. 27–42).

Lateral Transcranial Projection: Oblique Lateral Views of Temporomandibular Joints. The views are taken by the lateral transcranial projection and demonstrate the temporomandibular joints in open and closed mouth positions. The closed mouth view demonstrates the temporomandibular joint, the relation of the mandibular condyle to the fossa, and the width of the joint cartilage. The open mouth view demonstrates the excursion of the head of the condyle, downward and forward, in relation to the glenoid fossa and tubercle. This projection is useful in demonstrating fractures and dislocations of the mandibular condyle and the condylar process. The external auditory meatus and the mastoid processes are also shown (Fig. 27–43).

Mayer View. The temporomandibular joint, external auditory canal, mastoid process, and petrous pyramid are shown in the unilateral, superoinferior view (Fig. 27–44). Medial or lateral displacement of the bone fragments of the mandibular condyle can be shown by this projection. Fracture-dislocation of the bony portion of the external auditory canal can also be demonstrated by this technique.

Panoramic Roentgenogram. The panoramic roentgenogram (Fig. 27–45) is a helpful aid in defining the location and displacement of mandibular fractures. A study by Chayra, Meador, and Laskin (1986) showed that it is the most accurate view from which approximately 92 per cent of mandibular fractures were diagnosed. A diagnostic accuracy rate

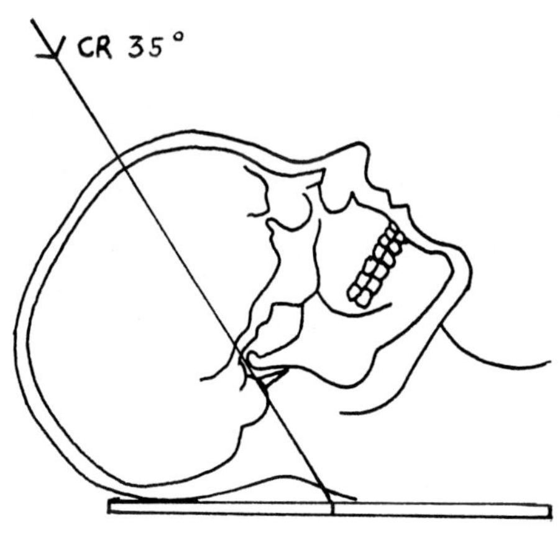

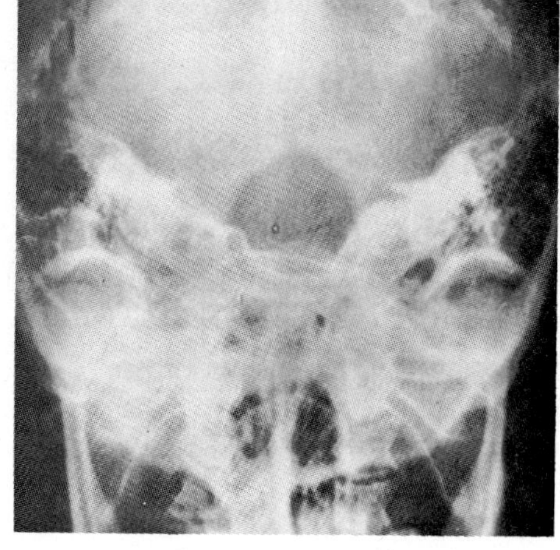

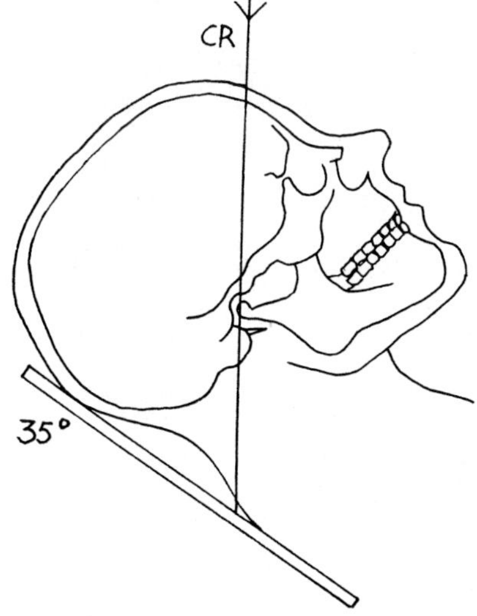

Figure 27–42. Oblique anteroposterior fronto-occipital view of the temporomandibular joints. The view is helpful in the study of fractures of the condyle of the mandible and in demonstrating medial or lateral displacement.

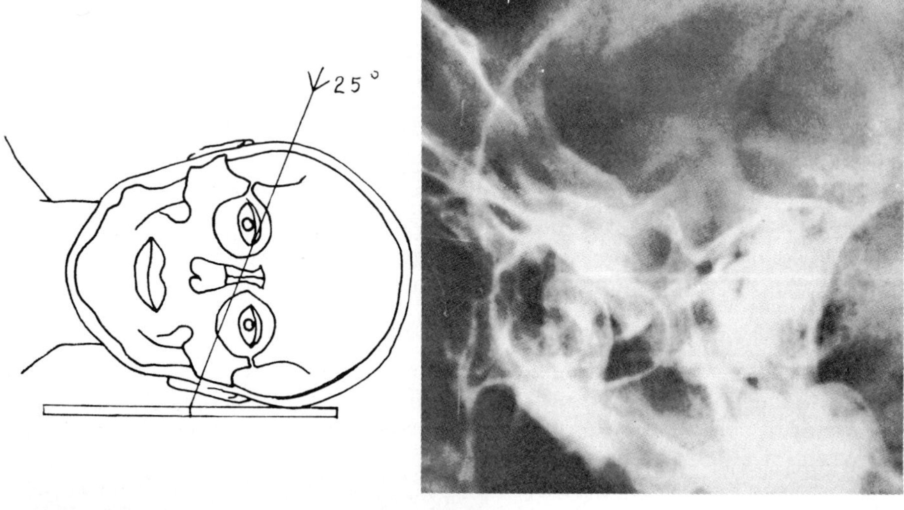

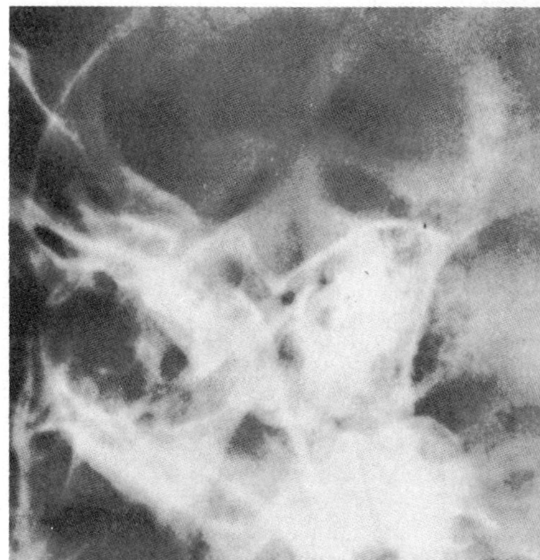

Figure 27–43. Lateral transcranial projections of the temporomandibular joints taken in the open and closed positions are useful in demonstrating motion of the mandibular condyle in relation to the glenoid fossa. The view may show fractures of the condylar process.

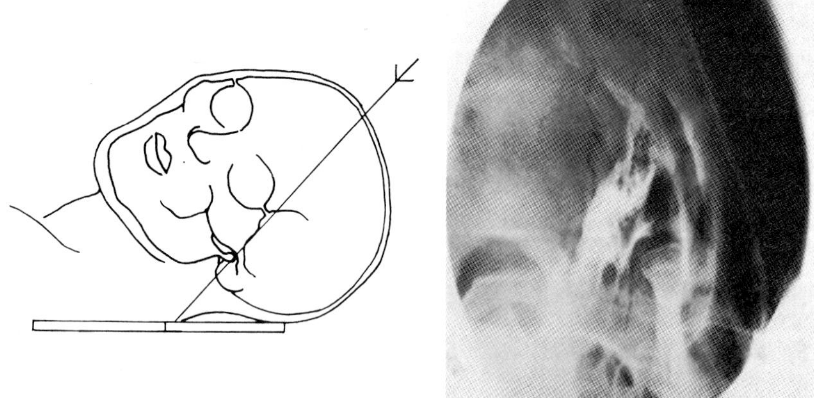

Figure 27–44. The Mayer view gives a unilateral superoinferior view of the temporomandibular joint, external auditory canal, mastoid, and petrous processes. This view is helpful in the demonstration of fractures and malformations of the temporomandibular joint and in the study of bony atresia of the external auditory canal.

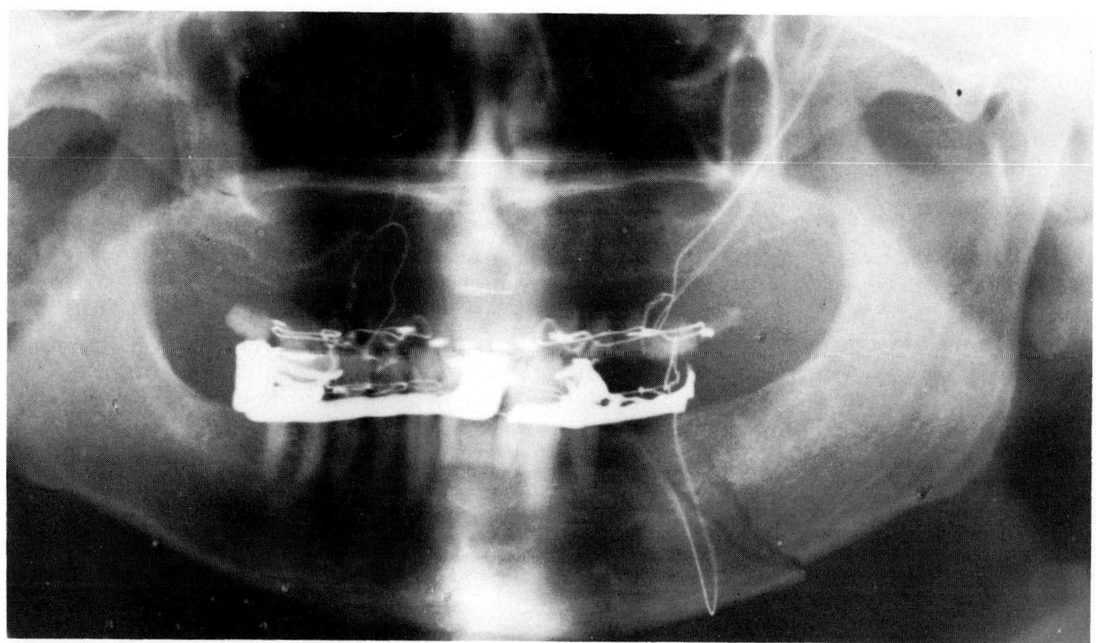

Figure 27–45. Panoramic postreduction roentgenogram showing a fracture of the mandibular body treated by circumferential wiring of the partial denture.

of 92 per cent for the panoramic roentgenogram and 67 per cent for the traditional mandibular series was reported. The sites in which fractures were most commonly undiagnosed on the panoramic were the condylar, angle and symphyseal regions, especially if there was some blurring. In the traditional mandibular series, fractures were missed in every site except the ramus.

Computed Tomographic (CT) Scans

Computed tomographic (CT) evaluation of the temporomandibular joint is discussed in Chapter 30. Computed tomography of the face is discussed under the regional anatomy of each fracture. Articles by Gentry and associates (1983), Kreipke and associates (1984), and Rowe, Miller, and Brandt-Zawadzki (1981) are especially recommended.

TREATMENT OF SOFT TISSUE WOUNDS

Tetanus Prophylaxis

All facial wounds are potentially contaminated and, even though they occur under what might seem to be clean conditions, it is advisable to take active measures against the possibility of the development of tetanus. The efficacy of immunization with toxoid was well demonstrated by the low incidence of tetanus reported by the U.S. Army in World War II; only one case developed in the European theater by February, 1945 (Graham and Scott, 1946). In the civilian population, most individuals have been actively immunized by their family physician or in the military service; many should have their serum antibody levels raised by the administration of a toxoid booster. If a patient has not been immunized, simultaneous intramuscular injection of 250 units of Hyper-Tet (tetanus immune globulin) and 0.50 ml of tetanus toxoid is recommended. Two additional tetanus toxoid boosters should be given at monthly intervals to complete the immunization. In general, tetanus toxoid is given to individuals who have been previously immunized if the interval between their last booster and the injury is greater than five years. In tetanus-prone wounds, a two year interval is recommended (these wounds are extremely contaminated).

Contusions, abrasions, and lacerations are not life threatening, with the exception of uncontrolled hemorrhage. Many facial wounds are complex and compound. The more serious ones not only may involve the superficial structures, but also may extend to the intracranial contents, the orbit, nose, sinuses, intraoral structures, and floor of the mouth. Cranial nerves V and VII may be affected. The salivary glands and salivary ducts may be injured. Soft tissue wounds may be associated with fractures of the mandible, maxilla, zygoma, nasal bones, orbit, frontal bone, or cranial vault. Most civilian wounds occur under relatively clean circumstances, and, with modern techniques of debridement and antibiotic coverage, can be treated with primary closure at literally any interval after injury. Because of the excellent blood supply of the face, the period from injury to surgery can be exempted from the usual 6 to 24 hour limits applied to the repair of lacerations in other areas of the body. The timing and technique of closure depend on the condition of the patient, the judgment of the surgeon, and the ability to establish a surgically clean wound. Tissue that is obviously contaminated and damaged by crushing and contusion presents more of a hazard for infection if primary repair is undertaken. In these situations, the surgeon may elect to perform either a delayed primary repair or a primary repair with serial interval operative examinations of the wound ("second look procedures") for further cleansing and debridement.

The probability of contamination increases rapidly and is directly proportional to the length of time that has elapsed since the time of the injury. It is known that organisms inoculated into a wound become encased in a protein fibrin coagulum within a few hours. It is thus necessary either to debride the wound edge surgically to remove the "lodged" organisms or to forcefully remove the protein-fibrin coagulum with a pressure irrigation or scrubbing technique. Organisms or contaminants may be driven into the wound. They may not be obvious on inspection of the wound edge, and in fact it may be inevitable that some foreign materials (such as wood splinters) that are driven into the soft tissue by injury forces may be overlooked. Such an occurrence should be considered in patients who present with infection after initial wound closure. The history and circumstances of the injury provide the most reliable evidence signaling the possibility of deeply imbedded foreign material.

Careful examination and evaluation of the wound should be made before any treatment is undertaken. Fractures of the underlying bone should be detected, and in many cases treated, before the soft tissue management. Treatment of the fracture after the soft tissue management (e.g., the application of arch bars for mandibular fractures) in many cases disrupts the soft tissue closure and further damages the soft tissue. Lacerations or contusions should be considered evidence of underlying bone injury and their presence should alert the clinician to inspect the radiographs of the bone in that area. If the fractures are exposed through soft tissue lacerations, it may be advisable to perform fixation of the fractures through the open wound rather than to utilize the standard incisions for facial fracture treatment. Injuries to important nerves, ducts, glands, and sinuses require consideration, and a thorough investigation of the function of structures in the vicinity of the laceration should be undertaken.

Delayed Primary Wound Closure

When the patient is seen late with extensive tissue edema, subcutaneous hematoma, and crushing, or when the wound edges are badly contused and some tissue is devitalized, it may be preferable to delay wound closure until conditions for primary healing are more favorable. Limited debridement to remove devitalized tissue, wet dressings, and antibiotic therapy should be the program of treatment until the resolution of edema and acute inflammation and a cleaner appearance of the wound indicate that delayed primary closure will be successful. Primary closure under unsatisfactory conditions can contribute to increased soft tissue loss with tension, infection, and tissue necrosis. If, after the program of open treatment, the wound edges cannot be approximated because of contracture, the wound may be covered with a skin graft, which may be secondarily excised in serial fashion.

The large canine population has resulted in a number of animal bites, particularly in children. An essential precaution, before primary suture, is the surgical creation of a clean wound. Irrigation of the wound with large amounts of saline may be successful. Alternatively, surgical debridement and excision of the wound edges can convert the wound into a clean injury. Canine saliva contains necrotizing enzymes; the latter produce continuing necrosis of the tissue in the wound if they are not evacuated. There have been various recommendations regarding the efficacy of antibiotic therapy for dog bites. It would seem that if a truly clean wound can be established surgically, antibiotics are not necessary (Haines, 1982; Lindsey, Nava, and Marti, 1982). Alternatively, if there is any chance that areas were overlooked on debridement, infection in these areas might be avoided by the use of antibiotics. In practice a "prophylactic" antibiotic seems reasonable. In cat bites, *Pasteurella multocida* is present and should be treated with prophylactic penicillin. There is a potential for cat scratch fever, presenting as lymphadenopathy subsequent to an injury. With human bites, contamination with more virulent organisms is encountered, and appropriate antibiotic treatment may require drugs that cover the gram-positive, gram-negative, aerobic and anaerobic spectrum. Because the risk of infection from human bites is much greater, some surgeons perform only secondary closures in these injuries.

Cleaning of the Wound

All wounds should be carefully inspected for foreign material. Removal is imperative to prevent separation, infection, delayed healing, and subsequent pigmentation of skin. The presence of foreign material reduces the bacterial inoculum necessary to cause infection. In general, greater than 10^5 organisms per gm of tissue are required to produce clinical infection. With the presence of foreign material, this number is reduced to 10^2. Hemostasis must be meticulous, as the presence of hematoma reduces the bacterial inoculum necessary to result in infection. The hematoma represents an ideal culture medium and is a "nonvascularized" area. The use of drains may be indicated in lacerations of the parotid gland or in extensive injuries where tissue fluid may accumulate, producing a dead space, which again reduces the bacterial inoculum causing infection.

The tissue edges can be cleansed with antiseptics, detergent soaps, and water. In rare cases, solvents such as ether, benzene, and alcohol may be necessary to remove materials not soluble in water or not removable by scrubbing or debridement. Scrubbing with a brush under adequate anesthesia is required to remove foreign material and prevent the development of infection and "traumatic tattoo." In some areas, immediate dermabrasion has been suggested. It is absolutely essential (see Fig. 27–8) to remove all materials in the wound at the time of initial treatment. They cannot be satisfactorily removed by any procedure, even secondary dermabrasion, once healing has occurred. The material can be removed initially with scrubbing, or the point of a No. 11 blade or a small dermatologic curette may help dislodge material.

Photography

Modern methods of photography make it simple to obtain an accurate photographic record of the patient throughout the course of treatment. Such records are important for insurance and for legal purposes. Photographs supplement the written evaluations and enhance the value of medical records. They help the surgeon assess the effectiveness of the therapy by providing a means of review of each case at its termination. The patient can appreciate the severity of the injury by reviewing initial photographs.

It is important also to include *preinjury* photographs for the purpose of identifying abnormalities present *before* the injury: developmental abnormalities, asymmetry, malocclusion, and previous scars. Old photographs document the facial features to be reconstructed and demonstrate the facial height and projection to be achieved (see Fig. 27–21*B*).

Preoperative Considerations

The patient should be in optimal condition for operative procedures on the facial structures. Correction of shock, hypovolemia, dehydration, and electrolyte imbalance should precede all surgical procedures except those necessary for emergency care. Conditions such as diabetes should be under control. A Foley catheter, arterial and venous pressure lines, an intracranial pressure monitor, and an oxygen saturation monitor provide reliable evidence of organ function during surgery. Some patients may be treated with steroids for head injuries. Those with rheumatic or valvular heart disease should be protected by perioperative antibiotic treatment.

Anesthesia

The extent of the injuries, the general condition of the patient, and the psychologic reaction to surgery in most cases dictate the use of a general anesthetic. General anesthesia is usually indicated because the tissues are hypersensitive, and prolonged operative procedures or manipulation of the facial structures may be distressing to the patient under local anesthesia. Although general anesthesia is preferable for the management of extensive facial trauma, there may be competition for working space presented by the necessity to perform simultaneous operative procedures or the presence of anesthetic or x-ray equipment adjacent to the operative field. A skilled anesthesiologist is needed to administer the general anesthesia under these difficult circumstances. Frequently, when local anesthesia is utilized, he can offer assistance by providing monitoring and judicious use of intravenous sedative drugs as a supplement to local anesthesia.

Nasotracheal anesthesia is usually satisfactory for the reduction and fixation of fractures of the maxilla or mandible, in which the nasal passages are not involved. Endotracheal anesthesia with oral intubation may be possible for maxillary or mandibular fractures if the tube can be placed behind the last molar tooth. The requirement for placing the patient in intermaxillary fixation before fracture fixation may prevent the use of oral intubation in some cases. Oral intubation is, however, satisfactory for fractures of the upper face when it is not necessary to establish intermaxillary fixation. When there is combined involvement of the mandible, maxilla, and nasal or other facial bones, a preoperative tracheotomy performed under local or general anesthesia and the administration of an anesthetic agent through the tracheostomy tube may be the method of choice. This is especially true if the patient has an accompanying head or chest injury, since tracheostomy makes pulmonary management easier. Anesthesia by a transtracheal route permits unobstructed reduction and fixation of facial fractures, placement of intermaxillary fixation, intranasal packing, and application of splints, head frames, and other appliances without the need to worry about airway obstruction. Postoperative edema of the floor of the mouth, neck, and hypopharyngeal area is not a concern if a tracheostomy has been performed. On the other hand, one must be alert to these conditions in the postoperative period. The use of a tracheostomy rather than prolonged nasotracheal intubation is dictated by the experience of the surgeon and of the team that is to provide postoperative monitoring and nursing care. Inadvertent extubation of an endotracheal tube when intermaxillary fixation and swelling of the floor of the mouth and pharynx are present may be a disaster causing the patient's death.

LOCAL ANESTHESIA

An attitude of reassurance, understanding, and sympathy, together with adequate premedication, permits extensive operations under local anesthesia (see Chap. 4). Nerve blocks may be performed to establish regional anesthesia in a wide field with reduced dosage of medication and less discomfort. Less complicated wounds, such as small cuts, bruises, lacerations, and some uncomplicated fractures of the facial bones (e.g., the nose), may be treated under local anesthesia, either in the operating room or in an outpatient treatment area, such as the emergency room.

Debridement and Care

Thorough, careful cleansing of all soft tissue wounds is imperative before any definitive treatment is attempted. All blood and debris should be carefully washed from the tissues with copious amounts of water and mild detergents. Foreign materials, such as glass, hair, clothing, tooth structures, pieces of artificial dentures, paint, grease, gravel, and dirt, should be removed (Fig. 27–46).

Except for the removal of obviously devitalized portions of tissue, extensive debridement of soft tissue has little place in the management of facial injuries. All tissues that may participate in a satisfactory repair should be retained. It is usually preferable to err on the side of retaining tissues that may not survive than to debride or destroy any tissues that might be important in a final result. The excellent blood supply of the face makes extensive debridement unnecessary. Often, critical tissue that is supplied by only a small pedicle will survive. Wounds of the same magnitude in other areas of the body necessitate more extensive surgical debridement.

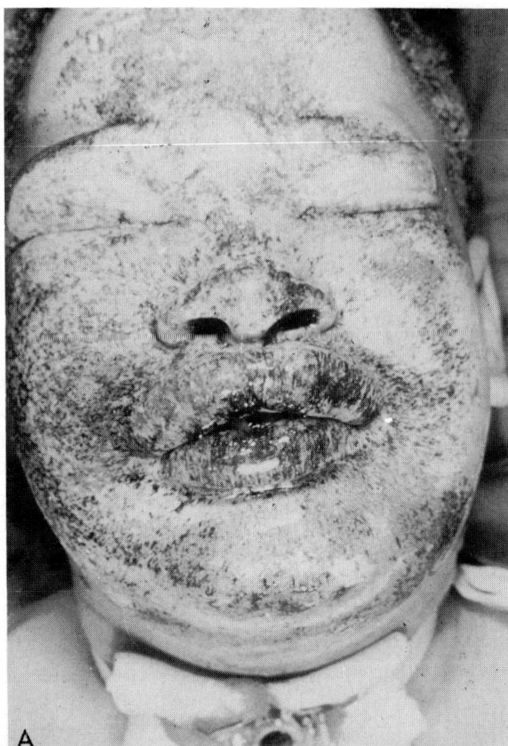

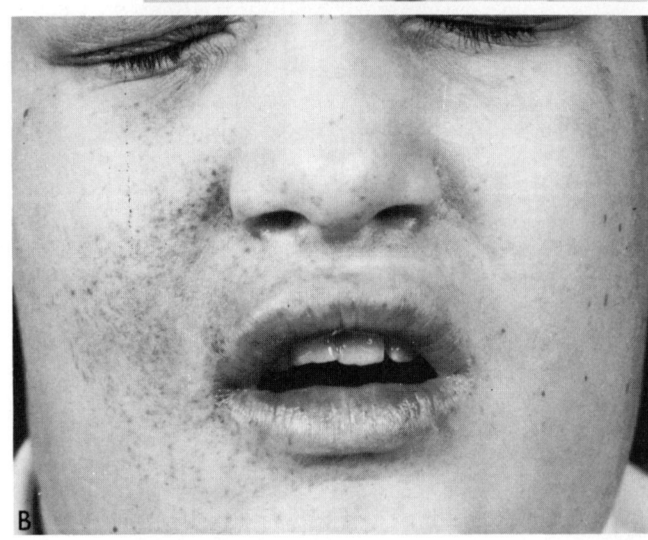

Figure 27–46. *A,* Injury in a 14 year old boy two hours after explosion of a homemade bomb. Inhalation of flame and hot gases resulted in severe edema and obstruction of the upper airway requiring either emergency intubation or tracheotomy. Superficial skin wounds were treated by scrubbing the powder particles away and curetting any remains. *B,* Three months after the injury. Much of the pigment could be subsequently removed by dermabrasion. It is always preferable to remove foreign material thoroughly at the time of original treatment.

ABRASIONS

Care should be exercised in the management of abrasions, even though the injury may be superficial, since many contain dirt. When first seen, a child with superficial abrasions may not appear to have any injury of consequence. Upon healing, however, a pigmented residual defect may be discovered. Dirt, grease, carbon, and other pigments should be carefully scrubbed out of the wound and a light lubricating dressing applied. Moist compresses (wet to wet) or the application of an antibacterial ointment will prevent drying and desiccation of the exposed wound surfaces. It cannot be overemphasized that the character of a fresh abrasion often masks the perception of retained dirt. Accidental or traumatic tattoo results in considerable cosmetic disability.

CONTUSED WOUNDS

Contusions usually result in extensive edema, ecchymosis, and hematomas that generally subside without active treatment. Subcutaneous hematomas are either localized or diffuse. Most hematomas are diffuse and absorb gradually. Occasionally an eyelid, cheek, or forehead hematoma requires drainage (Fig. 27–47). Contusions are often associated with lacerations or abrasions. Damaged contused tissue appears to heal more slowly than tissues suffering a clean laceration. Pigmentation changes, such as hyperpigmentation or hypopigmentation, may result from contusion. There may also be soft tissue atrophy following the blunt injury, and the final results of healing may be less desirable than anticipated.

LACERATED CONTUSED WOUNDS

The contused margins of lacerations should be excised unless they occupy the areas previously mentioned (lips, ears, ala of the nose, eyebrow, eyelid). The crushed tissue margin results in less satisfactory healing if allowed to remain. The removal of 1, or perhaps 2, mm of tissue creates a surgically clean wound with healthier tissue. If the contused marginal tissues are of anatomic importance, it is best to avoid debridement and consider secondary reconstructive surgery, if required.

DEEP LACERATIONS

Lacerations caused by sharp, clean objects, such as a knife, a windshield, flying glass, or sharp metal, may extend through all layers of the soft tissues and involve important muscles, nerves, glands, and ducts (Fig. 27–48). The muscles of facial expression are so closely associated with the skin that careful closure of the wound in layers gives adequate approximation of the muscle. If possible, facial muscle layers should be identified and closed separately with fine absorbable sutures. Partial lacerations of the muscles of mastication occur, but complete severance is uncommon. Closure of the muscle and fascia in layers, including the subcutaneous tissue, restores adequate function and prevents adherence of cheek skin to the muscle (Fig. 27–49).

FACIAL NERVE

It is often impractical and usually unnecessary to identify and suture the terminal branches of the facial nerve. The plexus of nerve fibers makes regeneration of activity a common occurrence despite the absence of direct facial nerve suturing. Reasonably ac-

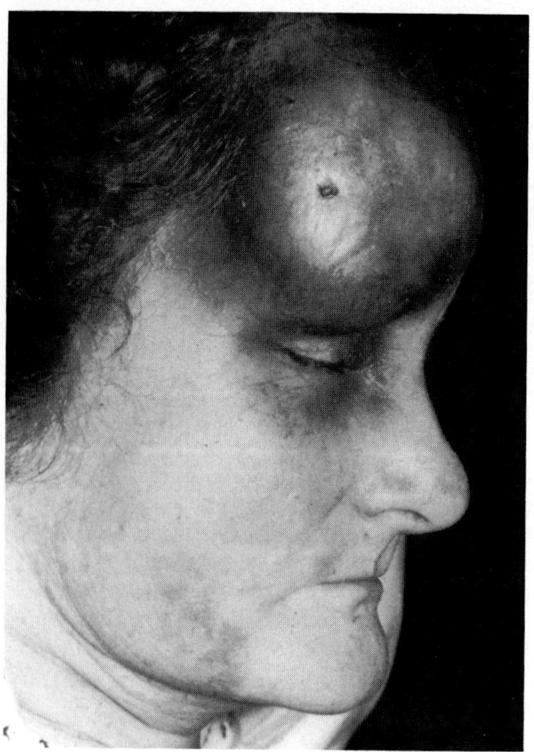

Figure 27–47. A forehead hematoma from a blunt injury to the supraorbital region. The supraorbital artery has been lacerated. Skin necrosis is occurring. The hematoma should be aspirated and the blood thoroughly removed with an operative irrigation.

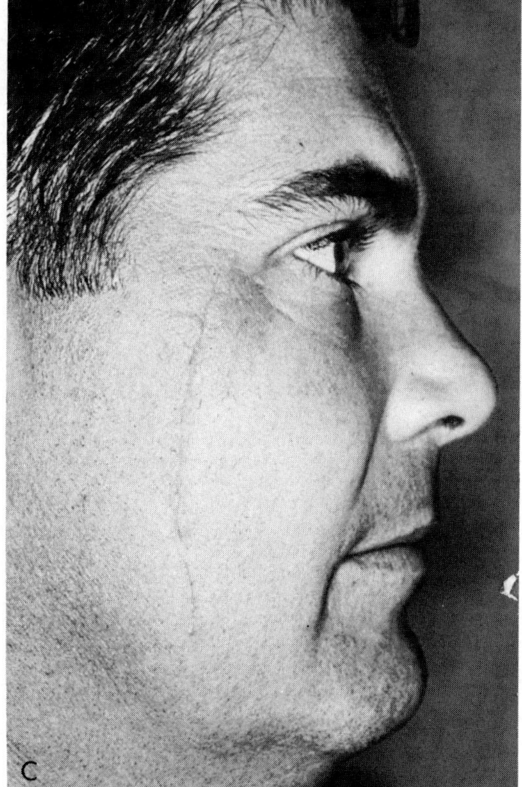

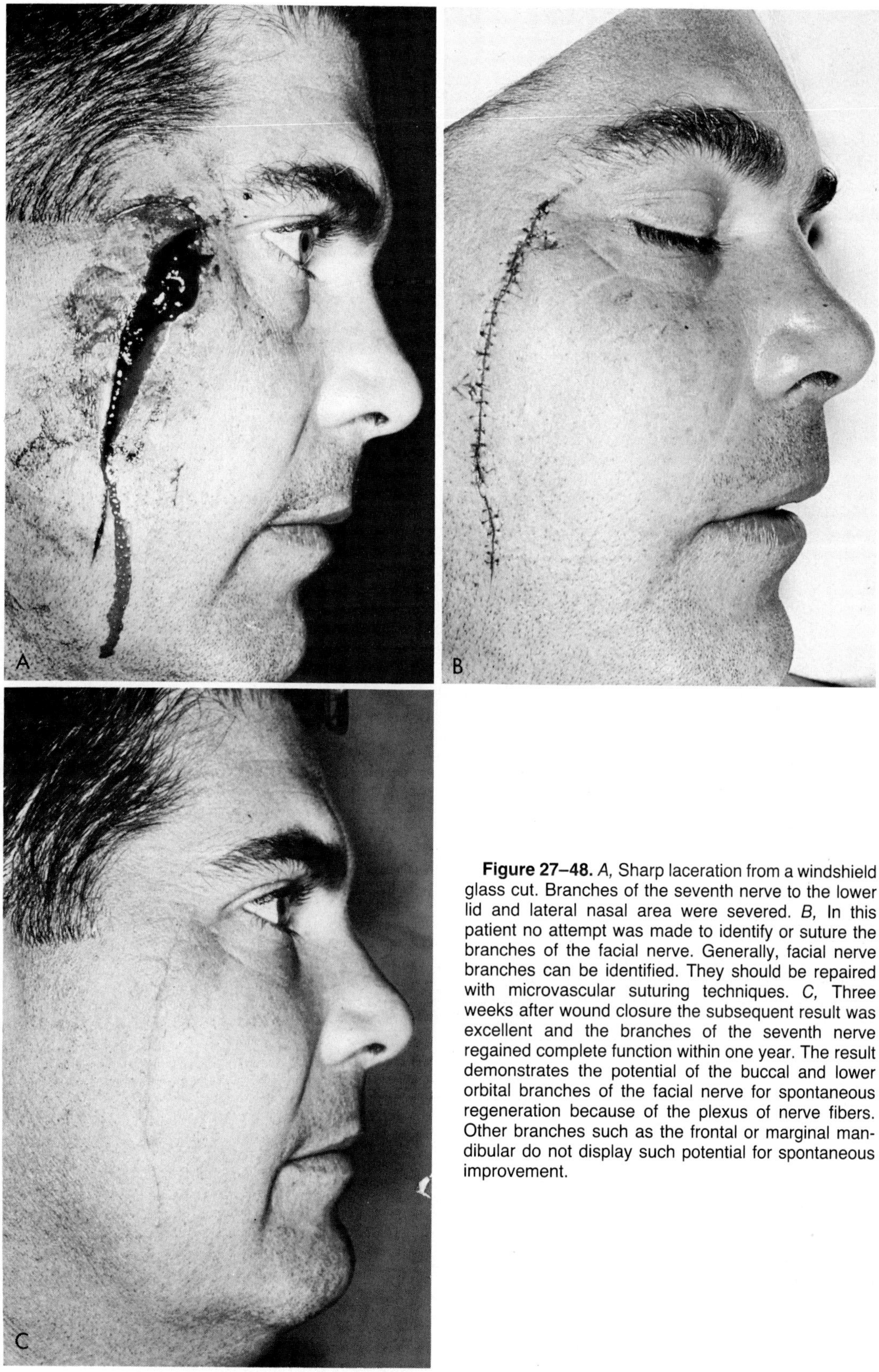

Figure 27–48. *A,* Sharp laceration from a windshield glass cut. Branches of the seventh nerve to the lower lid and lateral nasal area were severed. *B,* In this patient no attempt was made to identify or suture the branches of the facial nerve. Generally, facial nerve branches can be identified. They should be repaired with microvascular suturing techniques. *C,* Three weeks after wound closure the subsequent result was excellent and the branches of the seventh nerve regained complete function within one year. The result demonstrates the potential of the buccal and lower orbital branches of the facial nerve for spontaneous regeneration because of the plexus of nerve fibers. Other branches such as the frontal or marginal mandibular do not display such potential for spontaneous improvement.

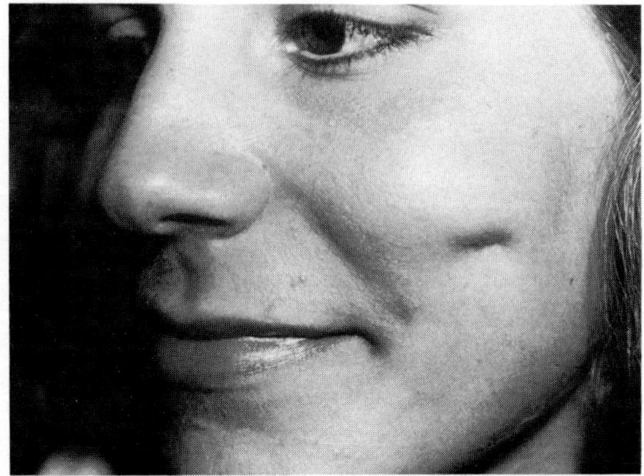

Figure 27–49. Adhesion of the skin to the underlying facial muscles following a small laceration produces an unsightly dimple. Reapproximating the fat with a scar revision can improve the appearance.

curate approximation of the tissues usually allows some element of nerve regeneration by neurotization of muscle. It is stated in the literature that nerve repair need not be performed anterior to a line drawn at the lateral canthus of the eyelids. In practice, the author repairs any identifiable branch of the facial nerve in the wound. Suture of named branches of the facial nerve should be performed and the branches should be searched for. Within two days, stimulation of the distal branch is not effective, and primary repair at the time of initial treatment is recommended. If the repair is delayed two to three days beyond injury, the distal branches of the nerve do not respond to faradic nerve stimulation. The nerves must be located through knowledge of their position and careful dissection with the aid of magnifying loupes. Repair under the microscope, utilizing the principles stressed for peripheral nerve repair, is recommended. If the seventh nerve has been injured within the parotid gland, a formal exposure and resuturing of the major branches should be performed. Dissection of the proximal portion of the nerve is necessary in order to identify it accurately and to allow approximation with fine sutures without tension.

TRIGEMINAL NERVE

The sensory branches of the trigeminal (fifth cranial) nerve in the region of the skin are small, and approximation is impractical and unnecessary. Partial or complete recovery of sensation usually occurs within a few months to a year. Slight hypoesthesia is the rule. Contusion of trigeminal nerve branches also occurs as a result of fractures. For example, the infraorbital nerve is often crushed at its exit from the infraorbital foramen in zygomatic or maxillary fractures.

PAROTID DUCT LACERATIONS

Lacerations of the parotid duct should be repaired at the time of wound closure to prevent parotid fistula to the skin surface or to the mucous membrane of the mouth. The latter is not significant, but a parotid fistula to the skin is an annoying problem (Fig. 27–50). To identify the course of the parotid duct, a line is drawn from the tragus of the ear to the midportion of the upper lip. The duct traverses the middle third of the line (Line *A–B* in Fig. 27–51). The parotid duct travels adjacent to the buccal branch of the facial nerve. Buccal branch paralysis with an overlying laceration should suggest the possibility of a parotid duct injury. The parotid, or Stensen's, duct empties into the mouth opposite the maxillary second molar. Injury can be identified by first gently dilating the orifice of Stensen's duct with a small lacrimal dila-

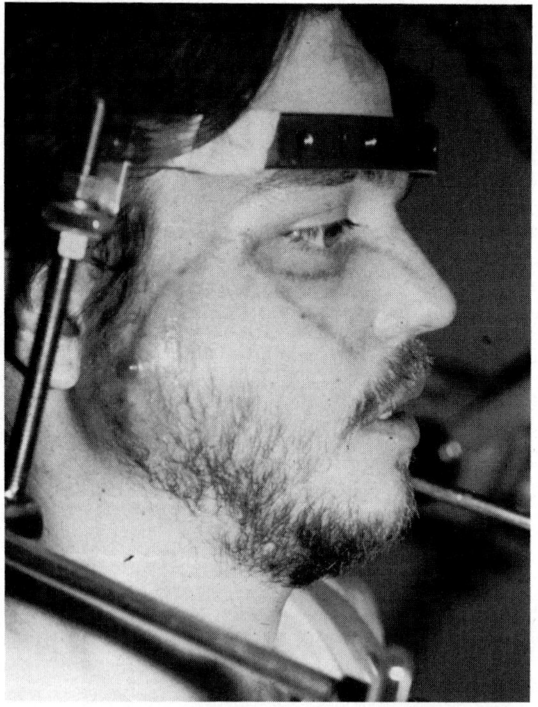

Figure 27–50. A transection of the parotid gland. Healing was followed by the development of a transient cutaneous fistula. Fistulas such as this one invariably close in the absence of major duct (distal) obstruction.

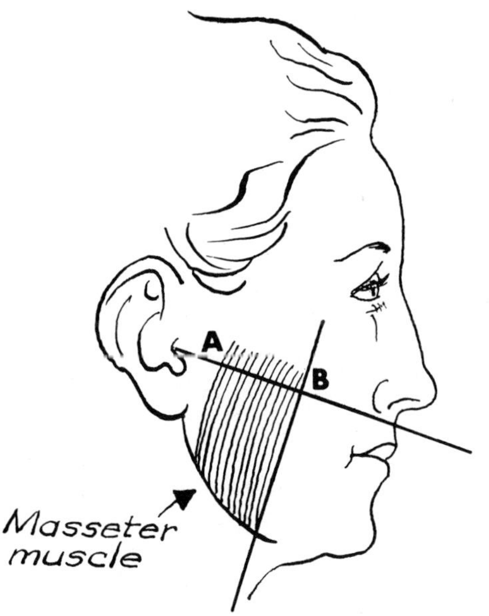

Figure 27–51. The course of Stensen's duct from the parotid into the upper buccal area is deep to the middle third of the line drawn from the tragus of the ear to the midportion of the upper lip. This corresponds roughly to the anterior limits of the masseter muscle. The hilus of the gland is at approximately point *A*, and the opening of the duct into the mouth is opposite the second maxillary molar tooth deep to point *B*. The buccal branch of the facial nerve crosses Stensen's duct near point *B*.

tor. Care must be taken not to injure the duct with the pointed tip of the dilator. A Silastic tube or silver probe may be inserted into the opening of the duct and the course of the duct followed. The duct can be irrigated with saline with a No. 22 Angiocath sleeve. The appearance of saline in the wound indicates that the duct is severed or partially transected. The proximal end of the duct may be identified in the wound expressing secretion of saliva. A Silastic catheter is placed in the duct and a repair with fine sutures is performed (Fig. 27–52). The use of loupe magnification is recommended. The tube is left in for a two week period as tolerated. The stent tubing may be trimmed with the end protruding into the mouth and anchored to the mucous membrane to prevent accidental dislodgement.

Lacerations of the gland that occur in the absence of major duct lacerations do not require treatment other than the routine management of the soft tissue. A drain should be left in place. No permanent fistulas have been observed from glandular lacerations in the absence of major duct involvement (see Fig. 27–50).

If the parotid duct cannot be repaired, there are several choices available: ligation, which produces a great deal of temporary swelling and has the possibility of late chronic infection of the gland; diversion of the proximal duct stump into the mouth at a more proximal location (often difficult); and radiation of the gland to destroy function. All these options are less desirable than primary repair. Lacerations of the gland frequently result in delayed fluid accumulation, even after drain removal. The fluid may be treated by intermittent aspiration, compression, creation of an area for dependent drainage, or reinsertion of a vacuum-aspirated drain. When the skin has become adherent to the gland, the drain is removed and the fistula closes.

SUBMAXILLARY DUCT INJURIES

The submaxillary duct is not often injured in fractures or soft tissue injuries unless there is a comminuted type of mandibular fracture with a laceration of the floor of the mouth or a gunshot injury that involves the floor of the mouth. Repair of the submaxillary duct is unnecessary. If it is unrepaired, a fistula into the floor of the mouth usually results. Scar with obstruction of the duct may require consideration for reestablishing a duct opening. Obstruction or chronic fistula of the duct is, however, usually treated by submaxillary gland excision.

LACRIMAL SYSTEM LACERATIONS

Lacerations near the medial canthus may sever the canaliculi or damage the lacrimal sac or other parts of the lacrimal system (see also Chap. 34). If a canaliculus is severed, the severed ends are sutured over a fine Silastic tubing utilizing microsurgical techniques (Callahan, 1979). The upper and lower lacrimal system should be intubated with fine Silastic tubing. The upper canaliculus alone is insufficient to drain the lacrimal secretion properly and the failure to repair a severed lower canaliculus results in epiphora. The duct ends can be identified by dilating the orifice of the lacrimal duct and irrigating with saline with a fine catheter. Saline in the wound identifies a lacrimal transection. Most late lacrimal obstruction is due to bone injury and compression of the nasolacrimal duct, and is treated by dacryocystorhinostomy (see Chap. 34).

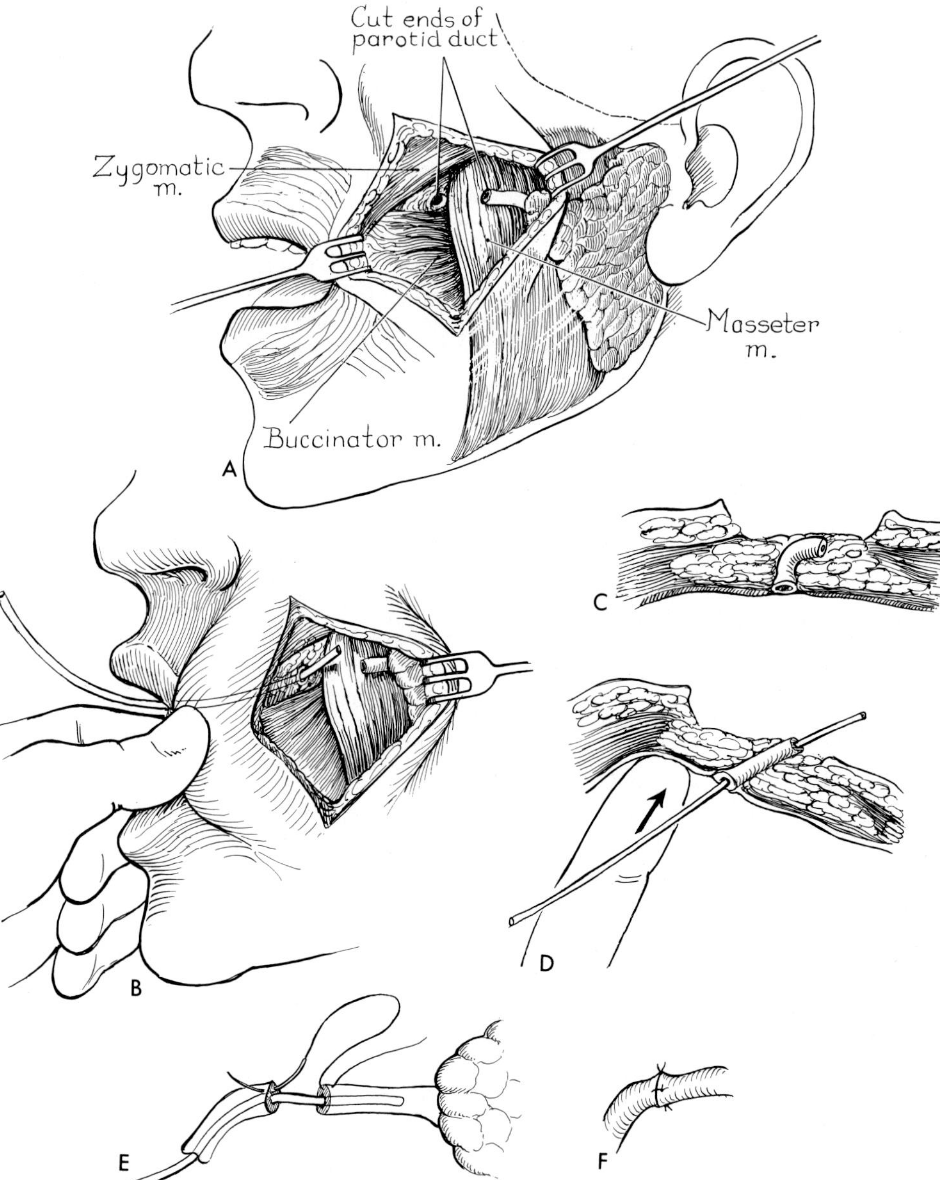

Figure 27–52. Repair of a severed parotid duct. *A,* Severed duct at the anterior border of the masseter muscle. *B,* A fine caliber Silastic catheter is threaded through the buccal opening of Stensen's duct. *C,* Angulation of Stensen's duct as it penetrates through the cheek wall. The angulation renders difficult the penetration of the catheter into the duct. *D,* Outward stretching of the cheek wall tends to straighten the duct and facilitates threading of the catheter through it. *E,* Direct anastomosis of the cut ends of the duct using a catheter as a splint. *F,* After suture of the cut ends of the duct. The stint should be left in the duct for a 10 to 14 day period.

INJURY TO SOFT TISSUES OF ORBIT

The eyes should be carefully inspected for abrasions, lacerations of the cornea, or puncture of the globe. Low pressure (soft globe) is indicative of a globe rupture. Many ruptures of the globe from blunt injury are accompanied by lid margin lacerations. Eyelid and associated ocular injuries deserve priority in the scale of the patient's wounds, including those away from the facial area. Lacerations through the eyelid margins require specialized repair if a serious esthetic and functional disability is to be avoided. The globe must be protected from drying until the repair can be performed. The skin wound that accompanies a penetrating injury of the globe may be quite trivial in appearance. The presence of fat in a wound in the periorbital region may indicate a penetrating globe injury. Protrusion of the fat into the wound also indicates the possibility of extraocular muscle transection. In all severe injuries in the periorbital area, consultation with an ophthalmologist may be desirable in order fully to evaluate globe injury, such as retinal detachment. If an ophthalmologist is not available, visual function should be ascertained *before any* treatment *is undertaken*. The minimal examination should include an assessment of vision (Rosenbaum pocket card), the degree of extraocular motion, an evaluation for diplopia, a funduscopic examination and a measurement of intraocular pressure (Barton and Berry, 1982). Visual acuity *must* always be ascertained before a deep laceration or fracture in the orbital region is treated. Pupillary inequality should be assessed. Miller and Tenzel (1967) suggested a number of simple tests that may be made in the emergency room. Reading a newspaper (elderly patients should wear their presbyopic correction glasses), the finger counting test (in four quadrants), and the Marcus Gunn pupillary sign are practical means of determining visual function. The Marcus Gunn test is discussed in detail later in the chapter (see Fig. 27–298). The direct and consensual response of the pupil to light is noted and the response of the contralateral eye documented. Any decrease or loss of visual function should be documented preoperatively and the patient should be asked about any history of visual loss. Litigation after treatment is common and visual loss may be inappropriately ascribed to a surgical procedure in the absence of a proper preoperative examination.

LACERATIONS OF NOSE

Lacerations of the nose may involve the skin, the lining in the vestibule of the nose, or the mucous membrane of the nasal cavity, most commonly at the junction of the bone and the cartilages (Fig. 27–53). The blow may produce sudden telescopic movements of the soft tissues, which are sheared off their attachments at the bony nasal margin. A thick, boggy, edematous septum may indicate a hematoma and a septocartilage laceration may be seen through a tear in the mucoperichondrium. Intranasal suturing of the laceration after reduction of the soft tissue and bone structures is performed accurately. Some intranasal lacerations do not require suture approximation. Intranasal packing may be utilized to approximate soft tissues and to prevent the accumulation of hematoma. The skin of the nose heals rapidly and sutures may be removed early. Early suture removal in lacerations of the skin of the nasal tip prevents unsightly scarring. The glandular structure of the skin of the nasal tip usually produces scars more prominent than those obtained in lacerations of the proximal portion of the nose.

Avulsions of the section of the nose near the tip and ala are repaired by using the original piece of skin and cartilage as a composite graft, if it is available. If the severed tissue is not available, skin to mucosa closure or a dressing technique may be utilized until soft tissue reconstruction is accomplished. In many cases, use of severed tissue is followed by uneventful healing. An important anatomic structure that is otherwise difficult or impossible to reconstruct can thus be saved.

AVULSED WOUNDS OF FACIAL AREA

If the wounds cannot be closed because of the avulsion and loss of soft tissue, a split-thickness skin graft provides immediate wound closure, avoiding infection and the use of dressings (Fig. 27–54). Full-thickness losses of nasal alar tissue may be repaired by the use of composite grafts from the ear margin as a primary reconstruction in selected circumstances (Fig. 27–55). The grafts usually survive if clean margins of soft tissue are established with surgical debridement. No part of the composite graft should be more than 1 to 1.5 cm away from its nutrient bed. Use of a larger skin to cartilage component

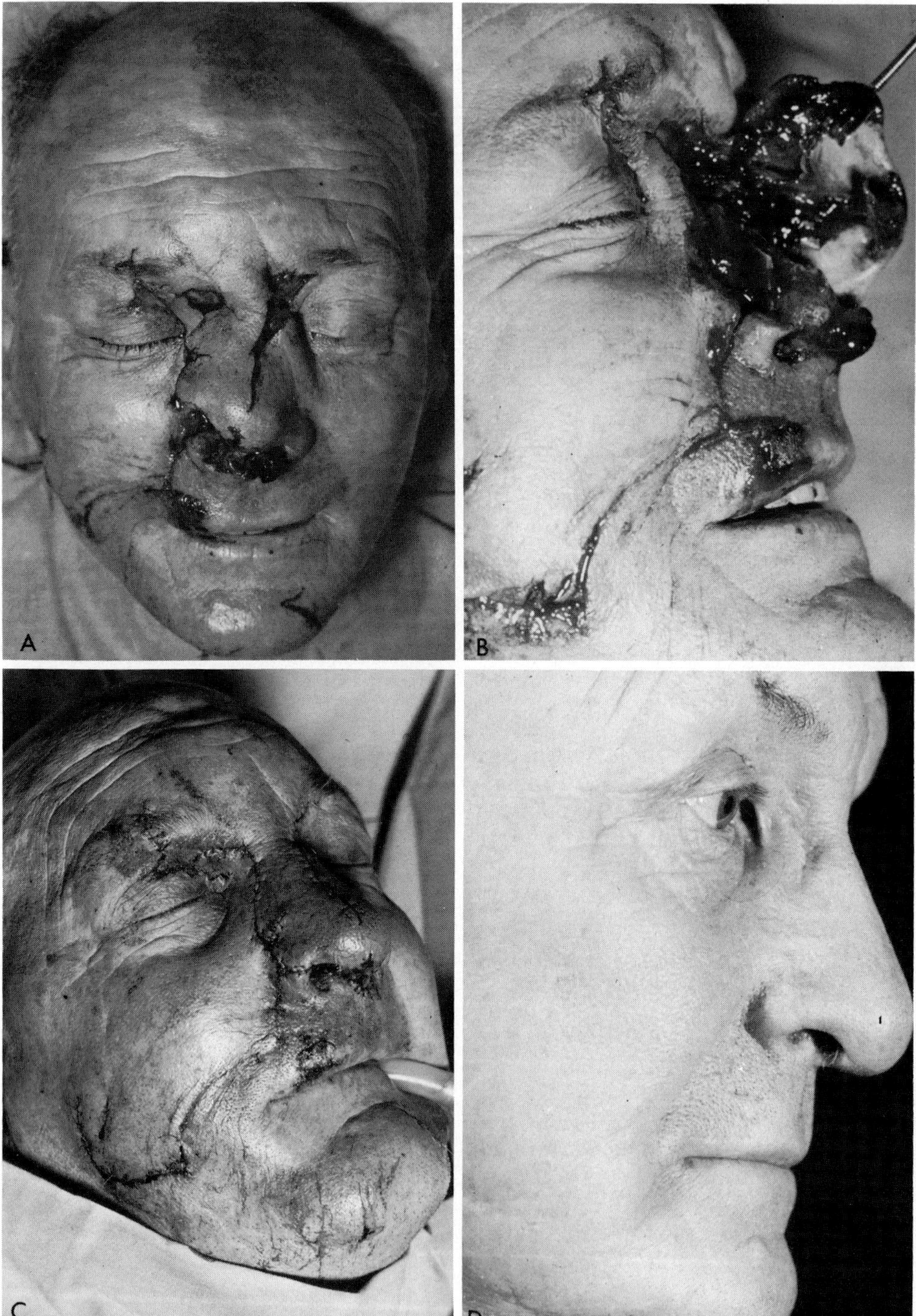

Figure 27–53. Facial wounds may be much more extensive than they appear on initial examination. The lacerated tissue should be retracted and the wound thoroughly irrigated, and cleansed of clots, and debrided after careful inspection. *B,* Retraction of the flaps demonstrates extensive injury to the nasal bones and cartilage. *C,* The fractured nasal bones are reduced and held by direct open wiring technique. The cartilaginous structures should be reapproximated to the bones with either sutures or fine wires. The mucous membrane of the nose is resutured before the wires are tightened. An immediate nasal bone graft may be performed for severe destruction of the nasal pyramid. *D,* Six months after operation, the patient has a patent nasal airway with minimal scarring after a single primary procedure.

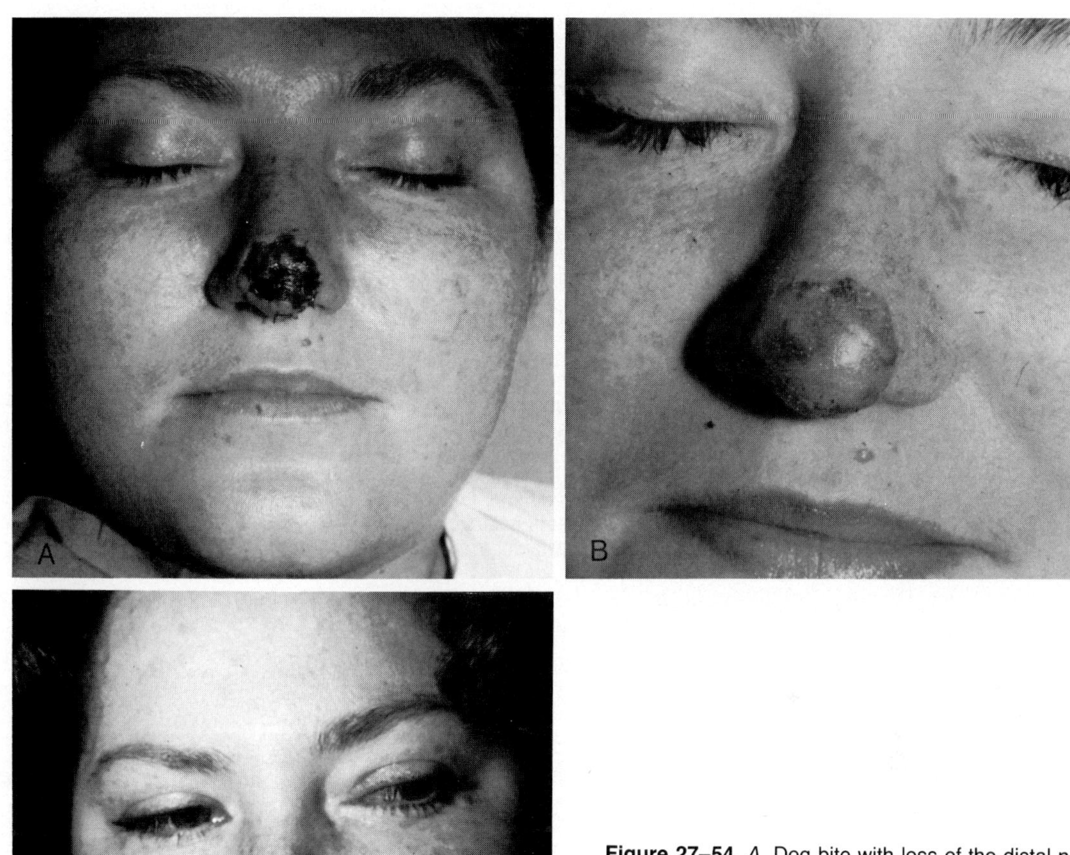

Figure 27–54. *A,* Dog bite with loss of the distal nose. *B,* Full-thickness skin graft applied for coverage. *C,* The result obtained after one year.

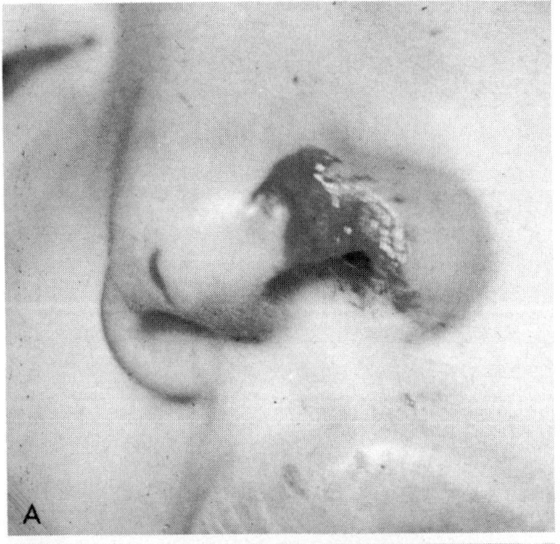

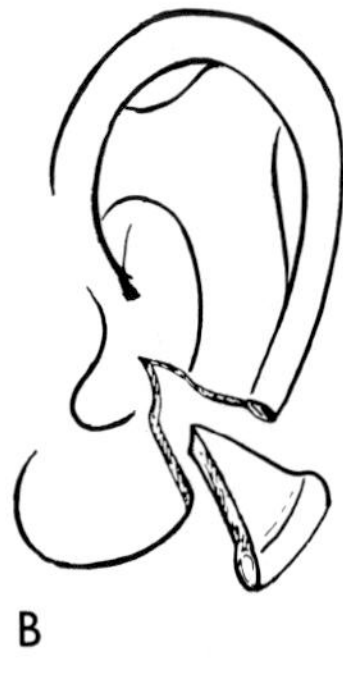

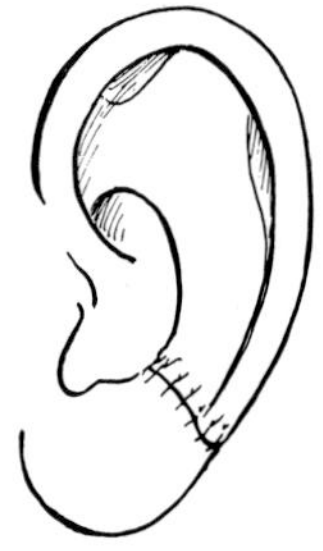

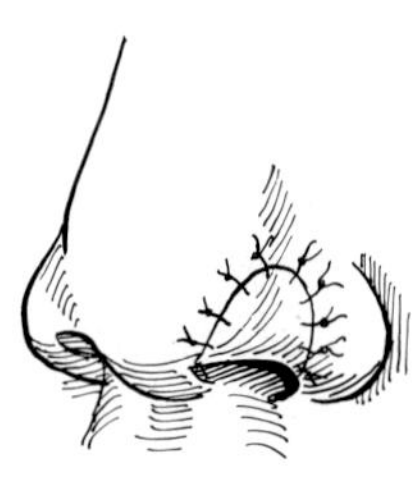

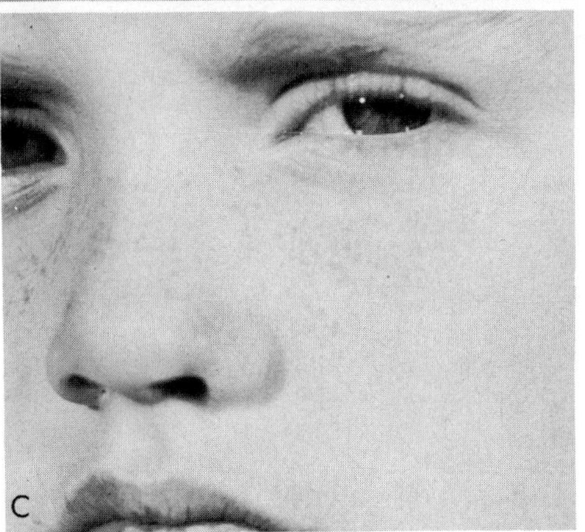

Figure 27–55. *A,* Six hours after full-thickness avulsion of the lateral nasal area by a dog bite. *B,* Early repair with a composite graft from the left ear. The graft contains skin for covering, cartilage for support, and skin for the lining. The auricle provides an excellent graft material for repair of nasal tip defects. The resultant auricular defect is minimal. *C,* The result one year after repair demonstrates a satisfactory reconstruction of the alar margin.

in the composite graft is also thought to increase the chance of survival.

LACERATIONS OF LIPS

Lacerations of the lips may involve only the superficial skin and subcutaneous tissues or may extend into the orbicularis oris muscle. Full-thickness lacerations can also be encountered. Bleeding may be profuse if the labial artery is severed. Local pressure or hemostatic ligation of the vessel controls the bleeding. The repair of a full-thickness lip laceration employs absorbable sutures in the mucosa and muscular layers. Accurate approximation of the muscle assists alignment of the vermilion-cutaneous junction. The vermilion-cutaneous margin and the vermilion-mucosal margin provide accurate landmarks, which should be precisely approximated (Fig. 27–56). Avoiding the use of vasoconstrictor agents allows more accurate identification of the vermilion-cutaneous margin. Debridement should be minimal. After careful and thorough cleansing of the wound, the lip structures may be closed in layers, beginning with the deepest and working out to the skin. The vermilion-cutaneous margin and the mucosal margins are landmarks from which to begin suturing of the skin.

INJURIES OF AURICLE

The ear may be involved in abrasions, contusions, lacerations, and hematomas. Abrasions heal with the continued application of light dressing and ointment. A well-designed dressing, suitably padded (with mineral oil–soaked cotton), minimizes edema and hemorrhage. Care must be taken that this does not exert inordinate pressure preventing circulation to a portion of the auricle. Appropriate debridement and cleansing of the wound minimize the sequelae of chondritis and deformity.

Lacerations of the auricle are usually as-

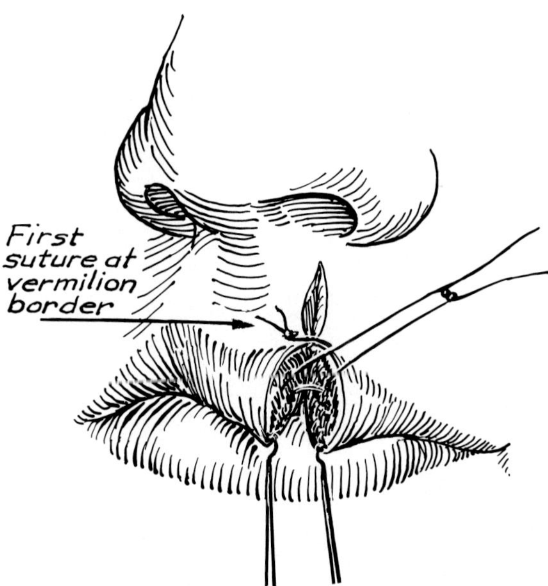

Figure 27–56. Repair of a vertical laceration of the vermilion-cutaneous margin. The first suture should be used for approximation of the vermilion-cutaneous border. Injection of a local anesthetic containing epinephrine might diminish the ability to align this suture. Both edges of the vermilion, including that adjacent to the skin and white roll of the lip and that adjacent to the mucous membrane, should be carefully aligned.

sociated with lacerations of the cartilage. The ear may be totally or incompletely avulsed, but is often viable when even a small pedicle remains. The ear should be carefully sutured into place and adequately supported with dressings. The ear canal can be stented with Xeroform gauze. Several fine chromic or Dexon sutures may approximate the cartilage and provide additional stability to the cutaneous repair. The cartilage should be trimmed accurate to the skin margin. The auricle has numerous landmarks that allow the accurate placement of skin sutures providing excellent realignment and minimal deformity (Fig. 27–57).

Avulsion of small or moderate-sized segments of auricle (missing tissue) can be adequately repaired by replacement with composite grafts or with a local flap. In general, existing skin should be closed and the defect reconstructed secondarily when a clean healed wound has been obtained. Hematomas of the ear and total avulsion of the skin or auricle are also discussed in Chapter 40.

CARE OF EXTENSIVE SOFT TISSUE WOUNDS WITH LOSS OF STRUCTURE AND TISSUE

Loss of tissue may preclude wound closure. If an extensive wound, such as one produced by an avulsive injury, cannot be treated by means of a skin graft or by a local rotation or advancement of tissue in the immediate area, the mucous membrane of the mouth or nasal cavity should be advanced to the skin margin and approximated with sutures. Primary closure prevents contracture, allows healing, and decreases infection. Early healing facilitates the definitive repair and minimizes the use of postoperative dressings. Every effort should be made to cover exposed bone with soft tissue to prevent desiccation and necrosis.

The most satisfactory scars after repair of facial lacerations are seen in cases in which the laceration parallels the relaxed lines of skin tension. These parallel the expressive skin folds of the face. Fortunate is the patient who has lacerations running in the proper direction. The final results may be less than optimal when the lacerations occur at right angles or at variance with the relaxed lines of skin tension.

Undermining should not produce distortion of adjacent facial features, such as the angle of the mouth or the ala of the nose. Undermining may be more extensive on one side of the wound than on the other to avoid damage to vessels, nerves, and other important structures. The degree of undermining should not be such as to interfere with the vascularity of partially avulsed flaps. Judicious excision of excess fat and subcutaneous tissues in selected cases may relieve tension on the wound margins and permit proper eversion of skin edges. Contused fat often heals with fibrosis and thickening.

Fine nylon or polyglycolic acid suture materials provide subcutaneous fixation with minimal reaction. Sutures should be placed close enough to relieve all surface wound tension. The cutaneous sutures should merely ensure epithelial approximation. Interrupted sutures, if utilized, are carefully placed and tied without excess tension; in this manner, suture marks are avoided. Interrupted surface sutures should be used cautiously in patients who are subject to hypertrophic scar formation. The subcuticular suture (Fig. 27–58) is excellent for skin closure in these

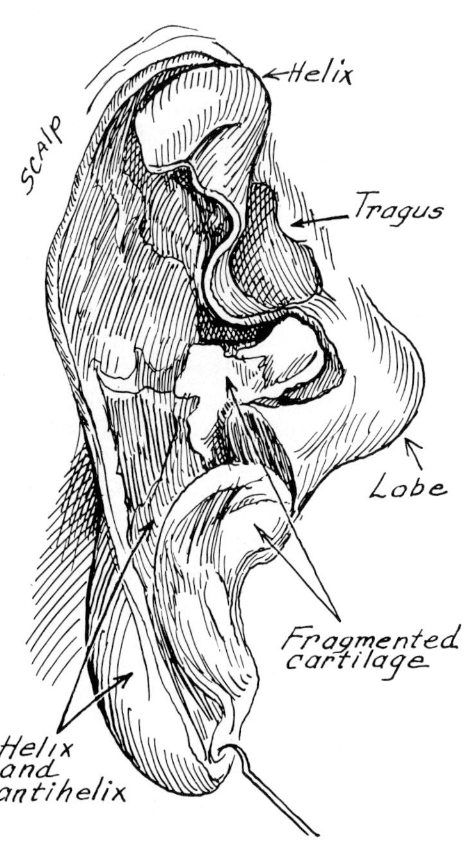

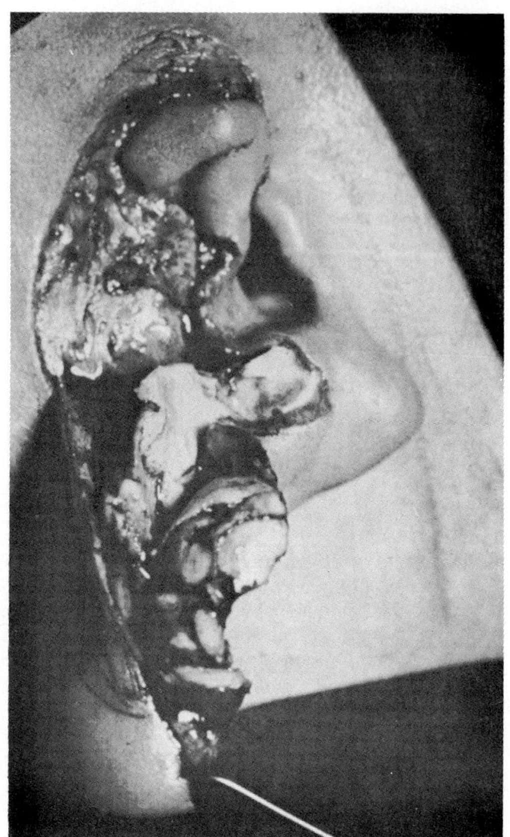

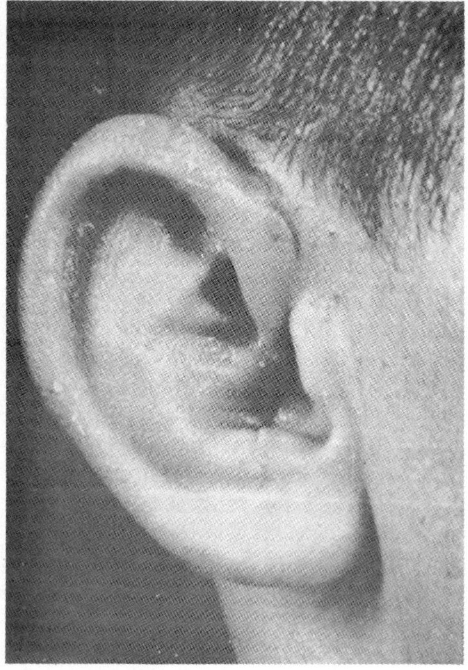

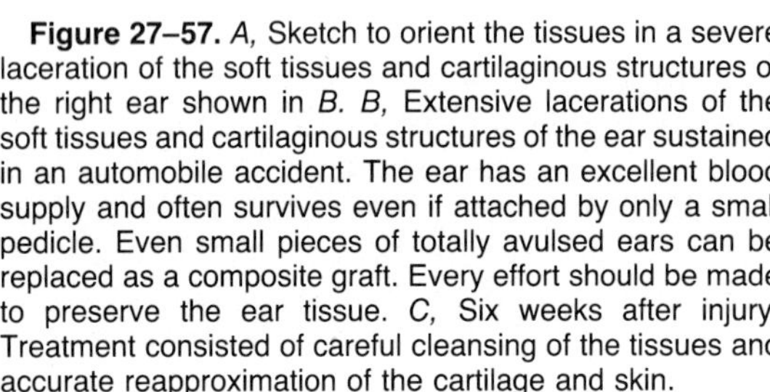

Figure 27–57. *A,* Sketch to orient the tissues in a severe laceration of the soft tissues and cartilaginous structures of the right ear shown in *B. B,* Extensive lacerations of the soft tissues and cartilaginous structures of the ear sustained in an automobile accident. The ear has an excellent blood supply and often survives even if attached by only a small pedicle. Even small pieces of totally avulsed ears can be replaced as a composite graft. Every effort should be made to preserve the ear tissue. *C,* Six weeks after injury. Treatment consisted of careful cleansing of the tissues and accurate reapproximation of the cartilage and skin.

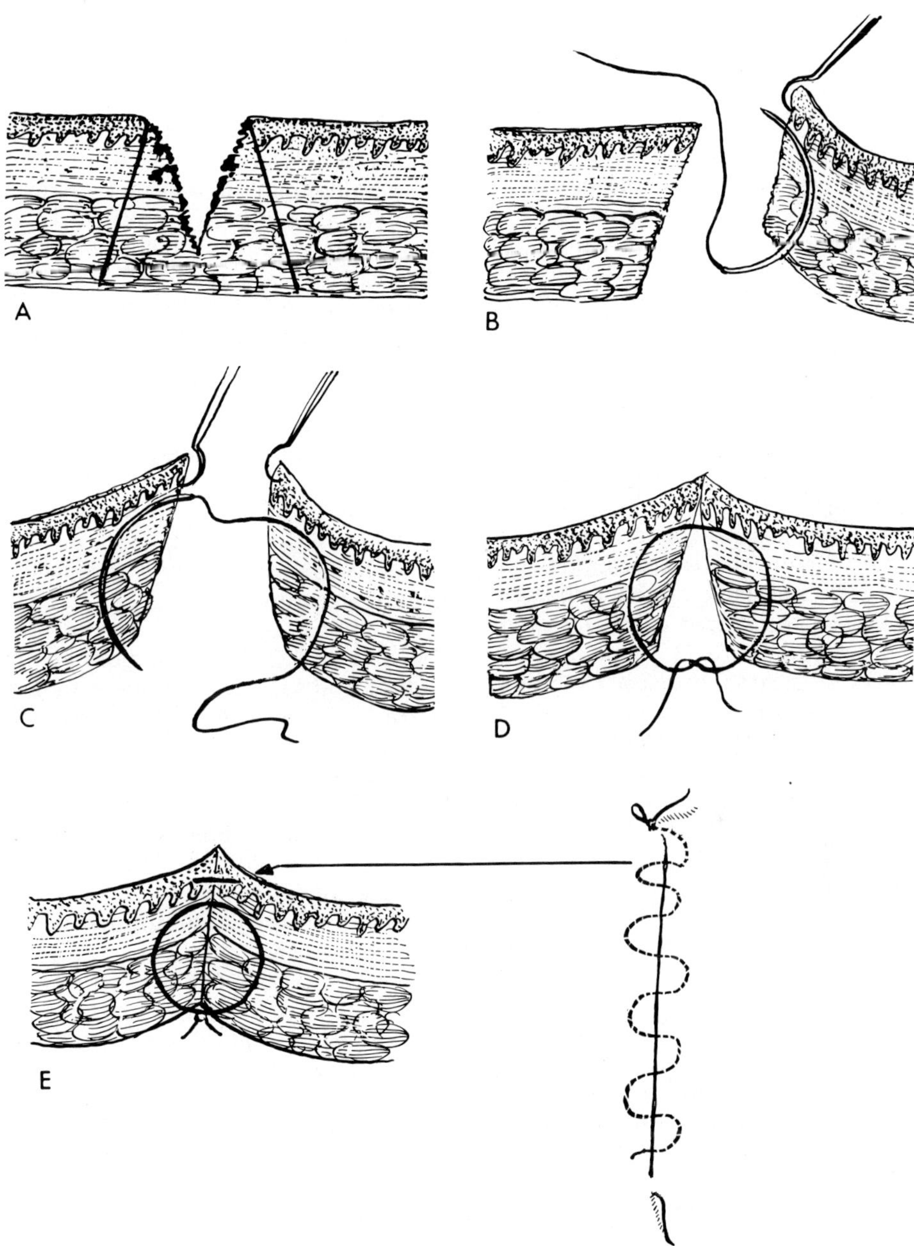

Figure 27–58. Method of debriding and suturing of a surface laceration. *A,* Slight undermining of the cut skin edges provides optimal surfaces for repair. *B,* After undermining the wound margins, the deep structures are closed in layers utilizing fine synthetic or catgut sutures with buried knots to provide subcutaneous fixation and elimination of dead space. *C,* A method of passing the needle to permit tying of the knot in the deep portion of the wound. Some eversion of the wound edges is accomplished by the direction of the bite of the suture. *D,* When the knot is tied, there is eversion of the tissues at the line of closure. *E,* Eversion of the skin edges along the line of closure obtained by the use of subcutaneous sutures, and final skin coaptation by means of a subcuticular monofilament nylon suture. The subcuticular suture provides accurate skin closure and may be left in place for three to four weeks. Fine cutaneous suture may be used to provide more precise skin alignment.

patients: it provides adequate approximation of the tissue margin and can be left in place for three to four weeks without the fear of a reaction or "suture tracks."

NONSUTURE TECHNIQUE OF WOUND CLOSURE

Gillman and associates (1955) proposed that simple approximation of wound margins by the use of adhesive tape would be an atraumatic, biologically sound method of wound closure. The nonsuture technique would eliminate the usual disadvantage of surface sutures, such as scarring. The technique has been applicable to the small superficial wound for many years, but lack of a suitable material for firmly approximating wound edges in the face of abrasions or desquamation has prevented its application to larger wounds or to those with significant tension. Some superficial wounds, especially in children, respond well to approximation with commercially available sterile adhesive strips. Benzoin can be placed on the wound edges to assist tape adherence. Dunphy and Jackson (1962) advocated the use of Steri-Strips, whose porosity and semitransparency are desirable qualities. The tape is reinforced and provides strong resistance to traction in the lateral direction. Adhesive strapping can provide uniform approximation of tissue margins and eliminates trauma from sutures. The disadvantage is possible uneven alignment of the wound edges. Adhesive straps may be left in place for two to three weeks if indicated and the wound, thus reinforced, prevents lateral pull on the incision.

Healing after sharp lacerations is predictable and generally complete at one year (Fig. 27–59). Even wounds with tissue loss demonstrate remarkably satisfactory healing (Fig. 27–60). In other cases, uneven flaps, "trapdoor" deformity (Fig. 27–61), or loss of structure (Fig. 27–62) mar the final result.

FRACTURES OF THE CRANIOFACIAL SKELETON

Fractures of the jaws invariably produce alterations in the relationship of the upper and lower teeth. In the case of the edentulous patient, the relationships alter the occlusal relations between the dentures. A knowledge of the dentition is requisite for the proper treatment of jaw fractures.

Dentition

The deciduous teeth begin to erupt at 5 to 6 months of age. The lower central incisors are generally first to be noted. By the age of 20 to 24 months, the child has a total of 20 teeth, 10 in the upper and 10 in the lower dental arch. The teeth consist of the incisors, the cuspid teeth, and the deciduous molars. This complement of teeth is known as the *deciduous* or temporary dentition. At the age of 6 years, in addition to the temporary dentition, the first permanent or six year molars erupt behind the second deciduous molars. At age 6 years, the maxillary and mandibular central incisor teeth are replaced by the permanent teeth. At age 9 years, the permanent lateral incisors have erupted. At age 10 to 11 years, the deciduous molar teeth are replaced by the permanent premolar teeth. At ages 12 and 13 years, the second permanent molar teeth come into position and the deciduous canine teeth are lost and replaced by the permanent canine teeth. At age 14 years, all the deciduous teeth usually have been exfoliated and replaced by the permanent teeth. The first and second permanent molars in all quadrants are present. The third molars are missing, impacted, or unerupted in some, but erupt in most persons over the age of 16 years. When all the permanent teeth have erupted, the adult has 32 permanent teeth, eight in each quadrant. The teeth are numbered as indicated: maxillary dental arch, right to left—1 to 16; mandibular dental arch, left to right—17 to 32.

The incisors and cuspid teeth have sharper edges, which are fitted for incising or tearing. The molars have broad surfaces suitable for grinding. The grinding and incising surfaces of the teeth fit or mesh together into what has been termed an *occlusal pattern.* In normal occlusion, the lower mandibular dental arch is slightly smaller than the upper maxillary dental arch. The lower teeth fit just inside the outer surface of the upper teeth. A knowledge of dental occlusal relationships (Fig. 27–63) is essential to the management of facial injuries involving the jaws. Abnormal relationships occur often enough for a knowledge of the usual deviations to be imperative.

A brief study of the mouth of a normal patient will orient the surgeon to the average occlusal relationships. The occlusal relationships between the first molar and cuspid teeth are indicated in Figure 27–63. The Angle

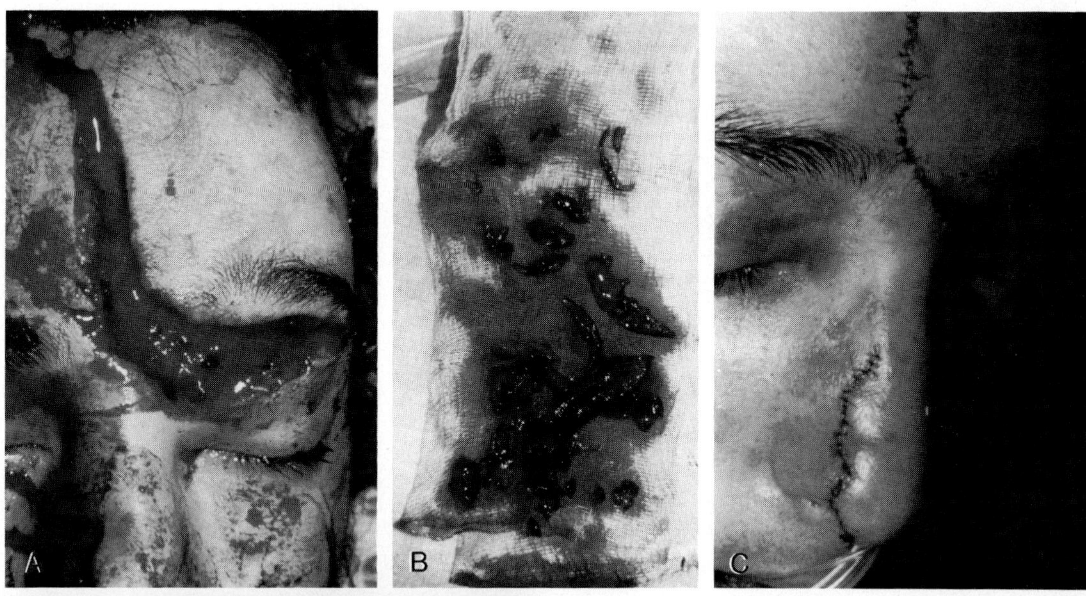

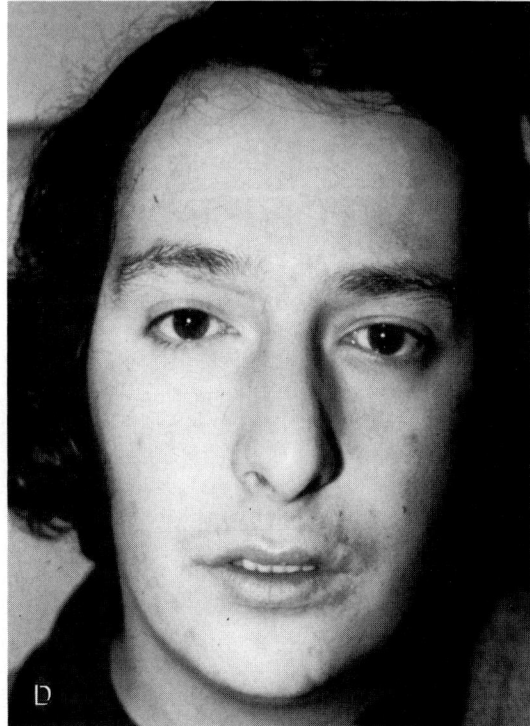

Figure 27–59. Facial lacerations. *A,* Avulsive laceration of the forehead and eyebrow. *B,* A margin of tissue (1 to 2 mm) was debrided from the entire wound. *C,* Closure was accomplished with fine suture material (cutaneous) and a secure dermal layer. *D,* The result obtained one year later.

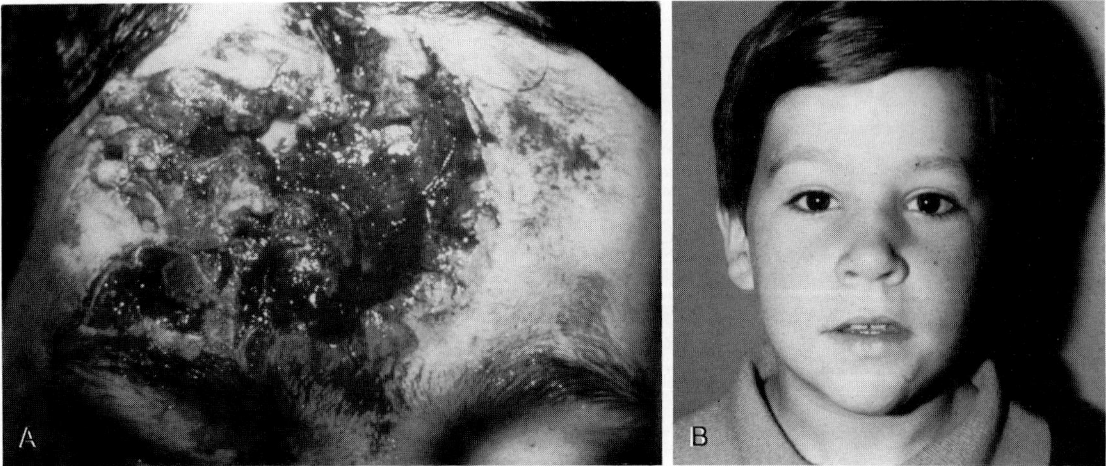

Figure 27–60. Avulsive laceration of the forehead. *A,* Initial appearance. Minimal debridement was performed to conserve tissue. *B,* The result obtained after one year.

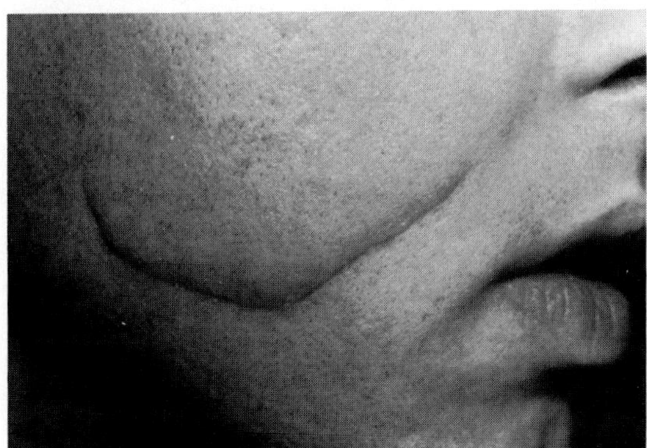

Figure 27–61. Trapdoor-type scarring in an avulsive laceration of the cheek.

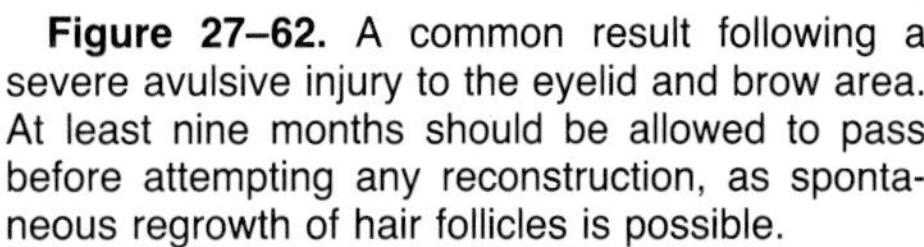

Figure 27–62. A common result following a severe avulsive injury to the eyelid and brow area. At least nine months should be allowed to pass before attempting any reconstruction, as spontaneous regrowth of hair follicles is possible.

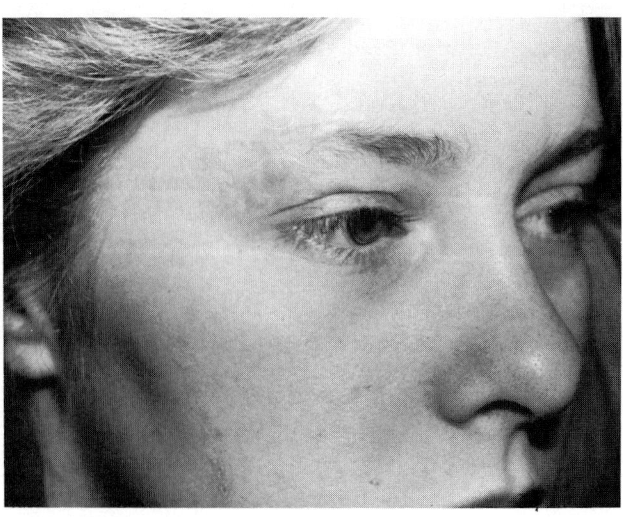

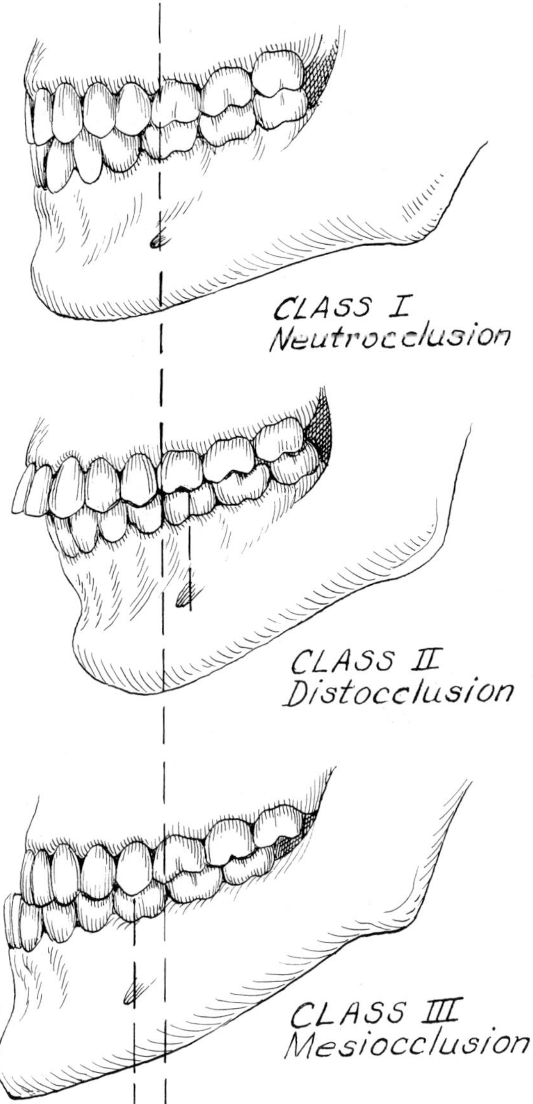

Figure 27–63. The classification of occlusion includes three main types (after Angle). The classification is based on the position of the mesial buccal cusp of the maxillary first molar in relation to the mesial buccal groove of the mandibular first molar. The position of the cuspid teeth should also be noted. Subdivisions of the three main classes are identified by differences in the mesial or lateral positioning of the teeth in the dental arches.

classification of malocclusion (Angle, 1899) describes the skeletal relationship between the maxilla and the mandible. The examining physician must be alert for abnormalities or deviations from the normal. Missing teeth in the partially dentulous patient can produce changes in dental relationships. Teeth that have not developed can also produce changes in the usual dental relationships. The first step in identifying abnormal occlusal patterns is to count the teeth, identifying those that are present. Impressions and models may be obtained and they allow a leisurely study of dental relationships. The relationships between the central incisors of the mandible and maxilla (the midline relationships of the jaws) and the relationships of the cuspid and first molar teeth serve as guides to the establishment of proper occlusion. The preexisting occlusion often is easily recognized. Wear facets indicate where the teeth have come together. A patient who had a Class III occlusal relationship (malocclusion) before injury would be impossible to treat by attempting to force the teeth into a neutral occlusal relationship. A Class I (neutral) occlusion is one in which the mesial buccal cusp of the upper first molar occludes with the mesial buccal groove of the mandibular first molar. The protruding or jutting type of jaw is known as Class III malocclusion (mesial occlusion), and the retrusive or underdeveloped jaw is termed Class II malocclusion (distoclusion). In addition, there are abnormalities in a lateral direction referred to as crossbite or laterognathism. Open bite or absence of occlusal contact in any area is also noted. An open bite may occur laterally (Fig. 27–64), anteriorly (Fig. 27–65), or anterolaterally.

In the injured patient in whom teeth or segments of bone are missing, it may be difficult to determine what the normal occlusal relationship should be. Usually the patient is helpful in advising the physician about the preexisting occlusal pattern, and

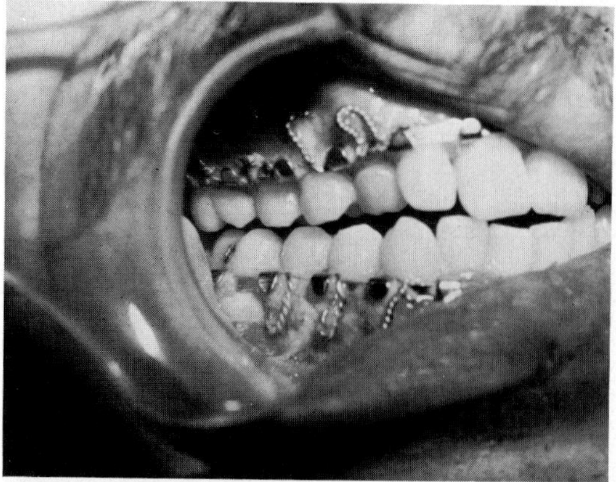

Figure 27–64. Open bite developing after release of intermaxillary fixation in a complicated panfacial fracture. The open bite was subsequently closed and the occlusal realignment obtained with light intermaxillary elastic traction for a brief period.

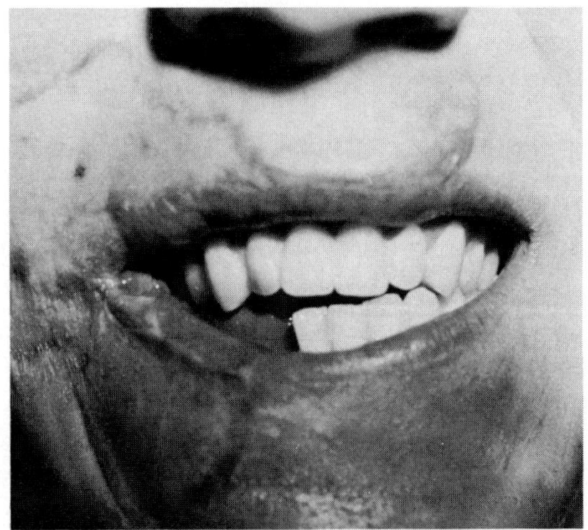

Figure 27–65. Malocclusion due to lingual rotation of fragments in a right parasymphyseal fracture. The lingual rotation of the left fragment created an anterior open bite and lingual version of the left side of the mandible.

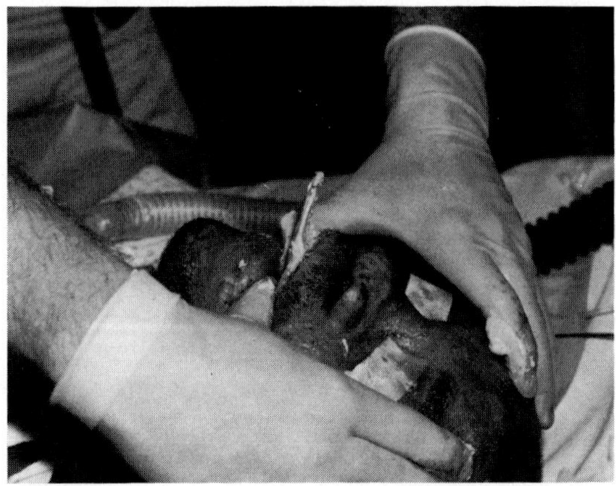

Figure 27–67. Impressions of the dental arches are taken in any fracture involving the occlusion, to serve as a record and study model. Experienced practitioners may find this unnecessary but the practice is useful for those with less experience and always provides a useful record guide to the preinjury occlusion by a study of the wear facets.

can comment on whether or not he feels his teeth are coming together properly. This is often one of the most sensitive indices of proper alignment of a fracture involving the occlusion. Slight differences in the way the teeth fit together are usually perceived by the patient without difficulty. Information may be obtained also from the patient's family, from old photographs, or from dentists or orthodontists who may have taken x-ray films or may provide models (Figs. 27–66, 27–67) of the previously existing dental relationships. In older patients, wear facets on the teeth give clues to preexisting relationships. A patient in neutroclusion, for instance, often shows worn surfaces on the outer (labial) edges of the lower anterior teeth and on the under (lingual) surfaces of the maxillary anterior teeth. The wear facets show that the teeth previously occluded in a normal relationship. The patient with a severely retruded jaw usually has no wear facets on the incisal edges of the lower anterior teeth. The patient who has a protruding lower jaw may have worn surfaces on the outer anterior edge of the maxillary teeth. If the patient has premolar and molar teeth in large segments of the upper jaw, these teeth usually fit into the contours of the opposing teeth. Dental consultation may be helpful when the apparent occlusion does not fit a precise preexisting pattern. It is important to restore the occlusion in fractures of the jaws to the preexisting relationships. Alternatively (and less desirably), the occlusion should be brought into a range where it can be easily corrected with orthodontic manipulation. It is necessary that the teeth be brought into the best possible occlusal relationship so that adequate chewing surface and joint function occur after the reduction, fixation, and consolidation of the jaw fractures.

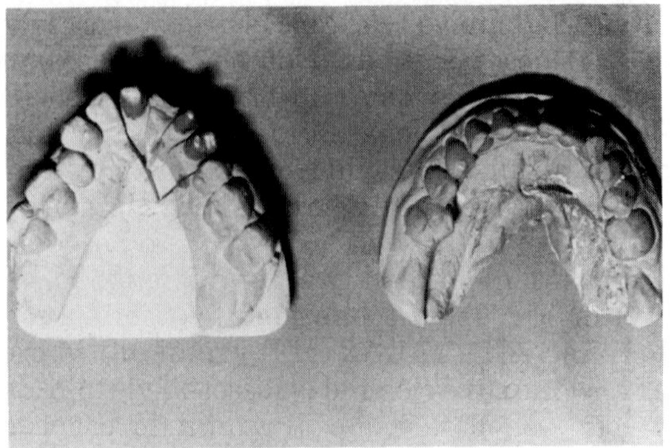

Figure 27–66. Models used for the construction of crowns or bridgework are often useful in defining the previous dental relationships.

DENTOALVEOLAR PROCESSES

The teeth are intimately associated with the main body of the mandible and maxilla and are held in place by a supporting projection called the alveolar bone. The alveolar bone is dense on its cortical surface, with a medullary portion supporting the teeth that is highly vascular and spongy in character. After loss of the permanent teeth by extrac-

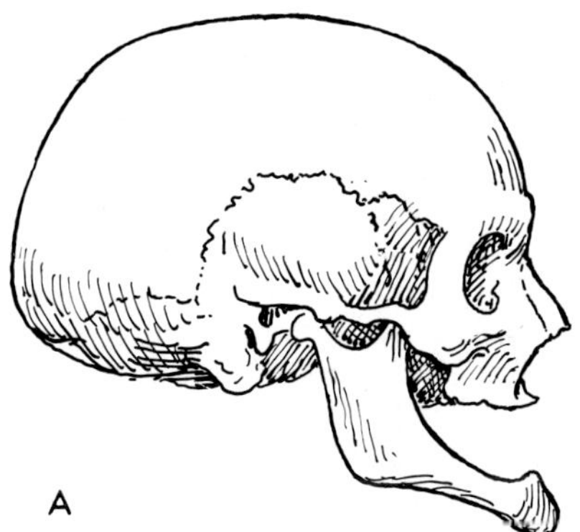

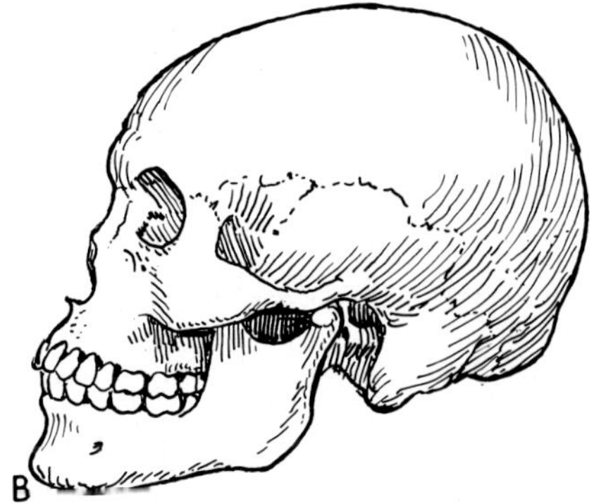

Figure 27–68. An edentulous skull is seen in *A* and a skull containing natural dentition in *B*. Note the structural changes in the edentulous skull due to loss of the teeth and atrophy of the maxillary and mandibular alveolar processes.

tion or through gum disease, the alveolar portion of the bone atrophies (Fig. 27–68). The final reduction in the size of the maxilla and mandible may be dramatic. The mandible, for example, may be reduced to a pencil-sized thinness in the elderly patient. Recession of the maxillary alveolar process to the nasal and maxillary sinus cavities may also occur. The edentulous mandible often displays poor healing characteristics. It is important in fractures of the edentulous mandible and maxilla to restore their relationships also. The prosthetic rehabilitation of a patient with dentures cannot tolerate large discrepancies in the relationship of the mandible and maxilla. One cannot ignore fractures in the edentulous patient, assuming that a prosthodontist can reconstruct a satisfactory occlusal pattern with an alteration in the design of an appliance.

DENTITION AS A GUIDE IN REDUCTION AND FIXATION OF JAW FRACTURES

Normal teeth are intimately associated with the mandible and maxilla, and restoration of the occlusion in fractured jaws usually indicates anatomic reduction of the fractured segments. In many cases of fracture, simple wiring of the teeth together in occlusion provides a satisfactory reduction and fixation of the jaw fracture. The restoration of the occlusion is a guide to the proper positioning of the maxilla in upper facial bone structures. When the mandible and maxilla are involved, ligation of the teeth in occlusion maintains fixation of the fractured segments. It is essential that surgeons who treat patients with facial bone fractures be acquainted with the normal anatomic structure of the teeth and tissues of the mouth.

DENTAL WIRING AND INTERMAXILLARY FIXATION TECHNIQUES

Gilmer Technique. The simplest way to establish intermittent fixation is by the Gilmer method of 1887. It was not until that year that the importance of the teeth and the fixation of fractures was recognized and described in the American literature. The technique is simple and effective, but has the disadvantage that the mouth cannot be opened for inspection of the fracture site without removing the wire fixation. This method consists of passing wire ligatures around the necks of all the available teeth and twisting in a clockwise direction until the wire is tightened around each tooth. After an adequate number of wires have been placed on the upper and lower teeth, the teeth are brought into occlusion and the wires are twisted, one upper to one lower wire. To be consistent and avoid difficulty in removal, it is always advisable to twist the wires in one direction, and the usual direction is clockwise. Twisted wires are cut short and the ends turned in against the necks of the teeth to avoid puncture of the mucous membranes and irritation to the patient (Fig. 27–69). Stainless steel wire of 24 or 26 gauge is usually employed. With the Gilmer method, the wires are twisted in a vertical direction or crisscrossed to prevent slipping in an anteroposterior direction.

Eyelet Method. The eyelet method (Eby, 1920; Ivy, 1922) of intermaxillary fixation is useful and has the advantage that the jaws

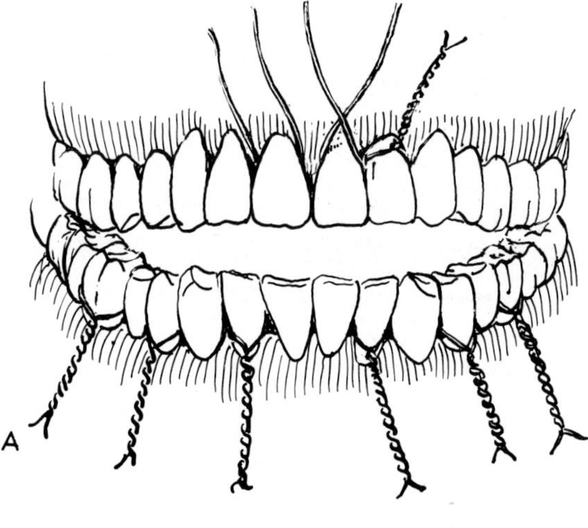

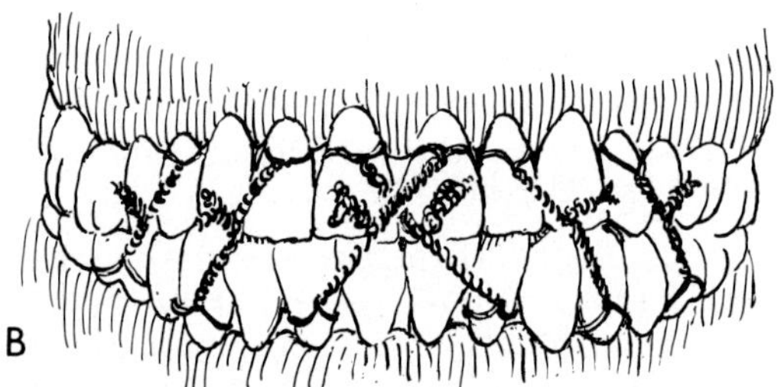

Figure 27–69. The Gilmer method of intermaxillary fixation of the teeth in occlusion by intermaxillary wiring.

may be opened for inspection by removal of only the intermaxillary ligatures (Fig. 27–70). This method consists of twisting a 20 cm length of 22 or 24 gauge wire around an instrument to establish a loop. Both ends of the wire are passed through the interproximal space from the outer surface. One end of the wire is passed around the anterior tooth and the other around the posterior tooth. One end of the wire may be passed through the loop. In the upper jaw the eyelet should project above, and in the lower jaw below, the horizontal twist to prevent the ends from impinging upon each other. After the establishment of a sufficient number of eyelets, the teeth are brought into occlusion and ligatures are passed loop fashion between one upper and one lower eyelet. The wires are twisted tightly to provide intermaxillary fixation. If it is necessary to open the mouth for inspection, the ligature loop wires may be cut, and if needed, replaced without difficulty. If heavy wire is used to form the eyelets, they may be turned to form hooklike projections to which intermaxillary orthodontic rubber bands are attached to provide occlusion between the jaws.

Arch Bar Method. Prefabricated arch bars are commercially available (Figs. 27–71, 27–72). These represent the usual method of establishing intermaxillary fixation. They are ligated to the external surface of the dental arch by passing 24 gauge steel wires around the arch bar and around the necks of the available teeth. The wires are twisted tightly to hold the arch bars in the form of an arc completely around the dental arch. The arch bars have hooklike projections, which are placed in a downward direction on the lower jaw and in an upward direction on the upper jaw. If an adequate number of teeth are present, the arch bar may be simply ligated to the teeth. If segments of teeth are

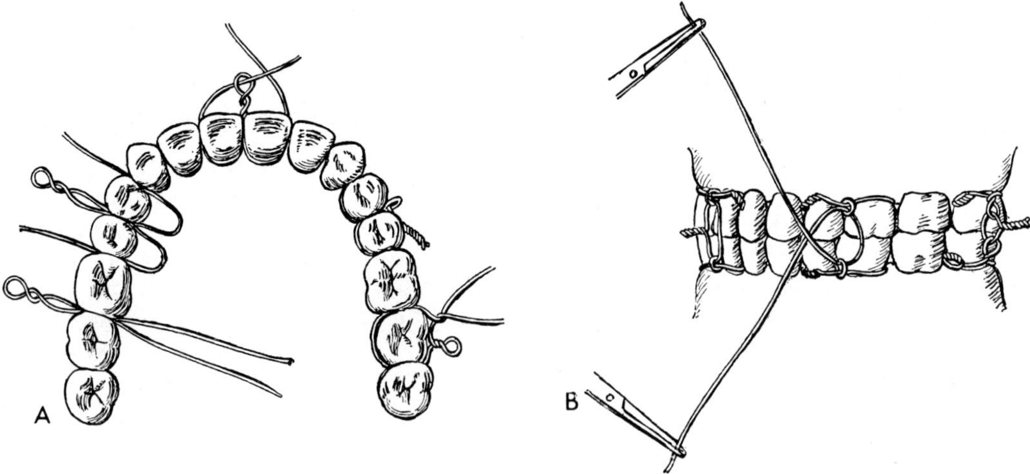

Figure 27–70. The eyelet method of intermaxillary fixation popularized by Ivy.

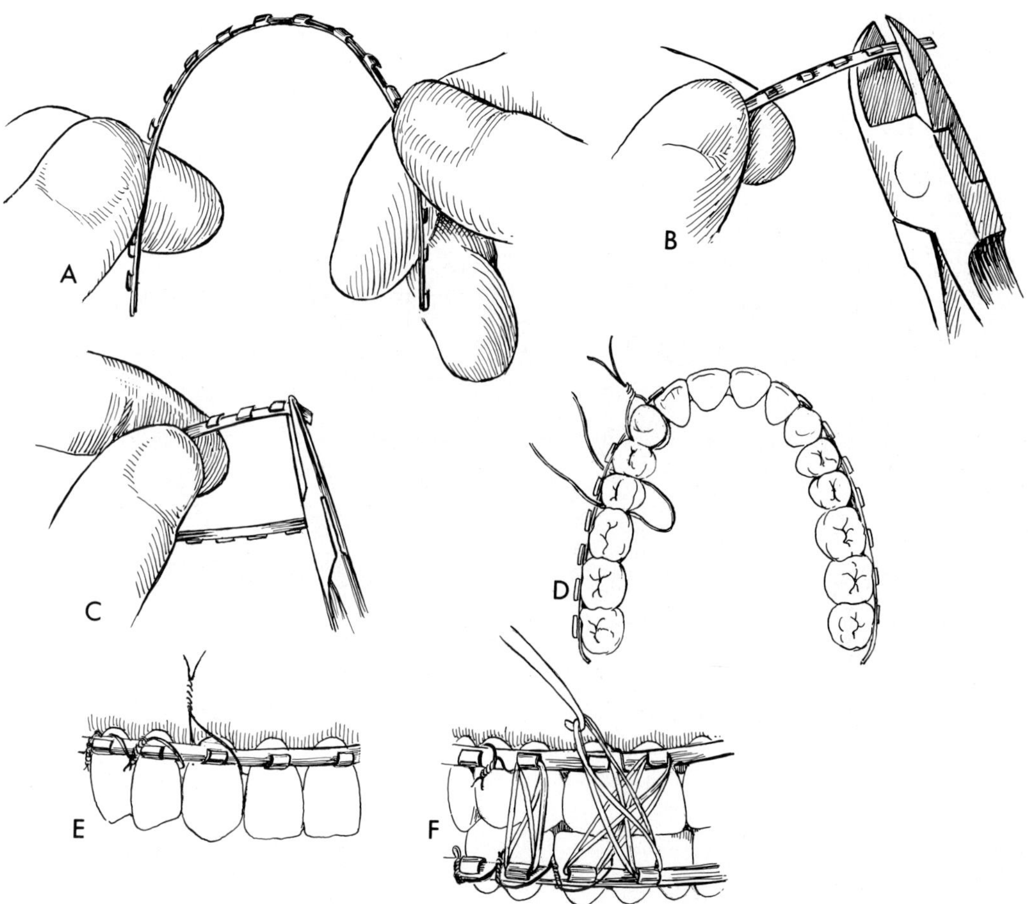

Figure 27–71. Method of adapting and ligating a prefabricated Ernst arch bar to the upper teeth and applying rubber bands for intermaxillary traction.

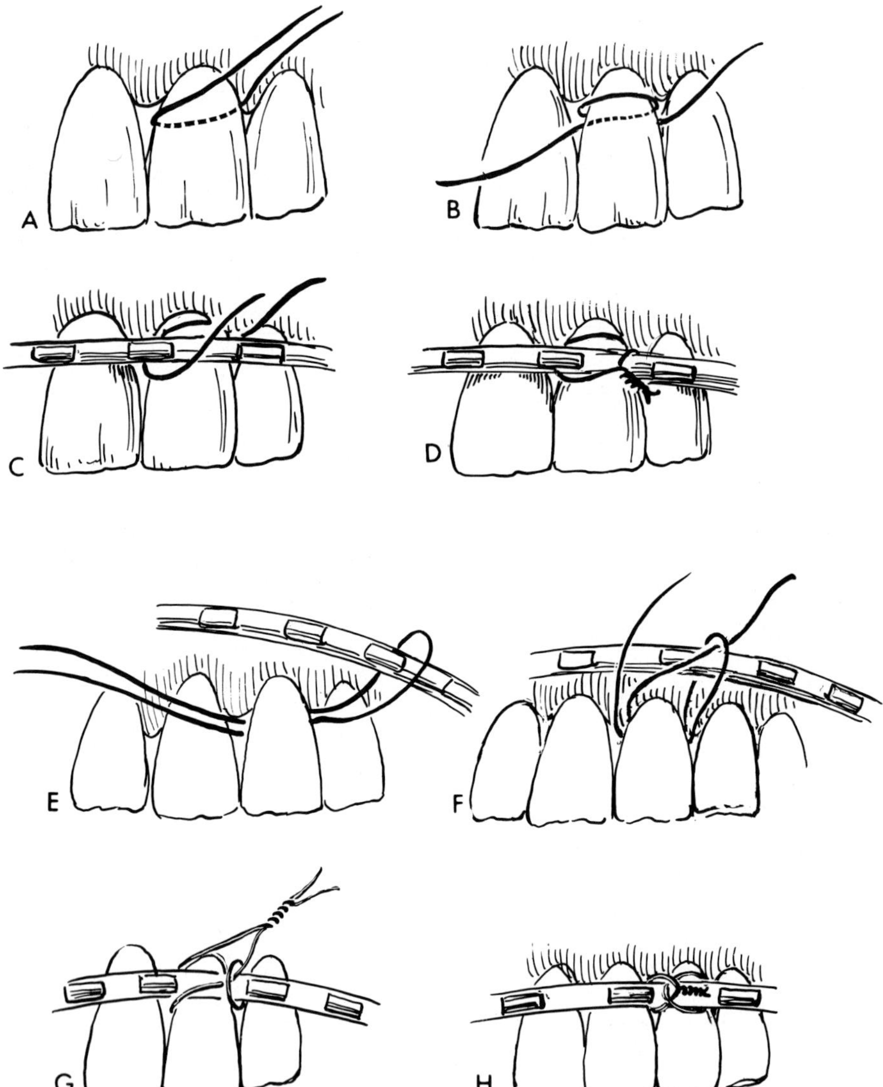

Figure 27–72. The conical shape of the maxillary anterior teeth requires special wiring techniques to keep the wire and arch bar from slipping. The method of Rowe and Kiley provides secure fixation of the arch bar in the maxillary incisor and cuspid area.

missing, or if the condition of the dentition indicates that additional support for the arch bar is necessary, the arch bar may be stabilized by the use of acrylic splint or additional wires. This is sometimes necessary even if there is a full complement of teeth when traction is to be exerted in the anterior section of the mandible or maxilla. Such traction may result in loosening of the incisor teeth, whose roots are not as stable as the molar teeth. Greater stability may be obtained by suspension of the maxillary arch bar from the margin of the piriform aperture and anterior nasal spine of the maxilla (Fig. 27–73); a gingivobuccal sulcus incision allows visualization of the piriform aperture. A small drill hole can be placed and a wire anchored through the drill hole and connected to the arch bar. The stability can be increased by drilling through the piriform aperture on each side and leading these wires down to the arch bar (Fig. 27–74). The mandibular arch bar can be stabilized by one or more circumferential wires passed around the mandible (see Fig. 27–73). It is helpful to have a special instrument set for arch bar application.

After the arch bars are secured, wire ligatures are passed between the two arches to bring the teeth into occlusion. The ligatures are usually applied opposite the mandibular molar, bicuspid, and cuspid teeth. Wires or elastics are not utilized anterior to the cuspid teeth unless specific precautions have been taken to prevent incisor extrusion from anterior traction. These precautions include the use of an occlusal wafer or piriform aperture and circum-mandibular wires. Since the incisor teeth do not oppose one another, one can extrude them from the socket with strong anterior traction. The use of an occlusal wafer allows an occlusal surface to be developed between the teeth, and this opposes the forces of extrusion. Rubber orthodontic bands (Fig.

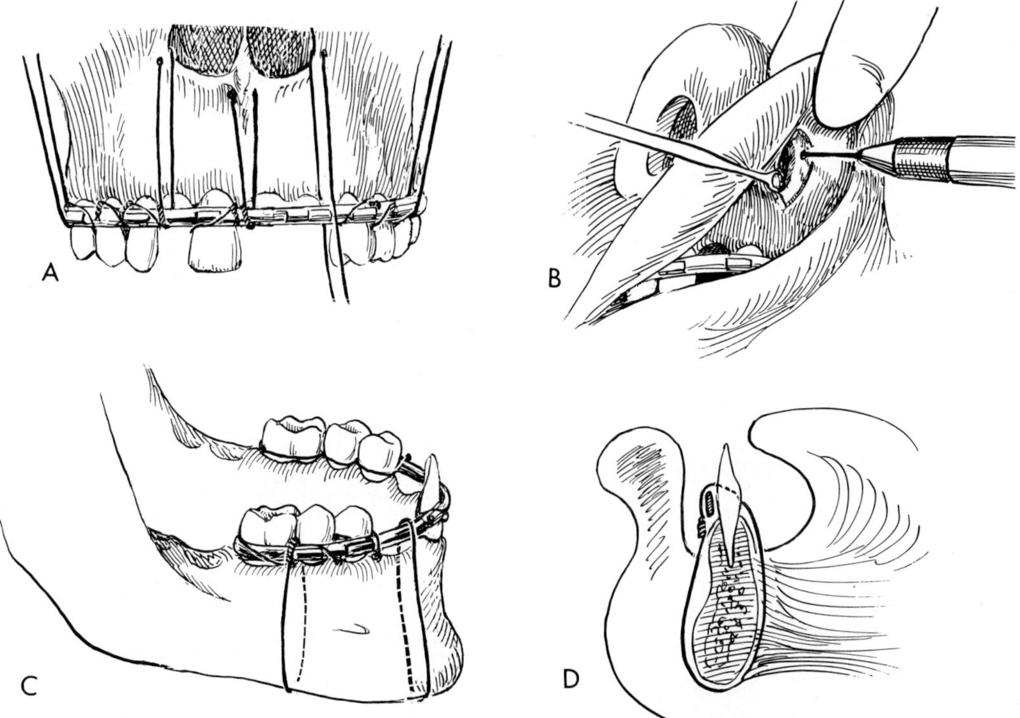

Figure 27–73. Supplementary fixation of arch bars is necessary in partially edentulous jaws. Teeth may be missing owing to previous extraction or injury and may be insufficient in number to secure the arch bar adequately. *A,* Support in the maxillary anterior region can be obtained by passing wires through small drill holes at the piriform aperture at the nasal cavity or through the anterior nasal spine. Additional wires may be suspended around the zygomatic arches or to the orbital rims. *B,* The approach to the piriform margin is through a small vertical incision in the labial vestibule of the upper lip. *C, D,* Circumferential wires may be used to give stability to the lower arch bars when an insufficient number of teeth are available for attachment of the bar. The bar can also be strengthened by the application of a small amount of acrylic, following the initial wiring, to increase its rigidity.

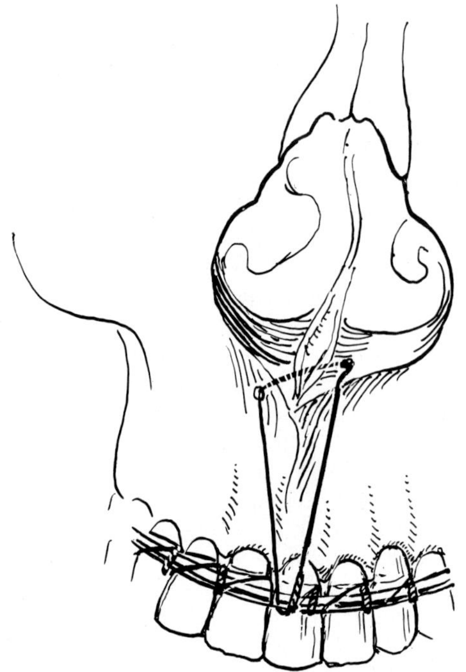

Figure 27–74. Alternative technique of passing the wire through the nasal spine at the margin of the piriform aperture.

27–75) can be used to oppose the two dental arches by applying the rubber bands between the arch bar. The rubber bands exert constant traction, which will oppose the teeth in their proper relationship. The elastic fatigues and the rubber bands must be replaced. Rubber bands are useful if one is trying to move a dental segment into another occlusal relationship. They can be applied, for example, in Class III or Class II relationships to provide traction anteriorly or posteriorly on the jaws. Dental relationships should be used to describe movements of teeth and interdental relations (Figs. 27–76, 27–77). In this manner, a malocclusion can sometimes be corrected by the simple use of orthodontic rubber bands. Once the proper occlusal relationship of the teeth has been obtained, the rubber bands are replaced with wires. In some patients who have concomitant fractures of the condyle area, it is desirable to allow the patient to begin motion and yet reapply rubber band traction at night to reestablish occlusal relationships. This technique allows mobilization of the temporomandibular joint and yet continues to reestablish occlusal relationships with interval elastic traction. Patients can learn to apply the elastics at home. They are often sensitive to minor changes in occlusal relationships. Mobilization additionally improves dental hygiene. The use of rubber bands is advantageous because they are more easily removed than wires. Wires are frequently less bulky than rubber bands and easier to clean with a tooth brush or Water-Pik appliance. At the end of the usual course of treatment, if there is any mobility at the site of fracture, fixation is easily reestablished for a short period.

Stout Method. This method (Stout, 1942)

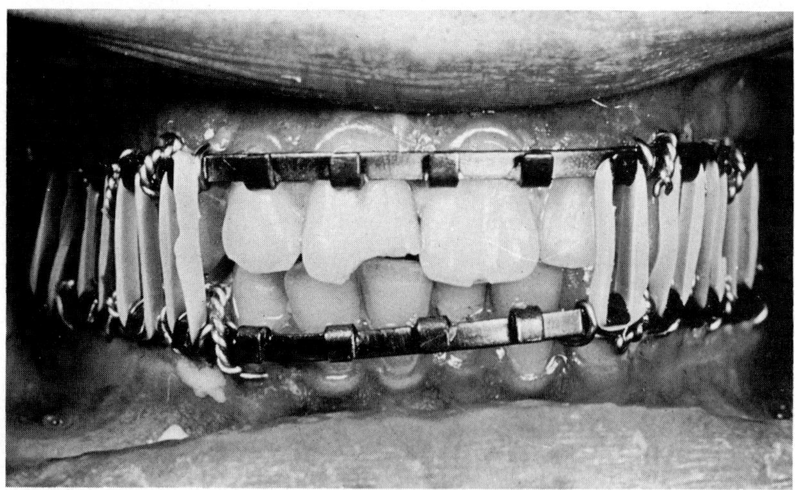

Figure 27–75. Intermaxillary fixation with rubber band traction. If a sufficient number of posterior teeth are present to give stability to the arch bars, the anterior teeth are not ligated. Heavy traction on the anterior teeth may loosen the teeth from the alveolar bone. This method provides a quick, easy, and effective means of intermaxillary fixation that exerts constant slight traction. The author prefers wire for most patients because no traction is necessary.

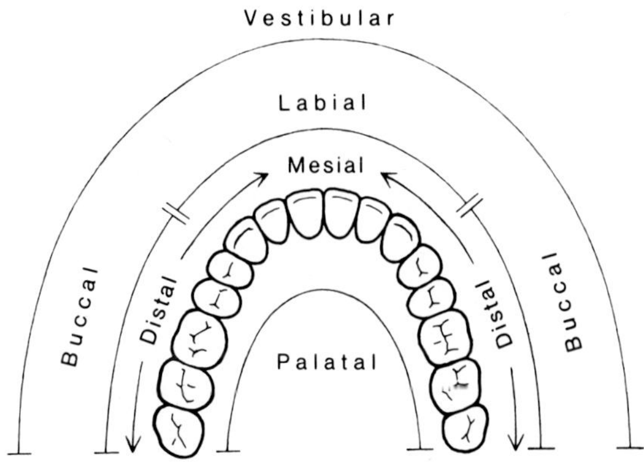

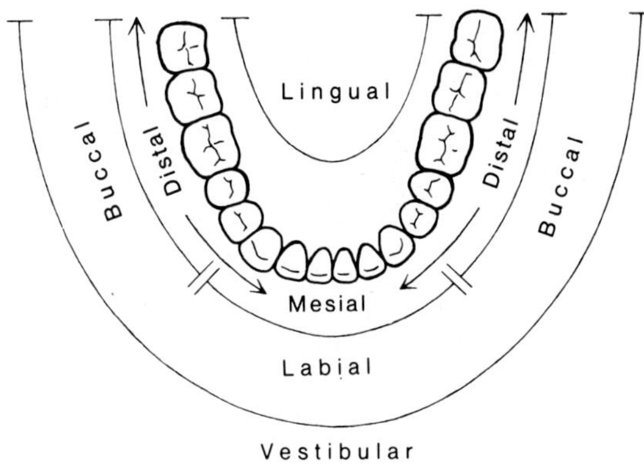

Figure 27–76. Dental terminology describing maxillary and mandibular relationships. (From Texhammar, R., and Schmoker, R.: Stable Internal Fixation in Maxillofacial Bone Surgery—Manual for Operating Room Personnel. New York, Springer-Verlag, 1984, p. 12.)

consists of the formation of small wire loops around the upper and lower dental arches, to which rubber band traction is applied (Fig. 27–78).

Other Methods. There are other ways to use wire appliances with rubber bands. An effective method for isolated teeth is that of Kazanjian (1933): a heavy gauge wire is twisted around the neck of the tooth in a very firm fashion, leaving a "button" of wire at the neck of the tooth for the attachment of a rubber band (Fig. 27–79).

The arch bar may be attached to the teeth by means of orthodontic bands. This is a precise and accurate method of securely holding the bar (Fig. 27–80). The appliance is

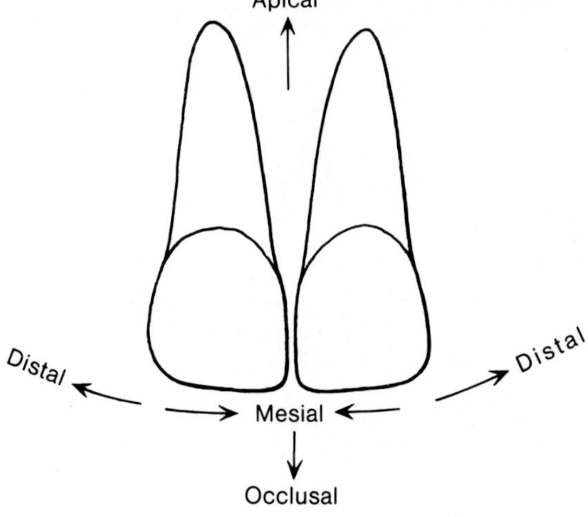

Figure 27–77. Dental terminology describing the relationships of teeth. (From Texhammar, R., and Schmoker, R.: Stable Internal Fixation in Maxillofacial Bone Surgery—Manual for Operating Room Personnel. New York, Springer-Verlag, 1984, p. 12.)

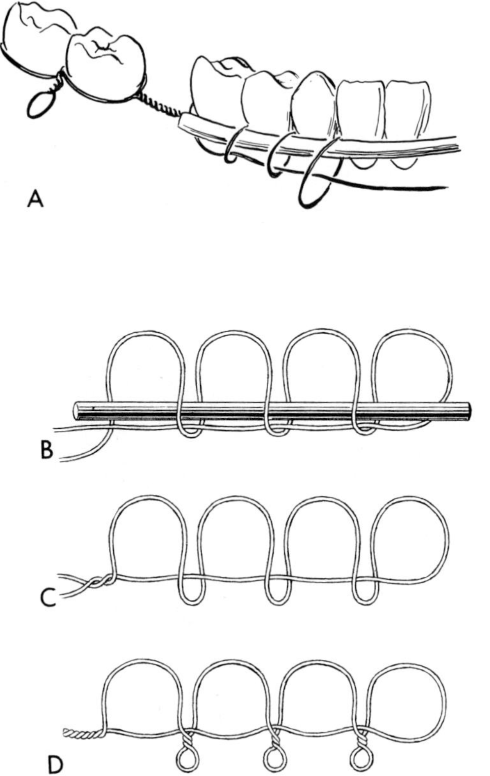

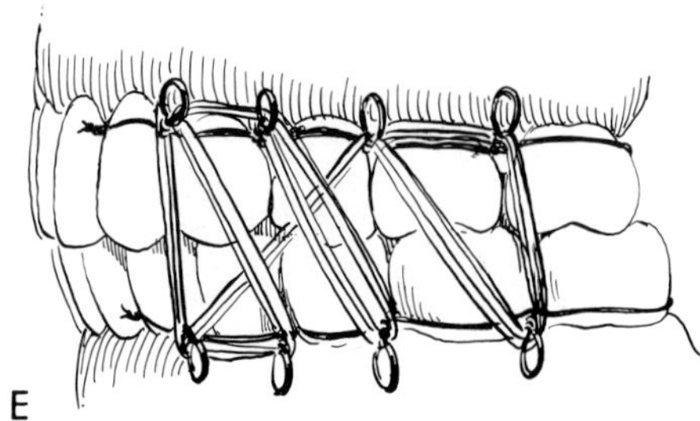

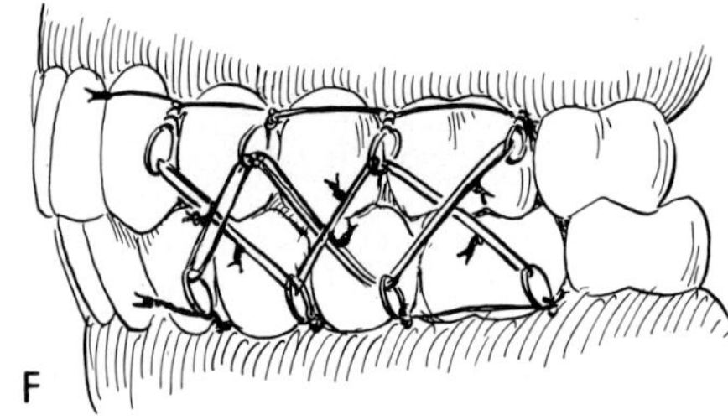

Figure 27–78. Stout's modification of the eyelet technique of intermaxillary fixation. The eyelets are formed by a continuous wire threaded around the teeth and over a soft metal bar, which is removed before the eyelets are twisted. *A* to *D,* Method of application of the Stout wire. In *E,* the eyelets may be used as hooks to which the rubber bands are applied or, as in *F,* they may be used for maxillary wire fixation. (From Kazanjian and Converse.)

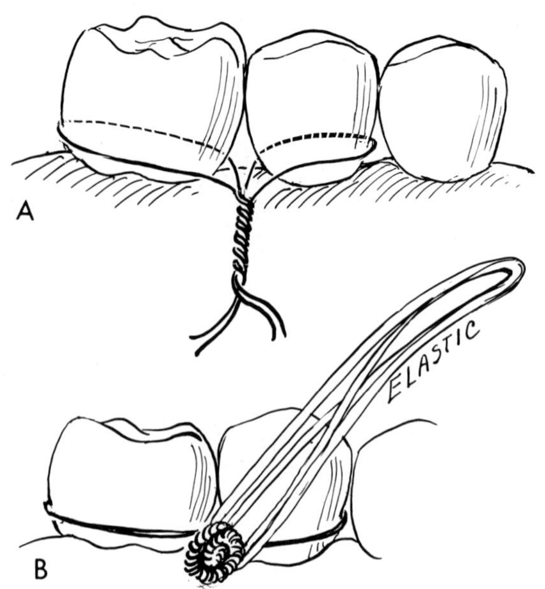

Figure 27–79. The Kazanjian button. This method is useful in providing attachment for rubber band traction in cases in which single or insufficient teeth are present in the fragment to permit the application of an arch bar.

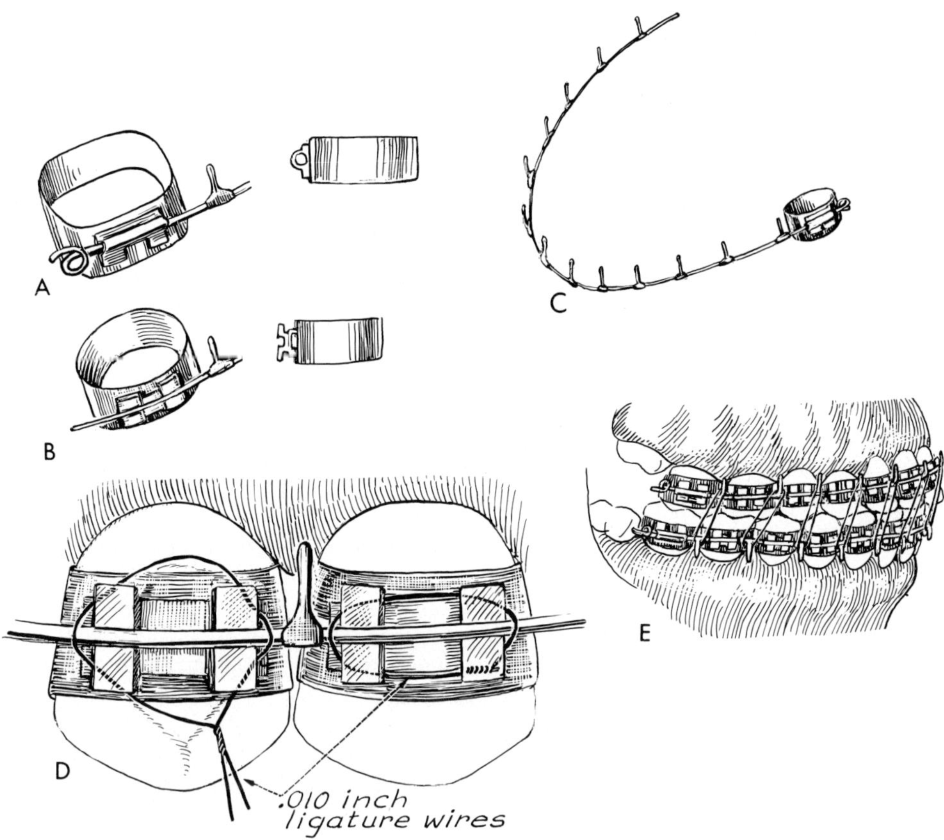

Figure 27–80. Edgewise orthodontic and fixation appliance. *A,* Edgewise appliance consists of molar bands with rectangular sheaths (internal dimensions 0.022 × 0.028 inch) through which an edgewise arch wire is inserted at each end. *B,* Remaining teeth in each dental arch carry bands with "twin brackets" (slot dimensions 0.022 × 0.028 inch) to permit insertion of edgewise wire (0.021 × 0.025 inch) and secure it in position with ligature wires (0.010 inch). *C,* Arch wire with spurs soldered to the gingival side is as it appears before final insertion and planned surgery. *D,* Arch wiring and position are maintained with wire ligatures placed around brackets. *E,* Appliance as it appears at the time of surgery with intermaxillary wires (0.028 inch) placed between the arches to fix one jaw to the other. (From Kazanjian and Converse.)

time consuming to construct, is expensive to use in fractures, and requires the presence of an orthodontist as a member of the team.

Adaptations of the use of wire ligatures are many. A fracture in which there is a stable complement of teeth on each side can be secured with a single wire circling the teeth across the line of fracture, or with several wires twisted around the adjacent teeth and twisted together. Sometimes these wires are helpful in the initial establishment of occlusion and are then supplemented by the placement of a full arch bar.

Splints in Maintenance of Intermaxillary Fixation. Acrylic splints are useful in the maintenance of intermaxillary fixation and in the continuity of the maxillary or mandibular dental arch. Segments of missing teeth can be compensated for with a suitably designed maxillary or mandibular splint. Alternatively, a fracture can be reduced and stabilized by the proper application of a palatal or a lingual splint. Appliances of this type are effective but require detailed dental knowledge for construction. Their use is routine in more complicated fractures of the jaws (Fig. 27–81). The splints can be fabricated by properly educated personnel; alternatively, a prosthodontic laboratory may be able to fabricate acrylic splints for those less familiar with the intricacies of fabrication. Acrylic splints provide precise dental alignment during healing, which often cannot be obtained with any other technique. They prevent fracture segment rotation or telescoping of fragments; they also provide an occlusal "stop" for missing teeth. An acrylic splint is occasionally placed to facilitate dental occlusion

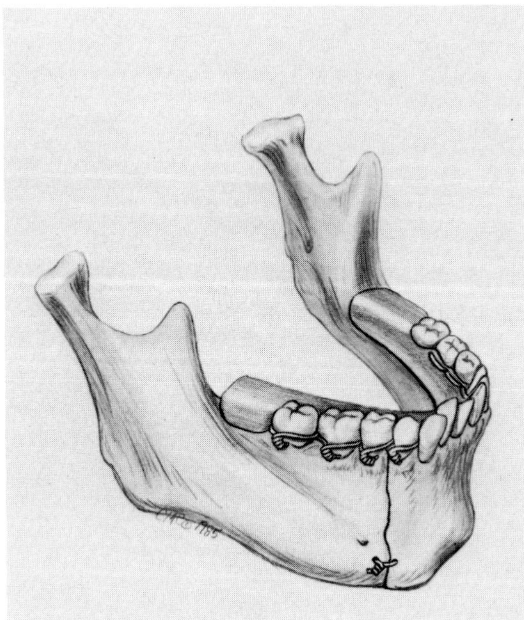

Figure 27–81. The application of a lingual splint supports an open reduction of a parasymphyseal fracture. The action of the splint prevents lingual rotation of the upper border of the mandible. It is most often used together with arch bars, which are omitted in the illustration for clarity.

while plate and screw fixation of a fracture is employed, and it is then removed.

Monomaxillary vs. Bimaxillary Fixation. When several teeth are present on each side of a fracture line, the use of a suitable splint or prefabricated arch bars augmented by acrylic stabilization may obviate the need for bimaxillary fixation, to the considerable increase of the patient's comfort and nutrition. A wiring technique for monomaxillary fixation with the use of a splint is indicated in Figure 27–81.

Fractures of the Mandible

The prominence, position, and anatomic configuration of the mandible are such that it is one of the most frequent facial bones, like the nose and zygoma, to be fractured. In automobile accidents, the mandible is the most commonly encountered fracture at major trauma centers. The mandible is a movable, predominantly U-shaped bone consisting of horizontal and vertical segments. The horizontal segments consist of the body on each side and the symphysis area centrally. The vertical segments consist of the two rami, which articulate with the skull at the temporomandibular joints. The mandible is attached to other facial bones by a complex system of muscles and ligaments. The mandible articulates with the maxilla through the teeth.

The mandible is a strong bone but has several areas of weakness (Kruger and Schilli, 1982). The body of the mandible is composed principally of dense cortical bone with a small substantia spongiosa through which blood, lymphatic vessels, and nerves pass. The mandible is thin at the angles where the body joins with the ramus, and can be further weakened by the presence of an unerupted third molar in this area. The mandible is also weak at the neck of the condyle. The root of the cuspid tooth, the longest root, and the mental foramen, through which the mental nerve and vessels extend into the tissue in the lateral aspect of the face and lower lip, both weaken the area of the distal body. Fractures frequently traverse the mandible adjacent to the mental foramen. The weak areas for fractures are thus the subcondylar angle and distal body areas.

With the loss of teeth from the mandible, atrophic changes occur in the alveolar bone and alter the structural characteristics of the mandible. Fractures often occur in the partially dentulous mandible through edentulous areas rather than through areas better supported by adequate tooth structures (Hagan and Huelke, 1961). Mandibular movements are determined by the action of reciprocally placed muscles attached to the bone. When fractures occur, displacement of the segments is influenced by the pull of the muscles attaching to the segments. The direction of the fracture line can also oppose the pull of the muscles. The mandible may be fractured by any external force. The most common causes are automobile accidents, falls, fist fights, missile injuries, and sporting accidents. Fractures may occur in the course of a difficult tooth extraction or during conditions such as electroshock therapy.

CLASSIFICATION

Mandibular fractures are classified according to the location (Fig. 27–82), the condition of the teeth (Fig. 27–83), the direction of the fracture and its favorability for treatment, the presence of a compound injury through

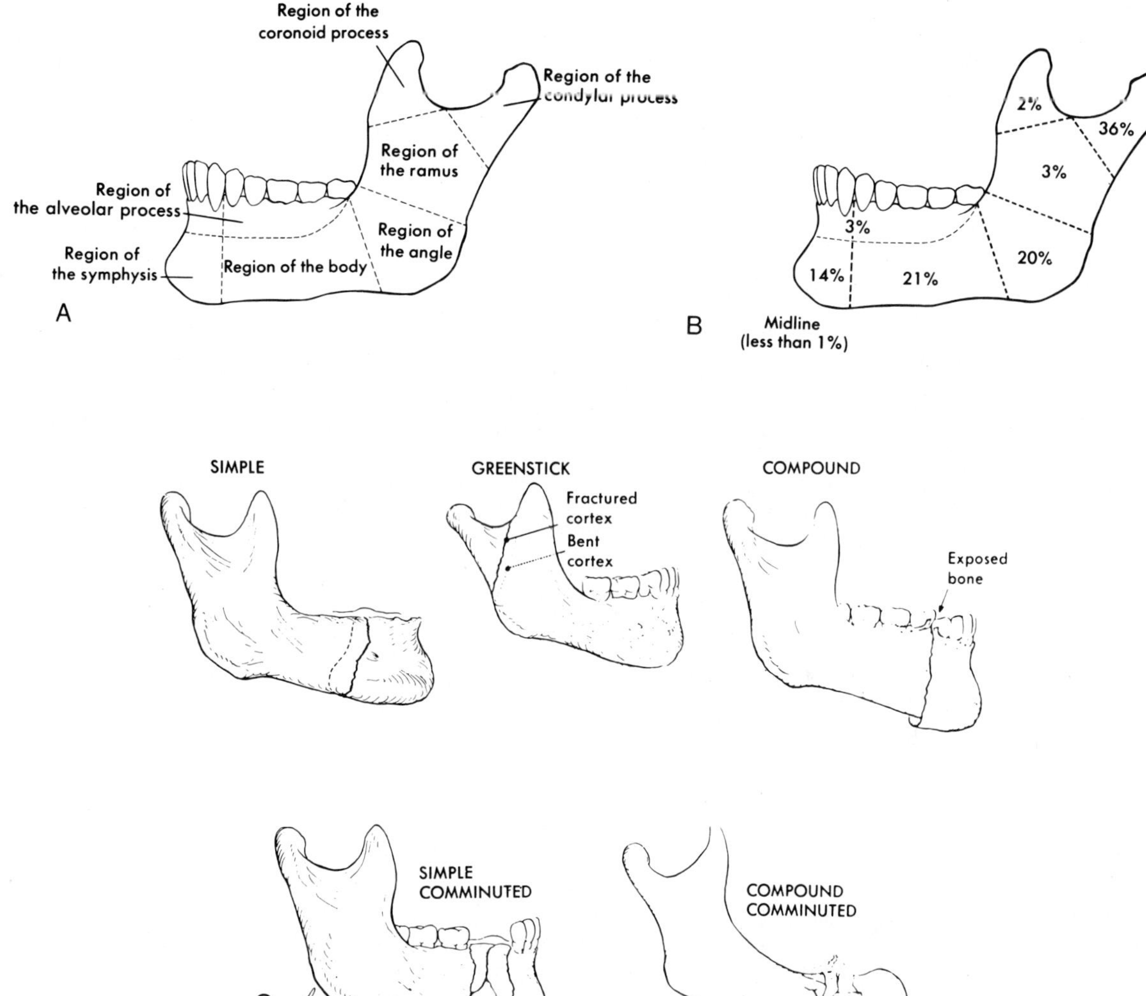

Figure 27–82. *A,* The regions of the mandible. *B,* The percentage of fractures occurring within each region. (From Dingman, R.O., and Natvig, P.: Surgery of Facial Fractures. Philadelphia, W.B. Saunders Company, 1964.) *C,* Types of mandibular fractures. (From Kruger, G. O.: Textbook of Oral and Maxillofacial Surgery. 6th Ed. St. Louis, MO, C.V. Mosby Company, 1984.)

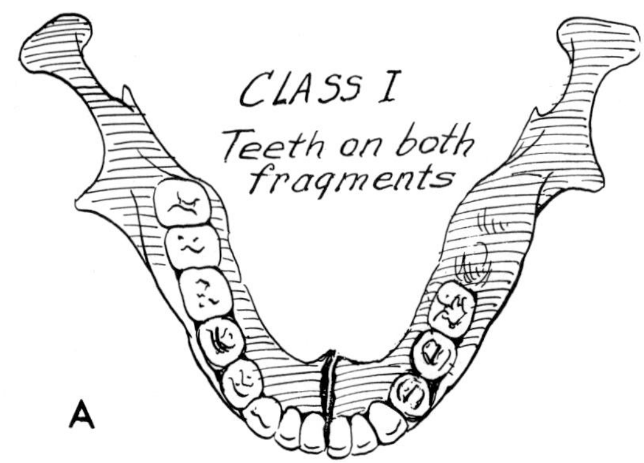

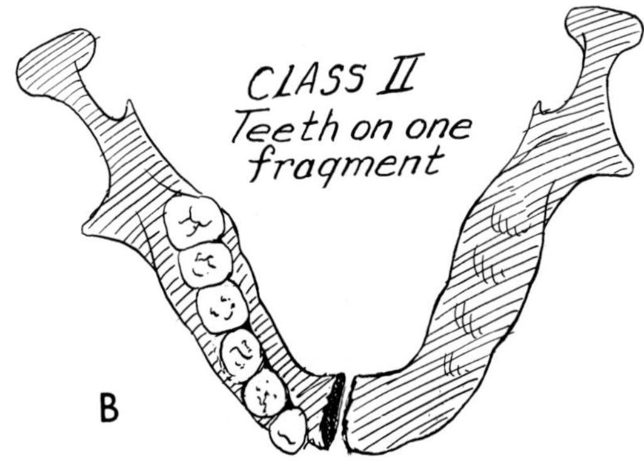

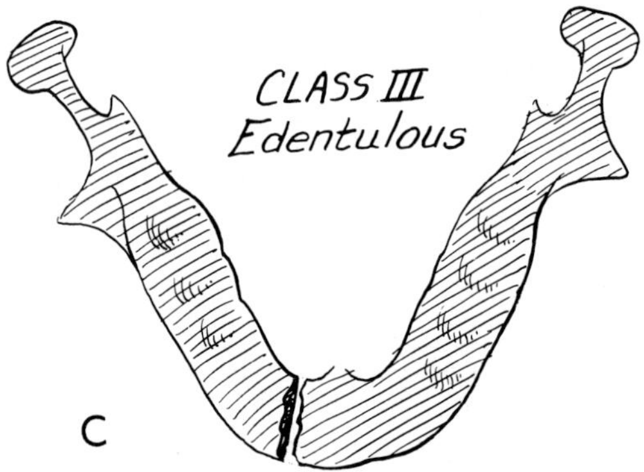

Figure 27–83. Classification of mandibular fractures according to the presence or absence of teeth on the fragments. *A,* Class I fracture, teeth on both fragments. *B,* Class II fracture, teeth on only one fragment. *C,* Class III fracture; both fragments are edentulous. (After Kazanjian and Converse.)

the skin or the mucosa, and the characterization of the fracture pattern (Rowe and Killey, 1968; Kazanjian and Converse, 1974; Kruger and Schilli, 1982; Kruger, 1984).

Direction of Fracture and Favorability for Treatment

Horizontal

Favorable.

Unfavorable.

Vertical

Favorable.

Unfavorable.

Severity of Fracture (see Figure 27–82*C*)

Simple Fractures. In this type of fracture, there is no contact of the fracture site with the outside environment. There is no discontinuity of the overlying soft tissue structures.

Compound Fractures. In these fractures, there is a break through the overlying skin or mucosa. There is direct communication of the fracture site through the laceration; thus, the potential for contamination is increased. In practice, most fractures in the horizontal portion of the mandible are compound into the mouth. More rarely, the fractures are compound through the skin.

Variety of Fracture (see Figure 27–82*C*)

"Greenstick" Fractures. In "greenstick" fractures, there is incomplete discontinuity of the bone. The mandibular bone structure may be bent or partially fractured to resemble a greenstick that has been forcibly bent and only partially broken.

Simple Fractures. In simple fractures, there is no communication with the outside environment. The fracture is a linear fracture that usually shows little displacement.

Compound Fractures. In these, there is a communication with the outside environment.

Complex Fractures. In these fractures, there are multiple segments, the fracture lines occurring in various directions; sometimes these extend into a joint or into adjacent tooth or bone structures. These fractures usually indicate a more severe degree of injury.

Comminuted Fractures. In these fractures, there are many small fragments, some of which may be devitalized by the injury. The fractures may be simple or compound.

Impacted Fractures. In these fractures, the bone ends are driven firmly together out of position.

Forces Required to Disengage Fragments and Restore Fracture Segment Position

Depressed Fractures. These fractures have depression and dislocation of the segments.

Conditions Predisposing to Fracture. Any generalized bone disease, such as rickets, osteomalacia, metastasis, infection, and fragilitas ossium, can produce bone weakness that predisposes to a fracture. The loss of teeth predisposes to fracture.

Localized Bone Disease. Any localized bone disease, such as a benign or malignant neoplasm, a cyst, local infection such as osteomyelitis, or a tumor of the bone such as a hemangioma, produces an area of weakness that predisposes to a fracture. Such conditions must be searched for and possibly treated during the reduction of a fracture.

Causes of Mandibular Fractures

Trauma. Direct trauma indicates that a force at the site of the fracture has resulted in discontinuity of the bone.

Indirect. A blow on the opposite side of the jaw or at a distance from the fracture site may produce a fracture in the contralateral portion of the mandible. This is seen in fractures of the condyle, which may occur from a blow on the chin or the contralateral side.

A blow on the symphysis may result in a fracture of both mandibular condyles but no fracture of the symphysis. A fracture of the left body, the result of a direct blow, may be accompanied by a contralateral fracture of the right subcondylar area.

Presence or Absence of Serviceable Teeth in Segments of Mandible. Kazanjian and Converse (1949) proposed a classification describing the presence or absence of teeth adjacent to each side of the fracture. This classification has a relationship to the management of the fracture (see Fig. 27–83).

Class I. Teeth are present on both sides of the fracture line. The teeth can be used as a guide to anatomic reduction and can be utilized for the attachment of wires or appliances to maintain the fragments in position during healing. One or more teeth on each side of the fracture may be sufficient, even though the upper teeth are not present to permit intermaxillary fixation.

Class II. Teeth are present on only one side of the fracture line. The teeth are used for a fixation of the mandibular to the maxillary teeth. In many cases, it would be wise to utilize a splint, a dental appliance, or open reduction to stabilize the edentulous segment and to ensure proper occlusion with the maxilla.

Class III. The fracture fragments contain no teeth. The teeth may have been dislodged or fractured at the time of injury, or may have been previously removed. Such a fracture would be stabilized entirely with a splint, with internal fixation, or with a combination of a splint and internal fixation.

Mandibular Fracture Classified as to Location. Dingman and Natvig (1964) classified mandibular fractures as to location, being the location most commonly involved (see Fig. 27–82*A*,*B*). Alternatively the fracture pattern and the presence of an open wound may be utilized (Fig. 27–82*C*).

Parasymphyseal and Symphyseal. Fractures that occur between the mental foramen are usually classified as symphyseal and parasymphyseal fractures. They are usually present vertically or obliquely. Often, the fracture may be comminuted with triangularly shaped bone fragments displaced from the inferior, lingual border of the mandible.

Canine. These fractures occur through or around the cuspid teeth and may travel adjacent to the mental foramen. Every effort should be made to retain the cuspid tooth, as it is a key tooth in the restoration of occlusion and stability of the dental arch.

Body of Mandible. This area includes fractures occurring from the cuspid tooth to the angle of the mandible.

Angle. In this region, fractures of the mandible that occur behind the second molar tooth are classified. The region of the angle is weaker and is further weakened by the presence of an unerupted third molar tooth.

Ramus of Mandible. These fractures occur between the angle of the mandible and the sigmoid notch.

Coronoid Process. These involve fractures of the coronoid that may be broken off at a level above or below the mandibular sigmoid notch.

Subcondylar Area. This area includes fractures below the anatomic neck of the condyle. The fracture may extend into the ramus.

Alveolar Fractures. These fractures involve the disconnection of a segment of alveolar bone with or without attached teeth. The teeth may be avulsed from the fragment, fractured separately, or present in the bone fragment. Alveolar fractures may occur separately or in association with other fractures of the mandible.

CLINICAL EXAMINATION

The clinical examination of the mandible is the most important diagnostic measure used to identify a fracture. In most cases, radiographs should support the clinical findings.

The following clinical symptoms and signs of fracture of the jaw are important:

Pain is usually present on motion and may be noted immediately as a result of injury.

Fractures occurring along the course of the inferior alveolar nerve may produce *numbness* in the distribution of the mental nerve and *numbness* of the ipsilateral teeth.

There is usually exquisite *tenderness* over the site of the fracture. This is helpful in localizing the fracture site.

The patient is *unable to open* the mouth or to bring the teeth into proper occlusion. He often refuses to eat or to brush his teeth, which causes discomfort and an abnormal odor.

Excessive saliva is often produced as a result of local irritation.

Edema and *ecchymosis* indicate the site of the fracture. Enlargement of the soft tissues at the fracture site is a result of hemorrhage and may be the result of contamination and the development of an infection. Immediately after the injury, there usually is distortion and enlargement of the overlying soft tissues. Hemorrhage may appear as ecchymosis or may produce a hematoma, and may extend into the floor of the mouth area.

If dislocation of the fracture segments has occurred, the patient may demonstrate *physical deformity.* The jaw may deviate to one side or there may be an abnormal contour to the jaw line. The patient may be unable to open or close the mouth, depending on the position and site of the fracture. An open bite deformity, for example, may be present, a finding that indicates that the patient cannot bring the teeth into proper occlusion in the anterior portion of the dentition. The mandible may be shifted to one side or the other or posteriorly, giving a bizarre appearance to the lower facial area.

In fractures of the condyle with displacement, the mandible may shift toward the involved side as the patient attempts to open the mouth. This is caused by nonfunction of the lateral pterygoid muscle on the ipsilateral side with unopposed activity on the intact side. On protrusive motion, the jaw shifts to the side of the fracture. *Abnormal mobility* may be present on manual distraction of the sides of the dental alveolar arches. A gap or level discrepancy may be present in the dentition.

The patient may notice a grating sound (*crepitus*) on movement of the mandible. This is caused by the movement of the fracture segments against one another.

Because of the absence of the normal cleansing activity of mastication, an odor (*fetor oris*) may be present. After a day or two, debris often accumulates in an intraoral laceration with food, blood clots, and devitalized tissue undergoing bacterial putrefaction. This situation results in an offensive breath, which is indicative of the onset of a localized infectious process.

DIAGNOSIS

The diagnosis of a mandibular fracture is made on the basis of one or more of the following findings:

Bimanual manipulation of the mandible causes *mobility* or distraction at the site of the fracture, especially when the fracture occurs in the body or the parasymphyseal area. One hand should stabilize the ramus while the other manipulates the symphysis or the body area. The fracture will be demonstrated by abnormal movement, and the condition and the symptom reinforced by the presence of discomfort.

The mandible should be pulled forward with a finger in the ear canal and a finger over the condyle (see Fig. 27–13). Abnormal mobility or crepitus indicates a fracture in the subcondylar area or ligament laxity indicating a temporomandibular joint injury.

The most reliable finding in fractures of the mandible in dentulous patients is the presence of any *malocclusion*. Often the most minute dislocation caused by the fracture is quite obvious to the patient inasmuch as the teeth do not mesh or come together in the proper manner.

The patient is unable to move the jaw (*dysfunction*) and requests solid foods that require minimal movement of the jaw in mastication. Speech is difficult because of pain on motion of the mandible.

Crepitation may be noticeable by manipulation of the fracture site. Often the necessary manipulation produces such discomfort that it is not wise to demonstrate this sign on physical examination.

Swelling is usually quite obvious and is frequently associated with ecchymosis and a hematoma. Often an intraoral laceration is present over fractures in the horizontal portion of the mandible.

There is frequently *deviation* to one side or the other, a finding that supports the diagnosis of a fracture.

Tenderness over the fracture site is present, especially in the region of the temporomandibular joint. Such tenderness is highly suggestive of the presence of a fracture.

Roentgenographic Examination

Roentgenographic examination is imperative, but should support the clinical diagnosis of a fracture. One study (Chayra, Meador, and Laskin, 1986) indicated that the clinical examination was responsible for the diagnosis of a fracture in 10 per cent of cases in which the diagnosis could not be supported by roentgenograms obtained at the time of the injury. Thus, the patient should be treated for a fracture if there is sufficient clinical indication.

Careful roentgenograms should be taken on all suspected fractures as indicated, with particular attention to the condyle and subcondylar area. The panoramic roentgenogram is especially helpful but may not be obtainable in patients with multiple trauma. Specialized examinations, such as occlusal films, palatal films, and apical views of the teeth are helpful in detecting fractures or in analyzing the degree of tooth root injury (see Figs. 27–34, 27–35, 27–36, and 27–37).

Muscles Influencing Movement of Mandible

Muscle function is an important variable influencing the degree and direction of displacement of fractured mandibular segments. Overcoming the forces of displacement is also important in reduction and fixation of mandibular fragments.

Posterior Group of Mandibular Muscles. The posterior group of muscles is commonly referred to as the "muscles of mastication." The muscles are short and thick and are capable of exerting extremely strong forces on the mandible. The muscles of mastication are the temporalis, the masseter, and the medial (internal) and lateral (external) pterygoid muscles. The overall activity of this group is to move the mandible in the general upward, forward, and medial direction (Fig. 27–84).

Masseter Muscle. This is a thick, short, powerful, heavy muscle attached to the inferior portion of the zygomatic eminence and to the zygomatic arch. It arises from tendinous fibers in the anterior two-thirds of the lower border of the zygomatic bone, and from the medial surfaces of the zygomatic arch, and inserts into the lateral surface of the ramus and densely onto the bone along the inferior border of the mandible at the region of the angle. The masseter muscle is an elevator of the jaw and functions to pull the mandible upward and forward.

Temporalis Muscle. This muscle arises from the limits of the temporal fossa. It is a broad, fan-shaped muscle whose fibers converge to descend under the zygomatic arch and insert on the coronoid process, the lateral and medial surface of the coronoid, and the anterior surface of the ramus as far down as the occlusal plane of the third molar tooth. The anterior fibers are elevators and the posterior fibers are retractors of the mandible.

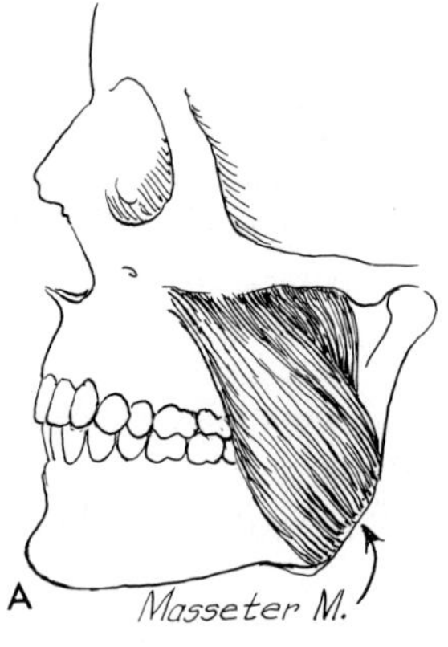

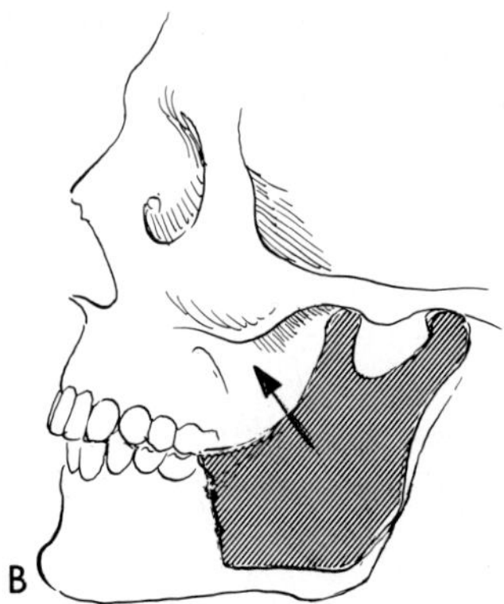

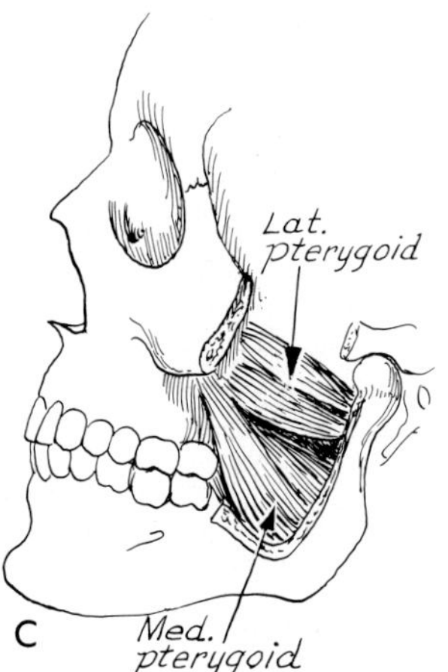

Figure 27–84. The posterior group of muscles attached to the mandible. The overall force from the activity of this group of muscles is movement of the mandible upward, forward, medially, or laterally. *A,* The masseter muscle. *B,* Upward displacement in a fractured mandible produced by a pull of the masseter muscle on the edentulous proximal fragment. *C,* The medial and lateral pterygoid muscles. *D,* Directional pull of the medial and lateral pterygoid muscles. *E,* The temporalis muscle and the direction of pull. (From Kazanjian and Converse.)

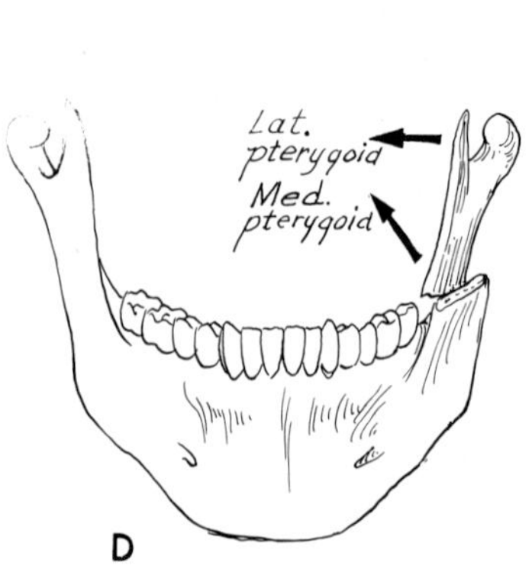

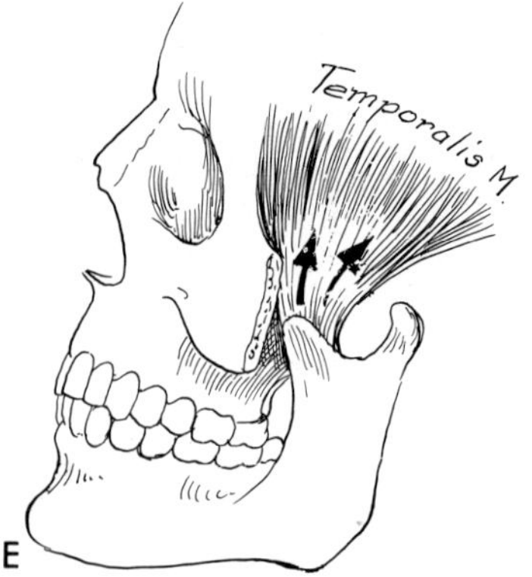

Medial Pterygoid Muscle. This muscle originates in the pterygoid fossa, mainly from the medial surface of the lateral pterygoid process, and from the pyramidal process of the palatine bone and maxillary tuberosity. It inserts into the medial surface of the ramus and angle of the mandible. The fibers of the medial pterygoid muscle pass in a downward, posterior, and lateral direction to the angle of the mandible. The function of the medial pterygoid muscle is to exert upward, medial, and forward traction on the mandible.

Lateral Pterygoid Muscle. This muscle has two heads of origin. The upper head arises from the infratemporal crest, the infratemporal surface of the greater wing of the sphenoid bone, and a small area of the squamous part of the temporal bone. The lower head arises from the lateral surface of the lateral pterygoid plate. The upper head inserts into the capsule of the joint and into the articular disc of the temporomandibular joint. The lower head inserts into the anterior surface of the neck of the condyle. The innermost or upper portion pulls the mandible upward, medially, and forward; the external portion pulls the condyle downward, medially, and forward. Contraction of the muscle on one side pulls the mandible to the opposite side. Contraction of both lateral pterygoid muscles simultaneously protrudes the mandible.

Anterior or Depressor Group of Mandibular Muscles. These are considered the opening muscles of the mandible (Fig. 27–85). With the hyoid bone fixed, they depress the mandible. When the mandible is fractured, they displace the fractured segments downward, posteriorly, and medially. This group is made up of the geniohyoid, genioglossus, mylohyoid, and digastric muscles.

Geniohyoid Muscle. This muscle arises from the inferior medial spine of the mandible and passes downward and posteriorly to insert into the body of the hyoid bone. Its function is to elevate the hyoid and to depress the mandible.

Genioglossus Muscle. This is the main muscle of the tongue and is attached to the genial tubercles on the inner, inferior surface of the anterior mandible. Its fibers pass primarily into the substance of the tongue and into the upper surface of the hyoid bone. Its function is to protrude the tongue, elevate the hyoid, and depress the mandible.

Mylohyoid Muscle. This fan-shaped muscle acts as a diaphragm for support of the floor of the mouth. It arises from the mylohyoid line on the inner surface of the body of the mandible. Its fibers pass medially to insert into a median raphé and posteriorly to insert into the hyoid bone. Its function is to elevate the hyoid bone and to depress the mandible. Its fibers pull medially, posteriorly, and downward.

Digastric Muscle. The digastric muscle arises from the digastric fossa at the inferior, medial portion of the mandible bilaterally and extends posteriorly to pass beneath the fibrous sling, attached near the lesser cornu of the hyoid bone. Its tendon is continuous with that of the posterior portion, which originates from the digastric fossa of the temporal bone. The function of this muscle is to elevate the hyoid and depress the anterior portion of the mandible.

THE TEMPOROMANDIBULAR JOINT

The function and anatomy of this joint (see Chap. 30) are important in considering injuries of the mandibular condyle (Fig. 27–86). The temporomandibular joint is known as a ginglymoarthrodial joint; it is capable of a hingelike action, as well as a gliding and rotating action. The joint is composed of the articular head of the condyle of the mandible and the glenoid fossa of the squamous portion of the temporal bone. The glenoid fossa forms a portion of the floor of the middle cranial fossa. The articular surface of both the condyle and the temporal fossa is covered with a thin smooth layer of cartilage surrounded by connective tissue, which differentiates into an inner and outer layer. The inner layer, which is known as the synovial membrane, secretes a viscid fluid lubricant that minimizes friction and aids smooth functioning of the joint. The outer layer of the connective tissue is intimately associated with ligaments that surround the joint and provide an enveloping capsule within which the articular surfaces function. The temporomandibular joint is a compound joint. It is separated into two distinct chambers, one above and the other below an articular disc composed of fibrocartilage known as the meniscus. Movement of the articular disc is controlled by the attachments of the lateral pterygoid muscle that insert, through the capsule of the joint, into the anterior edge of the disc, and by the attachment of the disc to the posterior portion of the joint capsule. The hinge, rotating, and

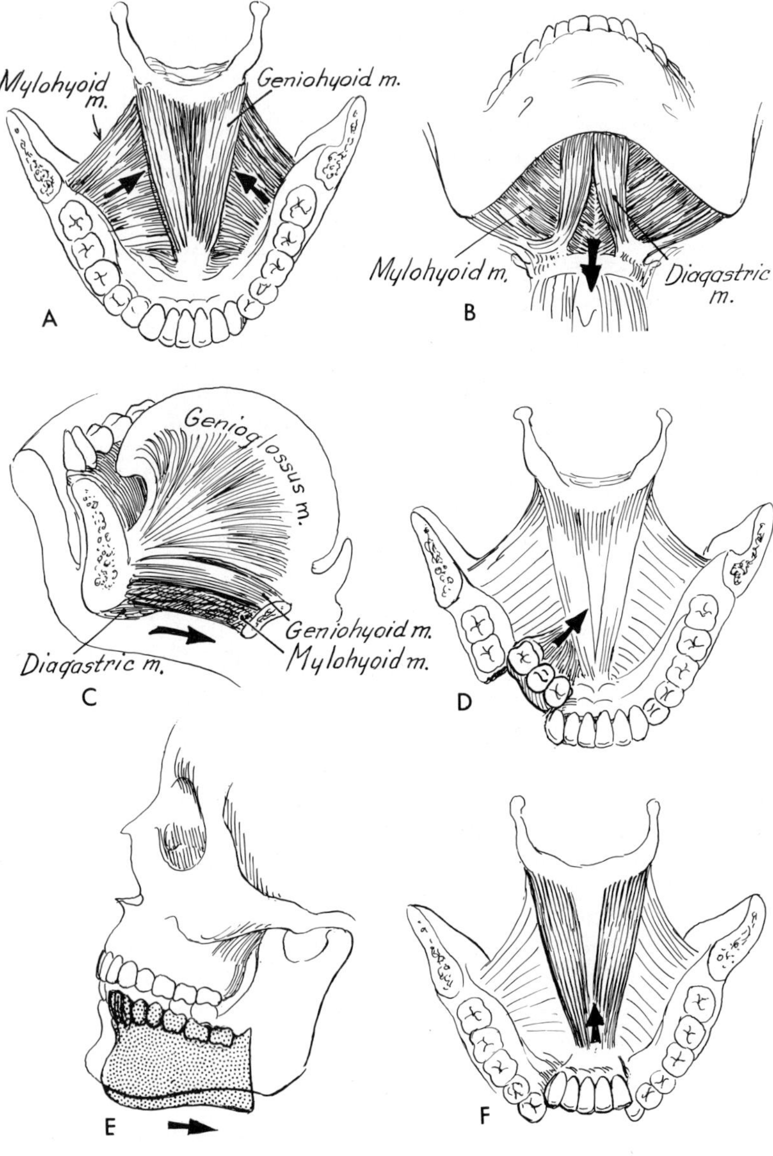

Figure 27–85. The anterior or depressor group of muscles of mastication, the suprahyoid muscles. The arrows indicate the direction of pull and the displacement of the fragments in fractures of the mandible. (From Kazanjian and Converse.)

gliding movements of the temporomandibular joint are controlled by the muscles attached to the mandible. The movement of the disc is regulated by its ligaments, and injuries to the ligaments allow abnormal motion of the disc, which produces clicking, locking, or pain.

Factors Influencing Displacement of Fractured Mandibular Segments

The direction and extent of displacement of fragments depend on the site of the fracture, the direction of the fracture, the direction of pull of the muscles attached to the mandible, the direction and intensity of force, the presence of overlying muscle, and the presence or absence of teeth in the fragments. In fractures of the mandible, the segments may be displaced in the direction of the strongest muscular action.

Direction and Angulation of Fracture Line. Kelsey Fry (Fry and associates, 1942) pointed out that fractures may be favorable or unfavorable for displacement according to their direction and bevel. The muscular force on some fracture fragments is opposed by the direction and bevel of the fracture line. Thus,

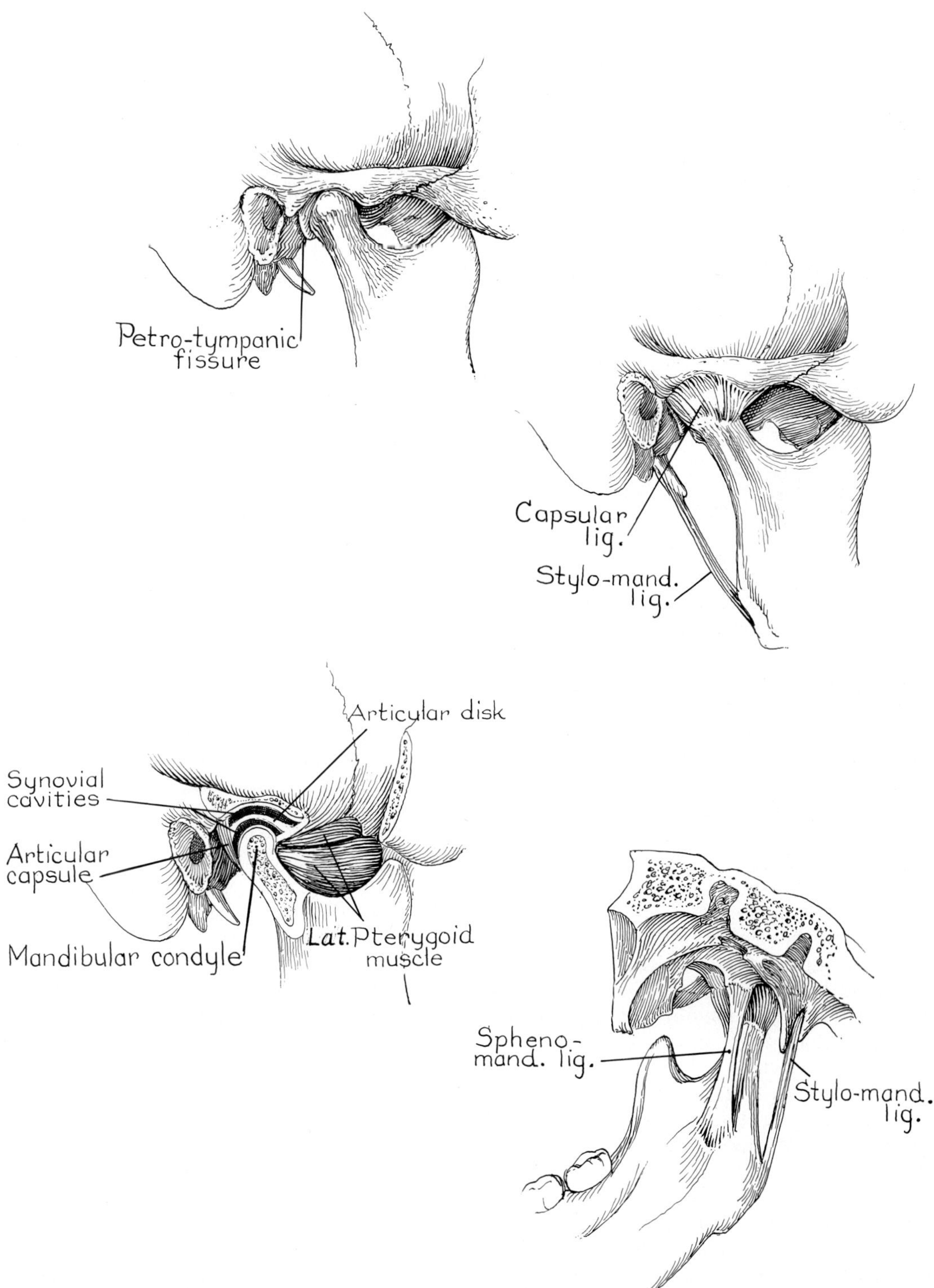

Figure 27–86. The temporomandibular joint and its associated ligaments. (From Kazanjian and Converse.)

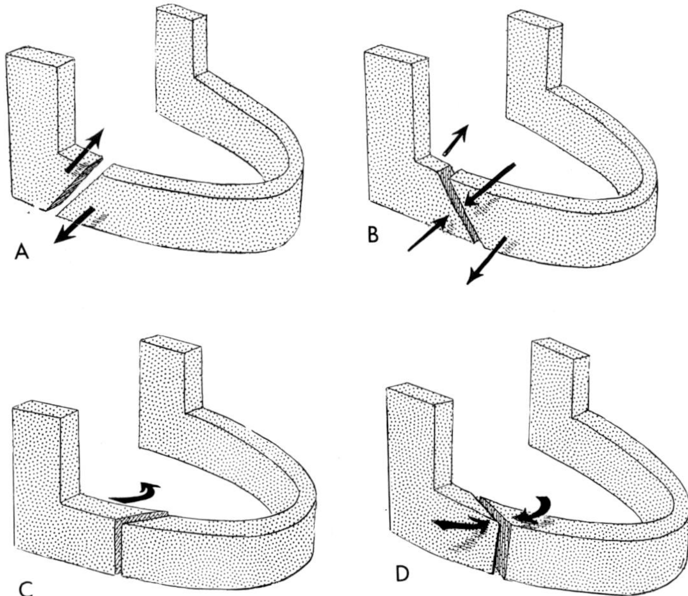

Figure 27–87. In *A* and *C* the direction and bevel of the fracture line do not resist displacement due to muscular action. The arrows indicate the direction of muscle pull. In *B* and *D* the bevel and direction of the fracture line resist displacement and oppose muscular action. The direction of the muscle pull in fractures beveled in this direction would tend to impact the fractured bone ends. (After Fry, W. K., Shepherd, P. R., McLeod, A. C., and Parfitt, G.J.: The Dental Treatment of Maxillofacial Injuries. Oxford, Blackwell Scientific Publications, 1942.)

the muscular force would pull the fragments into a position favorable for healing, whereas in other fractures the muscular pull is unfavorable and separation of the fracture fragments occurs by action of the muscular force (Fig. 27–87). Mandibular fractures that are directed downward and forward are classified as horizontally favorable (*H.F.*) because the posterior group of muscles and the anterior group of muscles pull in antagonistic directions favoring stability at the site of the fractures. Fractures running from above, downward, and posteriorly are classified as horizontally unfavorable (*H.U.*). The bevel of the fracture may also influence the displacement medially. If a fracture runs from posteriorly, forward, and medially, displacement would take place in a medial direction, because of the medial pull of the elevator muscles of mastication (vertically unfavorable or *V.U.*). The fracture that passes from the lateral surface of the mandible posteriorly and medially is a favorable fracture, because the muscle pull tends to prevent displacement. It is called a vertically favorable fracture (*V.F.*) (Fig. 27–87).

Presence or Absence of Teeth in Fractured Segments. Upper displacement of the posterior segment is prevented by the occlusal contact of the lower against the upper teeth. The elevator muscles of the mandible pull the posterior fragment forward. The anterior group of muscles depresses the anterior segments of the mandible, separating the teeth anterior to the fracture from the upper teeth. A single tooth in the posterior fragment may be extremely important and should be retained. This tooth acts as an "occlusal stop" and, even if damaged, will contribute to stability of the posterior fragment in the reduction (Figs. 27–88, 27–89).

Soft Tissue at Site of Fracture. Fractures of the ramus of the mandible, even though extensively comminuted, have very little displacement because of the splinting action of the medial and lateral pterygoid and masseter muscle attachments (Fig. 27–90). Some degree of stability is also provided by the periosteum and soft tissue attachments surrounding the body of the mandible, but these are usually weak, and very little stability is offered by their presence. In extensive soft tissue wounds, such as gunshot injuries, no stability is offered by the torn tissues. Some degree of stability is provided to the fragments by the replacement of soft tissues if accurate suturing returns them carefully into their original position.

Direction and Intensity of Traumatic Force. The force on the mandible may directly or indirectly influence the site of fracture and the amount of displacement. Direct lateral force in the region of the premolar teeth may result in a fracture of the involved

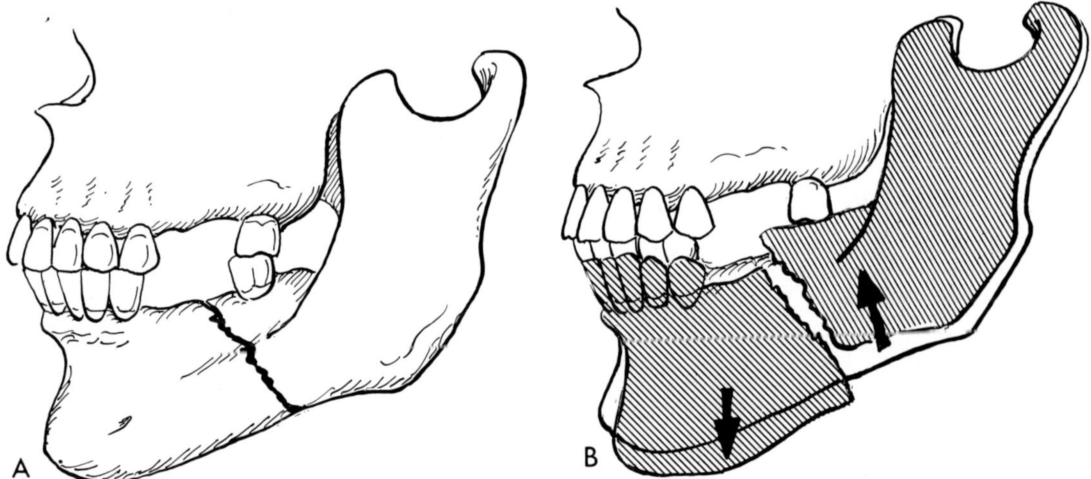

Figure 27–88. *A,* Upward displacement of the posterior segment of the mandible can be prevented by the presence of a tooth on the posterior fragment occluding against a maxillary tooth. *B,* When these teeth are not present, displacement of the posterior fragment occurs because of the absence of occluded teeth. A splint might prevent this displacement; however, open reduction is preferred.

side and a fracture of the condyle on the contralateral side. Traumatic forces applied to the anterior portion of the mandible may produce a fracture of the symphyseal or parasymphyseal areas. A fracture fragment, often a triangular fracture fragment at the base of the mandible, may be driven posteriorly into the floor of the mouth. Symphyseal or parasymphyseal fractures are frequently accompanied by a laceration of the floor of the mouth. Displacement of these fragments is exaggerated by the muscles of the floor of the mouth, which exert a downward and posterior force. Blows to the anterior portion of the mandible (symphyseal and parasymphyseal area) may cause bilateral or unilateral condylar fractures, or may force the condyle into the middle cranial fossa or ear canal. The condyle may be fractured or dislocated, or may be both fractured and dislocated. If the condyles are forced into the external auditory canal, a fracture of the tympanic plate occurs. Displacement of the condyle may lacerate the ear canal, producing bleeding.

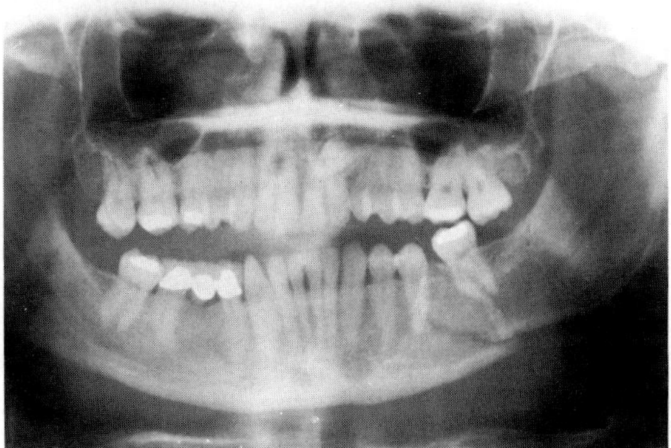

Figure 27–89. Fracture of the body of the mandible. The presence of a tooth on each side of the fracture line makes control of the proximal fragment somewhat easier.

Fractures of Alveolar Structures and Damage to Teeth. Damage of the anterior teeth occurs more often than damage of the posterior teeth because of their forward position and single conical root structure. Teeth may be completely avulsed from the bone or may fracture at the gingival line with the roots remaining in the bone, or segments of the alveolar bone may be fractured with the teeth remaining firmly attached. The fracture line may traverse the tooth at any level. The fracture line may parallel the border of the tooth, or if a fracture of the crown and edges of the tooth occurs, exposure of the dental pulp is produced (Schneider and Stern, 1971; Neal, Wagner, and Alpert, 1978; Kahnberg and Ridell, 1979; Kahnberg, 1979; Amaratunga, 1987a).

Reimplantation of avulsed teeth may be successful and is reportedly more appropriate in children. Presumably, the open structure of the root apex in children allows for more successful reestablishment of blood supply. Reimplantation is most successful if the tooth is reimplanted within one-half to one hour and if the tooth is firmly supported. In adults, the pulp is occasionally removed and the

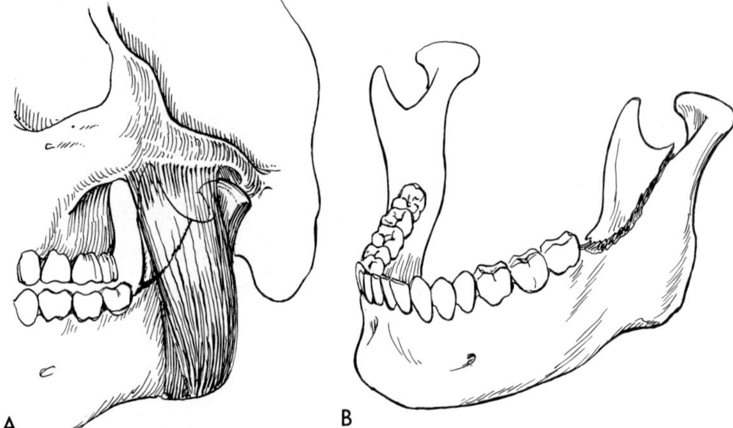

Figure 27–90. In ramus fractures, the heavy musculature and the periosteum surrounding the ramus of the mandible provide protection and tend to prevent displacement of fractured segments. *B,* Fractures of the coronoid process are uncommon and displacement is usually minimal.

canal filled and treated before the tooth is reimplanted. These teeth "ankylose" to the alveolar structures of bone. If a crown of a tooth has been fractured with exposure of the dental pulp, it may be advisable to protect the pulp in some way at the time of establishing intermaxillary fixation. If this is not done, infection and severe pain may be troublesome. If segments of alveolus that contain teeth have been fractured and have an adequate blood supply by virtue of the soft tissue attachments, attempts should be made to replace the segments along with their contained teeth and to fix them securely into position with wires or small screws. The arch bar and dental ligatures assist positioning of the dental segment. Most of these tooth-bearing segments survive and provide a satisfactory masticatory surface. One should presume that some of the teeth in this segment will ultimately need root canal therapy, and care should be taken not to strip surrounding soft tissues and devascularize the segment.

Injury to the teeth without avulsion or fracture may result in devitalization owing to hemorrhage in the dental pulp. The teeth become insensitive and discolored as a result of infiltration of the blood pigments into the tooth structure. If infection occurs, the teeth must be treated, the infection drained, or the tooth extracted. Some, even though discolored and nonvital, remain as asymptomatic and useful teeth (Schneider and Stern, 1971; Neal, Wagner, and Alpert, 1978; Kahnberg and Ridell, 1979; Kahnberg, 1979; Amaratunga, 1987a). As mentioned, teeth in the line of fracture should be retained if they offer any degree of stability to the bone fragments and if they have solid attachments. It is important that loose teeth with extensive periodontal disease be considered for removal or that steps be taken to prevent infection. Antibiotic therapy protects against infection, and some studies have demonstrated a twofold advantage against infection if antibiotics are employed when teeth are involved in the fracture. If teeth are loose, or interfere with reduction, they should be removed. In general, third molars in a fracture line are removed if an open reduction is required. If the fracture would otherwise be amenable to closed reduction, the tooth may be left, employing antibiotic therapy, until healing has occurred and the third molar can be removed (Fig. 27–91). The removal of a third molar tooth from a fracture of the angle, which would not otherwise need an open reduction, often precipitates the need for an open reduction (Neal, Wagner, and Alpert, 1978). After the mandibular fracture has healed or the patient has begun mobilization, the teeth should be given the necessary attention by the patient's dentist. Apical views of the teeth and sensory stimulation studies detect apical pathology or devitalization. Such teeth must be carefully observed for periapical abscess and they may require root canal treatment.

Principles of Treatment of Mandibular Fractures

Primary consideration in the management of fractures of the mandible is to restore the function of the mandible and the masticatory efficiency of the dentition (Rowe and Killey, 1968; Kazanjian and Converse, 1974; Irby, 1979; Kruger and Schilli, 1982; Kruger, 1984). To accomplish this, the principles of

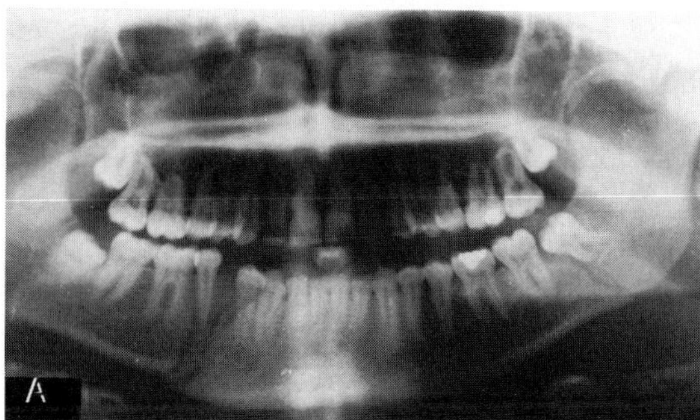

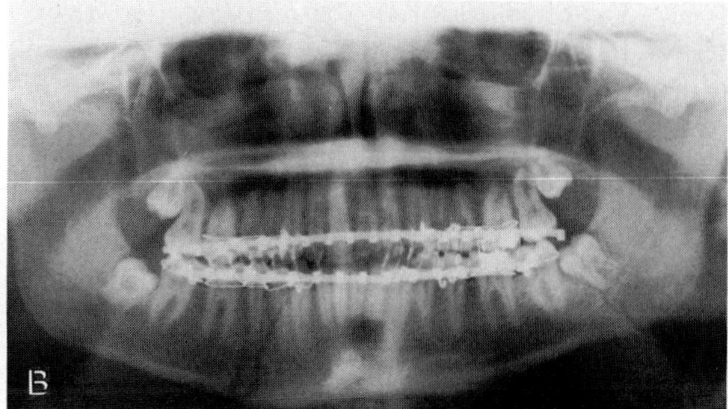

Figure 27–91. *A,* A fracture of the right body and left angle of the mandible. *B,* The fracture was treated by closed reduction and immobilization. The third molar in the left-angle fracture, partially erupted, was extracted after healing. Extraction of this molar at the time of closed reduction would have precipitated an open reduction.

fracture management must be applied. These are:

1. Reduction of the fractured bone segments into their anatomic position.

2. Production of the proper occlusal relationships.

3. Establishment of a fixation technique that will hold both the fractured bone segments and occlusion in position until healing has occurred.

4. Control of infection.

In general, the simplest method of attaining and satisfying these requirements is the best method. The methods of fixation employed may vary with the age of the patient, his general state of health, the training of the surgeon, the facilities and circumstances available, and the conditions under which the patient is to be treated. The satisfactory end result may be accomplished by the use of any one of a number of methods, and no method is without its complications, advantages, or disadvantages.

Treatment of Class I Fractures. Class I fractures are those in which there are teeth on each side of the fracture (Fig. 27–92). These fractures can often be managed by the application of intermaxillary fixation. If the fracture is favorable vertically and horizontally, this may be all that is necessary. The patient is kept in intermaxillary fixation for a four to six week period (Amaratunga, 1987b,c). Some fractures are best managed by open reduction and direct interosseous wiring in combination with dental appliances or intermaxillary fixation. Alternatively, a dental splint or plate and screw fixation can be employed (Spiessl, 1976; Schilli, 1977; Champy and associates, 1978; Rowe, Miller, and Brandt-Zawadzki, 1981; Ewers and Härle, 1985; Klotch and Bilger, 1985; Schilli, Ewers, and Niederdellmann, 1985), either with or without intermaxillary fixation (monomaxillary fixation). These techniques are especially appealing to the patient because it is unnecessary to wire the teeth in occlusion postoperatively, and they permit intake of solid foods, oral hygiene, and often an early return to work. These aspects of convenience should not influence the treatment if a satisfactory result can be obtained simply by intermaxillary fixation. The use of solid as opposed to liquid food for a period of four to six weeks is not of great overall significance and should not always influence the surgeon to use more complicated methods. During the

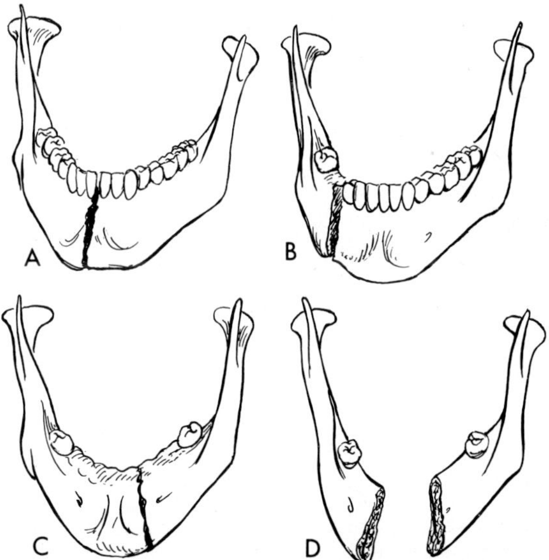

Figure 27–92. Class I fractures of the mandible. Teeth are technically present on both sides of the fracture site, but the fractures in *B, C,* and *D* would require open reduction for stability. The author feels that any displaced parasymphyseal fracture(s) should have an open reduction.

four to six weeks of intermaxillary fixation, the patient often loses 15 lb. Appropriate dietary counseling and the use of vitamins and supplements are important to provide proper nutrition.

Horizontal Interdental Wiring. The fracture can be reduced manually and held together with 25 gauge stainless steel wires twisted around the necks of selected teeth on both sides of the fracture site, and twisted to a wire on the opposite side of the fracture site (Fig. 27–93). This method is simple and expedient and can be utilized on any Class I fracture to position the segments before a more definitive reduction. The wire may be angulated or passed in such a way that it produces the leverage that attempts to reduce and maintain the alignment of the fracture (Fig. 27–94). It is inadvisable to use only the teeth immediately adjacent to the fracture site, since their attachments may be loosened and they may be dislodged by the force of the ligature wire.

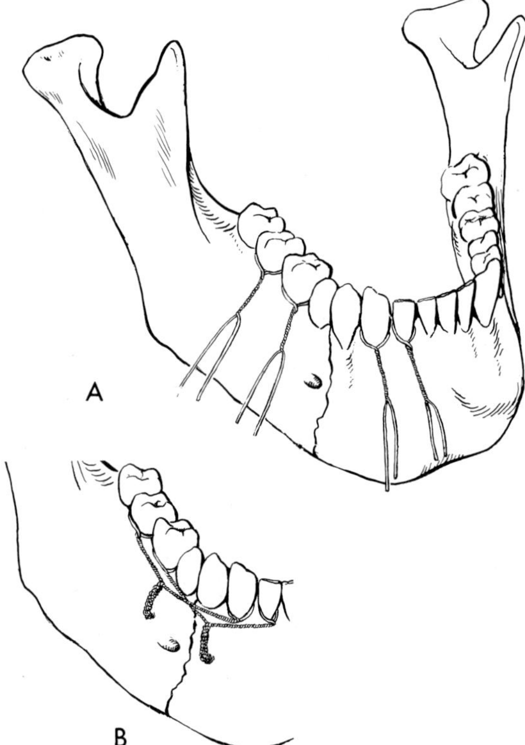

Figure 27–93. Horizontal interdental wiring of mandibular fragments. *A,* In fractures with minimal displacement, the wires may be twisted around the teeth on each side of the fragment and twisted across the fracture site. In practice it is much easier and more stable to use an arch bar and open reduction. *B,* Wires are twisted together across the fracture site. Acrylic can be applied to increase stability. This fracture is probably better treated with an open reduction at the lower border to accompany the intermaxillary fixation. In practice open reduction usually is also necessary.

Prefabricated Arch Bars. The Erich modification of the Winter-type arch bar is used routinely by many surgeons. These are made of semirigid pliable metal and can be easily contoured to the dental arch, cut to length, and carefully fitted to the necks of the teeth without a great deal of special equipment. Arch bars are generally used for intermaxillary fixation, but a single arch bar attached to the lower teeth for support of the Class I–type fracture may be used for monomaxillary fixation. This is done by shaping a bar long enough to pass completely around the dental arch. The arch bar is securely ligated to the necks of the teeth in the larger fragment, and the wires are loosely placed around the teeth and the arch bar on the displaced fragment. The fracture is reduced manually and held firmly in position by instrumental or digital manipulation. An assistant tightens the wires in an effort to maintain the reduced position of the jaw segments (Fig. 27–95).

Sections of arch bars attached to the teeth of the posterior segment can be ligated in the anterior region after reduction of the fracture (Fig. 27–96). This provides adequate fixation and holds the fractured segments together. If maxillary teeth are present, supplementary fixation with intermaxillary rubber band traction will bring the teeth into optimal occlusion. An open reduction at the inferior border is also usually required.

Cable Arch Wires. If no arch bars are available, a cable wire can be fashioned to provide stability across the site of the fracture and a means of intermaxillary fixation. The cable wires are fabricated by using a long length of 22 gauge stainless steel wire, which is passed around the last tooth on each quadrant of the dental arch and twisted up tightly to the teeth but left long. The wire from the right side is twisted to the wire on the left side at the midline and the excess cut and removed. Ligature wires are then passed around the necks of the teeth and around the cable arch bar until all the available teeth have been ligated. The teeth can be wired into occlusion by passing small wires around the upper and lower cable and twisting these tightly to provide a perpendicular force to achieve intermaxillary fixation.

The Banded Dental Arch. Angle (1899) devised a banded arch wire for fixation of

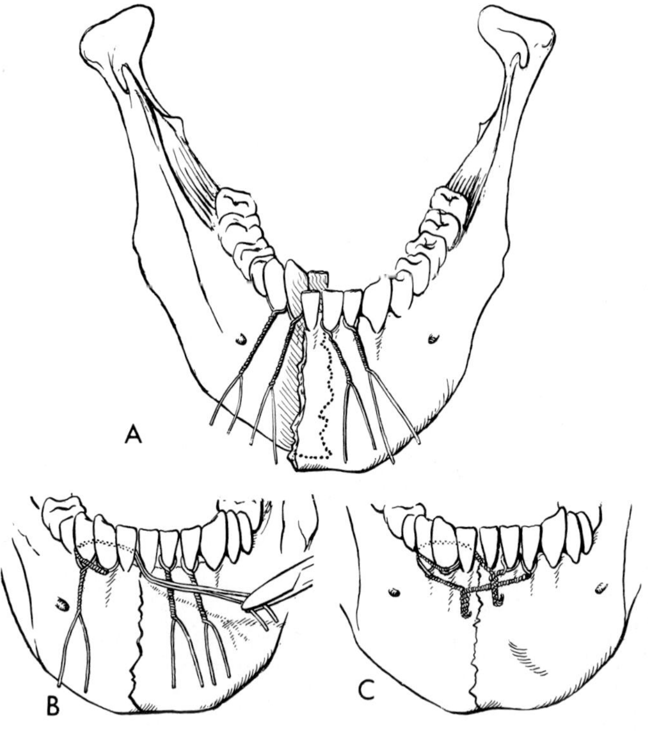

Figure 27–94. The wiring of an overriding fragment in a mandibular fracture. *A,* Wires are anchored to selective teeth on each side of the fracture site. *B,* The fracture is reduced by using the teeth on the overriding fragment to force the other fragment into apposition. *C,* The wires are twisted together across the fracture line. An open reduction at the inferior border is also preferred because the wiring technique serves only for initial positioning. (From Kazanjian and Converse.)

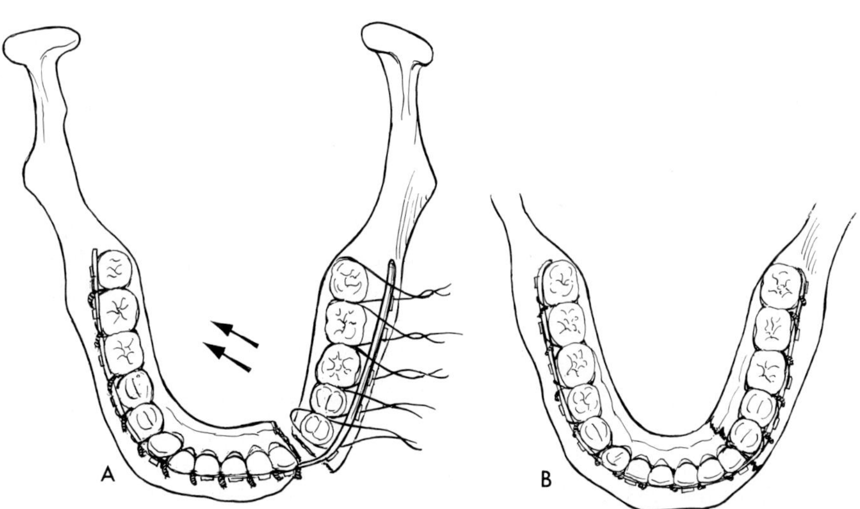

Figure 27–95. The application of an arch bar to a parasymphyseal fracture of the mandible. *A,* The arch bar is ligated to one side and wires are placed about the remaining teeth. *B,* After reduction of the fracture, the remaining wires are tightened. This fracture frequently requires the use of inferior border wiring or a plating technique or possibly the application of a lingual splint to support the reduction obtained with the arch bar.

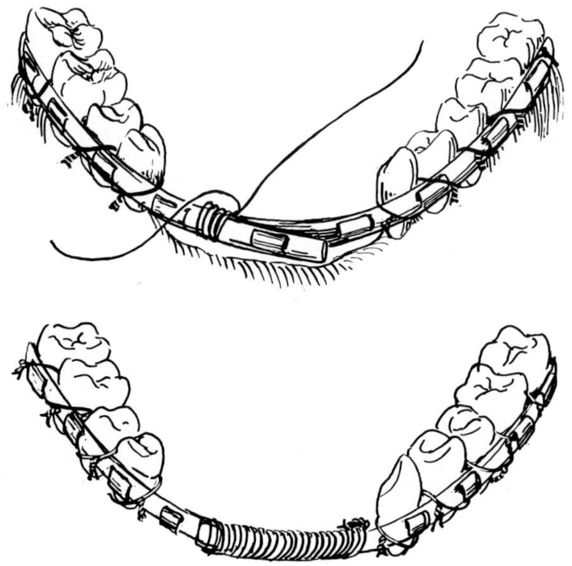

Figure 27–96. Fractured fragments of the parasymphyseal region may be supported by an arch bar attached to the segments on each side and wired together securely at the midline after reduction. This technique provides only temporary support before an open reduction. (After Kazanjian and Converse.)

mandibular fractures. These consist of prefabricated bands in sizes to fit the molar or bicuspid teeth. The bands are held with a jack screw and nut attachment, and twisted tightly until the band is securely opposed to the tooth. A long section of 14 gauge annealed brass wire flattened to 19 gauge is soldered to the band. The malleable brass wire is contoured along the lateral surface of the teeth to which it is ligated with fine stainless steel wire. These cumbersome methods are now seldom used.

The orthodontist also may be helpful in applying bands to the teeth and an interconnecting bar. Banded appliances on the upper and lower teeth serve quite adequately as fixation devices for intermaxillary fixation. Because they are more complicated and expensive, they are seldom utilized. The use of bonded appliances does not provide enough strength for the usual patient with a mandibular fracture. In general, the preferred method is the application of an Erich arch bar.

Cast Cap Splints. Cast cap splints are utilized extensively in some countries. They require sophisticated dental assistance since the appliances are designed to cover the occlusal surfaces and exposed portions of the teeth, and require the services of skilled technicians. They are often made of German silver and are expensive. Cast splints are especially useful when a strong appliance is needed. The cast cap splint is cemented to the occlusal surfaces of the teeth. Any splint that prevents observation of the occlusion is a disadvantage, as the exact occlusion cannot be determined with the splint in position.

Effective, equally useful, and less expensive splint appliances can be constructed by a dental laboratory or a properly trained physician. The acrylic splint is the most useful and is a strong, thin, easily fabricated splint that provides excellent stabilization; also, the technique can be easily learned. The technique requires moderate sophistication in the knowledge of occlusion (Fig. 27–97).

External Pin Fixation. External pin fixation is principally used for complications of mandibular fractures or for injuries in which segments of bone are missing (see Chap. 72). The use of external pin fixation can allow immediate motion. The disadvantage of scarring and the cumbersome character of the appliance prevent its routine application in fracture management (Fig. 27–98).

Treatment of Compound Comminuted Fractures of Anterior Portion of Mandible. Many fractures of the mandible, because of the intimate attachment of the thin overlying periosteum and mucosa, are usually compound into the mouth. They may also be compound through the skin. Antibiotics seem to reduce the complications of infection, and an agent appropriate against oral flora is generally used. The antibiotic, however,

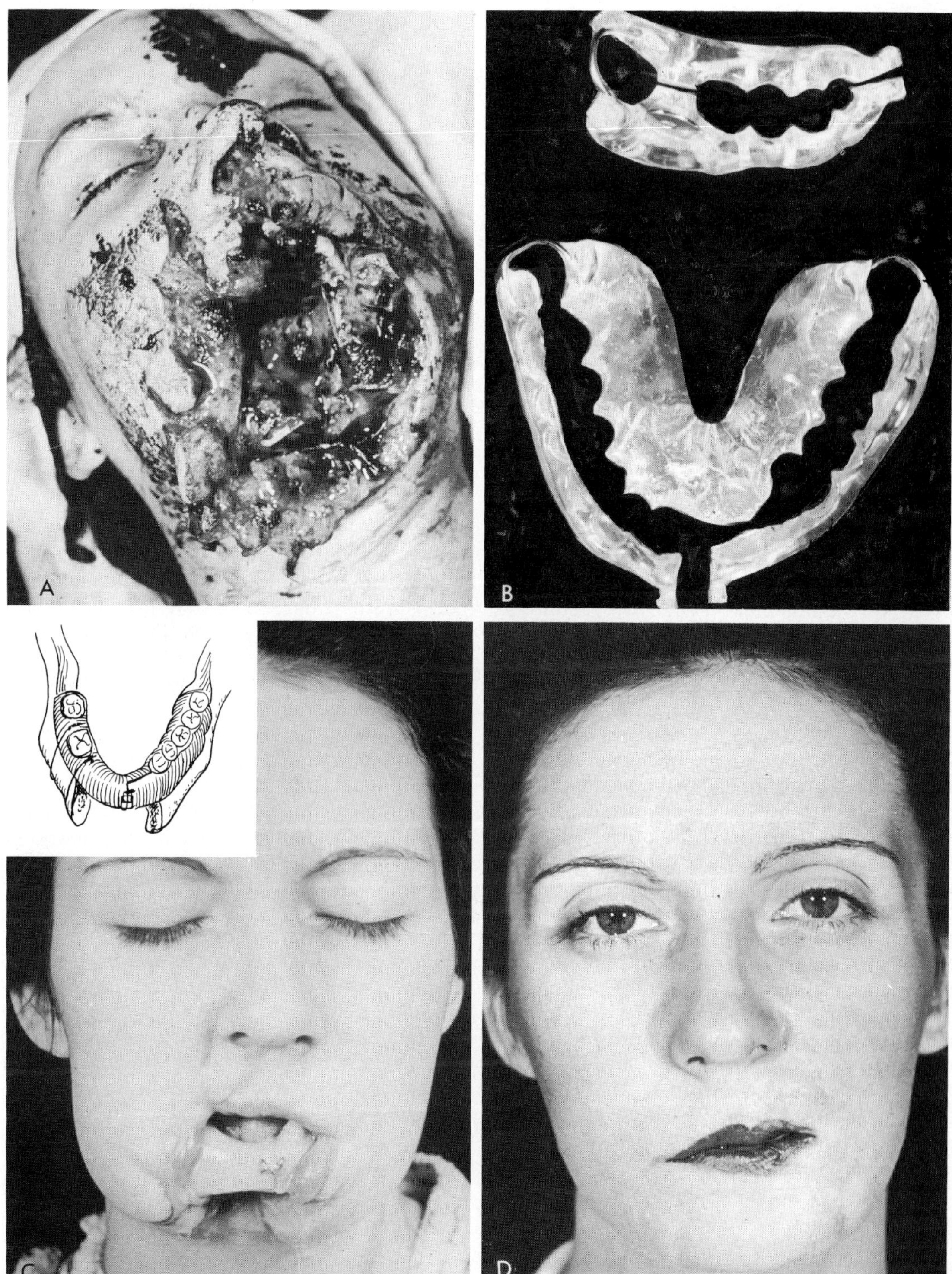

Figure 27–97. *A,* Gunshot wound with extensive destruction of soft tissue and bone. *B,* Acrylic splints made from a reconstructive model of the patient's dentition are used to stabilize the fractured mandibular segments after the method of Stout. *C,* Gunshot wound of the mandible with loss of bone from the right first molar to the left cuspid teeth. The segments of the mandible are held by an acrylic splint with circumferential wires around the mandible. *D,* Results after restoration of soft tissue by a cervical thoracic flap and bone grafting. Modern techniques would utilize mandibular external fixation.

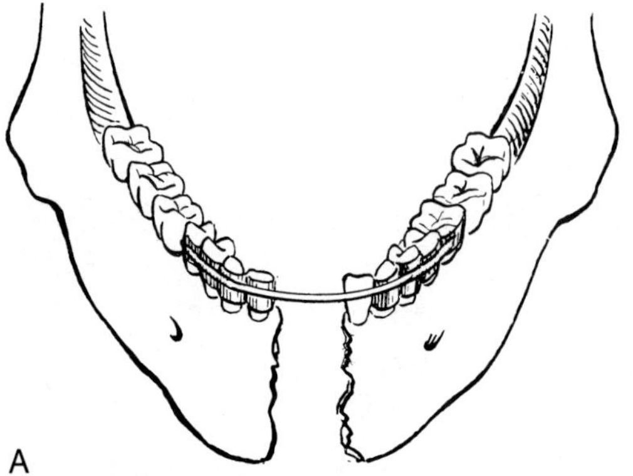

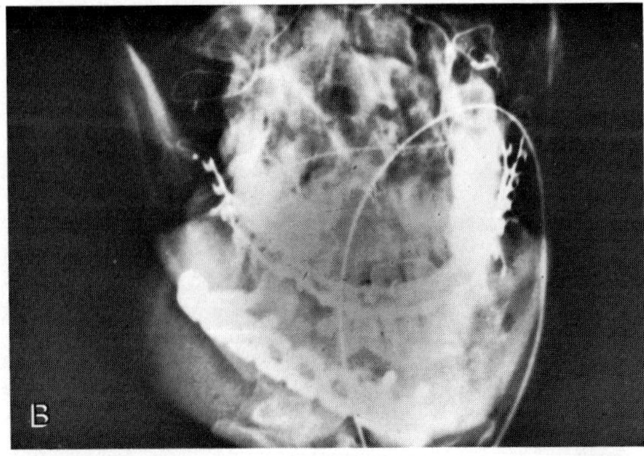

Figure 27–98. In fractures with loss of bone or extensive comminution in the anterior region, segments previously were held in alignment by means of an arch bar attached to orthodontic bands on each side of the fracture site *(A)*. Currently, a reconstruction plate *(B)* can be used to bridge the defect and provide a secure positioning. External fixation is an alternative approach.

should not be a replacement for proper surgical technique, absolute immobilization of the fracture, and adequate cleansing and debridement of the compound fracture. Conservative management generally results in healing of compound fractures with bone continuity if the bone fragments are stabilized and covered by soft tissue with sufficient blood supply.

Adequate fixation of bone fragments is imperative. This may be accomplished with intermaxillary fixation alone between the retained mandibular and maxillary teeth. Alternatively, a lingual splint may be utilized to stabilize the segments of the mandible and prevent lingual rotation, which can be aggravated by the forces of intermaxillary fixation (Fig. 27–99). In general, fractures of the anterior portion of the mandible are approached with a gingivobuccal sulcus degloving incision for open reduction (Fig. 27–100). They may also be approached through an existing laceration or an external incision. The fracture fragments are identified and the soft tissue is removed from the fracture site. The latter is especially important, since the inclusion of even a small amount of soft tissue in a fracture site prevents the bone ends from being accurately coapted. The soft tissue may die, providing a nidus for infection. The general method of fixation of fractures involves placing an arch bar at the superior border, and the inferior border of the mandible is aligned and approximated by a direct wiring technique (Fig. 27–101) or plate and screw fixation (Fig. 27–102). Periosteal attachments should be retained where possible, but adequate exposure often demands a wide mobilization. Bone fragments survive if stabilization is sufficient and if they are covered by soft tissue with sufficient blood supply. The periosteum thus should not prevent proper fracture reduction and stabilization. It is more important to stabilize the fracture rigidly than to preserve periosteal attachments.

Some surgeons (Brown, Fryer, and McDowell, 1949) have preferred the use of Kirschner wires if fracture fragments are large enough for immobilization with this technique. Fragments are skewered in a "shish kabob" fashion, with the wire attached to the solid proximal segments.

If there has been extensive loss of soft tissues of the lip, chin, and floor of the mouth, along with bone, the posterior bone segments should be covered with skin and mucosa and properly splinted into position to prevent displacement by scar tissue contraction in the floor of the mouth. The use of an acrylic prosthetic mold to provide support to soft tissues can be a helpful addition to the intermaxillary fixation device applied (see Fig. 27–97). These extra appliances to stabilize soft tissue are individually designed to fit specific needs. It is important to preserve all bone fragments, as they can often be stabilized, especially with the use of a rigid fixation technique, such as plate and screw fixation. They should never be discarded despite the virtual absence of soft tissue attachment. The bone fragments, in these conditions, are bone grafts, but they often reestablish continuity of the bone without the addition of any bone from other areas.

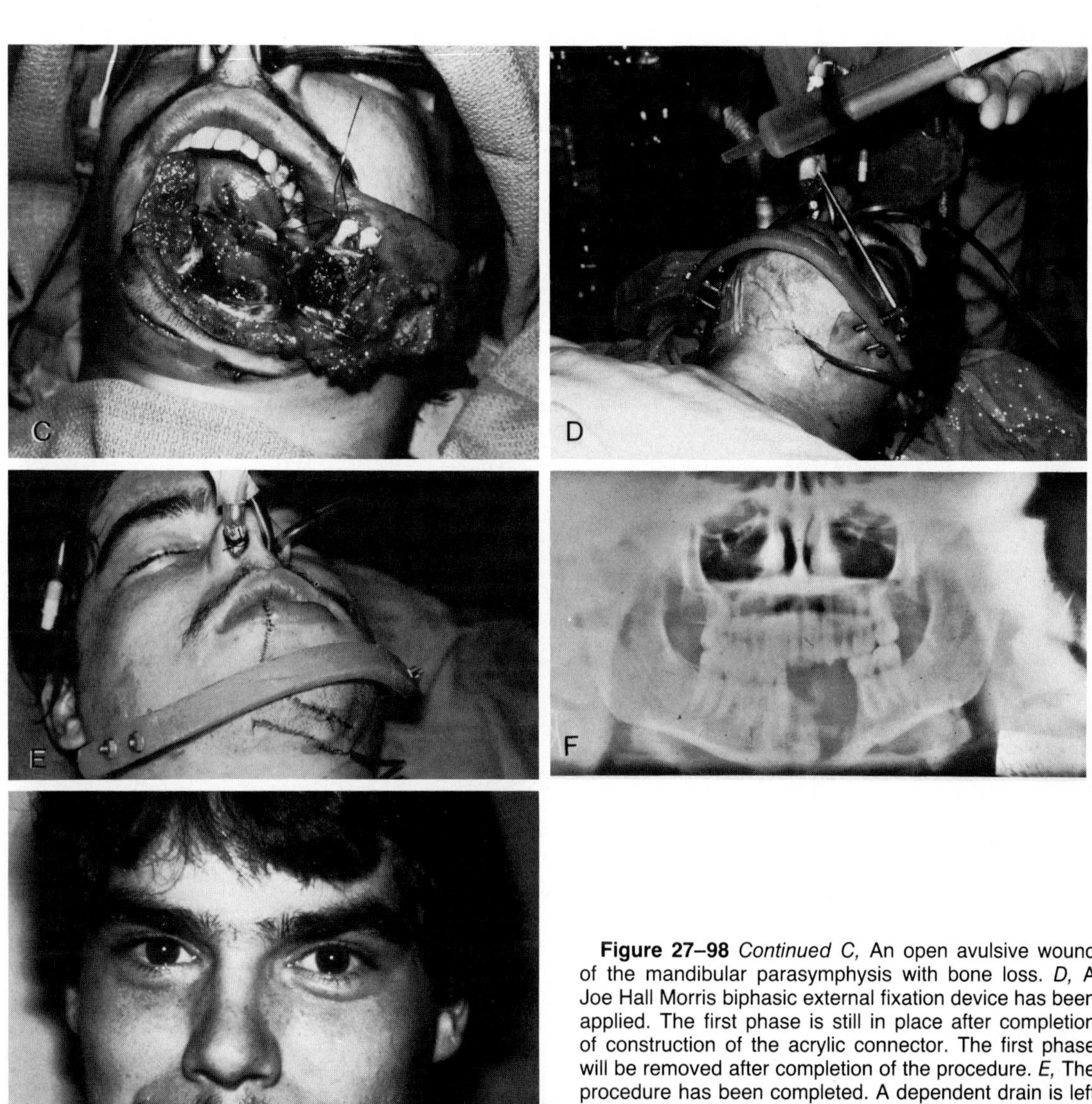

Figure 27–98 *Continued C,* An open avulsive wound of the mandibular parasymphysis with bone loss. *D,* A Joe Hall Morris biphasic external fixation device has been applied. The first phase is still in place after completion of construction of the acrylic connector. The first phase will be removed after completion of the procedure. *E,* The procedure has been completed. A dependent drain is left in the neck. The acrylic connector holds the lateral mandibular fragments in a stable relationship. Interfragment wiring was also used across the symphyseal area. *F,* Postreduction panoramic roentgenogram. Some bone may need to be added to the symphyseal area. *G,* Postoperative appearance.

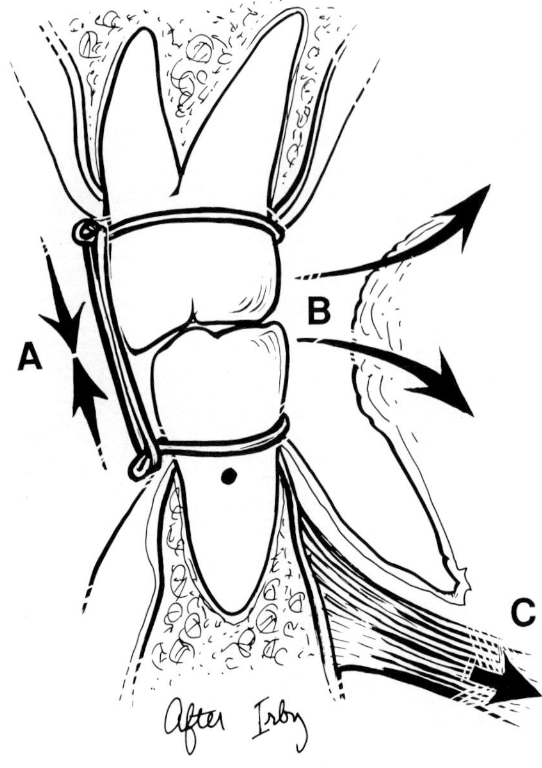

Figure 27–99. The force of intermaxillary elastic traction *(A)* is seen applied on one surface of the teeth. This creates a force that acts to tip the segments palatally or lingually *(B)*. Additionally, the mylohyoid muscle tends to tip the fragments lingually *(C)*. (From Irby, W.B.: Facial Trauma and Concomitant Problems. St. Louis, MO, C.V. Mosby Company, 1974, p. 35.)

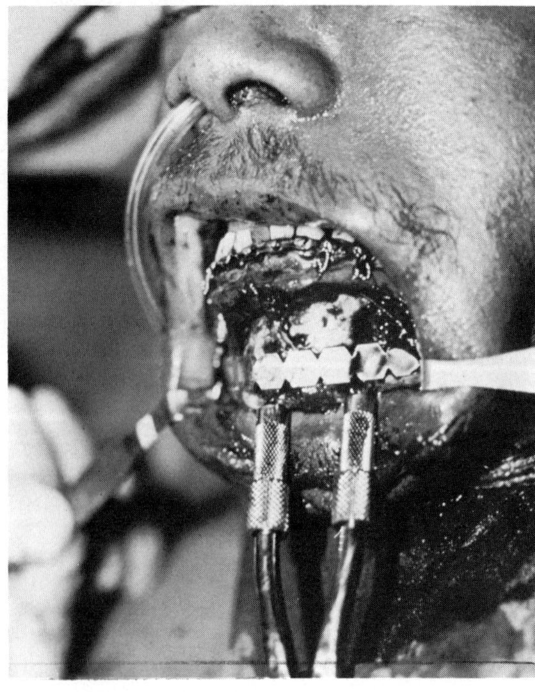

Figure 27–100. Open reduction of a mandibular parasymphyseal fracture is being performed through an intraoral degloving incision. A compression forceps (applied with screws to the inferior border) is holding the fragments together. A template is applied across the fracture, and a compression plate will be molded to the same curvature as the template and applied to the buccal cortex with bicortical screws.

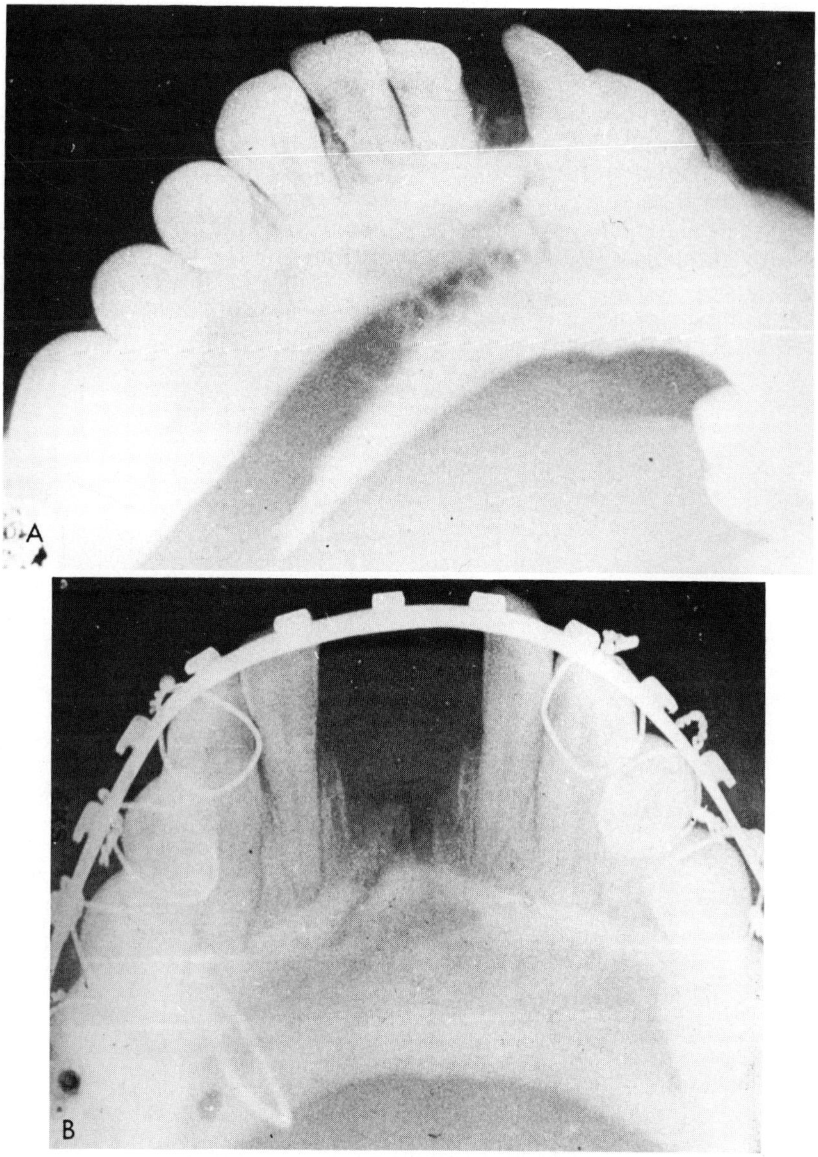

Figure 27–101. Oblique fracture through the symphyseal region. *A,* Displacement from the pull of the mylohyoid muscle. This type of fracture does not respond well to intermaxillary fixation alone, and interosseous wiring or plating is indicated. A complete exposure of the inferior border of the mandible is necessary to permit accurate alignment of this "lingual split" fragment. A "lag screw" is ideal. *B,* Symphyseal fracture fixation by interosseous wiring supplemented by arch bar intermaxillary fixation.

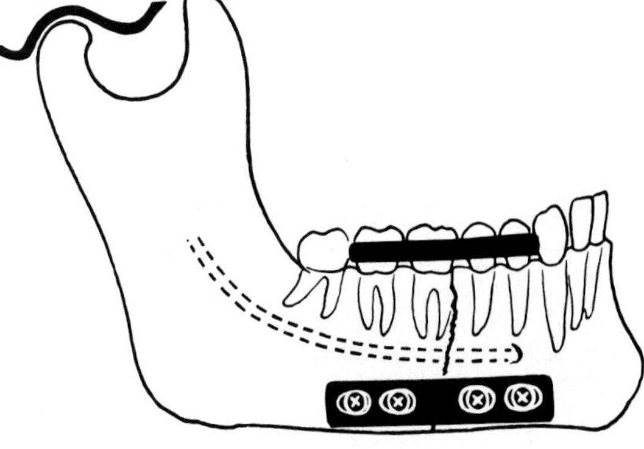

Figure 27–102. Mandibular body fracture. A tension band at the upper border of a body fracture and a dynamic compression plate at the inferior border. (From Spiessl, B.: New Concepts in Maxillofacial Bone Surgery. New York, Springer-Verlag, 1976.)

Treatment of Class II Fractures. In Class II fractures, teeth are present on only one side of the fracture site (Fig. 27–103). The fracture may occur in any portion of the body of the mandible. The problems of control of the edentulous fragment vary according to the direction and bevel of the fracture and the position of the teeth. The presence of comminution also influences the degree of displacement.

Open reduction and direct interosseous wiring is indicated rather than the use of appliances in most fractures with displacement where teeth are absent in the posterior segment. The patient is often more comfortable, oral hygiene is improved, and the anatomic results are superior.

Fractures Horizontally and Vertically Favorable. If a fracture occurs from above, downward and forward, the forces resist separation and the fracture is favorable from the standpoint of treatment (Fig. 27–104*A*). If the fracture is directed, as in Figure 27–104*A*, but is oblique along the frontal plane,

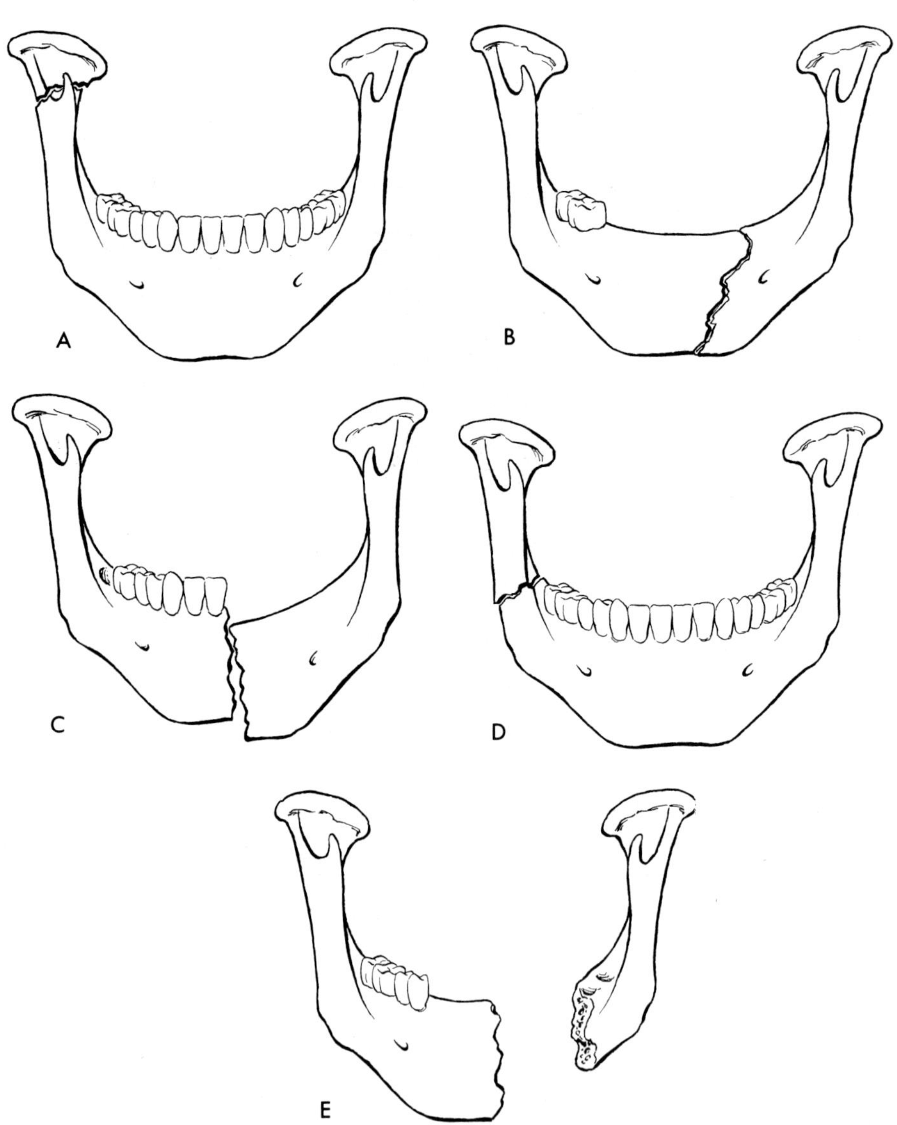

Figure 27–103. Class II fractures. Various types of fractures of the mandible with teeth on only one side of the fracture line. In *A* the fracture might be treated by intermaxillary fixation alone. In *B* and *C* the fracture would require open reduction with interosseous wire or plate and screw fixation. In *D* the fracture might be treated by intermaxillary fixation alone, depending on displacement of the fragment. In *E* the fracture would require open reduction. (From Kazanjian and Converse.)

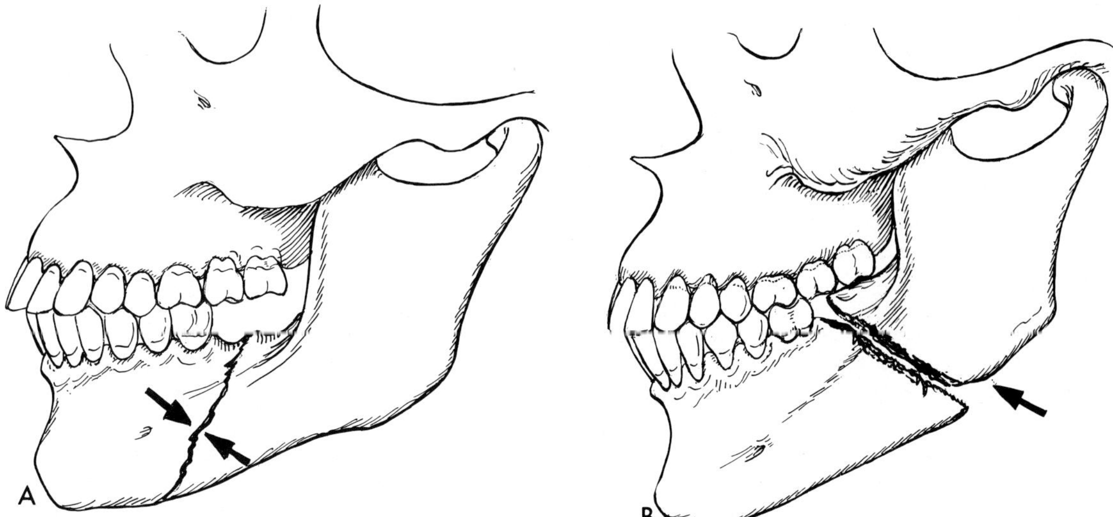

Figure 27–104. *A*, Favorable and unfavorable direction of the line of Class II fracture. In *A* the line of fracture is directed downward and forward, which is favorable. In *B* the line of fracture is directed downward and backward, which is unfavorable.

upward displacement of the posterior fragment will occur. When the line of fracture is directed downward and backward (Fig. 27–104*B*), the elevator (or posterior) muscles displace the posterior fragment upward and medially. In this situation, fixation of the teeth in intermaxillary occlusion alone does not suffice to give stability at the fracture site.

Fixation in favorable Class II fractures can be accomplished by arch bars and intermaxillary fixation or with another intermaxillary fixation technique such as a splint (see Fig. 27–97).

Fractures in which the angle is unfavorable do not resist displacement. The pull of the elevator muscle attached to the posterior segment displaces the proximal segment upward and laterally. Wiring of the remaining teeth does not control the edentulous posterior fragment. A number of methods can be used to control the posterior fragment; however, open reduction is usually preferred. Techniques that can be utilized other than open reduction include those described below.

USE OF A SPLINT IN EDENTULOUS POSTERIOR SEGMENT. A splint with an occlusal block (Fig. 27–105) placed between the maxillary

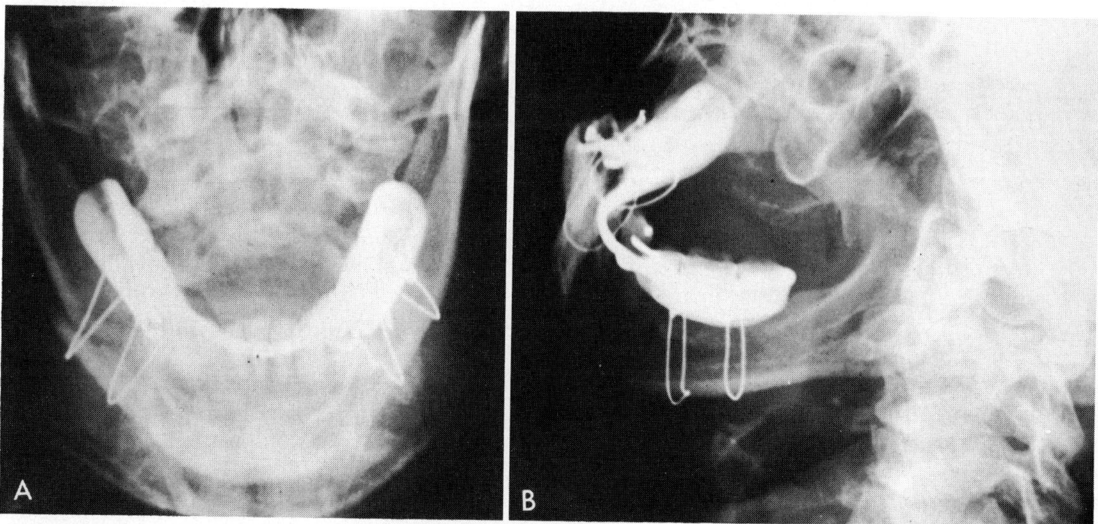

Figure 27–105. *A*, Stabilization of a mandibular fracture by use of the patient's partial denture and circumferential wires around the mandibular segments. *B*, Lateral view of the circumferential wires around the denture.

and mandibular teeth may immobilize the posterior segment. A sufficient alveolar ridge is required for purchase of the splint to control the position of the fragment. It is difficult to control rotation of this fragment and the technique is often unsuccessful. A splint, if utilized, may be fabricated into an upper or lower denture, or a lingual splint with occlusal stops. Such splints, placed in an attempt to control posterior segment position, often cause irritation to the gingival tissue, and if sufficient force is applied they may result in pressure necrosis of soft tissue and bone.

FORKED WIRE EXTENSION. A band with a bar appliance attached to the teeth, with a 14 gauge wire prong projecting posteriorly across the fracture line and pressing down against the bony ridge of the posterior fragment, may prevent upward displacement. This type of appliance also is usually ineffective. It provides questionable stability of the proximal fragment and may cause irritation of the soft tissues and the bone. The modern preferred technique is open reduction with direct interosseous wiring or plate and screw fixation (see Figs. 27–102, 27–106).

USE OF A SPLINT FOR DENTURES WITH CIRCUMFERENTIAL WIRING. If the patient is wearing a partial denture and the fracture is through a portion of the mandible in the saddle of the denture, it may be used to maintain fixation of the fractured segments. An adequate intraoral ridge of bone should be present and the technique is not applicable to the atrophic mandible. This is done by applying circumferential wires on each side of the fracture around the mandible. The denture can be incorporated in these wires with a drill hole or the wire can be simply passed around the occlusal surface of the bone. The circum-mandibular wires approximate the mandibular segments to the denture (see Fig. 27–105). Excess pressure causes soft tissue necrosis. The degree of fixation employed is not great and the technique demands that an adequate intraoral ridge of bone be present for the flange of the denture to have purchase on the mandibular segments. In general, open reduction results in improved anatomic alignment and greater patient comfort (see Figs. 27–102, 27–106).

Open Reduction and Interosseous Wiring. It is important that the bone ends at the fracture site be securely united, since movement of the bone edges predisposes to infection and delayed union. For open reduction, an incision is chosen and marked with brilliant green to correspond to a relaxed line of skin tension at least 1 to 2 cm below the inferior border of the mandible. The skin creases in the neck serve as guides to the location of the incisions. The incision should be only long enough to provide adequate exposure of the fracture site for the length of the plate to be used. Interfragment wire fixation utilizes a smaller incision than does the plate and screw fixation technique. The incision is extended through skin, subcutaneous tissue, and platysma. The position of the marginal mandibular branch of the facial nerve is recalled (Dingman and Grabb, 1962) with the dissection, protecting this nerve and exposing the inferior border of the mandible. A subperiosteal dissection technique is then employed, which protects nervous and vascular structures.

Careful subperiosteal dissection establishes the extent and pattern of the fracture, confirming the impression from previous radiographs. Alignment of the basal bone by visualization of the inferior border is critical. Fracture fragments can be conveniently grasped and reduced with a Dingman bone forcep. A 1.5 mm wire passing bit in a rotating drill is used to make holes drilled on each side of the fracture site. Generally, one or two wires or a figure-of-eight crisscross wire is used to provide an initial reduction (Figs. 27–106, 27–107). The occlusion should be checked before and after the wires are tightened. It is occasionally necessary to place a single wire at the upper level, avoiding the tooth structures. Care must be taken to recall the position of the inferior alveolar nerve and artery and the position of roots of adjacent teeth when placing wires above the inferior border of the mandible. The occlusion is again checked and the alignment of the fracture is checked, as well as the stability of the fixation. If all these criteria are satisfied, the twisted end of the wire is tucked along the inferior border of the mandible or twisted into one of the drill holes alongside the area of reduction. The musculature, if possible, is reunited by sutures at the inferior border of the mandible placed through the fascia. Care must be taken to avoid the marginal mandibular branch of the facial nerve. The platysma is closed and the drain, if utilized, is brought out either through a small counterincision or through a dependent portion of the wound. The wound is closed in layers.

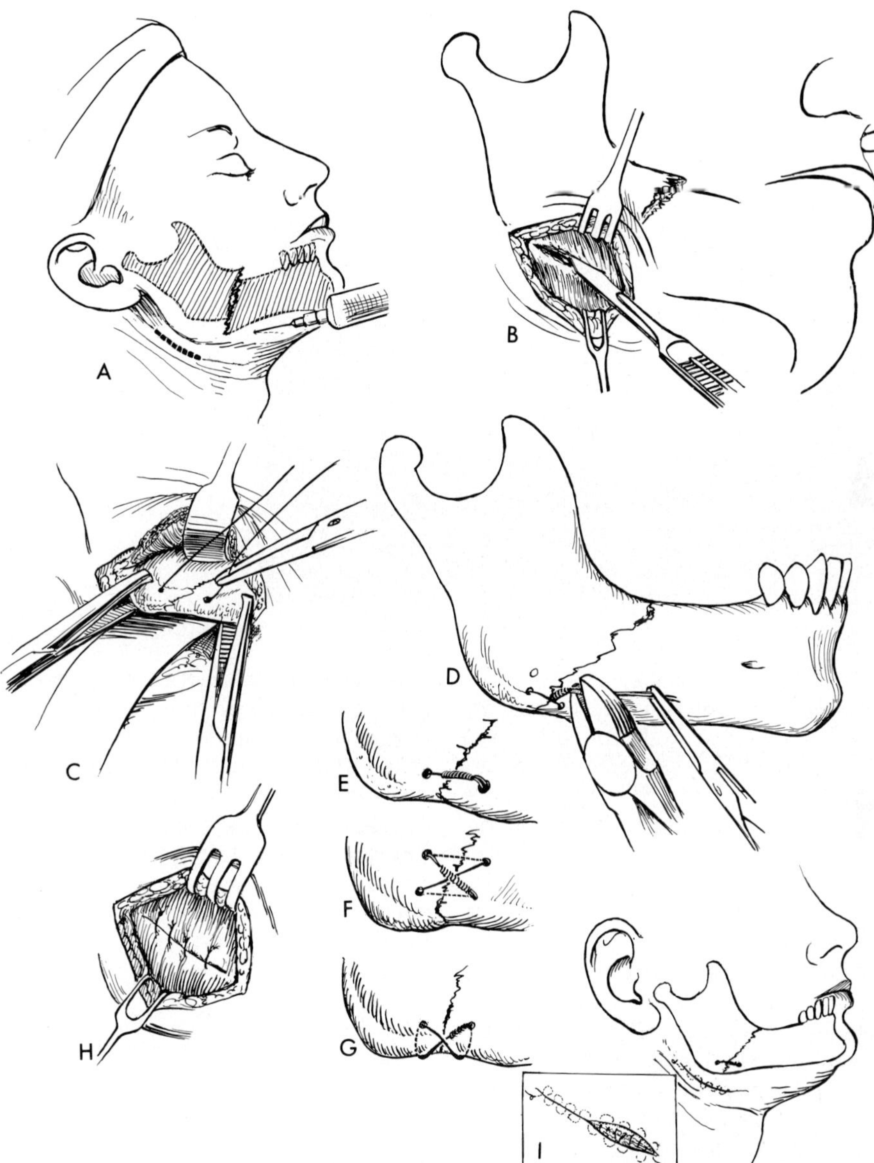

Figure 27–106. Open reduction and interosseous wiring for fracture of the angle of the mandible. *A*, The incision is made 1 cm or more below the border of the mandible. *B*, The attachments of the masseter muscle are divided and elevated. *C*, Small drill holes are passed through the bone, one on each side of the fracture site. The drill holes should be as perpendicular to the fracture plane as possible. *D*, No. 24 stainless steel wires are used for fixation. *E*, The cut end of the wire is tucked into the drill hole on one side. *F, G*, A "crosswire" (figure-of-eight type) may be used since there is a tendency for dislocation of fragments if only a single wire is used. Alternatively, two separate wires should be placed to prevent or limit the dislocation. *H*, The wound is closed in layers. A dependent or suction drain is often used. *I*, A continuous subcuticular suture is an excellent means of skin approximation.

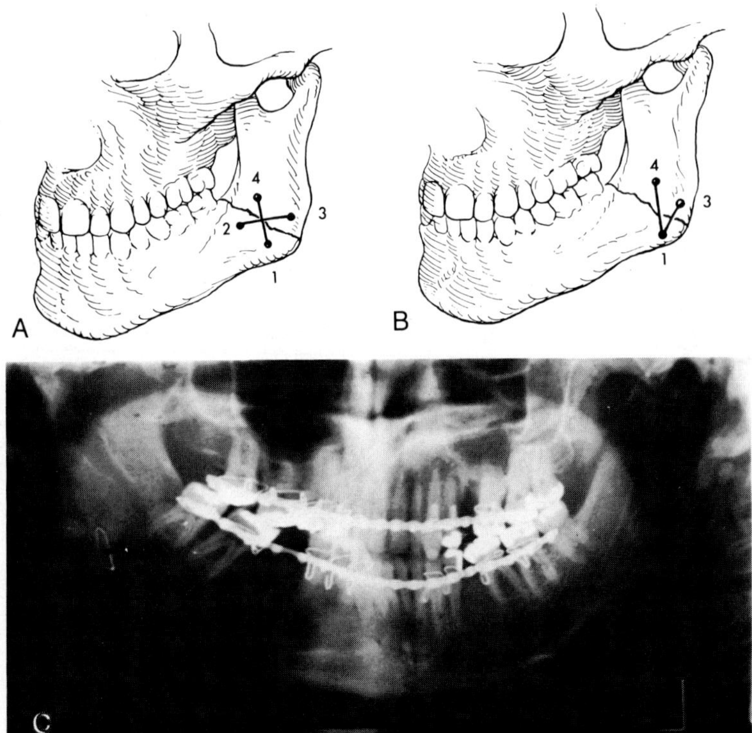

Figure 27–107. The use of a figure-of-eight or crossed wiring technique to increase the stability in lower border mandibular fracture with open reduction. Since this is difficult to determine, a crossed wiring technique *(A)* or multiple wires *(B)* are often utilized. (From Kruger, G. O.: Oral and Maxillofacial Surgery. 6th Ed. St. Louis, C. V. Mosby Company, 1984, p. 398.) *C*, Treatment of a mandibular angle fracture with open reduction and interfragment wiring accompanied by intermaxillary fixation. A single wire has been used at the lower border. Usually two wires are preferred.

INTRAORAL APPROACH TO OPEN REDUCTION. Either interosseous wiring or plate and screw fixation may be done through the intraoral route (Paul and Acevedo, 1968; Chuong and Donoff, 1985) in appropriate patients. This is often the preferred exposure of the symphyis/parasymphysis and can also be utilized for fractures about the angle of the mandible. Fractures of the body region are more difficult to expose with this technique, and more devascularization of the bone fragment occurs from stripping of the soft tissues. When the fracture lines run in horizontally unfavorable directions, interosseous wiring at the alveolar ridge (the upper border of the mandible) uses the muscular forces to best advantage. The wire or plate fixation provides a fulcrum at the crest of the ridge, and the muscle pull is most effectively opposed through the longest "lever arm" (Fig. 27–108).

For the use of the intraoral approach, the fracture site is exposed through an appropriately placed incision (Fig. 27–109). In the edentulous mandible with reduced bone height, the inferior alveolar nerve and artery may be located in soft tissue external to the remaining bone. An incision off the crest to the buccal side provides protection of these structures. The fracture site is exposed with subperiosteal dissection. The wire is passed through the drill holes and twisted tightly, impacting the edges of the bone as the wire is twisted (Fig. 27–109*C*). With practice, the intraoral approach is much more rapid than the extraoral approach for open reduction. The most important patient benefit is that it avoids a scar. With the intraoral approach, one must exercise care to design the incision to provide optimal vascular supply to the

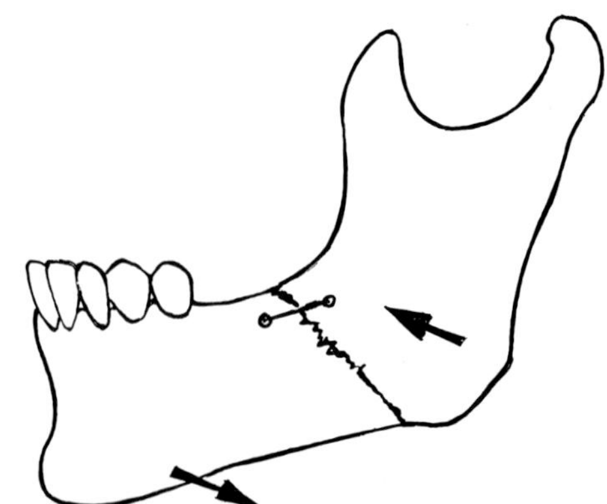

Figure 27–108. Fixation of a fracture with a wire near the upper border of the bone placed through an intraoral approach. Symphyseal and angle fractures are particularly amenable to intraoral exposure.

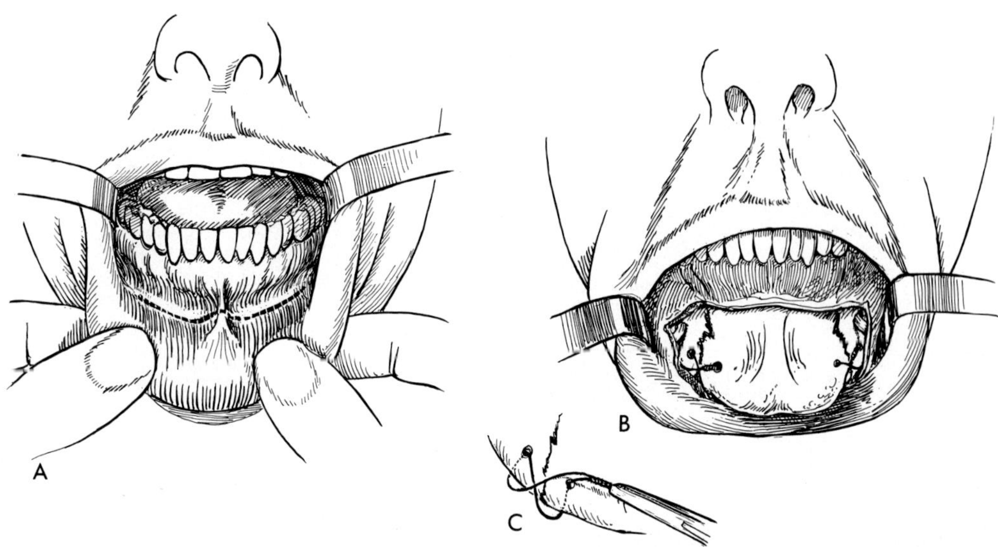

Figure 27–109. *A*, Location of the incision for the symphysis and parasymphysis "degloving" technique. *B*, Subperiosteal exposure is obtained, and wire fixation after reduction provides accurate alignment of the fragments. *C*, Figure-of-eight wire fixation.

mucosal flaps. The mucosal incision, if anterior, should be kept slightly out of the inferiormost extent of the buccal sulcus "gutter" to keep the suture line free from the pool of secretions that occurs anteriorly. After healing of the incision, some contracture of the vestibule is also noticed. If possible, a two-layer closure involving muscle and mucosa is most effective. Generally, nonabsorbable sutures, such as nylon, are preferred for intraoral closure over areas of open reduction. The use of absorbable sutures, like chromic catgut, predisposes to early wound breakdown at the time when the wound has not healed sufficiently to prevent this.

In intraoral open reductions, the basal bone of the mandible is not observed as precisely as with extraoral open reductions. There will be lingual gaps or rotation of the mandibular segments if care is not used in the reduction (Fig. 27–110). If skin lacerations are present, they may be utilized for the reduction. An extraoral approach (Fig. 27–111) may also be preferred.

EXTERNAL FIXATION. Previous methods of managing fractures with bone loss were cumbersome. These injuries are now easily managed with external fixation. In some fractures with an edentulous posterior segment, pins with an external connector (Morris, 1949) may be used to provide proper reduction (Fig. 27–112). This technique is especially helpful in fractures with comminution and those with

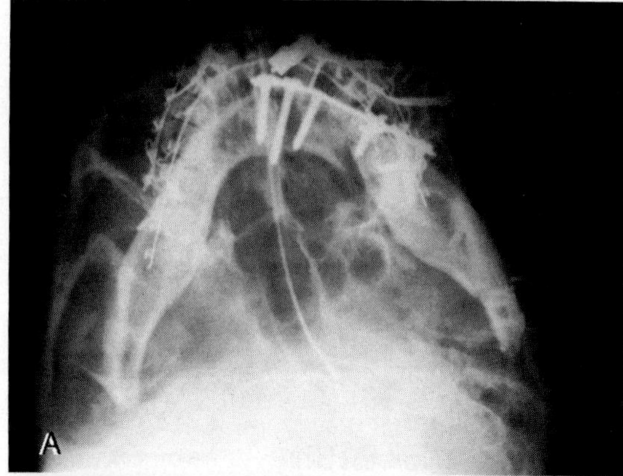

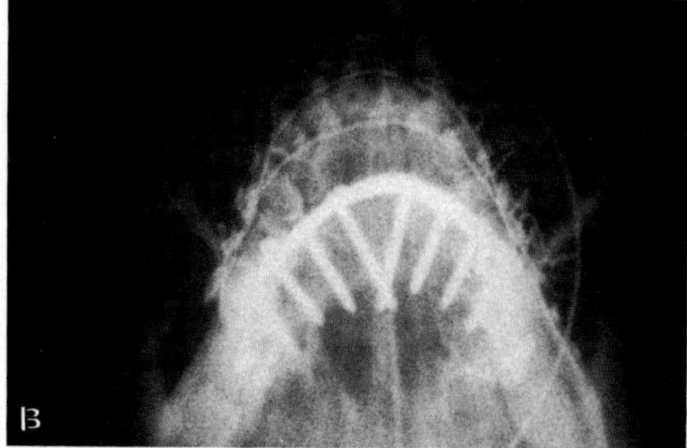

Figure 27–110. *A*, Malalignment of a distal body fracture is seen from the submental vertex view. This view is helpful in assessing alignment of the lingual cortex. Malalignment is prone to occur in intraoral open reductions in which full visualization of the basal bone of the mandible is not achieved. *B*, Another fracture demonstrating correct alignment. Note the combination of plate, interosseous wiring, and intermaxillary fixation.

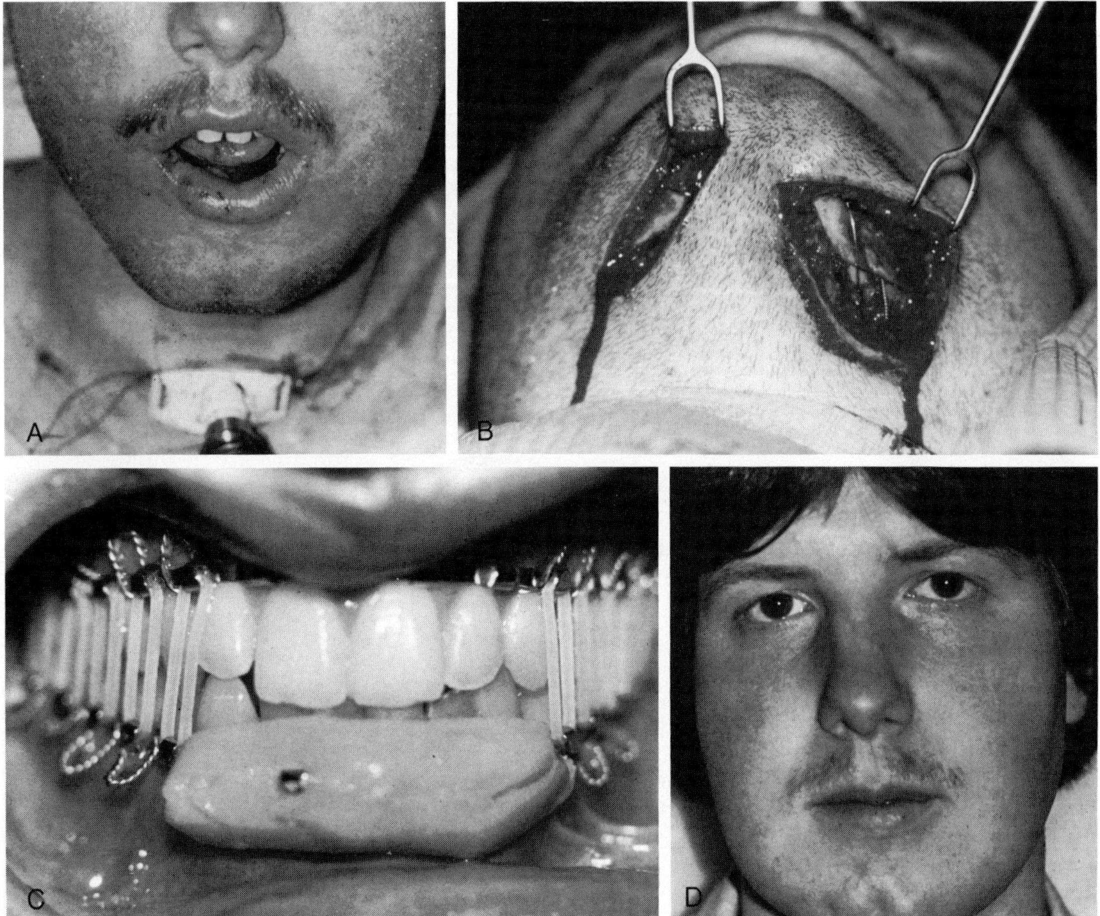

Figure 27–111. *A*, Bilateral body fracture in a young male. *B*, Open reduction with figure-of-eight and multiple wires through extraoral incisions. *C*, Intermaxillary fixation with an acrylic arch bar to support an alveolar fracture of the mandibular incisor teeth. The occlusion was maintained and the esthetic result is acceptable *(D)*.

reduced bone height that demonstrate substantial atrophy of the alveolar ridge. The external device may be maintained until the consolidation of the fracture segments has taken place.

KIRSCHNER WIRE FIXATION. Brown, Fryer, and McDowell (1949) described the use of intramedullary Kirschner wires (K-wires) to immobilize fractures. They favored this technique in the mandible for the immobilization of Class II and Class III fractures. Manual reduction of the fracture is obtained; the bones are held securely in position by an assistant or the operator; and a K-wire is directed through a small skin incision and driven through the bone with an electric drill. The wire should be driven across the fracture site and through the cortex of the opposite fragment. The wire ends are cut at the skin level and left in place for six to eight weeks, or the same period for which intermaxillary fixation would be applied. Supplementary intermaxillary fixation may be necessary in some cases, depending on the stability. One should realize that alignment is probably achieved by this technique, but impaction and fixation are not. Nerve and tooth root damage are possible complications of this technique.

METAL PLATES AND SCREWS FOR FIXATION. Plate and screw fixation results in an anatomic reduction with absolute immobility. Thus, it is "unforgiving" in that the occlusion cannot be changed by rubber band therapy.

The indications for plate and screw fixation of mandibular fractures by open reduction are:

1. Complex fractures with comminution. (In these injuries, the teeth and lower border wiring alone do not provide sufficient points of fixation.)

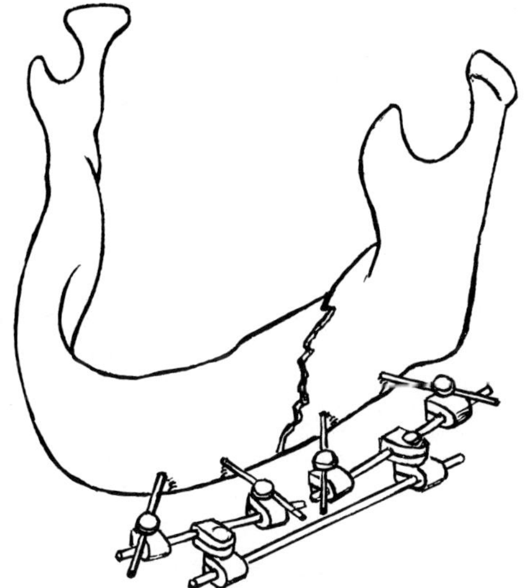

Figure 27–112. External pin fixation (Roger-Anderson) for stabilization of a mandibular fracture. (From Kazanjian and Converse.)

2. Fractures with extreme displacement, which are subject to rotation (comminuted parasymphyseal fracture with bilateral subcondyle fracture).

3. Fractures in the edentulous jaw exhibiting displacement.

4. The desire to avoid intermaxillary fixation in the postoperative period.

The principles of rigid intermaxillary fixation have been described by the Association for the Study of Internal Fixation (A.S.I.F.) (Spiessl, 1976; Souyris, Lamarche, and Mirfakhrai, 1980; Kruger and Schilli, 1982; Tu and Tenhulzen, 1985). The objectives of the procedure are the reduction and fixation of the fractured segments. In some cases, the objective can also be the achievement of sufficient rigidity to obtain active and pain-free mobilization of the mandible without jeopardizing the healing process. The latter aim is achieved by:

1. Accurate anatomic reduction of the fracture with the patient in proper occlusion. The emphasis is thus on *occlusal* and *basal* repositioning (upper border and lower border alignment).

2. The absolute stabilization of bone fragments.

3. A surgical technique that emphasizes protection of soft tissue and minimizes esthetic deformity.

OCCLUSAL REPOSITIONING. Rigid internal fixation requires a mastery of nonsurgical fracture treatment involving manual repositioning of the fractured fragments and the restoration of proper occlusal relationships by intermaxillary fixation. Arch bars or intermaxillary ligatures (Ernst ligatures) are applied to the maxillary and mandibular dentition. Acrylic can be used to make the intermaxillary fixation more rigid. In most cases, arch bars and intermaxillary fixation are recommended.

BASAL REPOSITIONING. With the patient in intermaxillary fixation, an extra- or intraoral exposure of the mandibular fracture site is performed and a basal reduction employed. A compression of the fracture may be achieved by the use of compression forceps, which are anchored to the basal mandibular bone with the insertion of screws (see Fig. 27–100). The fracture is held in absolute rigid approximation. A template is contoured to the surface of the mandible (see Fig. 27–100) and the plate to be used is bent to the exact contour of the template. It is then placed on the lower external surface of the mandible and the contour checked. Care is taken to position the plates so that damage to the apices of teeth and the inferior alveolar canal structures is avoided (Fig. 27–113). The plate is anchored to the mandible by the placement of bicortical screws (Figs. 27–114, 27–115). Drill holes of the minor diameter of the screw are placed through both cortices of the mandible, utilizing soft tissue protection. A tap threads the bone, and a screw with a major diameter larger than the minor diameter is selected of a length based on a pretap measure of the depth of the mandible in that location with the depth gauge. The screw is tightened into position. A compression mode can be utilized by drilling the hole at the outer margin of the drill holes in the plate (Fig. 27–115).

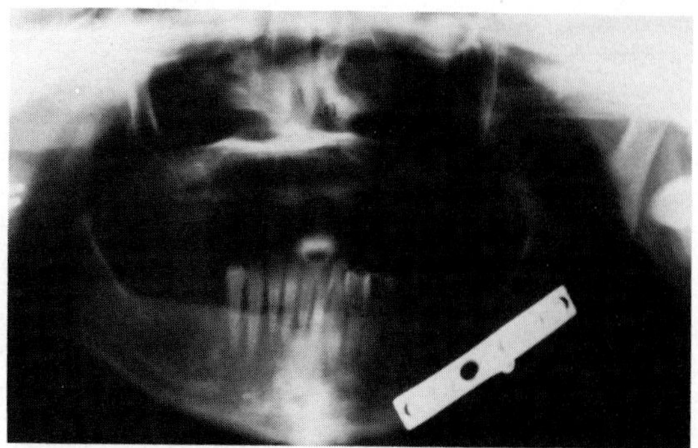

Figure 27–113. Treatment of a left mandibular angle fracture in an edentulous segment with a compression plate.

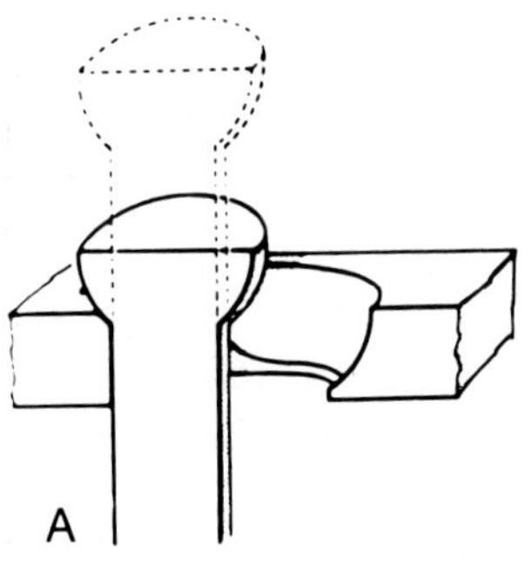

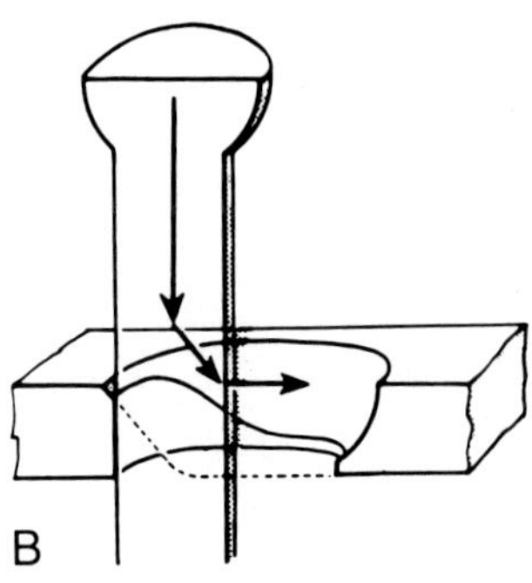

Figure 27–114. The spherical gliding principle with the dynamic compression plate (after Allgöwer and associates, 1970). *A*, A spherically shaped screw head is caused to move down an inclined plane (hole) in a dynamic compression plate. When the spherical screw head is turned, it glides in the section of the inclined plane. The bone fragment grasped by the screws is thus moved horizontally (spherical gliding principle) toward the fracture gap. By the horizontal movement, a locking action between the screw and the plate is avoided. The bone is compressed across the fracture site by this application of force. *B*, The path taken by the screw in the vertical and horizontal direction as it is tightened (Spiessl and Schroll, 1972). (From Spiessl, B.: New Concepts in Maxillofacial Bone Surgery. New York, Springer-Verlag, 1976.)

Drilling the drill hole at the inner margin provides a "neutral phase," whereas drilling at the outer margin allows the screw to slip down an inclined plane toward the fracture site as tightening occurs. In this case, the screw and bone move toward the fracture site, achieving compression at the fracture site, as the screw is tightened. This motion occurs because of the inclined plane in the screw holes of the plate (see Fig. 27–114). This is the so-called "spherical gliding principle" as indicated in Figure 27–114. As the screw is tightened, the screw bone unit moves in a horizontal direction with the vertical tightening of the screw. It is important that two screws be used per main fracture fragment.

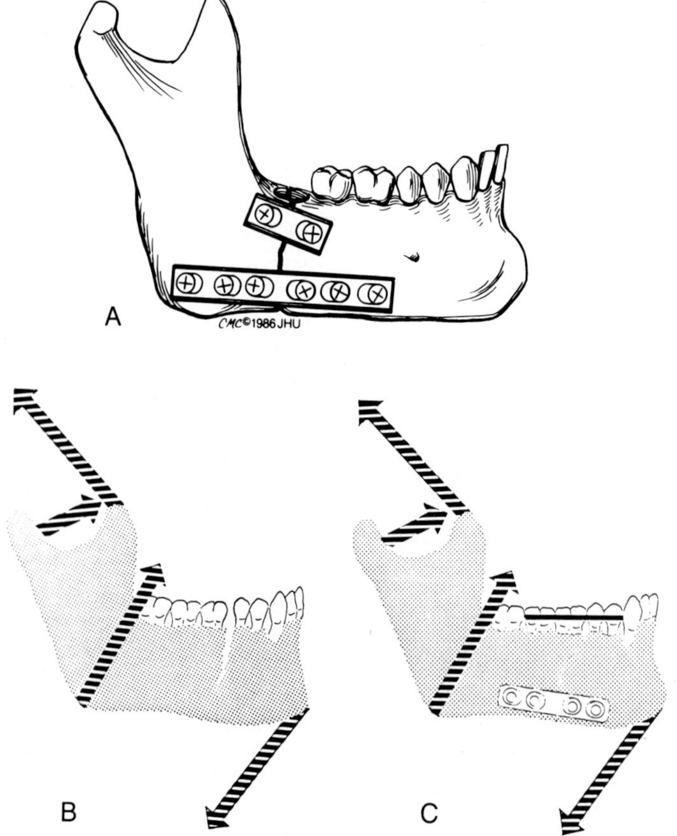

Figure 27–115. *A*, A body fracture treated by the application of a dynamic compression plate at the inferior border and a dynamic compression plate at the upper border, which acts as a tension band in the edentulous region. *B, C*, Muscular forces on a body fracture, and the action of a tension band and dynamic compression plate. In *B* the muscular forces are indicated by arrows and they tend to open the fracture at the superior border. In *C* the fracture is closed and securely reduced by the tension band at the upper border (arch bar) and the action of a dynamic compression plate at the inferior border. (From Spiessl, B.: New Concepts in Maxillofacial Bone Surgery. New York, Springer-Verlag, 1976.)

In practice, because of the frequent incidence of comminution along the lingual surface of the mandible, it is preferable to use three screws per fragment. For rigid internal fixation, it is necessary to have two tight screws in each major bone fragment; if one of the screws became loose, the rigidity of the fixation would be lost.

Incorrect internal fixation can result from poor plate adaptation (Fig. 27–116). This causes malalignment at the site of the fracture. In practice, the plate should be slightly "overbent" over the fracture (1 to 2 mm) to prevent gapping along the lingual cortex of the mandible. This achieves an even compression throughout the width of the fracture site. For the horizontal portion of the mandible, the principle is that a tension band must be placed along the upper mandibular border; this can either be a small tension band plate or an arch bar (see Fig. 27–115). Thus, both the superior and inferior surfaces of the mandible are kept in approximation. The forces are thus balanced and the following formula is applied:

Fractures within the dental arch:
Tension band plate or arch bar
plus
stabilization plate (dynamic compression plate).

Fractures beyond the dental arch:
Compression-tension band plate (dynamic compression plate)
plus
stabilization plate (dynamic compression plate)
(see Fig. 27–115*C*)
or eccentric dynamic compression plate.

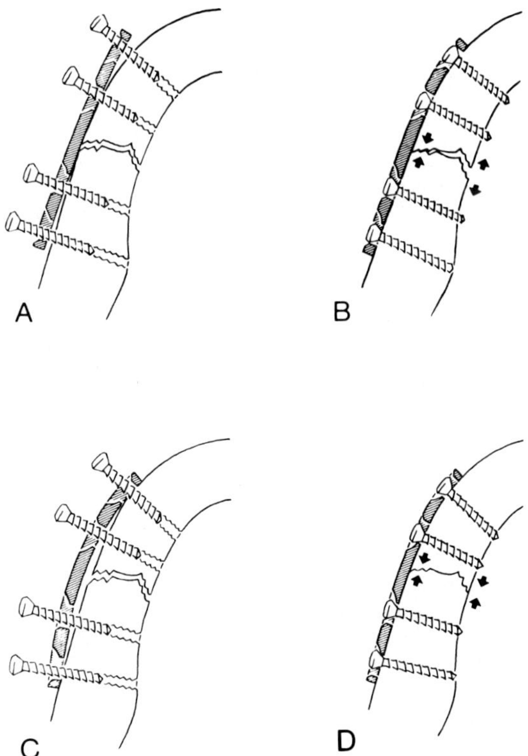

Figure 27–116. Incorrect internal fixation due to the use of a poorly adapted dynamic compression plate in the form of an insufficiently bent plate *(A)*. *B*, After tightening of the screws, there is complete adaptation of the plate against the surface of the bone. The result is distraction of the fragments on the lingual cortex. Compression is acting on only part of the fractured area. *C*, Correct application of the dynamic compression plate, taking the curve shape of the jaw into consideration. The plate is slightly overbent (1 mm). *D*, After tightening of the screws, the overbent plate produces compression over the whole fracture area. (From Spiessl, B.: New Concepts in Maxillofacial Bone Surgery. New York, Springer-Verlag, 1976.)

ECCENTRIC DYNAMIC COMPRESSION PLATE. In the case of the edentulous jaw or of a fracture in the dentulous portion of the jaw where it is desirable not to use an upper border tension band plate, an eccentric dynamic compression plate can be used (Fig. 27–117). In this plate, the lateral holes are beveled in such a way that compression at the superior border of the mandible results from tightening of the screws along the inferior border, and that the bevel tends to close the gap at the alveolar margin. Examples of the use of the eccentric plate are seen in Figure 27–118.

USE OF A LAG SCREW (Nicholson and Guzak, 1971; Niederdellmann and associates, 1976; Niederdellmann and Akuamoa-Boateng, 1981). In some cases of oblique fracture of the mandible, it may be desirable to use a "lag" screw for fixation. A lag screw is not a special screw; the term merely refers to the use of the screw to achieve compression by using the gliding hole in the outer cortex. This screw engages only the distal cortex (Fig. 27–119). A hole is drilled in the desired direction, utilizing the minor (shank) diameter of the screw. A hole through the proximal cortex is then drilled equal to the major (flange) diameter of the screw. The threads of the screw thus engage only the distal cortex of the mandible, drawing it toward the proximal cortex. Considerable compression is achieved with this technique, and in some cases of mandibular fracture lag screws *only* may suffice for complete fixation. This is an excellent technique with great applicability in facial bone surgery (Fig. 27–120).

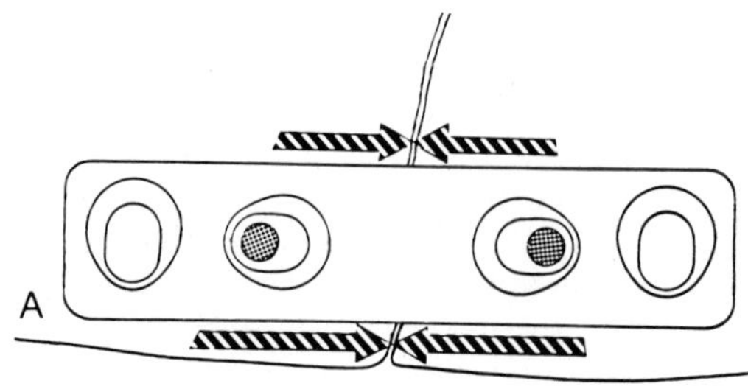

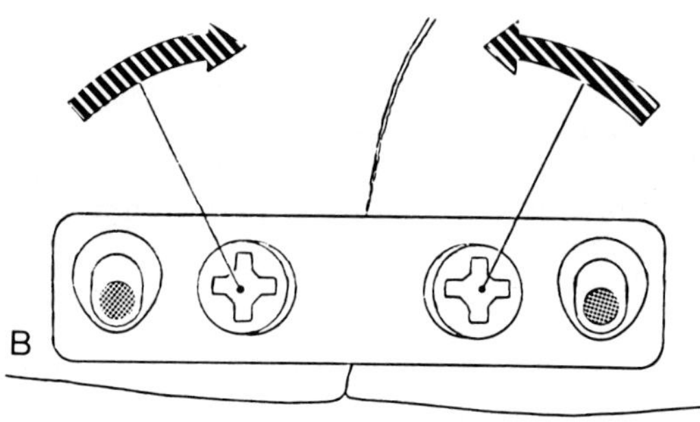

Figure 27–117. Eccentric dynamic compression plate: the inner holes are transverse and the outer holes are vertical or oblique. *A*, When the screws are driven next to the fracture in the inner holes, a compression arises at the lower margin of the jaw. *B*, When the screws are driven toward the margin of the lower jaw in the outer holes, a rotation of the fragments about the inner screw occurs, as the axis of rotation results in a compression in the alveolar process. (From Spiessl, B.: New Concepts in Maxillofacial Bone Surgery. New York, Springer-Verlag, 1976.)

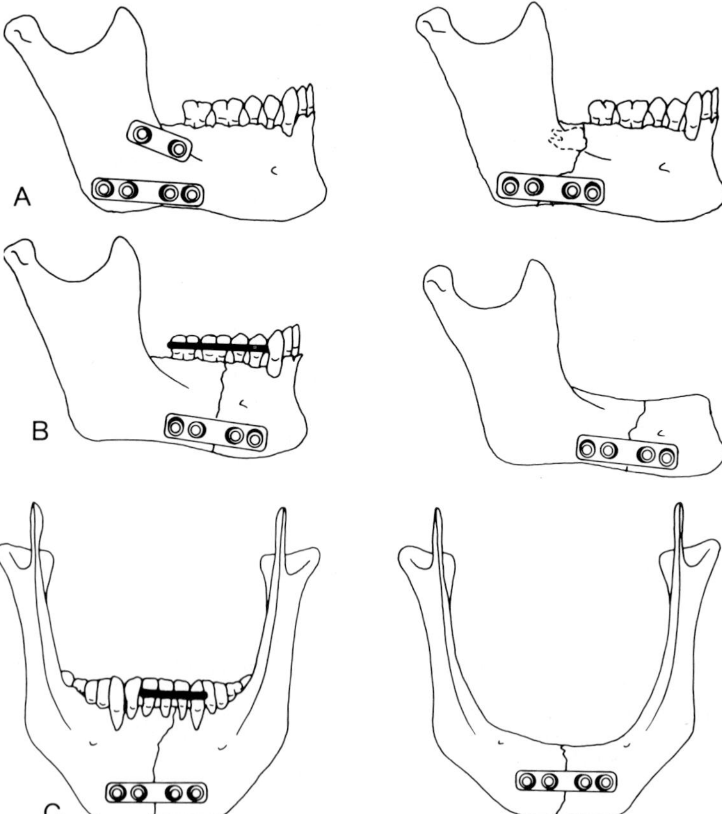

Figure 27–118. Indications for different plate fixation techniques. *A*, At the angle of the mandible: compression tension band plate and stabilization plate. If there is lack of space, an eccentric dynamic compression plate should be utilized. B, In the area of the lateral teeth: eccentric dynamic compression plate with an arch bar functioning as a tension band for a dentulous jaw. It can be used without an arch bar for the edentulous jaw. *C*, In the area of the front teeth: dynamic compression plate with an arch bar functioning as a tension band for the dentulous jaw. It can be used without an arch bar for the edentulous jaw. (From Spiessl, B.: New Concepts in Maxillofacial Bone Surgery. New York, Springer-Verlag, 1976.)

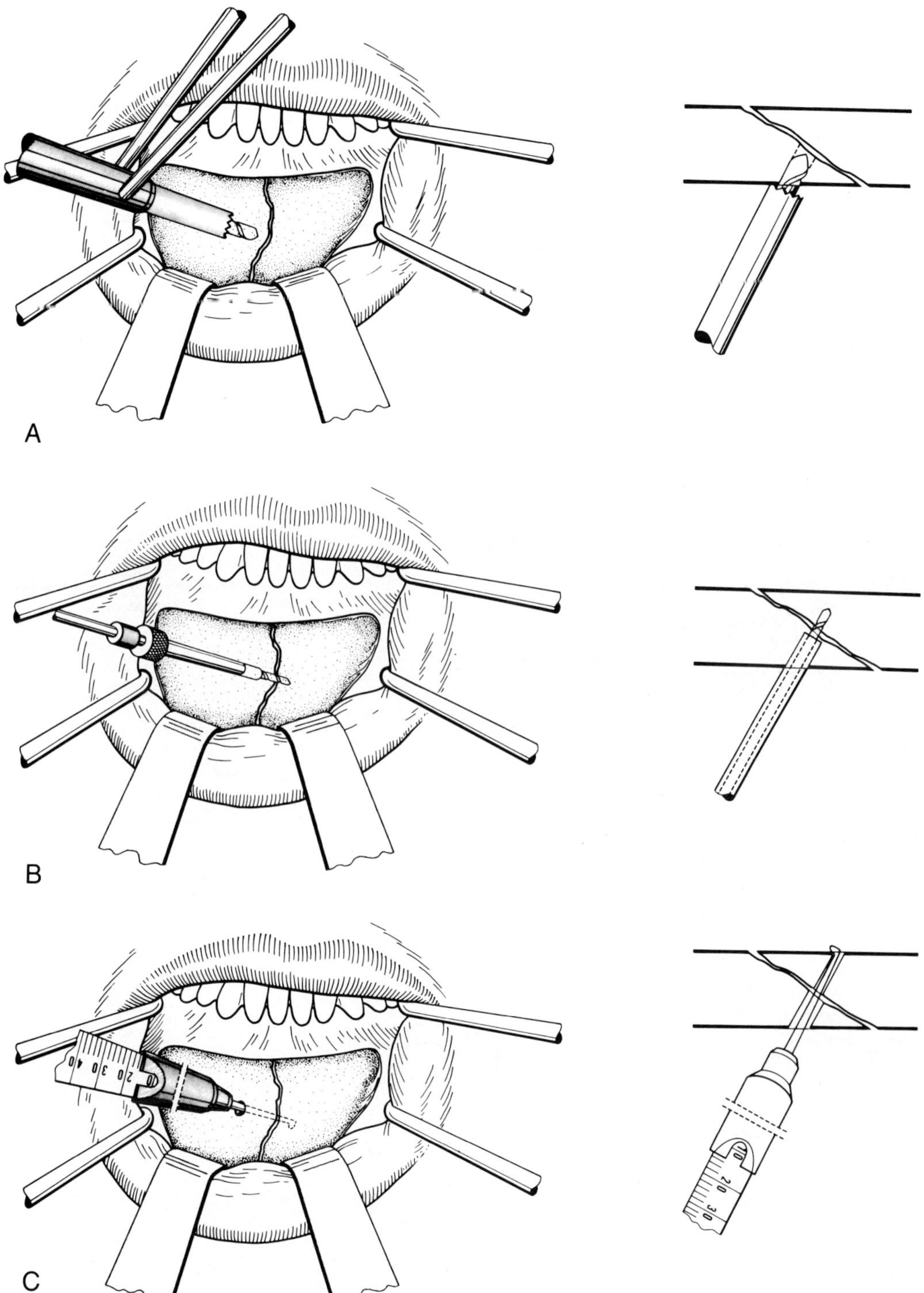

Figure 27–119. The lag screw concept involves drilling a "gliding hole" in the outer cortex. The screw does not engage the outer cortex but engages the inner cortex, pulling the inner cortex to the outer cortex. *A*, A gliding hole is drilled in the outer fragment. The gliding hole is the same size as the flange of the screw. *B*, A guide is placed hrough the gliding hole and a smaller drill bit, the size of the core diameter of the screw to be utilized, drills a hole in the inner cortex. *C*, The screw length is determined by a depth gauge.

Illustration continued on following page

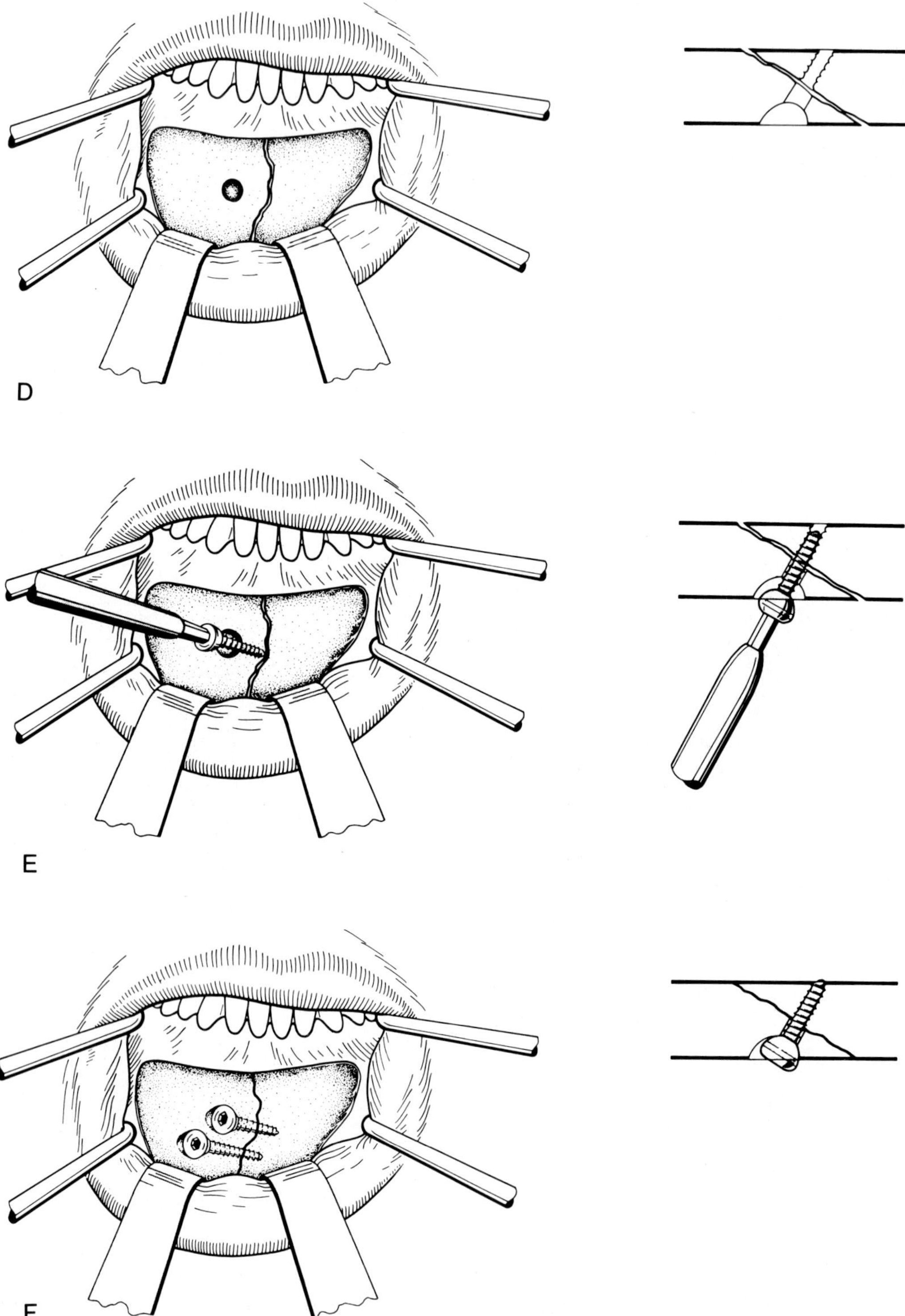

Figure 27–119 *Continued D*, The prepared gliding hole and thread hole and bed for the screw head are seen. The bed has been shaved with a counter sink. Care should be taken not to drill this too deeply or the entire thickness of the cortical bone of the outer surface of the mandible will be penetrated. *E*, Placement of the first lag screw. *F*, Final fixation of the fracture by the lag screws demonstrated. They engage the inner cortex and pull it to compress against the outer cortex. This technique either may be used alone or may also be used with a plate angling one of the screws as a lag screw. (From Niederdellmann, H.: Rigid internal fixation by means of lag screws. *In* Kruger, E., and Schilli, W. (Eds.): Oral and Maxillofacial Traumatology. Vol. 1. Chicago, Quintessence Publishers, 1982, p. 376.)

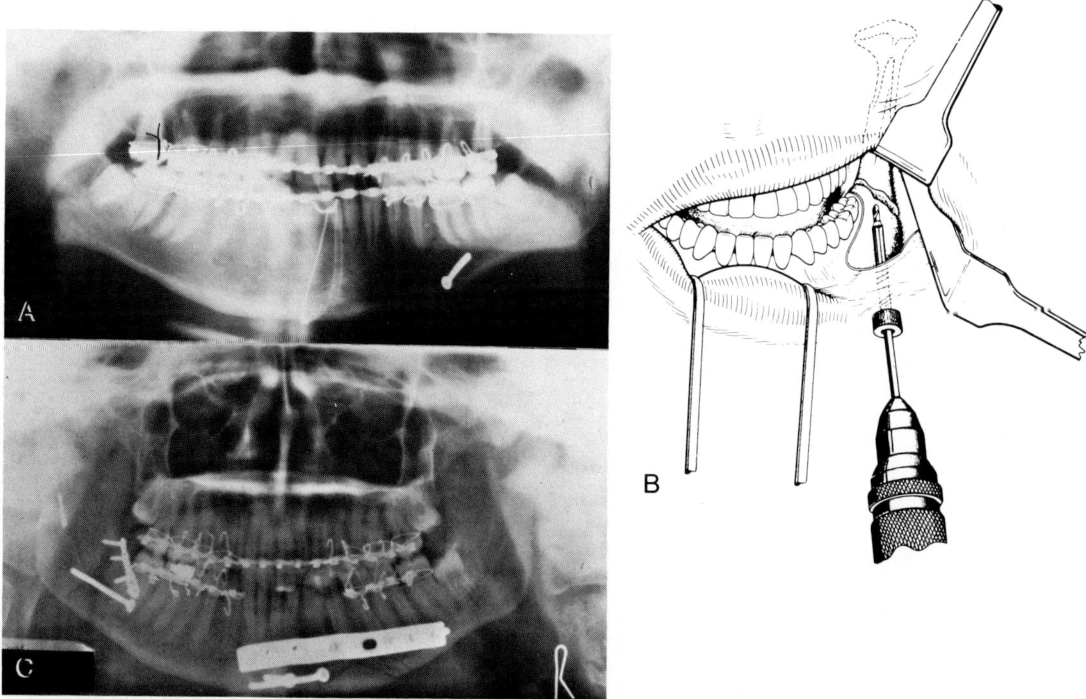

Figure 27–120. Use of lag screws. *A*, Treatment of a sagittally oriented fracture of the left mandibular body with a lag screw. *B*, The combined intraoral and transbuccal approach for placing a lag screw at the mandibular angle. (From Niederdellmann, H., and Shetty, V.: Solitary lag screw osteosynthesis in the treatment of fractures of the angle of the mandible: a retrospective study. Plast. Reconstr. Surg., *80*:68, 1987.) *C*, A lag screw utilized for fixation of a mandibular angle fracture. Lag screws have also been used to reduce a component of symphysis and body fractures. Note also the plate and intermaxillary fixation.

COMPLICATIONS OF RIGID INTERNAL FIXATION. In most series, rigid internal fixation results in a lower incidence of non-union and in more accurate and secure bone union. In some cases, plate exposure has occurred, especially when this approach is used in the intraoral reduction of mandibular body fractures. The original European literature always recommended an extraoral approach that requires a cutaneous incision. In one study (Prein, Eschmann, and Spiessl, 1976), scars after open reduction were very good in one-third of cases, satisfactory in one-half of cases, and poor or disturbing in the remainder. Thus, the author's preference has been for the use of intraoral approaches (Fig. 27–121).

LUHR SELF-TAPPING SYSTEM. In order to avoid the use of cumbersome clamps and tapping, simpler systems have been devised which utilize a self-tapping screw. In these cases a hole is drilled equal to the minor diameter of the screw, and the screw has cutting threads that obviate the necessity to tap the hole (Figs. 27–121, 27–122). Obviously, a self-tapping screw cannot be removed and reinserted without cutting a new group of threads that may render the screw unstable. For the Luhr system, the plates are smaller than those used in the AO-ASIF system and can be adapted quite favorably for intraoral approaches throughout the horizontal portion of the mandible. The use of smaller miniplates such as the Champy (Champy and associates, 1978) for mandibular fractures speeds exposure and fixation, but may not result in sufficient rigidity for mobilization without movement at the fracture site. This factor must be assessed carefully according to the experience of the surgeon and according to his technical skill and choice of plate. For the Luhr system, there is a midface and a mandibular system similar to the midface and mandibular systems existing within the AO system. In the Luhr system, the plate material is made of Vitallium, which is a cobalt-chromium-mollybdenum alloy. Stainless steel is subject to corrosion when in contact with electrolytes containing hydrogen and oxygen. This kind

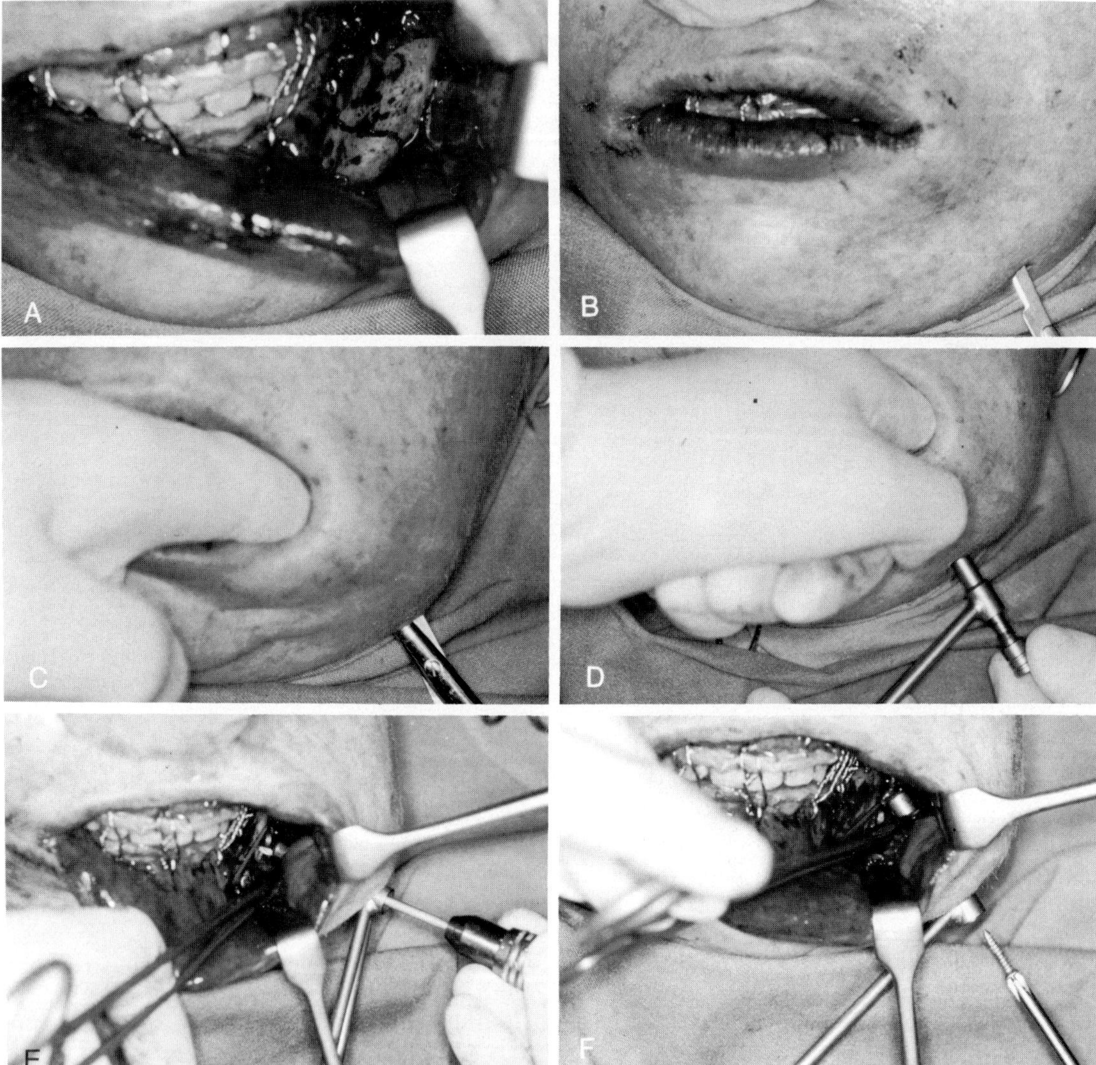

Figure 27–121. *A*, Exposure of the fracture by an intraoral incision over the mandibular inferior border. The occlusion is secured during the operation *only* by means of dental splints and intermaxillary wire fixation. (Subsequent to the osteosynthesis, the intramaxillary immobilization may be removed). *B*, Corresponding to the intraoral exposed fracture, a 4 mm stab incision is made in the skin. *C*, A blunt scissors is introduced into the stab incision, and the tissue spread in the direction of the facial nerve fibers. The tip of the blunt scissors must become intraorally visible. *D*, The protection sleeve with mandrel is inserted into the soft tissue canal, which has been opened by blunt dissection. The intraorally visible end of the bore sleeve is fixed by means of a special holding forceps. The mandrel is removed. *E*, The drill is inserted intraorally through the bore sleeve, and drilling is performed at the desired part of the mandible. *F*, The screw of the desired length (the length can be measured by the depth gauge transbuccally via the bore sleeve) is attached to the screwdriver and inserted through the bore sleeve.

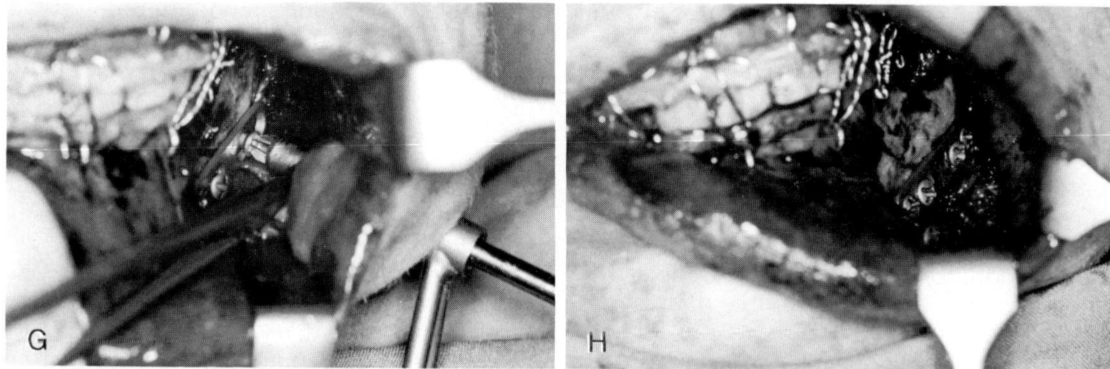

Figure 27–121 *Continued G*, The screw is inserted transbuccally into the predrilled bone, cutting its own thread. *H*, Subsequent to tightening of both compression screws in the compression holes, the fragments are repositioned. In addition, two outer retention screws are inserted through the same approach (the bore sleeve is moved medially or distally). The fracture is stabilized by means of compression osteosynthesis. (Courtesy of Hans Luhr, M.D., and Howmedica Co.)

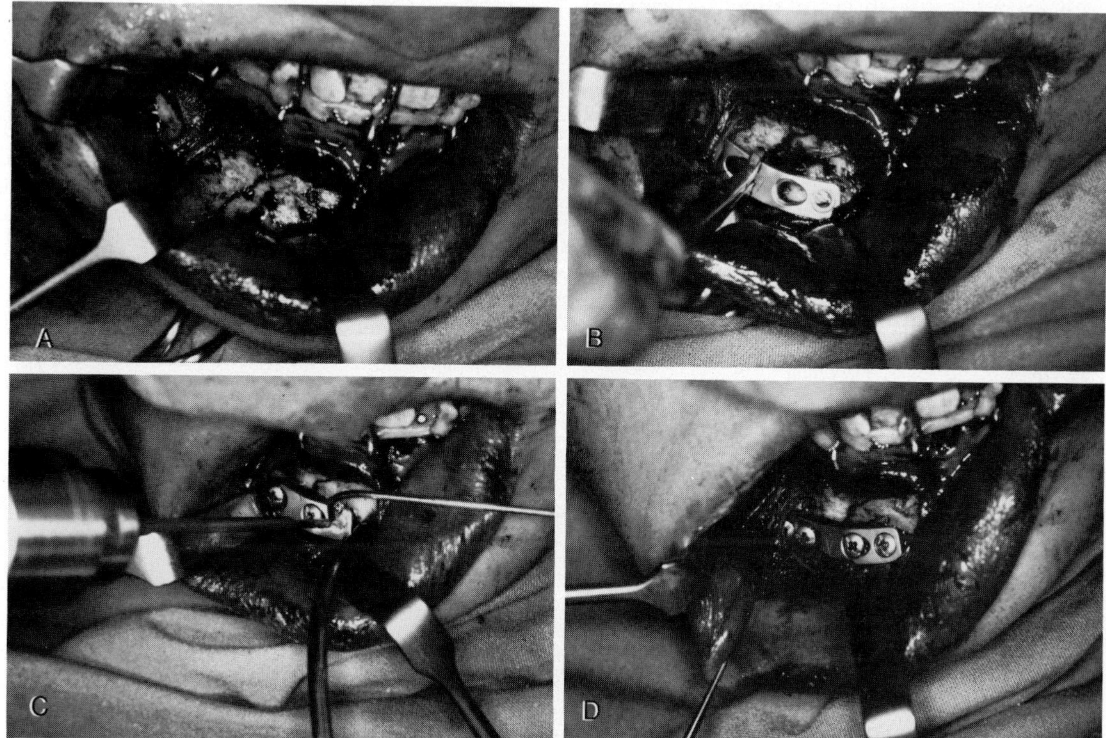

Figure 27–122. *A*, Exposure of the fracture by an intraoral incision. *The occlusion is ensured by means of dental splints and intermaxillary wires during the surgical procedure* (after the osteosynthesis has been performed, they can be removed). *B*, The mandibular compression-screw (MCS) plate is shaped to the bone surface by means of a bending tong. The mental nerve has been carefully exposed by blunt dissection and the plate is placed beneath the nerve, using a plate-holding clamp. *C*, In an organized operating field, drilling of holes and insertion of screws can easily be performed. First the compression screws are inserted. Only then is the underlying bone within the outer centric holes perforated by a surgical drill. *D*, After insertion of the outer screws the fracture is stabilized by the MCS plate and intermaxillary fixation is released. In patients with a dentulous mandible, the lower arch bar—acting as a tension band—should be left in situ for three to four weeks. (Courtesy of Hans Luhr, M.D., and Howmedica Co.)

of corrosion may occur after several years and carries the risk of localized metallosis. Some manufacturers recommend removal of stainless steel implants after two to five years. In addition to the localized metallosis, a different type of corrosion can occur owing to tissue contact and friction (*fretting* corrosion).

TITANIUM MESH TRAY (Zallen and Fitzgerald, 1976). Titanium mesh is available that can be contoured to the lower border of the mandible and anchored to the main fragments (Fig. 27–123). The mesh can be contoured to provide a basket for the comminuted fragments, anchoring them with appropriately placed screws. This method may require the supplemental use of intermaxillary fixation with arch bars.

It has usually been preferable to provide direct secure internal fixation than to use insecure dental appliances (splints). When associated with soft tissue loss, complicated fractures of the mandible should be stabilized by external fixation in preference to circumferential wiring with splints on the remaining teeth. Most small segments of bone and soft tissue that are useful in the reconstructive period should be saved and incorporated into the type of fixation employed.

Fixation in Class II Fractures when Maxilla is Edentulous. Intermaxillary fixation of Class II fractures with an edentulous maxilla is accomplished by using either splints or the patient's dentures (see Fig. 27–105*A*). In some cases, the splint may be chosen as a single "bite block"–type splint, which maintains position of the lower jaw as related to the upper dental edentulous alveolar segment. The bite block is maintained in position by internal wiring. Generally the use of separate maxillary and mandibular splints is preferable to the use of a single bite block. The upper and lower splints are wired with either circumzygomatic and piriform aperture wires for the upper splint, or circummandibular wires for the lower splint. A circumpalatal wire or wires to the inferior orbital rim or frontal bone may occasionally be employed.

Fractures of Condyle. Fractures of the condyle are discussed in Chapter 30.

Fractures of Coronoid Process. The coronoid process of the mandible is sheathed by overlying musculature (Natvig, Sicher, and Fodor, 1970). The temporalis muscle has broad attachments all along the anterior surface of the ramus and the coronoid area. The coronoid process fits up under the overlying zygomatic arch so that it is protected from frequent injury. Fractures of the coronoid may involve only the tip of the coronoid process (Natvig, Sicher, and Fodor, 1970; Frim, 1978), may involve the whole process, or may extend down the surface of the mandible to separate the whole anterior portion of the ramus from the rest of the mandible. They generally show little dislocation because of the broad, dense insertions of the temporalis muscle and fascia. In many cases, treatment is unnecessary because little displacement has been produced. If displacement is observed, open reduction via a Risdon or retromandibular approach is recommended. The use of interfragment wires and plate and screw fixation can prevent recurrent displacement. Most fractures of the coronoid are accompanied by other fractures of the mandible or zygoma (Natvig, Sicher, and Fodor, 1970; Frim, 1978; Rapidis and associates, 1985).

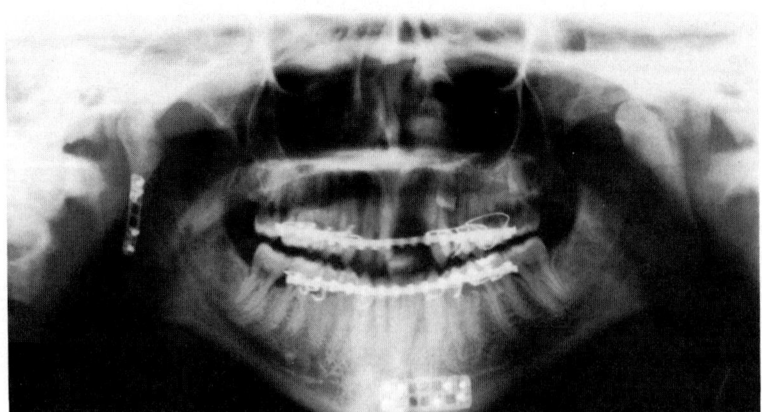

Figure 27–123. Titanium mesh and unicortical screws to reduce a parasymphyseal right subcondylar fracture. The left high condylar fracture was not opened. A satisfactory result in terms of occlusion and range of motion was achieved.

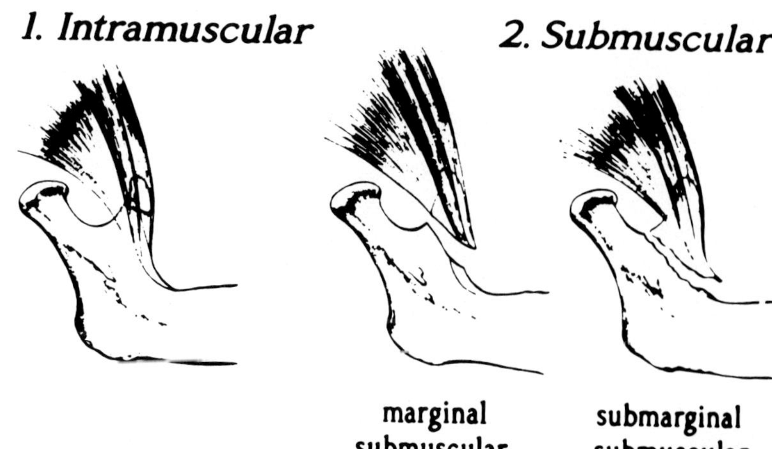

Figure 27–124. Classification of fractures of the coronoid process of the mandible. Displacement does not usually occur unless submarginal, submuscular fractures are present. (From Natvig, P., Sicher, H., and Fodor, P. B.: The rare isolated fracture of the coronoid process of the mandible. Plast. Reconstr. Surg., *46*:168, 1970.)

The classification of Natvig, Sicher, and Fodor (1970) is employed for describing coronoid fractures (Figs. 27–124, 27–125).

Fractures in Edentulous Mandible. Fractures of the edentulous mandible are seen less commonly than fractures of the dentulous or partially dentulous mandible (Marciani and Hill, 1929; Berry, 1939; Obwegeser and Sailer, 1973; Welsh and Welsh, 1976; Levine and Goode, 1982; Zachariades and associates, 1984). They represent less than 5 per cent of the mandibular fractures seen in most series. The fractures occur through the portions of bone where atrophy is the most advanced or where the bone is thin and weak. Some fractures are bilateral and displacement may range from minimal to moderate. The fractures may be closed or open to the oral cavity. Some closed fractures demonstrating minimal displacement may be treated with a soft diet (Fig. 27–126). In these cases, healing generally occurs within several weeks. The edentulous mandible is characterized by the loss of the alveolar ridge. The atrophy of the bone may be minimal, and in these cases there is sufficient height of the mandibular body (over 20 mm). In cases with moderate atrophy, the height of the mandibular body ranges from 10 to 20 mm. In cases in which the mandibular height is less than 10 mm, the atrophy is described as severe. Complications following fracture of the edentulous mandible directly parallel the extent of mandibular atrophy (Obwegeser and Sailer, 1973) since 20 per cent of the complications are seen in the 10 to 20 mm mandibular height group and 80 per cent of the complications (poor union) are experienced in cases demonstrating a mandibular height of less than 10 mm (Obwegeser and Sailer, 1973). This finding has caused some authors (Obwegeser and Sailer, 1973) to recommend immediate bone grafting for the severely edentulous mandible that requires open reduction (Fig. 27–127). It should be emphasized, however, that some fractures of the severely atrophic edentulous mandible may be treated without fixation or with only closed reduction techniques; an operation and bone grafting can be avoided in patients who demonstrate multiple health problems.

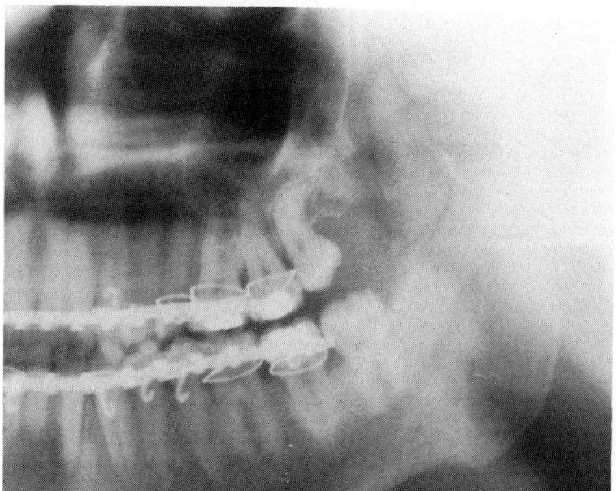

Figure 27–125. An isolated fracture of the coronoid process of the mandible. Treatment involved a brief period of intermaxillary fixation for control of pain. The patient was then allowed to function. Many coronoid fractures require no period of immobilization.

OPEN REDUCTION OF EDENTULOUS MANDIBLE. The usual methods of fixation of mandibular fractures are not applicable in the case of the edentulous mandible because intermaxillary fixation is more difficult to util-

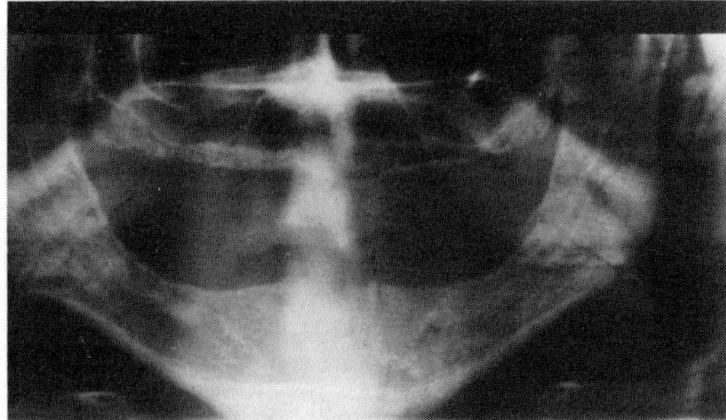

Figure 27–126. Bilateral angle and parasymphyseal fracture in an edentulous mandible. Periosteal continuity prevented much displacement. The patient could be adequately treated with soft diet alone.

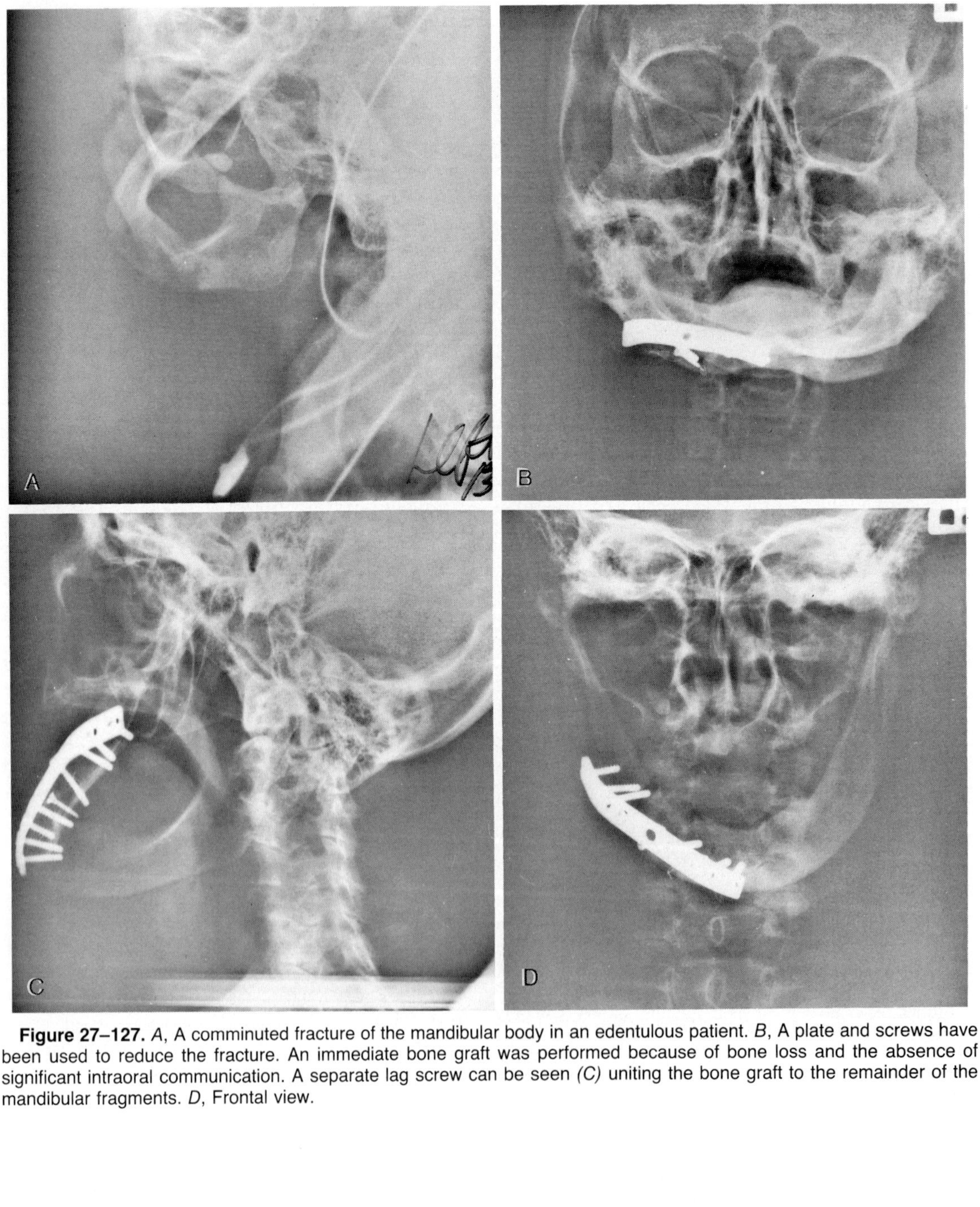

Figure 27–127. *A*, A comminuted fracture of the mandibular body in an edentulous patient. *B*, A plate and screws have been used to reduce the fracture. An immediate bone graft was performed because of bone loss and the absence of significant intraoral communication. A separate lag screw can be seen *(C)* uniting the bone graft to the remainder of the mandibular fragments. *D*, Frontal view.

ize. The treatment options for patients requiring an open reduction include the use of *intraoral appliances, circumferential wiring* techniques, *interfragment wires, external pin fixation appliances,* and *plate and screw fixation.*

Intraoral appliances are quite useful in simple fractures in which displacement is minimal or absent (Fig. 27–128). In some cases, one may desire to put the patient's mandible at rest with the use of splints or dentures modified to maintain stability of the mandibular segments. If displacement is minimal, the patient's dentures may be placed in the mouth and support obtained with a headwrap or chinstrap. This method, however, does not provide any rigidity. If displacement is more than minimal, the denture may be modified and relined with a soft dental compound to compensate for any change of contour of the alveolar process caused by the fracture or atrophy occurring in the preinjury period. It is necessary to avoid excessive pressure on the alveolar process to prevent tissue necrosis. Broken dentures may be repaired and the fragments utilized in fracture fixation. The splints may be left in place for a six to eight week period until consolidation of the fracture fragments has occurred. Alternatively, impressions of the alveolar ridges are taken, and models prepared and sectioned, and suitable splints or bite blocks constructed. The splints can be secured into position with circumferential wiring techniques (see Fig. 27–105*A*, *B*).

Baudens (1840) was the first to utilize *circumferential wiring* techniques for the reduction of mandibular fractures. He described the use of a wire inserted around the mandible in the molar area. Robert (1852) used a single circumferential wire to reduce a mandibular fracture, twisting the wire close to the bone and approximating the segments of an oblique fracture (Fig. 27–129). The circumferential wiring technique can be used alone or in combination with a bite block or dentures.

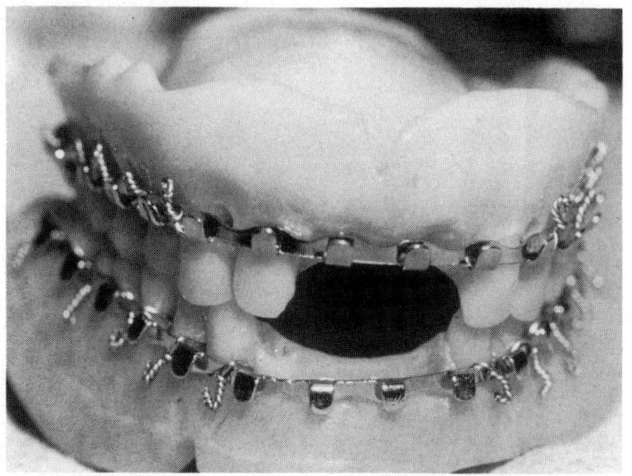

Figure 27–128. Modification of dentures for their use with intermaxillary fixation. The central teeth have been removed to provide an airway and facilitate feeding.

Interosseous wiring may be employed at the upper or lower border of the mandible to approximate fracture fragments. As previously emphasized, the use of one or two interosseous wires assists stability. For fractures in the body of the mandible, the upper portion of the mandible is used (Fig. 27–130), as this location more effectively counteracts the pull of the muscles causing mandibular displacement. The location of the inferior alveolar nerve and canal should be noted. In the severely atrophic mandible, the nerve may be in soft tissue directly on the surface of the superior border of the mandible because of bone atrophy. The open reduction may be performed through either intraoral (Paul and Acevedo, 1968; Chuong and Donoff, 1985) or extraoral routes.

Extraoral open reduction utilizes an incision in the upper portion of the neck about 1 to 2 cm below the inferior border of the mandible. The incision should be just long enough to give adequate exposure to the fractured segments. The soft tissues are divided and the branches of the facial nerve identified and protected. The periosteum is incised and the fracture reduced and held in position with bone forceps. Drill holes are placed through the bone on each side of the fracture site, and figure-of-eight or multiple wiring technique (Fig. 27–131), using 24 gauge stainless steel wire or plate and screw fixation, is employed. The fixation at the fracture site should be as positive as possible. The wound is closed in layers and the use of a suction drain is employed at the discretion of the surgeon.

Intraoral open reduction is effective in fractures of the edentulous mandible. The fracture is exposed through an incision lateral or medial to the crest of the alveolar ridge. The mucoperiosteum is reflected on both the buccal and lingual surfaces of the mandible. In severely atrophic mandibular fractures, the attachment of the mylohyoid muscles is near the crest of the alveolar ridge. It should also be recalled that the inferior alveolar nerve and artery may be located on the superior surface of the mandible. Interference with

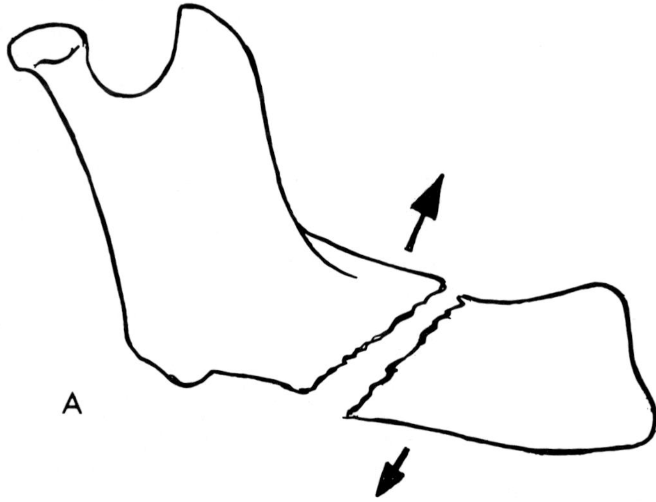

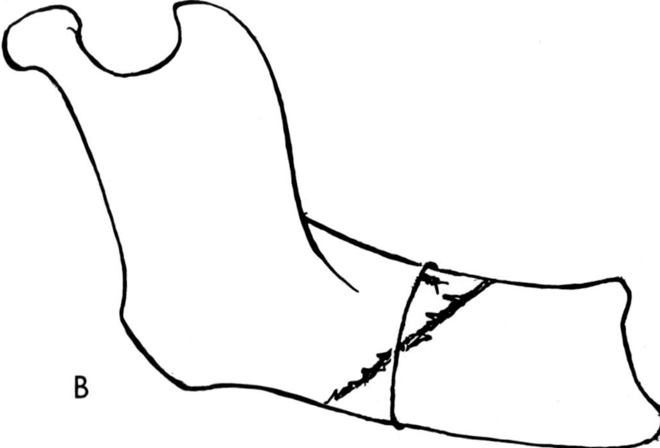

Figure 27–129. Fixation of an oblique mandibular fracture with a single circumferential wire. Arrows indicate the direction of the muscle pull.

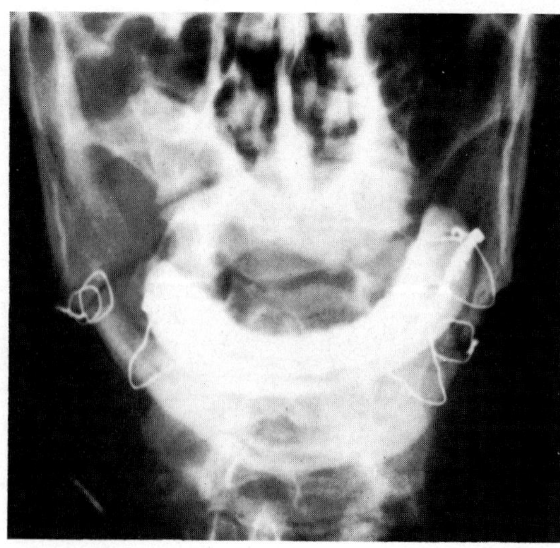

Figure 27–130. Direct interosseous wiring and circumferential wiring around the mandible and a prosthodontic appliance for treatment of a fracture of the edentulous mandible.

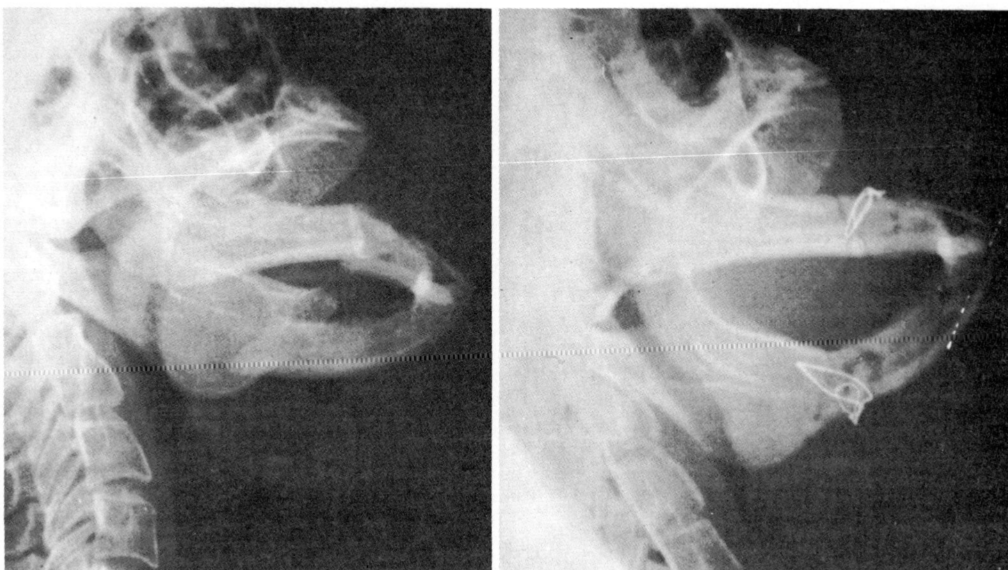

Figure 27–131. Bilateral fractures in an edentulous mandible. *A*, Preoperative roentgenogram showing overriding of the fragments, and downward and forward displacement in the anterior segment. *B*, Postoperative view after open reduction and direct wire fixation through an extraoral approach. Plate and screw fixation would be the preferred current method of treatment.

these muscular attachments results in swelling of the floor of the mouth and postoperative pain and discomfort on swallowing or chewing. Anesthesia in the distribution of the mental nerve may be produced by a section of the inferior alveolar nerve. After exposure of the fracture, a drill is used to prepare the bone for open reduction. Drill holes are placed and 24 gauge stainless steel wire may be passed from the buccal to the lingual surface and back through the other hole to the buccal surface area. One or two wires are utilized with the wire ends twisted so that the fragments are firmly and positively fixed into position. The wires are cut short and the cut end is pressed against the bone or tucked into a drill hole. Preferably, a plate may be used. Soft tissue should be securely closed over the fracture site. The wires used for open reduction may require removal after healing. However, many display little, if any, reaction and are not uncomfortable for the patient who wears dentures.

The use of plating through the intraoral approach (Paul and Acevedo, 1968; Chuong and Donoff, 1985) is simple and direct and provides a mechanical advantage over wiring techniques. Plates placed near the upper border of the fracture provide a fulcrum against which the muscle forces are most effectively neutralized. The posterior fragment of the mandible is tracked upward by the posterior muscles (Fig. 27–132). The anterior fragment of the mandible is tracked downward by the pull of the anterior mandibular muscles. Wires placed in the inferior portion of the mandible for fractures of the mandibular body do not oppose the tendency of the superior border to "gap." The unfavorable situation creates a tendency for the fracture fragments to separate at the superior border.

Antibiotics should be employed for either intraoral or extraoral open reduction in mandibular fractures (Zallen and Curry, 1975). Infection is not common and generally relates to inadequate fixation, excessive motion, soft tissue damage, and comminution in the area of the fracture site.

The advantages of the intraoral approach for the open reduction of mandibular fractures include the fact that (1) it is more easily accomplished than extraoral open reduction and (2) there is no danger to the facial nerve, submaxillary gland, or external maxillary artery. The approach is accomplished with a minimum of instrumentation, and healing is usually rapid and uncomplicated.

Multiply Fractured or Comminuted Edentulous Mandible. Kazanjian and Converse (1974) described the management of severe fractures of the anterior portion of the mandible in which only fragments of bone

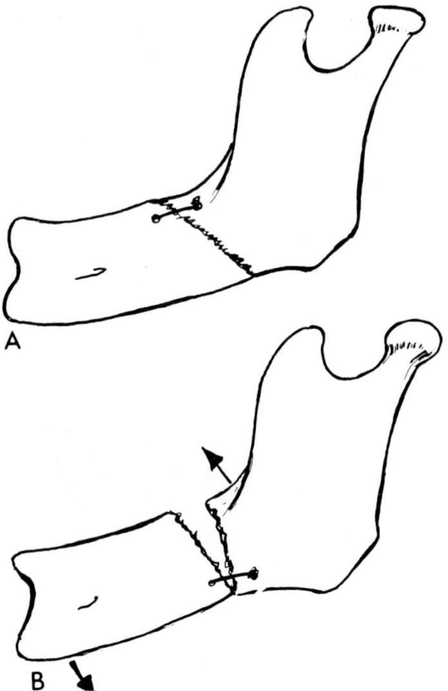

Figure 27–132. Interosseous fixation of the edentulous mandible. *A*, Correct location for the interosseous wire. The fulcrum is near the upper portion of the fracture, and the muscular forces favor bone contact. *B*, With the interosseous wire near the inferior border of the mandible, displacement may occur through the pull of the muscles (indicated by arrows).

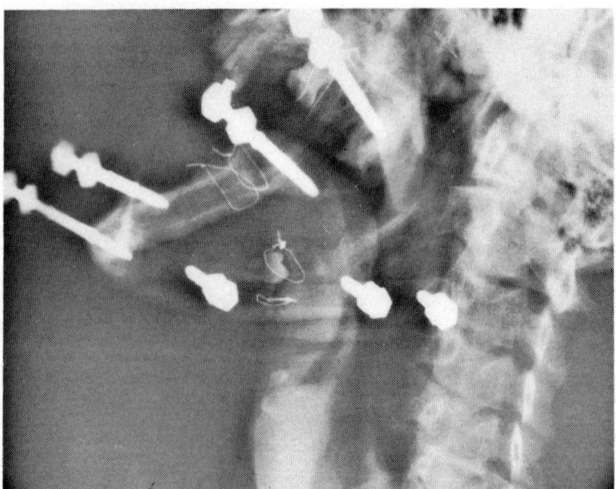

Figure 27–133. Reduction of a bilateral body fracture with wires and stabilization by a Morris external fixation device. Postoperative radiograph. A molar tooth is seen in the fracture site. No infection resulted. It could be argued that this tooth should have been removed at the time of fracture reduction.

remained; a horseshoe-shaped heavy wire conforming to the dental arch was used. Drill holes were placed in the proximal segments of bone, and smaller fragments were fixed by suspension with fine steel wires to the heavier arch wire. This technique was the forerunner of the current use of external fixation to span large areas of bone comminution (Fig. 27–133). Fixation may be obtained on the posterior segments and the plate contoured to reconstruct the mandibular form anatomically (Fig. 27–134). Smaller fragments can be screwed to the plate and soft tissues reapproximated to provide a blood supply to cover the bone fragments. In some cases the bone fragments may be united by direct interosseous wiring to each other. It is difficult to achieve enough stability utilizing wiring technique alone to maintain the form of the arch, and plate or external fixation provides stability. The author performs initial interfragment wiring and then stabilizes the interfragment wired pieces with an external fixation or a plate device to maintain arch form. If segments of the mandible are missing, the gaps may also be spanned by plates or external fixation devices, maintaining the form and structure of the remaining mandibular arch and permitting function. Bone defects may be primarily bone grafted if the oral mucosa closure is secure.

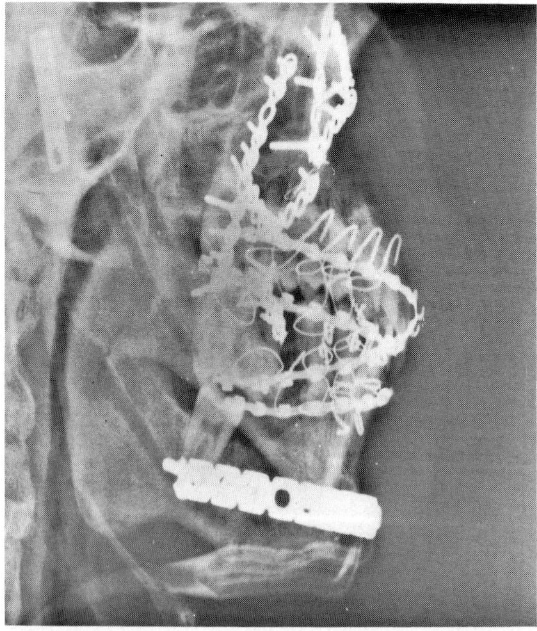

Figure 27–134. The application of a reconstruction plate for a comminuted fracture of the mandible. Care should be taken to place the plate as low as possible on the bone, otherwise the inferior alveolar canal and tooth roots are in jeopardy.

The importance of maintaining the exact anatomic position of bone fragments despite missing bone cannot be overemphasized. If the segments are allowed to displace, they become united by scar tissue in a dislocated position. Soft tissue and scars contract and later reconstruction is not as easily or effectively accomplished if the position of the bone fragments has not been preserved. Some authors used titanium trays or mesh to stabilize these complicated mandibular fractures. These devices are placed along the inferior border of the mandible and screwed into position to intact bone. The smaller bone fragments can be anchored to the titanium tray.

Some authors recommend immediate bone grafting for mandibular fractures demonstrating bone loss where adequate soft tissue closure can permit safe, immediate reconstruction. Obwegeser and Sailer (1973) advocated this method, using circumferential split rib grafts bound to the fracture in the severely atrophic edentulous mandible. Gruss and associates (1985b) utilized immediate bone grafting for some severe mandibular fractures. The technique provides a one-stage reconstruction and should be employed in situations in which soft tissue is adequate to permit bone grafting with safety. Soft tissue integrity is often insufficient to permit immediate bone grafting.

External Fixation of Mandibular Fractures. An external pin fixation device has been used for long bone fractures since the nineteenth century, and was described by Lambotte (1913). Roger Anderson popularized its use in fractures of the facial bones in 1936. At present, the most popular technique involves the use of a Morris biphasic fixation appliance (Morris, 1949). This is a stable, easily utilized device that employs an acrylic connector between Vitallium bone pins. External fixation was popularized in the 1936 to 1945 period. The popularization of open reduction techniques by Adams (Adams, 1942; Adams and Adams, 1956) and Dingman and Alling (1954) then resulted in the decreased use of pin fixation appliances in favor of open reduction and direct wire fixation.

The indications for external fixation include the multiply fractured mandible in which interosseous or interfragment wires do not provide sufficient stability. Fractures in the edentulous mandible can also be treated with immediate mobilization. In mandibular fractures demonstrating complications of non-union or infection, the mandibular fragments can be stabilized at a point remote from the wound or fracture site. Mobilization can be accomplished. In some cases, wiring of the jaws is contraindicated and the presence of an external pin appliance accomplishes fracture immobilization. Finally, when a stable mandibular base is required for the reduction of complicated maxillary fractures, it may be of advantage to ensure mandibular stability by the use of a mandibular biphasic appliance.

Little can be added to Morris's (1949) excellent original description of the technique, which involves the use of a primary connector (reduction phase), a mechanical appliance or metal rig that is in use for 25 to 30 minutes until the secondary phase is constructed. The secondary phase employs a small acrylic connector bar. The external splint can then be worn for the four to six week period of fixation usually required. The external fixation device makes possible better oral hygiene and diet, improved speech, and decreased periods of intermaxillary fixation. The disadvantages include the conspicuous nature of the appliance, the postoperative scarring relative to the pin sites, damage to the parotid gland or facial nerve from the placement of the pins, and the possibility of less accurate occlusal relationships if the surgeon is not careful in the reduction. The technique is described in detail in Chapter 72.

Complications in Treatment of Mandibular Fractures

Hemorrhage. The early complications seen in the treatment of mandibular fractures include hemorrhage into soft tissues. Extensive bone and soft tissue injury may accompany these fractures. Generally, blood loss is not excessive, but if major arteries are divided in open lacerations, it can be significant.

Airway. When mandibular fractures are bilateral, posterior displacement of the structures of the tongue and floor of the mouth is possible. In grossly displaced fractures, the tissues of the tongue and floor of the mouth can fall back to occlude the pharynx. Anterior traction on the tongue, repositioning of the anterior mandible bone fragments, or intubation or tracheostomy will protect the airway.

Following intermaxillary fixation, patients may have respiratory complications if vomiting or aspiration of stomach contents occurs. The stomach contents should be evacuated with nasogastric suction. This is an essential precaution for patients placed in intermaxillary fixation and can easily be accomplished at the time of surgery. It is sometimes desirable to remove the intermaxillary elastics or wire fixation so that the airway can be protected. When the patient is sufficiently awake and provided there is no nausea, the intermaxillary fixation may be reestablished. The presence of marked swelling can be an additional reason to release intermaxillary fixation until the swelling has subsided and the airway is protected. A nasopharyngeal airway can be an important protective device in some patients. It cannot be overemphasized that patients in intermaxillary fixation who are emerging from an anesthetic need close observation of the airway to prevent respiratory complications.

Infection. Modern methods of fracture treatment and the availability of antibiotics have greatly reduced the incidence of infection in mandibular fractures (Schneider and Stern, 1971; Neal, Wagner, and Alpert, 1978; Kahnberg and Ridell, 1979; Kahnberg, 1979; Amaratunga, 1987a). Most complications from infection can be avoided by appropriate debridement, accurate and secure fixation, and antibiotic treatment (Frim, 1978; Olson and associates, 1982; Chuong, Donoff, and Guralnick, 1983; Winstanley, 1984; Bochlogyros, 1985; Ellis, Moos, and Attar, 1985). Foreign bodies in the area of the fracture include segments of devitalized bone or fractured teeth, dirt, metal, glass, or other materials introduced into the fracture at the time of injury (Eid, Lynch, and Whitaker, 1976; Giordano and associates, 1982). Any devascularized tissue acts as a foreign body predisposing to infection.

Inadequate fixation is a frequent contributor to infection, as it allows movement of the fracture fragments. Healing is delayed and the pumping action at the site of the fracture forces foreign material, saliva, and bacteria into the fracture site, especially in compound fractures. Continuous damage to emerging granulation tissue and organizing bone occurs from this movement. The process of repair is diminished. Nonvital, loose, or abscessed teeth in the line of fracture lead to infection of the bone and adjacent soft tissue. It is desirable to retain teeth that are stable; however, root tips or root fragments in the line of fracture merely provide a focus for infection (see Fig. 27–133) (Schneider and Stern, 1971; Neal, Wagner, and Alpert, 1978; Kahnberg and Ridell, 1979; Kahnberg, 1979; Amaratunga, 1987a). In most cases, it is desirable to remove a loose tooth that puts the fracture at hazard for infection and to proceed to an alternative method of reduction, even though the tooth might allow a simpler reduction. Teeth present in the line of fracture are preserved if they have secure attachments. The presence of any preexisting disease in the area of the fracture, such as an abscessed tooth, periodontitis, or irradiated tissue, predisposes to infection.

Once established, an infection should be appropriately drained and purulent collections removed. Extraoral drainage may be necessary if the process is extensive and penetrating into the deep tissues of the neck. Any procrastination in instituting drainage of an abscess leads to the spread of infection through the bone and into the soft tissues of the neck. Devitalized fragments of bone are removed. It often is not necessary to remove any internal devices, such as wires or plates and screws, or bone. In mandibular fractures demonstrating osteomyelitis (Giordano and associates, 1982), the removal of plates and screws or wires is accomplished only after the application of an external fixation device. This maneuver allows control of the fracture site and bone position by utilizing areas of the mandible remote from the site of infection.

Avascular Necrosis and Osteitis. When bone is denuded of its periosteal and muscular attachments, it is deprived of its blood supply. Fractures often damage the medullary blood supply of the mandible (the inferior alveolar artery and vein). The stripping of soft tissues to accomplish fracture reduction also deprives the mandible of its secondary (cortical) blood supply through the branches of the facial artery entering the soft tissue attachments. The bone may undergo avascular necrosis. This type of osteitis may progress to osteomyelitis in the presence of bacterial colonization. Complications of avascular necrosis can be minimized by early coverage of exposed bone with well-vascularized soft tissue, by limiting the amount of soft tissue dissection, and by accurately reapproximating soft tissues so that they can again provide blood supply to the underlying bone.

Osteomyelitis. True osteomyelitis in the mandible is a relatively uncommon complication in the management of facial fractures

(Giordano and associates, 1982). Although localized infections occur with some frequency, the condition rarely progresses to true osteomyelitis. The use of antibiotics and the prompt drainage of any areas of suppuration prevent invasive colonization of bone. If osteomyelitis has occurred, it is usually demonstrable on x-ray. All sequestra of devitalized bone and any internal fixation devices should be removed. Management to control soft tissue spread of infection is indicated by appropriate drainage and antibiotic treatment. The bone should be stabilized with an external fixation device, and after soft tissue improvement and closure, the bone may be reconstructed with grafts under antibiotic coverage.

Late Complications of Mandibular Fractures. Late complications of mandibular fractures include delayed union and non-union, malunion, ankylosis of the temporomandibular joint, ankylosis of the coronoid process of the mandible, anesthesia of the inferior alveolar nerve, scar tissue contractures within the mouth, malocclusion, and facial deformity (Larsen and Nielsen, 1976).

Ankylosis of Temporomandibular Joint. Ankylosis of the temporomandibular joint (Ostrofsky and Lownie, 1977) may follow fractures or dislocations of the mandibular condyle. The process may be difficult to differentiate from ankylosis of the coronoid process of the mandible. The ankylosis may be fibrous or bony in character. Ankylosis of the temporomandibular joint most commonly follows intracapsular fractures involving the articular surface of the head of the condyle. After severe fracture, there may be aseptic necrosis with loss of the articular surface and destruction of the fibrous meniscus. Scarring and bone proliferation that occur may yield to fibrous or osseous ankylosis of the condyle to surrounding structures, such as the glenoid fossa and zygomatic arch. Fibro-osseous ankylosis may also occur. Since the joint capsule is weaker medially than laterally, bone proliferation may occur more commonly on the medial aspect. Occasionally, infection is a complicating factor. In these cases, any devitalized fragments of bone must be removed, and condylectomy is usually required. The patient should be studied preoperatively with axial and coronal CT scans of the temporomandibular joint area. A panoramic roentgenogram is also helpful. The coronoid process should also be seen, to exclude processes involving this structure.

Non-union of Mandibular Fractures (Bochlogyros, 1985). In most instances healing of the site of a mandibular fracture is accomplished within a short period of four to eight weeks (Amaratunga, 1987c). In several studies, healing was found to be sufficient to permit guarded motion after three weeks for most fractures. Healing in bone structures of the mandible, however, has been found to progress histologically for 26 weeks. Remodeling should be complete at this time. Older patients require longer periods of fixation. Healing in membranous bones is affected by the degree and type of fracture, the blood supply to the area, the age and general condition of the patient, the presence of other conditions such as atrophy of the alveolar process, and the dental condition of the patient. Motion at the fracture site is an important determinant of healing.

In some cases, a fracture may be prevented from uniting by the interposition of foreign substances, such as muscle and soft tissue between the fractured bone ends. Sometimes the mandibular body area splits in a sagittal plane, as an accompanying injury to a parasymphyseal fracture. Unless a full inspection of the mandible is performed, it is easy to miss the "sagittal split" of the mandibular body and fail to position the buccal and lingual cortices in proper approximation.

Poor position of fracture fragments predisposes to delayed non-union. One of the most common predisposing factors is improper immobilization with motion at the fracture site. In fractures that are comminuted, the loss or devascularization of portions of bone may result in sequestration of bone fragments, which contributes to delayed union or infection (Fig. 27–135). In patients who are debilitated, one can expect healing to be slower. If one examines series describing the non-union of patients with fractures of the mandible, the "body" is the site most often affected.

Healing of a mandibular fracture is best assessed by clinical examination, since roentgenograms may show persistent radiolucency of the fracture site, even in the presence of solid bone union. In membranous bones, it is not necessary to demonstrate the radiopacity through a fracture site as a criterion of bone union.

Nutrition is important in achieving fracture union. One patient was found to have lost 30 lb during a period of eight weeks' fixation. She disliked liquid foods and refused to take sufficient material to provide an ad-

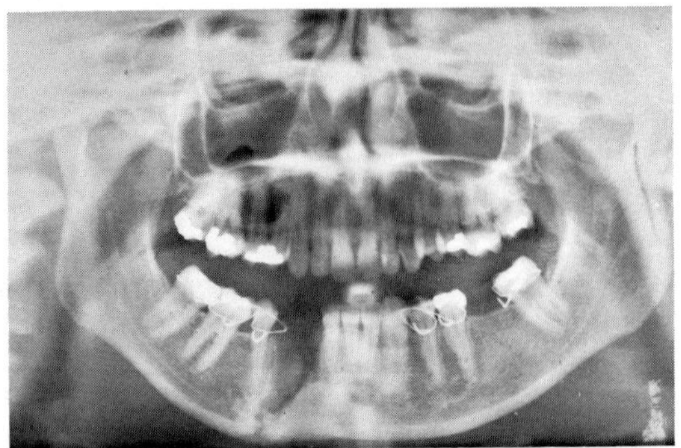

Figure 27–135. Developing nonunion in a parasymphyseal fracture. Bone loss is evident. Rounding and eburnation of the bone ends are apparent.

equate oral intake. When she was placed on a therapeutic feeding schedule, consolidation of the fracture occurred rapidly.

In most instances, "non"-union is really a "delayed" union and responds to a short period of increased immobilization. A thorough assessment of the fracture area should be performed radiologically and clinically. The degree of motion in three planes (transverse, vertical, and anteroposterior) should be assessed. In most cases, some motion is observed in one or two planes but not in all three. This finding indicates the potential for union, and a brief period of immobilization should be employed. A thorough radiologic examination of the fracture site should be performed to detect the presence of root tips, periapical infection in fractured teeth, and other factors that might predispose to poor bone healing. Rounded sclerotic bone ends indicate nonunion. In more advanced cases, dense eburnated bone is noted covering the ends of the fracture segments.

The management of non-united fractures is surgical. The bone ends should be exposed through an extraoral approach and the eburnated bone removed with bone burs or rongeurs. Any evidence of infection should be eradicated and, depending on the extent of the infection in the soft tissue, it may be elected to place the patient in external fixation or resort to internal fixation, such as plate and screw fixation. If the conditions are surgically adequate, the bone should be reconstructed with a bone graft, and in most cases cancellous bone can be used to pack the area between the bone ends. It is preferable to use an external fixation device or plate and screw approximation rather than interosseous wires and intermaxillary fixation. Mobilization of the mandible can be achieved by the first two techniques. When surgical treatment is employed, however, it is important that the patient be temporarily placed in intermaxillary fixation, so that the proper relationships between the mandible and maxilla are guaranteed. In most cases of nonunion, there is insufficient bone present to bridge the gap between the bone ends without forming a defect in the dental arch. Bone grafts are always preferable to questionable bone contact. In all cases, consideration should be given to the adequacy of soft tissue, which determines the blood supply for healing.

Malunion. Malunion of mandibular fractures occurs as a result of inadequate reduction and healing of the bone in an abnormal position. In most cases, malunion results from inadequate fixation. During the period of healing, the mandibular fragments can dislocate out of position and thus heal in malalignment. Rotation of the mandible in a lingual direction at the alveolus is a common occurrence in comminuted fractures, such as the parasymphyseal and bilateral subcondylar fracture. The use of a splint opposed against the lingual surface of the teeth prevents rotational displacement. Alternatively, plate and screw fixation can provide more secure apposition of bone fragments than wire interfragment fixation. Telescoping of bone segments in the ramus of the mandible also results from the strong muscle pull of the muscles of mastication. Shortening of the ramus occurs and a premature contact in the molar area may give rise to an open bite deformity.

When malunion is observed and ossification is not complete, it may be overcome by strong orthopedic traction with arch bars and rubber bands between the mandible and maxilla. This is effective only if the union is incomplete. In cases in which the union is more complete, such traction only extracts teeth from the sockets; it is emphasized that traction should never be applied anterior to the cuspid without some protection for the more delicate incisor teeth.

The treatment of established non-union consists of a planned osteotomy at the site of malunion, repositioning of the bones, and fixation by either direct bone plating or interosseous wiring. Bone plating or external fixation is preferable to techniques requiring further intermaxillary fixation. Bone grafts, again, are usually employed to supplement local bone conditions.

Fractures of the Nasal Bones and Cartilages

The external nose is a triangular pyramid composed of cartilaginous and osseous structures that support the skin, musculature, mucosa, nerves, and vascular structures. The upper third of the nose is supported by bone, and the lower two-thirds gains its support from a complicated interrelationship of the upper and lower lateral cartilages and the nasal septum (Fig. 27–136). The skin in the upper portion of the nose is freely movable and thin; in the lower portion the skin is thick and has prominent sebaceous glands. In the distal nose the attachment of the skin to the underlying cartilaginous structures is more intimate. The entire nose has an excellent blood supply, which permits extensive dissection with safety and results in early, rapid healing. The supporting framework of the nose is made up of semirigid cartilaginous structures that are attached to the solid and inflexible bone structure of the nose (Fig. 27–136). The cartilaginous tissues include the lateral nasal cartilages, the alar cartilages, and the septal cartilage. There are several sesamoid cartilages in the lateral portions of the ala and in the base of the columella. The cartilaginous structures support the overlying subcutaneous tissue, skin, mucosa, and lining of the nose. The cartilages are intimately attached to the bony structures, which consist of the frontal process of the maxilla, the nasal spine of the frontal bone, the pair of nasal bones, and the bones of the septum, the vomer, and the perpendicular plate of the ethmoid (Fig. 27–137). The paired nasal bones articulate in the midline with each other, and are supported laterally by the frontal processes of the maxilla and superiorly by the "nasal spine" of the frontal bone. The lower third of the nasal bones is thin and broad. In the proximal position the nasal bones are thicker and narrow in their articulation with the frontal bone. The thin por-

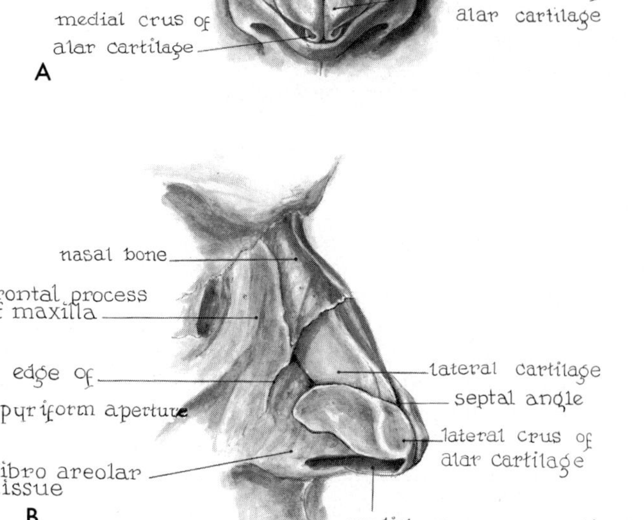

Figure 27–136. Anatomy of the nasal framework. *A*, Anterior view. *B*, Lateral view. (From Converse, J. M.: Cartilaginous structures of the nose. Ann. Otol. Rhinol. Laryngol., *64*:220, 1955.)

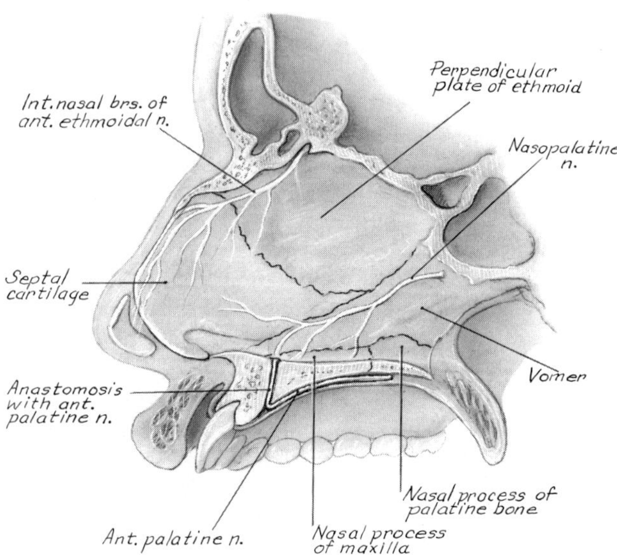

Figure 27–137. The bony and cartilaginous nasal septum and its innervation. (From Kazanjian and Converse.)

tion of the nasal bones is subject to fracture, whereas the thicker portions are more difficult to injure. The nasal bones seldom fracture in the upper portions, but fractures often occur in the lower half. In the upper portions the bones are also firmly supported by an intimate articulation with the frontal bone and frontal process of the maxilla.

TYPES AND LOCATION OF FRACTURES

Fractures in adults vary with the site of the impact and with the direction and intensity of force. Direct frontal blows over the nasal dorsum result in fracture of the thin lower half of the nasal bones, or if more severe may cause separation at the nasofrontal suture (Fig. 27–138). The margin of the piriform aperture is thin and may be fractured. Such piriform aperture fractures may be associated with fractures of the nasal bones and may extend to the frontal process of the maxilla (Fig. 27–138).

Lateral forces (Fig. 27–139) (Stranc and Robertson, 1979) account for most nasal fractures and produce a wide variation, depending on the age of the patient and the intensity and direction of force. Younger patients tend to have fracture-dislocations of larger segments, whereas in older patients with more dense brittle bone, comminution is observed more frequently. Kazanjian and Converse (1959) and Murray and associates (1984) confirmed that most nasal fractures occur in the thin portions of the nasal bone. In the Kazanjian and Converse series, 80 per cent in a series of 190 nasal fractures occurred at the junction of the thick and thin portions of the nasal bones. A direct force of moderate intensity from the lateral side may fracture only one nasal bone with displacement into the nasal cavity. If the force is of increased intensity, some displacement of the contralateral nasal bone occurs. In more severe frontal impact injuries, the frontal process of the maxilla may begin to fracture and may be depressed on one side. The depression first arises at the piriform aperture and then involves the entire structure of the frontal process of the maxilla; in effect, a heminasoethmoidal fracture at the lower two-thirds of the medial orbital rim is involved with the attached canthal ligament (Fig. 27–139*C*).

Violent blows result in fracture of the nasal bones and the frontal processes of the maxilla, lacrimal bones, septal cartilage, and ethmoidal area. The bones are driven into the ethmoidal area, and displaced fractures occur with damage to the bony portion of the nasolacrimal system, the perpendicular plate of the ethmoid, the ethmoid sinuses, the cribriform plate, and the orbital plate of the frontal bone. Displacement in these severe comminuted fractures results in broadening and widening of the interorbital space with displacement of the bones to which the medial canthal ligaments attach, producing a posttraumatic telecanthus (Fig. 27–140). This is

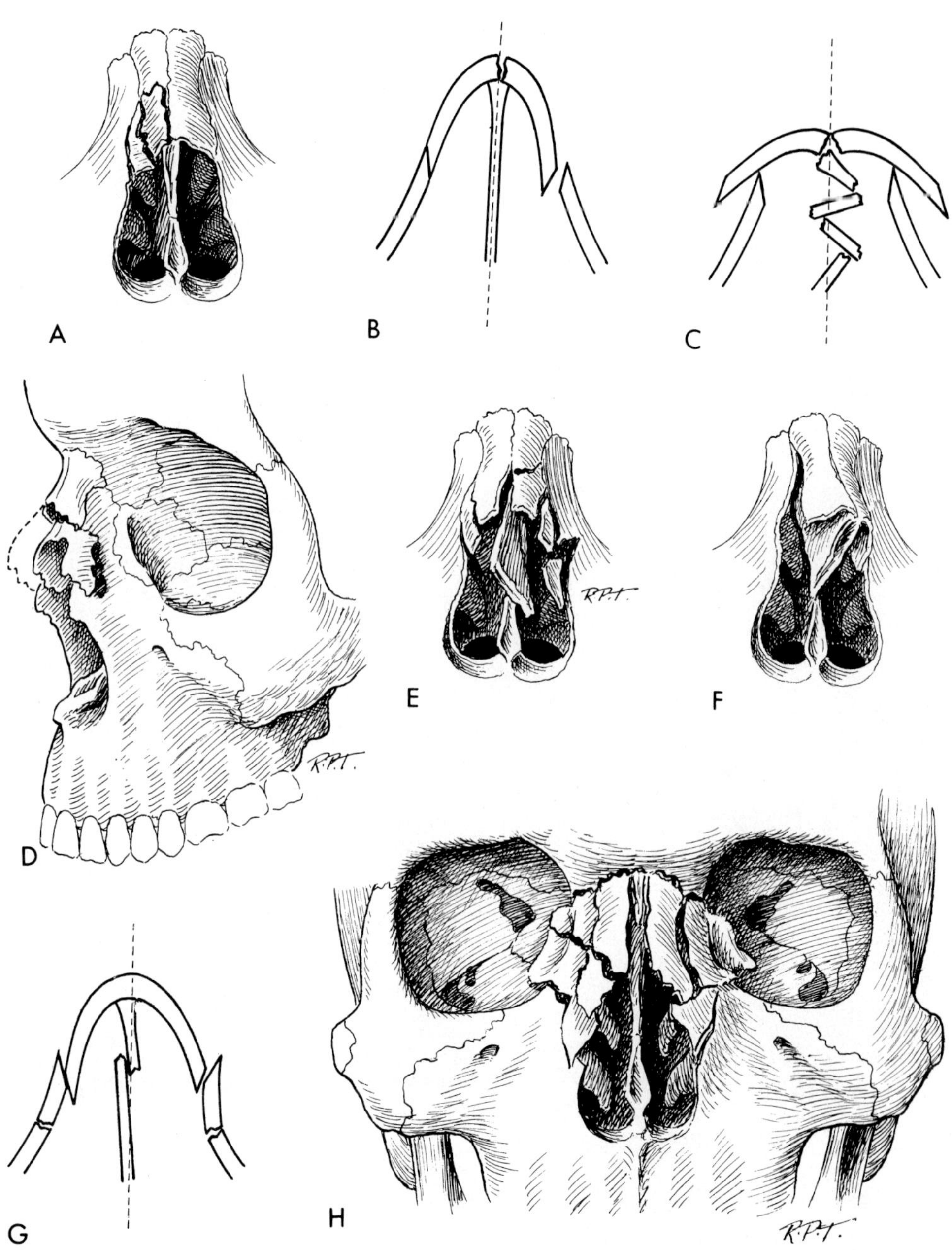

Figure 27–138. Various types of fractures of the nasal bones. *A, B*, Depressed fracture of one nasal bone. *C*, Open book type of fracture as seen in children. *D*, Fracture of the nasal bones at the junction of the thick upper and thin lower portions. *E*, Comminuted fracture of the nasal bone. *F, G*, Fracture-dislocation of the nasal bone. *H*, Comminuted fracture of the nasal bones involving the frontal process of the maxilla. (From Kazanjian and Converse.)

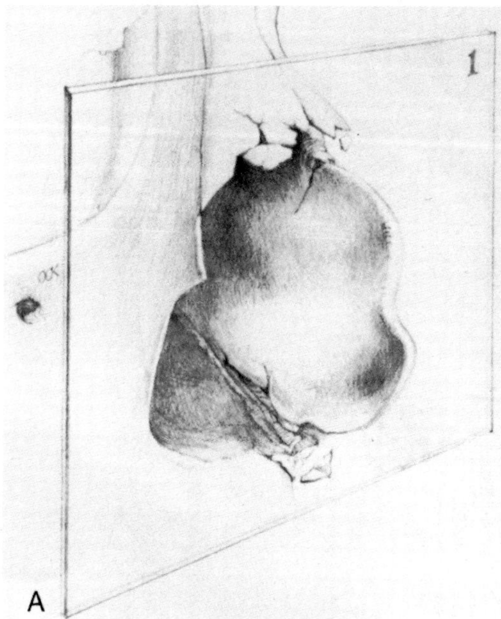

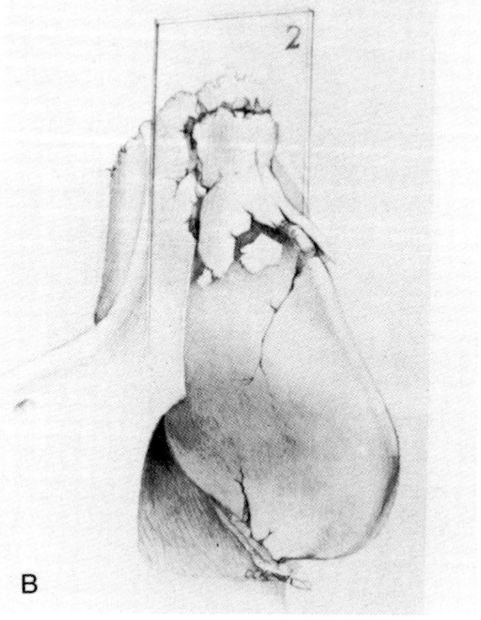

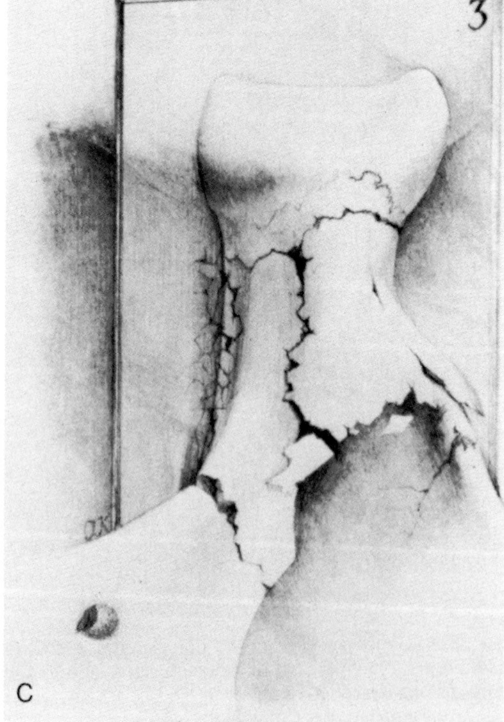

Figure 27–139. Stranc classification of displacement following a nasal fracture. Displacement is analyzed in terms of (1) lateral deviation and (2) anteroposterior displacement (frontal impact nasal fracture). Frontal impact nasal fractures are characterized by degrees of displacement: *A*, Plane 1 frontal impact nasal fracture. The end of the nasal bones and the septum are injured. *B*, Plane 2 frontal impact nasal fracture. The injury is more extensive, involving the proximal portion of the nasal bones and the frontal process of the maxilla at the piriform aperture. *C*, Plane 3 frontal impact nasal fracture involving one or both frontal processes of the maxilla extending up to the frontal bone. This is in reality a nasoethmoido-orbital fracture since it involves the lower two-thirds of the medial orbital rim. (From Stranc, M. F., and Robertson, G. A.: A classification of injuries of the nasal skeleton. Ann. Plast. Surg., 2:468, 1979.)

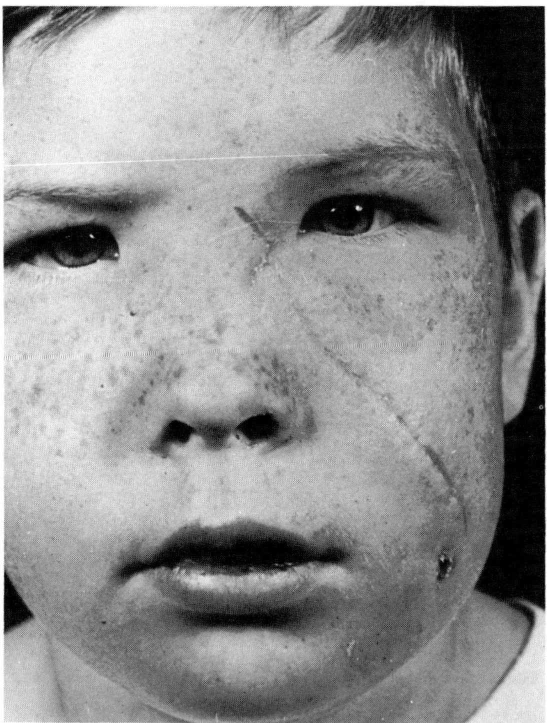

Figure 27–140. Post-traumatic telecanthus and widening of the interorbital space due to fracture of the nasal bones and frontal processes of the maxilla.

the nasoethmoido-orbital fracture, which occurs in a wide variety of combinations with associated fractures of adjacent bones, such as the frontal bone, zygoma, and maxilla.

Fractured bone segments in more severe injuries may be driven into the nasolacrimal system at various levels, resulting in an obstruction. Permanent epiphora may occur. Telescoped, comminuted nasal fractures involving the nasoethmoidofrontal area are commonly seen after severe frontal impact injuries. Frequently the entire central middle third of the face has struck an object, such as an instrument panel or some other projecting object inside an automobile. These fractures are not isolated nasal injuries, but represent the end stage of the frontal impact central midfacial fracture, i.e., the nasoethmoido-orbital injury.

FRACTURES AND DISLOCATIONS OF NASAL SEPTUM

Fractures and dislocations of the septal cartilage may occur independently or concomitantly with fractures of the nasal bone framework. Because of the intimate association of the bones of the nose with the nasal cartilages and bony nasal septum, it is unusual to observe fractures of either structure without damage to the other. In particular, the caudal (cartilaginous) portion of the nasal septum is almost always injured in nasal fractures. This caudal portion of the septum has a certain degree of flexibility and bends to absorb moderate impact. In more severe injuries, the septum fractures, often with a C-shaped or transverse component, in which the septum is fractured and dislocated from the vomerine groove. Displacement occurs with partial obstruction of the airway. The cartilage may be fractured in any plane, but the most frequent location of the fracture is that described with the horizontal and vertical components separating the anterior portion of the septum from the posterior. As the cartilage heals, it can also exhibit progressive deviation. Cartilage is thought to possess an inherent springiness, which can be released by tearing of the perichondrium on one side of the fracture. If the perichondrium and cartilage are torn, the septum tends to deviate away from the torn area toward the intact perichondrial side. Fractures of the septum are often associated with a "telescop-

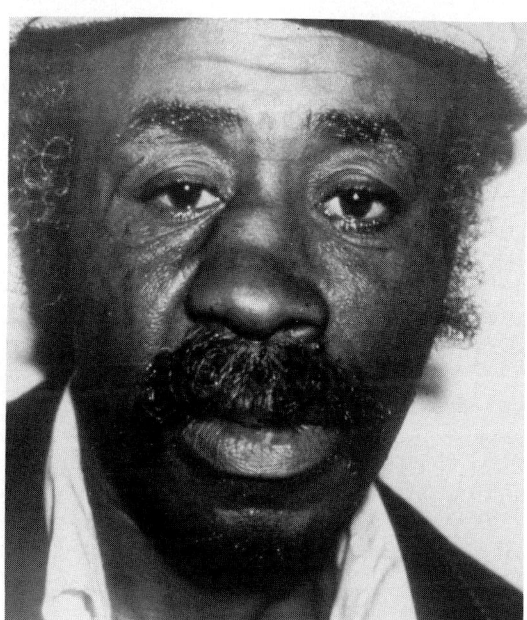

Figure 27–141. A combination of a frontal impact and laterally deviated nasal fracture. The nose displays deviation to the right, flattening and widening of the nasal pyramid, and a moderate posterior displacement of the distal end of the nasal bones and the septum. Reduction must involve correction of the lateral deviation and packing of the nasal bones into position to support the reduction of the posteriorly displaced distal nasal fragments.

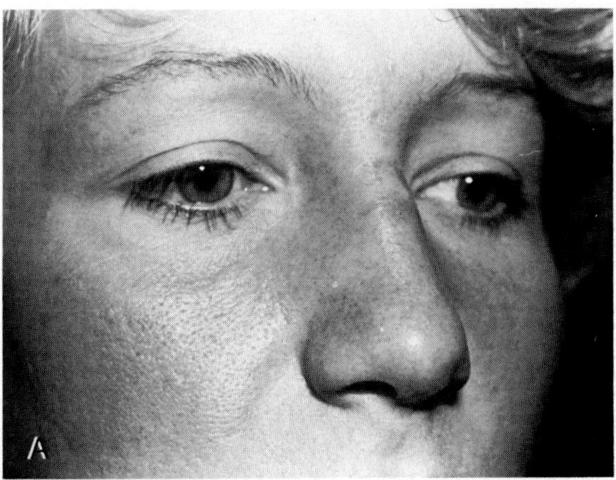

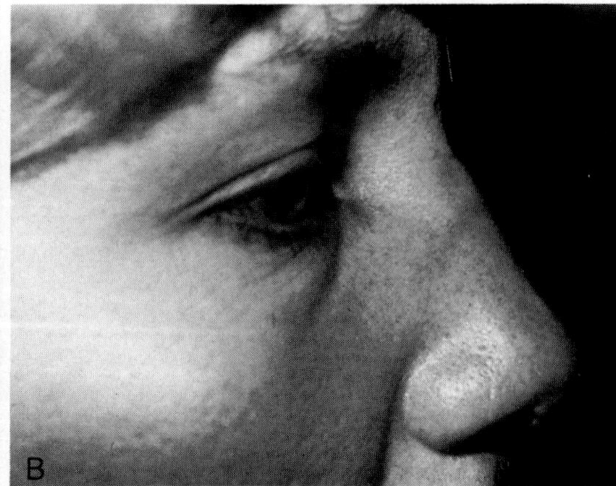

Figure 27–142. Loss of height of the septal structures after a nasal fracture. There is slight telescoping of the septal fragments, resulting in loss of nasal height. The appearance is that of a small dorsal hump in the bony portion of the nose. The loss of septal height is best seen from *(A)* oblique or *(B)* lateral views of the nose.

ing" type of displacement with overlapping of the fractured edges (Fig. 27–141). The septum can be shortened, giving rise to a slightly retruded appearance of the cartilaginous portion of the nose. Slight loss of dorsal nasal height can give rise to a nasal hump (Fig. 27–142) at the junction of the septum with the nasal bones. A slight loss of columellar projection produces a retraction in that area. Angulation of the caudal border of the septum can be indicative of a septal fracture.

Diagnosis

On physical examination (Fig. 27–143), there is mobility and crepitus on palpation with tenderness over the areas of the fracture site. On intranasal examination, there is deviation of the septum with laceration of the mucosa or hematoma. Periorbital and nasal edema, ecchymoses, and dislocation may mask the displacement. The intranasal findings are more accurately evaluated if the mucosa is shrunk with a vasoconstrictor. Blood clots should be removed, and any hematoma of the septum should be evacuated or aspirated to prevent cartilaginous deformity and septal necrosis from pressure of the hematoma.

Roentgenograms are helpful in the diagnosis and treatment and provide a legal record of the injury (Fig. 27–144). They are not absolutely necessary, but serve to confirm the absence of injury to adjacent bones and to diagnose the pattern of the nasal fracture. The usual facial radiographs may not clearly reveal a nasal fracture. Gillies and Millard (1957) recommended increasing the backward tilt of the occipitomental view from 15 to 30 to 45 degrees to illustrate fractures not apparent in the usual occipitomental projection. Soft tissue techniques on profile views demonstrate fractures of the thin anterior edge of the nasal bones and the nasal spine. CT scans accurately demonstrate most nasal fractures (Fig. 27–145) and their displacement, but should principally be employed to confirm the

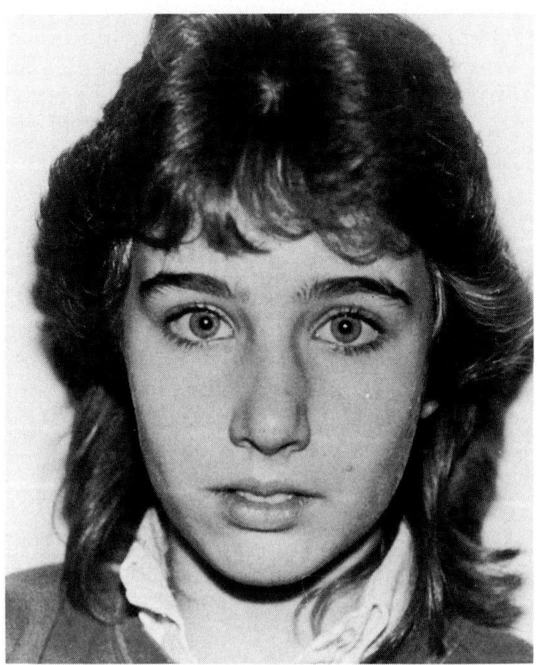

Figure 27–143. Laterally deviated nasal fracture. The right nasal bone is displaced medially and the left (greenstick) is displaced laterally.

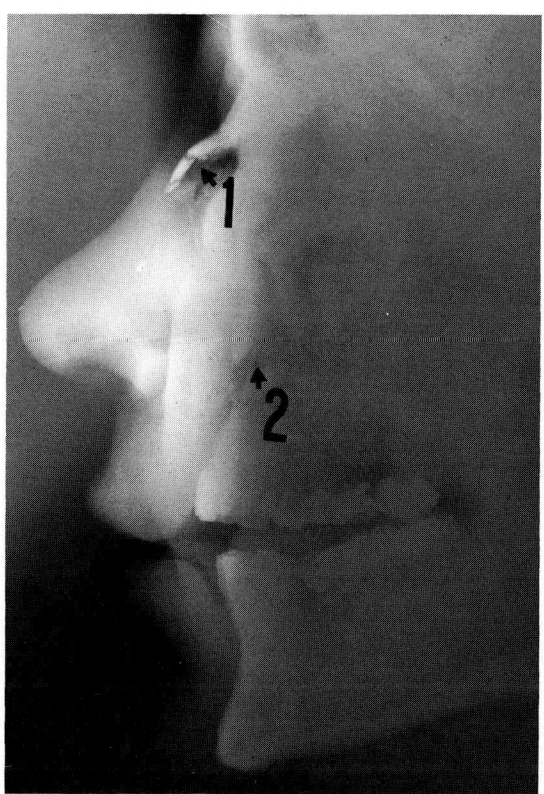

Figure 27–144. Lateral low density, soft tissue roentgenograms are the best to demonstrate the small bones of the nasal dorsum. Fractures of the nasal bones are seen *(1)* along with a fracture of the anterior nasal spine *(2)*.

absence of injury to adjacent structures, such as the orbit and nasoethmoidal area.

Treatment of Nasal Fractures

Fractures of the nasal bones may be reduced by means of a closed reduction technique. It is helpful to perform this reduction before edema prevents accurate palpation and visual inspection. Most simple fractures can be managed on an outpatient basis. More extensive comminuted fractures or compound fractures may be treated with open reduction if the lacerations are appropriate. In severe injuries of the nose, i.e., the Plane 2 nasal injury (see Fig. 27–139), an open reduction with bone grafting to restore nasal height may be required. In practice, the closed reduction of most nasal fractures is deferred until the edema has subsided and the accuracy of the reduction may be confirmed by visual inspection or palpation. Treatment may be postponed for five to seven days.

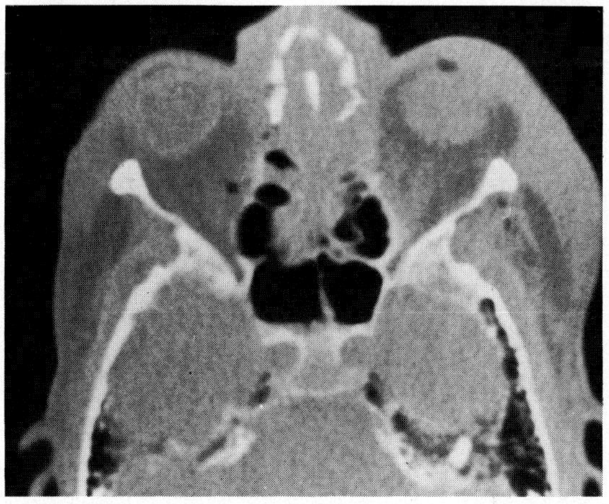

Figure 27–145. CT scan of a severe fracture of the nasal bones. The nasal bones are comminuted.

Anesthesia. Nasal fractures in children are best managed under general anesthesia. In both children and adults, the operation is facilitated by packing the nose with cotton pledgets that have been soaked in vasoconstricting drugs for seven to ten minutes. The preference of the author is to utilize 5 per cent cocaine on 1:100,000 epinephrine-soaked pledgets. The vasoconstriction shrinks the mucosal structures of the nose in order that an accurate intranasal examination can be performed. Most nasal fractures in adults can be successfully reduced with the aid of an intranasal topical and external nasal field block (see Chap. 35).

Instrumentation for Reduction of Simple Nasal Fractures. The fiberoptic headlight is an essential instrument for intranasal illumination. Intranasal specula of various sizes and lengths are essential for adequate intranasal visualization. Almost all nasal fractures can be reduced by upward and outward forces with an instrument placed in the nose under the nasal bones. The preference of the author is to use the handle of a No. 3 scalpel (Fig. 27–146). There are forceps designed for intranasal use, such as the Asch (Fig. 27–147) and the Walsham (Fig. 27–148) types. Inappropriate use of the forceps can cause damage to the skin or to a nonfractured portion of the nose. The mucosa can be lacerated without reducing the fracture. Depressed nasal bones are manipulated upward and outward with an instrument in one hand, as the other hand is used either to apply external pressure or to palpate the proper reduction of the nasal bone fragments. In practice, it is the author's usual preference to dislocate both nasal bones outward (see Fig. 27–146), completing the fracture, and then to remold them inward with digital pressure.

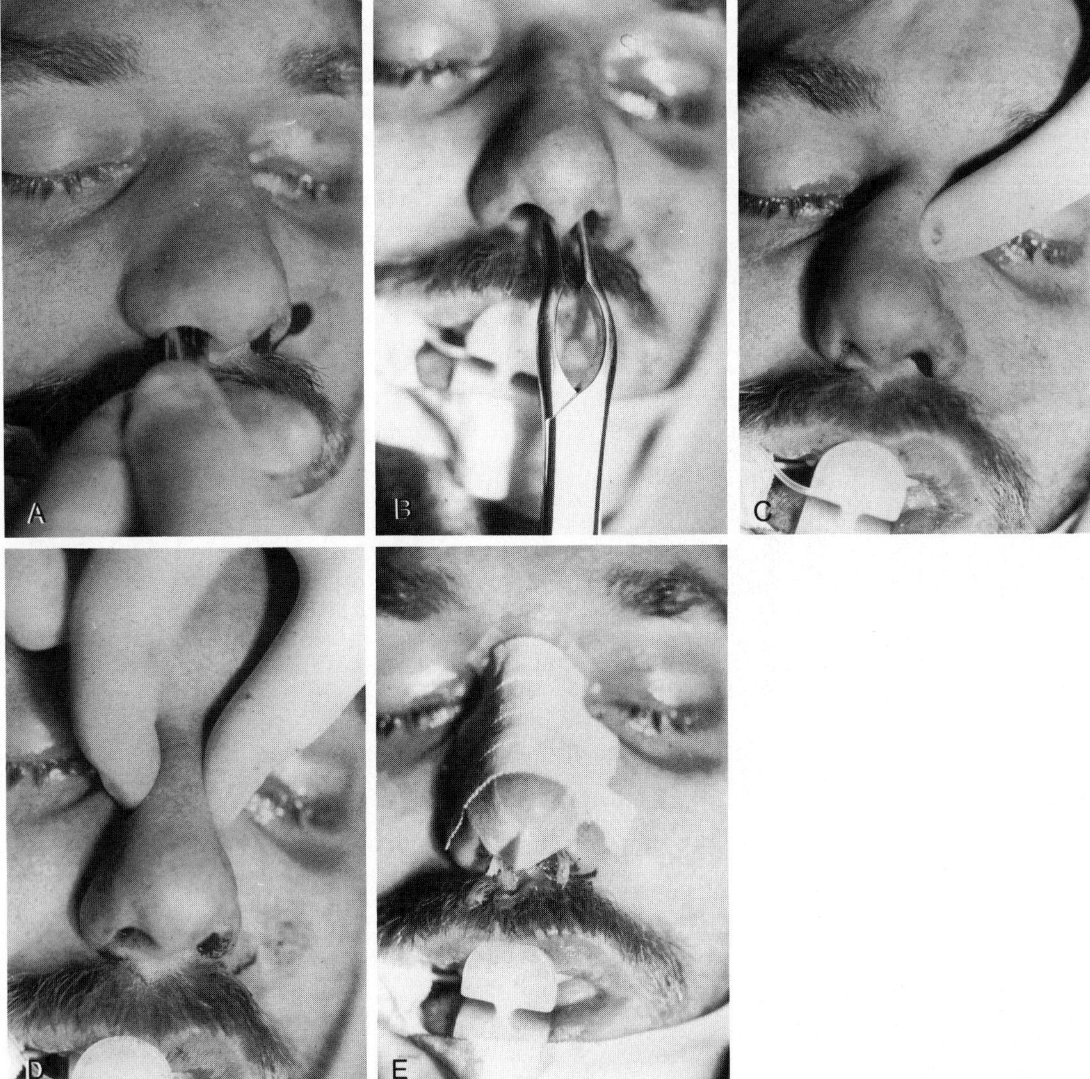

Figure 27–146. Reduction of a nasal fracture. After vasoconstriction of the mucous membrane, the nasal bones are outfractured with the handle of a No. 3 scalpel blade *(A)*. *B*, The septum is straightened with an Asch forceps. Both the nasal bones and septum should be able to be freely deviated in each direction *(C)*. If the fracture has been reduced, the nasal bones are molded back into the midline *(D)*. Steri-Strips and adhesive tape are applied to the nose *(E)* and a metal splint is applied over the tape. The tape prevents the edges of the metal splint from damaging the skin. A light packing is placed inside the nose to support the septum, minimize hematoma, and (in certain cases) support the distal end of the nasal bones.

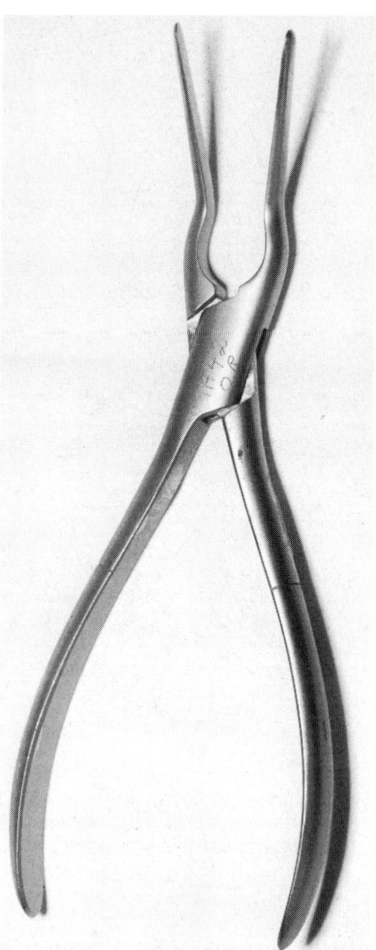

Figure 27–147. Asch forceps.

The septum may be replaced into the midline by use of the Asch forceps. Reduction of the bony nasal pyramid often facilitates the reduction of the septum. If the nasal bones are comminuted or loose, it is preferable to support them and the septum by means of intranasal antibiotic-soaked gauze packing and an external nasal splint (see Fig. 27–146). Simple nasal fractures may remain in position without the need for nasal packing or splints.

After the nasal, bony, and cartilaginous structures have been reduced and manipulated into position, intranasal packing is used to splint the nasal septum into position and to keep the mucosa of the septum approximated to the cartilage. This is an important maneuver following drainage of a septal hematoma. In the case of a depressed fracture of the distal portion of the nasal bones, a small amount of intranasal packing may be utilized to support that fragment in order to prevent recurrent displacement. If desired, a small length of Silastic tubing may be placed in each nostril floor as an airway and the packing placed around it. This maneuver adds considerably to the comfort of the patient. The tubes may not provide a satisfactory airway alone, but do permit equalization of pressure in the nasopharynx during the act of swallowing and prevent the discomfort of negative pressure in the middle ear.

The external splint may be either metal, plaster, or dental compound (Fig. 27–149). The end of the nose is cleaned several times a day with peroxide-soaked cotton-tipped applicators. The intranasal packing may be removed in two to seven days, depending on the function of the packing.

Treatment of Fractures and Dislocations of Septal Framework

The septum should be straightened and repositioned as soon after the injury as possible. With fractures of the nasal bones and the septum, it is important at the time of reduction that the displaced fragments can

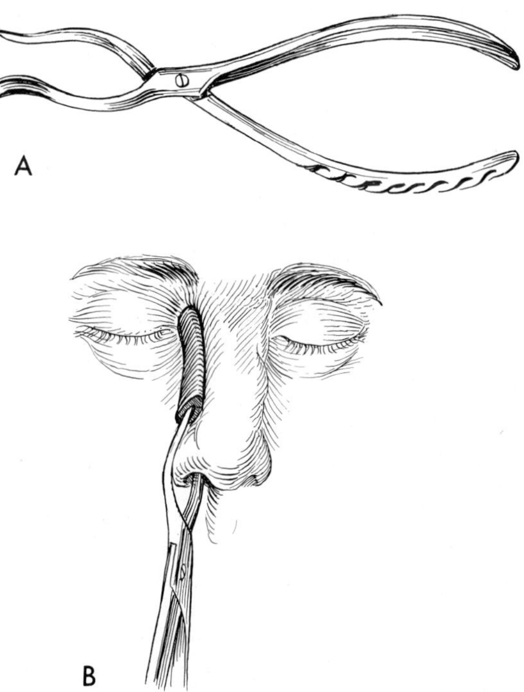

Figure 27–148. *A*, The Walsham forceps. *B*, Reduction of the fractured bone. Note the rubber tubing over the blade of the forceps. Care must be taken not to injure the skin by crushing.

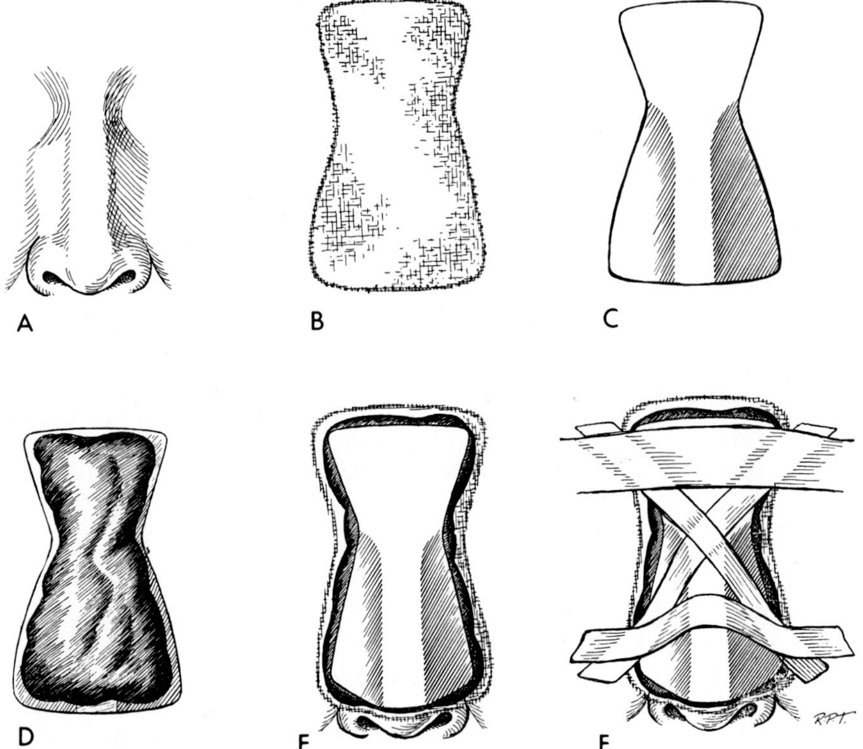

Figure 27–149. The nasal splint. *A*, The nose. *B*, A piece of fine mesh gauze is applied over the nose to protect the skin. *C*, A piece of soft metal, 22 gauge, is cut and shaped. (Often the gauze has been previously applied to the back of a nasal splint.) *D*, Softened dental compound is spread over the metal splint. *E*, The splint is applied to the nose. *F*, The splint is retained with pieces of tape. (From Kazanjian and Converse.)

be deviated freely in both lateral directions to indicate satisfactory completion of the fracture. Uncompleted "greenstick" fractures account for some cases of late deviation. In these cases, the reduction was incomplete and there is a recurrence of the displacement (Fig. 27–150). When the nasal bones are reduced, the intimate relationship of the nasal bones with the upper and lower lateral cartilages tends to reduce the septal cartilage also. Displacement of the cartilaginous septum out of the vomer will not be reduced with this maneuver alone. The correction of the position of the septum is completed with an Asch forceps. The septal fragments, thus realigned, are maintained by light intranasal packing. Some authors prefer Silastic or acrylic splints held by mattress sutures through the septum. Tears in the mucoperichondrium need not always be sutured; they may be dressed into proper position and they heal rapidly.

With some nasal fractures that are seen late, it may not be possible to obtain the desired result. Partial healing may make reduction of the displaced or overlapped fragments difficult. Such patients are best treated by a rhinoplasty after complete healing has occurred. Although some authors (Mayell, 1973; Harrison, 1979; Murray and associates, 1984) indicated that more satisfactory results in nasal fractures can be obtained by imme-

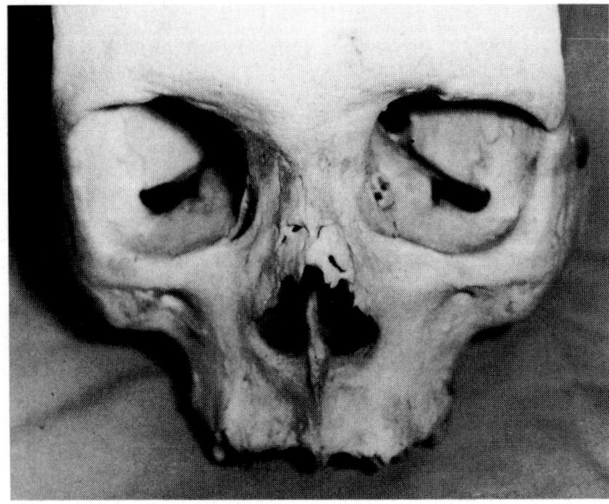

Figure 27–150. A healed fracture of the distal portion of the nasal bones in a skeleton.

diate submucous resection of the nasal septum in the area of the C-shaped fracture, this has the potential danger of loss of nasal height. It is the author's practice to obtain the best result possible with a closed reduction, and to warn the patient that a late rhinoplasty may be indicated for correction of residual deviation of the nasal septum with airway obstruction, residual deviation of the nose, or a dorsal nasal hump. Dorsal nasal humps may result from slight loss of the dorsal height of the septum or from excess bone proliferation around the distal end of the nasal bone, where the more common fractures occur.

Hematoma of Nasal Septum. Hematomas develop between the septal mucoperichondrium and the cartilage in fractures or dislocations of the septum as a result of bleeding. The mucoperichondrium of the nose is profusely supplied with blood vessels, and bleeding is common. Indeed, if bleeding from the nose has not occurred, the diagnosis of a nasal fracture should be in question. Hematomas of the septum are often bilateral, since fractures within the cartilaginous septum permit the passage of blood from one side to the other. Undrained septal hematomas may lead to fibrosis or to organization of the hematoma as a thick section of cartilage material (Fig. 27–151). If excess pressure occurs, the septum can undergo necrosis, and a perforation of the septum can result. Permanent thickening of the septum may obstruct the nasal airway. The condition is similar to the subperichondrial thickening of the auricle, commonly referred to as "cauliflower ear," which is observed following undrained hematomas of the auricle. Loss of the septum is usually associated with complete collapse of the cartilaginous dorsum of the nose. In septal hematomas, both surgical and antibiotic therapy should be routine.

A septal hematoma may be treated by incising the mucoperichondrium. Suction is employed. A horizontal incision is made through the mucoperiosteum at the base of the septum to prevent refilling of the cavity with blood or serum. This incision continues to drain and is located in a dependent position. In

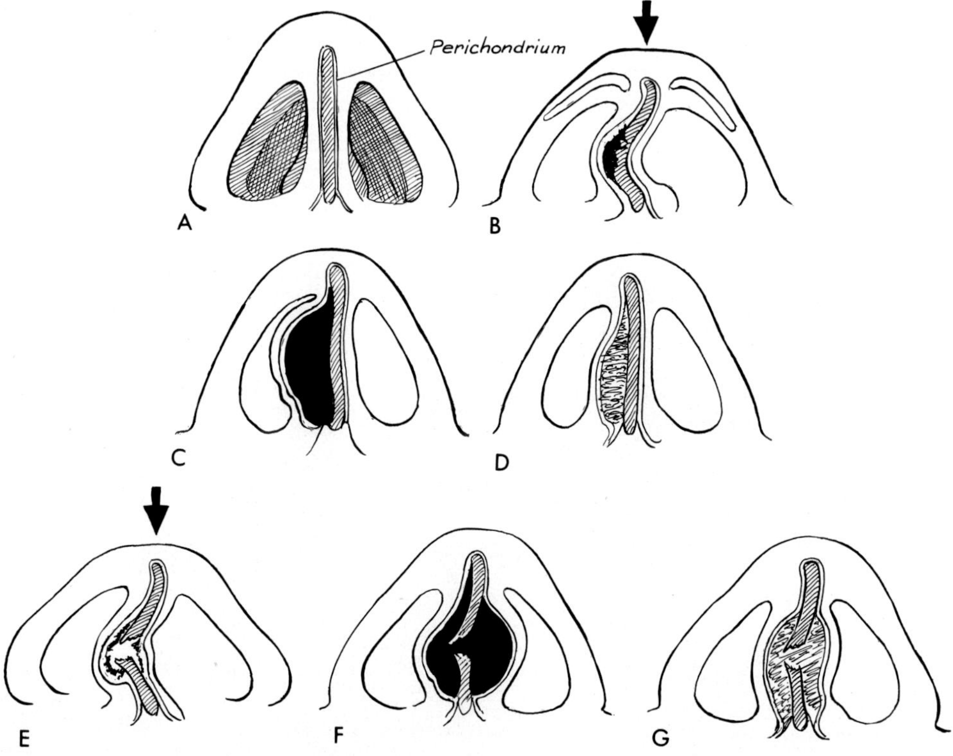

Figure 27–151. Hematoma of the septum. *A, B, C,* Mechanism of formation of a hematoma as a result of excessive bleeding of the septal cartilage without fracture. *D,* Thickening of the septum resulting from fibrosis when the hematoma is not evacuated. *E, F, G,* Fracture of the septal cartilage with formation of a bilateral hematoma and thickening of the septum from fibrosis. (From Kazanjian and Converse.)

bilateral hematoma, it is preferable to resect a portion of the septal cartilage in order to allow the two areas of hematoma to communicate if one-sided drainage is to be utilized. If both sides are to be incised, the septal cartilages should be preserved. A light nasal packing is usually advisable to prevent the accumulation of further bleeding beneath the flaps.

Comminuted Nasal Fractures. More comminuted nasal fractures can usually be reduced without too much difficulty if seen immediately after the injury. Intranasal packing and intranasal splinting may provide adequate fixation. If not, there is an indication to open some Plane 2 nasal fractures in which there is a loss of septal height (see Fig. 27–139). In these injuries, there is severe telescoping and depression of the cartilage fragments and a tendency to sink posteriorly. A sunken or flat nasal dorsum will occur after healing without open reduction. The author has *rarely* opened Plane 2 nasal injuries but has used dorsal bone grafts in the same manner as for treatment of a nasoethmoido-orbital fracture.

Compound Nasal Fractures. Lacerations frequently accompany injuries to the bony and cartilaginous structures of the nose. If the external wound is utilized for the open reduction, the nasal fracture may be more accurately reduced than is possible with a closed reduction technique. Fine (30 or 32) wires are used for interosseous wiring of the nasal bone fragments. The cartilaginous septum can be reunited to the dorsal bony framework. Careful repair of the nasal lining and muscular and subcutaneous layers accompanies skin closure. One is often impressed at the dramatically superior result that can be obtained from such open reduction techniques in contrast to closed reduction.

Transnasal Wiring with Plastic or Metal Plates. Support may be obtained for some nasal fractures demonstrating severe comminution by the use of small plates applied to the side of the nose. They should be padded with orthopedic felt wrapped in a layer of Xeroform gauze. The Xeroform prevents the felt from crusting with bloody secretions. The plate should extend the length of the nasal bones, and wires are passed through the nose with a straight or curved needle (Fig. 27–152). The plates prevent hematoma from occurring between the skin of the nose and they also serve to narrow the nasal dorsum. It should be emphasized that nasoethmoidal fractures (fractures involving the medial rim of the orbit) *cannot* be treated by this method alone. They *always* require a complete open reduction with interfragment wiring or plate and screw fixation. External plates can serve only to narrow the nose, to conserve nasal height, and to prevent hematoma and thickening of the skin.

Complications of Nasal Fractures. Early

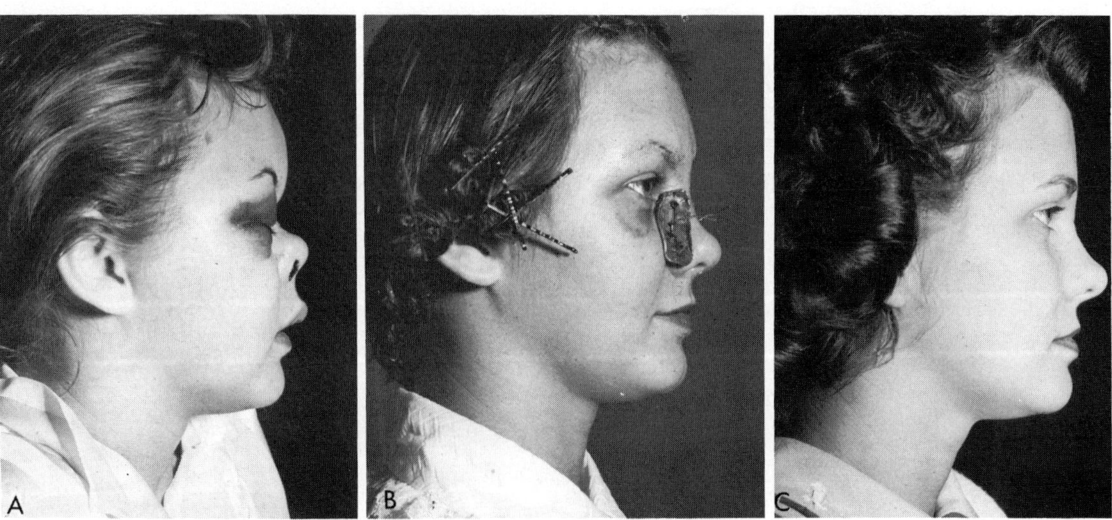

Figure 27–152. *A*, Backward and upward telescoping of the nasal bones into the ethmoid region due to a blow at the nasal tip. *B*, Reduction of fragments and fixation by the wired plate method. *C*, Result after consolidation of the fractured fragments and healing of soft tissues. These injuries are presently managed by open reduction and immediate bone grafting. (From Kazanjian and Converse.)

complications following nasal fractures are rare. They include bruising and ecchymosis of the skin and the eyelids, nasal bleeding, and hematoma of the nasal septum with the possibility of infection. Swelling after nasal fractures is temporary and usually disappears within a few days. Bleeding from the nose is usually of short duration, but some patients may experience rebleeding seven to ten days after the initial injury. Nasal bleeding usually ceases spontaneously or may be controlled with light intranasal packing. In rare cases, an anteroposterior pack may be required.

Hematoma under the soft tissue of the nasal septum is controlled by evacuation with proper incision and drainage. Infection is best treated by drainage, warm compresses, and appropriate antibiotics. Emphysema of the face and neck after the displacement of air into soft tissues rarely results in infection. It resolves spontaneously and the patient should be warned not to partially obstruct the nose as it is "blown."

Late Complications of Nasal Fractures. Untreated hematomas of the nasal septum may become organized, resulting in subperichondrial fibrosis and thickening with partial nasal airway obstruction. The septum may be as thick as 1 cm, and in cases of repeated trauma the cartilaginous septum may be largely replaced with calcified or chondrified material. Submucous resection of the thickened portion of the nasal septum may be required, and in some patients a partial turbinectomy may be advisable.

Synechiae may form between the septum and the turbinates in areas where soft tissue lacerations occur and the tissues are in contact. If bothersome, these may be treated by division with the placement of nonadherent, petrolatum-impregnated material between the cut surfaces for a period of five days. During this time, epithelization occurs.

Obstruction of the nasal vestibule may occur as a result of malunited fractures of the piriform margin or scar tissue contracture from loss of vestibular lining. Osteotomy of the bone fragments corrects the former; however, the contracture due to loss of soft tissue or scar contraction may require excision of scar, and replacement with skin or composite grafts within the nasal vestibule.

Residual osteitis is seen occasionally in compound fractures of the nose or in fractures associated with infected hematomas. Rarely a portion of the bony nasal framework may be lost as a result of infection and may require late replacement with bone grafts. In these cases, appropriate debridement with antibiotic therapy constitutes the preferred regimen of treatment.

Slight malunion of nasal fractures is common after closed reduction, since the exact anatomic position of the fragments can be difficult to detect by palpation alone, especially in the presence of edema. Residual deviation also occurs owing to release of "interlocked stresses" (Fry, 1966, 1967) following fracture of the cartilage. If troublesome, the resulting external deformities may require reconstructive rhinoplasty.

Treatment of a nasoethmoido-orbital fracture as a nasal fracture will produce a severe deformity. *It is essential that these fractures be excluded on the initial examination.* Treatment of a nasoethmoido-orbital fracture always requires an open reduction technique.

Fractures of the Zygoma

The zygomatic bone is a major buttress of the midfacial skeleton. It forms the malar eminence and gives prominence to the cheek area (Fig. 27–153). More important, it forms the lateral portion of the orbit and a major portion of the inferior orbit. The zygomatic bone is commonly called the malar bone and has a quadrilateral shape with frontal, maxillary, temporal (arch), and orbital processes. The zygomatic bone articulates with the external angular process of the frontal bone superiorly, with the maxilla in the medial orbit, with the temporal bone (arch) adjacent to the ear, and with the greater wing of the sphenoid in the lateral orbit. On its outer surface, it is convex and forms the malar eminence. On its inner surface, it is concave and participates in the formation of the temporal fossa. The bone has its broadest and strongest attachment with the frontal bone and maxilla. Thinner and weaker attachments occur with the sphenoid and the zygomatic arch. The zygoma forms the greater portion of the lateral floor and lateral wall of the orbit. In most skulls, the zygoma forms the lateral and superior wall of the maxillary sinus. This area may be partially pneumatized with air cells connecting with the maxillary sinus. The bone furnishes attachments for the masseter, temporalis, zygomaticus,

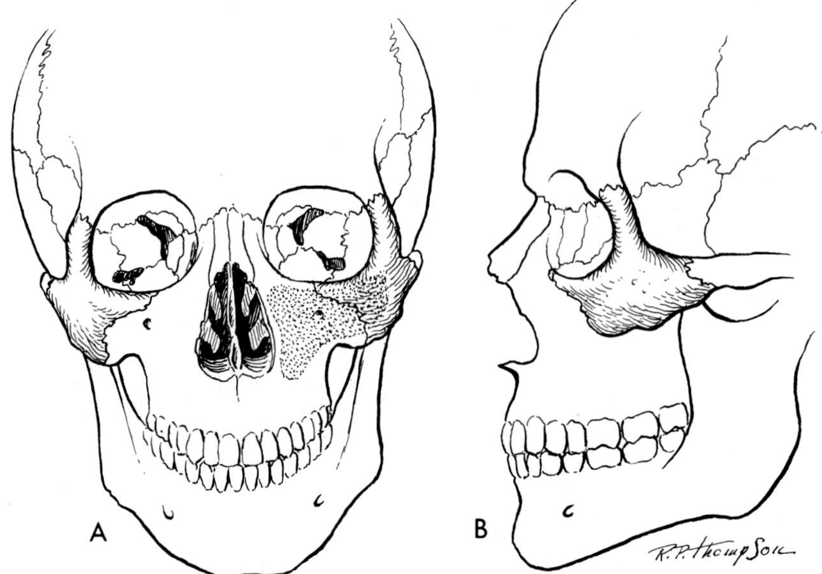

Figure 27–153. The zygoma and its articulating bones. *A*, The zygoma articulates with the frontal, sphenoid, and temporal bones and the maxilla. The dots show the portion of the zygoma and the maxilla occupied by the maxillary sinus. *B*, Lateral view of the zygoma. (From Kazanjian and Converse.)

and zygomatic head of the quadratus labii superioris muscles. The zygomaticotemporal and zygomaticofacial nerves pass through small foramina in the zygoma to innervate the soft tissues over the malar eminence and in the region of the zygomaticofrontal junction.

SURGICAL PATHOLOGY

The zygoma, although a sturdy bone, is frequently injured because of its prominent lateral location (Nysingh, 1960; Ellis, Attar, and Moos, 1985). Moderately severe blows are absorbed by the bone in its buttressing attachments. Severe blows, such as from a fall or a fist, may cause separation of the zygoma at its articulating surfaces. It is usually separated and displaced in a downward, medial, and posterior direction. The direction of displacement, however, varies with the direction of the injuring force and with the pull of the muscles, such as the masseter. The zygoma may be shattered, resulting in extensive comminution of the body of the zygoma and its attachments, as well as separation at the suture lines with the frontal bone, maxilla, and maxillary alveolus.

The zygoma is the principal buttressing bone between the maxilla and the cranium. Fractures usually involve the orbital rim, resulting in hematoma or extravasation of blood into the tissue near the lateral canthus. A periorbital and subconjunctival hematoma is the most accurate sign of an orbital fracture, which often includes a fracture of the zygoma (Fig. 27–154). Direct lateral force may result in fractures of the temporal portion of the zygoma and the zygomatic process of the temporal bone, which together make up the zygomatic arch. The latter may be fractured in the absence of a fracture of the remainder of the zygoma (Fig. 27–155). Medial displacement of the isolated arch fracture is usually observed, and if the displacement is sufficient the arch may impinge against the temporal muscle and the coronoid process of the mandible (Fig. 27–156). This may cause a restriction of mandibular motion. With lesser injuries, the swelling and bruising in this area often temporarily impair motion of the mandible or restoration of full intercuspation with regard to occlusion. Difficulty or inability to open the mouth because of interference with the forward and downward movement of the coronoid process may occur from either soft tissue swelling or bone obstruction. Accurate CT examination will disclose the nature of the problem. Fragments of bone driven through the temporal muscle may make contact with the coronoid process and precipitate the formation of a fibrous or

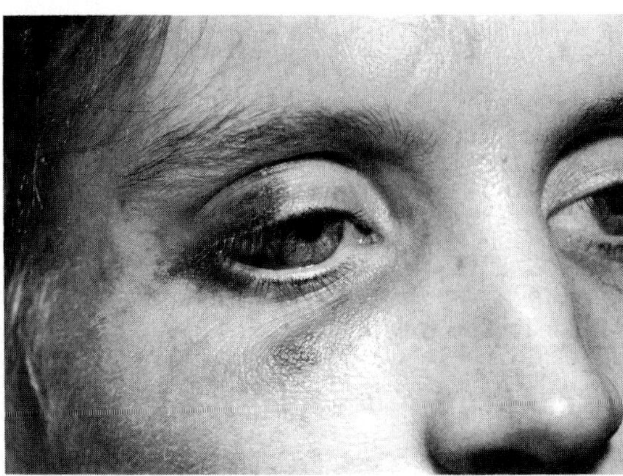

Figure 27–154. The combination of a palpebral and subconjunctival hematoma is suggestive of a fracture somewhere within the orbit. There is frequently a zygomatic fracture.

fibrosseous ankylosis, necessitating excision of the coronoid process as a secondary procedure.

Fracture-dislocation of the zygoma with sufficient displacement to impinge on the coronoid process requires a backward dislocation (see Fig. 27–156). Fracture-dislocation of the zygoma frequently results in separation at the zygomaticofrontal suture line, which is palpable through the skin over the upper and lateral margin of the orbit (Fig. 27–157). A steplike deformity at the infraorbital margin can often be palpated (Fig. 27–158). The lateral and superior walls of the maxillary sinuses are involved in fractures of the zygoma, and the resulting tear of the maxillary sinus lining results in accumulation of blood within the sinus with unilateral epistaxis, which usually clears after a short time. The lateral canthal mechanism is attached to Whitnall's tubercle approximately 10 mm below the zygomaticofrontal suture. When the zygoma is displaced inferiorly, the lateral attachment of the eyelids is also inferiorly displaced, giving rise to the visible deformity of an antimongoloid slant to the palpebral fissure (Fig. 27–159). The globe often participates in this displacement with an inferior position after fracture-dislocation. The displacement of the orbital floor in addition to displacement of the ligaments supporting the orbital soft tissue and globe allows the orbital dystopia (Mathog, Archer, and Nesi, 1986). The septum orbitale, which attaches to the inferior orbital rim, is displaced following zygomatic fracture. The lower eyelid may be shortened and displaced in reference to its position with the globe. Dysfunction of the extraocular muscles may be noted as a result of disruption of the floor and lateral portion of the orbit (Barclay, 1958, 1960, 1963). The mechanism is usually contusion. Displacement of the globe and orbital contents may also occur as a result of downward displacement of the suspensory ligament of Lockwood, which forms an inferior "sling" for the globe and orbital contents (Manson and associates, 1986a,b). Lockwood's ligament attaches to the lateral wall of the orbit adjacent to Whitnall's ligament. Fragmentation of the bony orbital floor may disrupt the continuity of the suspensory ligaments of the globe and orbit, and orbital fat may be extruded from the intra-

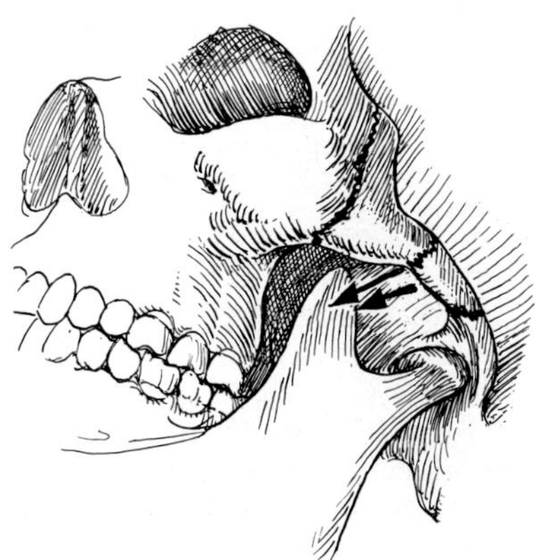

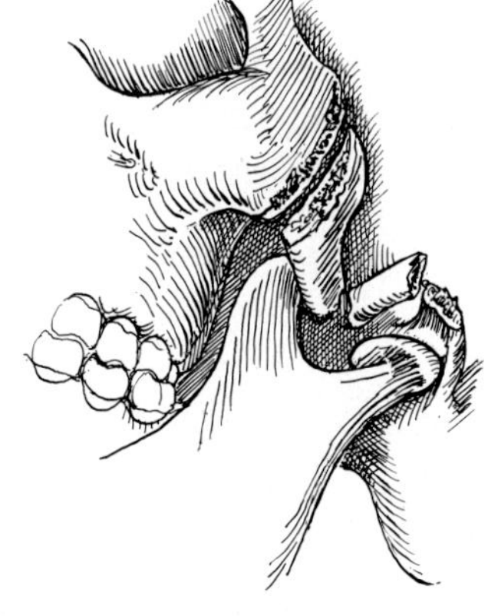

Figure 27–155. Fracture of the zygomatic arch with medial displacement against the coronoid process of the mandible, limiting mandibular motion.

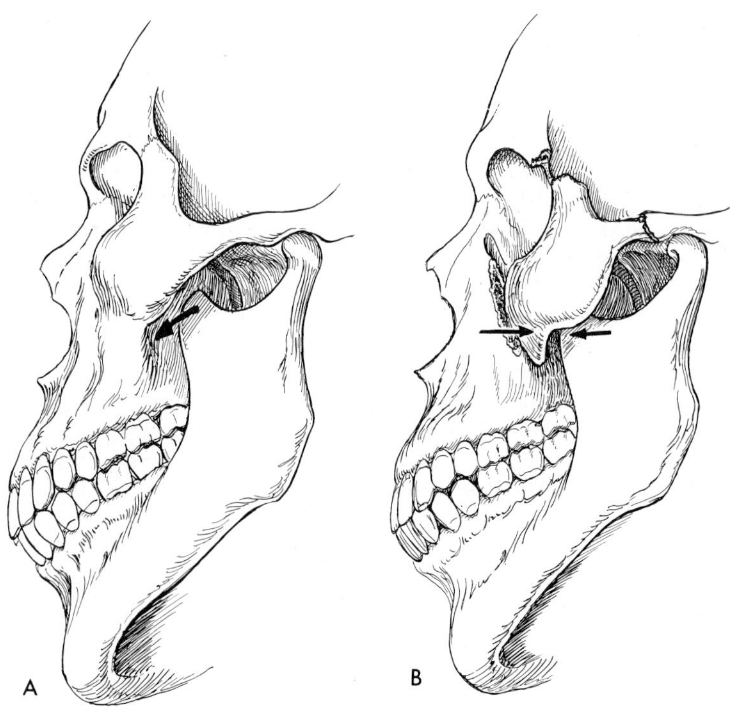

Figure 27–156. *A*, The intimate anatomic relationship between the zygoma and coronoid process. *B*, If the fractured zygoma is displaced backward sufficiently to impinge on the coronoid process, movement of the mandible is impaired.

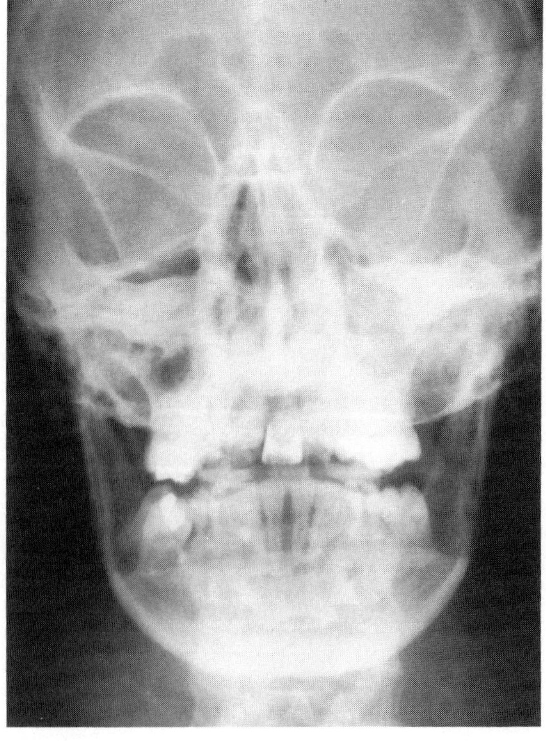

Figure 27–157. Markedly displaced zygomatic fracture. There is also a fracture of the external angular process of the frontal bone at the zygomaticofrontal suture.

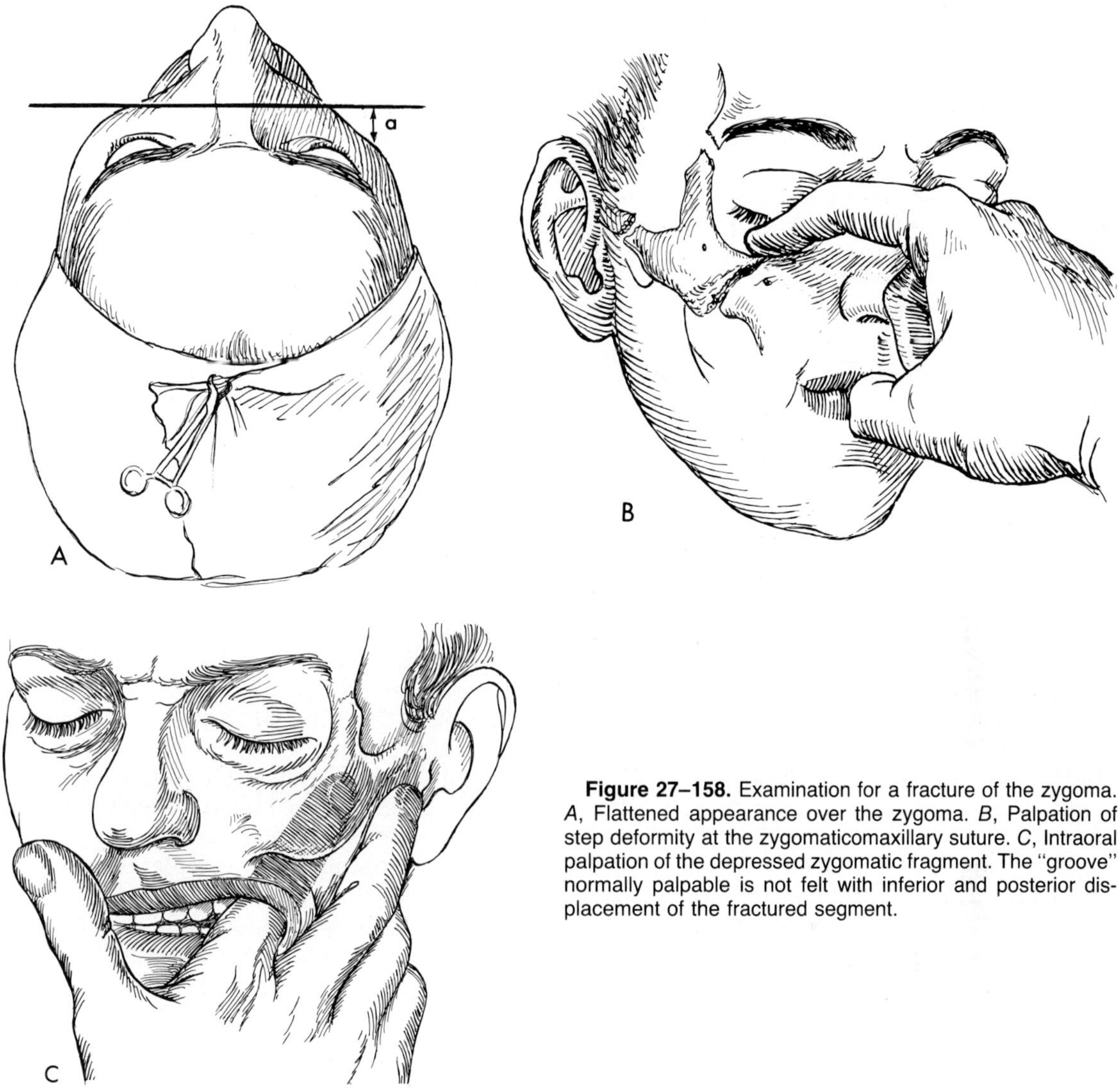

Figure 27–158. Examination for a fracture of the zygoma. *A*, Flattened appearance over the zygoma. *B*, Palpation of step deformity at the zygomaticomaxillary suture. *C*, Intraoral palpation of the depressed zygomatic fragment. The "groove" normally palpable is not felt with inferior and posterior displacement of the fractured segment.

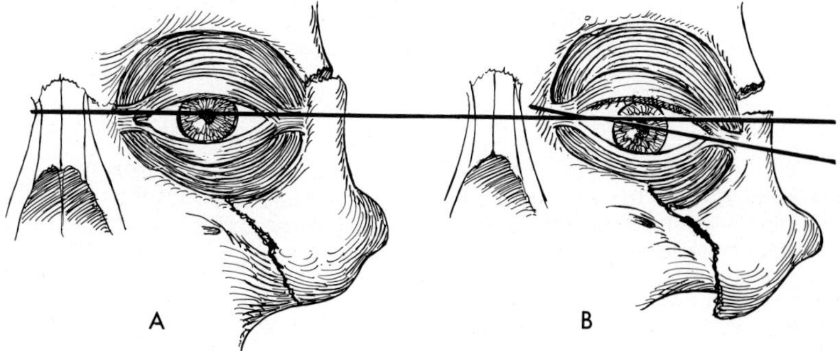

Figure 27–159. When the frontal process of the zygoma is depressed downward, the lateral canthal mechanism and the canthus of the eye follow. *A*, Normal position of the lateral canthus and a fracture without displacement. *B*, Downward displacement of the globe and lateral canthus as a result of frontozygomatic separation and downward displacement of the zygoma and the floor of the orbit.

muscular cone, herniating into the maxillary sinus, where it may become incarcerated between fractured bone segments or attached to sinus tissues by adhesion. Although double vision is usually transient in uncomplicated fractures of the zygoma (which always involve the orbital floor), it may persist when the fracture is more extensive, especially if the fracture extends to comminute the whole inferior orbital floor.

The orbital portion of the fracture is also complicated by fractures of the inferior rim of the orbit. Frequently a small medial fragment of the maxilla is fractured adjacent to its junction with the zygoma. The rim fractures result in instability of the rim with inferior and posterior displacement. The orbital septum, attached to the orbital rim, is also displaced downward and backward. This creates a downward pull on the lower eyelid, which has a tendency to eversion, resulting in further anatomic derangement produced by the fracture.

The infraorbital nerve (Fig. 27–160) travels in the floor of the orbit. In the posterior portion of the orbit, the nerve is in a groove, and in the anterior portion of the orbit, it is located in a canal. Adjacent to the orbital rim, the canal turns downward and exits approximately 10 mm from the upper edge of the orbital rim in a line parallel to the medial margin of the cornea when the eye is in straightforward gaze. The infraorbital nerve is often involved in fractures, since the canal and groove represent a weak portion of bone. Laceration of the nerve in the canal or crushing by impaction of bone fragments may result in permanent anesthesia. The nerve is frequently contused and although temporary symptoms of infraorbital nerve hypoesthesia are present, they usually disappear progressively. After zygomatic fracture, sensory disturbances of a more minimal nature have been detected in up to 40 per cent of patients (Yanagisawa, 1973; Altonen, Kohonen, and Dickhoff, 1976; Nordgaard, 1976; Tajima, 1977; Larsen and Thomsen, 1978). Persistent anesthesia following fracture (Yanagisawa, 1973; Altonen, Kohonen, and Dickhoff, 1976) may represent an indication for exploration and decompression of the infraorbital nerve with neurolysis to free it from scar tissue. The nerve enters the pterygoid space through the back of the orbit adjacent to the posterior aspect of the inferior orbital fissure.

Knight and North (1961) proposed a classification of fractures of the zygoma based on the anatomic displacement created by the fracture. This classification, which has been used for planning the efficacy of closed reduction treatments (Gillies, Kilner, and Stone, 1927), is presented for completeness; however, the usual surgical practice currently is to explore fully the zygoma and its articular processes to confirm direct anatomic alignment.

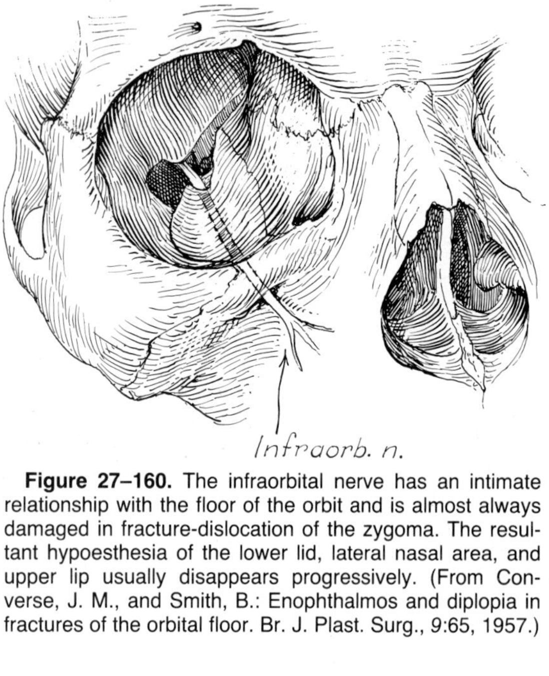

Figure 27–160. The infraorbital nerve has an intimate relationship with the floor of the orbit and is almost always damaged in fracture-dislocation of the zygoma. The resultant hypoesthesia of the lower lid, lateral nasal area, and upper lip usually disappears progressively. (From Converse, J. M., and Smith, B.: Enophthalmos and diplopia in fractures of the orbital floor. Br. J. Plast. Surg., *9*:65, 1957.)

Knight and North Classification

Group I. No significant displacement; fractures visible on roentgenogram, but fragments remain in line: 6 per cent.

Group II. Arch fractures; inward buckling of the arch; no orbital or antral involvement: 10 per cent.

Group III. Unrotated body fractures; downward and inward displacement, but no rotation: 33 per cent.

Group IV. Medially rotated body fractures; downward, inward, and backward displacement with medial rotation: 11 per cent.

Group V. Laterally rotated body fractures; downward, backward, and medial displacement with lateral rotation of the zygoma: 22 per cent.

Group VI. Includes all cases in which additional fracture lines cross the main fragment: 18 per cent.

DIAGNOSIS OF FRACTURES OF ZYGOMA

A history of the injury can provide an indication of the direction and magnitude of force. Such information may be helpful in arriving at a diagnosis, but the main findings are identified on clinical examination. Fractures of the zygoma may result from altercations, such as a fist striking the malar eminence, or from a fall against a hard object, again striking the malar prominence. Zygomatic fractures may result from shattering wounds, such as those produced by automobile accidents.

Fractures of the zygoma, with the exclusion of fractures of the arch, are invariably accompanied by periorbital ecchymosis, edema, and hematoma. The ecchymosis is also present in the subconjunctival and scleral areas. Swelling of the face and cheek is variable. With direct blows to the cheek, physical findings may be more difficult to elicit because swelling obscures inspection of the globe after several hours (Karlan and Cassisi, 1979). The lateral canthal ligament may be displaced, producing a downward slant to the palpebral fissure (antimongoloid slant) (see Fig. 27–159). Retraction of the lower lid may be observed because of the same mechanism. If the orbital floor is lowered, the globe may follow the downward displacement, producing, on resolution of the swelling, a deeply sunken upper lid. Unilateral epistaxis occurs on the involved side, indicating a fracture in the maxillary sinus. The patient may demonstrate a malocclusion or difficulty in moving the lower jaw because of swelling about the coronoid process of the mandible, or because of direct mechanical interference with coronoid excursion. He may complain of pain on movement of the mouth and may demonstrate only a short distance of mandibular movement.

Hypoesthesia or anesthesia of the ipsilateral upper lip, eyelid, medial cheek, and lateral nose is almost always present in zygomatic fractures requiring reduction. Depending on the extent of involvement within the orbit, double vision may be noted.

Palpation of the zygoma may be helpful in documenting the degree of displacement (Karlan and Cassisi, 1979). With the patient seated or lying in a semirecumbent position, the inferior orbital rim on both sides is palpated and compared (Fig. 27–161). Similarly, the zygomaticofrontal suture should be palpated, as well as the external angular process of the frontal bone. The malar arch should be palpated and compared. Viewed from above, a finger resting on the malar eminence can compare malar prominence. Step or level discrepancies may be palpated in the inferior orbital rim. The medial portion of the inferior orbital rim displays a small fractured segment medial to the zygoma fracture extending to the area of the lacrimal fossa. Hematoma is often visible in the mouth. Intraoral palpation may demonstrate irregularity or a narrowing of the space between the malar eminence and the maxilla. The groove normally present between the undersurface of the zygoma and the maxilla may be narrow or absent if the zygoma is displaced downward, medially, and posteriorly.

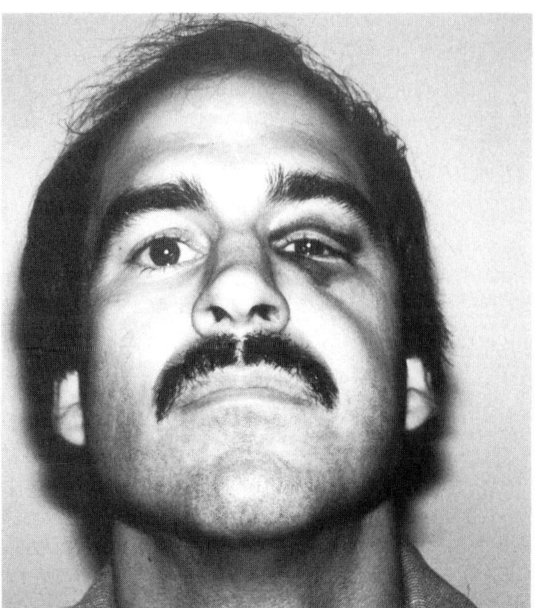

Figure 27–161. Posterior displacement of the malar eminence is seen from the worm's eye position. Note the step deformity of the inferior orbital rim.

Roentgenographic Evaluation. Confirmation of a zygomatic fracture may be documented by plain films, but a CT scan is required to demonstrate the intraorbital component accurately. The usual findings after zygomatic fracture are dysjunction at the zygomaticofrontal, zygomaticomaxillary, and zygomaticotemporal suture lines, as well as the lateral wall of the antrum. The maxillary sinus may be opaque because of the presence of blood. Depression of the orbital floor may be observed. The Waters view is the single best plain film; it demonstrates the fracture

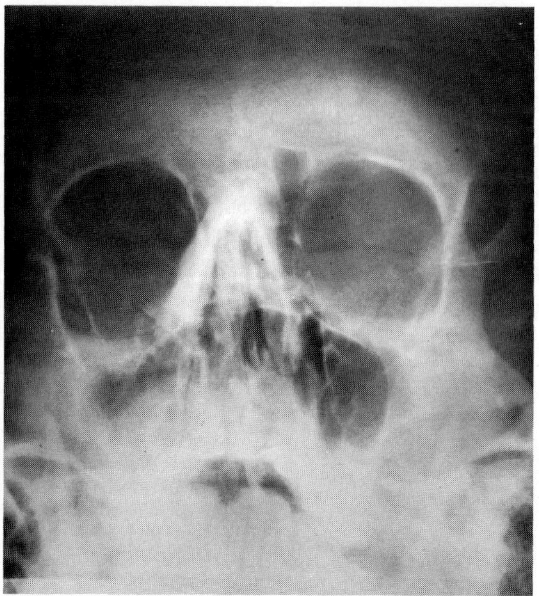

Figure 27–162. Fracture-dislocation of the zygoma showing inferior and posterior displacement (Waters view).

through the inferior orbital rim (Fig. 27–162) and zygomatic arch and lateral wall of the maxillary sinus. Displacement at the zygomaticofrontal suture can be accurately assessed only with a Caldwell radiogram (see Fig. 27–157). The zygomatic arches as well as the forward projection of the zygoma can be documented in the submentovertex view or by the Titterington position, the semiaxial superoinferior projection (see Fig. 27–27).

A CT examination accurately documents displacement of the zygoma, the degree of involvement of the orbital floor, and the status of the soft tissue contents of the orbit (Fig. 27–163). These views may be obtained in the axial or coronal plane and may also be helpful postoperatively (Fig. 27–164). Tomographic examination has been replaced by computed tomography.

TREATMENT OF FRACTURES OF ZYGOMA

In the past, the degree of fragmentation and the direction and amount of displacement influenced the operative management of fractures of the zygoma. Numerous approaches for reduction and fixation of zygomatic fractures have been described. Fixation was obtained by impaction against the adjacent articulating bones, by support from normal muscle and fascial attachments, by the use of packing, by cranial fixation appliances, or by direct fixation with interosseous wires. A plate and screw technique is now utilized.

Formerly, closed reduction techniques were employed for most zygomatic fracture reductions. In many cases of simple fracture without comminution in which the displacement involved areas other than the zygomaticofrontal junction, elevators were placed beneath the malar eminence, and the zygoma was "popped" back into position. The stability of this type of reduction depended on the integrity of periosteal attachments at all areas, but principally on "greensticking" at the zygomaticofrontal suture and the impaction against adjacent articulating bones such as the maxilla at the inferior orbital rim. Displacement at the zygomaticofrontal suture (Larsen and Thomsen, 1978), late presentation of the patient, and comminution of the zygoma were variables that ensured a poor result from closed reduction techniques. Disappointment and frustration in the management of the zygomatic fractures have been widely experienced after the use of closed methods. Complications include residual double vision, malunion, and deformity, all of which indicated either incomplete reduction or displacement following initial reduction (Fig. 27–165). It was obvious either that the reduction had been ineffective or that recurrent dislocation of the fracture occurred in the postoperative period. A careful study of the problem indicated that the fracture-dislocation was usually more severe than it had appeared from radiologic and clinical evaluation. It was difficult to document the type of displacement accurately because edema obscured the true condition and proper radiographs were often difficult to obtain. In the early stages, the intraorbital edema gave support to the globe. However, after the edema subsided, displacement of the globe and double vision would present. Blow-out fractures of the orbital floor frequently accompany zygomatic fractures, and these were often overlooked. The action of the masseter muscle resulted in displacement of the zygoma, as it has broad attachments to the malar eminence and arch.

Dingman (Dingman and Alling, 1954; Dingman and Natvig, 1964) investigated these problems by performing a clinical evaluation. In fractures of the zygoma, he first elevated them into what appeared to be a satisfactory position (closed reduction). The

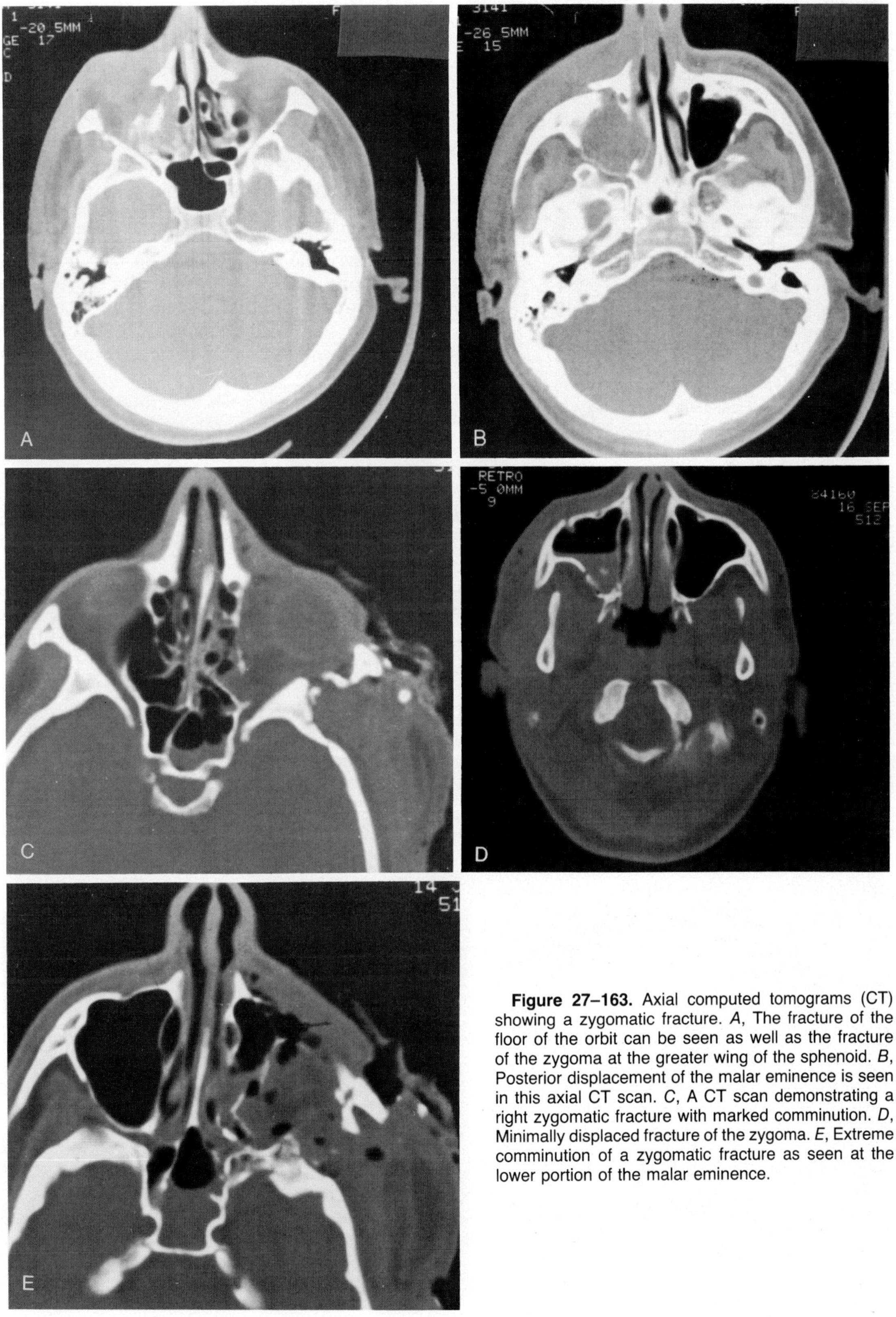

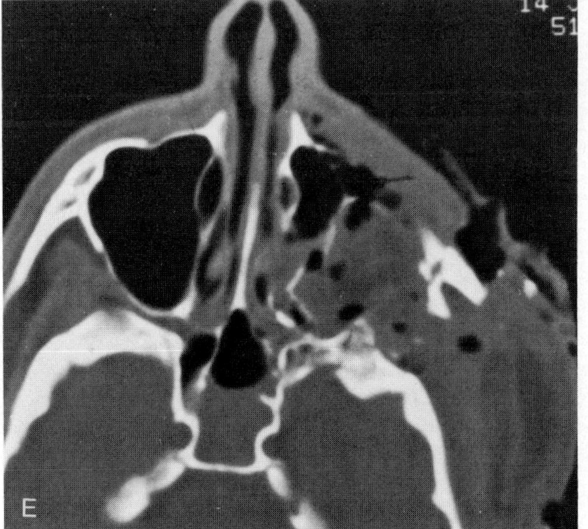

Figure 27–163. Axial computed tomograms (CT) showing a zygomatic fracture. *A*, The fracture of the floor of the orbit can be seen as well as the fracture of the zygoma at the greater wing of the sphenoid. *B*, Posterior displacement of the malar eminence is seen in this axial CT scan. *C*, A CT scan demonstrating a right zygomatic fracture with marked comminution. *D*, Minimally displaced fracture of the zygoma. *E*, Extreme comminution of a zygomatic fracture as seen at the lower portion of the malar eminence.

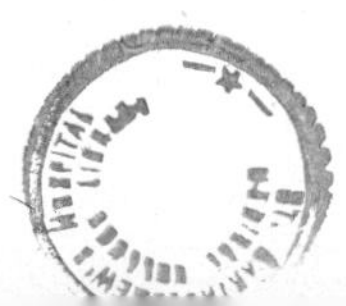

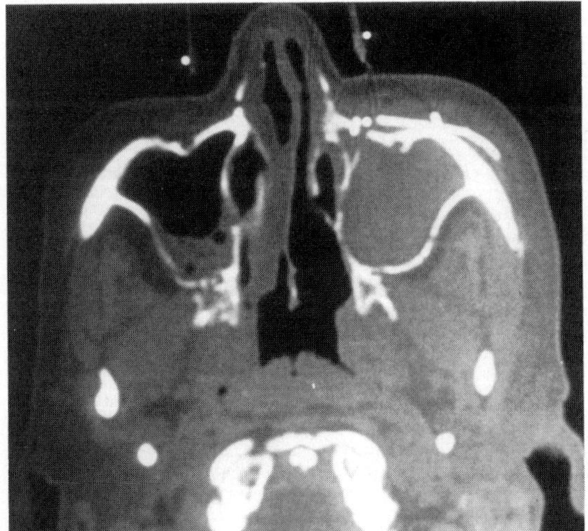

Figure 27–164. Postoperative CT scan demonstrating an onlay bone graft to the malar eminence.

fracture sites were exposed surgically in the zygomaticofrontal suture and zygomaticomaxillary areas. In many instances, the fractures had not actually been reduced adequately or soft tissue was interposed in the fracture sites. Investigation of the orbital floor showed depressed fractures, frequently with herniation of orbital contents into the maxillary sinus. Quite obviously, the fractures were not well addressed by the closed reduction technique. From these clinical studies, Dingman suggested that any significant fracture-dislocation of the zygoma should be treated by exposure of the fractured areas, open reduction, and direct wire fixation (Dingman and Alling, 1954). This method has proved to be the standard treatment resulting in a high degree of satisfaction. Subsequently, a more complete exposure of the fracture sites, including the zygomaticomaxillary buttress, has been provided (Gruss and associates, 1985b; Manson and associates, 1985). Such exposure contributes to the anatomic accuracy of the skeletal alignment. In zygomatic fractures accompanying Le Fort fractures, considerable displacement of the zygoma is often observed with comminution of the arch. Extreme anteroposterior depression of the zygoma can be observed. In these cases, exposure and anatomic reduction of the arch through a coronal incision is helpful in restoring proper anterior projection of the malar eminence. Thus, six points of alignment can be confirmed with craniofacial exposure techniques: the zygomaticofrontal suture, the infraorbital rim, the zygomaticomaxillary buttress, alignment with the greater wing of the sphenoid in the lateral portion of the orbit, the integrity of the orbital floor, and the alignment of the zygomatic arch.

Methods of Reduction

Keen (1909) described an intraoral approach for reduction of fractures of the zygoma. With the cheek retracted, a sharp elevator was passed through the buccal vestibule behind the tuberosity of the zygoma. An incision may be utilized, but a sharp, pointed, sturdy elevator was frequently used simply to puncture the mucosa and place the instrument on the posterior aspect of the malar

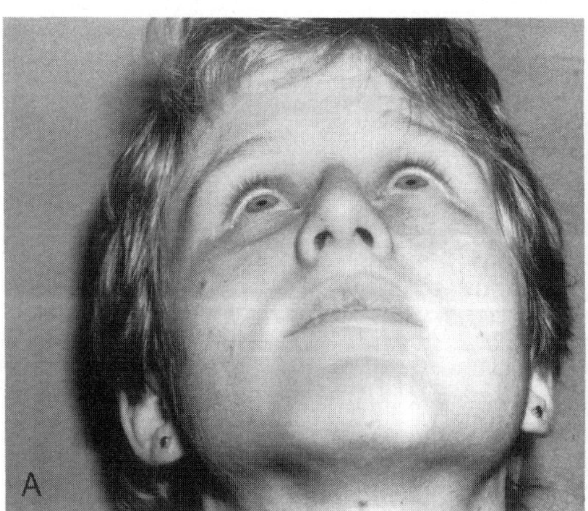

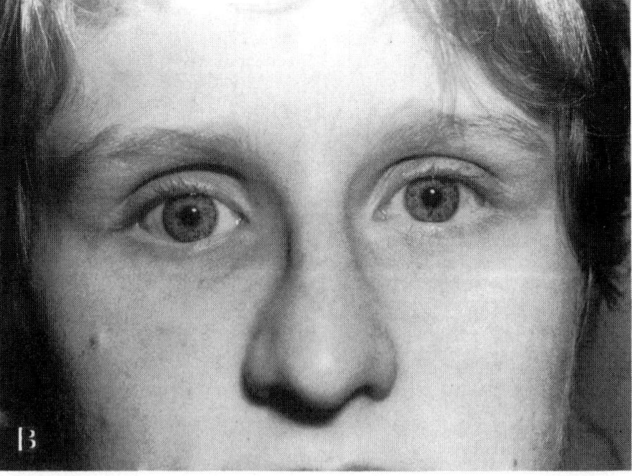

Figure 27–165. *A*, The result of a zygomatic fracture with malunion. The malar eminence is posteriorly displaced and the patient shows enophthalmos. In *B* the patient demonstrates inferior displacement of the globe and lateral canthus, and retrusion of the malar eminence.

eminence. Pressure applied in an upward, forward, and outward direction elevated the zygoma, which "snapped" back into its position and remained in position without fixation.

Reduction Through Maxillary Sinus. Lothrop (1906) employed a maxillary antrostomy as an approach. An elevator was placed under the inferior turbinate and passed by means of a curved trocar into the maxillary sinus. The elevator contacted the posterior wall of the malar eminence. Upward, outward, and superiorly directed force reduced the depressed fractured zygoma. An approach through a Caldwell-Luc antrostomy has also been utilized, again placing an elevator behind the malar eminence. It was emphasized that the elevator should be placed directly behind the malar eminence to avoid introducing the elevator into the orbit inadvertently.

Temporal Approach. A temporal approach for the reduction and fixation of zygomatic fractures was described by Gillies, Kilner, and Stone (1927). This approach was useful and effective, especially for "greensticked" or impacted fractures that demonstrated no displacement at the zygomaticofrontal suture. An incision behind the temporal hairline was employed and dissection accomplished to expose the temporalis muscle. An elevator was placed behind the zygomatic arch or under the malar eminence, depending on the area of reduction required (Fig. 27–166). A small 2 cm incision placed vertically within the temporal hairline healed with an inconspicuous scar. It is emphasized that the elevator had to be placed behind the deepest layers of the temporal fascia, so that it could be inserted beneath the arch and malar eminence (Fig. 27–166). The bone was palpated with one hand to document the reduction, while the other hand guided the elevator into position and corrected the displacement.

Dingman Approach. An incision is made in the lateral brow approximately 1.5 cm in length (Fig. 27–167). Another incision is made in the lower eyelid in either a rim or a subciliary location. Dissection exposes the zygomaticofrontal and zygomaticomaxillary suture lines. A moderately heavy periosteal elevator is passed through the upper incision behind the malar eminence and into the temporal fossa. The elevator is used to control the position of the zygoma and to reduce it

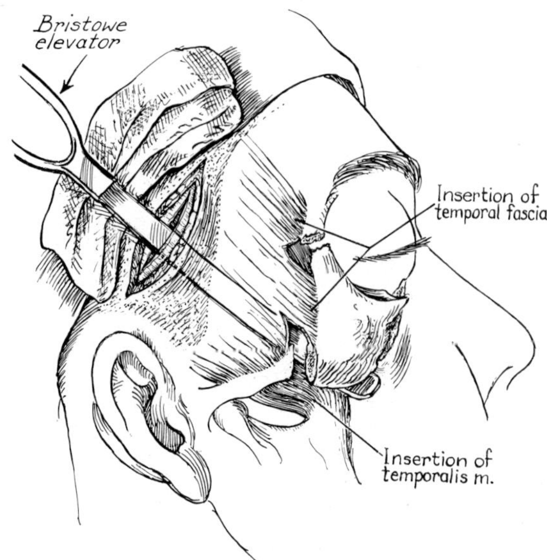

Figure 27–166. The temporal fascia is inserted onto the margin of the zygoma. In order to penetrate the temporal fossa, the elevator must be inserted deep to the temporal fascia. Forces are applied in an upward and forward direction protecting the temporal skull. (From Kazanjian and Converse).

by upward, forward, and outward force. Depending on the displacement of the fracture segments, the bone can be elevated into position. After the reduction of the zygoma, the orbital floor can be explored and any herniation of orbital contents reduced. The defect in the orbital floor is corrected by means of autogenous or alloplastic material.

Dingman and Natvig (1964) recommended that the drill holes be placed through the bone 5 mm to each side of the fracture site. Interosseous wires were utilized to secure the position by means of interfragment wiring.

It should be emphasized that the zygomatic arch fracture is a component of significant zygomatic fractures and can usually be reduced through any one of the approaches described by passing the elevator beneath the arch. Frequently, the heavy fascial and muscular attachments to the arch hold it in relative position unless displacement or comminution has been extreme. In these cases an open reduction through a coronal incision is required.

Comminuted Fractures of Zygoma

Violent injury to the zygoma results in shattering of the bone into multiple fragments. The approaches described above are

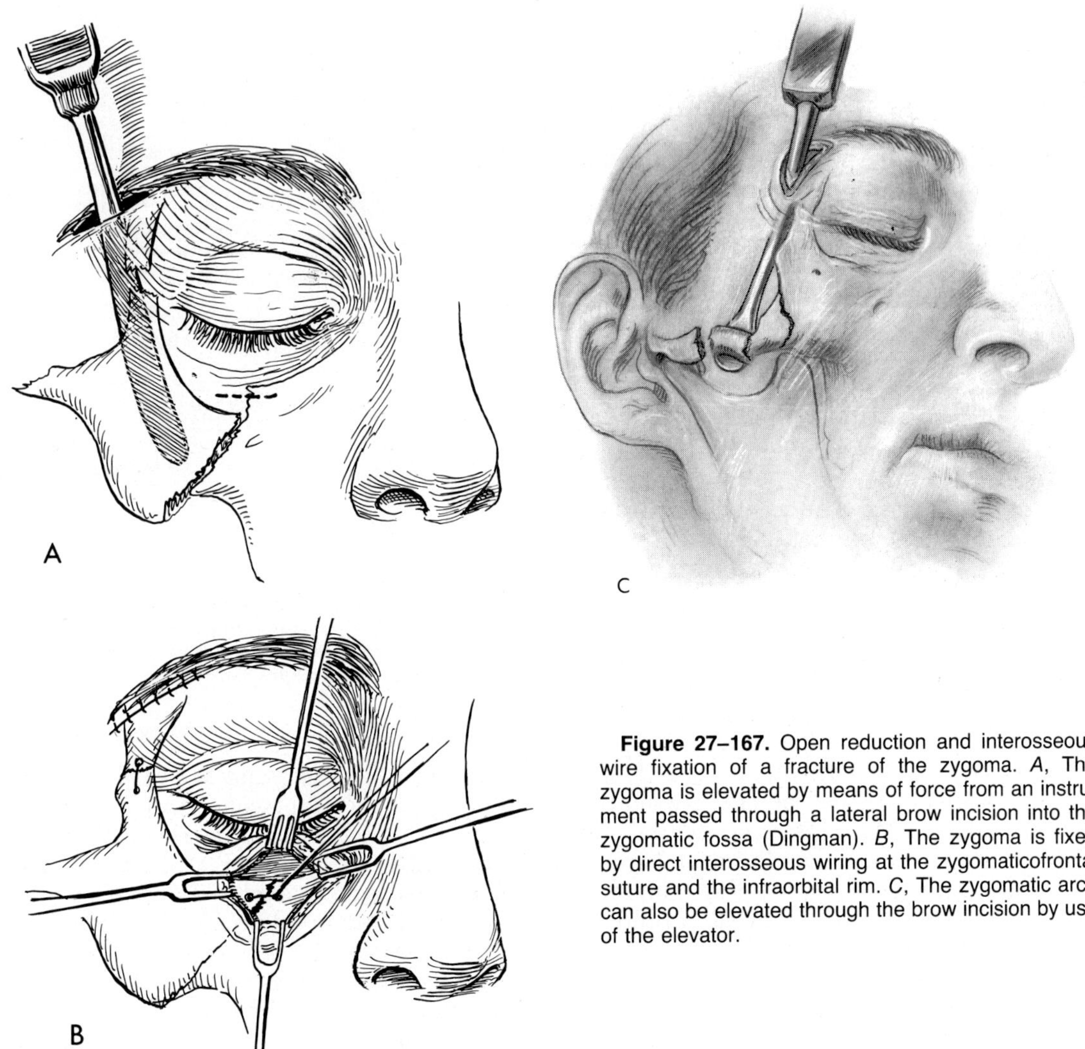

Figure 27–167. Open reduction and interosseous wire fixation of a fracture of the zygoma. *A*, The zygoma is elevated by means of force from an instrument passed through a lateral brow incision into the zygomatic fossa (Dingman). *B*, The zygoma is fixed by direct interosseous wiring at the zygomaticofrontal suture and the infraorbital rim. *C*, The zygomatic arch can also be elevated through the brow incision by use of the elevator.

unsatisfactory for fractures other than simple noncomminuted injuries. The method of management of these types of fracture must include a thorough visualization of the body and frontal and maxillary processes of the zygoma. The zygomaticomaxillary buttress is restored by direct (intraoral) interfragment wiring (Fig. 27–168) or plate and screw fixation. The entire zygoma can be exposed with a subciliary incision and skin-muscle flap (Fig. 27–169). The lateral canthal ligament must be dissected to allow visualization of the zygomaticofrontal suture. The lateral wall of the orbit can be inspected, including the alignment with the greater wing of the sphenoid. The orbital floor can also be dissected and its integrity confirmed.

Packing the Maxillary Sinus. The maxillary sinus approach to comminuted fractures of the zygoma should never be utilized alone. It involved exposure of the anterior maxilla and bone reduction through an intraoral incision. Further support was obtained by packing the maxillary sinus, which acted to restore the position of the orbital floor and the anterior projection of the malar eminence. The maxillary sinus packing was removed after one to three weeks. It should be emphasized that manipulation of the orbital floor through the maxillary sinus alone is dangerous, producing the possibility of damage to the soft tissue contents of the orbit. Packing may be done through a Caldwell-Luc intraoral incision, but only after direct visu-

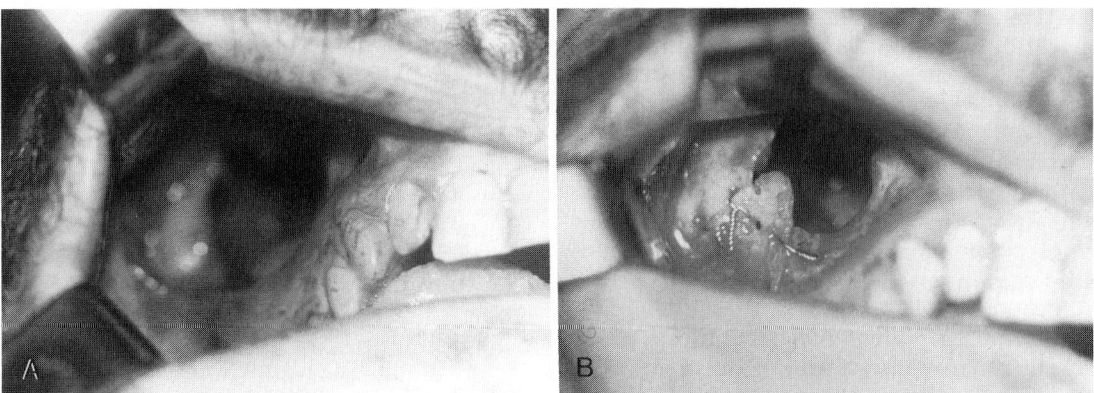

Figure 27–168. Exposure of the zygomaticomaxillary buttress through an intraoral incision. *A*, Intraoral view of the fracture segments. *B*, Interfragment wiring has united the zygomaticomaxillary buttress.

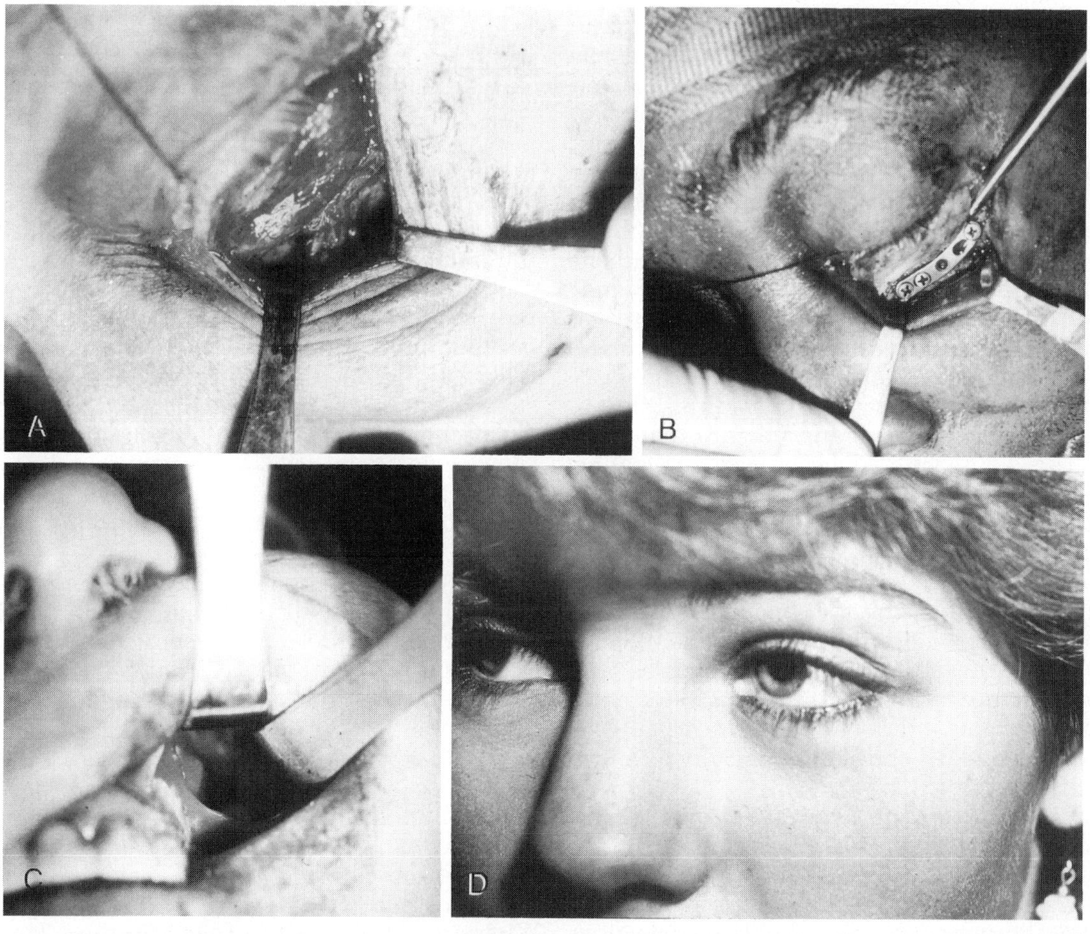

Figure 27–169. Use of a subciliary incision to expose a zygomatic fracture. *A*, Exposure of the orbital floor and anterior face of the zygoma. The infraorbital nerve is seen between the two refractors. *B*, The application of a Luhr plate along the infraorbital rim. *C*, Before application of the plate, alignment was confirmed intraorally with a separate upper gingivobuccal sulcus incision exposing the zygomaticomaxillary buttress. *D*, Result obtained six months after the use of a single subciliary incision for exploration and reduction of a fracture-dislocation of the zygoma with plate and screw technique.

alization of the floor of the orbit through a separate lower eyelid incision. Fragments of the orbital floor can be repositioned and held in position with sinus packing but only under direct vision, protecting the orbital contents.

Intraoral Approach as an Ancillary Point of Stabilization. The proper reduction of displaced zygomatic fractures may be confirmed by intraoral observation of the zygomaticomaxillary buttress (see Fig. 27–168). A mucoperiosteal flap is reflected following a gingival buccal sulcus incision. In this manner, the entire lateral wall of the maxilla is exposed, including the zygomaticomaxillary buttress. The maxilla may be exposed medially to the piriform aperture as required. Dissection progresses superiorly and the malar eminence is also exposed. The infraorbital foramen may be reached. A Kelly clamp may be placed through a Caldwell-Luc exposure or through the fractured site under the malar eminence to elevate the body of the zygoma. An elevator may be passed intraorally underneath the arch if desired. Impacted or partially healed fractures may be dislodged by an elevator or osteotome passed through the line of fracture. The zygomaticomaxillary buttress may be reconstructed using direct wire fixation, spanning any gap with a bone graft (see Fig. 27–168*B*). A bone graft may be "lag screwed" to the upper intact buttress and the maxillary alveolus. Alternatively, a plate and screws can be used to fix this area. Such fixation supports and confirms the remainder of the zygomatic fracture reduction.

This approach should be used in conjunction with a subciliary skin-muscle flap exposure (see Fig. 27–169). The intraoral approach alone is not an effective method because the entire fracture is not visualized, specifically the orbital component. Blindness is a risk if the orbital component is reduced with a Caldwell-Luc exposure alone. The upper fracture sites, i.e., the zygomaticofrontal junction and inferior orbital rim, should be exposed and realigned anatomically as a first maneuver.

Pin Fixation of Zygoma. Brown, Fryer, and McDowell (1949) devised a technique using one or more stainless steel pins (Kirschner wire or Steinmann pin) for fixation. Through the use of a hand-driven or electric drill, stainless steel pins were driven through the zygoma in a transverse or oblique direction and into the bones of the maxilla or zygoma on the contralateral side, care being taken to avoid the contralateral orbit. The pins are cut at skin level or in the mouth and left in for a period of four weeks during which the fracture fragments consolidate. This technique was often used as a closed reduction technique. Its accuracy is enhanced if the fracture sites are exposed and the zygoma is K-wired (Fig. 27–170). Although effective results have been reported in the hands of experienced surgeons, this technique has been replaced by open reduction and direct wiring or plate and screw fixation. Some advocates of wiring at the infraorbital rim and zygomaticofrontal suture area have used an additional K-wire in the body of the zygoma and passed it through the contralateral maxilla to provide a third point of fixation and stabilize unstable zygomatic fractures. The technique has its greatest use in cases with bone loss in which plate and screw fixation is not utilized. Complications in the form of scars, osteomyelitis, malunion, nonunion, and facial deformity have been reported after the use of this method by inexperienced operators.

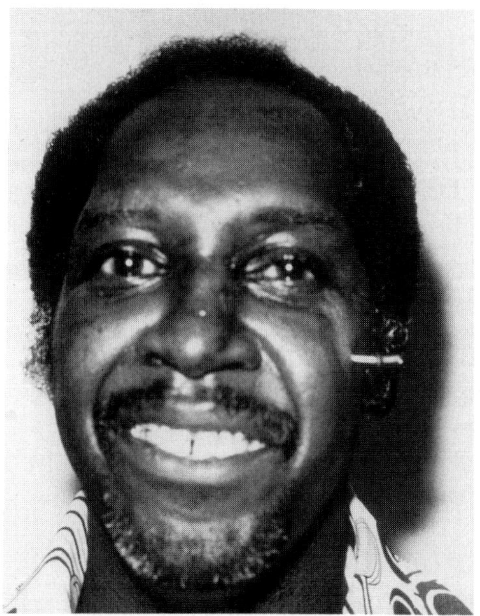

Figure 27–170. The use of a K-wire for zygomatic stabilization following zygomatic reduction. Note that the K-wire exits the left cheek region.

Open Reduction with Interfragment Wiring or Plate and Screw Fixation. This technique is effective in obtaining accurate reduction and positive fixation. Absolute anatomic accuracy may be achieved and the zygomaticofrontal suture and infraorbital rim

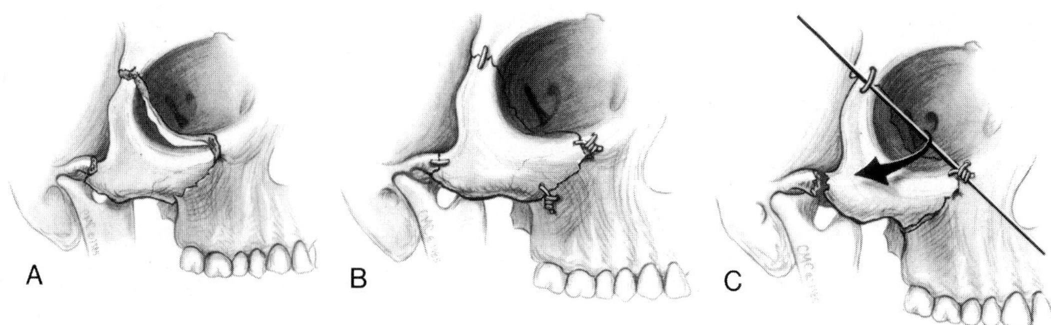

Figure 27–171. *A*, The typical zygomatic fracture is displaced at multiple areas where it articulates with the remainder of the craniofacial skeleton. Displacement is observed at the zygomaticofrontal suture and the greater wing of the sphenoid laterally. The floor of the orbit may display variable comminution. Displacement is observed in the zygomatic arch and at the junction of the zygoma with the maxillary alveolus (zygomaticomaxillary buttress). *B*, Wiring at the multiple points prevents displacement. Currently, plate fixation is preferred. *C*, After interfragment wiring of the orbital rim alone, the zygoma may not be stable. It may display inward and posterior displacement because of the pull of the masseter muscle that attaches to the zygomatic arch and malar eminence. Posterior displacement of the malar eminence is seen impinging on the coronoid process of the mandible. This problem is obviated by wiring (or plating) across the zygomaticomaxillary buttress.

are exposed through a single subciliary skin-muscle flap incision. The body of the zygoma is exposed and any fractures in the medial area of the infraorbital rim can also be approached. The entire orbit (inferior, lateral, and lower portion of the medial orbit) may be exposed and inspected through this single incision. After anatomic realignment of the zygomaticofrontal suture, the infraorbital rim and the lateral orbit are inspected to ensure alignment of the zygoma with the greater wing of the sphenoid. The floor is reconstructed anatomically either by positioning of the bone fragments, by the use of a small plastic plate, or by a form fitted bone graft from the skull, rib, or iliac crest (Fig. 27–171). Alignment of the zygomaticomaxillary buttress area is confirmed intraorally. Depending on the extent of arch displacement, these maneuvers often will have already reduced the arch. In cases of medial displacement of the arch, an elevation is accomplished with a "closed" reduction. An elevator is placed through a Gillies approach (see Fig. 27–166) and the arch is reduced. A towel clamp can also be placed about the arch and the arch "pulled" into position. After reduction of the principal fragments, small drill holes are placed through the margins of the bone adjacent to the fracture sites, at a distance of 4 to 5 mm from the site; 26 or 28 gauge stainless steel wire is used to secure the fragments with interfragment wiring technique. A small plate and screws can be used to span the fracture site and provide more positive fixation. Two screws per fragment provide solid immobilization (Figs. 27–172, 27–173). If the infraorbital rim is comminuted, the bone fragments are wired together sequentially before plating.

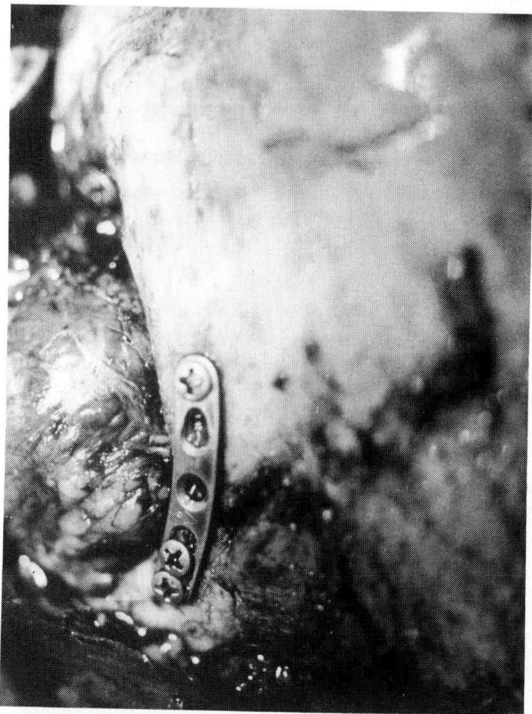

Figure 27–172. The application of a Luhr plate at the zygomaticofrontal suture. Another screw is about to be placed in the external angular process of the frontal bone. At least two screws per fragment are required for stability.

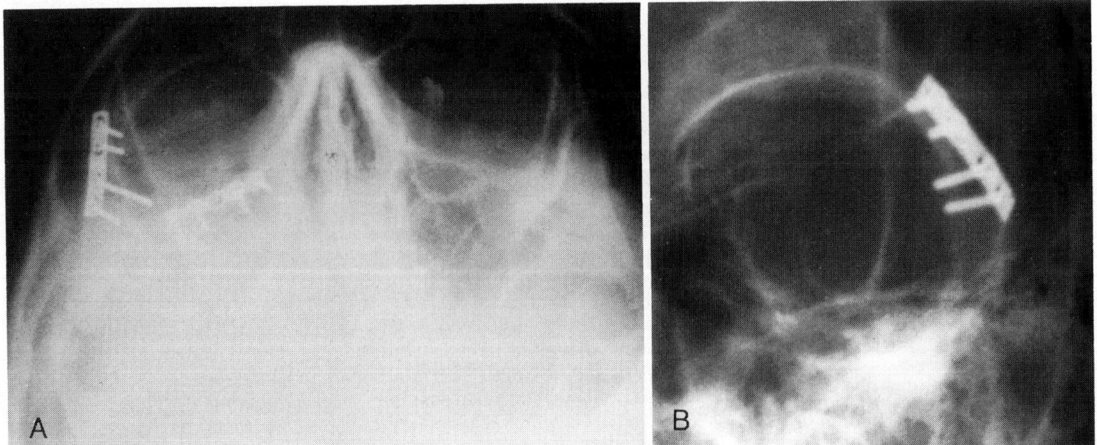

Figure 27–173. *A*, Plate and screw fixation of a zygomatic fracture at the frontozygomatic suture and the infraorbital rim. Alignment was obtained by visualization of all fracture sites, including an intraoral exposure. *B*, The bicortical strong structure of the frontal process of the zygoma allows reasonably secure fixation by the application of a single plate at the zygomaticofrontal suture. The zygoma must be explored, however, in its other articulations to confirm alignment before this reduction. In practice, the author prefers at least two plates, one at the zygomaticofrontal suture and the other at the infraorbital rim following full exposure of all articulations of the zygoma with the remainder of the facial bones.

Compound Comminuted Fractures of Zygoma

Fractures of the zygoma may be compounded intraorally or extraorally when the force is severe enough to cause soft tissue wounds. These wounds may or may not extend to the bone. A thorough inspection of the wound should be made to rule out the presence of foreign bodies, debris, and blood clots. Wood fragments are especially hazardous since they are often driven into soft tissue, a fact not easily perceived at the time of wound inspection. Fractured zygomatic fragments are reconstituted by direct multiple interosseous wiring technique (see Fig. 27–171) or plate and screw fixation. Frequently it is helpful to wire the fragments together before stabilizing them with a plate and screws. This maneuver positions them for stable reduction.

Careful cleansing, debridement, and closure of the soft tissues over the comminuted fracture usually result in satisfactory healing. Antibiotics may be used at the discretion of the surgeon and tetanus prophylaxis is indicated in open injuries.

In zygomatic fractures involving the arch that demonstrate the tendency to medial displacement, the segments may be supported after reduction by placing packing under the medial surface of the arch (Natvig, 1962). The fragments are elevated through the Gillies approach; packing is inserted, which is removed after several days; and a protective splint may be applied externally.

Delayed Treatment of Fractures of Zygoma. The best results are obtained when cases are treated relatively early. Consolidation begins to occur in the fracture site within one week and is reasonably well organized at three weeks, at which time it may be difficult to mobilize and reposition the bone. Repositioning may require an osteotomy. The latter can be accomplished by a thorough exposure of the bone to include the zygomaticofrontal area, the infraorbital rim, and the intraoral route as well. The malunited bone is mobilized by osteotomies (Perino, Zide, and Kinnebrew, 1980; Kawamoto, 1982) through the old fracture lines and the area of fibrous/bony ankylosis. After the bone has been mobilized, it should be held with a direct interosseous wiring technique or preferably plate and screw fixation (Fig. 27–174). The masseter muscle may need to be mobilized from the inferior surface of the malar eminence and arch in order to allow the bone to be repositioned. The masseter muscle contracts in length in a state of malreduction.

It must be emphasized that this procedure is performed with direct visualization of *all* fracture sites. A precise exposure of the orbital floor is required. Blind reductions or forceful reductions performed without a precise osteotomy of the fracture sites carry the risk of radiating fractures extending into the

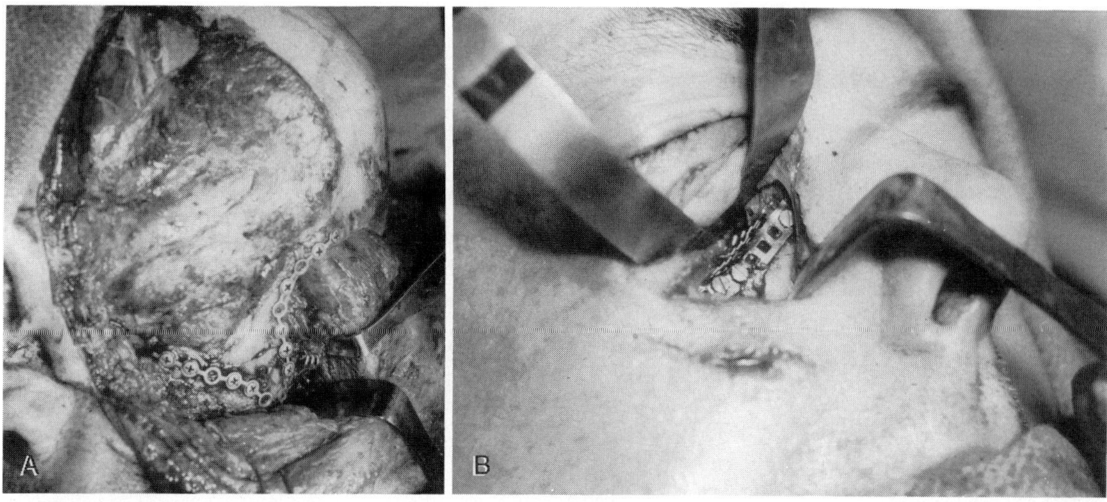

Figure 27–174. A "high energy" zygoma fracture with extreme comminution and depression. Shattering of the malar body and arch was present. *A*, A coronal incision was used to restore the proper projection of the arch by circumferential plating of the orbital rim and arch. *B*, The infraorbital rim and orbital floor are reconstructed with a titanium plate contoured to the proper curvature of the orbit and extending back 35 to 38 mm within the orbit.

apex of the orbit, with subsequent loss of vision.

COMPLICATIONS OF FRACTURES OF ZYGOMA

Zygomatic fractures are occasionally accompanied by complications. Bleeding into the maxillary sinus is usually of short duration. It may be necessary to remove the blood clots from the antrum in order to prevent a sinus infection; however, most clots disintegrate and drain spontaneously without producing infection. Infection in zygomatic fractures is rare and usually follows the compound comminuted fracture in which some debris has been overlooked. Such cases should be managed by debridement of soft tissue and bone, the establishment of drainage, and the administration of antibiotics. Secondary wound closure is performed. Acute exacerbation of a preexisting sinus disease may be a complicating factor. In these cases, a proper opening into the nose should be confirmed by free irrigation of saline into the nose with a Caldwell-Luc exposure, otherwise a persistent oro-antral fistula may be the result. Malfunction of extraocular muscles as a result of damage from fractured segments or floor injury is commonly observed. Several cases of blindness have occurred after malar reduction (Ketchum, Ferris, and Masters, 1976).

Late Complications. The late complications of zygomatic fractures include nonunion, malunion, diplopia, persistent infraorbital nerve anesthesia/hypoesthesia, and chronic maxillary sinusitis (Perino, Zide, and Kinnebrew, 1980). Scarring may result from a malpositioned incision (Fig. 27–175). Ectropion usually resolves spontaneously. Gross downward dislocation of the zygoma may result in diplopia and orbital dystopia (Fig. 27–176). Usually an excess of 5 mm of inferior repositioning is required to produce diplopia. Treatment (Perino, Zide, and Kinnebrew, 1980; Kawamoto, 1982) involves zygomatic mobilization, or osteotomy and bone grafting

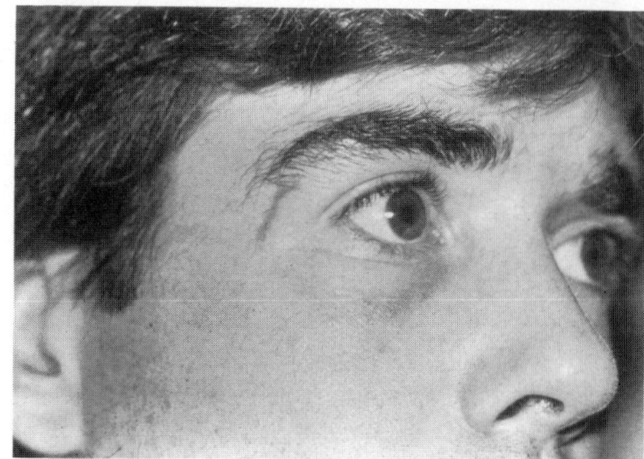

Figure 27–175. Malposition of incisions used for zygomatic fracture reduction. The brow and the subciliary incisions are improperly placed.

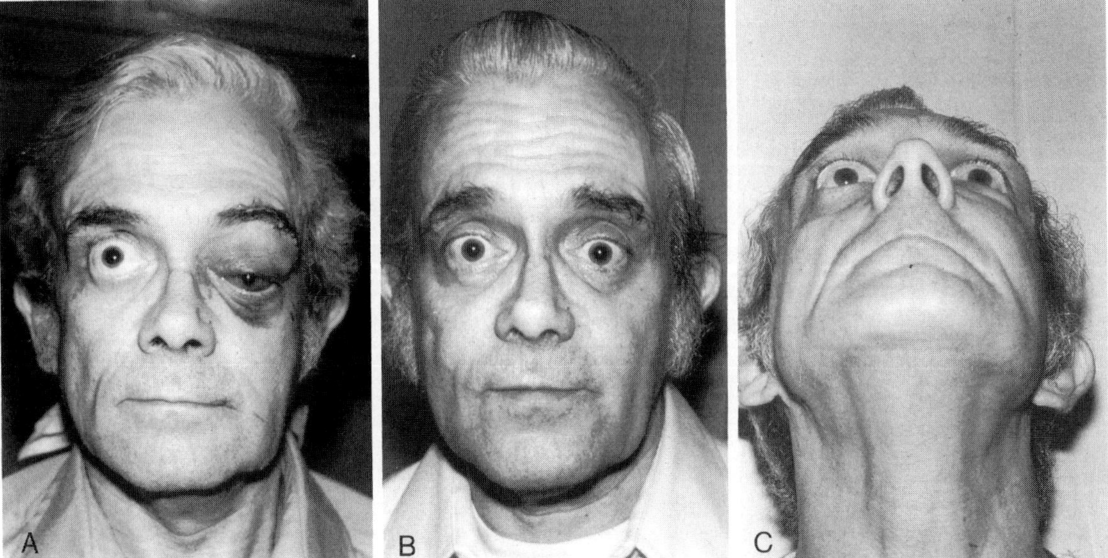

Figure 27–176. Fracture-dislocation of the zygoma with severe comminution of the orbit *(A)*. *B, C,* Result obtained after interfragment wiring and bone grafting.

to restore the proper position of the eye. Infection is rare (Fig. 27–177) and responds to simple drainage. Usually a preexisting maxillary sinusitis is responsible.

The late complications result mainly from malposition (Perino, Zide, and Kinnebrew, 1980). In these cases, correction is obtained either by osteotomy or by onlay bone grafts. In the case of osteotomy, the zygoma should be directly aligned and plate and screw fixation utilized. Onlay bone or cartilage grafts are usually necessary to supplement the result, overcoming the loss of bone that occurs in displaced fractures.

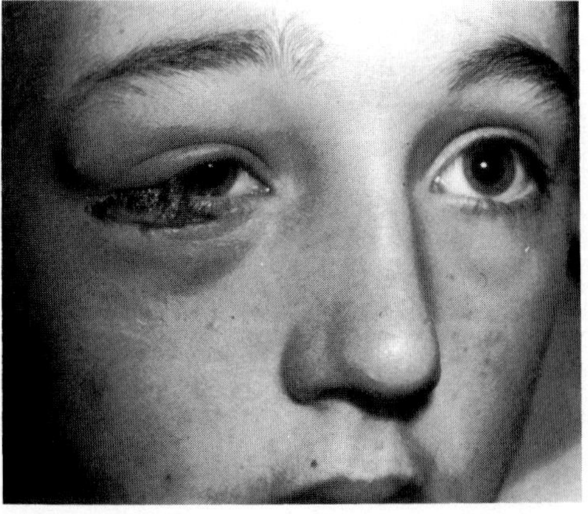

Figure 27–177. Infection after the reduction of a zygomatic fracture. The infection resolved following simple wound drainage, irrigation of the maxillary sinus, and drainage of the abscess in the upper eyelid. The plates used for the reduction did not require removal.

Orbital blow-out fractures and the ocular complications resulting from them are discussed in the section on fractures of the orbit (p. 1043).

Malposition of the arch or body of the zygoma may interfere with mandibular motion and require osteotomy. In such cases, the reduction has usually been performed in closed fashion and perhaps with excessive vigor in an attempt to mobilize a partially consolidated fracture.

Impacted fractures of the zygomatic arch against the coronoid process may result in fibro-osseous ankylosis with limited motion of the mandible (Ostrofsky and Lownie, 1977). If the zygoma cannot be adequately repositioned, resection of the coronoid process through an intraoral route usually frees the mandible from the fibrous ankylosis and permits normal function. It is important that the patient vigorously exercise to preserve and improve the range of movement obtained.

Persistent anesthesia or hypoesthesia in the distribution of the infraorbital nerve usually lasts only a short time. If total anesthesia exists for over six months, it is likely that the nerve is severely damaged or perhaps transected. If the nerve is impinged upon by bone fragments, especially in the medially displaced zygoma, decompression of the infraorbital canal and neurolysis are indicated.

Bone spurs or constricting portions of the canal should be removed so that the nerve will have an adequate opportunity for regeneration. Permanent anesthesia is temporarily annoying but patients finally become accustomed to the deficit. Drooling and difficulty with lip position may occur secondary to the hypoesthesia.

Fractures of the Maxilla

Maxillary fractures are encountered far less commonly than fractures of the mandible, zygoma, or nasal region (Morgan, Madan, and Bergerot, 1972; Kuepper and Harrigan, 1977; Luce, Tubbs, and Moore, 1979). The ratio appears at least to exceed that of 4:1 between mandibular and maxillary fractures as stated by Rowe and Killey in 1955. Some more recent series from trauma units have a higher incidence of maxillary fractures in relation to mandibular fractures (Manson, Su, and Hoopes, 1980; Manson and associates, 1985).

The maxilla forms a large part of the bone structure in the middle third of the facial skeleton. The maxilla itself is attached to the cranium through the zygomatic bone and, medially, the nasoethmoidal area. There is a strong vertical and horizontal system of "buttresses" or thick sections of bone that architecturally and structurally arrange the bones into a mass capable of resisting considerable violence (Fig. 27–178). The midfacial and orbital areas form an important protection to the brain case and intracranial structures. Violent forces and injuries of the midface are dissipated and absorbed by the alternating thin and thick structure of the bones of the midfacial skeleton (Fig. 27–179).

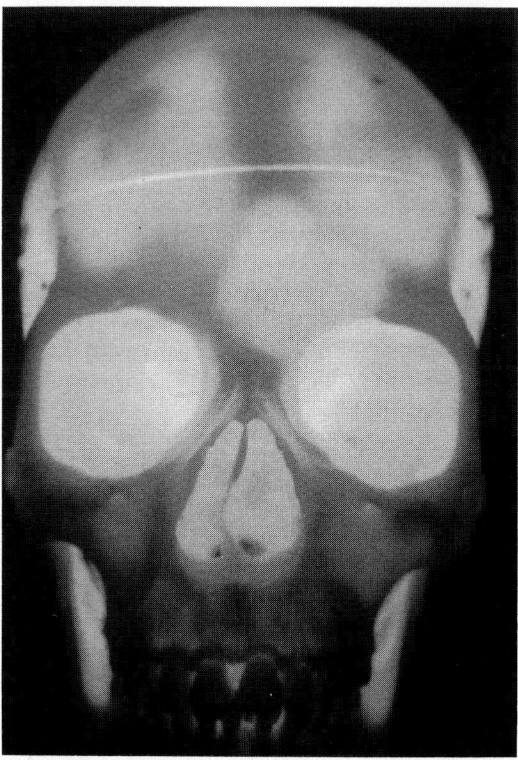

Figure 27–178. The midface is composed of alternating thick and thin portions of bone. The thick portions represent the buttresses of the midfacial skeleton.

ANATOMIC CONSIDERATIONS

The maxilla is formed from two irregular pyramidal component parts. It contributes to the formation of the midportion of the face and forms part of the orbit, nose, and palate. It is hollowed on its anterior aspect to provide space for the maxillary sinuses (Fig. 27–180). The maxilla thus forms a large portion of the orbit, the nasal fossa, the oral cavity, and a major portion of the palate, the nasal cavity, and the piriform aperture. The frontal processes of the maxilla provide anchorage for the canthal ligaments, and support the nasal bones and nasal cartilages. The maxilla is attached to the cranium by strong buttresses. These include the nasal bones and frontal processes of the maxilla at the glabella medially, and the zygoma and its articulations laterally. The zygoma articulates with both the frontal cranium and the greater wing of the sphenoid (see Fig. 27–179); it also attaches to the temporal bone through the arch. The maxilla contributes to stability only by its intimate association with the other bones of the midface and basal cranium.

The maxilla consists of a body and four processes—frontal, zygomatic, palatine, and alveolar. The body of the bone contains the large maxillary sinuses (Fig. 27–180). In childhood the sinuses are small, but as the adult structure is reached they become large and penetrate most of the central structure of the midface. Only a thin orbital floor and thin anterior and posterior medial wall of the maxilla remain. The growth of the sinus occurs in combination with the development of the permanent dentition. Tooth buds, present in the infant and young maxilla, are absent in adult structures, which results in further weakening of the bone. The overlying bone is thus thinned to eggshell thickness.

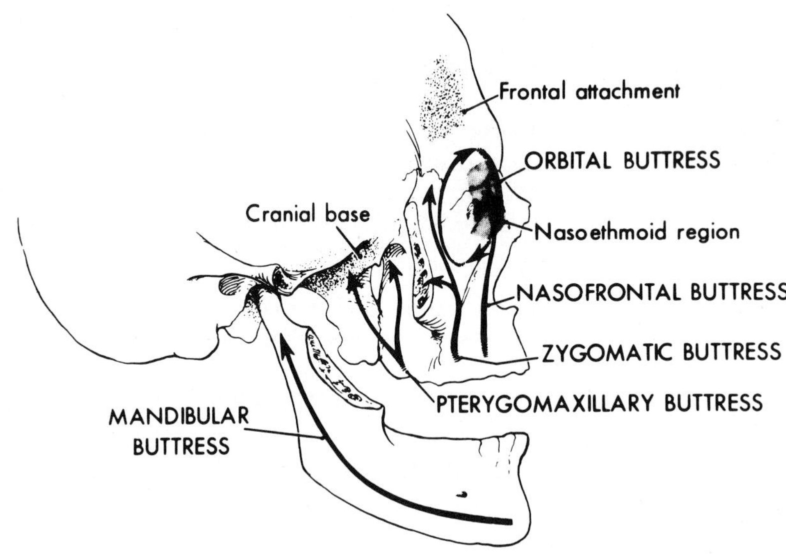

Figure 27–179. The vertical buttresses of the midfacial skeleton. Anteriorly, a nasofrontal buttress runs along the piriform aperture and the medial orbital rim. Laterally, the zygomatic buttress extends to the zygomatic process of the frontal bone from the midmaxillary area. An additional buttress is present along the zygomatic arch extending to the temporal bone. Posteriorly, the pterygomaxillary buttress is seen. The mandibular buttress forms a strong structural support for the lower midface in fracture treatment. Transverse buttresses include the palate, the orbital rims, and the frontal bar (supraorbital regions).

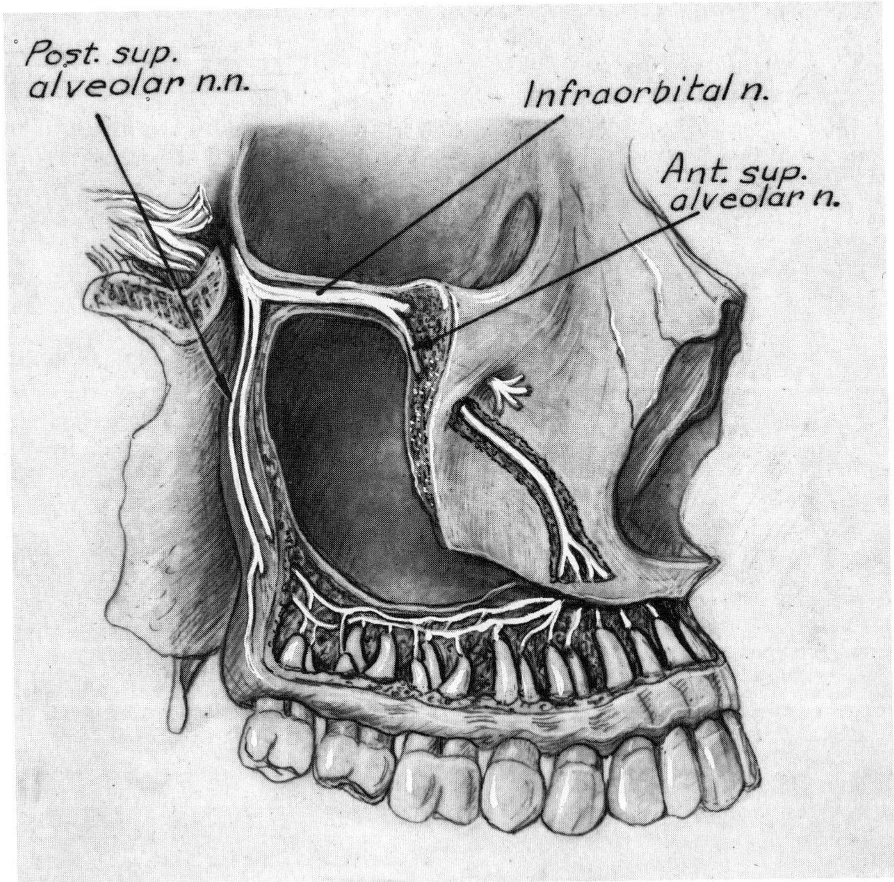

Figure 27–180. The maxilla. The maxillary sinus is open, showing the relationship with the floor of the orbit. Note also the interface between the pterygoid plates and the tuberosity of the maxilla. The sensory nerves are outlined. (From Kazanjian and Converse.)

The alveolar processes of the maxilla are quite strong and thick, giving excellent support to the horizontal processes of the mandible and protection to the upper portion of the bone. As the teeth are lost, this structure weakens and the alveolar process thins, becoming more atrophic. The entire maxilla thus becomes weaker and recession may occur. The entire alveolar portion of the bone may recede to the extent that the nasal spine is evident, and the bone may recede to the level of the floor of the maxillary sinuses. Accompanying resorption of the anterior surfaces of the maxilla may occur.

The nerves to the teeth pass through the anterior wall of the bone, and the infraorbital nerve passes through the infraorbital canal of the maxilla to supply the soft tissues of the upper lip and lateral aspect of the nose (Fig. 27–180). The mucosa overlying the bony palate and the mucosa of the soft palate are innervated by the palatine branches of the second division of the trigeminal nerve. These branches pass through the palatine canal between the maxilla and the palatine bones in the posterior portion of the palate. The nasopalatine nerves traverse each side of the vomer and pass from the nasal cavity through a small incisive foramen to provide the innervation of the mucoperiosteum of the anterior third of the hard palate.

SURGICAL ANATOMY

The maxilla is designed to absorb the forces of mastication and to provide a vertical buttress for occluding teeth. By virtue of the buttresses the load is distributed over the entire craniofacial skeleton (Fig. 27–181). Forces are distributed through the arch of the palate and the articulation of the maxilla against the frontomaxillary, zygomaticomaxillary, and ethmoidomaxillary sutures. The palatine bone and pterygoid plates of the sphenoid give additional stability posteriorly. These structures extend to the strong buttresses of the sphenoid bone in the skull base. The vomer, the perpendicular plate of the ethmoid, and the zygoma distribute the load to the temporal and frontal bones. The upper half of the nasal cavity, situated below the anterior cranial fossa and between the orbits, is designated as the interorbital space (Fig. 27–182) (see the section on Nasoethmoido-orbital Fractures).

Fractures of the maxilla are usually the result of a direct impact to the bone (Stanley, 1984; Stanley and Nowak, 1985). They vary from simple fractures of the alveolar process of the maxilla to comminuted fractures of the entire midface area. Their pattern and distribution depend on the magnitude of the force and on the direction (from a frontal or a

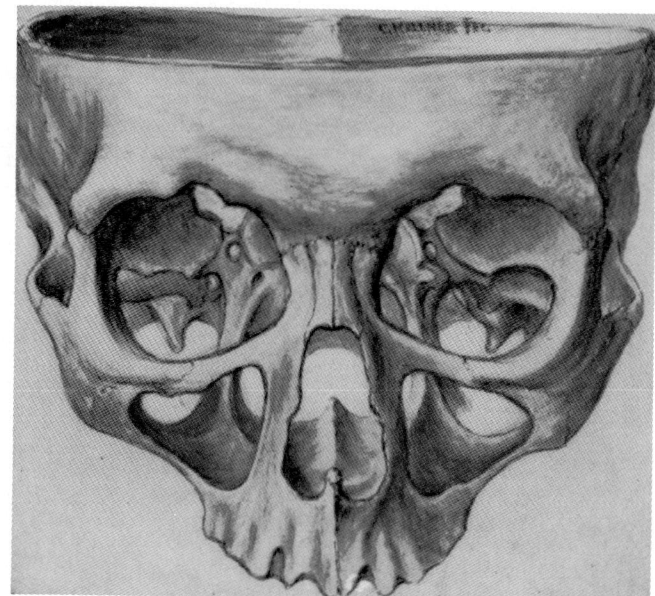

Figure 27–181. Drawing of a dissected skull. The thinner bony portions have been removed, leaving the heavier parts intact. (From Shapiro, H. H.: Applied Anatomy of the Head and Neck. Philadelphia, J. B. Lippincott Company, 1947.)

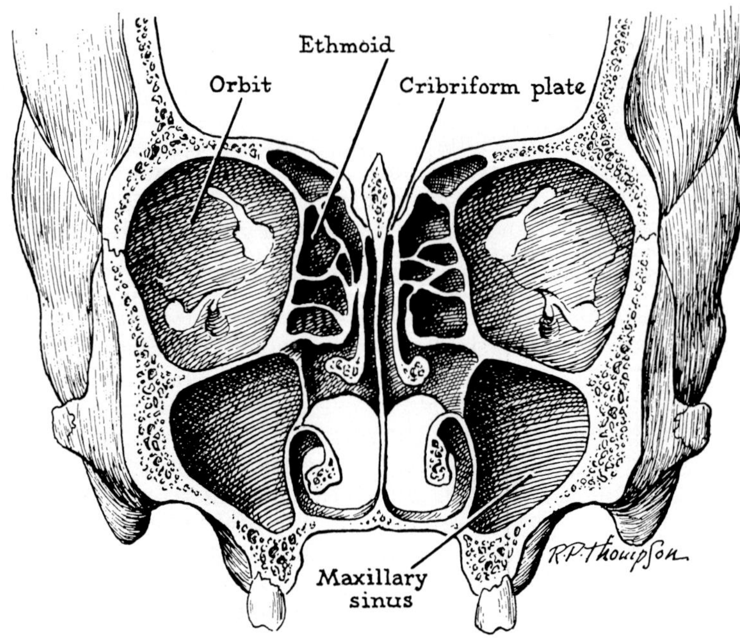

Figure 27–182. Frontal section through the skull showing the interorbital space, the ethmoid sinuses, and the relationship of the cribriform plate with the floor of the anterior cranial fossa. (From Kazanjian and Converse.)

lateral impact) (Rowe, 1982; Stanley, 1984; Stanley and Nowak, 1985).

Muscular contraction plays a less important role in displacement in maxillary than in that involved in mandibular fractures. Muscles attaching to the maxilla include the muscles of facial expression anteriorly, and the pterygoid muscles posteriorly. The muscles of facial expression have weaker forces and have little influence on the displacement of the fractured maxillary segments. A so-called "sagittal" fracture of the maxilla (fractured longitudinally along the palate) can be pulled laterally by these muscular attachments (Fig. 27–183). The pull of the pterygoid muscles posteriorly exerts downward and backward displacement in high maxillary fractures. When maxillary fractures are associated with fractures of the zygoma, the muscular action of the masseter may be a factor in displacement through its strong attachments to the body of the zygoma.

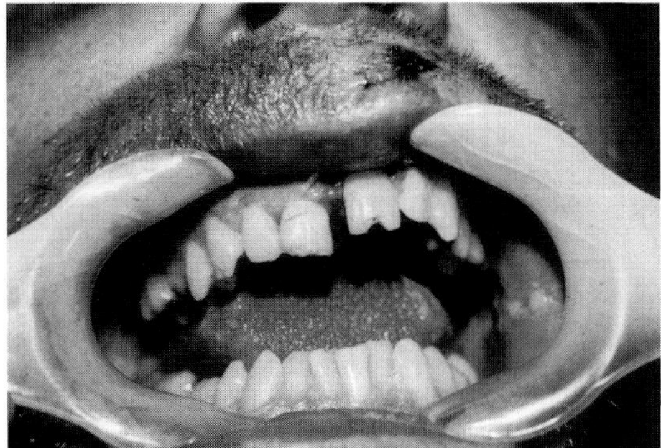

Figure 27–183. A sagittal fracture of the maxilla with displacement anteriorly and superiorly.

In upper Le Fort fractures, the nasolacrimal system may be involved in the fractured segments. The nasolacrimal canal is often traversed by the fracture lines. Function is frequently satisfactory; in some cases, however, function of the lacrimal drainage system may be impaired by either malalignment of the fractures or bone proliferation secondary to the healing processes. High maxillary fractures may involve the cranial fossa through extension of fractures into the frontal bone or anterior cranial floor. The high (Le Fort II and III) fractures may be associated with dural lacerations, cerebrospinal fluid fistula, pneumocephalus, and damage to the anterior portions of the brain.

LE FORT CLASSIFICATION OF FACIAL FRACTURES

The heavier portions of the maxilla give strength to the bone, while the thinner areas represent weakened sections through which fracture lines are most likely to occur. The fracture lines travel adjacent to thicker portions of bone. Le Fort (1901) completed experiments that determined the areas of structural weakness of the maxilla, which led to

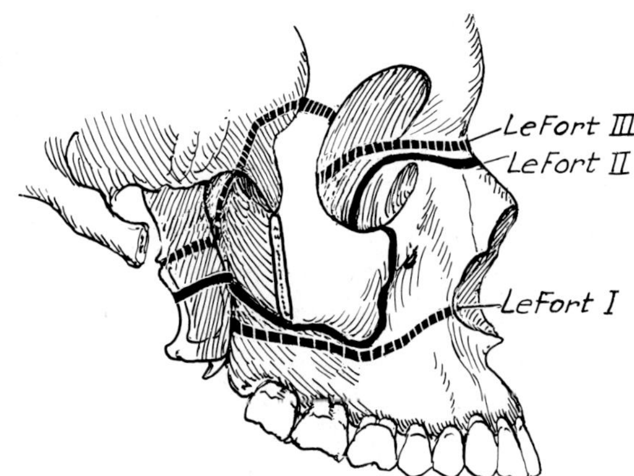

Figure 27–184. Le Fort lines of fracture. (From Kazanjian and Converse.)

the Le Fort classification of maxillary fractures (Fig. 27–184). This classification identifies the pattern of midfacial fractures. It should be emphasized that the usual Le Fort fracture consists of combinations and permutations of these patterns (Le Fort, 1901; Swearingen, 1965; Rowe and Brandt-Zawadzki, 1972; Stanley, 1984; Stanley and Nowak, 1985; Manson, 1986); frequently the highest level of fracture is different on one side from the other, and usually the comminution is more extensive on one side (Sofferman and associates, 1983).

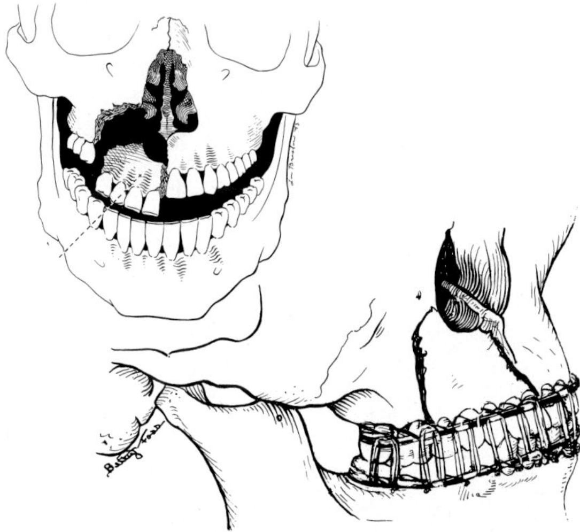

Figure 27–185. Fracture-dislocation of a large segment of alveolar bone and palate. Reduction and fixation is accomplished by rubber band traction between the mandibular teeth and maxillary teeth after manual repositioning of the fragments and application of the arch bars. The force of elastic traction can assist alignment in fracture reduction. The direction of the elastics occasionally needs to be changed and daily observation is required. If desired, an open reduction with plate and screw fixation at the margins of the piriform aperture may be performed.

Alveolar Fractures. The dentoalveolar portion of the maxilla may be fractured by direct force or by indirect force against the mandible, as a result of an injury. A portion of the alveolar process may be fractured (Fig. 27–185). In some cases this includes only the posterior molar teeth on one side, forming a "tuberosity" segmental alveolar fracture. In some cases an entire portion of an alveolus on one side may be fractured. This segment usually involves the teeth posterior to the cuspid. Lateral displacement of these fragments is often seen. Reduction usually is simply achieved by manual repositioning and fixation by the use of a palatal splint.

Transverse (Guérin) Fractures or Le Fort I Level Fractures. Fractures above the level of the apices of the teeth include essentially the entire alveolar processes of the maxilla, the vault of the palate, and the pterygoid processes in a single block. This type of injury is known as the Le Fort I or Guérin fracture (Fig. 27–186).

The fracture extends transversely across the base of the maxillary sinuses across the floor of the piriform aperture. High Le Fort I level fractures are observed similar to those in a high Le Fort I osteotomy.

Pyramidal Fractures (Le Fort II Fractures). Blows to the upper maxilla or blows involving a frontal impact result in fractures with a pyramidally shaped central maxillary segment (see Figs. 27–184, 27–186). The fracture begins above the level of the apices of the teeth laterally and extends through the pterygoid plates in the same fashion as the Le Fort I fracture. Traveling medially it extends to involve a portion of the medial orbit, extending across the nose to separate a pyramidally shaped maxillary segment from the superior cranial and midfacial structures. This fracture, because of its general shape and configuration, has become known as the "pyramidal" fracture of the maxilla or the Le Fort II fracture. The degree of variability of the fracture in terms of the level at which it crosses the nose is extreme. It may extend through the cartilages on one side and through the distal nasal bone on the other side, or may separate the nasal bones from the glabella at the junction of the nasal bones and frontal bone. Damage to the ethmoidal area is routine in pyramidal fractures; this is a weak area through which fracture lines

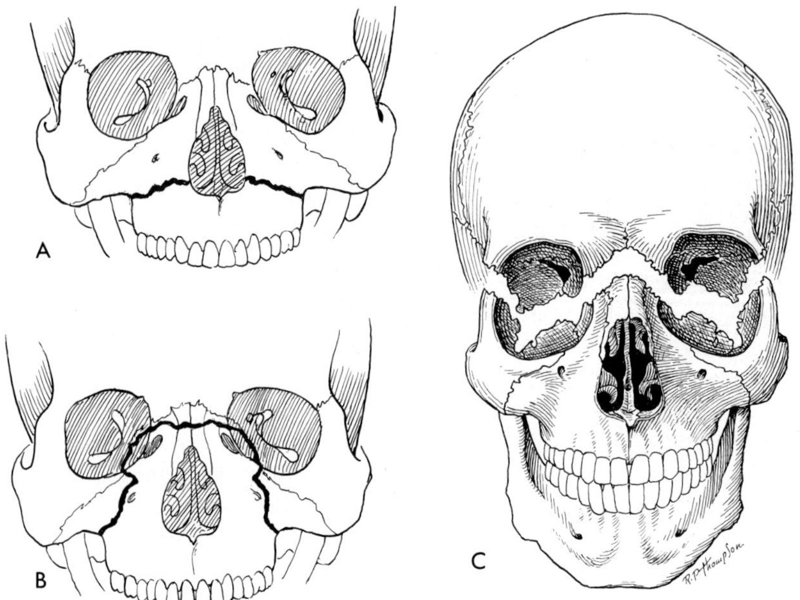

Figure 27–186. Le Fort classification of midfacial fractures. *A*, Le Fort I horizontal or transverse fracture of the maxilla, also known as Guérin's fracture. *B*, Le Fort II or pyramidal fracture of the maxilla. *C*, Le Fort III or craniofacial dysjunction. (From Kazanjian and Converse.)

traverse. The lacrimal system may be involved in the fractures.

Craniofacial Dysjunction or Le Fort III Fractures. Craniofacial dysjunction may occur when the fracture extends through the zygomaticofrontal suture and the nasofrontal suture and across the floor of the orbits to effect a complete separation of the midfacial structures from the cranium (see Fig. 27–186). In these fractures, the maxilla may not be separated from the zygoma or from the nasal structures. The entire midfacial skeleton is completely detached from the base of the skull and suspended only by soft tissues.

Vertical or Sagittal Fractures of Maxilla. Fractures of the maxilla may occur in a sagittal direction, and thus section the maxilla in a sagittal plane (Manson and associates, 1983). A common fracture splits the maxilla longitudinally along the junction of the maxilla with the vomer (Fig. 27–187). The fracture exits anteriorly between the cuspid teeth. The sagittal fractures are usually associated with other fractures of the

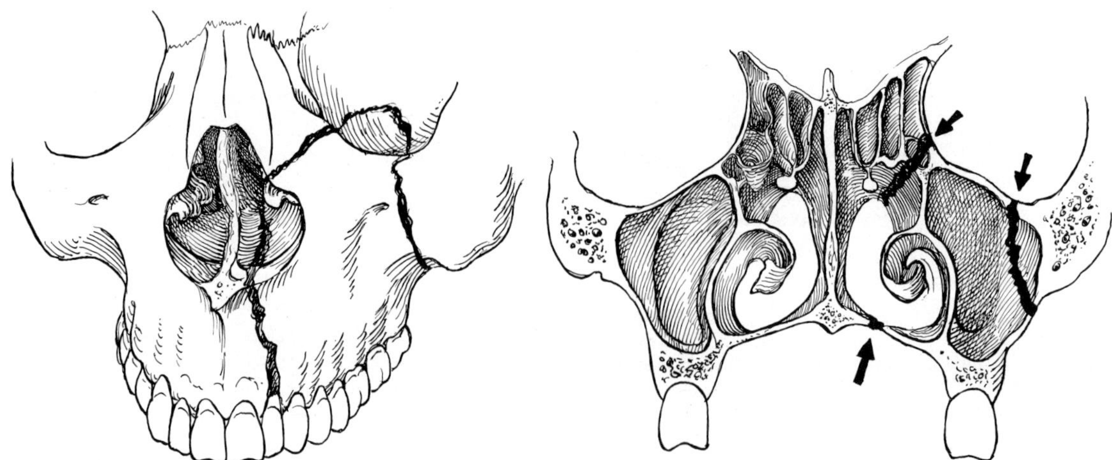

Figure 27–187. Sagittal fracture of the maxilla occurring through the thin portion of the hard palate lateral to the vomer. It is associated with fractures of the orbital floor and lateral maxillary wall in this patient. More often, these fractures cross at the Le Fort I level. (From Kazanjian and Converse.)

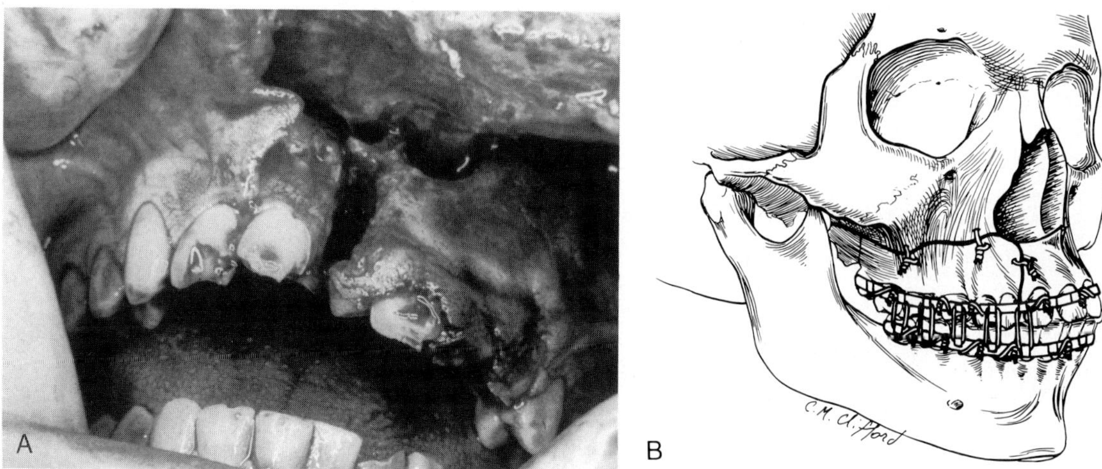

Figure 27–188. *A*, Many sagittal fractures of the maxilla are accompanied by a laceration into the piriform aperture. This finding should serve as a clue to a fracture. The piriform aperture can be reduced with interfragment wires *(B)* or plate and screw fixation.

maxilla. They increase comminution and make the treatment of Le Fort fractures considerably more difficult. The potential exists for transverse (facial and dental arch width) problems, as well as vertical and anteroposterior displacement. Displacement depends on the direction and degree of force involved. Some fractures can have such periosteal integrity that they can be quite stable even though a fracture can be demonstrated on CT scan or radiographs of the palate. Such fractures usually are not accompanied by the characteristic laceration in the upper buccal sulcus and along the roof of the palate (Fig. 27–188).

ETIOLOGY

The most common cause of fractures of the maxilla is a frontal or lateral impact. The victim of an accident is thrown forward, striking the middle third of the face against an object such as the instrument panel or steering wheel of an automobile. If the force is sustained on the lower maxilla in the region of the upper lip, an alveolar or a transverse fracture of the maxilla is likely to occur. If the force is more violent and sustained at a higher level, comminuted fractures of the maxilla may be expected. If the force is largely from a frontal impact, the fragment carrying the maxillary dentition is frequently a Le Fort II fracture. If the force is sustained from a lateral direction, the patient often has a Le Fort III level fracture on one side and a Le Fort II level fracture on the other side. The fragment of the maxilla that carries the maxillary dentition may be a "Le Fort I" or a "Le Fort II" fragment in its shape.

Although most traumatic forces are directed from the anterior or lateral direction, there may be upward forces on the anterior portion of the maxilla. It is possible to fracture the maxilla by upward force on the mandible alone.

Displacement in Maxillary Fractures. Displacement after maxillary fracture is generally posteriorly and downward. The patient has an elongated, retruded appearance in the middle third of the facial skeleton. Overall elongation of the facial structures occurs (Fig. 27–189). The maxillary fragment tilts downward, causing a premature contact in the molar occlusion. An anterior open bite is present, often more prominent on one side than on the other (Fig. 27–190). The pterygoid musculature aids the posterior and downward forces of maxillary displacement. Partial fracture of the maxilla or alveolar processes, with displacement of the segments into the sinus or region of the palate, may occur from laterally directed impacts (see Fig. 27–188). Sagittal fractures of the maxilla may result from forces transmitted through the mandible or the maxilla, or by direct frontal impact on the anterior maxilla. Impacted fractures of the maxilla are infrequent, but in some cases the entire maxilla is driven upward and backward into the interorbital space or pharyngeal region, and

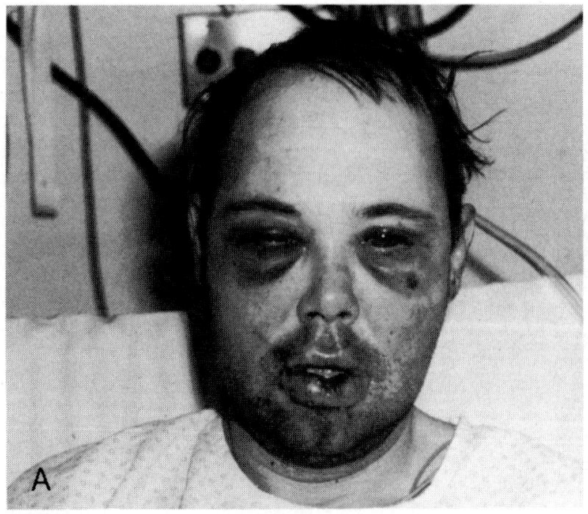

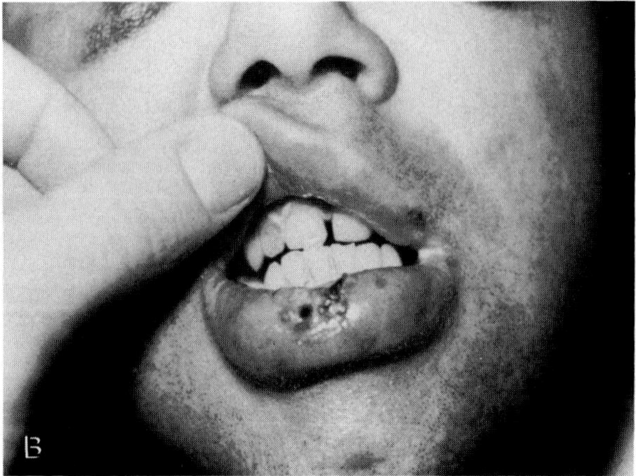

Figure 27–189. *A*, A patient with a Le Fort fracture who has not been placed in intermaxillary fixation. The midface is elongated and retruded—a flattened, donkey-like facies. *B*, Malocclusion is evident.

may be so securely impacted that no movement can be elicited on clinical examination.

Fracture of Maxilla without Maxillary Mobility. Mobility of the maxillary dentition is the hallmark of diagnosis of a maxillary fracture. It is exceeded only by malocclusion in diagnostic sensitivity. Certain fractures of the maxilla are "greensticked" and incomplete, and may display little or no maxillary mobility. Characteristically, a pure Le Fort III level fracture without comminution reveals only the presence of bilateral periorbital ecchymosis and malocclusion. Little, if any, maxillary mobility is present in this rare type of fracture. Maxillary sinus fluid is present on CT scans, and the fracture lines may be difficult to demonstrate on CT.

EXAMINATION AND DIAGNOSIS

Inspection. Epistaxis, ecchymosis (periorbital, conjunctival, and scleral), edema, and subcutaneous hematoma are suggestive of fractures involving the maxillary bone. The swelling is usually moderate, indicating the severity of the fracture. Malocclusion with an anterior open bite suggests a fracture of the maxilla. The maxillary segment is frequently displaced downward and posteriorly, resulting in premature occlusion in the posterior dentition. On intraoral examination, there may be tearing of the overlying soft tissues in the labial vestibule or the palate, findings that indicate the possibility of an underlying sagittal fracture of the maxilla. Hematoma may be present in the buccal mucosa. The face, after several days, may have an elongated, retruded appearance, the so-called "donkey-like" facies (see Fig. 27–189), suggestive of a craniofacial dysjunction.

Palpation. Bilateral palpation may reveal step deformities at the zygomaticomaxillary sutures, indicating fractures of the inferior orbital rims. These findings suggest a pyramidal fracture of the maxilla or a zygomatic component of a more complicated injury. Intraoral palpation may reveal fractures of the anterior portion of the maxilla or fractured segments of alveolar bone. Fractures at the junction of the maxilla and zygoma may be detected by digital palpation along the inferior rim of the orbit. Movement of the nasal bones by palpation suggests that a nasal fracture is associated with the maxillary fractures.

Digital Manipulation. Force applied by grasping the anterior portion of the maxilla between the thumb and index finger demonstrates mobility of the maxilla (Fig. 27–191). Zygomatic mobility may also be shown. The manipulation test for mobility is not entirely reliable because impacted or greensticked fractures may exhibit no movement. These fractures can be overlooked unless a specific careful examination of the occlusion is performed. The occlusal discrepancy may be minor, i.e., within one-half to one cusp displacement; curiously, the patient may be unable to discern this degree of occlusal discrepancy as abnormal. Manipulation of the anterior maxilla may show movement of the entire middle third of the face, including the bridge of the nose. This movement is appreciated by holding the head and moving the maxilla

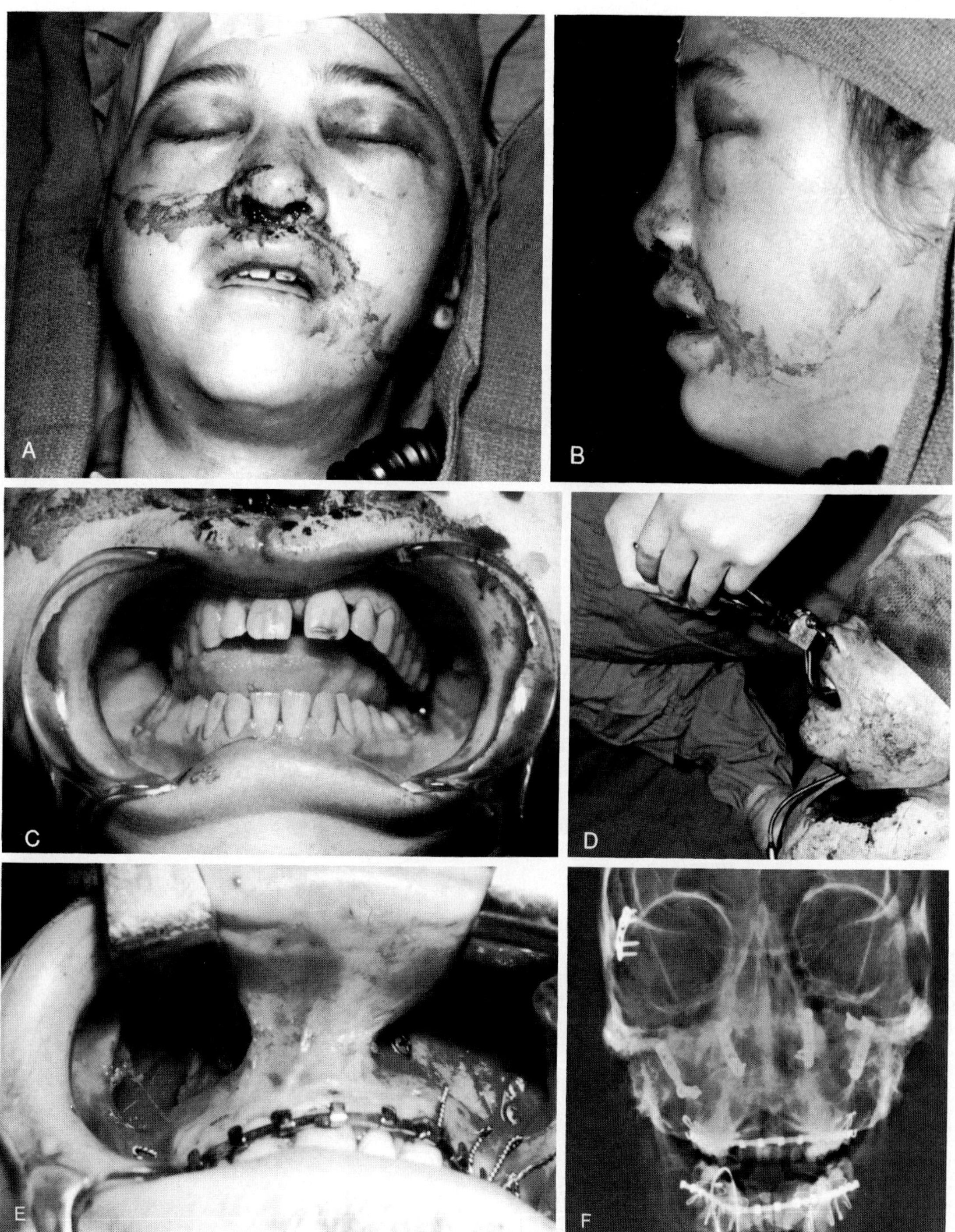

Figure 27–190. A patient with a Le Fort III level fracture on one side and a Le Fort I level fracture bilaterally. *A*, *B*, Frontal and lateral views demonstrating midfacial retrusion and elongation. *C*, Prereduction occlusion. *D*, Reduction of the fracture by means of Rowe forceps. *E*, Open reduction at the Le Fort I level through a gingivobuccal sulcus incision. Plate and screw fixation can be visualized. *F*, Postoperative radiograph demonstrating the plate and screw fixation.

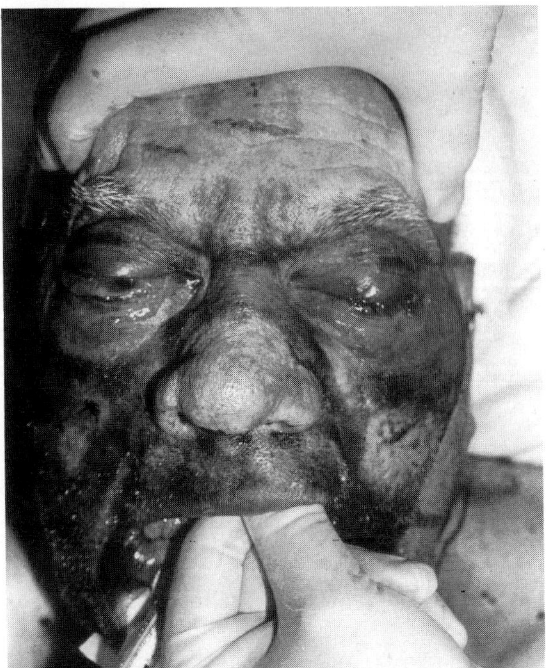

Figure 27–191. Maxillary mobility is determined by firmly grasping the upper jaw while holding the head steady.

with the other hand. Crepitation may be heard when the maxilla is manipulated.

Cerebrospinal Rhinorrhea or Otorrhea. Cerebrosinal fluid may leak from the anterior or middle cranial fossa and is apparent in the nose or ear canal. A fluid leak signifies the presence of a fistula extending from the intracranial subarachnoid space through the skull and into the nose or ear. Frequently the drainage is obscured by bloody secretions in the immediate postinjury period. Fractures of the anterior and middle cranial fossa frequently accompany severe midfacial injuries, and the presence of a cerebrospinal fluid leak or pneumocephalus should be diligently sought on physical examination and by appropriate radiographs.

Malocclusion of Teeth. If the mandible is intact, malocclusion of the teeth is highly suggestive of a maxillary fracture. It is possible, however, that the malocclusion relates to a preinjury condition. A thorough study of the patient's dentition with reference to previous dental records is helpful. Impressions can be taken and wear facets of the teeth studied to determine the preinjury occlusal pattern. It is possible to have a high craniofacial dislocation and still have reasonable occlusion of the teeth (high Le Fort III level fracture, single fragment). If the maxilla is rotated and markedly displaced backward and downward, there is a complete disruption of occlusal relationships with failure of any teeth to contact.

Roentgenographic Examination. The diagnosis of a fracture of the maxilla should be suspected clinically and confirmation obtained by careful roentgenographic examination. Maxillary fractures may be difficult to demonstrate on routine radiographs. While plain films can be utilized, craniofacial CT scan (Fig. 27–192) is required for diagnostic examination of maxillary fractures. The Waters, Caldwell, and submentovertex views, as well as those of the lateral skull, are required to document fractures of the maxilla in plain films. The presence of bilateral maxillary sinus opacity suggests a maxillary fracture. Separation at the inferior orbital rims, zygomaticofrontal suture, and nasofrontal area may be noted, as well as fractures through the lateral portion of the maxillary sinus. On lateral films, fractures of the pterygoid plates can be diagnosed by careful examination of the radiograph. Fractures of the palate are best viewed in plain films (occlusal).

Fractures of the maxilla are best documented by careful axial CT scans (Fig. 27–192). They should be taken from the palate through the anterior cranial fossa. The presence of bilateral maxillary sinus fluid should be suspected of representing a maxillary fracture until it is proved otherwise.

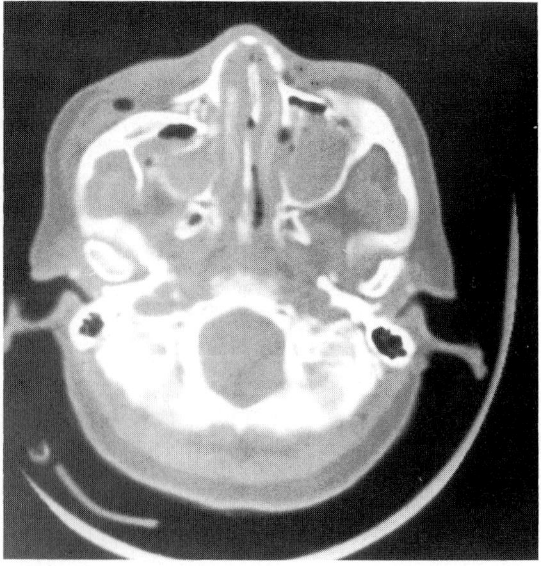

Figure 27–192. Axial CT scan of a bilateral Le Fort fracture at the Le Fort II level.

TREATMENT OF MAXILLARY FRACTURES

Treatment should be directed toward the establishment of an airway, control of hemorrhage, closure of soft tissue wounds, and placement of the patient in intermaxillary fixation.

With a fractured maxilla, considerable displacement can occur. Hemorrhage, swelling, and secretions may make breathing difficult. The upper airway may be blocked by structures forced into the pharyngeal region or by loose teeth, pieces of broken bone, broken dentures, or other foreign material. These must be removed, and if an adequate airway cannot be established, endotracheal intubation or tracheotomy should be performed.

Some maxillary fractures are associated with deep lacerations of the overlying skin and oral mucosa. Shearing fractures involving the bones of the sinuses result in profuse hemorrhage from the vessels within the mucosal structures. The greater palatine vessels may be lacerated on occasion. The wounds may involve the internal maxillary artery or its branches in the pterygoid space. Severe hemorrhage may occur into the nasal and pharyngeal airways. The bleeding may threaten exsanguination and may respond only to nasopharyngeal packing and placement of the patient in intermaxillary fixation. Anteroposterior nasal tamponade may fail to control the bleeding in more difficult cases. Rarely, angiographic embolization and ligation of the external carotid and superficial temporal artery on one or both sides may be indicated.

The simplest treatment of a maxillary fracture, and one of the most effective, is to place the patient in occlusion in intermaxillary fixation. This should be done as soon after the injury as possible. Much of the deformity of a midfacial fracture can be eliminated by the simple act of placing the patient in intermaxillary fixation and the fractured fragments at rest. When the mandible is intact, this maneuver limits the downward and posterior displacement of the lower portion of the midface. The elongated, retruded midface is effectively avoided because of the tendency of the mandibular musculature to assume a "balanced" or "rest" position (close to "centric rest").

Alveolar Fractures. Simple fractures of portions of the maxilla involving the alveolar bone and the teeth can usually be digitally reduced and held in position while an arch bar is applied (see Fig. 27–185). In some cases an open reduction of that portion of the alveolus may be performed with wire or plate and screw fixation. Sometimes an occlusal splint across the palate is necessary to provide additional stability for loose teeth in an alveolar fracture. The position of the teeth can also be maintained by ligating the teeth in the fracture segment to adjacent teeth with the use of an arch bar or interdental wiring technique. The arch bar can be acrylated for additional support. The fabrication of a splint or the acrylating of an arch bar can be accomplished with quick-curing acrylic resin molded to a model or the teeth and alveolus. The material should be cooled as it cures. If the fragments cannot be adequately reduced manually, or if there is consistent premature contact between the teeth of the maxilla and the mandible, the teeth of the fractured segment are in jeopardy by this premature contact. A more definite reduction of the area should be considered that allows the segment to be seated in proper position. Fixation of the alveolar segment should be maintained for at least four to 12 weeks or until clinical immobility has been achieved. Teeth involved in the fractured alveolar segments may be subject to damage of the neurovascular structures within the pulp, and appropriate endodontic evaluation should be obtained.

Treatment of Major Midfacial Fractures. Few advances in the conceptualization of Le Fort fracture patterns have occurred since Le Fort (1901) described his cadaver experiments in 1900. Until recently, few advances have been made in the treatment of Le Fort fractures since Adams (Adams, 1942; Adams and Adams, 1956) described internal fixation, suspension, and open reduction. Adams advocated open reduction and internal fixation of the orbital rims in midfacial fractures by a combination of closed reduction of the lower midface involving the placement of intermaxillary fixation devices and suspension wires leading to a point above the highest level of the fracture on each side (Fig. 27–193). His principles were welcomed because external fixation was avoided in most patients. The limitations of the Adams technique relate to the incomplete exposure and fixation of all fractured fragments and the use of compression with suspension wires as a means of facial fracture fixation. Although this technique served to simplify and improve the results of treatment and was satisfactory

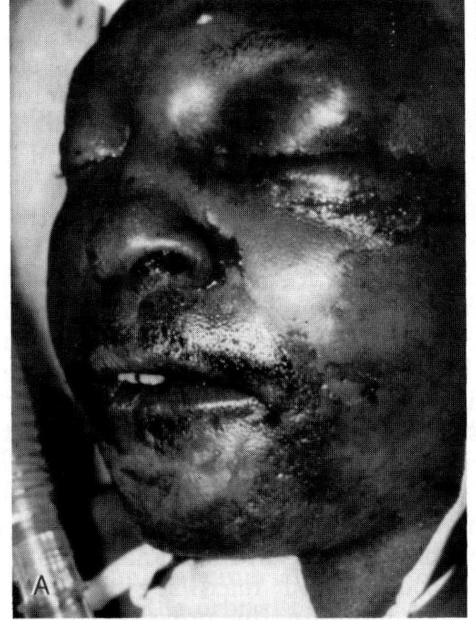

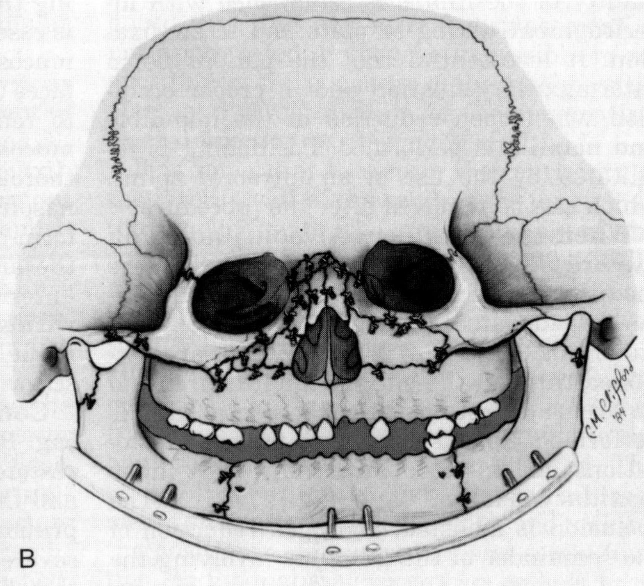

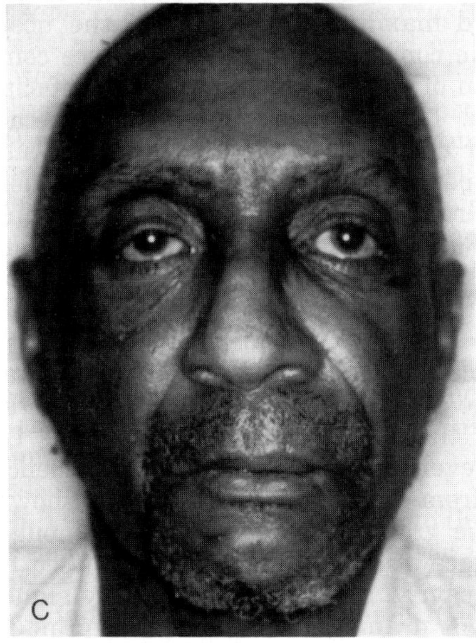

Figure 27–214. *A*, Panfacial fractures with mandibular body and bilateral subcondylar fractures. Retrusion of the lower midface and jaw can be seen. A bilateral nasoethmoido-orbital fracture is also present. *B*, Stabilization was accomplished by interfragment wiring and stabilizing the mandible by the application of a Morris external fixation device. *C*, *D*, The result obtained following extensive open reduction. *E*, Range of motion at 12 weeks post fracture. *D* and *E* are on page 1041.

dorsal height, prevents saddling of the dorsum, restores septal support, and prevents shortening of the nose, a most difficult post-traumatic deformity to correct. A thin bone graft often smoothes the nasal dorsum and produces a more satisfactory contour.

In severely comminuted midfacial fractures, after reduction and fixation by the usual methods of interfragment wiring, plate and screw fixation can be employed to increase stability if mobility is still present. Alternatively, the use of onlay bone grafts as "buttresses" can increase stability (Fig. 27–217). The supportive bone grafts increase the adequacy of stabilization. Bone grafts provide buttresses to maintain the facial height and projection. They also fill a structural void, and the additional bone graft may aid the rapidity and strength of bone consolidation during the weeks of intermaxillary fixation. Restoration of critical buttresses may prevent secondary recession of the maxilla.

Bone grafting of nasoethmoido-orbital fractures, restoring the medial orbital walls and floors in conjunction with bone grafting of the nasal dorsum, assists the correction of traumatic telecanthus and enophthalmos.

The indications for primary bone grafting

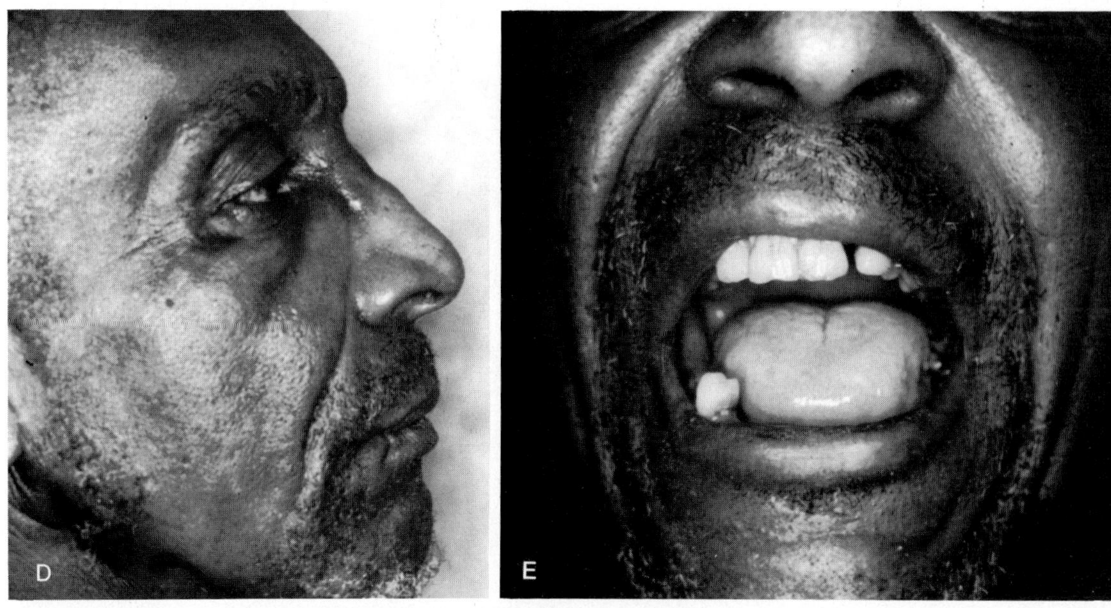

Figure 27–214. *Continued*

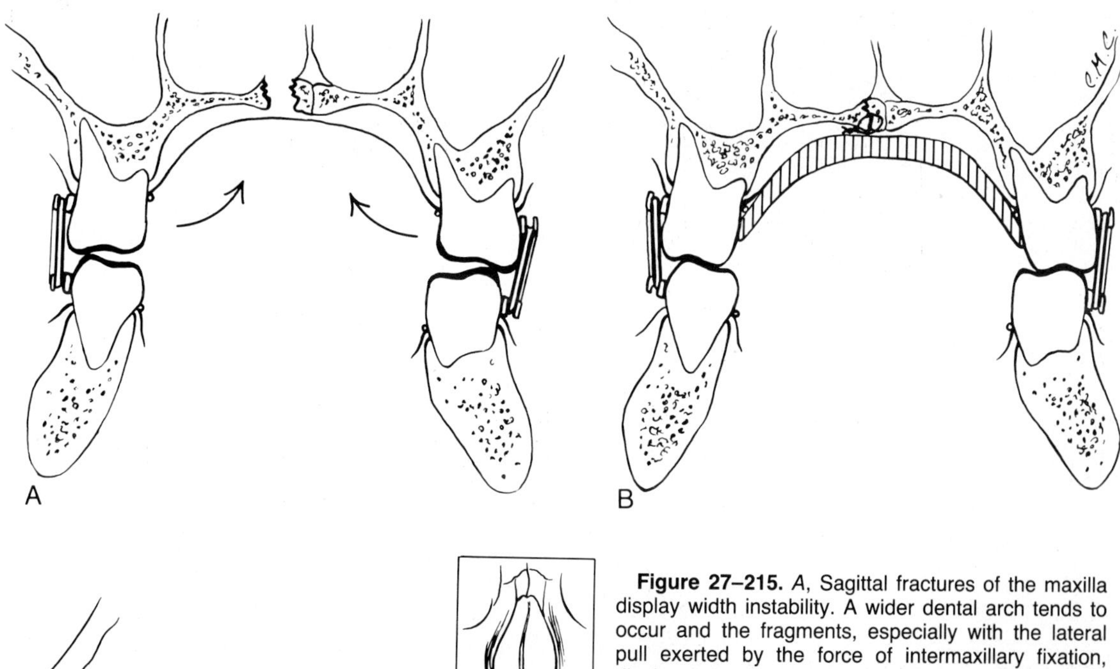

Figure 27–215. *A*, Sagittal fractures of the maxilla display width instability. A wider dental arch tends to occur and the fragments, especially with the lateral pull exerted by the force of intermaxillary fixation, display palatal rotation. *B*, A splint opposed to the palatal surface of the teeth assists alignment of the dental arches and prevents palatal rotation of the maxillary fragments. Note the palatal wiring between the fragments. *C*, The palatal splint is best secured with either interdental wires or a circumpalatal wire passed across the floor of the nose and through the soft palate.

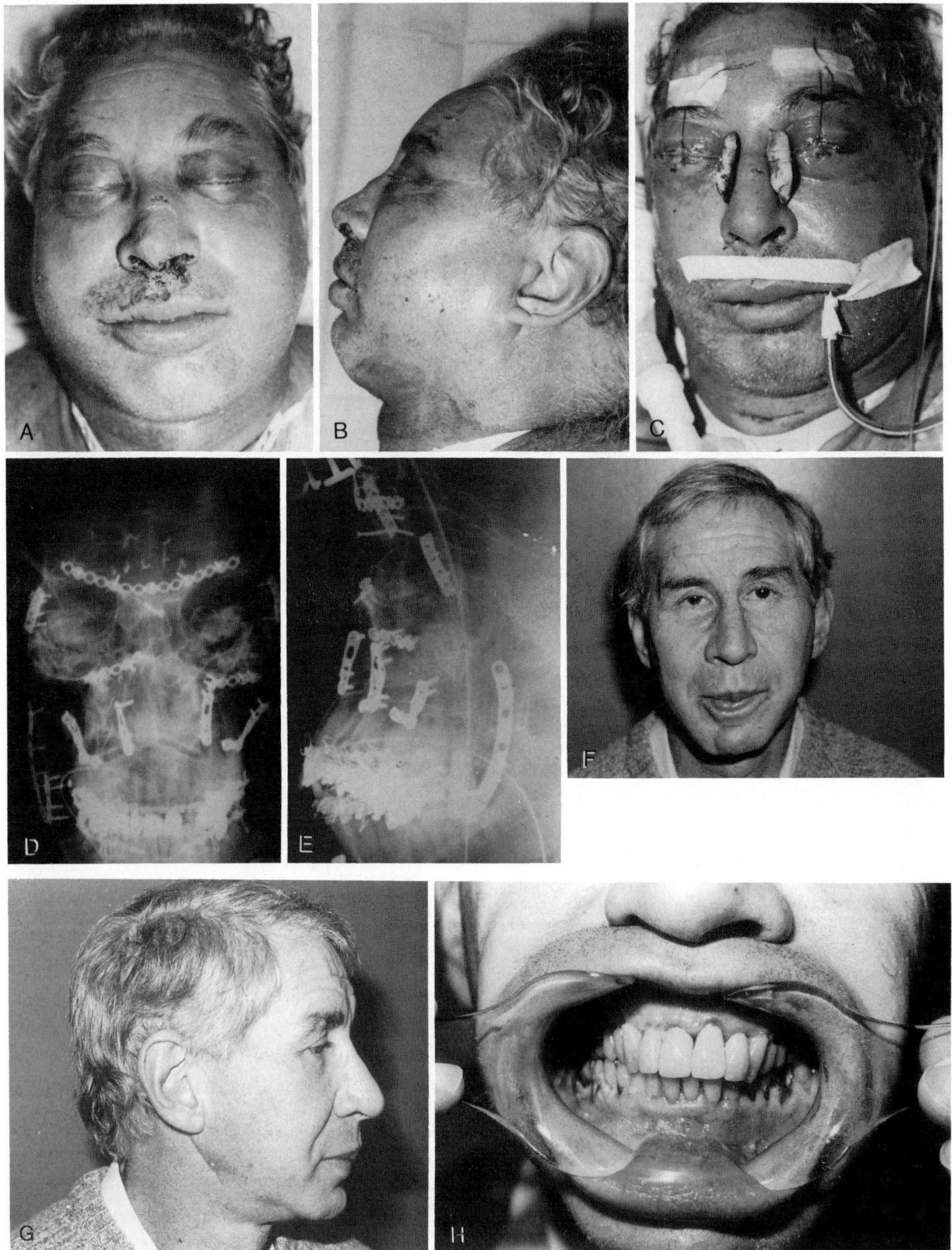

Figure 27–216. *A*, *B*, Panfacial fracture including the frontal sinus, nasoethmoido-orbital complex, bilateral comminuted Le Fort, and mandibular fractures. *C*, The result immediately after extensive open reduction. *D*, *E*, Design of fixation used for fracture reduction. *F*, *G*, Postoperative frontal and lateral views. *H*, Postoperative occlusion.

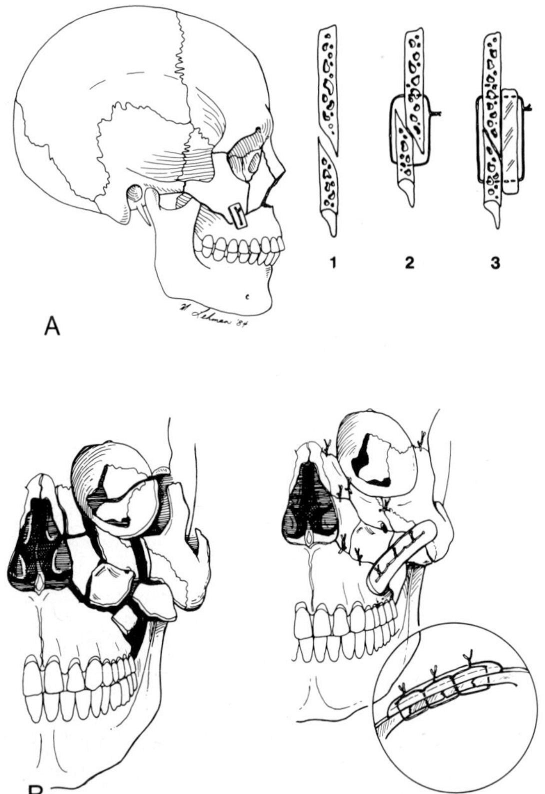

Figure 27–217. *A*, Buttress stabilization. Unstable oblique fracture of the anterior maxillary buttress stabilized by the incorporation of a small bone graft at the wiring site. *B*, Incorporation of a carefully contoured and measured bone graft into the site of a comminuted or segmental fracture of the anterior buttress produces buttress reinforcement and stabilization and reestablishment of correct maxillary height. For both *A* and *B*, similar stabilization can be accomplished by a miniplate. (From Gruss, J. S., and MacKinnon, S. E.: Complex maxillary fractures: role of buttress reconstruction and immediate bone grafts. Plast. Reconstr. Surg., *78*:9, 1986.)

include the need to replace critical structural supports. Extensive fractures without soft tissue coverage problems are the most common indication for primary bone grafting. Despite the presence of extensive soft tissue wounds, bone grafting is a successful technique provided that the wounds can be surgically cleansed by debridement and proper soft tissue coverage of most of the bone graft can be ensured. Contraindications include infected or severely contaminated soft tissue wounds that cannot be properly cleansed.

Bone grafts can also be anchored either within the orbit or to the anterior maxillary area with lag screws, or united to a reconstruction plate. Plates and screws should extend over fractured areas with at least two screws per main fragment.

Orbital and Nasoethmoido-orbital Fractures

Orbital fractures may occur as isolated fractures, but more commonly they are associated with other facial fractures. Patients presenting with orbital injuries, periorbital ecchymosis, or lacerations around the eye should have a thorough ophthalmologic examination to exclude the possibility of globe injury, globe rupture, or damage to the soft tissue contents of the orbit (Milauskas and Fueger, 1966; Miller and Tenzel, 1967; Milauskas, 1969; Petro and associates, 1970; Fradkin, 1971; Jabaley, Lerman, and Sanders, 1975; Holt and Holt, 1983).

Before the physical examination, a history should be obtained when possible. Specific details of the accident and how it occurred, and of any visual disturbance such as blurring, loss of vision, or diplopia, should be recorded. Previous visual loss or a history of a "lazy eye" is noted. Bleeding from the nose or a period of unconsciousness are important clues to the diagnosis of ancillary injuries. Any prior medical evaluation or surgical treatment involving the eye is also important. Diminished vision is often present as a result of previous conditions such as amblyopia.

The ophthalmologic examination should be performed routinely in patients with orbital injuries, to verify the presence of vision and light perception, to record the visual acuity, and to assess the possibility of intraocular or corneal injury. If the patient is unconscious, this examination may be performed despite the absence of a clear history. In conscious patients, their cooperation facilitates the examination. For some routine orbital injuries, it may be advisable to wait several days before proceeding with the fracture reduction to assess more accurately the progression of retinal or globe injury or the resolution of diplopia. Rarely, orbital fractures displace the globe to an extent that the lids do not adequately protect the cornea from drying (Raflo, 1984; Godoy and Mathog, 1985). This is an emergent condition that requires either a temporary lid occlusion or reduction of the fracture, preferably the latter.

The treatment of orbital fractures should not be delayed more than absolutely necessary. As soon as an injury has occurred, the process of an inflammatory reaction begins and ultimately results in fibrosis of any contused or entrapped orbital soft tissue. It seems reasonable, therefore, to replace orbital contents into their proper position so that any scarring occurs in an anatomically correct position.

The globe should be inspected for edema, corneal abrasion, and laceration or contusion. Extraocular muscle movements should be checked as far as possible. This can be checked in cooperative patients, both at near and far distance. A gross visual field examination is performed by having the patient stare at a fixed point and noting peripheral vision for an object, such as a cotton-tipped applicator. Globe pressure may be assessed and the results of a fundus examination recorded. Diminished vision may be assessed by recording the patient's ability to read print on an ophthalmic examination card. The presence of diminished vision without light perception indicates optic nerve damage or globe rupture. Light perception without usable vision indicates the possibility of an anterior chamber hemorrhage (hyphema) or vitreous hematoma. Such conditions require expert ophthalmologic treatment.

In lacerations that occur adjacent to the medial canthus or in nasoethmoido-orbital fractures having canthal ligament avulsion, the integrity of the lacrimal system should be assessed. The lacrimal punctum can be dilated with a pediatric punctum dilator, and a small irrigating cannula may be used to irrigate the drainage system (see Chap. 34). It may be helpful to occlude the opposite punctum with finger pressure. Drainage of fluid into the nose indicates the continuity of the lacrimal system. The appearance of fluid in the laceration indicates a divided lacrimal system.

Fractures of the orbit frequently occur in association with zygomaticomaxillary, nasoethmoido-orbital and high Le Fort (II and III) fractures. In these injuries, the lines of fracture traverse the medial and lateral orbit and the orbital floor. These fractures may be linear, simple injuries or may comminute the thin portions of the floor. When they are accompanied by displacement of sections of the orbit, such as the zygoma, discontinuity may occur in the area of the lateral orbital wall adjacent to the greater wing of the sphenoid, producing herniation of orbital contents into the temporal fossa. The most frequent displacement observed involves the medial orbital wall and the portion of the floor medial to the infraorbital groove and canal. These thin sections of bone are easily displaced inferiorly and posteriorly, allowing displacement of orbital soft tissue. In injuries that displace the inferior orbital rim posteriorly, there generally is comminution of the thin portion of the orbital floor. In fractures of the zygoma, downward displacement results in a separation of the lateral and inferior portions of the floor, with a lowering of the orbital floor and an outward rotation of the lateral orbit.

Many orbital fractures are complicated by double vision (Barclay, 1958, 1960, 1963), the usual cause of which is contusion of an extraocular muscle. In some cases, actual incarceration of orbital soft tissue has caused limitation of extraocular muscle excursions. McCoy and associates (1962) found a 15 per cent incidence of ocular complications in a series of 855 patients with facial fractures. Morgan, Madan, and Bergerot (1972), in a review of 300 cases of midfacial fractures, noted persistent diplopia in 11 per cent of the patients.

THE ORBIT—ANATOMIC CONSIDERATIONS

The orbits are paired bone structures separated in the midline by the interorbital space (Fig. 27–218). The interorbital space, the portion of the nasal and sinus cavity situated between the orbits, is delimited above by the floor of the anterior cranial fossa. This anterior cranial fossa partition is formed by the roof of each ethmoid sinus laterally and by the cribriform plate medially. The orbits are situated immediately below the floor of the anterior cranial fossa, a portion of the fossa being formed by the roof of the orbits.

The orbital contents are protected by strong bone structures. These include the nasal bones, the nasal spine of the frontal bone, and the frontal processes of the maxilla medially. Above, they include the supraorbital arches of the frontal bone. Laterally, the frontal process of the zygoma and the zygomatic process of the frontal bone constitute the lateral orbital rim. Inferiorly, the thick infraorbital rim is formed by the zygoma laterally and the maxilla medially.

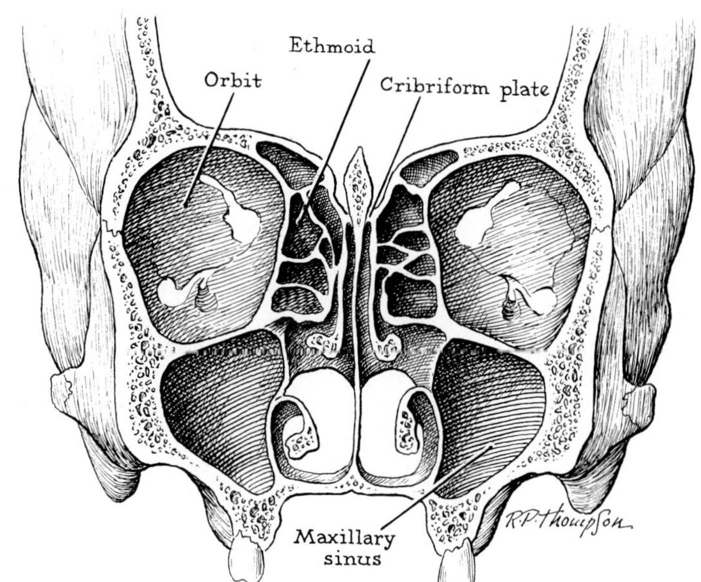

Figure 27–218. The interorbital space.

The skeletal components of the orbital cavity are the frontal bone, the lesser and greater wing of the sphenoid, the zygoma, the maxilla, the lacrimal bone, a small portion of the palatine bone, and the ethmoid bones (Fig. 27–219).

The bony orbit is described as a conical or pyramidally shaped structure. Actually, both of these comparisons are somewhat inaccurate. The widest diameter of the orbit is located just behind the orbital rim approximately 1.5 cm within the orbital cavity. From this point posteriorly, the orbit begins to narrow quite dramatically in its middle and posterior thirds (Fig. 27–220). The orbital rim is an elliptically shaped structure, whereas the orbit immediately behind the rim is more circular in configuration. The medial wall has a quadrangular, rather than a triangular, configuration. The optic foramen lies on a medial and slightly superior plane in the apex of the orbit. In children, the orbital floor is situated at a lower level in relation to the orbital rim because of the incomplete development of the maxillary sinus.

The orbits may be conceptualized in thirds progressing from anterior to posterior. Anteriorly, the orbital rims consist of thick bone. The middle third of the orbit consists of relatively thin bone, which thickens again in the posterior portion of the orbit (Fig. 27–221). The structure is thus analogous to a shock-absorbing device in which the middle portion of the orbit frequently breaks first, followed by the anterior portions of the rim. The two combinations of fractures thus protect the important nervous and vascular structures in the posterior orbit from severe displacement.

The floor of the orbit is a frequent site of fracture. It has no sharp line or demarcation with the medial wall, but proceeds into the wall by tilting upward in its medial aspect at a 45 degree angle. The lower portion of the medial orbital wall has a progressively lateral inclination. The floor is separated from the lateral wall by the inferior orbital fissure (sphenomaxillary). The floor of the orbit (the roof of the maxillary sinus) is composed mainly of the orbital plate of the maxilla, a

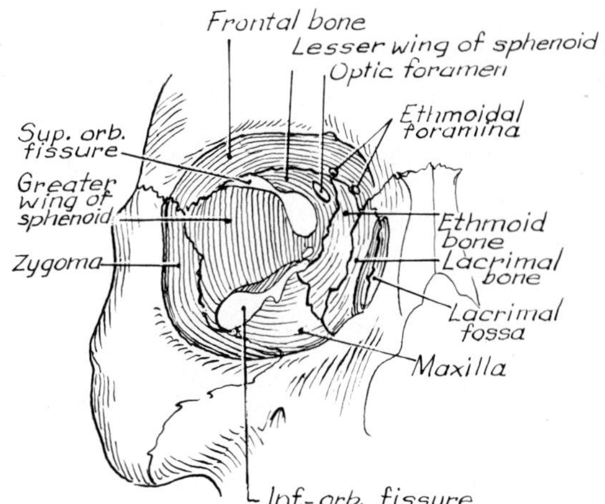

Figure 27–219. Frontal view of the right orbit.

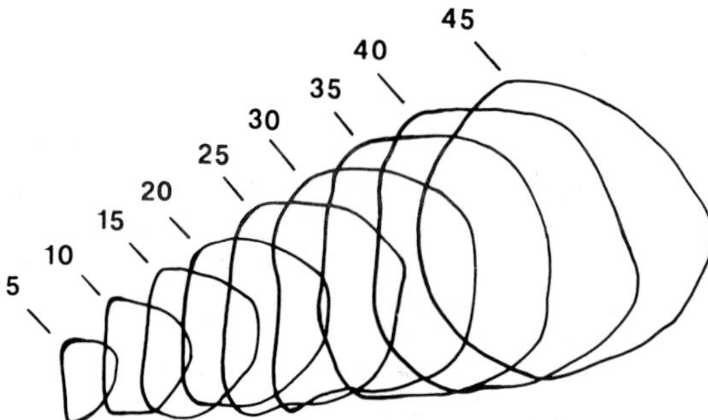

Figure 27–220. The size of the orbit decreases in diameter as one progresses posteriorly.

paper-thin structure medial to the infraorbital groove, and partly of the zygomatic bone anterior to the inferior orbital fissure. The inferior orbital groove or canal traverses the floor of the orbit from medial to lateral. The nerve canal begins anteriorly about the middle of the inferior orbital fissure and the nerve lies in a groove in the posterior portion of the orbit (Fig. 27–222). Anteriorly, it penetrates a canal and turns downward to pass through the thick inferior orbital rim, finally opening on the anterior surface of the maxilla as the infraorbital foramen.

The orbital floor bulges upward behind the globe, providing anterior globe support. The anterior portion of the floor (the first 1.5 cm) is concave and the remainder of the orbital floor is convex. In "blow-out" fractures, the force transmitted by the incompressible orbital contents tends to fracture and displace the convex portion of the floor with the concave portion inferiorly and posteriorly. The fractures first occur at the weakest points in the floor and medial orbital wall, i.e., in the convex portion of the orbital floor adjacent to the infraorbital nerve and in the medial (ethmoid) orbit (see Fig. 27–221). In the posterior portion of the orbit, the inclined plane of the orbital floor presents an especially thin area of bone. This "weak area" (see Fig. 27–221) represents some of the thinnest bone of the orbit. It extends directly into the thin bone of the medial ethmoid in the lamina papyracea, which is a "paper-like" plate of bone that is easily fractured. Fractures in the lamina papyracea of the ethmoid generally compress the bone symmetrically rather than displace

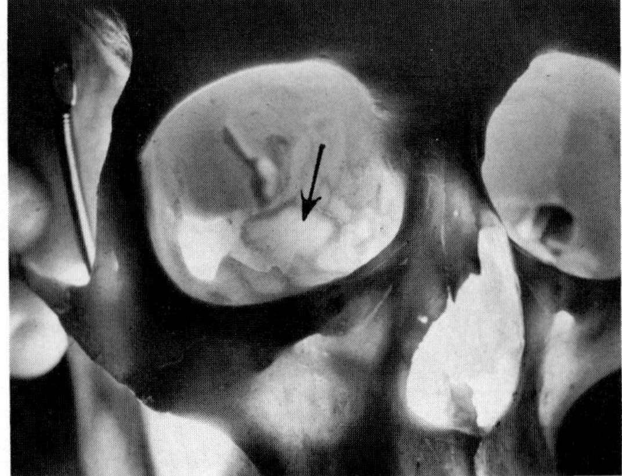

Figure 27–221. A transilluminated dried skull. The area of thin bone in the floor of the orbit is indicated by the arrow. Note the inferior orbital fissure posterolaterally, the lacrimal groove and lamina papyracea medially, and the wide angle of junction between the floor and medial wall. The weak area is further weakened by the infraorbital groove or canal.

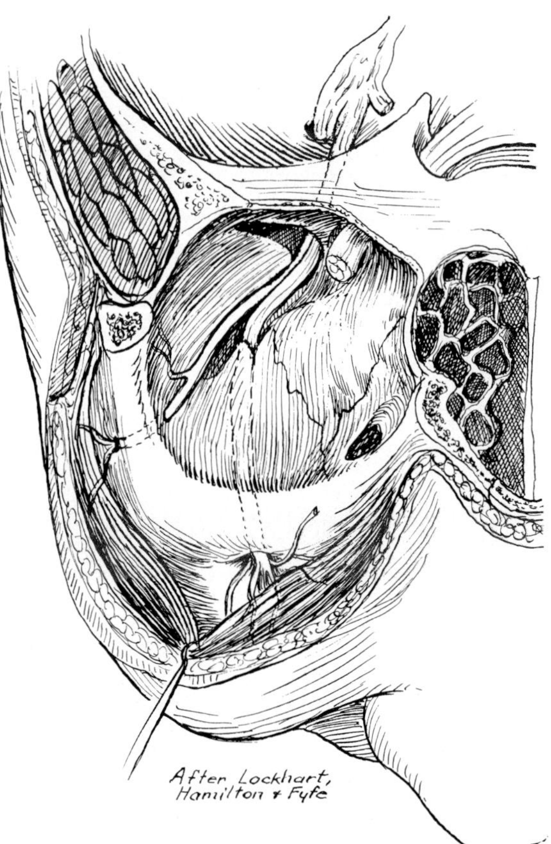

Figure 27–222. The trajectory of the maxillary nerve, which takes its origin as the second division of the trigeminal nerve (fifth cranial nerve). When it enters the infraorbital canal (or groove), it assumes the name "infraorbital" nerve and exits at the infraorbital foramen. The nerve exiting through the malar eminence is the zygomaticofacial nerve. Note the small twig ascending to the temporal area, the zygomaticotemporal nerve. Following zygomatic fractures, patients often have persistent pain adjacent to the zygomaticofrontal suture, a symptom probably related to an injury to this small nerve branch.

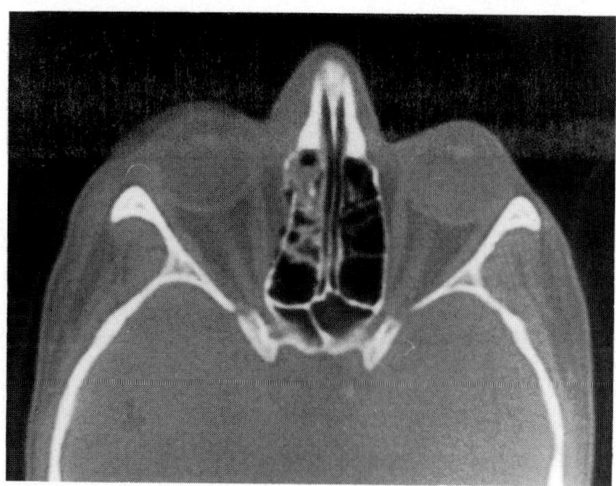

Figure 27–223. Unilateral compression of the medial ethmoidal cells (lamina papyracea), the usual medial orbital "blow-out" fracture.

small pieces (Fig. 27–223). Surgeons must be aware of this symmetric displacement as a mechanism of orbital enlargement, rather than comminution resulting in missing or dislocated smaller sections of bone fragments.

The inferior oblique muscle arises from the medial aspect of the orbital floor adjacent to the lacrimal groove at the anterior margin of the orbit immediately behind the rim. If necessary, subperiosteal dissection may free its origin. The location of this muscle should be recalled when performing orbital dissection.

The medial wall of the orbit is reinforced anteriorly by the frontal process of the maxilla (Fig. 27–224). The wall is relatively fragile and is formed by the frontal bone, the lacrimal bone, the lamina papyracea, the ethmoid, and part of the lesser wing of the sphenoid around the optic foramen (Fig. 27–225). The lamina papyracea is the largest component of the medial orbital wall and accounts for the structural weakness of the area. The lesser wing of the sphenoid and the optic foramen are posterior to the lamina papyracea. The optic foramen is located close to the posterior portion of the ethmoid sinus, not at the true apex of the orbit (Fig. 27–225). Consequently, in severe fractures involving the medial wall in its posterior portion, fracture lines may extend through the optic canal.

The groove for the lacrimal sac is a broad vertical fossa lying partly on the anterior aspect of the lacrimal bone and partly on the frontal process of the maxilla; the anterior and posterior margins of the lacrimal groove form the respective lacrimal crests. The groove is continuous with the nasolacrimal duct at the junction of the floor and medial wall of the orbit, passing down into the inferior meatus of the nose. Between the roof and the medial wall of the orbit are the anterior and posterior ethmoid foramina, which lead into canals communicating with the medial portion of the anterior cranial fossa, the ethmoid sinus, and the nose.

The lateral wall of the orbit (Fig. 27–226)

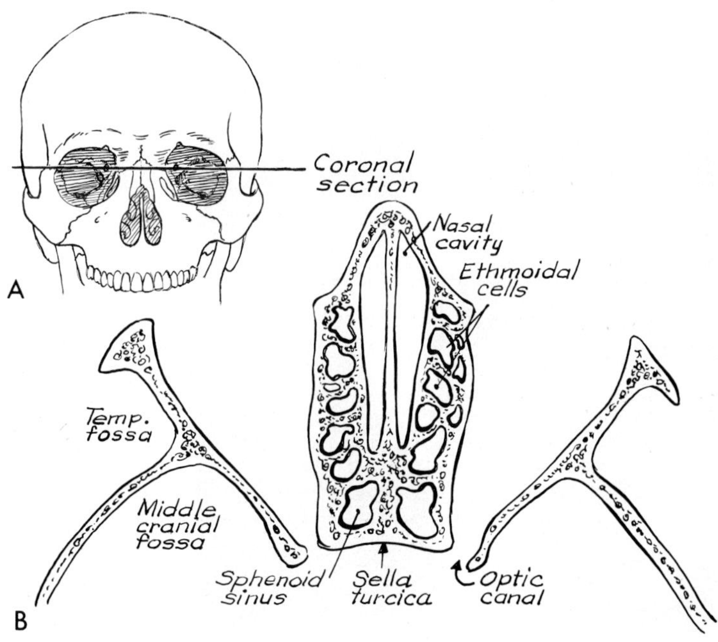

Figure 27–224. Transverse section showing the relationship of the orbit to the temporal fossa and middle cranial fossa. *A*, The level of section is indicated by the horizontal line. *B*, Note that the lateral wall is inclined from lateral to medial as far as the optic foramen; it is thus situated along an oblique frontal-sagittal plane.

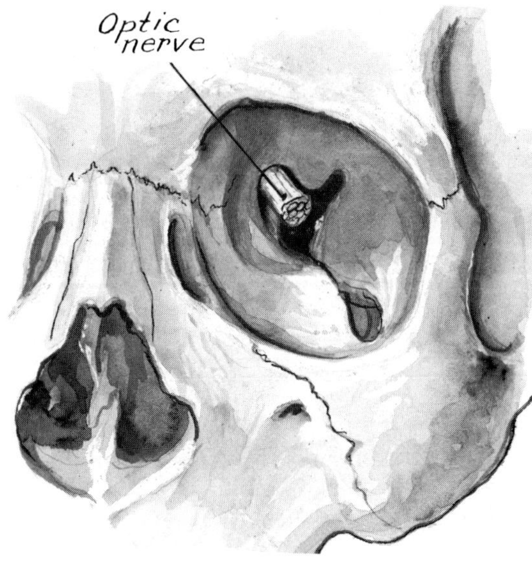

Figure 27–225. The relationship of the optic nerve and the orbital cavity. Note the high position of the optic foramen in relation to the floor of the orbit and the close proximity of the optic foramen with the posterior portion of the medial wall of the orbit. When one encounters the posterior ethmoidal vessels, one is within 5 mm of the optic nerve. The optic nerve is usually located 40 to 45 mm from the anterior orbital rim.

is relatively stout in its anterior portion. It is formed by the greater wing of the sphenoid, the frontal process of the zygomatic bone, and the lesser wing of the sphenoid lateral to the optic foramen. The superior orbital fissure is a cleft that runs outward, forward, and upward from the apex of the orbit, between the roof and the lateral wall. This fissure, which separates the greater and lesser wings of the sphenoid, gives passage to the three motor nerves to the extraocular muscles of the orbit (cranial nerves III, IV, and VI). The ophthalmic division of the trigeminal nerve also enters the orbit through this fissure. The fissure leads into the middle cranial fossa. The lateral wall of the orbit is situated in an anterolateral and posteromedial plane (Fig. 27–226). It is related to the temporal fossa; posteriorly, a small part of the wall lies between the orbit and the middle cranial fossa and the temporal lobe of the brain. Between the floor and the lateral wall of the orbit is the inferior orbital fissure, which communicates with the infratemporal fossa. The inferior orbital fissure has divisions of the maxillary portion of the trigeminal nerve and veins communicating with the infratemporal area.

The roof of the orbit is composed mainly of the orbital plate of the frontal bone, but

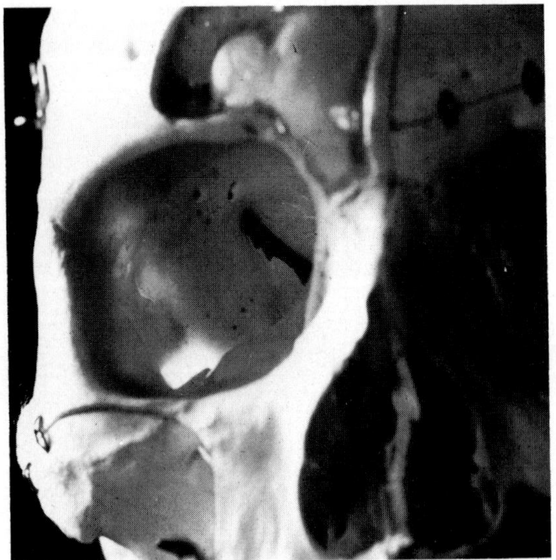

Figure 27–226. Transilluminated orbit demonstrating the thin posterior portion of the lateral orbital wall, contrasting with the strong abutment of its anterior portion and rim.

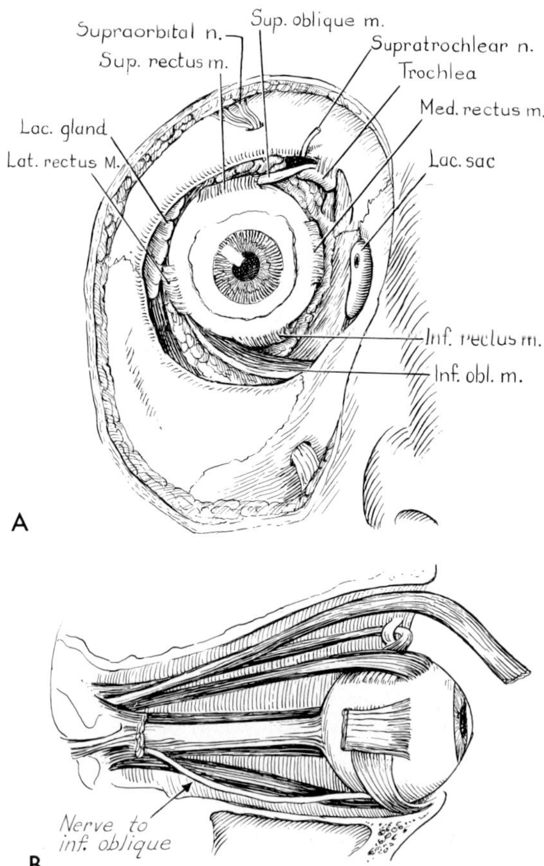

Figure 27–227. The extraocular muscles. *A*, Frontal view. The position of the inferior rectus and inferior oblique muscles on the undersurface of the ocular globe. *B*, Sagittal view. Relation of the nerve to the inferior oblique muscle. The nerve may be injured in blow-out fractures. (From Converse, J. M., and Smith, B.: Blow-out fracture of the floor of the orbit. Trans. Am. Acad. Ophthalmol. Otolaryngol., *64*:676, 1960.)

posteriorly it receives a minor contribution from the lesser wing of the sphenoid. The fossa lodging the lacrimal gland is a depression situated along the anterior and lateral aspect, which is sheltered by the zygomatic process of the frontal bone. The anterior and medial portions of the roof can be invaded by the supraorbital extension of the frontal sinus, or by extensions of the ethmoid sinus or frontoethmoidal air cells. The roof separates the orbit from the anterior cranial fossa and from the middle cranial fossa on the posterolateral aspect.

The roof often consists of thin, brittle bone; it is especially thin in its medial portion. The supratrochlear and supraorbital nerves and, more medially, the trochlea or "pulley" of the superior oblique muscle are located along the superior rim of the orbit. The tendon of the superior oblique muscle functions as a cartilaginous pulley or trochlea, which is fixed by ligamentous fibers immediately behind the superomedial angle of the orbital rim. Fractures involving the superomedial portion of the rim may result in compression of the supraorbital nerve within its foramen, with the development of anesthesia in the area of distribution of this sensory nerve. Diplopia may also result from injury to the superior oblique muscle, thus affecting the balance of extraocular muscle movement (Fig. 27–227).

Orbital Fat and Ocular Globe. The ocular globe is surrounded by a cushion of orbital fat within the orbital cavity. The ocular globe occupies only the anterior half of the orbital cavity. The posterior half of the orbital cavity is filled with fat, muscles, vessels, and nerves that supply the ocular globe and extraocular muscles, and provide sensation to tissues about the orbit (Fig. 27–227). The orbital cavity may thus be conceptualized in two halves from anterior to posterior. They are separated by Tenon's capsule, a fascial structure that subdivides the orbital cavity into an anterior (or *precapsular*) segment and a posterior (or *retrocapsular*) segment.

Throughout the extraocular fat there are fine septal communications that diffusely divide the fat into small compartments and provide ligament structures that attach to the bony orbital walls, to the extraocular muscles, and to Tenon's capsule. Thus, the fine ligamentous structures of the orbit provide a network of support for the soft tissue contents. These structures decrease in density as one progresses from anterior to posterior (Fig. 27–228).

The orbital fat can be divided into anterior and posterior portions. The anterior, extraocular fat is largely *extraconal*, which means that it exists outside the muscle cone. Posteriorly, the muscle cone is an approximate, rather than an exact, anatomic structure, as there are only fine fascial communications separating the *extraconal* from the *intraconal* fat compartments. Intraconal fat constitutes three-fourths of the fat in the posterior orbit (Fig. 27–229), and may be displaced *outside* the muscle cone, contributing to a loss of globe support from loss of soft tissue volume. The cushion of fat above the levator muscle is extraconal, as is the fat on the anterior portion of the orbital floor. The latter fat does not contribute to globe support.

Septum Orbitale. The orbital contents are maintained in position by the septum orbitale

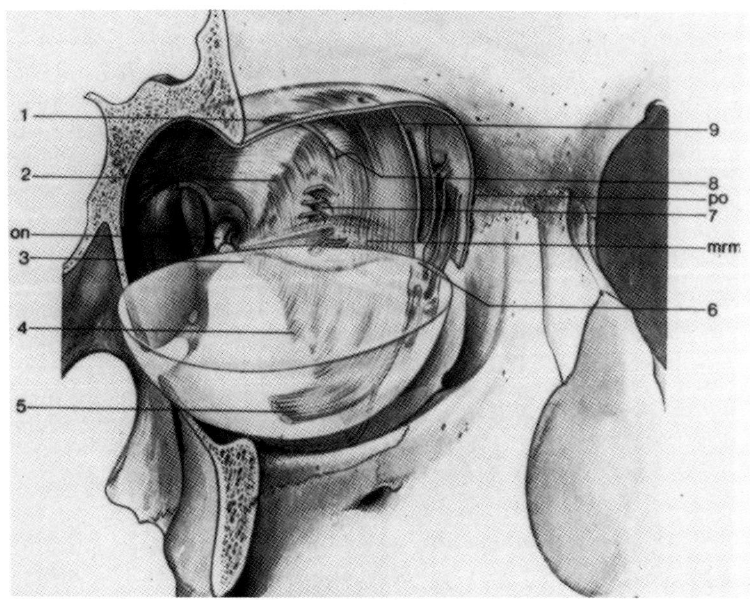

Figure 27–228. Some of the components of the fine ligament system running within the soft tissue of the orbit. An intricate network has been described by Koornneef. (From Koornneef, L.: Current concepts in the management of orbital blow-out fractures. Ann. Plast. Surg., 9:185, 1982.)

(orbital septum), a fascial structure inserting on the inner aspect of the orbital rim. The septum orbitale attaches to and blends with the levator aponeurosis in the upper eyelid for a distance of a few millimeters above the upper border of the tarsus. In the lower eyelid, the septum orbitale is attached to the lower border of the tarsus (Fig. 27–230).

Periorbita. The periosteum lining the periphery of the orbit is also known as the periorbita. The periorbita is continuous with the dura at those sites where the orbit communicates with the cranial cavity, i.e., the optic foramen, the superior orbital fissure, and the anterior and posterior ethmoidal canals.

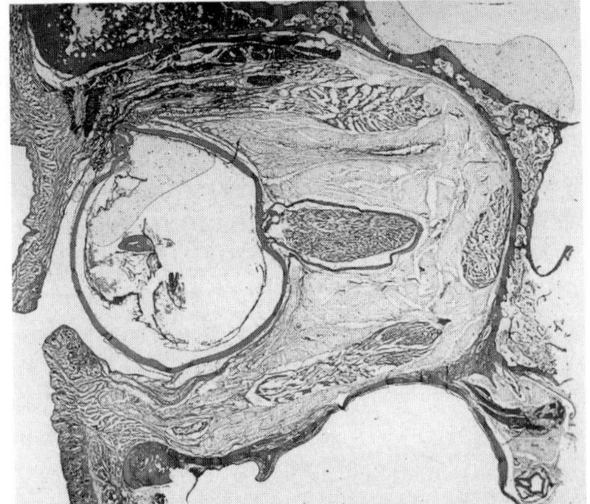

Figure 27–229. Sagittal section through the orbit. The muscles run close to the orbital walls, especially behind the globe. Most of the fat is intraconal.

Optic Foramen and Optic Canal. The optic foramen is situated at the junction of the lateral and medial walls of the orbit in its far posterior portion (see Fig. 27–225). The foramen is not on a horizontal plane with the orbital floor, but above the horizontal plane. The foramen is located 40 to 45 mm behind the inferior orbital rim. Inferior orbital dissection should be performed with precise knowledge of this position and location. The optic canal is 4 to 10 mm in length and is the passage through which the optic nerve and ophthalmic artery pass from an intracranial to an intraorbital position (see Fig. 27–224). The canal is framed medially by the body of the sphenoid and laterally by the lesser wing. It is thus in close approximation to the sphenoid sinus and the posterior ethmoidal air cells. The bony optic canal forms a tight sheath about the optic nerve, and fractures with swelling predispose to vascular compression of the nerve in the canal.

BLOW-OUT FRACTURES OF FLOOR OF ORBIT

A blow-out fracture is caused by the application of a traumatic force to the rim or the soft tissues of the orbit; it is usually accompanied by a sudden increase in intraorbital pressure. Converse and Smith (1957, 1960) postulated that the fracture occurs from transmission of force directly to the soft tissue contents of the orbit. The incompressible soft

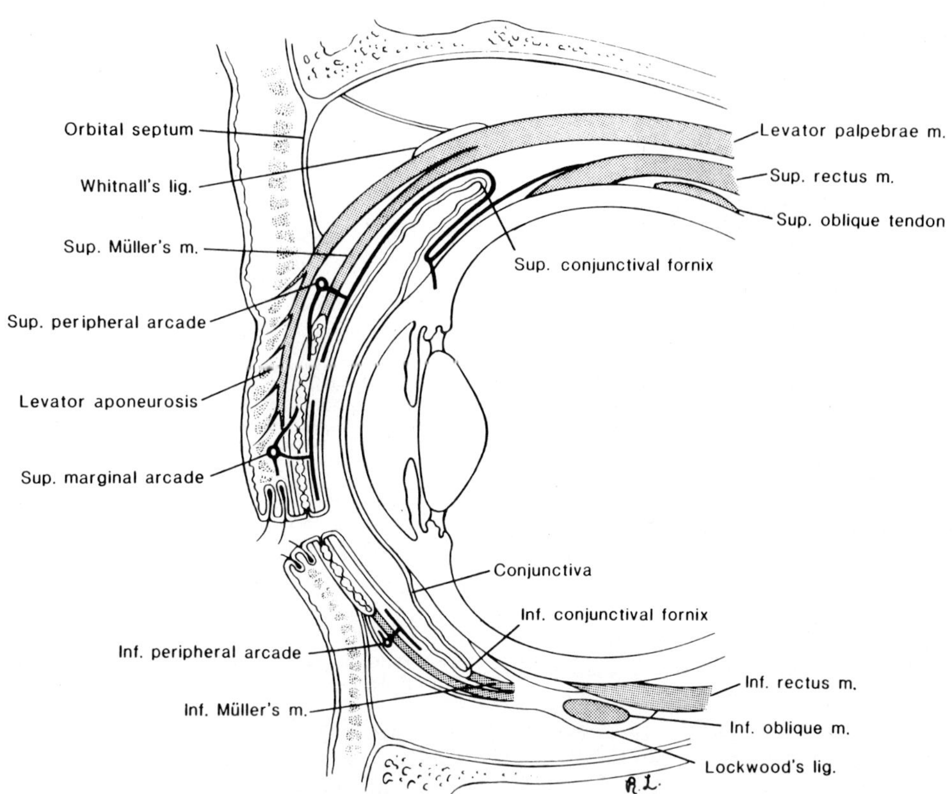

Figure 27–230. Sagittal view of the eyelids, globe, and arterial system.

tissues are displaced posteriorly, applying this force to the thin portions of the orbital floor and medial orbital wall, which are the first to fracture as a result of this force application. Soft tissue contents of the orbit are extruded through the fractured area, and incarcerated by the edges of the fracture or by a "trapdoor" displacement of a thin orbital bone plate. Orbital fractures are often complicated by diplopia, which usually consists of a vertical muscle imbalance produced by contusion of muscles or entrapment of soft tissue around the inferior rectus and inferior oblique muscles. The muscles and their surrounding fascial expansions are tethered to the orbital fat, which is the most common soft tissue extruded into the maxillary sinus. The escape of orbital fat outside the normal bony boundaries of the orbit and the displacement of intramuscular cone (intraconal) fat to an extramuscular position are responsible for loss of globe prominence or enophthalmos.

William Lang (1889) first described a depressed fracture of the orbital floor and the associated condition of post-traumatic enophthalmos. In this century the condition was again described by Pfeiffer (1943) and Converse and Smith (1957). The term "blow-out fracture" was coined by Converse and Smith (1957). They agreed with Pfeiffer (1943) and disagreed with Le Fort (1901) and La Grange (1918), believing that the mechanism of the orbital fracture was produced by a hydraulic force (Smith and Regan, 1957) of increased intraorbital soft tissue pressure, rather than a "buckling force" delivered to the rim, producing a fracture in the thin portion of the orbit. In 1967, Jones and Evans used fresh cadavers to evaluate the proposed mechanism of orbital floor fractures. They produced fractures of the floor of the orbit in 70 per cent of the specimens, isolated medial wall fractures in 20 per cent, and combined fractures of the floor and medial wall in 10 per cent. Most fractures occurred medial to the posterior part of the orbital groove where the orbital floor is the thinnest. In 1964, Dingman and Natvig described a patient with a "blow-in" fracture of the orbit. This fracture mechanism was assumed to be the result of the buckling effect of a strong blow to the orbital rim.

One of the early descriptions of a blow-out fracture was given by King and Samuel (1944): "We would like to add one other type of fracture of great importance which is not infrequent. In this, there is a downward displacement of a part of the orbital floor, unassociated with any damage to the margin of the orbit surrounding the facial bones. The cause of such a fracture is difficult to visualize. The most ready explanation is trauma transmitted through the eye to the orbital floor."

After the application of a traumatic force over the orbital contents by a nonpenetrating object, such as a round tennis ball (Fig. 27–231) or the human fist (Fig. 27–232), the orbital contents are forced backward into the narrower portion of the orbit (Table 27–2). The increased intraorbital pressure thus exerted causes a blow-out at the weakest area of the orbital floor without fracturing the orbital rim. This type of fracture may be referred to as a "pure" blow-out fracture (Table 27–3) (Converse and Smith, 1957). The strong rim of the orbit protects against objects with a radius of curvature greater than 5 cm.

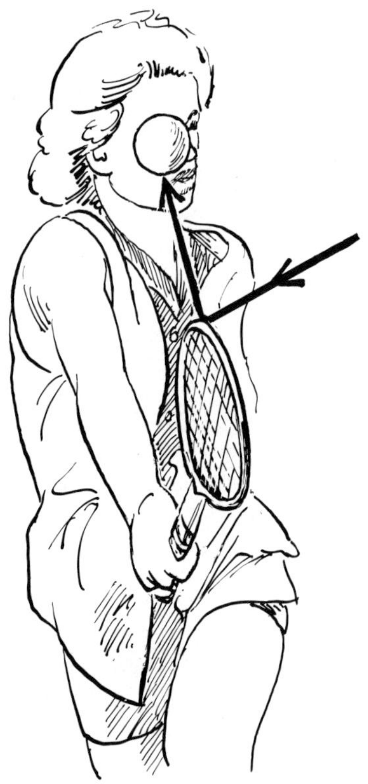

Figure 27–231. The tennis ball has a diameter in curvature greater than 5 cm and thus does not penetrate the protective barrier of the orbital rim.

Table 27–2. Etiologic Features in 100 Blow-out Fractures

Automobile	49
Human fist	18
Human elbow	4
Wooden plank	1
Ball	5
Snowball	2
Skin pole	2
Edge of table	1
Blunt object	1
Shoe kick	2
Steel bar	1
Machinery	2
Boxing glove	1
Mop handle	1
Human buttock	1
Airplain accident	1
Water ski accident	1
Ice bank	1
Fall on face	4
Iatrogenic (surgical)	1
Military casualty (shell fragment)	1

From Converse, J. M., Smith, B., O'Bear, M. F., and Wood-Smith, D.: Orbital blow-out fractures: a ten-year survey. Plast. Reconstr. Surg., *39*:20, 1967. Copyright 1967, The Williams and Wilkins Company, Baltimore.

An object having a curvature of less than 5 cm may penetrate this protective barrier and damage the globe. Such objects as golf balls, hockey pucks, or the tip of a football can result in this type of injury.

A champagne bottle cork may damage the globe, because its radius is less than 5 cm. Its less propulsive force is a less common

Table 27–3. Classification of Orbital Fractures

1. ***Orbital Blow-out Fractures***
   A, Pure blow-out fractures: fractures through the thin areas of the orbital floor, medial and lateral wall. The orbital rim is intact.
   B, Impure blow-out fractures: fractures associated with fracture of the adjacent facial bones. The thick orbital rim is fractured, and its backward displacement causes a comminution of the orbital floor; the posterior displacement of the orbital rim permits the traumatizing force to be applied against the orbital contents, which produces a superimposed blow-out fracture.
2. ***Orbital Fractures Without Blow-out Fracture***
   A, Linear fractures, in upper maxillary and zygomatic fractures. These fractures are often uncomplicated from the standpoint of the orbit.
   B, Comminuted fracture of the orbital floor with prolapse of the orbital contents into the maxillary sinus is often associated with fracture of the midfacial bones.
   C, Fracture of the zygoma with frontozygomatic separation and downward displacement of the zygomatic portion of the orbital floor and of the lateral attachment of the suspensory ligament of Lockwood.

From Converse, J. M., Smith, B., O'Bear, M. F., and Wood-Smith, D.: Orbital blow-out fractures: a ten-year survey. Plast. Reconstr. Surg., *39*:20, 1967. Copyright 1967, The Williams and Wilkins Company, Baltimore.

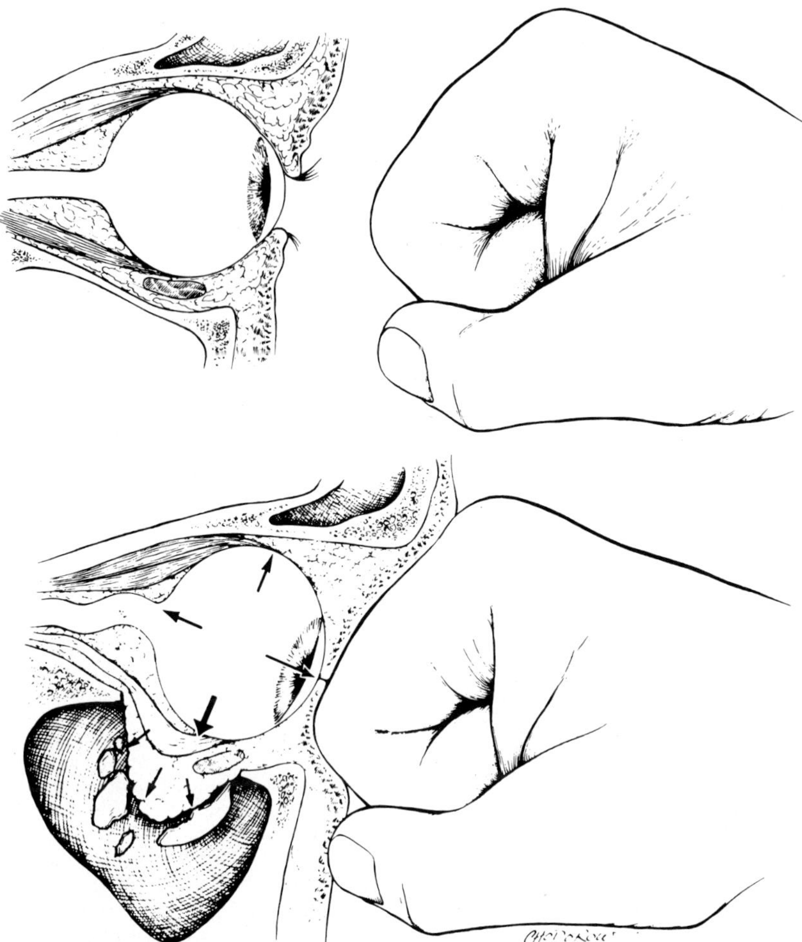

Figure 27–232. A frequent cause of blow-out fractures is the human fist, which penetrates the protective barrier formed by the rim of the orbit, causing increased intraorbital pressure. A blow-out fracture occurs at the weakest portion of the orbital floor. (Mechanism suggested by Converse and Smith.)

cause of blow-out fractures but more frequently the globe ruptures.

Larger objects cannot enter the orbital opening and may cause direct injury to either the eye or the bones of the rim. Fragile spectacle lenses, which can shatter, may be interposed between the traumatizing object and the globe. An evaluation for globe rupture or globe injury is thus imperative when any fractures about the orbit are suspected.

Blow-out fractures are more frequent on the right than on the left side, because most individuals are right-handed and many blow-out fractures are caused by the human fist in altercations.

Mechanism of Production of a Blow-Out Fracture

After the clinical description of the findings of fracture of the orbital floor, entrapment of the structures, and diplopia without fracture of the rim (Converse and Smith, 1957), one mechanism of production of the orbital blow-out fracture was demonstrated experimentally. It was verified in a cadaver by duplicating a force similar to that which had produced a blow-out fracture in one of Converse's patients, who had been hit by a ball used in the Irish game of hurling (Fig. 27–233) (Smith and Regan, 1957). The dried-out condition of the cadaver globe was corrected by the intraocular injection of normal saline solution. A hurling ball was placed over the closed lid of the cadaver orbit and the ball was struck sharply with a mallet. A cracking sound was heard and was interpreted as having been caused by a fracturing bone. An exploratory incision through the skin of the infraorbital margin and elevation of the orbital contents from the floor exposed a depressed comminuted fracture of the floor of

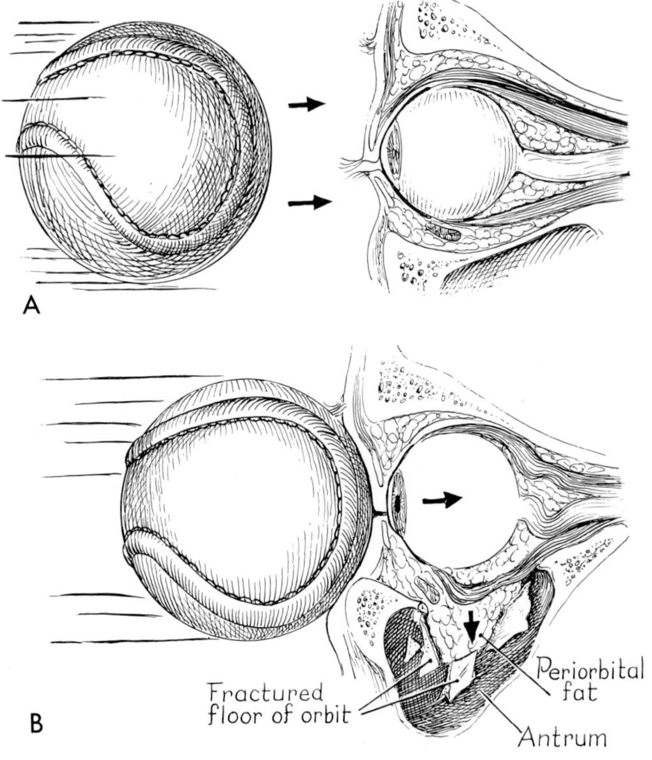

Figure 27–233. External pressure striking the globe and orbital rim produces a fracture of the globe of the orbit with entrapment of orbital soft tissue contents. The inferior oblique and inferior rectus muscles and their fascial expansions (in the adjacent fat) are incarcerated in the fractures. (From Converse, J. M., and Smith, B: Enophthalmos and diplopia in fractures of the orbital floor. Br. J. Plast. Surg., *9*:265, 1957.)

the orbit. Exenteration of the orbital contents exposed the fracture in its entirety. The result was a comminuted fracture involving the lamina papyracea of the ethmoid bone. No fracture of the orbital rim or zygomatic arch was observed.

In a second experiment, the opposite orbit of the cadaver was exenterated. The soft tissue covering the orbital rim was excised to allow direct contact of the bony orbital rim with the surface of the hurling ball. Repeated blows of similar force with a hammer failed to fracture either the floor or the rim of the orbit. However, when the striking force was sufficiently increased, the orbital rim and the floor were comminuted simultaneously.

The mechanism of a blow-out fracture relating to increased hydraulic pressure has been questioned by a number of authors (Rény and Stricker, 1969; Fujino, 1974a,b). Rény and Stricker suggested the following hypothesis. A traumatic force striking the inferior orbital rim, which is sufficiently resilient to transmit the force to the orbital floor, fractures the latter, while the rim rebounds without fracturing. Fujino (1974a,b) in a series of experiments in collaboration with engineers, demonstrated on a dried human skull, without orbital contents, that a brass striker weighing 120 gm with a flat silicone plate, when dropped on the infraorbital margin from a height of 15 cm, produced a linear fracture of the orbital floor (Fig. 27–234). When the weight was dropped from a height of 20 cm, a punched-out fracture in the convex portion of the orbital floor was produced (Fig. 27–235).

Fujino proved that increased hydraulic pressure within the orbit was not essential for the development of a blow-out fracture. He produced linear fractures of the orbital floor with a blow to the orbital rim, and with increased force a typical punched-out fracture of the posterior orbital floor occurred. Fujino also produced linear fractures by striking the eyeball alone in experiments. Less force is necessary to produce an orbital floor fracture when the impact point is the rim than when the impact point is the eyeball alone. Thus, the experiments imply that orbital floor fractures can be produced by either eyeball or rim impacts; however, less force is necessary when rim impacts occur. The role of increased intraorbital pressure is implicated in soft tissue incarceration in the fracture site. During high speed photographic analysis of the

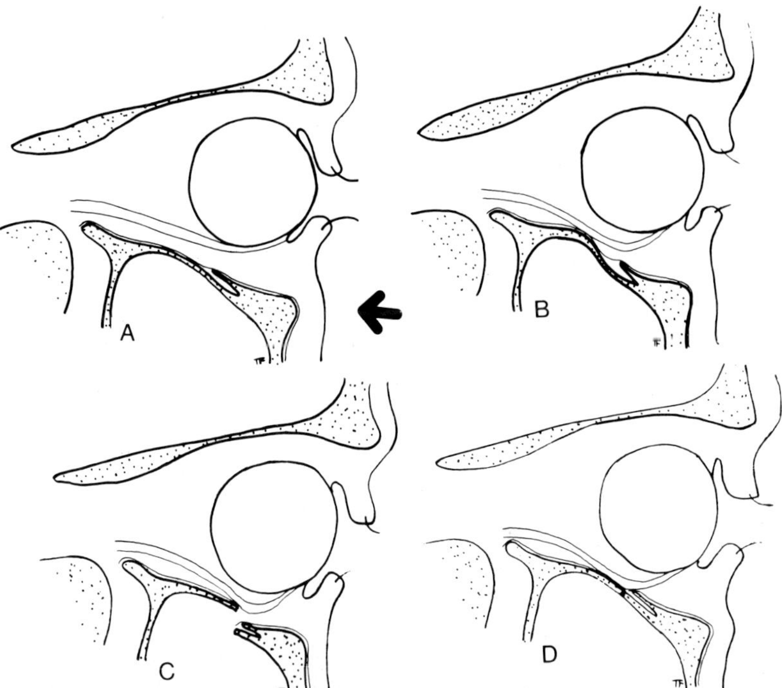

Figure 27–234. Mechanism of orbital blow-out fracture. A deforming force to the rim *(A)* creates a buckling of the orbital floor *(B)*. In *C* a fracture has occurred. After relief of the deforming force, the anterior fragment returns to its original position *(D)*. Soft tissue orbital contents may be trapped in the fracture site. (From Fujino, T.: Experimental "blow-out" fracture of the orbit. Plast. Reconstr. Surg., *54*:81, 1974.)

fractures, the deformity of the soft tissue in the orbit recovers much more slowly than the deformity of the bone structure. Thus, the soft tissue tends to be entrapped in bone fragments. Fujino (Fujino, 1963, 1974a,b; Fujino and Makino, 1980) also observed that in orbits that did not fracture the orbital contents distorted as in the case of fractures. This produced clinical symptoms noted by Milauskas (Milauskas and Fueger, 1966; Milauskas, 1969), mimicking blow-out fractures in which only soft tissue contusion has occurred, and further emphasizes the mechanisms described by Koornneef (1977, 1982) in his sectional anatomic specimens of the orbit. Koornneef documented the role of fine connective tissues septa enveloping the globe, muscles, and intraorbital contents within the periorbita. The connective tissues septa become involved in traumatic injury and fracture sites, and because of the delicate intraconnections of all orbital structures, produce motility problems after either fractures or blunt injuries. Thus, diplopia without incarceration of orbital soft tissue is explained by the connective tissue septa. Fujino (Fujino, 1963, 1974a,b; Fujino and Makino, 1980) further emphasized that in the case of a blow-out fracture, the anterior edge of the posterior segment of the orbital floor, after the development of a first fracture, pushes against the posterior part of the anterior segment until a second fracture occurs (see Fig. 27–234). They noted that a blow-out fracture by globe pressure alone required a force ten times greater than the force necessary to produce buckling of the orbital floor. Thus, these authors emphasized that if increased globe pressure were the primary causative factor, one would expect a higher incidence of ocular injuries than that observed. The incidence of ocular injuries accompanying globe fractures is 10 to 30 per cent.

Whatever the theory of the mechanism of blow-out fractures, the fact remains that in the presence of double vision due to entrapment and the inability to rotate the globe by means of a forced duction test, release of the entrapment is the only means of relieving the extraocular muscle imbalance and double vision. Tables 27–2 and 27–3 set out the etiologies and classification of orbital fractures. Types and complications are detailed in Tables 27–4 and 27–5.

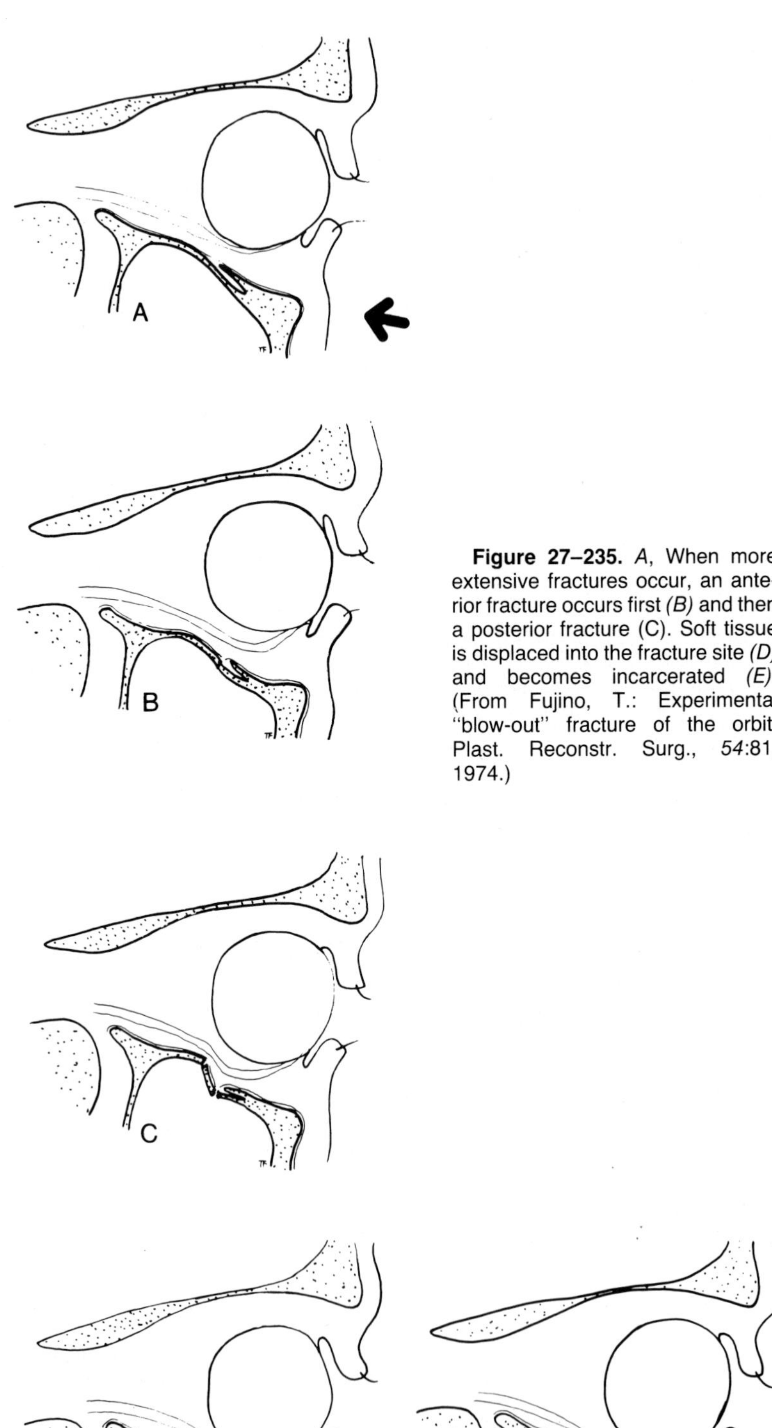

Figure 27–235. *A*, When more extensive fractures occur, an anterior fracture occurs first *(B)* and then a posterior fracture (C). Soft tissue is displaced into the fracture site *(D)* and becomes incarcerated *(E)*. (From Fujino, T.: Experimental "blow-out" fracture of the orbit. Plast. Reconstr. Surg., *54*:81, 1974.)

Table 27–4. Diplopia and Enophthalmos in Orbital Fractures

1. With diplopia, with enophthalmos. This condition results from incarceration of the orbital contents into the area of the fracture and from tearing of the periorbita and escape of the orbital fat.
2. With diplopia, without enophthalmos.This condition may occur with fixation of the orbital contents in a linear fracture. There is no escape of orbital fat, no enlargement of the orbit, and no enophthalmos.
3. Without diplopia, with enophthalmos. There is no fixation of the inferior orbital contents into the area of the fracture. The periorbita is torn and an opening has occurred that allows escape of orbital fat, or the orbital cavity is sufficiently enlarged to result in enophthalmos.
4. Without diplopia, without enophthalmos. This condition occurs when the fracture does not cause fixation of the orbital contents or disturb the anatomy of the periorbita or orbital cavity.

Impure Blow-Out Fractures

According to Garrett (1963), oculo-orbital damage occurs in approximately 10 per cent of all head injuries sustained in automobile accidents in the United States. In the typical high energy injury, the passenger's face is projected against a hard object, such as the dashboard or the steering wheel. The thick orbital rim is fractured and displaced backward, resulting in an eggshell comminution of the thin "middle" portion of the orbit. Because of the continuing momentum and the pressure against the soft tissue orbital contents, a portion of the contents is extruded through fracture sites, creating incarceration or prolapse of orbital contents. These fractures have been termed *impure* blow-out fractures, as suggested by Cramer, Tooze, and Lerman (1965). In the series studied by Emery, Noorden, and Sclernitzauer (1971), the human fist was the principal factor causing *pure* blow-out fractures. In the series of Converse and associates (1967), automobile accidents were responsible for the large proportion of injuries. Most of the patients demonstrated complicated fractures, such as pyramidal maxillary fractures (Le Fort II) and craniofacial dysjunction (Le Fort III), which involve the orbit by definition. The characteristic fracture lines may travel in a variety of patterns, but the orbital floor, lateral orbit, and medial orbit are frequently involved.

Table 27–5. Analysis of Complications in Orbital Fractures Persistent after Floor Repair (50 cases)*

		Postoperative	
	Preoperative	*3 Months*	*1 Year*
Extraocular muscle imbalance	43	30	20
Enophthalmos	27	15	11
Ptosis	12	3	2
Medial canthal deformity	12	12	9
Lacrimal obstruction	3	3	0
Vertical shortening of lower lid	4	4	2
Visual impairment	5	5	5
Trichiasis–symblepharon	2	1	0

*These complications were observed in patients referred to the author after unsuccessful treatment.

From Converse, J. M., Smith, B., O'Bear, M. F., and Wood-Smith, D.: Orbital blow-out fractures: a ten-year survey. Plast. Reconstr. Surg., *39*:20, 1967. Copyright 1967, The Williams and Wilkins Company, Baltimore.

Orbital Expansion/Contraction Secondary to Fractures

The space occupied by the soft tissue contents of the orbit may expand or contract secondary to fracture displacement. The term "blow-out" actually describes orbital expansion secondary to fracture displacement. Fractures have been described with an inward displacement, which actually reduces the space available to soft tissue contents (Godoy and Mathog, 1985). The term "blow-in" fracture has been used to describe the orbital volume contraction that occurs secondary to some types of bone displacement. A typical fracture causing orbital contraction would be an orbital roof fracture in which the displacement of the roof is downward and backward, creating a downward and forward displacement of the globe. The term "blow-out" actually applies to destruction of the floor and medial wall of the orbit, and signifies the potential for displacement of orbital contents into the sinus cavities. In the typical blow-out fracture, displacement of the globe posteriorly, medially, and inferiorly is seen. This occurs because of the prolapse of orbital soft tissue into the maxillary and ethmoid sinuses. Orbital fractures of the floor and the lateral portion of the orbit accompany zygomatic fractures, with the exclusion of the isolated zygomatic arch fracture.

Blow-Out Fractures in Children

Sinus development in children is incomplete and progresses as the tooth buds of the permanent dentition erupt. The floor of the

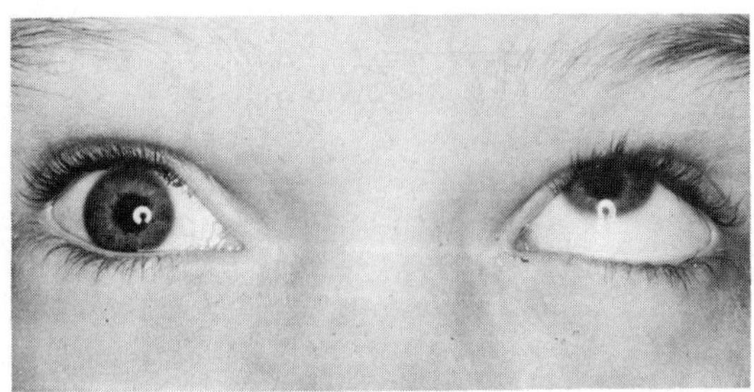

Figure 27–236. Blow-out fracture in a child produced by the striking force of a snowball. Note the near-complete immobility of the ocular globe and the enophthalmos.

maxillary sinus is seen to occupy a progressively lower level until ages 9 to 10 years when the development of the maxillary sinus is largely complete. As a result of the underdevelopment of the maxillary sinus in children, the floor of the orbit is more resilient than in adults. Blow-out fractures are thus less common in young children (Panagoupolous, 1957; Graham and Peltier, 1960; Bales, Randall, and Lehr, 1972; Hall, 1972; Reil and Kranz, 1976; Kaban, Mulliken, and Murray, 1977; Fortunato, Fielding, and Guernsey, 1982). The floor of the orbit is situated in a rather low position, dipping downward from the orbital rim. Children's bones are resilient and elastic, an additional factor accounting for the reduced frequency of fractures (see also Chap. 28). In children, the mechanism of entrapment is similar to that seen in adults, and the author has observed true muscle incarceration (as opposed to incarceration of fat adjacent to the inferior rectus muscle) more frequently in children than in adults (Fig. 27–236). This may be determined on CT scan, and surgery should be considered at the earliest opportunity in cases of muscle incarceration.

Surgical Pathology

Diplopia. Extraocular muscle imbalance and subjective diplopia are the result of muscle contusion or incarceration of the soft tissue adjacent to the muscles. Deviation of the visual axes can account for diplopia. The major cause is contusion, which must be differentiated from entrapment of the soft tissue structures in the blow-out fracture area. Both may produce findings of vertical muscle imbalance. The patient may have diplopia on looking upward or downward, actions of the inferior rectus muscle. Soft tissue structures involved include the inferior rectus muscle, inferior oblique muscles, suspensory ligament of Lockwood, periorbita, fascial expansions, and fat with the fine musculofacial ligamentous system described by Koornneef (1977, 1982) adjacent to the muscle.

The downward displacement of an ocular globe does not always result in double vision. Several authors have indicated that the displacement must exceed 5 mm for diplopia to be reasonably attributed to globe displacement. The eye is able to accommodate to a range of superoinferior displacement without diplopia, and indeed severe displacement occurring slowly is often asymptomatic. Massive comminution of the orbital floor accounts for downward and posterior displacement of the ocular globe. Frequently, there is no entrapment unless the action of the muscle is severely limited by contusion.

The inferior oblique muscle arises from the maxillary portion of the orbital floor immediately behind the rim and lateral to the lacrimal groove. The inferior rectus muscle is situated immediately above the infraorbital canal and the undersurface of the orbital contents. Both can be easily visualized in CT scans. It is not surprising, therefore, that these two muscles are often involved in fractures involving the *medial* floor and the rim of the orbit (see Fig. 27–227). The absence of elasticity in the impounded inferior rectus muscle would restrict rotation in the field of action of its antagonist, the superior rectus. Because the muscles are intimately connected at the point where the inferior oblique crosses beneath the inferior rectus, disturbance of the function of the inferior oblique muscle is usually observed in blow-out fractures. When the fracture is located *lateral* to the infraorbital groove or canal, the inferior rectus and inferior oblique muscles may not be involved. These variations in the site of the blow-out fracture explain variations in the symptoms and clinical signs of these fractures.

Injury to the cranial nerves supplying the inferior oblique and inferior rectus muscles must also be considered as an etiology in diplopia. The inferior oblique and inferior rectus muscles are innervated by the inferior division of cranial nerve III. The branch to the inferior rectus muscle passes along its upper surface to pierce it at the junction of the posterior and middle thirds of the muscle (see Fig. 27–227). The branch to the inferior oblique muscle runs along the lateral edge of the inferior rectus muscle and can be clearly seen in orbital dissections, entering the ocu-

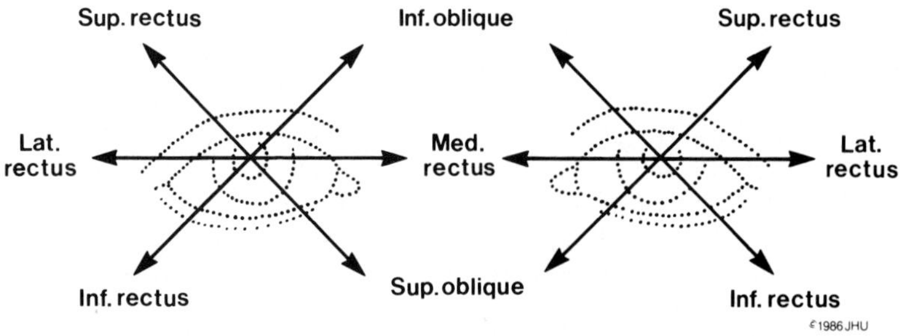

Sup. rectus
Inf. oblique
Sup. rectus
Lat. rectus
Med. rectus
Lat. rectus
Inf. rectus
Sup. oblique
Inf. rectus
©1986 JHU

Figure 27–237. The dominant field of action of each of the extraocular muscles.

lar surface of the inferior oblique muscle in the anterior third of the orbit. It is therefore exposed to injury by comminution or contusion in blow-out fractures. The relatively short course of the nerve to the inferior rectus muscle with its superior location renders it less vulnerable to injury. Visual field examination will help to determine whether muscle function is disturbed. Saccadic velocities can assess the acceleration of extraocular movement and can sometimes distinguish muscle contusion from actual entrapment.

Injury to cranial nerves III, IV, and VI or direct injury to the extraocular muscles may occur secondary to laceration by bone fragments, disruption of muscle attachments, contusion, and hemorrhage. Alternatively, it has been postulated that a change in muscle balance can be caused by a change in orbital shape. Muscle imbalance occurs when ptosis of the globe is associated with enophthalmos. Secondary deviations are caused by overaction of the "yolk" or "conjugate muscles" of the opposite eye. A factor to be remembered is that no extraocular muscle acts alone to produce ocular movements. Ocular rotation is the sum of the action, counteraction, and relaxation of the 12 extraocular muscles (six per globe). The subject of the physiology of the ocular rotatory muscles is complex and exceeds the scope of this chapter. The dominant actions of each of the extraocular muscles are indicated in Figure 27–237.

The etiology of muscle imbalance may include paralytic problems, tropias (constant imbalance), or phorias (latent imbalance occurring only with disruption of fusion). Phorias occur after temporary immobilization of the injured eye and are usually horizontal in nature.

Enophthalmos. Enophthalmos, the second major complication of a blow-out fracture, has a number of causative factors (Fig. 27–238). The major cause, as documented by three studies (Bite and associates, 1985; Manson and associates, 1986a,b; Stahlnecker and associates, 1985), is orbital enlargement with the escape of orbital soft tissue into an enlarged orbital cavity (Fig. 27–238*C*). The mechanism involves rupture of the periorbita and of the fine ligaments connecting the or-

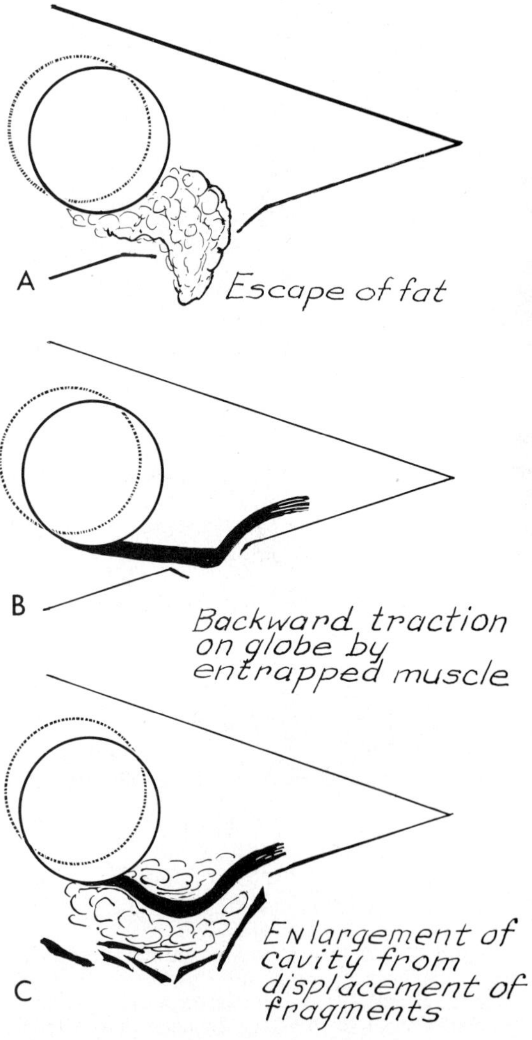

Figure 27–238. Three causes of enophthalmos in blow-out fractures. *A*, Escape of orbital fat into the maxillary sinus. *B*, Entrapment maintaining a backward position of the ocular globe. *C*, Enlargement of the orbital cavity. Some authors have also suggested that fat atrophy occurs, which would lessen the size of the orbital contents. In practice, fat atrophy is not the usual cause of the enophthalmos observed in the post-traumatic patient.

bital soft tissue structures. This allows their displacement with a remodeling of the shape of the soft tissue contents into a spherical configuration (Fig. 27–239). A postulated mechanism of enophthalmos is the retention of the ocular globe in a backward position when structures are entrapped in a fracture site. Another postulated factor is fat necrosis.

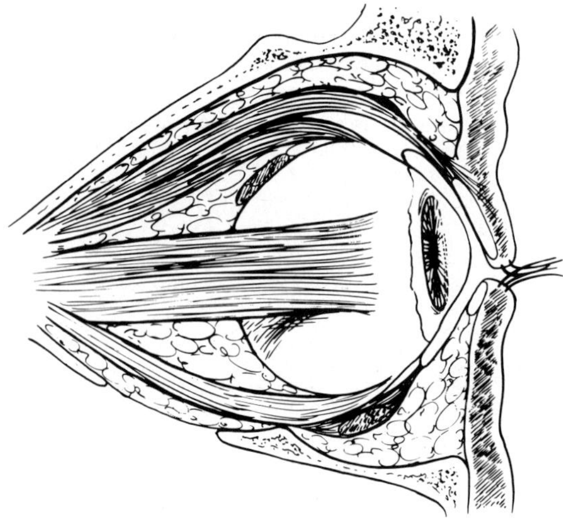

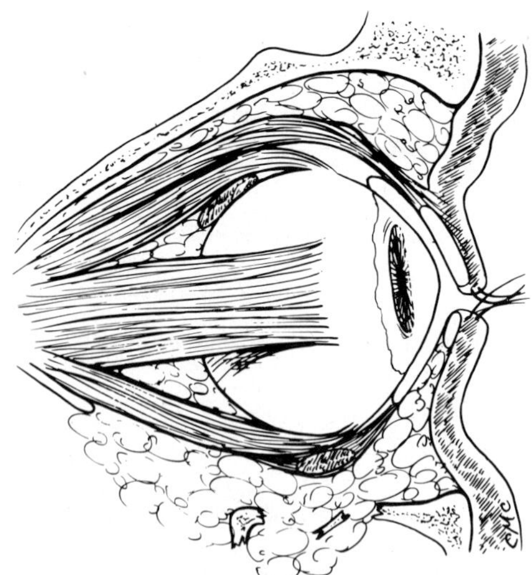

Figure 27–239. Loss of bony orbital support and disruption of the ligament system allow displacement of central (intraconal) orbital fat to a more peripheral position. The geometric shape of the orbit changes from a modified pyramid to more spherical configuration under the influence of gravity and the forces of fibrous scar contracture. The globe sinks backward, downward, and medially. (From Manson, P. N., Grivas, A., Rosenbaum, A., Vannier, P. M., Zinreich, J., and Iliff, N.: Studies on enophthalmos: II. The measurement of orbital injuries and their treatment by quantitative computed tomography. Plast. Reconstr. Surg., 77:203, 1986.)

Although fat necrosis has been shown to occur in some orbital injuries, the above studies indicated that this is not the major mechanism in the production of enophthalmos. Other mechanisms put forward include neurogenic theories of fat atrophy secondary to nerve disruption. It has been shown by Manson and associates (1986a,b) that part of the support of the globe is produced by the quantity and position of intramuscular or intraconal fat. In the anterior portion of the orbit, fat is located in an extraconal, as well as an intraconal, position. In the posterior position of the orbit, very little of the fat is extraconal. The intraconal fat, following fracture, is dislocated, and can be extruded to an extraconal location, thus contributing to a lack of globe support and enophthalmos.

Enophthalmos, when it is conspicuous and particularly when orbital contents are downwardly displaced, results in a ptosis of the upper eyelid and a deepening and hollow appearance of the supratarsal fold (Fig. 27–240). A shortening of the horizontal dimension of the palpebral fissure often accompanies the enophthalmos. This is especially so when nasoethmoido-orbital fractures are associated with significant fractures of the deep orbit.

Lower animals possess an orbital muscle that spans the area corresponding to the inferior orbital fissure. In some animals, this occupies a major portion of the lateral portion of the floor and lateral wall of the orbit. This is the orbitalis muscle and it is under sympathetic innervation. When the animal is frightened, the muscle contracts, protruding the eyeball for the purposes of focusing vision. In man this muscle is vestigial, and most anatomists discount its importance. It has sometimes been claimed that this muscle is a factor in the enophthalmos of Horner's syndrome, caused by paralysis of cranial nerve III. Most authors feel that the appearance of enophthalmos in this condition is actually for the most part due to the ptosis produced by the sympathetic denervation. It is possible that atrophic changes that occur in orbital fat may be responsible for the positional change of the globe. Some rare factors that have been held responsible for the development of post-traumatic enophthalmos are dislocation of the trochlea and superior oblique muscle, cicatricial contraction of the retrobulbar tissue, and rupture of the orbital ligaments or fascial bands. Koornneef (1977, 1982) postulated that downward

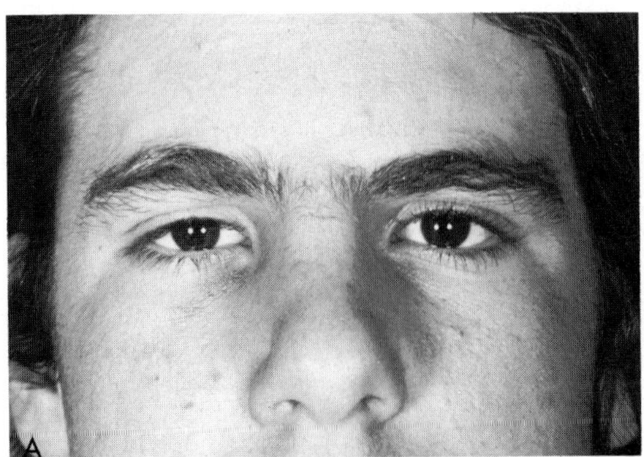

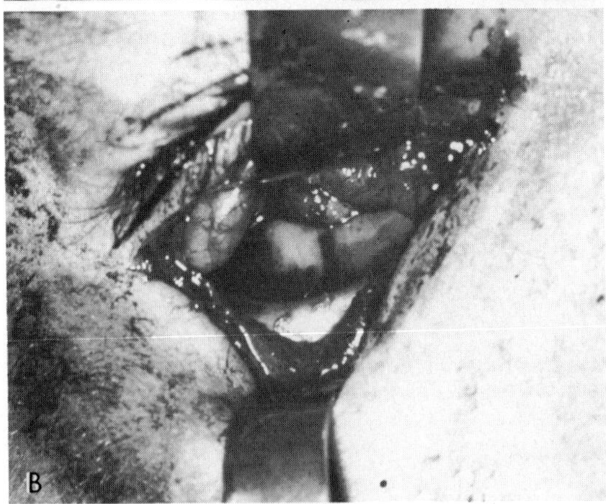

Figure 27–240. Enophthalmos produced by entrapment. *A*, Typical appearance of enophthalmos produced by entrapment of the orbital contents. *B*, The inferior orbital rim is intact. A linear fracture was located in the posterior reaches of the floor of the orbit. The photograph shows the entrapment.

traction on the globe by entrapped orbital contents contributes to the production of globe positional change (Fig. 27–241). Actually, as time passes, the soft tissue of the orbit is "contracted" and pulled backward by its adherence to displaced bone fragments.

Lang (1889) proposed enlargement of the orbital cavity as a factor in the production of enophthalmos:

I suggest that the injury may have produced a fracture and a depression of a portion of the orbital wall; the orbital fat would then no longer be sufficient in quantity to fill this enlarged postocular area without a sinking in of the globe from atmospheric pressure and a resulting limitation in ocular movements.

The enlargement of the orbital cavity from the depression of the floor is a frequent factor in the production of enophthalmos. However, there may be no entrapment of the orbital structures and no diplopia in severe enophthalmos because of a lack of incarceration of the ocular muscles or of the fat adjacent to the muscles, which are tethered to the muscles by fine ligaments.

Enophthalmos frequently accompanies major injuries involving the orbit, such as Le Fort II and III fractures. In these injuries, fractures occur through the lateral wall and floor and medial orbital walls and there may be no evidence of a blow-out fracture.

Examination and Diagnosis

In the typical blow-out fracture, the patient is aware of double vision. This may be present in the primary position (looking straight ahead), but it increases in upward gaze. The patient may not recognize double vision early if the eye is temporarily closed by edema of the eyelids or a dressing. When examined during the first hours after a fracture, the ocular globe may not appear to be displaced, and in fact, owing to the swelling and hemorrhage in the periorbital tissues, the later findings of enophthalmos, backward and downward displacement of the globe, and deepened supratarsal sulcus may be absent (Fig. 27–242). The patient should be examined for the possibility of ocular globe injury, eyelid damage, lacerations, and hematoma in

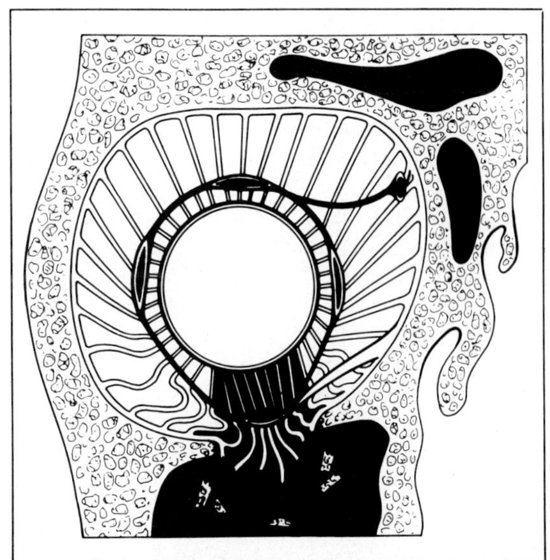

Figure 27–241. After fracture, the fine ligament system can be entrapped within the fracture site, creating a tethering of extraocular muscle motion. (From Koornneef, L.: Current concepts in the management of orbital blow-out fractures. Ann. Plast. Surg., 9:185, 1972.)

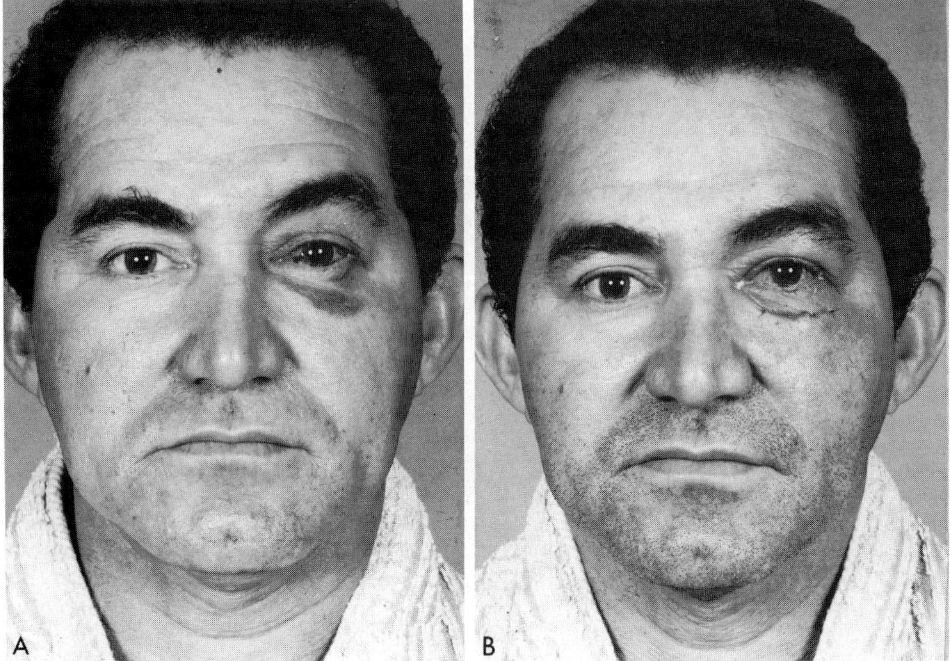

Figure 27–242. Blow-out fracture of the left orbit. *A*, Forward gaze. Note the enophthalmos. *B*, Forward gaze after release of the herniated structures and restoration of the continuity of the orbital floor. Note the low eyelid incision (a higher incision is now preferred). The enophthalmos has been corrected.

the levator muscle or aponeurosis. Globe injury or retinal detachment can accompany severe blunt injury to the periorbital structures.

When an object is held approximately 2 feet from the patient's eye and the patient is asked to look at the object, the affected eye is not able to rotate upward in the normal range as does the unaffected eye; restriction in rotation in other directions is also observed (Fig. 27–243). The function of the inferior rectus and inferior oblique muscles may be restricted by entrapment of structures or contusion and fibrosis. The superior rectus may not be able to rotate the globe because of the resistance offered by the short rein of the entrapped structures. After any entrapped structures are released, the globe is then able to rotate upward if contusion has not limited the range of extraocular motion. In children's fractures with muscle incarceration, the author has observed near-complete fixation of the globe.

In some fractures in which the infraorbital rim is comminuted, one can observe that the lower lid is vertically shortened with a tendency toward eversion. The inferior orbital rim is frequently displaced downward and backward and, in its forced retreat, carries with it the insertion of the septum orbitale. This mechanism may account for vertical shortening of the lower eyelid (Fig. 27–244).

Indications for Surgical Treatment. Although double vision is the most frequent complaint of the patient, this is not an indication for surgery in itself. Double vision may be caused by hematoma, edema, and neurogenic factors.

Indications for operation are:

1. Limitation of forced rotation of the eyeball.

2. Radiographic evidence of extensive fracture.

3. Enophthalmos or significant globe positional change.

Limitation of Forced Rotation of Eyeball. The *forced duction test*, or eyeball traction test, provides a means of differentiating entrapment of the ligaments of the inferior rectus muscle from weakness, paralysis, or contusion of the muscle with lack of muscle function. The incarceration of the inferior rectus muscle fascial system produces limitation to forced rotation of the globe, which is a pathognomonic sign of a blow-out fracture of the orbital floor (Fig. 27–245). In late

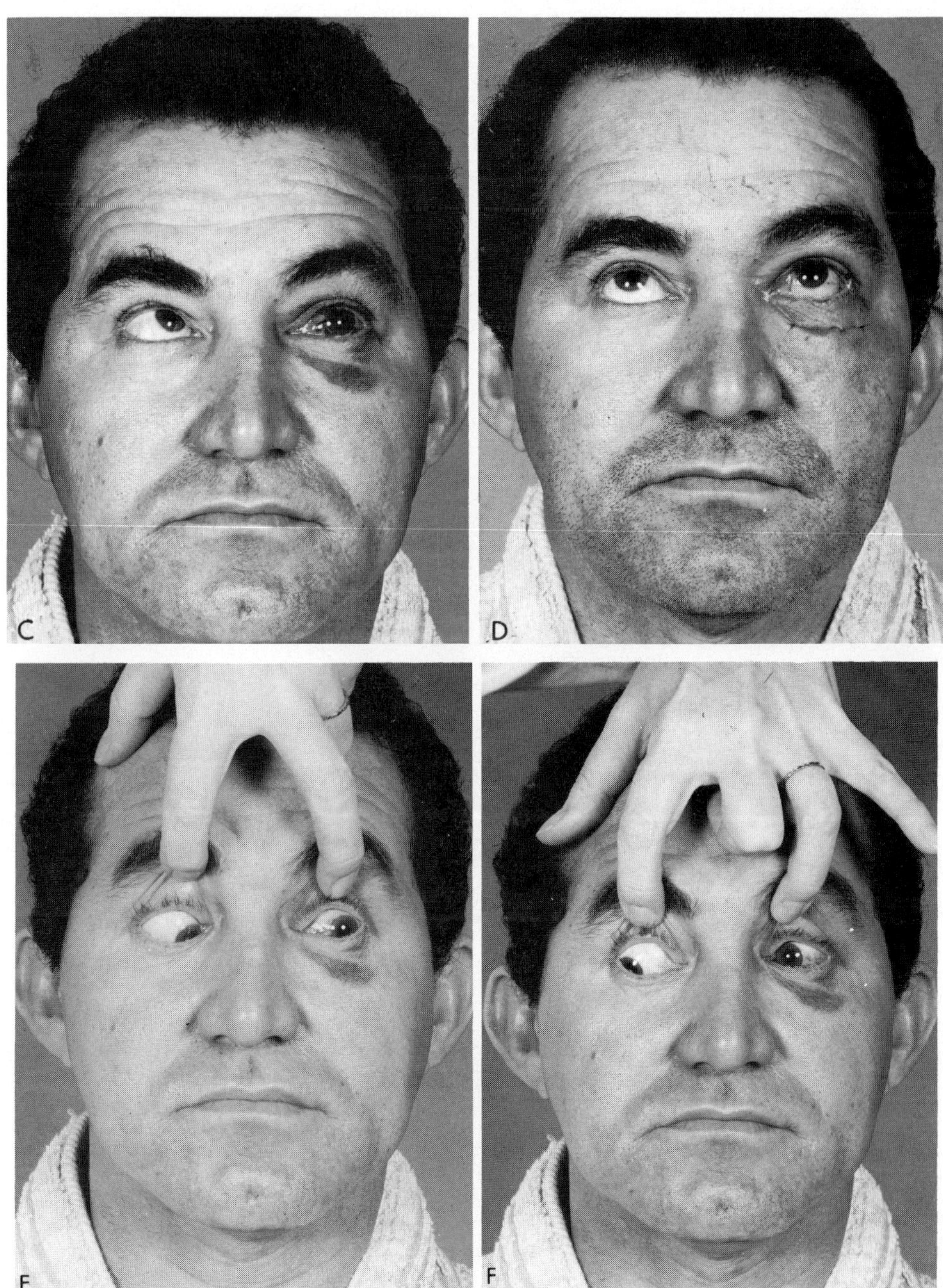

Figure 27–242 *Continued C*, Restriction in the upward and lateral gaze before operation. *D*, Upward gaze after surgery, demonstrating the release of the entrapment of orbital structures. *E*, The restriction in the dominant lateral gaze of the left ocular globe before the operation. *F*, The restriction of a downward and inward gaze before surgery. This patient was one of the first to be treated for a blow-out fracture. (From Converse, J. M., and Smith, B.: Blow-out fracture of the floor of the orbit. Trans. Am. Acad. Ophthalmol. Otolaryngol., *64*:676, 1960.)

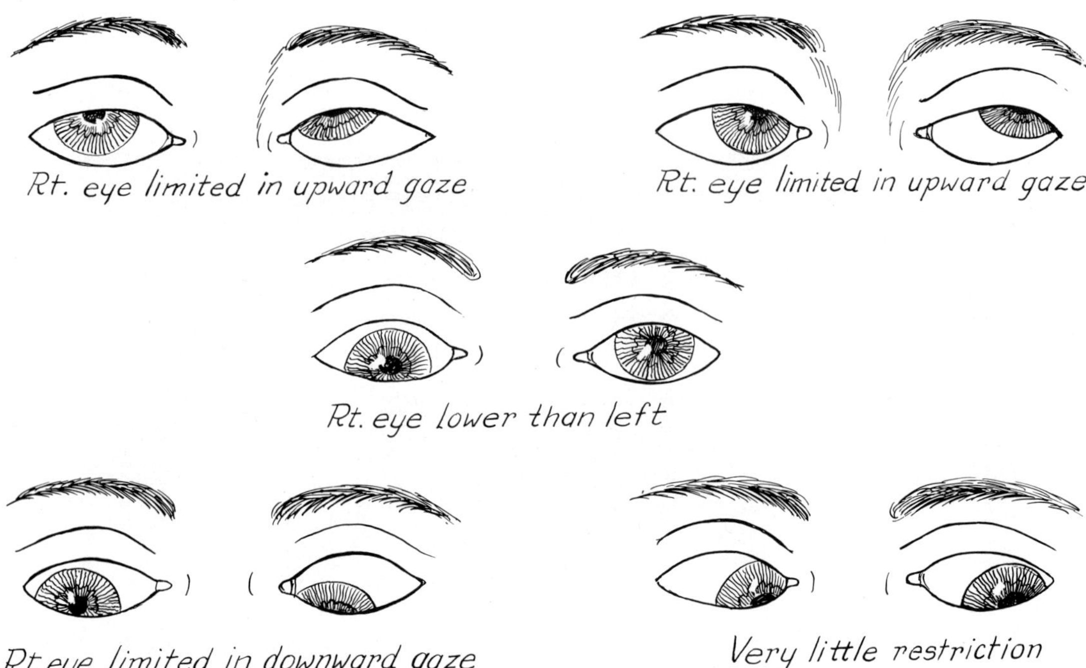

Figure 27–243. The limitation of oculorotatory movements following a blow-out fracture of the right orbit.

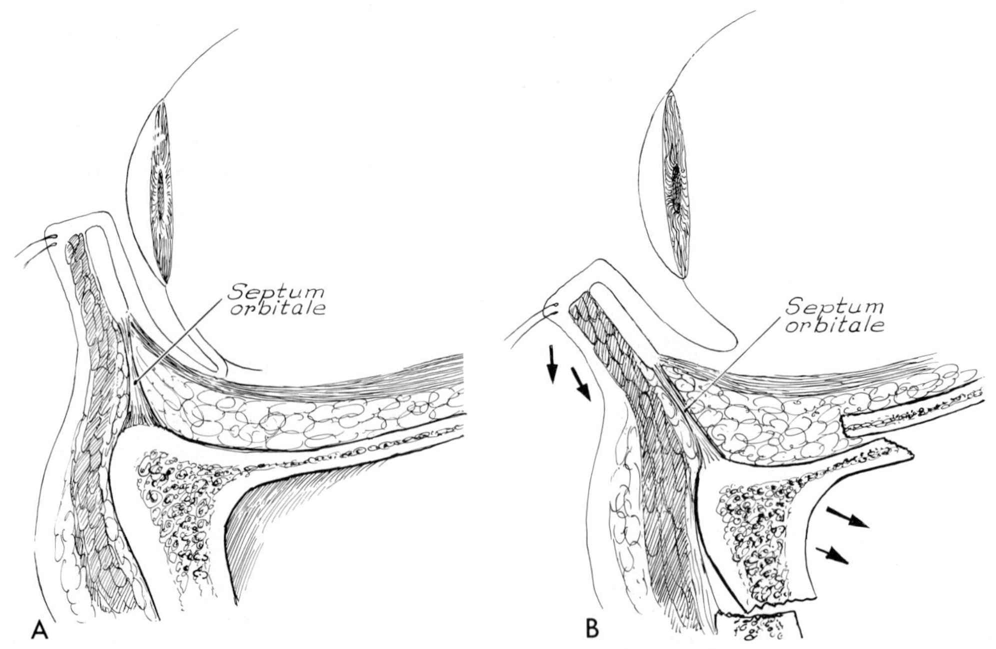

Figure 27–244. Shortening of the lower lid associated with an orbital rim fracture. *A*, Sagittal section illustrating insertion of the septum orbitale on the orbital rim. *B*, When the orbital rim is fractured and displaced backward, the septum exerts a downward and backward traction on the lower lid, causing vertical shortening and eversion. In comminuted fractures of the rim, there is a tendency of the reconstructed rim to be slightly posterior and inferior to the desired position, especially if interfragment wires are used.

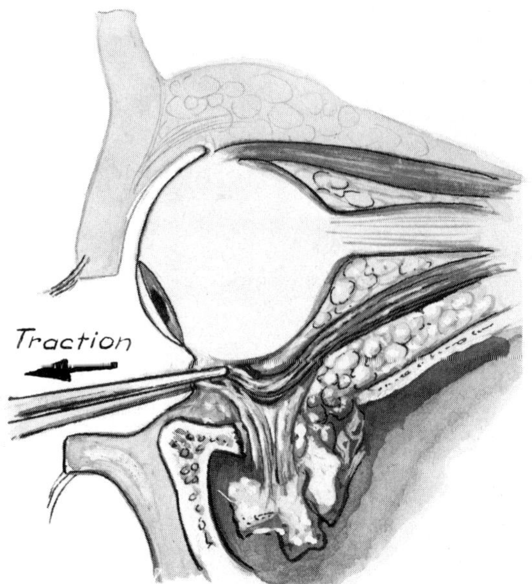

Figure 27–245. The forced duction test. Forceps grasp the ocular globe at the insertion of the inferior rectus muscle approximately 7 mm from the limbus.

injuries, fibrosis may produce limitation of motion (Figs. 27–246, 27–247). Fibrosis should be absent in early examinations, but severe edema and hemorrhage in the muscle may produce limited movement. To perform the test, a few drops of local anesthetic solution are instilled into the conjunctival sac. Sufficient anesthesia is provided to permit grasping of the insertion of the inferior rectus muscle onto the eyeball, which is accomplished with forceps inserted at a point 7 mm from the limbus. The globe should be gently rotated upward and downward, medially and laterally, confirming any resistance to motion. The motion should be free and unencumbered.

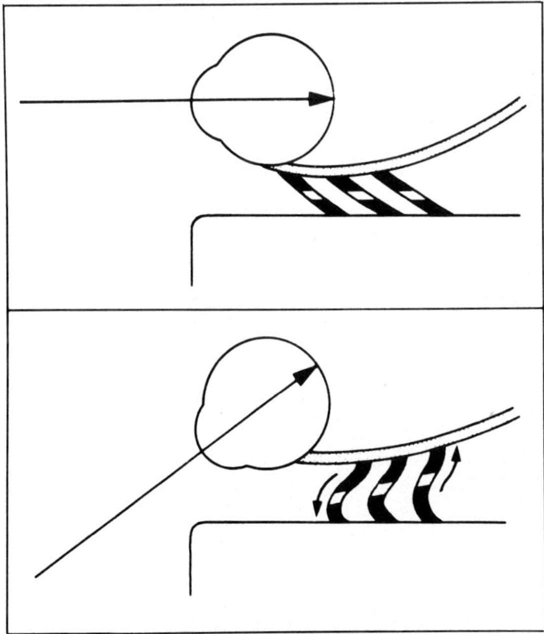

Figure 27–246. Normal excursion of the globe requires that the fine ligament system be able to move freely. (From Koornneef, L.: Current concepts in the management of orbital blow-out fractures. Ann. Plast. Surg., *9*:185, 1972.)

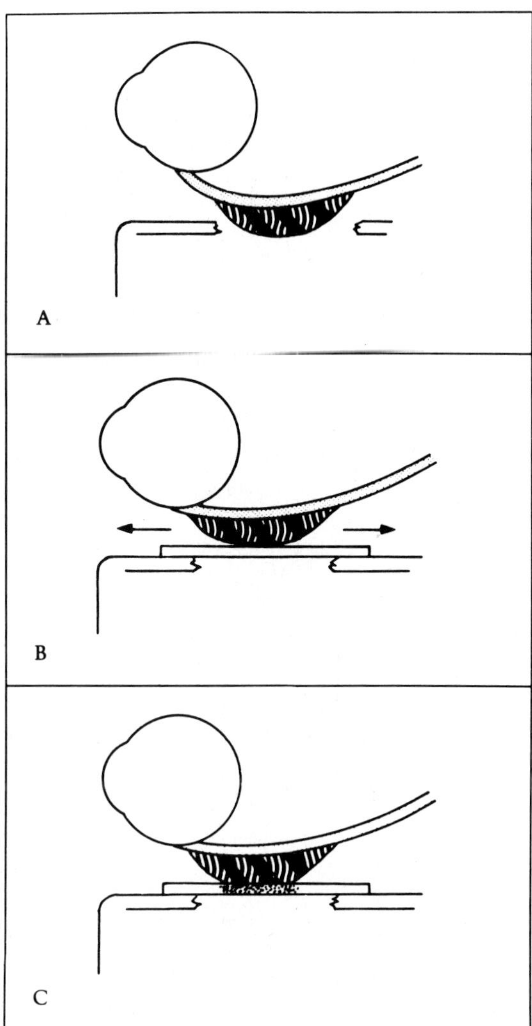

Figure 27–247. Incarceration of the fine ligament system *(A)* within the fracture site would prevent a full range of motion. *B*, The full range of motion might be restored by releasing the incarcerated structures from the fracture site. *C*, Adherence of the fine ligament system to the orbital floor reconstruction might result in decreased extraocular motion. (From Koornneef, L.: Current concepts in the management of orbital blow-out fractures. Ann. Plast. Surg., *9*:185, 1972.)

Radiographic Evidence of Fracture. Radiographic evaluation of any significant

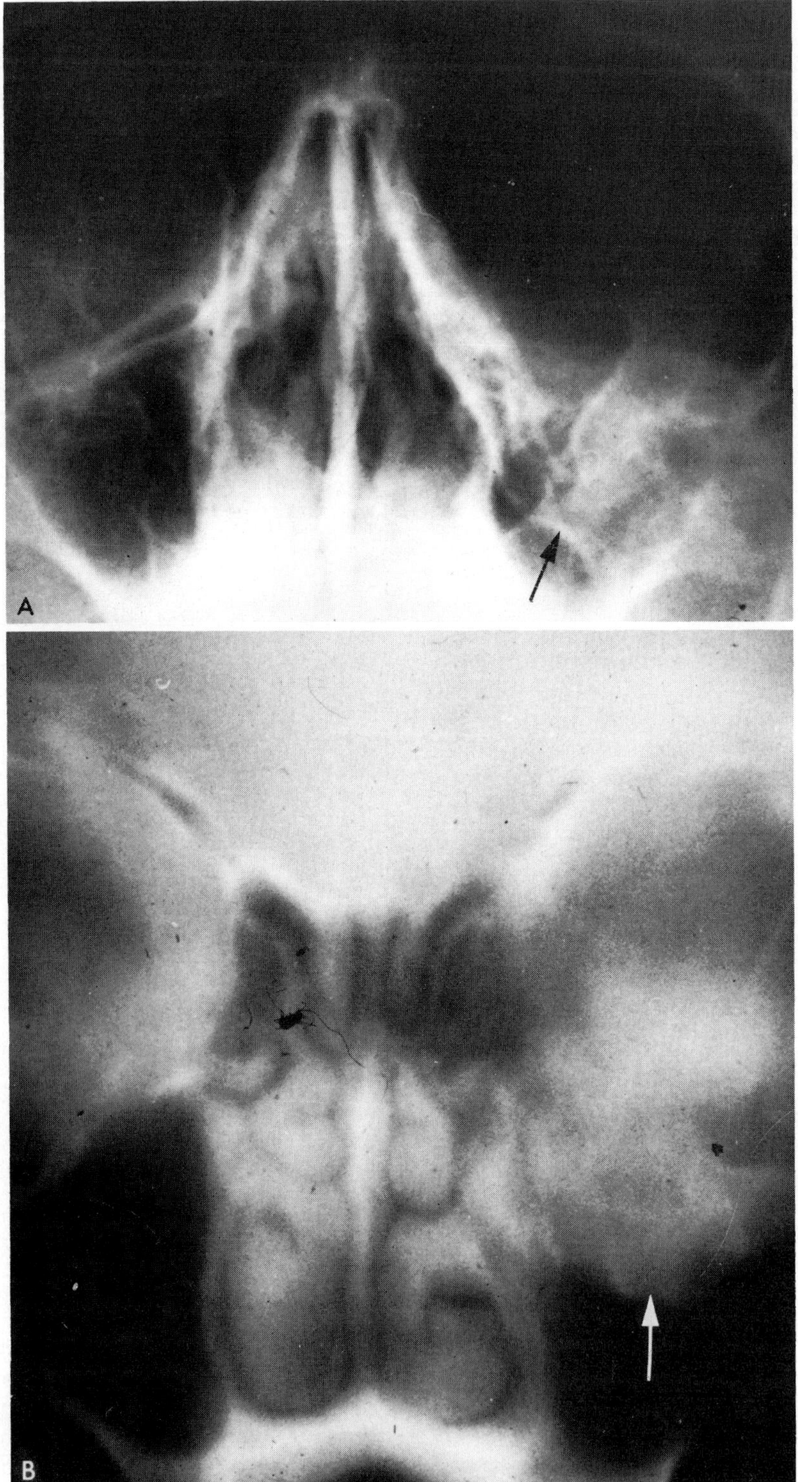

Figure 27–248. Roentgenogram showing a blow-out fracture. *A*, Waters view documenting blow-out fracture of the orbital floor *(arrow)*. *B*, The tomogram shows the prolapse of the orbital contents into the maxillary sinus *(arrow)* (Courtesy of Dr. J. Zizmor).

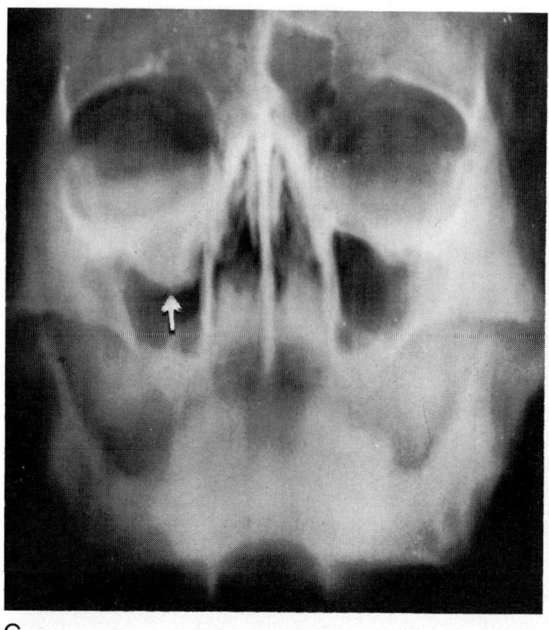

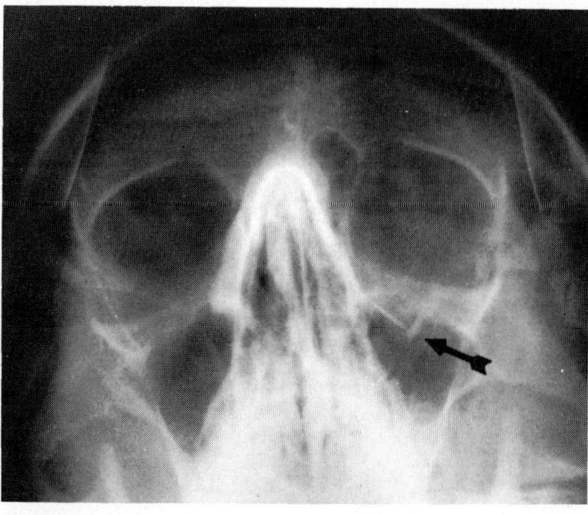

C D

Figure 27–248 *Continued C*, The tomogram shows prolapse of the orbital contents into the maxillary sinus *(arrow)*. *D*, Roentgenogram showing blow-out fracture *(arrow)* with fragments hanging on "periosteal hinges" into the maxillary sinus.

orbital fracture is essential. Plain films and tomography have been replaced by a CT scan in the axial and coronal planes. In the author's experience, actual coronal cuts, rather than reconstructions, are most helpful. A careful roentgenographic examination reveals a variety of findings and defines the location, size, and type of the fracture site.

Because of the superimposition of thick and thin bones, the roentgenographic picture on plain films is apt to be difficult to interpret. Such films should not be cited as evidence that a blow-out fracture does not exist. Rather, the clinical examination is the most important evidence of a blow-out fracture. Almost all significant orbital fractures involve periorbital and subconjunctival hematoma and anesthesia. The absence of such signs should make the diagnosis questionable.

Plain roentgenograms can suggest the presence of a fracture in the internal portion of the orbit by means of a variety of positions: the Caldwell position, the Waters position, the fronto-occipital position, the anteroposterior projection, the reversed Waters position, and the oblique orbital optic foramen view (Figs. 27–248, 27–249).

The diagnosis of a blow-out fracture is frequently missed if the radiographic examination does not include a CT scan. Fracture lines on plain films may be mistaken for superimposed bony septa or suture lines, or may be hidden by disease processes in the underlying maxillary sinus. The thin orbital floor, partially transparent on radiographs, may be obscured against the background of other bones of the skull. CT scans disclose the presence of a blow-out fracture and its location (Figs. 27–250, 27–251).

With adequate technique, blow-out fractures of the orbit can be radiologically confirmed in over 98 per cent of cases with conventional films supplemented by CT scan analysis.

The type of blow-out fracture varies. Lowering of the orbital floor may produce a "hanging drop" seen in a blow-out fracture through which the orbital fat has been extruded into the maxillary sinus (see Fig. 27–248*B*). A "trapdoor" fracture (see Fig. 27–251) may involve one or two bone fragments hanging into the sinus on a periosteal hinge. Massive extrusion of orbital contents into the maxillary sinus produces a characteristic depression. Associated fractures of the medial wall (see Fig. 27–249) frequently occur. Radiographic signs such as maxillary sinus fluid combined with the clinical examinations are taken as supportive evidence for the di-

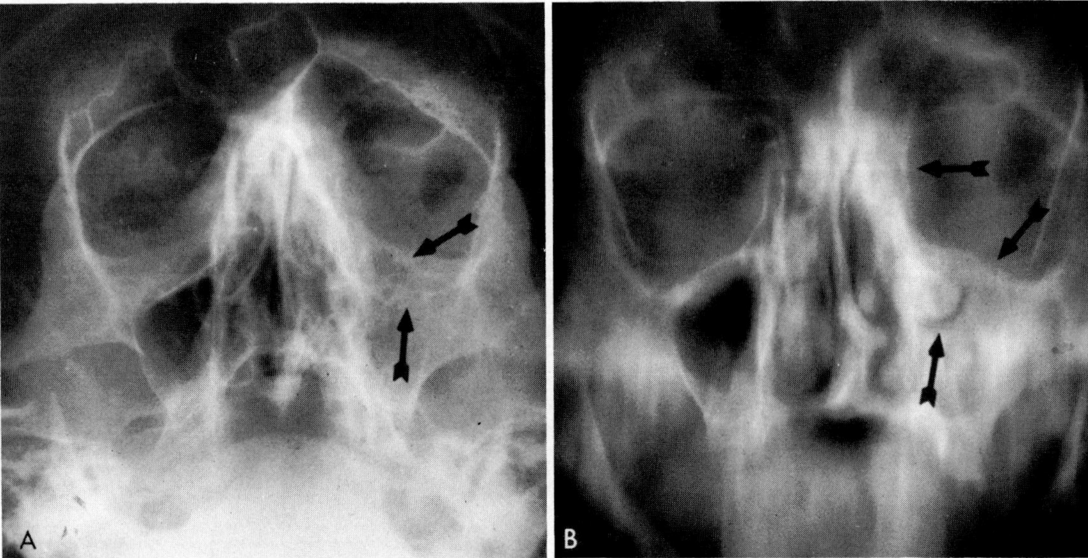

Figure 27–249. Waters view showing fracture of the floor of the left orbit. Tomogram showing fracture of the medial wall of the orbit. *A*, Before radiographic examination, blood in the left maxillary sinus was aspirated and air was substituted. The Waters view shows a depressed fracture of the left orbital floor with downward herniation of the orbital tissues *(arrows)*. *B*, The tomogram shows the fracture and a downward herniation of the orbital tissue profiled by a trace of air in the opaque left maxillary sinus. The tomogram also documents a fracture of the medial orbital wall, as indicated by opacification of the ethmoidal cells. There is emphysema in the left orbit *(arrows)*, which is usually present in a medial orbital fracture.

agnosis. Massive protrusion of soft tissue contents out of the usual confines of the bone cavity may be an indication for surgical exploration, as enophthalmos and globe positional change are likely. Crikelair and associates (1972) drew attention to the danger of "over-operating" when only presumptive radiographic signs (such as opacity of the maxillary sinus) are present. In the absence of positive clinical signs suggesting the need for surgical intervention, it should be postponed while the patient's course is kept under a period of observation. Diplopia with an initially equivocal forced duction examination often resolves after a short (seven day) period of observation.

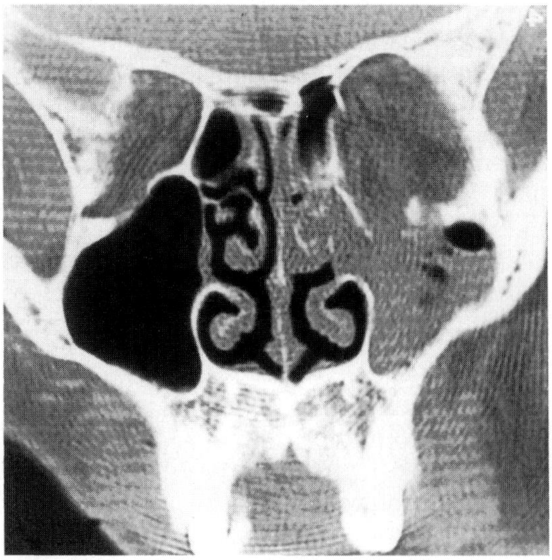

Enophthalmos. Clinically obvious globe

Figure 27–250. A fracture of the medial and inferior orbit (severe blow-out fracture). Coronal CT scans indicate incarceration of fat or muscle, which requires surgical release if diplopia with a positive force duction test is present.

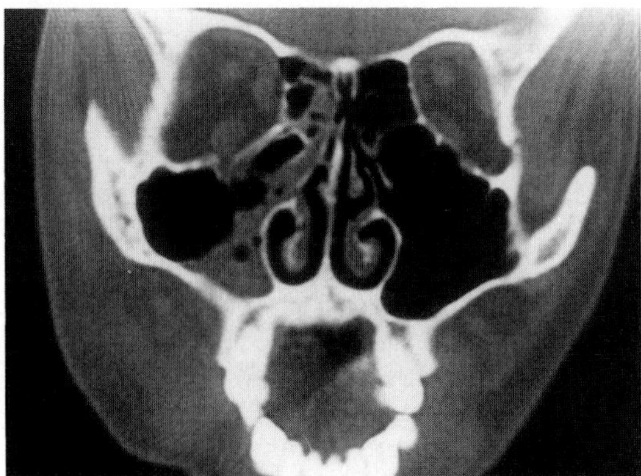

Figure 27–251. Fracture of the floor of the orbit with slight displacement. The inferior rectus muscle is actually incarcerated in the fracture site, an unusual occurrence, as it is usually fat that is incarcerated.

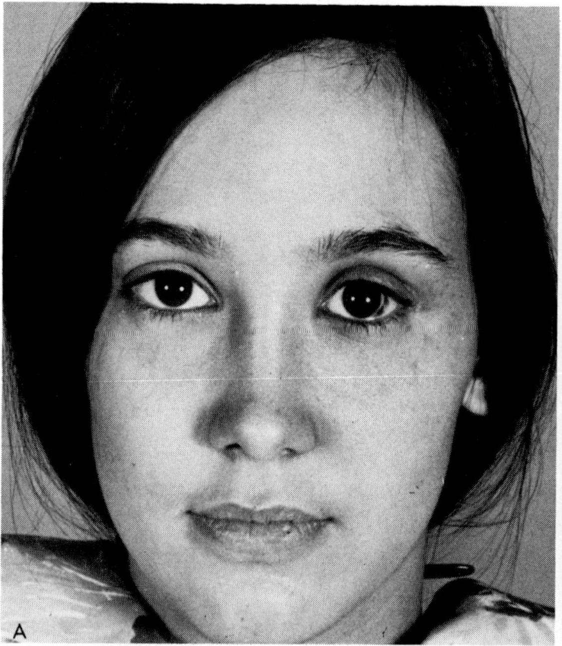

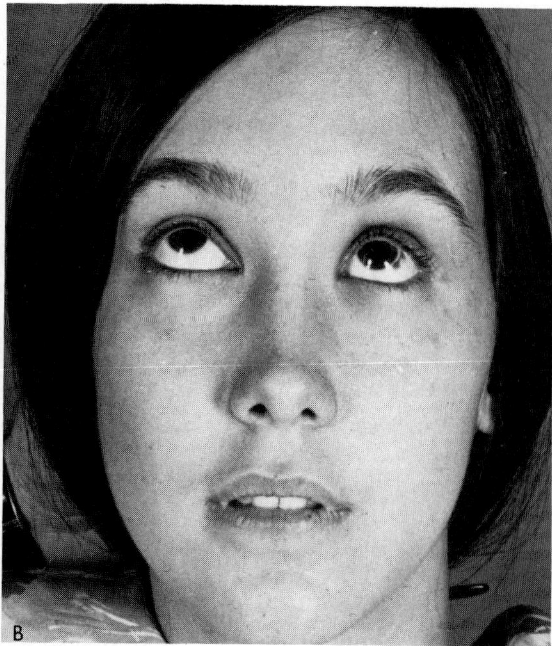

Figure 27–252. Orbital blow-out fracture without gross entrapment. *A*, Appearance of the patient after receiving a blow over the left eye. Note the subconjunctival ecchymosis. *B*, Despite some restriction in the upward gaze, the forced duction test was negative. Exploration of the floor of the orbit showed comminution of a major portion of the orbit with collapse of the floor into the maxillary sinus. This is an example of a case in which the patient had no diplopia and a negative forced duction test; severe enophthalmos would have developed had the orbital floor and the architecture of the orbit not been restored by bone grafting.

positional change, such as enophthalmos or vertical positional change of the ocular globe, is an indication for surgical exploration (Fig. 27–252). A globe positional change suggests gross derangement of the orbit with enlargement of bone volume, resulting in a change in the soft tissue shape and position of orbital contents. It usually is not apparent acutely because of swelling.

Sensory Nerve Conduction Loss. In a suspected orbital floor fracture, anesthesia or hypoesthesia in the area of distribution of the orbital nerve is suggestive evidence of a blow-out fracture involving the infraorbital groove or canal. This finding almost invariably accompanies blow-out fractures of the floor of the orbit; its absence should make the diagnosis questionable. Absence of infraorbital anesthesia implies that a fracture present is either lateral, medial, or posterior to the infraorbital groove or canal. In practice, the infraorbital groove or canal is almost always involved and the sign is present in 90 to 95 per cent of orbital floor fractures. In a patient with hypoesthesia or anesthesia who does not have other evidence for surgical exploration and whose fractures do not involve the orbital rim, a surgical exploration need not be performed, since improvement in nerve conduction accompanies spontaneous healing. If a rim fracture is demonstrated, especially with medial displacement of a rim fragment into the infraorbital canal, exploration is recommended to relieve any pressure on the nerve.

Treatment

The surgical treatment of blow-out fractures has three goals: (1) to disengage entrapped structures and restore oculorotatory functions, (2) to replace orbital contents into the usual confines of the bony orbital cavity, and (3) to restore orbital cavity size (volume) and replace the tissues into their proper position. The third attempts to minimize extraocular muscle imbalance and enophthalmos.

The primary objectives of treatment are achieved by the release of soft tissue contents, the accurate definition of the extent of the bone fracture, and the reconstruction of the bony wall of the orbit in its anatomic position. If there are indications for surgery, its timing should be as early as is practical. Early restoration prevents soft tissue scarring and contracture occurring in a nonanatomic position.

Timing of Surgical Intervention. For isolated blow-out fractures, it is not necessary to operate immediately, particularly if post-traumatic edema, retinal detachment, or other significant globe injuries such as hyphema are present. It is advisable to wait a few days, especially if the clinical signs indicating the necessity for surgery are equivocal. They often subside if a period of a few days is allowed to elapse. On the other hand, major significant orbital fractures are best treated with early surgical intervention, and the author believes that the earlier a significant derangement can be corrected, the better is the functional result. The clinician is thus responsible for making a clear evaluation of the extent of the injury and determining the necessity for surgical correction. In children, delay of operation can be less desirable, since bone regeneration is rapid and the freeing of incarcerated orbital soft tissue contents becomes more difficult. Scarring occurring in an abnormal position can persist after release of incarcerated orbital contents. Late motility problems from significant incarceration persist if treatment is postponed for two to three weeks despite the late release of orbital contents. Undue delay, therefore, is *not* advocated; judicious consideration of all aspects of operative versus nonoperative treatment is required.

In a large series of facial fractures studied by Hakelius and Ponten (1973), 22 per cent of the patients with midfacial fractures had diplopia. In comparing a series of cases treated within two weeks after the accident with another series in which treatment was delayed, Hakelius and Ponten in a follow-up study found that 16 per cent of the patients in the first group reported the presence of diplopia only when tired (93 per cent were completely free of diplopia). In the second group, 24 per cent still had unchanged diplopia. As a result of this study, an early active surgical approach was recommended for significant fractures. These can be assessed by accurate CT scan examinations. It is the author's impression that disruptions of the orbital floor exceeding an area of 2 sq cm set the stage for globe positional change; thus, fractures that exceed this dimension can be considered for surgical treatment. It is also significant that in a series of 50 patients referred with blow-out fracture and other complications after unsuccessful and delayed treatment (mean time between trauma and surgery, 3½ weeks), 43 patients showed extraocular muscle imbalance (Converse and associates, 1967). Emery, Noorden, and Sclernitzauer (1971) also reported the clinical findings in 159 patients with orbital floor fractures. They noted late diplopia in 60 per cent of patients with untreated blow-out fractures when diplopia was still present 15 days after the injury. However, the etiology of the diplopia can vary according to the mechanisms previously described.

The author occasionally observed that the forced duction test will "free" an entrapment; such cases do not require further treatment. It is difficult to agree with the advice of Putterman, Stevens, and Urist (1974), who advocated nonsurgical management of all isolated blow-out fractures of the orbital floor. These authors reported 25 per cent residual diplopia in a retrospective study and 27 per cent residual diplopia in a prospective study. Enophthalmos occurred in 65 per cent of the patients in the retrospective study and 36 per cent of those in the prospective study. Each case should be considered individually, and the decision for or against exploratory surgery should be made on the basis of the criteria outlined above. Diplopia in a functional field of gaze with positive evidence of muscle incarceration should be treated surgically. It is much more difficult to correct enophthalmos as a secondary than as a primary procedure, and certainly muscle damage is a more frequent accompaniment of secondary corrections for enophthalmos when scar tissue and contracture are present. The extraocular muscles travel close to the orbital walls in the posterior orbit and are vulnerable to surgical injury.

Operative Technique. A number of methods have been advocated for the treatment of blow-out fractures. The surgical approach has involved either the eyelid or the canine fossa through the maxillary sinus. The eyelid or conjunctival approach to the orbital floor is preferred because it facilitates the disengagement of any entrapped or prolapsed orbital tissues under direct vision. Other approaches do not provide the operating surgeon with a precise view of the orbital contents in order to ensure their protection. The author recognizes that the approach through the canine fossa and maxillary sinus is indicated in many blow-out fractures as an *adjunct* to the eyelid or conjunctival approach. It is helpful as a means of removing bone fragments from the sinus cavity, and is important in the management of comminuted fractures of the maxilla and other bones of the midfacial area. Some authors have recommended that gauze packing or inflatable balloons be inserted in the maxillary sinus to provide support for comminuted orbital floor fragments. They have also advocated that "trapdoor"-type fractures can be supported by gauze packing after the entrapment has been relieved. The author does not advocate gauze packing or an inflatable balloon to maintain the contour of the orbital floor when these bones are fragmented into small pieces. Rather, the replacement of the bone with a bone graft is the preferred technique. Many of the cases of blindness described after fracture reduction have resulted from an approach to the orbital floor solely through the canine fossa and maxillary sinus. In the patient shown in Figure 27–253, the globe was pushed upward under considerable pressure. Simultaneous observation of the floor of the orbit through the eyelid approach at the time of maxillary sinus packing would have prevented this complication. Suppuration has also been observed after gauze packing of the maxillary sinus. McCoy and associates (1962) reported a case in which packing of the maxillary sinus caused fragments of bone to damage the optic nerve, leading to blindness.

The maxillary sinus approach is also unsatisfactory for the release of entrapped orbital soft tissues or for the proper reconstruction of the orbital floor. In one follow-up study of a series of 50 complicated cases, eight patients whose fractures had been repaired through the maxillary sinus alone required the transeyelid approach to release the incarcerated orbital contents from the surrounding impacted healed bone fragments (Table 27–5).

Exposure of Orbital Floor. Various types of incisions have been employed to approach the orbital floor through the lower eyelid. The "one-stroke incision" to the orbital rim has the disadvantage of causing a unified line of cicatricial tissue, which can result in a retracted, scarred lower eyelid with vertical shortening.

The subciliary skin muscle flap incision near the margin of the lid leaves an inconspicuous scar. It should begin about 2 to 3 mm below the lash line and extend 8 to 10

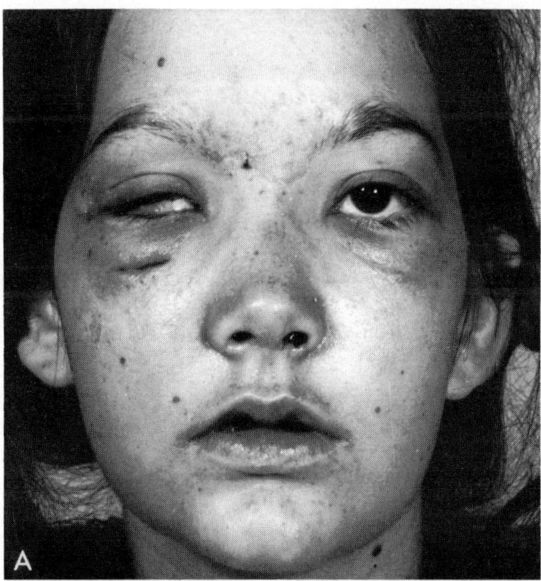

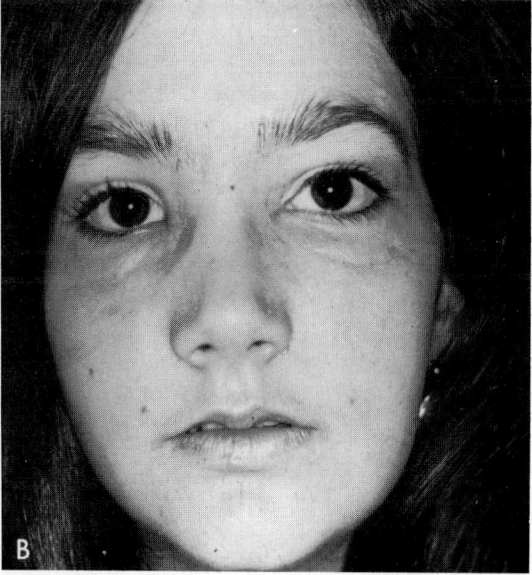

Figure 27–253. Excessive elevation of the orbital floor after maxillary sinus packing. *A*, Blow-out fracture of the right orbit treated by gauze packing placed in the maxillary sinus. The ocular globe has been pushed upward to the point where the pupil is hidden by the upper eyelid. *B*, After removal of the maxillary sinus packing, exploration of the floor of the orbit through an eyelid incision and restoration of the continuity of the fractured orbital floor. This case demonstrates the danger of attempting to restore the level of the orbital floor by packing without direct observation of the orbital floor through an eyelid incision. Excessive compression by packing may also cause blindness.

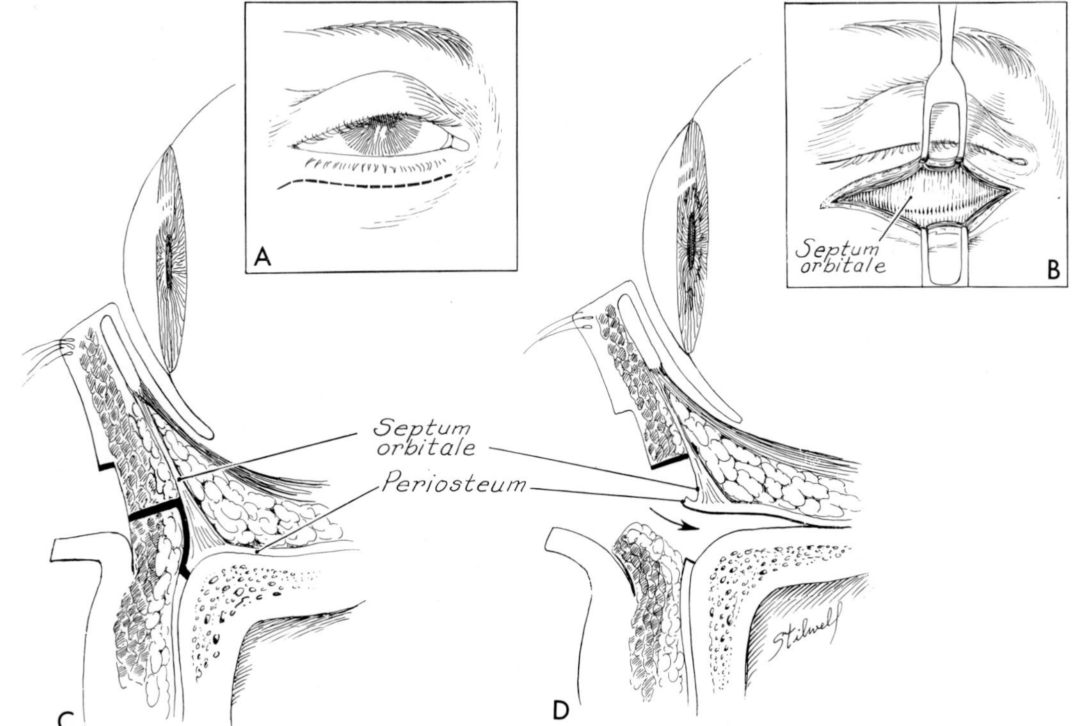

Figure 27–254. Technique of exposure of the orbital floor. *A*, Outline of the lower eyelid incision. *B*, The septum orbitale exposed. *C*, Sagittal section showing the skin incision through the orbicularis oculi muscle and the path of dissection over the septum orbitale to the orbital rim. *D*, The periosteum of the orbit (periorbita) is raised from the orbital floor. (From Converse, J. M., Cole, J. G., and Smith, B: Late treatment of blow-out fracture of the floor of the orbit. Plast. Reconstr. Surg., *28*:183, 1961.)

mm lateral to the lateral canthus (see Fig. 27–211). Incisions through lower lid skin folds require less dissection and the scar is usually not very conspicuous. It should be emphasized, however, that the least noticeable scar occurs from the subciliary or the transconjunctival approach with lateral canthotomy (see Fig. 27–211).

The Converse subciliary incision is made through the skin, and dissection is continued until the inferior edge of the tarsus is reached (see Fig. 27–211). At this point, a skin-muscle flap is raised from the tarsus and the septum orbitale is followed below the tarsus until the rim of the orbit is reached. An incision is made on the anterior aspect of the orbital rim to avoid damaging the septum, which inserts on the anterior face of the orbital rim in the lateral portion of the orbit (recess of Eisler) (see Fig. 27–211). Incisions on the rim of the orbit should always be in the periosteum below the insertion of the septum orbitale to minimize vertical shortening of the lid.

Incisions in the midlid crease (Fig. 27–254) may be deepened through the orbicularis, and the dissection plane is identical to that utilized for the subciliary incision (see Fig. 27–211).

The conjunctival approach is another incision advocated by Tessier (1973) for correction of craniofacial anomalies and by Converse and associates (1973) for post-traumatic deformities. If careful dissection is performed according to the techniques shown in Figure 27–255, it permits the surgeon to avoid perforating the septum orbitale with a consequent extrusion of orbital fat. The incision, if combined with a lateral canthotomy, provides exposure equal to that of the subciliary incision, which exceeds that of any other lid incision.

The conjunctival incision avoids an external scar except in the skin lateral to the lateral canthus. It is therefore inconspicuous; in the author's experience, it is accompanied by slightly more septal shortening than a properly performed subciliary approach. With either approach, some lagophthalmos may be noted in the lower lid in upward gaze. Increased scleral show can also be noted. These

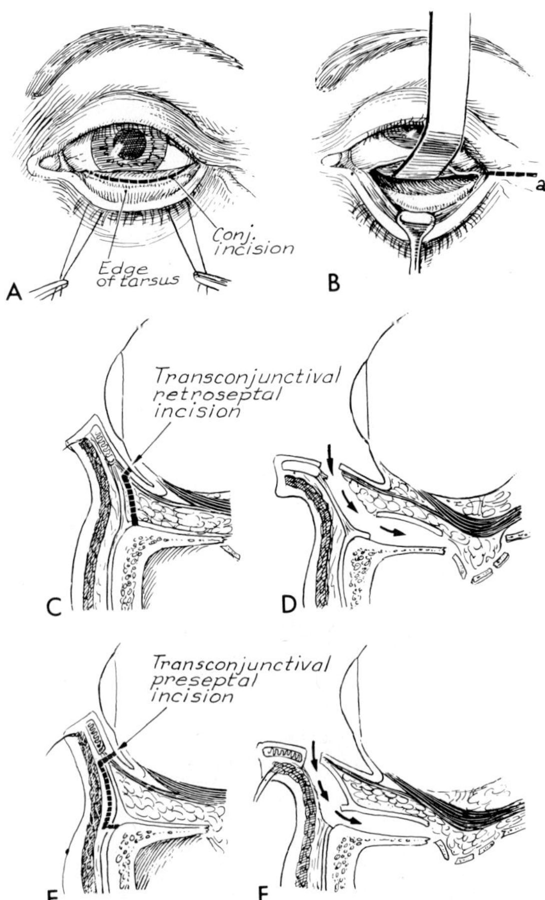

Figure 27–255. Transconjunctival approach. *A*, Conjunctival incision below the lower border of the tarsus. *B*, Subperiosteal exposure of the orbital floor. The dotted line shows the lateral canthal extension for additional exposure. *C*, Retroseptal approach. *D*, Sagittal view of the retroseptal approach to the fracture. *E*, Preseptal approach. *F*, Sagittal view of the preseptal approach to the fracture.

are usually temporary conditions that resolve after resolution of any mild cicatricial contraction.

The author prefers to avoid incisions in the lower septum orbitale whenever possible because of the need to restore fat to its proper location in the orbit. Extrusion of fat through septal incisions makes dissection more difficult.

When the orbital rim has been reached by following the septum orbitale, an incision through the periosteum is made several millimeters below the superiormost portion of the rim. Subperiosteal dissection is begun by first clearing the anterior face of the orbital rim, then extending backward over the edge of the orbital rim following the floor downward and posteriorly (Fig. 27–256). The subperiosteal dissection should begin in areas where the bone is more normal and extend to identify the area of fracture first from one side, and then the other. If the orbital contents are incarcerated, they should be gently replaced in the orbit rather than tugged with strong traction movements. In some cases, it may be preferable to enlarge the opening into the maxillary sinus with a small chisel or rongeur to allow the replacement of orbital soft tissue with less traction. Frequently, the infraorbital nerve is visualized as the bone is fractured around it. The infraorbital nerve should be respected. It is often helpful to aid visualization with loupe magnification. A small branch of the infraorbital artery extends from the infraorbital neurovascular bundle to the inferior rectus muscle. This can be divided. In the posterior half of the orbit, the inferior rectus muscle travels close to the orbital floor. It can be injured in the dissection and one must be careful to avoid blunt dissection within orbital fat. This can damage the muscular attachments and fascial connections within the orbit and can result in postoperative double vision. The author prefers to place a small retractor over the lid while an assistant holds the lower lid inferiorly. A Freer periosteal elevator is held in one hand and a small suction in the other. This maneuver allows visualization of the area of dissection; a headlight and loupe magnification are essential. One or two malleable retractors should be used to provide retraction of the orbital soft tissue contents without *any* pressure on the ocular globe. These can be gently placed in the proper location and held in position with light finger pressure by an assistant. Exposure of the lower medial, lateral, and floor portions of the orbit is provided by a properly performed subciliary skin-muscle flap approach or the conjunctival approach with lateral canthotomy.

If the inferior orbital rim is also fractured (an *impure* blow-out fracture), the fragments are realigned and fixation is maintained by the placement of interosseous wiring. After the interosseous wires have been linked, a small plate can be placed across the area if desired. If the orbital rim has been displaced backward, it is essential that the fragments be realigned in their former anterior and superior position. This measure is necessary not only to restore cheek prominence, but to prevent any vertical shortening of the lower

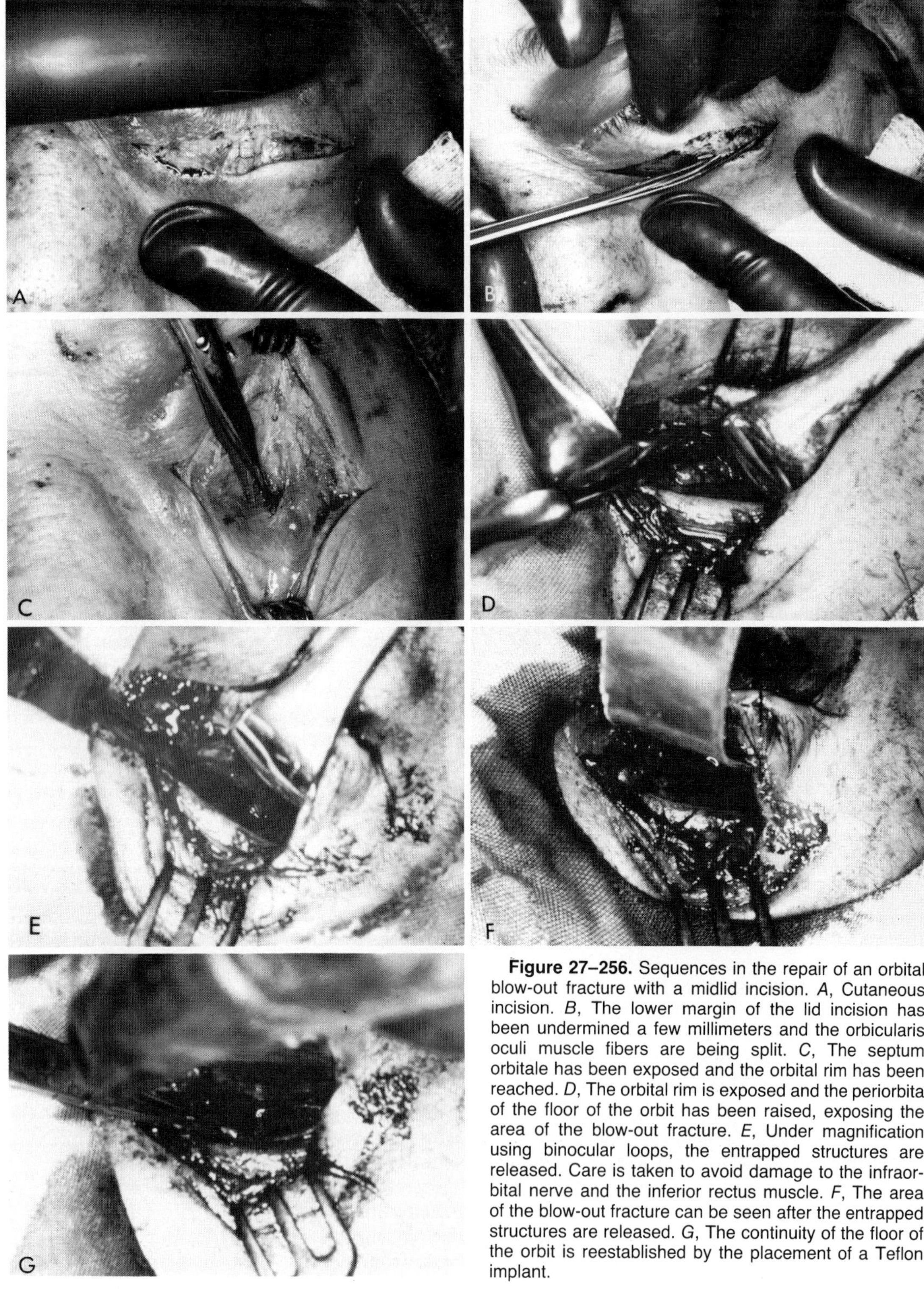

Figure 27–256. Sequences in the repair of an orbital blow-out fracture with a midlid incision. *A*, Cutaneous incision. *B*, The lower margin of the lid incision has been undermined a few millimeters and the orbicularis oculi muscle fibers are being split. *C*, The septum orbitale has been exposed and the orbital rim has been reached. *D*, The orbital rim is exposed and the periorbita of the floor of the orbit has been raised, exposing the area of the blow-out fracture. *E*, Under magnification using binocular loops, the entrapped structures are released. Care is taken to avoid damage to the infraorbital nerve and the inferior rectus muscle. *F*, The area of the blow-out fracture can be seen after the entrapped structures are released. *G*, The continuity of the floor of the orbit is reestablished by the placement of a Teflon implant.

eyelid. The tendency of a comminuted fracture of the orbital rim to assume an inferior and posterior displaced position should be avoided.

The inferior rectus muscle, the orbital fat, and any orbital soft tissue structures should be dissected free from the areas of the blow-out fracture. The intact floor should be located and traced around the edges of the blow-out. The floor must be explored sufficiently far back into the orbit for the posterior edge of the defect to be identified. In major blow-out fractures, this area is often a small ledge at the posterior portion of the orbit and can be located 35 to 38 mm behind the orbital rim. Identification of the intact ledge is verified on CT scan (longitudinal projection in the plane of the optic nerve). The ocular globe and its surrounding structures must be freed from any fracture sites. Proper rotation of the ocular globe after freeing of this orbital soft tissue may be confirmed by an intraoperative forced duction test. This test should be performed (1) before dissection, (2) after dissection, and (3) again after the insertion of any material used to reconstruct the orbital floor. It is vital that this reconstructive material not interfere with globe movement in any way, and it is absolutely essential to prove this before any incisions are closed. The full range of all ocular rotatory movements must be demonstrated. The most common cause of failure to release the entrapped structures is inadequate exposure of the floor in the posterior portion of the orbit.

Restoration of Continuity of Orbital Floor. Restoration of the continuity of the orbital floor is required in all orbital floor fractures, except in small fractures in which the entrapped structures can be freed readily and the forced duction test shows that the free rotation of the eyeball has been reestablished. In practice, the author reconstructs any orbital floor fracture that demonstrates (1) a bone defect or (2) a malpositioned, comminuted, or weakened orbital floor.

BONE GRAFTS. Split calvarial, iliac, or split rib bone grafts provide proper material for reconstruction of the orbital floor fracture. It is sometimes difficult, in extensive orbital fractures, to contour iliac or calvarial bone grafts as easily as a split rib can be molded to conform to the curvature of the posterior orbit (Figs. 27–257 to 27–259).

It is not necessary to have sinus lining present when there is a wide area of com-

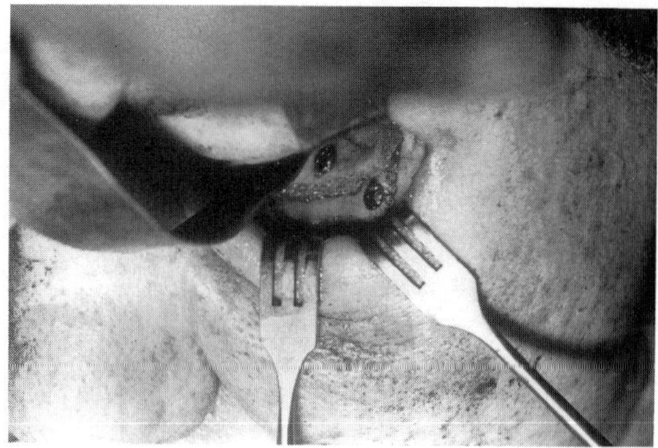

Figure 27–257. Orbital bone grafts can be "lag" screwed to intact portions of the orbital floor.

munication between the orbit and the maxillary sinus. Rather, the bone graft becomes a scaffold for the reconstitution of the sinus lining. As it becomes vascularized, the bone graft is better able to resist bacterial invasion than inorganic implants. The author prefers bone graft reconstruction in all major fractures in which the orbital floor is disrupted. Bone grafts can be tailored to fit the precise contour of the orbital floor more accurately and easily than can alloplastic materials (Fig. 27–260). It is also easier to anchor them with either a wire to the orbital rim or a "lag" screw (see Fig. 27–257) to the thicker bone of the orbit. Other bone graft donor sites, such as the anterior wall of the maxillary sinus, the ramus of the mandible, the perpendicular plate of the ethmoid, or septal or ear cartilage provide sufficient material only for small defects. The material is too thin, small, or brittle to be of much use. Costal cartilage has also been employed and constitutes a satisfactory, but seldom used, transplant material, which it is more difficult to carve and shape. Dingman and Grabb (1961) also described the use of irradiated cartilage allografts, and some authors have used irradiated bone.

INORGANIC IMPLANTS. The inorganic implant offers the advantage of obtaining the material necessary for reconstruction of the orbital floor without the need for removal of a bone graft. It is satisfactory for simple fractures. Many authors emphasize successful results in large defects that have wide areas of communication with the maxillary sinus (Mauriello, Flanagan, and Peyster, 1984; Amaratunga, 1987b). In a course of secondary operations, the regeneration of the maxillary sinus lining has occurred under the implant,

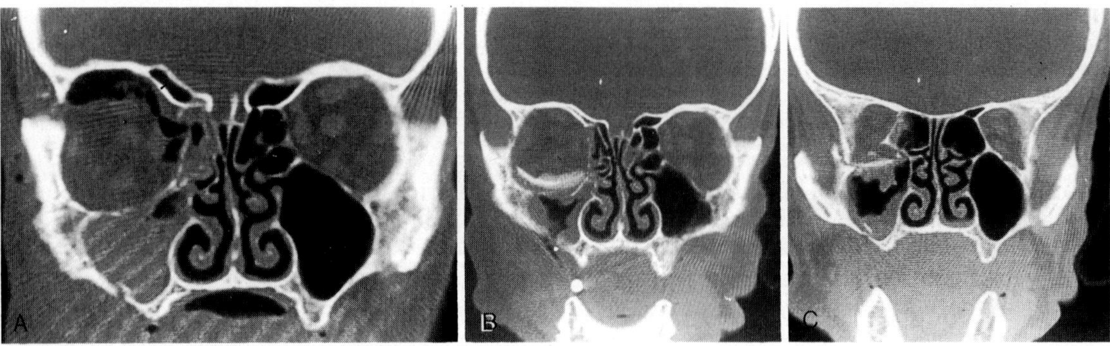

Figure 27–258. *A*, Fracture of the zygoma, floor, and medial portion of the orbit. The extraocular muscles are clearly visible and no incarceration is seen. Coronal CT scans provide direct evidence of muscle or fat incarceration, which should be used as an objective guide to the need for surgery for diplopia. Herniation of orbital fat has occurred outside the muscle cone. *B*, Restoration of the position of the zygoma and reconstitution of the orbital floor with a form-fitted bone graft. The volume is approximately that of the intact side. *C*, The volume of the posterior orbit must also be reconstituted. The bone graft must extend far posteriorly.

and in some cases bone regeneration has also been observed.

Inorganic implant materials employed in the orbital region have included Silastic metals, solid sponges, tantalum, stainless steel, vitallium, methylmethacrylate, polyvinyl sponge, polyurethane, polyethylene, Teflon, and Supramid. The author's preference for an inorganic implant material is either polyethylene (Medpor) or Supramid.

Ballen (1964) employed Cranioplast, a rapidly polymerizing methylmethacrylate, which is prepared by mixing powdered acrylic with a liquid catalyst. The material is molded in situ and hardens by a process of polymerization that gives off considerable heat. Ballen used this material in 31 patients but does not mention complications. Miller and Tenzel

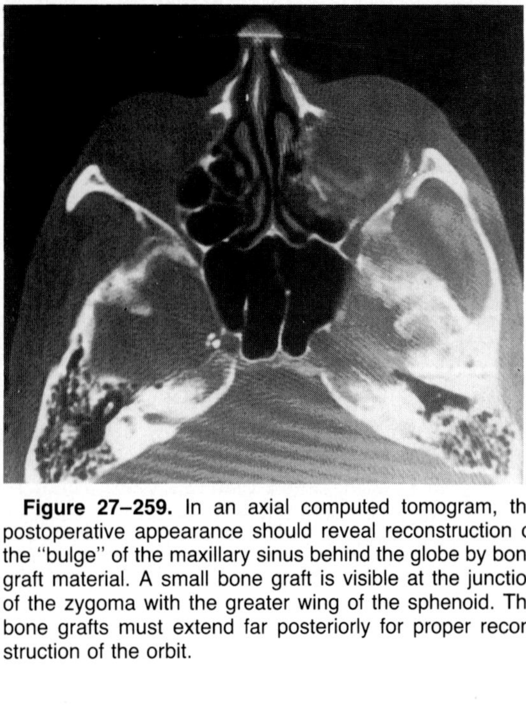

Figure 27–259. In an axial computed tomogram, the postoperative appearance should reveal reconstruction of the "bulge" of the maxillary sinus behind the globe by bone graft material. A small bone graft is visible at the junction of the zygoma with the greater wing of the sphenoid. The bone grafts must extend far posteriorly for proper reconstruction of the orbit.

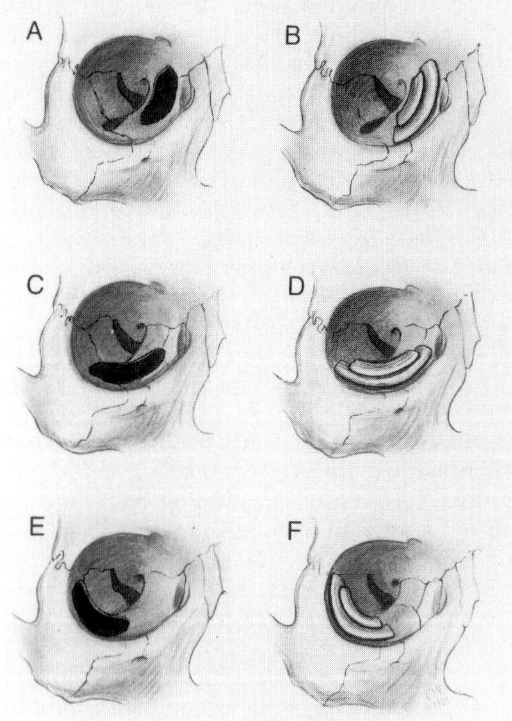

Figure 27–260. *A, B,* A medial blow-out fracture, treated with a bone graft. *C, D,* Fracture involving the floor of the orbit, treated with a bone graft. *E, F,* Fracture of the lateral portion of the orbit, treated with a bone graft. (From Manson, P. N., and French, J. A.: Fractures of the midface. In Georgiade, N. G., Riefkohl, R., Georgiade, G. S., and Barwick, W. I. (Eds.): Essentials of Plastic, Maxillofacial and Reconstructive Surgery. Baltimore, MD, Williams & Wilkins Company, 1987.)

(1967) employed prefabricated Cranioplast implants, which are prepared in various sizes and thicknesses, in over 300 patients (Tenzel, 1974). The prefabrication has the advantage of eliminating the time interval required for polymerization of methylmethacrylate.

Freeman (1962) described implanting sheets of Teflon in 36 patients with orbital floor fractures despite communication with the maxillary sinus in several. Browning and Walker (1965) reported the successful use of Teflon in 45 patients with orbital blow-out fractures.

The author's experience with artificial materials confirms that most patients do very well. The incidence of late infection is 1 to 2 per cent (Aronowitz, Freeman, and Spira, 1986), and displacement should not occur if the material has been properly anchored to the orbital rim to prevent dislodgement. Teflon, polyethylene, and Supramid are available in sheets 0.6 to 1 mm thick, and Silastic can also be carved to fit a specific defect. A proper thickness is required to provide support for soft tissue. The use of thin (< 0.6 mm) sheets does not usually provide proper orbital floor support.

The purpose of the orbital floor insert, whether a bone graft or an inorganic implant, is to *reestablish the size of the orbital cavity.* Less importantly, it begins to seal off the orbit from the maxillary sinus. This places the orbital soft tissue contents in their proper anatomic position and allows the occurrence of scar tissue in an anatomic position. The author prefers to place the smooth side of bone graft materials or implants toward the orbital contents. Any material used for floor reconstruction should be anchored or placed so that displacement is unlikely, in order to prevent extrusion of the material under the skin of the eyelid. Converse described a technique to secure the implant material (Fig. 27–261). The tongue is introduced under the anterior edge of the bone defect in the orbital floor, thus maintaining it in position and avoiding forward displacement and extrusion. In practice, it is easier simply to wire the implant to the orbital rim with a fine wire in a horizontal mattress fashion. The orbital implant should conform to the proper contour of the floor and not provide a place where dead space causes fluid accumulation. The maxillary sinus should be drained and any devitalized bone fragments or mucosa removed. Infection usually accompanies improper surgical cleansing of the maxillary sinus or blocked drainage.

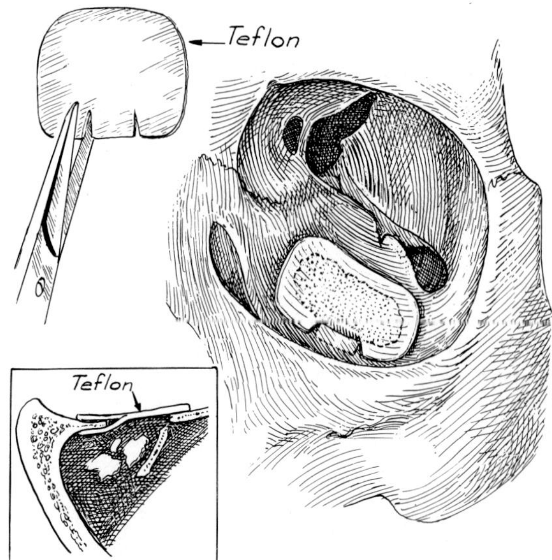

Figure 27–261. Technique to prevent foward displacement of a Teflon implant. The tongue is slipped under the anterior border of the bony defect and it blocks the forward migration of the implant. It is the author's preference to use fine wire to anchor the implant.

The failure to identify displacement in the absence of bone defects is a frequent cause of residual enophthalmos. The medial orbital wall and floor must be reconstructed in their proper location. Small fragments of bone may be present, all connected but displaced in location. Pressing on these with an elevator convinces the surgeon that their attachments are too weak to provide structural support to the soft tissue contents of the orbit. Their replacement with a bone graft, which may be inserted over existing fragments between the soft tissue contents of the orbit and the remaining bone, is the proper surgical procedure. It cannot be overemphasized that the remaining bone is often depressed into the sinus despite its continuous appearance in "eggshell" fractures.

ORBITAL FLOOR FRACTURES WITHOUT BLOW-OUT FRACTURE (LINEAR FRACTURES)

The symptoms and signs of fracture of the orbital floor without blow-out fracture are similar to those of a blow-out fracture. Usually, there is less effect on the ocular rotatory movements. It has been demonstrated, however, that a simple contusion and hematoma without fracture can produce the same symptoms as a blow-out fracture (Milauskas, 1969). There is numbness in the infraorbital nerve distribution and a disturbance of ocular rotatory movements. It would not facilitate the management of a case to perform a surgical exploration. It is thus imperative that accurate CT scans demonstrate the exact nature of the fracture and the soft tissue involvement in the fracture site. In a contusion without a fracture, the forced duction test should be negative in early stages. If there is hematoma, edema, or fibrosis in an extraocular muscle, the forced duction test may be positive. Transient diplopia usually accompanies hematoma, edema, and muscular contusions and usually the diplopia partially resolves with time.

Computed tomography in the axial and coronal plane fails to reveal the characteristic dehiscence of the floor of the maxillary sinus and medial orbital area. CT scans do not demonstrate the prolapse of orbital soft tissue contents into the maxillary or ethmoid sinuses. A simple crack may be demonstrated along the floor of the orbit, which, if not indicative of significant displacement, does not require treatment. It should be recalled that approximately one-third of zygomatic fractures are undisplaced or only minimally displaced, and a careful examination would be required to estimate the benefit that might be provided by surgery. Maxillary and zygomatic fracture lines always involve the orbital floor, and irregularity in the contour of the orbital rim is apparent on roentgenograms in this type of fracture.

Linear fractures of the orbital floor occurring in zygomatic and maxillary fractures often do not require orbital intervention, other than realignment and fixation of the orbital rim (the treatment is the same as that required for maxillary and zygomatic fracture). The orbital floor is always visualized and its integrity verified. Simple linear fractures do not require any treatment in the absence of displacement. Careful checking of the oculorotatory movements under anesthesia confirms the absence of any significant tethering of the extraocular muscle apparatus. Again, the radiographic examination by CT scan confirms the nature of the bone injury preoperatively.

In fractures with bone displacement, the risk of enlargement of the orbital cavity and consequent enophthalmos is an important consideration. The treatment of an orbital fracture must be performed in conjunction with the reduction and fixation of fractures of the orbital rim and the bones of the midfacial area. The only measure that can adequately restore the bone continuity of the displaced or fragmented bones is a full exploration of the usual sites of fracture, including the medial, inferior, and lateral orbit. Anatomic alignment of the bone skeleton and reconstitution of bone defects must occur in these areas. This is best done by direct exposure of the fractured area with bone graft reconstruction of the orbit in conjunction with reduction of the rim fractures. When there is doubt as to the integrity of the orbital floor, an exploration is indicated in order to prevent an occult comminuted depressed fracture being missed. It is easy to underestimate the extent of an orbital fracture if only axial CT scans are obtained.

Comminuted Fractures of Orbital Floor

In cases of exceptionally severe "crush" and "crash" injuries after accidents in automobiles, airplanes, or other high speed vehicles, the orbital injury is associated with other fractures of the frontal and midfacial skeleton. In these situations, the orbital rim and floor may be completely demolished. Fragments of bone, most of them suspended hammock-like from the periosteum, and the orbital contents sink into the maxillary sinus. The soft tissue, which normally has a pyramidal or cone-shaped configuration, remodels into a spherical shape with a loss of supporting bone in the medial, inferior, and lateral orbit (see Fig. 27–239). In order to undergo soft tissue remodeling, the ligaments holding the orbital soft tissue structures in approximation, including Lockwood's ligament (Koornneef, 1977, 1982; Manson and associates, 1986a), and the fine ligaments connecting the extraocular muscles with the periosteum and extending through intramuscular cone fat are disrupted by the force of the injury. Ligament disruption allows the soft tissue to remodel to whatever shape the underlying bone fragments provide in terms of structure. After remodeling has occurred, the soft tissue scarring is "fixed" and opposes anatomic repositioning despite bone reconstruction in the proper location. It is thus emphasized that early treatment of significant orbital fractures obtains superior esthetic results, as soft tissue scarring occurs in an anatomic position.

The orbital bones are pulverized and reduced to small particles. Fragments are displaced into the maxillary sinus. These should be removed, as they represent devascularized particles that provide a nidus for infection. If bone fragments can be salvaged, they are used to reconstruct the orbital rim. The lateral wall must be stabilized by interosseous fixation before the orbital floor is reconstructed. The orbital floor is usually intact laterally, adjacent to the greater wing of the sphenoid; posteriorly, a small ridge is present 35 to 38 mm behind the orbital rim. This ridge forms a guide for the reconstruction of the orbit, as the bone grafts should be placed on a 30 degree inclined plane from intact rim to the posterior ledge. Medially, the bone graft curves upward at 45 degrees to meet the medial orbital wall. Since bone graft displacement occurs in the absence of structurally sound fixation, the author has used a metal mesh platform for stabilization of the intraorbital bone grafts.

FRACTURES OF MEDIAL ORBITAL WALL

Medial orbital wall fractures usually occur in conjunction with an orbital floor fracture or a nasoethmoido-orbital fracture. The special etiologic factor is a small object such as a stick or ski pole, the tip of which may have struck the globe or medial canthal area.

Rougier (1965) reported tethering of the medial rectus muscle after a blow-out fracture, strongly suggesting an associated fracture of the medial orbital wall into the ethmoid sinus with entrapment of the medial rectus by a mechanism similar to that which occurs in the orbital floor. Fractures of the medial orbital wall were described by Miller and Glaser (1966), Edwards and Ridley (1968), Trokel and Potter (1969), Dodick and associates (1971), and Rumelt and Ernest (1972). The clinical signs included progressively increasing enophthalmos, narrowing of the palpebral fissure, horizontal diplopia with restriction of abduction, an increasing enophthalmos on abduction, and orbital emphysema.

It has been suggested that medial orbital wall fractures are associated with orbital floor fractures most commonly, and several authors demonstrated an incidence varying from 5 to 70 per cent (Gould and Titus, 1966; Jones and Evans, 1967; Dodick and associates, 1971; Pearl and Vistnes, 1978; Pearl, 1987). This relationship is explained by the structural relationships between the orbital floor and the medial orbital wall, described in an earlier section of this chapter. In the author's experience, as well as that of Prasad (1975), the entrapment of the medial rectus muscle is rare, and many of these fractures on radiographic examination are found to demonstrate little displacement. Frequently they show a moderate amount of orbital emphysema, but need no surgical reduction. The cellular structure of the ethmoid bone offers resistance that the hollow maxillary sinus beneath the orbital floor does not. The possibility of a concomitant blow-out fracture of the medial orbital wall should be suspected and identified in each case of orbital fracture; however, enophthalmos does not follow a medial orbital fracture to the same extent or frequency as it does an orbital floor fracture. Isolated medial blow-out fractures often require no treatment.

Radiographic Findings

Diagnosis is often made after proper roentgenologic examination of the orbit. The presence of air within the orbit (Fig. 27–262) is suggestive of a medial orbital fracture. One

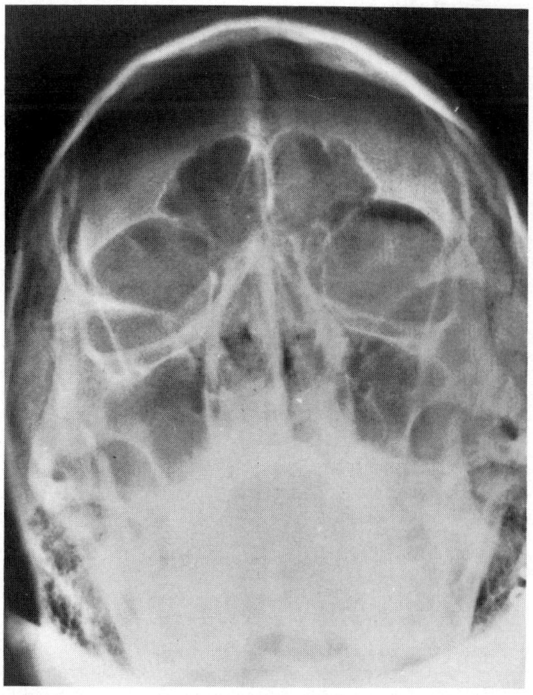

Figure 27–262. Plain radiograph demonstrating a medial blow-out fracture. Air is noted in the roof of the orbit.

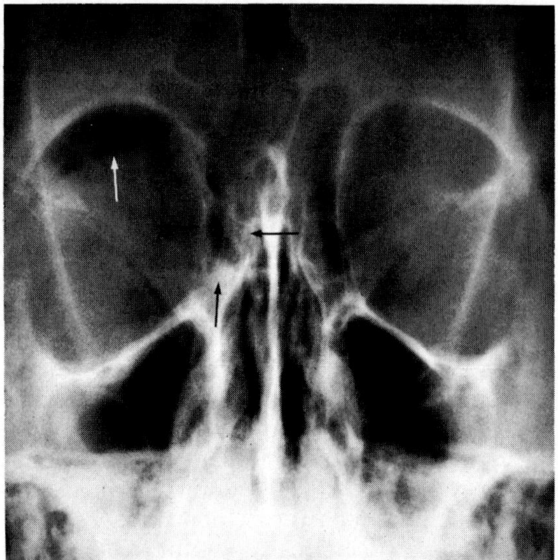

Figure 27–263. Radiograph showing displaced fragments *(black arrows)* in the medial orbital wall, clouding of the ethmoid sinus, and medial displacement of a portion of the medial orbital roof. Note also the fracture of the orbital roof *(white arrow)*.

can identify clouding of the ethmoid and maxillary sinuses (Fig. 27–263) and medial displacement of the medial orbital wall or displaced bone fragments (Fig. 27–263). Computed tomography demonstrates medial wall fractures with clarity (Fig. 27–264). The radiographic examination is invaluable in verifying the integrity of the medial orbital wall preoperatively so that adequate measures can be taken at the time of surgery.

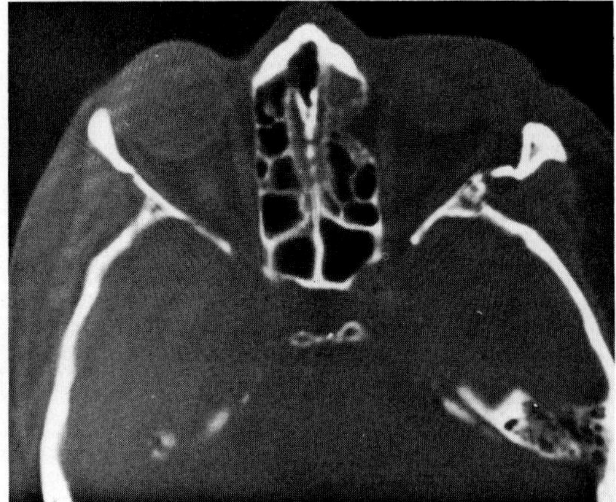

Figure 27–264. Fracture of the medial orbit occurring with a zygomatic fracture. The depression into the ethmoids is clearly visible. Note the close approximation of the medial rectus muscle to the fracture site.

Treatment

The proper treatment of medial orbital wall fractures depends on the anatomic location of the displaced bone and the extent of the fracture. The lower medial orbital wall can be exposed, freeing any soft tissue contents through lower eyelid incisions by retracting the orbital soft tissue contents upward and laterally. One can easily expose halfway up the medial orbital wall by means of this technique. If higher sections of the orbital wall need to be exposed, the approach can utilize a local incision (for naso-orbital fractures) or a coronal (scalp) incision. The coronal incision is necessary for the reduction of deep medial orbital fractures and it provides optimal visualization of the upper portion of the medial orbital wall. After the displacement of any soft tissue contents from the fracture, the exact contour of that portion of the orbit should be reconstructed with a properly curved bone graft (see Fig. 27–260). Small fractures do not require surgical treatment.

FRACTURES OF LATERAL ORBITAL WALL

The lateral orbital wall consists of a strong, resistant anterior frontozygomatic rim, which is exposed to frequent trauma. The wall becomes thinner behind the rim and consists of a thin posterior zygomatic portion that joins the greater wing of the sphenoid at the orbital process. Severe fractures of the lateral wall of the orbit occur in conjunction with high energy trauma to the zygomatic area and the frontozygomatic junction, with downward displacement of the lateral portions of the orbital floor. The fracture extends along, and sometimes involves, the anterior portion of the greater wing of the sphenoid, and travels through the inferior orbital fissure to comminute the orbital floor. In these fractures, the lateral canthus is dislocated downward with ectropion of the lower eyelid.

This type of fracture requires a direct approach exposing all fracture sites, similar to that employed in multiple fractures of the midfacial skeleton. Direct interosseous wiring of the fragments and primary bone grafting to restore the orbital floor, lateral wall, and zygomatic osseous framework are indicated. After the interfragment wiring, additional stability and stabilization of the forward projection of the malar eminence can be

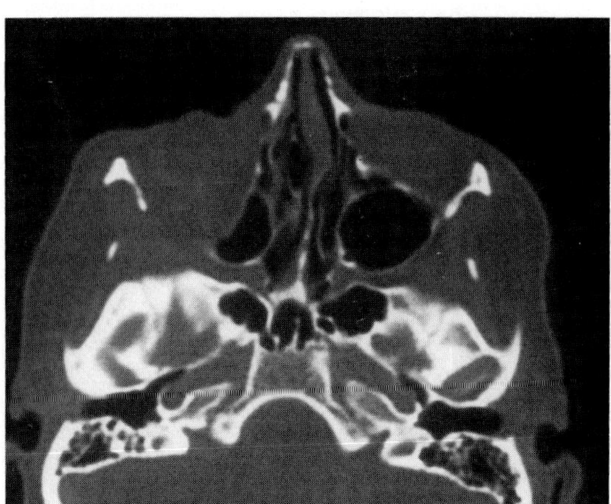

Figure 27–265. Loss of a portion of the greater wing of the sphenoid with herniation of the orbital soft tissue into the temporal fossa.

achieved with plate and screw fixation. In such severe fractures, the ocular globe suffers injury of varying degree, and loss of vision may be frequent. It is imperative that visual examination, so far as possible, precede any surgical manipulation.

Fractures of the lateral orbital wall are more frequent than is generally assumed. They can accompany zygomatic fractures (Fig. 27–265). Simple fractures of the zygoma involve the lateral orbital wall with a linear fracture; the displacement is minimal and is usually corrected by open reduction of the rim. In more severe fractures, the greater wing of the sphenoid is involved as well as the junction of the sphenoid with the zygoma. The author has noted the frequency of such fractures during fracture treatment through a coronal incision and in the correction of grossly malunited fractures of the zygoma and orbit. In these cases, orbital fat prolapses into the temporal fossa, suggesting a blow-out fracture of the posterior portion of the lateral orbital wall. There is a thin area of bone immediately behind the thick lateral orbital rim, which extends through the anterior portion of the greater wing of the sphenoid. A fracture of the rim may comminute this thin portion of the lateral orbital wall, facilitating orbital enlargement and a blow-out in this area. Such soft tissue displacement is a cause of postoperative enophthalmos.

FRACTURES OF ORBITAL ROOF

LaGrange (1918), in his classic monograph, showed that the thin medial portion of the orbital roof is fractured and displaced in its posterior part in the region of the superior orbital fissure and optic foramen. A fracture of this type can lead to serious complications, such as optic nerve ischemia and injury, and to damage to the nerves that travel through the superior orbital fissure. Dodick and associates (1971), in a series of 22 cases of suspected blow-out fractures of the orbit, obtained radiologic evidence of fracture of the orbital floor in 15 cases; in two cases, there was a comminuted fracture of the orbital roof.

A fracture of the orbital roof may also occur in conjunction with frontal bone, nasoethmoido-orbital, or zygomatic fractures. The medial portion of the orbital roof is thinner than the lateral portion and thus more susceptible to fracture.

If the superior rim of the orbit is fractured and the trochlea of the superior oblique muscle is damaged, impairment of function of the superior oblique muscle may result in double vision, which is often temporary.

Fractures of the orbital roof may involve only the thin portion of the roof, in which displacement is limited. They may involve the orbital rim, and occur either medially in the region of the frontal sinus or laterally in the supraorbital area. The lateral orbital rim fractures usually occur in conjunction with more extensive fractures of the frontal bone and temporal area, the so-called "fronto-temporo-orbital" fracture. The combined craniofacial (coronal) approach is required in these patients for proper neurosurgical exposure, repair of dural tears, and debridement of any damaged frontal lobe. The dura is often torn or penetrated by comminuted fragments. Splintered bone fragments are removed and the anterior cranial fossa and frontal region exposed. The orbital roof defect should always be repaired by a thin bone graft.

The displacement of the orbital roof is generally downward and inward, producing a concomitant forward and downward displacement of the globe and orbital soft tissue. Ptosis is present and, depending on the degree of involvement of the extraocular muscles and structures in the superior orbital fissure, paralysis of cranial nerves III, IV, and VI may occur. There may be anesthesia in the supraorbital branches of the ophthalmic division of the trigeminal nerve. When the fractures involve cranial nerves III, IV, and VI and the ophthalmic division of the trigeminal nerve, the *superior orbital fissure syndrome* is present (Kurzer and Patel, 1979; Zachariades, 1982). If the condition also involves the optic nerve (visual loss), the *orbital apex syndrome* is present (Miller and Tenzel, 1967; Miller, 1968; Ketchum, Ferris, and Masters, 1976; Manfredi and associates, 1981), which implies involvement of the posterior portion of the orbit by fracture.

NASOETHMOIDO-ORBITAL FRACTURES

Fractures of the maxilla, nasal bones, zygomas, and orbits are frequently complicated by fractures of the bones of the frontonasoethmoidal area and the central midfacial skeleton (nasoethmoido-orbital fractures) (Fig. 27–266). The bones of the middle third of the face are also in close anatomic relationship to the floor of the anterior cranial fossa and the frontal lobes of the brain, through the frontal and ethmoid sinuses and the cribriform plate. The certainty of concomitant orbital floor and medial wall blow-out fractures in these injuries has been discussed. The orbital roof also is frequently comminuted in its medial portion.

Fracture of the anterior cranial fossa usually accompanies frontoethmoido-orbital injuries. There is a possibility of brain damage and cerebrospinal fluid rhinorrhea with dural tears. The presence of depressed skull fractures should signal the need for neurologic evaluation and operative treatment. The signs of frontal lobe injury are often less obvious than in other areas of the brain, such as the motor cortex. They can include confusion, loss of consciousness, and inappropriate behavior. Physical signs may be noted on radiographs, such as epidural hematoma, pneumocephalus, subdural hematoma, or depressed skull fracture. The association of frontal and facial injuries with cervical fractures has been reported previously. Head injury is often complicated by other conditions, such as pulmonary edema and a disturbance of coagulation. A full evaluation of such patients is thus mandatory before any operative treatment is undertaken.

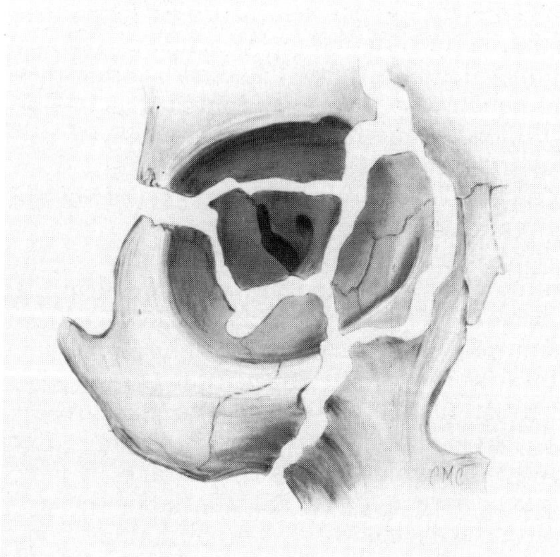

Figure 27–266. The orbital rim may be divided into thirds for the purpose of classifying fractures of the orbit. The superior portion is the *supraorbital* section. The *infralateral* portion is the zygoma. The *nasoethmoidal* area is represented by the lower two-thirds of the medial orbital rim.

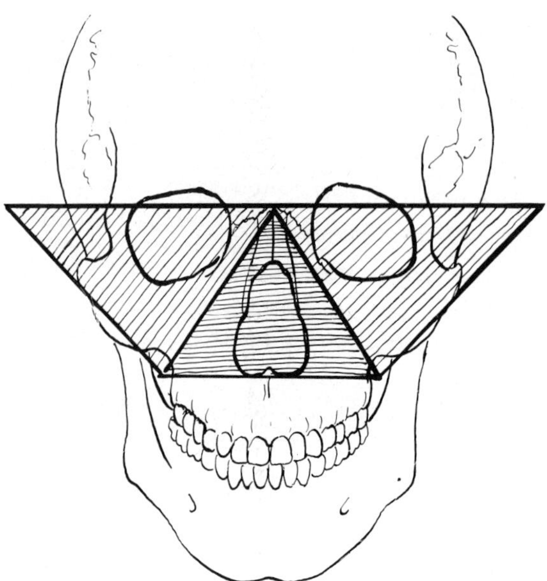

Figure 27–267. The bones forming the skeletal framework of the nose are situated in the upper and central portion of the midfacial skeleton. The diagram illustrates the concept by which the middle third of the face is divided into three triangles—a central nasal maxillary triangle and two lateral orbitozygomatic triangles.

Structural Aspects

The nasoethmoido-orbital area forms the central third of the upper midfacial skeleton (Fig. 27–267). The thin areas of the medial orbital walls transluminate readily and thus contrast with the heavier abutments formed by the nasal process of the frontal bone, the frontal process of the maxilla, and the thick upper portions of the nasal bones. Posteriorly the frontal process of the maxilla, the thinner lacrimal bone, and a delicate lamina papyracea are vulnerable to trauma (Fig. 27–268). The anterior and posterior ethmoidal fora-

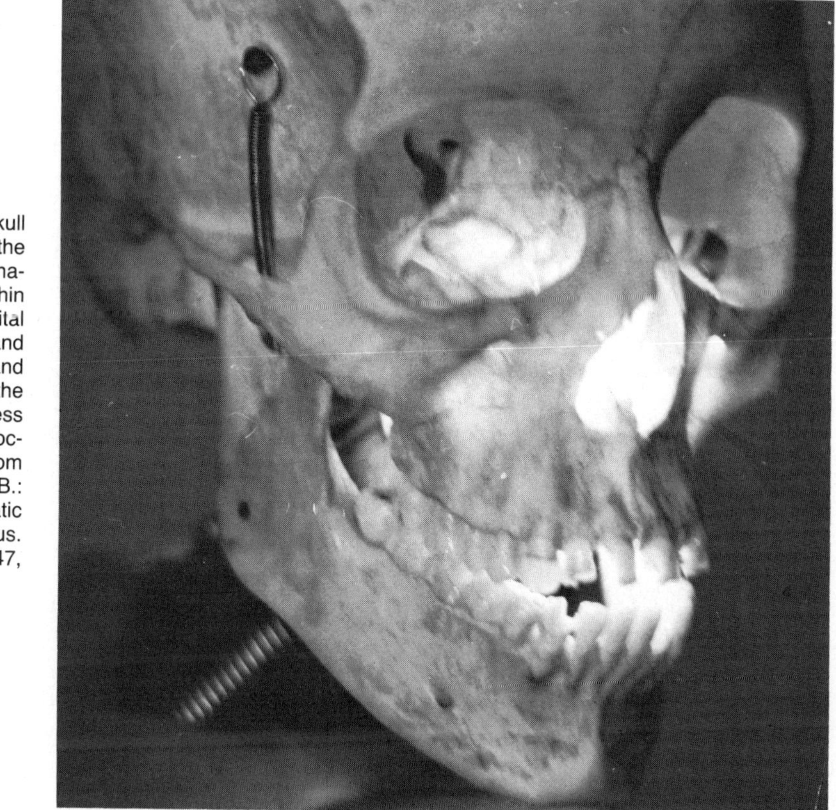

Figure 27–268. *A*, Human skull with a light source placed at the base of the skull behind the nasoethmoido-orbital region. Thin bony areas of the medial orbital wall transilluminate readily and thus contrast with the thick and heavier abutments formed by the nasal bones, the frontal process of the maxilla, and the nasal process of the frontal bone. (From Converse, J. M., and Smith, B.: Naso-orbital fractures in traumatic deformity of the medial canthus. Plast. Reconstr. Surg., *38*:147, 1966.)

mina are situated along the upper border of the lamina papyracea and the frontal ethmoidal suture, where the orbital plate of the frontal bone and lamina papyracea of the ethmoid are joined. The anterior ethmoidal foramen transmits the nasociliary nerve and the anterior ethmoidal vessel; the posterior ethmoidal foramen gives passage to the posterior ethmoidal nerves and vessels. These vessels frequently rupture in significant nasoethmoido-orbital fractures. Bone fragments can penetrate the soft tissue of the orbit, and the vessels may be lacerated. More often a symmetric medial compression of the ethmoidal labyrinth of sinuses is produced. The rupture of these vessels in nasoethmoido-orbital fractures is one of the causes of orbital hematoma. Usually, the comminution of the bone fragments lacerates the periosteum, and the intraorbital pressure is increased by a retrobulbar hematoma. It is unusual for a retrobulbar hematoma, despite its invariable presence in these injuries, to cause a significant problem or require decompression in itself.

The most medial posterior portion of the medial orbital wall is formed by the body of the sphenoid immediately in front of the optic foramen. In severe skeletal disruption of this area, the fracture lines involve the optic foramen and superior orbital fissure. This can produce a disturbance of circulation to the optic nerve or a pressure effect, which might result in blindness. It is unusual for the bones in the posterior third of the orbit to undergo significant displacement.

The term *interorbital space* designates an area between the orbits and below the floor of the anterior cranial fossa. The interorbital space contains two ethmoidal labyrinths, one on each side (Fig. 27–269).

The interorbital space is roughly pear shaped in transverse section, being wider in the middle than in the posterior portion. It is limited above by the cribriform plate in the midline and by the roof of each ethmoidal mass on the sides, and it is divided into two approximately equal halves by the nasal septum. The interorbital space is limited below at the level of the horizontal line through the

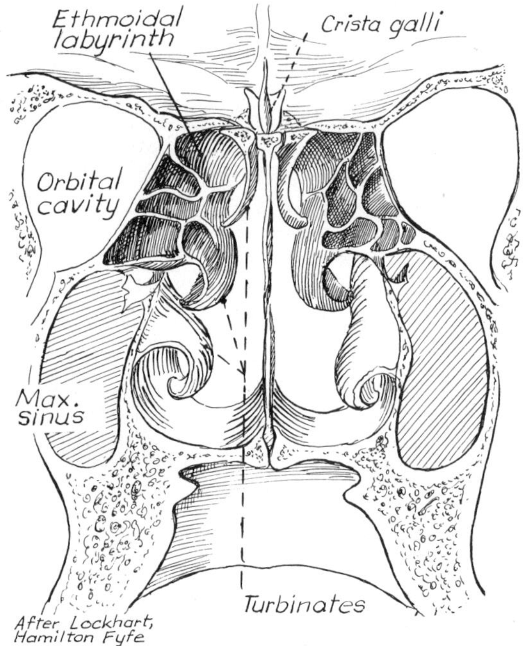

Figure 27–269. The interorbital space seen from behind. A frontal section through the ethmoids showing the relationship of the orbits with the interorbital space.

lower border of the ethmoidal labyrinth. The lateral wall is the medial wall of the orbit. Anteriorly, the interorbital space is limited by the frontal process of the maxilla and by the nasal process and spine of the frontal bone.

The interorbital space contains cellular bone structures lined by mucosa. These include the ethmoid cells, the superior and middle turbinates, and a median thin plate of bone, the perpendicular plate of the ethmoid, which forms the posterosuperior portion of the nasal septal framework.

The size of the *frontal sinus* varies greatly. It may occupy most of the frontal bone or only a small portion of the lower central portion. Developing in teenage years to reach its full size, it may be the size of an ethmoid cell or may be quite large, pneumatizing the entire frontal bone; often it is much larger on one side than on the other. Occasionally, it may be absent. It contains variable partial and complete septa.

The sinus has the shape of a pyramid with inferior, anterior, and posterior walls (Fig. 27–270). The inferior wall or floor of the frontal sinus corresponds to the roof of the orbit and is the thinnest portion of the frontal sinus. The anterior wall is thickest and composed of compact and some cancellous bone; the amount of cancellous bone is variable. The posterior wall is thinner than the anterior wall and is composed almost entirely of compact bone, which separates the sinus from the frontal lobe. A median partition is usually present. The nasofrontal ducts descend from the posteroinferior portion of the sinus through the ethmoidal labyrinth to exit into the nose somewhat posteriorly at the level of the middle turbinate.

The *ethmoid bone* occupies the lateral portion of the interorbital space. Below the interorbital space, the lower half of the nasal cavity is flanked by the maxillary sinuses. Each lateral mass of the ethmoid is connected medially to the cribriform plate; the roof of each ethmoidal mass is inclined upward from the cribriform plate and projects in its lateral portion approximately 0.25 cm above it. The level of the cribriform plate is variable and must be individually identified on radiographic examination.

The ethmoid area is pyramidal or cuboidal in shape and is 3.5 to 5 cm long and 1.5 to 2.5 cm wide. It is cellular in structure and contains eight to ten cells with thin lamellar walls. They are usually divided into anterior and posterior sections. These cells drain into the medial meatus of the nose. The frontal sinus drains through the ethmoid either as a distinct nasofrontal duct or by emptying into an anterior ethmoidal cell and into the middle meatus. There is thus an intimate anatomic

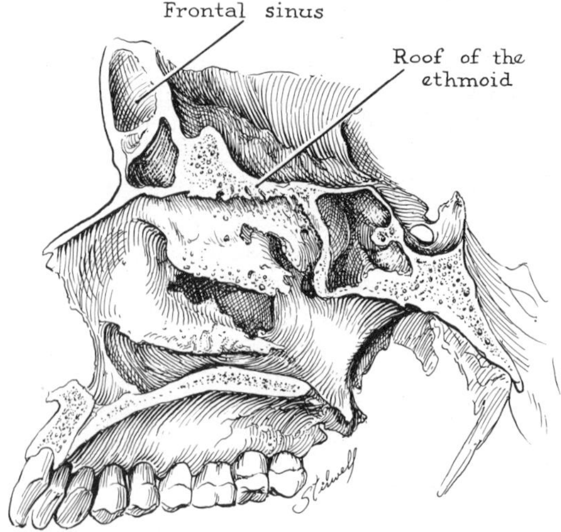

Figure 27–270. Sagittal section showing the lateral wall of the nose, the turbinates, and the frontal sinus with a frontoethmoidal cell behind it.

relationship with the frontal and ethmoid areas via the nasofrontal duct. A large ethmoidal cell, the frontoethmoidal, may be seen in the frontal bone between the frontal sinus and the roof of the orbit (Fig. 27–270). The extension of the "supraorbital ethmoidal cells" may be quite dramatic, pneumatizing the orbital roof, and they are a frequently neglected problem in fractures involving the frontal bone and anterior cranial fossa. Proper management of ethmoidal injuries should include the same treatment applied to fractures of the frontal sinus.

Surgical Pathology

The bones that form the skeletal framework of the nose are projected backward between the orbits when subjected to strong traumatic forces. The term "naso-orbital" was employed to designate this type of fracture and was suggested by Converse and Smith (1963). These bones are situated in the upper central portion of the middle third of the face anterior to the anatomic crossroads between the cranial, orbital, and nasal cavities (see Fig. 27–267). A typical cause of a nasoethmoido-orbital fracture is a blunt impact applied over the upper portion of the bridge of the nose caused by projection of the face against a blunt object such as the steering wheel or dashboard. The occupant of the automobile is thrown forward, striking the nasofrontal area. A crushing injury with comminuted fracture is thus produced. Bursting of the soft tissues due to the severity of the impact, and penetrating lacerations of the soft tissues resulting from projection through the windshield, may transform the closed fracture into an open compound comminuted injury (Fig. 27–271). If the impact force suffered by the strong anterior abutment is sufficient to cause backward displacement of these structures, no further resistance is of-

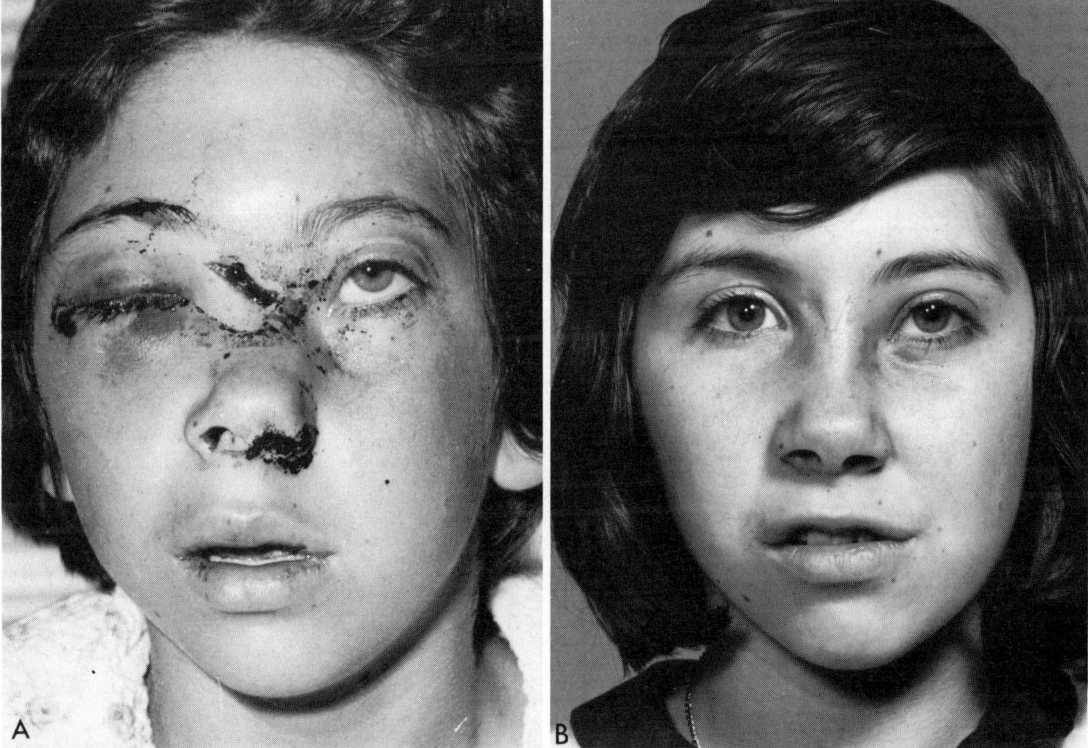

Figure 27–271. *A*, A 12 year old victim of an automobile accident with a typical nasoethmoido-orbital fracture. The patient had cerebrospinal fluid rhinorrhea, which subsequently ceased spontaneously. Note the flattened nasal dorsum, hematoma of the right orbit, and displacement of the left medial canthus. The initial treatment consisted of interfragment wiring to maintain the reduction of the comminuted bone fragments. *B*, After reconstructive surgery, a left medial canthoplasty was performed. A large portion of the left nasal bone and frontal process of the maxilla was extruded into the nasal cavity at the time of the accident. A bone graft was required to restore the nasal contour. (From Converse, J. M., and Smith, B.: Naso-orbital fractures and traumatic deformities of the medial canthus. Plast. Reconstr. Surg., *38*:147, 1966.)

fered by the delicate, matchbox-like structures of the interorbital space; indeed, these structures collapse and splinter, like a pile of matchboxes struck by a hammer (Converse and Smith, 1963). The roof of the interorbital space is frequently involved in these fractures and the anterior cranial fossa is thus penetrated, fractures occurring either adjacent to or through the cribriform plate area. Laterally, these structures involve the roofs of the ethmoidal sinuses in the medial portion and the lateral walls of the ethmoid sinuses.

Some of the neurologic complications resulting from naso-orbital fractures are laceration of the dura covering the frontal lobes, laceration of the tubular sheaths enveloping the olfactory nerves as they perforate the cribriform plate, penetration of the brain by sharp-edged ethmoidal or frontal cell walls, and necrosis or contusion of brain tissue.

An additional point of interest in the skeletal structure of this area is the continuity of the thin lamina papyracea of the medial orbital wall with a thin portion of the floor of the orbit. Splintering of the lamina papyracea also facilitates a blow-out fracture in this area (Fig. 27–272). Fractures of the medioinferior orbital rim and orbital floor are invariably present.

Lacerations of the soft tissue may sever the levator palpebrae superioris or penetrate through the medial canthal area. In some cases, the medial canthal tendon may be severed and the lacrimal system (canaliculi or upper portion of the sac) divided or avulsed from bone fragments.

Fractures of the other facial bones, particularly the midfacial skeleton, are frequently seen. In many patients, the frontal bone and other bones of the orbit are involved.

NASAL AREA: WEAKEST PORTION OF FACIAL SKELETON

Studies confirm that the nasal area is the weakest portion of the facial skeleton; fractures occur in this area with an impact load of 35 to 80 G. In Swearingen's study (1965), 45 impacts were made on cadaver heads to determine the fracture points of various portions of the facial skeleton. The comparative forces that can be tolerated over the various facial areas without fracture are illustrated in Figure 27–273. With the exception of the neck of the condyle, the zygomatic area is the next weakest area, being unable to sustain impact forces of greater than 50 G. The upper

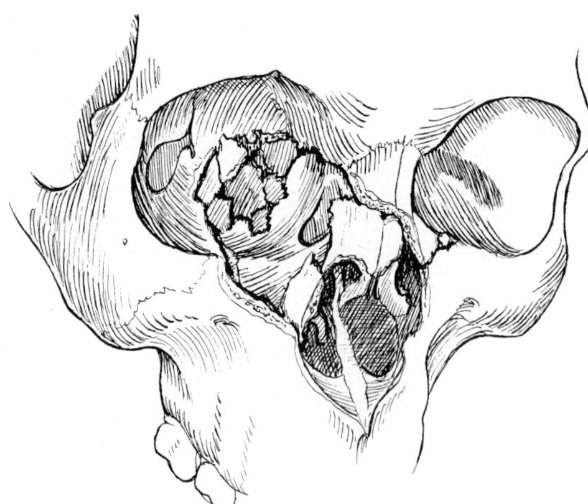

Figure 27–272. Unilateral nasoethmoido-orbital fracture. Because of the backward displacement of the skeletal structures, the lacrimal bone and the lamina papyracea and orbital floor have been severely comminuted. Primary bone grafting is indicated in such cases to restore the orbit.

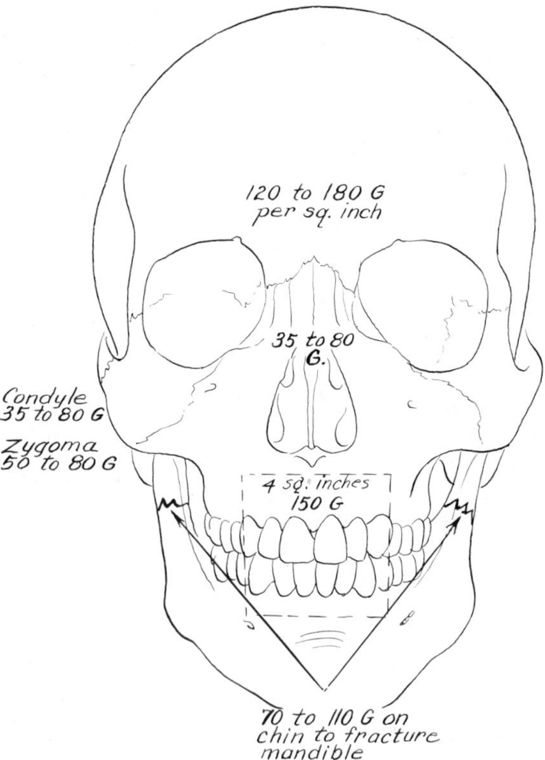

Figure 27–273. Summary of the maximal tolerable impact on a padded deformable surface. The schema illustrates the comparable forces that can be tolerated over various facial areas without fracture. (After Swearingen, J. J.: Tolerances of the Human Face to Crash Impact. Oklahoma City, Federal Aviation Agency, 1965.)

portion of the middle third of the face, which includes both the nasal and the orbital areas, is structurally susceptible to fracture. In contrast, the lower portion of the maxilla sustains impact forces of up to 150 G, and the major portion of the body of the frontal bone, with the exception of the central portion, which is weakened by the frontal sinus cavities, sustains impact forces of up to 120 G.

Although padding of the rigid dashboard decreases the severity of injuries sustained by the right front seat passenger, the padded dashboard lip in many automobiles has a contour suitable for the production of the "pushback" of the nasal structures between the orbits. Such fractures occur even though the passenger is wearing a lap seat belt; they occur less frequently when he is protected by the shoulder harness type of belt. The passenger without a seat belt is often projected through the windshield and suffers various types of soft tissue lacerations, which occur concomitantly with facial fractures. These include penetrating lacerations of the nasal and orbital areas.

It should be emphasized that the forces described by Swearingen (1965) are the minimal forces necessary for fracture. In practice, the actual force delivered to the area in many of these injuries exceeds the minimal forces for fracture by a multiple almost exceeding comprehension. Thus, the force is sufficient to comminute the bones of the facial skeleton.

Traumatic Telecanthus

In many nasoethmoido-orbital fractures, the patient has a characteristic appearance (Figs. 27–274, 27–275). The bony bridge of the nose may be depressed and widened, and the angle between the lip and the columella may be opened into an obtuse relationship. The eyes may appear far apart as in orbital hypertelorism. This may simply be due to a traumatic telecanthus or, in the presence of bilateral zygomatic fractures, there may be a true hyperteloric appearance. Traumatic telecanthus implies an increase in the distance between the medial canthi. This may not be present acutely in many nasoethmoido-orbital fractures, but may be noted with the bone displacement that occurs as time passes. Swelling may mask the exact discovery of bone displacement. Nasoethmoido-orbital

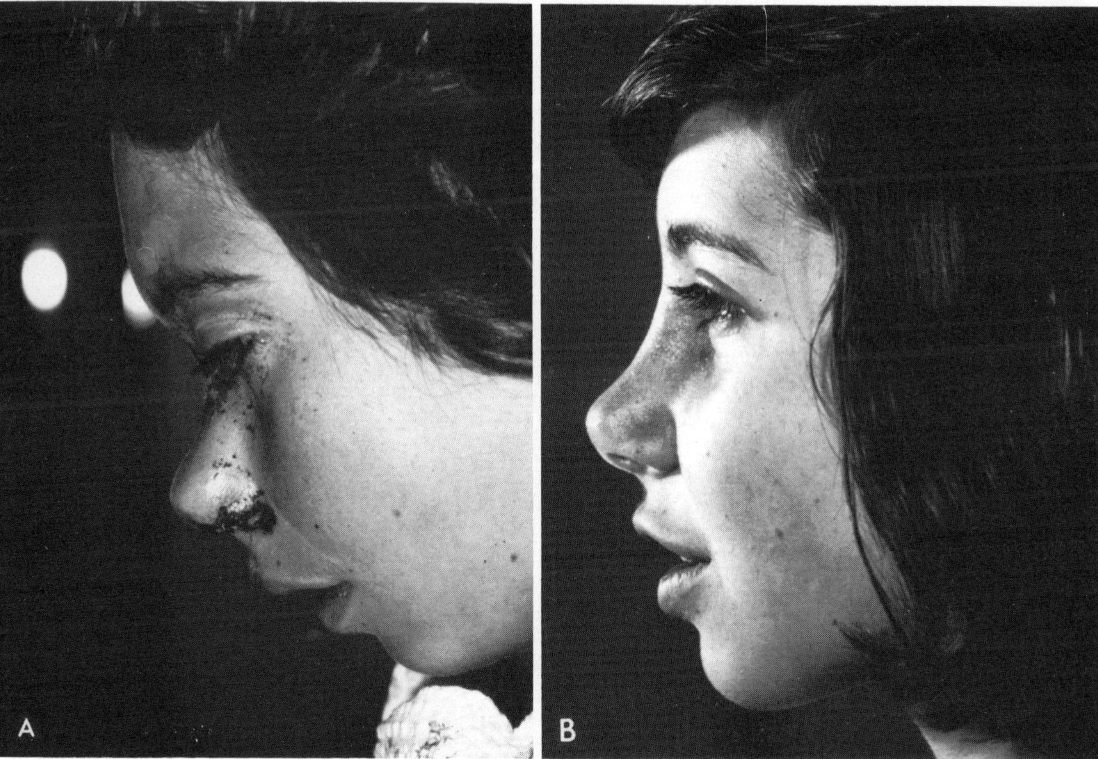

Figure 27–274. *A*, A patient with backward displacement of the nasal skeletal structures into the interorbital space (see Fig. 27–271). *B*, After completion of treatment.

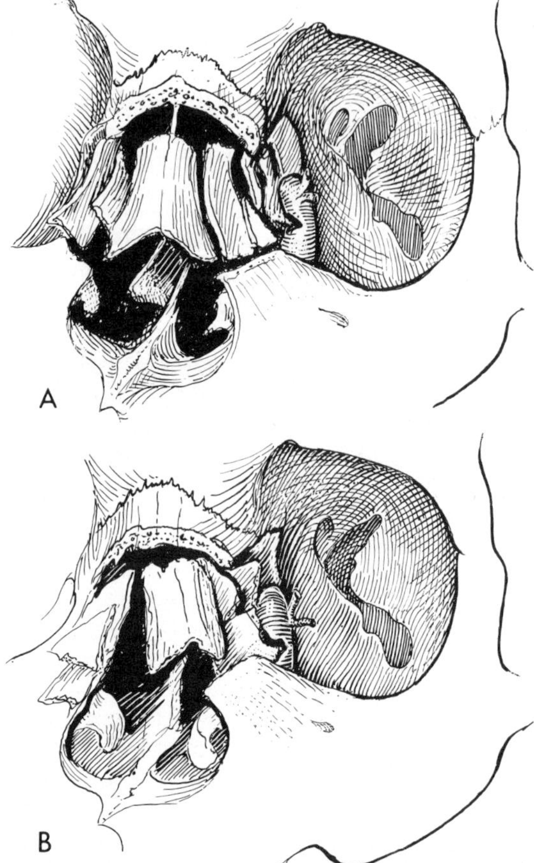

Figure 27–275. Two mechanisms for the production of traumatic telecanthus resulting from backward telescoping of the nasoskeletal structures and comminution of the medial wall of the orbit. (After Converse.) *A*, Backward displacement of the nasal bones and frontal processes of the maxilla into the ethmoid, resulting in displacement of the medial wall of the orbit laterally. *B*, Bone fragments displaced backward, lateral to the medial wall of the orbit, penetrating the lacrimal sac.

fractures may be unilateral (36 per cent) (Fig. 27–276) or bilateral (64 per cent) (Fig. 27–277). The unilateral type is common in upper Le Fort II and III injuries or in fractures involving the frontal area on one side progressing into the nasoethmoidal region. The final type of common unilateral nasoethmoidal fracture involves the zygoma and the medial orbit. Traumatic orbital hypertelorism (as opposed to telecanthus) is a deformity characterized by an increase in the distance between the orbits and ocular globe; it occurs rarely in massive disruption of the midfacial skeleton and frontal bone (Converse, Smith, and Wood-Smith, 1975).

According to Converse and Smith (1966), traumatic telecanthus is produced by two varieties of backward and lateral displacement of the bone structures (see Fig. 27–275). In the first, the frontal process of the maxilla and nasal bones penetrate the interorbital space, comminuting the ethmoid cells, and outfracturing the medial wall of the orbit. The medial canthal tendon attachments are displaced with the bone, and the medial canthus is displaced laterally and may be deformed, assuming a rounded shape. It is rare for the medial canthus to be avulsed from a significant-sized bone fragment in the absence of lacerations near the medial canthal area.

In the second type of fracture (see Fig. 27–275), the nasal bones and the frontal processes of the maxilla are splayed outward and projected backward into the medial portion of the orbital cavity along the lateral surface of the medial orbital wall. Again, the medial canthal tendon usually is not severed from bone, nor is the lacrimal or canalicular system transected in the absence of lacerations. Traumatic telecanthus may be contributed to by an increase in the thickness of the medial orbital wall from the overlapping bone fragments.

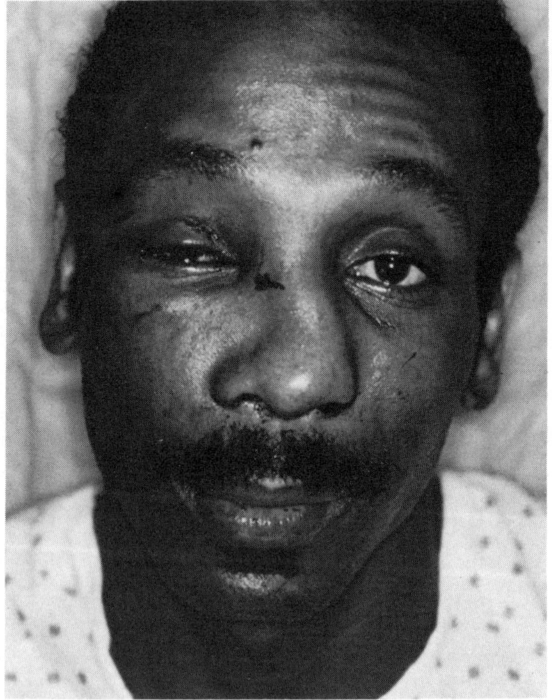

Figure 27–276. Unilateral nasoethmoido-orbital fracture. Lateral deviation of the nose is seen and lateral displacement of the right medial canthus is noted. A zygomatic fracture is also present.

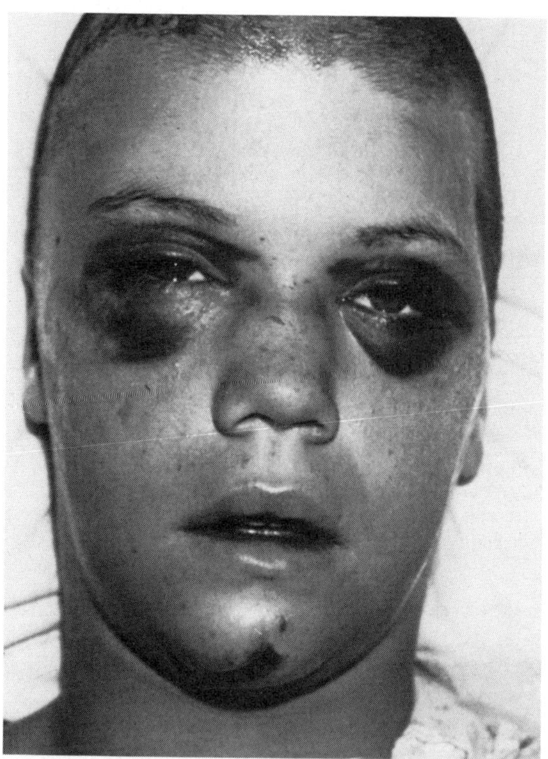

Figure 27–277. The typical appearance of an isolated central midfacial fracture. A bilateral nasoethmoido-orbital fracture is present. Bilateral palpebral ecchymosis and subconjunctival hematoma, with a posterior displacement of the nose and widening of the intercanthal distance, are seen. Telecanthus may not be apparent acutely.

Loss of bone in the area results from the splintering of small bone fragments. They may disappear following this injury or some may have been removed with debridement. Expulsion of bone fragments into the nasal cavity can occur at the time of fracture. Fragments can be displaced into the maxillary sinus. These small bone fragments often are not usable for reconstruction.

The superior and medial portions of the orbital rim are usually fractured and displaced.

Clinical Examination. The appearance of the patient who has suffered a naso-orbital fracture is typical (see Figs. 27–276, 27–277). A frontal impact nasal fracture is present, with the nose flattened and appearing to have been pushed between the eyes. There is a loss of dorsal nasal prominence, and an obtuse angle is noted between the lip and columella. Finger pressure on the nose documents the inadequate septal and bony support. The medial canthal areas are swollen and distorted with palpebral and subconjunctival hematoma. The lacrimal caruncles and plicae semilumares may be covered by the edematous and displaced structures. Ecchymosis and subconjunctival hemorrhage are usual findings. Directly over the canthal ligaments, crepitus or movement may be palpated with external pressure alone or with a bimanual examination (Fig. 27–278). Bimanual examination of the medial orbital rim is helpful if the diagnosis is uncertain.

Intranasal examination shows the findings observed in a fracture of the nasal bones and the septum. Fracture of the septum is suggested by displacement, swollen mucous membranes, and septal hematoma. Nasoethmoido-orbital fractures are often accompanied by the signs of orbital blow-out fracture or fracture of the frontal bone, maxilla, or zygoma. Edema and hematoma often mask the extent of the skeletal distortion in this area, particularly if the patient is not seen during the first hours after the accident.

The patient may be unconscious or may have had a loss of consciousness of long or

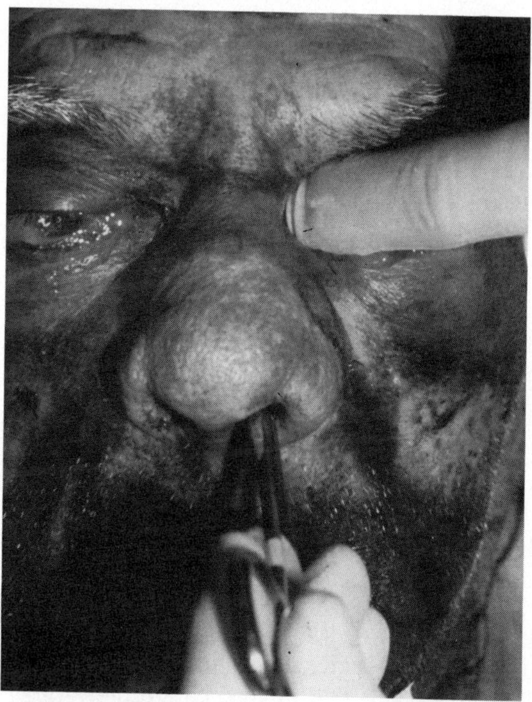

Figure 27–278. To determine the mobility of the canthal-bearing fragment (usually a portion of the lower two-thirds of the medial orbital rim), a clamp is placed intranasally directly under the frontal process of the maxilla, and the bone is moved between an external palpating finger and the clamp. Care must be taken not to misdiagnose a nasal fracture for a nasoethmoido-orbital fracture. The palpating finger should be placed deeply over the canthal tendon.

short duration. This is suggestive of brain injury. The patient may be irritable, restless, or even thrashing about after a severe injury. As in other fractures of the orbit, extensive edema of the periorbital structures and the lids may cause mechanical limitation of eyelid or extraocular movement.

There may be little evidence of skeletal deformity because of the hematoma or swelling. In some cases, the deformity is evident when the frontal bone has been crushed inward and the nasal structures have been projected into the interorbital space (see Fig. 27–275). The bones may be loose, and crepitation may be felt when they are mobilized. The entire upper jaw may be movable, and motion may be felt in the bones of the interorbital space. A portion of the forehead skin may be avulsed in compound fractures, exposing the bone or revealing the site of the fracture.

Clear fluid escaping from the nose is strongly suggestive of cerebrospinal fluid rhinorrhea. In acute injuries, this is often masked by bloody drainage, and cerebrospinal fluid rhinorrhea should be expected in any nasoethmoido-orbital injury because of the extension of the fracture to the cribriform plate area. Patients with cerebrospinal fluid rhinorrhea always show an initial escape of blood from the fracture sites. Over several days, the fluid becomes brownish in color, and finally clear. The cerebrospinal fluid may be distinguished from blood by the "double ring test," in which a small amount of nasal drainage is placed on a paper towel. The blood remains toward the center, whereas the cerebrospinal fluid migrates laterally, forming an inner-red and outer-clear ring, the "double ring" sign.

Roentgenographic Examination. Computed tomography is essential to document the injury. Plain radiographs often mask the fractures, as detail is obscured. Careful CT shows the suggestive signs of a nasoethmoidal fracture. Fractures are present across the frontal process of the maxilla, the nose, the orbital rims, and the orbital walls (Fig. 27–279). The fracture pattern may extend into adjacent structures, but in its simplest form the fractures surrounding the entire medial orbit rim *must* be documented to have a nasoethmoido-orbital fracture. Fractures of the anterior cranial fossa may be difficult to detect in ordinary axial CT. The presence of air in the subdural or subarachnoid space or in the ventricle is a sign of communication with the nasal cavity or sinuses. A direct pathway for infection has been established and is an indication for considering neurosurgical intervention. Fractures of the frontal sinus are frequent, and an air fluid level is often observed in the frontal sinus. Displacement of the anterior and posterior walls of the frontal sinus may be observed.

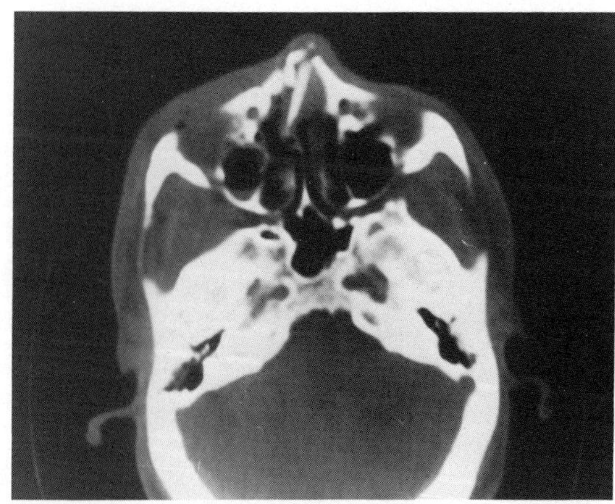

Figure 27–279. A computed tomogram (CT) demonstrating a bilateral nasoethmoido-orbital fracture with displacement and telecanthus. The injury is more extensive on one side than on the other.

Fragmentation and a buckled appearance of the cribriform plate are suggestive of penetration of bone fragments into the brain. This finding is an indication for neurosurgical exploration.

A CT examination in both the axial and coronal planes defines the extent of the fracture unilaterally and bilaterally, and documents any associated fractures, such as zygomatic, frontal, cranial, or Le Fort. In the author's series, 36 per cent of nasoethmoido-orbital fractures were unilateral (Fig. 27–280). These are usually associated with zygomatic or supraorbital fractures, or may involve circumferential fractures around one orbit. Occasionally, a point blow may fracture only the frontal process of the maxilla on one side. A high Le Fort (II or III) fracture often contains a unilateral nasoethmoido-orbital component.

Bilateral fractures of the nasoethmoido-orbital region are either isolated to the central midface area or extended to other areas. The bilateral injury may accompany a Le Fort II and frontal bone fracture, and as such represents a craniofacial injury. Often, the bilateral "extended" nasoethmoido-orbital

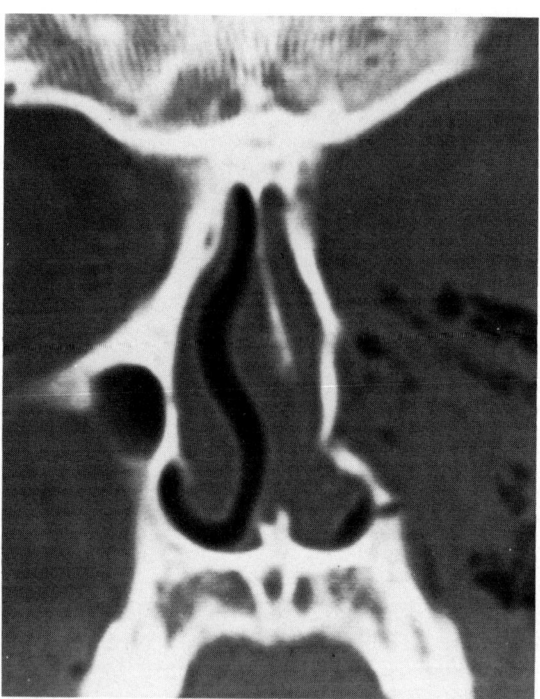

Figure 27–280. Coronal computed tomogram of a unilateral "greensticked" nasoethmoido-orbital fracture. The frontal process of the maxilla is greensticked at the junction of the frontal bone.

fracture is a part of a craniofacial injury consisting of a Le Fort IV level fracture on one side (frontal bone involvement) and a Le Fort III level fracture on the other (less involved) side. In its simplest form, the nasoethmoido-orbital fracture must involve one medial orbital rim; the base of the frontal sinus and the nasofrontal ducts are in close proximity. With extension of fractures into the frontocranial area, the anterior and posterior walls of the frontal sinus become involved in the fracture.

The fracture lines must separate the lower two-thirds of the medial orbital rim from the adjacent bones. This produces a bone segment to which the canthal ligament is attached, and which can displace, depending on periosteal continuity. In some cases, fracture lines may be observed on a radiograph; however, there is sufficient periosteal continuity to prevent displacement. No surgery is required. As the zygomatic fracture demonstrates "greensticking" at the zygomaticofrontal suture, a nasoethmoido-orbital fracture may reveal "greensticking" at the junction of the frontal process of the maxilla with the frontal bone. Characteristically, the first fractures occur through the piriform aperture and the medial orbital rim, with the frontal bone–frontal process of the maxilla displacing last.

The diagnosis of a nasoethmoido-orbital fracture on radiographs requires at a minimum four fractures that isolate the frontal process of the maxilla from adjacent bones. These include: (1) fractures of the nose, (2) fractures of the junction of the frontal process of the maxilla with the frontal bone, (3) fractures of the medial orbit (ethmoidal area), and (4) fractures of the infraorbital rim extending to the piriform aperture. These fracture lines define this bone segment as "free," and, depending on periosteal integrity, the medial orbital rim can displace.

Fractures can be seen extending into adjacent areas, as described above.

Treatment. Brain trauma should always be suspected in these injuries (Becker and associates, 1977). Brain is occasionally observed in the nose despite fractures being not easily visible on radiographic examination. This finding signifies a large discontinuity in the anterior cranial base, which requires neurosurgical repair. Neurosurgical intervention is required in patients who have depressed or open frontal skull fractures. The isolated nasoethmoido-orbital fracture may demonstrate fractures adjacent to the cribriform plate, and a CSF leak may persist for several days. The presence of such a CSF leak must be assumed in *any* patient with a nasoethmoido-orbital fracture. It has been the author's experience that, in the absence of frontal bone or frontal sinus involvement, cranial fossa fractures are minimally displaced and do not require a separate procedure to close the dural fistula. Few patients with simple linear basilar fractures accompanying isolated nasoethmoidal fractures required neurosurgical intervention. The need for such intervention should thus depend on the presence of depressed fractures involving the frontal bone, orbital roofs, or frontal sinus. The presence of pneumocephalus implies a communication from the nasal cavity or sinuses to the subarachnoid space, and these patients should receive careful evaluation for possible neurosurgical exploration. Careful neurologic examination is based on the level of consciousness, motor response, and eye movements. Any patient with a possibility of brain injury requiring observation may receive immediate surgical treatment by monitoring of the intracranial pressure with a Richman screw. In practice,

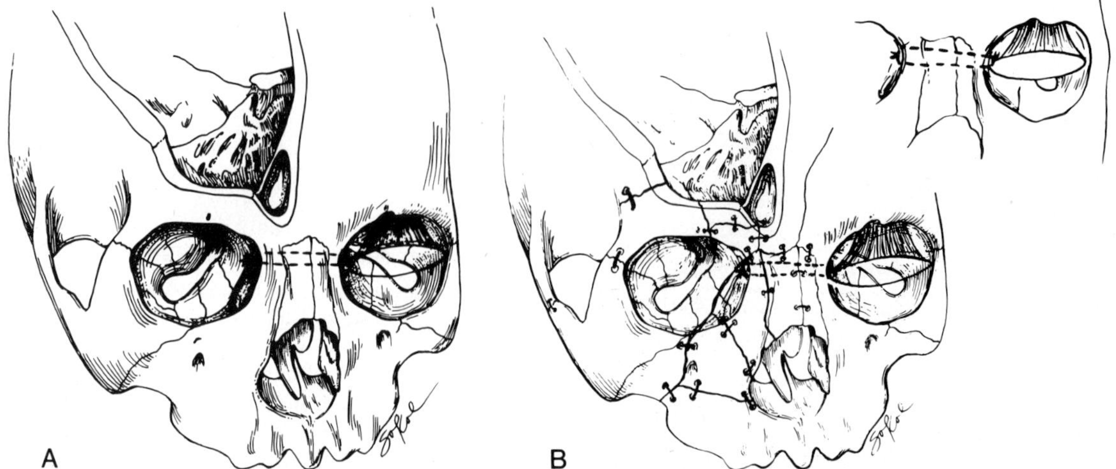

Figure 27–281. *A*, Telecanthus is prevented only by proper transnasal reduction of the medial orbital rims performed posterior and superior to the lacrimal system. Interfragment wiring must be used, however *(B)*, to link all bone fragments.

any patient receiving general anesthesia who does not have an examination and a history that excludes the possibility of brain injury should be so monitored. In this manner, it is not necessary to delay surgical treatment to clarify the neurosurgical status of the patient. This type of monitoring allows the earliest repair to be achieved with safety.

The technique of the treatment of nasoethmoido-orbital fractures consists of a thorough exposure of the nasoorbital region by means of a coronal or local incision. In some cases (the author's series), a laceration may be present over the forehead or nose. Such a laceration, although common, may not provide sufficient exposure. The ipsilateral inferior orbital rim and floor must also be exposed in unilateral nasoethmoido-orbital fractures, and the bilateral lower orbital rims in bilateral orbital fractures. There is *no* place for closed treatment in nasoethmoido-orbital fractures by external or intranasal manipulation. The surgical treatment of nasoethmoido-orbital fractures consists of (1) a thorough exposure of all fracture sites, (2) a transnasal wire reduction of the medial orbital rim (Fig. 27–281), and (3) the linking of all bone fragments to adjacent bones with interosseous wiring (Fig. 27–282). The most essential feature of the reduction is the transnasal reduction of the medial orbital rims (see Fig. 27–281). This can be performed without detaching the canthal ligament by mobilizing the bone anteriorly and laterally.

Surgical Approaches

USE OF A LACERATION. In many nasoethmoido-orbital fractures, a laceration is present (Fig. 27–283). In isolated injuries, this laceration might be appropriate for the reduction. If the fractures extend into the frontal sinus or frontal bone area, a coronal incision is usually required.

OPEN-SKY OR VERTICAL NASAL MIDLINE INCISION. Converse and Hogan (1970) described the "open-sky" technique. In compound nasoethmoido-orbital fractures, the external wound permits direct inspection of the area and the comminuted fragments can be realigned under direct vision (Figs. 27–284 to

Text continued on page 1097

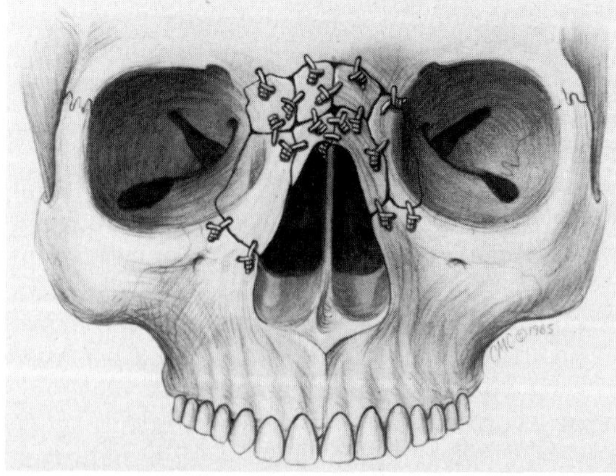

Figure 27–282. The bone fragments must be linked by interfragment wires from stable bone proceeding to stable bone inferiorly. The transnasal wire (see Fig. 27–281) reducing the orbital rims has been omitted for clarity. In practice, *it* is the most important step in nasoethmoido-orbital fracture reduction. The inferior fracture reduction is performed through a gingivobuccal sulcus incision.

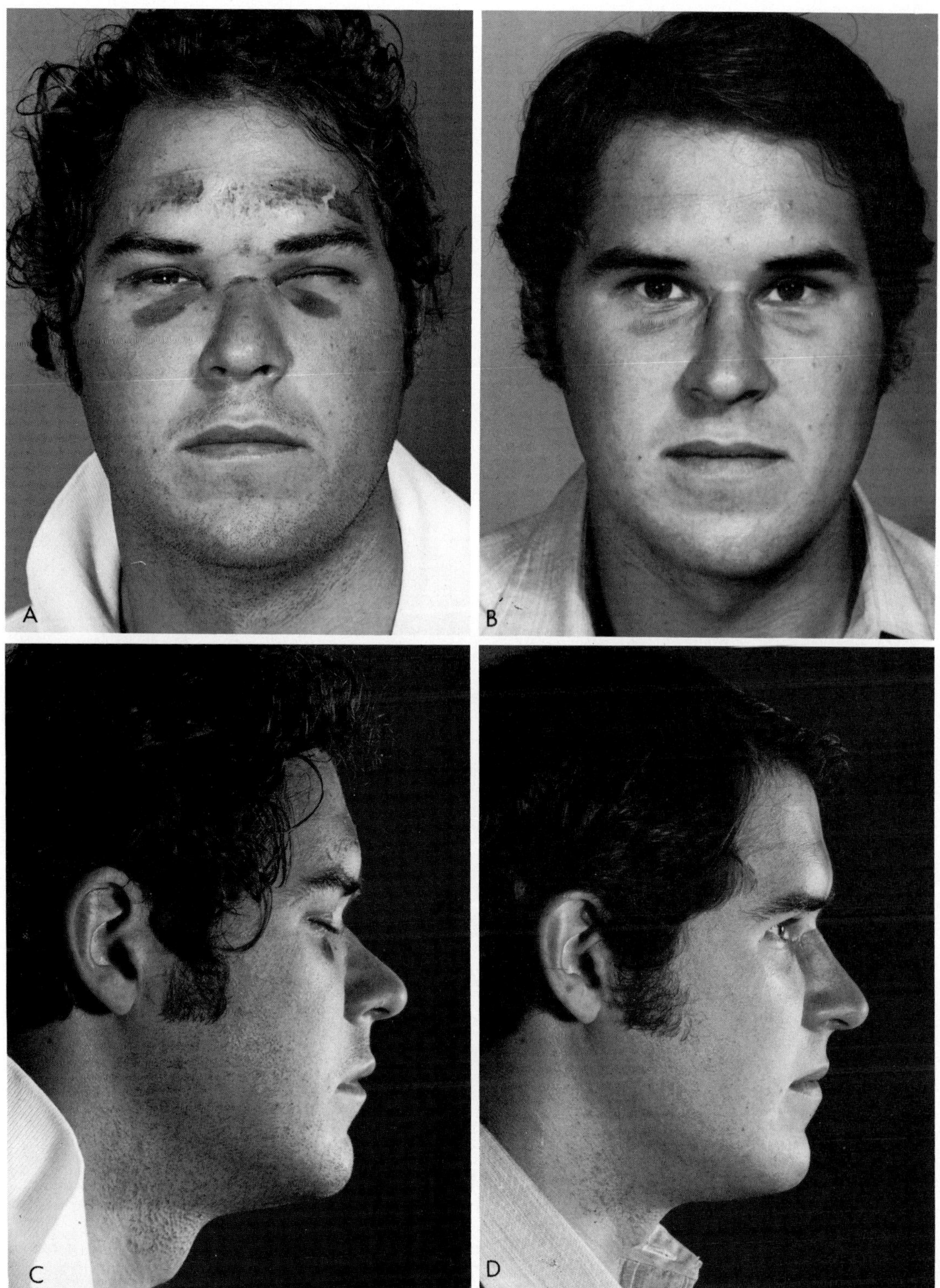

Figure 27–283. Primary bone grafting following treatment of nasoethmoido-orbital fracture and comminuted blow-out fractures of the orbital floor. *A, C,* Appearance of the patient nine days after trauma. The patient, an automobile racing driver, was involved in a crash. The helmet descended over his face, and the rim of the helmet struck the dorsum of his nose. This caused the fracture with backward recession of the bones of the nasal framework into the interorbital space with the splaying apart of the medial orbital walls, telecanthus *(A)*, depression of the root of the nose *(C)*, and bilateral orbital floor blow-out fractures. *B, D,* Appearance four months postoperatively. A "trap-door" flap was raised at the laceration site and the comminuted fragments were reassembled and wired. The orbital fractures were treated by disentrapment of the orbital fragments and placing of a Teflon implant over the blow-out defects. A primary bone graft restored the nasal contour.

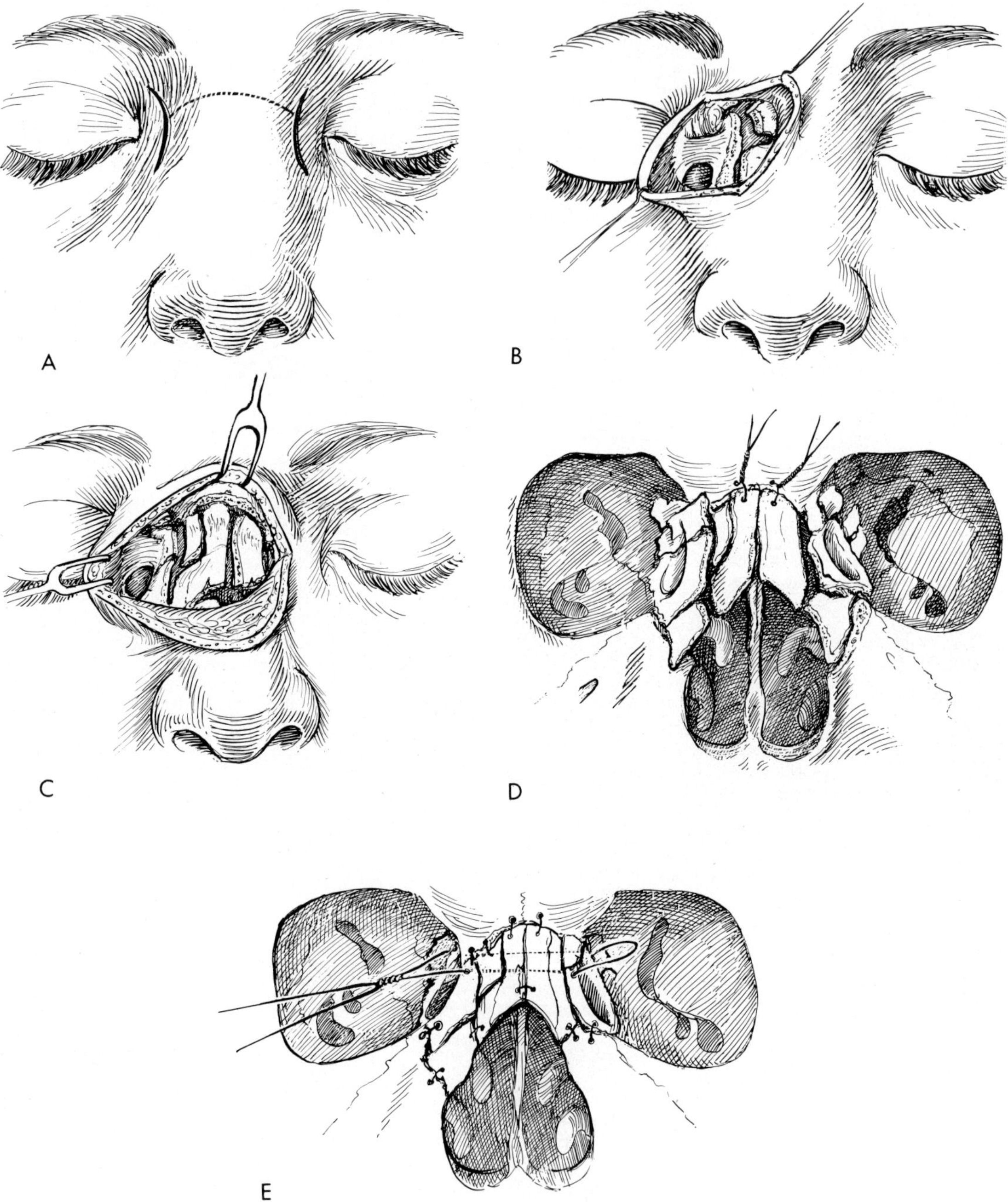

Figure 27–284. Open-sky technique in the treatment of nasoethmoido-orbital fractures. *A*, In practice, the lateral nasal incisions are seldom necessary. The transverse component is the most important. *B*, Exposure obtained through the external incision. *C*, Comminuted fragments, the lacrimal sac, and the medial canthal tendon are examined. *D*, Interosseous wiring of the main fragments of the nasal bones is established, providing initial stability. *E*, Other fragments have been joined by interosseous wiring, and a through-and-through transnasal wire maintains the anatomic position of the medial orbital walls. This is the most important feature of a nasoethmoido-orbital fracture repair. (After Converse, J. M., and Hogan, V. M: Open-sky approach for reduction of naso-orbital fractures. Case report. Plast. Reconstr. Surg., *46*:396, 1970.)

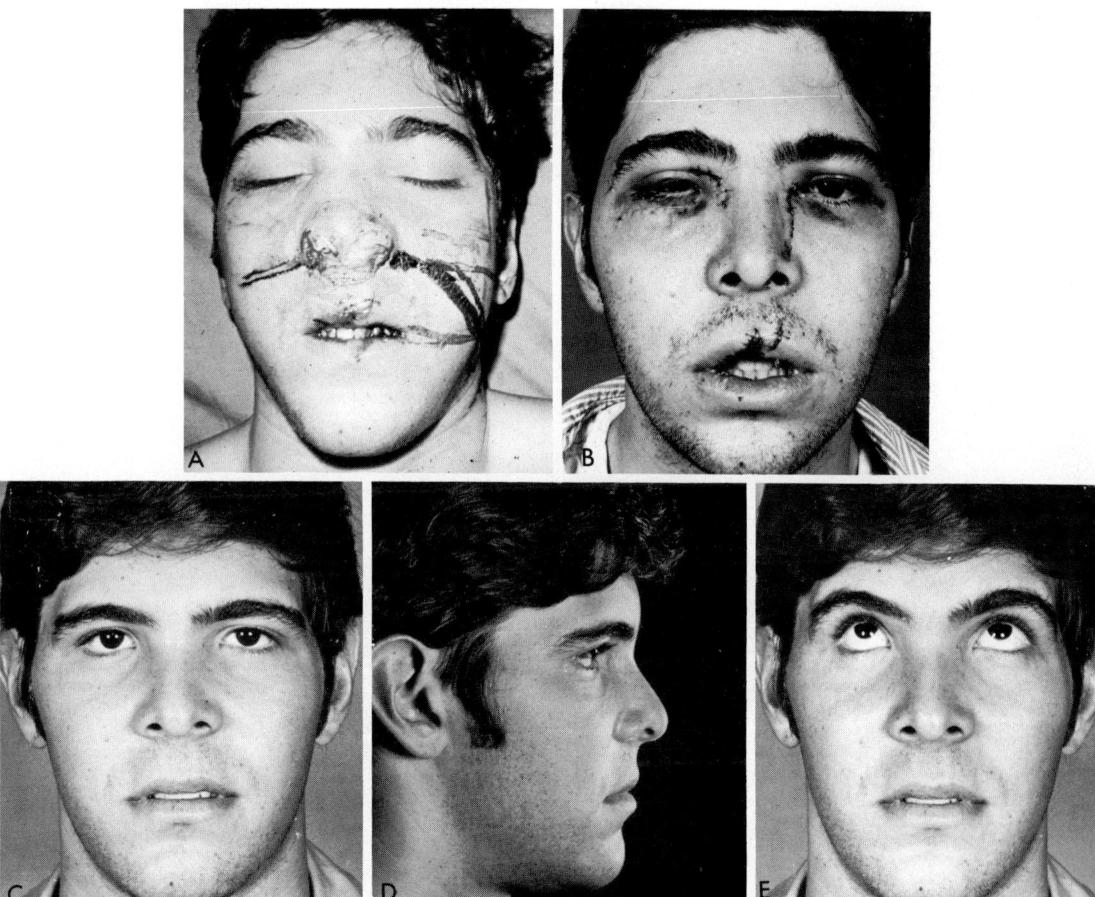

Figure 27–285. Open-sky technique in the treatment of nasoethmoido-orbital fractures. *A*, Facial injury resulting from projection of the face on the steering column of an automobile. The patient is suffering a nasoethmoido-orbital fracture, a blow-out fracture of the right orbital floor, and a Le Fort II fracture of the maxilla. *B*, 48 hours after treatment. The comminuted fragments of the fracture were reduced, realigned, and maintained in fixation by direct interosseous wiring through skin incisions. Through a lower eyelid incision, the contents entrapped in the blow-out fracture were released, and an inorganic implant restored the orbital floor continuity. *C, D*, Appearance after one month. *E*, Oculorotatory movements of the right eye have been reestablished; the fractured maxilla was reduced by intermaxillary fixation. (*A* to *D* from Converse, J. M., and Hogan, V. M.: Open-sky approach for reduction of naso-orbital fractures. Case report. Plast. Reconstr. Surg., *46*:396, 1970.)

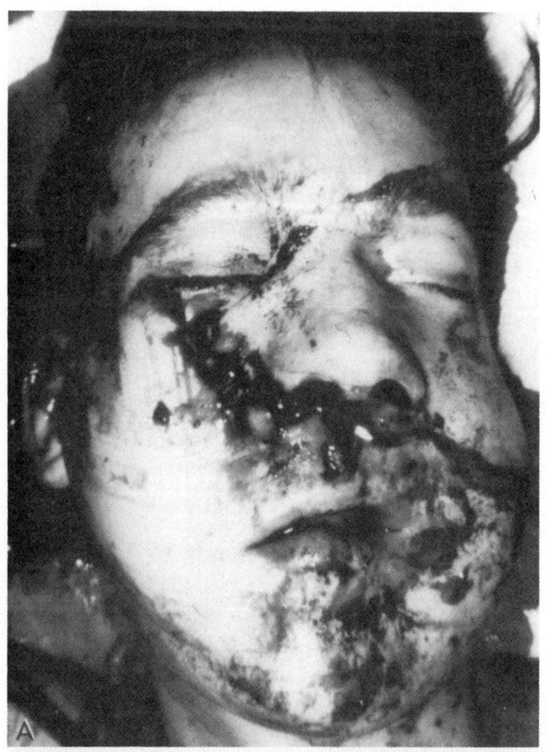

Figure 27–286. *A*, Appearance of a patient after an automobile accident with nasoethmoido-orbital and midfacial fractures (Le Fort I and II). The left ocular globe has been penetrated by a piece of glass and it required enucleation. The traumatic telecanthus was corrected by the open-sky method. There was considerable loss of nasoskeletal structures due to the severe comminution. A primary bone graft was performed. B, C, Appearance of the patient after completion of the repair. She was provided with a prosthetic ocular globe. (From Converse, J. M., and Bonanno, P. C.: *In* Kazanjian and Converse.)

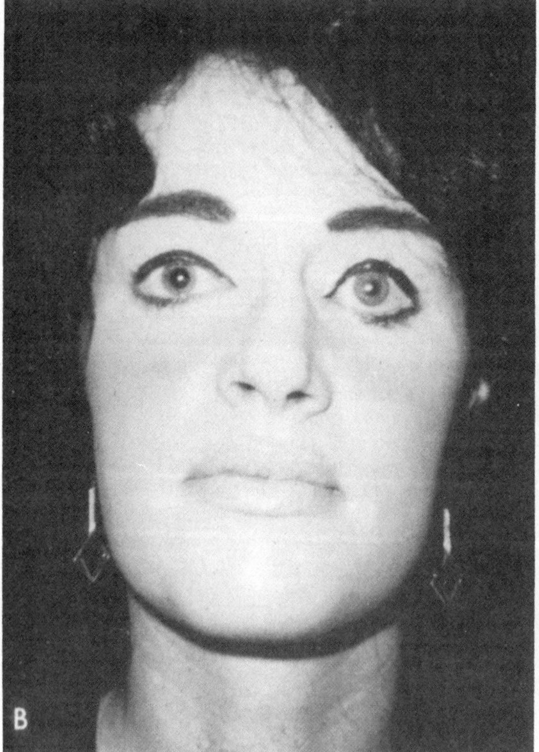

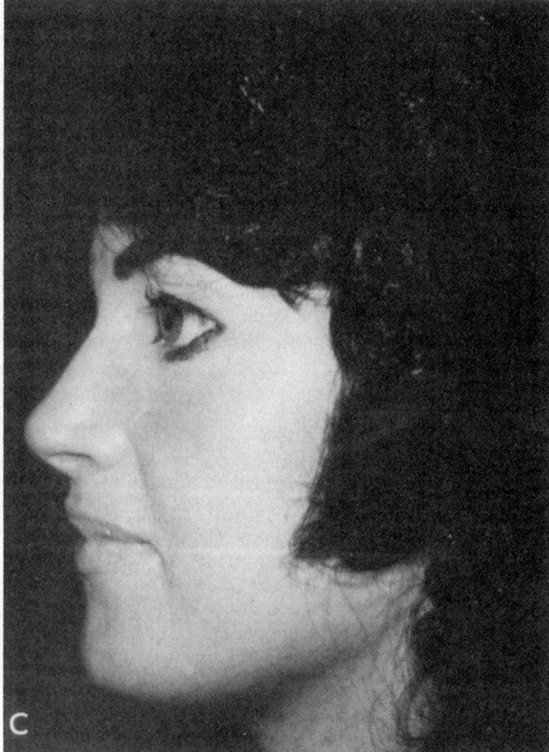

27–286). In severely comminuted nasoethmoido-orbital fractures that are not compound, an open reduction is indicated. The open-sky technique utilizes bilateral vertical incisions through the skin over the lateral wall of the nose, accompanied by a horizontal connecting limb across the junction of the nose with the forehead. In most cases, the horizontal portion of the incision extending from canthus to canthus is all that is necessary. In closing these incisions, it is essential that the subcutaneous tissue be properly aligned to avoid the tendency to form a depressed scar. The minimal dissection that must be accomplished includes the anterior portion of the frontal process of the maxilla. The medial canthal tendon should be identified and its attachments preserved. The lacrimal sac and nasolacrimal duct are not detached from bone. Subperiosteal exposure should include the inferior rim of the orbit, the orbital floor, and the medial orbit by dissecting behind the bone fragments. The medial orbital rim or bone fragments can be dislocated to allow satisfactory visualization. In some cases, an instrument placed intranasally is useful to elevate the fracture fragments into position (Fig. 27–287). The lacrimal system generally is not transected unless lacerations involve the skin adjacent to the canthus. Rarely, the canthus is detached from bone, but a detached canthus is usually the product of dissection and the canthus is generally attached to a sizable bone fragment. It is the author's impression that the esthetic results are improved if the canthal ligament is not detached from bone in the dissection. Repair of a severed lacrimal apparatus (Callahan, 1979), although seldom required, may be done under direct vision after the initial interfragment wires are placed and before their tightening. The fragments of the nasal bones and the frontal process of the maxilla should be joined to each other as well as to remaining fragments of the frontal bone (Fig. 27–287). In this manner, the proper anatomic alignment of the bone skeleton is ensured. Such alignment facilitates restoration of the anterior cranial fossa, which in turn promotes closure of the cerebrospinal fluid fistula. The principle of the open treatment in nasoethmoido-orbital fractures involves the preservation of all fragments of bone even when they are detached from soft tissues. Primary bone grafting, however, is usually necessary to restore the height or preserve the contour of the nose. Additionally, the medial wall of the orbit and the lower orbit generally must be reconstructed with bone grafts to achieve the integrity required to prevent enophthalmos.

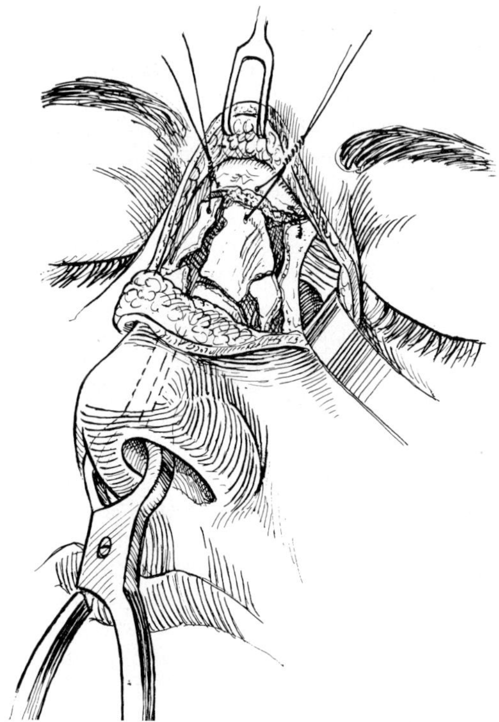

Figure 27–287. Elevation of retroposed comminuted fragments in a nasoethmoido-orbital fracture by means of an Asch forceps. The position of the fragments is maintained by wiring all fragments to one another with the addition of a transnasal reduction of the medial orbital rims.

Primary bone grafting is essential to restore the orbital and nasal bone continuity and contour. When the cartilaginous septum is destroyed and does not provide support, this area should be strengthened by a cantilever bone graft attached to the proximal portion of the nasal bones (Fig. 27–288). In some cases, a cartilage graft may be placed in the columella for columellar support as well. In severely telescoped nasoethmoido-orbital fractures, the cartilaginous support of the columella is destroyed. Bone grafting is esential to restore the shape and size of the orbit. Usually the fractures begin in the medial portion of the orbital roof and extend lateral to the infraorbital nerve on each side. A properly curved bone graft can be used to replace missing floor segments or strengthen comminuted fragments.

VERTICAL MIDLINE NASAL INCISION. The vertical midline nasal incision is also used to expose the nasoethmoido-orbital region.

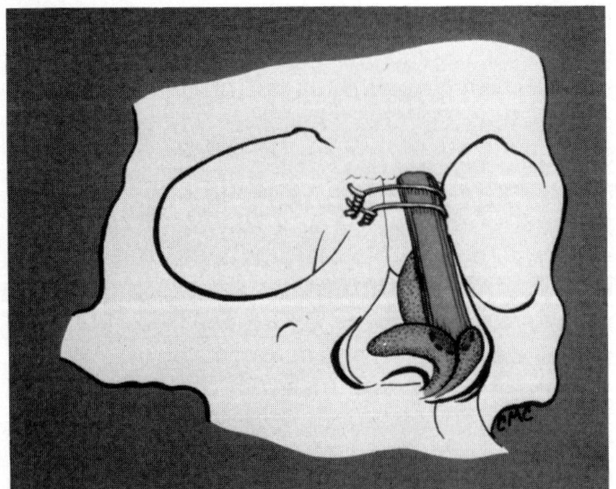

Figure 27–288. A doral nasal bone graft may also be wired or screwed to the nasal bone fragments. The dorsal nasal bone graft increases nasal height and produces a smooth dorsum.

Healing usually occurs as a fine line scar. Separate canthal incisions are not required. This incision is appropriate in older or bald patients with glabellar rhytids for the treatment of localized fractures confined to the nasoethmoido-orbital area. The incision should not extend beyond the finely textured skin on the proximal portion of the nose; the skin of the distal two-thirds responds poorly to elective incisions.

CORONAL INCISION. A coronal incision is the most appropriate one to expose the nasoethmoido-orbital region, especially in young patients who have no suitable lacerations. The incision provides unexcelled exposure of the frontal, temporal, zygomatic, and orbital regions.

In order to expose the medial orbital rims, the periosteal attachments of the orbital soft tissue should be freed from the roof of the orbit and the entire frontal process of the maxilla with subperiosteal dissection. This maneuver allows exposure of the nose and the nasal and medial orbital rim areas. The medial orbital rims are dislocated laterally and anteriorly to facilitate drilling and wire passing. The nasal bone fragments are dislocated or temporarily removed to allow better exposure of the medial orbital rim segments. The medial orbital rims are linked to adjacent bone fragments with wiring, and the essential step, which is the performance of a transnasal reduction of the medial orbital rims posterior and superior to the canthal tendon and lacrimal fossa, creates the proper intercanthal dimensions. Plate and screw fixation may be employed after the initial wiring (Fig. 27–289). It should be emphasized that the transnasal reduction should be posterior and superior to the lacrimal fossa in order to provide the proper direction of force to recreate the preinjury bony architecture of the region (Figs. 27–290, 27–291). The transnasal reduction is not a "transnasal canthopexy," as it does not involve the canthal ligament. If the canthal ligament requires reattachment (the canthal tendon is rarely stripped from a sizable bone fragment), the canthal tendon is grasped with one or two passes of a 2-0 nonabsorbable suture adjacent to the medial commissure of the eyelid through a separate 3 mm incision (Fig. 27–292). Probes can be used to avoid the lacrimal system, or the system may be intubated if repair is required. This is passed through and connected to the transnasal reduction of the medial orbital rims.

The medial canthal tendon (see also Chap. 34) is a somewhat triangular band attached to the frontal process of the maxilla from the anterior lacrimal crest to the nasal bone (Robinson and Stranc, 1970; Anderson, 1977; Zide and McCarthy, 1983; Manson and associates, 1986a). It has a distinct lower free border and superiorly becomes continuous with the periosteum. The posterior portion of the medial canthal tendon functions as the cover for the lacrimal sac, and posteriorly becomes continuous with the lacrimal fascia. The commissure of the eyelids is only several millimeters from the canthal apex. Branches of the canthal tendon divide to extend through the upper and lower eyelids and to attach to the medial margin of the tarsal plate. There is a complicated relationship of the parts of the orbicularis muscle, the lacrimal sac, the divisions of the canthal tendon, and the attachment to the bone. Both Anderson (1977) and Zide and McCarthy (1983) stressed the importance of a vertical component of the medial canthal tendon. Surgeons have for some time appreciated that the force direction of the posterior and superior limbs of the medial canthal tendon is important in procedures that reposition the canthal apparatus. The medial canthal tendon exerts a force that keeps the eyelids tangent to the globe. Thus, redirecting the canthal tendon posteriorly acts to maintain the position of the rest of the medial canthus after either accidental or surgical disinsertion of the tendon. Both Anderson (1977) and Zide and

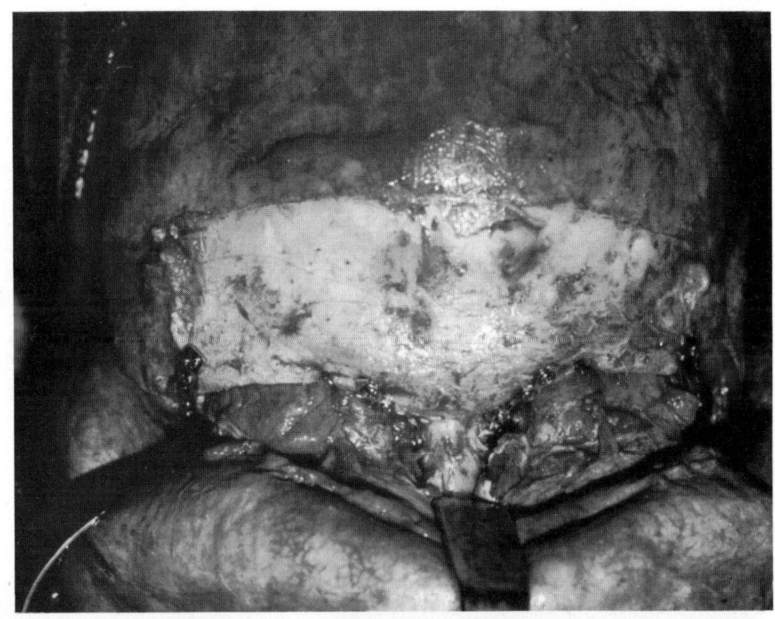

Figure 27–289. Reduction of a nasoethmoido-orbital fracture with plates and screws. The initial position was achieved by interfragment wires, including a transnasal reduction wire for the medial orbital rims. The nasoethmoidal area was reduced first and the zygomatic fractures were then plated. Note the retracted scalp (coronal) flap.

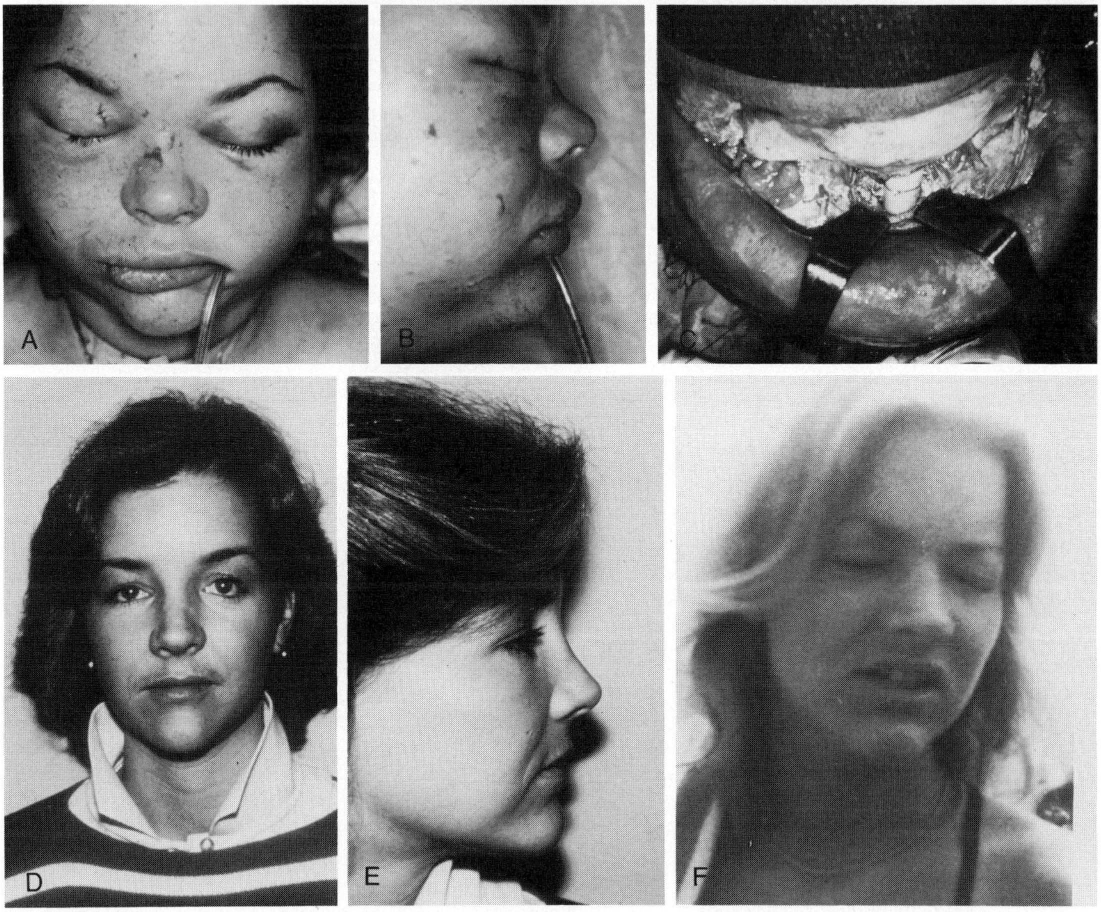

Figure 27–290. Bilateral nasoethmoido-orbital fracture *(A, B)* with a Le Fort and mandibular fracture. Open reduction was performed with coronal, bilateral subciliary, and gingivobuccal sulcus incisions. A dorsal bone graft is seen through the coronal incision *(C)*. *D*, *E*, Postoperative views demonstrating the result obtaned by a single procedure. It compares favorably with the preinjury photograph *(F)*.

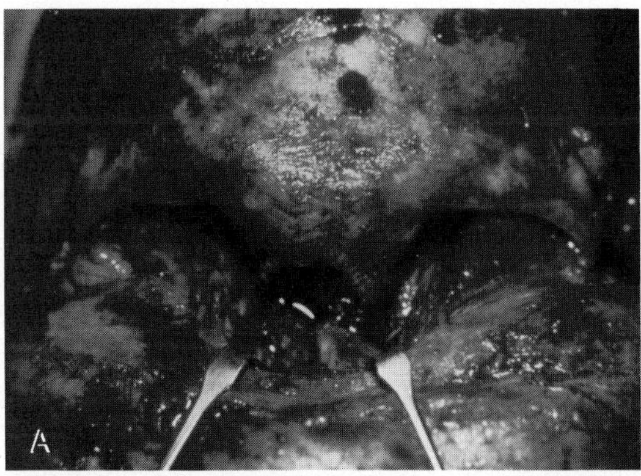

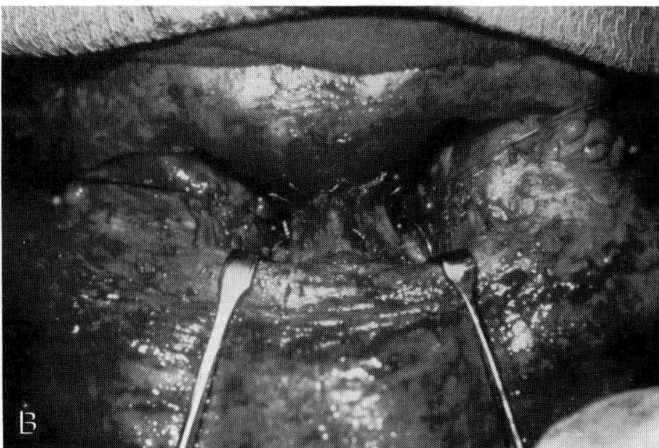

Figure 27–291. *A*, Coronal incision demonstrating the exposure of a bilateral nasoethmoido-orbital fracture. *B*, Following reconstruction by interfragment wiring of the central midface.

McCarthy (1983) felt that the strong superior branch that travels along the orbital rim to the frontonasal suture acts to maintain vertical canthal position in these cases. The posterior branch is actually weak and is not capable of much structural integrity.

Following disinsertion of the canthal apparatus, one must create, by canthal reattachment, a vector of force components that resuspends the entire complex and provides the optimal architecture and position. Converse (1976) empirically determined that the optimal position for surgical repositioning was posterior and superior to its normal insertion. Most anatomic texts overemphasize the anterior limb of the medial canthal tendon and its attachment onto the frontal process of the maxilla and anterior lacrimal crest, thus distorting the true nature of the entire canthal apparatus. The author's preferred surgical technique for reattachment involves placing a suture through the canthal ligament immediately adjacent to the eyelid commissure; this is similar to the technique described by Zide and McCarthy (1983) (Fig. 27–293). This is best accomplished with a 3 mm horizontal incision immediately adjacent to the medial commissure of the eyelid (see Fig. 27–292). The lacrimal system may be avoided by the insertion of fine probes. A braided suture is passed at least twice in the tendon and passed through to the inside of the coronal exposure (Fig. 27–294) medial to the orbital soft tissue where a complete subperiosteal dissection has been performed (Fig. 27–294). In most cases, it is necessary to

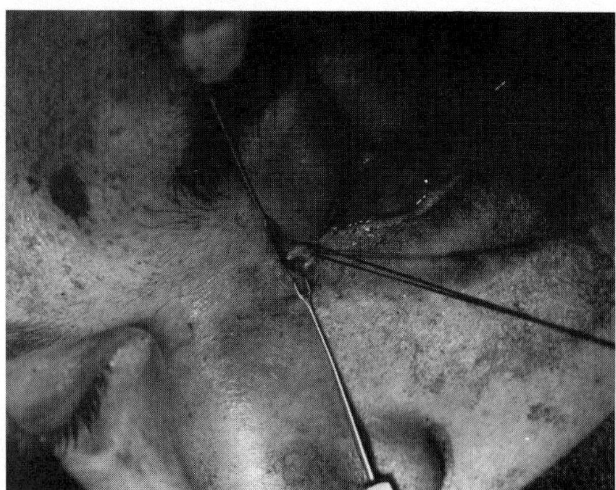

Figure 27–292. If canthal reattachment is required, a separate incision is made horizontally, 3 mm in length, at the medial canthus of the eyelids. The lacrimal system may be protected by fine probes. A suture is passed twice through the tendon and connected to the transnasal reduction wire.

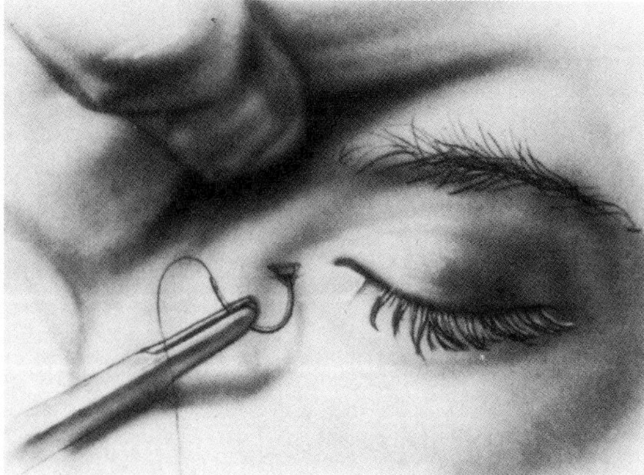

Figure 27–293. Through a small horizontal incision, a suture is passed at least twice through the portion of the tendon immediately adjacent to the eyelid commissure. The lacrimal system may be avoided with fine probes if desired. (From Zide, B. M., and McCarthy, J. G.: The medial canthus revisited—an anatomic basis for canthopexy. Ann. Plast. Surg., *11*:1, 1983.)

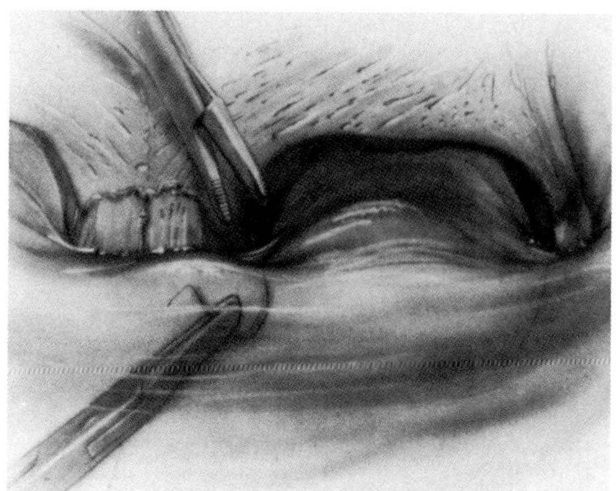

Figure 27–294. The passing needle is grasped behind the scalp (coronal) flap. The transcutaneous suture (see Fig. 27–293) aids in identification of the suture. (From Zide, B. M., and McCarthy, J. G.: The medial canthus revisited—an anatomical basis for canthopexy. Ann. Plast. Surg., *11*:1, 1983.)

mobilize most of the soft tissue contents of the orbit merely to allow an *unstressed* repositioning of the canthal ligament. Cutaneous incisions, such as Z-plasties, W-plasties, and other repositioning flaps, are *seldom* necessary when proper mobilization of all the orbital soft tissue has been performed. Indeed, the thickness of the soft tissue adjacent to the medial portion of the nose and orbit may have to be thinned to recreate the normal skin thickness. Skeletonizing the skin by excision of excess scar tissue increases the mobility of the dissected canthus. In some post-traumatic cases, the thickness is impressive and represents a proliferation of scar tissue after hemorrhage and edema. The braided suture in the canthus is attached to a transnasal wire positioned *posterior* and *superior* to the edge of the lacrimal groove (Fig. 27–295). The wire can be pulled tight to check the alignment, released, and then tightened finally at the close of the procedure.

Complications of Orbital and Nasoethmoido-orbital Fractures

The early diagnosis and adequate treatment of nasoethmoido-orbital fractures produce optimal esthetic results with the least number of late complications. Depending on the quality of the initial treatment and the result of healing, further reconstructive surgery may be required in some cases. Late complications, such as frontal sinus obstruction, occur in some situations. Converse and associates (1966, 1975, 1976) and Kazanjian and Converse (1974) discussed in detail the

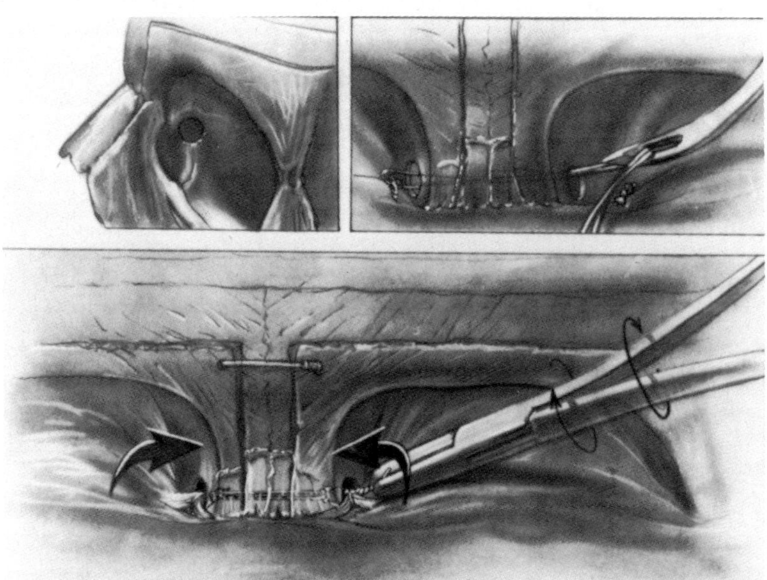

Figure 27–295. *Left top*, Preferred site (circle) of bone fenestration. *Right top*, The wire is passed through the space left in the knot of the braided wire. The free ends are passed transnasally after one free end is passed through the contralateral knot. The wire is tightened. *Bottom*, Assistance facilitates this key manuever to ensure seating of the tendons into the bone fenestrations. Overgrafting the medial wall of the orbit anteriorly widens the intercanthal distance. Posterior to the canthus is the area where most bone grafting is required. (From Zide, B. M., and McCarthy, J. G.: The medial canthus revisited—an anatomical basis for canthopexy. Ann. Plast. Surg., *11*:1, 1983.)

treatment of the sequelae of nasoethmoido-orbital fractures.

Deformities and *functional impairment* are late complications that can be reduced by early diagnosis and treatment. A nasoethmoido-orbital fracture may be obscured by swelling or other facial injuries, or may escape detection. An unconscious patient cannot volunteer information about diplopia or cooperate for examinations. The diagnosis of a nasoethmoido-orbital fracture should be suspected and confirmed by a bimanual examination in questionable cases. After several weeks, deformity and enophthalmos are more evident. At this time, fibrous cicatrization is established, and the reconstruction of the orbital cavity and restoration of symmetric ocular function and proper soft tissue position in the fracture must be undertaken in the presence of scarred skin and soft tissue strictures. Soft tissue when injured assumes the configuration of the underlying unreduced bone fragments. The soft tissue tends inexorably to return to this position despite the late reconstruction of the bone in a more acceptable anatomic position. A scheme of late or delayed fracture reconstruction is illustrated in Figure 27–296 (see Chap. 33).

Dead space between the *inorganic implant* and the bone of the orbital floor should be avoided, since accumulated fluid in the dead space constitutes a favorable medium for the growth of bacteria. In many cases the orbital floor is opened to the maxillary sinus, providing a mechanism for drainage. Orbital infection and suppuration are indications for incision, drainage, and removal of any foreign material. The orbital floor can be reconstructed later after resolution of the infection. In some cases sufficient scarring has occurred to support the orbital soft tissue in the proper anatomic position. Antibiotic therapy should be routinely employed in all patients to avoid this complication.

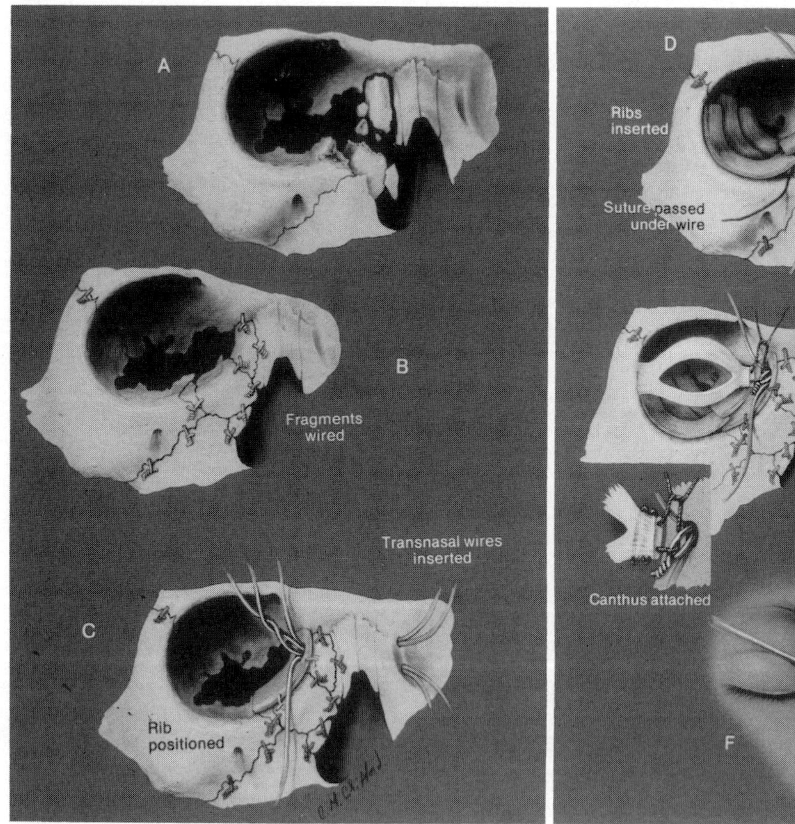

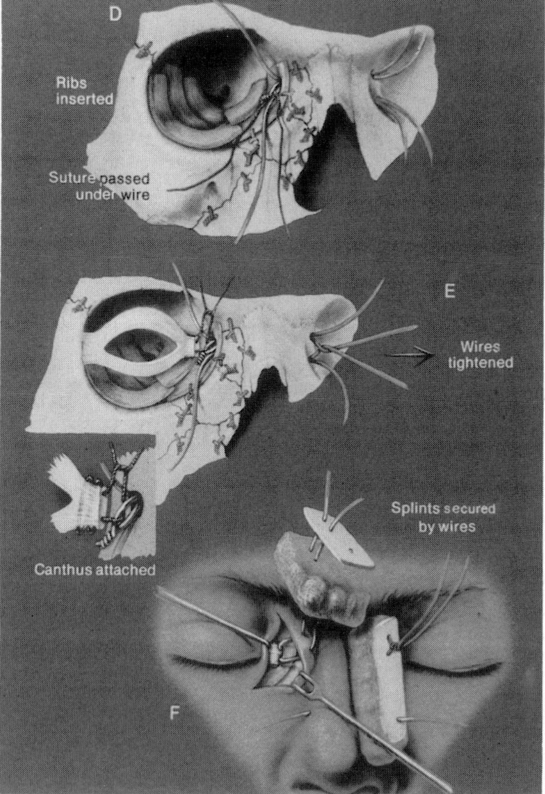

Figure 27–296. Delayed fracture reconstruction. *A*, Missing bone after a nasoethmoido-orbital fracture. *B*, The fragments are repositioned with interfragment wiring. *C*, A transnasal canthopexy is performed. *D*, Rib grafts are inserted to restore the size of the orbit to the correct dimensions. *E*, The transnasal canthopexy wires are tightened, uniting the canthus to the transnasal reduction wire with a separate suture. *F*, Splints, well padded, assist in approximating the canthus to the reconstructed medial orbital rim.

In the typical blow-out fracture caused by a fist punch, a 1 mm Teflon implant or a 0.6 to 0.8 mm Supramid implant is adequate to restore the continuity of the orbital floor. Excessive thickness of the implant may cause the globe to be elevated or proptotic. In the early postoperative period, proptosis and elevation of the globe are *expected.* As the swelling subsides, the globe should assume a more anatomic position. If the globe remains displaced by the implant, the latter should be removed and replaced by one either thinner or more properly conformed to the desired orbital shape. Improperly designed implants can place excessive pressure on the optic nerve posteriorly.

In severe trauma, *retrobulbar hematoma* may displace the ocular globe. The globe displacement may be superior or inferior. Drainage of the hematoma usually occurs at the time of orbital exploration, otherwise spontaneous resorption occurs. In rare cases decompression is required.

An implant of excessive anteroposterior dimensions may compress the structures of the superior orbital tissue, infraorbital nerve, or optic nerve. Symptoms will result. The implant must be designed to avoid such excesses of pressure. Extrusion of the implant anteriorly may occur with forward migration if the implant is not secured to the orbital rim or orbital floor. The technique most often used by the author is a simple horizontal mattress wire to the rim. Converse advocated the technique described in Figure 27–261. The author recommends a curved bone graft as the most satisfactory substitute for the orbital floor (see Fig. 27–296*D*). Rib grafts are easy to structure to the exact curvature of the desired orbital segment requiring replacement. The grafts are well tolerated by the patient and sufficiently strong to support the orbital contents, and yet malleable enough to bend properly. More brittle types of bone, such as calvarium and iliac crest, are more difficult to contour to the posterior dimensions of the orbit.

While autogenous bone is well tolerated by the patient and is the most physiologic substitute, it is not immune to resorption or infection and it requires the use of a donor site. Teflon, Silastic, Supramid, and Cranioplast implants have been described for orbital reconstruction and provide suitable inorganic implant materials. A newer material, polyethylene (Medpor), can be contoured and it assumes the desired curvature, much as a rib graft. Any of these materials can be bent, shaped, shaved, or carved and fitted to the orbital floor without preliminary preparation or much delay. They are entirely satisfactory in simple, isolated orbital floor blow-out fractures.

Despite early treatment of orbital fractures, *ocular muscle imbalance and enophthalmos* may occur (Barclay, 1958, 1960; Bartkowski and Krzystkowa, 1982; Smith and associates, 1984). Many adequately treated orbital floor fractures do not recover complete extraocular muscle function; however, they usually cause no double vision in functional fields of gaze. Double vision present only at the extremities of gaze is not a functionally limiting problem and does not generally require surgery. Double vision is most limiting when it occurs inferiorly and the patient cannot properly observe walking or reading; this type is more incapacitating than double vision occurring superiorly. Extraocular surgery on the affected eye or on the contralateral unaffected eye is necessary in some patients to restore eye muscle balance. Prisms can also be employed.

Complicated blow-out fractures are often accompanied by multiple fractures of the facial bones and injuries of the soft tissues. Many of these fractures with complications fall into this category. Patients show some residual impairment of ocular rotatory action and diplopia, and sometimes demonstrate globe positional change, enophthalmos, and depression of the zygomatic prominence despite the best efforts at primary reconstruction (Rény and Stricker, 1969; Tajima and associates, 1974). Enophthalmos correction may be required (Collin, 1982; Pearl, 1987). The treatment of enophthalmos is discussed in Chapter 33. Ptosis of the upper eyelid, downward displacement of the orbital contents, medial canthal deformities, shortening of the horizontal dimension of the palpebral fissure, reduction of the vertical dimension of the lower eyelid, saddle deformities, or widening of the nasal bony bridge may also occur. Depression or lowering of the supraorbital arch is also present. In these complicated orbital fractures, surgical reconstruction is required months after the initial injury.

Ocular injury following orbital fracture has been reported as varying between 14 per cent (Milauskas and Fueger, 1966), 17 per cent (Miller and Tenzel, 1967), and 29 per cent

(Jabaley, Lerman, and Sanders, 1975) in various series (Jones, 1961; Milauskas and Fueger, 1966; Converse and Hogan, 1970; Petro and associates, 1970; Fradkin, 1971; Jabaley, Lerman, and Sanders, 1975; Holt and Holt, 1983). Ocular globe injury also varies in severity from a corneal abrasion to loss of vision due to a ruptured globe, retinal detachment, vitreous hemorrhage, or a fracture involving the optic canal. Blindness or loss of an eye is remarkably infrequent despite the severity of some of the injuries sustained.

The importance of the ophthalmologic examination in all fractures of the orbit has already been discussed. Vitreous hemorrhage, dislocated lens, rupture of the sclera, traumatic cataract, choroidal rupture, retinal detachment, anterior or posterior chamber hemorrhage, rupture of the iris sphincter, glaucoma, and retinal detachment are only some of the complications that follow blunt or penetrating injury to the globe, resulting in diminution or loss of vision. Many complications may be avoided, minimized, or at least not aggravated if early treatment and protection are instituted.

It cannot be overemphasized that verification of vision is essential in the course of an ophthalmologic examination. An excellent prognostic sign is the Marcus Gunn pupillary test. A light is moved rapidly from one eye to the other alternately (Figs. 27–297, 27–298). If a conduction defect of the optic nerve is present, the pupil on the involved side appears to dilate as the light is brought from the unaffected eye to the involved eye. Preinjury monocular vision should also be considered.

Ocular globe injury varies in severity from a corneal abrasion to anterior or posterior chamber hematoma (hyphema or vitreous hematoma) and may include a detached retina or ruptured globe. The posterior third of the orbit is frequently involved by linear fractures, which usually show little displacement. Such fractures, however, may compromise the

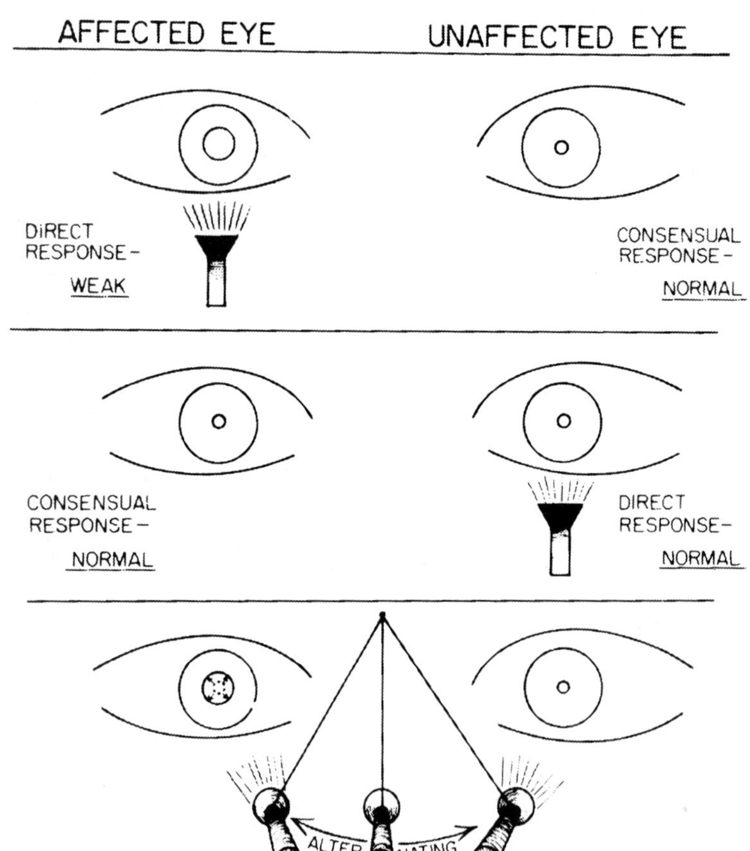

Figure 27–297. The Marcus Gunn test for pupillary response. The test should be conducted in a dark room with the patient's eyes fixed on a distant object *(above)*. Shining a light in the affected eye produces minimal or no constriction of that pupil *(center)*. Shining a light in the unaffected eye produces normal constriction of the pupils of both eyes (consensual response) *(below)*. When the light is moved from the unaffected eye to the affected eye, a paradoxical dilatation, rather than a constriction, of the affected pupil designates a positive test. (From Jabaley, M. E., Lerman, M., and Sanders, H. J.: Ocular injuries in orbital fractures: a review of 119 cases. Plast. Reconstr. Surg., *56*:410, 1975.)

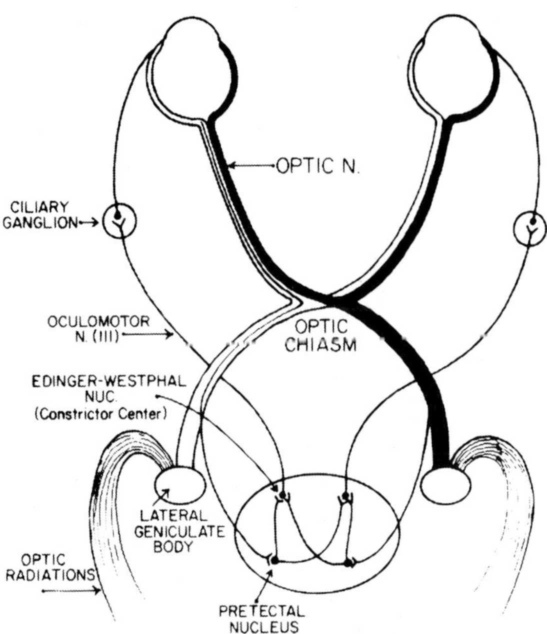

Figure 27–298. The normal pupillary reflex pathway and the relationship to the Marcus Gunn pupil. In the normal eye, light striking the retina produces an impulse in the optic nerve that travels to the pretectal nucleus, both Edinger-Westphal nuclei, via nerve III to the ciliary ganglion and the pupillary constrictor muscles. In lesions involving the retina or the optic nerve back to the chiasm, a light in the unaffected eye produces consensual constriction of the pupil of the affected eye, but a light in the affected eye produces a paradoxical dilation of the affected pupil. (From Jabaley, M. E., Lerman, M., and Sanders, H. J.: Ocular injuries in orbital fractures: a review of 119 cases. Plast. Reconstr. Surg., *56*:410, 1975.)

circulation to the intracanalicular portion of the optic nerve as it travels through the optic canal (Manfredi and associates, 1981). Blindness or loss of the eye is remarkably infrequent in view of the severity of some of the injuries sustained, a finding that attests to the great capacity of the structure of the orbital bones to absorb force without serious ocular injury.

The need for preliminary ophthalmologic examination (Barton and Berry, 1982) is often dramatically illustrated by cases that demonstrate *decreased vision* although no operation has been performed. Such a case was reported by Miller (1968). The patient with a midfacial fracture in whom vision in the left eye was 20/70 a few hours after the injury dropped to no light perception by the fifth day. No surgery had been performed. If surgery had taken place before the fifth day, the resulting blindness would probably have been attributed to the operation. Deterioration of vision is common in facial injuries several days after the initial event, even when no surgery is performed (Miller and Tenzel, 1967; Weymuller, 1984).

Blindness never resulted from repair of the orbital floor in any of the patients treated by Converse and associates (1967). The author had one patient who lost vision after a nasoethmoido-orbital repair. The patient was placed on systemic heparin on the second postoperative day for a subclavian vein thrombosis. The anticoagulation was extreme and the patient developed severe bilateral periorbital hematoma with increased pressure. Despite decompression of the orbit, vision was permanently lost in one eye. Nicholson and Guzak (1971) reported six cases in which vision was lost in a series of 72 patients who underwent orbital floor repair by means of silicone implants inserted by various surgeons in the same hospital. This extreme rate of visual loss, occurring in a reputable hospital, is unexplained, since most competent experienced specialists have not encountered visual loss after orbital fracture repair (Wilkins and Havins, 1982). A summary of the literature has demonstrated that the incidence of blindness or visual damage following orbital fracture repair should be much less than 0.1 per cent (Lederman, 1981; Wilkins and Havins, 1982). It may, however, exceed the incidence in other periorbital operations, such as blepharoplasty, for which the incidence is one in 10,000.

Interruption of the continuity of the *lacrimal apparatus* (Stranc, 1970b; Gruss and associates, 1985a), a chronic inflammatory condition of the lacrimal sac, or cystic dilatation (known as a mucocele) with epiphora requires late dacryocystorhinostomy or other surgical procedures. If transection of the canalicular lacrimal system has occurred, it should be repaired over fine tubes (see Chap. 34) (Callahan, 1979).

Hematoma is unusual. It occurs if continuous bleeding from arteries within the orbit, such as the infraorbital or anteroposterior ethmoidal arteries, is not spontaneously arrested at the time when the fractures are reduced. Partially lacerated arteries have a tendency to continue bleeding, and in some fractures involving the medial orbital wall a retrobulbar hematoma may occur. Increased orbital pressure may be produced, resulting in reflex loss of flow in the ophthalmic artery or diminution of flow because of pressure. Usually the fractures, lacerating the periorbita, have decompressed the hematoma. Blindness may be a consequence of a hematoma occurring under firm pressure dressings. Hematomas within the orbit inevitably accompany fractures, and the management of most hematomas should be conservative. The vision must be examined before and after surgery, and pressure dressings, although necessary, should be large and well padded by bulky soft material. All patients should be checked for light perception immediately after orbital surgery and twice daily for the first several days.

True *ptosis* of the upper lid should be differentiated from pseudoptosis resulting from the downward displacement of the eyeball in enophthalmos. True ptosis results from loss of action of the levator palpebrae superioris. This may occur as a result of an injury to or dehiscence of a thinned section of tendon, a transection of the levator aponeurosis, hematomas within the muscle, or damage to the superior divisions of cranial nerve III. Intramuscular hematomas may progress to fibrosis with loss of function of a portion of the muscle. In cases of levator aponeurosis transection, usually only a portion of the aponeurosis has been divided. These cases can be improved by late repair. In general, a period of six months or more is allowed to elapse to see how much function is recovered before surgery is undertaken. Appropriate procedures are employed, depending on the amount of eyelid motion. Levator adjustment should be deferred until proper globe position has been obtained and is stable.

Vertical shortening of the lower eyelid with exposure of the sclera below the limbus of the globe in the primary position (*scleral show*) may result from downward and backward displacement of the fractured inferior orbital rim. In extreme comminution of the inferior orbital rim, there is a tendency of fractured segments connected by interfragment wiring to sink downward and posteriorly. The septum and lower lid are dragged downward (see Fig. 27–244). Release of the septum orbitale attachment from the orbital rim and restoration of the position of the orbital rim by osteotomy may be required. If such operative procedures fail, the lid position may be improved by grafts involving either tarsus and conjunctiva or skin, following release (see Chap. 34). Canthal repositioning (Couly, Hureau, and Tessier, 1976; Zide and McCarthy, 1983) and lid shortening procedures improve lower lid position in some patients (see Chap. 34). These procedures generally do not elevate the lower lid more than 3 to 4 mm. Pseudoptosis and depression of the supratarsal fold often accompany vertical shortening of the lower lid. These problems must be addressed individually after proper globe and canthal position has been obtained.

Some authors believe that vertical shortening of the lower lid is more common after subciliary incisions than after midtarsal or inferior rim incisions. It should be emphasized that the subciliary incision with a skin flap not only is hazardous but has a disturbing 40 per cent incidence of complications (Manson and associates, 1987). A skin muscle flap is preferred. The condition of lower lid shortening relates both to contracture of the soft tissue and to the proper position of the inferior orbital rim. Converse (Kazanjian and Converse, 1974) adopted a lower lid incision utilizing a subtarsal division of the orbicularis to reduce such complications. Careful avoidance of injury to the orbital septum also seems to decrease the incidence of these problems.

Infraorbital nerve anesthesia is disconcerting to patients who experience it. The area of sensory loss usually extends from the lower lid over the cheek and lateral ala to the upper lip. Release of the infraorbital nerve from the pressure of the bone fragments within the canal may be indicated. Zygomatic fractures demonstrating medial displacement are especially liable to produce disturbances of sensation (Nysingh, 1960; Nordgaard, 1976; Larsen and Thomsen, 1978). It should be recalled that the anterior and middle divisions of the superior alveolar nerves pass through the anterior wall of the maxilla and are thus liable to injury in fractures that comminute this area. In any orbital floor or zygomatic fracture exploration, the inferior orbital nerve should be visualized on the anterior aspect of the maxilla as it exits from the canal, and any pressure on the nerve within the bone canal should be relieved as a routine part of the procedure. Since the infraorbital nerve is in a groove along the floor of the orbit in the middle and posterior portions of the orbit before it exits the middle portion of the inferior orbital fissure, it must be avoided in orbital dissections. After blunt injury by fracture, sensation usually improves spontaneously over a one to two year period following nerve injury. Recovery may be expected to some extent; however, complete return is often not obtained (Nysingh, 1960; Nordgaard, 1976; Larsen and Thomsen, 1978).

Cerebrospinal fluid rhinorrhea occurs as a routine finding of a nasoethmoido-orbital fracture. In experimental fractures, isolated fractures of the nasoethmoido-orbital region are invariably accompanied by a longitudinal fracture paralleling the cribriform plate. Such limited fractures may be managed conservatively: repositioning the components of the nose and orbit is all that is required. It has not been necessary to operate on patients for control of the CSF leak alone. Some authors prefer antibiotic therapy (which has been thought to protect the patient from meningitis), but its value has not been demonstrated in control or double-blind studies (Lewin, 1954; Raaf, 1957; Mincy, 1966; Brawley and Kelly, 1967; Jefferson and Reilly, 1972; Leech, 1974; Ignelzi and VanderArk, 1975; Klastersky, Sadeghi, and Brihaye, 1976; Dagi, Meyer, and Poletti, 1983).

There have been occasional reports of cases of late post-traumatic cerebrospinal fluid rhinorrhea occurring up to 15 to 20 years after remote injuries (Schneider and Thompson, 1957). These patients generally have more significant fractures extending along the anterior cranial base. In the author's experience, more significant cranial base fractures are accompanied by fractures of the frontal bone and frontal sinus, and benefit from operative repair.

In cerebrospinal fluid rhinorrhea, radiologic evaluation and metrizamide contrast (see under Frontobasilar Fractures) can often document the site of the leak. If only a simple fracture is observed, the leak may close on conservative treatment. The patient should be observed for signs of impending complications such as meningitis or extradural or intradural abscess (Donald and Bernstein, 1978; Remmler and Boles, 1980; Donald, 1982; Schilli, Ewers, and Niederdellmann, 1985). It is recommended that no packing be placed in the nasal fossa and that smoking be forbidden. The head of the bed should be elevated to an angle of 60 degrees. Some neurosurgeons prefer lumbar drainage to decrease the pressure in the cerebrospinal fluid, in the belief that this will assist closure of the leak. The patient should be warned against blowing his nose because the material may be forced up into the cranial cavity. If cerebrospinal fluid rhinorrhea is prolonged, an operation to close the fistula should be considered. This may be either extracranial or intracranial. Because of the high incidence of bilateral injuries and the exposure provided by an intracranial procedure, this approach is preferred by the author. Considerable success, however, has been obtained by extracranial approaches to correct localized, documented fistulas. A metrizamide contrast study can delineate the area of involvement. Collins (1982) stated that spinal fluid drainage is confirmed by the presence of glucose in amounts of more than 30 mg of glucose per 100 ml of fluid. The amount of glucose must be related to the serum concentration of glucose. The use of glucose oxidase paper is not reliable as a test for glucose. As many as 75 per cent of positive reactions have been obtained when the oxidated paper test is made in patients with normal secretions. Fistulas may be documented by isotope dyes placed in the lumbar or ventricular cerebrospinal fluid spaces.

Early reduction of facial fractures in the presence of cerebrospinal fluid rhinorrhea is one of the best methods of treatment for a cerebrospinal fluid fistula (Collins, 1982; Dingman, 1974). The objective is to obtain reduction and fixation of the fractured bones in order to provide support for the area of injury and anatomic repositioning of the bone fragments. In cases in which significant frontal fractures are present or fractures of the base of the skull are extensive, an intracranial repair is recommended with exposure of the anterior portions of the cranial fossa. Frequently, the dural tear not only is present in the frontal lobe but extends along the cranial base. It is unlikely that significant dural tears could be repaired through a frontal sinus or extracranial approach.

Fractures of Frontobasilar Region

Fractures of the frontal bone, frontal sinus, orbital roofs, and nasoethmoidal area (Fig. 27–299) are encountered less often than other facial fractures, and practitioners therefore are less familiar with the symptoms, diagnosis, and management. Unlike orbital floor fractures, orbital roof fractures are rarely isolated and they usually coexist with other fractures in adjacent areas, such as the frontal bone and the frontal sinus (Fig. 27–300). Because of the high energy necessary to pro-

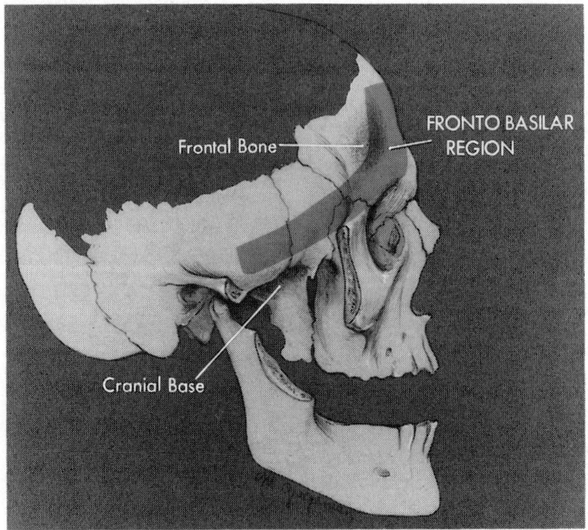

Figure 27–299. The frontobasilar region of the skull.

duce a frontal bone fracture, they frequently occur in the setting of severe generalized trauma in which regional and remote injuries to other organ systems accompany the fractures. The fractures usually are not isolated to the superior orbital rim but extend throughout the orbit and into the nose and midface. Complications from acute or delayed injuries to the visual system further complicate the management of these fractures.

The anterior cranial fossa forms the boundary between the midface and the cranial cavity. Injuries to the frontobasilar region (see Fig. 27–299) provide an area of interface for multiple surgical specialties. The available literature presents varying opinions regarding the type and timing of treatment.

Classification

Experimental data and clinical experience indicate that fractures of the frontal skull correspond to patterns, as do midfacial fractures, which have been organized according to the Le Fort classification. The frontal skull (the "Le Fort IV" fracture) contains areas of thick and thin bone, and the thicker "ridges" describe a system of "buttresses" as in midfacial fractures (Figs. 27–301, 27–302). The thinner areas transilluminate (see Fig. 27–178). Fractures tend to extend within the thinner areas until they reach the next thicker area or buttress. Areas of the frontal skull include the temporal, the lateral (extending from the supraorbital frontal area up to the coronal suture), and the central (low) frontal sinus section (see Fig. 27–300). The frontal sinus is surrounded by a semicircular buttress at its periphery (see Fig. 27–178). Localized fractures of the supraorbital rim occur, such as rim fractures or fractures of the external angular process of the frontal bone (accompanying high energy zygoma

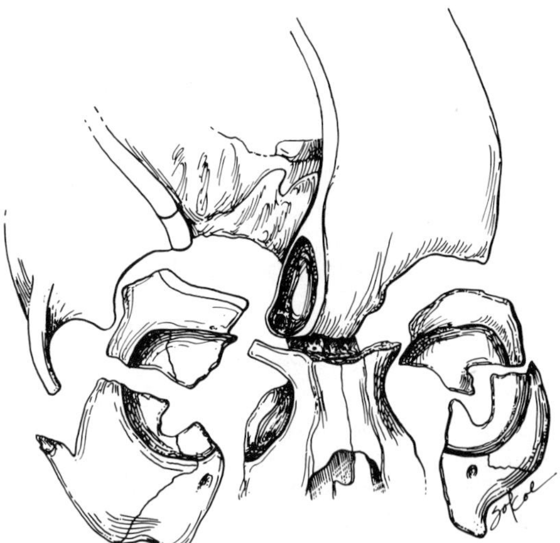

Figure 27–300. The component parts of the frontobasilar region. The supraorbital, zygomatic, and nasoethmoidal areas make up the three sections of the orbital rim. The frontal bone and frontal sinus areas make up the anterior cranium. The anterior cranial fossa is always involved in severe injuries of the frontobasilar region.

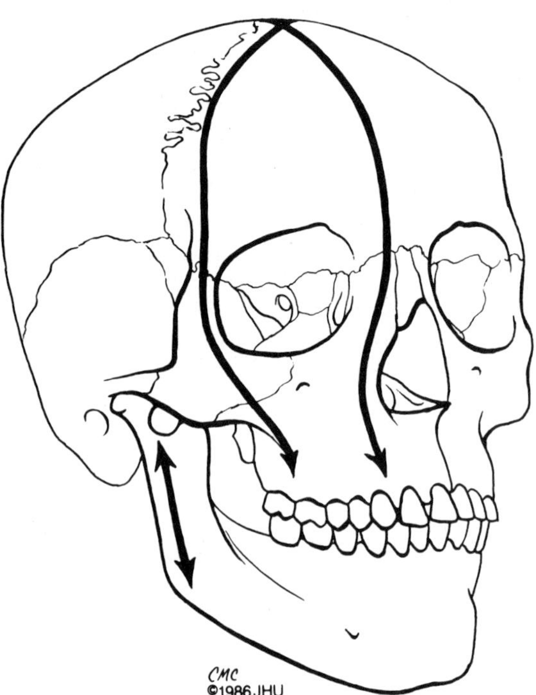

Figure 27–301. The vertical buttresses of the skull extend into the frontal area.

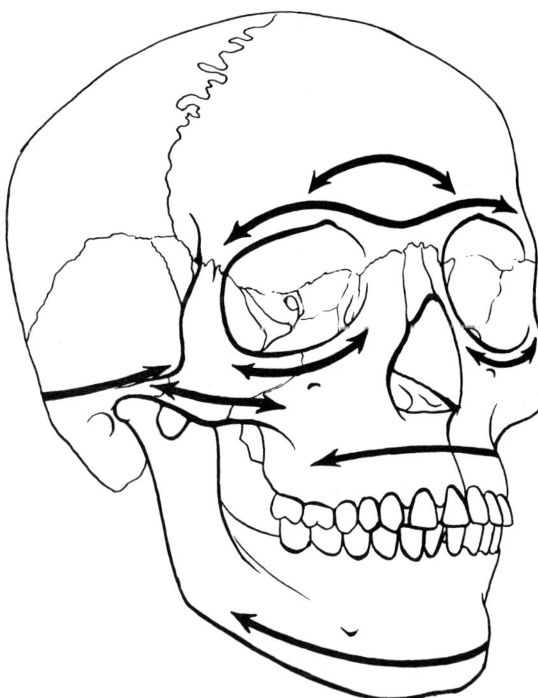

Figure 27–302. The horizontal buttresses of the skull, midface, and mandible.

fractures), but more extensive fractures usually involve two to three areas of the larger section of the frontal bone. A common fracture pattern involves the temporal, lateral, and frontal sinus components of the above-described area pattern. At lower energy impacts, simple linear fractures occur within the weaker areas and extend to involve an entire area with comminution. "Areas of weakness" are described in the frontal skull that correspond to areas circumscribed by the buttresses. These areas correspond to the "lines of weakness" in the Le Fort midfacial fracture classification. The frontal skull may be conceptualized as the Le Fort IV facial injury level. Facial injuries are often more severe on one side than the other, and it is common to see a Le Fort IV level injury on one side and a Le Fort III injury on the other.

Anatomic Characteristics

The bicortical structure of the frontal bone is thick and represents one of the stronger areas of the skull. The central inferior portion of the frontal bone is weakened by the frontal sinus structures, which are unequal in size. The frontal bone becomes unicortical at the rim of the orbit, turning posteriorly to form the orbital roof, which consists of compact bone, a unicortical extension of the bicortical structure of the frontal bone. At the junction of the medial and middle thirds of the supraorbital rim, a small notch or foramen is present for the supraorbital nerve and artery. The orbital roof posterior to the rim is a thin plate of bone that separates the anterior cranial fossa from the orbital contents. It turns upward immediately behind the rim. It is thinnest in the central portion, like the orbital floor. Medially, the orbital roof becomes quite thin and is only slightly stronger than the medial portion of the orbital floor. The orbital roof also consists of the sphenoid bone, its greater and lesser wings. Posteriorly, the orbital roof slopes downward to abut the orbital portion of the zygomatic bone laterally, and the ethmoid and frontal process of the maxilla medially. The orbital roof is often extremely thin beneath the large frontal sinus, whose extent is quite variable. The frontal sinus may occupy only a small portion of the frontal bone or it may extend to pneumatize almost the entire structure. The floor of the frontal sinus thus forms the medial portion of the orbital roof. Radiographic confirmation of the extent of the frontal sinus on each side is important when plans are being formulated for the treatment of frontobasilar fractures. The periosteum of the orbital roof is firmly adherent anteriorly at the rim, but more loosely adherent posteriorly. Thus, subperiosteal hemorrhage may dissect rather freely in the superior portion of the orbit, displacing the soft tissue downward and forward. A small fossa exists at the nasal aspect of the orbital roof just behind the orbital rim for the trochlea of the superior oblique tendon. The trochlea is located approximately 4 mm behind the rim at its anterior aspect. Medially, the supratrochlear and dorsal nasal arteries pierce the septum orbitale above and below the trochlea. The infratrochlear branch of the nasociliary nerve accompanies the arteries in this area. The supraorbital, supratrochlear, and infratrochlear nerves are branches of the ophthalmic division of the trigeminal nerve. The septum orbitale is continuous with the periosteum overlying the orbital rim, fusing inferiorly with the levator aponeurosis just above the tarsus. The superior transverse ligament of Whitnall attaches to the supraorbital rim temporally between the lobes of the lacrimal gland and medially to the fascia surrounding the trochlea.

The levator muscle originates just above the optic foramen near the superior oblique muscle, which originates just medial to the origin of the levator. Both proceed anteriorly beneath the periosteum of the orbital roof, the former turning inferiorly at Whitnall's ligament and the latter becoming tendinous, passing through the trochlea, and then passing backward to attach to the globe. The levator muscle is separated from the periorbita by a thin layer of fat in which the frontal nerve travels.

The optic foramen is the vertically ovoid anterior opening of the optic canal and measures 6 × 5 mm. The optic nerve and ophthalmic artery, which are situated inferior and lateral to the nerve, pass through the canal, which enters just above and medial to the apex of the orbit. The optic canal is bounded superiorly by the lesser wing of the sphenoid, and inferiorly and medially by the sphenoid body. It is bounded anteriorly and medially by the posterior ethmoidal air cells, and laterally by the bony connection between the lesser sphenoid wing and the sphenoid body.

The superior orbital fissure is formed by the greater and lesser wings of the sphenoid. Through the superior orbital fissure pass the superior and inferior divisions of the third nerve, cranial nerves IV and VI, and the ophthalmic divisions of cranial nerve V (Fig. 27–303).

The dural sheath of the optic nerve is firmly attached to the rim of the foramen and fuses with the periosteum within the canal. The nerve is suspended from the periosteum by the arachnoid. A small vascular network accompanies the nerve through the foramen, and compression accounts for a compromised circulation.

Injury Patterns

The dense structure of the frontal bone makes it the strongest of the bones of the face, requiring 150 gm per sq. inch (Swearingen, 1965) for the production of a fracture (see Fig. 27–273). Forces often greatly exceed the minimal force necessary for a fracture to occur. These forces in the frontal bone are four to five times the minimum required to produce fractures in the zygomatic, nasal, or mandibular subcondylar areas.

Fractures of the orbital roof may occur from either direct or indirect mechanisms. Direct roof fractures result from the extension of fractures of the frontal bone, orbital rim, and frontal sinus area. The consistent feature is thus a fracture of the superior orbital rim. These direct fractures either may be localized, involving a small section of the rim and an

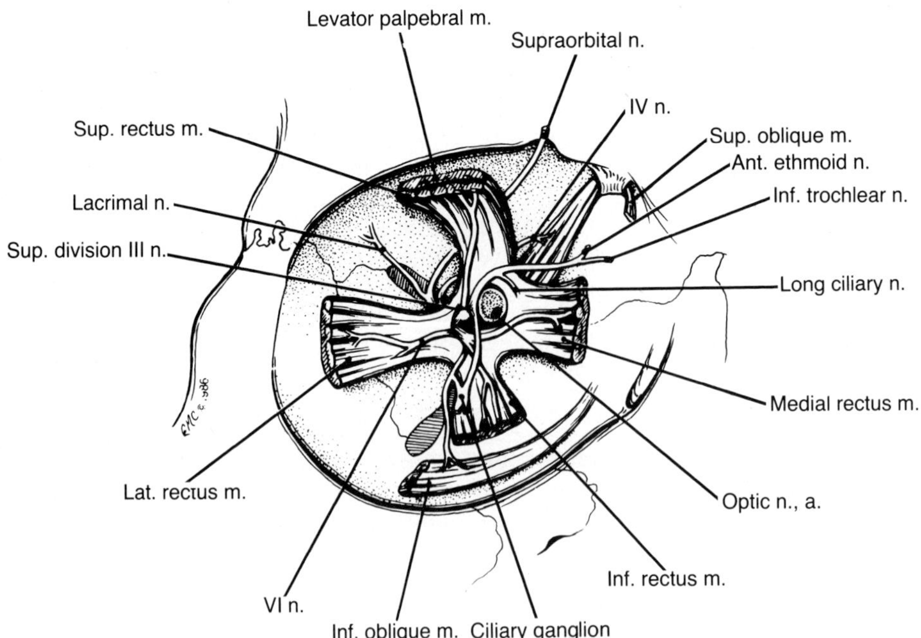

Figure 27–303. The contents of the superior orbital fissure and orbital apex.

anterior portion of the orbital roof, or involve large segments of the frontal bone, such as the lateral frontotemporo-orbital fracture (Fig. 27–304), including an entire lateral segment of the frontal bone, the entire orbital roof, the squamous portion of the temporal bone, and the frontal sinus. In the larger fractures, there is greater displacement of the fragments, and the orbital roof may be comminuted in its anterior and middle sections. This comminution rarely extends to involve the posterior third of the orbit.

Indirect fractures can be produced in the same manner as a "blow-out" fracture of the orbital floor. They result from a mechanism similar to that described by Smith and Regan (1957) and Fujino (Fujino, 1963, 1974a; Fujino and Makino, 1980). In these injuries, a buckling force occurs that causes a fracture in an area of "least resistance." Indirect orbital roof fractures have been reported to occur with a transmission of forces from distant fracture sites, such as the nasal bones, the frontal process of the maxilla, the caudal part of the maxillary process of the frontal bone (nasoethmoidal area), and the frontal skull. Exceptional trauma to the zygoma (Vondra, 1965) has also been known to cause fracture lines that pass through the roof of the orbit and extend to the superior orbital fissure and optic foramen.

Incidence

In a review of 1031 consecutive fractures, Schultz (1967) found that fewer than 5 per cent had supraorbital fractures. Most of these fractures resulted from automobile accidents (72 per cent) or motorcycle accidents (14 per cent). There was a 2:1 predominance of male patients.

Signs and Symptoms

The most common signs and symptoms of a fracture in the frontobasilar region are a bruise or laceration in the area of the brow or the orbit. Such a physical finding should prompt an examination for any evidence of an underlying fracture. For the orbital component of the fracture, the most reliable sign is the combination of a palpebral and a subconjunctival hematoma. The palpation or the visualization of a step deformity in the rim is helpful, although it often is not apparent because of swelling and bruising. Swelling may produce upper lid ptosis from contusion, levator damage, or simply hemorrhage. In such cases, the lid should be manually opened so that the globe can be fully inspected and a proper ocular and visual examination performed.

Evaluation of the visual system is critical and should be performed as soon as the patient is stabilized. Petro and associates (1970) found that supraorbital fractures represented 14 per cent of the total number of periorbital fractures but accounted for one-fourth of eye injuries. In their study, one-half of the patients with ocular injuries had decreased vision. The most common injury to the globe was laceration or rupture. The treatment of this complication must take precedence over other reconstructive maneuvers, even though the prognosis for vision may be poor. Retinal contusion, intraocular hemorrhage, and intraocular evidence of optic nerve damage may all be present and must be documented, for they all have an impact on the evaluation of the vision and the visual potential. In particular, it is extremely important to document light perception, pupillary light reflex, or the visual acuity present before treatment, so that the treatment cannot be blamed for the

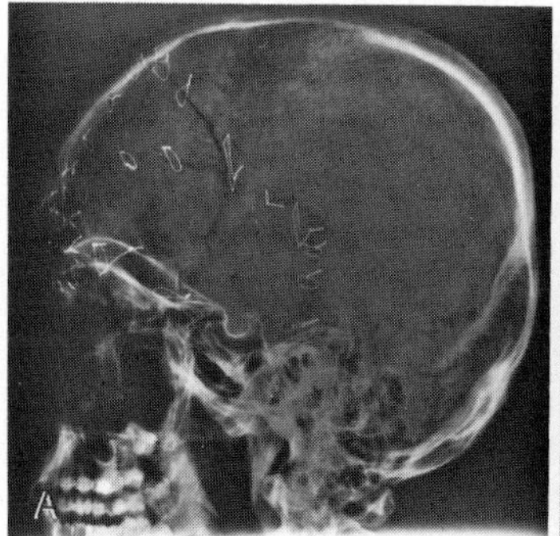

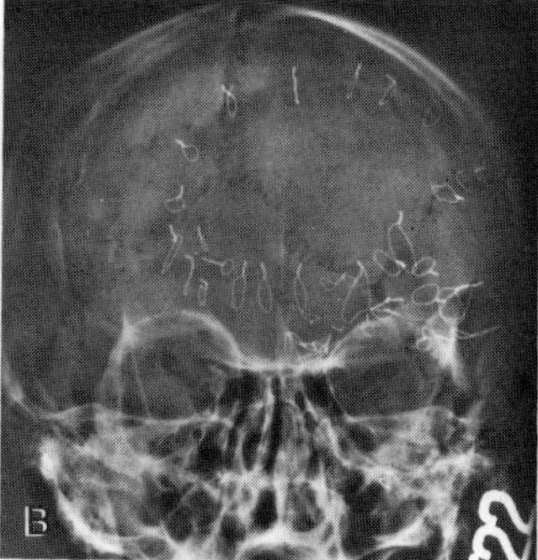

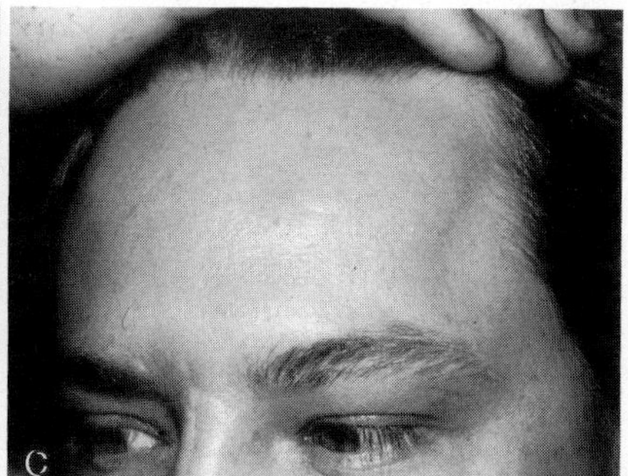

Figure 27–304. *A, B,* Interfragment wiring of a complicated fracture of the frontal bone, frontal sinus, and laterofrontal temporo-orbital region. *C,* The result following that procedure.

visual damage produced by the fracture. If the patient is not able to cooperate for visual testing, evaluation of the pupillary response is all that is possible, but is extremely important. Evidence of paresis in a field of gaze indicates involvement of a cranial nerve or extraocular muscle. Fractures of the orbital roof commonly produce temporary palsy of the levator muscle. They less commonly cause a paresis of the superior rectus muscle, which can mimic incarceration of the inferior rectus muscle. The two conditions may be differentiated by a thorough radiographic and clinical examination, including forced duction testing. The author has not observed incarceration of the levator and superior rectus muscle in an orbital roof fracture. Fracture fragments of the roof, however, may be displaced downward (Fig. 27–305), impinging on the action of these muscles. A CT scan demonstrates bone fragments pressing into the muscles and the globe, nerve, and adnexal structures.

Hypoesthesia in the distribution of the supraorbital nerve accompanies larger supraorbital fractures, especially those that involve the supraorbital foramen (usually the direct "lateral frontotemporo-orbital" fractures). The hypoesthesia is usually temporary and secondary to nerve contusion.

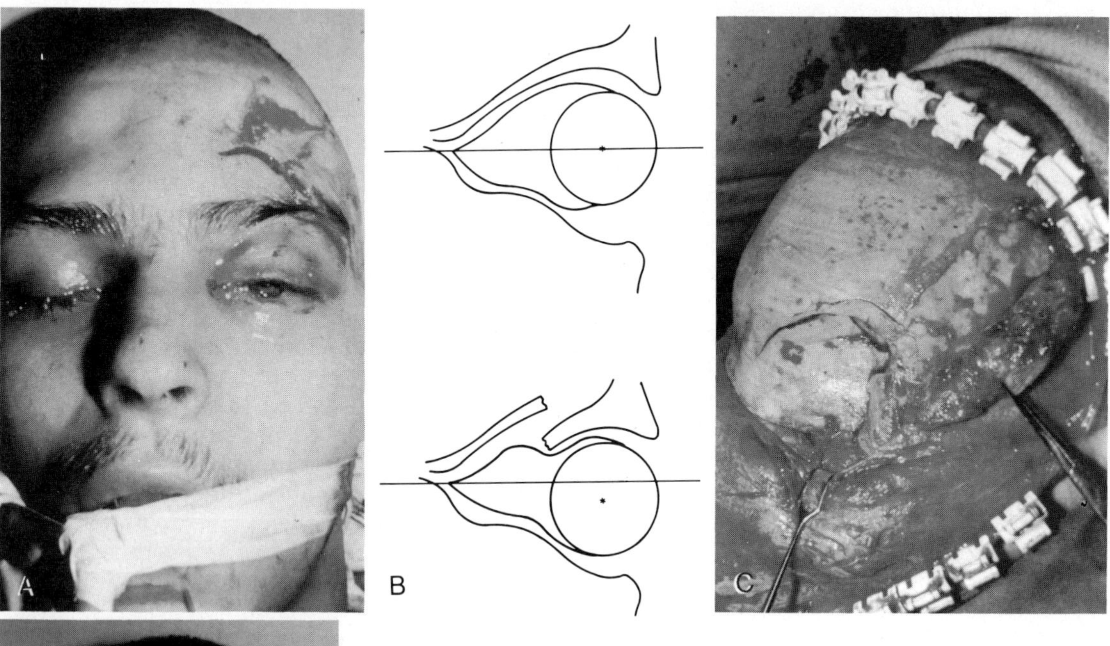

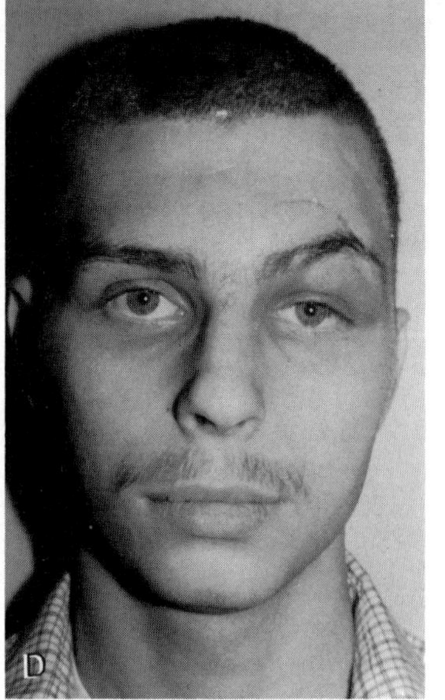

Figure 27–305. *A*, A fracture involving the lateral frontotemporo-orbital region. There is depression of the fractures with an accompanying laceration. The eye is displaced downward and forward via the mechanism seen in *B*. *C*, The depressed bone fragments of the frontotemporo-orbital fracture at operation. *D*, The result following primary reconstruction.

Swelling in the roof of the orbit causes a downward displacement of the roof and rim of the orbit. It produces a characteristic downward and forward position of the globe (Fig. 27–305). This is one of the most accurate clinical signs of a displaced roof fracture. The lids may not close completely over this displaced globe, resulting in corneal exposure.

Upper lid ptosis (see Fig. 27–305*A*) may be produced by either direct nerve damage, muscle contusion, or hematoma. A spectacle hematoma (one confined to the distribution of the orbital septum) is strong evidence of a supraorbital fracture. A high index of suspicion of a supraorbital fracture should exist when lacerations involve the brow or upper lid area, or when there is significant contusion. Appropriate radiographic examination (a carefully performed CT scan in axial and coronal planes) must be carried out to confirm the presence of a fracture.

Frontal Lobe and Cranial Nerve Injuries. The frontal lobe is often contused after significant supraorbital fractures and is assessed by clinical examination and CT scans. More severe brain injuries produce confusion, coma, personality change, irritability, or inappropriate affect. It must be emphasized, however, that many patients have few symptoms. Cranial nerve palsies exist by extension of the fractures to the cribriform plate and the superior orbital fissure. The silent nature of frontal lobe symptoms does not allow one to easily detect the full extent of the underlying cerebral injury on clinical examination. Significant frontal lobe contusion can occur with few, if any, symptoms present. Confusion, somnolence, and personality change are the first symptoms produced. Evaluation with a Glasgow Coma Scale (see Table 27–1) documents the patient's ability to talk, move extremities, and open the eyes according to a graded response system. Lowered scores emphasize the need for precise radiologic evaluation and continuous intracranial pressure monitoring, which must be performed if anesthesia is required. Patients with significant fractures or brain injury are at risk of rapid neurologic decompensation, and require intracranial pressure monitoring whether or not anesthesia is to be provided. Intracranial pressure monitoring allows the immediate detection and treatment of increased intracerebral pressure, and it can significantly increase survival. Intracranial pressures of greater than 25 mm Hg usually contraindicate nonemergent fracture treatment.

Fractures involving the orbital roof and anterior cranial fossa have a high frequency of dural and arachnoid lacerations, which allow cerebrospinal fluid to leak into either the nose or the orbit (Fig. 27–306). Leaks into the orbit (orbitorrhea) rarely cause any symptomatic problem other than swelling and they are frequently undetected. Infection (meningitis) is unusual with orbitorrhea. If the leak communicates with the nose or sinuses, cerebrospinal fluid rhinorrhea exists and may be detected by examination of the fluid dripping from the patient's nose in a head forward position. A double ring sign may be present when nasal secretion is examined following its absorption on a white paper towel.

The incidence of meningitis and cerebrospinal fluid rhinorrhea ranges between 5 and 10 per cent in those who have a fistula. The frequency of meningitis increases with the duration of the leak. Although many authors favor the administration of a "prophylactic" antibiotic to protect against meningitis, it has not been demonstrated that these offer a

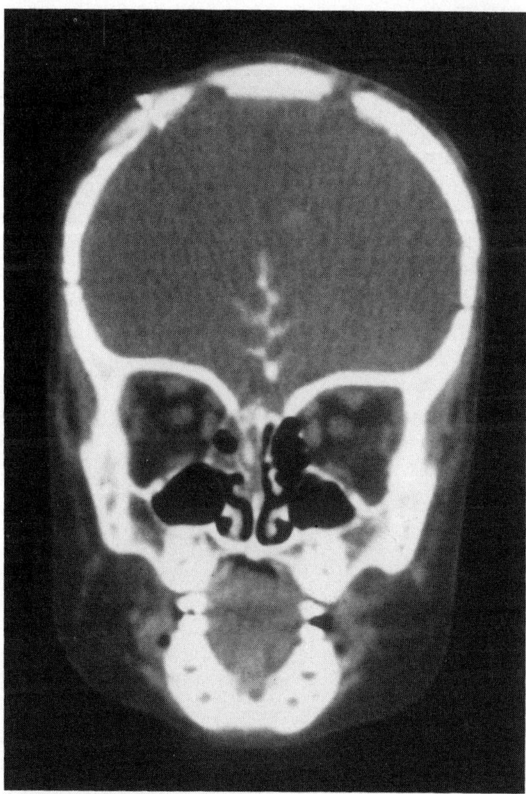

Figure 27–306. A cerebrospinal fluid leak demonstrated by metrizamide scanning. The leak is seen through the right cribriform plate and it extends through the ethmoid sinus.

clear advantage (see Complications of Orbital and Nasoethmoido-orbital Fractures). An antibiotic is merely effective in eliminating a select range of bacteria, and the emergence of resistant organisms occurs quickly in multiply traumatized patients. Thus, little long-term protection is achieved by antibiotic therapy in the presence of a persistent cerebrospinal fluid fistula.

Pneumocephalus and Orbital Emphysema. Communication of the orbit with the paranasal sinuses by fracture allows the escape of air into the orbit or into the cranial cavity, producing orbital emphysema or pneumocephalus (Fig. 27–307) (Jacobs and Persky, 1980). These conditions are observed in significant fractures of the frontal bone and orbital roof, and resolve with reduction of the fracture, closure of the dural laceration, and healing of the sinus mucosa. There is a difference of opinion as to whether prophylactic antibiotics should be administered. The presence of air in the orbit or within the cranium is evidence of contamination with nasal or sinus organisms. It has been difficult to demonstrate, however, that the administration of antibiotics on a prolonged basis is effective in preventing meningitis when pneumocephalus or orbital emphysema is present. Each of these has the same clinical significance as a cerebrospinal fluid fistula and implies a communication between the cranial cavity and the nasal environment.

Absence of Orbital Roof and Pulsating Exophthalmos. Fracture-dislocation or loss of the orbital roof from post-traumatic atrophy of thin bone fragments or from neurosurgical debridement following a compound skull

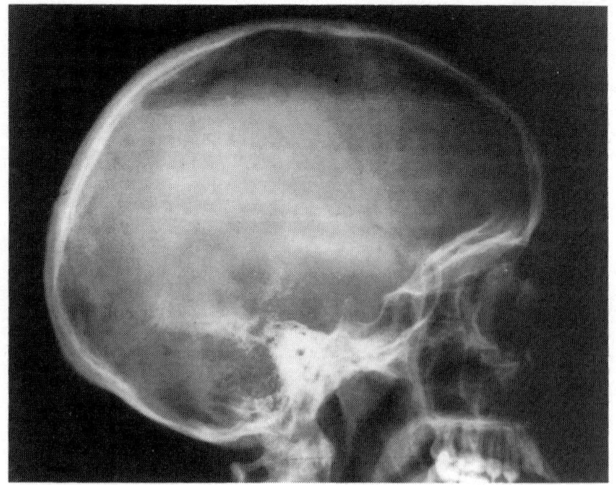

Figure 27–307. Pneumocephalus is well visualized in the lateral skull film.

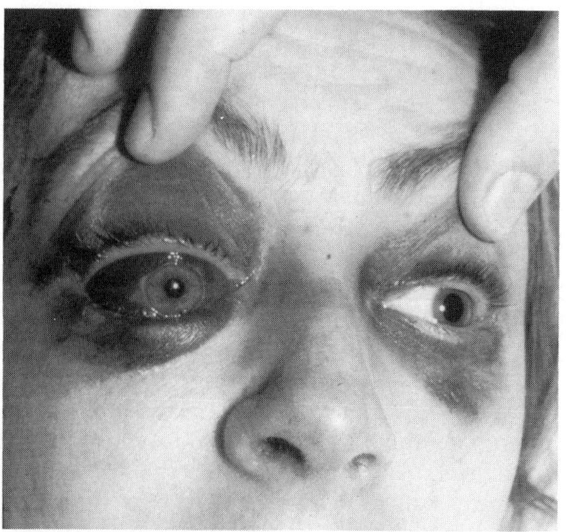

Figure 27–308. Superior orbital fissure syndrome. The globe is displaced downward and forward owing to a hematoma within the superior portion of the orbit. The patient is unable to open her right eye. Paralysis of extraocular motion is present and anesthesia is present in the first division of the trigeminal nerve.

fracture may produce a syndrome of pulsating exophthalmos, which is due to cerebral pulsations transmitted to the globe and adnexal structures. There is usually a downward and forward protrusion of the globe exaggerated by the pulsation. These symptoms are corrected by reconstruction of the orbital roof.

Carotid Cavernous Sinus Fistula. Some severe fractures involving the roof and middle cranial fossa may result in a communication between the carotid artery and cavernous sinus (Cahill, Rao, and Ducker, 1981), which produces a syndrome of pulsating exophthalmos. A bruit may be detected by auscultation over the globe. The syndrome is frequently accompanied by blindness and is usually treated by embolization under radiographic control.

Superior Orbital Fissure Syndrome and Orbital Apex Syndrome. Significant fractures of the orbital roof extend posteriorly to involve the superior orbital fissure and optic foramen. Involvement of the structures of the superior orbital fissure produces a symptom complex known as the *superior orbital fissure syndrome* (Kurzer and Patel, 1979; Zachariades, 1982). This consists of involvement of the following structures (see Figs. 27–303, 27–308): the two divisions of cranial nerve III (producing paralysis of the levator, superior rectus, inferior rectus, and inferior oblique muscles); cranial nerve IV, causing paralysis of the superior oblique muscle; cranial nerve VI, producing paralysis of the lateral rectus muscle; and the ophthalmic division of the trigeminal nerve, causing anesthesia in the brow, upper lid, medial upper nose, and ipsilateral forehead area. The symptoms of the superior orbital fissure syndrome accompanied by blindness imply concomitant involvement of the superior orbital fissure and optic foramen. If involvement of the optic nerve accompanies this syndrome, the symptom complex is called the *orbital apex syndrome* (Fig. 27–309).

Visual Loss. Visual loss is a common complication of cerebral or significant facial injuries. It occurred in 6 per cent of patients with Le Fort II and III (Miller and Tenzel, 1967; Weymuller, 1984), frontal bone (Elisevich and associates, 1984; Kline, Morawetz, and Swaid, 1984), frontal sinus, severe zygomatic (Vondra, 1965), or severe orbital fractures. Approximately 5 per cent of patients with head trauma manifest an injury to some portion of the visual system (Kline, Morawetz, and Swaid, 1984). About 70 per cent of injuries involve the anterior visual pathways alone, damage to the optic nerve accounting for one-third (Elisevich and associates, 1984). Fractures of the sphenoid bone, particularly of the body, accompany optic nerve and chiasmal injuries (Elisevich and associates, 1984). While large series of head injury showed a 0.5 to 1.5 per cent incidence of visual impairment (Elisevich and associates, 1984; Kline, Morawetz, and Swaid, 1984), other authors demonstrated that the optic nerve is one of the most frequently injured cranial nerves, affecting 15 per cent of survivors of major head injury (Elisevich and associates, 1984; Kline, Morawetz, and Swaid, 1984). In an autopsy review of patients dying of acute closed head injury, ischemic necrosis and shearing lesions of the anterior visual pathways were present in one-half and one-quarter had bilateral lesions (Elisevich and associates, 1984). Its mechanisms are multiple and complex and deserve careful consideration. Because of early aggressive management of the trauma victim with successful control of intracranial pressure, there has been a significant drop in the mortality rate (50 to 25 per cent) of patients with severe head injuries (Teasdale and Jennett, 1974; Becker and associates, 1977). Consideration of the visual injury demands priority. Of survivors of significant brain injury, 45 per cent are capable of returning to their preinjury occupation, while an additional 45 per cent are able to perform activities of daily living. The great variety of residual visual abnormalities in this expanding survival population is currently being recorded. Assessment of visual function is often difficult in an individual with an altered state of consciousness. If the vision is found to be impaired, decisions must be made regarding further evaluation and management based on the site of the injury. Visual impairment is defined as a visual acuity of less than 20/60, and blindness as less than 20/200. When less than 20 per cent of the visual field remains, the condition is classified as blindness.

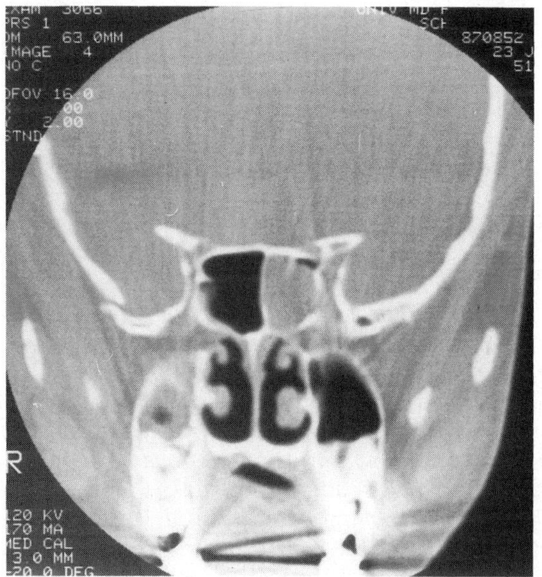

Figure 27–309. A coronal CT scan demonstrating a sphenoid sinus hematoma and fractures in the posterior portion of the orbit adjacent to the superior orbital fissure and optic canal. An orbital apex syndrome (blindness and the superior orbital fissure syndrome) was present.

Optic Nerve Anatomy

The optic nerves are 50 mm in length and extend from the chiasm to the posterior aspect of the globe (Fig. 27–310). For purposes of analysis, four segments are identified: the intracranial, intracanalicular, intraorbital, and intraocular portions (Kline, Morawetz, and Swaid, 1984). The smallest part of the optic nerve is the *intraocular portion,* which exits the globe nasal to and slightly above the fovea. The nerve travels through a rather rigidly confined scleral canal where a watershed area (Elisevich and associates, 1984; Kline, Morawetz, and Swaid, 1984) between

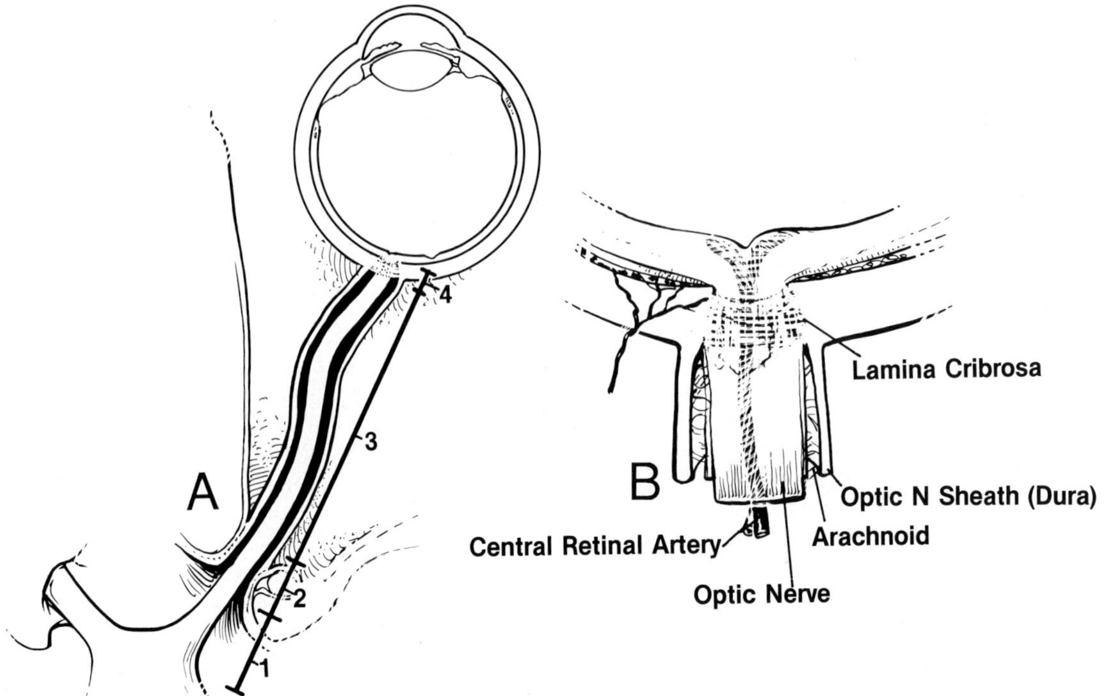

Figure 27–310. *A*, The optic nerve and the four segments. *B*, Close-up view of the intraocular portion.

the retinal and ciliary microcirculations exists in the immediate retrolaminar portion of the optic nerve. This section is thus susceptible to infarction from swelling or interstitial hemorrhage within the rigid confines of the scleral canal. In addition, transmission of raised intracranial pressure into the optic nerve sheath can rupture intradural vessels and produce ischemia. A 32 per cent incidence of intraocular hemorrhage was reported in cases of subarachnoid hemorrhage (Elisevich and associates, 1984). Preretinal hemorrhages that have broken into the vitreous through the internal limiting membrane (Terson's syndrome) have been described in cases of severe cerebral trauma with intracranial hypertension (Elisevich and associates, 1984; Kline, Morawetz, and Swaid, 1984).

The *orbital portion* of the optic nerve extends from the posterior aspect of the globe to the optic canal. It is somewhat longer than the actual straight line distance involved, and thus has a loose, slightly circuitous course through the orbit. The optic nerve is covered by the dura, arachnoid, and pia mater from the brain. The nerve is surrounded by orbital fat and extraocular muscles. The central retinal artery and vein course forward in the orbit below the optic nerve. At a point 10 mm posterior to the globe, the vessels enter the optic nerve, piercing the dura mater and arachnoid. The anterior intraorbital portion of the optic nerve is vascularized by centrifugal branches of the central retinal artery, whereas the remainder of the intraorbital portion receives only pial circulation.

The *intracanalicular portion* of the optic nerve measures 10 mm in length and 4 mm in diameter. It traverses the optic canal, which is formed by the union of the two roots of the lesser wing of the sphenoid bone. The canal, averaging 5 to 10 mm in length and 4 to 6 mm in width, travels posteriorly and medially. The canal contains the ophthalmic artery, as well as fibers of the sympathetic plexus and an extension of the sheaths of the meninges. The intracanalicular optic nerve is tightly fixed within the optic canal by the dura mater, which divides into two layers as it enters the orbit. One remains as the outer sheath of the optic nerve and the other becomes the orbital periosteum. The subarachnoid space communicates through the optic canal and around the optic nerve to the posterior aspect of the globe.

The *intracranial portion* of the optic nerve is 10 mm in length. It is located in the diaphragma sellae. Lateral to the optic nerve is the internal carotid artery, which gives off the ophthalmic artery just inferior to the nerve. On the ventral surface of each frontal lobe, the olfactory tract is separated from the optic nerve by the anterior cerebral and anterior communicating artery. The intracranial portion of the optic nerve terminates at the optic chiasm.

Types of Optic Nerve Injury

From a practical standpoint, indirect injury to the optic nerve can be divided into two categories: anterior, in which the funduscopic abnormalities are evident, and posterior, in which the fundus initially appears normal. Anterior injury denotes involvement of the intraocular optic nerve and that portion of the intraocular segment containing the central retinal artery. In all instances, ophthalmoscopic abnormalities are visible. Central retinal artery occlusion produces an edematous retina, a pale optic disc, threadlike arterioles, and visible sludging of blood within the retinal vasculature (Elisevich and associates, 1984; Kline, Morawetz, and Swaid, 1984). Traumatic ischemic optic neuropathy results in a diffusely swollen disc, with the remainder of the fundus normal in appearance (Elisevich and associates, 1984; Kline, Morawetz, and Swaid, 1984).

The diagnosis of posterior indirect optic nerve injury is based on evidence of optic nerve dysfunction in the *absence* of funduscopic abnormalities on initial examination and *no* evidence of chiasmal injury. Optic disc pallor and loss of the retinal nerve fiber layer become apparent over a four to eight week period. It is presumed that the lesion lies somewhere between the entry of the central retinal artery and the optic nerve and optic chiasm (Elisevich and associates, 1984; Kline, Morawetz, and Swaid, 1984). The intracanalicular portion of the optic nerve is by far the most frequent site of injury. Visual field defects may be total or partial. Partial visual field defects fall into two main categories, central scotomas and nerve fiber bundle defects (Elisevich and associates, 1984; Kline, Morawetz, and Swaid, 1984).

The mechanisms of indirect optic nerve injury include complete or incomplete lacerations of the optic nerve and lesions produced by bone deformation or fracture, including those in the optic canal, and those secondary to fractures of the orbital roof or the anterior clinoid process (Kline, Morawetz, and Swaid, 1984). Vascular insufficiency may be produced by either ischemia or infarction (Kline, Morawetz, and Swaid, 1984). Concussion and contusion of nerve fibers cause temporary or permanent nerve damage. Hemorrhage into the optic nerve sheath or intraneural hemorrhage also produces a nerve deficit.

The degree of recovery depends on the extent of nerve damage and the mechanism of nerve injury. For example, ischemia produced by an accumulation of hematoma within the optic canal might be capable of relief by decompression (Fukado, 1975). Tearing of nerve fibers within the optic canal would not be improved by decompression of the canal. Concussion, a transient disturbance, usually recovers spontaneously, whereas contusion of the nerve is identified by a histologic structural alteration of neural tissue characterized by extravasation of blood and cell death (Elisevich and associates, 1984; Kline, Morawetz, and Swaid, 1984). The lesion on histologic examination has a characteristic triangular shape, with the apex internal to its base (Kline, Morawetz, and Swaid, 1984). Necrosis of some nerve fibers follows and the ensuing visual loss is permanent.

Visual Examination Techniques

Visual Acuity. Visual acuity in each eye should be assessed using a Snellen Visual Acuity chart or a Rosenbaum pocket vision card. Alternatively, printed material can be shown to the patient and the response noted. In an uncooperative patient, response to a light stimulus, such as photophobia, pupillary constriction, or lid closure, indicates probable light perception.

Pupillary Reactivity. An assessment of pupillary reactivity is of critical importance, because the direct pupillary response to light is thought by many to be the most reliable sign of the extent of optic nerve injury. Roentgenographic studies, a history of accompanying head trauma, and ophthalmoscopic findings are all considerably less valuable than the status of the pupillary light reflex. After an ipsilateral optic nerve injury the pupil on the side of the injured nerve is equal in size to the opposite pupil but less reactive to direct light stimulation. The pupil on the side of the optic nerve lesion, however, usually reacts consensually. This indicates the presence of an afferent lesion in the pupillary light reflex pathway, specifically a conduction defect involving the optic nerve on the side of the less reactive pupil (Elisevich and associates, 1984; Kline, Morawetz, and Swaid, 1984). The difference in pupillary reactions, with the light first in one and then in the other, may be enhanced by swinging a flashlight back and forth from one eye to the other (see Figs. 27–297, 27–298). When the light is moved from the intact eye to the abnormal eye, a paradoxical dilatation of the abnormal eye is seen, the Marcus Gunn pupillary phenomenon (Jabaley, Lerman, and Sanders, 1975).

Visual Field Testing. Visual field testing may reveal a complete or partial lesion. Central scotoma or nerve fiber bundle defects are identified (Elisevich and associates, 1984; Kline, Morawetz, and Swaid, 1984). The discovery of a hemianopic defect (either bitemporal or homonomous) excludes consideration of optic nerve decompression. Documentation of a deteriorating unilateral visual field defect may be an indication for optic nerve decompression.

Funduscopic Examination. In posterior indirect optic nerve injury, the optic disc and entire fundus initially appears normal (Elisevich and associates, 1984; Kline, Morawetz, and Swaid, 1984). Within several weeks, optic atrophy becomes apparent. An abnormal fundus initially signifies optic nerve injury, either at its junction with the globe or along the intraorbital portion containing the central retinal artery and central retinal vein. The spectrum of funduscopic abnormalities accompanying other globe injuries should be considered.

Visual Evoked Response (VER). Examination of the visual system during the acute phase of head injury with the unconscious patient is difficult. The visual evoked response (VER) to fast stimulation in some cases provides valuable objective data. Patients with unrecordable visual evoked responses have not experienced a return of vision after optic nerve decompression. The limited availability and impracticality of performing the VER testing limit its usefulness, however.

Neuroradiologic evaluation with high resolution CT performed in both the axial and coronal planes is the optimal radiographic evaluation (Manfredi and associates, 1981; Guyon, Brant-Zawadzki, and Seiff, 1984). Not all fractures involving the optic canal are demonstrable on radiography. In a study of 379 patients with facial fractures, Manfredi and associates found that 16 patients had evidence of sphenoid and ethmoid sinus hemorrhage on routine skull and facial radiographs (Fig. 27–311). In five of these patients (31 per cent) there was CT evidence of an optic canal fracture and the clinical findings of optic nerve injury. The authors concluded that any head trauma patient with sphenoethmoid sinus hemorrhage on conventional radiography or loss of visual acuity should undergo a detailed cranial CT scan as well as a complete ophthalmologic examination. The CT scan can provide valuable information about soft tissue structures, to confirm such findings as stretching, edema, or transection of the optic nerve (Stuzin and associates, 1988).

Optic Chiasm. The optic chiasm may be injured in head or facial trauma. Bilateral optic disc pallor and Wernicke's hemianopic pupillary reaction are early clues of chiasmal injury (Elisevich and associates, 1984). Diabetes insipidus has been found to accompany these cases (25 to 50 per cent) (Elisevich and associates, 1984). Patients with traumatic chiasmal syndromes have either bitemporal hemianopias or monocular blindness with contralateral temporal hemianopia. Some authors have suggested vascular injury, infarction, contusion, hemorrhage, rupture, or contusion necrosis as the mechanisms of this phenomenon (Elisevich and associates, 1984).

Optic Radiations and Calcarine Cortex. Injury of the occipital cerebral cortex produces temporary hemicortical and opticortical blindness that is often delayed hours or days after the injury and frequently overlooked (Elisevich and associates, 1984). Ischemia from focal vasospasm is favored as the pathogenic mechanism (Elisevich and associates, 1984). Contusion of the temporoparietal area produces expected homonomous quadrantic or hemianopic visual field defects (Elisevich and associates, 1984).

Carotid Cavernous Sinus Fistulas. Fistulas between the carotid artery and the cavernous sinus produced impaired vision in 90 per cent of cases and blindness in one-third (Cahill, Rao, and Ducker, 1981; Elisevich and associates, 1984). The superior ophthalmic vein conducts the abnormal flow, resulting in ischemic retinopathy from venous congestion. Reduced ophthalmic pres-

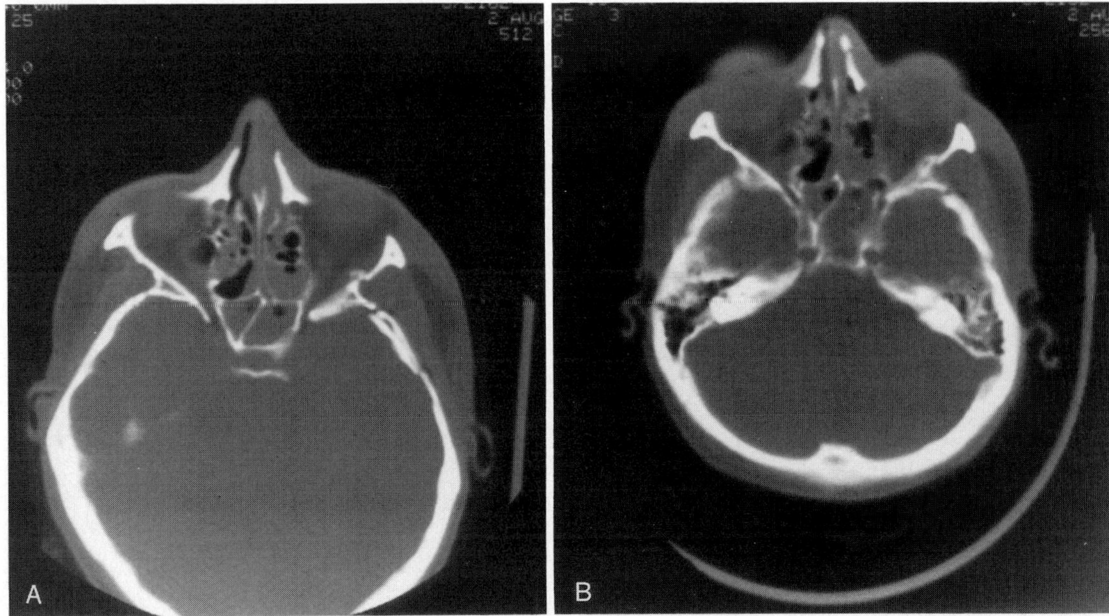

Figure 27–311. Fracture of the greater wing of the sphenoid with displacement can be seen. A sphenoid and ethmoid sinus hematoma is present *(A)*. *B*, Another view of the fracture showing displacement of the greater wing of the sphenoid in the posterior portion of the orbit.

sures are noted and they also contribute to the anoxia.

Treatment of Optic Nerve Injury. It is obvious that multiple conditions contribute to an indirect optic nerve injury. Some of these might be amenable to surgical decompression (Fukado, 1975) but many would not (Elisevich and associates, 1984; Kline, Morawetz, and Swaid, 1984). This accounts for some of the confusion in the literature, which expresses widely divergent opinions about the advisability of decompression of the optic canal. A comparison of series in which most patients are stated to improve after surgical decompression (Fukado, 1975) shows that only a few had no light perception whatsoever before the operation; most had "impaired vision." Most authors have experienced fewer successes after decompression of the optic nerve for blindness (Elisevich and associates, 1984; Kline, Morawetz, and Swaid, 1984).

The following guidelines were suggested by Walsh (Kline, Morawetz, and Swaid, 1984):

Optic nerve decompression should not be undertaken as an elective procedure or on an unconscious patient; if the loss of vision is associated with a nonreactive pupil and the loss occurred at the moment of impact, the procedure is probably not indicated; if the loss of vision or the loss of pupillary response to light develops after the moment of impact, the possibility of an operation improving the situation should be considered; if it cannot be determined if the loss of vision or pupillary response was delayed, a period of 4–6 days should elapse, and if spontaneous improvement occurs, no surgery should be undertaken. If improvement does not occur, it might be reasonable to decompress the optic canal.

Most authors administer megadose steroids when optic nerve injury is apparent. There are several operative approaches for optic nerve decompression. The two most commonly employed use the transorbital and transethmoidal routes; the transfrontal approach requires a full craniotomy.

Treatment of Fractures of Frontal Area. Fractures of the lower portion of the frontal bone (Finney, Reynolds, and Yates, 1964; Hamberger and Wiesall, 1969) and supraorbital and glabellar regions are less frequent, occurring either independently or in conjunction with nasoethmoido-orbital fractures. Schultz (1970) noted that patients suffering supraorbital and glabellar fractures required a longer average hospital stay than other facially injured patients irrespective of the cause.

After fracture displacement, the rim and roof of the orbit tend to flatten, whereas they normally constitute a doubly arched structure that bows both superiorly and anteriorly (Fig.

27–312). Thus, the fractured supraorbital rim tends to assume a flattened anteroposterior projection and a flattened roof, which is accompanied by lower globe position.

The author has observed concomitant fracture of the supraorbital arch, depressed fracture of the glabellar region, and nasoethmoido-orbital fractures in many patients. These can occur either independently or concurrently in the same patient (Fig. 27–313).

When bone fragments are missing, the frontal bone flap can be split and used as a graft. Grafts are also useful to reconstruct badly comminuted segments of the orbital roof and orbital floor (Fig. 27–314). In former times it was fashionable to remove comminuted bone fragments, allowing healing to occur, and to present the patient for secondary reconstruction. The appearance in Figure 27–315 is typical of these patients and makes proper reconstruction difficult.

The roentgenographic diagnosis requires axial and coronal CT scans that demonstrate the frontal and ethmoid sinuses, the frontal bone, the anterior cranial base, the orbit, and the nasoethmoido-orbital regions (Figs. 27–316, 27–317). Only with a thorough CT examination can the extent of soft tissue and bone damage be evaluated. Both bone and soft tissue windows are essential for the evaluation of the brain and the bones.

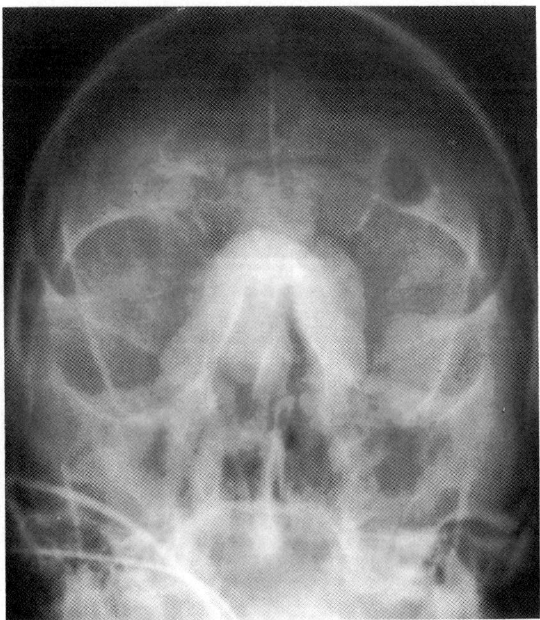

Figure 27–313. Fractures of the frontal sinus extending into the nasoethmoidal area and maxilla.

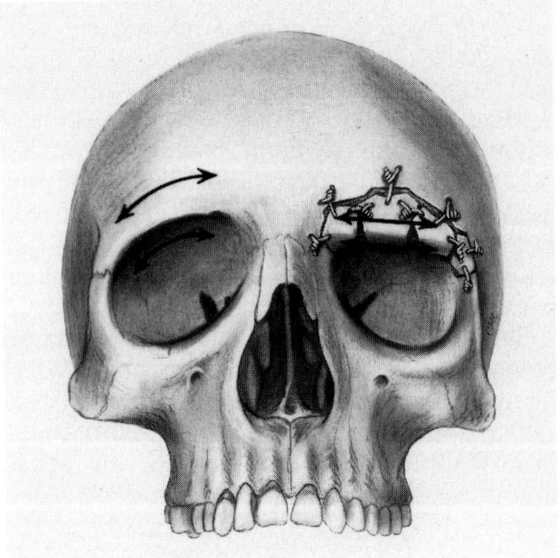

Figure 27–312. In fractures of the supraorbital rim and orbital roof, one must recreate the "double arches" (see right orbit). The orbital rim arches anteriorly and the roof arches superiorly. After a comminuted fracture and interfragment wiring of multiple segments, there is a tendency for depression of the multiply wired pieces to occur in an anteroposterior plane and for a flattening of the roof to occur in a vertical plane (see left orbit). The use of plate and screw fixation prevents these two movements.

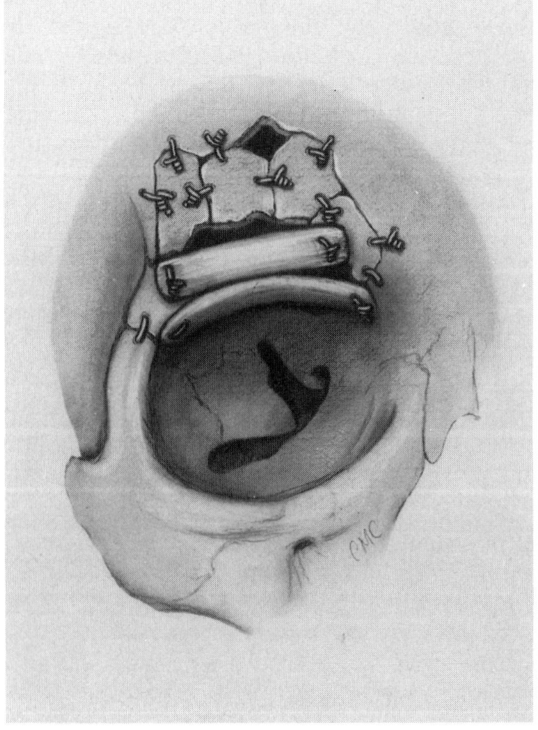

Figure 27–314. Grafts are used to replace the missing bone in a frontotempo-orbital fracture.

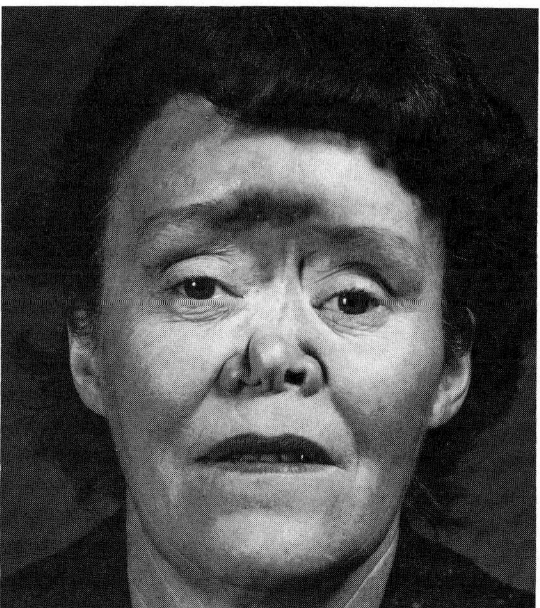

Figure 27–315. Example of the deformity resulting from a severe nasoethmoido-orbital fracture and fracture of the glabellar portion of the frontal bone involving the frontal sinus. The patient suffered severe head injury and was in a coma for 72 hours; neurosurgical intervention was required for brain damage (removal of bone fragments penetrating into the frontal lobes and arrest of cerebrospinal rhinorrhea).

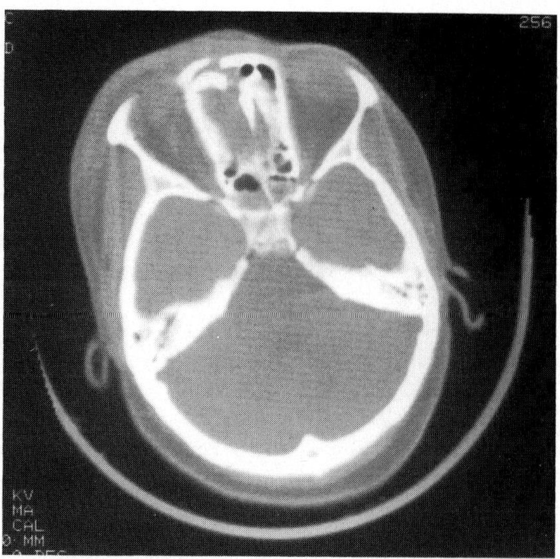

Figure 27–317. CT scan showing a fracture involving the cranial base and nasoethmoidal area.

Treatment nearly always involves open reduction through a laceration or a surgical incision. Exposure for a localized supraorbital fracture can be achieved through a laceration or an incision immediately above the eyebrow if the incision is correctly placed. The result of the supraorbital eyebrow exposure is a scar that *is* perceptible. Incisions within the eyebrow produce a noticeable, hairless scar separating the upper and lower follicles of eyebrow hair.

The best technique of exposure in major fractures involving the frontal bone is the coronal incision advocated by Tessier and associates (1977). This allows a combined intracranial and extracranial approach, making possible visualization of all fragments, repair of all dural tears, and debridement of any necrotic portion of the frontal lobe. Reduction and alignment of fracture fragments are performed, linking the fragments together with multiple interfragment wires (Fig. 27–318)—the chain-link fence technique after Munro and Chen (1981) and Gruss and associates (1985b)—and stabilizing the united bones with a plate to reconstruct the continuity of the frontal bar and supraorbital arch. Although large fragments of a skull fracture occasionally may be levered upward and remain in position without interosseous wire fixation, it is better to stabilize the fragments with either direct interosseous wiring or a plate and screw fixation technique. Plate and screw fixation (Jackson, Somers, and Kjar, 1986) can be accomplished using holes through the anterior table and 4 or 5 mm screws. The calvarial bone fragments also provide a bone graft donor site, if split.

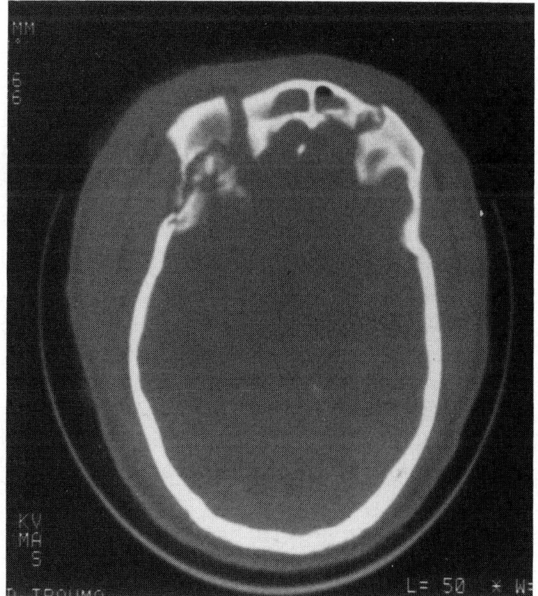

Figure 27–316. Complicated fracture of the frontal sinus (bilateral) and cranial base.

Frontal Sinus Fractures. The frontal si-

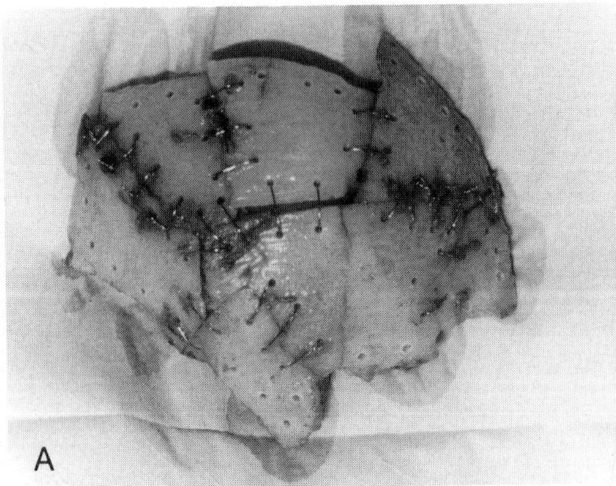

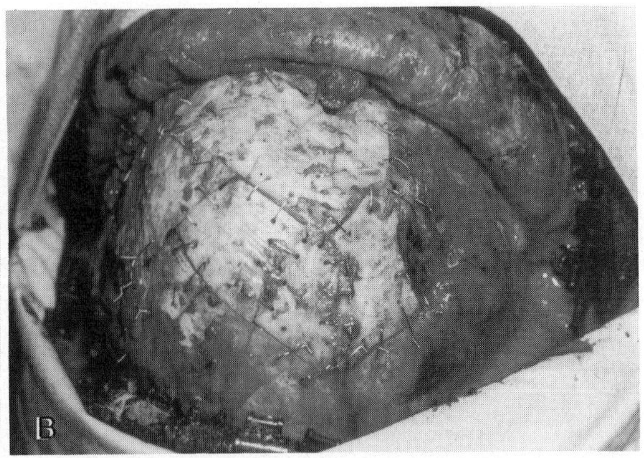

Figure 27–318. *A*, A mosaic of cranial bone fragments is reunited with interfragment wires. *B*, The fragments are replaced after completion of the neurosurgical portion of the procedure.

nuses are paired structures that have only an ethmoidal anlage at birth. They have no frontal bone component. They start to be detectable at 3 years of age but pneumatic expansion does not begin until approximately age 7 years; their full development is complete by the ages of 18 to 20 (Sataloff and associates, 1984) They are lined with respiratory epithelium, which consists of a ciliated membrane and mucus-secreting glands; the blanket of mucin is essential for normal function. The exact function of the paranasal sinuses is still incompletely determined. They serve as a focus for infection and protect the intracranial contents from injury (Sataloff and associates, 1984).

The predominant form of frontal sinus injury is fracture. Fracture involvement has been estimated to occur in 2 to 12 per cent of all cranial fractures, and severe fractures occur in 0.7 to 2 per cent of patients with cranial or cerebral trauma (Sataloff and associates, 1984). Approximately one-third involve the anterior table alone, and two-thirds involve the anterior table, posterior table, and/or ducts (Sataloff and associates, 1984). Forty per cent of frontal sinus fractures have an accompanying dural laceration (Sataloff and associates, 1984).

The signs that should signal frontal sinus injury include any blunt blow to the forehead. These are signified by lacerations, bruises, or hematoma. Anesthesia of a supraorbital nerve may be present. Cerebrospinal fluid rhinorrhea may occur. There may be subconjunctival ecchymosis with or without air in the orbit. In some cases a depression (Fig. 27–319) may be observed over the frontal sinus, but swelling is usually predominant in the first days after the injury. The fractures are demonstrated on radiographic examination; an air fluid level (Fig. 27–320) in the frontal sinus level may be observed, or pneumocephalus may occur. Small fractures may be difficult to detect on plain films; the first presentation of a frontal sinus fracture may be a frontal sinus obstruction (Fig. 27–321) with abscess formation (Donald and Bernstein, 1978; Remmler and Boles, 1980; Schilli, Ewers, and Niederdellmann, 1985).

Infection in the frontal sinus may produce quite serious complications (Donald and Bernstein, 1978; Remmler and Boles, 1980; Schilli, Ewers, and Niederdellmann, 1985), such as meningitis, extradural or intradural abscess, intracranial abscess, or osteomyelitis of the frontal bone.

The prevention of infectious and obstructive complications is emphasized in the management strategies for frontal sinus injury (Lehman, 1970; Hybels and Newman, 1977; Adkins, Cassone, and Putney, 1979; Peri and associates, 1981; Donald, 1982; Donald and Ettin, 1986). Close communication of the intracranial venous sinus system with the mucous membrane of the frontal sinus is a significant factor in both the production of osteomyelitis and the extension of the infectious processes into the intracranial cavity, cavernous sinus, and brain substance (Donald and Bernstein, 1978; Remmler and Boles, 1980; Schilli, Ewers, and Niederdellmann, 1985). The development of a frontal sinus mucocele is linked to obstruction of the nasofrontal duct, which is involved with fracture in over one-third to one-half of the cases of frontal sinus injury (Donald, 1979; Adekeye and Ord, 1984; Sataloff and associates, 1984). The duct passes through the anterior ethmoidal air cells to exit adjacent to the

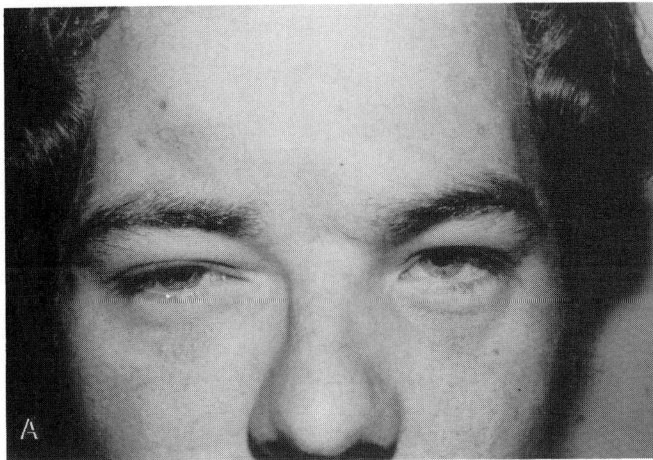

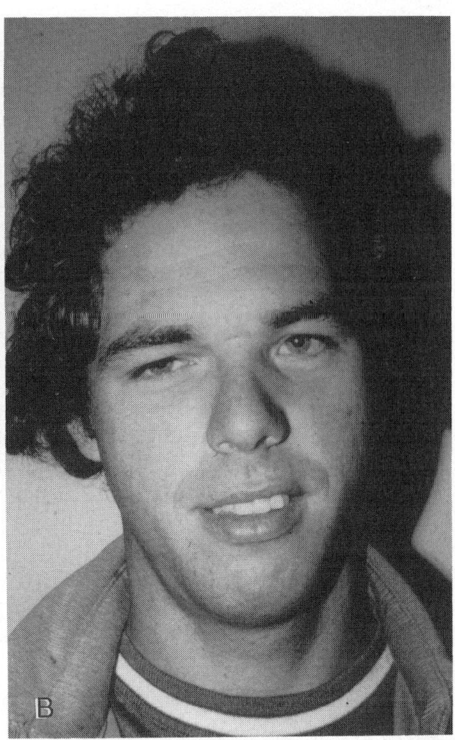

Figure 27–319. *A*, Depressed frontal sinus fracture that was not apparent because of overlying edema. The patient noticed the forehead depression several weeks after the injury. *B*, The result obtained following a coronal incision and primary reconstruction.

ethmoidal infundibulum. Blockage of the nasofrontal duct prevents adequate drainage of normal mucosal secretions and predisposes to the development of obstructive epithelia-lined cysts or mucoceles. Mucoceles may also develop when islands of mucosa are trapped by scar tissue or within fracture lines. When the mucous membrane of the sinus is eradicated except for the region of the duct, the sinus rapidly acquires a new mucosal cover (Schenck, 1975; Donald, 1979). The sinus is completely obliterated only when the duct is also deprived of its lining. With partial mucosal removal (Schenck, 1975; Donald, 1979), mucoceles form rapidly on the sinus walls or in the cavity, suggesting growth of loose frag-

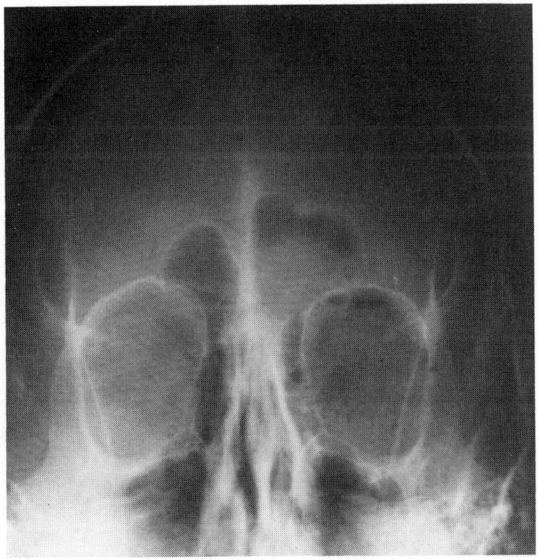

Figure 27–320. Unilateral fracture of the frontal sinus with obstruction and an air fluid level.

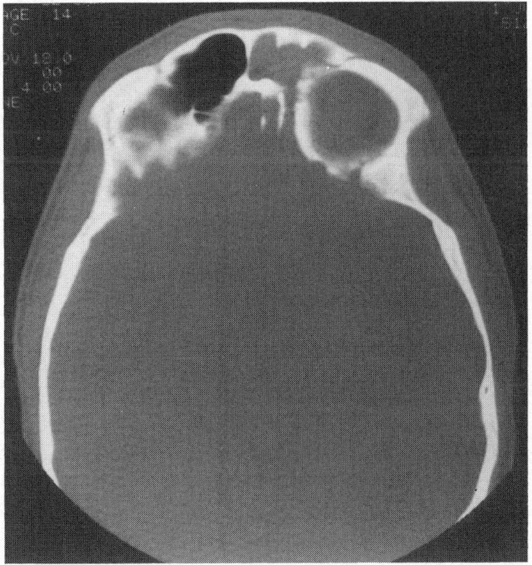

Figure 27–321. Fracture of the frontal sinus with evidence of obstruction.

ments of epithelium originating in the duct or from the sinus. Investigators consider that invaginations of mucosa along the channels of veins extending into the bone are the nidus for regrowth of the epithelium (Lehman, 1970; Donald, 1979). Thus, they recommend not only stripping of the mucoperiosteum, but burring of the surface of the bone to eliminate the mucosal invaginations.

Surgical Treatment of Frontal Sinus Fractures. In previous years a rather radical removal of bone or mucosal membrane was performed collapsing the skin against the dura (see Fig. 27–315). Indications for surgical intervention include depression of the anterior table, radiographic demonstration of involvement of the nasofrontal duct, obstruction of the duct, and fractures of the posterior table that may have lacerated the dura. Some authors recommend exploration of any posterior table fracture or any fracture in which an air fluid level is visible; others have a more selective approach. Simple linear fractures of the anterior or posterior sinus walls may be observed if undisplaced and there is no evidence of any air fluid accumulation or central nervous system involvement.

Any depressed fracture requires exploration, and obliterative procedures are recommended. The sinus is usually explored via a local laceration or a coronal incision. The anterior wall is removed and the mucous membrane thoroughly eradicated down into the nasofrontal duct area. The nasofrontal duct is occluded with a well-designed, "formed to fit" calvarial bone plug. If much of the bone wall is intact, the cavity can be filled with either fat (Larrabee, Travis, and Tabb, 1980; Donald and Ettin, 1986) or cancellous bone. Alternatively the cavity can be left vacant (the author's usual treatment); it fills with a combination of bone and fibrous tissue, a process called "osteoneogenesis." If the posterior table is missing, no grafting is performed, but it is emphasized that the floor of the anterior cranial fossa should be reconstructed with bone. Any involved ethmoidal sinus areas should be treated in the same fashion, removing abnormal injured mucosa and bone grafting the defect. Although some authors have found muscle and artificial material, such as methylmethacrylate, to be successful in frontal sinus treatment, the author prefers bone, and perhaps fat in *selected* cases in which the sinus walls are relatively intact. Fat acts to prevent the regrowth of epithelium and to fill the dead space. The fat is taken atraumatically from a remote donor site. The anterior wall of the sinus is replaced (Fig. 27–322), supplementing any bone defects with bone grafts. The final brow contour is dependent on the accuracy of the rim and frontal bone reconstruction and bone resorption (Fig. 27–323). The orbital roof should be accurately reconstructed with thin bone grafts. Primary reconstruction produces a more superior esthetic result than secondary reconstruction in most cases.

GUNSHOT WOUNDS OF THE FACE

The treatment of gunshot and shotgun wounds of the face remains controversial, many authors suggesting that immediate soft tissue closure and bone reconstruction be performed (Mladick, Georgiade, and Royer, 1970). Other authors have recommended that delay in closure and treatment is advisable (Broadbent and Woolf, 1972; May and associates, 1973; Finch and Dibbell, 1979; Goodstein, Stryker, and Weiner, 1979). Some have even questioned the possibility of effective rehabilitation of affected individuals (Goodman and Kalsbeck, 1965; May and associates, 1973; Hubschmann and associates, 1979). Recent experience has emphasized the safety and efficacy of immediate soft tissue closure and bone reconstruction in an anatomically correct position. Improved functional and esthetic results are obtained with shorter periods of disability and an improved potential

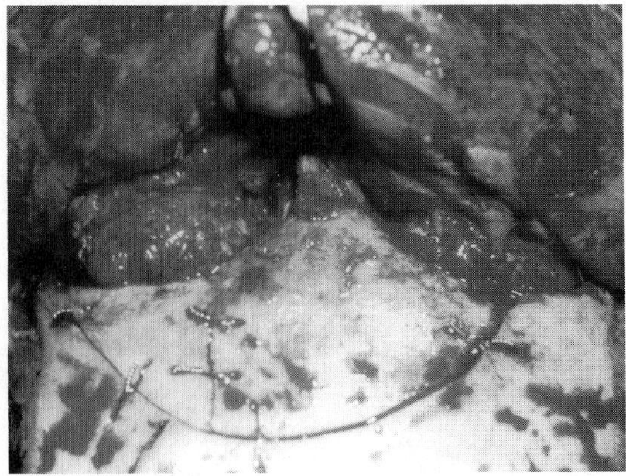

Figure 27–322. Frontal bone fragments are replaced with interfragment wiring after reconstruction of the cranial base with a bone plug. The frontal sinus mucosa has been thoroughly removed and the bone edges burred to eliminate microscopic invaginations of frontal sinus mucosa. Note the reflected scalp (coronal) flap.

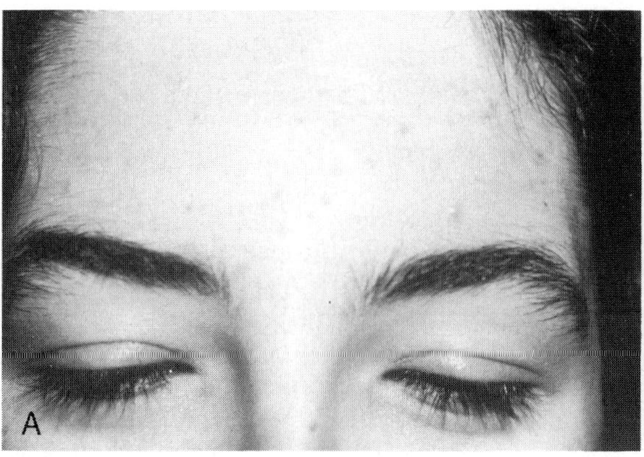

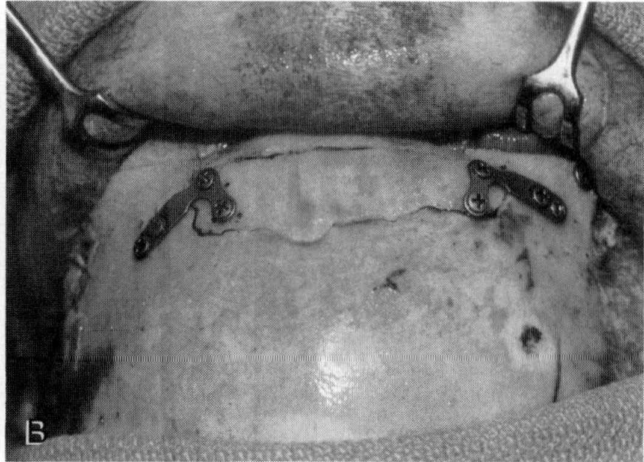

Figure 27–323. *A*, The result obtained after reconstruction of the frontal sinus. *B*, The anterior wall of the frontal sinus may be replaced with plate and screw fixation.

for rehabilitation. When proper surgical judgment is exercised, significant complications are not increased by an emphasis on early definitive treatment (primary soft tissue closure and immediate bone reconstruction).

All ballistic injuries to the face involve both soft tissue and bone injury. The degree of injury depends on the mass and speed of the projectile. Other factors can affect the injury, but the energy relates principally to the mass and speed of the projectile by the formula:

$$\text{Kinetic energy} = \text{mass} \times \text{velocity}^2 / 2\ \text{G}$$

If one doubles the velocity of a missile, one squares the kinetic energy. Mass is also important, since doubling the mass doubles the kinetic energy. Other factors influence tissue damage, such as tumbling of the projectile, the presenting area of the missile, drag, the density of the tissue, and the distance penetrated.

For ballistic weapons, "low energy deposit" projectiles have a limited mass and travel at speeds of less than 1000 feet per second. These include civilian hand guns, which create limited soft tissue injury. Shotgun pellets have a larger mass and are considered intermediate energy deposit projectiles. They travel at speeds of approximately 1200 feet per second, and when grouped in a close distribution at close ranges, are capable of causing considerable injury. If the pellets have spread apart (far distances), the soft tissue injury sustained is much reduced.

It should be emphasized that ballistic injuries often represent either assault or suicide attempts (Epsteen, 1958; Goodman and Kalsbeck, 1965; Broadbent and Woolf, 1972; May and associates, 1973). The pattern of injury is thus dependent on the location of the gun muzzle and the path of the projectile.

In *low velocity* injuries, the entrance wound of a bullet is generally a puncture hole corresponding roughly to the size of the projectile. When the bullet enters the tissue, it is deflected. The *yaw* (the angle between the axis of symmetry of the bullet and its line of flight) increases after deflection, and kinetic energy is transferred from the bullet to the tissue in all directions. The tissue continues to move outward until all the energy deposited by the bullet has been absorbed. Bullets approach a sidewise orientation at 90 or 270 degrees of yaw. The maximal *drag* and the greatest deposit of energy occur when a bullet is moving sideways. A pistol bullet with a sidewise orientation experiences three to five times the drag it has moving point first. Thus, as tissue density and resistance cause deflection and slowing of the bullet, energy is transferred to the tissue, and tissue damage increases as the drag increases. For these reasons, the path of the injury may enlarge as the bullet travels through tissues. Exit wounds may be larger than entrance wounds, depending on the velocity and orientation of the bullet. Tissue damage may increase along the tract of the projectile, depending on where the projectile deposits the energy. If the bullet path is short, entrance and exit wounds may be of similar size, as there has been little deflection of the bullet relative to its longitudinal axis or absorption of energy.

For low and intermediate velocity gunshot wounds, the kinetic energy imparted is smaller. The wound produced is associated with a zone of soft tissue and a zone of bone injury, and there is little significant tissue loss except in the exact path of the bullet. For high velocity wounds, the amount of tissue injury greatly increases, and both tissue and bone loss are present.

In formulating a treatment plan for ballistic injuries, it is helpful to identify the entrance and exit wounds and the path of the bullet, and to appreciate the mass and velocity of the projectile, so that the extent of the areas of tissue injury and tissue loss can be assessed. Both soft tissue and bone injury and loss must be assessed (four components), and the areas of injury and loss outlined precisely (Fig. 27–324).

LOW VELOCITY GUNSHOT WOUNDS

In general, low velocity gunshot wounds involve little soft tissue and bone loss and limited associated injury outside the exact path of the bullet. It is thus appropriate that they be treated with immediate stabilization of bone and primary soft tissue closure. In some cases, small amounts of bone may need to be debrided or replaced with primary bone grafting. Because of the lack of significant associated soft tissue injury, and little potential for progressive death and necrosis of soft tissue parts, these injuries may be treated as "facial fractures with overlying lacerations," both conceptually and practically. Four general anatomic injury types were realized after a review of patients experiencing low velocity wounds of the facial area (Fig. 27–324).

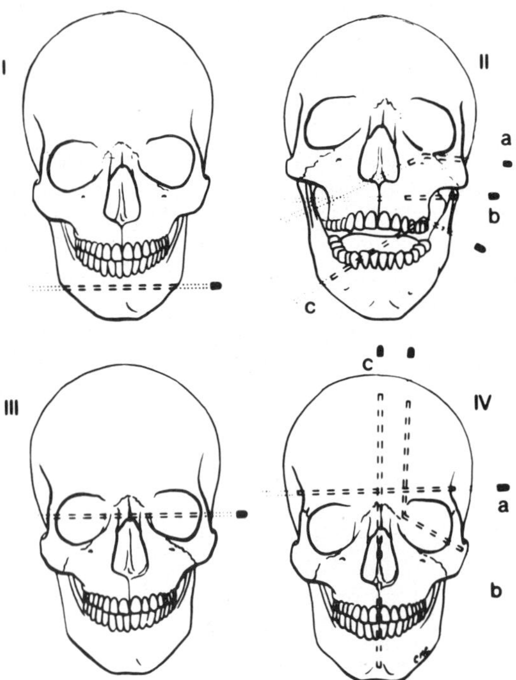

Figure 27–324. The patterns of gunshot wounds of the face. *I,* Lower facial wounds involve the mandibular area and tongue. *II,* Involvement of the lower midface and lower orbit constitutes the second pattern. *III,* The third pattern is involvement of the bilateral orbit and temporomandibular joint. *IV,* The final pattern involves the frontal bone and the orbit. Two characteristics should be determined: (1) the area of tissue loss and bone loss and (2) the area of tissue injury. Fractures in the area of tissue injury are managed as routine facial fractures. Those in the area of bone loss are managed with external fixation or primary bone replacement. The tracts *(interrupted lines)* described in a, b, and c are representative variations.

Lower Face. Injuries in this classification involve the tongue and the mandible (15 per cent of all facial gunshot wounds involve soft tissue alone). There is usually limited loss of mandibular structure, a finding that makes closed reduction and intermaxillary fixation feasible in one-half of the patients. Ramus and condylar injuries are well managed by a brief period of intermaxillary fixation with early mobilization. "Training" or nighttime elastics are sometimes used to maintain occlusion when simultaneous mobilization is necessary in the face of a tendency to malocclusion. One-fourth of the patients sustain sufficient injury to the tongue and floor of the mouth, along with marked edema, to threaten the airway. Either prolonged intubation or tracheostomy should be considered. Soft tissue injury is usually minimal in this classification. Entrance and exit wounds are excised and closed primarily with limited debridement of soft tissue along the bullet tract. Drainage of the tract is provided to limit infection. When open reduction is required, small fragments of bone are removed and interosseous wire or plate and screw fixation is used as part of the open reduction techniques (Fig. 27–325). In some patients, bone grafting may be necessary to strengthen the amount of bone present when a comminuted injury occurs. The decision to bone graft the defect either primarily or secondarily depends on the ability to establish a surgically clean wound without significant intraoral communication.

Midface. Gunshot injuries in this classification involve the lower midface. The maxillary alveolus and maxillary sinuses and lower portion of the nose and zygoma are often the only structures affected. In some cases, only a simple drainage of the maxillary sinuses is required. In other cases, open reduction and internal fixation of a limited maxillary or zygomatic fracture are necessary. Injuries to

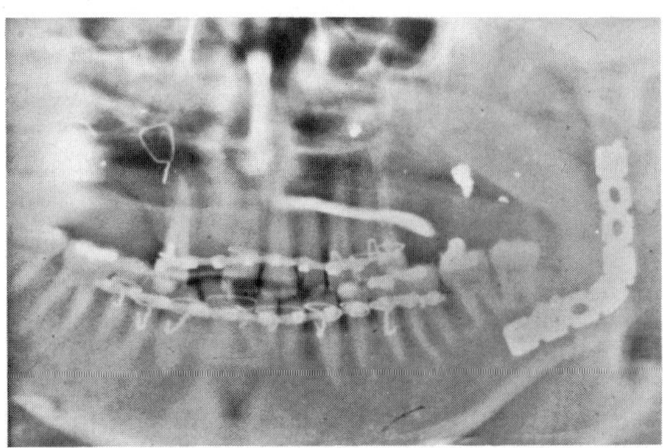

Figure 27–325. A reconstruction plate spans the bone fragments in a gunshot wound of the mandibular angle. The bone fragments can be "lagged" to the reconstruction plate, which extends from the condyle to the distal body.

the palate are closed with local flaps. Airway management must again be considered, depending on the degree of nasal and oral swelling. No bilateral maxillary fracture with mobility of the entire maxillary alveolus (Le Fort) is produced by a low velocity gunshot wound.

Orbital. Injuries in this classification involve the orbits and nasoethmoidal complex. The bullet often exits through the contralateral temporomandibular joint. All injuries are treated by open reduction and immediate bone grafting for replacement of significant orbital bone loss or support of orbital soft tissue. The thin structure of the orbital bones makes them less desirable than bone grafts after their crushing by a ballistic injury. Damage to the globe is present in almost 90 per cent of cases, with bilateral blindness in 50 per cent and unilateral blindness in 40 per cent. Careful ocular examination is thus imperative to detect fragments in the globe and periorbital soft tissue. Injury of the lacrimal system occurs in one-third and the disruption has been managed by primary simple intubation (Callahan, 1979) and secondary reconstruction. The temporomandibular joints are treated by open exploration or closed early fixation, depending on the presence of bullet fragments and the degree of comminution.

Craniofacial. Intracranial involvement characterizes this classification type. The supraorbital, orbital, frontal bone, and frontal sinus structures are involved. Appropriate neurosurgical debridement of dural or cerebral lacerations is important, with frontal sinus elimination by mucosal stripping and bone grafting of the nasofrontal duct. Immediate bone grafting of frontal defects should be performed. Globe or optic nerve injury is present in 40 per cent, with blindness in 25 per cent.

INTERMEDIATE AND HIGH VELOCITY BALLISTIC INJURIES TO THE FACE

Intermediate and high velocity ballistic injuries to the face must be managed with a specific treatment plan that involves stabilization of existing bone in an anatomic position and maintenance of this bone stabilization throughout the period of soft tissue and bone reconstruction. Wounds from intermediate and high energy missiles usually demonstrate areas of both soft tissue and bone loss as well as areas of soft tissue and bone injury. Usually, less loss is present than is first suspected. It is important to have a low threshold for "second look" surgical procedures in order to define additional soft tissue necrosis and reassess the absence of hematoma or developing areas of abscess formation. These procedures are imperative for high velocity injuries if primary reconstruction is attempted. Thus, the emphasis is on primary soft tissue closure and stabilization of existing bone fragments, with reexploration for possible additional debridement at 48 hour intervals until the soft tissue loss ceases and the entire wound is controlled. Many of these injuries in civilian practice represent shotgun wounds, and they frequently result from suicide attempts. Close range shotgun wounds are often characterized by extensive soft tissue and bone destruction. The management depends on the anatomic area of the injury, and four specific patterns have been recognized (Fig. 27–326).

Central Lower Face. This injury is characterized by loss of the central portion of the mandible, maxilla, and skin of the lips. The mandibular bone loss should be managed by external fixation or plate and screw reconstruction of the remaining portions of the mandible in anatomic position. The plate and screw fixation technique can be utilized if soft tissue cover of the plate can be obtained. Usually, soft tissue closure can be accomplished primarily with some decrease in the length of the lip structure. At a later time, local flap replacement of lip structure provides the best esthetic result. If local flaps are not possible, regional flaps can be employed. After the soft tissue has been repaired, the maxillary and mandibular bone deficiencies may be reconstructed. It is im-

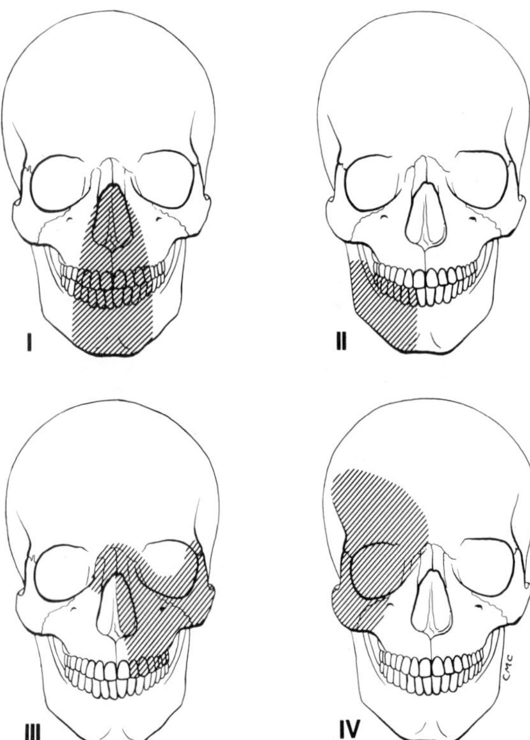

Figure 27–326. Patterns of soft tissue and bone loss in shotgun injuries. The extent of tissue injury actually extends far beyond the areas of tissue loss, here demonstrated by shaded areas. *I*, Central mandibular and midface soft tissue and bone loss. *II*, Lateral mandibular soft tissue and bone loss. *III*, Maxillary and orbital soft tissue and bone loss. *IV*, Orbital and cranial soft tissue and bone loss.

portant that the anatomic position of the remaining segments of the maxilla and the mandible be held throughout the period of soft tissue and bone reconstruction in order to limit the magnitude of the deformity. In extensive soft tissue loss, when primary skin and mucosal repair cannot be accomplished, a skin to mucosa closure is recommended for wound closure. Reexploration may be necessary at 48 hour intervals to identify additional devitalized tissue, remove hematoma, and prepare the wound for reconstruction.

Lower Lateral Face. The most frequently observed shotgun injury is characterized by loss of a lateral mandibular segment and surrounding soft tissue (Fig. 27–327). These patients can usually be managed by primary soft tissue closure by advancement flaps after limited debridement. Nylon should be used for intraoral closure. External fixation or reconstruction plate and screw fixation can be used to span the mandibular bone gap or comminuted mandibular segments. After intraoral soft tissue closure is completed, the bone can be reconstructed by bone grafting. Facial nerve injuries should be repaired primarily or as soon as feasible.

Midface. Injuries in this classification type involve the maxilla, zygoma, orbits, and maxillary sinuses. The nasoethmoido-orbital region is involved in all cases. When fractures are present, they are managed as routine facial fractures with bone loss. Immediate bone grafting of the orbital and nasal defects is recommended. There is rarely significant loss of skin preventing primary closure, but there is often significant loss of maxillary sinus lining. The reconstruction can involve either interosseous wire or plate and screw fixation.

In each classification a zone of injury is identified where fractures are present *without* significant bone or soft tissue loss. Fractures in this area are managed as routine facial fractures. When soft tissue and bone loss are present, it is important to stabilize existing bone in its anatomic position until soft tissue reconstruction can be accomplished. In some cases, it may be possible to plan more complex reconstruction of soft tissue and bone by a single procedure with free composite tissue transfer (Fig. 27–328). The use of local tissue for soft tissue reconstruction (such as a local flap) usually provides the best esthetic result. Distant flaps tend to have a less satisfactory color and contour match.

Significant wounds of the maxillary sinus are subject to skin breakdown after primary closure under tension. When there is considerable destruction of the maxillary sinus area, consideration should be given to obliteration of this area with a flap reconstruction (Fig. 27–328). A distant flap, like an omental flap, can be used to fill in defects so that the remaining soft tissue can be brought over this well-vascularized bed. When both lining and bone in the maxillary sinus are significantly destroyed, the underlying oronasal fistula usually erodes through the less vascularized skin eventually unless proper lining is present. The soft tissue flap obliteration of the maxillary sinus area provides this type of lining. Persons who sustain significant injury to the midface should be considered candidates for arteriography to define carotid artery integrity. The emphasis remains on primary closure of soft tissue and primary reconstruction of the existing bone in its anatomic position. Nonabsorbable intraoral sutures are recommended.

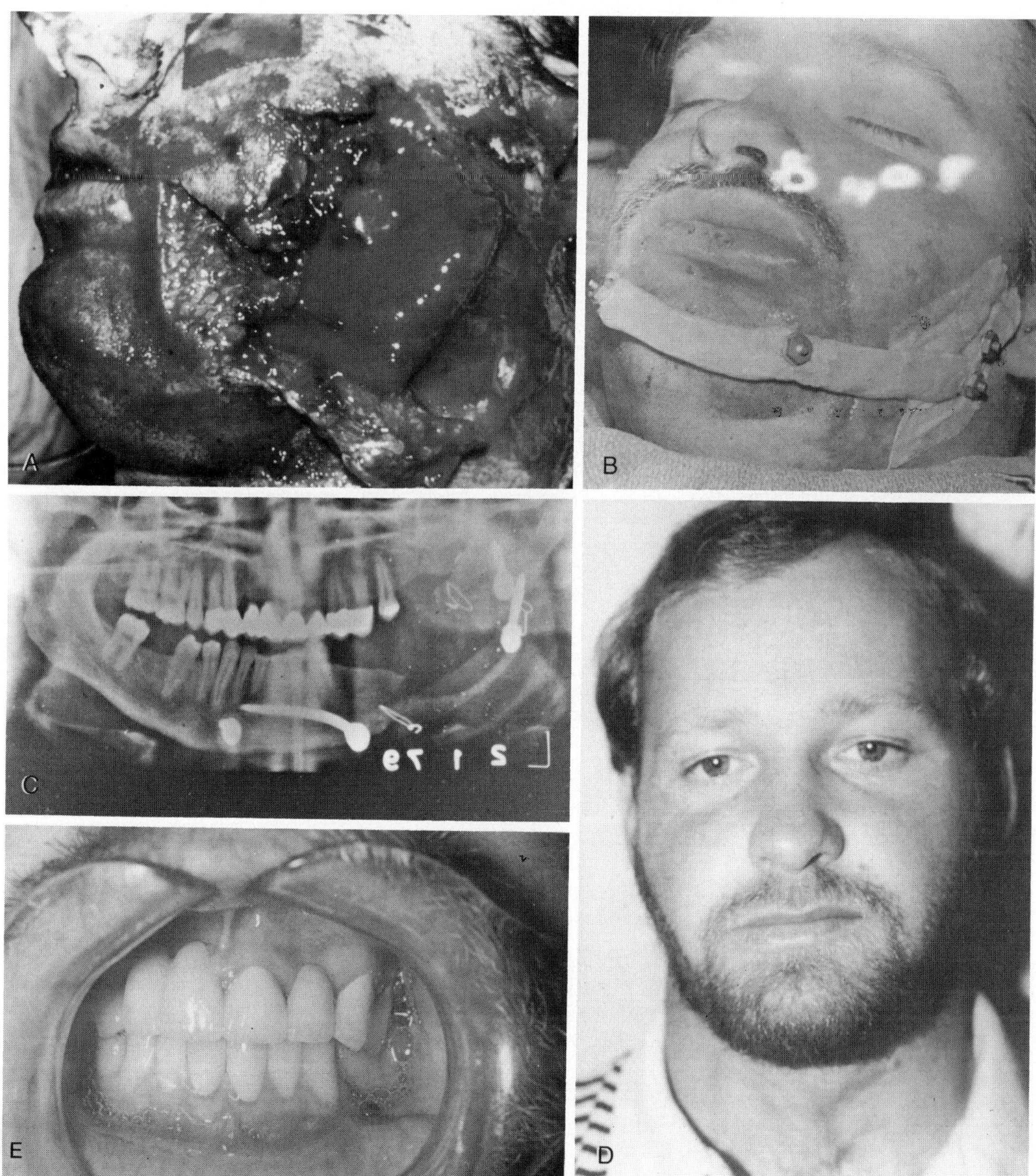

Figure 27–327. *A*, Shotgun wound of the left cheek and mandible with bone loss. *B*, Closure of the wound accomplished and the remaining mandibular fragments stabilized with an external fixation device (Morris biphasic appliance). *C*, Reconstruction of the missing segment of the mandible with an iliac bone graft. *D*, Postoperative appearance. *E*, Restoration of the occlusion.

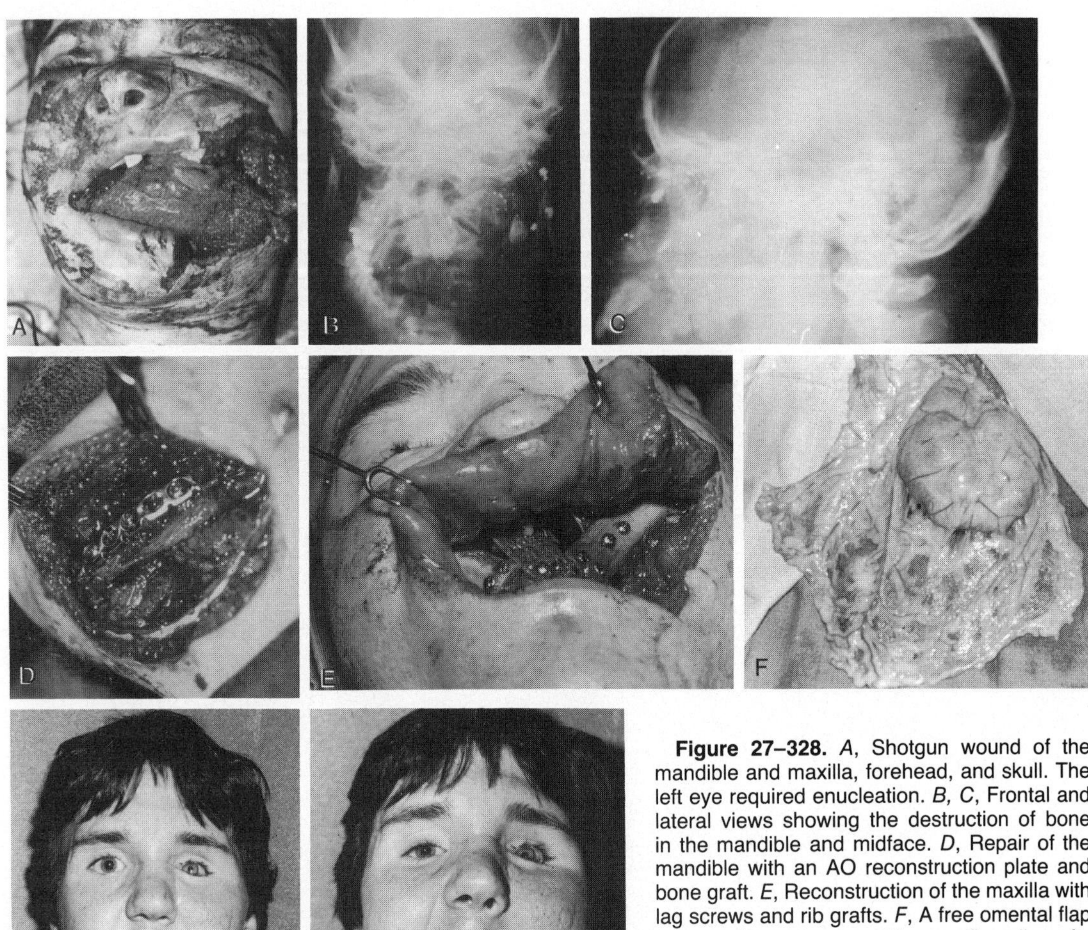

Figure 27–328. *A*, Shotgun wound of the mandible and maxilla, forehead, and skull. The left eye required enucleation. *B, C*, Frontal and lateral views showing the destruction of bone in the mandible and midface. *D*, Repair of the mandible with an AO reconstruction plate and bone graft. *E*, Reconstruction of the maxilla with lag screws and rib grafts. *F*, A free omental flap was used to wrap around the maxillary rib grafts in this patient with a severe deficit of maxillary sinus lining. *G, H*, Result obtained.

Craniofacial Injuries. Injuries in this classification type involve the cranium and the upper third of the face, including the orbit, globe, frontal bone, and frontal sinus area. They may be characterized by intracranial involvement, and thus carry a worse prognosis. There may be associated injuries of the nasoethmoido-orbital complex and frontal sinus. A primary reconstruction by open reduction and bone grafting and sinus elimination is recommended. The involved globe may need to be enucleated. The actual soft tissue skin deficit is usually less extensive in the upper facial injuries, but in some patients flap reconstruction of significant orbital skin and bone loss is required to "blank out" the defect.

Patients with gunshot or shotgun wounds of the face are often presumed to have significant soft tissue and bone injury that precludes immediate reconstruction. In fact, while the zone of soft tissue and bone injury is quite extensive, the area of actual loss is limited with little tissue injury and loss in low velocity injuries. It is reasonable and effective to approach low velocity injuries in the same manner as comminuted facial fractures with overlying facial lacerations. Fractures in the zone of injury are managed with early or immediate internal fixation, using interosseous wires or plate and screw fixation. Bone grafting in the middle and upper face is successful in almost any injury. This treatment plan has not resulted in an increased infection rate or in dramatically increased complications. In low velocity injuries, the lacerations (entrance and exit wounds) are excised and closed over a drain.

Intermediate velocity gunshot or shotgun wounds benefit from a limited initial debridement with frequent "second look" operations for debridement at 24 or 48 hour intervals, to ensure that all soft tissue is viable and that no hematoma, abscess, or progressive tissue necrosis exists. In more extensive injuries, a larger zone of soft tissue and bone injury is defined, and treatment can be accomplished in the usual manner as for comminuted facial fractures with overlying lacerations. The zones of soft tissue and bone loss should also be identified. The treatment should emphasize anatomic stabilization of existing bone fragments in the correct position and early soft tissue reconstruction by local or regional flap transfer. Bone reconstruction can then proceed. Such operative management is successful in reducing the ultimate disability of patients sustaining these severe injuries.

After successful reconstruction, it is unusual for any patients to pursue another suicide attempt. They benefit from constant psychiatric monitoring during periodic manifestations of the problems that led to the suicide attempt. The prognosis with regard to a return to a functional role in society depends on the psychiatric rehabilitation and on the limitation of facial deformity. For these reasons, it is imperative that consideration be given to maximizing the esthetic result, which requires primary definitive soft tissue and bone reconstruction.

POST-TRAUMATIC FACIAL PAIN

(Rewritten from Crockford, 1977)

Pain is an uncommon chronic symptom following repair of facial trauma; it often represents a complication of treatment. Pain may be persistent and disabling and may result in drug addiction.

Nerve injuries invariably accompany facial fractures. The nerves pass through bone, creating areas of weakness that are the sites of fracture. Various types of nerve injuries can result, and correspond to Seddon's (1943) classification of neuropraxia, axonotmesis, and neurotmesis. It is likely that facial pain is produced by mechanisms similar to those described for peripheral nerves (Melzack and Wall, 1965; Wilson, 1974; Speculand and associates, 1979). Cranial nerves may be cut, crushed, or otherwise injured by facial fractures. Traction injuries produced by the traumatic injury are conceivable. After fracture, bone proliferation and scar tissue formation may further compromise the injured nerve. A nerve frequently subjected to injury is the inferior alveolar, passing through the mandible, and exiting at the mental foramen. Most mandibular angle and body fractures result in trauma to this nerve. If transection has not occurred, considerable recovery can be anticipated (90 to 95 per cent).

The external nasal nerve may be injured as it emerges between the nasal bone and upper lateral cartilage (McNeill, 1963).

The infraorbital nerve is invariably injured in orbital floor and zygomatic fractures. The zygomaticofacial or zygomaticotemporal nerve may be injured as well and result in pain experienced near the superior portion of the orbit, in the temple, or in the malar eminence. The pain can be disabling. Barclay (1960) documented infraorbital nerve damage in over 80 per cent of fractures of the zygoma. Persistent sensory disturbance has been documented by Tajima (1977) and Nordgaard (1976), frequently involving the anterior maxillary teeth. Although recovery of sensation occurs after fracture, the recovery is usually incomplete.

The supraorbital and supratrochlear nerves are also at risk as they pass through a groove or canal in the superior portion of the orbit. Frontal contusions often damage these nerves, impacting them between the injuring object and the unyielding frontal bone.

Considering the frequency of facial fractures, it is truly remarkable that pain is not a more prominent chronic symptom of facial injuries. In fractures demonstrating nonunion or malposition, one can understand how nerve function may be disturbed. On histologic examination, intraneural fibrosis and axonal disturbances have been documented following trauma to peripheral nerves. Intraneural scarring is common; however, it has not been possible to correlate fibrosis and axonal disturbances with the severity of clinical symptoms.

Melzack and Wall (1965) emphasized the distinctions between central and peripheral pain, and postulated a "gate theory" that explains the electrophysiologic manifestation of pain. Neuromas or nerve entrapment obviously may produce pain by the pressure or constriction of sensory axons by collagen. Peripheral nerves have been demonstrated to be inflamed and swollen to several centimeters proximal to the site of such injuries. Histologic examination confirms scar tissue between the nerve fibers. Peripheral pain, uncontrolled for several months, usually spreads centrally to become established in a self-perpetuating neuronal circuit that makes relief very challenging.

The usual patient with chronic facial pain has a history of a well-defined injury that is capable of producing sensory disturbance in an anatomic distribution of a sensory nerve. An occasional patient does not remember a trivial injury, and thus presents more diagnostic difficulty.

In the great majority of patients with damage to the facial sensory nervous system, there is a history of a recognizable event, with anesthesia or hypoesthesia in the anatomic distribution of a cutaneous sensory nerve. Sensation may be partially recovered or accompanied by paresthesias.

The dysesthesias may become more severe, preventing the patient from touching the affected area. The pain precipitated may be by physical or psychologic stimuli. Attacks of pain may occur with response to cold or wind, or to touching the affected point. They may be spontaneous with no precipitating cause. The pain may spread to involve areas other than the original area affected. In some patients, the skin may have a reddish-bluish cast and be cool to the touch, with hyperactive vasomotor activity simulating the causalgia that occurs in peripheral extremities. The onset of pain may be immediate, but in most cases it develops as a slow, chronic sequela to the original injury. Most patients are able to relate a slow exacerbation of the pain over a period of weeks after their injury.

Recent developments bring new understanding to the physiology of pain pathways and to the complex interrelationships that neurotransmitters provide regarding the nature of chronic pain and the potential for medical intervention. Because the roots of sensory nerves transmit pain impulses in serial fashion to the brain, neurotransmitting chemicals can mediate the impulses. Thus, they represent specific targets for intervention within the nervous system. Chronic pain physiology overlaps into spheres of perception and complex bichemical mechanisms, such as the indolamine-catecholamine balance and endogenous opioid system. These biochemical systems modulate pain and its emotional components (Hendler, 1982; Hendler and associates, 1987).

For many years it was felt that there were no specific nerves for the mediation of pain. Pain was thought to result from overstimulation of nerve receptors. It is now conceived that small, unmyelinated C-fibers and A-delta fibers carry pain impulses from specialized nerve endings that function as pain sensors in skin, blood vessels, muscles, and other organs (Hendler, 1982; Hendler and associates, 1987). Two types of pain have been identified: "fast" and "slow," constituting the initial pain felt acutely by patients. The described afferent pain fibers travel to the spinal cord, where they synapse with chemical transmitters involved in the relay of neural signals. The free nerve endings are unmyelinated and are extremely sensitive to mechanical, thermal, or chemical signals. In damaged tissue, "pain" messages may be transmitted. The substances (such as histamine, serotonin, and prostaglandin) are released following injuries and may make sensory nerves more excitable. The A-delta and C-fibers travel in myelinated bundles of 10 to 50 nerves from visceral receptors to reach the dorsal horn (Hendler, 1982; Hendler and associates, 1987). They relay their messages into one of six laminae, usually laminae 1 and 5, and possibly 4 and 6 (Hendler, 1982; Hendler and associates, 1987). In these laminae, there is a mixture of visceral and cutaneous pain signals that may serve as the basis for referred pain. Ascending fibers travel across the gray matter of the spinal cord to the lateral spinothalamic tract in the white matter. Descending excitatory fibers also travel from the lamina. The lateral spinothalamic tract transmits pain signals from the dorsal horn via the medial lemniscus to the thalamus, and fibers ascend to the cortex. Synapses are involved in the medulla, the reticular activating system, the thalamus, and the hypothalamus and in other parts of the limbic system (Hendler, 1982; Hendler and associates, 1987). As pain evolves from an acute to a chronic prolonged state, various ancillary fiber pathways are utilized, and diverse areas of the brain become involved in the perception and modulation of the pain response.

Synapses are a junction point between two nerves. They consist of a presynaptic portion of a nerve that transmits the incoming signals, a synaptic cleft or gap, and a postsynaptic receptor area, which is connected to another nerve cell. Neurosynaptic transmitter factors are manufactured in synaptic vesicles. The nerve electrical impulses change membrane permeability, allowing neurotransmitters to diffuse across the synaptic cleft to affect the receptor sites. These activate an area of the next nerve cell. Some chemicals mimic the action of neurosynaptic transmitters and are called agonists, occupying the same receptor site as the neutrally occurring chemical. Substances that block or otherwise inhibit the production, transmission, or reception of the neurosynaptic transmitters are called antagonists.

Although numerous neurotransmitter substances are known to exist, indolamines, catecholamines, and enkephalin-endorphins are compounds considered important in the psychopharmacology of chronic pain. The biogenic amines (such as norepinephrine, dopamine, and L-dopa), and the endolamines, such as serotonin, account for 2 to 5 per cent of the neurotransmitters in the nervous system. Most biogenic amine transmitters are found in the hypothalamus, the median forebrain, and the reticular activating system. These structures, as part of the limbic system, are believed to play an important role in the mediation and emotional perception of chronic pain. The enkephalins are endogenous pentapeptides that act on the morphine receptors within the central nervous system. They are also found in high concentration within the limbic system. Specific receptors for the endogenously produced substances have been localized to the spinal cord and brain. Stimulation of areas known to be high in the neurotransmitter enkephalins produces analgesia (Hendler, 1982; Hendler and associates, 1987). The effect persists beyond the time of stimulation, indicating that enzyme induction has been involved. The compound serotonin is also associated with the activity of the enkephalins. The "pain threshold" has been raised by blocking the reuptake of serotonin with tricyclic antidepressants, such as doxepin or amytriptyline or by augmenting the production with a precursor (L-tryptophan) (Hendler, 1982; Hendler and associates, 1987). Catecholamines, such as norepinephrine, are also involved in analgesia. When dopamine, a direct precursor of norepinephrine and itself a neurotransmitter, is increased, analgesia is enhanced. If a dopamine antagonist is used, analgesia is diminished (Hendler, 1982; Hendler and associates, 1987). Dopamine appears to be a component in the enkephalin-associated analgesia, and it antagonizes the activity of norepinephrine.

Methods of pain treatment may be surgical or medical. In each case, the effects and the treatment may be either local, systemic, or central. Before specific pain treatment is continued on a chronic basis, it must be understood that other causes of pain (such as a fracture non-union) have been removed as obvious excitatory conditions.

TREATMENT

The most important responsibility of the physician is that patients developing chronic pain syndromes be recognized and given the appropriate specialized careful management that can abort the "vicious cycle" pain syndrome. Patients with pain confined to a specific area of the face are relatively easy to recognize as their pain increases. A second group have diffuse pain that spreads to adjacent areas and is not confined to a specific anatomically identifiable distribution, and these tend to be more anxious and difficult. It is absolutely essential to incorporate a competent and understanding psychologist or psychiatrist in treatment. It is also essential to rule out causes of pain that might be alleviated by medical or surgical means and that do not have an entirely psycho-physiologic basis for the exacerbation. Some simple treatments should be begun that may start the cycle of relief. All aggravating factors, medical, psychologic, financial, and emotional, must be taken into account when decisions are made about the treatment plan.

Nerve Block. Diagnostically and therapeutically, a local nerve block in the anatomic distribution of an affected sensory nerve is one of the most helpful maneuvers. These injections, if effective, have prognostic value, as they indicate that the performance of successive blocks may decrease the symptomatic reaction to the pain. The self-perpetuating pain cycle may be alleviated and the patient provided with much needed rest. The relief often occurs for a longer period than may be expected from the effect of the local anesthetic alone. The use of long-acting anesthetics, such as bupivacaine (Marcaine) with epinephrine, is worthwhile. Some clinicians prefer to add a small amount of soluble steroid to the pain medication to decrease inflammation. Crockford (1977) administered small doses of a soluble steroid (triamcinolone hexacetonide) to treat painful neuromas of the hand. Other clinicians considered the steroid compounds to be more active against immature than against mature collagen (Pataky, Graham, and Munger, 1973). The emphasis should be on early treatment. The series of injections are usually given at biweekly to monthly intervals until sufficient relief is obtained and the cycle is broken. Even if a first injection does not have much activity, a second may sometimes have a greater effect. In patients who demonstrate coolness or sweating of the affected area, a diagnostic and therapeutic trial of sympathetic block (stellate ganglion block) is indicated. A course of several blocks in two weeks should be given. Although surgical treatment of the superior cervical sympathetic ganglion has been described, the use of serial blocks is equally effective. Most clinicians have avoided the use of more active therapies, such as phenyl alcohol block of peripheral nerves involved in post-traumatic pain, believing that these agents cause further damage to the affected cutaneous nerves.

Medical systemic treatment is a necessary accompaniment to the injections. The patient should be immediately started on a regimen consisting of a minor analgesic, an antihistamine such as diphenhydramine hydrochloride (Benadryl), and a medication for sleep. Sleep is essential and may require the use of an antidepressant with a marked hypnotic effect. Some clinicians give carbamazepine (Tegretol) for its effect in trigeminal neuralgia and migraine, but the possibility of serious side effects, such as liver damage and blood dyscrasias, must be considered before resorting to its use.

Surgery. Occasionally, neurolysis of a nerve, such as might be involved in an area of fracture compression, is of value, even years after the injury. The author has decompressed infraorbital nerves years after the zygomatic fracture, releasing the nerve completely from the foramen and into the orbital groove by completing the decompression through the canal. This operation should always be considered in patients in whom disabling painful total anesthesia persists a year or more after the injury. The decompression should be accompanied by neurolysis, and some clinicians prefer to apply a local steroid to the nerve.

Neurotomy has also been used to treat chronic pain, although a high recurrence rate is reported in most series. Some clinicians have given a local steroid to decrease the inflammatory response (Pataky, Graham, and Munger, 1973).

In cases in which the symptoms mimic causalgia, a chemical block sympathectomy of the affected area has been employed. More complex neurosurgical procedures, such as are used for trigeminal neuralgia, may be successful in selected cases.

REFERENCES

Adams, W. M.: Internal wiring fixation of facial fractures. Surgery, *12*:523, 1942.

Adams, W. M., and Adams, L. H.: Internal wire fixation of facial fractures: a 15 year follow-up report. Am. J. Surg., *92*:12, 1956.

Adekeye, E. O., and Ord, R. A.: Giant frontal sinus mucocoele. J. Maxillofac. Surg., *12*:184, 1984.

Adkins, W. Y., Cassone, R. D., and Putney, F. J.: Solitary frontal sinus fracture. Laryngoscope, *89*:1099, 1979.

Allgöwer, M.: Progress in Surgery. Vol. 9. Basel, Karger, 1970.

Altonen, M., Kohonen, A., and Dickhoff, K.: Treatment of zygomatic fractures: internal wiring-antral-packing-reposition without fixation. J. Maxillofac. Surg., *4*:107, 1976.

Amaratunga, N. A.: The effect of teeth in the line of mandibular fractures on healing. J. Oral Maxillofac. Surg., *45*:312, 314, 1987a.

Amaratunga, N. A.: Mouth opening after release of maxillomandibular fixation in fracture patients. J. Oral Maxillofac. Surg., *45*:383, 1987b.

Amaratunga, N. A.: The relation of age to the immobilization period required for healing of mandibular fractures. J. Oral Maxillofac. Surg., *45*:111, 1987c.

Anderson, R.: An ambulatory method of treating fractures of the shaft of the femur. Surg. Gynecol. Obstet., *62*:865, 1936.

Anderson, R. L.: The medial canthal tendon branches out. Arch. Ophthalmol., *95*:2051, 1977.

Anderson, R. L., Panje, W. R., and Gross, C. E.: Optic nerve blindness following blunt forehead trauma. Ophthalmology, *89*:445, 1982.

Angle, E. H.: Classification of malocclusion. Dent. Cosmos, *41*:240, 1899.

Aronowitz, J. A., Freeman, B. S., and Spira, M.: Long-term stability of Teflon orbital implants. Plast. Reconstr. Surg., *78*:166, 1986.

Ayella, R. J.: The face. *In* Ayella, R. J.: Radiologic Management of the Massively Traumatized Patient. Baltimore, The Williams & Wilkins Company, 1978, p. 33.

Babcock, J. L.: Cervical spine injuries. Diagnosis and classification. Arch. Surg., *111*:646, 1976.

Bales, C. R., Randall, P., and Lehr, H. B.: Fractures of the facial bones in children. J. Trauma, *12*:56, 1972.

Ballen, P. H.: Further experiments with rapidly polymerizing methylmethacrylate in orbital floor fractures. Plast. Reconstr. Surg., *34*:624, 1964.

Barclay, T. L.: Diplopia in association with fractures of the zygomatic bone. Br. J. Plast. Surg., *11*:147, 1958.

Barclay, T. L.: Four hundred malar-zygomatic fractures. Trans. Int. Soc. Plast. Surg. 2nd Congress. Edinburgh, Livingstone, 1960, pp. 259–265.

Barclay, T. L.: Some aspects of treatment of traumatic diplopia. Br. J. Plast. Surg., *16*:214, 1963.

Bartkowski, S. B., and Krzystkowa, K. M.: Blow out fracture of the orbit. Diagnostic and therapeutic considerations, and results in 90 patients. J. Maxillofac. Surg., *10*:155, 1982.

Barton, F. E., and Berry, W. L.: Evaluation of the acutely injured orbit. *In* Aston, S. J., Hornblass, A., Meltzer, M. A., and Rees, T. D. (Eds.): Third International Symposium of Plastic and Reconstructive Surgery of the Eye and Adnexa. Baltimore, Williams & Wilkins Company, 1982, p. 34.

Baudens, J. B.: Fracture de la machoire inférieure. Bull. Acad. Med. Paris, *5*:341, 1840.

Becker, D. P., Miller, J. D., Ward, J. D., Greenberg, R. P., Young, H. F., and Sakalas, R.: The outcome from severe head injury with early diagnosis and intensive management. J. Neurosurg., *47*:491, 1977.

Berry, H. C.: Fractures of the edentulous maxilla and mandible. J. Ark. Dent. Assoc., *10*:7, 1939.

Bite, U., Jackson, I. T., Forbes, G. S., and Gehring, D.: Orbital volume measurements using three-dimensional CT imaging. Plast. Reconstr. Surg., *75*:502, 1985.

Block, M. S., Zide, M. F., and Kent, J. N.: Proplast augmentation for posttraumatic zygomatic deficiency. Oral Surg. Oral Med. Oral Pathol., *57*:123, 1984.

Bochlogyros, P. N.: A retrospective study of 1,521 mandibular fractures. J. Oral Maxillofac. Surg., *43*:597, 1985a.

Bochlogyros, P. N.: Non-union of fractures of the mandible. J. Maxillofac. Surg., *13*:189, 1985b.

Bonanno, P. C., and Converse, J. M.: Primary bone grafting in management of facial fractures. N.Y. State J. Med., *75*:710, 1975.

Bowsher, D.: Central mechanisms of orofacial pain. Br. J. Oral Surg., *17*:185, 1979.

Brawley, B. W., and Kelly, W. A.: Treatment of basal skull fractures with and without cerebrospinal fluid fistulae. J. Neurosurg., *26*:57, 1967.

Broadbent, T. R., and Woolf, R. M.: Gunshot wounds of the face: initial care. J. Trauma, *12*:229, 1972.

Brown, J. B., Fryer, M. P., and McDowell, F.: Internal wire-pin immobilization of jaw fractures. Plast. Reconstr. Surg., *4*:30, 1949.

Browning, C. W., and Walker, R. V.: The use of alloplasties in 75 cases of orbital floor reconstruction. Am. J. Ophthalmol., *60*:684, 1965.

Bucholz, R. W., Burkhead, W. Z., Graham, W., and Petty, C.: Occult cervical spine injuries in fatal traffic accidents. J. Trauma, *19*:768, 1979.

Cadenat, H., Combelles, R., Boutault, F., and Hemous, J. D.: Osteosynthesis of subcondylar fractures in the adult. J. Maxillofac. Surg., *11*:20, 1983.

Cahill, D. W., Rao, K. C., and Ducker, T. B.: Delayed carotid-cavernous sinus fistula and multiple cranial neuropathy following basal skull fracture. Surg. Neurol., *16*:17, 1981.

Callahan, M. A.: Silicone intubation for lacrimal canaliculi repair. Ann. Plast. Surg., *2*:355, 1979.

Cambell, D. A.: Discussion. *In* Glas, W. W., King, O. J., Jr., and Lui, A.: Complications of tracheostomy. Arch. Surg., *85*:156, 1962.

Champy, M., Lodde, J. P., Schmidt, R., Jaeger, J. H., and Muster, D.: Mandibular osteosynthesis by miniature screwed plates via a buccal approach. J. Maxillofac. Surg., *6*:14, 1978.

Chan, R. N., Ainscow, D., and Sikorski, J. M.: Diagnostic failures in the multiply injured. J. Trauma, *20*:684, 1980.

Chayra, G. A., Meador, L. R., and Laskin, D. M.: Comparison of panoramic and standard radiographs in the diagnosis of mandibular fractures. J. Oral Maxillofac. Surg., *44*:677, 1986.

Christian, M. S.: Non-fatal injuries sustained by seatbelt wearers: a comparative study. Br. Med. J., *2*:1310, 1976.

Chuong, R., and Donoff, R. B.: Intraoral open reduction of mandibular fractures. Int. J. Oral Surg., *14*:22, 1985.

Chuong, R., Donoff, R. B., and Guralnick, W. C.: A retrospective analysis of 327 mandibular fractures. J. Oral Maxillofac. Surg., *41*:305, 1983.

Collin, J. R. O.: Management of established enophthalmos with a seeing eye. Trans. Ophthalmol. Soc. U.K., *102*:98, 1982.

Collins, W. F.: Physiology of pain. *In* Youmans, J. R. (Ed.): Neurological Surgery. 2nd Ed. Vol. 2. Philadelphia, W. B. Saunders Company, 1982.

Converse, J. M.: Orbital and naso-orbital fractures. *In* Tessier, P., Callahan, A., Mustardé, J. C., and Salyer, K. E. (Eds.): Symposium on Plastic Surgery in the Orbital Region. St. Louis, C. V. Mosby Company, 1976, p. 79.

Converse, J. M., and Bonanno, P. C.: *In* Kazanjian, V. H., and Converse, J. M.: Surgical Treatment of Facial Injuries. 3rd Ed. Baltimore, The Williams & Wilkins Company, 1974, p. 354.

Converse, J. M., Cole, G., and Smith, B.: Late treatment of blow-out fracture of the floor of the orbit. Plast. Reconstr. Surg., *28*:183, 1961.

Converse, J. M., Firmin, F., Wood-Smith, D., and Friedland, J. A.: The conjunctival approach in orbital fractures. Plast. Reconstr. Surg., *52*:656, 1973.

Converse, J. M., and Hogan, V. M.: Open-sky approach for reduction of naso-orbital fractures. Case report. Plast. Reconstr. Surg., *46*:396, 1970.

Converse, J. M., and Smith, B.: Reconstruction of the floor of the orbit by bone grafts. Arch. Opthalmol., *44*:1, 1950.

Converse, J. M., and Smith, B.: Enophthalmos and diplopia in fracture of the orbital floor. Br. J. Plast. Surg., *9*:265, 1957.

Converse, J. M., and Smith, B.: Blowout fracture of the floor of the orbit. Trans. Am. Acad. Ophthalmol. Otolaryngol., *64*:676, 1960.

Converse, J. M., and Smith, B.: Naso-orbital fractures (symposium: midfacial fractures). Trans. Am. Acad. Ophthalmol. Otolaryngol., *67*:622, 1963.

Converse, J. M., and Smith, B.: Naso-orbital fractures and traumatic deformities of the medial canthus. Plast. Reconstr. Surg., *38*:147, 1966.

Converse, J. M., Smith, B., O'Bear, M. F., and Wood-Smith, D.: Orbital blow-out fractures: a ten year survey. Plast. Reconstr. Surg., *39*:20, 1967.

Converse, J. M., Smith, B., and Wood-Smith, D.: Deformities of the midface resulting from malunited orbital and naso-orbital fractures. Clin. Plast. Surg., *2*:107, 1975.

Couly, G., Hureau, J., and Tessier, P.: The anatomy of the external palpebral ligament in man. J. Maxillofac. Surg., *4*:195, 1976.

Cramer, L. M., Tooze, F. M., and Lerman, S.: Blowout fractures of the orbit. Br. J. Plast. Surg., *18*:171, 1965.

Crikelair, G. F., Rein, J. M., Potter, G. D., and Cosman, B.: A critical look at the "blowout" fracture. Plast. Reconstr. Surg., *49*:374, 1972.

Crockford, D. A.: Posttraumatic facial pain. *In* Converse, J. M. (Ed.): Reconstructive Plastic Surgery. 2nd Ed. Philadelphia, W. B. Saunders Company, 1977, p. 741.

Crumley, R. L., Leibsohn, J., Krause, C. J., and Burton,

T. C.: Fractures of the orbital floor. Laryngoscope, *87*:934, 1977.

Dagi, T. F., Meyer, F. B., and Poletti, C. A.: The incidence and prevention of meningitis after basilar skull fractures. Am. J. Emerg. Med., *1*:295, 1983.

Dawson, R. L., and Fordyce, G. L.: Complex fractures of the middle third of the face and their early treatment. Br. J. Surg., *41*:255, 1953.

Dingman, R. O.: Personal communication, 1974.

Dingman, R. O., and Alling, C. C.: Open reduction and internal wire fixation of maxillofacial fractures. J. Oral Surg., *12*:140, 1954.

Dingman, R. O., and Grabb, W. C.: Costal cartilage homografts preserved by irradiation. Plast. Reconstr. Surg., *28*:562, 1961.

Dingman, R. O., and Grabb, W. C.: Surgical anatomy of the mandibular ramus of the facial nerve based on the dissection of 100 facial halves. Plast. Reconstr. Surg., *29*:266, 1962.

Dingman, R. O., Grabb, W. C., and O'Neal, R. M.: Management of injuries of the naso-orbital complex. Arch. Surg., *98*:566, 1969.

Dingman, R. O., and Natvig, P.: Surgery of Facial Fractures. Philadelphia, W. B. Saunders Company, 1964.

Dodick, J. M., Galin, M. A., Littleton, J. T., and Sod, L. M.: Concomitant medial wall fracture and blowout fracture of the orbit. Arch. Ophthalmol., *85*:273, 1971.

Donald, P. J.: The tenacity of the frontal sinus mucosa. Otolaryngol. Head Neck Surg., *87*:557, 1979.

Donald, P. J.: Frontal sinus ablation by cranialization. Arch. Otolaryngol., *108*:142, 1982.

Donald, P. J., and Bernstein, L.: Compound frontal sinus injuries with intracranial penetration. Laryngoscope, *88*:225, 1978.

Donald, P. J., and Ettin, M.: The safety of frontal sinus fat obliteration when sinus walls are missing. Laryngoscope, *96*:190, 1986.

Dulley, B., and Fells, P.: Long term follow-up of orbital blow-out fractures with and without surgery. Mod. Prob. Ophthalmol., *14*:467, 1975.

Dunphy, J. E., and Jackson, D. S.: Primary applications of experimental studies in the care of the primarily closed wound. Am. J. Surg., *104*:273, 1962.

Eby, J. D.: Principles of orthodontia in the treatment of maxillofacial injuries. Int. J. Orthod., *6*:273, 1920.

Edwards, W. C., and Ridley, R. W.: Blowout fracture of the medial orbital wall. Am. J. Ophthalmol., *65*:248, 1968.

Eid, K., Lynch, O. J., and Whitaker, L. A.: Mandibular fractures: the problem patient. J. Trauma, *16*:658, 1976.

Elisevich, K. V., Ford, R. M., Anderson, D. P., Stratford, J. G., and Richardson, P. M.: Visual abnormalities with multiple trauma. Surg. Neurol., *22*:565, 1984.

Ellis, E., III, Attar, A., and Moos, K. F.: An analysis of 2067 cases of zygomatic-orbital fracture. J. Oral Maxillofac. Surg., *43*:417, 1985.

Ellis, E., Moos, K. F., and Attar, A.: Ten years of mandibular fractures: an analysis of 2137 cases. Oral Surg. Oral Med. Oral Pathol., *59*:120, 1985.

Emery, J. M., Noorden, G. K., and Sclernitzauer, D. A.: Orbital floor fractures: long-term follow-up of cases with and without surgical repair. Trans. Am. Acad. Ophthalmol. Otolaryngol., *75*:802, 1971.

Epsteen, C.: Psychological impact of facial deformities. Am. J. Surg., *96*:745, 1958.

Ewers, R., and Härle, F.: Experimental and clinical results of new advances in the treatment of facial trauma. Plast. Reconstr. Surg., *75*:25, 1985.

Ferraro, J. W., and Berggren, R. B.: Treatment of complex facial fractures. J. Trauma, *13*:783, 1973.

Finch, D. R., and Dibbell, D. G.: Immediate reconstruction of gunshot injuries to the face. J. Trauma, *19*:965, 1979.

Finney, L. A., Reynolds, D. H., and Yates, B. M.: Comminuted subfrontal fractures. J. Trauma, *4*:711, 1964.

Fortunato, M. A., Fielding, A. F., and Guernsey, L. H.: Facial bone fractures in children. Oral Surg. Oral Med. Oral Pathol., *53*:225, 1982.

Fradkin, A. H.: Orbital floor fractures and ocular complications. Am. J. Ophthalmol., *72*:699, 1971.

Freeman, B. S.: Direct approach to acute fractures of the zygomatic-maxillary complex and immediate prosthetic replacement of the orbital floor. Plast. Reconstr. Surg., *29*:587, 1962.

Friedman, W. H., Katsantonis, G. P., Rosenblum, B. N., Cooper, M. H., and Slavin, R.: Sphenoethmoidectomy: the case for ethmoid marsupialization. Laryngoscope, *96*:473, 1986.

Frim, S. P.: Fracture of the coronoid process. Oral Surg. Oral Med. Oral Pathol., *45*:978, 1978.

Fry, H. J. H.: Interlocked stresses in human nasal septal cartilage. Br. J. Plast. Surg., *19*:276, 1966.

Fry, H. J. H.: Nasal skeletal trauma and the interlocked stresses of the nasal septal cartilage. Br. J. Plast. Surg., *20*:146, 1967.

Fry, W. K., Shepherd, P. R., McLeod, A. C., and Parfitt, G. J.: The Dental Treatment of Maxillofacial Injuries. Oxford, Blackwell Scientific Publications, 1942.

Fueger, G. F., Bright, J., and Milauskas, A.: The roentgenological anatomy of the floor and of the orbit. In Bleeker, G. M., and Lyle, T. K. (Eds.): Fractures of the Orbit. Baltimore, The Williams & Wilkins Company, 1970.

Fujino, T.: Mechanism of orbital injuries in automobile accidents. Bull 4. Automotive crash injury research of the Cornell Aeronautical Laboratory, Buffalo, NY, 1963.

Fujino, T.: Experimental "blowout" fracture of the orbit. Plast. Reconstr. Surg., *54*:81, 1974a.

Fujino, T.: Mechanism of orbital blowout fracture. Jpn. J. Plast. Surg., *17*:427, 1974b.

Fujino, T., and Makino, K.: Entrapment mechanisms and ocular injury in orbital blow-out fracture. Plast. Reconstr. Surg., *65*:571, 1980.

Fukado, Y.: Results in 400 cases of surgical decompression of the optic nerve. *In* Bleeker, G. M., et al. (Eds.): Proceedings of Second International Symposium on Orbital Disorders. Basel, Karger, 1975.

Garrett, J. W.: Ocular-orbital injuries in automobile accidents. Bull. 4. Automotive Crash Injury Research of the Cornell Aeronautical Laboratory, Buffalo, NY, 1963.

Gentry, L. R., Manor, W. F., Turski, P. A., and Strother, C. M.: High-resolution CT analysis of facial struts in trauma: 2. Osseous and soft tissue complications. AJR, *140*:533, 1983.

Gillies, H. D., Kilner, T. P., and Stone, D.: Fractures of the malar-zygomatic compound with a description of a new x-ray position. Br. J. Surg., *14*:651, 1927.

Gillies, H. D., and Millard, D. R.: The Principles and Art of Plastic Surgery. Vol. 2. Boston, Little, Brown & Company, 1957.

Gillman, T., Penn, J., Bronks, D., and Roux, M.: Closure of wounds and incisions with adhesive tape. Lancet, *2*:945, 1955.

Gilmer, T. L.: A case of fracture of the lower jaw with remarks on treatment. Arch. Dent., *4*:388, 1887.

Giordano, A. M., Foster, C. A., Boles, L. R., Jr., and Maisel, R. H.: Chronic osteomyelitis following mandibular fractures and its treatment. Arch. Otolaryngol., *108*:30, 1982.

Godoy, J., and Mathog, R. H.: Malar fractures associated with exophthalmos. Arch. Otolaryngol., *111*:174, 1985.

Goodman, J. M., and Kalsbeck, J.: Outcome of self-inflicted gunshot wounds of the head. J. Trauma, *5*:636, 1965.

Goodstein, W. A., Stryker, A., and Weiner, L. J.: Primary treatment of shotgun injuries to the face. J. Trauma, *19*:961, 1979.

Gould, H. R., and Titus, C. O.: Internal orbital fractures: the value of laminagraphy in diagnosis. Am. J. Roentgenol. Radium Ther. Nucl. Med., *97*:618, 1966.

Graham, G. G., and Peltier, R. J.: Management of mandibular fractures in children. J. Oral Surg., *18*:416, 1960.

Graham, J. R., and Scott, T. M.: Notes on the treatment of tetanus. N. Engl. J. Med., *235*:846, 1946.

Gruss, J. S.: Naso-ethmoid-orbital fractures: classification and role of primary bone grafting. Plast. Reconstr. Surg., *75*:303, 1985.

Gruss, J. S., Hurwitz, J. J., Nik, N. A., and Kassel, E. E.: The pattern and incidence of nasolacrimal injury in naso-ethmoidal orbital fractures: the role of delayed assessment and dacryocystorhinostomy. Br. J. Plast. Surg., *38*:116, 1985a.

Gruss, J. S., MacKinnon, S. E., Kassel, E., and Cooper, P. W.: The role of primary bone grafting in complex craniomaxillofacial trauma. Plast. Reconstr. Surg., *75*:17, 1985b.

Gurdjian, E. S., and Webster, J. E.: Head Injuries: Mechanisms, Diagnosis, and Management. Boston, Little, Brown & Company, 1958, p. 58.

Guyon, J. J., Brant-Zawadzki, M., and Seiff, C. R.: C.T. demonstration of optic canal fractures. A.J.R., *143*:1031, 1984.

Gwyn, P. P., Carraway, J. H., Horton, C. E., Adamson, J. E., and Mladick, R. A.: Facial fractures—associated injuries and complications. Plast. Reconstr. Surg., *47*:225, 1971.

Hagan, E. H., and Huelke, D. F.: An analysis of 319 case reports of mandibular fractures. J. Oral Surg., *19*:93, 1961.

Haines, S. J.: Topical antibiotic prophylaxis in neurosurgery. Neurosurgery, *11*:250, 1982.

Hakelius, L., and Ponten, B.: Results of immediate and delayed surgical treatment of facial fractures with diplopia. J. Maxillofac. Surg., *1*:150, 1973.

Hall, R. K.: Injuries of the face and jaws in children. Int. J. Oral Surg., *1*:65, 1972.

Hamberger, C. A., and Wiesall, J.: Disorders of the Skull Base Region. Diagnosis and Treatment. New York, John Wiley & Sons, 1969.

Harrison, D. H.: Nasal injuries: their pathogenesis and treatment. Br. J. Plast. Surg., *32*:57, 1979.

Hayward, J. R.: Treatment methods for jaw fractures. J. Oral Surg., *20*:273, 1962.

Hendler, N.: The anatomy and psychopharmacology of chronic pain. J. Clin. Psychiatry, *43*:15, 1982.

Hendler, N., Viernstein, M., Schallenberger, C., and Long, D.: Group therapy with chronic pain patients. Psychosomatics, *22*:333, 1987.

Holt, G. R., and Holt, S. E.: Incidence of eye injuries in facial fractures: an analysis of 727 cases. Otolaryngol. Head Neck Surg., *91*:276, 1983.

Hubschmann, O., Shapiro, K., Baden, M., and Shulman, K.: Craniocerebral gunshot injuries in civilian practice—prognostic criteria and surgical management: experience with 82 cases. J. Trauma, *19*:6, 1979.

Huelke, D. F., O'Day, J., and Mendelsohn, R. A.: Cervical injuries suffered in automobile crashes. J. Neurosurg., *54*:316, 1981.

Hutcherson, R. R., and Krueger, D. W.: Accidents masking suicide attempts. J. Trauma, *20*:800, 1980.

Hybels, R. L., and Newman, M. H.: Posterior table fractures of the frontal sinus: I. An experimental study. Laryngoscope, *87*:171, 1977.

Ignelzi, R. J., and VanderArk, G. D.: Analysis and treatment of basilar skull fractures with and without antibiotics. J. Neurosurg., *43*:721, 1975.

Irby, W. B.: Facial Trauma and Concomitant Problems. 2nd Ed. St. Louis, C. V. Mosby Company, 1979.

Ivy, R. H.: Observations of fractures of the mandible. J.A.M.A., *79*:295, 1922.

Jabaley, M. E., Lerman, M., and Sanders, H. J.: Ocular injuries in orbital fractures. A review of 119 cases. Plast. Reconstr. Surg., *56*:410, 1975.

Jackson, I. T., Somers, P. C., and Kjar, J. G.: The use of Champy miniplates for osteosynthesis in craniofacial deformities and trauma. Plast. Reconstr. Surg., *77*:729, 1986.

Jacobs, J. B., and Persky, M. S.: Traumatic pneumocephalus. Laryngoscope, *90*:515, 1980.

James, R. B., Frederickson, C., and Kent, J. N.: Prospective study of mandibular fractures. J. Oral Surg., *39*:275, 1981.

Jeckel, N., Rakosi, T., and Joos, U.: The neuromuscular reaction to continuous dynamic jaw extension in cases with restricted mouth opening. J. Craniomaxillofac. Surg., *15*:94, 1987.

Jefferson, A., and Reilly, G.: Fractures of the floor of the anterior cranial fossa: the selection of patients for dural repair. Br. J. Surg., *59*:585, 1972.

Jones, D. E., and Evans, J. N.: "Blow-out" fractures of the orbit: an investigation into their anatomical basis. J. Laryngol. Otol., *81*:1109, 1967.

Jones, L. T.: An anatomical approach to problems of the "eyelids and lacrimal apparatus." Arch Ophthalmol., *66*:111, 1961.

Jones, L. T., and Wobig, J. L.: Surgery of the Eyelids and Lacrimal System. Birmingham, AL, Aesculapius Publishing Company, 1976.

Jones, W. D., III, Whitaker, L. A., and Murtagh, F.: Applications of reconstructive cranio-facial techniques to acute craniofacial trauma. J. Trauma, *17*:339, 1977.

Kaban, L. B., Mulliken, J. B., and Murray, J. E.: Facial fractures in children. Plast. Reconstr. Surg., *59*:15, 1977.

Kahnberg, K. E.: Extraction of teeth involved in the line of mandibular fractures. I. Indications for extraction based on a follow-up study of 185 mandibular fractures. Swed. Dent. J., *3*:27, 1979.

Kahnberg, K. E., and Ridell, A.: Prognosis of teeth involved in the line of mandibular fractures. Int. J. Oral Surg., *8*:763, 1979.

Karlan, M. S., and Cassisi, N. J.: Fractures of the zygoma—a geometric, biomechanical, and surgical analysis. Arch. Otolaryngol., *105*:320, 1979.

Kawamoto, H. K., Jr.: Late posttraumatic enophthalmos: a correctable deformity? Plast. Reconstr. Surg., *69*:423, 1982.

Kazanjian, V. H.: Treatment of automobile injuries of the face and jaws. J. Am. Dent. Assoc., *20*:757, 1933.

Kazanjian, V. H., and Converse, J. M.: The Surgical Treatment of Facial Injuries. Baltimore, Williams & Wilkins Company, 1949; 2nd Ed., 1959; 3rd Ed., 1974.

Keen, W. W.: Surgery, Its Principles and Practice. Philadelphia, W. B. Saunders Company, 1909.
Ketchum, L. D., Ferris, B., and Masters, F. W.: Blindness in midfacial fractures without direct injury to the globe. Plast. Reconstr. Surg., *58*:187, 1976.
King, E. F., and Samuel, E.: Fractures of the orbit. Trans. Ophthalmol. Soc. U.K., *64*:134, 1944.
Klastersky, J., Sadeghi, M., and Brihaye, J.: Antimicrobial prophylaxis in patients with rhinorrhea or otorrhea: a double blind study. Surg. Neurol., *6*:111, 1976.
Kline, L. B., Morawetz, R. B., and Swaid, S. N.: Indirect injury of the optic nerve. Neurosurgery, *14*:756, 1984.
Klotch, D. W., and Bilger, J. R.: Plate fixation for open mandibular fractures. Laryngoscope, *95*:1374, 1985.
Knight, J. S., and North, J. F.: The classification of malar fractures: an analysis of displacement as a guide to treatment. Br. J. Plast. Surg., *13*:325, 1961.
Koornneef, L.: Spatial Aspects of the Orbital Musculofibrous Tissue in Man: A New Anatomical and Histological Approach. Amsterdam, Swets & Zeitlinger, B. V., 1977.
Koornneef, L.: Current concepts on the management of blowout fractures. Ann. Plast. Surg., *9*:185, 1982.
Kreipke, D. L., Moss, J. J., Franco, J. M., Maves, M. D., and Smith, D. J.: Computed tomography and thin-section tomography in facial trauma. AJR, *142*:1041, 1984.
Kruger, E., and Schilli, W. (Eds.): Oral and Maxillofacial Traumatology. Chicago, Quintessence Publishers, 1982.
Kruger, G. O.: Textbook of Oral and Maxillofacial Surgery. 6th Ed. St Louis, C. V. Mosby Company, 1984.
Kuepper, R. C., and Harrigan, W. F.: Treatment of midfacial fractures at Bellevue Hospital Center, 1955–1976. J. Oral Surg., *35*:420, 1977.
Kurzer, A., and Patel, M. P.: Superior orbital fissure syndrome associated with fractures of the zygoma and orbit. Plast. Reconstr. Surg., *64*:715, 1979.
La Grange, F.: De l'anaplerose orbitaire. Bull. Acad. Med. Paris, *80*:641, 1918.
Lambotte, A.: Chirurgie Opératoire des Fractures. Paris, Masson & Cie, 1913.
Lang, W.: Traumatic enophthalmos with retention of perfect acuity of vision. Trans. Ophthal. Soc. U.K., *9*:41, 1889.
Lange, W. E.: Fractures of the orbit. Plast. Reconstr. Surg., *35*:26, 1965.
Larrabee, W. F., Jr., Travis, L. W., and Tabb, H. G.: Frontal sinus fractures—their suppurative complications and surgical management. Laryngoscope, *90*: 1810, 1980.
Larsen, O. D., and Nielsen, A.: Mandibular fractures. I. An analysis of their etiology and location in 286 patients. Scand. J. Plast. Reconstr. Surg., *10*:213, 1976.
Larsen, O. D., and Thomsen, M.: Zygomatic fractures. I. A simplified classification for practical use. Scand. J. Plast. Reconstr. Surg., *12*:55, 1978.
Lederman, I. R.: Loss of vision associated with surgical treatment of zygomatic-orbital floor fracture. Plast. Reconstr. Surg., *68*:94, 1981.
Leech, P.: Cerebrospinal fluid leakage, dural fistulae and meningitis after basal skull fractures. Injury, *6*:141, 1974.
Le Fort, R.: Etude expérimentale sur les fractures de la machoire supérieure. Rev. Chir. Paris, *23*:208, 360, 479, 1901.
Lehman, R. H.: Frontal sinus surgery. Acta Otolaryngol. [Suppl.], *270*:1, 1970.
Leibsohn, J., Burton, T. C., and Scott, W. E.: Orbital floor fractures: a retrospective study. Ann. Ophthalmol., *8*:1057, 1976.
Levine, P. A., and Goode, R. L.: Treatment of fractures of the edentulous mandible. Arch. Otolaryngol., *108*:167, 1982.
Lewin, W.: Cerebrospinal fluid rhinorrhea in closed head injuries. Br. J. Surg., *42*:1, 1954.
Lewis, V. L., Jr., Manson, P. N., Morgan, R. F., Cerullo, L. J., and Meyer, P. R., Jr.: Facial injuries associated with cervical fractures: recognition, patterns, and management. J. Trauma, *25*:90, 1985.
Lindsey, D., Nava, C., and Marti, M.: Effectiveness of penicillin irrigation in control of infection in sutured lacerations. J. Trauma, *22*:186, 1982.
Lothrop, H. A.: Fractures of the superior maxillary bone, caused by direct blows over the malar bone. A method for the treatment of such fractures. Boston Med. Surg. J., *154*:8, 1906.
Luce, E. A., Tubbs, T. D., and Moore, A. M.: Review of 1,000 major facial fractures and associated injuries. Plast. Reconstr. Surg., *63*:26, 1979.
Manfredi, S. J., Raji, M. R., Sprinkle, P. M., Weinstein, G. W., Minardi, L. M., and Swanson, T. J.: Computerized tomographic scan findings in facial fractures associated with blindness. Plast. Reconstr. Surg., *68*:479, 1981.
Manson, P. N.: Some thoughts on the classification and treatment of Le Fort fractures. Ann. Plast. Surg., *17*:356, 1986.
Manson, P. N., Clifford, C. M., Su, C. T., Iliff, N. T., and Morgan, R.: Mechanisms of global support and posttraumatic enophthalmos: I. The anatomy of the ligament sling and its relation to intramuscular cone orbital fat. Plast. Reconstr. Surg., *77*:193, 1986a.
Manson, P. N., Crawley, W. A., Yaremchuk, M. J., Rochman, G. M., Hoopes, J. E., and French, J. H.: Midface fractures: advantages of immediate extended open reduction and bone grafting. Plast. Reconstr. Surg., *76*:1, 1985.
Manson, P. N., Grivas, A., Rosenbaum, A., Vannier, M., Zinreich, J., and Iliff, N.: Studies on enophthalmos: II. The measurement of orbital injuries and their treatment by quantitative computed tomography. Plast. Reconstr. Surg., *77*:203, 1986b.
Manson, P. N., Ruas, E., Iliff, N., and Yaremchuk, M.: Single eyelid incision for exposure of the zygomatic bone and orbital reconstruction. Plast. Reconstr. Surg., *79*:120, 1987.
Manson, P. N., Sargent, L., Rochman, G., Morgan, R., and Hoopes, J. E.: 162 Nasoethmoidal-orbital fractures: technical consideration in immediate reconstruction. Submitted to Plast. and Reconstr. Surg.
Manson, P. N., Shack, R. B., Leonard, L. G., Su, C. T., and Hoopes, J. E.: Sagittal fractures of the maxilla and palate. Plast. Reconstr. Surg., *72*:484, 1983.
Manson, P. N., Su, C. T., and Hoopes, J. E.: Structural pillars of the facial skeleton. Plast. Reconstr. Surg., *66*:54, 1980.
Marciani, R. D., and Hill, O.: The treatment of the fractured edentulous mandible. J. Oral Surg., *37*:569, 1979.
Mathog, R., Archer, K. F., and Nesi, F.: Posttraumatic enophthalmos and diplopia. Otolaryngol. Head Neck Surg., *94*:69, 1986.
Matras, H., and Kuderna, H.: Combined craniofacial fractures. J. Maxillofac. Surg., *8*:52, 1980.
Mauriello, J. A., Jr., Flanagan, J. C., and Peyster, R. G.: An unusual complication of late orbital floor fracture repair. Ophthalmol., *91*:102, 1984.

May, M., West, J. W., Heeneman, H., Gowda, C. K., and Ogura, J. H.: Proceedings: Shotgun wounds to the head and neck. Arch. Otolaryngol., *98*:373, 1973.

May, M.: Nasofrontal-ethmoidal injuries. Laryngoscope, *87*:948, 1977.

Mayell, M. F.: Nasal fractures. Their occurrence, management and some late results. J. R. Coll. Surg. Edinb., *18*:31, 1973.

McCoy, F. J., Chandler, R. A., Magnan, C. G., Jr., Moore, J. R., and Siemsen, G.: An analysis of facial fractures and their complications. Plast. Reconstr. Surg., *29*:381, 1962.

McDonald, J. V.: The surgical management of severe open brain injuries with consideration of the long-term results. J. Trauma, *20*:842, 1980.

McNeill, R. A.: Traumatic nasal neuralgia and its treatment. Br. Med. J., *2*:536, 1963.

Meade, J. W.: Tracheostomy—its complications and their management. N. Engl. J. Med., *265*:519, 1961.

Mektubjian, S. R.: Operative policy in severe facial trauma in combination with other severe injuries. J. Maxillofac. Surg., *10*:14, 1982.

Melmed, E. P., and Koonin, A. J.: Fractures of the mandible. A review of 909 cases. Plast. Reconstr. Surg., *56*:323, 1975.

Melzack, R., and Wall, P. D.: Pain mechanisms: a new theory. Science, *150*:971, 1965.

Merville, L.: Multiple dislocations of the facial skeleton. J. Maxillofac. Surg., *2*:187, 1979.

Merville, L. C., and Derome, P.: Concomitant dislocations of the face and skull. J. Maxillofac. Surg., *6*:2, 1978.

Merville, L. C., and Real, J. P.: Fronto-orbital-nasal dislocations. Initial total reconstruction. Scand. J. Plast. Reconst. Surg., *15*:287, 1981.

Michelet, F. X., Deymes, J., and Dessus, B.: Osteosynthesis with miniaturized screwed plates in maxillofacial surgery. J. Maxillofac. Surg., *1*:79, 1973.

Milauskas, A. T.: Diagnosis and Management of Blowout Fractures of the Orbit. Springfield, IL., Charles C Thomas, 1969.

Milauskas, A. T., and Fueger, G. F.: Serious ocular complications associated with blow-out fractures of the orbit. Am. J. Ophthalmol., *62*:670, 1966.

Miller, G. R.: Blindness developing a few days after a midfacial fracture. Plast. Reconstr. Surg., *42*:384, 1968.

Miller, G. R., and Glaser, J. S.: The retraction syndrome and trauma. Arch. Ophthalmol., *76*:662, 1966.

Miller, G. R., and Tenzel, R. R.: Ocular complications of midfacial fractures. Plast. Reconstr. Surg., *39*:117, 1967.

Miller, S. H., Lung, R. J., Davis, T. S., Graham, W. P., and Kennedy, T. J.: Management of fractures of the supraorbital rim. J. Trauma, *18*:507, 1978.

Mincy, J. E.: Posttraumatic cerebrospinal fluid fistula of the frontal fossa. J. Trauma, *6*:618, 1966.

Mladick, R. A., Georgiade, N. G., and Royer, J.: Immediate flap reconstruction for massive shotgun wound of face. Plast. Reconstr. Surg., *45*:186, 1970.

Morgan, B. D., Madan, D. K., and Bergerot, J. P.: Fractures of the middle third of the face—a review of 300 cases. Br. J. Plast. Surg., *25*:147, 1972.

Morgan, P. R., and Morrison, W. V.: Complications of frontal and ethmoid sinusitis. Laryngoscope, *90*:661, 1980.

Morley, T. P., and Hetherington, R. F.: Traumatic cerebrospinal fluid rhinorrhea and otorrhea, pneumocephalus and meningitis. Surg. Gynecol. Obstet., *104*:88, 1957.

Morris, J. H.: Biphase connector, external skeletal splint for reduction and fixation of mandibular fractures. Oral Surg., *2*:1382, 1949.

Munro, I. R., and Chen, Y. R.: Radical treatment for fronto-orbital fibrous dysplasia: the chain link fence. Plast. Reconstr. Surg., *67*:719, 1981.

Murray, J. A., Maran, A. G., Mackenzie, I. J., and Raab, G.: Open vs. closed reduction of the fractured nose. Arch. Otolaryngol., *110*:797, 1984.

Nahum, A. M.: The biomechanics of maxillofacial trauma. Clin. Plast. Surg., *2*:59, 1975.

Natvig, P.: Personal communication, 1962.

Natvig, P., Sicher, H., and Fodor, P. B.: The rare isolated fracture of the coronoid process of the mandible. Plast. Reconstr. Surg., *46*:168, 1970.

Neal, D. C., Wagner, W. F., and Alpert, B.: Morbidity associated with teeth in the line of mandibular fractures. J. Oral Surg., *36*:859, 1978.

Nicholson, D. H., and Guzak, S. W.: Visual loss complicating repair of orbital floor fractures. Arch. Ophthalmol., *86*:369, 1971.

Niederdellmann, H., and Akuamoa-Boateng, E.: Lag-screw osteosynthesis: a new procedure for treating fractures of the mandibular angle. J. Oral Surg., *39*:938, 1981.

Niederdellmann, H., and Shetty, V.: Solitary lag screw osteosynthesis in the treatment of fractures of the angle of the mandible; a retrospective study. Plast. Reconstr. Surg., *80*:68, 1987.

Niederdellmann, H., Schilli, W., Düker, J., and Akuamoa-Boateng, E.: Osteosynthesis of mandibular fractures using lag screws. Int. J. Oral. Surg., *5*:117, 1976.

Nordgaard, J. O.: Persistent sensory disturbances and diplopia following fracture of the zygoma. Arch. Otolaryngol., *102*:80, 1976.

Nysingh, J. G.: Zygomatico-maxillary fractures with a report of 200 cases. Arch. Chir. Neerl., *12*:157, 1960.

Obwegeser, H. L., and Sailer, H. F.: Another way of treating fractures of the atrophic edentulous mandible. J. Maxillofac. Surg., *1*:213, 1973.

Olson, R. A., Fonseca, R. J., Zeitler, D. L., and Osbon, D. B.: Fractures of the mandible. J. Oral Maxillofac. Surg., *40*:23, 1982.

Ostrofsky, M. K., and Lownie, J. F.: Zygomatico-coronoid ankylosis. J. Oral Surg., *35*:752, 1977.

Panagoupolous, A. P.: Management of fractures of the jaws in children. J. Int. Coll. Surg., *28*:806, 1957.

Pataky, P. E., Graham, W. P., III, and Munger, B. L.: Terminal neuromas treated with triamcinolone acetonide. J. Surg. Res., *14*:36, 1973.

Paul, J. K., and Acevedo, A.: Intraoral open reduction. J. Oral Surg., *26*:516, 1968.

Pearl, R. M.: Surgical management of volumetric changes in the bony orbit. Ann. Plast. Surg. *19*:349, 1987.

Pearl, R. M., and Vistnes, L. M.: Orbital blow-out fractures: an approach to management. Ann. Plast. Surg., *1*:267, 1978.

Peri, G., Chabannes, J., Menes, R., Jourde, J., and Fain, J.: Fractures of the frontal sinus. J. Maxillofac. Surg., *9*:73, 1981.

Perino, K. E., Zide, M. F., and Kinnebrew, M. C.: Late treatment of malunited malar fractures. J. Oral Maxillofac. Surg., *42*:20, 1980.

Petro, J., Tooze, F. M., Bales, C. R., and Baker, G.: Ocular injuries associated with periorbital fractures. J. Trauma, *19*:730, 1970.

Pfeiffer, R. L.: Traumatic enophthalmos. Arch. Ophthalmol., *30*:718, 1943.

Prasad, S. S.: Blow-out fracture of the medial wall of the orbit. *In* Bleeker, G. M., et al. (Eds.): Proceedings of Second International Symposium on Orbital Disorders. Vol. 14. Basel, Karger, 1975.

Prein, J., Eschmann, A., and Spiessl, B.: Results of follow-up examinations in 81 patients with functionally stable mandibular osteosynthesis. Fortschr. Kiefer Gesichtschir., *21*:304, 1976.

Putterman, A. M., Stevens, T., and Urist, M. J.: Nonsurgical management of blow-out fractures of the orbital floor. Am. J. Ophthalmol., *77*:232, 1974.

Putterman, A. M., and Urist, M. J.: Treatment of enophthalmic narrow palpebral fissure after blow-out fracture. Ophthalmic Surg., *6*:45, 1975.

Raaf, J.: Post-traumatic cerebrospinal fluid leaks. Arch. Surg., *95*:648, 1967.

Raflo, G. T.: Blow-in and blow-out fractures of the orbit: clinical correlations and proposed mechanisms. Ophthalmic. Surg., *15*:114, 1984.

Rapidis, A. D., Papavassiliou, D., Papadimitriou, J., Koundouris, J., and Zachariadis, N.: Fractures of the coronoid process of the mandible. An analysis of 52 cases. Int. J. Oral Surg., *14*:126, 1985.

Reil, B., and Kranz, S.: Traumatology of the maxillofacial region in childhood. J. Maxillofac. Surg., *4*:197, 1976.

Remmler, D., and Boles, R.: Intracranial complications of frontal sinusitis. Laryngoscope, *90*:1814, 1980.

Rény, A., and Stricker, M.: Fractures de L'Orbite. Indications Ophthalmologiques dans les Techniques Opératoires. Paris, Masson et Cie, 1969.

Reynolds, J. R.: Late complications vs. method of treatment in a large series of mid-facial fractures. Plast. Reconstr. Surg., *61*:871, 1978.

Rish, B. L., Dillon, J. D., Meirowsky, A. M., Caveness, W. F., Mohr, J. P., et al.: Cranioplasty: a review of 1030 cases of penetrating head injury. Neurosurgery, *4*:381, 1979.

Robert, C. A.: Nouveau procédé de traitment des fractures de la portion alvéolaire de la machoire inférieure. Bull. Gen. Ther., *42*:22, 1852.

Robinson, T. J., and Stranc, M. F.: The anatomy of the medial canthal ligament. Br. J. Plast. Surg., *23*:1, 1970.

Rougier, M. J.: Résultats fonctionnels du traitement chirurgical des paralysies oculaires secondaires aux tramatismes de la face. Bull. Soc. Ophthalmol. Fr., *65*:502, 1965.

Rougier, J., Freidel, C., and Freidel, M.: Fractures of the orbital roof and ethmoid region. *In* Bleeker, G. M., and Lyle, T. K. (Eds.): Proceedings of the Symposium on Orbital Fractures. Amsterdam, Excerpta Medica, 1969.

Rowe, L. D., and Brandt-Zawadzki, M.: Spatial analysis of midfacial fractures with multidirectional and computed tomography: clinicopathologic correlates in 44 cases. Otolaryngol. Head Neck Surg., *90*:651, 1982.

Rowe, L. D., Miller, E., and Brandt-Zawadzki, M.: Computed tomography in maxillofacial trauma. Laryngoscope, *91*:745, 1981.

Rowe, N. L., and Killey, H. C.: Fracture of the Facial Skeleton. Baltimore, Williams & Wilkins Company, 1955; 2nd Ed., 1968.

Rubin, L. R.: Langer's lines and facial scars. Plast. Reconstr. Surg., *3*:147, 1948.

Rumelt, M. B., and Ernest, J. T.: Isolated blowout fracture of the medial orbital wall with medial rectus muscle entrapment. Am. J. Ophthalmol., *73*:451, 1972.

Sataloff, R. T., Sariego, J., Myers, D. L., and Richter, H. J.: Surgical management of the frontal sinus. Neurosurgery, *15*:593, 1984.

Schaefer, S. D., Diehl, J. T., and Briggs, W. H.: The diagnosis of CSF rhinorrhea by metrizamide CT scanning. Laryngoscope, *90*:871, 1980.

Schenck, N. L.: Frontal sinus disease. III. Experimental and clinical factors in failure of the frontal osteoplastic operation. Laryngoscope, *85*:76, 1975.

Schilli, W.: Compression osteosynthesis. J. Oral Surg., *35*:802, 1977.

Schilli, W., Ewers, R., and Niederdellmann, H.: Bone fixation with plates and screws in the maxillofacial region. Int. J. Oral Surg., *10*:329, 1985.

Schmitz, J. P., and Hollinger, J. O.: The critical size defect as an experimental model for craniomandibulofacial nonunions. Clin. Orthop., *205*:299, 1986.

Schmoker, R., Von-Allmen, G., and Tschopp, H. M.: Application of functionally stable fixation in maxillofacial surgery according to ASIF principles. J. Oral Maxillofac. Surg., *40*:457, 1982.

Schneider, R. C., and Thompson, J. M.: Chronic and delayed traumatic cerebrospinal rhinorrhea as a source of recurrent attacks of meningitis. Ann. Surg., *145*:517, 1957.

Schneider, S. S., and Stern, M.: Teeth in the line of mandibular fractures. J. Oral Surg., *29*:107, 1971.

Schultz, R. C.: Facial injuries from automobile accidents: a study of 400 consecutive cases. Plast. Reconstr. Surg., *40*:415, 1967.

Schultz, R. C.: Supraorbital and glabellar fractures. Plast. Reconstr. Surg., *45*:227, 1970.

Seddon, H. J.: Three types of nerve injury. Brain, *66*:237, 1943.

Smith, B., Lisman, R. D., Simonton, J., and Della-Rocca, R.: Volkmann's contracture of the extraocular muscles following blowout fracture. Plast. Reconstr. Surg., *74*:200, 1984.

Smith, B., and Regan, W. F., Jr.: Blowout fracture of the orbit: mechanism and correction of internal orbital fracture. Am. J. Ophthalmol., *44*:733, 1957.

Smith, R. R., and Blount, R. L.: Blowout fractures of the orbital roof with pulsating exophthalmos, blepharoplasties, and superior gaze paresis. Am. J. Ophthalmol., *71*:1052, 1971.

Sofferman, R. A., Danielson, P. A., Quatela, V., and Reed, R. R.: Retrospective analysis of surgically treated Le Fort fractures. Arch. Otolaryngol., *109*:446, 1983.

Souyris, F., Lamarche, J. P., and Mirfakhrai, A. M.: Treatment of mandibular fractures by intraoral placement of bone plates. J. Oral Surg., *38*:33, 1980.

Speculand, B., Goss, A. N., Hallett, E., and Spence, N. D.: Intractable facial pain. Br. J. Oral Surg., *17*:166, 1979.

Spiessl, B. (Ed.): New Concepts in Maxillofacial Bone Surgery. New York, Springer-Verlag, 1976.

Spiessl, B., and Schroll, K.: Naso-ethmoidal injuries. Osterr. Z. Stomatol., *70*:2, 1973.

Stader, O.: A preliminary announcement of a new method of treating fractures. North Am. Vet., *18*:37, 1937.

Stahlnecker, M., Whitaker, L., Herman, G., and Katowitz, J.: Evaluation and secondary treatment of post-traumatic enophthalmos. Presented at the American Association of Plastic Surgeons, Coronado Beach, CA, Apr. 29, 1985.

Stanley, R. B., Jr.: Reconstruction of midface vertical dimension following Le Fort fractures. Arch. Otolaryngol., *110*:571, 1984.

Stanley, R. B., and Mathog, R. H.: Evaluation and correction of the combined orbital trauma syndrome. Laryngoscope, *93*:856, 1983.

Stanley, R. B., Jr., and Nowak, G. M.: Midfacial fractures: importance of angle of impact to horizontal craniofacial buttresses. Otolaryngol. Head Neck Surg., *93*:186, 1985.

Stout, R. A.: *In* Manual of Standard Practice of Plastic and Maxillofacial Surgery. Philadelphia, W. B. Saunders Company, 1942.

Stranc, M. F.: Primary treatment of nasoethmoid injuries with increased intercanthal distance. Br. J. Plast. Surg., *23*:8, 1970a.

Stranc, M. F.: Pattern of lacrimal injuries in nasoethmoid fractures. Br. J. Plast. Surg., *23*:339, 1970b.

Stranc, M. F., and Gustavson, E. H.: Plastic surgery. Primary treatment of fractures of the orbital roof. Proc. R. Soc. Med., *66*:303, 1973.

Stranc, M. F., and Robertson, G. A.: A classification of injuries of the nasal skeleton. Ann. Plast. Surg., *2*:468, 1979.

Sturla, F., Abnsi, D., and Buquet, J.: Anatomical and mechanical considerations of craniofacial fractures: an experimental study. Plast. Reconstr. Surg., *66*:815, 1980.

Stuzin, J. M., Cutting, C. B., McCarthy, J. G., and Dufresne, C. R.: Radiographic documentation of direct injury of the intracanicular segment of the optic nerve in the orbital apex syndrome. Ann. Plast. Surg., *20*:368, 1988.

Swearingen, J. J.: Tolerances of the human face to crash impact. Report from the Office of Aviation Medicine, Federal Aviation Agency, July, 1965.

Tajima, S.: Malar bone fractures: experimental fractures on the dried skull and clinical sensory disturbances. J. Maxillofac. Surg., *5*:150, 1977.

Tajima, S., and Nakajima, H.: The treatment of fractures involving the frontobasal region. Clin. Plast. Surg., *7*:525, 1980.

Tajima, S., Sugimoto, C., Tanino, R., Oshiro, T., and Harashina, T.: Surgical treatment of malunited fractures of zygoma with diplopia and with comments on blow-out fractures. J. Maxillofac. Surg., *2*:201, 1974.

Teasdale, G., and Jennett, B.: Assessment of coma and impaired consciousness. Lancet, *2*:81, 1974.

Tenzel, P. R.: Personal communication, 1974.

Tessier, P.: The conjunctival approach to the orbital floor and maxilla in congenital malformation and trauma. J. Maxillofac. Surg., *1*:3, 1973.

Tessier, P., Guiot, G., Rougerie, J., Delbet, J. P., and Pastoriza, J.: Ostéotomies cranio-naso-orbital-faciales. Hypertélorisme. Ann. Chir. Plast., *12*:103, 1967.

Tessier, P., Hervouet, F., Lekieffre, M., Rougier, J., Woillez, M., and Derome, P. (Eds.): Plastic Surgery of the Orbit and Eyelids. Translated by S. A. Wolfe. New York, Masson, 1977.

Trokel, S. L., and Potter, G. D.: Radiographic diagnosis of fracture of the medial wall of the orbit. Am. J. Ophthalmol., *67*:772, 1969.

Tu, H. K., and Tenhulzen, D.: Compression osteosynthesis of mandibular fractures: a retrospective study. J. Oral Maxillofac. Surg., *43*:585, 1985.

Vondra, J.: Fractures of the Base of the Skull. London, Iliffe Books, 1965.

Welsh, L. W., and Welsh, J. J.: Fractures of the edentulous maxilla and mandible. Laryngoscope, *86*:1333, 1976.

Weymuller, E. A., Jr.: Blindness and Le Fort III fractures. Ann. Otol. Rhinol. Laryngol., *93*:2, 1984.

Wilkins, R. B., and Havins, W. E.: Current treatment of blow-out fractures. Ophthalmology, *89*:464, 1982.

Wilson, M. E.: The neurological mechanisms of pain. A review. Anaesthesia, *29*:407, 1974.

Winstanley, R. P.: The management of fractures of the mandible. Br. J. Oral Maxillofac. Surg., *22*:170, 1984.

Wolfe, S. A.: Application of craniofacial surgical precepts following trauma and tumour removal. J. Maxillofac. Surg., *10*:212, 1982.

Yanagisawa, E.: Symposium on maxillofacial trauma. Pitfalls in the management of zygomatic fractures. Laryngoscope, *83*:527, 1973.

Zachariades, N.: The superior orbital fissure syndrome; report of a case and review of the literature. Oral Surg. *53*:237, 1982.

Zachariades, N., Papavassiliou, D., Triantafylou, D., Vairaktaris, E., Papademetriou, I., et al.: Fractures of the facial skeleton in the edentulous patient. J. Maxillofac. Surg., *12*:262, 1984.

Zallen, R. D., and Curry, J. T.: A study of antibiotic usage in compound mandibular fractures. J. Oral Surg., *33*:431, 1975.

Zallen, R. D., and Fitzgerald, B. E.: The treatment of mandibular fractures with use of malleable titanium mesh. J. Oral Surg., *34*:748, 1976.

Zide, B. M., and McCarthy, J. G.: The medial canthus revisited—an anatomical basis for canthopexy. Ann. Plast. Surg., *11*:1, 1983.

Zizmor, J., Smith, B., Fasano, C., and Converse, J. M.: Roentgen diagnosis of blowout fracture of the orbit. Trans. Am. Acad. Ophthalmol., *66*:802, 1962.

28

Craig R. Dufresne
Paul N. Manson

*Pediatric Facial Trauma**

DEVELOPMENTAL MALFORMATIONS OF THE FACIAL SKELETON
- Postnatal Growth of the Face
- Postnatal Growth of the Mandible
- Postnatal Growth of the Nasomaxillary Complex

CLINICAL EXAMINATION

RADIOLOGIC EVALUATION

EMERGENCY TREATMENT

PRENATAL, BIRTH, AND INFANT INJURIES

SOFT TISSUE INJURIES IN INFANTS AND CHILDREN

FACIAL FRACTURES
- Etiology
- Incidence
- Alveolar Fractures
- Mandibular Fractures
- Midfacial Fractures
- Zygomatic and Orbital Fractures
- Nasal and Nasoorbital Fractures
- Nasoethmoido-orbital Fractures
- Frontal Bone and Frontal Sinus Fractures
- Supraorbital Fractures
- Compound, Multiple, Comminuted Midfacial Fractures

COMPLICATIONS OF PEDIATRIC FACIAL TRAUMA

Facial injuries in children are considered separately because of special problems that arise in their treatment and management. Children, like adults, are subject to similar types of injuries and trauma. However, facial injuries are much less common in children, particularly during the first five years of life. By the age of puberty the frequency and the pattern of maxillofacial injuries begin to parallel those seen in adults. The principles of treatment of facial trauma in children are basically the same as those utilized in adults. However, the techniques must be modified by certain anatomic, physiologic, and psychologic factors specifically related to childhood.

The automobile is responsible for a large number of deaths and severe injuries in childhood. Children under 5 years of age account for 2 to 3 per cent of automobile occupant deaths. Children under 14 years of age account for approximately 6 per cent of automobile deaths. Of children between the ages of 5 and 14 years who are injured in automobile collisions, only 56 per cent were actual occupants of the automobiles (Burdi and associates, 1969; Adekeye, 1980; Agran and Dunkle, 1982; Agran, Dunkle, and Winn, 1985).

Other causes of accidents in children extend over a wide range from falls to thermal burns. Athletic activities are responsible for facial injuries in older children. The vast canine population in the United States subjects children to dog bites that often result in considerable soft tissue disorganization and loss.

Soft tissue injuries and fractures may require special therapeutic techniques owing to difficulties in obtaining the cooperation of young children. Another important aspect of facial injuries in children is the potential for later effects upon facial development. A posttraumatic facial deformity in the child is a result not only of the displacement of bony structures caused by the fracture, but also of faulty or arrested development stemming from the injury. Developmental malformations seen in young adolescents and adults are often secondary to early childhood injuries. A statement should always be made to the parents of a child, preferably in writing,

*Portions of this chapter are revised from sections of Chapter 26 in the predecessor of this book, Converse, J.M. (Ed.): *Reconstructive Plastic Surgery* (2nd ed., 1977), which was prepared by J.M. Converse and R.O. Dingman.

that maldevelopment in growth may occur as a result of facial fractures despite adequate treatment, particularly in injuries involving the nasomaxillary complex and the condylar region of the mandible. This is an essential medicolegal precaution.

DEVELOPMENTAL MALFORMATIONS OF THE FACIAL SKELETON

Many facial developmental malformations can be attributed to trauma in early childhood. Trauma may have a deleterious effect on the growth and development of facial bone structure in postnatal life similar to that of a defective gene during prenatal development. In many cases it is difficult to ascertain whether the disturbances occurred before or after birth.

Postnatal Growth of the Face

Knowledge about craniofacial growth (see also Chap. 47) has been determined by a variety of methods (Enlow, 1982). The cross sectional approach requires the use of large numbers of skulls of varying ages (Johnson, 1962; Harwood-Nash, 1970). Early growth of the face is rapid. At 3 months, the face is less than half the size of that an adult (approximately 40 per cent). At 2 years it has reached approximately 70 per cent and at 5.5 years it attains approximately 80 per cent of adult size (Scott, 1959; Enlow, 1982).

The proportions of the face change markedly during the period of postnatal growth (Fig. 28–1). The skull at birth presents a relatively large cranial portion and a small facial component as compared with an adult skull. The cranial-to-facial proportions are 8:1 at birth, but they fall to 4:1 by 5 years of age and 2:1 in the adult (Figs. 28–2 to 28–5) (Scott, 1959; Enlow, 1982).

These changes are due to two factors: (1) the actual growth of the face, and (2) the modification of the proportions that bring forth characteristics distinguishing the faces of males from those of females and establishing distinctive individual features (Enlow, 1982).

The overall facial skeleton is relatively small at birth. The nasal cavity and paranasal sinuses are also small. The nasal cavities are as wide as they are high. The piriform aperture is broad in its lower border, and the floor of the nasal cavities is on a level slightly

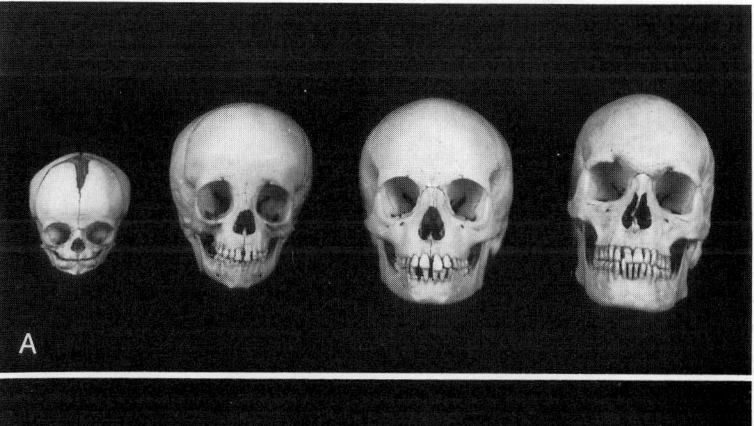

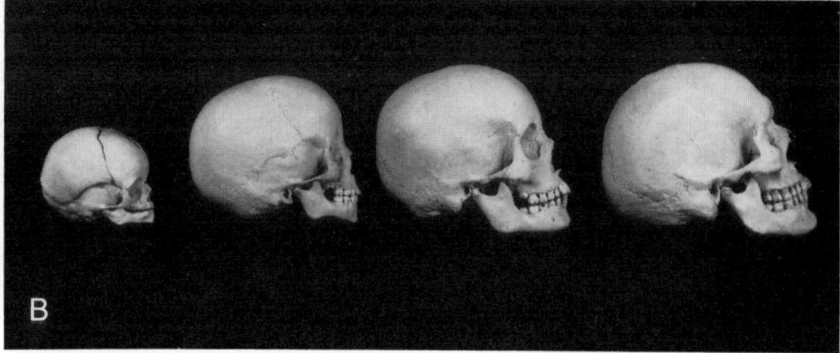

Figure 28–1. Series of skulls showing changes in the size of the face as well as the position of the face in relation to the cranium. Growth of the face is associated with growth of the jaws and eruption of the teeth. *A*, Frontal view. *B*, Lateral view.

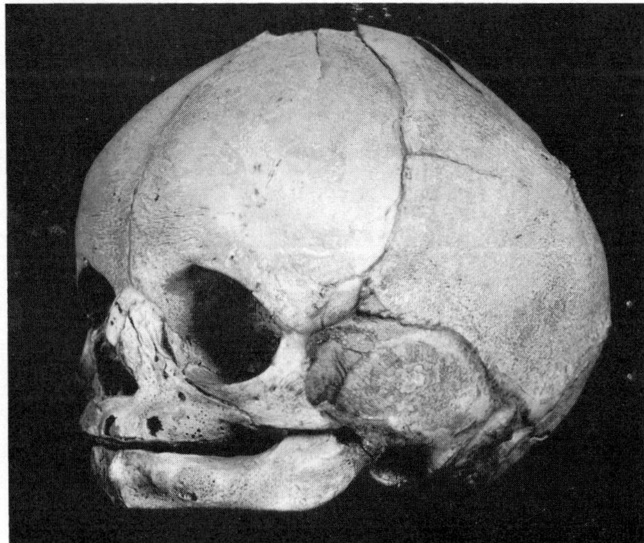

Figure 28–2. Skull of an infant in the first year of life.

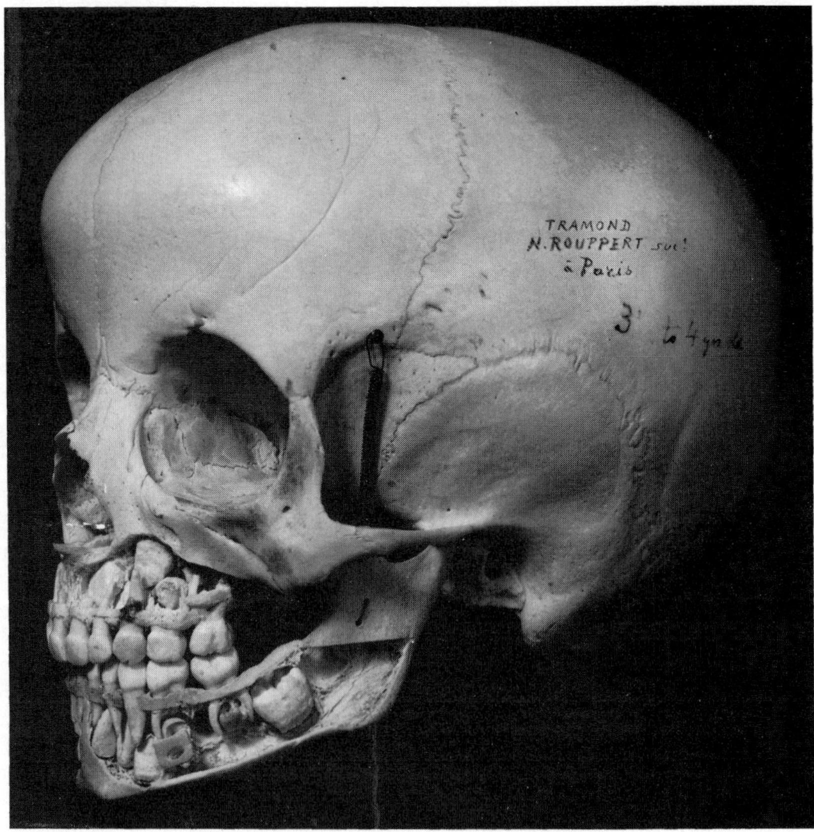

Figure 28–3. Skull of a 3 year old child showing the position of the permanent (secondary) teeth in relation to the deciduous (primary) dentition.

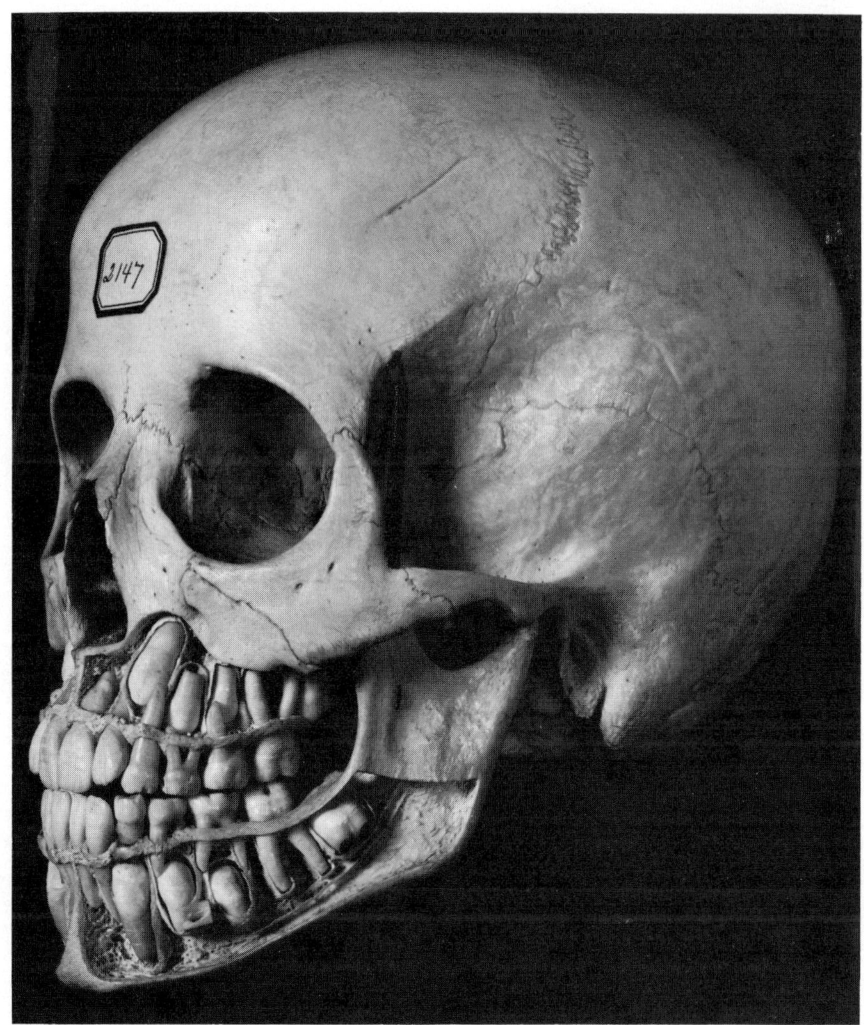

Figure 28–4. Skull of a child in the seventh year showing the position of the permanent teeth in relation to the deciduous dentition.

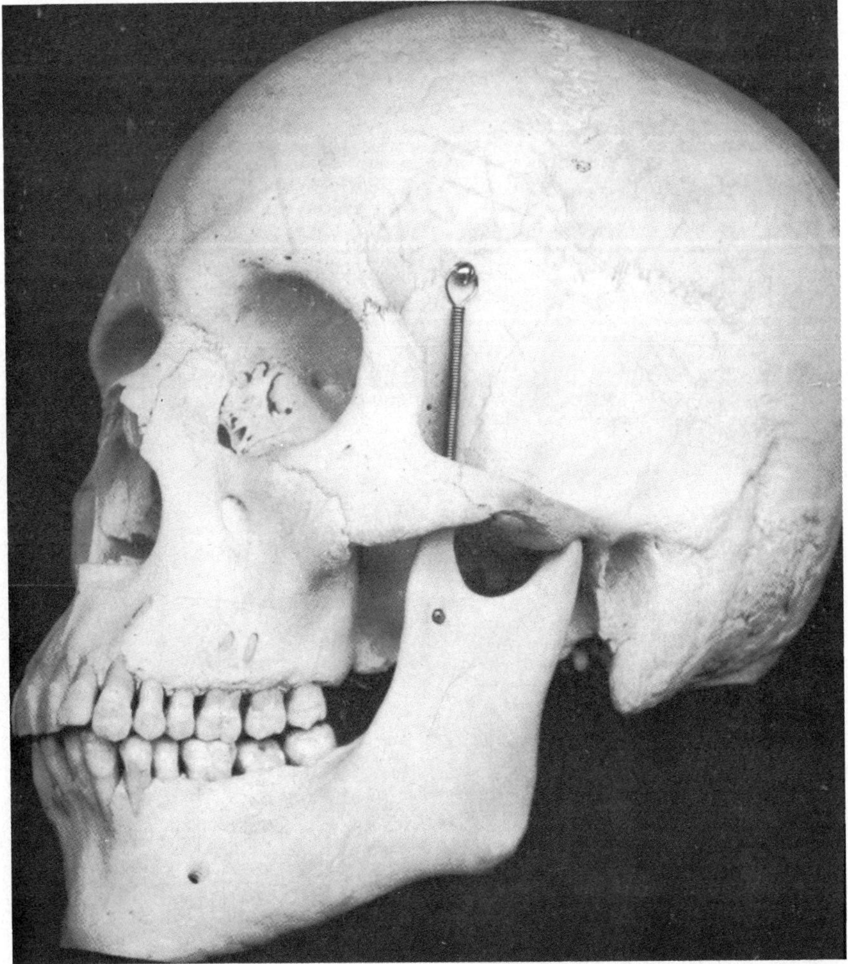

Figure 28–5. The adult skull.

below that of the lower rim of the orbit in a horizontal line passing approximately through the two infraorbital foramina (Fig. 28–6) (Scott, 1959; Enlow, 1982).

Children are further characterized from adults in that the nose and sinuses are essentially a single structure, the sinuses being small or absent. The ethmoid or maxillary sinuses begin to evaginate from the nasal cavity in the second trimester. They first present as separate recesses, with the ethmoid sinuses later growing into a honeycomb of cells. The growth of the maxillary sinus parallels that of the face. The maxillary sinuses are narrow in the newborn and not sufficiently developed to reach the area beneath the orbit. The sinus slowly increases in size and becomes quite large after age 5 years (Bernstein, 1971). During the first year the medial and lateral dimensions have reached beneath the orbit, but no farther laterally than the infraorbital foramen. During the third and fourth years, the mediolateral dimensions of the maxillary sinus increase considerably. By age 5 years it extends to a point lateral to the infraorbital canal. The floor of the maxillary sinus remains above the level of the floor of the nose in the child up to the age of 8 years. It is only after the eruption of the permanent dentition in the twelfth year and the development of the alveolar process that the maxillary sinus descends below the level of the floor of the nose. Eruption of the permanent maxillary teeth determines the inferior growth of the maxillary sinus and therefore the level of the sinus floor. By the age of 8 years, the floor is at the level of the inferior meatus and reaches the

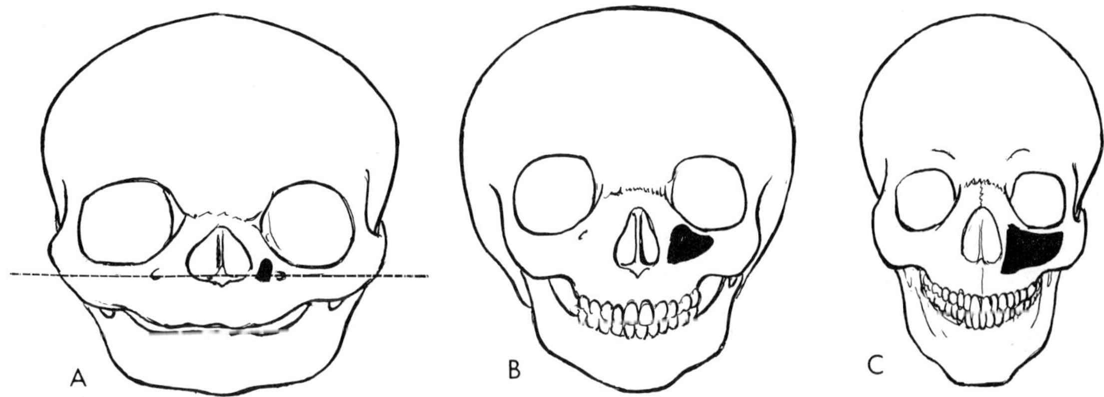

Figure 28–6. The skull at birth *(A)*, at 5 years *(B)*, and in the adult *(C)* has been drawn with the same vertical dimension to show the relative size increases of the maxillary sinus. Note the progressive increase in the size of the maxillary sinus, extending laterally beyond the infraorbital foramen *(B)* and descending below the level of the floor of the nose *(C)* after eruption of the permanent teeth. (From Kazanjian and Converse.)

level of the nasal floor by the age of 10 to 12 years. The maxillary sinus is fully developed by age 16 years (Bernstein, 1971; Fearon, Edmonds, and Bird, 1979; Brook and Friedman, 1982).

The frontal sinus develops as evaginations from the nose during the second trimester. It can be distinguished from the ethmoid sinuses after age 5 years. The sinus reaches adult size by late puberty. The frontal sinuses are seldom symmetric and vary greatly in size and shape. Occasionally they may be absent. The lining of the sinus cavities is respiratory mucous membrane that is continuous with the mucosal lining of the nasal cavity. Fractures may impair sinus drainage by blocking the sinusal ostia or interfering with the ciliary function of mucosa. Retained secretion, mucocele, or abscess may occur under these conditions and may require drainage procedures (Bernstein, 1971; Brook and Friedman, 1982).

In the early years of life the cranium is large in comparison with the size of the facial bones. A major increase in cranial size occurs in the first two years. The first six months of life are characterized by a period of generalized rapid growth, followed by a slower period of growth from age 6 months to 4 years. The increase in the vertical dimension of the face is due in part to the development and eruption of the dentition. In the newborn the crown portions of the upper and lower teeth or the alveolar process do not contribute to the vertical height, as the teeth have not erupted. A rapid phase of growth characterizes the period from 4 to 7 years and this rapid growth phase is followed by a slower period of growth from the ages of 9 to 15 years. From ages 15 to 19 years another period of rapid growth is observed. The facial bones continue to grow until the age of 21 in the male, but at different rates according to the area of the face. Much of the growth, however, is completed well before the teenage period. The orbits, for example, have usually obtained their full adult size by age 7 years and are similar in dimension to the adult by age 2 years. The palate and maxilla have achieved two-thirds of adult size by age 6 years. In contrast, the nasal bones show major growth in the adolescent period. A major proportion of cranial growth is completed by the age of 2 years. From birth to age 10 years the brain triples in size and is 90 per cent of its final size by the age of 10 years. From birth the cranium increases four times to its adult size, whereas the facial skeleton increases 12 times to obtain its adult proportions (Hellman, 1935; Scott, 1959; Enlow, 1982).

Increase in facial height is greater in the middle third of the face than in the lower third. The increase in the anteroposterior direction is greater in the lower jaw than in the upper jaw. The face also widens more in the lower jaw than in the upper jaw (Moss and Rankow, 1968).

At birth, the proportion of the nasal fossa occupied by the ethmoid bone is twice the height of the maxillary portion. During childhood the growth of the maxillary portion is

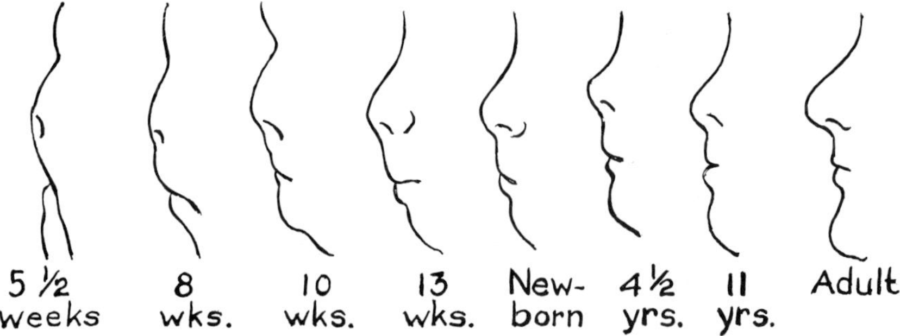

Figure 28–7. Series of profile outlines of the face from 5.5 weeks to adulthood. (After Peter and Schaefer.)

accelerated, approximating the ethmoidal portion at the seventh year when adult proportions are obtained. The growth of the maxillary portion of the nasal fossa is due in part to the increase in size of the maxillary sinus and to the eruption of the dentition and the supporting alveolar processes. Changes in the maxilla and mandible result in characteristic changes of profile (Hellman, 1935; Scott, 1959; Moss and Rankow, 1968; Enlow, 1982).

The peak rate of growth in the head and face occurs between 3 and 5 years. After this period, growth proceeds slowly, but an acceleration occurs again between the 13th and 15th years. Growth is greatly diminished after the age of 15 years. Growth of the nose is completed between the 18th and 25th years (Fig. 28–7). From a surgical standpoint, one may consider the growth of the nose completed at approximately the age of 16 years. Minor changes occur throughout life (Ortiz-Monasterio and Olmedo, 1981; Muller, 1983).

Postnatal Growth of the Mandible

The mandible is the facial bone most frequently involved in post-traumatic developmental malformations. Embryologically, the dorsal part of the first mandibular arch grows forward beneath the developing eye region to the olfactory area, forming the maxillary process (see Chap. 46). As a result of this formation, the mesenchymatous condensation, which gives origin to the first pharyngeal arch, becomes convex, and part of the dorsal portion becomes chondrified, forming a small cartilaginous mass that represents the pterygoquadrate bar of lower vertebrates. The remaining ventral and much larger portion of the pharyngeal arch chondrifies to form *Meckel's cartilage* (Enlow, 1982).

The posterior extremities of the pterygoquadrate bar of Meckel's cartilage articulate with each other. The intermediate portion of Meckel's cartilage retrogresses and its sheath becomes ligamentous, forming the anterior ligament of the malleus and the sphenomandibular ligament. The dorsal portion, in contact with the pterygoquadrate cartilage, becomes recognizable as a definitive cartilaginous rudiment of the malleus, whereas the ventral portion is involved in development of the incus (Fig. 28–8) (Moss and Rankow, 1968).

Later in development, two membranous bones are laid down on the outer side of Meckel's cartilage. The most anterior of these, which appears early, is related to the lateral aspect of the ventral portion of the cartilage and forms the mandible. At first it is a small covering of membranous bone. However, by growth and extension it soon surrounds Meckel's cartilage, except at its anterior extremity, where endochondral ossification occurs. Upward growth forms the mandibular ramus at the posterior end of the developing mandible. This portion of the mandible comes into contact with the squamous portion of the temporal bone to form the temporomandibular joint, in which a fibrocartilaginous articular disc develops. Part of the ramus of the mandible is transformed into cartilage before cartilage ossification occurs (Moss and Salentijn, 1969; Enlow, 1982).

In mammals, as in many other vertebrates, arches of the membranous bone are laid down lateral to the cartilages of the first pharyn-

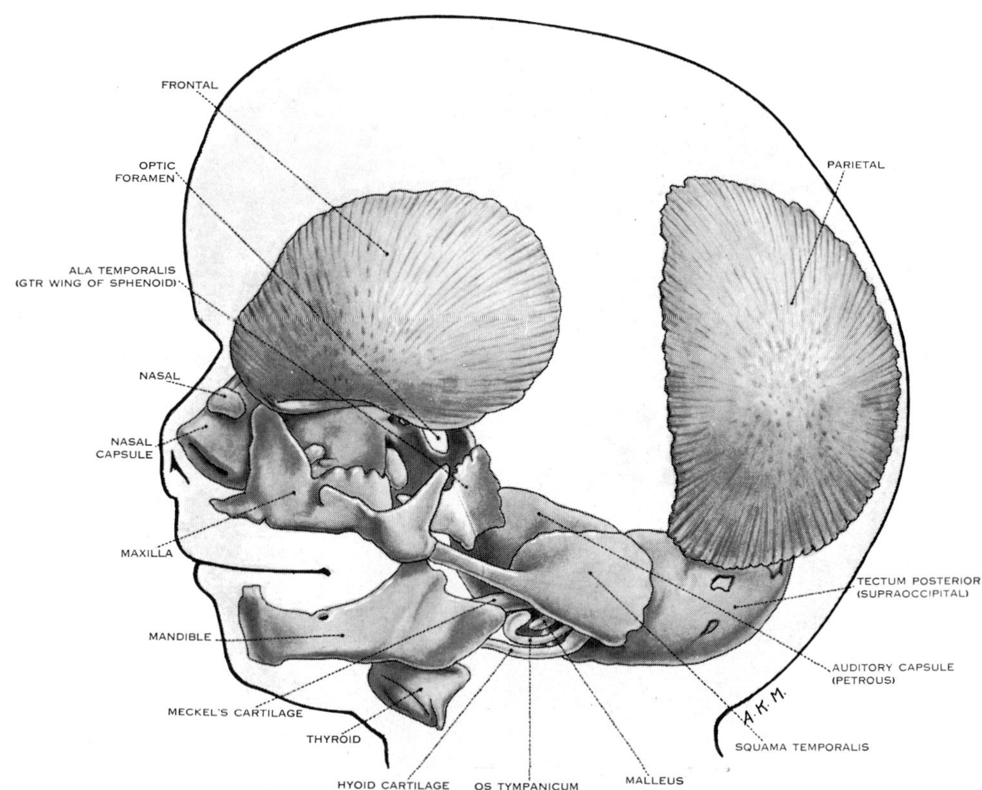

Figure 28–8. Lateral aspect of a model of the skull of an 80 mm human embryo. (Based on Hertwig's model, from Kollmonn's Handatlas, 1970.) (From Hamilton, W. J., Boyd, J. D., and Mossman, H. W.: Human Embryology. Copyright 1945, The Williams & Wilkins Company, Baltimore.)

geal arch and in the substance of the maxillary and mandibular processes. In the maxillary process of each side, four such ossification areas form the premaxilla, maxilla, and zygomatic and squamous portion of the temporal bones (Enlow, 1982).

The mandible, small at birth, is destined to grow both by bone growth and by development of the alveolar process, which accompanies teeth development. The recognition of condylar growth centers showed that the forward projection of the mandible is a consequence of this posterior growth. Elongation of the mandible involves continuous addition of bone at each condyle and along the posterior border of the ramus (see Chap. 47). Posterior appositional growth is only one of many movements associated with total mandibular growth, as all the different portions of the bone participate in the growth process. In addition to the centers of growth, increase in size is the result of surface apposition, the local contours of the mandible constantly undergoing changes as a result of remodeling, resorptive, and depository activities (Moss, 1968; Moss and Rankow, 1968; Moss and Salentijn, 1969; Enlow, 1982).

Growth of the condyle is the result of endochondral ossification in the epiphysis. Microscopic examination of human material showed chondrogenic, cartilaginous, and osseous zones. The condyle is capped by a narrow layer of a vascular fibrous tissue, which contains connective tissue cells and a few cartilage cells. The inner layer of this covering is chondrogenic, giving rise to hyaline cartilage cells that form the second or cartilaginous zone. Destruction of the cartilage and ossification around the cartilage scaffolding can be seen in the third zone. The cartilage of the head of the mandible is not similar to the epiphyseal cartilage of the long bone; it differs from articular cartilage in that the free surface bounding the articular spaces is covered by fibrous tissue. The role of trauma is particularly important to the condylar articular cartilage in that it may result in mandibular hypoplasia (Fig. 28–9), particu-

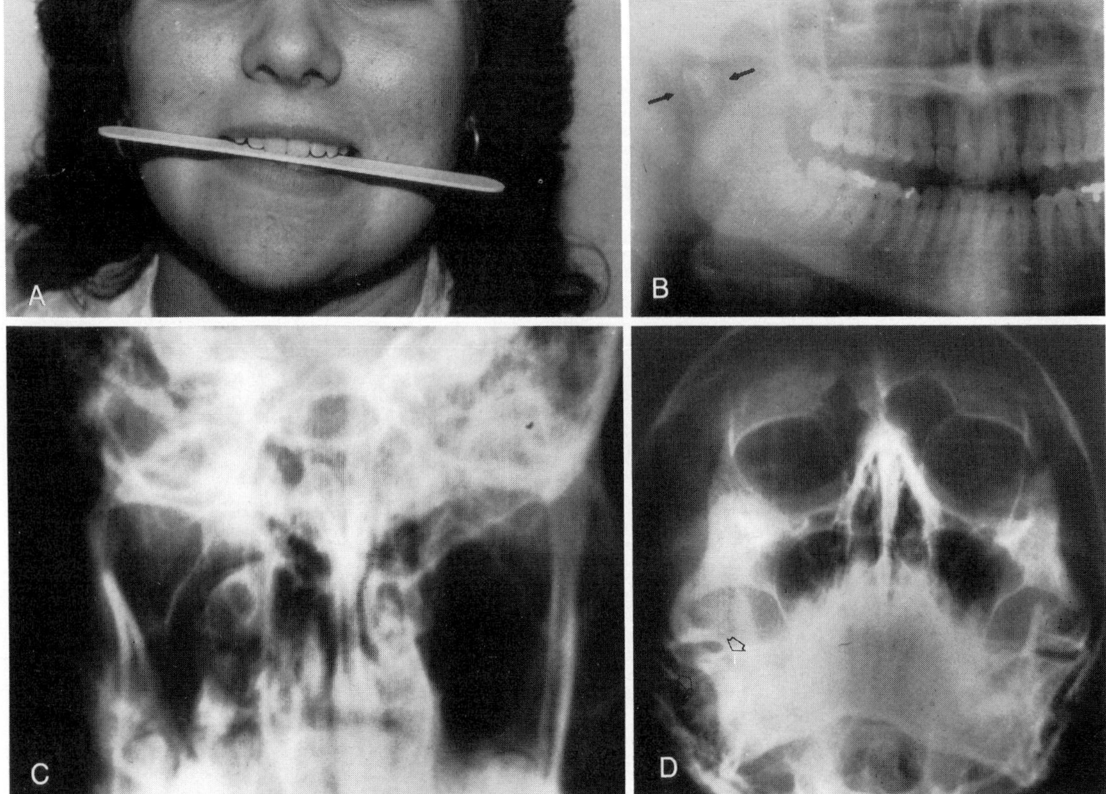

Figure 28–9. *A,* A 20 year old woman showing asymmetric facial growth after sustaining a right condylar fracture at age 5 years. Right maxillary and mandibular growth was affected, resulting in an occlusal cant and a 15 mm height difference between the two rami. *B,* Panoramic roentgenogram showing a shortened, deformed right condyle. *C,* Plain film revealing asymmetry of the rami and condyles. *D,* Waters view demonstrating the malformation of the right ramus and condyle.

larly if the trauma occurs before the age of 5 years (Moss, 1968; Moss and Rankow, 1968; Moss and Salentijn, 1969).

Postnatal Growth of the Nasomaxillary Complex

The skeleton of the midface area is formed from membranous bone, with the exception of the nasal cartilaginous capsule. These bones grow in a complex manner in a variety of regional directions. The growth and development of the nasomaxillary complex has been studied by numerous anatomists. The anteroposterior growth of the nasomaxillary complex is related in utero and also after birth to the growth of the cranial base cartilages and their synchondroses. The intersphenoidal and the septoethmoidal synchondroses show evidence of activity until adulthood. At birth the nasal septum is continuous with the cartilages of the cranial base. Around the first year, the perpendicular plate of the ethmoid starts to ossify from the nasoethmoidal center. At 3 years of age there is bony union between the ethmoidal and the vomer bones. The bony structures of the nasomaxillary areas follow a complex process of growth (Moss and Rankow, 1968; Enlow, 1982).

There is not only a forward and downward growth of the maxilla, but also a constant remodeling of the multiple regional parts. The main steps in development include a displacement away from the cranial base, a posterior enlargement corresponding to the lengthening of the dental arch, and an anterior resorption of the malar region. The nasal vaults grow forward and laterally, and the descent of the premaxillary area occurs by resorption on the superior and anterior surface of the nasal spine and by bony deposition on the inferior surface (Enlow, 1982).

Considerable controversy has arisen over the role of the septum in the growth of the nasomaxillary complex and over the implications of trauma causing abnormal growth of the area. The midfacial area is formed of membranous bone, with the exception of the cartilaginous nasal capsule. Some authors consider the septum to be the driving force in the growth of the midfacial area (Sarnat and Gans, 1952; Scott, 1959). Others feel that the role of the nasal septum in growth is of lesser importance (Moss and Rankow, 1968). According to Moss, facial growth is controlled by a *functional matrix*, which comprises the nonskeletal elements of the face, including spaces, muscles, and soft tissue (Moss, 1968; Moss and Rankow, 1968; Moss and Salentijn, 1969).

Others have concluded that the maxilla drifts forward as part of an overall genetic and environmental pattern of growth, bone being laid down in the sutures and on the maxillary tuberosity. The maxilla is thought to be more easily influenced in its growth than the mandible (May and associates, 1981; Enlow, 1982).

The role of trauma in interfering with the growth and development of the midfacial area seems to be difficult to determine. In making comparison with another facial area, namely, the mandible, one finds considerable disparity between the extent of the damage suffered by the condylar area and the extent of the ensuing maldevelopment. In some cases of fracture of the condylar area in children, complete restoration of anatomic form occurs without interference with growth and development; in other cases, which seem to be minor, damage results in mandibular hypoplasia. Much depends, apparently, on the extent of the damage to the condylar cartilage (Fig. 28–9) (Sarnat and Gans, 1952; Andreasen, 1970b; Andreasen and Ravn, 1971; Bales, Randall, and Lehr, 1972; Jazbi, 1977).

CLINICAL EXAMINATION

The clinical examination of children is often difficult. Pediatric patients are frequently unable or unwilling to provide a history and the parents may or may not be present to add detailed information. Children are often uncooperative and become easily frightened and apprehensive. The fears and anxiety of the parents are transmitted to the child and the clinical examination can be difficult in the absence of cooperation. If the parents are contributing to the anxiety of the child, they should be removed from the examination area. This is an individual choice and depends very much on individual circumstances. The proper assessment of a particular child and his or her parents demands an individual evaluation, considerable patience, some psychiatric qualifications, and a gentle but firm determination. Children should be warned of pain and they should be told the truth if they ask questions. Patience and time spent in obtaining their confidence can be helpful. However, they often remain unwilling to cooperate and the examination must then proceed. Sedation may be necessary in patients in whom the observation of a head injury is not a concern, and general anesthesia may sometimes be required for adequate examination and treatment.

Other injuries outside the facial region are observed in 60 per cent of patients with minor trauma. Skull fractures and cervical spine injuries accompanying facial fractures are frequent in childhood. The identification of a head injury is particularly important in that children are often frightened and the physician may easily overlook confusion or confuse the subtle symptoms of a cerebral injury with the emotional reaction to the accident (Freid and Baden, 1954; McCoy, Chandler, and Crow, 1966; Bales, Randall, and Lehr, 1972; Hall, 1974; Kaban, Mulliken, and Murray, 1977; Adekey, 1980; Mayer and associates, 1980).

The clinical examination consists of an orderly inspection of all facial areas, including observation, palpation, and a functional examination. Areas in which lacerations or bruises are present are identified as specific areas of concern. Frequently, an underlying fracture is present. An orderly palpation of all bony surfaces should be performed by beginning in the skull and forehead area and by palpating the rims of the orbits and the nose, in order to identify any evidence of tenderness, irregularity, or step or "level" discrepancy in the bony structure. Crepitus may be present, particularly over a nasal or orbital rim fracture. The examination is continued over the zygomatic arches, the cheeks, and the surface of the mandible. An intraoral examination is performed to demonstrate loose teeth and identify intraoral lacerations or hematomas. Lateral pressure on the mandibular and maxillary dental arches is necessary to determine instability or pain in fractures involving the midline of the mandible or maxilla. A common fracture in the child's Le Fort injury, for instance, is a "sagittal" fracture of the palate and maxilla. The fracture may easily be missed in the absence of a mucosal laceration if the segments of the maxilla are not examined for lateral instability as well as for anteroposterior movement. The presence of avulsed, loose, or missing teeth should signal the possibility of a significant fracture of the mandible or maxilla (Dingman and Natvig, 1964; Georgiade and Pickrell, 1967; Converse, 1979; Rowe and Williams, 1985).

A cooperative child may be examined for such conditions as double vision. A visual acuity may be recorded and visual fields assessed. The child may volunteer that mandibular motion is painful or that the "bite" is not correct. Such details help to provide additional evidence of fracture and point to the anatomic location to be examined more carefully and evaluated radiographically.

RADIOLOGIC EVALUATION

The standard radiologic evaluation previously consisted of plain films: Caldwell, Waters, submentovertex, Towne, and lateral skull views. The quality of films is directly proportional to the child's cooperation. Frightened and apprehensive children move during the examination and produce blurring of the radiograph. In children, the bone structures are sufficiently cancellous that fracture lines are difficult to observe (Dingman and Natvig, 1964; Georgiade and Pickrell, 1967; Rowe and Williams, 1985). These conditions complicate the radiographic evaluation of pediatric fractures.

Failure to confirm a suspected fracture on radiography should not always deter treatment. Clinical judgment should overrule other considerations. The advent of computerized tomographic (CT) scanning has improved the radiologic diagnosis of mid- and upper facial fractures. Fractures of the frontal area, orbit, and maxilla are precisely demonstrated, although the examination may require sedation. In addition, concomitant brain injury can be evaluated with suitable techniques in a single examination, taking facial and cranial views (Georgiade and Pickrell, 1967; Rowe and Williams, 1985).

The management of major injuries in children thus challenges the clinician to achieve a rapid, accurate alignment of facial bone fragments to minimize functional disturbances and permit maximal future growth and development (Freid and Baden, 1954; Freihofer, 1977).

Children are often subjected to injuries from falls and accidents. The frequency of fractures, however, is small and children's bones, which are soft and resilient, are protected by both anatomic and environmental factors. The larger cancellous-to-cortical structural ratio makes the bones bend and resist injury. The incomplete ("greenstick") fracture is common (Fig. 28–10). Children, having a smaller face-to-head size ratio, pro-

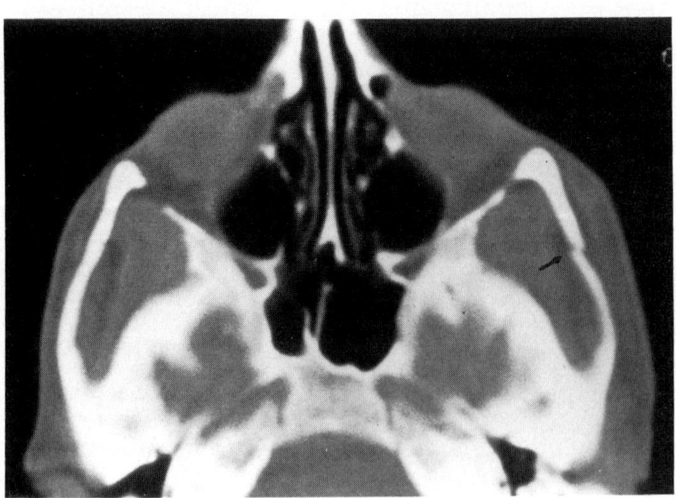

Figure 28–10. An example of a "greenstick", nondisplaced zygoma fracture on CT scan *(arrow)*.

tect their faces by the protruding frontal skull. The soft tissues are proportionately thicker in children and thus provide for more padding (Dingman and Natvig, 1964; Georgiade and Pickrell, 1967).

EMERGENCY TREATMENT

The control of hemorrhage, the provision of an adequate airway, and the prevention of aspiration are the major considerations that demand emergency management in facially injured children. In young children, the dimensions of the trachea and pharynx are small, and as such can easily be obstructed by blood clots, mucus, fractured teeth, or foreign objects. Provision of an adequate airway is initiated by the removal of such material from the oropharynx. Obstruction of the hypopharynx may be relieved simply by forward traction on the tongue or mandible. Tracheostomy usually is not necessary in children, and protection of the airway can be achieved by orotracheal or nasotracheal intubation (Oliver and associates, 1962; Bridges and associates, 1966; Othersen, 1979).

Pediatric endotracheal tubes are not "cuffed," and thus material from the oropharynx may enter the trachea around the tube. The use of a throat pack helps to protect the trachea from aspiration. The small size of the trachea makes obstruction by retained mucous secretions a constant threat, even in the face of endotracheal intubation. Appropriate management with humidification, suction, and mucolytic agents is required. Tracheostomy complications or decannulation problems occur in one-half of those who undergo the procedure, and practically all the complications occur in patients under 5 years of age. Complications include pneumothorax, emphysema, bleeding, infection, tracheal erosion or stenosis, occlusion of the cannula, displacement of the tube, and difficulty in decannulation (Oliver and associates, 1962; Bridges and associates, 1966).

The blood volume of children is small, and significant circulatory compromise occurs with the loss of 20 per cent or less of total blood volume. The blood volume is 90 ml/kg before the age of 1 year. Hemorrhage from lacerations associated with closed fractures must be treated immediately. The control of significant hemorrhage from cutaneous lacerations may usually be achieved with digital pressure. Precise identification of the bleeding vessel before ligation facilitates the avoidance of facial nerve injury. For significant nasopharyngeal hemorrhage from closed maxillofacial fractures, a nasopharyngeal packing is used. Intranasal tamponade is generally successful in the management of profuse nasopharyngeal hemorrhage associated with severe facial fractures. A posterior pack is placed in the back of the nose through the mouth and pulled into place with strings led through the nose (Rasmussen, 1965; Reil and Kranz, 1976). Alternately, small Foley catheter balloons can be inflated in the nasopharynx after a catheter has been passed through each nostril, and then pulled anteriorly and secured. Anterior packing is placed within the recesses of the nasal cavity to provide the pressure necessary to tamponade the hemorrhage. Care should be taken in patients with injuries to the cranial base that the packing is not inadvertently placed intracranially (Rasmussen, 1965).

Aspiration is frequent with significant injuries of the mandible and maxilla, and contributes to rapid respiratory obstruction or impairment of respiratory gas exchange. In the series of McCoy and associates (1962, 1966), it was found to be the most frequent complication. It can be prevented by intubation and the use of a pharyngeal pack. Aspiration can also be minimized by oronasopharyngeal suctioning in patients in whom the use of an endotracheal tube is undesirable. The prolonged use of an endotracheal tube carries with it the complication of tracheal stenosis. This can be minimized by appropriate attention to detail and possibly by the use of steroids. Roentgenographic studies of the airway can be used to identify patients with a constriction of the tracheal lumen. Those in whom tracheal narrowing is identified are treated with bronchoscopy, removal of granulation tissue, systemic steroids, and a tracheal stent for the acute tracheal intubation injury (McCoy and associates, 1962; Oliver and associates, 1962; McCoy, Chandler, and Crow, 1966; Othersen, 1979; McCoy, 1980).

PRENATAL, BIRTH, AND INFANT INJURIES

Intrauterine compression is thought to be the cause of prenatal deformities, although evidence of this type of injury has never been substantiated. Clinically anecdotal reports have described instances in which positioning or crowding of multiparous siblings resulted in facial deformities.

Birth injuries may result from prolonged labor with difficult passage through the birth canal and delivery by obstetric forceps. Most of the injuries due to obstetric forceps are minimal, and recovery usually takes place without residual deformity. Infant and child skulls are pliable because of the segmental arrangement, flexibility, resilience, and relative softness of the bones. The bones develop as a loosely joined system found in the matrix surrounding the brain. They are separated by fontanelles and sutures covered by thin fibrous sheaths. These characteristics explain the malleability of the cranial and facial bones and the fact that they are subject to distortion in crushing injuries, which may have subsequent developmental repercussions (Hellman and Pritchard, 1971).

Fractures of the skull are occasionally encountered, usually after forcible attempts at delivery, although they may occur spontaneously. There are two presentations: (1) an appearance of a shallow groove and (2) an elliptic or round depression posterior to the coronal suture. The former is common and has few sequelae. The latter, if not operated on, results in death in over half of the cases secondary to increased intracranial pressure or hemorrhage (Hellman and Pritchard, 1971).

Deviation of the septum has been attributed to forced deflection during birth. More severe injuries have been attributed to forceps compression of the soft tissues and bones of the face, which may cause permanent facial scars or osseous deformities in the region of the zygomatic arch and temporomandibular joint. The latter result in temporomandibular ankylosis with subsequent developmental hypoplasia of the mandible. The lack of development of the mastoid process at birth and the subcutaneous position of the seventh cranial nerve predispose to facial paralysis by pressure from delivering forceps. Such injuries are, in fact, observed when the posterior blade of the forceps places pressure over the stylomastoid foramen as the seventh nerve exits. Spontaneous recovery in a few days is the general rule (Hellman and Pritchard, 1971).

Injuries to the eye or its adnexa, such as damage to the extraocular musculature, may be caused by intraorbital hemorrhage. Fractures of the body of the mandible due to birth injury are rare. They usually are linear fractures with little, if any, displacement. Healing occurs in a short time without manipulative treatment. Cases have been reported of newborn babies having sustained separation of the two halves of the mandible at the symphysis following a maneuver by the obstetrician, who placed his finger in the child's mouth and used forceful manipulation to deliver the baby (Mauriceau's maneuver).

Injury to the sternocleidomastoid muscle may occur, particularly during a breech delivery with lateral hyperextension. There may be a tear of the muscle or fascia, resulting in a hematoma and eventual cicatricial torticollis deformity. If not corrected or released, this may lead to craniofacial asymmetry (Roemer, 1954).

It has long been suspected that infants fall much more frequently than is generally known. Of 536 infants involved in the study sponsored by the National Safety Council, 47.5 per cent fell from a high place such as an adult bed, a crib, or an infant dressing table during their first year of life (Keith and Campion, 1922). Some of the infants in the study suffered cranial, intracranial, and facial injuries. It can be assumed that facial trauma occurring in such falls in infants, although it does not often result in fractures because of the elasticity of the neonatal bones, may be sufficient to interfere with the growth centers and may explain some of the developmental malformations of the face observed in later years (Lindenberg and associates, 1955; Jazbi, 1977).

SOFT TISSUE INJURIES IN INFANTS AND CHILDREN

Maxillofacial soft tissue trauma and injuries in the pediatric population range from contusions and abrasions to massive avulsive injuries. As with any injury, the return to normal function and appearance is the paramount aim of treatment. The basic fundamentals of management of such injuries are similar to those pertaining to adults. Debridement of tissues should be restricted to that which is clearly devitalized. Careful cleaning and irrigation of wounds should be carried out in order to remove dirt and any foreign bodies. On occasion, a stiff nylon or wire brush, needle, or blade is required to remove small embedded particles that would result in tattooing of the soft tissues (Bernstein, 1969; Mustardé, 1971).

Contusions and ecchymosis usually require only symptomatic treatment. When these are combined with an underlying hematoma, open drainage may have to be performed. When still in the "currant jelly" stage, a hematoma can easily be drained by incision. After further liquefaction, aspiration may be performed. Hematomas of the external ears present special problems: if not evacuated, they organize into residual subcutaneous and perichondrial scar tissue and result in the "cauliflower ear" deformity (Tate, 1971; Reil and Kranz, 1976).

Lacerations may be of the simple, beveled, torn, burst, or stellate type. Repair should be undertaken after the underlying structures have been cleaned and debrided and the foreign bodies removed. The wound edges should be debrided conservatively, but adequately. Suturing should be meticulous. When lacerations through soft tissue containing cartilage are being repaired, as in the ear or nose, stabilizing stitches using absorbable material should be used to stabilize the cartilage in its proper place, followed by layer closure. Lacerations in special regions of the face require particular attention to realignment of the anatomy, e.g., the vermilion border of the lips, eyelids, and eyebrows. The eyebrow should never be shaved before its alignment (Converse and Dingman, 1977; Converse, 1979).

Soft tissue wounds in children heal rapidly and therefore require primary suture. Lacerations repaired at an early age tend to become less conspicuous with the passage of time. Pediatricians often advise parents to wait until the child has reached adolescence before the repair is effected. This is poor advice, because many scars repaired in infancy and childhood are inconspicuous if not invisible in adolescence (Converse and Dingman, 1977).

Some wounds tend to heal with considerable hypertrophic scarring. These discouraging results often require later surgical repair, and this possibility should be mentioned to the parents. Densely scarred areas may require reconstructive procedures, for such untreated areas may interfere with subjacent bony growth, particularly in the area of the chin and mandible (Converse and Dingman, 1977; Converse, 1979).

Loss of soft tissue of the face by avulsion or thermal burns is remedied by skin transplantation. Defects of the nose are adequately repaired in many cases by composite auricular grafts, which show a high success rate in children. Subtotal or total loss of the nose is quite rare (Converse and Dingman, 1977).

Intraoral lacerations usually are loosely sutured to help reduce the healing time. Lacerations of the tongue are sutured in several layers to lessen the chance of hematoma formation.

When a major salivary gland duct is lacerated, both ends must be located and sutured together. In the case of the parotid duct, the distal end is usually first found by placement of a probe or a catheter through the oral opening. This is then brought out through the laceration and used as a stent for the anastomosis. The stent is left in place for 24 hours and removed. It has not been proved whether leaving the stent in place guarantees the success of the anastomosis. After repair of the duct, the overlying soft tissue is closed in three layers, a maneuver that prevents formation of a fistulous tract and helps to avoid the formation of a sialocele. If one develops, it may be treated by aspirations and pressure dressings (Converse and Dingman, 1977; Converse, 1979).

If branches of the facial nerve are divided, the nerve can often be repaired primarily if the wound is clean and the laceration relatively sharp. In more destructive injuries such as avulsions or gunshot wounds, nerve repair is usually done secondarily with nerve grafts. As a rule, facial nerve injuries should be repaired surgically if they occur posterior to a vertical line drawn from the lateral canthus. Injuries occurring anterior to this line usually do not need to be repaired (Reil and Kranz, 1976; Converse and Dingman, 1977).

FACIAL FRACTURES

Etiology

The causes of children's fractures are varied. In the infant, falls, toy injuries, and animal bites are common. One should also be aware of the "battered baby" syndrome in which lacerations (particularly in the frenulum of the upper lip), facial or skull fractures, and cervical spine and cerebral injuries can be observed (Caffey, 1946; Silverman, 1953; Tate, 1971; Caffey, 1974; Teasdale and Jennett, 1974; Cohen and associates, 1986). Vehicular trauma (either from motor vehicle or bicycle), athletic injuries, sporting accidents, and injuries occurring from airborne objects are often observed in children over 5 years of age. Unrestrained children in motor vehicles (guest passenger injuries) are a frequent problem. Males are more subject to injury than are females in almost all age groups after age 5 years. In infants, falls are frequent after they have begun to walk, and occur from strollers, baby seats, and dressing tables before that time (Burdi and associates, 1969; Caffey, 1974). Birth injuries frequently dislocate the nasal septum or injure the facial nerve (May and associates, 1981) or temporomandibular joint (Moffett, 1966; Hellman and Pritchard, 1971; Steinhauser, 1973).

The history of the injury may indicate the mechanism and direction of force of the injury and may provide clues for the focus of the clinical examination. Such symptoms may include swelling, pain, numbness in a cranial nerve distribution, or a visual disturbance consisting of either diminished vision, double vision, or inability to open the eyelid. Nasal or oral bleeding, tooth displacement, difficulty in eating, malocclusion, decreased excursion of the jaw, bruising, and ecchymosis point to a skeletal injury. Exophthalmos or enophthalmos may be present. A cerebrospinal fluid (CSF) leak may indicate involvement of the cranial base. Subcutaneous emphysema is seen in the periorbital area when air enters the tissues from fractures of the nose, orbit, or sinuses.

Incidence

Fractures of the facial bones are less frequent in children than in adults. Except in large medical centers, the total experience of any surgeon in managing facial fractures in children is limited.

During their early years, children live in a protected environment under close parental supervision. The resilience of the developing bone, the short distance of the falls, and the thick overlying soft tissue enable the child to withstand forces that in the adult would result in extensive comminution rather than in the greenstick fractures seen most frequently in children. The tooth to bone ratio in the developing mandible is comparatively high, and the bone has a more elastic resistance. The rudimentary paranasal sinuses, the large cartilaginous growth centers, and the small volume ratio between the jaws and the cranium are factors providing additional protection to the facial bone structures.

The incidence of facial bone fractures in children varies according to different reports. In a series of mandibular fractures reviewed by Kazanjian and Converse (1974), children between 4 and 11 years of age represented approximately 10 per cent of the group. In a series reported by Panagopoulos (1957), fractures of facial bones in children represented only 1.4 per cent of the entire series. Pfeifer (1966), in a review of 3033 cases of facial bone fractures, noted that 4.4 per cent had occurred in children in the age group from birth to 10 years; in the age group extending to 14 years the incidence was 11 per cent, and in the age group from 11 to 20 years of age the incidence was 20.6 per cent.

Rowe (1968) summarized his data by stating that 1 per cent of all facial fractures occur before the 6th birthday, and a total of 5 per cent occur in children under the age of 12 years. Approximately one in ten fractures in children under 12 years involves the midfacial skeleton. Rowe noted that midfacial fractures are uncommon before the age of 8 years.

One of the principal causes cited for the rarity of fractures of the facial skeleton in children is the large size of the cranium in relation to the facial skeleton. McCoy, Chandler, and Crow (1966), in an analysis of 1500 cases of facial fractures, reported 86 children of whom 35 (40.8 per cent) had associated skull fractures.

Facial fractures are infrequent before the age of 5 years but become more common up to the age of 10 years when the frequency, pattern, and distribution of fractures tend to parallel that observed in adults. The two peaks of fracture incidence in children are in the 5 to 8 and 10 to 12 age groups. Around the age of 5 years, children enter school and are exposed to a new life style with participation in contact sports. They are subject to physical acts of violence such as fighting. Sports and bicycle activities are no longer

Table 28–1. Facial Fractures Observed in Children

Panagopoulos (1957)	1.4
Pfeifer (1966)	4.4
Rowe (1968, 1969)	5
Converse (1979)	10
McCoy et al. (1966)	6

Figures expressed in percentages.

Table 28–2. Le Fort, Midfacial, and Alveolar Fractures

Author	Le Fort	Maxillary Alveolar
MacLennan (1957)	0.25	
Rowe (1968, 1969)	0.2	
Hall (1972)	6	
Kaban et al. (1977)	0	3
Converse (1979)	10	
Fortunato et al. (1982)	13	2
Reil and Kranz 1982)	6.5	9.5
Ramba (1985)	8	22

Figures expressed in percentages.

under close parental supervision and an increasing frequency of accidents is observed. In the early teenage years, the adventuresome spirit and energy again dominate activity and are unsuppressed by concerns about the consequences of actions. In comparison, infants and preschool children are protected by their parents and constantly supervised, and as a result few significant facial fractures are observed (Dingman and Natvig, 1964; Mustardé, 1971; Rowe and Williams, 1985).

The incidence of fractures of the midface and frontal region varies with the series reported, with the society or country surveyed, and with the characteristics of practice of the reporting author. Nasal fractures and alveolar fractures of the maxilla, for example, are the two most common midfacial injuries. Both are frequently managed on an outpatient basis and often escape hospital record keeping. Thus, the low incidence of midfacial fractures usually reflects only the group admitted to the hospital (Kaban, Mulliken, and Murray, 1977).

The period of childhood includes birth to the ages of 14 to 16 years. Several authors have indicated that the proportion of facial injuries observed in children accounts for 5 per cent of the total of facial fractures observed (Table 28–1). In general, 1 per cent of these injuries are observed in the zero to 5 year age group. Midfacial fractures are uncommon (Table 28–2) with no such injury reported by Kaban, Mulliken, and Murray (1977) in their series of 109 children. Hall (1972, 1974) found a 6 per cent incidence of middle third fractures. Rowe (1968) reported 0.5 per cent of the total of facial injuries in children to be midfacial fractures. At the Johns Hopkins Hospital a ten year survey has been completed and includes 300 patients a year admitted to the pediatric trauma center. Fewer than 5 per cent of these patients had a facial fracture (Table 28–3). Soft tissue injuries were frequent and usually were lacerations or contusions. On the other hand, over 60 per cent of these patients admitted to the hospital had a significant head injury. The protection of the facial bones achieved by the smaller face to head size ratio and the

Table 28–3. Johns Hopkins Series of Pediatric Trauma Admissions

	Total Admissions 3010			**Facial Fractures** 158		
Age	*0–3½ yrs* 11.8%	*4–7 yrs* 23.7%		*8–11 yrs* 26.7%	*12–16 yrs* 37.6%	
Etiology		**Motor vehicle accident** 49.5%		**Physical violence** 21.7%	**Sports** 15%	**Miscellaneous** 13.7%
Pattern	***Mandible*** 31.6%	***Nasal*** 26.7%	***Orbital*** 22.7%	***Zygomatic*** 7.9%	***Frontal*** 2.9%	***Le Fort*** 2.7%

Maxillary	**Fracture**	**Pattern**
Le Fort	I	1.9%
Le Fort	II	.9%
Le Fort	III	1.9%

Table 28–4. Distribution of Pediatric Facial Fractures

Author	Mandible	Nasal	Orbital	Zygomatic	Le Fort
Hall (1972)	20	60			6
Bales et al. (1972)	64.8		5.4	8	16.2
Reil and Kranz (1976)	87		2	4.5	6.5
Kaban et al. (1977)	35	50.4	17.4	5.5	0
Adekeye (1980)	86	5.3		5.3	2.7
Schultz and Meilman (1980)	14	64		15.5	6.5
Fortunato et al. (1982)	55		20	9	13
Ramba (1985)	65	5.8	7	17	8

Figures expressed in percentages.

resilient soft bone structure are emphasized by these statistics.

Other series figures are summarized in Table 28–4. In most patient series, fractures of the nasal bones and mandible account for the majority of injuries. The distribution of facial injuries is also seen in Table 28–4. As previously mentioned, the statistics do not reflect the true incidence of the anterior dental-alveolar fracture, which is usually managed without hospital admission, or the nasal fracture, which is also managed on an outpatient basis (see Table 28–2).

Alveolar Fractures

In the young child, teeth may be dislodged from a segment of the alveolar bone subjected to a labial, buccal, and lingual displacement (Figs. 28–11, 28–12). Frequently the fragments of bone can be molded into alignment, and the teeth survive if adequately supported for several months by wiring to an arch bar, by fixation with an acrylic splint, by threading wires between the teeth and wiring the fragment, or by fixation with a cable arch wire. In the child with incompletely developed roots, teeth may regain their blood supply and survive. In some instances, if treated within an hour and root canal therapy is instituted, the tooth can be replanted with success. If the teeth are fractured and the alveolar structures hopelessly damaged so that they cannot retain tooth structures, it is best to remove the teeth, trim the alveolar process, and suture the soft tissues over the retained injured bone. Bone fragments should not be dissected from the attached soft tissue. Even loose bone fragments, if covered with soft tissue, often survive as grafts (Roed-Petersen and Andreasen, 1970; Andreasen, 1971; Andreasen and Ravn, 1971; Andreasen, Sundstrom, and Ravn, 1971).

Fractured crowns of teeth without exposure

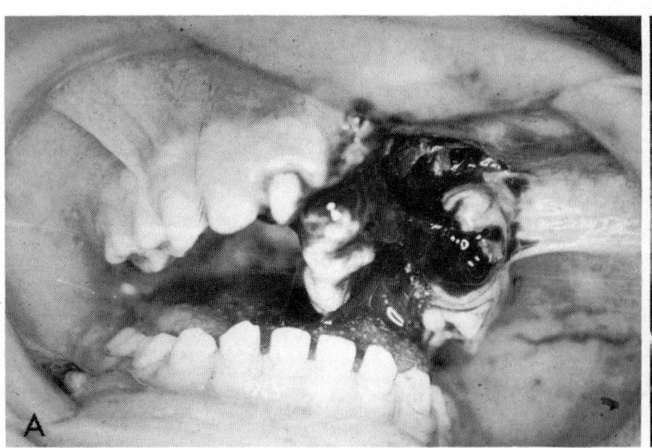

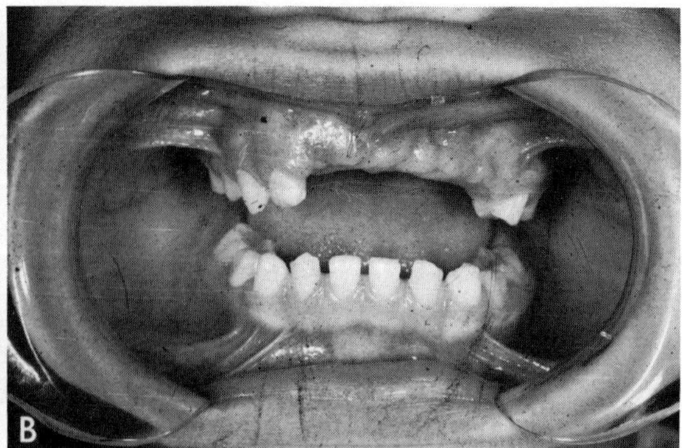

Figure 28–11. Maxillary alveolar fracture with dislocation and avulsion of several teeth. *A,* Preoperative appearance. *B,* Postoperative healing after removal of the deciduous teeth, replacement of the alveolar bone, and suture of the soft tissues.

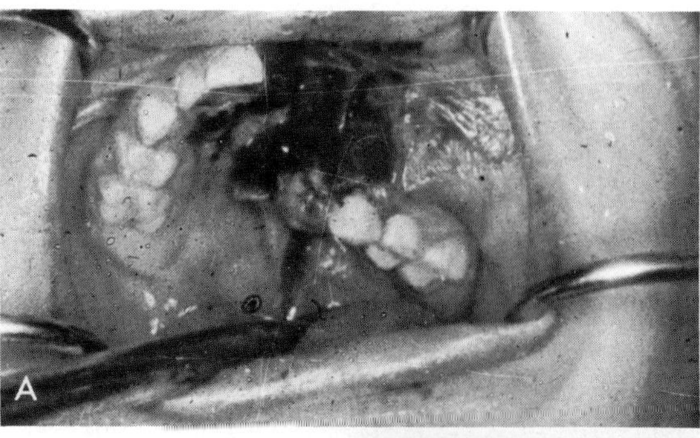

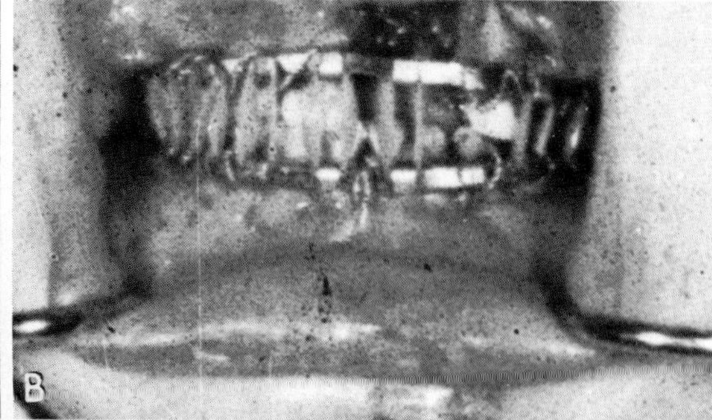

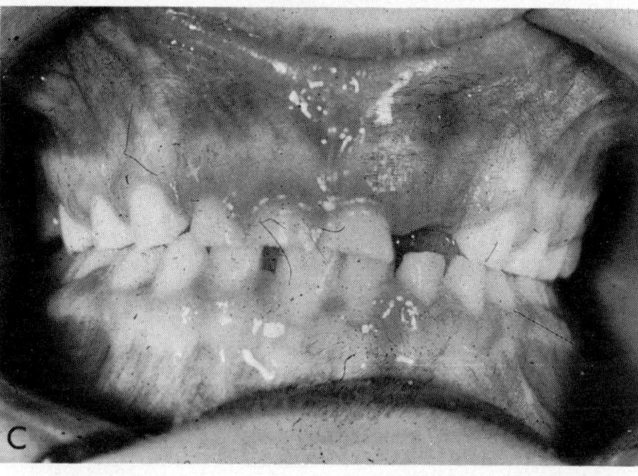

Figure 28–12. Compound maxillary fracture with displacement of fragments and avulsion of the teeth. *A,* Preoperative appearance. *B,* After reduction, the fractured segments were replaced, the remaining teeth were fixated with an arch bar and intermaxillary fixation was established. Note the circumferential wire reinforcing the lower arch bar. *C,* Satisfactory result with survival of the fragments and avulsed teeth.

of the pulp should be protected by dental methods, as they can usually be restored successfully. If the crown of the tooth is fractured and dental pulp exposed, the prognosis may be good if the tooth is capped or a partial pulpectomy is performed. This type of therapy is most successful in the tooth with an open apex. However, even in the more fully developed tooth, pulpectomy and root canal treatment may be effective in saving the tooth structures. Fracture of the root near the crown usually requires extraction. If teeth can be retained only a few months, they may be useful in maintaining space until prosthetic replacement can be provided. Damage to the permanent tooth buds may result in deformed tooth structures, false eruption, or irregular arrangement of the erupting teeth in the dental arch (Andreasen, 1970b,c).

Dental injuries traditionally have been divided into those that involve deciduous teeth and those that involve permanent dentition. Injuries to the deciduous dentition may often occur between the ages of 1 and 2½ years when children are learning to walk. Owing to the relative softness of the premaxilla at this age, the most common injury is one of displacement of the upper incisors. This may result in either an intrusion of the tooth into the premaxilla, a loosening or partial dislocation with lingual or buccal displacement, or a total tooth avulsion (Andreasen, 1970a,b,c; Roed-Petersen and Andreasen, 1970; Andreasen, 1971; Andreasen and Ravn, 1971; Andreasen, Sundstrom, and Ravn, 1971; Bales, Randall, and Lehr, 1972).

Intruded teeth frequently reerupt in the subsequent weeks and may reach full eruption in four to six months. In a child younger than 2½ years of age with incomplete root formation, intruded teeth may retain normal vitality after reeruption. In children older than 2½ or 3 years of age, calcific degeneration and necrosis of pulp are common sequelae to the reeruption of intruded teeth after root formation is mature (Andreasen, 1970c; Andreasen and Ravn, 1971; Andreasen, Sundstrom, and Ravn, 1971).

Elaborate methods for fixation of injured deciduous teeth are contraindicated. Partially dislocated deciduous teeth should be reoriented intraorally if sufficiently stable. Otherwise, they should be extracted, followed in some instances by placement of a space maintainer. The future of partially dislocated teeth is related to the maturity of the dental root at the time of injury. The capacity of teeth, particularly those with an open apex, to retain viability is considerable, given immobilization for three to four weeks and the prevention of infection. Total avulsion of deciduous teeth is less common than other forms of displacement, but it results in the greatest damage to the overlying permanent teeth (Andreasen, 1971).

Fractures of the crowns and roots of the deciduous teeth are comparably rare and far less common than fractures in the permanent teeth. Fractured crowns with exposed dentin but without pulpal involvement should be protected until definitive dental restoration can be completed. An extensive crown fracture invariably involves the pulp and the tooth should be extracted. Root fractures, particularly those involving the coronal portions of the root, also require extraction of the tooth. Surgical removal of the apical portions of the fractured deciduous tooth roots is necessary to prevent later interference in the eruption of the permanent teeth. Fractures in the apical portions of the root usually heal uneventfully (Andreasen and Ravn, 1971; Rowe and Winter, 1971).

Trauma to the deciduous teeth, because of the close anatomic relationships between the apices of the primary and the permanent teeth, may result in damage to the developing permanent dentition. The prevalence of such developmental disturbances ranges from 12 to 69 per cent (Andreasen and Ravn, 1971; Andreasen, Sundstrom, and Ravn, 1971; Berkowitz, Ludwig, and Johnson, 1980).

In one review of 103 patients with traumatized permanent dentition, white or yellow-brown discoloration of the enamel was observed in 23 per cent, and discoloration of the teeth and enamel associated with circular enamel hypoplasia in 12 per cent (Andreasen and Ravn, 1971). Other disturbances in morphology, such as crown dilaceration, late root angulation, and partial or complete arrestive root formation, were found in 6 per cent of patients. Disturbances in the permanent dentition were less frequent in patients whose injury occurred after they reached 4 years of age (MacLennan, 1957; Rowe, 1971; Berkowitz, Ludwig, and Johnson, 1980).

Subluxation of permanent teeth with the associated alveolar bone is treated by repositioning and splinting according to conventional methods. The teeth frequently become nonvital and require root canal therapy and root canal filling at a later date, particularly when the root formation is complete at the moment of injury. In cases of complete avulsion of the permanent tooth when the root is immature and the apex widely open, the tooth should be reimplanted and stabilized in the socket within a few minutes of injury (MacLennan, 1957; Berkowitz, Ludwig, and Johnson, 1980). In these instances the prognosis for pulp revitalization, revascularization, reinnervation, and continued root formation is good. Reimplantation of a complete avulsion when the root formation is mature, especially when the avulsion is over 30 minutes old, invariably leads to root resorption. The resorption may, however, be an exceedingly slow process, taking ten years or more. Reimplantation in such cases should include pulp removal, pulp space restoration, and splinting (Rowe, 1969, 1971; Rowe and Winter, 1971; Rowe and Williams, 1985).

Mandibular Fractures

Predisposition to greenstick or incomplete fractures in developing bone is attributed to two factors. The first is subcutaneous tissue, mainly adipose tissue, which increases rapidly in thickness during the nine months after birth. At the age of 5 years the subcutaneous layer is actually only half as thick as in a 9 month old infant. The second factor is the resilience of the developing bone. The line of differentiation between cortical bone and medullary bone is not sharply defined, and the resilience of the young bone explains the higher frequency of greenstick fractures in children. When fractures occur as in the body of the mandible, there is often a considerable degree of displacement. The fracture lines tend to be long and oblique, extending downward and forward from the upper border of the mandible. The obliquity of the fracture

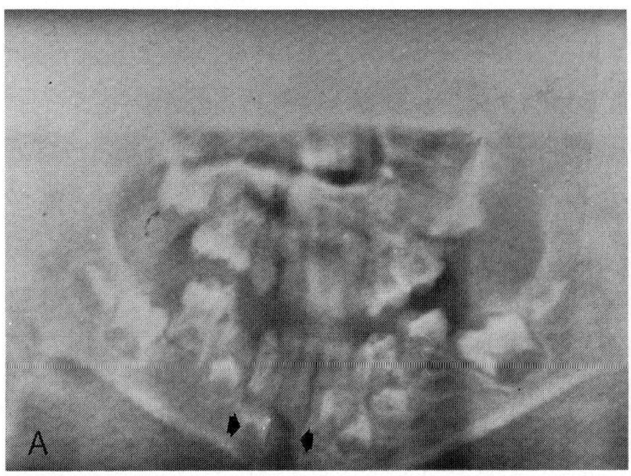

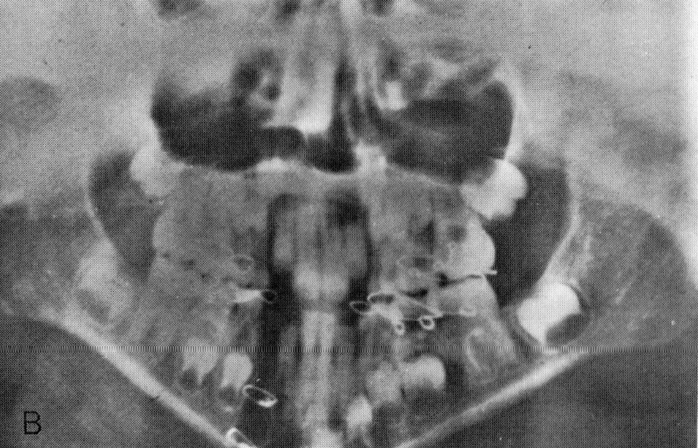

Figure 28–13. *A,* Preoperative panoramic roentgenogram of a parasymphyseal mandibular fracture and alveolar fractures in a child. *B,* Treatment included open reduction and stabilization with wire fixation. Note the close proximity of the secondary tooth follicles.

line is different from that observed in the adult, in whom the direction of the fracture line is usually downward and backward (Bernstein, 1969; Converse, 1979).

Before the eruption of the permanent or secondary dentition, the developing follicles occupy most of the body of the mandible. This anatomic characteristic must be considered if interosseous fixation is to be employed, in order to avoid injuring the tooth buds of the permanent dentition (Fig. 28–13). The wires must be placed near the lower border of the mandible. The roots of the deciduous teeth are gradually being resorbed, and between the ages of 5 and 9 years (a period of mixed dentition), because of the frequent absence of teeth and the poor retentive shape of the crowns of the deciduous teeth, it is often difficult to use the dentition for fixation (Converse and Dingman, 1977; Converse, 1979).

The teeth cannot be employed for fixation in the treatment of mandibular fractures in young infants in whom the teeth are unerupted or only partly erupted. An impression of the mandible can be taken under light anesthesia and an acrylic splint fabricated. After realignment of the fragments, the splint is placed over the mandibular arch, lined with softened dental compound for better adjustment, and maintained in position by circumferential wiring. This type of monomaxillary fixation may be adequate in selected cases (Graham and Peltier, 1960; Danforth, 1969; Kaban, Mulliken, and Murray, 1977).

Intermaxillary fixation is obtained by circumferential wiring around the body of the mandible, combined with circum-maxillary wiring where the wire is further passed into the floor of the nose and downward through the palate, thus surrounding the alveolar area of the maxilla without interfering with the tooth buds of the secondary dentition. Transalveolar wiring above the apices of the teeth can be used in the older child after the eruption of the secondary dentition. At the later age, however, the dentition may be adequate for intermaxillary dental fixation (Danforth, 1969; Converse and Dingman, 1977; Kaban, Mulliken, and Murray, 1977).

During the period when the deciduous dentition is being replaced by the permanent dentition, particularly in the period between the ages of 6 and 12 years, some difficulty may be experienced in obtaining interdental fixation. Acrylic splints may prove to be more useful in this age group (Danforth, 1969).

In older children in whom the dentition is more retentive, various types of fixation can be employed. A band and arch appliance can be employed if the teeth permit retention of the appliance (Fig. 28–14). Circumferential wires aid in stabilizing the mandibular appliance. Eyelet wiring may also be feasible. Direct interosseous fixation, placing the wire near the lower border of the mandible in order to avoid injuring the tooth buds, is of considerable assistance in maintaining the fixation when only deciduous teeth are present for fixation (see Chap. 27). The interosseous wires may be placed through an intraoral approach after the mandible is degloved. A circumferential wire around the mandible is also a useful adjunct in reinforcing the fixation established by arch bar fixation, and it

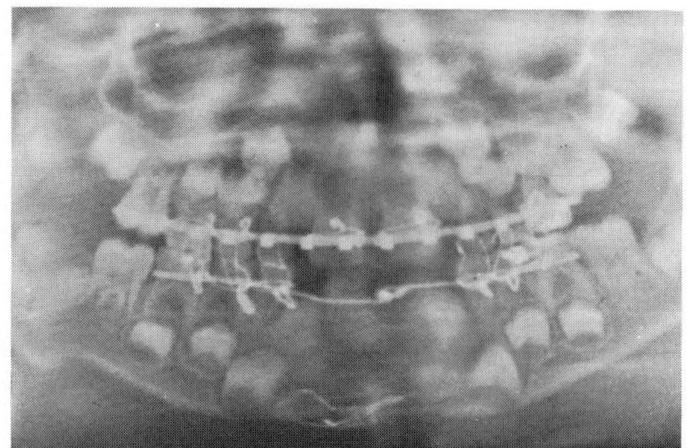

Figure 28–14. Panoramic roentgenographic view of a reduced symphyseal fracture stabilized with wire fixation and arch bars.

can be employed after exposing the ends of the fractured bone intraorally by the degloving procedure (Kazanjian and Converse, 1974; Converse and Dingman, 1977; Converse, 1979).

Fractures of the mandible, like those of other facial bones, must be recognized and treated early in children because of the rapid reparative process. The loose and displaced bony fragments become adherent to one another within three or four days after injury. At this time, fragments are difficult to manipulate and must be loosened under general anesthesia before reduction of the fragment is possible.

Minor degrees of malunion and malocclusion can be tolerated in the growing facial bones and mandible owing to the corrective adjustments that take place with the erupting teeth under normal masticatory stresses (Fig. 28–15) (Converse and Dingman, 1977).

Fractures or injuries to the articular surface of the temporomandibular joint should be suspected in all children who have suffered a severe blow to the chin. Radiographic studies may demonstrate fractures of one or both mandibular condyles with or without displacement. Condylar fractures and injuries should always be viewed with concern in the young child because of the possibility of secondary growth deformities resulting from damage to the condylar growth centers (Fig. 28–16). Injuries to the articular surface of the joint may result in hemarthrosis with cicatricial organization and subsequent bony ankylosis (see Chap. 30). This potential should always be considered and discussed with the parents in injuries of this type (Blev-

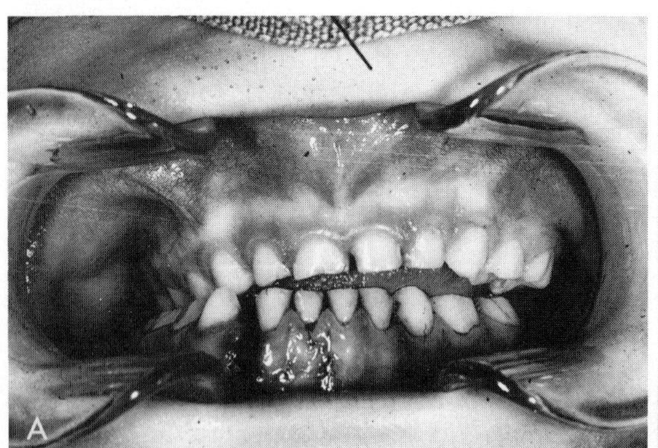

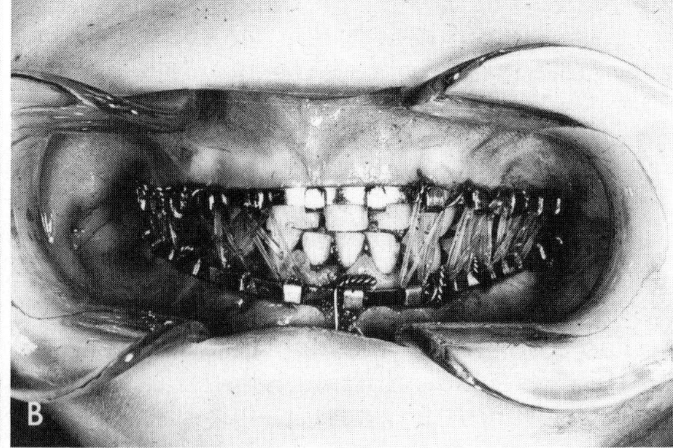

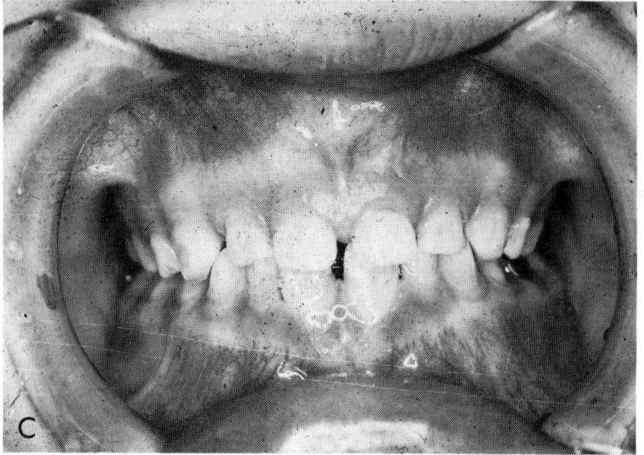

Figure 28–15. Band and arch appliance. *A,* Compound fracture of the mandible between the right deciduous lateral incisor and cuspid tooth. *B,* Closed reduction with arch bar fixation and a circumferential wire around the symphysis of the mandible to stabilize the lower arch bar. Note the circumferential wire twisted at the top of the arch bar. *C,* Occlusion of the teeth two years later.

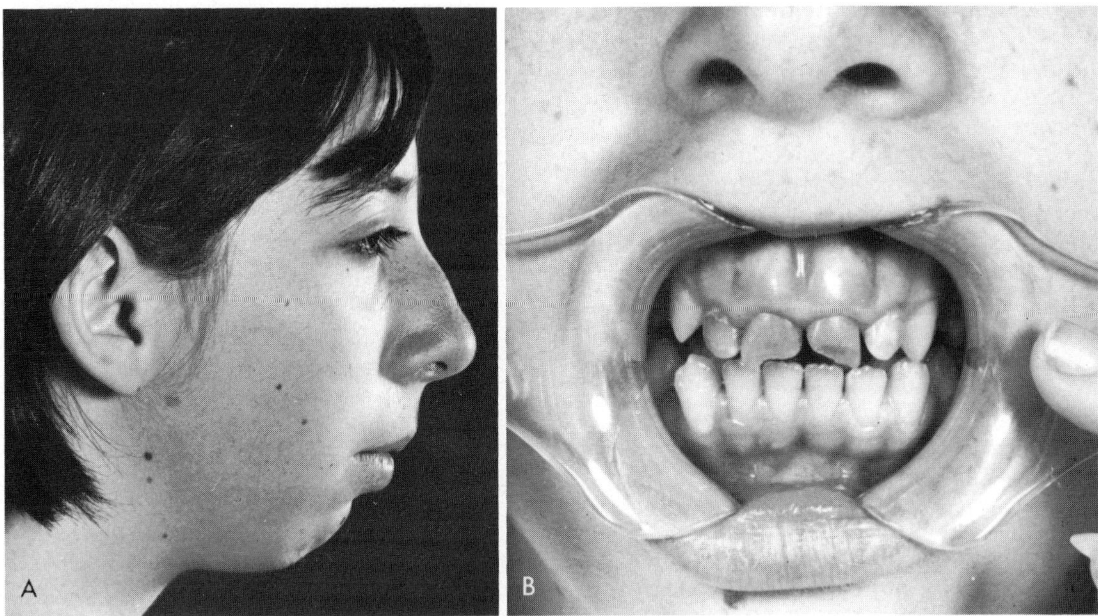

Figure 28–16. Typical mandibular deformity resulting from condylar injury in early childhood. *A*, Underdeveloped mandible in a patient with temporomandibular ankylosis. *B*, Maximal opening (1 to 2 mm) achieved by the patient. Note the hygienic status of the teeth.

ins and Gores, 1961; Boyne, 1967; Fortunato, Fielding, and Guernsey, 1982).

Condylar cartilage is first noted during prenatal life at the 12th week. Large vascular channels appear during the 20th week of fetal life and persist until the second or third year of postnatal life, when they progressively diminish in size. During this period the neck of the condyle progressively increases in length to form the long, slender condylar neck of the adult. Despite the fact that during the first three years of postnatal life the condyle is short and thick and thus less susceptible to fracture, it is also more vulnerable to a crushing injury because of its vascular trabecular structure. The crushing results in intra-articular and periarticular hemorrhage and osteogenesis, and progressive ossification results in temporomandibular ankylosis. Dufourmentel and Mouly (1969) noted that the condyle in the young child was more easily crushed than fractured. Early or immediate motion often prevents this complication (Blevins and Gores, 1961; MacLennan and Simpson, 1965; Boyne, 1967; Hall, 1972, 1974; Fortunato, Fielding, and Guernsey, 1982).

Condylar fractures that involve the bone of the neck of the condyle are often of the greenstick variety and are not usually accompanied by disturbances of the temporomandibular joint. Fortunately, many fractures in the condylar area of the mandible in children are not followed by ankylosis or growth disturbance (Graham and Peltier, 1960; MacLennan and Simpson, 1965).

Temporomandibular ankylosis may follow injury to the condyle. Often there is no history of injuries, and radiologic examination is unremarkable. Months later, the patient may develop limitation of motion of the mandible as a result of partial ankylosis. A progressive straightening of the neck of the condyle is observed after fractures in which bony contact between the fragments have been maintained (MacLennan, 1956; MacLennan and Simpson, 1965). Pfeifer (1966) noted that, in fracture dislocation with loss of contact between the fragments, there was a shortening of the ramus on the affected side and asymmetry of the mandibular arch. In these cases resorption of the condyle was observed, followed by the formation of a new joint. Ankylosis did not occur in any of these cases, although deviation on opening of the mouth was frequently observed owing to shortening of the ramus and dysfunction of the lateral pterygoid muscle.

Before the age of 5 years the condylar neck is less developed, and the bony tissues are soft and more susceptible to a "crush" type of injury. After the age of 5 years, the condyle in all probability fractures at the neck. The crush type of injury may cause the condylar cartilage to sustain the main damage. Because the condylar cartilage is one of several factors in mandibular growth, mandibular hypoplasia results when it is injured. The degree of deformity seems to be inversely proportional to the age at which the injury is sustained. The younger the patient at the time of injury, the more severe is the deformity (Panagopoulos, 1957; Rowe, 1969; Proffit, Vig, and Turvey, 1980).

There seems, therefore, to be a distinct difference in the results of a crushing injury in early childhood and a fracture of the condylar neck in later childhood. Whereas the crushing injury and the resultant damage to the condylar cartilage, as emphasized by Walker (1957, 1960), result in developmental arrest, the deformity arising from the condylar neck fractures, when treated by simple intermaxillary fixation, is self-correcting. However, the advisability of intermaxillary fixation in fractures of the condylar neck in children has been questioned by other authors, who observed spontaneous recovery of function and form in children with unilateral or bilateral condylar neck fractures treated by early motion and no immobilization (Rowe, 1971). Fractures of the condyle are also discussed in Chapter 30.

Midfacial Fractures

Midfacial fractures in children up to the age of 12 years have constituted less than 0.5 per cent of all facial fractures (Rowe, 1968). Because of the higher degree of elasticity of the facial bones, absence of sinus development, and the lesser degree of development of the midfacial skeleton in relation to the cranial area, midfacial fractures in children are less frequent than in adults. Maxillary, nasoorbital, and orbital blow-out fractures can occur, and in children submitted to an unusually strong traumatic force, frontal bone and telescoping nasoorbital fractures can be associated with the midfacial fractures (Rowe and Williams, 1985).

The typical Le Fort lines of fracture (see Chap. 27) are rarely seen in children's fractures. Low maxillary or Le Fort I types of fracture are not common until after the age of 10 years owing to the underdevelopment of the facial structures. Pyramidal or Le Fort II fractures are seen more commonly and sometimes unilaterally. The patients frequently present with a split palate owing to the weakness (incomplete fusion) of the midpalatal suture (Fig. 28–17*A*). Problems with fixation are similar to those encountered in the treatment of mandibular fractures because of the presence of poorly retentive teeth. In addition, alveolar fractures are associated with tooth loosening, luxation, avulsion, and fracture, particularly the anterior teeth, which are especially exposed to injury. A fixation appliance (cable arch, arch, or acrylic splint) may be attached to the remaining teeth, and in the older child to the selected erupted permanent teeth (Figs. 28–17*B,C,D*) (Schultz and Meilman, 1980; Schultz, 1982).

Careful internal interfragment wiring or compression plate fixation are means of fixation in the older child. In the young child, wire fixation to the frontal bone, the orbital rim, or the zygomatic arch may be unsatisfactory because the bone is soft and the wire, when placed under tension, tends to cut through the bone. Internal wire fixation to the edges of the piriform aperture, which consists of thicker and stronger bone, is a preferred method (Kazanjian and Converse, 1974).

Rapid fabrication of an acrylic splint can be achieved in the operating room with a quick curing acrylic resin. Other fractures of the midface are held by interfragment wiring fixation or plating to the edge of stable bony skeletal structures (Kazanjian and Converse, 1974; Converse and Dingman, 1977).

Even when properly reduced, midfacial fractures may eventually lead to a midfacial retrusion deformity or asymmetry because of the injury to the growth centers of the maxilla and nasal septum. With maxillary growth, there is not only a forward and downward component, but a concomitant remodeling of the multiple regional parts (see Chap. 47). The development includes a displacement away from the cranial base, a posterior enlargement corresponding to the lengthening of the dental arch, and an anterior resorption of the malar region. The nasal vaults grow forward and laterally, while descent of the premaxillary area occurs by resorption on the superior and anterior surface of the nasal spine, promoting bony deposition on the inferior surface. It is fortunate that this com-

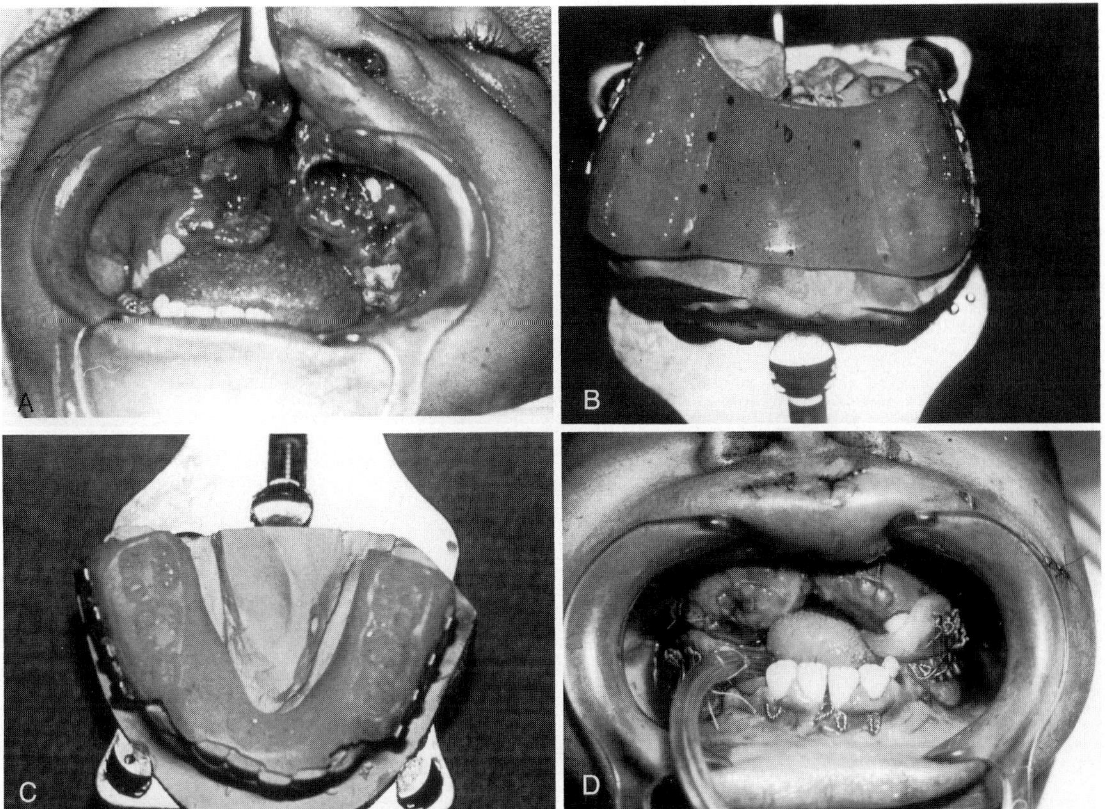

Figure 28–17. *A,* A 7 year old child with multiple facial fractures including a Le Fort II fracture, split palate, nasoethmoido-orbital fracture, right zygoma fracture, and dentoalveolar fractures. *B,* After mock model surgery to realign the split palatal fractures, the occlusal splint is fabricated. *C,* Mandibular splint. *D,* Appearance of the child after open reduction and wiring of the facial fractures, insertion of the occlusal splint, and circumpalatal wiring.

plex developmental scenario is seldom interrupted by maxillary fracture in childhood (Dawson and Fordyce, 1953; Bales, Randall, and Lehr, 1972; Converse, 1979; McCoy, 1980).

Incomplete reduction and immobilization of maxillary fractures, however, are the most frequent causes of malunion with elongation or reduction of the facial height and malocclusion in the pediatric age group. Malunion can best be prevented by immediate exploration and open reduction of the fractured segments. Timing of the reduction becomes critical, however, since bony healing occurs rapidly. Remobilization of a malunited maxillary fracture in children is extremely difficult two to three weeks after injury, as opposed to remobilization of a similar fracture in adults (Mustardé, 1971; McCoy, 1980).

Zygomatic and Orbital Fractures

Zygomatic fractures are rare in children and most commonly occur in the older child. Considerable force is required to fracture the resilient zygoma of the child and the fracture usually takes the form of a fracture-dislocation. Lack of complete union at the frontozygomatic suture also explains the infrequency of this type of fracture. Treatment is similar to that of adult zygomatic fractures (Fig. 28–18) (Schultz and Meilman, 1980; Schultz, 1982).

The incidence of pure pediatric zygomatic fractures has been reported as 4.7 per cent and zygomatic fracture with a significant orbital component as 16.3 per cent (McCoy and associates, 1962; McCoy, Chandler, and Crow, 1966; McCoy, 1980). In another series,

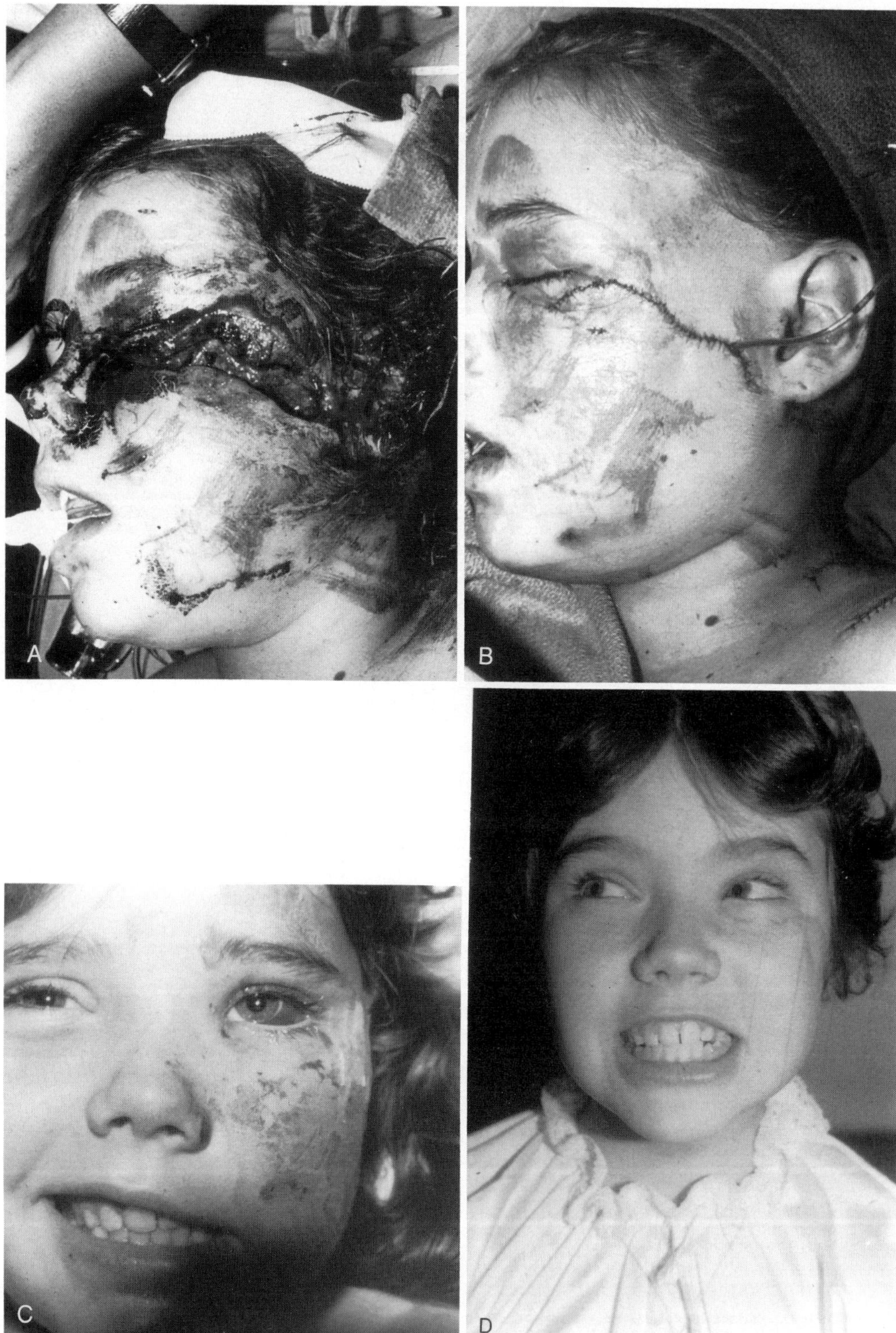

Figure 28–18. *A,* A 7 year old child after severe trauma to the left side of the face, with avulsion of soft tissues, open zygomatic fracture, and avulsion of the buccal branches of the facial nerve. *B,* Appearance at completion of open reduction and wire fixation of the zygomatic fracture, repair of the facial nerve, and approximation of the soft tissues. *C,* Early postoperative view demonstrating facial weakness and edema. *D,* One year follow-up demonstrating return of function and satisfactory facial symmetry.

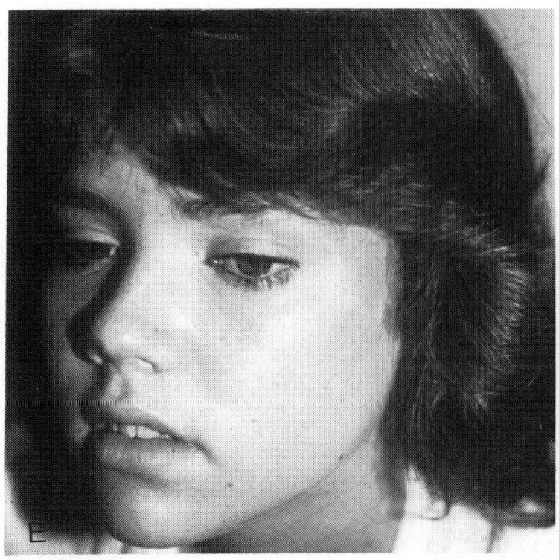

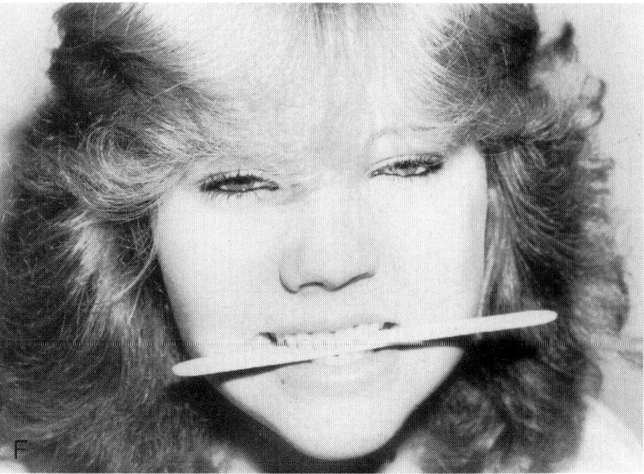

Figure 28–18 *Continued E,* Seven year follow-up showing return of function and satisfactory facial symmetry. *F,* Ten year follow-up showing developmental residua in the zygomatic area.

the incidence of zygomatic fracture necessitating operative treatment was only 0.3 per cent (Rowe, 1969; Rowe and Williams, 1985). Malar complex fractures with asymmetry and flattening of the eminence or fractures of the orbital rims with a palpable step-off deformity must be corrected accurately within the first five to seven days to avoid later dysfunction and deformity. Unlike the situation in the adult, after this type of fracture has healed it is not as amenable to correction by refracturing or bone grafting (Manson, Hoopes, and Su, 1980; Manson and associates, 1985).

Depressed malunited zygomatic fractures vary in their severity (see also Chap. 27). There is often a residual hypoesthesia of the upper lip, nose, and cheek or flatness of the cheek. The lateral canthus may be displaced inferiorly, giving an antimongoloid slant to the palpebral fissure. In addition, the inferior displacement of the fracture may impinge the zygoma against the coronoid process, resulting in an open bite (Rowe and Winter, 1971; Riefkohl and Georgiade, 1984; Rowe and Williams, 1985).

Orbital fractures in children are observed after automobile accidents and are often characterized by a separation of the frontozygomatic junction in the lateral orbital wall, with downward displacement of the floor. This type of unilateral craniofacial detachment is more frequent in the child than the Le Fort III bilateral craniofacial dysjunction.

The boundary of the zygoma forms the malar eminence and has five principal attachments to adjacent structures: the frontal bone, the zygomatic arch, the medial maxilla at the infraorbital rim, the maxillary alveolus inferiorly, and the greater wing of the sphenoid. Fractures of the zygoma always involve the orbital floor with exclusion of fractures isolated to the zygomatic arch. The infraorbital nerve is usually involved in its exit from the upper anterior maxillary wall adjacent to the infraorbital rim. The diagnosis of an "orbital" fracture is suggested by the presence of periorbital and subconjunctival hematomas and by hypoesthesia in the distribution of the infraorbital nerve. The "orbital" fracture frequently is a fracture-dislocation of the zygoma (Converse, 1976; Converse and Dingman, 1977; Converse, 1979). If the zygoma is dislocated inferiorly, the lateral canthus, attached to the zygoma at Whitnall's tubercle, is displaced inferiorly, causing an antimongoloid slant to the palpebral fissure. A step-off discrepancy may be palpable at the infraorbital rim or zygomaticofrontal suture. Tenderness may be present over these areas. A hematoma is often noted in the upper buccal sulcus, and zygomatic fractures are often accompanied by unilateral epistaxis, which occurs from bleeding within the fractured maxillary sinus. Depending on the extent of the orbital floor involvement, there may be extraocular muscle dysfunction, which results in diplopia. Difficulty in chewing or moving of the jaw or mild occlusal discrepancies of a temporary nature are secondary to swelling in the area of the zygomatic arch, with interference in excursion of the coronoid process of the mandible. Isolated zygomatic arch fractures are usually bowed inward. Following resolution of the swelling, a depression is seen in the lateral cheek in the upper preauricular area (Converse and Dingman, 1977; Converse, 1979).

The radiographic evaluation of a zygomatic fracture consists of Waters and Caldwell views to assess displacement. The Waters view defines the infraorbital rim and lateral wall of the maxillary sinus; the orbital floor is also visualized. The Caldwell view is used to assess displacement at the zygomaticofrontal suture (Roberts and Shopfner, 1972). Posterior displacement of the malar eminence and the zygomatic arch is assessed through the submentovertex skull films or axial CT scans (Roberts and Shopfner, 1972; Schultz, 1982).

A CT examination is routinely obtained in any patient in whom a maxillary or orbital fracture is suspected. Plain radiographs in children are difficult to interpret and the identification of fracture lines may be troublesome. Plain films do not display the bones, soft tissues, and contents of the orbit with the same accuracy and detail as can be obtained with a CT examination (Figs. 28–19, 28–20) (Tsai and associates, 1980; Cohen and associates, 1986).

The indications for open reduction are deformity, enophthalmos, persistent diplopia, vertical malposition of the globe, retrusion of the malar eminence, and anesthesia or hypoesthesia in the infraorbital nerve distribution (Converse, 1967, 1976; Fearon, Edmonds, and Bird, 1979). The last-named symptoms can, however, occur with a medially displaced zygomatic fracture. Significant fracture fragment displacement that is evident on radiographic examination is treated by open reduction and interfragmentary wiring at the frontozygomatic suture and the infraorbital rim (Dingman, 1953; Dingman and Natvig, 1964). The infraorbital rim and the zygomaticofrontal suture are exposed through a subciliary incision with a skin muscle flap. The lateral canthus may be detached to expose the zygomaticofrontal suture through this incision alone. This approach provides a wide exposure of the zygoma and orbital floor and leaves a barely perceptible scar. Holes may be drilled with a 1 mm drill bit 0.5 cm from the edges of the fracture line. Number 26 or 28 stainless steel wires are placed through the drill holes and, while the fragments are held in approximation, the wire is tightened snugly and tucked in such a way that it is no longer palpable. Alternatively, a small plate and 1.5 mm screws can be used to obtain stability at the zygomaticofrontal suture.

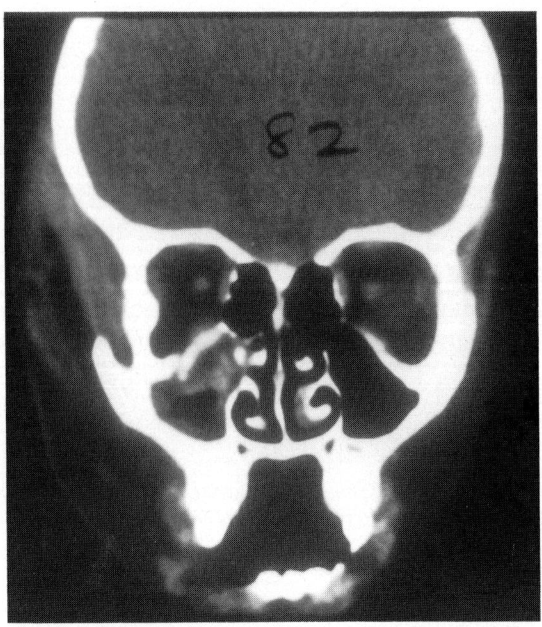

Figure 28–20. Coronal CT view of an orbital floor fracture entrapping the inferior rectus muscle between the two fracture segments.

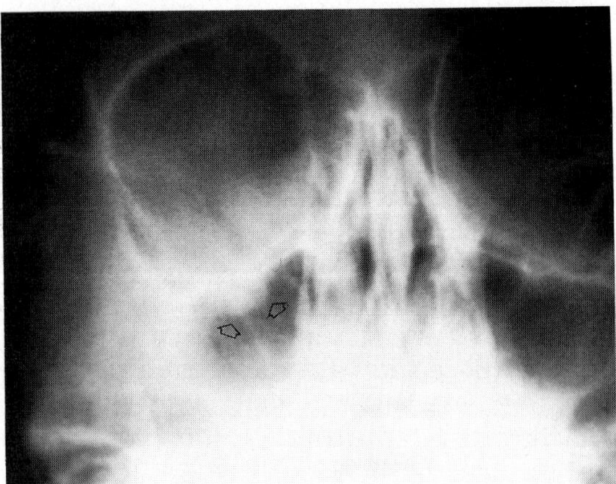

Figure 28–19. Waters view demonstrating a small "blow-out" fracture with herniation of the orbital contents into the maxillary sinus (the teardrop sign).

The intraoral visualization of the zygomaticomaxillary junction through an upper gingival buccal sulcus incision can ensure proper alignment in reduction of the zygoma at the zygomaticomaxillary buttress. In adults, routine placement of interfragmentary wires or plates are used in this area (see Chap. 27);

however, caution must be exercised in children because of the presence of unerupted permanent teeth. Interfragmentary wires can be placed at the Le Fort I level, but they must be carefully positioned to avoid injury to the developing tooth buds. In young children the maxillary sinus is not fully developed and the bone is soft. Caution must be observed when tightening wires so as not to pull the wire through the soft cancellous bone. As previously emphasized, fractures of the zygoma usually are not seen in small children because of the incomplete development of the maxillary sinus. The bone structure of the midface must be weakened by development of the sinus for the typical fracture lines to occur (Dingman, 1953; Converse and Dingman, 1977; Fearon, Edmonds, and Bird, 1979).

The orbital floor is explored routinely as part of the operative treatment of the zygomatic fracture. Depending on the integrity of the floor, a Supramid plate of 0.6 to 0.8 mm thickness can be used to cover a bone defect and wired to the infraorbital rim to prevent displacement. Linear cracks are usually aligned with reduction of the orbital rim, and an implant is not required. The orbital dissection should progress until the edges of an orbital defect are precisely located, so that the exact area of the defect may be covered by the reconstructive material. A split rib graft or a graft from the inner table of the iliac crest may be harvested. Care should be taken to spare the superior lip of the crest in children, and in young children the crest is of a cartilaginous consistency. If the child is old enough, a split calvarial graft may be taken. A Tessier rib contour forceps may be used to shape the graft to the exact curvature desired for orbital reconstruction. Bone grafts may be secured to the infraorbital rim with a small wire if desired, or anchored with a lag screw to the zygoma (Manson and associates, 1983, 1986a).

Malunited zygomatic fractures occur either because of an unstable reduction or because periorbital and cheek edema obscured the bony depression to the extent that reduction was not attempted. Occasionally, the fracture may be adequately reduced but accidental pressure on the face moves the fragments out of position. Some authors reported a 10 per cent incidence of malalignment in zygomatic fractures (Dingman, 1953; Dingman and Natvig, 1964). Dingman (1953) noted that complications are more common with conservative (closed) reduction of the fracture and advocated open reduction. Zygomaticocoronoid ankylosis may occasionally follow severe zygomatic or Le Fort fracture. It is often managed by intraoral coronoidectomy (Furnas, 1976; Fearon, Edmonds, and Bird, 1979; Manson and associates, 1983, 1986a,b).

"BLOW-OUT" FRACTURES

The etiology of "pure" orbital blow-out fractures in children, unassociated with zygomatic fracture, is similar to that in adults. They are caused by the patient being hit in the orbital region with a ball or another child's fist or by trauma received in automobile accidents. The maxillary sinus is small in the young child. The floor of the orbit is concave, dipping downward behind the rim of the orbit, an anatomic characteristic that can mislead the surgeon into an erroneous diagnosis of orbital floor collapse on plain radiographic films. Despite the small size of the maxillary sinus, orbital contents escape through the fractured floor and may cause enophthalmos (Converse and Dingman, 1977; Manson and associates, 1986a,b).

Restoration of the continuity of the orbital floor is the method of treatment, as in the adult. Comminuted fractures in children should be carefully reconstructed as soon as possible. The bone fragments consolidate rapidly in a malaligned position. The release of the entrapped orbital contents from the area of the blow-out fracture, which can be covered by small alloplastic implants or bone grafts, is usually followed by rapid return of ocular rotatory movements. Children seem to have rapid recuperative abilities after a blow-out fracture, usually achieving a functional range of extraocular muscle function. Proper positioning of these structures prevents adhesions between the globe, the periorbital fat, the inferior rectus and inferior oblique muscles, and the orbital floor (Manson and associates, 1986a,b).

Diplopia and enophthalmos are complications that may follow various types of orbital floor fracture (Fig. 28–21). Although infrequent, diplopia may present immediately after injury or may occur with resolution of the swelling. Later, enophthalmos becomes a more obvious sign. Injury to and entrapment of the periorbita may cause subsequent inflammation and fibrosis, with adherence to

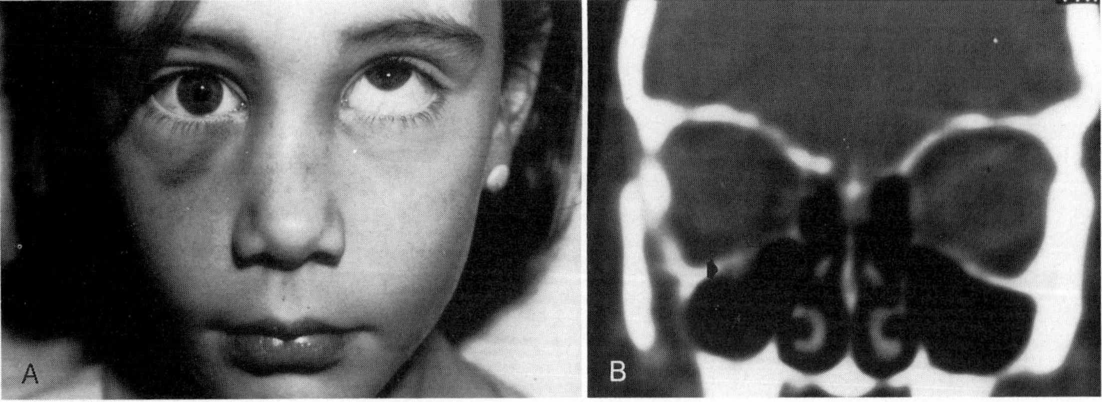

Figure 28–21. *A,* Appearance of an 8 year old girl who sustained a blow to the right eye with entrapment of the inferior rectus muscle. Note the limitation of upward gaze. *B,* Coronal CT view demonstrating *(arrow)* entrapment of the inferior rectus muscle in a linear fracture along the orbital floor.

the orbital walls and impairment of muscle function. Herniated, entrapped, ecchymotic orbital fat and muscle may undergo necrosis. Fracture expansion of the orbital floor increases orbital volume and makes the eye appear small.

Loss of vision can develop from postoperative orbital hemorrhage, trauma to the optic nerve, central artery occlusion, or thrombosis of the orbital vein. To prevent this complication, every effort should be made in a reduction to avoid excessive pressure or tension on the globe. Alloplastic material should be kept in a position that avoids pressure in the area of the optic nerve when placement is far posterior within the orbit (Converse, 1967, 1976; Furnas, 1976).

Complete correction of late enophthalmos caused by a healed, enlarged, and depressed bony orbit can seldom be accomplished by simple procedures such as alloplastic or bone graft supplementation of the orbital floor and side walls or relocation of the lateral and medial canthal ligaments. Complete relocation and recontouring of the entire bony orbital cone by marginal orbitotomy (see Chap. 33) and supporting bone grafts are usually required to correct such deformities (Furnas, 1976; Manson and associates, 1986a,b).

Nasal and Nasoorbital Fractures

Fractures of the nasal skeleton in children are more frequent than fractures of the maxilla and zygoma. In the early years of childhood, the nasal skeleton is proportionally more cartilaginous than bony, and the diagnosis of nasal fracture is more difficult. The nasal bones in children can separate in the midline along an open suture line. The "open book" type of fracture, with overriding of the nasal bones over the frontal processes of the maxilla, is a characteristic of significant fractures of the nasal bones in children (Converse and Dingman, 1977).

As with other types of childhood facial injuries, particularly more so in nasal injuries, the complicating factor is that growth and development may be affected even after accurate diagnosis and adequate treatment (Fry, 1967; Jazbi, 1977).

The first five years of postnatal life are years of rapid facial growth. After a period of moderately active growth, a second period of rapid growth occurs between the ages of 10 and 15 years. Growth of the nasomaxillary complex may be affected by trauma during the early postnatal years and may be more frequent than generally expected. Such injuries, as well as those suffered during delivery, may explain nasal deviation and nasomaxillary hypoplasia that have no other apparent cause (Mayell, 1973; Ortiz-Monasterio and Olmedo, 1981; Muller, 1983).

The diagnosis of nasal injury in a young child is difficult and may often require general anesthesia in order to permit careful intranasal, extranasal, and skeletal inspection and palpation. Roentgenographic examination is a prerequisite for diagnostic and medicolegal purposes.

The nasal bones are formed on the surface of the cartilaginous capsule and there is considerable overlap between the lateral cartilages and the nasal bones. The lateral cartilages may be detached from the undersurface of the nasal bones because of the relatively loose attachment in the child, and may collapse in conjunction with a fracture of the septum. A hematoma may form in any area between the lateral cartilages and the undersurface of the nasal bones. It should be evacuated through an intercartilaginous or subperiosteal incision (Stucker, Bryarly, and Shockley, 1984; Tucker, 1984).

Fractures and dislocation of the septal cartilage are frequent attendant injuries in fractures of the nasal bones, but they may occur independently. Hematoma of the septum, a collection of blood between the cartilages and the mucoperichondrium caused by rupture of the abundant vasculature of the area, manifests itself as a bluish-red bulging in the vestibule of the nasal fossa. One should be aware of the child who cannot breathe through the nose after a nasal injury (Converse and Dingman, 1977). Septal hematoma may also be caused by a single traumatic bending of the septal cartilage without fracture or dislocation. Hematoma of the septum is always a serious complication in children, not only because of the nasal obstruction that results from fibrous thickening of the septum, but also because of the possibility of collapse of the dorsum (saddle deformity) with loss of septal cartilage support through pressure necrosis from hematoma or abscess (Converse and Dingman, 1977; Stucker, Bryarly, and Shockley, 1984; Tucker, 1984).

Special care should be taken to drain the septal hematoma. An L-shaped incision, extending through the mucoperiosteum over the vomer, is made along the floor of the nose and extended vertically upward through the mucoperichondrium over the septal cartilage. The flap of mucous membrane is raised and the hematoma evacuated. The dependent position of the incision ensures drainage and thus prevents a recurring collection of blood. When the septal framework is fractured, the hematoma may collect bilaterally on both sides of the septal cartilage. A portion of the septal cartilage can be removed so that the two areas of hematoma communicate; alternatively, a bilateral septal incision through the mucoperichondrium provides dependent drainage and prevents recurrence of the hematoma (Converse and Dingman, 1977).

Treatment of nasal bone fractures in children is similar to that in adults (see Chap. 27). Under general anesthesia an elevator is placed into the nasal fossa, and the fractured fragments of nasal bones and frontal processes of the maxilla are elevated. Further alignment is obtained by external manual palpation. The septum, if fractured, is straightened and, if it is dislocated, the lateral cartilages are realigned and repositioned. A splint of dental compound or plaster is placed over the nose for five to seven days. Intranasal packing is often necessary, in conjunction with the external splint, to assist in the alignment of the bony and cartilaginous fragments (Stucker, Bryarly, and Shockley, 1984; Tucker, 1984).

Nasal bone fractures heal rapidly in children, frequently with overgrowth of bone, bony displacement, or hypertrophic callus. This results in a widening of the bony dorsum of the nose. Children who have suffered comminuted nasal bone fractures may show developmental deformities years later, even though they received adequate treatment after the accident, an important consideration from a medicolegal viewpoint. The deformities may include deviation and thickening of the septum, flattening of the nasal dorsum, widening of the bony skeleton by hypertrophic callus, and varying degrees of nasomaxillary hypoplasia (Stucker, Bryarly and Shockley, 1984; Tucker, 1984).

One should not hesitate to realign by osteotomy the nasal pyramid or septum in children who have suffered an injury resulting in malunited fracture and nasal obstruction. The risk of impairing growth is slight, as the growth potential has already been affected by the initial trauma. The deformity, characterized by depression of the dorsum and widening of the nasal bridge, may require correction for psychologic as well as functional reasons. A costal cartilage or bone graft (see Chap. 35) may be required, in the understanding that definitive surgery will be required during adolescence (Converse and Campbell, 1954; Converse, 1976; Converse and Dingman, 1977).

Nasoethmoido-orbital Fractures

Nasoorbital fractures, in which the bony structures of the nose are pushed backward into the intraorbital space along with the medial orbital walls, occur in automobile accidents and are treated by open reduction and interfragmentary wiring techniques (see

Chapter 27). The coronal incision provides optimal exposure for these fractures. Open reduction can prevent the subsequent sequelae of traumatic telecanthus, saddle nose deformity, and lacrimal apparatus disturbances. Nasoethmoido-orbital fractures are always associated with blow-out fractures of the orbital floor and medial orbital walls, and fractures of the orbital rims (Manson and associates, 1980, 1983, 1985, 1986a,b).

Nasoethmoido-orbital fractures result from a direct severe blow to the frontal, glabellar, or upper nasal region and frequently accompany frontal bone or high Le Fort II or III fractures. The nasal component of the nasoethmoido-orbital fracture is usually laterally and posteriorly displaced. Nasoethmoido-orbital fractures are characterized by retrusion and flattening of the nasal pyramid and an increase in the columella-lip angle. The fracture is not isolated to the nose, but involves the medial portion of the orbital rims and extends into the ethmoidal sinuses, orbital floors, and medial portion of the infraorbital rim on one or both sides, depending on the extent of the injury (Fig. 28–22). A small laceration is frequently present over the nasal bridge or forehead area. Epistaxis may be severe. The finding of bilateral periorbital hematoma signals not only the fracture of the nose and orbit but also the possibility of a fracture continuing into the anterior cranial fossa. Greenstick or incomplete nasoethmoido-orbital fractures or fractures with minimal displacement may be missed unless a high index of suspicion is present when patients with trauma to the frontonasal area are examined. Partial fractures are usually incomplete ("greensticked") at the nasofrontal suture (Mustardé, 1971; Reil and Kranz, 1976; Converse and Dingman, 1977; Riefkohl and Georgiade, 1984).

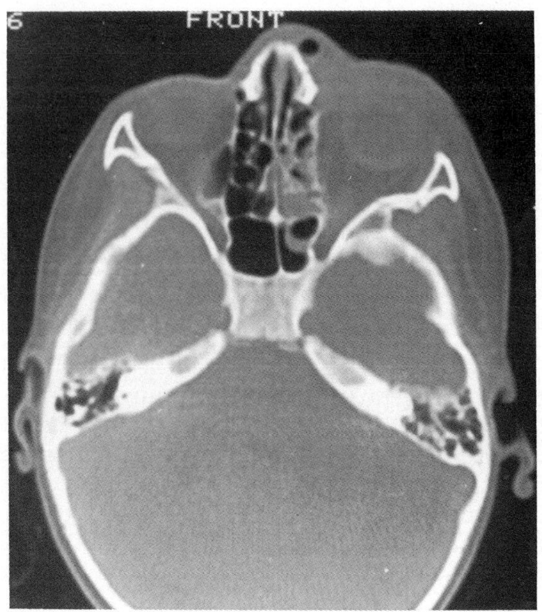

Figure 28–23. Fracture of the left zygoma extending to the greater wing of the sphenoid with a left-sided nasoethmoido-orbital fracture.

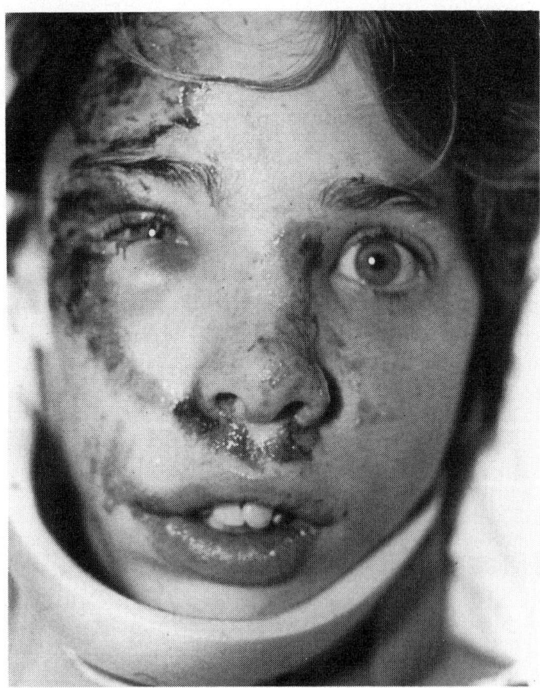

Figure 28–22. A 12 year old child who sustained a right-sided unilateral nasoethmoido-orbital fracture and a frontal bone fracture. Note the unilateral right-sided telecanthus.

The radiographic evaluation consists of views of the nose and Waters, Caldwell, and lateral skull films. The plain films do not demonstrate the fractures as clearly as does a CT (Fig. 28–23). Thin cuts should be taken through the area of interest, namely, the medial orbital rim (Schultz and Meilman, 1980).

Fractures that demonstrate isolation of the medial orbital rim with the attached medial canthal ligament document the injury and indicate the potential for instability. The necessity for a precise physical examination to determine the mobility of this fragment cannot be overemphasized. Tenderness over the medial orbital rim should signal the possible presence of a nasoethmoido-orbital fracture. A CSF leak or pneumocephalus may also be present (Converse and Dingman, 1977). A bimanual test for mobility of the medial orbital rim may be performed by inserting a clamp into the nose and pressing the tip intranasally against the medial orbital rim opposite the canthal ligament. Pressing a finger against the external surface of the canthal ligament, one can move the fractured medial orbital rim fragment between the clamp and the index finger. Any mobility signals the necessity for an open reduction. One-third of nasoethmoido-orbital fractures demonstrated on CT scan are not sufficiently mobile to require open reduction.

Nasoethmoido-orbital fractures often accompany other frontal bone or facial fractures. A linear fracture may extend up into the frontal bone, a common condition in children. In adults, fractures of the frontal sinus and supraorbital area frequently accompany a nasoethmoido-orbital injury. Nasoethmoido-orbital fractures often accompany high Le Fort II and III fractures and are frequently unilateral. In summary, one should suspect the presence of a nasoethmoido-orbital fracture when there are severe nasal fractures with anteroposterior displacement, lacerations of the frontal and nasal area, or bilateral periorbital ecchymosis. Traumatic telecanthus may be observed in the immediate postinjury period in severely displaced fractures, but often develops more slowly over a period of a week to ten days in those fractures demonstrating less comminution (Dingman and Natvig, 1964; McCoy, 1980; James, 1985). The eyelid traction test (lateral movement of the medial canthal ligament when traction is applied to the lower eyelid) is seldom useful in the evaluation of these injuries.

If the patient's neurologic condition is stable, the injuries should be treated by definitive open reduction if mobility is present. A Richman screw is used to monitor the intracranial pressure if anesthesia is required in the presence of a significant head injury (Fig. 28–24) (Miller and associates, 1977; Mayer and associates, 1980). The open reduction consists of an exposure of the frontal bone; upper, medial, and inferior aspects of the orbits; nose; and infraorbital areas through coronal and bilateral subciliary eyelid incisions (see also Chap. 27). The entire framework of the nasoethmoido-orbital area is exposed in a subperiosteal plane. Multiple drill holes are placed to wire each fragment to the adjacent fragment, proceeding from intact bone to intact bone. Frequently, the open reduction extends from the frontal bone to the upper portion of the Le Fort I level. The latter area may require exposure through gingivobuccal sulcus incisions. After the fragments have been linked with interfragmentary wires, bone grafts are placed to restore the continuity of the medial and inferior orbit. The fragments are held in reduction and the wires tightened. The most important principle in the treatment of nasoethmoido-orbital fractures is to restore the proper inner canthal distance by a transnasal reduction of the medial orbital rims. A wire is placed between the canthal ligament on the posterior edge of the medial orbital rim fragment and led to the other sides so that the distance between the medial orbital rims is limited by the tightening of the wire. It is not necessary to detach the medial canthal ligament to accomplish the reduction of a nasoethmoido-orbital fracture. In fact, the architecture of the canthus and the intercanthal distance are improved if the canthal ligament is not detached from the medial orbital insertion dur-

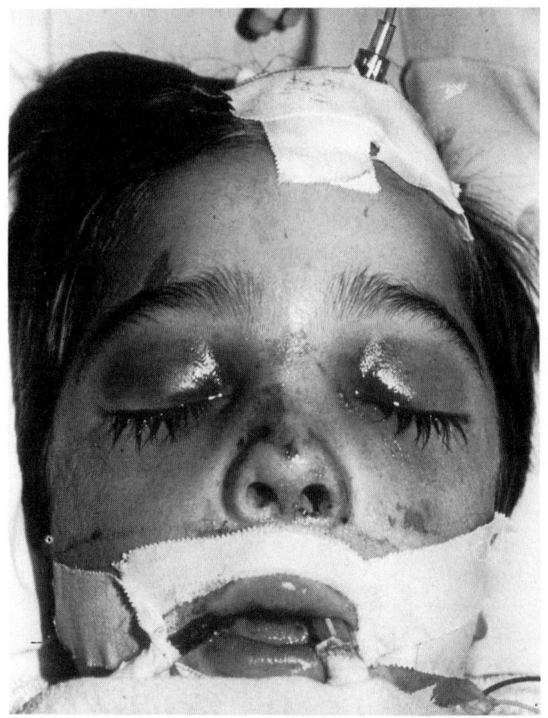

Figure 28–24. A young child after severe frontal-temporal-orbital fracture and a greenstick nasoethmoido-orbital fracture. The need for ventricular pressure monitoring (Richman screw) to prevent increased cerebral edema and possible herniation was evident on admission.

ing the reduction. A bone graft may be used to reconstitute nasal height and provide a smooth nasal dorsum or septal support. It is wired in cantilever fashion or anchored with a lag screw at the glabella area (Converse, 1976; Converse and Dingman, 1977; McCoy, 1980).

A fracture of the base of the frontal sinus always accompanies nasoethmoido-orbital injuries. Isolated basal frontal sinus fractures (see later sections) have not been routinely treated by frontal sinus manipulation or ablation, and most patients do not demonstrate late problems with mucocele formation or nasofrontal duct obstruction (Brook and Friedman, 1982).

Adjacent fractures of the supraorbital area or severe comminuted frontal bone or frontal sinus fractures are managed as described in later sections. The lacrimal system usually is not transected in the absence of lacerations near the medial canthus or avulsion of the ligament from the bone, which is not a common situation. Late lacrimal obstruction occurs in 5 per cent of patients having an open reduction, is usually located in the nasolacrimal duct, and may be treated by dacryocystorrhinostomy (see Chap. 33) (Furnas, 1976).

Frontal Bone and Frontal Sinus Fractures

Patients with head injuries should be evaluated by neurologic examination, CT scan, and the Glasgow coma scale (Teasdale and Jennett, 1974; Mayer and associates, 1980). The outcome of severe head injury is better in children (as far as survival is concerned) than in adults (Hendrick, 1959, 1964; Gruszkiewicz, Doron, and Peyser, 1973; Bruce and associates, 1978, 1981). The prognosis, however, for memory, intellect, and mental functions is not as hopeful (Berger and associates, 1985). Perhaps these findings reflect the peculiar sensitivity of the childhood nervous system (Lindenberg and associates, 1955; Levin and associates, 1982). There is high incidence of diffuse swelling and low incidence of mass lesions. It is important to keep the intracranial pressure below 20 torr (Miller and associates, 1977). Flaccidity, the absence of a gag reflex, lack of oculovestibular stimulation, and an abnormal respiratory pattern carry the worst prognosis.

The frontal skull in children is more prominent than the face and thus skull fractures are frequent. Many times the fracture line is vertical and linear and extends into the orbit near the supraorbital foramen. A CT scan evaluates displacement and the need for open reduction in closed injuries. In open injuries, debridement is necessary to ensure the absence of significant contamination. Neurosurgical criteria for open reduction of skull fractures include significant skeletal displacement, the presence of an accompanying dural tear, intracranial or extracranial hematoma, CSF leak, pneumocephalus, or frontal lobe contusion with mass affect (Fig. 28–25). A CSF leak may exit from the wound or may be manifest as CSF rhinorrhea. In patients with epistaxis, it may be difficult to document rhinorrhea for several days. The cranial base is cartilaginous in the central anterior sections in small children but heals quickly, as in adult fractures. Frequently the only sign of a closed skull fracture may be a contusion or bruise in the forehead area or, in basal skull fractures, an eyelid hematoma. There may be accompanying lacerations and, less commonly, depressions from displaced bone fragments. The radiographic examination includes Caldwell, Waters, and lateral skull films. The examinations are always supplemented by a craniofacial CT scan for precise evaluation (Schneider and Thompson, 1957; Carrington, Taren, and Kahn, 1960; Harwood-Nash, 1970; Caldicott, North, and Simpson, 1973).

Treatment consists of exposure of the fron-

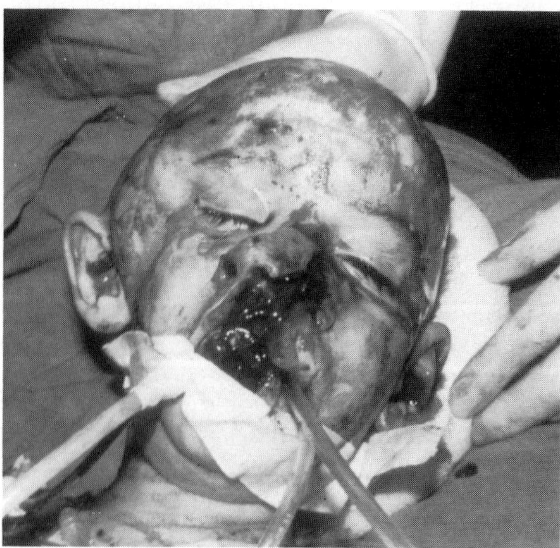

Figure 28–25. Severe childhood facial injuries resulting in a Le Fort II fracture, a nasoethmoido-orbital fracture, a CSF leak, and a right-sided epidural bleed after a four-story fall.

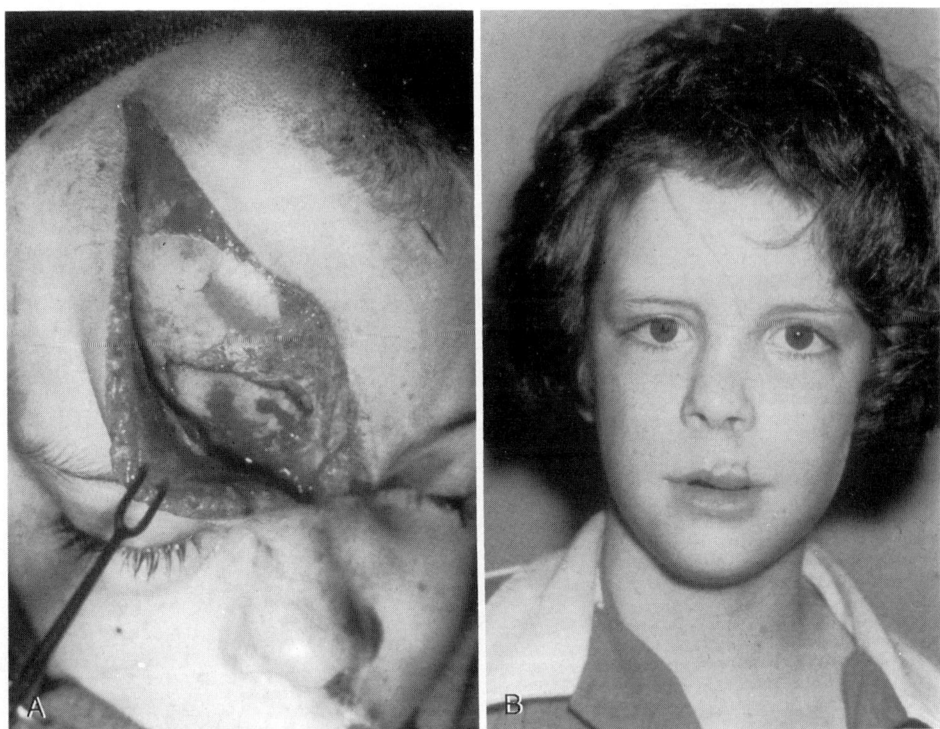

Figure 28–26. *A,* Appearance of a 9 year old boy with a soft tissue avulsion, a frontal bone fracture, and a left unilateral nasoethmoido-orbital fracture. *B,* One year after treatment, with evidence of mild telecanthus and facial asymmetry.

tal bone, frontal lobe, and fracture sites, either through a laceration (if convenient) or a coronal incision (Figs. 28–26, 28–27). The fractured area is exposed with subperiosteal dissection and the fracture fragments are repositioned or removed. A precise debridement is performed and any dural lacerations are closed following evacuation of epidural hematoma. Injuries to the underlying frontal lobe are appropriately managed. The bone fragments are cleared and any remnants of frontal sinus mucosa thoroughly removed. A light abrasive bur is used to remove any traces of frontal sinus mucosa from the frontal sinus walls. The bone fragments are replaced and connected with interfragmentary wires. The replacement of frontal bone fragments is successful in children and the risk of infection is not as high as that in adults. Replacement of frontal bone fragments avoids late cranioplasty. Both sequelae are avoided in children by primary reconstruction of the frontal skull (Gillingham, 1947; Lyerly, 1957; Carrington, Taren, and Kahn, 1960; Converse and Dingman, 1977).

An unusual phenomenon called "pseudogrowth" of skull fractures can occur in children. The skull fractures enlarge slowly over a period of one month after the fracture. Some patients develop a palpable bone defect with protrusion of the meninges and require bone replacement. In other cases, the pseudogrowth of skull fractures can be seen on radiographic study. The defect may not always be identifiable clinically by palpation. The radiographic appearance is not a guide to treatment. It is the clinical examination of the integrity of the skull that dictates the need for calvarial reconstruction (Goldstein and associates, 1970; Sekhar and Scarff, 1980).

The frontal sinus usually is not developed to any significant extent until the teenage years. Frontal sinus fractures may involve the anterior and posterior walls or the nasofrontal duct (Weber and Cohn, 1977). Frontal sinus fractures demonstrating significant displacement involving the anterior or posterior walls are treated by thorough removal of mucous membrane, light abrasion of the sur-

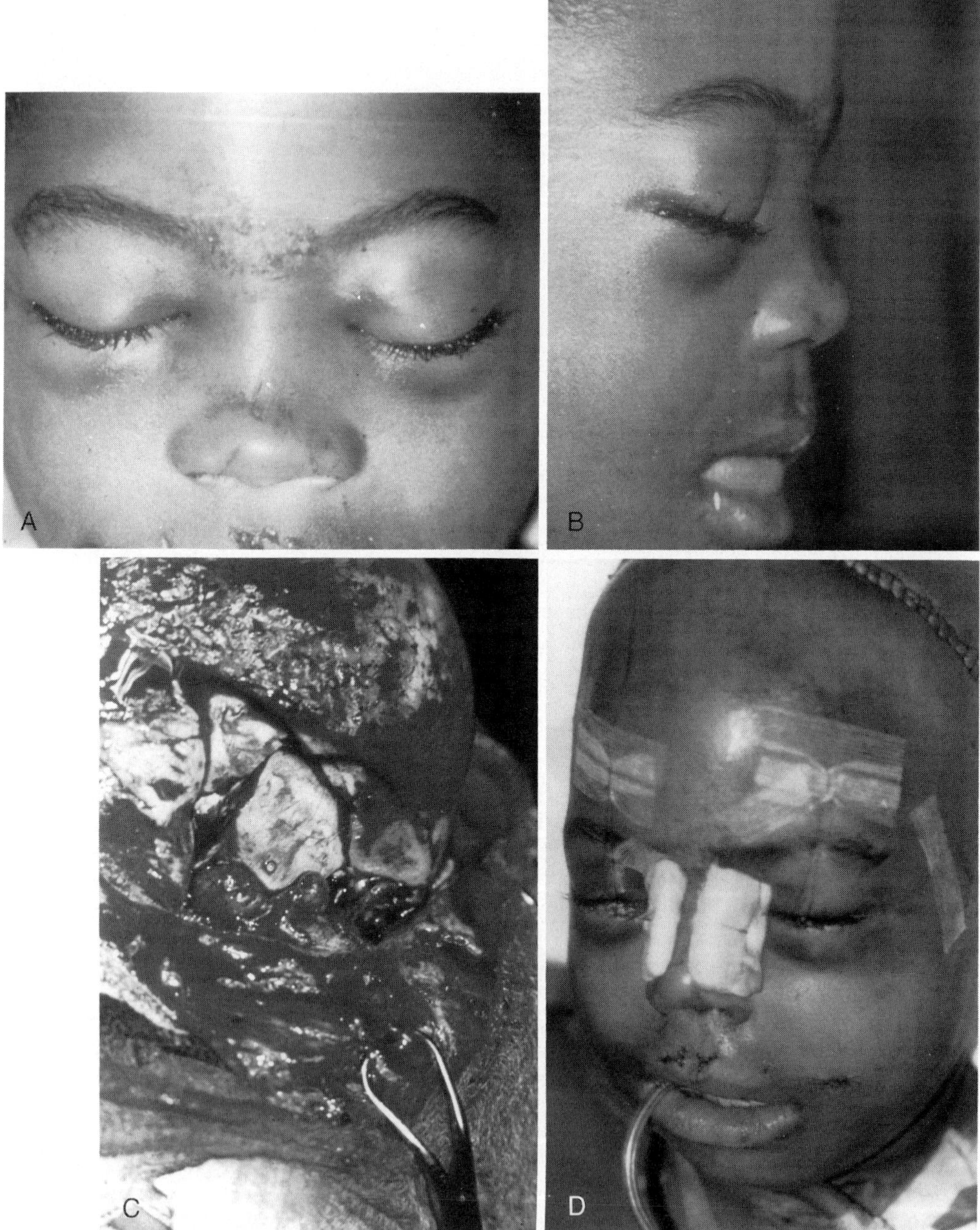

Figure 28–27. A young child with a severe bilateral nasoethmoido-orbital fracture with comminution of the frontal bone and telecanthus. *A,* Frontal view. *B,* Lateral view. *C,* Intraoperative view showing a comminuted frontal and nasoethmoid complex. *D,* Immediate postoperative appearance with nasal splints in place. Note the bicoronal and bilateral subciliary (eyelid) incisions. The eyelids are temporarily occluded and suspended to the forehead.

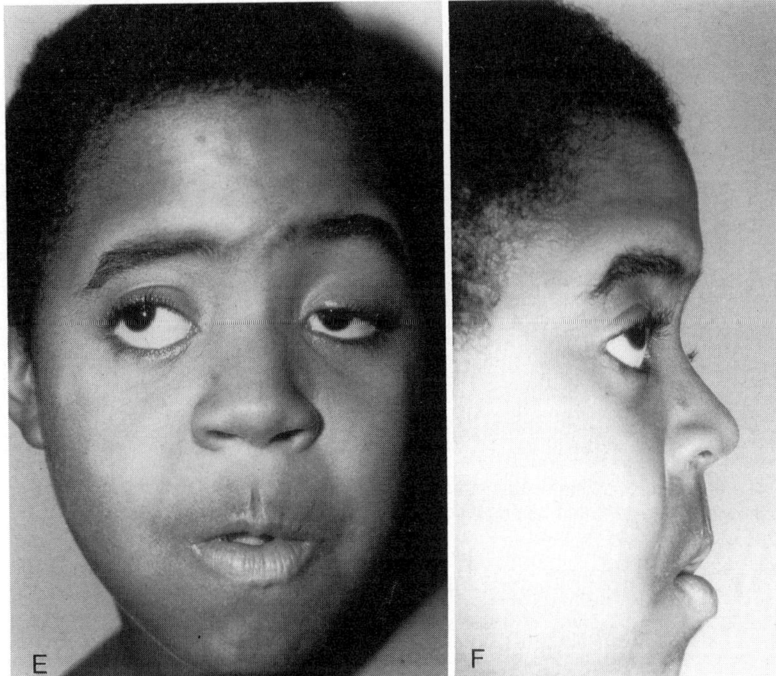

Figure 28–27 *Continued E,* Follow-up frontal view demonstrating satisfactory facial symmetry and nasal profile. However, the extraocular muscles require balancing. *F,* Follow-up lateral view.

face of the frontal sinus cavity to eliminate the microscopic evaginations of the mucous membrane, and replacement of the anterior bone fragments. Some prefer to insert cancellous bone graft material into the exenterated frontal sinus cavity. Bone plugs are used to plug the nasofrontal duct area. The open cavity becomes filled by a fibrous bony material over a period of time even if no material is placed to fill the frontal sinus cavity. Fractures of the frontal sinus that are not displaced but which demonstrate persistent air fluid levels should be managed by frontal sinus exploration through a coronal incision with removal of the mucous membrane, bone graft plugging of the nasofrontal duct, and obliteration of the cavity. Significantly displaced fractures of the anterior wall of the frontal sinus are managed by open reduction. The mucous membrane may be locally debrided or removed as necessary; sinus ablation may not be required. Linear undisplaced fractures without significant persistent fluid accumulation indicating obstruction may be managed by observation only. Posterior wall frontal sinus fractures are treated as depressed skull fractures, with repair of the dura and appropriate debridement of the frontal lobe (Converse and Dingman, 1977; Schultz and Meilman, 1980; Fortunato, Fielding, and Guernsey, 1982). The treatment of frontal sinus fractures is also discussed in Chapter 27.

Supraorbital Fractures

Supraorbital fractures involve the superior portion of the orbital rim and orbital roof. These either may be localized, involving small fragments of the superior orbital rim, or may extend to involve much of the lateral portion of the frontal bone and entire lateral two-thirds of the lateral frontal and temporal (supraorbital) area (Figs. 28–28, 28–29). This is the so-called "lateral frontal-orbital-temporal" fracture.

Supraorbital fractures may be diagnosed by identifying a depression, step, or level discrepancy in the contour of the supraorbital rim. Hypoesthesia may be present in the distribution of the supraorbital nerve. The roof of the orbit is generally involved and depressed inferiorly. The depression of the roof pushes the globe inferiorly and anteriorly and the patient demonstrates exophthalmos and inferior globe displacement (Fig. 28–30). Paralysis of the levator muscle may produce

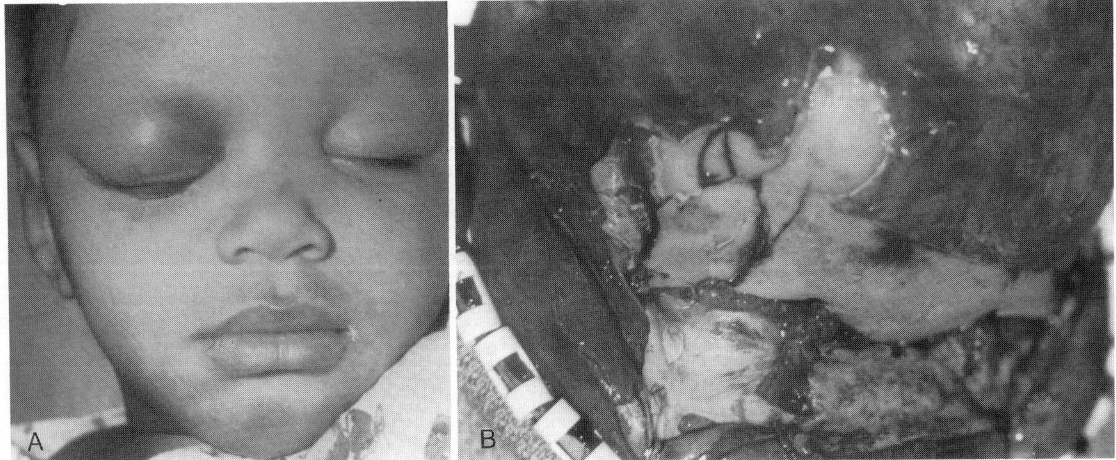

Figure 28–28. *A,* A 3 year old child who sustained a severe right-sided supraorbital fracture after a fall down stairs. *B,* Intraoperative view showing the extent and comminution of the frontal-orbital-temporal fracture.

a partial or complete ptosis. The patient may be unable to rotate the eye upward owing to direct muscle contusion or involvement of the motor nerves in the superior orbital fissure. Severe fractures extending into the superior orbital fissure may produce a *superior orbital fissure syndrome* (Fig. 28–31). When complete, the syndrome produces paralysis of all the extraocular muscles, complete ptosis, and anesthesia in the ophthalmic division of the trigeminal nerve. When the fracture extends to the optic foramen, the *orbital apex syndrome* may be produced, consisting of the superior orbital fissure syndrome and blindness (Converse, 1976; Furnas, 1976; Zachariades, 1982; Manson and associates, 1986a,b).

Radiographic evaluation of the supraorbital fracture consists of a plain skull film series using the Caldwell, lateral, and Waters views. A craniofacial CT scan is mandatory for the evaluation of the brain and orbit or for the exact determination of the pattern

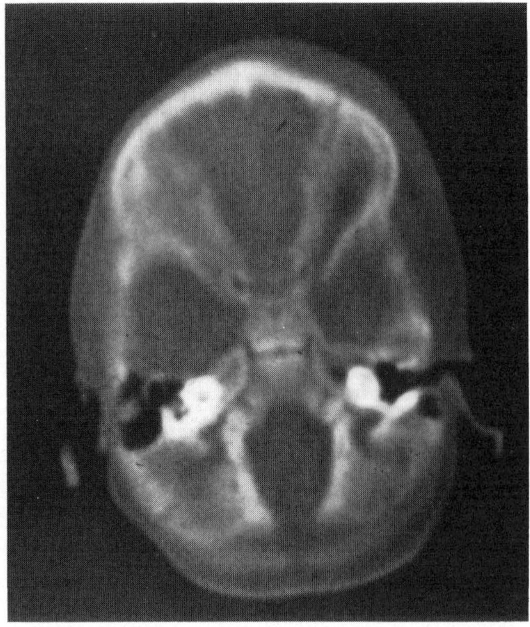

Figure 28–29. CT scan of a young child who sustained a right-sided supraorbital fracture.

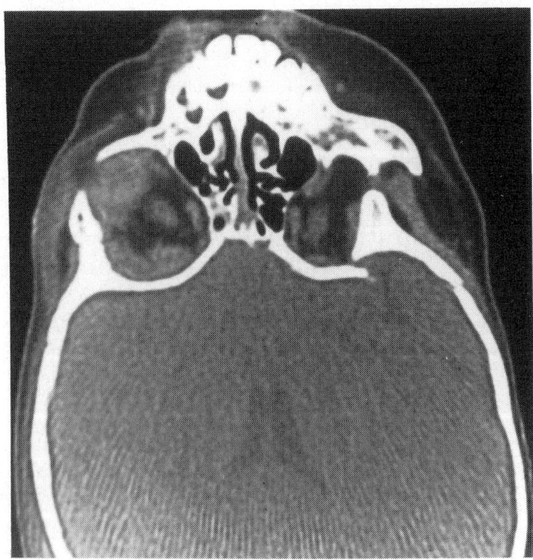

Figure 28–30. CT cross section demonstrating the mechanism by which a frontal-orbital-temporal fracture results in an ipsilateral exophthalmos. The lateral orbital wall compression results in extrusion of the orbit and the orbital contents.

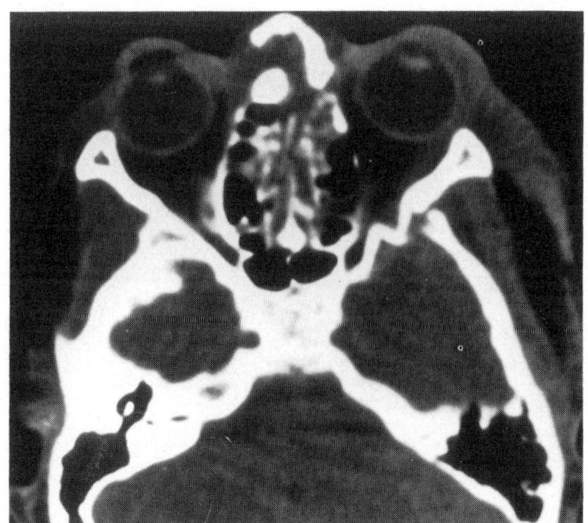

Figure 28–31. Frontal-orbital-temporal fracture that has resulted in collapse and compression of the structures of the superior orbital fissure (superior orbital fissure syndrome). Note the irregularities of the greater wing of the sphenoid.

of the frontal and orbital fractures and their displacement (Manson and associates, 1986a,b).

Open reduction of a supraorbital fracture may be accomplished through a laceration, where appropriate, but usually a coronal incision is required. The fragments are replaced in proper position and connected to adjacent intact bone with interfragmentary wires. If a bone graft is necessary to restore continuity in the supraorbital rim or orbital roof, it should be thin and may be placed under the edges of the adjacent, intact orbital roof. The pressure from the edematous soft tissue in the orbit usually holds a graft in place satisfactorily without fixation. Lateral frontal-orbital-temporal fractures require neurosurgical exposure and treatment of underlying epidural hematomas, brain injury, or dural lacerations (Schultz and Meilman, 1980; Schultz, 1982).

Whenever an orbital fracture or globe injury is suspected, a thorough visual screening examination should be performed. The basic screening consists of evaluation of visual acuity, confrontation fields, extraocular motion, pupil size and reactivity, and diplopia; examination of the anterior and posterior chambers; and a determination of intraocular pressure. The muscle involved in the production of diplopia may be identified by determining the field in which the diplopia is produced (Schultz and Meilman, 1980; Schultz, 1982).

Compound, Multiple, Comminuted Midfacial Fractures

In trauma of particularly severe violence, lacerations with partial avulsion of the soft

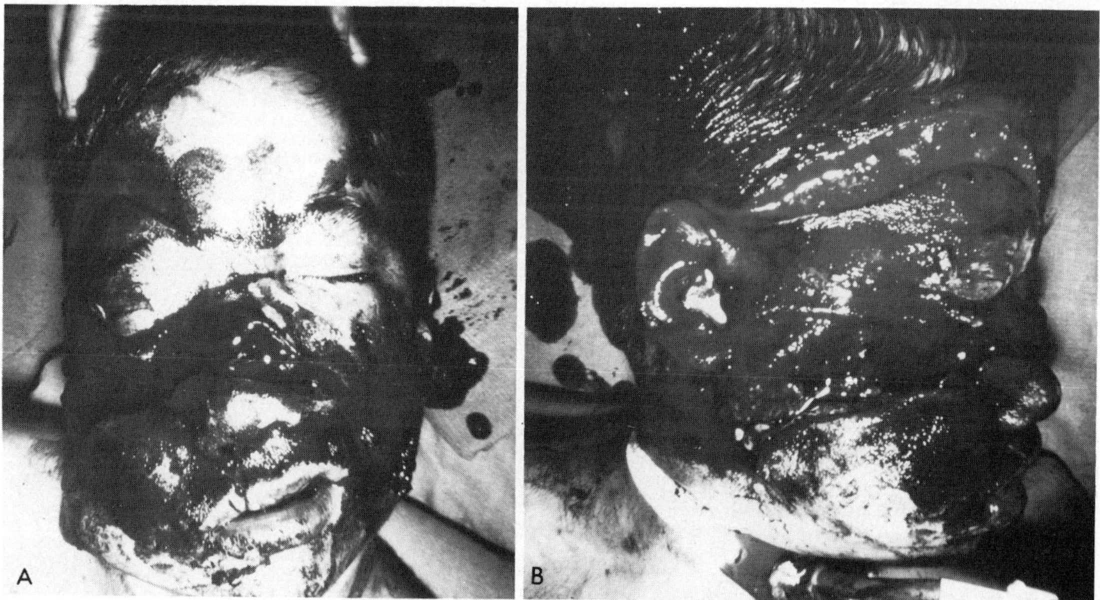

Figure 28–32. A 5 year old boy struck by a descending elevator. *A,* Extent of facial lacerations. *B,* Avulsed flaps of soft tissue. He also sustained partial laceration of the branches of the facial nerve and division of Stensen's duct.

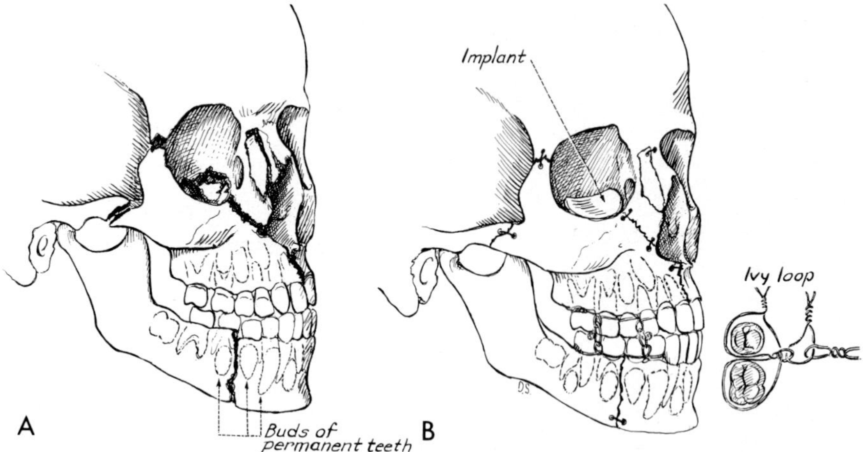

Figure 28–33. Multiple fractures suffered by the boy illustrated in Figure 28–32. *A,* Sites of fractures. The orbital blowout fracture was repaired by a Silastic implant. Other fractures were treated by realignment and interfragmentary wiring. Note the wire fixation of the mandible near the lower border.

tissues and multiple fractures of the facial bones require careful surgical care. The reward for adequate primary management is the prevention of severe facial disfigurement (Figs. 28–32 to 28–35).

Partly or nearly totally avulsed flaps of soft tissue and loose comminuted bone fragments should be preserved and replaced, as the blood supply of the face (particularly in children) ensures survival.

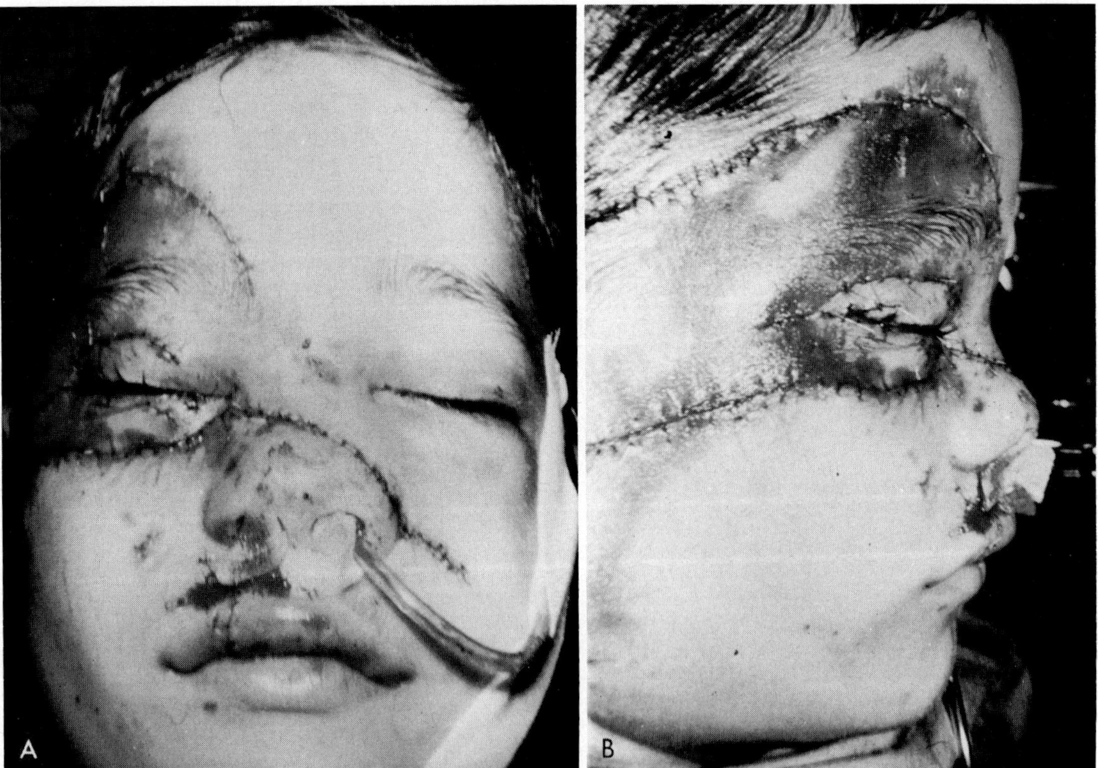

Figure 28–34. The child illustrated in Figure 28–32 at completion of surgery. *A,* A feeding tube has been placed through the left nasal fossa. *B,* Profile view following approximation of the flaps and open reduction and interfragmentary wiring of the fractures.

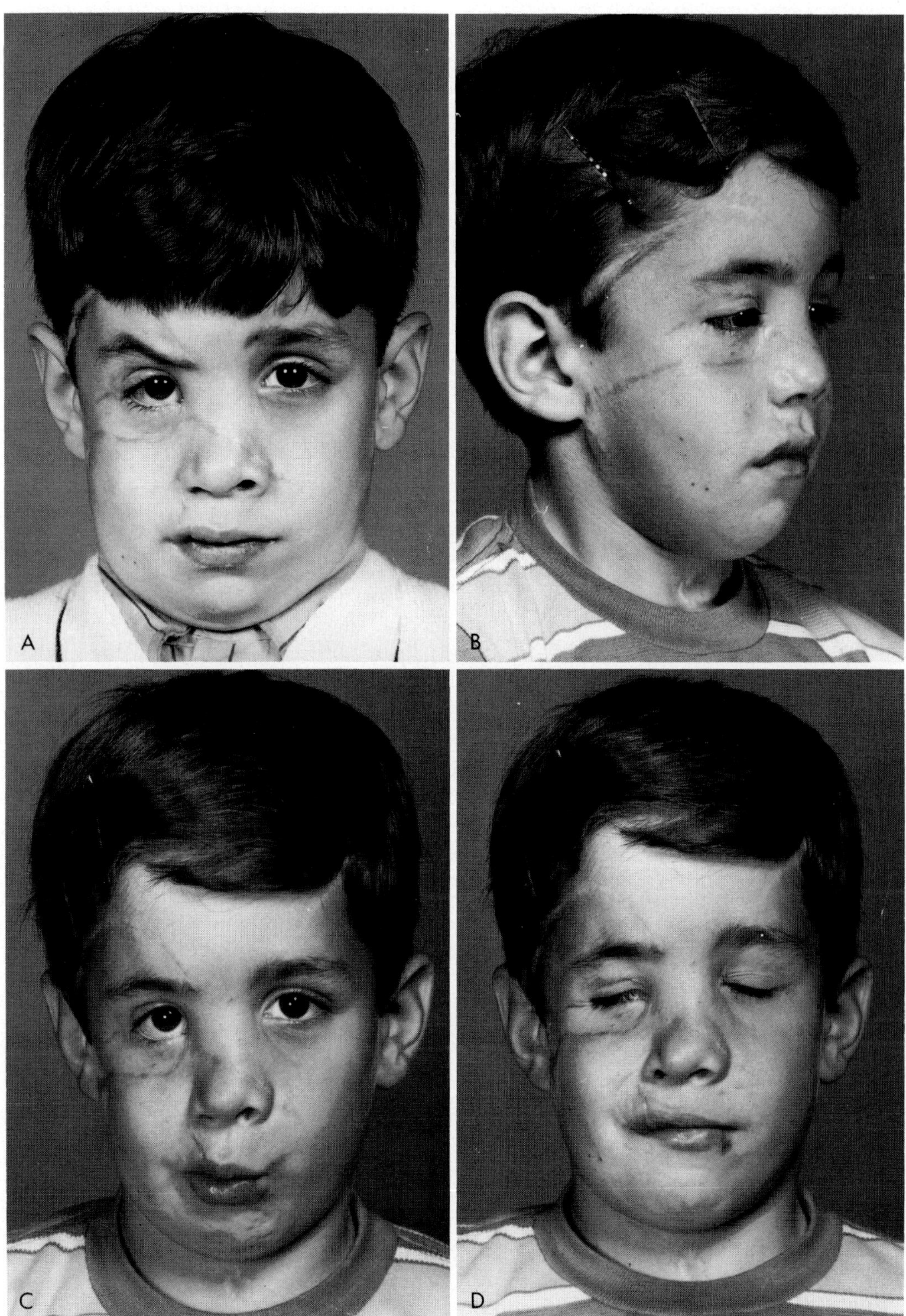

Figure 28–35. Follow-up views of the boy in Figure 28–32. *A, B,* One year after injury. *C,* The patient is able to whistle without associated movements of the eyelids. *D,* When the patient closes his eyelids, associated movement of the right upper lip is noted.

Maxillary fractures in children are classified as in adults (see Chap. 27). The level of separation between the upper midface and the lower maxilla is identified and forms the basis for the classification. The common terminology is consistent with that described by Le Fort. The Le Fort I (or horizontal maxillary fracture) separates the maxillary alveolus from the remainder of the upper midfacial skeleton. The fracture lines run horizontally from the base of the piriform aperture and extend across the nasomaxillary and zygomaticomaxillary buttresses. These fractures are infrequent in young children because of the absence of the maxillary sinuses. With the development of the permanent dentition, the tooth buds disappear and the floor of the maxillary sinus reaches the level of the floor of the nose. This weakens the bone structure at the Le Fort I level significantly and predisposes to the occurrence of a Le Fort I fracture (Dingman and Natvig, 1964; Converse and Dingman, 1977; Converse, 1979).

The Le Fort II, or pyramidal, fracture separates a central pyramidally shaped segment from the adjacent zygomatic portions of the facial skeleton. The maxillary alveolus, medial orbit, and nose thus move as a single segment (Dingman and Natvig, 1964; Converse and Dingman, 1977).

The Le Fort III fracture, or craniofacial dysjunction, separates the facial bones from the cranial skeleton through the orbits. The highest fracture lines extend from the zygomaticofrontal junction across the lateral orbit and orbital floor, and either enter the nasoethmoid area to cause a dysjunction of the nose from the frontal bone or comminute the nasoethmoid area to produce a nasoethmoido-orbital fracture. Le Fort III fractures are rarely a single fragment and exist as comminuted combinations of lesser Le Fort fragments such as a zygomatic fracture and a Le Fort II fracture. The superior level of the fracture observed is usually higher (in terms of Le Fort classification) on one side than the other. It is common, for example, to see a Le Fort III superior level on one side with a Le Fort II superior level fracture on the other. In this situation, the fractured fragments consist of a Le Fort II segment carrying the maxillary dentition accompanied by a zygomatic fracture on a Le Fort III side. The occurrence of a single fragment Le Fort III fracture can be identified when bilateral periorbital ecchymosis is accompanied by an occlusal abnormality (Dingman and Natvig, 1964; Converse and Dingman, 1977).

The palatal suture running sagittally does not complete ossification until the end of the second decade of life. It is thus common to see a hemipalatal fracture dividing the maxillary alveolus in segments. Hemi–Le Fort fractures may also accompany the split palatal fractures. Their occurrence is often suggested by an accompanying laceration. The fracture may be documented on a CT scan or on plain films of the palate taken with an occlusal dental radiograph (Manson and associates, 1983).

The diagnosis of a Le Fort fracture is confirmed by maxillary mobility. In rare cases, the maxilla is greensticked or impacted and is not mobile, but a malocclusion can be observed. It may be difficult to determine a minor malocclusion in the period of mixed dentition. Accompanying fractures such as zygomatic, orbital, or nasoethmoido-orbital fractures are commonly associated with Le Fort fractures and, as mentioned, the Le Fort III fracture usually consists of the upper fractures in association with a mobile maxillary alveolus at the Le Fort I or II level. If no primary treatment is rendered for several days, the midface is usually elongated and retruded. The maxilla drops downward and especially posteriorly, and an anterior bite is present. Profuse nasopharyngeal bleeding usually accompanies a Le Fort fracture. Facial swelling may be massive and impressive. A CSF leak may accompany high Le Fort II or III fractures, and pneumocephalus may be present if the fractures extend to the cranial base (Converse and Dingman, 1977; Manson and associates, 1983, 1985).

The radiographic evaluation of a Le Fort fracture consists of plain films (Waters, Caldwell, and lateral skull films), and a CT scan is recommended for more precise evaluation of the orbit, nasoethmoid, and maxillary areas.

The treatment of Le Fort fractures consists of placing the patient in intermaxillary fixation in occlusion for two to four weeks (see Chap. 27). The maxilla is usually stable within two to four weeks in children. In patients with a split palate, a palatal acrylic splint should be placed to ensure the precise relationship of the halves of the maxillary alveolus. Dental impressions are taken and stone models are prepared. The models are sectioned at the sites of the fracture and repositioned. A splint is made to fit the repositioned model. It may be necessary to retain the splint longer than four weeks if mobility is demonstrated in the fracture of the palate after release of intermaxillary fixation (Dingman and Natvig, 1964; Converse and Dingman, 1977; Manson and associates, 1985).

Open reduction and interfragmentary wiring or plating are preferred for the treatment of upper facial fractures involving the orbit and nasoethmoido-orbital area, as described in previous sections on zygoma and nasoethmoido-orbital and orbital floor fracture treatment (see also Chap. 27). The vertical buttresses of the mid- and upper face are restored by interfragmentary wiring or plate and screw fixation (Manson and associates, 1985). In general, exposure of the lower fractures at the Le Fort I level is performed to place interfragment wires to unite the fractured areas. Care must be taken to avoid the tooth buds. Alternately, suspension wires can be led to a point above the highest level of the fractures on each side, but their use is more cumbersome and fracture alignment is often inaccurate (Manson and associates, 1983).

In practice, suspension wires are rarely used for fracture alignment or maxillary immobilization, but are principally utilized for stabilization of the arch bar or splint in the period of mixed dentition (see Chap. 27). Increasing the extent of open reduction eliminates the need for suspension wires. Arch bars may require support with piriform aperture or circum-mandibular wires in patients with missing teeth, mixed dentition, or alveolar fractures. The difficulty of ligating deciduous teeth to an arch bar is secondary to the bulbous shape of the crowns of the primary teeth. The fact that the roots are frequently shallow or incomplete allows the teeth to be easily extracted. In the period of mixed dentition, the resorbing root structure makes extrusion a distinct possibility. In some cases the arch bar may be incorporated into a lingual or palatal splint, which assists stability, especially if alveolar fractures are present. Acrylic may be applied to the arch bars for additional stability. Again, the splints are secured with piriform aperture, inferior orbital rim, or circum-mandibular wires as necessary.

The treatment of most maxillary and mandibular fractures involves ligating arch bars to the maxillary and mandibular dentition. The bars are utilized to place the patient in occlusion, with the teeth in proper relationship and in maximal intercuspation. The relationship is held for a time until fracture healing has occurred. Because children heal more quickly than adults, the period rarely exceeds three or four weeks. In some patients the teeth may be held in occlusion with Ivy or wire loops (Kazanjian and Converse, 1974).

The care of the patient in intermaxillary fixation involves intermittent observation of the occlusal relationship and the adjustment of wires or elastic traction, as indicated. The use of a splint in the presence of an alveolar fracture prevents fracture segment tipping or collapsing. Overriding or telescoping of the segments of the dentition occurs when teeth are missing, and may be prevented with a splint with an occlusal stop to provide for the missing dentition. The range of mandibular excursion should exceed 35 mm after therapy and ideally should approach 45 to 55 mm (Schultz and Meilman, 1980).

COMPLICATIONS OF PEDIATRIC FACIAL TRAUMA

Multiple types of complications may follow pediatric facial trauma. Pulmonary complications include aspiration of stomach contents, since gastric dilation occurs in over 25 per cent of children in some series (McCoy and associates, 1962; Oliver and associates, 1962; McCoy, Chandler, and Crow, 1966; Othersen, 1979). Some authors note that tracheostomy does not prevent this complication and suggest that a cuffed tube should consequently be employed. Early evacuation of the stomach contents by nasogastric tube is indicated as a preoperative and postoperative measure (McCoy and associates, 1962; McCoy, Chandler, and Crow, 1966).

Ocular injuries, damage to the lacrimal system, and cerebrospinal fluid rhinorrhea are observed in children and must receive the same consideration as these complications in the adult patient (Schultz and Meilman, 1980). Nonunion occurs infrequently. Malunion is frequent in fractures undergoing late reduction. Osteomyelitis (which at one time was a serious complication of fractures) is rarely seen with modern antibiotic therapy

(Converse and Dingman, 1977; Schultz and Meilman, 1980).

Underdevelopment, maldevelopment, malocclusion, and ankylosis are all potential complications that can occur with facial trauma, particularly in facial bone fractures in children.

Complications from facial fracture treatment occur in 10 to 20 per cent of patients and relate to the organ system injured and the efficacy of treatment. Dental problems include delayed eruption of teeth, malformed teeth, loss of permanent teeth, and damage to tooth bud follicles (Gelbier, 1967). Cystic or malignant degeneration of a tooth bud has not been observed. Tooth buds in the line of fracture usually survive with a 20 per cent incidence of deformation of the crown (Andreasen, 1970a; Andreasen, Sundstrom, and Ravn, 1971; Schneider and Stern, 1971).

Other complications include double vision, reduction in visual acuity, and lacrimal system obstruction.

Cerebrospinal fluid rhinorrhea is managed as in adults with primary repair of the dural tear at the time of the bone or brain surgery, or delayed repair at one to three weeks if the CSF leak does not cease spontaneously (Rasmussen, 1965; Grote, 1966; Caldicott, North, and Simpson, 1973). Preoperative evaluation of the location of the CSF leak by metrizamide scan facilitates documentation of the injury (Schneider and Thompson, 1957) and surgical repair. Late CSF leaks are unusual but almost always require surgical repair.

REFERENCES

Adekeye, E. O.: Pediatric fractures of the facial skeleton: a survey of 85 cases from Kaduna, Nigeria. J. Oral Surg., *38*:355, 1980.

Agran, P. F., and Dunkle, D. E.: Motor vehicle occupant injuries to children in crash and noncrash events. Pediatrics, *70*:993, 1982.

Agran, P. F., Dunkle, D. E., and Winn, D. G.: Motor vehicle childhood injuries caused by noncrash falls and ejections. J.A.M.A., *253*:2530, 1985.

Andreasen, J. O.: Fracture of the alveolar process of the jaw. A clinical and radiographic follow-up study. Scand. J. Dent. Res., *78*:263, 1970a.

Andreasen, J. O.: Luxation of permanent teeth due to trauma. Scand. J. Dent. Res., *78*:273, 1970b.

Andreasen, J. O.: Etiology and pathogenesis of traumatic dental injuries. A clinical study of 1,298 cases. Scand. J. Dent. Res., *78*:329, 1970c.

Andreasen, J. O.: Treatment of fractured and avulsed teeth. J. Dent. Child., *28*:29, 1971.

Andreasen, J. O., and Ravn, J. J.: The effect of traumatic injuries to primary teeth on their permanent successors. II. A clinical and radiographic follow-up study of 213 teeth. Scand. J. Dent. Res., *79*:284, 1971.

Andreasen, J. O., Sundstrom, B., and Ravn, J. J.: The effect of traumatic injuries to primary teeth on their permanent successors. I. A clinical and histologic study of 117 injuries to permanent teeth. Scand. J. Dent. Res., *79*:284, 1971.

Bales, C. R., Randall, P., and Lehr, H. B.: Fractures of the facial bones in children. J. Trauma, *12*:56, 1972.

Berger, M. S., Pitts, L. H., Lovely, M., Edwards, M. S., and Bartkowski, H. M.: Outcome from severe head injury in children and adolescents. J. Neurosurg., *62*:194, 1985.

Bergland, O., and Borchgrevink, H.: The role of the nasal septum in midfacial growth in man elucidated by the maxillary development in certain types of facial clefts: a preliminary report. Scand. J. Plast. Reconstr. Surg., *8*:42, 1974.

Berkowitz, R., Ludwig, S., and Johnson, R.: Dental trauma in children and adolescents. Clin. Pediatr., *19*:166, 1980.

Bernstein, L.: Maxillofacial injuries in children. Otol. Clin. North Am., *2*:397, 1969.

Bernstein, L.: Pediatric sinus problems. Otol. Clin. North Am., *4*:126, 1971.

Blevins, C., and Gores, R. J.: Fractures of the mandibular condyloid process: results of conservative treatment in 140 patients. J. Oral Surg., *19*:392, 1961.

Boyne, P. J.: Osseous repair and mandibular growth after subcondylar fractures. J. Oral Surg., *25*:300, 1967.

Bridges, C. P., Ryan, R. F., Longenecker, C. G., and Vincent, R. W.: Tracheostomy in children: a twenty year study at Charity Hospital in New Orleans. Plast. Reconstr. Surg., *37*:117, 1966.

Brook, I., and Friedman, E. M.: Intracranial complications of sinusitis in children. Ann. Otol., *91*:41, 1982.

Bruce, D. A., Alavi, A., Bilaniuk, L., Dolinskas, C., Obrist, W., and Uzzell, B.: Diffuse cerebral swelling following head injuries in children: the syndrome of "malignant brain edema." J. Neurosurg., *54*:170, 1981.

Bruce, D. A., Schut, L., Bruno, L. A., Wood, J. H., and Sutton, L. N.: Outcome following severe head injuries in children. J. Neurosurg., *48*:679, 1978.

Burdi, A. R., Huelke, F., Snyder, R. G., and Lowry, A. H.: Infants and children in the adult world of automobile safety design: pediatric and anatomical considerations in design of child restraints. J. Biomech., *2*:267, 1969.

Caffey, J.: Multiple fractures in the long bones of infants suffering from chronic subdural hematoma. AJR, *56*:163, 1946.

Caffey, J.: The whiplash shaken infant syndrome: manual shaking by the extremities with whiplash-induced intracranial and intraocular bleedings, linked with residual permanent brain damage and mental retardation. Pediatrics, *54*:396, 1974.

Caldicott, W. J., North, J. B., and Simpson, D. A.: Traumatic cerebrospinal fluid fistula in children. J. Neurosurg., *38*:1, 1973.

Carrington, K. W., Taren, J. A., and Kahn, E. A.: Primary repair of compound skull fractures in children. Surg. Gynecol. Obstet., *110*:203, 1960.

Cohen, R. A., Kaufman, R. A., Myers, P. A., and Towbin, R. B.: Cranial computed tomography in the abused child with head injury. AJR., *146*:97, 1986.

Converse, J. M., Smith, B., Obear, M. F., and Wood-Smith, D.: Orbital blow-out fractures: a ten-year survey. Plast. Reconstr. Surg., *29*:20, 1967.

Converse, J. M.: Orbital and naso-orbital fractures. *In* Tessier, P., Callahan, A., Mustardé, J. C., and Salyer, K. E. (Eds.): Symposium on Plastic Surgery in the Orbital Region. Vol. 12. St. Louis. C. V. Mosby Company, 1976, pp. 79–106.

Converse, J. M.: Facial injuries in children. *In* Mustardé, J. C. (Ed.): Plastic Surgery in Plastic Surgery in Infancy and Childhood. Edinburgh, Churchill Livingstone, 1979.

Converse, J. M., and Campbell, R. M.: Bone grafts in surgery of the face. Surg. Clin. North Am., *34*:365, 1954.

Converse, J. M., and Dingman, R. O.: Facial injuries in children. *In* Converse, J. M. (Ed.): Reconstructive Plastic Surgery. Philadelphia, W. B. Saunders Company, 1977, pp. 794–821.

Danforth, H. B.: Mandibular fractures: use of acrylic splints for immobilization. Laryngoscope, *79*:280, 1969.

Dawson, R. I. G., and Fordyce, G. L.: Complex fractures of the middle third of the face and their early treatment. Br. J. Surg., *41*:254, 1953.

Dingman, R. O.: Symposium: malunited fractures of the zygoma. Repair of the deformity. Trans. Am. Acad. Ophthalmol. Otolaryngol., *57*:889, 1953.

Dingman, R. O., and Natvig, P.: Facial fractures in children. *In* Surgery of Facial Fractures. Philadelphia, W. B. Saunders Company, 1964, pp. 311–327.

Dufourmentel, C., and Mouly, R.: Facial traumas associated with traffic accidents. Mem. Acad. Chir. (Paris), *95*:558, 1969.

Enlow, D. H.: Handbook of Facial Growth. 2nd Ed. Philadelphia, W. B. Saunders Company, 1982.

Fearon, B., Edmonds, B., and Bird, R.: Orbito-facial complications of sinusitis in children. Laryngoscope, *89*:947, 1979.

Fortunato, M. A., Fielding, A. F., and Guernsey, L. H.: Facial bone fractures in children. Oral Surg., *53*:225, 1982.

Freid, M. G., and Baden, E.: Management of fractures in children. J. Oral Surg., *12*:129, 1954.

Freihofer, H. P., Jr.: Results of osteotomies of the facial skeleton in adolescence. J. Maxillofac. Surg., *5*:267, 1977.

Fry, H.: Nasal skeletal trauma and the interlocked stresses of the nasal septal cartilage. Br. J. Plast. Surg., *20*:146, 1967.

Furnas, D. W.: Emergency diagnosis of the injured orbit. *In* Tessier, P., Callahan, W., Mustardé, J. C., and Salyer, K. E. (Eds.): Symposium on Plastic Surgery in the Orbital Region. Vol. 12. St. Louis, C. V. Mosby Company, 1976, pp. 67–78.

Gelbier, S.: Injured anterior teeth in children. A preliminary discussion. Br. Dent. J., *123*:331, 1967.

Georgiade, N. G., and Pickrell, K. L.: Treatment of maxillofacial injuries in children. J. Int. Coll. Surg., *27*:640, 1967.

Gilbert, G. G.: Growth of the nose and the septo-rhinoplastic problem in youth. Arch. Otolaryngol., *68*:673, 1958.

Gillingham, F. J.: Neurosurgical experiences in northern Italy. Br. J. Surg., War Surg. Suppl., *1*:81, 1947.

Goldstein, F. P., Rosenthal, S. A., Garancis, J. C., Larson, S. J., and Brackett, C. E., Jr.: Varieties of growing skull fractures in childhood. J. Neurosurg., *33*:25, 1970.

Graham, G. G., and Peltier, R. J.: Management of mandibular fractures in children. J. Oral Surg., *18*:416, 1960.

Grote, W.: Traumatische Liquorfisteln im Kindes and Jurgendalter. Z. Kinderchir. Grenzgeb, *3*:11, 1966.

Gruszkiewicz, J., Doron, Y., and Peyser, E.: Recovery from severe craniocerebral injury and brain stem lesions in childhood. Surg. Neurol., *1*:197, 1973.

Hagan, E. H., and Huelke, D. F.: An analysis of 319 case reports of mandibular fractures. J. Oral Surg., *19*:93, 1961.

Halazonetis, J. A.: The "weak" regions of the mandible. Br. J. Oral Surg., *6*:37, 1968.

Hall, R. K.: Injuries of the face and jaws in children, Int. J. Oral Surg., *1*:65, 1972.

Hall, R. K.: Facial trauma in children. Aust. Dent. J., *19*:336, 1974.

Harwood-Nash, D. C.: Fractures of the petrous and tympanic parts of the temporal bone in children: a tomographic study of 35 cases. Am. J. Roentgenol., *110*:598, 1970.

Hellman, L. M., and Pritchard, J. A. (Eds.): William's Obstetrics. 14th Ed. New York, Appleton-Century-Crofts, 1971.

Hellman, M.: The face in its developmental career. *In* The Human Face: A Symposium. Philadelphia, Dental Cosmos, 1935.

Hendrick, E. B.: The use of hypothermia in severe brain stem lesions in childhood. Arch. Surg., *79*:362, 1959.

Hendrick, E. B., Harwood-Nash, D. C., and Hudson, A. R.: Head injuries in children: a survey of 4465 consecutive cases at the Hospital for Sick Children. Clin. Neurosurg., *11*:46, 1964.

Hoopes, J. E., Wolfort, F. G., and Jabaley, M. E.: Operative treatment of fractures of the mandibular condyle in children using the post-auricular approach. Plast. Reconstr. Surg., *46*:357, 1970.

Huang, C. S., and Ross, R. B.: Surgical advancement of the retrognathic mandible in growing children. Am. J. Orthod., *82*:89, 1982.

James, D.: Maxillofacial injuries in children. *In* Rowe, N. L., and Williams, J. I. (Eds.): Maxillofacial Injuries. Vol. I. London, Churchill Livingstone, 1985.

James, R. B., Fredrickson, C., and Kent, J. N.: Prospective study of mandibular fractures. J. Oral Surg., *39*:275, 1981.

Jazbi, B.: Subluxation of the nasal septum in the newborn: etiology, diagnosis and treatment. Otolaryngol. Clin. North Am., *10*:125, 1977.

Jennes, M.: Corrective nasal surgery in children. Arch. Otolaryngol., *79*:145, 1964.

Johnson, H. A.: A modification of the Gillies' temporalis transfer for the surgical treatment of lagophthalmos of leprosy. Plast. Reconstr. Surg., *30*:378, 1962.

Kaban, L. B., Mulliken, J. B., and Murray, J. E.: Facial fractures in children: an analysis of 122 fractures in 109 patients. Plast. Reconstr. Surg., *59*:15, 1977.

Kazanjian, V. H., and Converse, J. M.: The Surgical Treatment of Facial Injuries. 3rd Ed. Baltimore, Williams & Wilkins Company, 1974.

Keith, A., and Campion, C.: A contribution to the mechanism of growth of the human face. Int. J. Orthod., *8*:607, 1922.

Khosla, M., and Boren, W.: Mandibular fractures in children and their management. J. Oral Surg., *29*:116, 1971.

Koornneef, L.: Current concepts on the management of orbital blow-out fracture. Ann. Plast. Surg., *9*:185, 1982.

Kravits, H., Driessen, G., Gomberg, R., and Korach, A.: Accidental falls from elevated surfaces in infants from birth to one year of age. Pediatrics, *44* (Suppl.):869, 1969.

Landtwing, K.: Evaluation of the normal range of vertical mandibular opening in children and adolescents with special reference to age and stature. J. Maxillofac. Surg., *6*:157, 1978.

Leake, D., Doykos, J., III, Habal, M. B., and Murray, J. F.: Long-term follow-up of fractures of the mandibular condyle in children. Plast. Reconstr. Surg., *47*:127, 1971.

Lehman, J. A., Jr., and Saddawi, N. D.: Fractures of the mandible in children. J. Trauma, *16*:773, 1976.

Levin, H. S., Eisenberg, H. M., Wigg, N. R., and Kobayashi, K.: Memory and intellectual ability after head injury in children and adolescents. Neurosurgery, *11*:668, 1982.

Lindenberg, R., Fisher, R. S., Dunlacher, S., et al.: The pathology of the brain in blunt head injuries of infants and children. Proceed. 2nd Int. Cong. Neuropathology. Vol. 1. Amsterdam, Excerpta Med., 1955, pp. 477–479.

Lyerly, J. G.: The treatment of depressed fractures of the skull with special reference to the cranial defect. Am. Surg., *23*:1115, 1957.

MacLennan, W. D.: Fractures of the mandible in children under the age of six years. Br. J. Plast. Surg., *9*:125, 1956.

MacLennan, W. D.: Injuries involving the teeth and jaws in young children. Arch. Dis. Child., *32*:492, 1957.

MacLennan, W. D., and Simpson, W.: Treatment of fractured mandibular condylar processes in children. Br. J. Plast. Surg., *18*:423, 1965.

Manson, P. N., Clifford, C. M., Su, C. T., Iliff, N. T., and Morgan, R.: Mechanisms of global support and posttraumatic enophthalmos. I. The anatomy of the ligament sling and its relation to intramuscular cone orbital fat. Plast. Reconstr. Surg., *77*:193, 1986a.

Manson, P. N., Crawley, W. A., Yaremchuk, M. J., Rochman, G. M., Hoopes, J. E., and French, J. H., Jr.: Midface fractures: advantages of immediate extended open reduction and bone grafting. Plast. Reconstr. Surg., *76*:1, 1985.

Manson, P. N., Grivas, A., Rosenbaum, A., Vannier, M., Zinreich, J., and Iliff, N.: Studies on enophthalmos: II. The measurement of orbital injuries and their treatment by quantitative computed tomography. Plast. Reconstr. Surg., *77*:203, 1986b.

Manson, P. N., Hoopes, J. E., and Su, C. T.: Structural pillars of the facial skeleton: an approach to the management of Le Fort fractures. Plast. Reconstr. Surg., *66*:54, 1980.

Manson, P. N., Shack, R. B., Leonard, L. G., Su, C. T., and Hoopes, J. E.: Sagittal fractures of the maxilla and palate. Plast. Reconstr. Surg., *72*:484, 1983.

Mathog, R. H., and Boies, L. R., Jr.: Nonunion of the mandible. Laryngoscope, *86*:908, 1976.

Mathog, R. H., and Rosenberg, Z.: Complications in the treatment of facial fractures. Otolaryngol. Clin. North Am., *9*:533, 1976.

May, M., Fria, T. J., Blumenthal, F., and Curtin, H.: Facial paralysis in children: differential diagnosis. Otolaryngol. Head Neck Surg., *89*:841, 1981.

Mayell, M. J.: Nasal fractures: their occurrence, management and some late results. J. R. Coll. Surg. Edinb., *18*:31, 1973.

Mayer, T., Matlak, M. E., Johnson, D. G., and Walker, M. L.: The modified injury severity scale in pediatric multiple trauma patients. J. Pediatric Surg., *15*:719, 1980.

McCoy, F. J.: Late results in facial fractures. *In* Goldwyn, R. M. (Ed.): Long-term Results in Plastic and Reconstructive Surgery. Vol. II. Boston, Little Brown and Company, 1980, pp. 484–501.

McCoy, F. J., Chandler, R. A., and Crow, M. L.: Facial fractures in children. Plast. Reconstr. Surg., *37*:209, 1966.

McCoy, F. J., Chandler, R. A., Magnan, C. G., et al.: An analysis of facial fractures and their complications. Plast. Reconstr. Surg., *29*:381, 1962.

Miller, J. D., Becker, D. P., Ward, J. D., Sullivan, H. G., Adams, W. E., and Rosner, M. J.: Significance of intracranial hypertension in severe head injury. J. Neurosurg., *47*:503, 1977.

Mizuno, A., Nakamura, T., Kanabata, T., Shigeno, T., Motegi, K., and Watanabe, I.: Blow-out fracture of the orbit in 4 children. Int. J. Oral Surg., *14*:284, 1985.

Moffett, B.: The morphogenesis of the temporomandibular joint. Am. J. Orthod., *52*:401, 1966.

Morgan, B. D., Madan, D. K., and Bergerot, J. P.: Fractures of the middle third of the face—a review of 300 cases. Br. J. Plast. Surg., *25*:147, 1972.

Moss, M. L.: The primacy of functional matrices in orofacial growth. Dent. Pract. Dent. Rec., *19*:65, 1968.

Moss, M. L., and Rankow, R.: The role of the functional matrix in mandibular growth. Angle Orthod., *38*:95, 1968.

Moss, M. L., and Salentijn, L.: The capsular matrix. Am. J. Orthod., *56*:474, 1969.

Muller, D.: Long-term results after rhinoplasty of nose trauma in childhood. Laryngol. Rhinol. Otol., *62*:116, 1983.

Mulliken, J. B., Kaban, L. B., Evans, C. A., Strand, R. D., and Murray, J. E.: Facial skeletal changes following hypertelorbitism correction. Plast. Reconstr. Surg., *77*:7, 1986.

Mustardé, J. C.: Facial injuries in children. *In* Mustardé, J. C. (Ed.): Plastic Surgery in Infancy and Childhood. Philadelphia, W. B. Saunders Company, 1971, pp. 178–206.

Oliver, P., Richardson, J. R., Clubb, R. W., and Flake, C. A.: Tracheotomy in children. N. Engl. J. Med., *267*:631, 1962.

Ortiz-Monasterio, F., and Olmedo, A.: Corrective rhinoplasty before puberty: a long-term follow-up. Plast. Reconstr. Surg., *68*:381, 1981.

O'Ryan, F., and Epker, B. N.: Deliberate surgical control of mandibular growth. Oral Surg., *53*:2, 1982.

Othersen, H. B., Jr.: Intubation injuries of the trachea in children. Management and prevention. Ann. Surg., *189*:601, 1979.

Panagopoulos, A. P.: Management of fractures of the jaws in children. J. Int. Coll. Surg., *28*:806, 1957.

Pfeifer, G.: Kieferbruche im Kindesalter and ihre Auswirkungen auf das Wachstum. Fortschr. Kiefer Gesichtschir., *11*:43, 1966.

Precious, D. S., McFadden, L. R., and Fitch, S. J.: Orthognathic surgery for children. Int. J. Oral Surg., *14*:466, 1985.

Proffit, W. R., Vig, K. W., and Turvey, T. A.: Early fractures of the mandibular condyles: frequently an unsuspected cause of growth disturbances. Am. J. Orthod., *78*:1, 1980.

Putterman, A. M., Stevens, T., and Urist, M. J.: Nonsurgical management of fractures of the orbital floor. Am. J. Ophthalmol., *77*:232, 1974.

Ramba, J.: Fractures of the facial bones in children. Int. J. Oral Surg., *14*:472, 1985.

Rasmussen, P. S.: Acute traumatic liquorrhea. Acta Neurol. Scand., *41*:441, 1965.

Reil, B., and Kranz, S.: Traumatology of the maxillofacial region in childhood. J. Maxillofac. Surg., *4*:197, 1976.

Riefkohl, R., and Georgiade, N.: Facial fractures in children. *In* Serafin, D., and Georgiade, N. (Eds.): Pediatric Plastic Surgery. St. Louis, C. V. Mosby Company, 1984.

Roberts, F., and Shopfner, C. E.: Plain skull roentgenograms in children with head trauma. Am. J. Roentgenol., *114*:230, 1972.

Roed-Petersen, B., and Andreasen, J. O.: Prognosis of permanent teeth involved in jaw fractures. Scand. J. Dent. Res., *78*:343, 1970.

Roemer, F. J.: Relation of torticollis to breach delivery. Am. J. Obstet. Gynecol., *68*:1146, 1954.

Rowe, N. L.: Fractures of the facial skeleton in children. J. Oral Surg., *26*:505, 1968.

Rowe, N. L.: Fractures of the jaws in children. J. Oral Surg., *27*:497, 1969.

Rowe, N. L.: Injuries to teeth and jaws. *In* Mustardé, J. C. (Ed.): Plastic Surgery in Infancy and Childhood. Philadelphia, W. B. Saunders Company, 1971.

Rowe, N. L., and Williams, J. C.: Children's fractures. *In* Maxillofacial Injuries. New York, Churchill Livingstone, 1985, p. 538.

Rowe, N. L., and Winter, G. B.: Traumatic lesions of the jaws and teeth. *In* Mustardé, J. C. (Ed.): Plastic Surgery in Infancy and Childhood. Philadelphia, W. B. Saunders Company, 1971, pp. 154–175.

Sanders, B.: Pediatric Oral and Maxillofacial Surgery. St. Louis, C. V. Mosby Company, 1979.

Sarnat, B. G., and Gans, B. J.: Growth of bones: methods of assessing and clinical importance. Plast. Reconstr. Surg., *9*:140, 1952.

Schneider, R. C., and Thompson, J. M.: Chronic and delayed traumatic cerebrospinal rhinorrhea as a source of recurrent attacks of meningitis. Ann. Surg., *145*:517, 1957.

Schneider, S. S., and Stern, M.: Teeth in the line of mandibular fractures. J. Oral Surg., *29*:107, 1971.

Schultz, R. C.: Pediatric facial fractures. *In* Kernahan, D. A., Thompson, H. G., and Bauer, B. S. (Eds.): Symposium on Pediatric Plastic Surgery. St. Louis, C. V. Mosby Company, 1982.

Schultz, R. C., and Meilman, J.: Facial fractures in children. *In* Goldwyn, R. M. (Ed.): Long-Term Results in Plastic and Reconstructive Surgery. Boston, Little, Brown and Company, 1980.

Scott, J. H.: Further studies on the growth of the human face. Proc. R. Soc. Med., *52*:263, 1959.

Sekhar, L. N., and Scarff, T. B.: Pseudogrowth of skull fractures in childhood. Neurosurgery, *6*:285, 1980.

Silverman, F. N.: The roentgen manifestations of unrecognized skeletal trauma in infants. Am. J. Roentgenol. Radium Ther. Nucl. Med., *69*:413, 1953.

Sorensen, D. C., and Laskin, D. M.: Facial growth after condylectomy or ostectomy in the mandibular ramus. J. Oral Surg., *33*:746, 1975.

Steinhauser, E. W.: The treatment of ankylosis in children. Int. J. Oral Surg., *2*:129, 1973.

Stoksted, P., and Schonsted-Madsen, V.: Traumatology of the newborn's nose. Rhinology, *17*:77, 1979.

Stucker, F. J., Jr., Bryarly, C., and Shockley, W. W.: Management of nasal trauma in children. Arch. Otolaryngol., *110*:190, 1984.

Tate, R. J.: Facial injuries associated with the battered child syndrome. Br. J. Oral Surg., *9*:41, 1971.

Teasdale, G., and Jennett, B.: Assessment of coma and impaired consciousness. Lancet, *2*:81, 1974.

Tsai, R. Y., Zee, C. S., Apthorp, J. S., and Dixon, G. H.: Computed tomography in child abuse head trauma. J. Comput. Tomogr., *4*:277, 1980.

Tucker, C. A.: Management of early nasal injuries with long-term follow-up. Rhinology, *22*:45, 1984.

Waite, D. E.: Pediatric fractures of the jaw and facial bones. Pediatrics, *51*:551, 1973.

Walker, D. G.: The mandibular condyle: fifty cases demonstrating arrest in development. Dental Pract., *7*:160, 1957.

Walker, R. V.: Traumatic mandibular condylar fracture dislocations: effect on growth in the *Macaca* rhesus monkey. Am. J. Surg., *100*:850, 1960.

Washburn, M. C., Schendel, S. A., and Epker, B. N.: Superior repositioning of the maxilla during growth. J. Oral Maxillofac. Surg., *40*:142, 1982.

Weber, S. C., and Cohn, A. M.: Fracture of the frontal sinus in children. Arch. Otolaryngol., *103*:241, 1977.

Williams, A. F.: Children killed in falls from motor vehicles. Pediatrics, *68*:576, 1981.

Winters, H. P.: Isolated fractures of the nasal bones. Arch. Chir. Neerl., *19*:159, 1967.

Wolford, L. M., Schendel, S. A., and Epker, B. N.: Surgical-orthodontic correction of mandibular deficiency in growing children. J. Maxillofac. Surg., *7*:61, 1979.

Zachariades, N.: The superior orbital fissure syndrome. Review of the literature and report of a case. Oral Surg., *53*:237, 1982.

29

Joseph G. McCarthy
Henry Kawamoto
Barry H. Grayson
Stephen R. Colen
Peter J. Coccaro
Donald Wood-Smith

Surgery of the Jaws

INTRODUCTION
- Initial Assessment
- Preoperative Orthodontic Therapy
- Preoperative Planning
- Fixation Techniques
- Postoperative Care
- Postoperative Orthodontic Therapy and Retention
- Types of Osteotomies in Orthognathic Surgery

DEVELOPMENTAL DEFORMITIES
- Mandibular Deformities
  - Surgical approach
  - Prognathism
  - Micrognathism and hypoplasia
  - Laterognathism: lateral deviation of mandible
  - Condylar hypoplasia
  - Condylar hyperplasia and unilateral mandibular macrognathia
  - Hemifacial hyperplasia
  - Facial hyperplasia
  - Benign masseteric hypertrophy
- Chin Deformities
  - Microgenia
  - Macrogenia
- Maxillary and Mandibular Dentoalveolar Deformities
  - Maxillary dentoalveolar protrusion
  - Maxillary dentoalveolar retrusion
  - Mandibular dentoalveolar protrusion
  - Bimaxillary dentoalveolar protrusion
  - Open bite deformity
- Maxillary Deformities
  - Classification
  - Preoperative planning
  - Surgical approach to midface
  - Micrognathia-retrognathia
  - Vertical excess
  - Vertical deficiency
- Nasomaxillary Hypoplasia
- Maxillomandibular Disharmonies
- Complications of Orthognathic Surgery

ACQUIRED DEFORMITIES
- Mandibular Defects
- Maxillary Defects

INTRODUCTION

The mandible and the maxilla constitute a major portion of the facial skeleton. Because of their prominent location and the intimate interrelationships of the facial bones, small alterations can produce a wide range of facial deformities. Conversely, orthognathic surgery can yield profound changes in facial appearance. The deformities can be classified into three main groups.

Congenital Malformations. Congenital malformations of the jaws may be unilateral or bilateral. They are often associated with such conditions as mandibulofacial dysostosis (Treacher Collins syndrome), craniofacial dysostosis, and other types of anomalous development of the first and second branchial arches (see Chaps. 61, 62, and 63). Another example is the cleft of the alveolus and palate (see Chap. 55).

Developmental Malformations. Developmental malformations can be caused by several factors, including:

1. Congenital anomalies involving adjacent structures. Jaw malformations associated with congenital facial paralysis (Möbius), hemangioma, or muscular torticollis are examples of this type.

2. Trauma. Faulty development due to injury in early life results in varying degrees of deformity. These injuries can assume diverse forms. A fall on the chin can produce an unrecognized condylar fracture injury of the growth center (see Chap. 28). A facial burn with tight, deficient, and contracted soft tissues can compress and deform the underlying skeleton, especially the chin.

3. Abnormal neuromuscular patterns. Asymmetric maxillary and mandibular

growth following facial nerve paralysis sustained during the period of early mandibular growth is an example of this type of malformation. Another example is an open bite produced by faulty tongue (thrust) habits.

4. Infection. Osteomyelitis or adjacent soft tissue infection, particularly if it occurs early in life, may result in severe deformity.

5. Endocrine imbalance. The classic example of this type of deformity is mandibular prognathism associated with acromegaly.

6. Nutritional deficiencies. These are rare in developed countries. Vitamin D deficiency is an appropriate example.

7. Arthritis. Juvenile rheumatoid arthritis can result in temporomandibular joint ankylosis, micrognathia, and microgenia.

Acquired Deformities. Loss of bone as the result of partial or total resection of the mandible or maxilla in the treatment of malignant tumors produces severe deformities. The deformities and their repair are also discussed in Chapters 68, 69, and 70.

Traumatic deformities of the jaws are the result of (1) loss of bone, which is not replaced at or soon after the time of injury; (2) malunion secondary to improper primary care; or (3) temporomandibular joint derangement, with or without ankylosis.

These deformities may affect any portion of the jaw: the dentoalveolar process, the denser bone of the body, the ramus, or the mandibular condyle. Similarly, deformities of the maxilla can involve the central nasomaxillary complex, the dentoalveolar process, or the adjacent zygomas.

Malocclusion of the teeth is a frequent accompaniment of the deformity. Correction of the malocclusion often provides a guide for planning the reconstructive procedure.

Relationship Between Surgeon and Orthodontist. The value of an effective working relationship between the surgeon and the orthodontist in orthognathic surgery cannot be overemphasized (McCarthy, Grayson, and Zide, 1982). Now that the disciplines are integrated, therapeutic objectives are more easily reached, thereby avoiding the problems that occur when the patient is treated by isolated modalities.

When a complementary association exists between the surgeon and orthodontist, the patient benefits. The surgeon's concern may center on generalized facial esthetics and overlying soft tissue deformities, while the orthodontist may directly focus on obtaining optimal occlusal function, periodontal health, dentofacial esthetics, and function of the temporomandibular joint.

The interdisciplinary collaboration is practiced in five principal areas: initial assessment, preoperative orthodontic therapy, preoperative planning and preparation of the intraoperative occlusal splint, postoperative orthodontic therapy and retention, and longitudinal studies.

Initial Assessment

Planning the correction of craniofacial deformities requires data from various sources: the patient's description or perception of his problem (chief complaint); the medical and dental history; the clinical examination; the cephalometric analysis; examination of the panoramic or dental radiographs; and evaluation of the temporomandibular joint.

Chief Complaint. The patient's report of his problem provides vital information to the clinician. It should direct attention to the patient's perceived needs, which may or may not be those that appear most prominent to the clinician. Careful listening during the interview and the ensuing dialogue with the patient helps to assess the patient's motivation and expectations.

Medical and Dental History. Does the patient have medical risk factors that contraindicate surgical reconstruction? A review of the medical history should alert the clinician to, or rule out, potential medical problems. The dental history is obtained for similar reasons. Does the periodontal and restorative status, past and present, suggest that the patient is a candidate for perioperative orthodontic therapy? Does the patient provide evidence that he is capable of maintaining a level of oral hygiene and health that is acceptable for an operation? Periodontal disease, periapical pathology, and carious lesions must be treated before combined surgical-orthodontic therapy is begun. Is there a history of temporomandibular joint dysfunction?

Clinical Examination. The patient should first be examined in a neutral position with the Frankfort horizontal (a line from the upper acoustic meatus to the infraorbital rim) parallel to the floor and with the teeth and condyles in centric position (teeth in maximal intercuspation). The forehead and orbits are

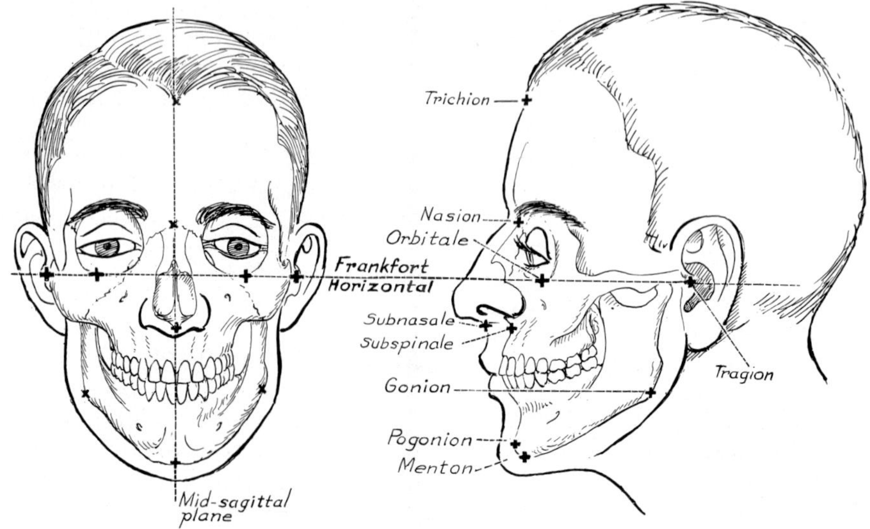

Figure 29–1. Anthropometric landmarks. The points of reference and planes are essential in orienting the face.

examined to rule out eyelid ptosis or any disparity or asymmetry of contour, such as plagiocephaly or orbital dystopia. Any exophthalmos, unilateral or bilateral, can be appreciated, and it can be determined whether it is attributable to a deficiency of the orbital roof or floor, or both. The interorbital distance is evaluated for signs of hypertelorism or hypotelorism.

At this point the head should be examined from above ("bird's eye") and below ("worm's eye"). Attention is also directed to an assessment of the malar eminences and the transverse dimensions of the midface. In addition, the malar eminences should be evaluated from frontal, lateral, and submental views. Examination of the nose includes evaluation of the dorsum, frontonasal angle, nasolabial angle, and alar base width and symmetry. A similar examination is performed in the subnasal region. The posture and competence of the lips are recorded. Abnormalities detected in this part of the examination may suggest an underlying dentofacial abnormality or skeletal malocclusion. The interlabial gap should not exceed 3.5 mm at rest, and there should not be more than 1 to 2 mm of gingival exposure on smiling. Maxillary incisor show with the lips in repose should not exceed 3.5 mm for males or 5 mm for females.

An intraoral examination follows, with particular care given to the status of the oral hygiene and the palatal, tonsillar, and lingual anatomy. The occlusion is studied with respect to its transverse and sagittal relationships. Lateral and protrusive excursions of the mandible, as well as the path of the mouth on opening and closing, are recorded. The presence of pain, clicking, and grating noises associated with the temporomandibular joint is sought. An evaluation of oral habits, deglutition, and respiration sometimes explains structural abnormalities such as open bite and vertical dysplasia of the facial skeleton.

It is also wise to examine the ears and neck region for abnormalities associated with various congenital syndromes.

Facial Proportions. Anatomic landmarks are displaced or absent in malformations of the craniofacial complex. Anthropometric points of the face are used in describing facial malformations (Fig. 29–1). Commonly used landmarks are the *trichion*, the midpoint at the hairline of the forehead; the *glabella*, the most prominent point in the midline between the brows; the *nasion*, the most anterior point of the midline of the frontonasal suture; the *subnasale*, the point beneath the nose where the columella merges with the upper lip in the midsagittal plane; the *stomion*, the interval between the lips; and the *menton*, the lowest median point of the mandible. The *pogonion* is the most anterior point on the chin. The *porion* is the highest point on the external auditory meatus; the *orbitale* is the lowest point on the infraorbital margin; and the *Frankfort horizontal* passes through the porion and orbitale.

The height of the face is divided in approximately equal thirds by horizontal lines

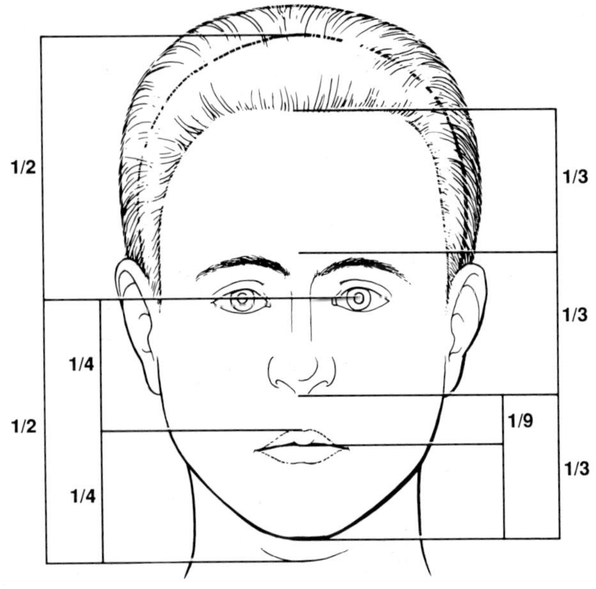

Figure 29–2. The divisions of the face. The face is divided into thirds by the trichion, nasion, subnasale, and menton (see Fig. 29–1). The distance between the vertex of the cranial vault and the midpupillary point defines the upper half, and that between the latter and the hyoid defines the lower half. Additional subdivisions are designated.

drawn through the nasion and subnasale (Fig. 29–2). The lower third of the face, subnasale to menton, can be further subdivided into three equal parts. The lips should meet near the junction of the upper and middle thirds. These subdivisions can be used as a general guide in classifying and assessing the degree of existing facial deformity.

Facial Profile. Various authors have attempted to define the "ideal" facial profile. Gonzalez-Ulloa and Stevens (1968) placed the anterior point of the chin (soft tissue pogonion, Po^s) on a vertical line beginning at soft tissue nasion (N^s) and drawn at right angles to the Frankfort horizontal plane (Fig. 29–3*A*).

Restricting his landmarks to the lower face, Ricketts (1968) recommended a line drawn from the nasal tip to the soft tissue pogonion (Po^s): the upper and lower lips should fall posteriorly 4 and 2 mm, respectively, from the line (Fig. 29–3*B*).

Burstone (1967) proposed a line from the subnasale (SN) to the soft tissue pogonion (Po^s) because the latter exhibited only half of the variability of the nasal height in his survey of "acceptable" adolescent faces (Fig. 29–3*C*). He contended that the upper and lower lips should extend 3.5 and 2.2 mm, respectively, anterior to this line. His sample also exhibited an interlabial gap of 1.8 mm with the teeth in centric occlusion.

According to Steiner (1959), a line through soft tissue pogonion and the inflection point of the "S" formed by the lower nose and upper lip profile should define the anterior extent of the upper lip (Fig. 29–3*D*).

Holdaway's model is illustrated in Figure 29–3*E*. The nasion–B point intercept forms an angle of 7 to 9 degrees with a tangent to the upper lip and chin. If the angle ANB is enlarged or reduced, the difference is added or subtracted to the "H" angle.

Lip posture is closely related to the position and forward inclination of the maxillary incisor teeth (Jackson, 1962). Changes in vertical intermaxillary distance influence lip posture. The anteroposterior skeletal jaw relationship alters the lip profile; a change in lip posture after correction of a prognathic mandible is an example.

Evaluation of Dental Study Model. Evaluation of dental study models defines abnormalities in arch form, individual tooth position, occlusal planes, and transverse arch width. Preoperative resolution of these problems by orthodontic therapy, as later discussed, facilitates surgical correction, optimizes the intermaxillary fixation, and improves postoperative stability. Dental models not only are helpful in establishing the diagnosis or the degree of deformity but also are used to perform mock surgery. Execution of mock surgical procedures on the study models also permits the clinician to construct an interocclusal acrylic splint for use in fixation. In addition, model surgery provides an opportunity to evaluate the postoperative occlusion

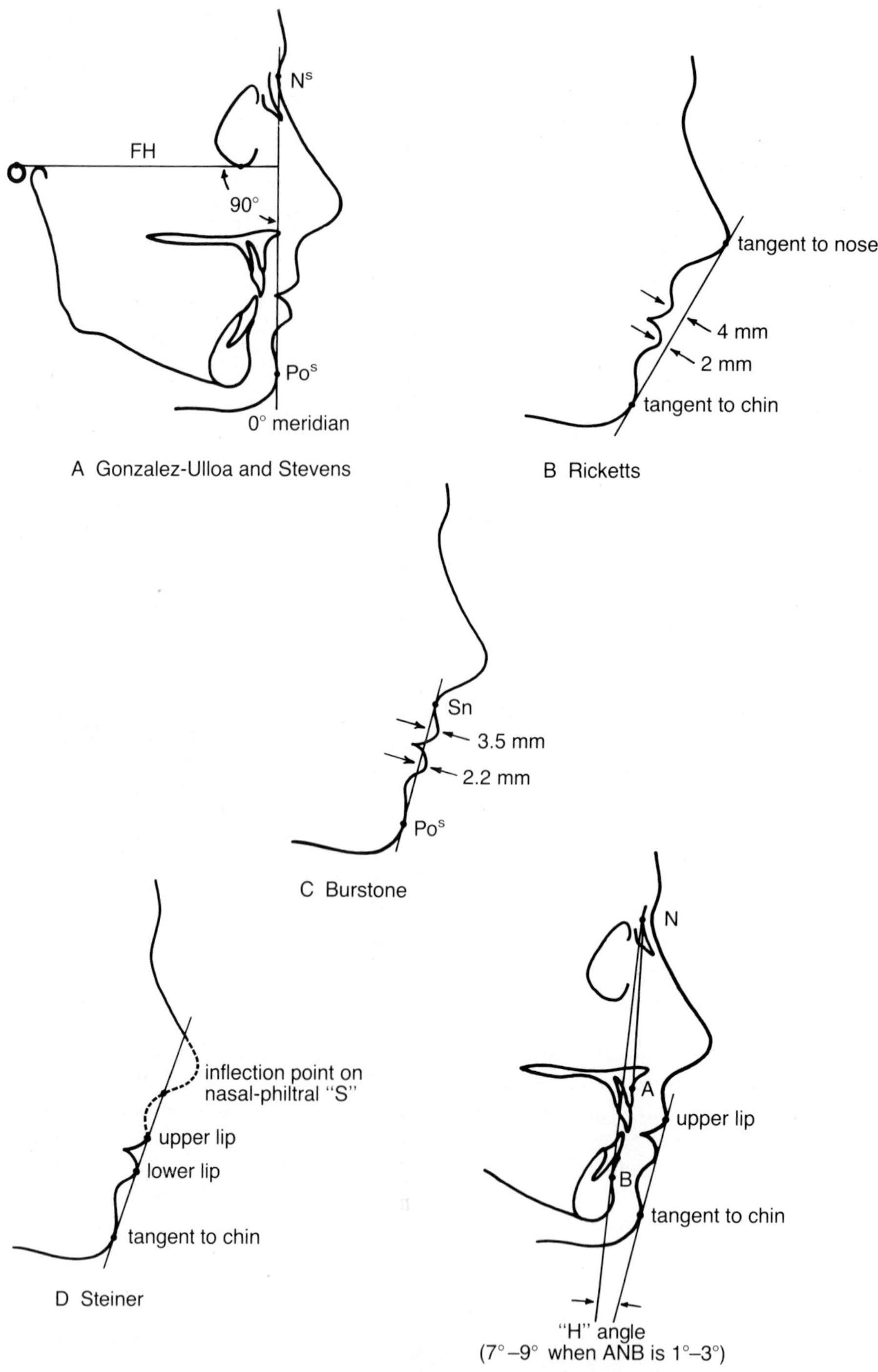

Figure 29–3. Various "ideal" facial planes. (From McCarthy, J. G., and Ruff, G.: The chin. Clin. Plast. Surg., *15*:125, 1988.)

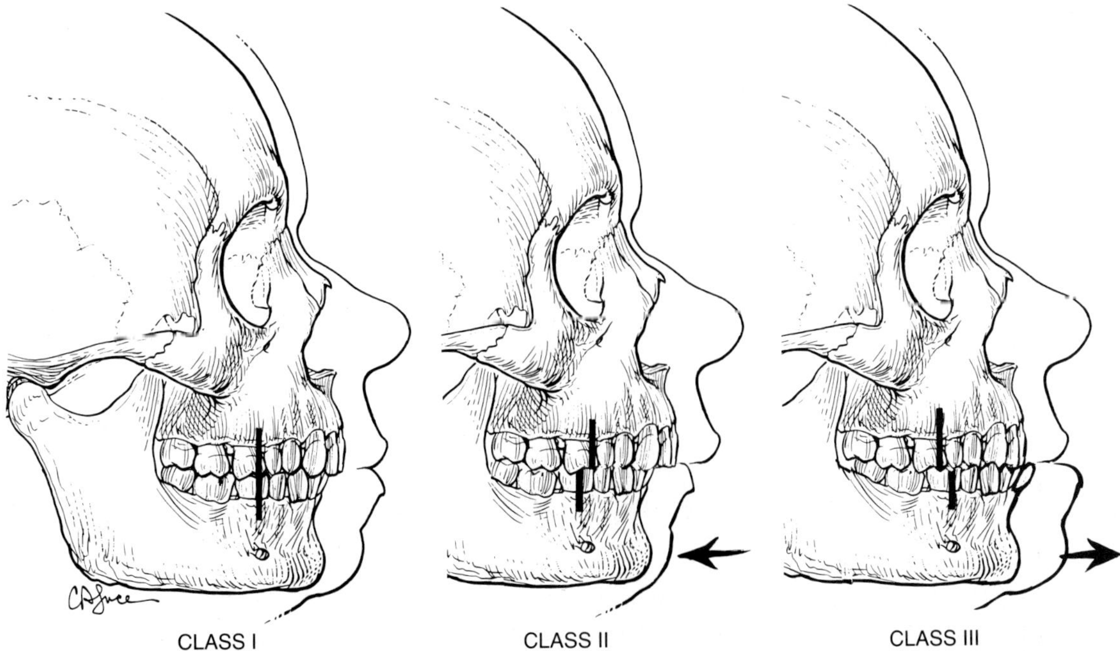

Figure 29–4. Angle's classification of malocclusion. The classification is based on the mesiodistal (anteroposterior) relationships of the maxillary and mandibular first permanent molar teeth. The relationship between the position of the jaws and the facial profile is also illustrated. *Class I (neutroclusion).* The facial profile falls within the normal range. The maxillary and mandibular first molar teeth are in an ideal anteroposterior relation. The mesiobuccal cusp of the maxillary first molar is aligned correctly with the mesiobuccal groove of the mandibular first molar tooth. *Class II (distoclusion).* The mandible is retrognathic and the lower face appears to be recessed. The mandibular first molar occupies a more posterior (distal) position than normal. *Class III (mesioclusion).* Dental occlusion found in mandibular prognathism. The mesiobuccal groove of the mandibular first molar is mesial (anterior) to the mesiobuccal cusp of the maxillary first molar.

anticipated from performing the surgical treatment plan.

Dentoalveolar Complex. Poor dentoalveolar relationship is a major cause of facial imbalance. The parts of the lower face most frequently affected by the position of the dentoalveolar structures are the upper and lower lips and the lower portion of the nose; these areas are bounded laterally by the nasolabial folds and below by the chin (Case, 1921).

The interdigitation of the cusps of the upper and lower teeth establishes what is known as the occlusal relationship, often referred to as the dental occlusion. The mandibular dental arch is normally posterior to and smaller than the maxillary arch. The buccal or lateral cusps of the upper teeth project laterally from the buccal cusps of the lower teeth. The upper incisor teeth and canines (cuspids) overlap the corresponding lower teeth anteriorly. The midsagittal line passes between the central incisors. The mesiobuccal cusp of the maxillary first molar is aligned axially with the mesiobuccal groove of the mandibular first molar. When these relationships are disturbed, a malocclusion is produced.

Classification of Malocclusion. Angle's (1899) classification of malocclusion is widely accepted in the United States. It is based on the *mesiodistal* (anteroposterior) relationship of the maxillary and mandibular first permanent molars (Fig. 29–4).

Class I (Neutroclusion). The mesiobuccal cusp of the maxillary first molar is aligned axially with the mesiobuccal groove of the mandibular first molar. However, irregularities of the anterior teeth may be present because a discrepancy between tooth size and arch length can cause a crowding and malocclusion of the anterior teeth.

Class II (Distoclusion). The buccal groove of the lower first molar is distal (posterior) to the mesiobuccal cusp of the upper first molar.

DIVISION 1. In addition to the distoclusion of the posterior teeth, the upper arch is narrow and the incisors protrude in a labial direction.

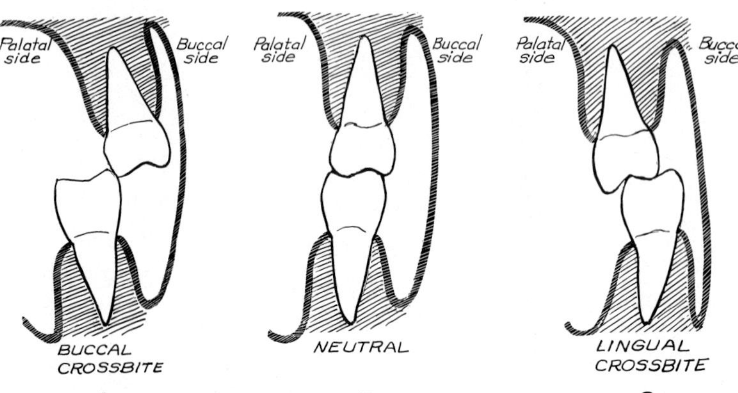

Figure 29–5. Buccolingual relationships of the teeth. *A,* Buccal version. Malocclusion is due to the tilting of the maxillary tooth toward the cheek. *B,* Neutral (centric) occlusion. Ideal relationship in which the buccal cusp of the upper tooth overlaps that of the lower tooth. *C,* Crossbite malocclusion caused by the lingual displacement of the upper teeth in relation to the lower teeth. Note that the buccal cusp of the upper tooth no longer overlaps that of the lower tooth.

DIVISION 2. The posterior teeth are in distoclusion. The upper incisors are inclined in a lingual direction and are also crowded.

Class III (Mesioclusion). The buccal groove of the lower first molar is mesial (anterior) to the mesiobuccal cusp of the upper first molar. The mandibular teeth are in an anterior relationship to the corresponding maxillary teeth.

The original Angle classification describes dental malocclusion between the mandibular and maxillary teeth. These anteroposterior *dentoalveolar* malocclusions are often reflected in the facial profile. A patient with a Class I occlusion generally has a satisfactory facial profile; a patient with a Class II, Division 1 malocclusion may have the typical "bird-face" profile; and a patient with a Class III malocclusion appears to have a protruding lower jaw. However, these correlations do not always exist, and not all types of malocclusion affect the facial profile. For this reason, the Angle classification is inadequate to appraise dentofacial balance; it is also misapplied to describe malocclusion caused by *skeletal* jaw deformities.

There can also be abnormalities in the buccolingual relationships of the teeth (Fig. 29–5) as well as the incisal edges (Fig. 29–6).

Skeletal Relations of Maxilla and Mandible (Cephalometric Analysis). The dentoalveolar structures are supported by the skeletal (or basilar) portion of the jaws. Changes in skeletal relationships have direct bearing on the dentoalveolar complex. Skeletal relationships are best studied with the aid of the cephalometric roentgenogram.

By means of cephalometric roentgenography, a simultaneous record of the *dental, skeletal,* and *soft tissue* components of the face is obtained, as well as a proper evaluation of the relationship of these elements. With this technique, the patient, the film, and the x-ray tube are positioned accurately in a fixed relationship within the cephalometric apparatus. Numerous efforts have been made to correlate certain dental and skeletal relationships seen on the cephalometric roentgenogram with the characteristics of a well-balanced face (Tweed, 1946; Downs, 1948; Steiner, 1953). Considerable variability is apparent even among individuals specifically selected for study because of satisfactory facial balance (Riedel, 1957; Burstone, 1958; Peck and Peck, 1970).

The use of cephalometric roentgenography was first proposed by Converse and Shapiro (1954) as an aid in the diagnosis and planning of surgical-orthodontic treatment of facial malformation.

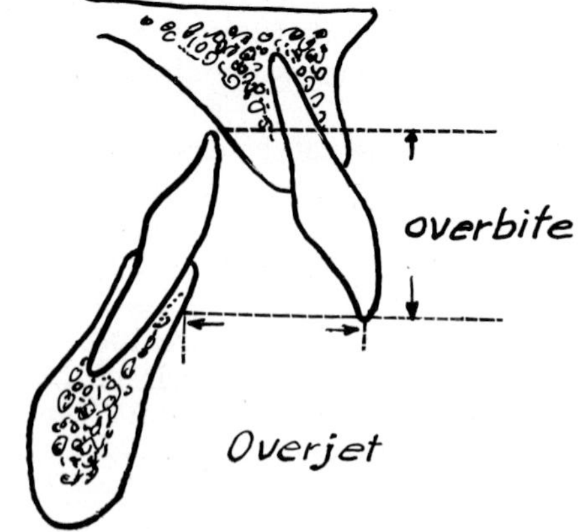

Figure 29–6. Relationship of the incisal edges. Overbite is the vertical overlap of the biting edges. Overjet refers to the labiolingual relationship of the incisal edges.

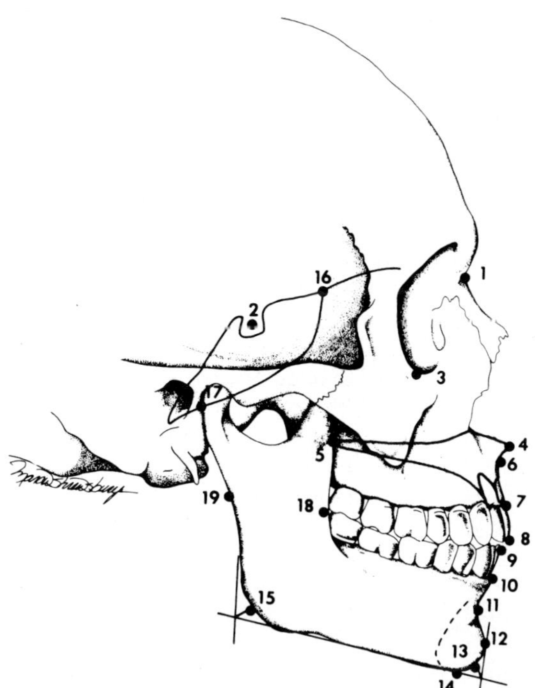

Figure 29–7. Key cephalometric landmarks. *1.* Nasion; *2.* sella; *3.* orbitale; *4.* anterior nasal spine; *5.* posterior nasal spine; *6.* point A; *7.* supradentale; *8.* upper incisal edge; *9.* lower incisal edge; *10.* infradentale; *11.* point B; *12.* pogonion; *13.* gnathion; *14.* menton; *15.* gonion; *16.* sphenoidal-ethmoid intersect; *17.* articulare; *18.* anterior border of mandible; *19.* posterior border of mandible. (Modified from Zide, B., Grayson, B., and McCarthy, J. G.: Cephalometric analysis: Parts I, II, and III. Plast. Reconstr. Surg., *68*:816, 1981.)

The Cephalostat. The cephalostat holds the head in a fixed and reproducible position. Stabilization is achieved by a pair of ear rods that enter the external auditory meatus and minimize changes in head position. A third point of fixation is achieved with a rod that rests passively on the soft tissue covering the inferior orbital rim or nasofrontal suture. The stabilization prevents head rotation along the sagittal plane. During the film exposure, the teeth must be in occlusion with the lips in repose. The x-ray cassette is held at a constant distance from the midline of the cephalostat and head. For purposes of longitudinal study, it is necessary to standardize distortion of the x-ray image by fixing the subject-to-film distance and the x-ray source-to-subject distance.

Cephalometric Tracings. By tracing the cephalogram on acetate film, one may objectively identify skeletal and soft tissue landmarks that are helpful in evaluating bone and soft tissue morphology and in planning the surgical correction. The clinician should be familiar with these landmarks and structures. Figure 29–7 outlines the specific landmarks that are commonly used.

Craniofacial anatomy should be radiographically assessed in the vertical and horizontal dimensions and compared with normative data, controlling for age and sex. The cephalometric analysis is divided into four parts: (1) vertical facial measurements, (2) horizontal midface measurements, (3) horizontal lower face measurements, and (4) dental measurements.

This segmental approach allows the clinician to view and evaluate each component alone and interrelate the various components to one another and to the entire craniofacial complex.

Vertical Facial Measurements. The following measurements are helpful in evaluating the face in the vertical dimension (Fig. 29–8):

1. N-Me (anterior total face height or TFH), which can be subdivided into

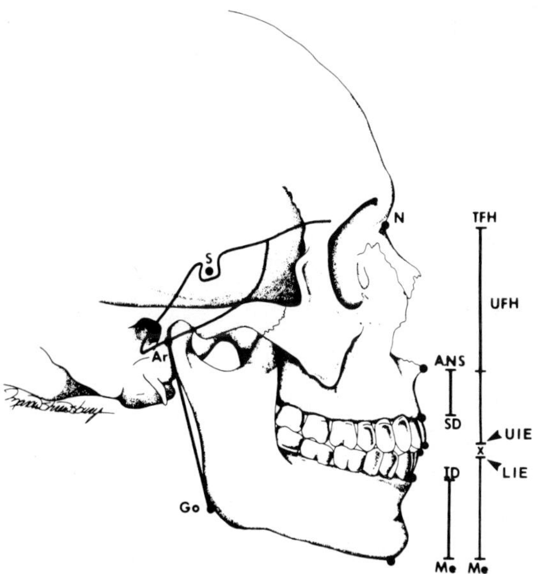

Figure 29–8. Vertical facial measurements. Total face height (Me-N) may be divided into upper face height (N-ANS) and lower face height (ANS-Me). Lower face height consists of five components: ANS-SD, ANS-UIE (upper incisal edge), interincisal gap (x), Me-LIE (lower incisal edge), and Me-ID. Posterior lower face height is defined as Ar-Go. (Modified from Zide, B., Grayson, B., and McCarthy, J. G.: Cephalometric analysis: Parts I, II, and III. Plast. Reconstr. Surg., *68*:816, 1981.)

a. N-ANS (anterior upper face height or UFH).
b. ANS-Me (anterior lower face height or LFH).

2. The ANS-Me measurement can be subdivided into
   a. ANS-SD (subpiriform maxilla), increased in vertical maxillary excess (long face syndrome) and reduced in short face syndrome and following dental extraction and alveolar remodeling.
   b. ANS-UIE (subpiriform maxilla plus height of upper incisal crown), which changes with dental extraction, abrasive incisal wear, and inclination of incisors.
   c. Me-LIE (height of anterior mandible).
   d. Me-ID (height of anterior mandible, exclusive of teeth), often increased in mandibular deficiency syndromes (dentoalveolar overbite) and reduced after extractions and resultant alveolar crest remodeling.
   e. Interincisal relationships.
3. Ar-Go (posterior lower face height).
4. SN-MP (angular relationship between inferior border of mandible and anterior cranial base (Fig. 29–9), often increased in skeletal open bite, micrognathia, and long face syndrome and frequently reduced in mandibular prognathism and short face syndrome.
5. Ar-Go-Me (angular relationship of mandibular ramus and body) or gonial angle.

Horizontal Midface Measurements. The following measurements are employed to evaluate the midface in a horizontal plane (Fig. 29–10):

1. SN (length of anterior cranial base). Ba-SN is the cranial base angle.
2. SNO (angular measurement defined by sella-nasion and nasion-orbitale lines), reduced in upper midface deficiency states. All angular measurements relating to the cranial base are affected by abnormalities of the latter.
3. O ⊥ NA (perpendicular distance from orbitale to facial plane line NA).
4. SNA (angular measurement defined by sella-nasion and nasion-A lines), generally increased in maxillary hyperplasia and reduced in maxillary hypoplasia.
5. ANS-PNS (anteroposterior depth of maxilla at palatal plane), increased in max-

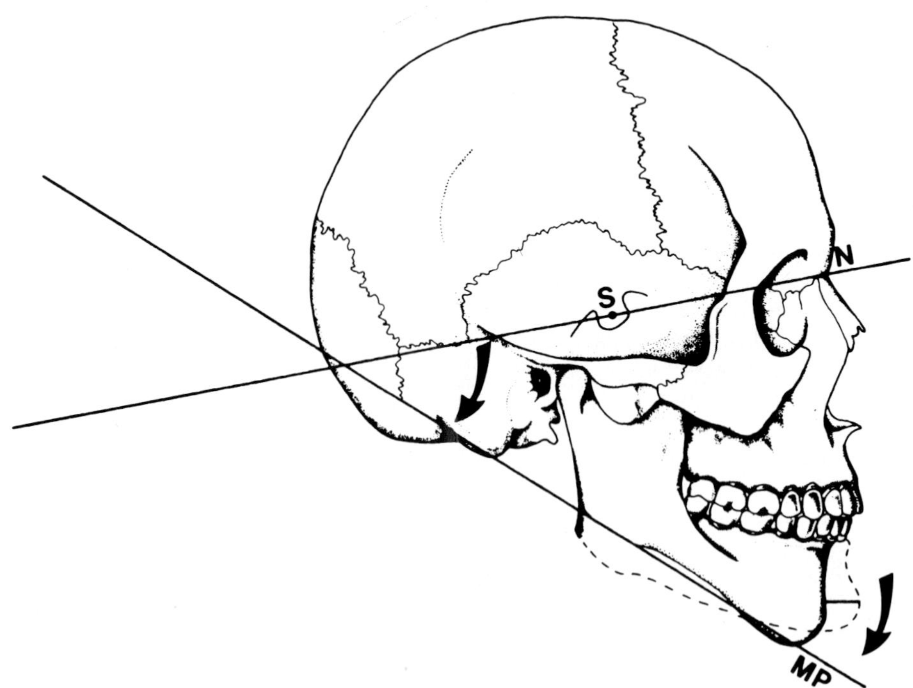

Figure 29–9. Mandibular plane angle. As the mandible rotates clockwise, the angle becomes higher as in cases of micrognathia. In low angle cases *(broken line),* the mandible often appears protrusive. (Modified from Zide, B., Grayson, B., and McCarthy. J. G.: Cephalometric analysis: Parts I, II, and III. Plast. Reconstr. Surg. *68*:816, 1981.)

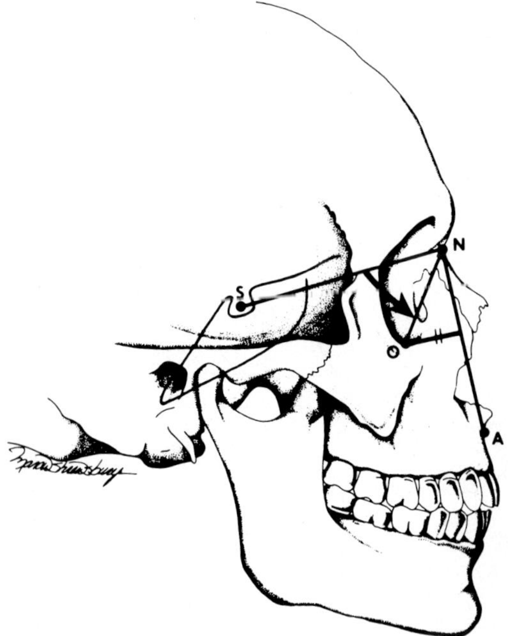

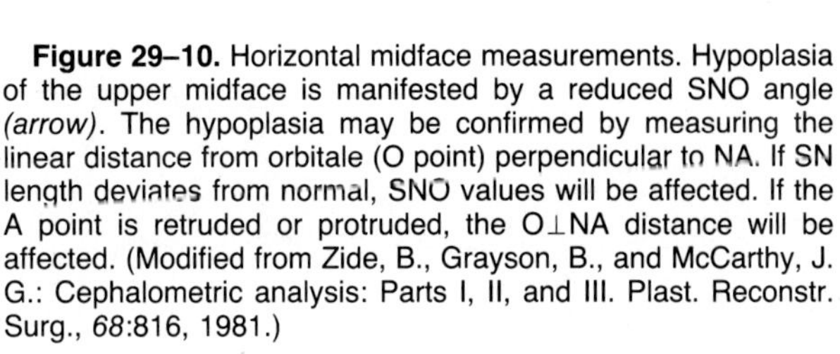

Figure 29–10. Horizontal midface measurements. Hypoplasia of the upper midface is manifested by a reduced SNO angle *(arrow)*. The hypoplasia may be confirmed by measuring the linear distance from orbitale (O point) perpendicular to NA. If SN length deviates from normal, SNO values will be affected. If the A point is retruded or protruded, the O⊥NA distance will be affected. (Modified from Zide, B., Grayson, B., and McCarthy, J. G.: Cephalometric analysis: Parts I, II, and III. Plast. Reconstr. Surg., *68*:816, 1981.)

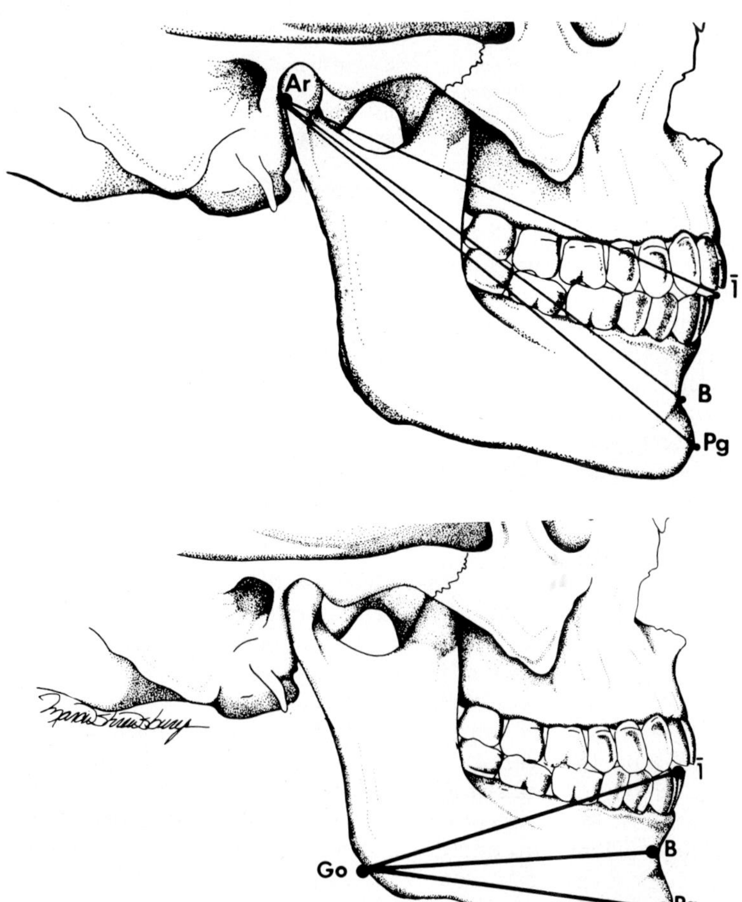

Figure 29–11. Horizontal lower face measurements. Measurements from AR to anterior points define the overall oblique length of the mandible, including the ramus. Measurements from Go to anterior points define the horizontal length of the body of the mandible. (Modified from Zide, B., Grayson, B., and McCarthy, J. G.: Cephalometric analysis. Parts I, II, and III. Plast. Reconstr. Surg. *68*:816, 1981.)

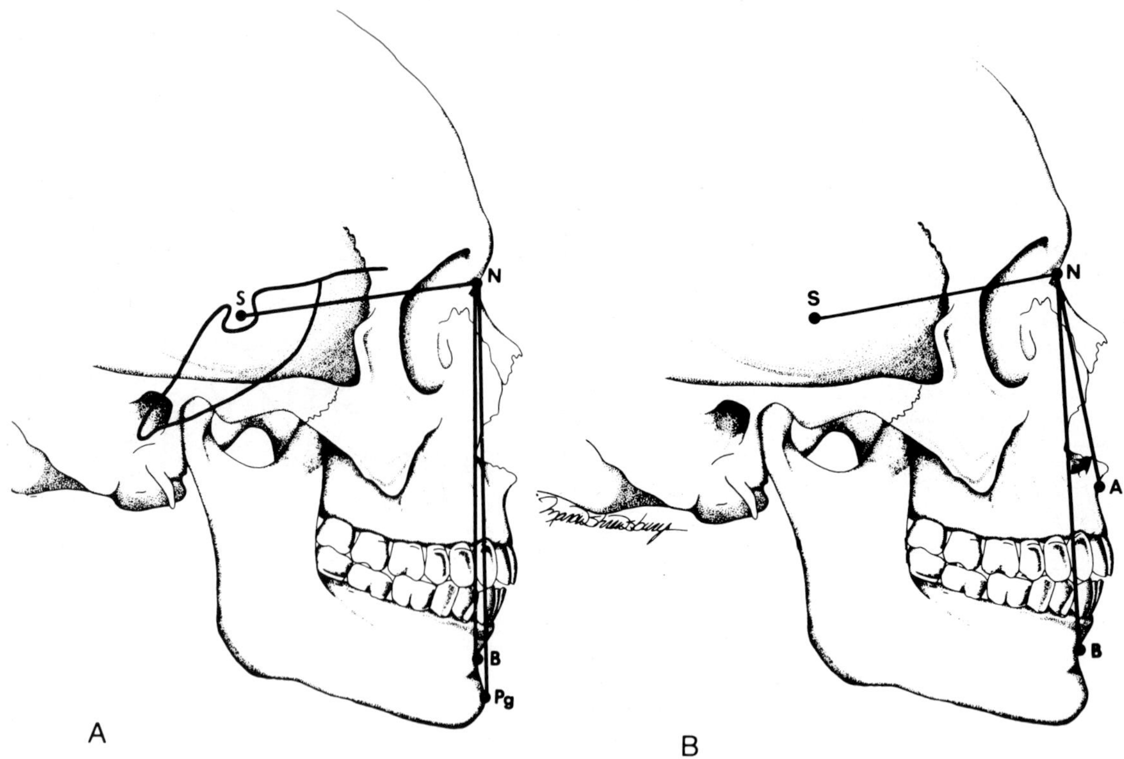

Figure 29–12. Horizontal lower face measurements. *A,* SNB defines the position of the mandible relative to the anterior cranial base. SN-Pg describes bony development at the symphysis and assists in determining the requirement for surgery at the symphysis. *B,* The anteroposterior position of the mandible relative to the maxilla is described by the ANB angle. (Modified from Zide, B., Grayson, B., and McCarthy, J. G.: Cephalometric analysis: Parts I, II, and III. Plast. Reconstr. Surg., *68*:816, 1981.)

illary hyperplasia and reduced in maxillary hypoplasia.

Horizontal Lower Face Measurements. The following values are important in the clinical assessment of the lower face in the horizontal plane (Figs. 29–11 and 29–12):

1. a. Ar-Pg
   b. Ar-B
   c. Ar-LIE ($\overline{1}$)
   } Oblique mandibular measurements from articulare at three planes.
2. a. Go-Pg
   b. Go-B
   c. Go-LIE ($\overline{1}$)
   } Linear measurements from gonion describing mandibular body length at three levels.
3. a. SNB (angular relationship of point B to anterior cranial base, increased in mandibular protrusion and reduced in mandibular micrognathia.
   b. SNPg (angular relationship of pogonion to anterior cranial base), increased in macrogenia and reduced in microgenia.
4. ANB (angular relationship of points A, N, and B), increased in maxillary protrusion or mandibular retrusion and decreased in maxillary retrusion or mandibular protrusion.

Dental Measurements. These values are helpful in determining dental stability and orthodontic management.

1. $\underline{1}$-SN, inclination of maxillary incisor with respect to anterior cranial base (SN).
2. $\overline{1}$-MP, angle of lower incisor with respect to inferior border of mandible.
3. $\overline{1}$ to $\underline{1}$, angular relationships of maxillary and mandibular incisors to one another.

CEPHALOMETRIC CONTROL DATA

Individual patient data should be compared with considerable caution to the data of a well-selected control population. One should control for race, sex, age, and overall scale or size of the craniofacial complex. An example of control data is that derived from the University of Michigan Growth Study, published as *An Atlas of Craniofacial Growth* by Riolo and associates (1974). The data were scaled up and down from normal in increments of 5 per cent (Table 29–1). This permits controlling for the proportions or scale of the patient independent of size. The data are available

Table 29–1. Control Cephalometric Data Sheet, Institute of Reconstructive Plastic Surgery New York University Medical Center (see Riolo and associates, 1974)

Name of Patient ______________________ Date of Cephalogram ______________

#	**Age: 16** Variable	Mea.	−20%	−15%	−10%	−5%	** Sex: Female ** Norm	+5%	+10%	+15%	+20%
0	*Height (cm)*	____	130.4	138.6	146.7	154.9	163.0	171.2	179.3	187.5	195.6
	Midface Height										
130	ANS-N (mm)	____	44.6	47.3	50.1	52.9	55.7	58.5	61.3	64.1	66.8
162	SE-PNS (mm)	____	40.9	43.4	46.0	48.5	51.1	53.7	56.2	58.8	61.3
132	ANS-SD (mm)	____	14.5	15.4	16.3	17.2	18.1	19.0	19.9	20.8	21.7
9	SN-ANS-PNS (deg)	____					8.0				
	Total Face Height										
160	Me-N (mm)	____	98.6	104.7	110.9	117.0	123.2	129.4	135.5	141.7	147.8
158	Me-ANS (mm)	____	55.4	58.9	62.4	65.8	69.3	72.8	76.2	79.7	83.2
131	ANS-UIE (mm)	____	24.1	25.6	27.1	28.6	30.1	31.6	33.1	34.6	36.1
104	Me-LIE (mm)	____	33.8	36.0	38.1	40.2	42.3	44.4	46.5	48.6	50.8
103	Me-ID (mm)	____	25.0	26.6	28.2	29.7	31.3	32.9	34.4	36.0	37.6
88	Ar-Go (mm)	____	39.7	42.2	44.6	47.1	49.6	52.1	54.6	57.0	59.5
13	SN/MP (deg)	____					31.2				
98	6 cusp MP (mm)	____	26.1	27.7	29.3	31.0	32.6	34.2	35.9	37.5	39.1
	Dental										
53	⊥SN (deg)	____					103.1				
71	T-MP (deg)	____					92.1				
61	⊥T (deg)	____					133.6				
	Midface Horizontal										
149	S-N (mm)	____	61.5	65.4	69.2	73.1	76.9	80.7	84.6	88.4	92.3
102	SNO (deg)	____	42.8	45.5	48.2	50.8	53.5	56.2	58.9	61.5	64.2
101	O ⊥ NA (mm)	____	13.1	13.9	14.8	15.6	16.4	17.2	18.0	18.9	19.7
116	ANS-PNS (mm)	____	45.6	48.5	51.3	54.2	57.0	59.9	62.7	65.6	68.4
117	PNS-A (mm)	____	41.4	44.0	46.6	49.2	51.8	54.4	57.0	59.6	62.2
119	PNS-UIE (mm)	____	50.2	53.4	56.5	59.7	62.8	65.9	69.1	72.2	75.4
2	SNA (deg)	____					81.8				
	Lower Face Horizontal										
85	Ar-Pg (mm)	____	92.2	97.9	103.7	109.4	115.2	121.0	126.7	132.5	138.2
84	Ar-B (mm)	____	84.5	89.8	95.0	100.3	105.6	110.9	116.2	121.4	126.7
82	Ar-LIE (mm)	____	79.4	84.3	89.3	94.2	99.2	104.2	109.1	114.1	119.0
92	Go-Pg (mm)	____	65.2	69.3	73.4	77.4	81.5	85.6	89.7	93.7	97.8
91	Go-B (mm)	____	61.4	65.2	69.0	72.9	76.7	80.5	84.4	88.2	92.0
89	Go-LIE (mm)	____	64.3	68.3	72.4	76.4	80.4	84.4	88.4	92.5	96.5
95	AB-PB (mm)	____	28.5	30.3	32.0	33.8	35.6	37.4	39.2	40.9	42.7
3	SNB (deg)	____					79.2				
4	ANB (deg)	____					2.6				
5	SN-Pg (deg)	____					80.2				
50	Ar-Gol-Me (deg)	____					122.2				

in this manner for each age and sex from ages 6 through 16 years. The data allow the clinician to study the unique shape differences that characterize a deformity as a separate issue from the size difference when compared with "normal."

Postsurgical skeletal relocation is not necessarily associated with a comparable amount of soft tissue change. Moreover, in the preoperative period one cannot precisely predict the amount of skeletal relapse or regression that may be seen over the long run after a surgical advancement or recession. In the growing child, the effects of natural development on the mobilized skeletal segment cannot be accurately foreseen. There are few studies in the literature that accurately deal with this subject. It is known that mandibular advancement procedures associated with closure of a large anterior open bite result in a high degree of postoperative relapse. Similarly, the higher the level of the osteotomy in the midface advancement (Le Fort III versus Le Fort I), the greater is the degree of relapse.

The effect of maxillary advancement on the size of the nasolabial angle is variable. Dann, Fonseca, and Bell (1976) reported a reduction of 1.2 ± 0.3 degrees per 1 mm advancement of the central incisor after Le Fort I osteotomy (Fig. 29–13). There is also an associated elevation of the nasal tip. However, any discussion of change in the nasolabial angle after maxillary advancement must consider the following: the inclination of the incisors, the preservation or excision of the anterior nasal spine, the height of the osteotomy, and a history of previous lip and palate surgery. The soft tissues of the lip also project less forward than the skeletal advancement. With the Le Fort II and III osteotomies there can be lengthening of the nasal dorsum, particularly when an interposition bone graft is placed at the nasofrontal junction. In the correction of the long face syndrome, in which the maxilla is elevated (Le Fort I), the position of the upper lip relative to the maxillary incisor is affected. If the maxillary alveolus is displaced 1 mm posteriorly, there is an associated 0.5 mm posterior and 0.5 mm inferior repositioning of the upper lip (Fig. 29–14).

Preoperative Orthodontic Therapy

The goal of preoperative orthodontic tooth movement is to change the position of the teeth and the shape of the dental arches in order to obtain a stable and functional occlusal relationship in the operating room. Achieving the optimal anteroposterior (Fig. 29–15*A*) and transverse (Fig. 29–15*B,C*) den-

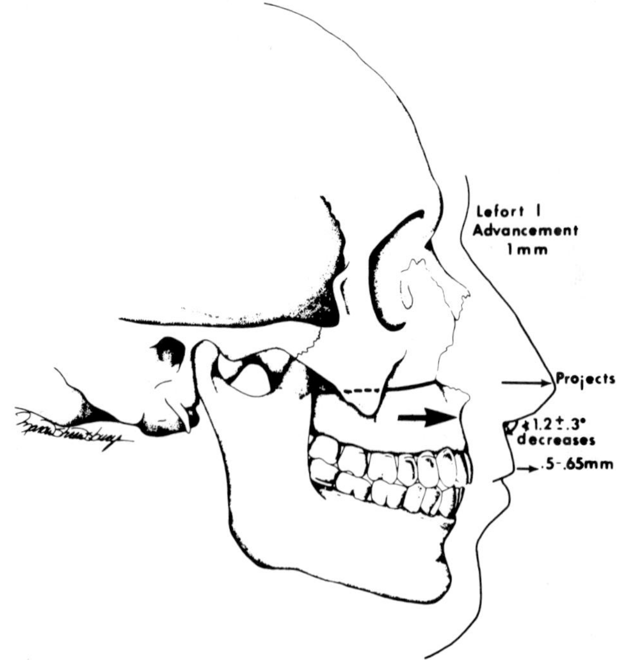

Figure 29–13. The soft tissue of the upper lip moves forward less than the skeletal translocation. The nasolabial angle is reduced and the nasal tip is projected forward. The nasolabial angle change depends to some degree on soft tissue scars and the presence or absence of the anterior nasal spine. (Modified from Zide, B., Grayson, B., and McCarthy, J. G.: Cephalometric analysis: Parts I, II, and III. Plast. Reconstr. Surg., *68*:816, 1981.)

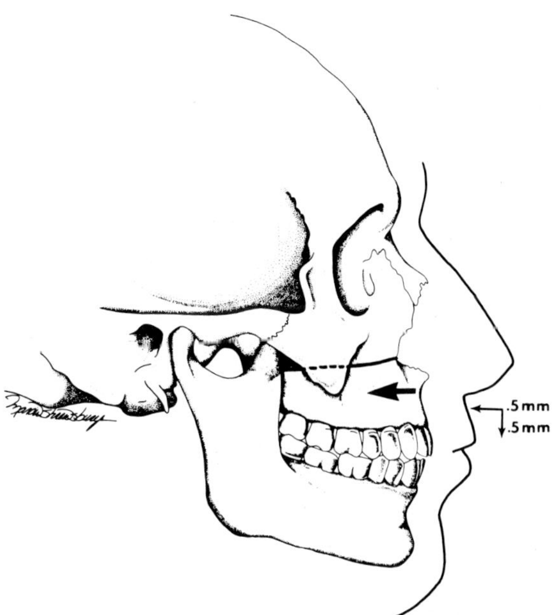

Figure 29–14. The upper lip is repositioned 0.5 mm posteriorly and 0.5 mm inferiorly for each 1.0 mm of maxillary retrodisplacement. The values vary if the maxilla is concomitantly raised or lowered. (Modified from Zide, B., Grayson, B., and McCarthy, J. G.: Cephalometric analysis: Parts I, II, and III. Plast. Reconstr. Surg., *68*:816, 1981.)

tal relationships at the time of the osteotomy contributes to long-term stability of the mobilized skeletal segment.

Some of the more commonly encountered presurgical orthodontic procedures will be discussed.

Coordination of Maxillary and Mandibular Arch Width. The presurgical clinical picture of a patient with Class II skeletal malocclusion is characterized by anterior overjet and maxillary incisor procumbency (Fig. 29–16*A*). Despite the reduced mandibular dimension, a normal buccolingual relationship of the posterior teeth may be observed (Fig. 29–16*B*,*C*).

Surgical advancement of the mandible without previous orthodontic treatment of maxillary arch width corrects the incisal relationships (protrusion and overjet) but disturbs the posterior occlusion (Fig. 29–17). This may be demonstrated by hand-holding the models and advancing the lower cast to mimic the operation. Mandibular advancement without surgical or orthodontic expansion of the maxillary arch would result in a posterior crossbite. Both arches can be described in a somewhat oversimplified manner as being V shaped, with the greatest width posteriorly. As the mandible is advanced, the widest portion of the lower dental arch is brought under the narrower portion of the maxilla (Fig. 29–17*C*), resulting in a severe occlusal instability. If left unattended in this occlusal relationship, the patient may change his mandibular occlusal position (mandibular shift) to improve function. Presurgical orthodontic expansion of the maxilla should be planned to accommodate the wider portion of the advancing mandibular arch (Fig. 29–17*B*).

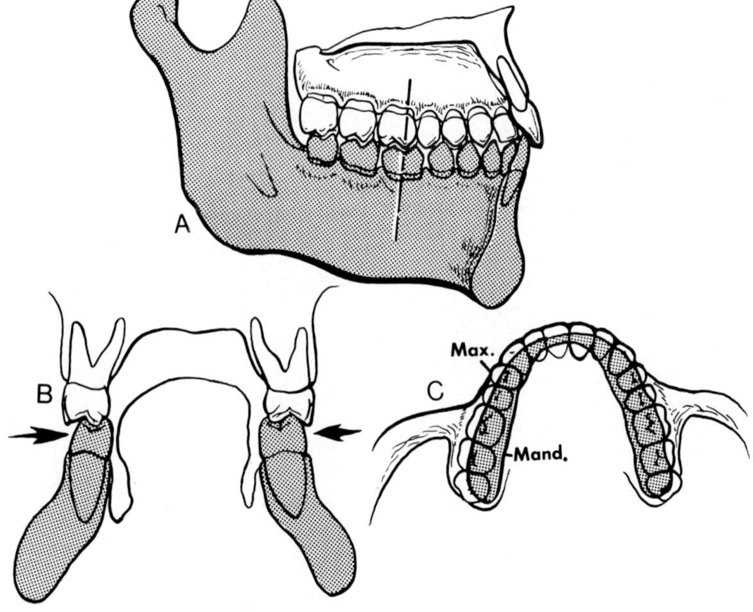

Figure 29–15. *A,* The normal anteroposterior dental relationships showing Class I intercuspation of the molars and cuspids. *B,* Coronal cross section showing normal buccolingual relationship of the posterior teeth. Note that the maxillary teeth are slightly buccal to the mandibular teeth. *C,* The maxillary and mandibular dentoalveolar complex may be described as congruent V-shaped arches. Note that the maxillary arch is slightly wider than the mandibular arch *(stippled area).*

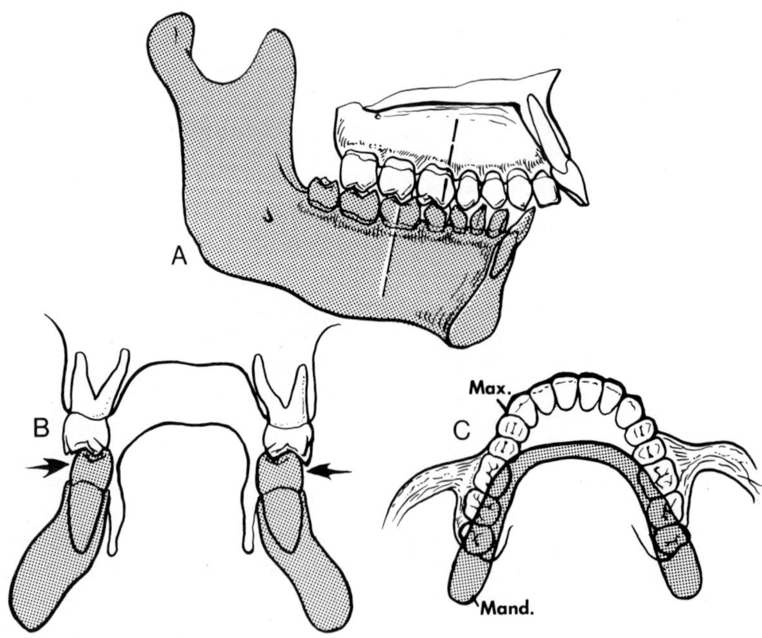

Figure 29–16. *A,* The retropositioned mandibular arch shows Class II intercuspation of the molars and cuspids. *B,* Coronal cross section of the molar region in skeletal Class II malocclusion frequently shows normal transverse arch width (maxillary posterior teeth slightly buccal to mandibular teeth). *C,* The maxillary and mandibular arch form shows the abnormal anteroposterior discrepancy between the incisors but relatively normal transverse relationships of the posterior teeth (maxillary posterior teeth slightly buccal to the lower posterior teeth).

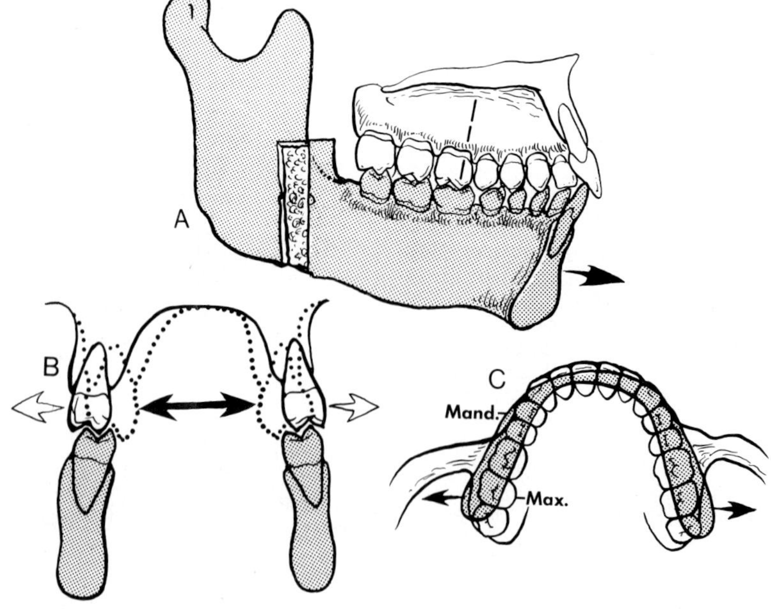

Figure 29–17. *A,* Surgical advancement of the mandible without correction of the width of the maxillary transverse arch may correct the incisal relationships (protrusion and overjet). *B,* The presurgical orthodontic treatment of this case would include expansion of the maxillary dentoalveolar arch *(solid line). C,* Advancement of the mandible to a position under the more narrow anterior portion of the maxillary arch often results in disharmony of the buccolingual relationships of the posterior teeth (mandible *stippled).* Note that mandibular advancement without maxillary expansion in this case results in bilateral posterior crossbites (mandibular teeth occluding buccal to maxillary teeth).

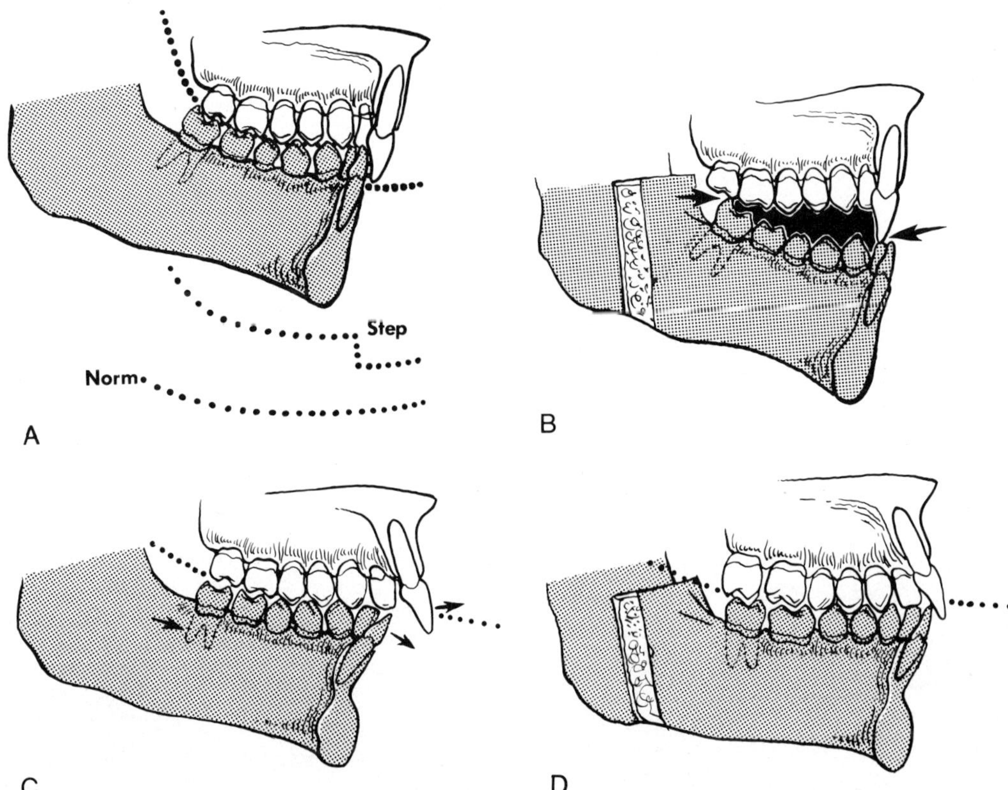

Figure 29–18. *A,* Observe the irregularities in the mean occlusal plane *(dotted line).* The normal occlusal plane is flat anteriorly with a moderate curve upward in the molar region (curve of Spee). *B,* Surgical repositioning of the maxilla or mandible without presurgically achieving leveling of the occlusal planes often results in an unstable occlusion, premature dental contacts, trauma, interocclusal space, mandibular shifts, and crossbites. *C,* Using fixed orthodontic bands and wires, the occlusal planes are leveled in this case by labial tipping of the maxillary and mandibular incisors and uprighting of the molars. *D,* The postsurgical maxillary-mandibular change is achieved and the occlusal planes are compatible, providing for stable dental intercuspation and satisfactory function.

Leveling of Occlusal Plane and Elimination of Occlusal Interferences. The planes described by the occlusal surfaces of opposing dental arches (occlusal plane) can be severely curved and irregular (Fig. 29–18*A*). Surgical reposition of the maxilla or mandible without orthodontic leveling of the occlusal plane (Fig. 29–18*B*) can result in lack of occlusal contact (open bite) or areas of premature contact, causing excessive trauma, dental crossbites, or muscular and temporomandibular joint disturbances.

In the example illustrated, the orthodontist, using fixed orthodontic bands and wires, leveled the occlusal planes by tipping the incisors labially (toward the lips) and repositioning the molars (Fig. 29–18*C*). The postsurgical maxillomandibular change is achieved, and the occlusion is functional and contributory to the stability of the surgical change (Fig. 29–18*D*).

Repositioning Incisors to Improve Prediction of Postsurgical Lip Position. Abnormal incisor position often appears as a compensation to an underlying skeletal deformity. In the case illustrated in Figure 29–19*A*, the maxillary incisors are tipped toward the lips (labially) and the mandibular incisors are tilted toward the tongue (lingually). Presurgical orthodontic correction of these abnormal incisor inclinations affects the position of the lip, the amount of incisor show at rest and on smiling, the nasolabial angle, and the labiomental (mandibular) soft tissue contours.

The amount of skeletal change can most accurately be planned only after the optimal intra-arch position of the incisors is obtained (Fig. 29–19*B*). Achieving correct intra-arch incisor position before surgery results in postsurgical soft tissue lip relationships that are more predictable (Fig. 29–19*C*); failure to

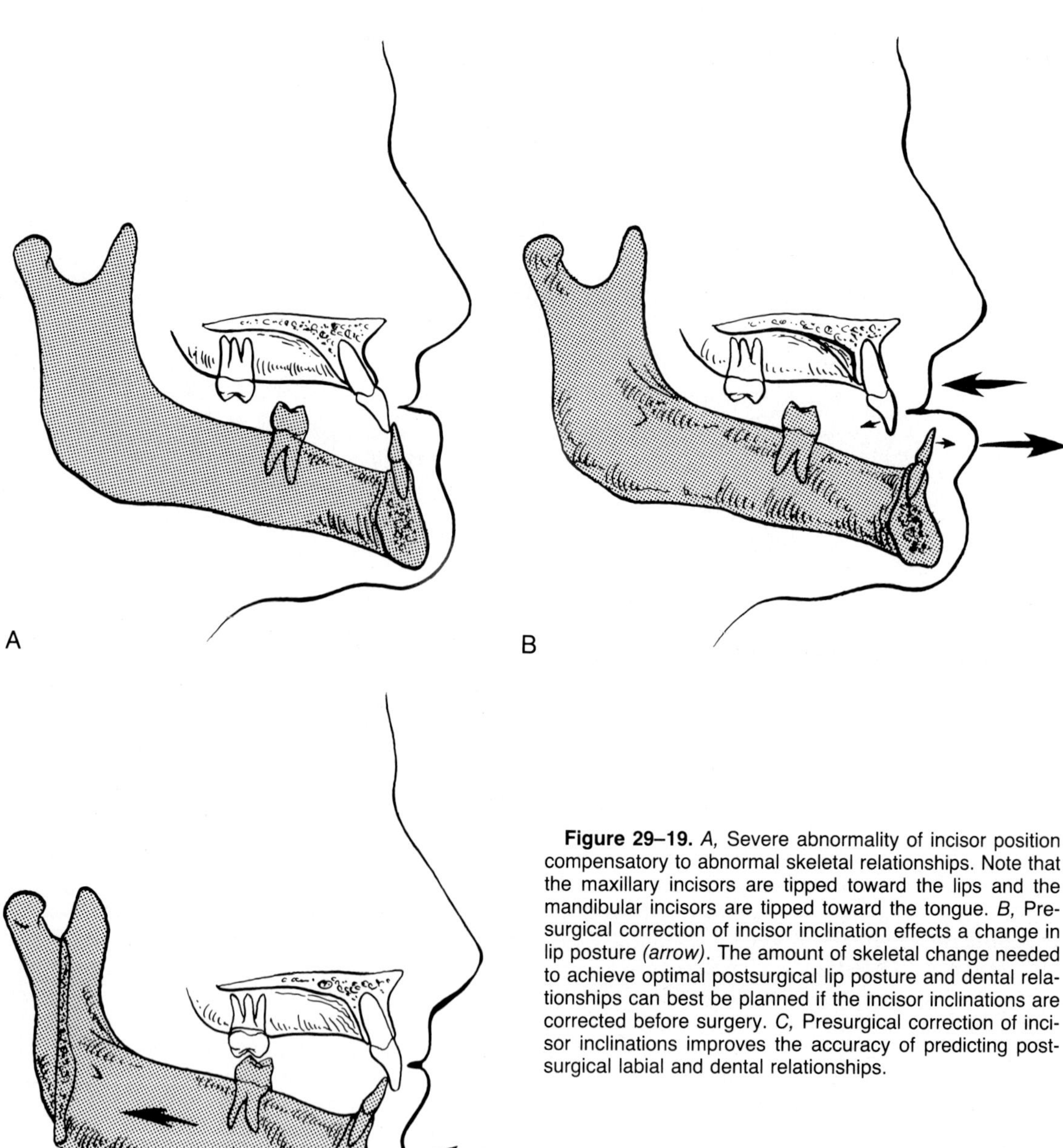

Figure 29–19. *A,* Severe abnormality of incisor position compensatory to abnormal skeletal relationships. Note that the maxillary incisors are tipped toward the lips and the mandibular incisors are tipped toward the tongue. *B,* Presurgical correction of incisor inclination effects a change in lip posture *(arrow)*. The amount of skeletal change needed to achieve optimal postsurgical lip posture and dental relationships can best be planned if the incisor inclinations are corrected before surgery. *C,* Presurgical correction of incisor inclinations improves the accuracy of predicting postsurgical labial and dental relationships.

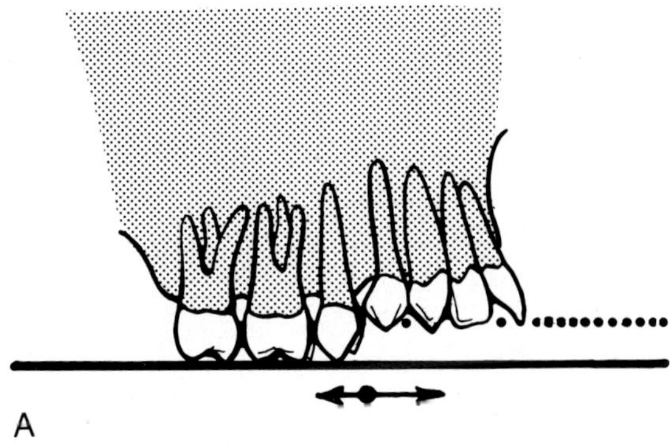

A

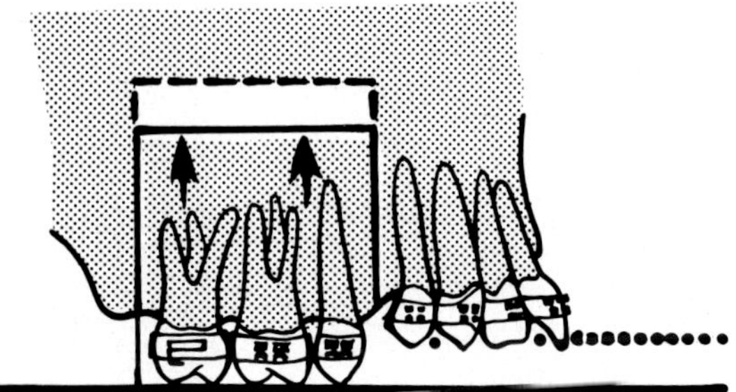

B

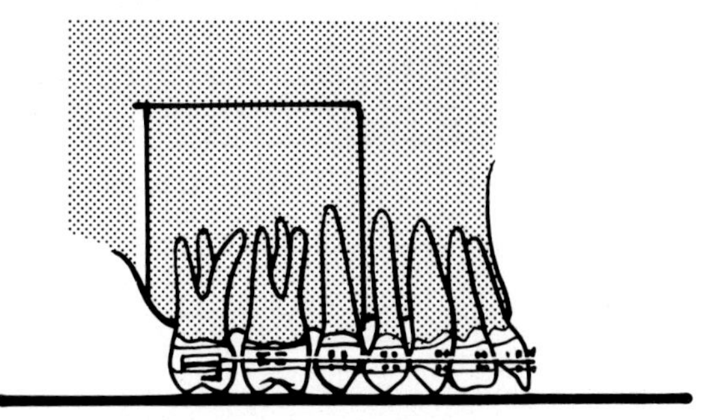

C

Figure 29–20. *A,* Maxillary arch with a marked step in the occlusal planes. Note the absence of the interdental space needed for osteotomy site between the bicuspids. *B,* Note the space produced between the first and second bicuspid by orthodontic movement of the teeth. The segmental osteotomy is performed without the need for tooth extractions. *C,* The posterior segment is repositioned superiorly and the interdental space is closed. The orthodontic appliance also contributes to the postsurgical fixation of the osteotomized segment.

obtain presurgical orthodontic correction of intra-arch incisor position may result in undesirable postsurgical change in lip posture as the teeth are corrected. Moreover, failure to correct an abnormal incisor tipping preoperatively can prevent the possibility of significant segment movement in some cases.

Creating Interdental Space for Segmental Osteotomies. Correction of certain severe malocclusions and maxillomandibular relationships may be achieved by movements of block segments of the dentoalveolar complex. Such procedures require space on the dental arch at the site at which the osteotomy is performed (Fig. 29–20*A*). In lieu of elective extraction of teeth, space may be created by orthodontic tooth movement or root tipping (Fig. 29–20*B*). Repositioning of the segment may thus be accomplished with preservation of valuable dental units and minimizing the possibility of injury to adjacent dental roots (Fig. 29–20*C*).

Preoperative Planning

Before the operation, progress records of the patient are obtained. The evaluation and manipulation of these records are in effect mock surgical procedures attempting to predict the outcome and define the operative plan. Simulated surgical procedures can be performed on

1. Dental study models.
2. Cephalometric tracings.
3. Photographic records.
4. Computed three-dimensional cephalometric and CT images.

Mock Surgery on Dental Study Models and Preparation of Intraoperative Occlusal Splint. A set of dental study models, mounted on an articulator (Fig. 29–21*A*), enables the clinician to plan the surgical correction and construct an acrylic bite registration (splint) of the desired occlusal and skeletal change. The casts are cut and repositioned to mimic the surgical procedure (Fig. 29–21*B*). The bite splint is fabricated directly on the occlusal surfaces of the repositioned casts. The "occlusal index" should be thin, yet of sufficient strength to tolerate stress (Fig. 29–22*A*). After the surgical osteotomies are completed, the maxillary and mandibular teeth are keyed into the occlusal splint, simultaneously establishing the planned change in both dental and skeletal relation-

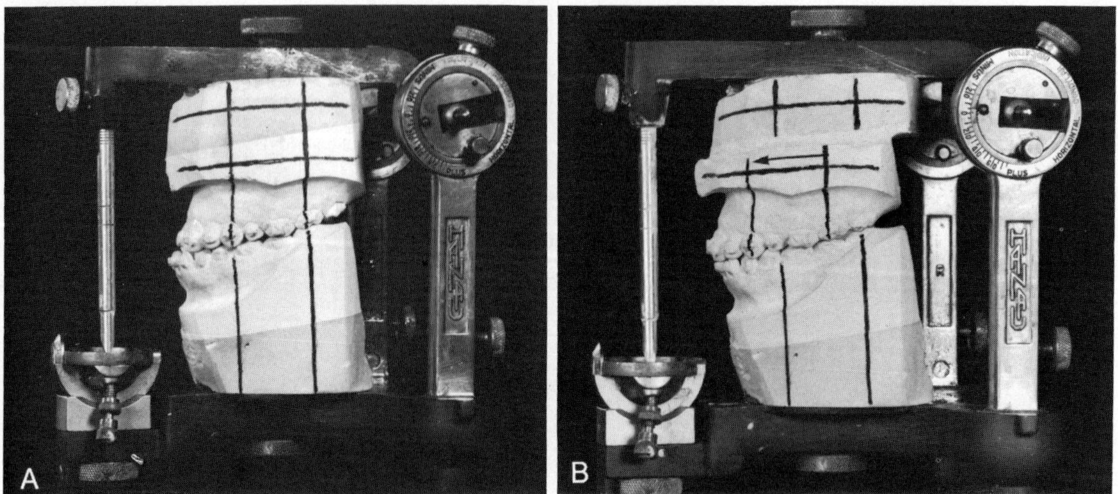

Figure 29–21. *A,* Dental study models mounted on an articulator that simulates the path of mandibular excursions and facilitates presurgical orthodontic planning. *B,* The maxillary cast is cut and advanced into the "ideal" occlusion. Markings drawn on the cast bases may be used to measure the amount of advancement needed to achieve the planned occlusal relationships.

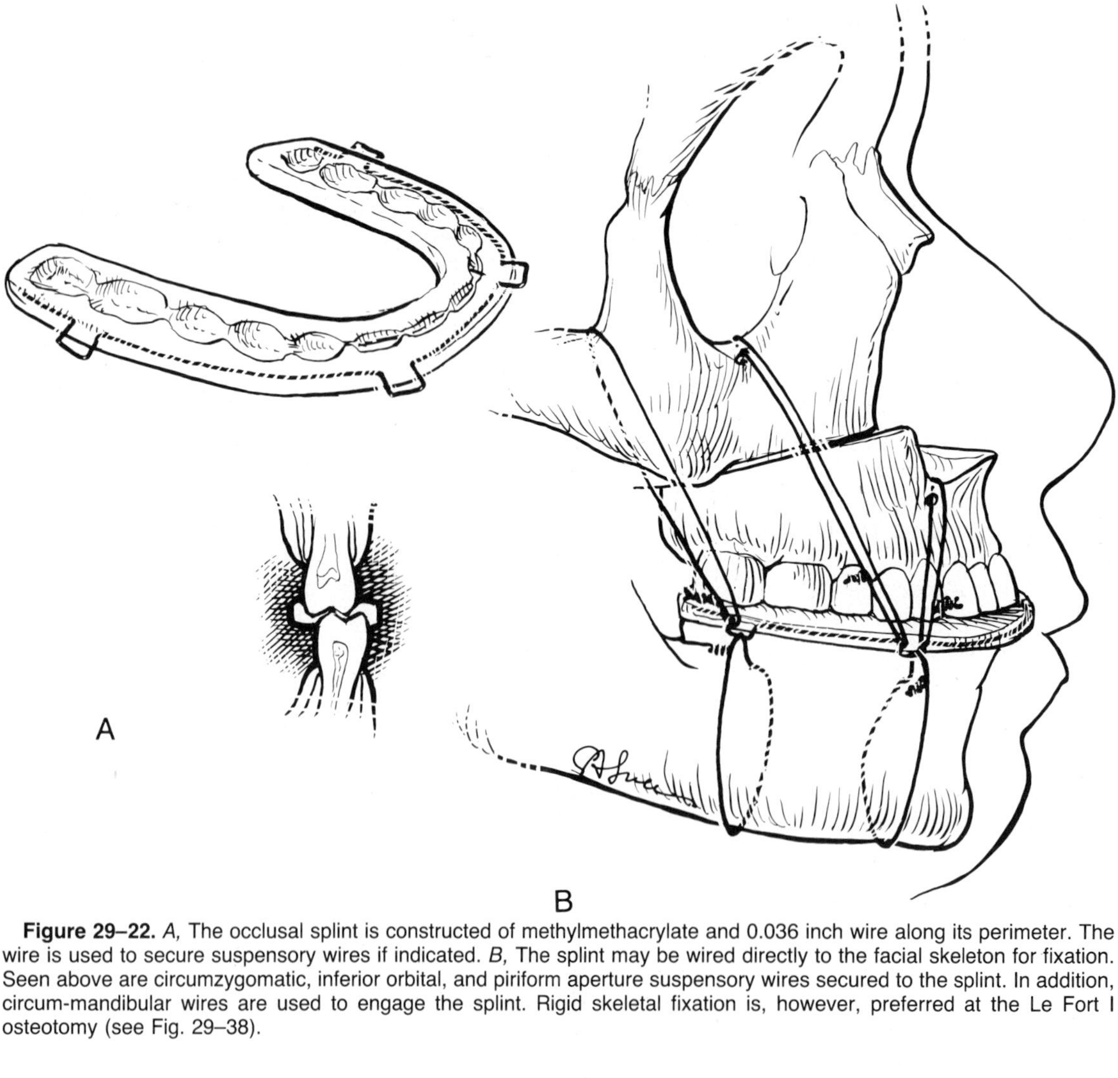

Figure 29–22. *A,* The occlusal splint is constructed of methylmethacrylate and 0.036 inch wire along its perimeter. The wire is used to secure suspensory wires if indicated. *B,* The splint may be wired directly to the facial skeleton for fixation. Seen above are circumzygomatic, inferior orbital, and piriform aperture suspensory wires secured to the splint. In addition, circum-mandibular wires are used to engage the splint. Rigid skeletal fixation is, however, preferred at the Le Fort I osteotomy (see Fig. 29–38).

ships. The custom-made splint also contributes to stabilization during the fixation period. The splint may also serve for attachment of circumzygomatic, infraorbital, zygomaticofrontal, or circum-mandibular suspensory wires (Fig. 29–22*B*). Rigid skeletal fixation is, however, preferred.

An intermediate splint should be employed during two-jaw surgery. In these cases, the study models are mounted on an articulator in proper spatial relation with the hinge "condyle" of the articulator. In order to achieve this, a "face bow" registration must be made. The face bow is a metal frame that is used to relate the position of the maxilla via an occlusion bite impression to the condylar head and infraorbital rims of the patient. The face bow is mounted on the articulator and used to position the dental study models to the hinge of the articulator ("face bow transfer").

The intermediate splint is used to reposition the maxilla in a two-jaw case. The maxilla study model is cut and repositioned on its plaster base. A simulated Le Fort I osteotomy vertically repositioned (more posteriorly than anteriorly to close the open bite and reduce overall vertical dimension) is illustrated in Figure 29–23. The intermediate splint is constructed on this model. It is removed and the mandibular model is cut and repositioned upward and forward to achieve the planned postsurgical occlusion (Fig. 29–23*E*). The model is now used for final splint construction.

Mock Surgery on Cephalometric Tracings. The lateral cephalogram is covered with a transparent sheet of matte acetate on which

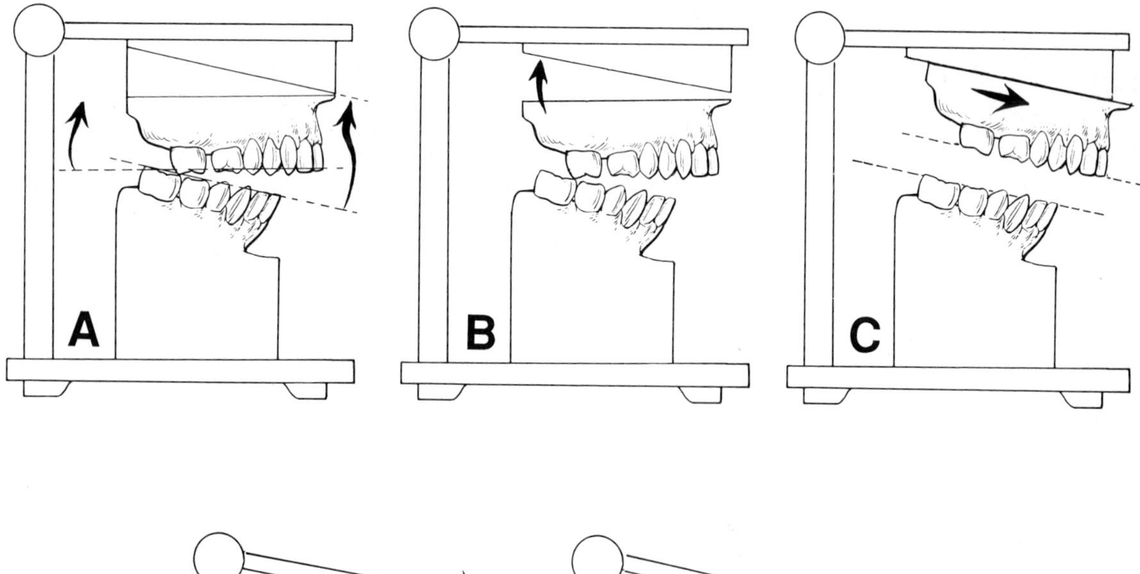

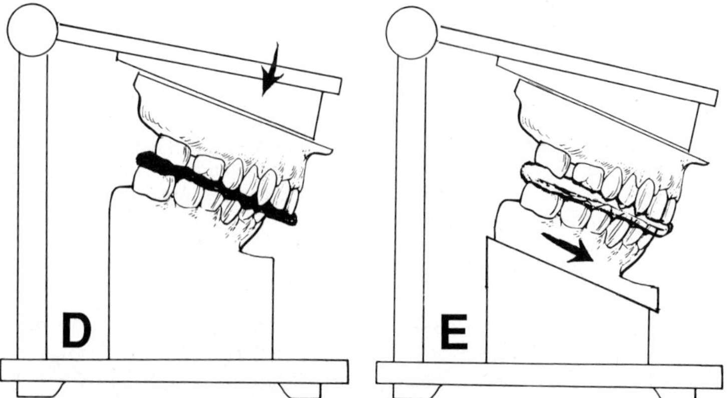

Figure 29–23. *A,* Preoperative occlusion as demonstrated on dental models. *B,* Projected posterior vertical maxillary impaction. Note the mock surgery *(arrow)* on the maxillary model. *C,* Associated advancement *(arrow)* of the maxillary cast. *D, Intermediate* splint constructed on a study model simulating posterior impaction and anterior advancement of the maxilla. *E, Final* or *definitive* splint constructed after advancement *(arrow)* of the mandibular cast.

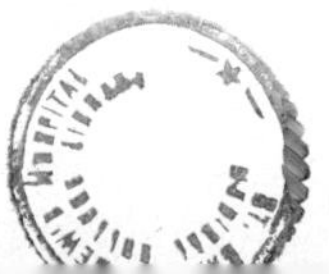

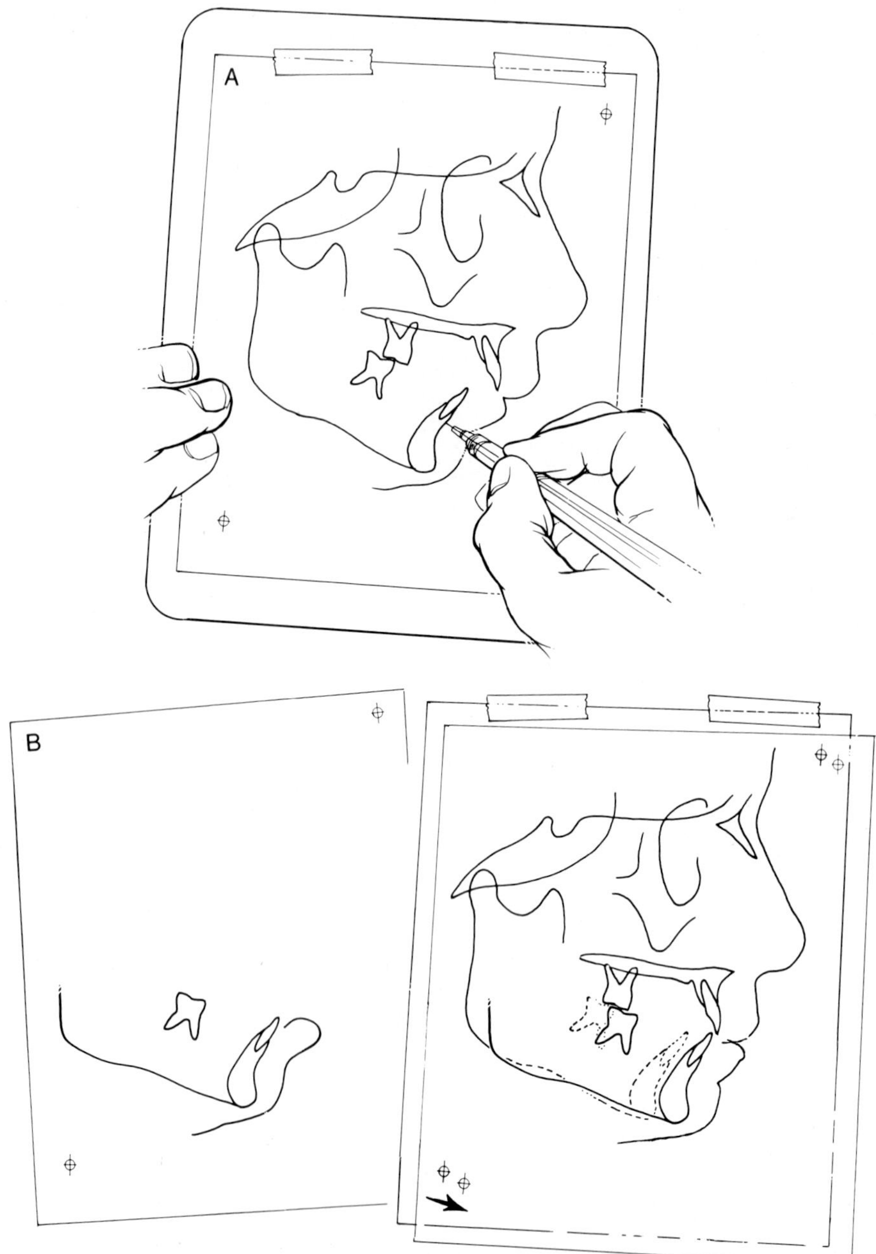

Figure 29–24. Mock surgery on cephalometric tracings. *A,* The relevant cephalometric anatomy and landmarks are traced on matte acetate overlaid on the cephalogram. *B,* Simulation of a mandibular advancement is achieved by marking a separate tracing of the mandible and soft tissue profile. The latter tracing is superimposed and advanced to show the estimated profile and skeletal configuration. It cannot be assumed that there is a 1:1 ratio of soft to hard tissue advancement.

the principal cephalometric anatomy and landmarks are traced (Fig. 29–24*A*). Additional acetate sheets are used to trace the bones and associated soft tissue that will be mobilized by the procedure (Fig. 29–24*B*). Figure 29–24*C* illustrates the composite of preoperative tracing and a tracing of the mandibular body showing advancement, with the resultant profile change. In the same way simulation of the Le Fort I, II, or III and various segmental osteotomies may be evaluated. The clinician utilizing this method must be acutely aware of the surgical and dental limitations surrounding each procedure. The ability to predict the soft tissue changes, as a result of cephalometric mock surgery, depends on an understanding of the ratio of change between bone movement, soft tissue movement, and relapse. Three variables that directly influence the ability to predict this ratio are the surgical technique, the intrinsic quality (quantity, density, presence of surgical scars) of the soft tissue, and the direction and magnitude of the skeletal change.

Mock Surgery on Photographic Records. The lateral photograph is enlarged to life size (Fig. 29–25*A*). This is done by first including in the photograph a ruler held at the midsagittal plane of the face. When the photograph is being printed, a ruler is placed on the enlarging table while the image is adjusted in size so that the projected ruler size is equal to that of the real ruler. The print produced has been enlarged so that the ruler and profile are precisely life size. This image is printed several times for use during mock surgery on the photograph.

A scissor is used to cut the portion of facial anatomy that corresponds to the planned bone surgery. In Figure 29–25*B* the midface, lip, and nose have been cut from the photograph of a young adult female with the long face syndrome. The mandible, lower lip, and chin have been cut to show the soft tissue change resulting from genioplasty and autorotation of the mandible, secondary to vertical maxillary impaction (Fig. 29–25*B*). Note the elevation of the nasal tip, closing of the nasolabial angle, lip competence, and anterior projection of the chin that is seen in the "paste-up" of mock surgery. A tracing of the profile in the original photo superimposed on the mock surgical photo allows the clinician to measure the amount of actual direction and magnitude of skeletal change needed (Fig. 29–25*C*). As in mock surgery on the cephalogram, the variables affecting the accuracy of this predictive activity are surgical technique, quality of the soft tissue, and the direction and magnitude of bone change.

Three-dimensional Computer-aided Planning. In addition to providing more detailed imaging of the craniofacial skeleton, computer graphics (Marsh and Vannier, 1983; Merz, 1983) offers the promise of planning craniofacial surgical procedures in three dimensions. Orthognathic surgery has traditionally been planned with a combination of cephalograms, photos, dental models, and data from the clinical examination (Zide, Grayson, and McCarthy, 1981a,b, 1982). This process requires considerable experience and is accurate for bilaterally symmetric deformities. True three-dimensional deformities, such as unilateral craniofacial microsomia, are not best approached by two-dimensional cephalometric modalities. Two-dimensional cephalometric data, however, may be used to create a three-dimensional data structure. By means of computer graphic techniques, a three-dimensional surgical simulation program is possible.

Computer-aided Surgical Planning with Three-dimensional Cephalometrics. Three-dimensional cephalometric landmark points are obtained by correlating corresponding points on posteroanterior (PA) and lateral cephalograms, as shown in Figure 29–26. Three numbers are required to specify a point in space (i.e., height, width, and depth measurements). The width component is determined primarily by the PA film, whereas the depth component can be determined from either view. Any point on a cephalometric film has a three-dimensional position in space when one remembers the precise way in which a cephalogram is taken (Broadbent, Broadbent, and Golden, 1975). The three-dimensional line from the PA cephalogram intersects the three-dimensional line from the lateral cephalogram at the location of the anatomic landmark in question (Grayson and associates, 1988). In this way the correlation of points between the PA and lateral cephalogram yields a distortion-free, three-dimensional data set for each patient. A similar process was carried out on the standard tracings of Bolton (Broadbent, Broadbent, and Golden, 1975) to create a numerical model of "normal." The data are imaged by connecting lines (Figs. 29–27, 29–28, and 29–29) or triangular tiles (Figure 29–27) between data points using standard computer graphic methods (Rogers and Adams, 1976; Foley and Van Dam, 1982).

Computer software allows the user to perform interactively a surgical simulation on the three-dimensional data structure. For each mobile osteotomy fragment, the user must specify rotational movements, i.e., one rotation about each of the x, y, and z axes and three positional movements (i.e., x, y, and z translations) to change the absolute location of the segment in three dimensions (Fig. 29–28). In this way the user has com-

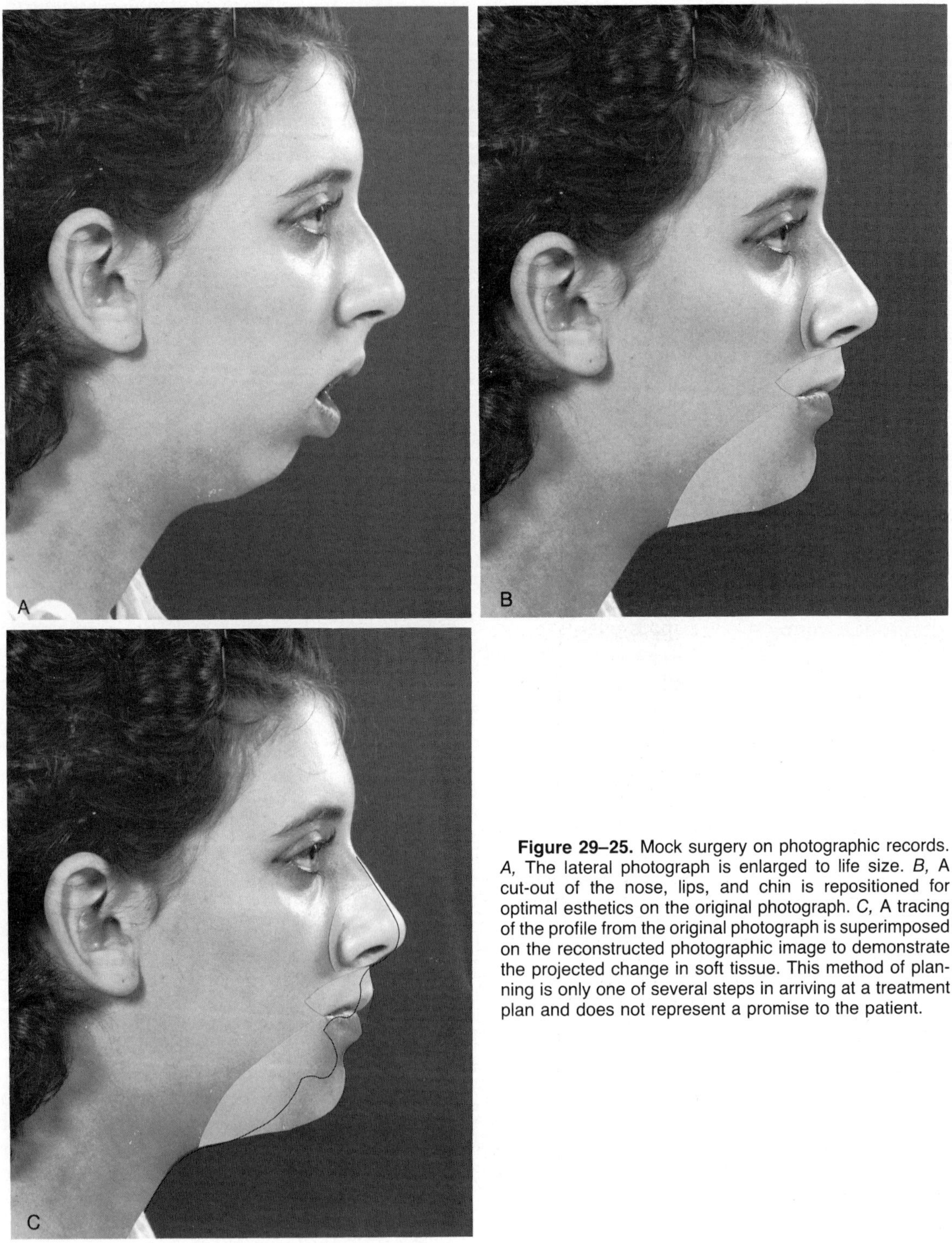

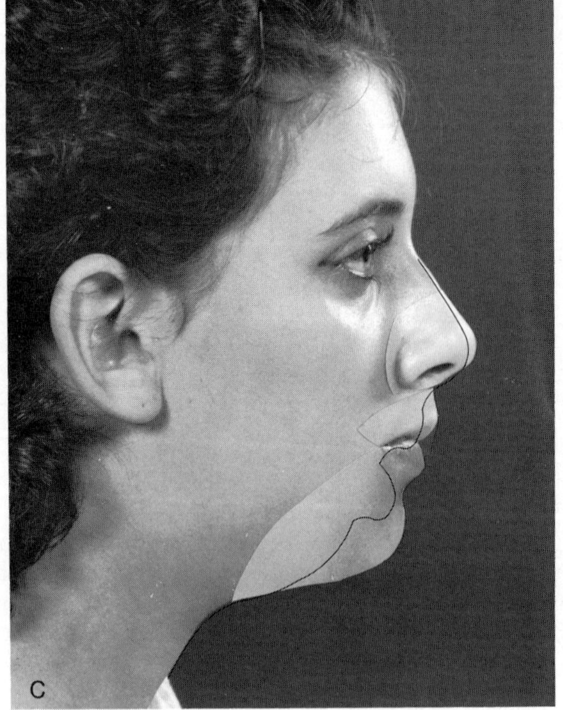

Figure 29–25. Mock surgery on photographic records. *A,* The lateral photograph is enlarged to life size. *B,* A cut-out of the nose, lips, and chin is repositioned for optimal esthetics on the original photograph. *C,* A tracing of the profile from the original photograph is superimposed on the reconstructed photographic image to demonstrate the projected change in soft tissue. This method of planning is only one of several steps in arriving at a treatment plan and does not represent a promise to the patient.

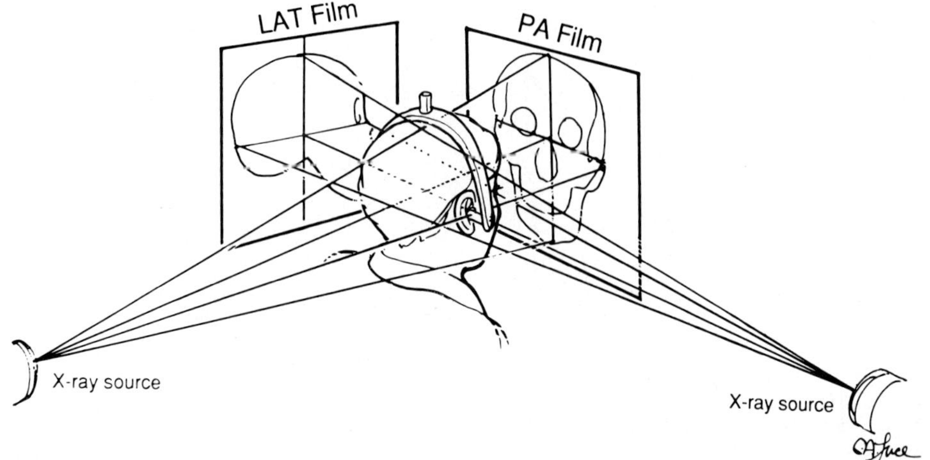

Figure 29–26. For both the posteroanterior and lateral cephalograms the three-dimensional positions of the x-ray source and the radiographic image of the anatomic point are known. Two three-dimensional lines that pass through the anatomic point are therefore defined. The intersection of the two lines gives the three-dimensional locus of the anatomic point.

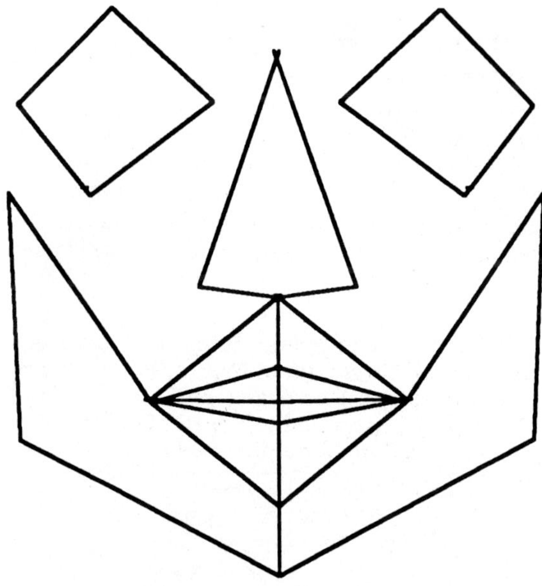

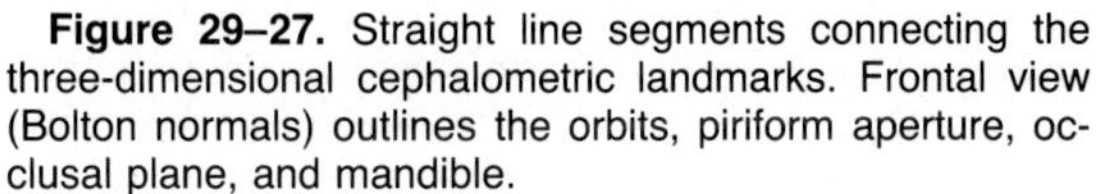

Figure 29–27. Straight line segments connecting the three-dimensional cephalometric landmarks. Frontal view (Bolton normals) outlines the orbits, piriform aperture, occlusal plane, and mandible.

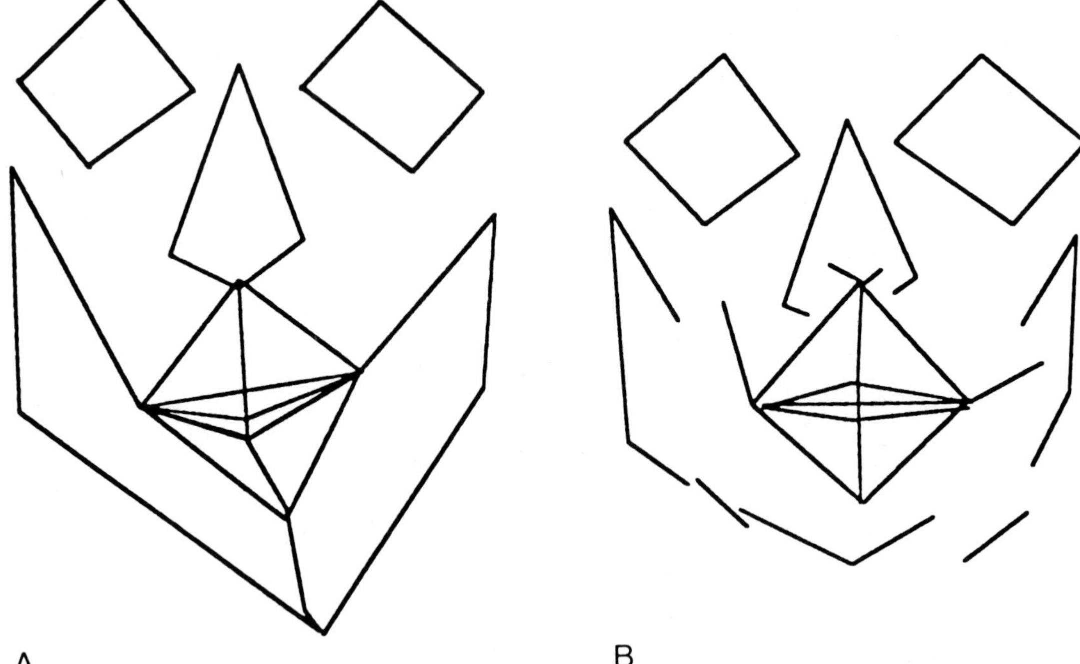

Figure 29–28. Triangular tiled image. *A,* A patient with severe unilateral craniofacial microsomia preoperatively. *B,* Corresponding view after simulated Le Fort I osteotomy, bilateral sagittal split (ramisection) of the mandible and genioplasty.

plete control of the position and orientation of each osteotomized segment in space (Grayson and associates, 1988). The visual feedback from the change in the resultant image is used by the operator to alter the design or to perform other osteotomies. After the surgical designer is satisfied with the plan, a numerical printout is generated that gives precise measurements of bone movements that may be taken to the operating room (Table 29–2).

An automated surgical simulation program was also written based on an optimization principle (Grayson and associates, 1988). The computer moves the mobile osteotomy fragments until the position of the patient's landmarks most closely approaches the positions of the normal landmark set. The distances between each of the patient's landmarks and their normal counterparts are computed.

The surgical designs for a patient with unilateral craniofacial microsomia are illustrated in Figure 29–29. The surgical simulation is a Le Fort I osteotomy, a sagittal split of the mandible, and a horizontal osteotomy (genioplasty) to alter the position of the chin point. This design was arrived at by first using the optimization program to put the osteotomy fragments in anatomic position. The clinician *must* interactively modify the design to account for the biologic variables of relapse, bone graft resorption, soft tissue characteristics, and occlusion.

Table 29–2. Computer Printout that Reports Amount of Movement of Right (RMT) and Left (LMT) Maxillary Tuberosities and Anterior Nasal Spine (ANS) Required to Specify Position of a Le Fort I Osteotomy Segment

RMT moved superiorly 8.12 mm
RMT moved left −1.34 mm
RMT moved anteriorly 2.04 mm
LMT moved superiorly 4.06 mm
LMT moved left −1.06 mm
LMT moved anteriorly 2.04 mm
ANS moved superiorly 6.09 mm
ANS moved left −1.20 mm
ANS moved anteriorly 2.04 mm

CT-based Surgical Simulation. Various hardware and software combinations are commercially available that create three-dimensional images from computed tomographic (CT) data provided by the original scanner. Numerous custom-editing features have been added to these devices that allow custom editing and image manipulation to

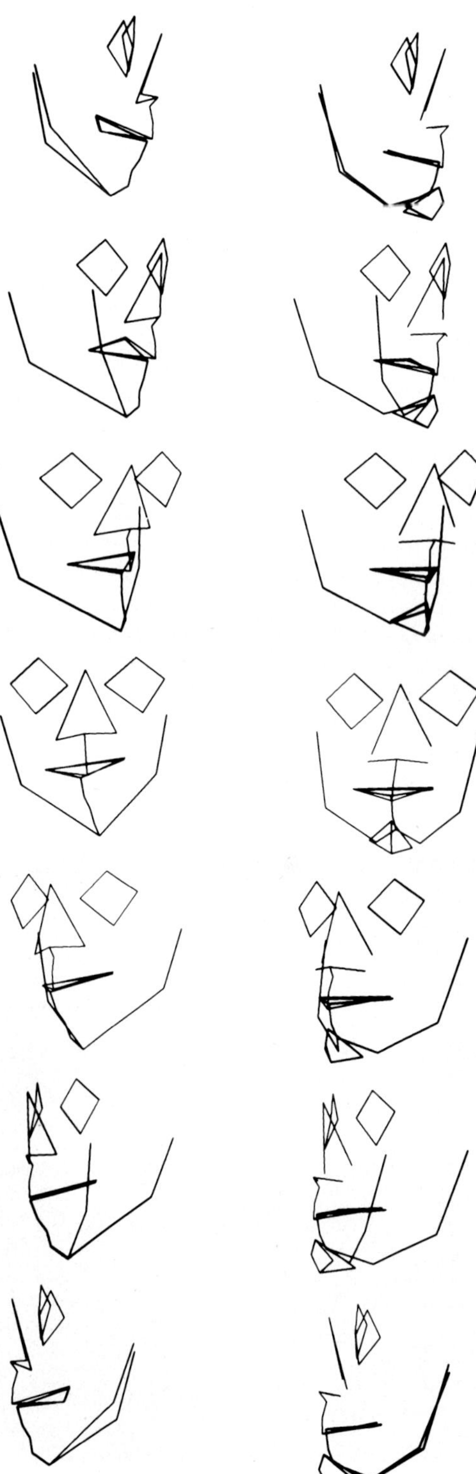

Figure 29–29. Rotation of cephalometric three-dimensional image. *Left column,* Preoperative views of a patient with unilateral craniofacial microsomia. *Right column,* Mock surgical correction for corresponding views (Le Fort I osteotomy, bilateral mandibular ramisection, and genioplasty).

produce highly synthesized images specifically designed to demonstrate a particular abnormality. This type of custom editing amounts to electronic dissection. Working in this manner, the clinician functions as though in an electronic anatomy laboratory. Examples of these images appear in Figure 29–30.

The first efforts in the direction of surgical simulation based on CT scan data were made by Marsh and associates (1983) and Vannier, Marsh, and Warren (1984). Their efforts involved three principal directions: mirror imaging, automated three-dimensional solid model making, and the adaptation of commercial computer-aided design (CAD) software. The most satisfactory approach to surgical simulation involves performing the simulation directly on a computer terminal (Cutting and associates, 1986). The user cuts and moves the osteotomy fragments in real time and measures the postoperative change, as illustrated in Figures 29–30 and 29–31.

After the bone movements under the skin have been modeled, it is desirable to evaluate their effect on the skin surface. Previous attempts to correlate soft tissue change with an underlying bone movement based on conventional cephalograms have been minimally satisfactory because of insufficient data collection (Wilmott, 1981). For example, estimates of the amount of soft tissue change in a genioplasty produce quite variable results. A patient with a wide face should experience more advancement of the soft tissue chin for an underlying bone advancement than would a patient with a narrow face. In a narrow face, the skin tends to be more tightly stretched over the bony prominence after the chin advancement. This results in much greater soft tissue compression. The eventual solution to predicting soft tissue responses to facial osteotomies may be found in the finite element method (Rice, 1983; Rockey and associates, 1983), which was developed in engineering for the modeling of the responses of a material to stress and strain under different circumstances. A continuous flexible structure is modeled as a set of finite elements. The characteristics of each of the elements are known. Stress is applied to the entire system, and the forces between elements are continually readjusted by the computer program until an equilibrium of forces occurs. This type of software is useful in modeling the skin surface response to underlying bone change.

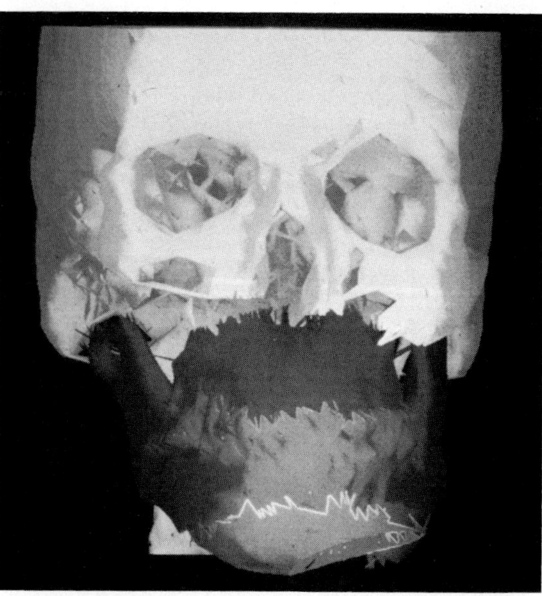

Figure 29–31. With interactive computergraphic technique the clinician can effect the necessary skeletal changes (Le Fort I osteotomy, asymmetric mandibular advancement, and genioplasty).

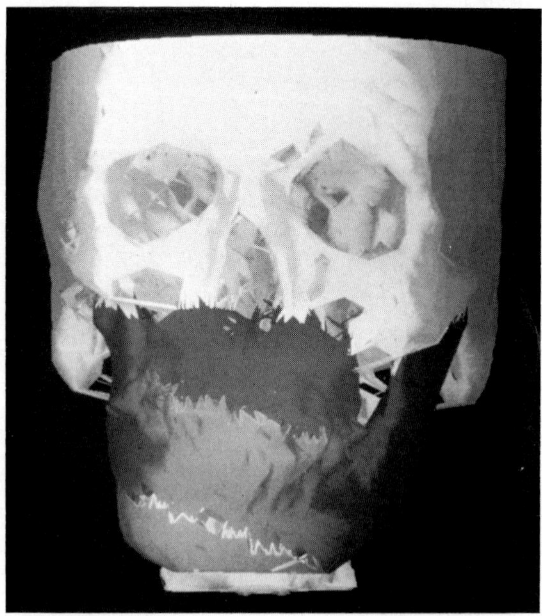

Figure 29–30. CT-based surgical simulation of a patient with unilateral craniofacial microsomia. Note the occlusal cant and underdevelopment of the maxilla and mandible on the affected side.

Laser Light Scanner. Two-dimensional photography has traditionally been the dominant method for reporting the result of orthognathic surgery. Unfortunately, foreshor-

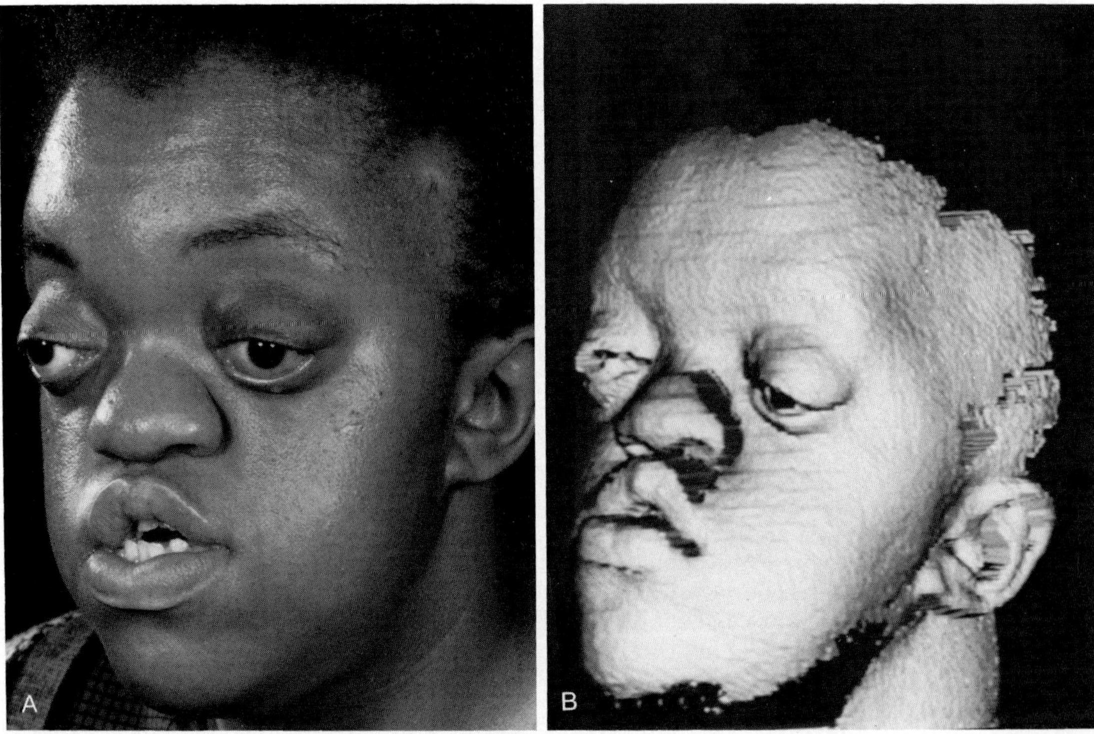

Figure 29–32. Laser light scanner. *A,* Adolescent female with craniofacial synostosis. *B,* Laser light scan image. (From Cutting, C. B., McCarthy, J. G., and Karron, D. B.: Three-dimensional input of body surface data using a laser light scanner. Ann. Plast. Surg., *21*:38, 1988.)

tening in photographs prevents the recording of three-dimensional distance and angle measurements. The three-dimensional laser light scanner makes possible the input and measurement of facial surface data. The current quantitative capabilities of this system are those of three-dimensional anthropometry (Cutting, McCarthy, and Karron, 1988).

A low energy laser light beam is projected as a vertical line onto the surface of the face. A video camera at an angle to the light source records the image of this line as it moves across the entire face. The video device and computer record the radius from the central axis of the head to the body surfaces that are scanned. The data are available immediately in digital form for computer reconstruction of the surface image and three-dimensional measurement (Fig. 29–32). A comprehensive morphometric system for quantitative analysis of this surface data is being developed. It may then be possible to perform statistical operations such as averaging and comparison between groups. This promises to advance the science of evaluating surface changes due to skeletal surgery. In addition it will provide the tools needed to study population averages for facial surface contour.

Fixation Techniques

Satisfactory fixation is absolutely essential to a successful result in orthognathic surgery. It cannot be overemphasized that *all osteotomized segments must be optimally immobilized in proper three-dimensional relationships.*

The fixation device appliances must satisfy several criteria: They must

1. Be as simple in application as possible.
2. Provide optimal immobilization.
3. Allow maintenance of oral hygiene.
4. Be made of relatively inert material.
5. Permit minor adjustments in the operating room.

Various types of fixation appliances have been used over the years and will be individually discussed.

Cast Cap Splints. The disadvantage of dental cast cap splints and other mechanical appliances rigidly conceived and constructed on the anatomic articulator is that complete accuracy cannot always be relied on. The appliance must often be adjusted in the operating room, because surgical movement cannot always reproduce the exact position that was preplanned on the articulator. Minor adjustments of this type of appliance are not always possible.

Acrylic Splints. Acrylic splints of various design are also used. In edentulous patients and in individuals in whom the teeth are not serviceable, prosthodontic appliances ensure fixation of the separated fragments of the jaws. Acrylic splints of the segmental type are joined after positioning of the fragments by the addition of quick-curing acrylic applied in the operating room (Fig. 29–33). The appliances are usually maintained by internal craniofacial suspension wiring or by circumferential (mandibular) wiring in edentulous patients; they can also be anchored with wires to the remaining teeth in partially edentulous patients. Dentures, biteblocks with biteguides, and flanges are also necessary accessories in some patients. The type of splint illustrated in Figure 29–34 is of particular value in a partially edentulous mandible.

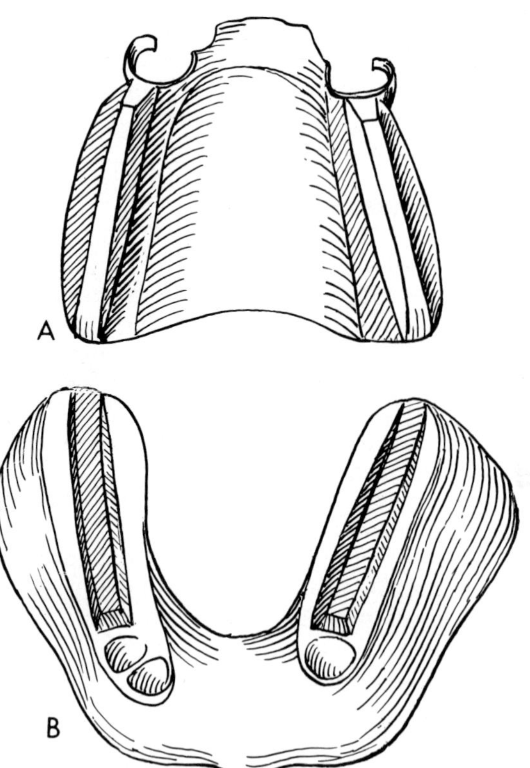

Figure 29–33. Maxillary and mandibular biteblocks (acrylic) for edentulous and partially edentulous patients.

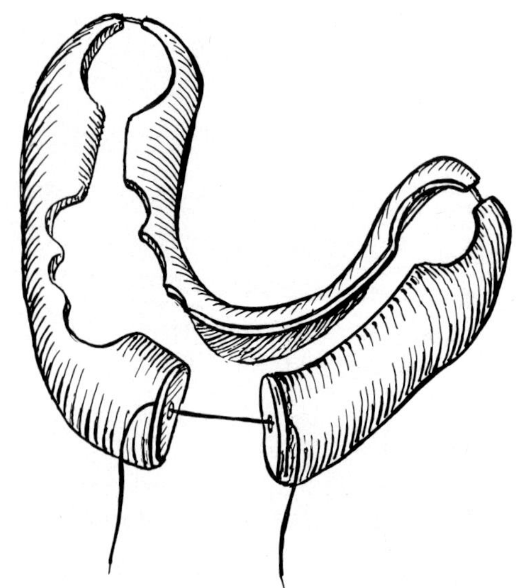

Figure 29–34. Acrylic splint to show how the splint is expanded to permit its placement over the dentoalveolar arch. The splint is tightened in position with an anterior stainless steel wire. Note the wire in the posterior end of the splint, which permits the splint to open.

Arch Bars. Arch bars (Erich) similar to those used for fixation purposes in facial bone fractures have also been employed in orthognathic surgery (Fig. 29–35). They have been traditionally used only when orthodontic support is not available. They suffer the disadvantages of preventing postoperative orthodontic adjustments and requiring a relatively full complement of teeth.

Orthodontic Appliances. These are preferred by many surgeons since they provide satisfactory fixation and are sufficiently flexible to allow dental adjustments at the time of operation and during the period after removal of intermaxillary fixation. The appliances are employed preoperatively (often to permit orthodontic therapy) and are used to establish intermaxillary fixation at the time of operation either by wires or by orthodontic rubber bands (Fig. 29–36).

RIGID SKELETAL FIXATION

This technique has only recently been adopted in North America despite extensive European experience in the treatment of jaw fractures and in fixation of osteotomized segments in orthognathic surgery (Champy and associates, 1978; Michelet, Deymes, and Desus, 1973; Drommer and Luhr, 1981; Rittersma and associates, 1981; Steinhauser, 1982). A miniaturized system (microplates)

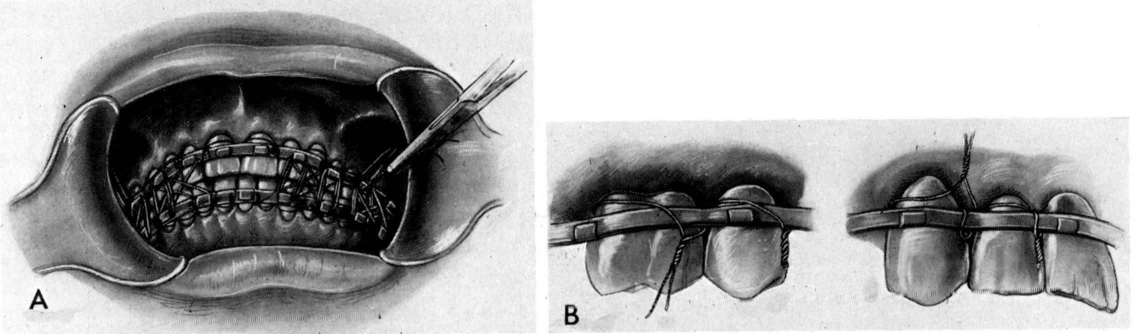

Figure 29–35. Application of arch bars. *A,* Prefabricated malleable arch bars are contoured to adapt to the curvature of the teeth, and fixation to the teeth is established by wires passed around the necks of the individual teeth. The wire is twisted to secure the arch bar to the teeth. Elastic bands can be used to provide intermaxillary traction to bring the teeth into occlusion. *B,* Note the technique used on the anterior teeth to avoid downward slippage of the arch bar.

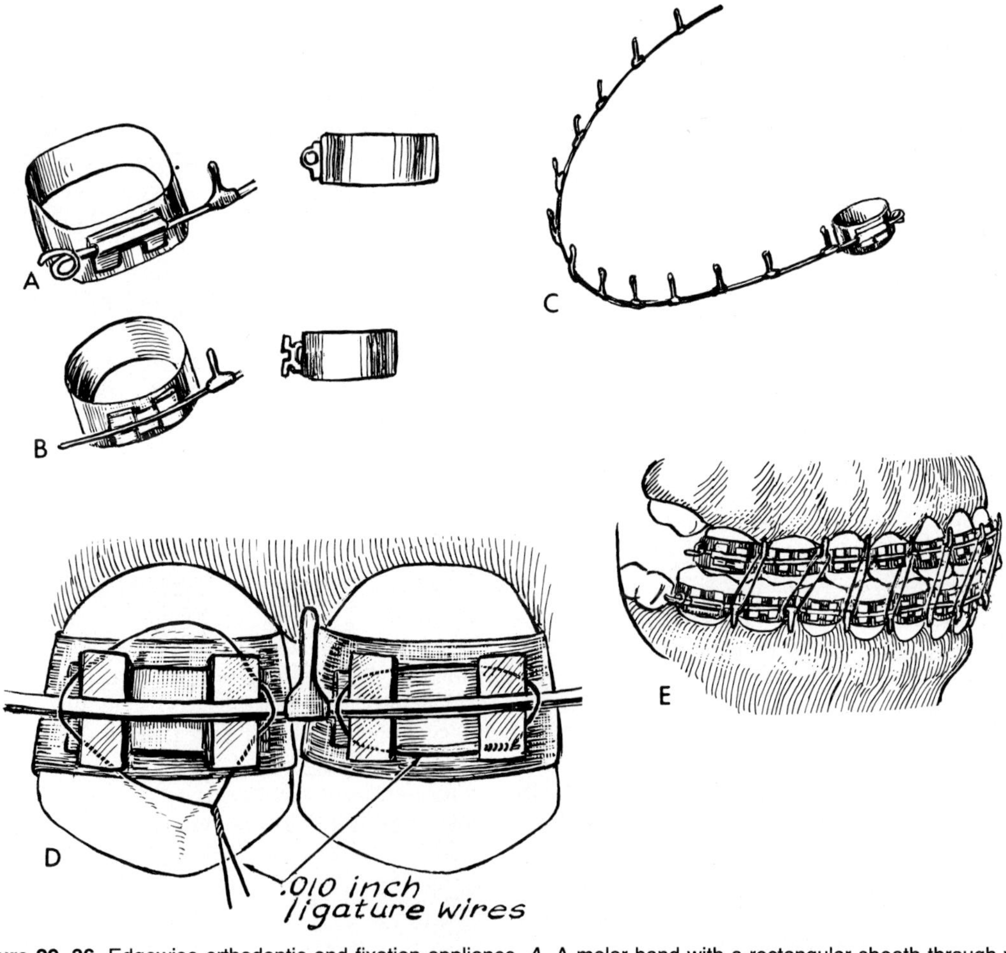

A
C
B
E
D
.010 inch
ligature wires

Figure 29–36. Edgewise orthodontic and fixation appliance. *A,* A molar band with a rectangular sheath through which the edgewise arch wire is inserted. *B,* Dental bands with "twin brackets" are placed on the remaining teeth. The brackets permit the insertion of the edgewise wire. *C,* Arch wire with spurs soldered to the gingival side as it appears prior to final insertion. *D,* The arch wire has been inserted in the "twin brackets" and is secured in position with wire ligature ties. *E,* The appliance in place with intermaxillary wires (0.028 inch) placed between the arches to fix one jaw to the other.

has also been developed for special situations, e.g., the nasoethmoidal area, the orbit, the wall of the frontal sinus, and the craniofacial skeleton of the infant (Luhr, 1988).

Advantages

The main advantage of the technique is a marked reduction in the length of intermaxillary fixation. Moreover, if the patient's comfort so dictates, light training elastics can substitute for wires in intermaxillary fixation. In addition, airway problems can be minimized since the elastics can be quickly cut without jeopardizing the skeletal stability. Oral intake should obviously improve with evidence of less weight loss. Oral hygiene is also improved. Patients who have periodontal pathology with bone loss, long considered poor candidates for orthognathic surgery, can be considered since intermaxillary fixation with its attendant forces on the teeth is no longer required. With a significant decrease in the length of intermaxillary fixation, there should also be less symptomatology in patients with intrinsic temporomandibular joint disease. After rigid skeletal fixation is established in the operating room, condylar position must be checked by releasing the intermaxillary fixation and observing the occlusion. If there is a problem, the fixation can be removed and reestablished. Rigid skeletal fixation in three dimensions should theoretically improve the long-term stability of mobilized segments, but confirmation of this awaits longitudinal studies (Rosen, 1986).

Disadvantages

One disadvantage is the increased cost of the appliances, which is considerable. In addition, the time spent in the operating room is increased. The cost factor is offset by reduced hospital stays and shortened disability time.

The most significant disadvantage is the absence of tolerance for error. It is difficult for the orthodontist to correct faulty skeletal position with elastic traction in the postoperative period because of the resistance offered by the plates and screws. Consequently, the surgeon must be meticulously exact in his preoperative planning and intraoperative technique if rigid skeletal fixation is used.

Technique. A variety of systems are available (Champy and associates, 1978; Drommer and Luhr, 1981; Steinhauser, 1982).

The Luhr system is composed of vitallium plates and self-tapping screws (Fig. 29–37). The miniplates are available in a variety of shapes and are molded to exact shape with two pairs of pliers. A malleable counterpart is available for shaping in the wound itself; it can be removed and used as a model for the vitallium plate (Fig. 29–38). The self-tapping screws are 2 mm in diameter and range in length from 4 to 28 mm. An important technical precaution is to avoid high-speed drilling (over 1000 rpm), which causes additional bone necrosis and results in "stripping" of the screw, especially in areas of thin bone as in the anterior maxilla. A drill hole not exceeding 1.5 mm in diameter provides maximal holding power for the screw. An "emergency" screw 2.4 mm in diameter can grasp the bone even in "stripped" screw holes.

Although the concept of axial compression at the fracture site favors bone healing, it is not always desirable in orthognathic surgery. For example, compression (and impaction) of mobilized tooth-bearing bony segments can result in occlusal disparities. Accordingly the *compression mode* should not be used in these circumstances (Fig. 29–39).

Finally, the manually modeled miniplates must fit the contours of the bone *accurately*. If the plate does not passively conform to the attached skeletal segment, the latter will move secondarily to the application of muscular and dental forces (Fig. 29–40).

Postoperative Care

Before fixation is established in the operating room, a No. 18 Fr nasogastric tube is inserted and its patency and position are verified. This maneuver should allow emptying of gastric contents and prevent vomiting of swallowed blood. The tube will also allow feedings if necessary. In general, it is usually removed by 24 hours or with evidence of the return of gastrointestinal function.

Maintenance of the airway is the critical factor in the postoperative management of the patient who undergoes orthognathic surgery. Usually, nasoendotracheal intubation is performed by the anesthesiologist. The tube can be secured by a heavy silk suture passed

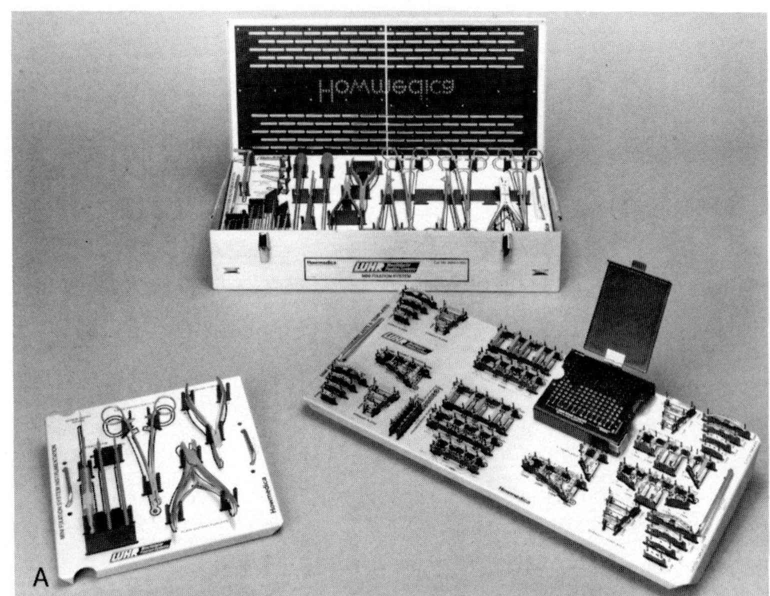

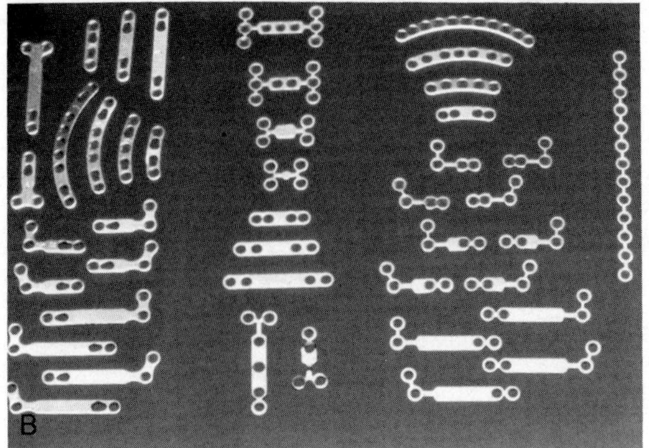

Figure 29–37. *A,* Rigid skeletal fixation set. *B,* Available types of plates.

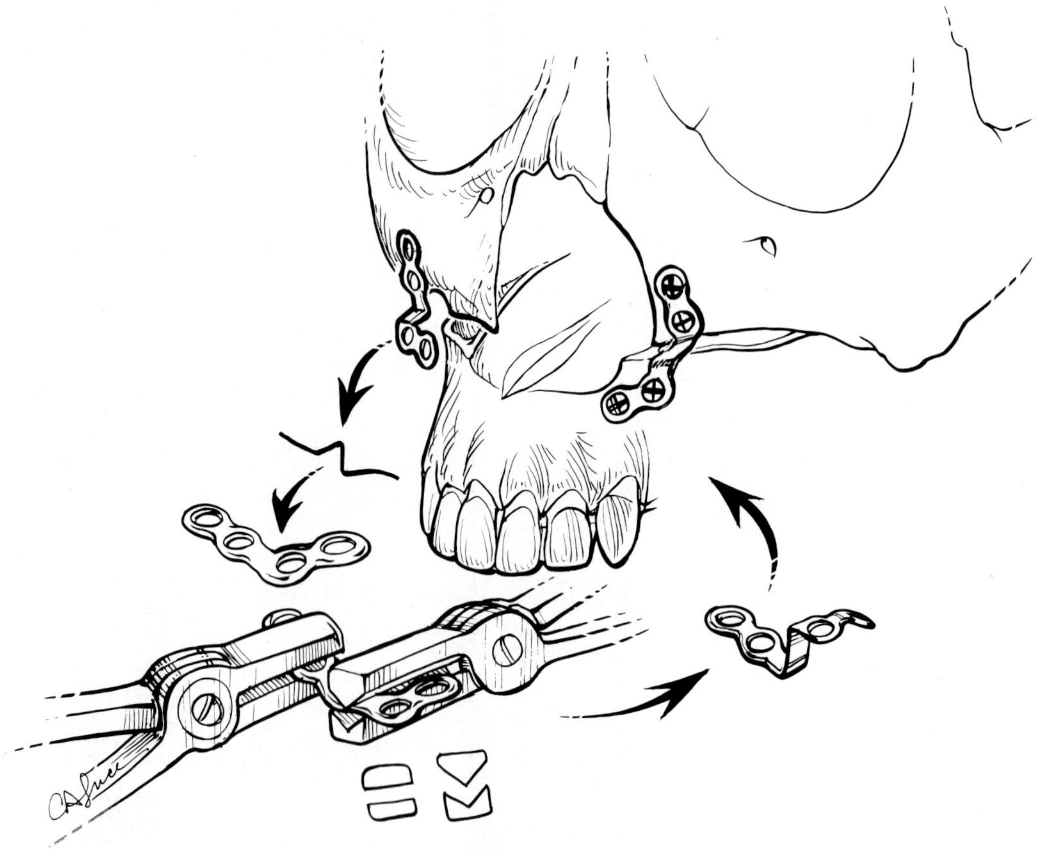

Figure 29–38. On the left, bending of the malleable template at the site of a Le Fort I osteotomy is illustrated. The template is used as a pattern for shaping the miniplate with either straight or angulated pliers as illustrated on the right.

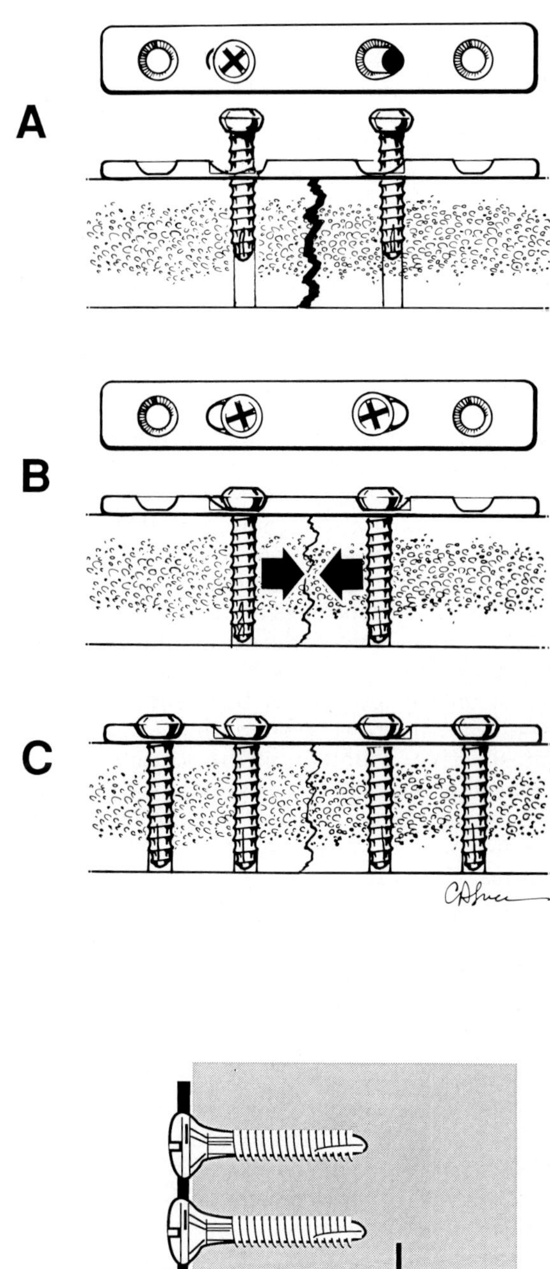

Figure 29–39. The compression mode of miniplate fixation. *A,* A four-hole plate. Note that the inner holes are eccentrically shaped so that, as the screws are tightened, the heads fall into the wider portion and compress the bony margins *(B)*. *C,* Completed view of the skeletal fixation.

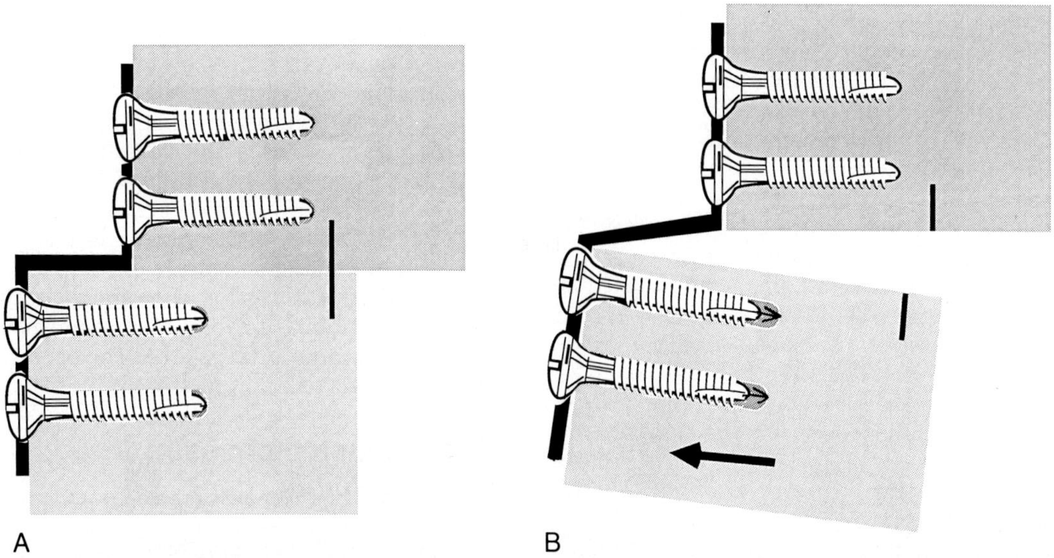

A

B

Figure 29–40. *A,* Accurate shaping of the miniplate to the skeletal contours. *B,* Failure to shape the miniplate accurately results in displacement of the bony segments on tightening of the screws. Note the disparity in the vertical line. (After Rosen, 1986.)

through the septum and multiply wrapped around the tube. Depending on the magnitude of the procedure and status of the patient, the tube can be removed at the conclusion of the operation, in the recovery room, or in the intensive care unit one or two days postoperatively.

When the nasoendotracheal tube is removed after the evaluation of pulmonary function studies, it is replaced by a soft rubber nasopharyngeal "trumpet." The latter ensures the airway but must be periodically removed and cleansed.

Elective tracheotomy is reserved for patients undergoing massive craniofacial reconstruction, especially those who have associated medical problems or who lack the ability to communicate adequately. Patients with severe mandibular hypoplasia may be candidates for elective tracheotomy if endotracheal intubation cannot be accomplished even with the aid of a flexible fiberoptic laryngoscope.

Parenterally administered steroids have traditionally been used to lessen postoperative edema after orthognathic surgery, but prospective, double-blind clinical studies are few. In a fairly well controlled study (Munro and associates, 1986) of pediatric patients undergoing maxillary or mandibular osteotomies, the administration of dexamethasone appeared to decrease postoperative swelling, but the difference was not statistically significant in comparison with the placebo group. Nevertheless, it is the routine of the authors to administer steroids during the perioperative period.

Probably the most frustrating aspect of orthognathic surgery for the patient is the diet. If intermaxillary fixation is employed, the experience can be extremely discouraging, especially with edematous and hypoesthetic cheeks and lips.

The patient usually is not allowed oral fluids for 24 to 48 hours after surgery. The first fluids are taken through a *Breck feeder*, which consists of a 60 ml syringe with an attached length of soft rubber tubing that is introduced into dental spaces or the retromolar space. It takes time for the patient to become comfortable with its use. The patient must be cautioned to check the temperature of all foods since the latter can be introduced directly into the posterior oropharynx and cause a burn.

The patient and family must experiment with tube feedings and begin with fluids, which are better tolerated than blenderized feedings. The blender is invaluable in providing palatable and tolerable feedings. Mashed potatoes can be combined with broth or milk, ice cream with milk, and thicker soups with water before being inserted into the blender. Cereals tend to clog the tubing. A *disposable cup* is preferable to one of glass or ceramic since it can be molded to the shape of the patient's lips. The use of the cup can be extremely messy and the patient should be advised to secure a bath towel around his neck. *Spoon* feeding must await the resolution of swelling of the lips and cheeks. It is best to plan four to six feedings per day, since each session tends to be prolonged, the feedings are not satisfying, and hunger returns quickly.

Oral hygiene should be of major concern to the patient. The teeth are at jeopardy because they are partially covered by appliances, and plaque accumulates rapidly. On the third or fourth day a Water-Pik can be used, initially at a low setting (2 to 3). Plax can eventually be added to the irrigant to decrease the build-up of dental plaque.

Postoperative Orthodontic Therapy and Retention

After release of surgical-orthodontic fixation, the repositioned dento-osseous units usually "settle in." This change generally occurs in the direction of the presurgical skeletal anatomy and thus may be termed "immediate relapse." Solid functional occlusion, characterized by stable incisal and posterior intercuspation, reduces the tendency for rapid postfixational skeletal change. The orthodontist can counter the musculocutaneous forces of relapse by the application of intermaxillary elastics and various extraoral appliances. Careful monitoring of occlusal and skeletal relationships is an intrinsic aspect of postsurgical orthodontic therapy. The process of balancing the forces of relapse with orthodontic appliances for up to one year after surgery contributes to long-term stability. It is during this time interval that the occlusion may be refined to its final state.

Types of Osteotomies in Orthognathic Surgery

In the surgical-orthodontic correction of jaw deformities, osteotomies are performed in three different ways.

Skeletal Osteotomy. The skeletal osteotomy is performed through the entire thickness of the body of the bone (the basilar portion). It can be either a simple cut with overlapping of the fragments, a resection of a segment, or a transection with addition of bone by grafting. The segments are repositioned and held securely by fixation in an improved dentoalveolar and skeletal relationship. Examples are the vertical osteotomy (see Fig. 29–55) and sagittal section of the ramus (see Fig. 29–65) or the Le Fort I osteotomy of the maxilla (see Fig. 29–196).

Dentoalveolar Osteotomy. In contrast, the dentoalveolar osteotomy can be confined to the tooth-bearing portion of the jaw. The bone is sectioned at the base of the dentoalveolar segment, leaving sufficient bone to protect the apices and vascular supply of the teeth. The dentoalveolar block containing several teeth and their supporting structures is moved to the planned new position (Fig. 29–41). Movement is directed vertically, anteriorly or posteriorly, or laterally. A combination of directions can be used to suit the needs dictated by the deformity (Fig. 29–42). In these procedures, the blood supply is maintained by the mucoperiosteal attachments.

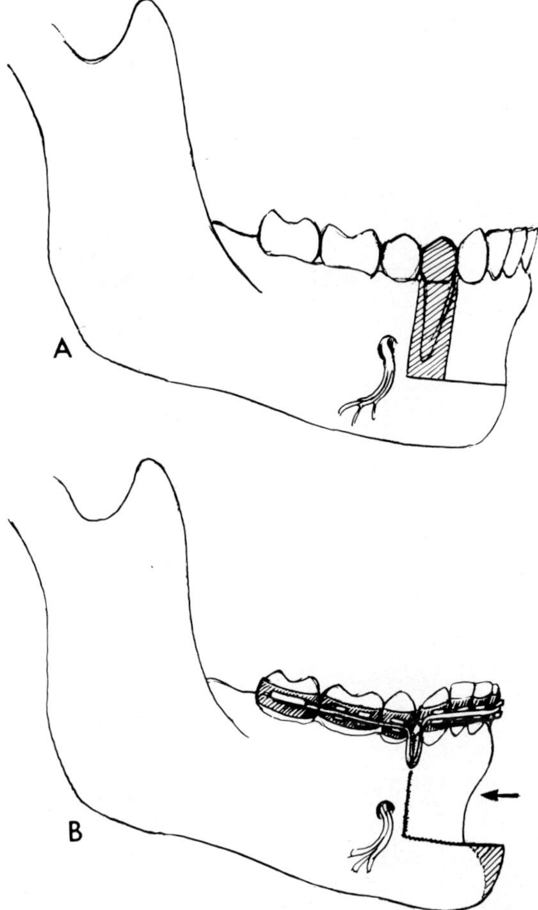

Figure 29–41. Dentoalveolar osteotomy. *A,* When the dentoalveolar segment is to be recessed, it may be necessary to remove a tooth as well as a portion of the alveolar bone. The line of the osteotomy extends vertically through the alveolus and horizontally below the apices of the teeth. *B,* The anterior dentoalveolar segment is repositioned and immobilized by a monomaxillary fixation appliance. The chin contour is improving by resecting the area represented by the shading. (From Converse, J. M., and Horowitz, S. L.: The surgical-orthodontic approach to the treatment of dentofacial deformities. Am. J. Orthod., *55*:214, 1969.)

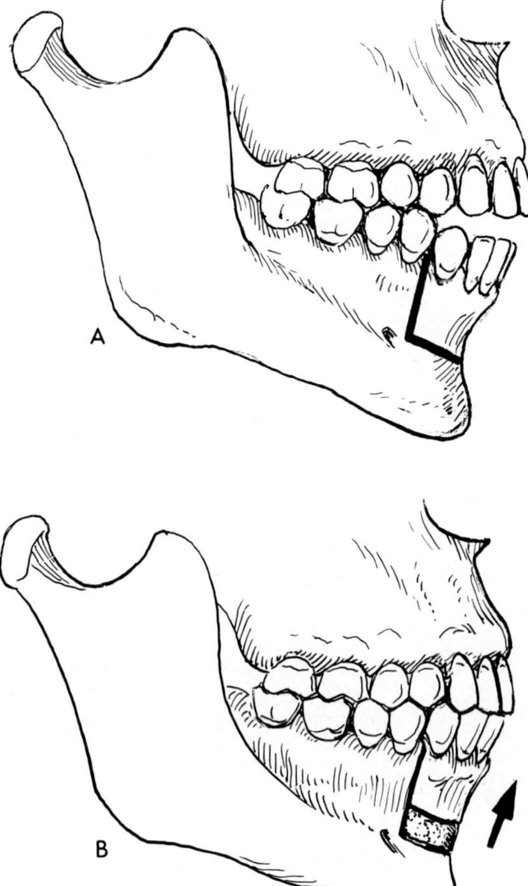

Figure 29–42. Dentoalveolar osteotomy for the correction of anterior open bite. *A,* Anterior dentoalveolar segment outlined. *B,* The segment is mobilized vertically, the open bite is closed, and bone grafts are placed in the resulting bone defect. A similar procedure can be used in the upper dentoalveolar process.

Cortical Osteotomy. The cortical osteotomy extends only through the cortical bone of the alveolar segment. It is of particular value in the maxillary arch and has its major application in the correction of the constricted

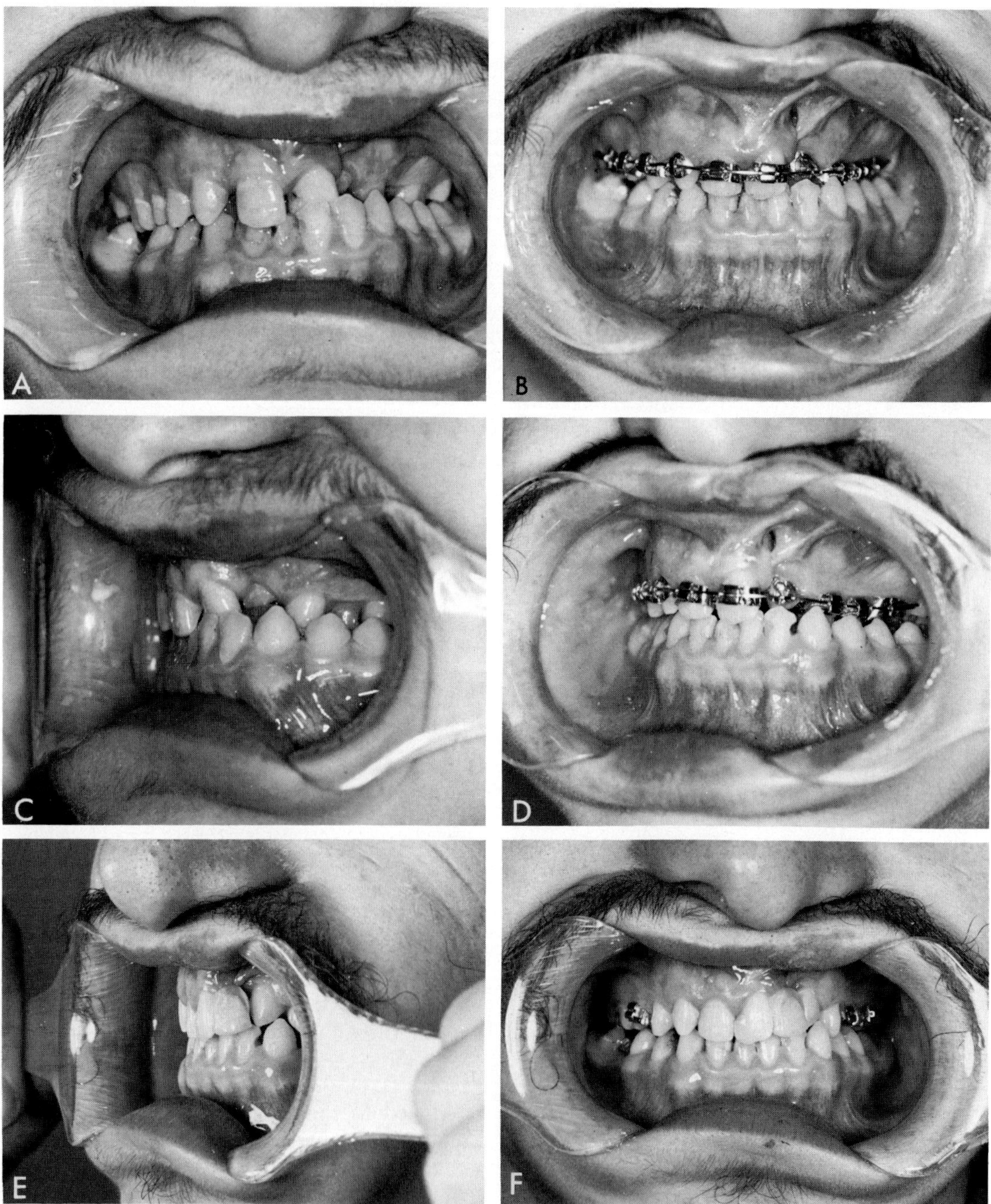

Figure 29–43. Maxillary arch expansion by cortical osteotomy. *A,* Malocclusion with crossbite before orthodontic therapy. *B,* After completion of orthodontic therapy. *C,* Oblique view before orthodontic therapy. *D,* Oblique view after orthodontic therapy. Note the inadequate result. Occlusal relationships have not been reestablished between the left maxillary and mandibular teeth because of the lingual displacement of the left maxillary arch. *E, F,* After cortical osteotomy and expansion by the appliance shown in Figure 29–44.

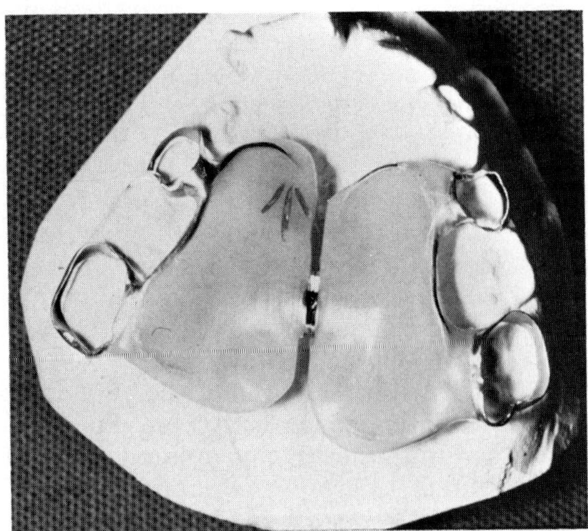

Figure 29–44. Palatal split-plate appliance activated by a jackscrew is used to expand the alveolar arch, which was weakened by a cortical osteotomy.

maxilla of the patient with cleft palate (Fig. 29–43). The technique includes placement of an orthodontic expansion appliance or a split palatal acrylic plate with a jackscrew that exerts continuous gentle expansion forces after the surgical weakening of the alveolar bone support by the cortical osteotomy (Fig. 29–44). This procedure produces rapid expansion by lateral displacement of the entire dentoalveolar segment, without tipping of the teeth (see Fig. 29–43*E,F*).

DEVELOPMENTAL DEFORMITIES

Mandibular Deformities

SURGICAL APPROACH

The entire mandible can be surgically altered by various types of osteotomies combined with the displacement of bone, the resection of bone, or the addition of bone by grafting. The mandible has been sectioned in practically every conceivable manner, and in some cases combinations are required in different regions.

Excellent exposure can be obtained by the use of various types of incision and various approaches. Dissection is facilitated and blood loss minimized if the area is infiltrated with a solution containing 1:100,000 epinephrine before the incision is made. Hypotensive anesthesia techniques can also be used but usually are not necessary.

Extraoral and Intraaoral Approaches to Body and Symphysis of Mandible

Extraoral Approach. Although cutaneous incisions have been largely supplanted by intraoral incisions, they still occasionally have a place. This approach should be avoided in patients who tend to form hypertrophic scars or keloids.

The body of the mandible can be exposed through a *submandibular skin incision* (Risdon) made approximately 1 to 2 cm below the inferior border in a natural submandibular crease (see Fig. 29–56). Accurate placement of the incision is best achieved by marking its path with the patient seated and before the administration of anesthesia. The dissection is continued through the platysma. Precaution must be taken to avoid injury to the marginal mandibular branch of the facial nerve as the dissection progresses down to the bone. The landmarks described by Dingman and Grabb (1962) should be observed.

The mental symphysis can be exposed through an incision in the *submental fold* or immediately below the chin along the *posterior edge of the inferior border of the symphysis*. The latter incision usually leaves a less conspicuous scar than one placed in the fold itself.

Intraoral Approach. The transoral route provides unrivaled exposure of the body, which can be matched only by the extraoral approach with an extensive submandibular incision. Furthermore, a visible external scar and the risk of injury to the facial nerve are avoided.

Converse (1950) was the first to use the intraoral approach to transplant contour-restoring bone grafts. Success depends on satisfactory soft tissue coverage of the osteotomy and bone graft site. Healing is compromised by a deficient blood supply and the absence of a protective seal. When the body of the mandible is greatly elongated or augmented, the soft tissue may not be adequate to provide coverage, since it is placed under tension. It is important, therefore, to design the incision so that a tension-free closure is ensured to protect the operative site. Infection, nonconsolidation of the fragments, necrosis of bone, and sequestration are complications that occur when the soft tissue is poor in quality or lacking in quantity.

The intraoral route has been employed not only for contour bone grafting of the skeletal framework of the face but also for osteotomies

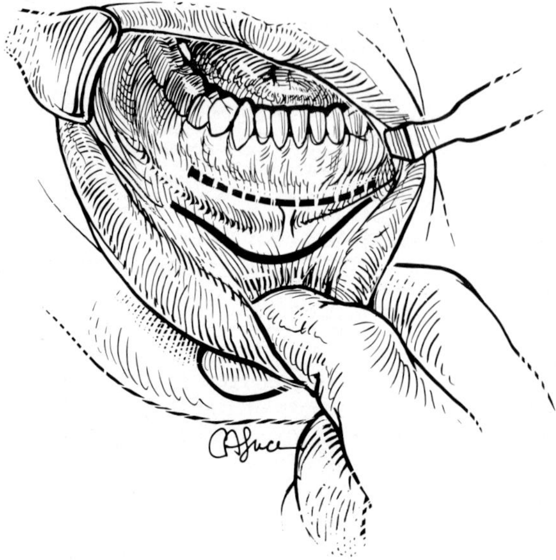

Figure 29–45. Intraoral incisions: the labiobuccal vestibular *(solid line)* and the mucogingival *(interrupted line)* incisions.

performed on both the ramus and body of the mandible (Converse and Shapiro, 1952; Converse, 1954; Kazanjian and Converse, 1959, 1974b; Obwegeser, 1957). Most jaw malformations can be corrected by the various intraoral approaches.

Labiobuccal Vestibular Incision. This incision is made on the labial aspect of the vestibule, at least 1 cm above the frenulum (Fig. 29–45). The frenulum should not be sectioned; it is difficult to restore and heals poorly. The length of the incision depends on the extent of the procedure. The mucosa is raised from the musculature of the cheek or the lip, and sharp dissection is continued until the mandible is reached. At this point the periosteum is incised and final exposure is obtained by mucoperiosteal elevation.

When the symphyseal area is to be exposed, the incision extends through the mucosa above the level of the frenulum. The mucosa is dissected from the orbicularis oris. The periosteum is incised and the symphysis is exposed in the subperiosteal plane.

The mental nerve must be respected at all times. Care should be taken to avoid injuring the nerve as it exits from the mental foramen near the apices of the premolar teeth and branches into the lip.

Mucogingival Incision. An incision is made approximately 5 mm below the mucogingival junction and on the dental aspect of the vestibule (Fig. 29–45). Again, the frenulum should be skirted. This approach provides rapid and excellent exposure of the mandible since the route is direct to the underlying bone. However, the incision should not be placed too close to the mucogingival junction because a short mucosa cuff holds sutures poorly. Furthermore, scar contraction may cause stripping of the nearby gingiva, especially when the health of the gingiva is poor. Nevertheless, when properly executed the mucogingival incision is preferable because of its direct approach qualities.

Placement of the incision at the very depth of the vestibule should be avoided. Food particles tend to gather in this area and healing of the wound suffers.

Degloving Procedure. The degloving procedure described by Converse (1959, 1964b) provides excellent exposure of the anterior portion of the mandible (Fig. 29–46). Either the labiobuccal or the mucogingival incision is extended across the midline from one canine-premolar region to the other; the entire symphysis and anterior portion of the body can be exposed when necessary. When an extensive augmentation of the chin is planned, the labiobuccal placement of the incision is recommended, because excessive soft tissue tension and possible disruption of the wound are lessened.

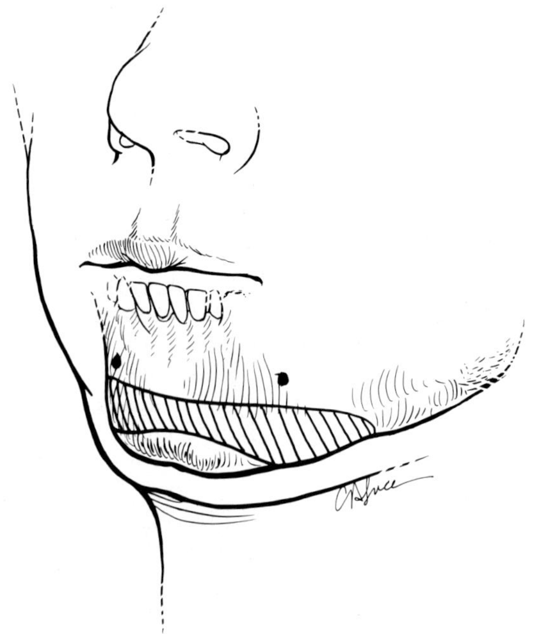

Figure 29–46. Extent of undermining *(diagonal lines)* or skeletal exposure with the degloving procedure. Note that the soft tissue over the pogonion is not disturbed. The mental foramina are designated.

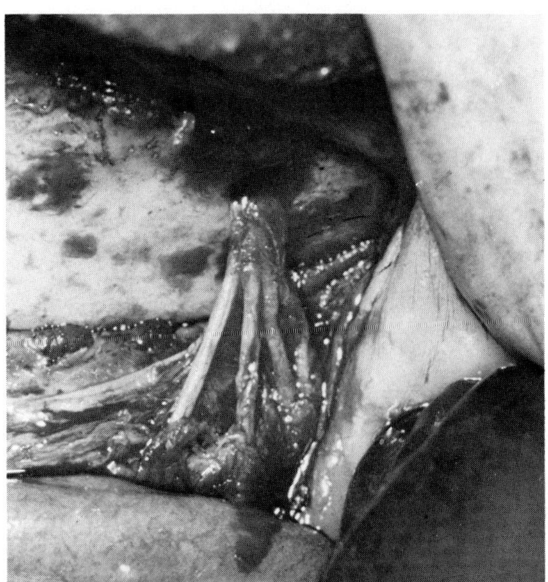

Figure 29–47. Dissection of the left mental nerve. To avoid avulsion of the mental nerve when the degloving technique is used, the three branches of the nerve can be dissected free of the soft tissues. This precaution permits the surgeon to work around and below the mental foramen and the inferior alveolar canal without endangering the nerve.

There is a real risk of injury to the mental nerve during the operative procedure. If the required amount of exposure is not great, a limited dissection about the mental foramen decreases the incidence of paresthesia. However, if a wide exposure is called for, the three branches of the mental nerve are carefully dissected free from the soft tissues (Fig. 29–47). Thus freed, the mental nerve and its branches are retracted and protected under direct vision, with less danger of tearing or sectioning as the subperiosteal exposure is continued posteriorly.

Extraoral and Intraoral Approaches to Mandibular Ramus

Extraoral Approach. The technique most frequently used is an incision below the angle of the mandible, occasionally referred to in the United States and Canada as the *Risdon approach* (see Fig. 29–56). The incision is marked with the patient in an upright position and is placed in or parallel to a skin fold of the neck, thus minimizing the noticeability of the subsequent scar. The angle of the mandible is reached by blunt dissection under the platysma in order to avoid injury to the marginal mandibular branch of the facial nerve. The systematic exposure of the marginal mandibular branch of the facial nerve as a protective measure has been abandoned by the authors because a number of patients developed unnecessary temporary paresis after this maneuver.

The *preauricular incision*, which curves into the supratragal notch or along the tragal rim, provides another route to the upper ramus and condyle; it is extended upward into the scalp or forward as a "hockeystick" into the sideburn for additional exposure. A combined preauricular and submandibular incision is particularly useful for working on both the upper and lower portions of the ramus; the parotid gland, facial nerve, and masseter are raised between the two incisions (see Chap. 30).

The preauricular incision can also be extended around the lobe of the ear, up into the retroauricular fold, and posteriorly over the mastoid process into the hairline. This extended incision is similar to that used in face lift operations. Excellent exposure of the parotid gland, masseter, and submandibular areas is gained.

Intraoral Approach. The intraoral approach to the mandibular ramus is through a *vertical incision* placed slightly laterally along the anterior border of the ramus (see Fig. 29–65*A*). The incision extends inferiorly and laterally to the molar region, following the bony oblique ridge, which continues from the anterior border of the ramus to the mental tubercle. Above the level of the occlusal plane, the incision should be made only through the mucosa and down to the buccinator. Below the level of the occlusal plane the cut is extended to the bone. A subperiosteal dissection can expose the entire ramus without the annoyance of having the buccal fat pad herniating into the wound. The incision can be prolonged anteriorly as a labiobuccal vestibular incision to expose the entire facial surface of the mandible.

Combined Extraoral and Intraoral Approach. In certain complex deformities, it may be advisable to use a dual approach to expose the body and ramus of the mandible. The mandibular body is exposed through the usual intraoral route; the ramus is uncovered through a submandibular or preauricular (extraoral) incision. The two dissections are joined after the periosteum of the bone has been raised.

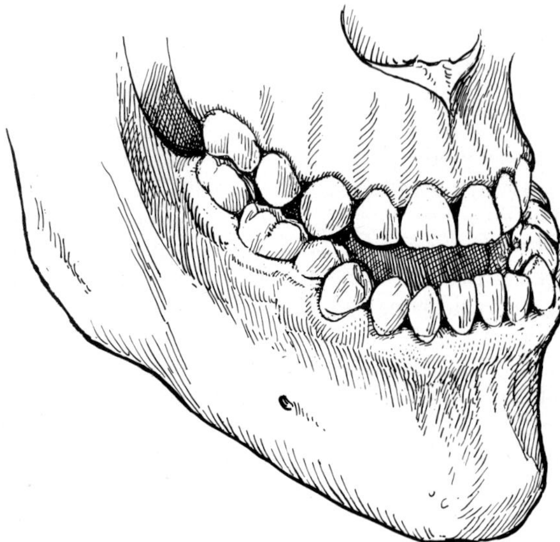

Figure 29–48. Mandibular prognathism with an anterior open bite. (After Hunter.)

PROGNATHISM

John Hunter in 1778 defined mandibular prognathism as follows: "the lower jaw projecting too far forwards so that the fore teeth pass before those of the upper jaw, when the mouth is shut; which is attended with inconvenience, and disfigures the face" (Fig. 29–48).

The basilar skeleton is oversized (macrognathia) and the lower jaw protrudes. The dentoalveolar structures are also anteriorly displaced in a characteristic Class III (Angle) malocclusion. Dentoalveolar relationships alone, however, cannot be used as the sole criterion in diagnosing mandibular prognathism, since a Class III malocclusion can also coexist upon a normal-sized mandible. Thus, the distinguishing feature is an enlarged mandibular skeleton. Cephalometric analysis confirms the relative anterior location of the mandible to the cranial base: the SNB angle is greater than normal.

Incipient mandibular prognathism can often be recognized early during the primary dentition stage. More frequently, evidence of the condition is not apparent until the second decade of life. The deformity and facial imbalance tend to increase in severity throughout adolescence. The dentoalveolar complex usually participates in the downward and forward facial displacement to create a Class III malocclusion.

Etiology

Mandibular prognathism can be hereditary or due to trauma or disease. The prevalence of prognathism in family members in certain ethnic groups is cited in support of the hereditary factor. The Habsburg royal family (of Spain) with its "Habsburg jaw" is a well-known historical example illustrated by Velasquez (Grabb, 1968). The family tree of many patients, however, is not similarly marked.

The role of trauma in mandibular prognathism is poorly defined. Early childhood injury to the condyles can induce growth (Jacobsen and Lund, 1972), usually unilateral in expression, rather than the more commonly observed inhibition of growth. This is probably the exception rather than the rule. Malunion following fractures of the jaw can lead to a prognathic deformity, abnormal occlusion of the teeth, and an open bite. Severe burn contractures of the neck in children can also cause protrusion of the anterior portion of the mandible. The first surgical correction of a lower jaw deformity described in the American literature (Hullihen, 1849) was performed to correct such a problem (see Fig. 29–181).

Patients with extensive lymphangiomas or hemangiomas that involve the lower face and tongue often have prognathism; this is due to the abnormally abundant blood supply, to involvement of the tongue, or both of these factors. Fibrous dysplasia is often associated with a prognathic mandible. Acromegaly is a well-known cause of prognathism due to endocrine imbalance. More esoteric examples are seen in patients with Klinefelter's syndrome or Paget's disease.

Underdevelopment of the maxilla can be associated in varying degrees with mandibular prognathism and it accentuates the mandibular deformity.

Classification

Because of numerous variations in size and shape of the mandibular body and ramus, many cephalometric studies have been made relating the jaws to the cranial base in order to define craniofacial patterns.

Prognathism theoretically can result from variations in either the dimension or the morphologic relationships of various craniofacial segments. Jaw length, for example, seems to be a less significant factor than the shape and size of the cranial base (Björk, 1947). In the typical case, the length of the body and the height of the ramus are not significantly greater than normal. Horowitz, Gerstman, and Converse (1969), reviewing 52 cases of mandibular prognathism, concluded that size discrepancy is not a primary problem, but is the result of a complex disturbance of the craniofacial relationships. Relative changes in the position and form of the mandible contribute to the deformity. Sanborn (1955) believed that the basic fault lies in the area of the gonial angle, as the angle is more obtuse than normal. He concluded that the Class III malocclusion is not mainly one of overgrowth but one of abnormal angulation between the ramus and the body. This conclusion may apply to the most common cases, but a review of the various types of mandibular prognathism confirms that the deformity can be produced by bone overgrowth; prognathism associated with acromegaly is such an example.

At least four distinct craniofacial patterns can be differentiated (Fig. 29–49):

1. A maxilla within the normal range of size associated with a mandible that is abnormally large. The result is a prominent appearance of the lower third of the face.

2. Underdevelopment of the maxilla coupled with an overdevelopment of the mandible. This is the finding in most cases of mandibular prognathism. An accentuated "underbite" is present, with the lower incisors overlapping the upper teeth in a Class III occlusal relationship.

3. An anterior open bite combined with mandibular prognathism. The clinical and cephalometric examination in most of these cases shows an abnormally wide (obtuse) gonial angle and inferior inclination of the mandibular body (steep mandibular plane). The prognathic deformity is compounded by the inability to occlude the anterior teeth.

4. Bimaxillary prognathism (or protrusion) in which both jaws are prognathic.

Sanborn (1955) (Fig. 29–50) classified mandibular prognathism according to anteroposterior jaw position: (1) the maxilla within and mandible anterior to the normal range; (2) the maxilla posterior to and mandible within normal range; (3) both maxilla and mandible within the normal range; and (4) the maxilla posterior to and mandible anterior to the normal range.

Pseudoprognathism of Mandible. In this condition the mandible is within the normal range of development but appears prognathic because of hypoplasia of the maxilla. The maxillary dentition is usually crowded into a constricted dental arch with a high arched palate. The pseudoprognathic appearance is alleviated by expanding the collapsed dental arch and surgically advancing the recessed maxilla.

Treatment of Mandibular Prognathism

Proper timing of the operation is essential. Correction of the mandibular prognathism should be delayed until the adolescent mandibular growth spurt is passed. In male patients the growth spurt is usually complete around the age of 17 or 18 years; females generally conclude this phase a few years earlier. An exact end point of growth is difficult to ascertain. However, serial lateral cephalograms spaced six months apart or radiograms of the wrist provide helpful information. In extreme cases with facial disfigurement, earlier operation can be recommended on the understanding that a second procedure may be required.

An unequivocal dividing line between a Class III dentoalveolar malocclusion (an orthodontic problem) and a mandibular skeletal prognathism (a surgical problem) cannot be declared. For practical purposes, the severity of the facial imbalance provides an acceptable guide to treatment, orthodontic management being reserved for the lesser deformities. The ideal goal is to achieve the maximal esthetic improvement commensurate with attainment of a stable functional occlusion.

Orthodontic Versus Surgical Treatment. As early as 1898, when discussing severe prognathism of the mandible, Angle condemned orthodontic interference as the sole method of treatment. He advised recognition of the limitations of orthodontic therapy. Orthodontic treatment produces changes in the relation and form of the dentoalveolar segment of the jaw, but it does not significantly influence the position and shape of the skeletal structures, i.e., the body and ramus of the mandible.

Although Angle's advice is heeded for the most part, growth predictions are not infallible. Thus, an uncomfortable situation can be created in which the orthodontist finds that years of childhood therapy may have gone for naught.

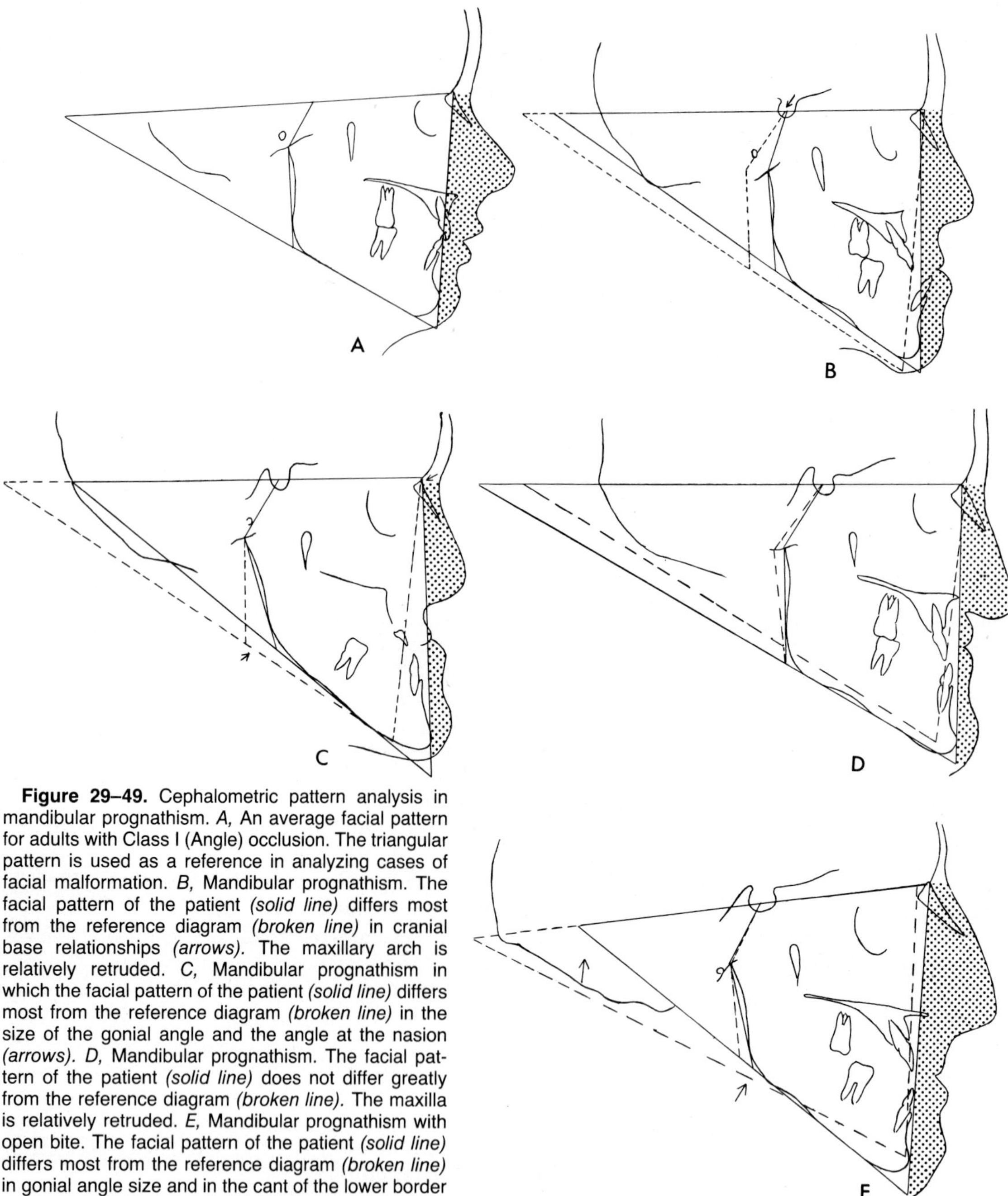

Figure 29–49. Cephalometric pattern analysis in mandibular prognathism. *A,* An average facial pattern for adults with Class I (Angle) occlusion. The triangular pattern is used as a reference in analyzing cases of facial malformation. *B,* Mandibular prognathism. The facial pattern of the patient *(solid line)* differs most from the reference diagram *(broken line)* in cranial base relationships *(arrows).* The maxillary arch is relatively retruded. *C,* Mandibular prognathism in which the facial pattern of the patient *(solid line)* differs most from the reference diagram *(broken line)* in the size of the gonial angle and the angle at the nasion *(arrows). D,* Mandibular prognathism. The facial pattern of the patient *(solid line)* does not differ greatly from the reference diagram *(broken line).* The maxilla is relatively retruded. *E,* Mandibular prognathism with open bite. The facial pattern of the patient *(solid line)* differs most from the reference diagram *(broken line)* in gonial angle size and in the cant of the lower border of the mandible to the cranial base line *(arrows).* (After Horowitz, Gerstman, and Converse, 1969.)

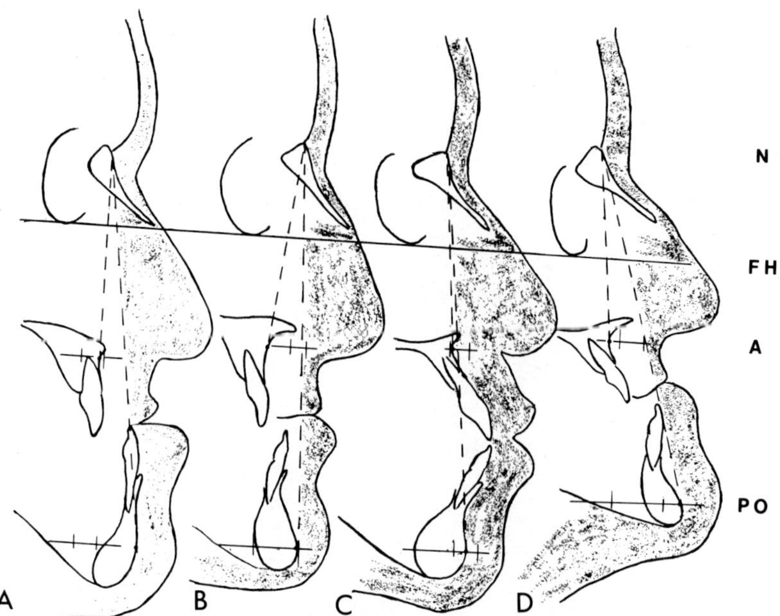

Figure 29–50. Cephalometric tracings representing the four main groups of Class III facial skeletal and soft tissue profiles. The short vertical lines at points A and PO designate the normal range or standard deviation of maxillary and mandibular prognathism. *A,* Those Class III patients presenting a maxilla within the normal range of prognathism but a mandible beyond the normal range of prognathism. *B,* Those with a maxilla below the normal range of prognathism and a mandible within the normal range of prognathism. *C,* Those with both maxilla and mandible within the normal range of prognathism. *D,* Those with a maxilla below the normal range of prognathism and a mandible beyond the normal range of prognathism. (After Sanborn, 1955.)

Orthodontic therapy, however, although incapable of completely correcting the skeletal deformity, is essential during the preoperative preparations and in the postoperative period to ensure a balanced, stable occlusion of the teeth.

Preoperative Planning. Preliminary planning is required to estimate the amount of recession of the mandible by either an operation on the ramus or the resection of a measured segment from the mandibular body. The differential diagnosis of prognathism is of practical significance in planning the operation, since one technique may be more appropriately applied to a particular problem than another.

Study of the dental casts is essential in analyzing the dentoalveolar relationships and evaluating the degree of required mandibular recession. Casts of the upper and lower teeth are placed in the existing occlusal relationship (Fig. 29–51). A vertical line is marked through the mesiobuccal cusp of the maxillary first molar and extended to the underlying mandibular tooth. The casts are then placed into the most ideal relationship, and the vertical line on the upper cast is again extended downward to cross the lower tooth (Fig. 29–51*B*). The distance between the lines on the lower cast indicates the extent of posterior displacement of the mandible required. The measurement should be made bilaterally; it is often necessary to recess one side more than the other when asymmetry is present.

In selected cases in which a mandibular deformation is responsible for an anterior open bite, the mandibular cast is cut at the appropriate level to allow for the correction. In other instances, however, the surgical correction of an anterior open bite should be directed at the maxilla (see p. 1358).

The interdigitation of the cusps of the teeth is studied. Preoperative and postoperative orthodontic therapeutic needs must also be determined. Proper orthodontic alignment reduces or eliminates the need for judicious spot grinding of interfering cusps to obtain the most favorable occlusion. An acrylic occlusal wafer (splint) may be required to overcome gross occlusal interferences.

The skeletal deformity is assessed on the

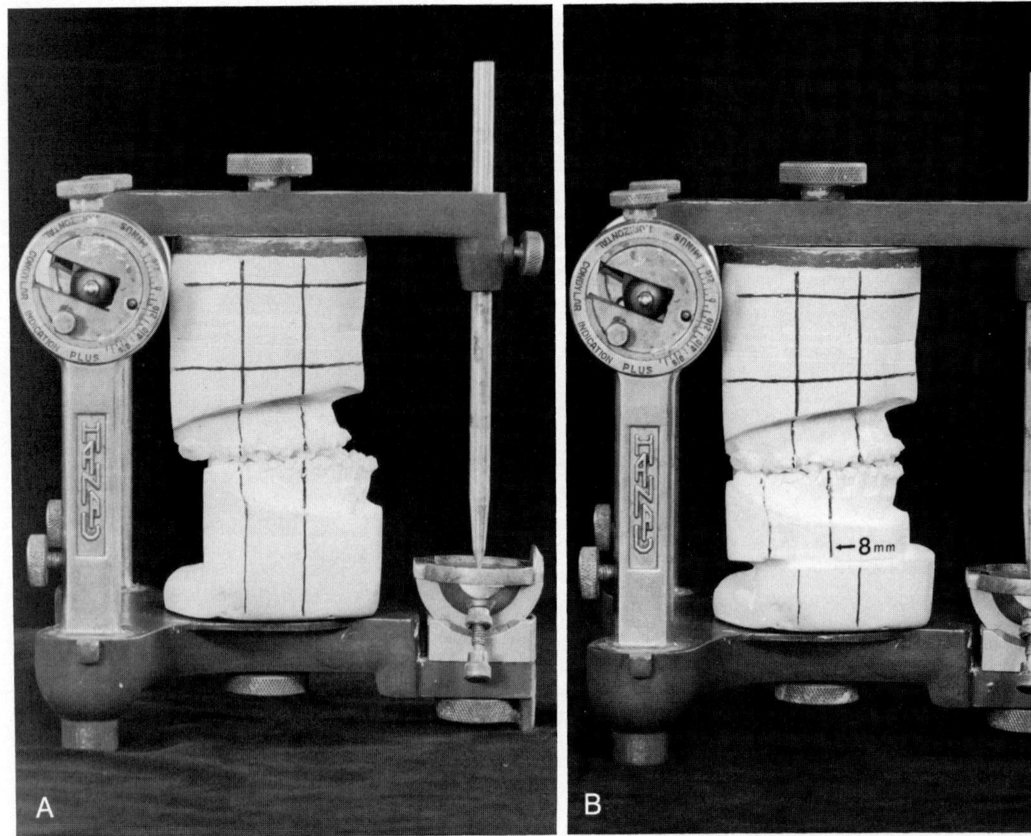

Figure 29–51. Dental cast study in a patient with mandibular prognathism. *A,* The casts of the upper and lower teeth are placed in existing occlusal relationships in an articulator. Note the vertical line marked through the mesiobuccal cusp of the maxillary first molar and extended to the underlying mandibular tooth. A second line passes through the maxillary canine and underlying mandibular tooth. *B,* The mandibular cast has been set back, placing the molars into a Class I relationship, and the incisors have been properly aligned. Note that the discrepancy in the lines represents the amount of surgical set-back (8 mm) needed to achieve this occlusion.

cephalometric roentgenogram and tracing. Cut-outs of the tracing are useful in the planning. Although in the last analysis the patient is usually more concerned about facial contour, the planning of the postoperative dental occlusion is a vital step in achieving a satisfactory long-term result.

Many variations in the deformity influence the choice of procedure. Precise definition of the problem permits the selection of the most desirable restorative measure.

Evolution of Techniques for Correction of Mandibular Prognathism. It is rewarding to review the operations that have been used in the past and to observe their gradual evolution toward present-day techniques.

Three approaches for the correction of mandibular deformities have been followed throughout the years. The first operation to correct a malocclusion, performed by Hullihen (1849), was focused on the mandibular body (see Fig. 29–181). The second approach by Jaboulay (1895) almost a half-century later was directed to the condylar area. The ramus was the last region to be explored; it was sectioned horizontally by Babcock (1910) to correct mandibular prognathism.

Evolution of Operations on Mandibular Body. Hullihen's patient was a young woman with a mandibular dentoalveolar deformity caused by scar contracture from a childhood burn of the lower face and neck. Using a hand saw, he sectioned the mandible transversely below the anterior teeth and removed a V-section from the premolar region. By tilting the anterior fragment backward and upward, the protrusion of the teeth and the open bite deformity were corrected. Blair was successful in performing a similar operation in 1887; his second attempt was a failure. The two operations were reported by Angle (1898). In the second case, total loss of the anterior fragment occurred through necrosis. This disaster was attributed to inadequate fixation; stabilization was limited to the use of a Barton bandage and direct interosseous wiring between the bone fragments. Angle emphasized the importance of postoperative fixation of the fragments, advice well heeded even to this day.

In 1906 von Eiselsberg described a step osteotomy of the body of the mandible to increase the surface of contact. Lane (1905), Pickrell (1912), and Pichler (1918) used vertical straight-line osteotomies. A curvilinear section was removed from the mandibular angle by Cryer (1913). Aller (1917) recommended the resection of a wedge of bone extending through the entire height of the mandibular body.

Little regard was given to protection of the inferior alveolar neurovascular bundle until Harsha (1912) preserved this structure while removing a vertical section of bone posterior to the molar teeth. New and Erich (1941) in one stage removed a segment of bone from a tooth-bearing portion of the mandible. Dingman (1944) advocated a two-stage straight-line osteotomy with preservation of the neurovascular bundle. In the first stage, the teeth in the line of the resection and surrounding dentoalveolar bone were removed through an intraoral approach down to the level of the inferior alveolar canal. Four weeks later, via an extraoral submandibular incision, the bone below the inferior alveolar canal was resected to complete the correction of the prognathism. A similar procedure performed in a single stage through an intraoral approach was suggested by Thoma (1948).

Converse and Shapiro (1952) developed a technique that combined the advantages of the step osteotomy, the intraoral approach, and a single operation. The step osteotomy was made anterior to the mental foramen, when possible, thus preserving the inferior alveolar nerve, the mental nerve, and the sensory innervation of the lower lip. When a resection behind the mental foramen was indicated, the neurovascular bundle was exposed by removing the outer cortical plate over the canal. The remaining bone was also removed, keeping the nerve protected under direct observation. The step osteotomy increased the bony surface of contact and thus decreased the risk of delayed union or nonunion, complications that occur more frequently with the straight-line resection.

A C-shaped variation of the step osteotomy of the mandibular body was described in 1966 by Toman. To provide additional contact between the fragments, Mayer (1971) reported a technique based on the sagittal splitting principle to shorten the body. All body osteotomies have limited application since they require the sacrifice of teeth.

Evolution of Operations on Mandibular Condyle. Bilateral condylectomy was advocated by Jaboulay (1895) for the correction of prognathism. Dufourmentel (1921) was a proponent of this method and resected a measured section of the condyle. Gonzalez-Ulloa (1951) and Merville (1970), using a similar technique, evaluated the amount of resection in the condylar area by cephalometric measurements. The predetermined amount of the head of the condyle was removed to permit correction of the prognathism. Because of the partial destruction of the temporomandibular joint and the associated secondary deformities and complications, condylectomy has been discontinued.

Section of the condylar neck with the Gigli saw (see Fig. 29–54) was popularized by Kostečka (1928). He later employed a similar technique to perform a horizontal osteotomy of the ramus. The blind operation, using the Gigli saw, has numerous disadvantages: soft tissue laceration, facial nerve injury, limited recession of the mandible, and frequent malunion and nonunion at the site of the osteotomy, establishing a pseudarthrosis and eliminating condylar function.

In 1945 Moose described an intraoral technique for subcondylar osteotomy, which he performed with a long-shank dental handpiece and a round bur. Smith and Robinson (1954) reported the extraoral removal of bone below the sigmoid notch and a section of the base of the condylar process. Satisfactory bone contact is obtained by this operation and the lateral pterygoid muscle, by its forward pull, assists in maintaining the bony contact.

Shortening the neck of the condyle is another technique that has been used for the unusual deformity characterized by elongation of this structure.

Evolution of Operations on the Mandibular Ramus. Lane (1905) used a horizontal osteotomy of the ramus for correction of retrognathism. Babcock (1909) applied this technique to the correction of mandibular prognathism. A Gigli saw was introduced through an intraoral puncture and passed through the skin posterior to the ramus. The other end of the saw was brought out through the skin anterior to the ramus. Ragnell (1938) and Hogeman (1951) made an opening through a postauricular incision to expose the posterior border of the ramus and section the ramus with a saw placed above the mandibular foramen.

Pichler and Trauner (1948) recommended an "inverted L" section of the ramus. The horizontal part of the "L" was made above the mandibular foramen, and the vertical limb was dropped down behind the foramen, parallel to the posterior border of the ramus.

A major contribution to the surgery of prognathism was made by Caldwell and Letterman in 1954. They described an operation for prognathism in which the ramus is split vertically from the sigmoid notch downward to a point just anterior to the mandibular angle (Fig. 29–52). The proximal (condylar) fragment laterally overlaps the distal (tooth-bearing) fragment when the mandibular body is recessed to correct the prognathic relationship. Robinson (1956) and Hinds (1957) made the osteotomy from the sigmoid notch to a point posterior to the mandibular angle: the oblique osteotomy of the ramus.

Kazanjian (1954) advocated direct exposure of the ramus through a submandibular inci-

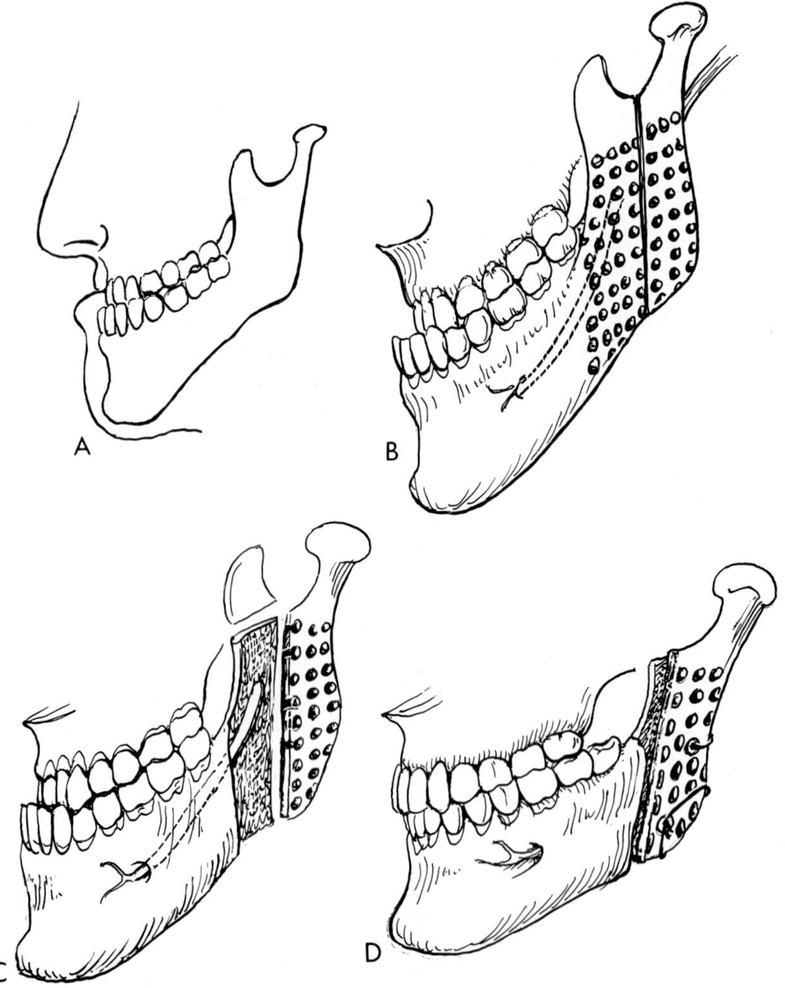

Figure 29–52. The operation of Caldwell and Letterman for the correction of prognathism. *A,* Outline of a prognathic mandible. *B,* The ramus is exposed and a series of drill holes are made through the outer cortex of the bone. The ramus is split by a vertical osteotomy. *C,* The outer table of the anterior fragment is removed, exposing the inferior alveolar neurovascular bundle. The coronoid process is amputated. *D,* The mandible is recessed; the fragments overlap. Care is taken to avoid compression of the inferior alveolar nerve. (After Caldwell and Letterman, 1954.)

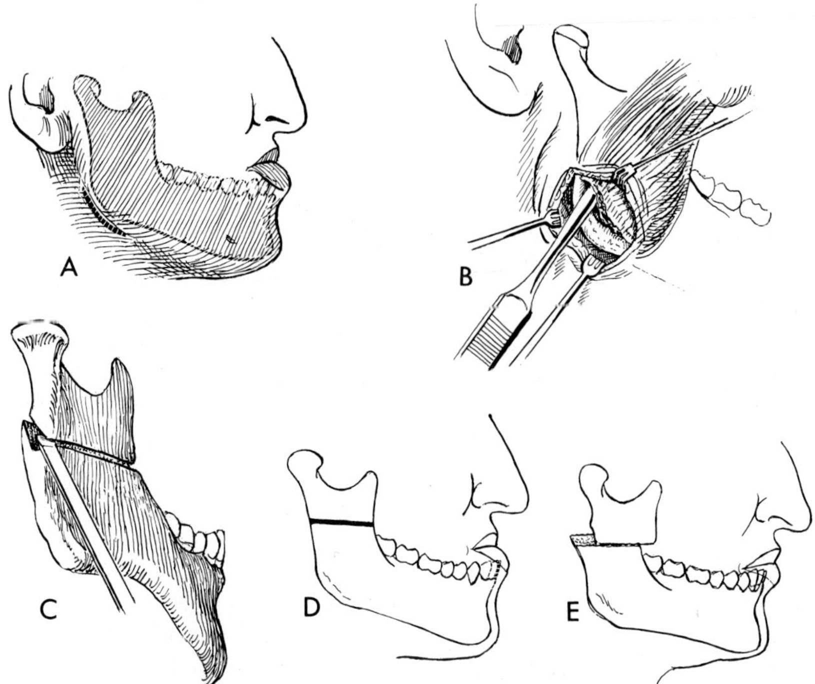

Figure 29–53. Technique of horizontal osteotomy of the ramus through the extraoral approach. *A*, The incision is made below the angle of the jaw. *B*, The periosteum and the masseter muscle are raised from the lateral aspect of the ramus. *C*, The osteotome cuts obliquely through the ramus of the mandible, above the level of entry of the inferior alveolar nerve. *D, E*, Backward displacement of the mandible after osteotomy. (After Kazanjian, 1954.)

sion and a beveled cut made with an osteotome above the mandibular foramen (Fig. 29–53). This method increased the surface of the contact between the bone fragments and decreased the tendency toward distraction of the segments by contraction of the lateral pterygoid muscle. Schuchardt (1954a), through an intraoral approach, used a step osteotomy that further increased the surface of contact.

In 1957 Obwegeser, enlarging upon the step osteotomy of Schuchardt and the bone surface of contact, introduced an intraoral splitting of the ramus in a sagittal plane. Dal Pont (1961) suggested an anterior extension of the osteotomy to include the lateral cortical plate over the posterior aspect of the mandibular body, thus further increasing the surface of contact between the fragments and aiding the stability of the fragments (see Fig. 29–65). Dautrey (1975) further modified the technique of the sagittal splitting of the ramus, performing a subcortical section, thus remaining lateral to the inferior alveolar canal (see Fig. 29–70).

At the present time, the most commonly used techniques to recess the mandible are the intraoral section of the ramus along the frontal plane *(the vertical or oblique osteotomy)* or along a sagittal plane *(the sagittal splitting osteotomy)*. Both procedures provide adequate bone contact between the fragments and rapid consolidation.

Surgical Correction of Mandibular Prognathism

Osteotomies of Condylar Region. Condylectomy has generally been abandoned as a technique for correction of mandibular prognathism. Destruction of a normal temporomandibular joint is a drastic procedure that is unnecessary now that simpler, less disabling corrective methods are available.

Osteotomies of the condylar neck are also historical procedures. Blind osteotomy (Kostečka, 1928) is needlessly dangerous in view of safer contemporary techniques (Fig. 29–54). In addition, the amount of mandibular recession is limited, the quantity of bone contact is sparse, and the small condylar fragments are difficult to control.

Osteotomies of Ramus

Horizontal Osteotomy of Ramus. The horizontal osteotomy was the first osteotomy of the ramus to be used to correct mandibular

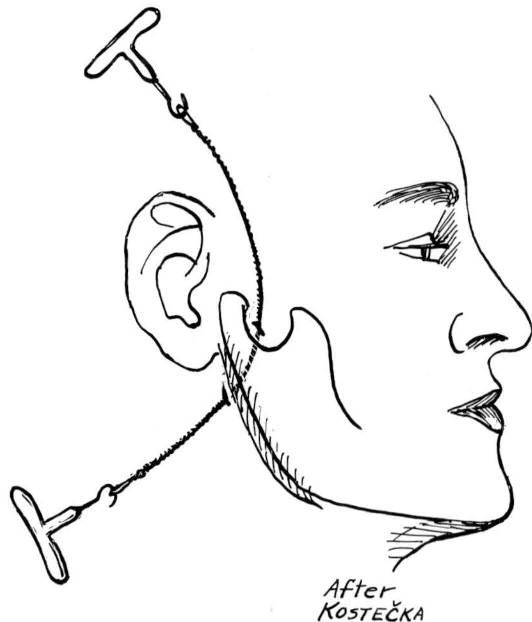

Figure 29–54. Kostečka's technique of osteotomy through the neck of the condyle with a Gigli saw. Kostečka used a similar technique to perform a horizontal osteotomy of the ramus.

prognathism (Babcock, 1909). A similar operation was performed by Blair (1915). An intraoral or extraoral approach can be used. Although the technique is simple, the number of complications are high; thus, it is rarely used.

The operation has several drawbacks. The area of contact between the fragments is small. Contraction of the temporalis and the lateral ptergyoid muscles tends to distract the proximal segment an average of 15 degrees away from the lower distal segment (Hogeman, 1951; Björk, Eliasson, and Sörensen, 1970). Muscle interposition into the gap leads to delayed union or nonunion. A long period (ten weeks) of intermaxillary fixation is necessary. Furthermore, Nordendram and Waller (1968) reported a relapse incidence of 52 per cent of patients, persistent paresthesia of the lower lip in 55 per cent, and 31 per cent root resorption of the mandibular incisors in patients followed postoperatively for at least one year. Injury to the facial nerve was also reported.

Vertical Osteotomy of Ramus. Caldwell and Letterman (1954) introduced the *vertical* osteotomy of the ramus to correct mandibular prognathism (Fig. 29–55). The ramus was split through an external (cutaneous) approach from the sigmoid notch to a point anterior to the mandibular angle (see Fig. 29–52). The cortical surface of the distal fragment was removed in the area of contact. The proximal segment was wired in position lateral to the distal fragment. To neutralize the pull exerted by the temporalis the coronoid process was detached at its base. Modifications were described by Georgiade and Quinn (1961), Smith and Chambers (1962), Van Zile (1963), and Converse (1964a).

Robinson (1956) and Hinds (1957) proposed a variation when they directed the osteotomy posterior to the mandibular angle: the *oblique* osteotomy (Fig. 29–55).

The techniques of vertical and oblique osteotomies of the ramus are essentially the same. The oblique section places the line of osteotomy further posterior to the mandibular foramen but furnishes a smaller proximal segment. The vertical cut theoretically provides a wider bone surface of contact, but the clinical implications are not significant.

TECHNIQUE OF VERTICAL–OBLIQUE OSTEOTOMY OF RAMUS (EXTERNAL APPROACH). Although this approach has been largely superseded by the intraoral route, it is still sometimes used. The cutaneous incision is made in one of the natural flexion creases of the neck below the angle of the mandible (Fig. 29–56*A*). When properly placed, the resulting scar is inconspicuous. Individuals predisposed to hypertrophic scar formation, black patients in particular, should be operated on by an intraoral technique.

The proposed incision should be marked with the patient upright, and the teeth should be in occlusion so that the mandibular angle

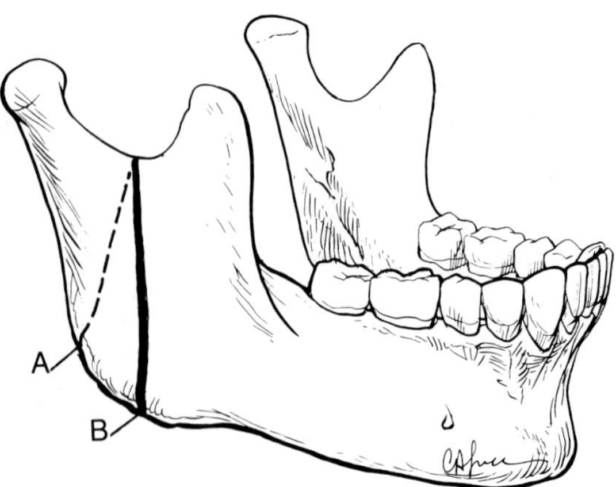

Figure 29–55. The oblique *(A)* and vertical *(B)* osteotomies of the mandibular ramus.

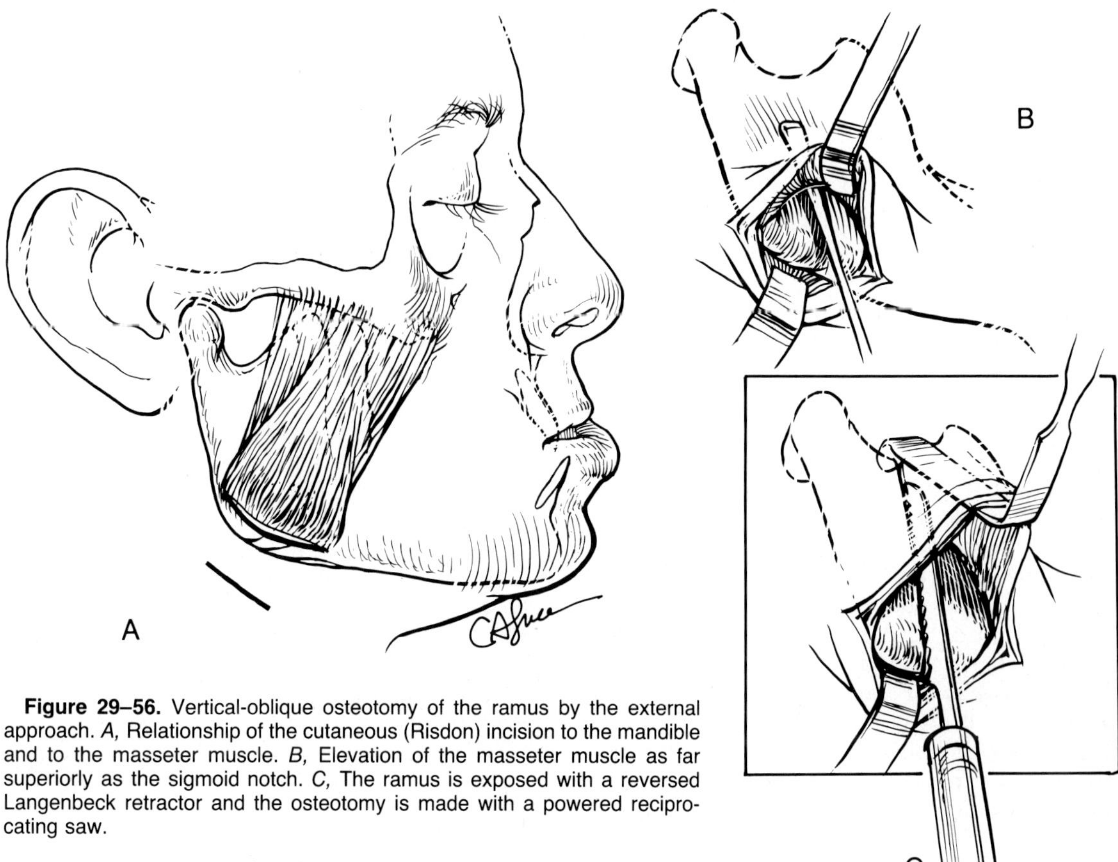

Figure 29–56. Vertical-oblique osteotomy of the ramus by the external approach. *A,* Relationship of the cutaneous (Risdon) incision to the mandible and to the masseter muscle. *B,* Elevation of the masseter muscle as far superiorly as the sigmoid notch. *C,* The ramus is exposed with a reversed Langenbeck retractor and the osteotomy is made with a powered reciprocating saw.

can be located by palpation. An incision 2 to 3 cm in length and a fingersbreadth below the inferior border of the angle usually provides sufficient exposure. Sharp dissection is carefully continued through the platysma. The tissues are then separated bluntly to expose the angle of the mandible without endangering the marginal mandibular branch of the facial nerve.

EXPOSURE OF LATERAL SURFACE OF RAMUS. Although the skin incision (Risdon) is short, careful retraction with appropriate retractors gives sufficient exposure (Fig. 29–56*B*). The periosteum is incised along the lower border of the mandible and posteriorly around the angle (Fig. 29–56*B*). The masseter muscle is raised from the bone with a periosteal elevator. The subperiosteal elevation is continued superiorly to the sigmoid notch and the base of the condylar and coronoid processes. Reflection of the periosteum from the posterior border should be limited to the inferiormost portion to maintain the greatest amount of soft tissue attachment to the proximal fragment.

Illumination is essential, and a fiberoptic lighted retractor or headlamp is particularly helpful. The angulated retractor should have a lip that fits into the sigmoid notch (Fig. 29–56*C*). The entire lateral surface of the ramus and the sigmoid notch are readily identified.

In cases of extreme prognathism, neutralization of the temporalis is advised. Caldwell (1964) stated that the coronoid process must be sectioned if the correction is greater than 10 mm, to allow unrestricted posterior movement of the jaw. In contrast, according to Hinds and Kent (1972), section of the base of the coronoid is rarely required; they have recessed the mandible for up to 23 mm without freeing the coronoid process. However, Hinds and Girotti (1967) recommended resection of the coronoid process to overcome the pull of the temporalis when an associated anterior bite is closed. This point may be moot since, in general, ramal sectioning procedures to close anterior open bite deformities are rarely indicated now because of the problem of relapse.

EXPOSURE OF MEDIAL SURFACE OF RAMUS.

In the past a medial ramal subperiosteal dissection along the path of the osteotomy was performed. If a reciprocating powered saw is used instead of a drill to make the cut, this dissection can be omitted. The reciprocating saw works on a vibrating principle and, when properly used, does not lacerate the underlying soft tissue. A rotating drill, however, can readily catch the underlying soft tissue on contact.

Osteotomy. For reasons listed above, the osteotomy is best made with a powered reciprocating saw (Fig. 29–56*C*). The sigmoid notch and the angle of the mandible are the key landmarks. In addition, on some mandibles an antilingual prominence may be present that provides a clue to the location of the mandibular foramen.

The cut should begin slightly posterior to the deepest portion of the sigmoid notch. If a vertical path is chosen, it will end just anterior to the angle. An oblique osteotomy terminates just posterior to the angle and has the advantage of carrying the cut further posterior and away from the mandibular foramen. Nevertheless, in either case the inferior alveolar neurovascular bundle should be free of damage if the osteotomy is properly executed.

The saw blade should also be directed posteriorly to create a bevel that further carries the osteotomy away from the mandibular foramen. In addition, such a bevel increases the area of cancellous bone exposure, which encourages bone healing and also decreases the protrusion of the tip of the proximal segment. The working surface of the saw should be generously irrigated with normal saline to minimize the heat production that is detrimental to healing.

REPOSITIONING OF FRAGMENTS. After both ramal sections are completed, the distal segment can be displaced posteriorly with ease to the desired occlusion (Fig. 29–57). Intermaxillary fixation is achieved to maintain the desired position. Despite careful presurgical orthodontic alignment, residual occlusal interferences may remain. These can be detected on dental models made before the operation. An acrylic occlusal splint can be fabricated preoperatively to compensate for these dental irregularities.

After the jaws are indexed, the proximal fragments must be positioned laterally to overlap the distal segment, and a check must be made to ensure that the condyles are seated well into the glenoid fossa. Furthermore, in order to provide bone to bone contact, the insertion of the medial pterygoid muscle as well as any intervening adjacent soft tissues must be stripped from the medial surface of the proximal fragment.

Coaptation of the two bone surfaces is afforded by continuous traction of the lateral pterygoid muscle and the remaining attached portions of the medial pterygoid muscle, which exert a forward and medial pull and maintain firm contact between the bone fragments (Fig. 29–58). Because of this favorable adducting influence and the propensity of the condylar segment to self-settle in the glenoid fossa, it has been said that interosseous wir-

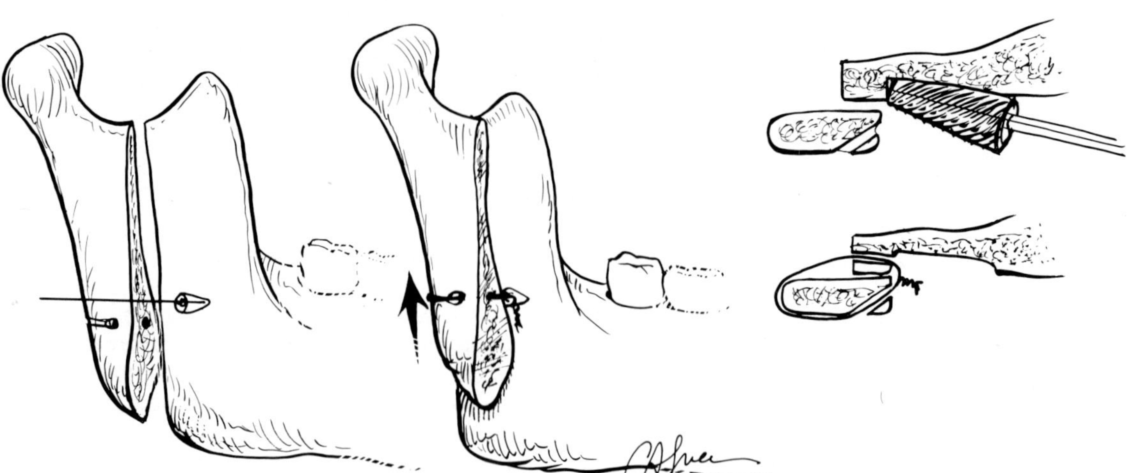

Figure 29–57. Set-back of the distal segment with overlapping of the ramal fragments. Contouring of the condylar fragment may be indicated, and removal of the attached medial pterygoid is necessary to ensure bone to bone apposition. Note the technique of interosseous wire fixation of the ramal fragments.

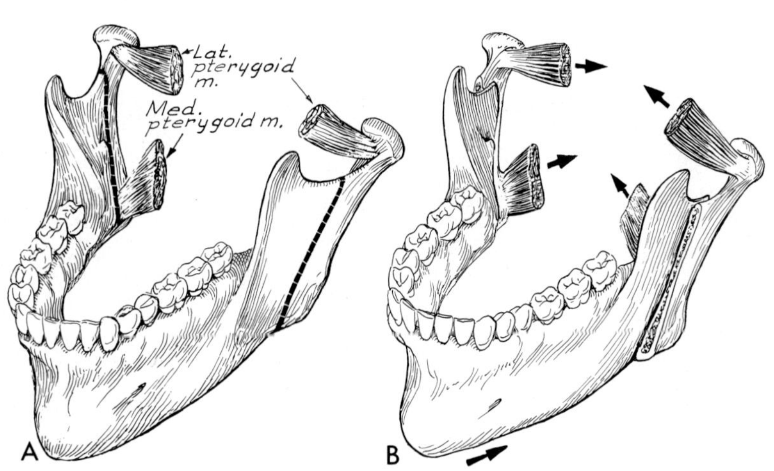

Figure 29–58. Direction of pull of lateral pterygoid muscle. *A,* Note the insertion and the direction of pull exerted by the lateral pterygoid muscle. *B,* The lateral pterygoid muscle tends to exert medial traction upon the condylar fragment, thus maintaining the fragments in close apposition after vertical section of the ramus. Direct interosseous wiring or fixation usually is not required.

ing of the fragments is not necessary. For the most part, this is true; however, there is also a tendency for the proximal segment to descend (condylar sag) out of the fossa. With the external approach, securing the fragments with a No. 26 or 28 gauge interosseous wire is a simple matter. Thus, a few extra moments spent seem to be worthwhile. The drill hole in the proximal segment should be placed at a lower position than that in the distal fragment. With this arrangement, the condylar segment is pulled into the glenoid fossa as the wire is loosely twisted (see Fig. 29–57). It should be recalled that the purpose of the wire is to prevent caudal drift of the condyle-bearing fragment; thus, it should not be overtightened in order not to create excessive pressure in the joint and produce temporomandibular joint pain.

The wound is irrigated and closed in layers. The use of a drain and a head dressing is optional, and for the most part unnecessary. Rigid internal fixation with miniplates and screws cannot be effectively applied.

Greater bone surface contact has been recommended as a theoretical advantage of using the vertical osteotomy. The trade-off is that the line of section is closer to the mandibular foramen. Clinically, the difference in the rate and quality of osseous union between the vertical and oblique osteomies is insignificant. Nonunion is rare after six weeks of intermaxillary fixation (Fig. 29–59).

TECHNIQUE OF OBLIQUE OR VERTICAL OSTEOTOMY OF RAMUS (INTRAORAL APPROACH). The intraoral approach avoids a cutaneous scar and possible injury to the marginal mandibular branch of the facial nerve. Winstanley (1968) described an intraoral oblique subcondylar osteotomy approached from the lateral surface of the ramus. Herbert, Kent, and Hinds (1970) and Wilbanks (1971) brought the osteotomy further down, posterior to the mandibular angle (oblique osteotomy). A similar technique can be employed to bring the line of osteotomy anterior to the angle (vertical osteotomy) (see Fig. 29–55).

The lateral surface of the ramus is exposed through an incision from the midramal region to the buccal sulcus opposite the second mandibular molar. Above the level of the occlusal plane, the incision should be confined to the mucosa and the underlying buccinator should be left intact. By sparing the buccinator, the annoying herniation of the buccal fat pad (Bichat) into the wound is prevented. Below the level of the occlusal plane, the cut is extended to the bone.

A subperiosteal dissection reflects the soft tissues off the anterior and lateral surface of the ramus. Detachment of the remaining insertion of the masseter and the internal pterygoid muscles along the posterior and inferior border of the mandible is completed with a sharply curved pterygomasseteric sling periosteal stripper (Fig. 29–60). The entire lateral surface of the ramus below the level of the sigmoid notch can be exposed by inserting a Bauer intraoral sigmoid notch retractor into the sigmoid notch and engaging a Le Vasseur-Merrill retractor around the posterior border of the mandible (Fig. 29–61*A*,*B*). The retractor has an incorporated fiberoptic bundle.

The osteotomy is performed with an offset oscillating saw (Fig. 29–61*C*). The saw blade

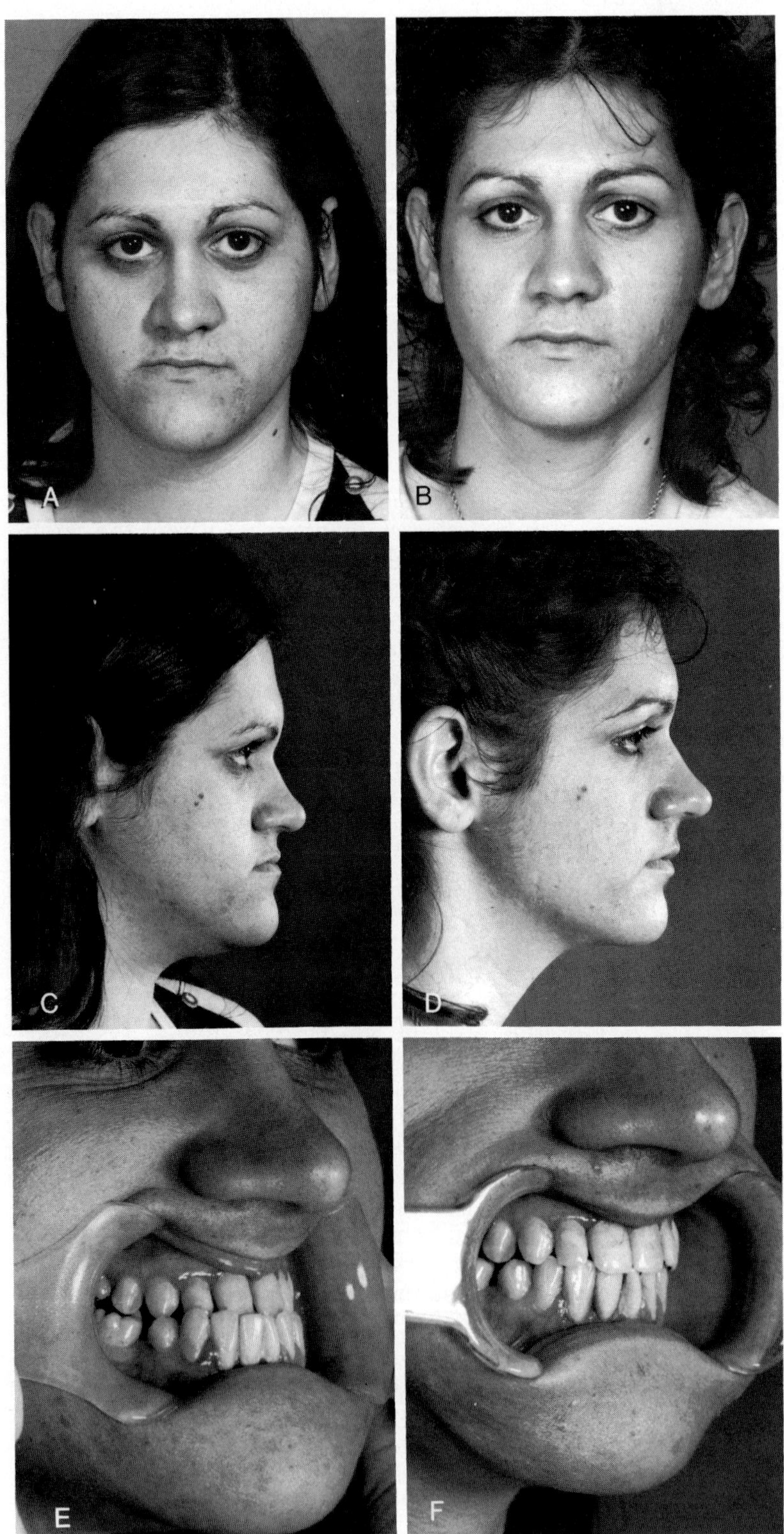

Figure 29–59. Vertical osteotomy of the ramus through a cutaneous incision. *A, C, E,* Preoperative views. *B, D, F,* Postoperative views. Note the inconspicuous skin scar. The patient also underwent preoperative and postoperative orthodontic therapy.

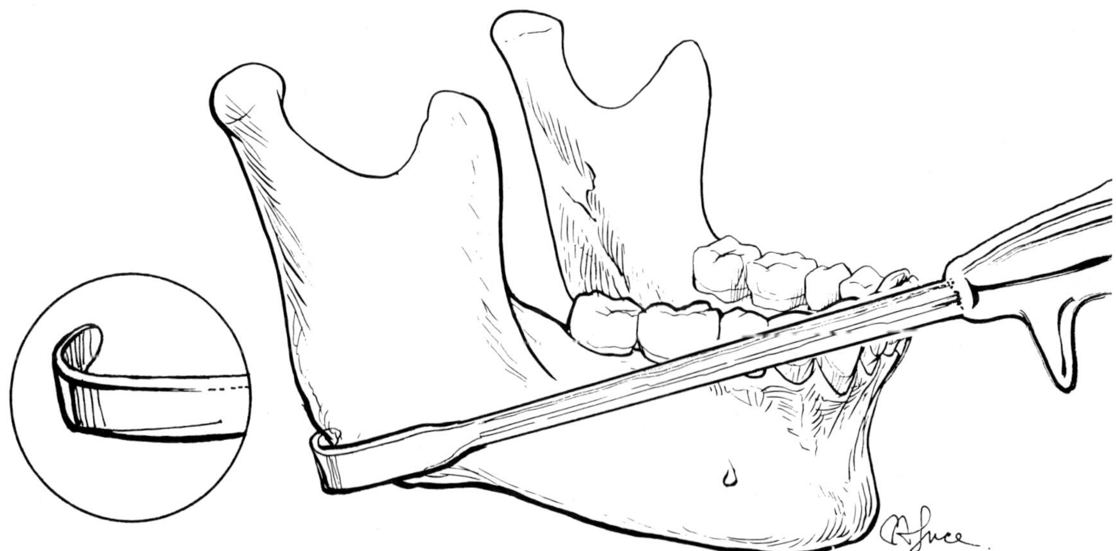

Figure 29–60. Elevation of the soft tissues with a sharply curved pterygomasseteric sling periosteal elevator. Inset shows curved end.

is 10 to 12 mm in length and, when properly used, does not usually harm soft tissue because of its oscillating cutting principle. Either the oblique or the vertical osteotomy path can be used (see Fig. 29–55), depending on the preference of the surgeon, for reasons stated earlier. It is best to begin the osteotomy at the midvertical level of the ramus behind the mandibular foramen. On some mandibles, a slight bone elevation (antilingular prominence) is present on the lateral surface of the ramus, which corresponds to the location of the mandibular foramen on the medial surface. After the saw blade penetrates the medial cortical plate, the blade is turned 45 degrees and directed slightly posterior to the midsigmoid notch. After this, the blade is redirected toward the anterior (vertical osteotomy) or posterior (oblique osteotomy) region of the mandibular angle. Throughout the cutting, saline irrigation should be provided to prevent burning of the bone by the saw.

The proximal fragment is now loose and is displaced laterally as the mandible is retruded. As the posterior fragment is rotated laterally, the medial pterygoid muscle is stripped off, and the segment is allowed to find its position over the lateral aspect of the distal fragment. After the contralateral osteotomy is completed in a similar manner, intermaxillary fixation is established. The lateral position of the proximal segments is confirmed. The intraoral wounds are irrigated with normal saline solution and closed by catgut sutures. Drains and pressure dressing are not required (Fig. 29–62).

TECHNIQUE OF INVERTED L-OSTEOTOMY. A variation of the vertical-oblique osteotomy is an inverted L cut. A chief advantage of this osteotomy is that the path of pull of the temporalis is not altered since its insertion remains with the proximal fragment. It should be considered when the mandible must be moved in a posterior direction in excess of 10 mm. Greater displacement could create an unfavorable relationship between the coronoid process and the condyle.

The procedure is similar to that of the vertical-oblique osteotomy. Additional dissection is required on the medial aspect of the ramus above the level of the mandibular foramen. The same retractors can be used for exposure. After the vertical component of the osteotomy is made, a horizontal cut is performed with a side-cutting Lindemann bur or a reciprocating saw (Fig. 29–63). The proximal fragment is managed in a similar manner as that of the vertical/oblique osteotomy but wiring of the fragments is required to combat the pull of the temporalis muscle.

Advantage and Disadvantage of Vertical and Oblique Osteotomies of Ramus (Extraoral and Intraoral Approaches). The main advantages of these techniques are the facility of execution and avoidance of injury to the inferior alveolar nerve. Teeth

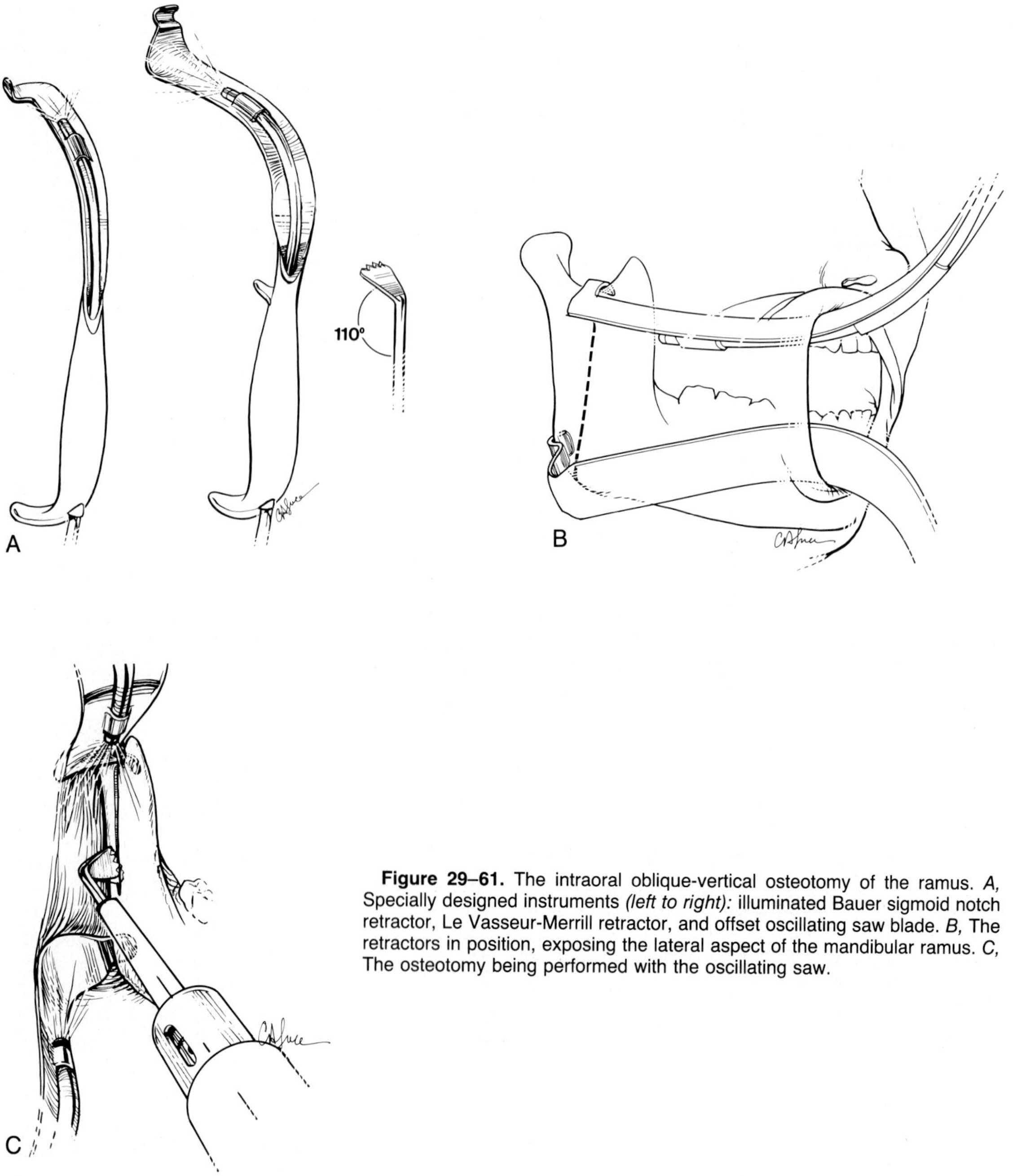

110°

A

B

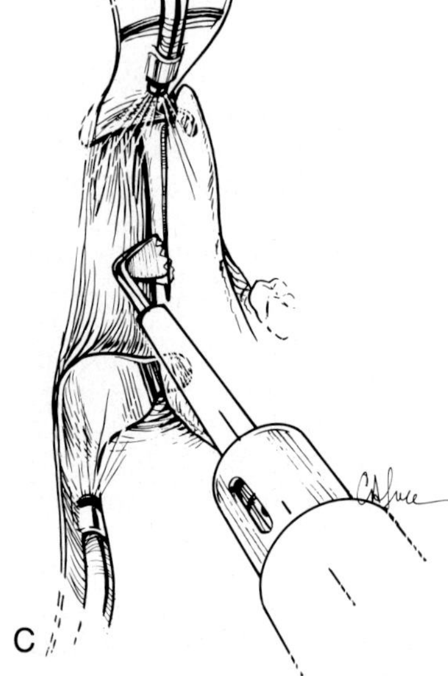

Figure 29–61. The intraoral oblique-vertical osteotomy of the ramus. *A,* Specially designed instruments *(left to right):* illuminated Bauer sigmoid notch retractor, Le Vasseur-Merrill retractor, and offset oscillating saw blade. *B,* The retractors in position, exposing the lateral aspect of the mandibular ramus. *C,* The osteotomy being performed with the oscillating saw.

do not have to be sacrificed as is sometimes required in body section techniques.

The disadvantage of the extraoral approach is the cutaneous scar; however, if the incision is properly placed the mature scar is difficult to detect. The intraoral approach should be used in patients with tendencies toward hypertrophic and keloidal scar formation and in those who object to an external scar. Furthermore, the external approach incurs the risk of injury to the marginal mandibular branch of the facial nerve.

The intraoral approach is more difficult to perform. Special instrumentation is necessary to provide the required exposure and to execute the osteotomy. Since access is limited, the procedure may not be applicable to patients with restricted jaw opening and to those with heavy masseteric musculature. In addition, it has been recommended that the intraoral approach be avoided when the angle of mandibular divergence as measured on a submental vertex roentgenogram is less than 130 degrees (Massey and associates, 1974). However, in the authors' experience the submental roentgenogram represents a needless step (Niebergall and Mercuri, 1985). Only rarely is it not possible to perform the osteotomy with present-day equipment. After the dissection of the lateral surface of the ramus is completed, the feasibility of the technique can be determined. If the exposure is deemed to be inadequate, one could immediately change to a sagittal splitting osteotomy of the ramus (see p. 1247).

Another disadvantage of the vertical or oblique osteotomy is the need for continuous postoperative intermaxillary fixation. Rigid internal fixation with miniplates and screws cannot be effectively applied.

Shape of Mandible After Vertical or Oblique Osteotomy of Ramus. Patients with mandibular prognathism generally have a mandibular angle that is more obtuse than normal. This gives an unpleasant "straight-line" appearance from the condyle to the chin of the lower jaw. It is widely believed that the vertical and oblique sections of the ramus will improve this contour defect. This precept is not confirmed by longitudinal data. During the immediate postoperative period, the gonial angle is less obtuse and the mandibular contour has a more acceptable appearance. However, cephalometric follow-up studies (Kelsey, 1968: Cunat and Gargiulo, 1973) made one to two years after the operation showed that the angle remodels itself to its preoperative configuration.

Postoperative Condylar Changes. Temporomandibular joint dysfunction has not been a postoperative problem. When the proximal (condylar) fragment is overlapped laterally over the distal fragment, a change in relation and a torquing force between the condyle and the glenoid fossa are produced. Ware and Taylor (1968) studied this problem with serial roentgenography (Fig. 29–64). Three months after the operation, the condylar head was found to be displaced downward and forward out of the glenoid fossa. The displacement is probably due to gravity and the unopposed action of the lateral pterygoid muscle. The condyle, then, slowly moves in an upward and posterior direction toward a normal position. At the end of one year, the condyle was found to be in its preoperative location. It was concluded that the postoperative condylar change was most likely due to remodeling. Because of the positive remodeling of the condylar region, wiring the fragments is not thought to be important (Isaacson and associates, 1978; Johanson and associates, Lilja, 1979; Åstrand, Eckerdal, and Sund, 1983).

Others feel that control of the proximal fragment by wire fixation is a worthwhile additional step to stabilize the occlusal relationships (Thoma, 1961; Hall, Chase, and Payor, 1975; Egyedi, Houwing, and Juten, 1981). In this regard, the time of treatment also deserves to be considered. If the operation is performed toward the end of the orthodontic treatment, the orthodontist would prefer to complete the case as soon as possible and remove the braces so that the patient can be placed in retention. Ideally, the dental arches should be aligned with the teeth in centric occlusion and the jaws in centric relation. However, with the condyles in a downward and forward position, centric relation is not achieved. Thus, wiring the fragments to prevent condylar sag is frequently a worthwhile extra step.

Via an extraoral approach, wiring the two segments is not a difficult task. Through the intraoral approach, it is a challenging feat. Circumramal wires (Indresano, 1975) and percutaneous pins (Joy and Cronan, 1983) can be used.

Interosseous wire fixation still allows a little play between the fragments and permits the muscular forces to help settle the seg-

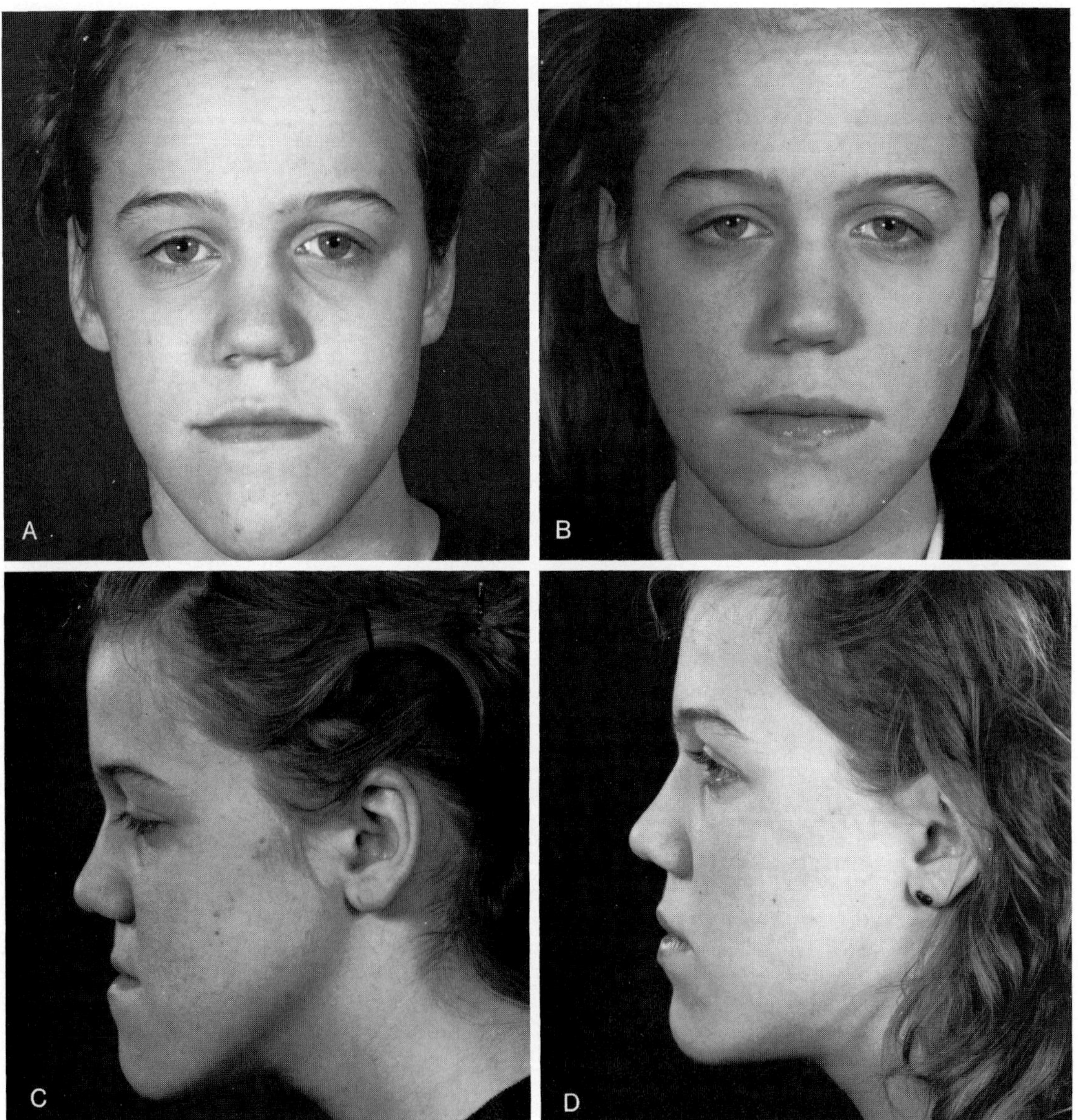

Figure 29–62. Correction of mandibular prognathism by an intraoral vertical-oblique osteotomy of the ramus (see Fig. 29–61) and orthodontic therapy. *A, C, E,* Preoperative views of a 15 year old girl with mandibular prognathism, Class III malocclusion, and occlusal disparities. *B, D, F,* Appearance after completion of treatment.

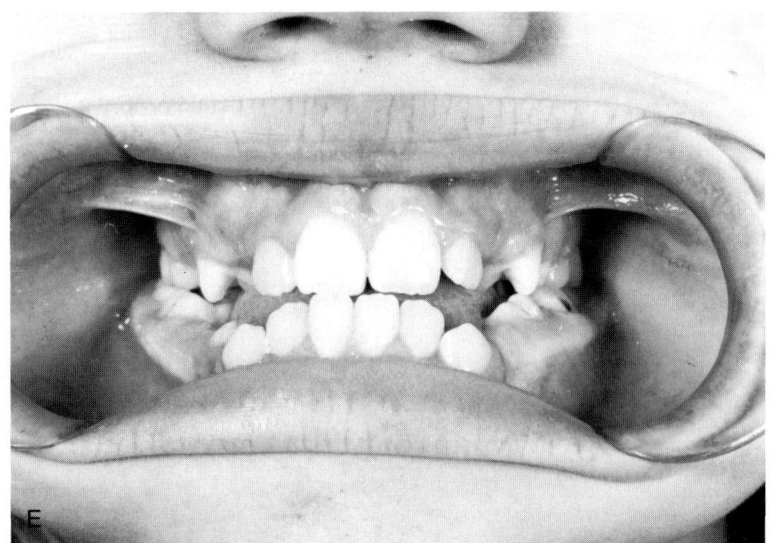

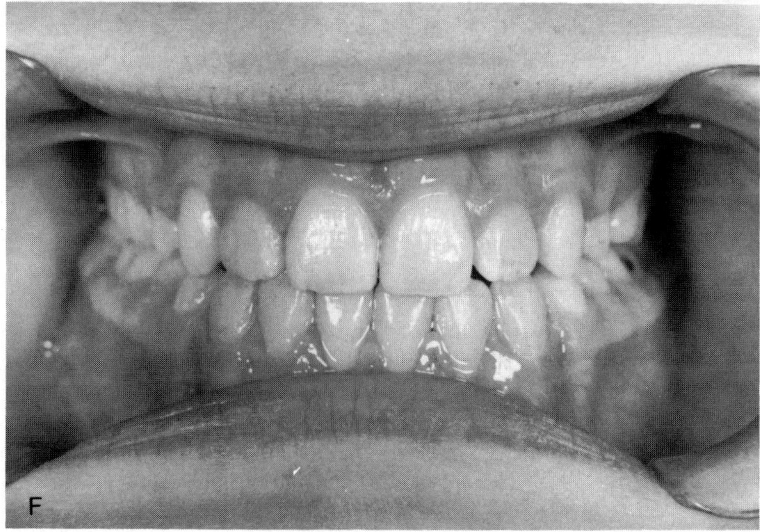

Figure 29–62 *Continued*

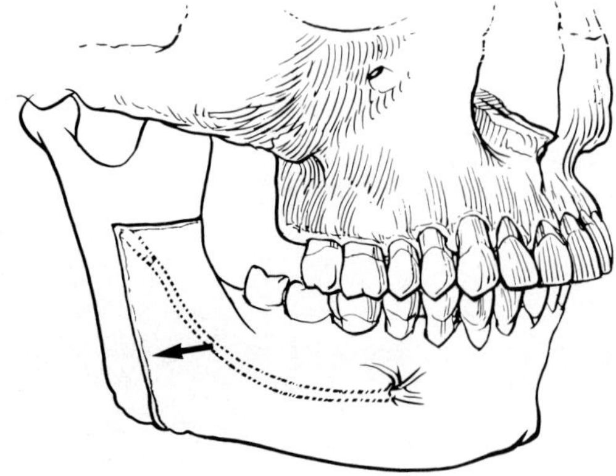

Figure 29–63. Inverted L osteotomy. Lines of osteotomy and the planned direction *(arrow)* of the mandibular recession. The condylar fragment will be buccal to the tooth-bearing segment.

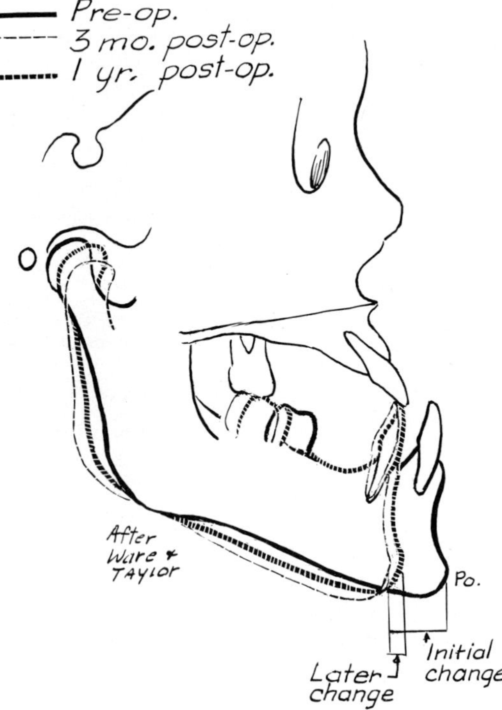

Figure 29–64. Cephalometric tracing showing changes of the mandible after vertical osteotomy of the ramus. Three months postoperatively, the condylar head is out of the glenoid fossa, and pogonion (Po) is in the most retruded position. One year postoperatively, the condylar head returns to a more normal relationship with the glenoid fossa. A small degree of relapse has occurred at pogonion. Note also that the mandibular angle contour remains essentially unchanged. (After Ware and Taylor, 1968.)

ments. The disadvantage of using a pin is that it prevents this self-adjustment feature. To simplify the intraoral wire fixation, Ricketts and Kawamoto (1980) advocated a technique that uses a large cross-cut fissure bur to place a countersink in the distal fragment (see Fig. 29–57). A 1 mm wire passing drill is used to create a tunnel from the depth of the countersink through the posterior border of the distal segment. The same drill is used to place a similar passage, which is more inferiorly placed, through the proximal fragment. A 28 gauge stainless steel wire is threaded through both drill holes and loosely tightened to return the condyle into the glenoid fossa and to prevent condylar sag.

Relapse. Postoperative cephalometric studies (Poulton, Taylor, and Ware, 1963; Hinds and Kent, 1972; Bell and Creekmore, 1973) show an anterior movement of pogonion of 1 to 3 mm. The skeletal relapse becomes stabilized during the first year. The dentoalveolar intermaxillary relationship does not appear to be unfavorably changed, probably because of the improved cuspal interdigitation and accommodation of the pliable alveolar bone. Whether the fragments are wired together has no effect on relapse (Åstrand, Eckerdal, and Sund, 1983).

Nerve Injury. Injury to the marginal mandibular branch of the facial nerve is always a possibility if the dissection is continued deep to the platysma muscle. The auriculotemporal (Frey) syndrome (Kopp, 1968) and parotid fistula formation (Goldberg, Marco, and Googel, 1973) have also been reported as complications following the extraoral approach. These complications, although rare when the technique is correctly performed, should not occur after the intraoral approach.

Technique of Sagittal (Sagittal-split) Osteotomy of Ramus. The technique of vertical section of the ramus divides this structure along a *frontal* plane. In contrast, the technique of sagittal section, as its name implies, divides the ramus along a *sagittal* plane.

As mentioned earlier in the chapter, Schuchardt (1954a) described a step osteotomy through the intraoral approach directed along the sagittal plane of the ramus, thus increasing the surface of contact between the fragments. Obwegeser (1957) refined this concept by increasing the surface of contact. He extended the vertical distance between the medial and lateral horizontal cuts of the ramus and created the sagittal split with an osteotome. Dal Pont (1959, 1961) increased the surface of contact still further by including the retromolar region and lateral cortical plate of the body of the mandible (Fig. 29–65). The wide surface of contact and the avoidance of an external incision have made the Obwegeser–Dal Pont sagittal-splitting osteotomy a popular technique; this is especially so with the use of rigid internal fixation.

The operation is performed through an incision made along the anterior border of the ramus and extended downward and laterally over the buccal surface of the body of the mandible, similar to that used in the intraoral vertical-oblique ramal osteotomy (Fig. 29–65*A*). The portion of the incision along the anterior border of the ramus should be kept lateral to the oblique line. Lateral placement of the incision facilitates wound closure after intermaxillary fixation is applied.

Subperiosteal dissection of the medial and lateral aspects of the ramus is begun (Fig. 29–65*B*). The masseter is disinserted from the lateral aspect of the ramus. The reflection of the soft tissue should be confined to that needed for exposure. After the sagittal splitting, the blood supply to the distal tip of the proximal fragment will be greatly diminished and preservation of the neighboring soft tissue attachments will be welcomed.

When the periosteum is being elevated over the medial aspect of the ramus, care must be taken in the area of the lingula to avoid injuring the inferior alveolar neurovascular bundle as it enters the mandibular foramen. The periosteum is carefully raised above the neurovascular bundles, which, with retraction and illumination, can readily be seen. The subperiosteal dissection extends to the posterior border of the ramus. Specially designed retractors, of which there are various models (Fig. 29–66), are hooked onto the posterior border of the ramus to provide additional exposure. Obwegeser advocated using a bur to remove some bone from the anteromedial aspect of the ramus, which is continuous with the oblique line. The lingula, the inferior alveolar neurovascular bundle, and the posterior portion of the medial ramus then come into the operator's line of vision as a result of the removal of bone.

The ramus is exposed and ready for the sagittal splitting procedure. A horizontal cut is made through the medial cortex approxi-

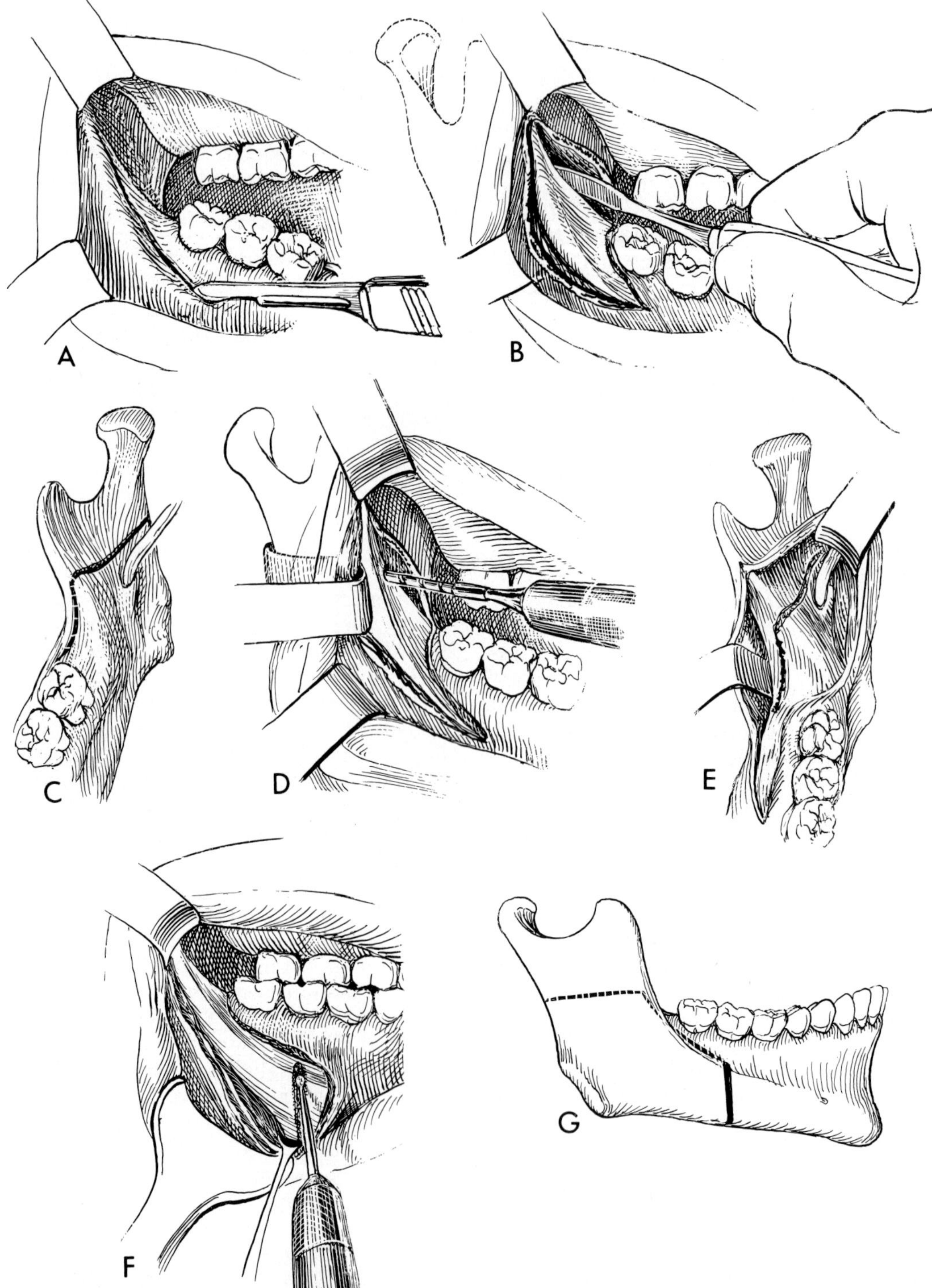

Figure 29–65. Technique of Obwegeser-Dal Pont sagittal osteotomy of the ramus. *A,* An incision is made along the anterior border of the ramus following the oblique line. *B,* Subperiosteal elevation of both the medial and lateral surfaces is begun. *C,* The medial cortical osteotomy is placed above the level of the mandibular foramen and is continued anteriorly along the oblique line. *D,* Bone can be removed from the medial aspect of the anterior border of the ramus to permit a better view of the lingula and the mandibular foramen region. The Lindemann spiral bur or reciprocating saw cuts the medial cortex above the foramen. *E,* The medial section of the cortex is completed. *F,* A vertical cut through the lateral cortex in the region of the second molar tooth is made with a small round bur. *G,* The cortical line of section is indicated by the broken line over the medial aspect of the ramus and along the anterior border. The solid line represents the vertical cut through the lateral cortex of the body of the mandible.

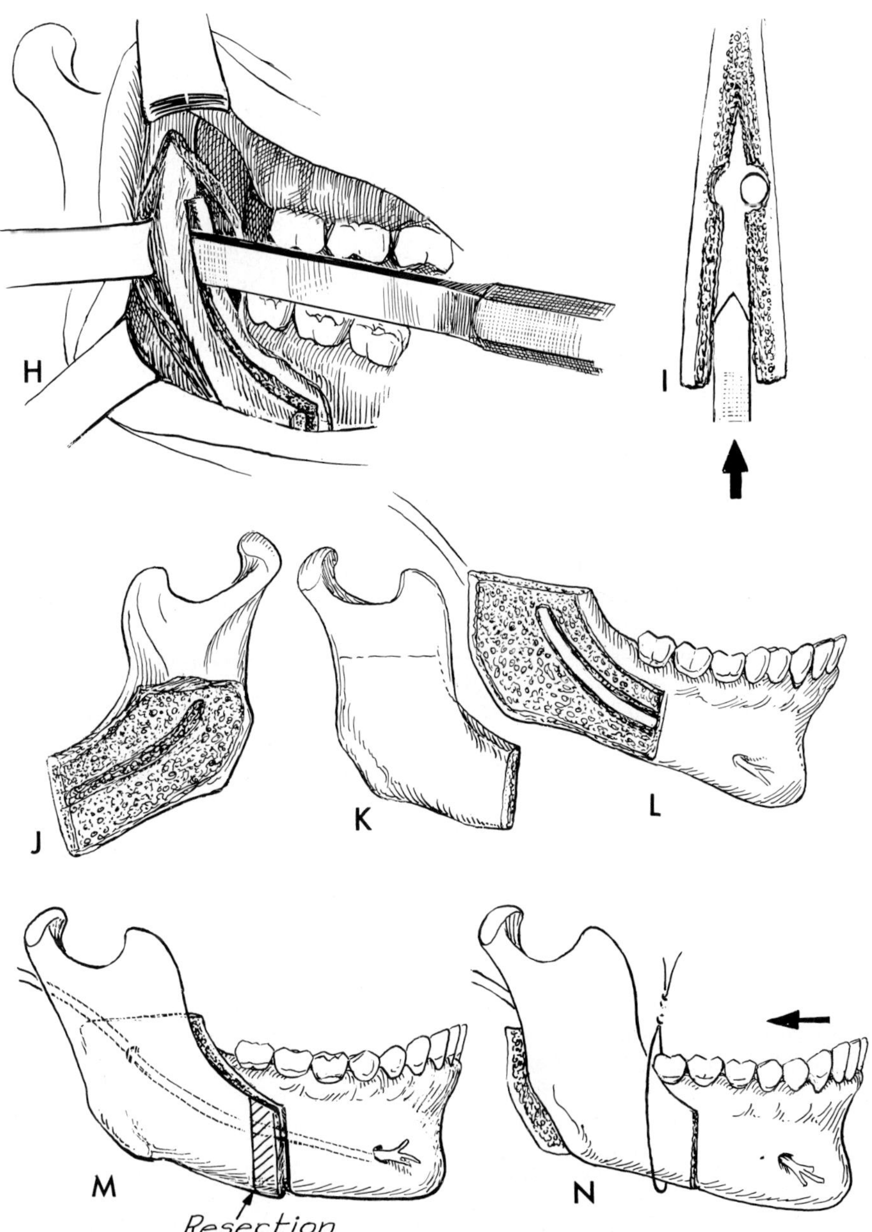

Figure 29–65 *Continued H,* The sagittal splitting of the ramus is performed with a thick osteotome. *I,* The thick osteotome also acts as a wedge as it splits the ramus. *J,* View of the medial aspect of the lateral (condylar) fragment. *K,* The lateral aspect of the lateral (condylar) fragment. *L,* The medial (tooth-bearing) fragment. *M,* Excess bone *(shaded area)* must be resected from the anterior portion of the lateral fragment to allow for bony apposition after posterior displacement of the tooth-bearing fragment. *N,* Final position of the tooth-bearing portion of the mandible. A buried circumferential wire around the fragments or an interosseous wire is placed to approximate the fragments. (After Obwegeser, 1957.)

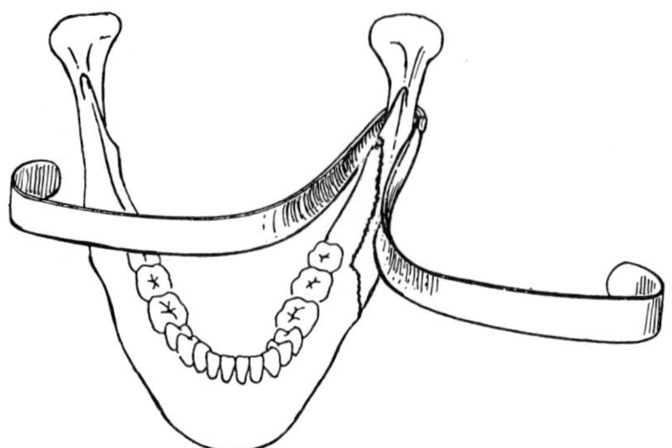

Figure 29–66. Obwegeser retractors facilitate exposure of the ramus in the sagittal splitting operation.

mately 1 cm above the lingula with a spiral Lindemann bur (see Fig. 29–65*C,D*) or a reciprocating saw. Bleeding from the cancellous bone can be used as a guide to determine whether the cortical bone has been penetrated. In the classical sagittal splitting procedure, this cut was carried to the posterior border of the ramus. Its extension can be limited to an area just beyond the mandibular foramen (Hunsuck, 1968), a maneuver that provides a smaller but adequate area of contact after the osteotomy. A series of drill holes placed along the anterior border of the ramus, medial to the oblique line, facilitate the sagittal osteotomy (see Fig. 29–65*E*). The tip of the reciprocating saw can be used for the same purpose. A second cut is made vertically through the lateral cortex of the body of the mandible in the area of the first or second molar (see Fig. 29–65*F*). Care should be taken not to endanger the roots of the teeth and to make sure that the cut extends through the inferior border of the mandible.

Obwegeser recommended the use of a thick osteotome to split the ramus before the neurovascular bundle is reached (see Fig. 29–65*H,I*). The stocky osteotome acts as a wedge to help cleave the ramus through its weakest plane, i.e., the cancellous bone and the inferior alveolar canal. The ramus is held by a retractor (Fig. 29–66) hooked around its posterior border during the splitting procedure. The retractor also acts to limit the backward trajectory of the osteotome, thus preventing injury to the soft tissue structures behind the ramus, notably the facial nerve.

It should be recalled that the inferior alveolar canal traverses obliquely through the ramus as it continues into the body; thus, its neurovascular bundle lies closer to the anterior border of the ramus as it descends through the ramus (Fig. 29–67). Care should therefore be taken as the osteotome is driven through the anterior one-third of the ramus to reduce the danger of direct injury to the neurovascular bundle. Because of the thick blade of the osteotome, most of the cleavage is caused by the wedging force of the blade. After the sagittal splitting, the medial tooth-bearing fragment contains the neurovascular bundle as it continues into the body of the mandible in the inferior alveolar canal; the lateral (proximal) fragment includes the condyle and the coronoid process (see Fig. 29–65*J* to *L*). The inferior alveolar nerve can be seen in its canal within the medial segment. Since the wedging action of the thick osteotome creates a major portion of the split through the weakest plane, on occasion the neurovascular bundle is seen to span the gap between the fragments. Thus, the segments must be separated slowly with a final, controlled twisting motion of the osteotome; if the neurovascular bundle is found to remain adherent to the lateral segment, it must be gently teased out of the canal with a small elevator.

Upon completion of the osteotomy, the body of the mandible is retruded into the predetermined occlusal relationship with the maxillary teeth (see Fig. 29–65*M*). The excess overlapping bone at the vertical body cut (the Dal Pont extension) is resected to establish a butt joint (Fig. 29–65*M*).

The condyle, under the influence of the lateral pterygoid muscular pull, has a tendency to drift forward and downward from its position in the glenoid fossa. Proper temporomandibular joint relationships should be reestablished before the fixation of the fragments.

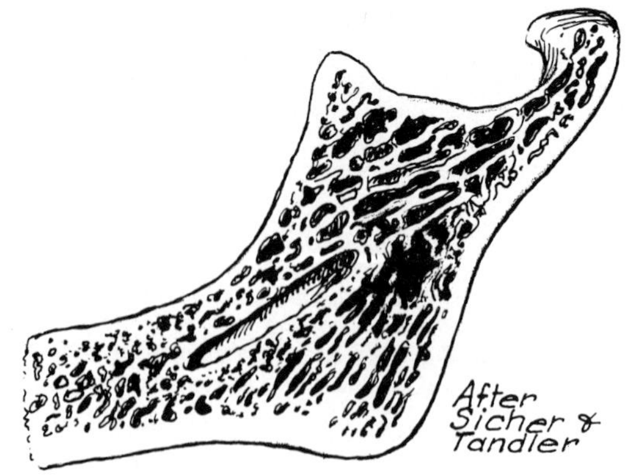

Figure 29–67. Sagittal section showing that the course of the inferior alveolar neurovascular bundle is closer to the anterior border of the ramus than is generally appreciated.

There are several methods of fixation of the fragments. Originally, Obwegeser employed a buried circumferential wire around the fragments in the retromolar area (see Fig. 29–65*N*). Direct interosseous wiring along the superior border of the Dal Pont extension is a popular alternative (Fig. 29–68). The drill hole is placed higher on the distal segment so that, when the wire is tightened, the condyle is elevated into the glenoid fossa (the "high to low" technique).

While postoperative intermaxillary fixation has traditionally been employed, the newer techniques of rigid internal fixation offer the advantage of minimizing or eliminating the period of intermaxillary fixation. The fragments are secured by three lag screws alone (Fig. 29–68*B, C*) (Spiessl, 1974, 1982) or by miniplates plus screws. Freihofer (1976, 1977), however, showed that a space is created between the proximal and distal segments as the mandible is moved into its new position. As the raw surfaces are coapted to eliminate this gap, unfavorable rotational changes are forced upon the condyle in its relation to the glenoid fossa. To prevent this geometric distortion, Luhr (1985, 1986) advocated the use of a positioning device to maintain the proper condylar relationships.

Regardless of the method of rigid fixation chosen, certain basic intraoperative steps must be followed. After the mandible is repositioned, intermaxillary fixation is established. If a miniplate is used, it must be contoured exactly to fit the bone. As the screws are applied in a poorly contoured miniplate, the latter will not adapt to the bone; instead, the bone moves toward the plate and the occlusion is adversely affected. In selecting the site of the drill holes, the inferior alveolar canal and the tooth roots must be avoided. The drill holes must be accurately

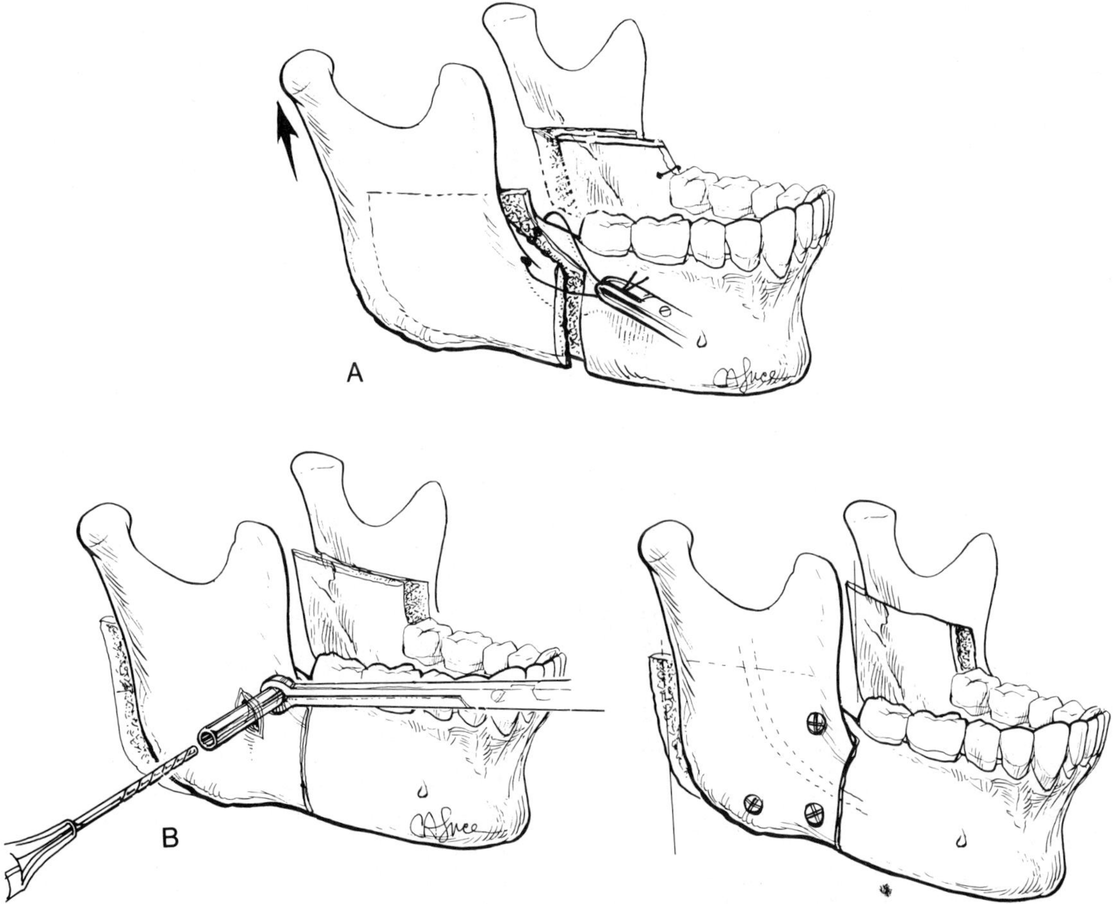

Figure 29–68. Techniques of fixation. *A,* The "high to low" technique. The hole in the distal segment is made higher so that when the wire is tightened the condyle is elevated *(arrow)* into the glenoid fossa. *B, C,* Insertion of lag screws after drill holes are made through a percutaneous trochar. The inferior alveolar nerve must be avoided.

placed with a slow-turning drill under constant irrigation. The drill hole should be oriented at right angles to the bone. It is not always possible to achieve such an alignment through a transoral route. The drill holes are then made via a trocar that is introduced through a percutaneous stab wound in the cheek, or preferably in a submandibular skin crease (Fig. 29–68*B*). If a miniplate is used, the compression mode must not be employed or the occlusion will be altered. If the miniplate is not used and rigid fixation is based on only screws, the lag screw principle is employed; i.e., the diameter of the drill hole must be larger than that of the screw in the proximal fragment and of the exact size in the distal fragment.

After the rigid fixation device is placed, the intermaxillary fixation is released. The occlusion is checked with the condyle properly seated in the glenoid fossa (centric relation). A light training elastic can be applied to keep the jaws properly aligned.

The intraoral wounds are irrigated and closed with absorbable sutures. Drains and dressing usually are not required. Some surgeons prefer to apply a compressive dressing to decrease the obligatory postoperative edema. Others argue that omission of the dressing permits undue swelling or hematoma to expand laterally away from the oropharyngeal space; the risk of possible embarrassment of the airway is lessened.

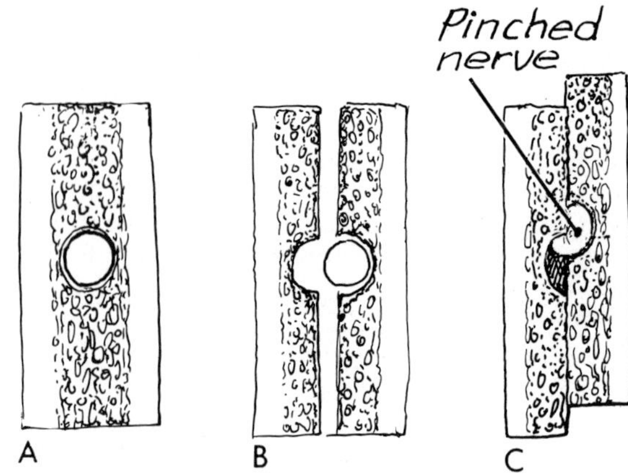

Figure 29–69. The mechanism by which the inferior alveolar nerve may be compressed by the split segments of the ramus, resulting in loss of the conductivity of the nerve.

THE DAUTREY MODIFICATION. The Dautrey (1975) modification of the Obwegeser–Dal Pont sagittal split of the ramus was devised to reduce the risk of injury or compression of the inferior alveolar nerve (Fig. 29–69).

The steps of exposure and the cortical portions of the osteotomy are essentially the same. The principal distinguishing feature of the modification is that the plane of separation through the cancellous bone is made directly beneath the lateral cortical plate and lateral to, instead of through, the inferior alveolar canal (Fig. 29–70).

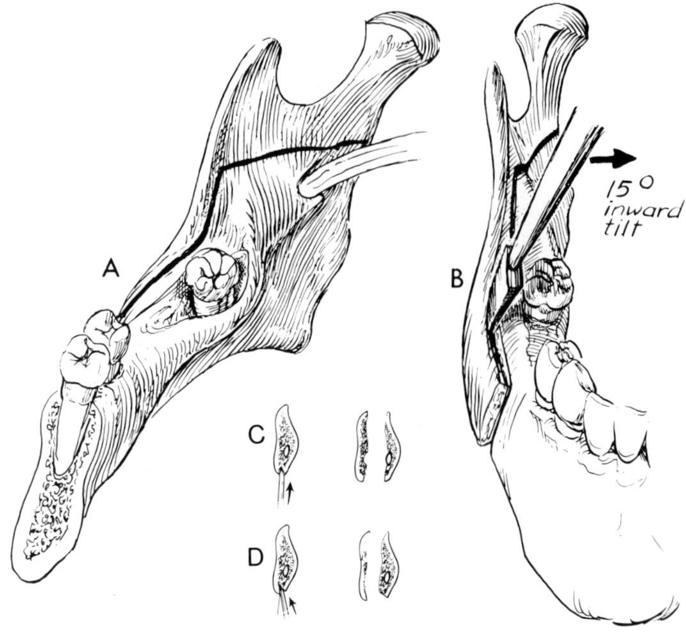

Figure 29–70. The Dautrey modification of the sagittal split of the ramus. *A,* A conscious effort must be made to keep the cutting edge of the osteotome against the lateral cortical plate. Note the tendency of the posterior border of the ramus to flare laterally. *B,* By passing laterally or tangentially to the inferior alveolar canal, the possibility of directly injuring the nerve is lessened. *C,* The osteotome should not enter the inferior alveolar canal. *D,* By remaining immediately under the lateral cortex, injury to the nerve is avoided.

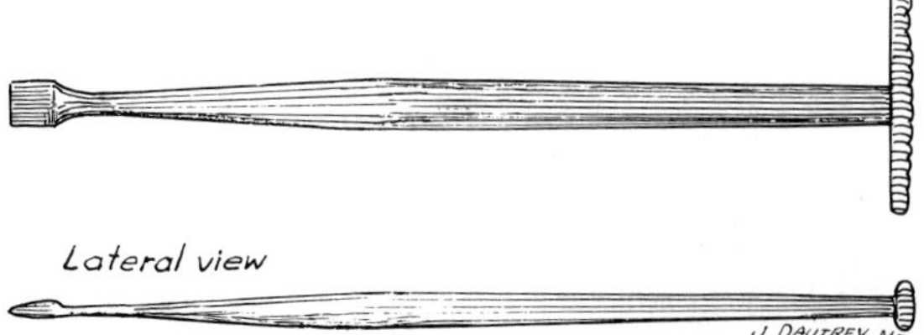

Figure 29–71. Dautrey's osteotome. The cutting edge is 1.5 mm thick.

The key instruments for the operation are the osteotomes, which are extremely thin and vary from 5 to 7 mm in width (Fig. 29–71). The thin blades act by cutting through the bone rather than creating a wedging force. The osteotomes are placed in series, much like splitting a log. Each is driven gradually into the bone in a direction parallel to and immediately deep to the lateral cortex. (See Fig. 29–70*D*). A rotation force on the osteotome should be avoided for fear of provoking a fracture of the lateral cortex. The osteotome gradually reaches the inferior border and more posterior aspect of the ramus, where it comes into contact with the broad hook of a stout retractor, which also stabilizes the jaw against the blow of the mallet.

The technique splits the entire ramus anteroposteriorly. Thus, the surface of contact between the fragments is maximal. An interosseous wire joins the cortices of the segment, and the anterior mortise provides additional stabilization by preventing any vertical tilt that can produce a posterior open bite (Fig. 29–72). Rigid fixation is an alternative method of stabilization (Fig. 29–73).

ADVANTAGES AND DISADVANTAGES OF SAGITTAL SECTION OF RAMUS. The intraoral approach and the avoidance of the external scar are favorable features of the technique. The distinct advantage is the wide surface of cancellous bony contact between the split fragments. Rapid bone consolidation is assured. The usual recommended period of intermaxillary fixation has been five to six weeks, but an interval as short as four weeks has been advocated (Hunsuck, 1968). Delayed union and nonunion are rare.

The wide surface of contact also allows great latitude in the positional change between the fragments. This versatility has contributed to the popularity of the sagittal section procedure. The tooth-bearing fragment can be retruded, advanced in cases of mandibular retrusion, and rotated to correct lateral deviations. However, it should not be used to close an anterior open bite because of the propensity for relapse. The broad surface of contact has also made it possible to use rigid internal fixation techniques.

Another advantage of the sagittal splitting technique is that spatial alteration between the condyle and the glenoid fossa is minimal. The muscles of mastication quickly adapt to their new anatomic and biomechanical relationships. Rusconi, Brusati, and Bottoli (1970) found no electromyographic changes of the masseter and temporalis immediately following the operation and one year thereafter. Nevertheless, on a clinical basis the ability to open the mouth is usually lessened after the operation and a trial of physical therapy is sometimes required.

The main disadvantage of the sagittal splitting procedure is the high incidence of loss of sensibility of the lower lip. Guernsey and DeChamplain (1971) reported an 80 per cent incidence of bilateral hypoesthesia immediately after the operation. With time, sensi-

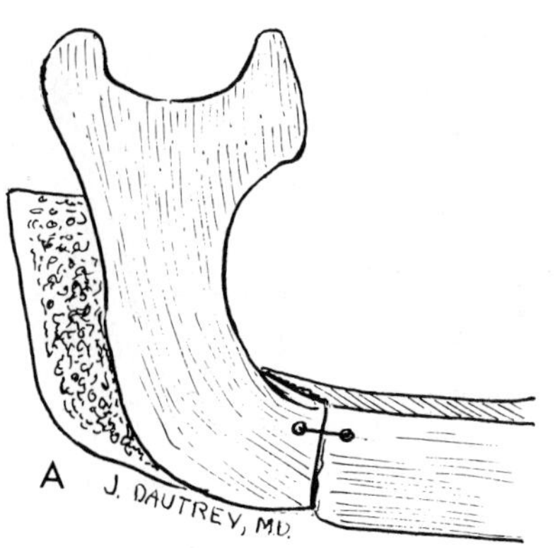

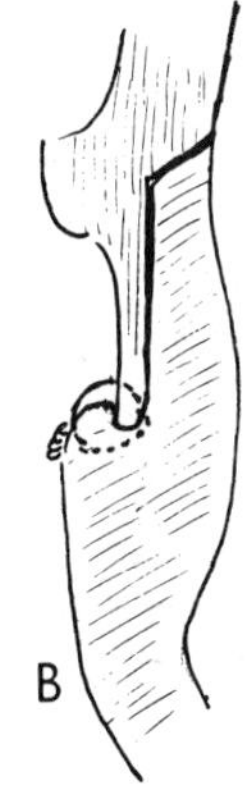

Figure 29–72. *A,* Final position of the fragments. An interosseous wire joins the two cortices. *B,* The anterosuperior angle of the condylar fragment joins the tooth-bearing fragment in a mortise-like fashion, preventing a lateral displacement and vertical tilt postoperatively.

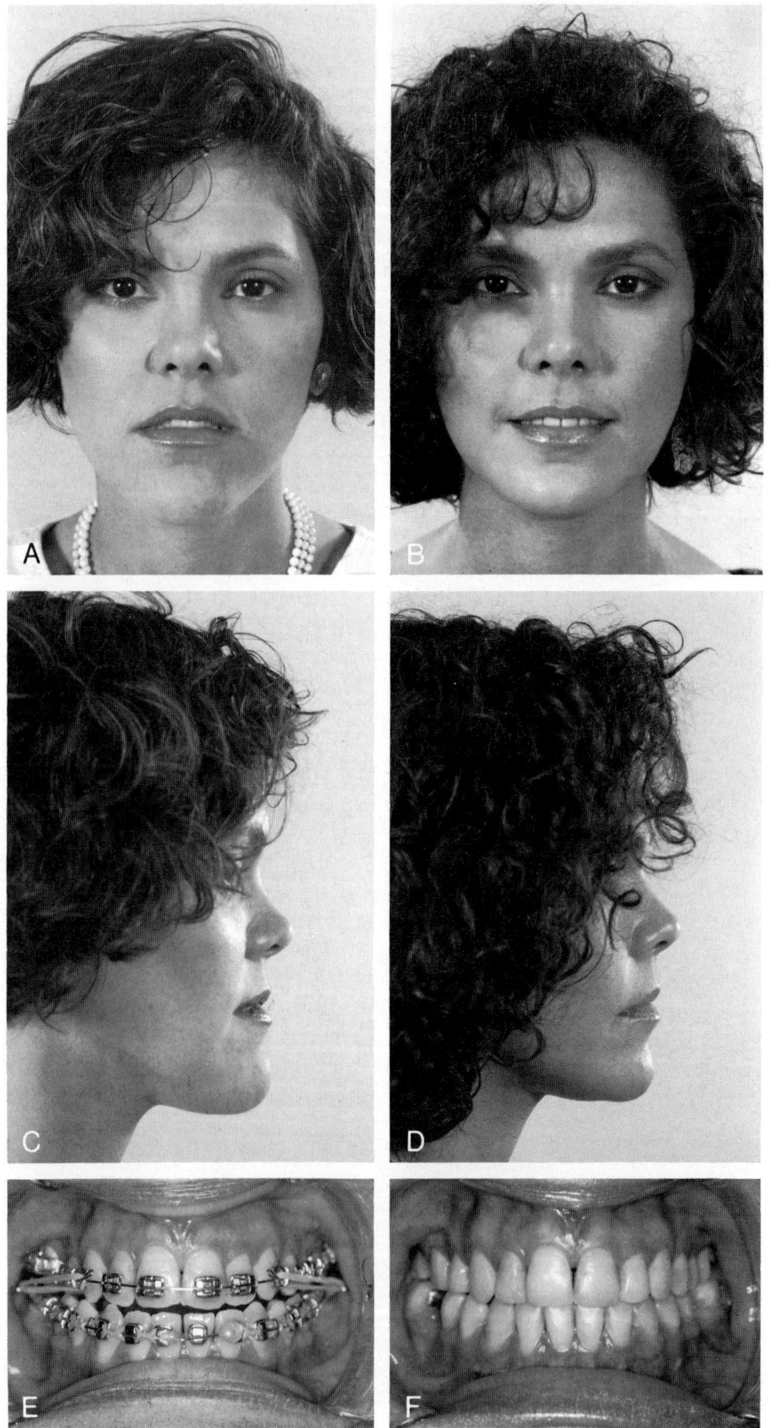

Figure 29–73. A female with mandibular prognathism and Class III malocclusion. *A, C, E,* Preoperative views. *B, D, F,* Postoperative views after combined orthodontic-surgical (intraoral sagittal split setback) therapy. Note the improvement in mandibular form and occlusion.

bility returns to all but 20 to 45 per cent of the patients (White and associates, 1969; Koblin and Reil, 1972; Pepersack and Chausse, 1974; Willmar, Hogeman, and Thiseus, 1979). All patients in the Pepersack and Chausse (1974) study were examined at least five years after their operations; in 45 per cent there was some degree of permanent decrease in sensibility of the lower lip. Both the teaching and the private cases of the University of Zurich were included in this report. A smaller incidence of diminished lip sensibility was present in the patients of more experienced surgeons.

Niederdellmann and Dieckmann (1974) warned of the dangers involved in exposure of the medial aspect of the ramus: direct injury or stretching of the inferior alveolar nerve, or hematoma formation in the area. Another possible cause of diminished lip sensibility is possible compression of the inferior alveolar nerve between the two fragments of the ramus because of the change in the relationships between the sections (see Fig. 29–69) (Converse, 1974b).

With the Dautrey modification the problem of lip paresthesia is significantly reduced, since the split occurs lateral to the inferior alveolar canal. The risk of direct nerve injury is decreased, since the canal is not purposely violated. The possibility of nerve compression between the two fragments is also eliminated. In Dautrey's experience, transitory loss of sensibility or paresthesia for a period of two to three months was noted in 10 per cent of the patients; none had permanent anesthesia of the lower lip (Dautrey, 1974).

Comminution of the proximal fragment can be a problem when the ramus is thin, especially when the Dautrey modification is used; extreme care must be exercised during the osteotomy to avoid this complication. Guernsey and DeChamplain (1971) recommended placing the medial horizontal osteotomy closer to the lingula instead of in the thinner subsigmoid region. Limiting this horizontal cut (Hunsuck, 1968) to an area just posterior to the mandibular foramen, instead of continuing it to the posterior border of the ramus, decreases the risk of comminution. Neuner (1976) proposed an oblique sagittal osteotomy, which is made with a reciprocating saw placed immediately posterior to the mandibular foramen and above the lingula.

Other complications of the Obwegeser–Dal Pont procedure reported in a survey by Behrman (1972) are hemorrhage, airway obstruction, necrosis or sequestration, infection, and injury to the facial nerve. In addition, decreased sensibility of the tongue can occur if the lingual nerve is traumatized during the medial dissection of the ramus.

Relapse. Relapse rate after the sagittal split technique is approximately the same as that observed after a vertical ramus section. A one year cephalometric roentgenographic follow-up study by Egyedi (1965) showed an average relapse of 2 mm. A longitudinal study of 100 patients who underwent sagittal split osteotomy at least three years earlier showed satisfacory maintenance of the corrected occlusion with only minimal evidence of skeletal relapse (Wilmar, Hogeman, and Thiésus, 1979).

Results. Examples of patients with correction of a pure mandibular prognathism deformity are shown in Figure 29–73. When the prognathic appearance is exaggerated by an accompanying hypoplastic maxilla, both jaws must be repositioned.

Edentulous Prognathic Patients

In edentulous patients the alveolar process is reduced in varying degrees (Fig. 29–74) and can complicate the correction of the man-

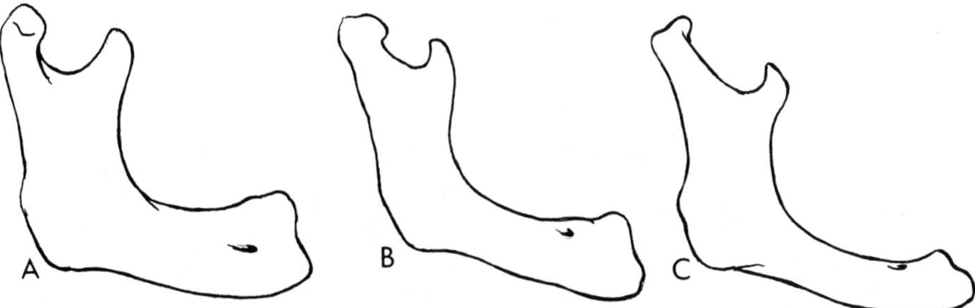

Figure 29–74. Progressive loss of height of the body of the mandible in the edentulous jaw. (After Grant, 1951.)

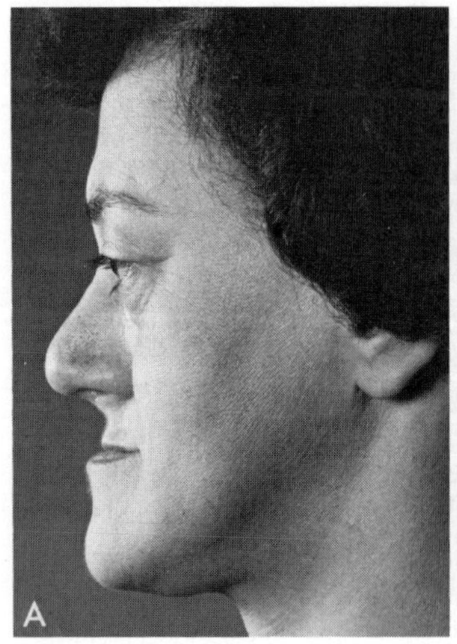

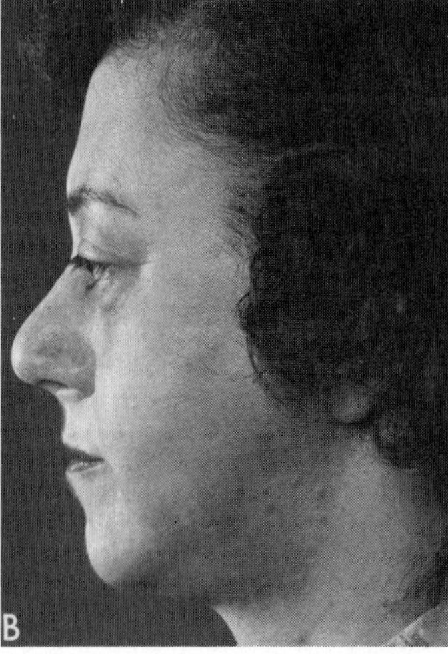

Figure 29–75. Mandibular prognathism in an edentulous patient treated by ramus section. *A,* Preoperative profile view. *B,* Result obtained after bilateral section of the ramus. The patient's upper denture was maintained in craniofacial fixation by internal suspension wires. The lower denture was maintained in intermaxillary fixation with the upper denture, and circumferential wiring was used to fix it to the mandible. (Patient of Dr. J.M. Converse.)

dibular prognathism. Resorption of the alveolar process results in a loss of vertical dimension, which in turn causes the mandible to rotate in a cephalad and anterior (counterclockwise) direction to aggravate the prognathic appearance. In certain patients the progressive resorption of bone results in exposure of the inferior alveolar nerve (Fig. 29–74*C*). Wearing a denture becomes a painful if not impossible, experience and additional reconstructive procedures are required (see p. 1455) after correction of the prognathic relationship.

In the mild to moderately prognathic edentulous patient, the prosthodontist can usually provide efficient dentures to compensate for the faulty relationship of the alveolar processes. Surgical correction is required, however, when mandibular prognathism is more severe. According to the deformity, either a body osteotomy or a ramal approach may be indicated. Strong preference should be given, whenever possible, to a ramal osteotomy. Stabilization of the osteotomy site of an atrophic mandible is a hazardous task that should not be chosen if alternatives exist.

Figure 29–75*A* shows an edentulous patient with mandibular prognathism in whom the deformity was corrected by bilateral osteotomies of the ramus. The patient had worn dentures for a number of years. Preliminary studies had shown that satisfactory jaw relationships could be obtained by bilateral vertical section of the ramus. The patient's dentures were used as fixation splints. The upper denture was maintained in fixation by internal circumferential inferior orbital rim and zygomatic arch suspension wiring, and the lower denture by circumferential mandibular wiring. A satisfactory correction was obtained.

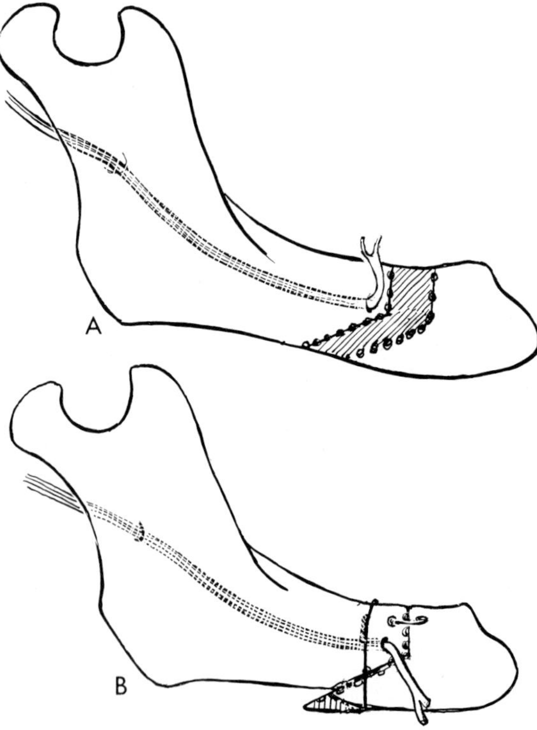

Figure 29–76. Technique for the correction of mandibular prognathism in an edentulous patient. *A,* Resection of bone after reverse L-shaped osteotomy of the body of the mandible. *B,* Circumferentialf and interosseous wiring is used to immobilize the fragments after the excess bone is resected. (After Kazanjian.)

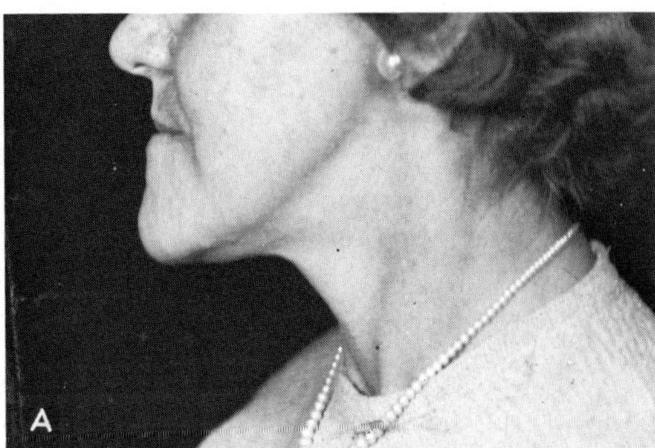

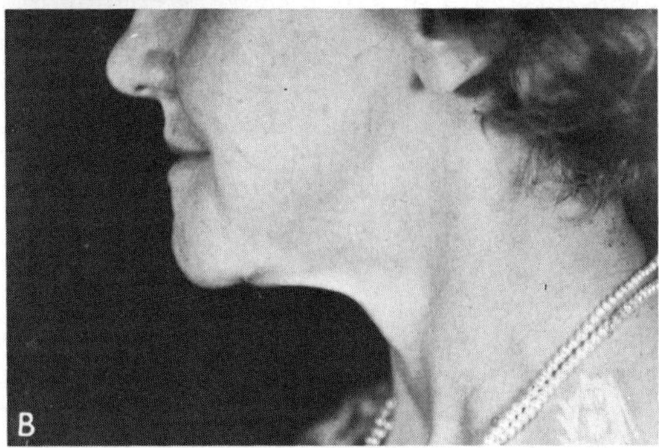

Figure 29–77. Mandibular prognathism in an edentulous patient treated by body section. *A,* Preoperative profile. *B,* Result obtained after resection of bone from the body of the mandible, as illustrated in Figure 29–76.

In the body osteotomy, the mental foramen and the lateral surface of the body of the mandible are exposed (Figs. 29–76, 29–77). When the inferior alveolar nerve in an edentulous mandible is being exposed before the osteotomy, a practical consideration to bear in mind is the superficial position of the mental foramen and inferior alveolar nerve due to resorption of the alveolar process. Furthermore, in cases of moderate to severe atrophy, body procedures should be avoided because of the real risk of nonunion.

A section of bone of predetermined size is removed. The anterior segment is recessed into its new position. Interosseous wires or miniplates are used to secure the fragments, but they must lie well inferior to the denture-bearing region.

Children and Adolescents with Prognathism

Adolescent patients with prognathic tendencies show a rapid accentuation of the mandibular prominence soon after the eruption of the permanent teeth. The deformity becomes more striking as the facial bones, particularly the mandible, attain full development (Fig. 29–78). Immediate improvement results if the deformity is corrected by early intervention. The growth of the mandible, however, is not arrested and recurrence of the prognathism can be expected with further growth. Thus, the major decision that must be made relates to the timing of the operation. A roentgenogram of the wrist for bone age, or serial lateral cephalograms spaced six months apart, can be used as a guide.

Children with extreme prognathism and an inadequate masticatory mechanism should

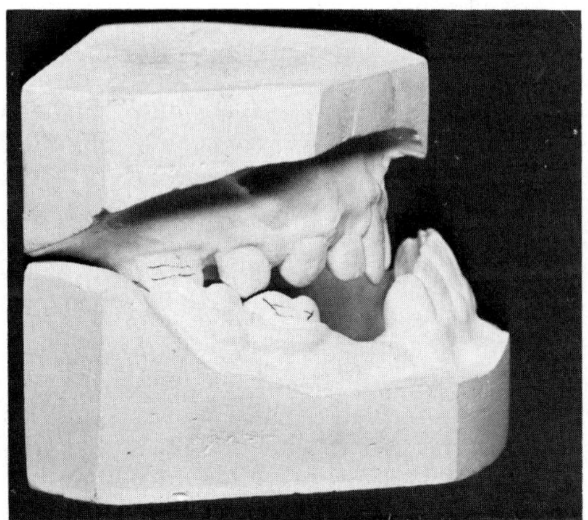

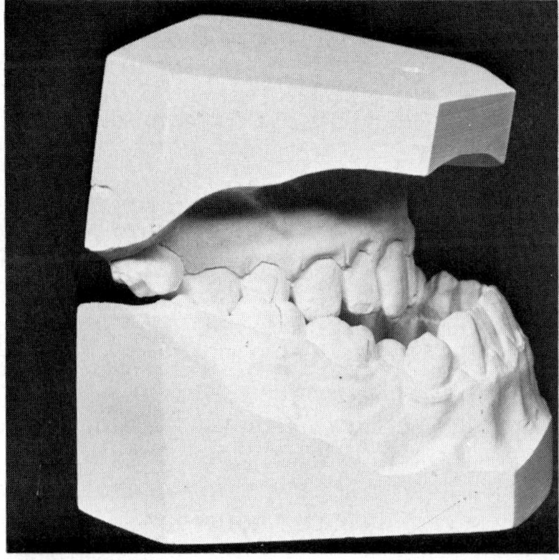

Figure 29–78. The upper set of casts show the dentoalveolar relationships in a 12 year old boy with mandibular prognathism. The lower dental models are of the same patient at the age of 16 years; the distance between the upper and lower incisors has increased by 5 mm. (From Kazanjian, V. H.: The surgical treatment of prognathism. An analysis of sixty-five cases. Am. J. Surg., *87*:691, 1954.)

not be neglected. A corrective procedure should be recommended on the understanding that an additional operation will be required after completion of mandibular growth. A vertical-oblique ramus section can be safely performed without jeopardizing the unerupted molar teeth, as might a sagittal splitting procedure. A body section cannot be performed in children because of the presence of unerupted permanent teeth.

Mandibular Prognathism with Open Bite

This type of mandibular deformity presents special problems of treatment, discussed later in the section concerned with the treatment of open bite problems (see p. 1351).

Mandibular Prognathism with Microgenia

It seems paradoxical that the chin of a large prognathic jaw can be excessively retruded. The large size of the jaw does not preclude an inadequate development of the mental symphysis. Furthermore, in some cases the chin is not only retruded but exaggerated in vertical dimension. Approximately one-quarter of patients with mandibular prognathism require modification of the mental symphyseal region. This should be kept in mind to prevent the anomalous clinical situation of a patient whose prognathism has been corrected and yet requires one of the procedures for increasing the chin projection described on page 1312.

Choice of Procedure in Correction of Prognathism

The advantages of sectioning the ramus are that (1) it is usually a relatively simple operation; (2) when it is correctly performed, there is no interference with the conduction of the inferior alveolar nerve; and (3) greater efficiency in mastication is obtained, since the teeth are not sacrificed.

The body section techniques are indicated in cases of mandibular prognathism with a severe change in the curve of the dental arch or with severe disparity between the mandibular and maxillary arch forms, and in some cases of anterior open bite deformity. Body section techniques allow changes to be made in (1) a selective segmental vertical direction, (2) arch length, and (3) arch width. A better mandibular arch can be obtained in the severely prognathic and hypertrophied jaw as a result of reducing jaw size and modifying the curve of the dental arch.

The disadvantages of the osteotomies through the body of the mandible include a more laborious surgical procedure, the possibility of nonunion, danger of injury to the inferior alveolar nerve, and the sacrifice of teeth. If the resection of bone is carefully planned, the chances of inadequate bone contact and nonconsolidation are slight. After a period of approximately eight to ten weeks, in the rare case in which there is no evidence of union, the area can be reinforced by bone grafts from the ilium or calvarium. If during the operation the area of contact between the fragments appears to be insufficiently intimate to ensure consolidation, chips of bone from the resected segments of the mandible can also be inserted into the defect at the osteotomy site.

Injury to the inferior alveolar nerve can be avoided if the resection is placed anterior to the mental foramen and the inferior alveolar canal is not penetrated. In body osteotomies posterior to the mental foramen, adequate exposure reduces the risk of nerve injury.

Body ostectomy procedures can be used advantageously in selected patients with missing teeth. As previously stated, many prognathic patients are partially edentulous. The gaps in the dental arch are convenient sites for osteotomies and bone resection; after reduction of the length of the body, the gaps are closed and the continuity of the dentition is restored.

One of the objections to the vertical-oblique ramus osteotomy has been that the normal line of action of the powerful muscles of mastication is disrupted. It is not possible to recess the mandible to any great degree without completely changing the vector forces and function of these muscles (see Fig. 29–58). This problem has been partially resolved by the subperiosteal elevation of the muscles from their insertions on the medial and lateral aspects of the ramus and, on rare occasions, section of the base of the coronoid process to release the traction of the temporalis. In extreme cases, an inverted L-osteotomy should be considered.

In certain cases of pronounced prognathism, the posterior displacement can result in excessive retrusion of the posterior border of the ramus with impingement on the facial nerve. The hazard is eliminated by resecting

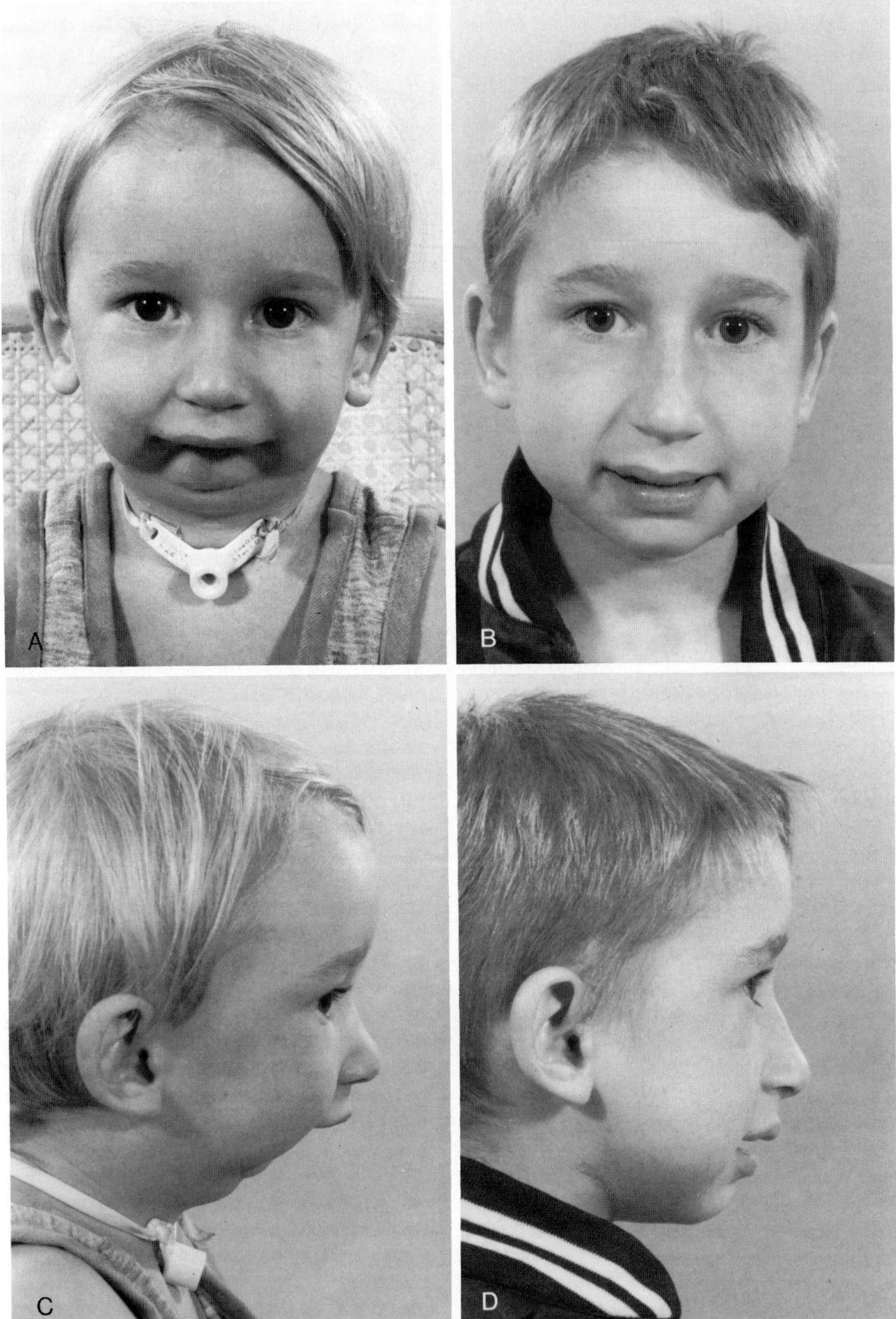

Figure 29–79. Severe mandibular micrognathism (bird face) and bilateral temporomandibular joint ankylosis secondary to trauma in infancy. *A, C,* Preoperative appearance. Tracheostomy was required. *B, D,* Appearance after release of the ankylosis and reconstruction of the joints and mandibular rami with rib costocartilage grafts.

the protruding posterior border of the ramus or removing a wedge of bone at the osteotomy site (Van Zile, 1963).

Because the sagittal split of the ramus (Obwegeser–Dal Pont procedure) is frequently complicated by the loss of sensibility in the lower lip, the Dautrey modification is superior, since it minimizes the risk of producing permanent lip paresthesia. It can also be employed for advancement procedures.

The sagittal split procedure is advantageous in that it causes only a minimal disturbance of the position of the condyle; the vertical section results in an outward rotation of the condyle in the glenoid fossa. Nevertheless, clinical observation of any dysfunction of the temporomandibular joint as a result of this rotation is rare. This finding is attributed to the ability of the condyle to adapt and remodel itself (Ware and Taylor, 1968). Lastly, if rigid fixation techniques are to be used, a sagittal splitting procedure is required.

The choice between an extraoral and an intraoral approach is determined by the possible contraindication of an external scar. In the patient who is predisposed to hypertrophic scars or keloids, the external incision is contraindicated. Female patients may object to an external scar; an intraoral approach is favored in such cases. In muscular male patients with hypertrophied masseteric muscles or in individuals with limited opening of the mouth, an intraoral procedure on the ramus is technically difficult. If a vertical-oblique intraoral osteotomy is being considered, a low angle of divergence may preclude the use of this method. Retraction of the soft tissue and muscles is difficult and the exposure of the bone is poor. In this group of patients, the vertical osteotomy through an external approach may be the technique of choice.

An additional minor advantage of the external approach is that antibiotic coverage can be dispensed with. Zallen and Strader (1971) believe that prophylactic antibiotics are not warranted when the extraoral approach is employed.

Regardless of the technique used, gratifying restoration of facial balance and harmony is obtained. The stigma of aggressiveness and belligerence associated with the face having a prominent lower jaw is eliminated. Natural fullness of both lips is obtained, and the upper lip assumes a more adequate length and anteroposterior position (Knowles, 1965; Aaronson, 1967). For psychologic reasons, prognathic patients tend to hold their head in a forwardly inclined position to minimize the chin prominence (Fromm and Lundberg, 1970). Postoperatively, the head is carried in a more normal upright position. Even with the change in suprahyoid muscle posture, the hyoid bone position remains the same (Takagi and associates, 1967), and disturbances in respiration, swallowing, and speech do not occur.

MICROGNATHISM AND HYPOPLASIA

Several terms have been used to denote a small lower jaw. From a literal sense, each has a slightly different connotation, but the terms are frequently used interchangeably. From its Greek derivation, the word *micrognathia* signifies a small jaw. *Mandibular hypoplasia* results in a small mandible due to failure of growth and development. *Retrognathia* is used to describe a jaw that is posteriorly displaced but not necessarily changed in size. The use of the term *mandibular atresia* should be discouraged; *atresia*, derived from the Greek, means "no perforation." *Microgenia* connotes a small chin.

Because of the characteristic appearance of the face, the Germans have used the term "Vogelgesicht" (bird face) to describe mandibular micrognathia. In the United States the deformity is familiarly referred to as the "Andy Gump" facies because of its identification with the well-known cartoon personality. The prominence of the lower third of the face is absent; the anteroposterior dimension and height of the lower face are decreased. Excessive forward and downward displacement of the anterior maxillary teeth and, in some cases, an accumulation of soft tissue under the micrognathic mandible complete the birdlike profile (Figs. 29–79, 29–80).

Etiology

Mandibular micrognathia can be classified according to its etiology as congenital, developmental, or acquired.

One of the most frequent causes of *congenital* mandibular hypoplasia is maldevelopment of the first and second branchial arches. Involvement can be unilateral or bilateral. A relatively frequent deformity of the congeni-

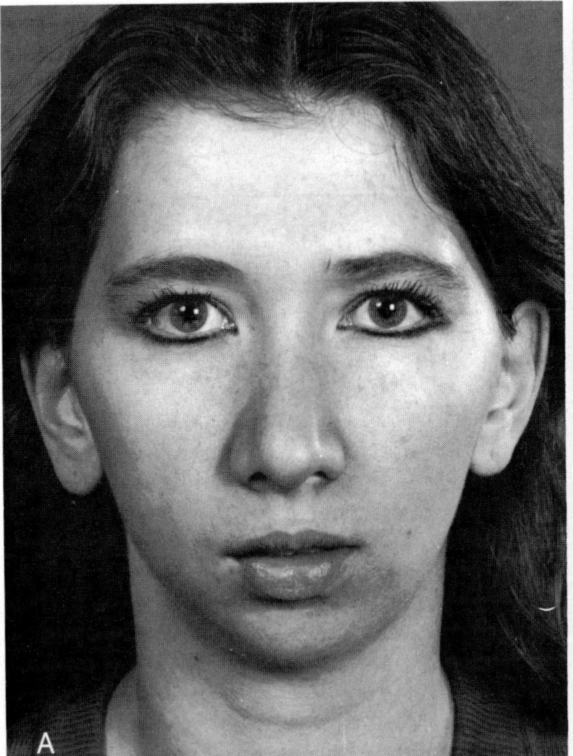

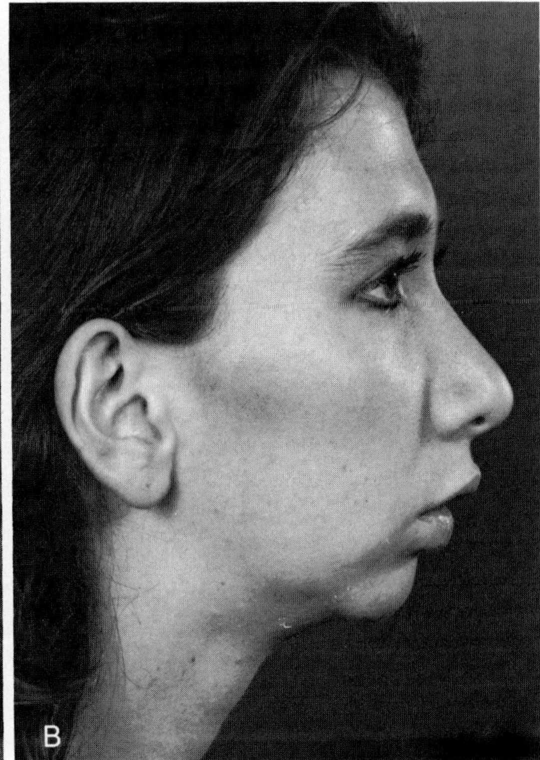

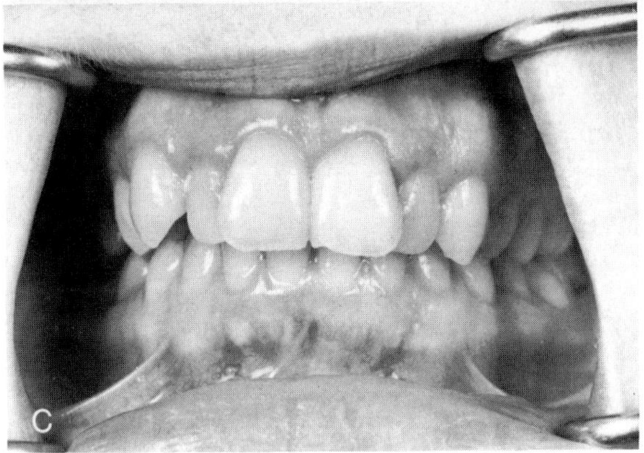

Figure 29–80. Mandibular micrognathia. *A,* Frontal view. Note the generalized underdevelopment of the mandible. *B,* Profile. *C,* Occlusal view demonstrating the marked overjet.

tal type is observed in craniofacial microsomia (Chap. 62) and mandibulofacial dysostosis (Chap. 63). The condyle, ramus, and body are small; the condyle is situated in a medial position in relation to the infratemporal space. Mandibular hypoplasia of the Robin sequence type may be the result of intrauterine compression; it is the only form of micrognathia that can be self-correcting as the individual grows (see Chap. 63). Fetal maldevelopment of the condylar region can result in temporomandibular ankylosis in newborns. Agenesis of the temporomandibular joint is a rare condition observed in severe forms of craniofacial microsomia.

The *developmental* type of mandibular hypoplasia is more common than is usually assumed. There are numerous patients who have the typical Class II malocclusion with underdevelopment of the mandible for unknown reasons. Injury caused by the application of forceps at birth can result in compression of the temporomandibular region and retardation of mandibular growth. A fall in infancy can cause damage to the condylar region and impair subsequent lower jaw development. In severe cases, temporomandibular ankylosis may follow, which adds a functional disability to the deformity. Causes other than trauma can also interfere with condylar growth: e.g., rheumatoid arthritis or suppurative disease originating in the mastoid process and extending into the temporomandibular joint, a rare complication since the advent of antibiotics. The injudicious use of radiation therapy is another source of condylar growth arrest.

Acquired mandibular hypoplasia is produced by bone resection for tumor or by the loss of bone due to trauma, when the fragments are allowed to collapse and the anterior portion of the mandibular arch is displaced posteriorly.

Variations of Mandibular Hypoplasia and Associated Functional Disturbances

Deficiencies in the length and width of any part of the lower jaw characterize mandibular hypoplasia. The degree of involvement of each section varies; unilateral and bilateral deformities occur.

When the deformity is *bilateral*, generalized micrognathia is observed (Fig. 29–80). The mandibular body is short and often thick, and shows a characteristic accentuated antegonial notch. The height of the ramus is decreased and the condyles are frequently deformed. In a number of patients with agenesis of the condyle or condylar destruction following a septic episode in infancy, the adaptive mandible may articulate with the calvarium by means of pseudarthrosis or even the coronoid process.

The chin of a patient with bilateral involvement is usually retruded in the midsagittal plane. The chin eminence is small and indistinct. With the lips in repose, the lower lip is retracted downward to produce a large intralabial gap. As the lips attempt to form a seal, hyperactivity and strain of the mentalis occurs. The chin pad puckers and rides cephalad to the bony chin prominence. The anterior teeth of the retruded mandible are more posteriorly located but labially inclined and overerupted compared with their maxillary counterparts.

Interference with the growth of one side of the mandible, the consequence of *unilateral* injury, occurs more frequently than bilateral impairment of growth. Although the initial site of disturbance is confined to one side, the entire mandible is eventually affected. The damaged side of the mandible is shorter and the chin also points toward the affected side. The uninjured side of the mandible is flat and to an uninitiated observer appears to be the deformed portion. The disparity between the two halves of the body of the mandible is evident when measurements are made from the midpoint of the chin to the mandibular (gonial) angle. The degree of mandibular hypoplasia depends on the age at which the injury to the growth centers is inflicted: the earlier the event, the greater is the ensuing deformity. The asymmetry is clinically insignificant and difficult to detect in early childhood, but becomes more apparent as growth progresses. When the jaw is severely retruded, the patient also suffers a serious disfigurement.

External facial asymmetry, due to the disproportionate growth of the two halves of the mandible, is accompanied by disturbed dental occlusion. The malocclusion is generally of the Angle Class II, division 1 type. Laterognathism (lateral deviation of the mandible) and posterior crossbite are usually present.

Disparity of ramus height is also a feature of unilateral underdevelopment of the mandible, the ramus on the affected side being shorter than that of the normal side. The discrepancy is clinically obvious; the mandibular angle on the affected side is situated at a higher level and in some cases is poorly defined. The commissure of the mouth is elevated in repose and reflects the malinclination of the occlusal plane as it assumes an oblique upward cant toward the ipsilateral maxilla. The body of the mandible curves cephalad to join the short ramus.

When ankylosis of the temporomandibular joint complicates the deformity, a serious functional disability is imposed. Restoring the ability to open the mouth and providing a functional joint become the paramount goal and should be undertaken as early as possible. Recapturing joint motion, however, does not solve all the patient's functional problems. Effective mastication is not achieved if the teeth of the posteriorly displaced mandible fail to occlude with the maxillary teeth. The mandible must be elongated surgically to reestablish satisfactory relationships between the maxillary and mandibular arches and efficient masticatory function. Ideally, function and form should be simultaneously reestablished (Munro, Chen, and Park, 1986).

Treatment of Mandibular Hypoplasia

Surgical elongation of the mandible can restore jaw relationships, correct the asymmetry in unilateral cases, and improve the appearance of the patient. When a normal complement of teeth is present, dental occlusion is improved and masticatory efficiency is increased.

Early Surgical-Orthodontic Planning. Early consultation with the orthodontist eliminates later misunderstandings (see p. 1189). One should particularly avoid and advise against untimely orthodontic therapy, which modifies the position of the dentition to conform to the malformed mandible and greatly complicates subsequent surgical treatment. Little is gained by achieving a forced occlusion between the teeth if the body of the jaw remains malformed. Later surgical procedures to elongate the mandible will, of necessity, produce malocclusion. Such ill-advised presurgical orthodontic treatment can be avoided by early coordinated observation and planning by the orthodontist with the surgeon. Conversely, no surgical interventions should be made without consultation with an orthodontist.

Although each case commands an individualized plan, the general preoperative goals of orthodontic treatment are to remove dental compensation, properly align the teeth to the underlying basilar bone of the jaws, and level the occlusal plane.

Preoperative Planning. Diagnosis and planning of surgical correction begin with clinical examination of the patient. A number of laboratory records are required to formulate a surgical strategy: photographs, cephalometric and panoramic roentgenograms, and dental study models. More complicated deformities may call for additional aids.

The clinical examination and the photographs are helpful in studying the soft tissue contour deficiency and the condition of the intraoral structures. The following must be particularly noted: (1) the vertical and horizontal facial balance and the patient's customary head posture; (2) the lateral shifting of the chin point when the mandible is opened or closed, movements indicative of temporomandibular joint dysfunction or neuromotor disability; (3) the orofacial musculature in repose and while functioning; and (4) the condition of the soft tissues of the mouth, especially any soft tissue lesions and periodontal disease.

The dentoalveolar relationships observed on the clinical examination are analyzed in detail using the dental casts. The casts provide a record of arch length, width, and form, as well as of individual tooth positions and occlusal relationships. Duplicate working casts are cut to simulate the line of osteotomy.

In mandibular hypoplasia, as in mandibular prognathism, an essential guide in preoperative planning is the condition of the dentition. A decision must be made as to whether adequate dental occlusal relationships between the mandible and the maxilla can be reestablished by osteotomies through the mandibular ramus, the body, or both.

The working set of casts is mounted on a dental articulator; the use of a face bow transfer may be required in particularly difficult cases. The anterior portion of the sectioned dental working cast is relocated to the desired position. The sections are temporary joined with dental wax and securely held together with a slab of plaster after the final position is established. The casts are used to fabricate a splint that will hold the various fragments together. In cases in which the osteotomies are confined to the ramus and the dental arch is kept intact, the cast can be simply related on an adjustable articulator (see Fig. 29–21).

In asymmetric deformities, more elongation is required on one side, and in some cases of mandibular asymmetry the contralateral side must be shortened to achieve symmetry. Realignment ot the midsagittal plane is used as a guide in positioning the anterior segment. In addition, a posteroanterior cephalometric roentgenogram can be used to determine the change required in the position of the chin point (see p. 1209). The analysis of mandibular skeletal deformity should include evaluation of the size, proportion, and position of the mandible with respect to midface and cranial base structures. This analysis proceeds by first selecting an age-, sex-, and where possible race-matched normative cephalometric population. The cephalometric data sheet (see Table 29–1) shows the University of Michigan normative values for a selected population. An individual whose cephalometric data aligned vertically in the central column would have cephalometric characteristics of normal size and shape. The data have been scaled, increasing in 5 per cent increments to the right and decreasing to the left of the central column. A patient whose overall size is small and of normal facial shape would

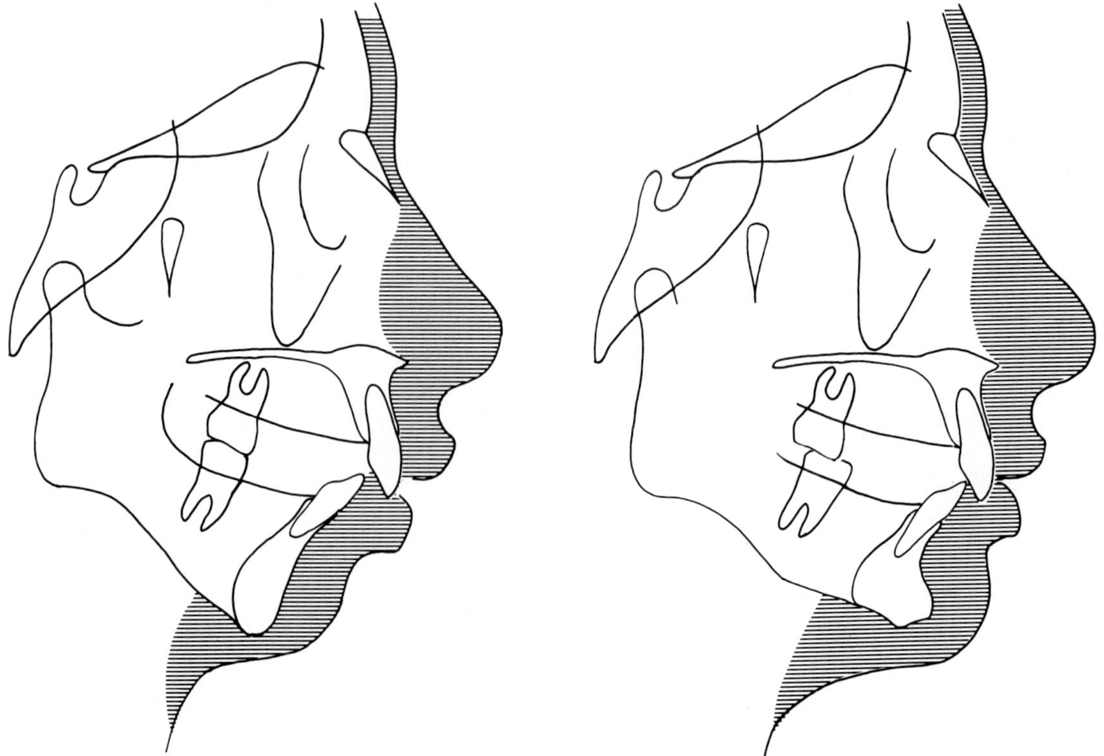

Figure 29–81. Mandibular advancement and genioplasty: cephalometric views. *Left,* preoperative. *Right,* postoperative. (See Fig. 29–80.)

display data aligned vertically in one of the columns to the left of normal.

When the cephalometric data are recorded on the sheet, the overall scale of the individual is determined. A patient with mandibular hypoplasia may also have small stature and facial dimensions. The midface and cranial base measurements may be 5 per cent smaller than normal, while the mandibular measurements appear 20 per cent below normal. In this case the mandible is viewed as dysmorphic and the midface and cranial base of small but normal proportion. In a patient whose overall stature and dimensions are large the cranial base and midface may be proportionately 15 or 20 per cent larger than normal, while the mandibular data are normal. The increased size of the cranial base and midface, consistent with the increased stature of the individual, would suggest the "normal" mandibular data to be proportionately small.

The anteroposterior position of the mandible with respect to the maxilla and anterior cranial base is evaluated by measuring the forward projection of these structures away from landmarks found in the posterior face (pterygomaxillary point), cranial base, sella turcica, and basion. The retropositioned mandible (independent of its size) would show reduced dimensions between basion, sella turcica, and pogonion, while the forward projection of midface structures (ANS, A-point, and orbitale) would be proportionately normal. A case study is illustrated in Figures 29–81 and 29–82.

The cephalometric roentgenogram is also helpful in determining the final position of the fragments after the osteotomy. The tracing is cut and the anterior portion is repositioned forward to simulate the amount of advancement (see Fig. 29–24) required to correct the deformity. The new facial contour can be estimated by tracing the soft and hard tissue outlines.

If the clinical and cephalometric analysis indicate an elongation osteotomy of the body of the mandible, the tracing is sectioned in the appropriate region and the anterior portion of the body is advanced to restore a

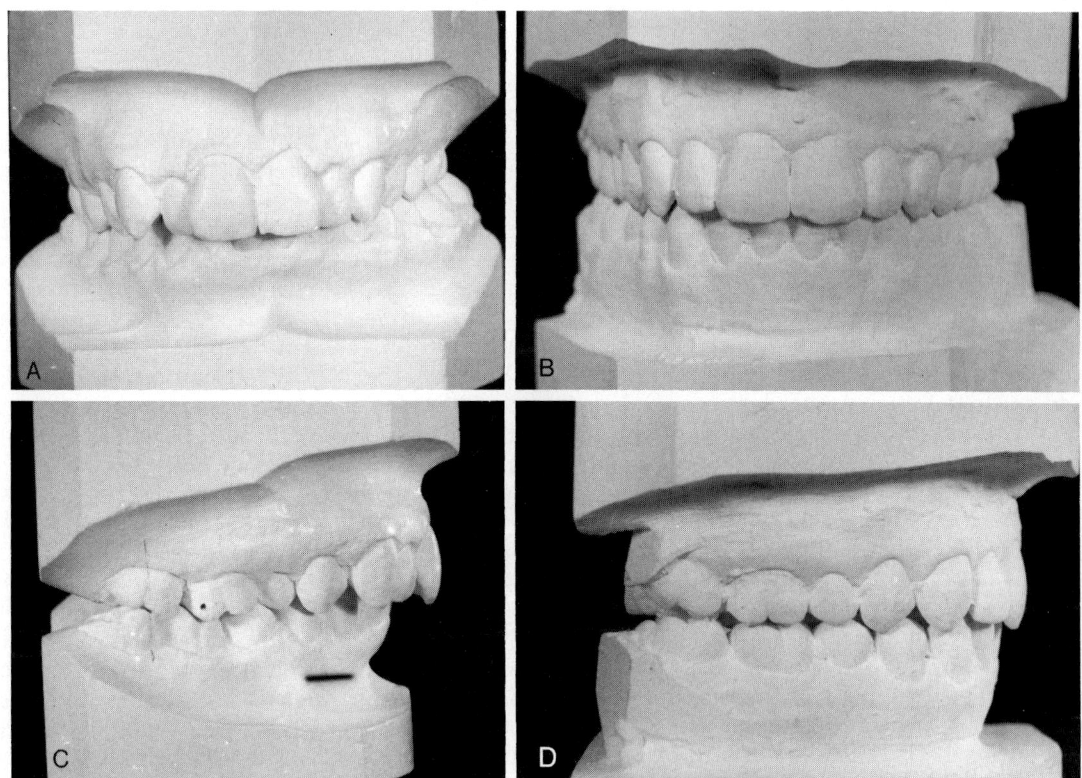

Figure 29–82. Dental models of the patient shown in Figures 29–80 and 29–81. *A, C,* Preoperative. *B. D,* Postoperative after sagittal split advancement of the mandible and genioplasty.

harmonious occlusal relationship with the maxillary teeth.

When a chin recontouring procedure (genioplasty) or a rhinoplasty is indicated to improve the patient's profile, a tracing of the correction should be made to assess its influence on the projected facial profile (see Fig. 29–25).

A panoramic roentgenogram is a valuable document to assess the structures supporting the dentition and the form of the jaws. It is especially informative in patients who have an associated temporomandibular ankylosis. Additional special views of the joint and computed tomographic (CT) scans are also worthwhile.

Throughout the preoperative planning period the orthodontist should be consulted. The cephalometric analysis, the timing of orthodontic movement of the teeth, and the type of fixation appliances require discussion.

An important part of treatment planning is the choice of the site of osteotomy, as well as of the type of osteotomy and the surgical approach to the mandible. For example, the anterior maxillary alveolar process and teeth, unopposed by the retruded mandibular teeth, tend to drift forward and downward. A segmental maxillary set-back (see p. 1336) may also be required.

Elongation Osteotomies of Body of Mandible: General Considerations. Although, in the vast majority of cases, the sagittal splitting procedure of the ramus is preferred to lengthen the mandible, there are special indications for the infrequently used body osteotomies. The line of osteotomy and its location in the body of the mandible vary according to the deformity and the status of the dentition. Gaps in the dental arch due to missing teeth offer a convenient site for the line of osteotomy, because possible injury to the adjacent teeth is avoided. Various types of osteotomy are available (Fig. 29–83), but the basic associated problems common to all body lengthening osteotomies require further consideration.

The surgical problems involved in mandibular body osteotomies include (1) maintenance of contact between the body fragments to ensure consolidation, (2) preservation of the continuity of the inferior alveolar neurovascular bundle, and (3) provision of soft tissue coverage over the area of the elongation.

Maintenance of Contact of Bony Fragments. The L-osteotomy (Fig. 29–83*A* to *D*), the step osteotomy (Fig. 29–83*E* to *H*), or sagittal splitting of the mandibular body (Fig. 29–84) are preferable to the straight vertical osteotomy because they provide an increased area of contact between the fragments. Maintenance of contact between the fragments is ensured by the fixation appliance and direct interosseous wiring or miniplate stabilization. If the surface of contact between the bone fragments is inadequate, bone grafts are placed in the line of osteotomy to facilitate consolidation.

Preservation of Inferior Alveolar Neurovascular Bundle. The inferior alveolar nerve divides into two terminal branches, the mental and incisive nerves. The mental nerve exits from the mental foramen and divides into three branches that provide the sensory innervation to the skin of the chin and the mucous membrane and skin of the lower lip. The other terminal branch, the incisive nerve, is an anterior extension of the nerve within the mandible. It supplies the sensory innervation to the canine and incisors. Whereas tearing or sectioning the mental nerve at the mental foramen results in permanent loss of sensibility of half of the lower lip, section of the incisive nerve abolishes the sensibility of the anterior teeth, a consequence of little clinical significance.

The mental foramen is the landmark used to determine the position of the osteotomy. Osteotomy of the body of the mandible is preferably made anterior and inferior to the mental foramen, and the step design is completed by a horizontal or oblique extension below the level of the inferior alveolar nerve and canal (Fig. 29–83*C,D*). The incisive nerve is sectioned but the mental nerve is preserved. However, when an osteotomy through the body must be performed posterior to the mental foramen, the inferior alveolar neurovascular bundle must be exposed to avoid severing it.

When the osteotomy line is located posterior to the mental foramen (Fig. 29–83*E,F*), continuity of the nerve is preserved by the following technique. The outer cortical plate, posterior to the mental foramen, is removed by a power-driven round bur. The nerve is thus decompressed. If a wide area must be exposed, the sagittal splitting technique affords the greatest exposure (Fig. 29–84). The

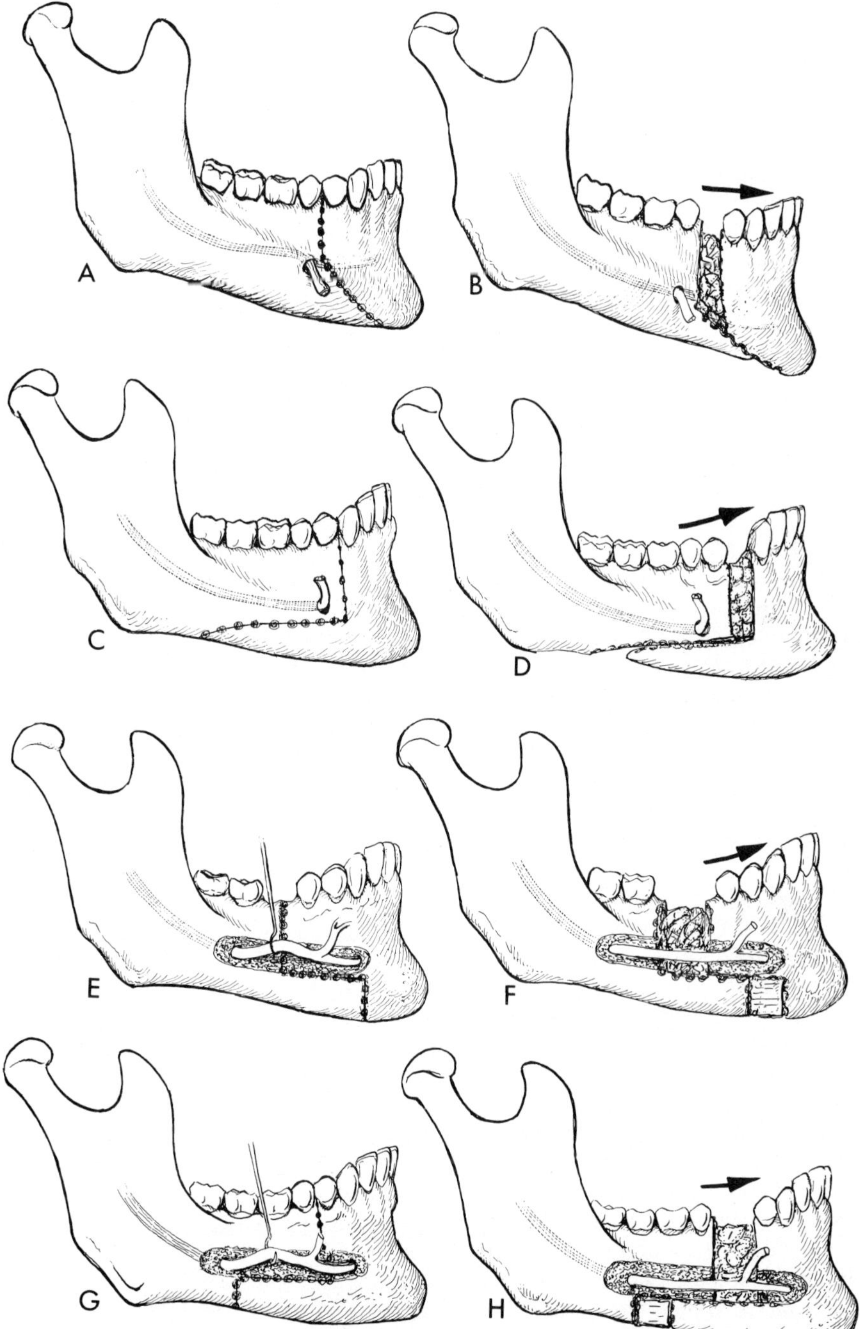

Figure 29–83. Four variations of osteotomy lines to lengthen the body of the mandible. *A,* L-osteotomy placed anterior to the mental foramen. *B,* Elongation obtained by the L-osteotomy. Bone chips fill the resulting gap. *C,* The reverse L-osteotomy is a preferred technique for elongation of the body of the mandible. It is designed in the shape of an L resting on its back. *D,* Elongation obtained by the reverse L-osteotomy. *E,* Step osteotomy placed posterior to the mental foramen with exposure of the inferior alveolar neurovascular bundle. *F,* Elongation obtained by the step osteotomy. A bone graft is wedged into the gap along the lower border of the mandible, and bone chips are placed in the upper gap. *G,* Reverse step osteotomy with exposure and preservation of the main trunk and also the incisive branch of the inferior alveolar nerve. *H,* Elongation obtained by the reverse step osteotomy.

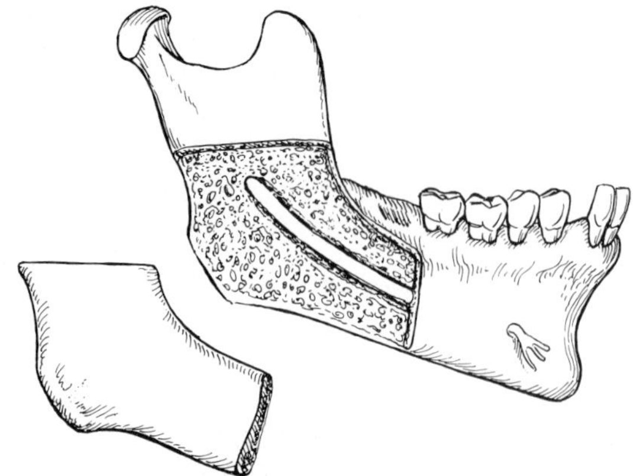

Figure 29–84. Sagittal splitting of the body of the mandible and ramus prior to the osteotomies required in a complex deformity. The outer table of the bone is removed, exposing the inferior alveolar neurovascular bundle, which is protected as the mandible is divided by an osteotomy (not illustrated). (After Obwegeser.)

resected outer cortex is replaced over the inferior alveolar canal after the procedure is completed. Care should be taken to avoid compression of the nerve.

When the osteotomy is performed anterior to the mental foramen, the conduction of the inferior alveolar nerve and of the mental nerve is generally preserved. Loss of sensibility in the anterior teeth has not been a notable cause of complaint on the part of patients. In cases when the osteotomy is performed posterior to the mental foramen, decompression of the nerve may suffice to preserve conduction when the lengthening of the mandibular body is moderate. However, if tension on the nerve becomes evident when considerable advancement is required, two techniques can be employed to decrease tension and prevent the loss of nerve conduction. The first consists of complete decompression of the neurovascular bundle from the mental foramen to the area of the osteotomy; the second method, indicated in cases requiring greater lengthening, is nerve grafting. The inferior alveolar nerve is separated from the vessels using visual magnification with binocular loupes or the operating microscope (Hausamen, Samii, and Schmidseder, 1973). The nerve is sectioned and allowed to retract, and a nerve graft is sutured to the sectioned ends of the nerve, applying Millesi's tension-free principle (see Chap. 19).

Preservation of Soft Tissue Coverage. The best technique of exposure is the degloving procedure (see Fig. 29–46). Excellent exposure of a major portion of the body is obtained and preservation of the mental nerves is facilitated.

The labiobuccal vestibular incision, made well above the cul de sac of the sulcus and continued backward over the inner aspect of the cheek, provides ample tissue to ensure coverage in the average elongation osteotomy and is preferable to the gingival incision. The rigid attachment of the gingiva to the underlying alveolar bone makes it more difficult to suture under tension and more apt to tear.

When an unusual amount of elongation is required (Figs. 29–85, 29–86), adjacent soft tissue must be used to cover the area of the osteotomy or the bone graft interposed between the fragments. Usually, as in the patient shown in Figure 29–85, the portion of the body to be elongated is edentulous. If the resulting bone defect is extensive, sufficient bone contact cannot be expected between the fragments if an L-shaped or step osteotomy is used; a bone graft must be interposed (see also the planning of the mandibular lengthening in Fig. 29–87).

Before the osteotomy of the mandibular body (Fig. 29–87*A*), a wide, rectangular, cheek-based flap is outlined to overlap the grafted area (Fig. 29–87*B*). The distal portion of the flap extends from the floor of the mouth and includes the mucoperiosteum over the bone and the mucosa of the sulcus and cheek. The base of the flap is on the cheek wall below the parotid duct orifice. The exposed mandible is sectioned and elongated; the fragments are placed in their new position and the resulting gap is filled with a bone graft (Fig. 29–87*C,D*). The flap is drawn lingually and sutured in position (Fig. 29–87*E,F*). To avoid tension, the buccal sulcus is bridged and thus temporarily obliterated (Fig. 29–87*E* to *H*).

The fragments are indexed to one another by a splint that has been fabricated preoperatively from the working dental casts. Interosseous wire or miniplates provide internal alignment. The jaws are held in intermaxillary fixation for approximately six to eight weeks, or a shorter period if miniplates are used. Primary healing is expected if the design of the flap is proper and tension is avoided. After the bone graft has healed, a

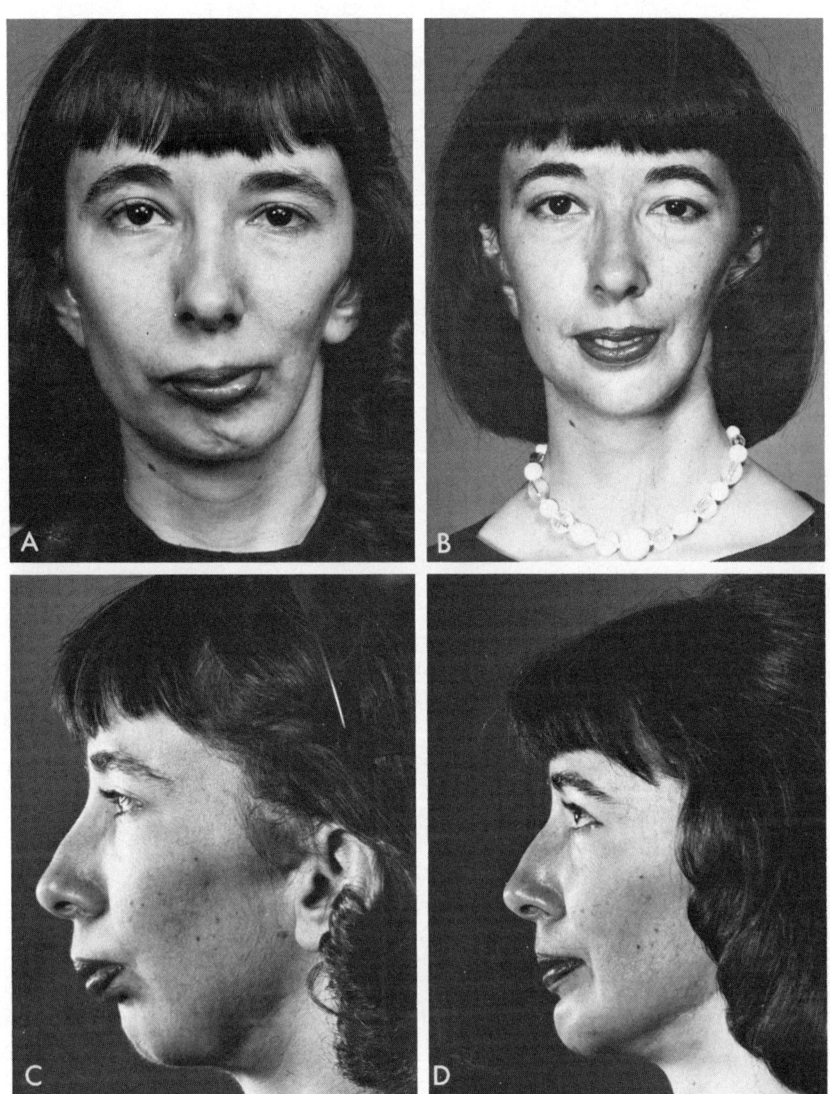

Figure 29–85. Micrognathia resulting from irradiation of the left side of the mandible in childhood. *A,* Appearance of the patient with micrognathia and considerable shortening of the left half of the mandible. *B,* Postoperative appearance after bilateral osteotomy and bone grafting of the body of the mandible through the intraoral approach. *C,* Preoperative profile. *D,* Postoperative profile showing elongation of the body of the mandible. (From Converse, J. M.: Micrognathia. Br. J. Plast. Surg., *16*:197, 1963.)

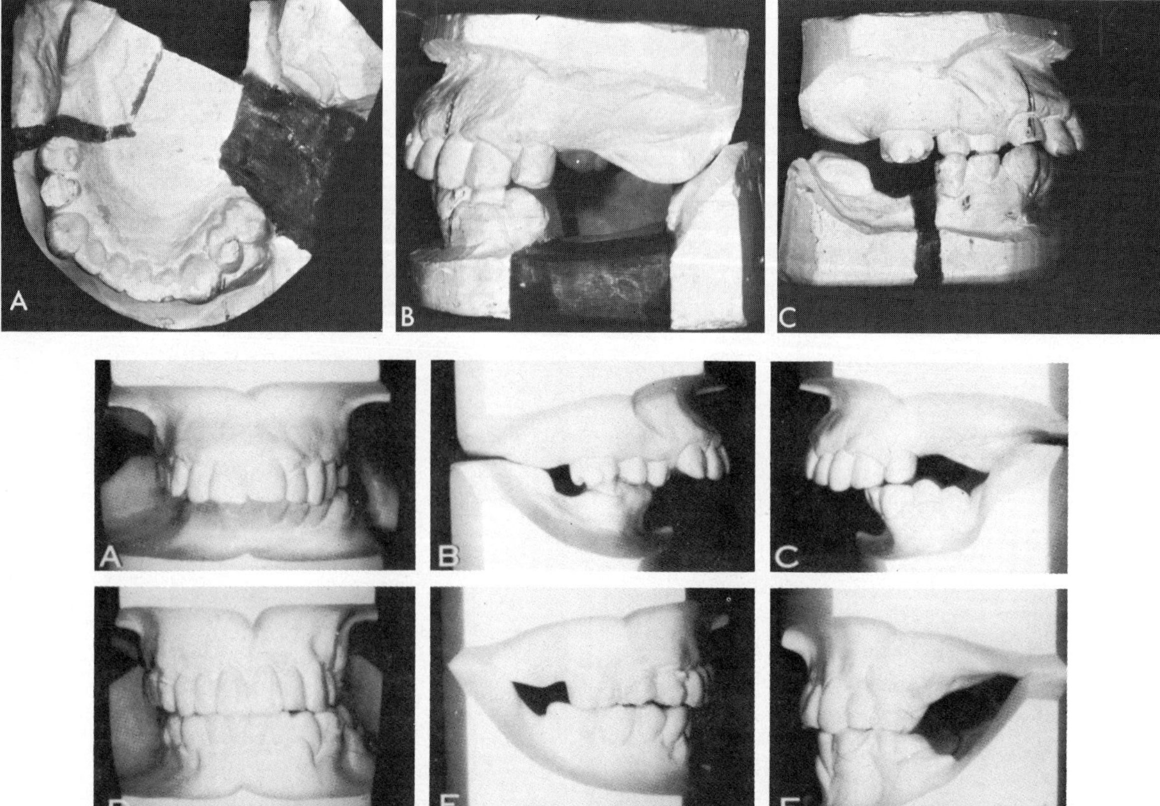

Figure 29–86. *Above,* Planning the osteotomies on the dental casts of the patient shown in Figure 29–85. The casts are sectioned, advanced, and rotated to correct the jaw and occlusal relationships. Wax is used to join the fragments and represents the amount of advancement required. Note the larger amount of advancement that is necessary on the left side and the lesser amount required on the right side. *Below,* Dental casts showing the occlusal relationships. *A* to *C,* Preoperative occlusal relationships of the patient shown in Figure 29–85. *D* to *F,* Postoperative relationships.

new buccal sulcus is established by the skin or mucosa inlay technique, which restores an alveolar ridge and sulcus for the support of a prosthesis (see Figs. 29–276, 29–277).

A transposition flap of mucoperiosteum and vestibular mucous membrane represents another technique for providing coverage of the exposed bone graft (Fig. 29–88). The flap will cover only narrow gaps but has the advantage of eliminating the need for a second operation to restore the buccal sulcus.

Techniques for Lengthening Mandibular Body. A step osteotomy can be used to lengthen the shortened body of the mandible (see Fig. 29–83). Bone contact is maintained between the fragments by the horizontal portion of the step. This method was employed by von Eiselsberg (1906) to lengthen the body of the mandible and by Blair (1907) to correct an open bite.

The simplest technique of elongation is the reverse L-osteotomy (see Fig. 29–83*C,D*). The design is that of an L reclining on its back. The vertical branch is placed anterior to the mental foramen, and the horizontal limb below and parallel to the inferior alveolar canal. The horizontal extension must be placed close to the lower border of the mandible because of the slight descent of the inferior alveolar canal before it turns cephalad to reach the mental foramen. Thus, if the horizontal cut is made too close to the mental foramen, there is a risk of penetrating the canal and injuring the neurovascular bundle. The panoramic roentgenogram is helpful in locating the canal and foramen.

Conduction can be reestablished through a partially divided inferior alveolar nerve. Furthermore, considerable overlap of the sensory innervation occurs in the denervated lower lip from the adjacent sensory nerves, but full sensibility is rarely recovered through this

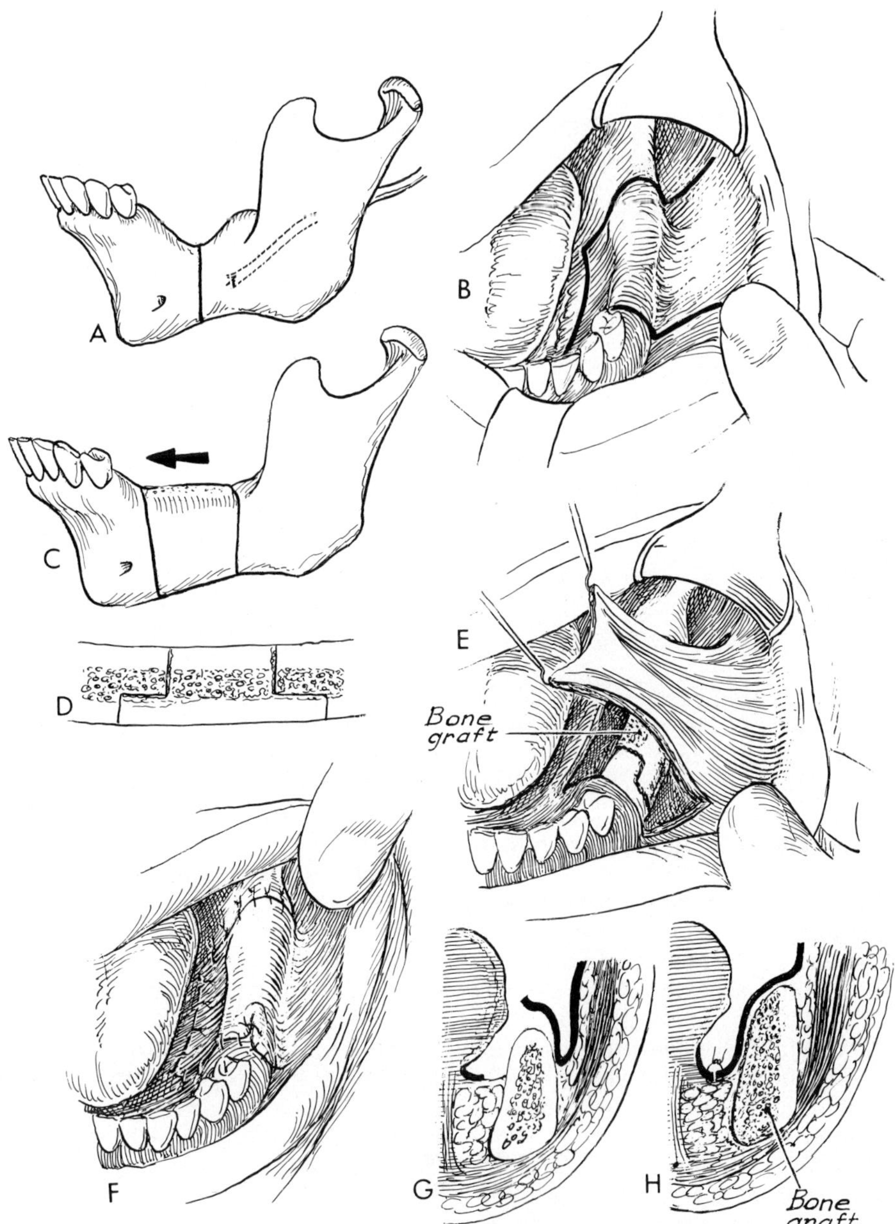

Figure 29–87. Covering a bone graft when an unusual amount of elongation is required. *A,* The line of osteotomy of the body of the mandible is indicated. *B,* Outlining of the cheek-based flap, which is raised prior to the osteotomy. *C,* The bone graft in position after the mandible has been lengthened. *D,* Cross section illustrating the greater surface of contact with the host bone achieved by the overlapping flanges of the bone grafts. *E,* Mucosal flap is advanced over the grafted area. *F,* Suturing is completed. *G,* Frontal section illustrating the flap being raised prior to the osteotomy. *H,* Flap suturing in a position to cover the bone graft. The buccal sulcus is obliterated and will be restored at a later date by the skin graft inlay technique.

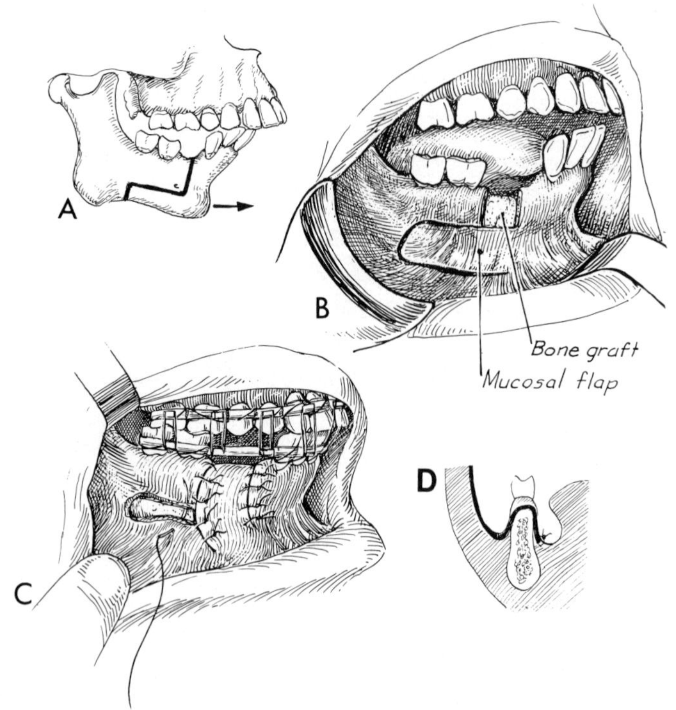

Figure 29–88. Vestibular-alveolar transposition flap for coverage of the area of osteotomy after elongation of the body of the mandible. *A,* Design of the step osteotomy for elongation of the body of the mandible. *B,* Vestibular-alveolar transposition flap and the exposed area to be covered. *C,* The transposed flap is sutured into place. The donor area is closed by direct approximation. *D,* Cross section showing the position of the flap. The distal portion is sutured to the mucous membrane of the floor of the mouth.

process. For this reason, preservation of the continuity of the inferior alveolar bundle should be a routine procedure.

The osteotomy is made by small, oscillating, and reciprocating saws or by a series of bur holes joined together by a fissure bur or an osteotome.

After completion of the osteotomy, the anterior segment is drawn forward to its new position. A splint made preoperatively from the working dental cast is applied to support the anterior fragment in its new position. Intermaxillary fixation or miniplates completes the dental immobilization of the fragments. The inferior border of the proximal segment tends to tilt lingually from the contraction of the medial pterygoid and mylohyoid muscles. Direct interosseous wire or miniplate fixation is required (1) to stabilize the posterior fragments, (2) to help maintain the forward position of the anterior fragment, and (3) to prevent a posterior and downward tilt (clockwise rotation of the mental symphysis under the displacing forces of the suprahyoid muscles).

Measured blocks of bone graft are wedged into the gaps left by the step osteotomies. Any remaining interstices are filled with cancellous bone chips. The intraoral soft tissues are closed with absorbable sutures. Six to eight weeks of postoperative intermaxillary fixation are usually required or a shorter period when miniplate fixation is used.

A patient with mandibular hypoplasia who underwent an elongation osteotomy of the body of the lower jaw is shown in Figure 29–89. Bone grafting for additional contour restoration followed. The occlusal relationship of the teeth before and after surgical and prosthodontic treatment is shown in Figure 29–90.

Interdental Osteotomy. The vertical branch of the step osteotomy can be made through the alveolar bone between two adjacent teeth without injuring the dental roots. The extraction of a tooth is thus avoided. Intraoral periapical dental and panoramic roentgenograms give a clear picture of the position of the roots of the teeth and the amount of intervening alveolar bone. Additional space, if needed, can be created by the orthodontist (see Fig. 29–20). The buccal and lingual cortical bone along the proposed line of osteotomy between the adjacent teeth is remove with a fine fissure bur or a reciprocating saw. Only the cortical plate is penetrated. After the remainder of the step osteotomy has been completed, a narrow, tapered

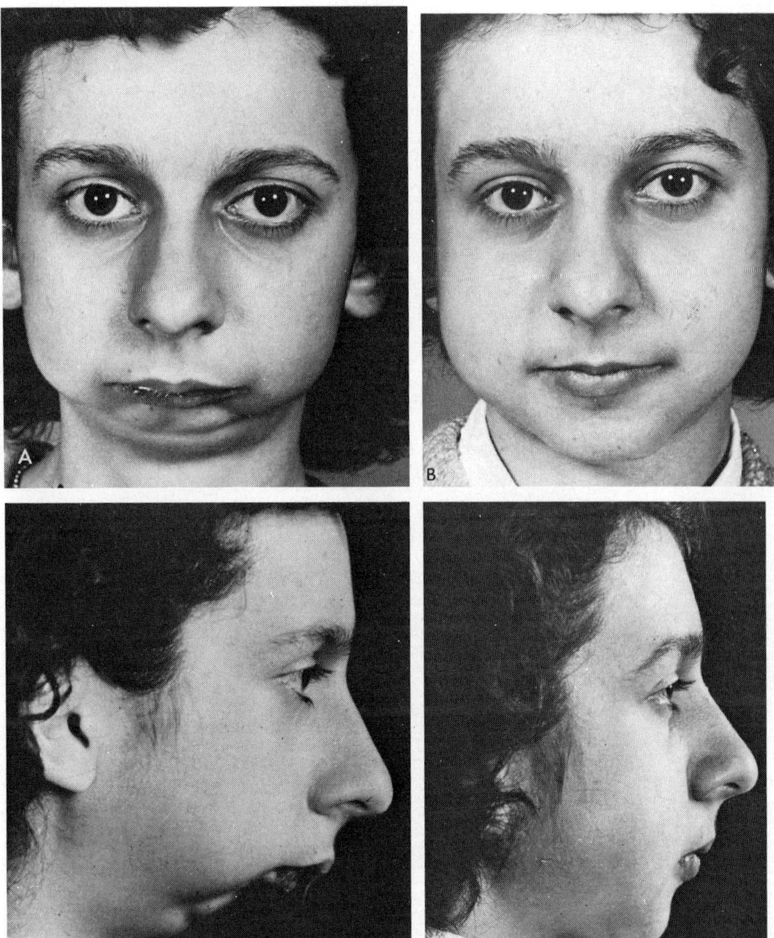

Figure 29–89. Bilateral temporomandibular ankylosis and mandibular micrognathia. *A, C,* Preoperative views. *B, D,* Postoperative appearance after (1) temporomandibular arthroplasty, (2) elongation osteotomy of the body of the mandible, and (3) restoration of mandibular contour by iliac bone grafting through the intraoral approach. (From Converse, J. M.: Micrognathia. Br. J. Plast. Surg., *16*:197, 1963.)

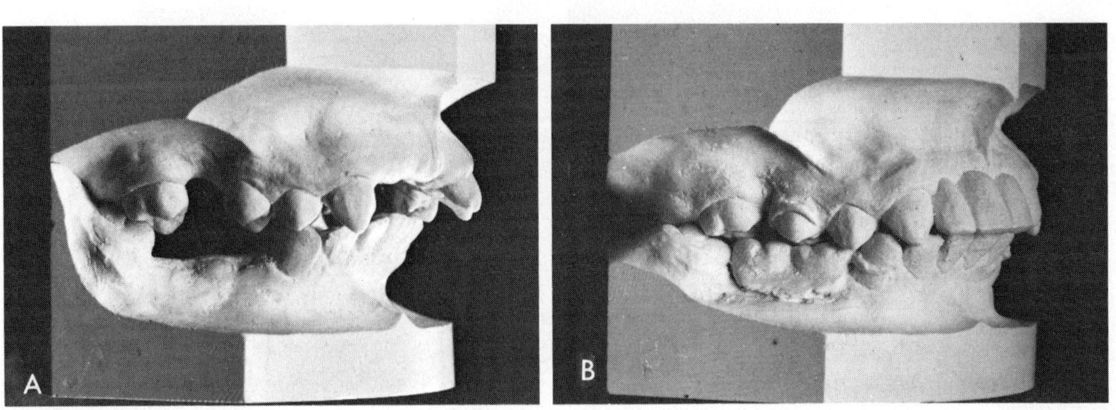

Figure 29–90. Dental casts of patient shown in Figure 29–89. *A,* Preoperative dentoalveolar relationships. *B,* Postoperative casts with improved occlusal relationships and prosthodontic restorations.

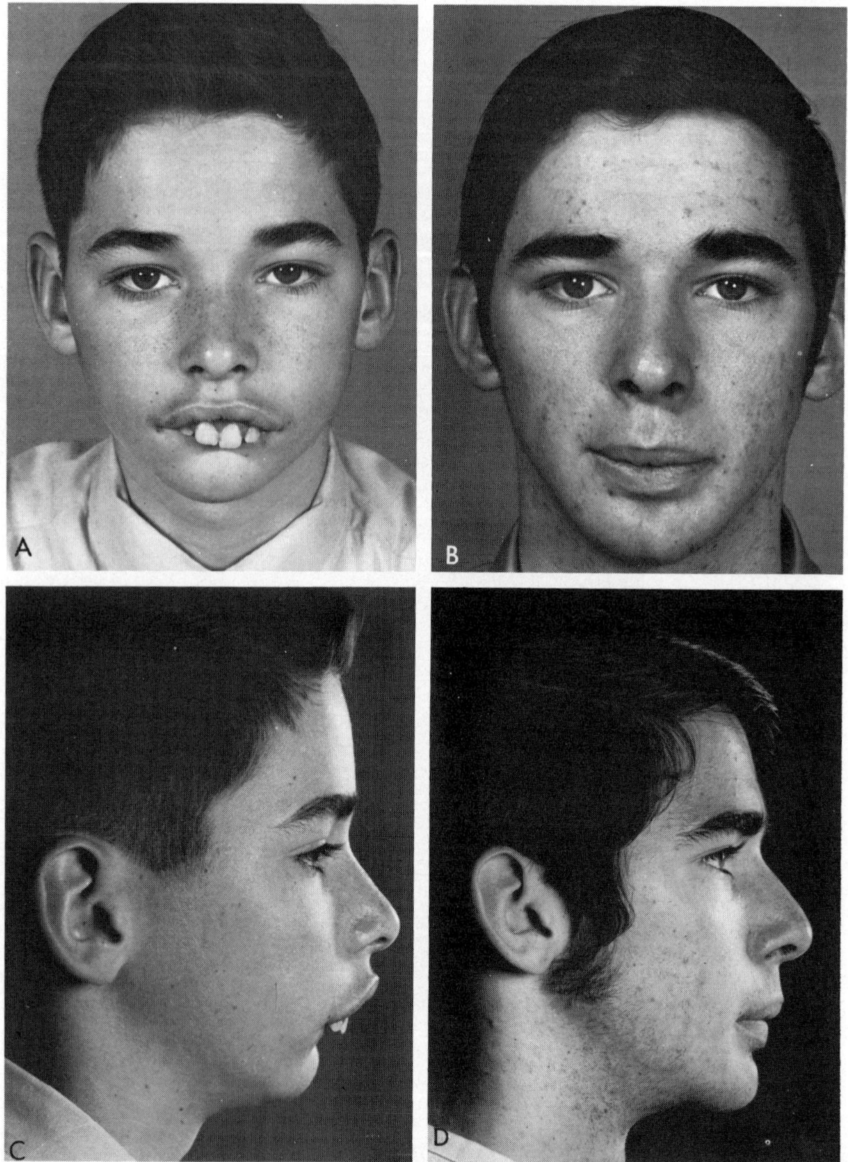

Figure 29–91. Mandibular micrognathia and maxillary protrusion treated by maxillary segmental premolar (set-back) osteotomy in a first stage, elongation osteotomy of the mandibular body in a second stage, and horizontal osteotomy of the mandible. *A,* Appearance before surgery. Note the downward and forward protrusion of the maxillary dentoalveolar segment. A premolar set-back maxillary osteotomy was required to correct this deformity (see Fig. 29–161). *B,* Four years later after completion of three operative stages. *C,* Preoperative profile. *D,* Postoperative profile. Note the adequate projection of the chin and the satisfactory lip seal.

osteotome severs the cancellous bone that remains between the teeth. It is best to start at the apical area where the roots are farthest apart and to work toward the alveolar crest.

Variations. When there are gaps in the posterior teeth, a step osteotomy posterior to the mental foramen can be used (see Fig. 29–83*E,F*). A bone graft is required to fill the void left by the elongation. The inferior alveolar nerve is decompressed and lengthened. Moderate elongation of the inferior alveolar bundle is not a problem, and lengthening can be done without causing excessive tension on the nerve if the nerve is widely decompressed. The inferior alveolar canal should be decompressed to the mental foramen.

An osteotomy in the shape of a widely angled L with its horizontal limb extending

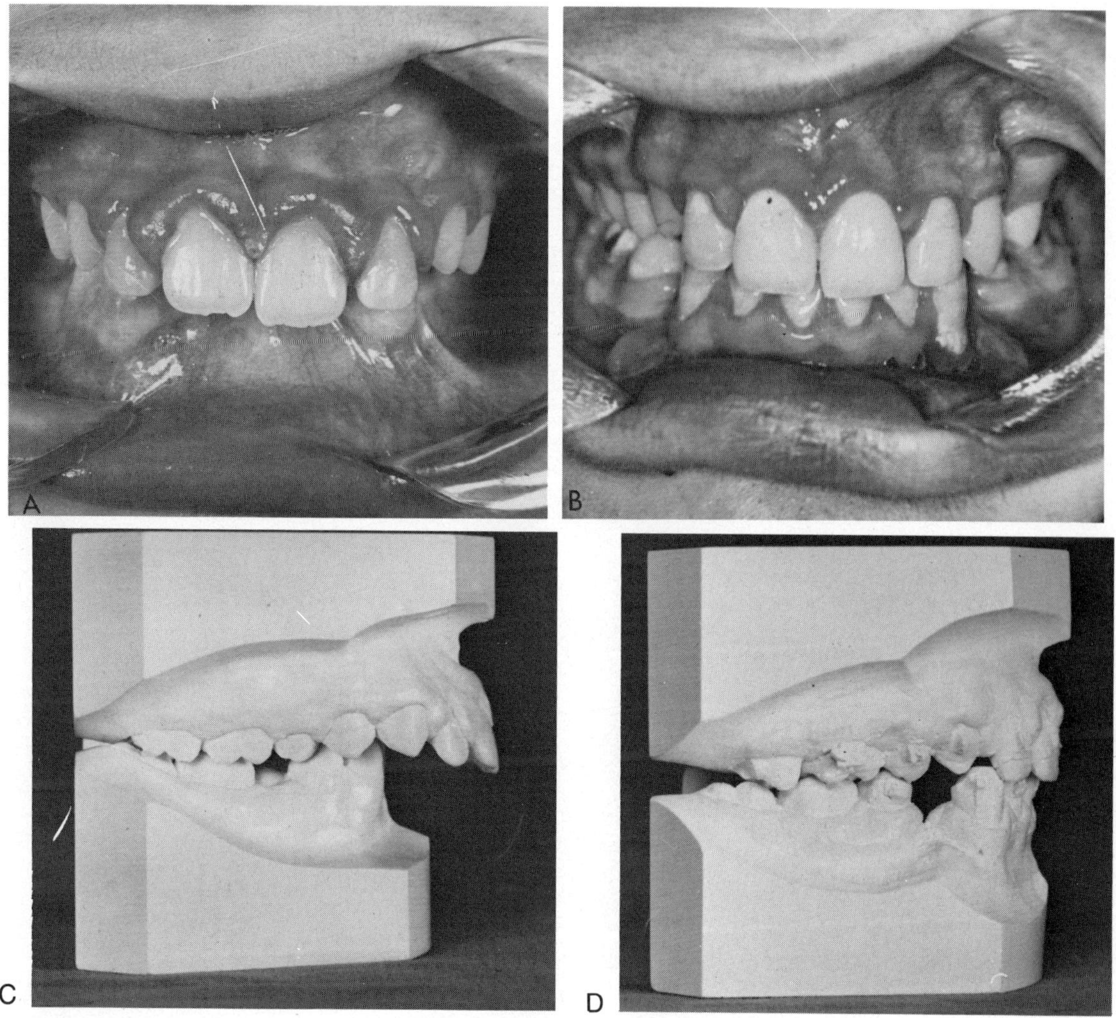

Figure 29–92. Intraoral views and dental casts (models) of the patient shown in Figure 29–91. *A*, Before surgical-othodontic treatment. *B*, After completion of treatment. *C*, Before. *D*, After.

forward and downward can be applied when lengthening of the mandible must be combined with correction of an anterior closed bite and there is a short lower facial height (see Fig. 29–83*A*,*B*).

Mandibular Hypoplasia Associated with Maxillary Dentoalveolar Protrusion. The problem of correction is illustrated by the patient shown in Figure 29–91, who was first examined at the age of 12 years. The mandibular hypoplasia was severe and the soft tissues over the mental symphysis were tight and unyielding. The anterior maxillary dentoalveolar process had drifted forward and downward, resulting in an accentuated overjet and overbite (Fig. 29–92*A*). There are several alternative ways to correct the deformity. The technique used in the patient illustrated produced an excellent result, but probably would yield to newer methods of treatment (discussed later).

Photographs, cephalometric tracings, and casts of the dentition were used to formulate a treatment plan. Because of the patient's young age, a three-phase surgical plan was chosen. The first phase consisted of a premolar segmental maxillary dentoalveolar (setback) osteotomy (see Fig. 29–161). After extraction of a premolar tooth on each side of the dental arch and removal of a transverse strip of bone, the anterior maxillary dentoalveolar segment was displaced backward and upward into the predetermined position. An edgewise orthodontic appliance maintained the fixation (monobloc), and intermaxillary fixation was not required because of the stable posterior segments (Fig. 29–93).

After exposure of the mandible by the de-

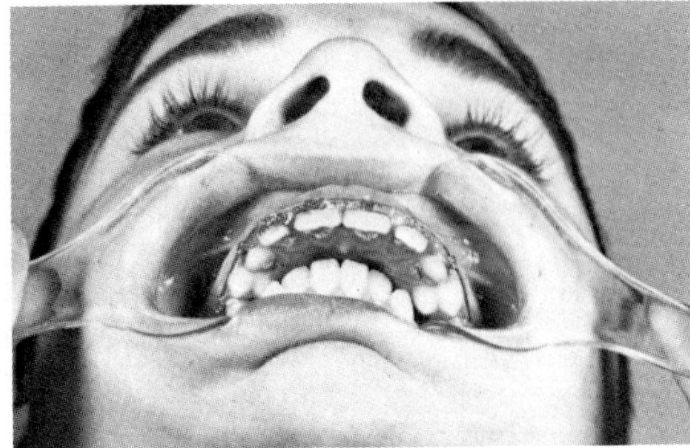

Figure 29–93. Edgewise orthodontic appliance for fixation after premolar set-back osteotomy.

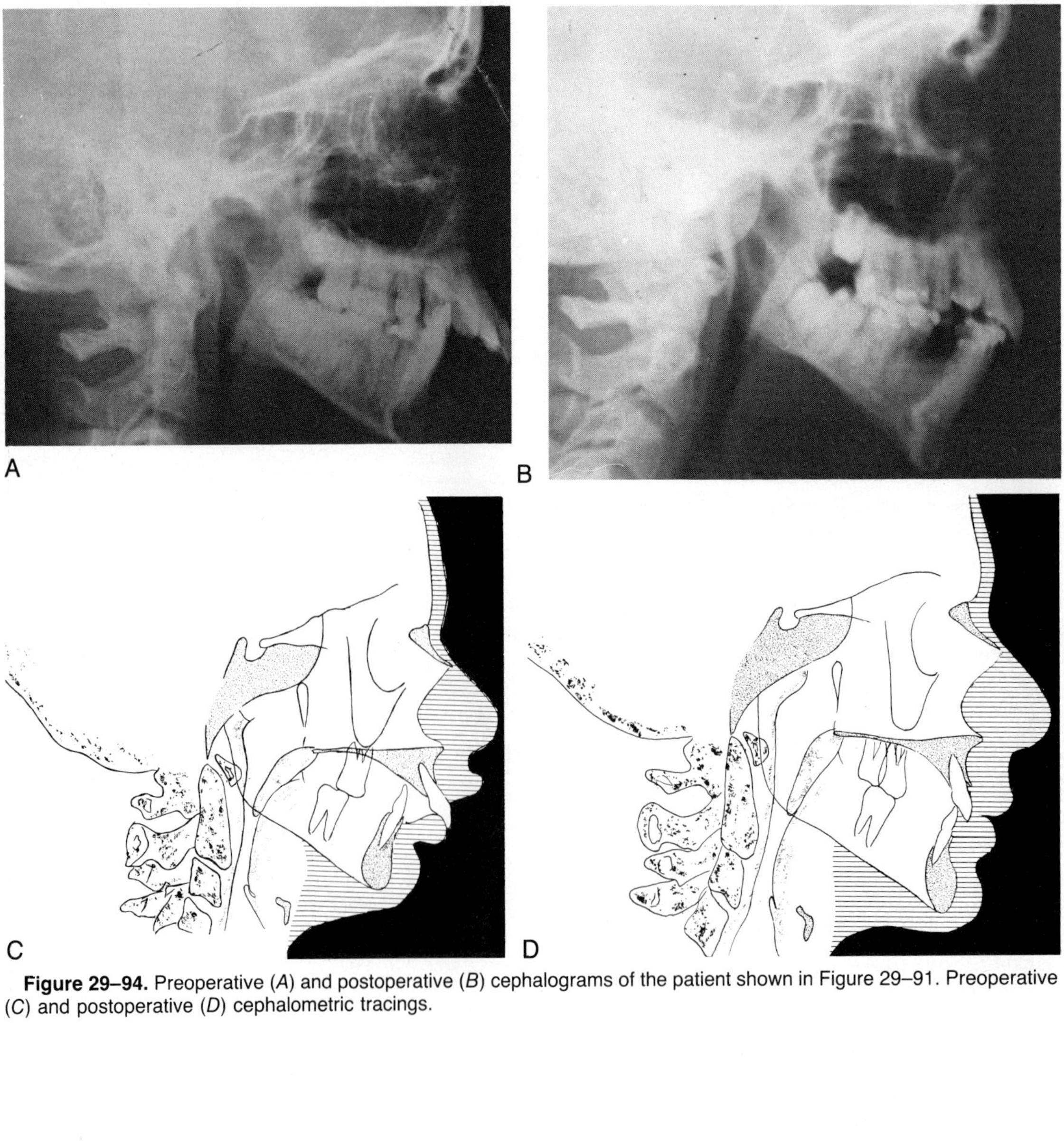

A B C D

Figure 29–94. Preoperative (*A*) and postoperative (*B*) cephalograms of the patient shown in Figure 29–91. Preoperative (*C*) and postoperative (*D*) cephalometric tracings.

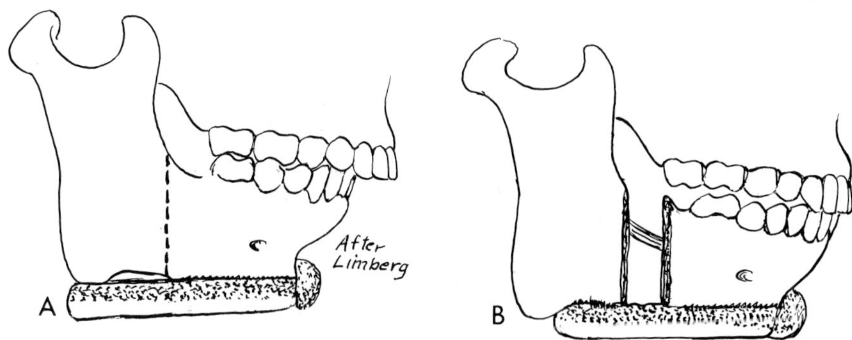

Figure 29–95. Limberg's technique using a retromolar lengthening osteotomy. *A,* A bone graft was initially placed along the lower border of the mandible to maintain bone continuity. *B,* Subsequent body advancement. (From Converse, J. M.: Micrognathia. Br. J. Plast. Surg., *16*:197, 1963.)

gloving technique, the body of the mandible was lengthened in a second stage by a step osteotomy (see Fig. 29–83*E,F*). A horizontal advancement osteotomy of the lower portion of the mandible (osseous genioplasty) was also performed (see p. 1312). The tight soft tissues over the mental symphysis prevented adequate projection of the chin. However, the step osteotomy of the mandibular body achieved sufficient lengthening and improved the occlusal relationships.

Three months later the mandible was again exposed by the degloving technique, and a second horizontal advancement osteotomy was performed. The resistance of the soft tissues, both intraoral and extraoral, was overcome with difficulty (see Fig. 29–91*B,D*). A comparison of the cephalograms and their tracings made before the onset and five years after completion of treatment (Fig. 29–94) illustrates the skeletal and soft tissue contour changes.

An alternative method to correct the combined problem of mandibular hypoplasia and maxillary protrusion in an adult or full-grown patient would be to advance the mandible using an intraoral sagittal splitting ramal procedure (see p. 1280) and perform a simultaneous maxillary anterior set-back (see p. 1336) and an osseous genioplasty (see p. 1312). Advancing the mandible through a ramal procedure avoids creating a gap in the dental arch, which is a major objection to the body section procedure. Furthermore, the body osteotomy makes it difficult to perform a simultaneous osseous genioplasty.

Retromolar Step Osteotomy. The retromolar osteotomy to lengthen the body of the mandible was employed by Limberg (1928). A bone graft was placed along the lower border of the mandible in a preliminary stage (Fig. 29–95*A*). In a second stage a vertical retromolar osteotomy was performed, the mandibular body was advanced, and the previously transplanted bone graft was used to maintain body continuity (Fig. 29–95*B*).

The retromolar step osteotomy has the advantage of not producing a gap in the dental arch when the body of the mandible is elongated, but it is more difficult to perform (Fig. 29–96). The vertical cut of the step is placed behind the last molar. Intraoral decompression of the inferior alveolar nerve is difficult in this area because of the lingual position of the nerve; an external approach may be required. However, because of the difficulties associated with the technique and the development of simpler procedures, the retromolar osteotomy is mainly of historical interest.

Bone Grafting Associated with Elongation Osteotomy. Iliac bone grafts, consisting mostly of cancellous bone, are used as flat pieces that cover the lines of osteotomy, and as blocks of bone and small chips that fill the gaps caused by the advancement. Calvarial bone grafts can also be used for lesser defects, but lack the volume of desired cancellous bone. Resected segments of the mandibular bone can also be employed. The bone grafts ensure bone continuity, increase the chances of successful consolidation at the osteotomy sites, and improve the size and contour of the mandible. They are successful only if covered with well-vascularized soft tissues.

Other Elongation Osteotomies of Mandibular Body. The oblique osteotomy through the body of the mandible was described by Blair (1907) and Kazanjian (1939). It is another technique that can be used in the edentulous mandible when the inferior

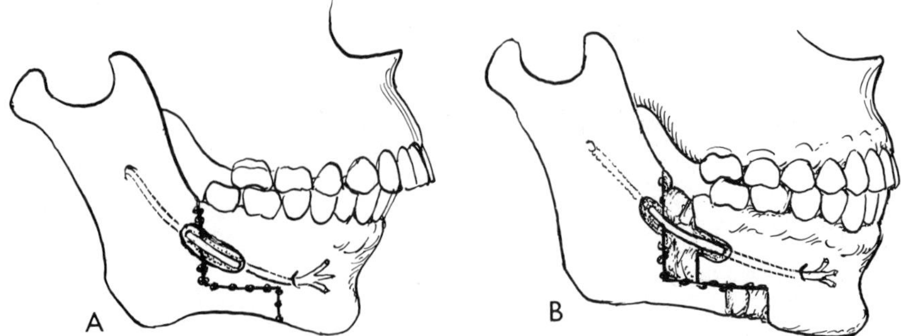

Figure 29–96. Retromolar step elongation osteotomy. *A,* Outline of the step osteotomy and exposure of the inferior alveolar nerve. *B,* Position of the fragments after the anterior segment of the mandible has been advanced. Bone grafts are placed in the bony gap.

alveolar nerve has been destroyed by trauma, disease, or ablative operations of the mandibular body (Fig. 29–97).

Advantages and Disadvantages of Body Elongation Osteotomies. The main indication for a body elongation osteotomy is the need to correct mandibular arch form as well as length. A mandible of unequal body length and distorted dental arch contour is a candidate for these techniques.

The disadvantages of mandibular body osteotomies are many and should make the surgeon pause before choosing to perform them. The main drawbacks of the technique are (1) possible injury to the inferior alveolar nerve when the osteotomy must be placed behind the mental foramen, (2) creation of gaps in the dental arch that require later dental prosthetic restoration, (3) technical difficulties, (4) the need to provide additional soft tissue to cover the osteotomy sites, and (5) the need for bone grafts to prevent delayed union and nonunion.

Operations on Mandibular Ramus to Increase Projection of Mandible. Horizontal osteotomies through the ramus above the inferior alveolar foramen to lengthen the mandible were practiced by Lane (1905) and Blair (1907). Such operations are subject to the three major complications previously enumerated with regard to mandibular prognathism: (1) distraction of the proximal fragment by the pull of the temporalis and lateral pterygoid muscles, with subsequent delayed union or nonunion; (2) occasional loss of the vertical dimension of the ramus through overlapping of the fragments, caused by the pull exerted by the masseter and medial pteryoid muscles on the distal fragment; and (3) relapse. These complications often result in an anterior open bite. Because of these problems, the horizontal osteotomy has been abandoned.

Wassmund (1927) described a ramal section in the shape of an inverted L; the vertical osteotomy, instead of reaching the sigmoid

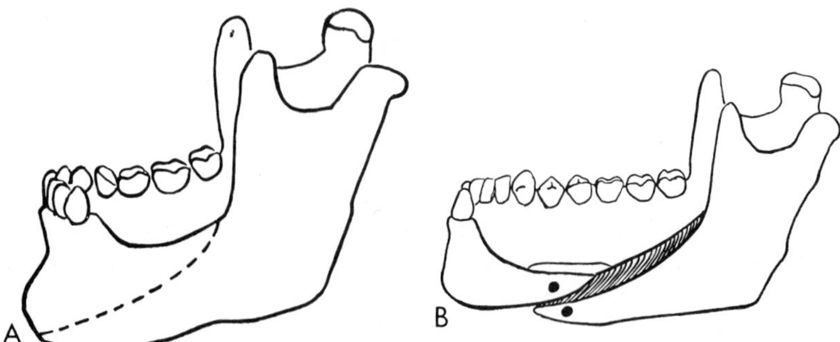

Figure 29–97. *A,* Oblique osteotomy of the mandible. The mandible is sectioned diagonally after its lateral surface has been exposed intraorally. *B,* A hole is drilled at each end of the bone segments, which are fixated with stainless steel wire after advancement. This type of osteotomy is indicated only when the inferior alveolar nerve has been destroyed.

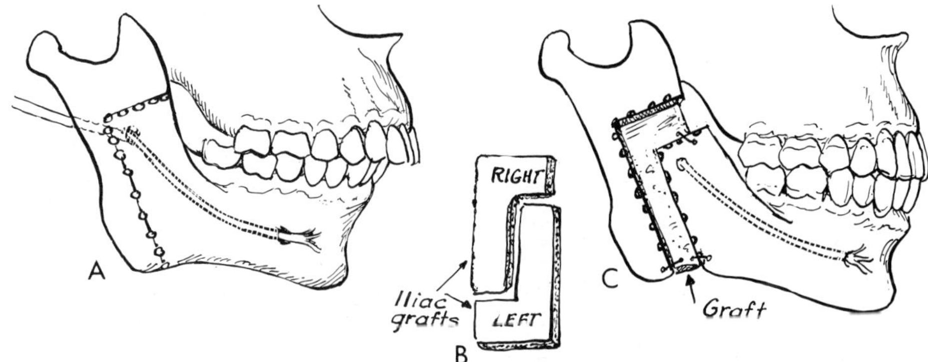

Figure 29–98. Wassmund's inverted L-shaped osteotomy of the ramus. *A,* Outline of the osteotomy. *B,* Bone grafts (right and left). *C,* Operation completed. Bone graft in position.

notch, took a sharp forward turn above the lingula and through the base of the coronoid process. Pichler and Trauner (1948) and Schuchardt (1958) also used this type of osteotomy to treat mandibular hypoplasia. In this technique, bone grafts are placed in the resulting defect to promote bony consolidation (Fig. 29–98).

The Babcock (1937) operation, consisting of insertion of cartilage into the temporomandibular joint posterior to the condyle, was revived by Trauner (1957). The entire mandible is forced forward to improved the mandibular position and the occlusal relationship of the teeth. It is doubtful whether surgical interference with the temporomandibular joint is now justified in view of the development of less destructive operations.

The evolution of surgical techniques to treat mandibular hypoplasia parallels that for the correction of mandibular prognathism. The basic surgical principles were also adapted to elongate the mandible through ramal osteotomies.

Robinson (1957) performed an oblique osteotomy of the ramus and bone grafted the gap. For children, Longacre (1957) recommended wedging split rib grafts between the fragments. Onlay bone grafts can also be added in an attempt to increase the bulk of the ramus and improve the overlying soft tissue contour (Fig. 29–99).

Caldwell and Amaral (1960) combined an iliac bone graft with a vertical section of the ramus. They resected the coronoid process to neutralize the pull of the temporalis and to eliminate possible impingement of the coronoid process on the posterior surface of the zygoma after advancement of the distal fragment. The lateral cortical bone over the lower portion of the ramus was removed to receive an iliac bone graft that bridged the gap (Fig. 29–100).

Robinson and Lytle (1962) reported a series of cases in which they omitted the section of the coronoid process and the addition of bone grafts. The V-shaped defect in the ramus is allowed to fill with bone formed by the investing periosteum. However, a 12 week period of intermaxillary fixation is required and the long-term stability is doubtful.

Increasing Vertical Dimension of Ramus. On occasions, as in craniofacial microsomia (see Chap. 62), it may be desirable to increase the vertical dimension of a hypoplastic ramus. The procedure should not be regarded lightly, since the powerful masseter and medial pterygoid muscles respond in an unkindly manner to being stretched. Relapse is a definite possibility.

Several methods can be considered, depending on the amount of ramus present. If the ramus is sufficiently well developed, a satisfactory choice would be the sagittal splitting osteotomy, since the harvest of a bone graft is avoided. Unfortunately the ramus is usually too small for this technique; an alternative is an inverted L-osteotomy with interposition of a bone graft (see Fig. 29–98). The ramus is exposed by a subperiosteal elevation of the masseter and the medial pterygoid muscles, and a division of their sling along the inferior border of the mandible. This step is essential if success is to be achieved. A block of iliac or calvarial bone is wedged into the interval between the fragments. The distal fragment must be maintained in its elongated position and an intraoral biteblock placed in the molar area. The proximal and distal fragments are held together with in-

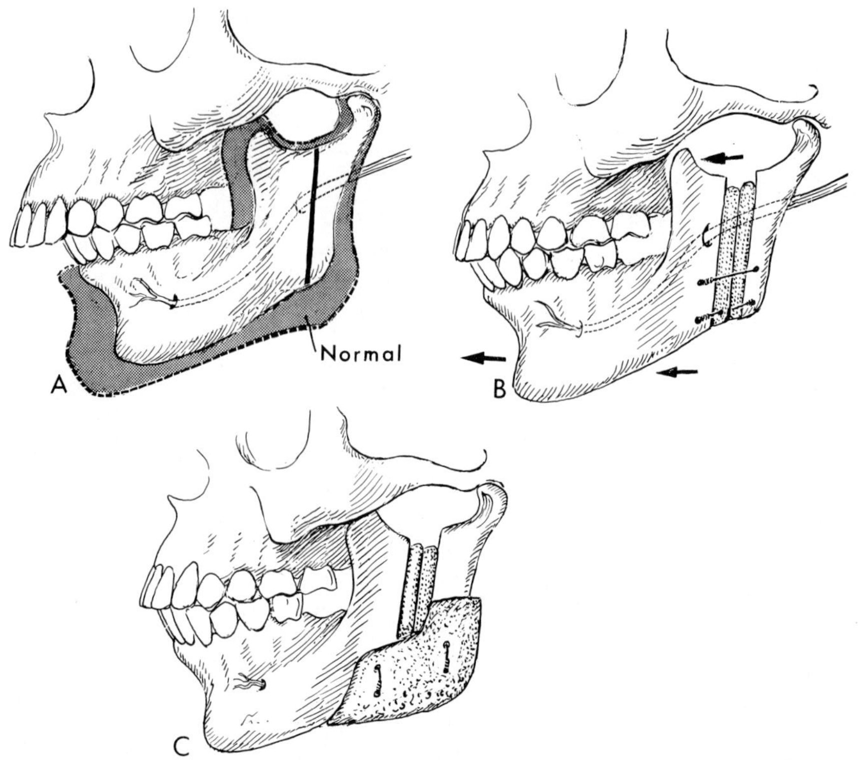

Figure 29–99. Elongation of the mandible by vertical section of the ramus and onlay and interposition bone grafting. *A,* Micrognathic mandible is contrasted to the normally developed mandible (*shaded*). *B,* After vertical section of the ramus, bone grafts are interposed between the fragments and maintained by interosseous wiring. *C,* An onlay bone graft is added to reinforce the interposed bone grafts and augment the contour of the mandibular angle. (From Converse, J. M., Horowitz, S. L., Coccaro, P. J., and Wood-Smith, D.: The corrective treatment of the skeletal asymmetry in hemifacial microsomia. Plast. Reconstr. Surg., *52*:221, 1973. Copyright 1973, The Williams & Wilkins Company, Baltimore.)

terosseous wires or, preferably, a miniplate; the stabilization is completed with intermaxillary fixation. This type of procedure was performed in 1941 by Converse and Rushton on a patient whose results were reported by Rushton (1942, 1944) and Gillies and Millard (1957). A similar technique was employed by Osborne (1964).

Advantages and Disadvantages of Vertical Osteotomy of Ramus. The principal advantage of the vertical section procedure of the ramus is its simplicity. Exposure is satisfactory, the osteotomy is easy to perform, and adequate advancement can be obtained. In contrast to body elongation techniques, the vertical osteotomy of the ramus presents minimal risk to the inferior alveolar nerve, edentulous areas are not produced in the dental arch, and soft tissue coverage of the osteotomy is not a problem. A small ramus can be increased in size and contour restoration with bone grafts is possible at the same time.

The disadvantages include inability to correct dental arch length discrepancies and severe posterior crossbite problems, the need to harvest a bone graft, and the frequent call for a cutaneous incision. The external scar is objectionable and injury to the marginal mandibular nerve is always a possibility. The amount of advancement is limited by the forward movement of the coronoid, which may impinge against the zygoma. The Wassmund inverted L (see Fig. 29–98) or the Hayes C-osteotomy (see Fig. 29–106) offers an alternative since the coronoid process does not participate in the advancement.

On balance, the vertical/oblique osteotomy suffers greatly in comparison with the sagittal splitting ramal osteotomy for the treatment of mandibular hypoplasia.

Elongation of Mandible by Sagittal Section of Ramus. *The ramal sagittal splitting technique is the most popular method used to increase the anteroposterior dimension of the*

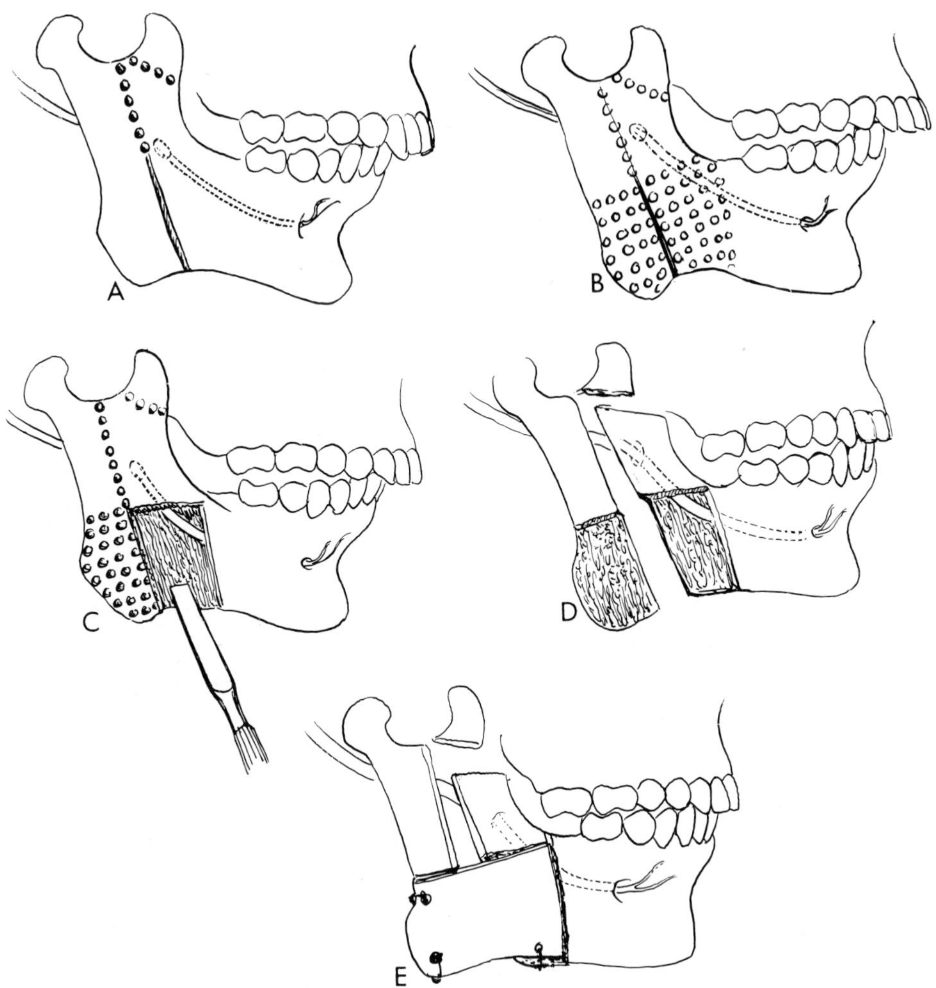

Figure 29–100. Vertical osteotomy of the ramus of the mandible combined with a bone graft for advancement of the body of the mandible. *A,* Lines of osteotomy. *B,* The outer cortex in the region of the angle is perforated by multiple drill holes. *C,* The outer cortex of the mandible is removed with an osteotome. *D,* The body of the mandible is advanced after completion of the osteotomy; the coronoid process is also detached. *E,* A bone graft is wired in position to maintain bony contact between the separated mandibular fragments. (After Caldwell and Amaral, 1960.)

mandible. A wide surface of contact between the fragments is provided (Fig. 29–101), and thus the addition of a bone graft is not required. The basic technique is similar to that used in the treatment of mandibular prognathism as described earlier (see Fig. 29–65). However, important points of difference do exist.

When the mandible is advanced, a muscular imbalance is created and unfavorable stretch is placed upon the attached muscles, especially the suprahyoid group. The body reacts to restore the equilibrium and the surgeon must successfully cope with these relapsing forces. The fixation of the fragments becomes critical.

The condyle must be properly seated in the glenoid fossa. If the proximal segment is inferiorly or anteriorly malpositioned, the condyle will be similarly displaced. At the end of the healing period when the lower jaw is released, the mandible is pulled upward and backward as the condyle attempts to find its seat in the glenoid fossa. The result is a relapse to an Angle Class II malocclusion with the addition of an anterior open bite. If an interosseous wire is used to approximate the fragment, the drill holes should be placed so as to produce an upward and backward force on the proximal segment as the wire is being twisted. The wire can be placed along either the inferior border (Booth, 1981) or the

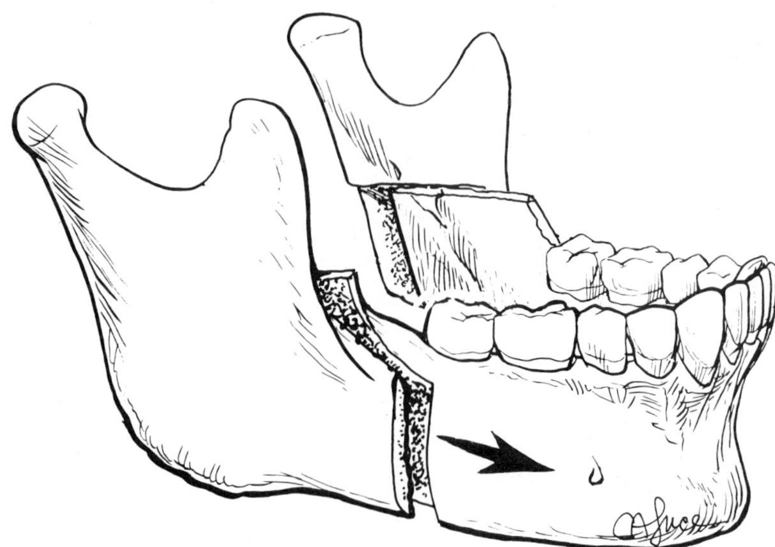

Figure 29–101. Advancement of the mandible by sagittal split osteotomy of the mandibular ramus (see Fig. 29–65 for details of the osteotomy). The various types of fixation are illustrated in Figure 29–68.

upper border of the fragments in the so called "high to low" position (Epker, 1977), with the drill hole placed higher on the distal segment and lower on the proximal one (see Fig. 29–68*A*).

Intermaxillary fixation that relies on binding the dentition together should be avoided (Schendel and Epker, 1980). Although the occlusion might be maintained because of the plasticity of the dentoalveolar complex, important relapse of the basilar mandibular skeleton will occur. A system of fixation using the basilar skeleton is therefore preferred. Small bilateral, maxillary vestibular incisions are made to expose the piriform aperture by subperiosteal dissection. A drill hole is made through the piriform rim to receive a stout (No. 24 or 26 gauge) wire loop. A similar pair of wire loops is passed around the mandibular symphyseal region with the aid of an awl. The two loops are secured to one other through an intermediary wire loop (Fig. 29–102). The jaws are held together for six weeks as bone consolidation takes place.

If rigid fixation techniques are used, the mandible should first be placed in intermaxillary fixation. The rigid fixation system is applied (see Fig. 29–68). If only screws are used, the lag screw principle should be incorporated when drilling the holes in the proximal segment. If miniplates are used, they are secured with monocortical screw fixation into each of the fragments. The compression mode should not be activated if miniplates with this feature are used. Intermaxillary fixation is released and the occlusion is checked, attention being directed to seating the condyle in the glenoid fossa in a proper fashion. Light training elastics can also be used to index the occlusion in the intervals between meals, which should consist of a mechanical soft diet.

The patient shown in Figure 29–103 had

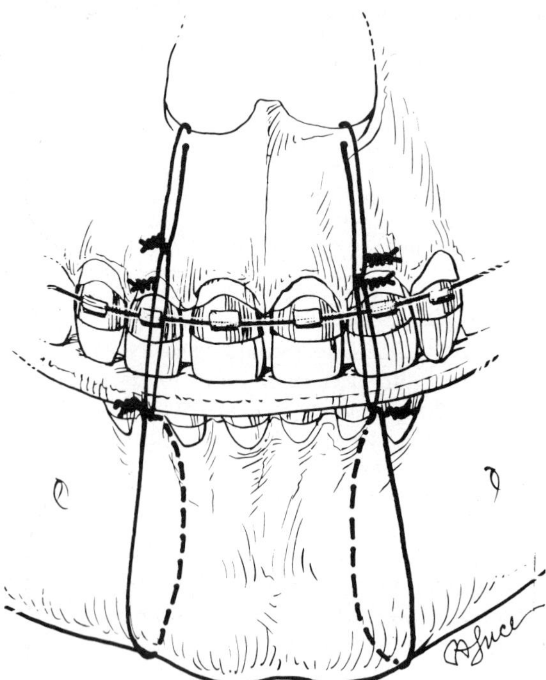

Figure 29–102. Technique of piriform aperture-circumferential wiring fixation after sagittal split osteotomy of the mandibular ramus. Note that intermediate wire loops connect the upper and lower sets of wires.

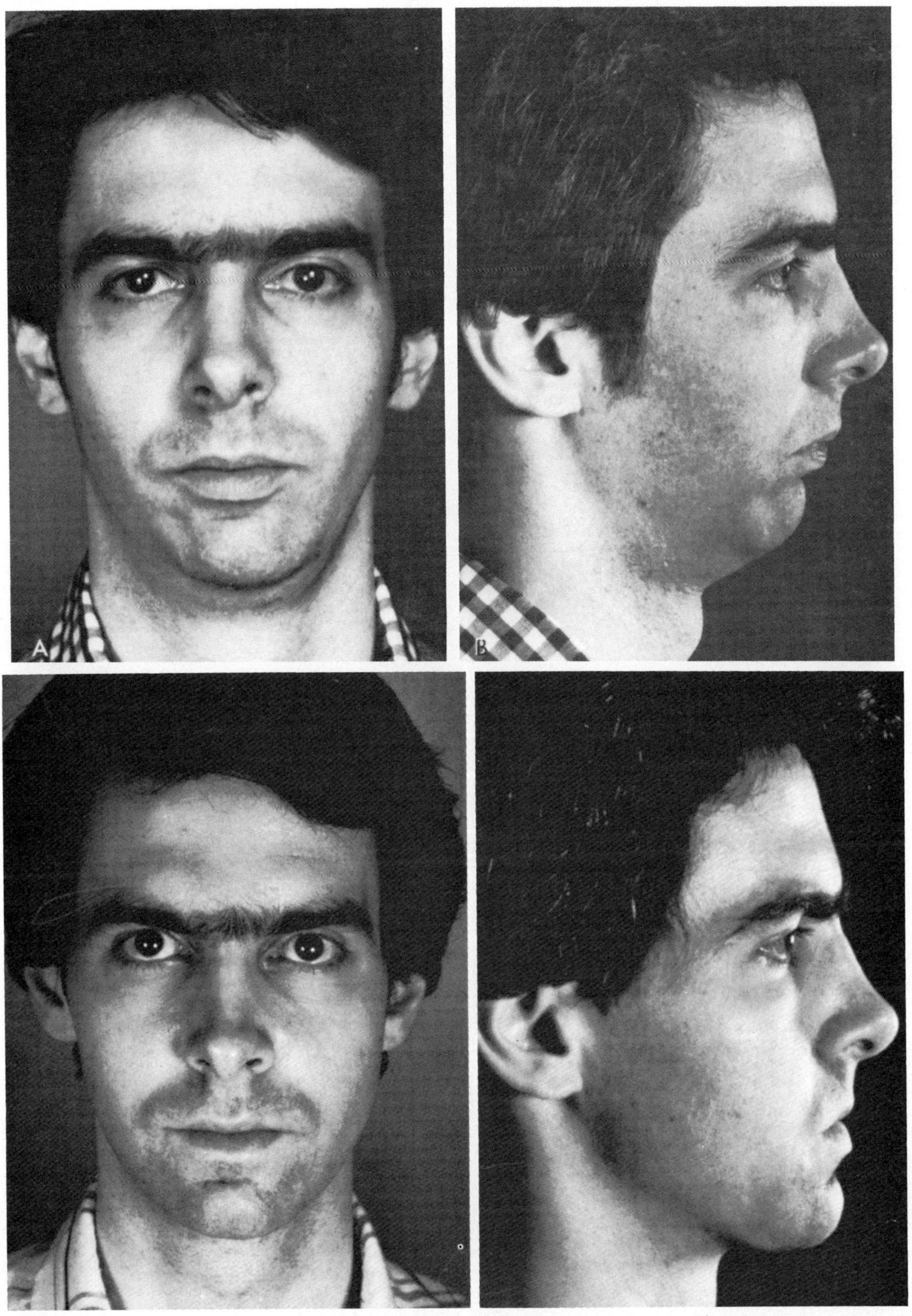

Figure 29–103. Mandibular advancement with the sagittal split osteotomy of the ramus. *A, B,* A 25 year old man who displays a mandible and chin that are deficient relative to the maxilla. *C, D,* Appearance after sagittal split osteotomy of the mandibular ramus, asymmetric genioplasty, and orthodontic therapy.

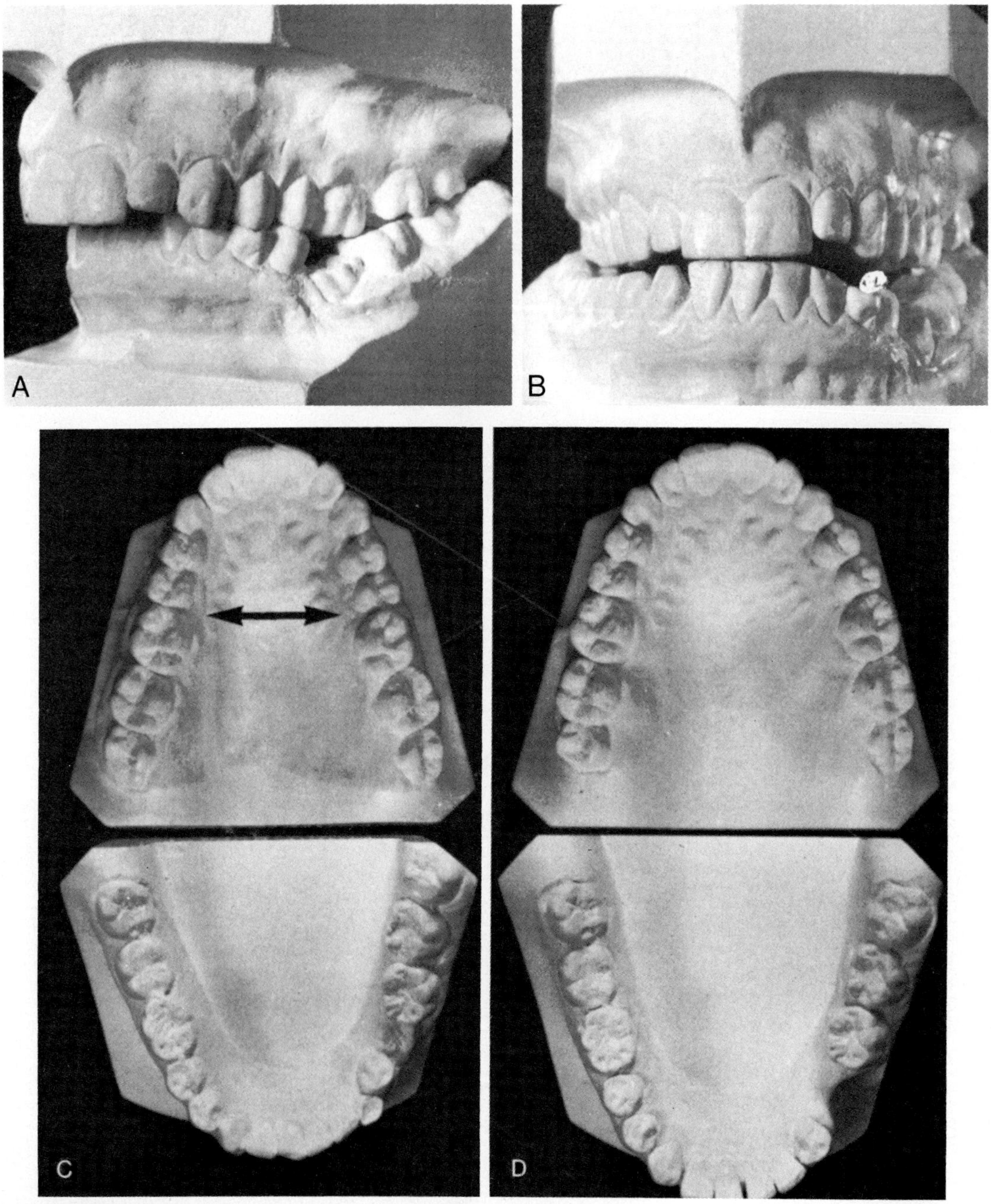

A

B

C

D

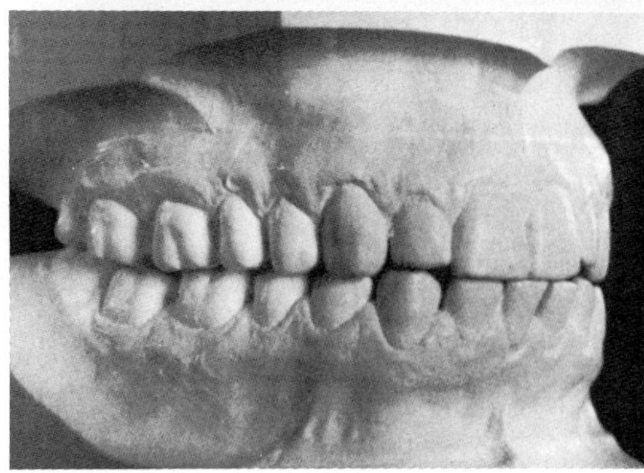

E

Figure 29–104. Dental models of the patient illustrated in Figure 29–103. *A,* Initial models showing anterior overjet, anterior crossbite, deep bite, and irregularities in the occlusal plane. *B,* As the mandible is advanced in the hand-held models, the transverse maxillary arch width deficiency is exposed and the posterior open bite is displayed. *C,* The narrow maxillary arch requires preoperative expansion (*arrow*) and the occlusal plane requires leveling. *D,* The occlusion immediately before mandibular advancement. Note the improved maxillary arch form and width, leveling of the occlusal planes, and extraction of the retained deciduous teeth. *E,* Postoperative occlusion.

his mandible elongated by means of the sagittal splitting ramal osteotomy. An ideal occlusal relationship was achieved (Fig. 29–104) and the cephalometric tracing shows the degree of advancement and the changes realized (Fig. 29–105).

Advantages and Disadvantages of Sagittal Section of Ramus. The intraoral approach eliminates the problem of an external scar. Gaps are not produced in the dental arch. The principal advantage of the technique, however, is the wide surface of bone contact afforded after advancement of the segments. Bone grafts are not needed to maintain bone contact. Consolidation of the fragments is rapid and nonunion is rare. Rigid fixation techniques can be used if the surgeon so desires.

The disadvantage are similar to those cited for the treatment of mandibular prognathism (see p. 1253). However, additional hazards are incurred when the ramal hypoplasia is more pronounced, as in cases of craniofacial microsomia. The chances of comminution of the proximal fragment and the risk of injuring the inferior alveolar nerve are greater. Severe degrees of hypoplasia may preclude the use of the technique. In such cases the inverted L section technique accompanied by an interposition bone graft is preferable (see Fig. 29–98).

Osteotomy of Ramus and Body of Mandible for Elongation of Mandible. A C-shaped osteotomy of the mandibular ramus was described by Caldwell, Hayward, and Lister (1968). It was originally referred to as an L-osteotomy, although the outline of the cut more resembles a C. The design of the osteotomy begins with a superior horizontal section placed above the level of the mandibular foramen. The vertical component runs behind the mandibular foramen and spares the mandibular angles. It extends forward below the inferior alveolar canal toward the body of the mandible as the inferior horizontal limb of the C. At the end of the C it angulates through the inferior border of the mandible.

A combined intraoral and extraoral approach is used. The insertions of the masseter and medial pterygoid muscles are reflected from the bone. The superior horizontal branch

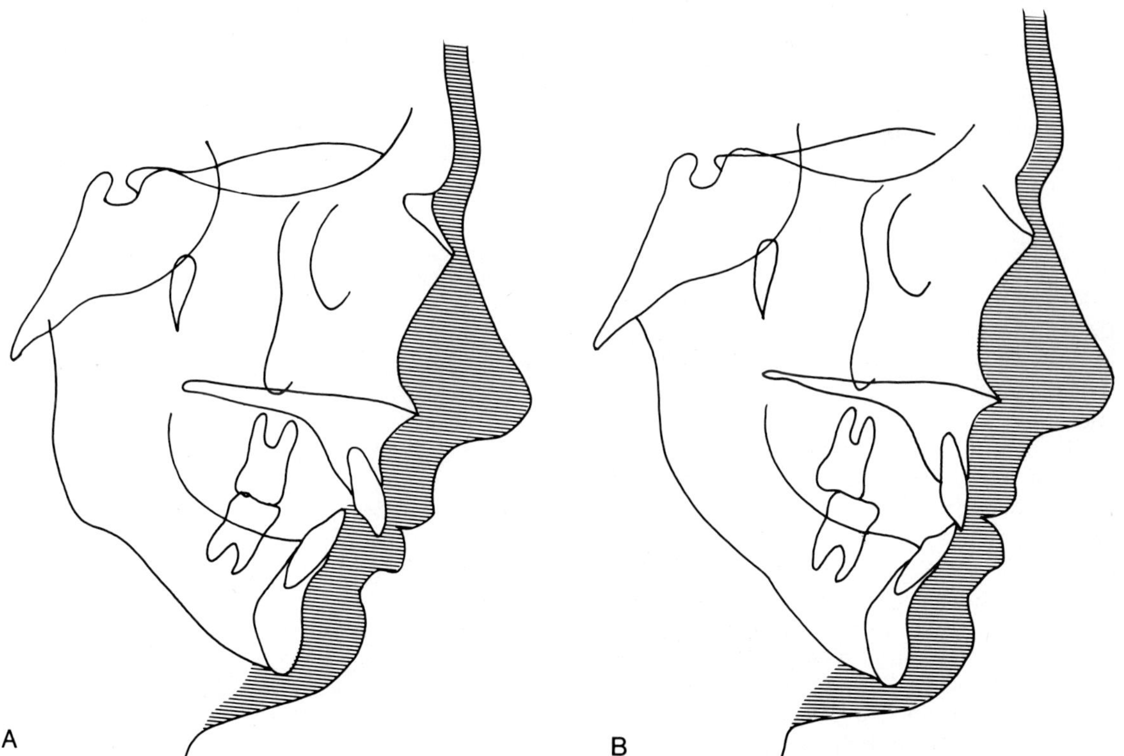

Figure 29–105. *A,* Preoperative lateral cephalogram. Note the skeletal and soft tissue (*shaded*) profile. *B,* After mandibular advancement.

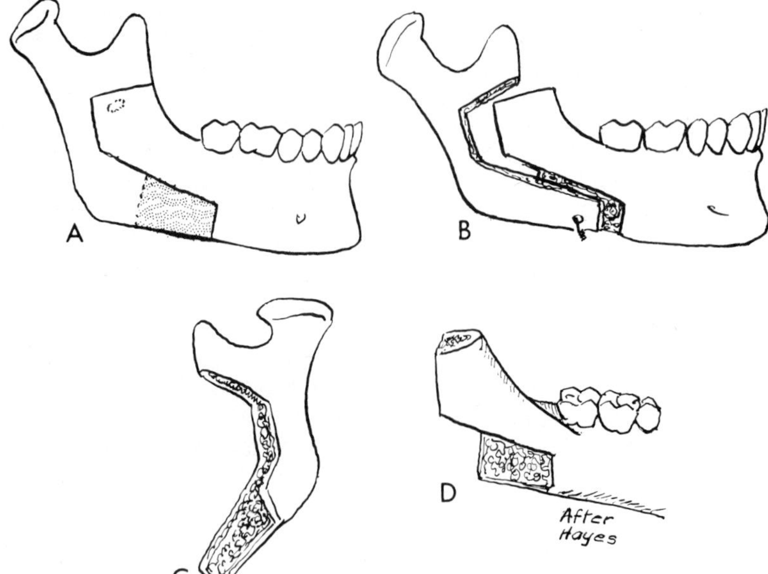

Figure 29–106. The C-shaped ramus osteotomy with an anterior extension. *A,* Design of the osteotomy. The shaded area indicates where the sagittal splitting of the body is made. *B,* After completion of the advancement, a single interosseous wire is placed at the inferior border. *C,* Lingual view of the condylar segment showing the osteotomy and the sagittal split of the body. *D,* The tooth-bearing segment: the outer cortex of the sagittal split rests with the condylar fragment. (After Hayes.)

of the C is made with a Lindemann bur via an intraoral approach. A reciprocating saw can also be used for this cut and it has the advantage of creating a thinner kerf. The remainder of the osteotomy is done through the extraoral incision. The horizontal sections should be kept parallel to the plane of advancement. After the osteotomy is completed, the tooth-bearing fragment is advanced to the desired location and intermaxillary fixation is applied. The condyle on the proximal fragment is returned to the glenoid fossa and the fragments are joined by an interosseous wire. There may be sufficient bony contact to dispense with bone grafts unless they are needed to add bulk and form.

Hayes (1973) incorporated the principle of the sagittal osteotomy to increase the surface of contact along the inferior portion of the mandibular body (Fig. 29–106). The steps of the operation are essentially the same as those of the C-osteotomy except along the inferior horizontal limb. After the lower horizontal branch of the osteotomy reaches the body, the bone cut is made only through the lateral cortical plate. The medial cut of the lower horizontal osteotomy is dropped vertically to the inferior border, where the mandibular body begins. The distance between the medial and lateral vertical cuts should be approximately double the amount of desired advancement to ensure adequate bone contact. The horizontal extension is then split in a sagittal plane (Fig. 29–106*B* to *D*). The fragments are separated and the tooth-bearing anterior fragment is held in its corrected relationship to the maxilla by intermaxillary fixation. A single interosseous wire or a miniplate can be placed at the inferior border (Fig. 29–106*B*).

Advantages and Disadvantages of C-Osteotomy. The advantage of the C-osteotomy is that it provides sufficient bone contact so that a bone graft is not needed. The body sagittal split modification further increases the surface of osseous contact. The technique can be used when the ramus is small, whereas the sagittal splitting technique is not always possible in such cases. In addition, injury to the inferior nerve is less likely to occur, unless the inferior horizontal section is unintentionally made too high through the inferior alveolar canal.

The external incision is a disadvantage. Care must also be taken when the sagittal splitting of the mandibular body is performed, because excessive force can produce a fracture at the critical junction between the lower horizontal and vertical sections. Comminution in the region of the sagittal split is also possible.

Lastly, the geometry of the cuts must be planned in such a way as to avoid unfavorable rotational forces on the proximal fragment due to bony interferences. Thus, on the whole, little is offered by the C-osteotomy that might favor its use over a conventional sagittal splitting procedure of the ramus.

Choice of Technique for Elongation and Advancement of Mandible. The availability of the many techniques to lengthen the mandible can be bewildering at first. Each has its strong and weak features. However, for the most part, *the sagittal splitting ramal osteotomy should be the procedure against which others are measured.* In analyzing the deformity, the surgeon must first ask in what part of the mandible the deficiency lies. If at all possible, procedures that will require bone grafts, placement of cutaneous scar, or creation of gaps in the dental arch should be avoided. Lastly, the inherent risk and the likelihood of relapse must be weighed for the individual patient.

Elongation osteotomy of the mandibular body is limited to patients with permanent dentition; the presence of tooth buds in the body precludes its use. Bilateral osteotomies of the ramus can be used in children to advance the body of the mandible since the ramus is free of tooth buds, except perhaps for the third molar.

When gross disparity and malalignment exist between the upper and lower dental arch forms, a body elongation osteotomy is indicated. Osteotomies of the ramus change the relative position of the mandibular dental arch but not its form. Dentoalveolar discrepancies can be corrected by the orthodontist, but an arch disparity due to skeletal deformities is best managed by surgical modification of the shape of the mandibular body.

In some asymmetric cases, a combination of osteotomies can sometimes be used. On the shorter side, a sagittal splitting osteotomy of the ramus can be used to advance the mandible and still maintain contact of the fragments. On the normal side, a vertical osteotomy is performed to facilitate rotation of the mandible without unduly disturbing the temporomandibular joint. The unaffected side behaves more like a pivoting center, and bone contact is preserved.

Age at Operation. A major problem that remains controversial is the age at which the corrective procedure should be performed in the developmental type of mandibular hypoplasia. Temporomandibular ankylosis should be relieved as soon as feasible. With the presently available means of fixation, an osteotomy to increase the size and anteroposterior dimension of the ramus can technically be performed at an early age. The unanswered question is whether the mandible will grow at a normal pace after the operation. Further longitudinal studies are needed.

Postoperative Relapse. Postoperative regression of the advanced segment of the mandible is a major problem. Cephalometric studies have provided valuable information. Poulton and Ware (1973) observed patients treated by the sagittal splitting procedure of the ramus over a three year period. Serial cephalograms documented 50 to 80 per cent skeletal relapse during the period of study. McNeill, Hooley, and Sundberg (1973) noted similar relapse in their postoperative cephalometric studies. The degree of relapse correlates with the amount of mandibular advancement (Ive, McNeill, and West, 1977). The major portion of the relapse occurs during the period of intermaxillary fixation. Faulty repositioning of the condyle in the glenoid fossa is a principal factor in the relapse, but mandibular regression can occur even when the anatomic position of the condyle in the glenoid fossa is verified by roentgenography during the immediate postoperative period.

An interesting observation is that the dentoalveolar relationships are maintained since the teeth are used for the intermaxillary fixation (Freihofer and Petresevic, 1975). The relapse occurs mainly in the basilar skeletal portion of the mandible, as indicated by the regression of pogonion (bony chin point) or reduction of the anterior and posterior facial height. For this reason, skeletal rather than interdental fixation is recommended (Schendel and Epker, 1980; Ellis and Gallo, 1986). Rigid fixation might also prove to be an aid in resisting the relapsing forces.

Counterclockwise rotation of the mandible, which increases the posterior facial height, is associated with a greater degree of instability (Schendel and Epker, 1980). This type of mandibular movement is often incurred in attempts to advance the lower jaw with a steep mandibular plane angle and to close an anterior open bite deformity.

Several soft tissue factors contribute to regression of the advanced mandibular skeleton: the suprahyoid musculature, soft tissue deficiency, and the sphenomandibular ligament.

Suprahyoid Musculature. The anterior belly of the digastric, the mylohyoid, and the geniohyoid muscles exert a strong rotatory downward and backward pull on the anterior fragment (clockwise rotation). The stretching of the muscles, as the advancement is made, contributes further to the muscle pull. Three methods of counteracting the effect of the muscular contraction are employed: (1) subperiosteal disinsertion of the suprahyoid musculature, (2) external mandibular supporting appliances, and (3) external traction devices.

Disinsertion of Muscle Attachments. Subperiosteal disinsertion of the anterior belly of the digastric and of the geniohyoid muscles from the lower mental spines was proposed as a method to combat the clockwise rotatory forces (Converse, 1963; Steinhauser, 1973). Tongue dysfunction and airway obstruction were not observed postoperatively. Disinsertion of the mylohyoid and the genioglossus muscles from the upper mental spine is not advised because it may interfere with swallowing and cause retroposition of the tongue and airway obstruction. Follow-up studies, however, failed to prove the merit of the extra step (Schendel and Epker, 1980) and the procedure has largely been abandoned.

External Mandibular Supporting Appliances. Regression of the advanced mandibular segment can also be minimized by the use of external mandibular supporting devices. Poulton and Ware (1973) employed a Pitkin cervical collar to help neutralize the relapsing forces. The line of force applied by the collar, however, does not completely counteract the pull exerted by the suprahyoid muscles. The cervical collar is worn throughout the intermaxillary fixation period and at night for six to 12 months along with an acrylic occlusal splint. The amount of relapse was reduced from 50 to 80 per cent to 10 to 30 per cent. The cervical brace also helped to correct the forward movement of the hyoid bone and cervical vertebrae that occurs because of the tendency to drop the head during the postoperative period. Both the hyoid bone and the cervical vertebrae return to their original preoperative positions as the muscles readapt to their new positions.

McNeill, Hooley, and Sundberg (1973) recommended prolonged maintenance of intermaxillary fixation combined with the use of the Pitkin cervical collar until the relapse forces are expended. Serial cephalography is used to judge the proper time to discontinue the fixation and the collar.

External Traction Devices. An external apparatus that exerts traction on the mandible can be used to neutralize the pull of the suprahyoid musculature. However, these are unsightly and cumbersome to wear. They were used mainly in the past for body osteotomy procedures and are now mostly of historical interest.

The external devices generally used the calvarium as a stable base from which outriggers were fashioned to combat the backward and downward rotation of the advanced anterior mandibular fragment. Animal studies have shown that it is actually possible to elongate the mandible by applying continuous external traction after the osteotomy (Snyder and Associates, 1973). Abbott (1927) had previously used a similar method to lengthen the tibia and fibula. New bone formation occurs at the osteotomy site without the placement of bone grafts.

The Kazanjian extraoral traction appliance used a plaster head cap as a base for its midline outrigger. A horizontal maxillary extension rests on the labial surfaces of the upper incisors to serve as a fulcrum. The mandibular arm of the apparatus is attached to the symphyseal region to provide the desired forward traction. The Georgiade halo or "crown of thorns" appliance dispenses with the plaster cap in favor of threaded calvarial screws that securely hold a prefabricated adjustable frame and its outriggers.

Fortunately for the patient, improved design of osteotomies, internal fixation, and a better understanding of the procedures have permitted the demise of external devices in general.

Soft Tissue Deficiency. A hypoplastic mandible not only has a deficient skeleton but is often surrounded by a deficient, tight, soft tissue envelope that resists attempts at skeletal advancement. Wide elevation of the soft tissue neighboring the osteotomy site may be helpful. Vertical parallel incisions through the periosteum assist in overcoming the restrictive force of the periosteal capsule and in allowing for a moderate degree of expansion.

Resistance to advancement can also be caused by a deficiency of intraoral mucosa. Releasing the mucous membrane requires introduction of local flaps or, in extreme instances, the skin graft inlay technique (see p. 1451).

When covering soft tissue deficiency is a problem, a chin implant of silicone or a small skin expander can be used to stretch the tissue before the advancement of bone. If a solid implant is used, it must not be left in position for more than one or two months, to avoid resorption of the underlying bone from the pressure exerted by the implant. The expanding device must be placed over the hard bone of the lower border of the symphysis, and not be allowed to drift upward into the soft dentoalveolar bone below the roots of the teeth (see p. 1411).

Sphenomandibular Ligament. The sphenomandibular ligament is a fibrous band extending from the angular spine of the sphenoid bone to the lingula of the mandibular ramus. In vertical and sagittal osteotomies of the ramus, the lingula remains on the advanced segment of the mandible. The inelastic ligament may hinder the anterior repositioning and play a role in producing relapse (Hovell, 1970). The vertical orientation of the ligament, however, would appear to offer little resistance to the advancement.

Other Techniques to Prevent Relapse. Overcorrection has been advocated for the treatment of mandibular hypoplasia. An acrylic occlusal splint is required to compensate for the dental intercuspal interferences. A posterior open bite should be incorporated in the design of the wafer (Poulton and Ware, 1973). The appliance helps to rotate the symphysis upward and anteriorly and provides more chin prominence. However, the posterior open bite increases the posterior facial height, which is usually short, and thus increases the propensity toward relapse. The increase in the posterior vertical facial dimension is maintained as the posterior maxillary teeth extrude downward to close the artificial posterior open bite.

Secondary Operations. If a relapse occurs, a secondary procedure usually achieves a satisfactory result. Further procedures may be required, such as an advancement osseous genioplasty.

Contour Restoration in Mandibular Micrognathia. After the mandible has been lengthened and advanced to correct the malocclusion, additional measures to improve the facial contour are often needed.

The contours of the mandible can be restored with bone grafts or alloplastic materials. Augmentation by inorganic implants generally fares poorly in these regions; however, in the area of the mental symphysis, such implants are widely used with success. Capsule formation, underlying bone resorption, and migration of the implant, if it is not deliberately fixed into place, are only a few of the problems shared by implants (see p. 1411). Hydroxyapatite holds promise since infiltration by bone occurs, but it is brittle, fragile, and difficult to work with.

Iliac, costal, and calvarial bone grafts are commonly used for contour restoration. They frequently work well on deformed mandibles (Fig. 29–107), but the success of onlay bone grafts is unpredictable. Partial absorption may require additional onlay bone grafting until the desired contour is obtained. Longacre and DeStefano (1957) showed that serial onlay bone overgrafting can produce satisfactory results.

Several measures can be used to decrease the resorption of the graft. The first is the selection of donor site; grafts from the cranium generally fare the best. Experimental data suggest that onlay bone grafts with attached periosteum enjoy a more favorable survival rate (Thompson and Casson, 1970; Knize, 1974). The periosteum of the onlay graft may encourage more rapid revascularization. The recipient site also influences the success of the graft. Wide subperiosteal contact between the bone grafts and the mandibular bone favors osteogenesis. Failures of contour restoration by bone grafting occur if the overlying soft tissues are under sufficient tension to cause pressure atrophy of the grafted bone.

Many techniques are available for contour restoration of the chin. They are discussed later in the section devoted to the management of microgenia.

LATEROGNATHISM: LATERAL DEVIATION OF MANDIBLE

A truly symmetric face does not exist. When carefully studied, the right and left halves of the average face show some degree of asymmetry. As the skeletal portion of the mandible deviates to one side beyond the average range, facial asymmetry becomes clinically pronounced and mandibular laterognathism is produced; the mental symphysis is lateral to the midsagittal plane of the face. The midlines between the upper and lower central incisors do not coincide; a posterior crossbite is usually present. In lesser deviations of the mandible, the dentoalveolar structures of the jaws achieve a compromised occlusal relationship to compensate for the skeletal deviation.

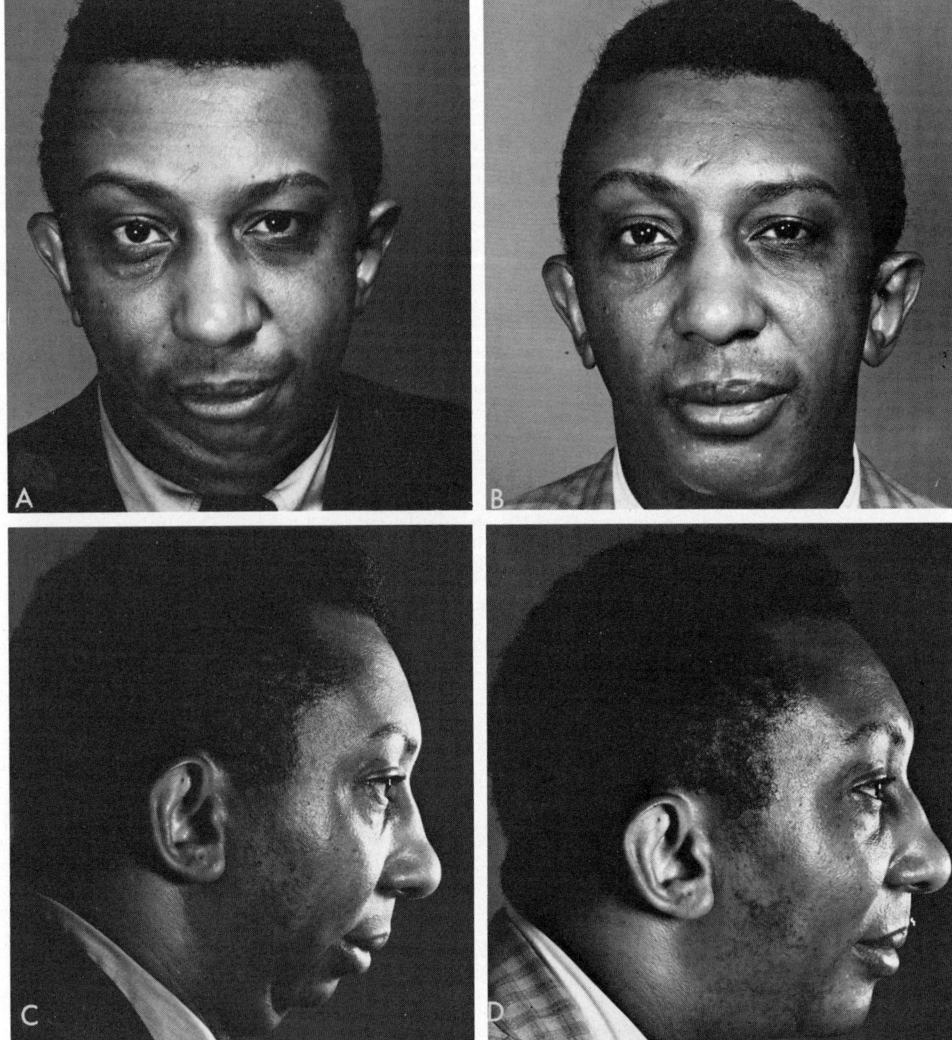

Figure 29–107. Onlay bone grafting for contour restoration of the mandible. *A,* A patient with temporomandibular ankylosis and micrognathia. The dental relationships were acceptable. *B,* Result four years after contour-restoring onlay bone grafts were placed through the intraoral approach. *C,* Preoperative profile. *D,* Postoperative view.

Etiology

Trauma plays an important role in the etiology of lateral deviation of the mandible. Unilateral underdevelopment is often the result of injury to one condyle in early life. Laterognathism is also of congenital origin, i.e., the deformity characteristic of the malformation of the first and second branchial arches (unilateral craniofacial microsomia, see Chap. 62). Conversely, it can be caused by unilateral condylar hyperplasia or congenital hemifacial hyperplasia. The deformity can also be acquired; traumatic loss of a portion of the mandible skews the jaw toward the deficient side. Another example is the loss of bone after resection of tumors.

Preoperative Planning

Asymmetry of the face is usually readily detected on clinical examination. Determination of the defective side of the face may not be so easy; on casual examination, the unaffected side may appear to be the involved side. The position of the chin is used as a rough clinical guide. When the deformity is caused by an underdevelopment or loss of a portion of the mandible, the chin assumes a retruded position and strays toward the affected side. Conversely, when the deformity is caused by unilateral hyperplasia, the chin appears to be more prominent and is deflected to the contralateral side. The lateral movement of the chin when the jaw is opened

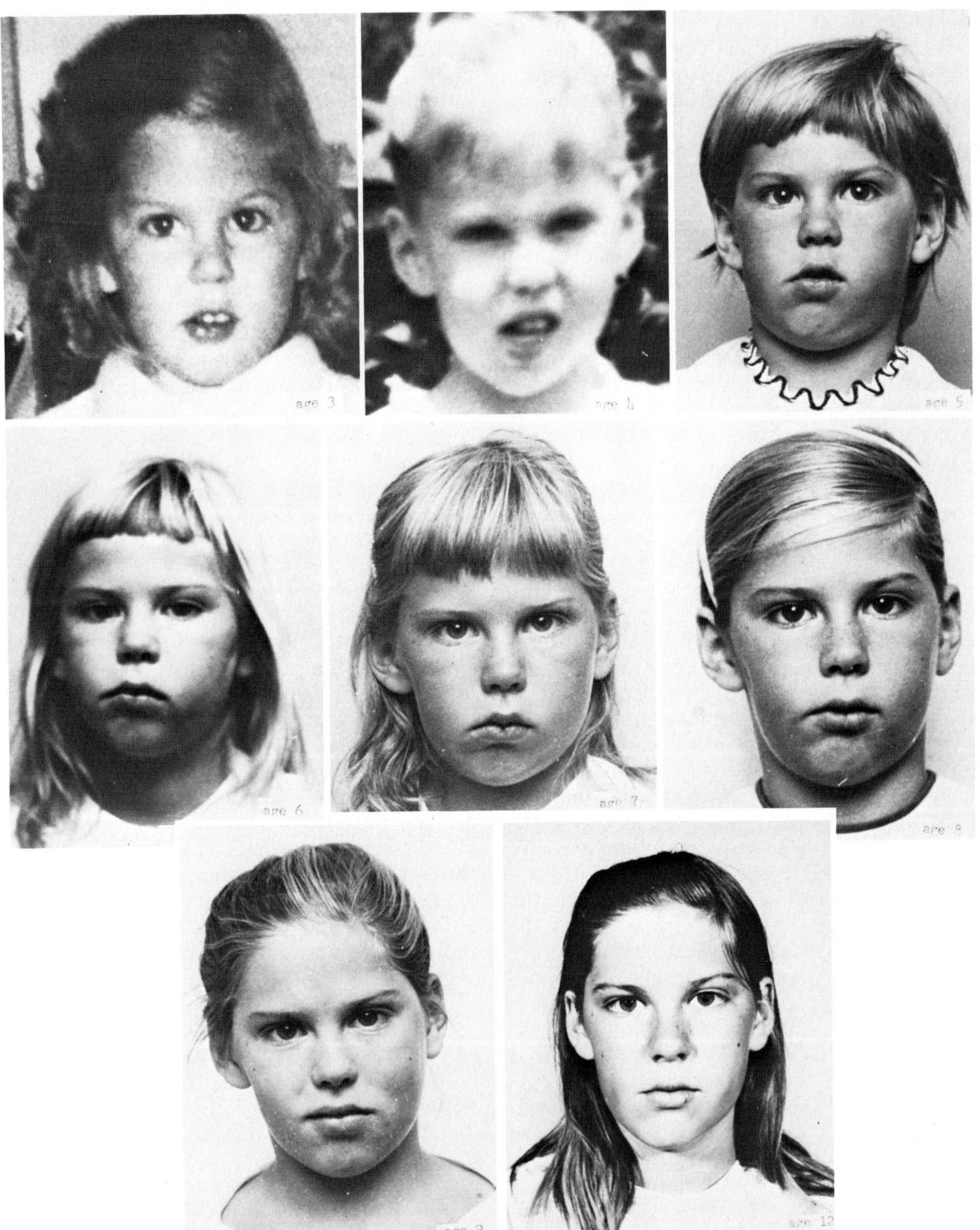

Figure 29–108. Reestablishment of mandibular symmetry by increased muscular activity. Asymmetry caused by a fall on the chin at the age of 2 years. The successive photographs show the improvement from the age of 5 years to the age of 12 years as a result of the treatment (see text). (From Coccaro, P. J.: Restitution of mandibular form after condylar injury in infancy (a 7-year study of a child). Am. J. Orthod., *55*:32, 1969.)

therefore cannot be used as a reliable guide. The chin always deviates to the shorter side, regardless of whether it is actually or relatively short. Panoramic and cephalometric roentgenograms confirm the clinical diagnosis and are invaluable in treatment planning (see Chap. 62). Dental casts should be trimmed to show any cant of the occlusal plane and anteroposterior mandibular asymmetry.

CONDYLAR HYPOPLASIA

Altered condylar growth is seen in many congenital malformations, but trauma is probably responsible for the vast majority. Injury to the condylar cartilage from delivery forceps at birth, a fall, other trauma, or sepsis in early childhood can lead to arrested growth. The degree of growth impairment is greater when the insult occurs early in life.

Although direct injury to the condyle usually results in impaired growth, just the opposite effect can also occur. Jacobsen and Lund (1972) reported a longitudinal study of patients with condylar neck fractures. Immediately after the injury, the chin deviated toward the affected side. After the adolescent skeletal growth spurt, the chin was displaced toward the contralateral side. The condylar heads were reformed (see also Chap. 30).

Altered Muscular Activity and Condylar Injury. The condylar growth center shows some form of activity until at least the 21st year and is generally regarded as one of the most active in the growing mandible (see also Chap. 47). When it is traumatized, there is a definite deceleration in growth due to the inhibitory effect on the proliferation of the cartilage and ossification, particularly during the preschool years. The progressive facial asymmetry that ensues is directly related to the damaging effect of the injury on the condylar growth center. There is radiographic evidence that the injury not only affects growth but also alters the anatomic relationships of the structures that give rise to the origin and insertion of the muscles of mastication. Thus, muscle length and vectors of force are involved, contributing to abnormal mandibular movements during mastication and at rest. Soon afterward, facial asymmetry inevitably results.

Alteration of the balanced neuromuscular relationships is a particularly serious condition. Stability and the functional movement of the mandible are disrupted. Hence, detrimental secondary skeletal changes follow to produce an asymmetry.

Symmetry can occasionally be restored by using the principles of myofunctional therapy. Coccaro (1969) showed that promoting muscular activity on the defective side helps the musculoskeletal system to achieve its maximal growth potential. The change in myofunction is directly reflected on the intimately related underlying bone. The patient, a 5 year old girl, had fallen on her chin at the age of 2 years. The examination showed a deviation of the chin to the right and a flattened appearance of the mandible on the left side (Fig. 29–108). When requested to move her jaw, the patient could move her mandible to the right with facility but had limited movement to the left. This finding suggested some disability of the right lateral pterygoid muscle. The posteroanterior cephalogram (Fig. 29–109) showed a hypoplastic and medially displaced condyle and ramus on the right side.

When the patient was 6 years old, a sectional orthodontic appliance was constructed to fit over the left deciduous cuspid and molars. An occlusal registration was obtained, with the patient shifting the jaw laterally as far to the left as possible. With the appliance in position, she was compelled to move the mandible from the affected to the unaffected side to achieve dental occlusion. The purpose of the appliance was to force the patient to use the muscles of mastication on the hypoplastic right side. She was instructed to wear the appliance at all times and to remove it only after meals for cleaning. Because of wear and changes in retention, the appliance was replaced periodically. At age 8 years, growth of the affected side appeared to be progressing favorably.

When the use of the appliance was finally terminated, the patient continued to move her jaw effectively to the unaffected side, even without the appliance. Restoration of symmetry continued as a result of the improved muscular function on the affected side. The discernible changes in ramal height and improved condyle-fossa relationships are documented in Figures 29–109*B* and 29–110.

Attempts have been made to replace the deficient or defective condylar head with a bone graft having an epiphyseal growth center. Metatarsal grafts have been used by Stuteville and Lanfranchi (1955), Stuteville

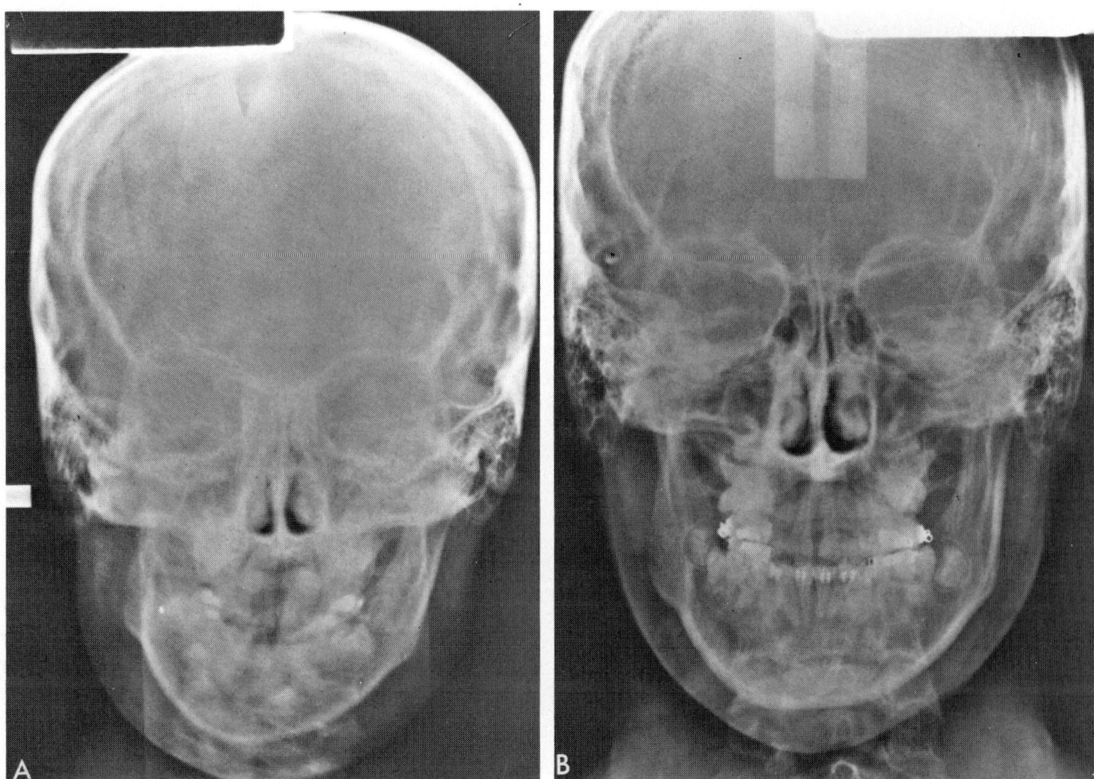

Figure 29–109. *A,* Posteroanterior cephalogram of the patient shown in Figure 29–108 at the age of 5 years. *B,* Cephalogram at the age of 12 years. Note the improvement in mandibular form and size. (From Coccaro, P. J.: Restitution of mandibular form after condylar injury in infancy (a 7-year-study of a child). Am. J. Orthod., *55*:32, 1969.)

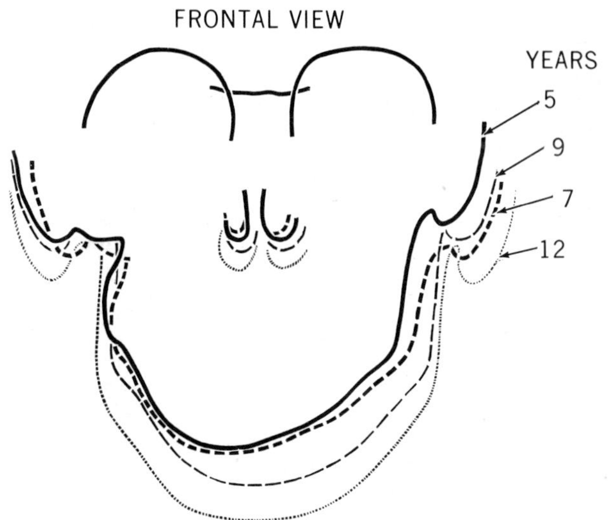

Figure 29–110. Serial tracings of posteroanterior cephalograms superimposed in the midline and on the lesser wings of the sphenoid bone, showing growth changes contributing to the improvement in facial symmetry. Note the degree of serial reduction of the asymmetry. (From Coccaro, P. J.: Restitution of mandibular form after condylar injury in infancy (a 7-year study of a child). Am. J. Orthod., *55*:32, 1969.)

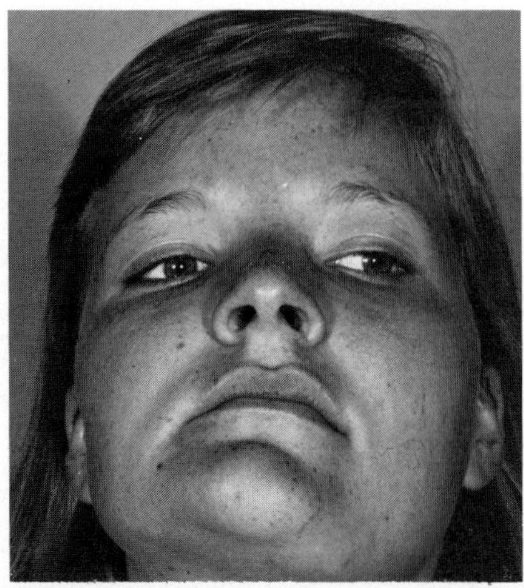

Figure 29–111. A patient with left-sided condylar hyperplasia. Note that the chin is deviated to the unaffected side.

(1957), Entin (1958), Bromberg, Walden, and Rubin (1963), Dingman and Grabb (1964), and Glahn and Winther (1965). Costochondral grafts were also employed by Bromberg, Walden, and Rubin (1963) and Ware and Taylor (1968), who also used the proximal head of the fibula. Longitudinal studies suggest that the epiphyseal growth center probably does not survive and that the growth observed is mainly appositional in nature (Munro, 1988). The graft serves to restore anatomic relationships and function rather than reestablish a growth center. This finding is in keeping with the *functional matrix theory* of Moss (1960).

In the adult, when the deformity is not excessively conspicuous and the deviation of the chin is the salient feature, an osseous genioplasty that repositions the mental symphysis toward the midline will restore symmetry (see Fig. 29–141).

It is possible to restore symmetry by bilateral ramal osteotomies combined with orthodontic therapy. Advancing the affected side and overlapping the ramal fragments on the longer side equalize mandibular length. More severe hypoplasia results in a unilateral hypoplastic deformity.

CONDYLAR HYPERPLASIA AND UNILATERAL MANDIBULAR MACROGNATHIA

Condylar hyperplasia can be idiopathic or the result of injury during childhood (see also Chap. 30). Gruca and Meiselles (1926), Ivy (1927), Rushton (1944), McNichol and Rogers (1945), Cernéa (1954), and others have reported on this condition. The condyle progressively increases in size and elongates, a characteristic finding in this type of hyperplasia.

A patient with the classical deformity is shown in Figure 29–111. The ramus and the body of the affected mandible are enlarged in all dimensions. The patient shows a shift of the midpoint of the mandible toward the contralateral side. The occlusal relationships of the teeth thus are also affected. The posterior maxillary teeth on the involved side are usually in a buccal crossbite relationship, and a posterior open bite is frequently present. Facial contour is prominent over the enlarged condylar head, and roentgenograms confirm its exaggerated size. No limitation of temporomandibular joint motion is observed, although pain is often present in the joint. The pain radiates in various directions and is more acute when the patient opens the mouth. Resection of the condylar head on the affected side, drastic as it may seem, may be the only way to interrupt progression of the asymmetry and relieve the symptoms.

A patient with the characteristic deformity of unilateral macrognathia of the mandible is shown in Figure 29–112. In addition to the condyle, the entire half of the mandible is hyperplastic. Progressive enlargement of the half of the mandible and elongation of the face on the same side was first noted at age 12 years and continued until the patient was 22 years old. The lower border of the affected hemimandible bows inferiorly; the chin deviates to the opposite side, and the angle of the mouth (commissure) on the same side appears elevated. The anterior open bite is pronounced and is accompanied by a lingual version of the mandibular teeth plane. The patient underwent preoperative orthodontic therapy, bilateral sagittal split ramisection of the mandible, and Le Fort I osteotomy to level the occlusal plane.

In the growing child, resection of the condylar head may be required. A preauricular approach is used to remove the enlarged condylar head (see Chap. 30) and, if necessary, portions of the neck.

In the exceptional case in which the neck of the condyle is unusually elongated and causing laterognathism, resection of a measured segment of the condylar neck can reestablish symmetry and adequate dental occlusion (Figs. 29–113, 29–114).

Text continued on page 1300

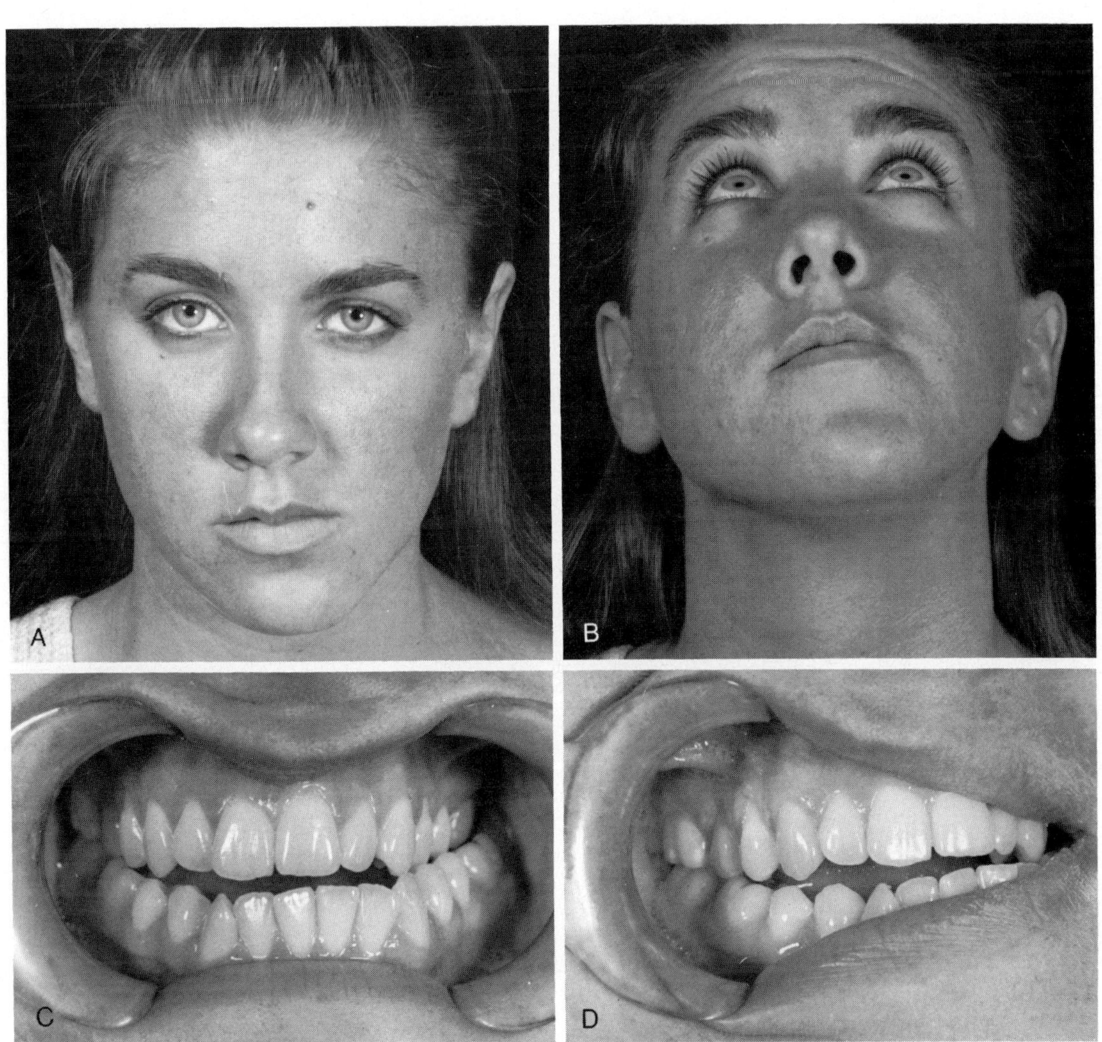

Figure 29–112. A 22 year old female with condylar hyperplasia and unilateral mandibular macrognathia. *A* to *D*, Preoperative views. Note the unilateral macrognathia, deviation of the chin to the opposite side, anterior open bite, and tilting of the occlusal plane.

Illustration continued on following page

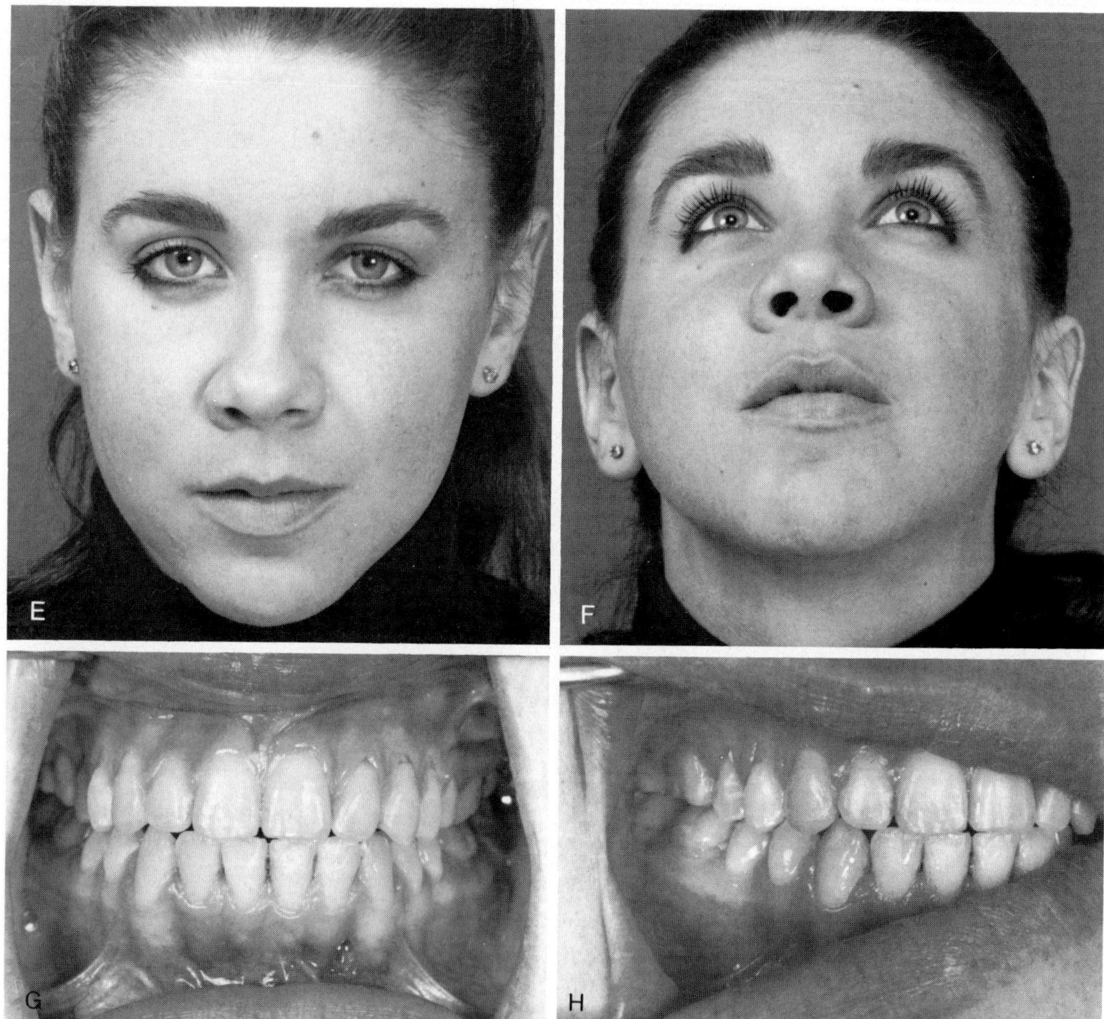

Figure 29–112 *Continued E* to *H,* After orthodontic therapy, mandibular rotation (bilateral sagittal split ramisection), and Le Fort I osteotomy. Note the improved relationship of the midline structures and restoration of a functional occlusion.

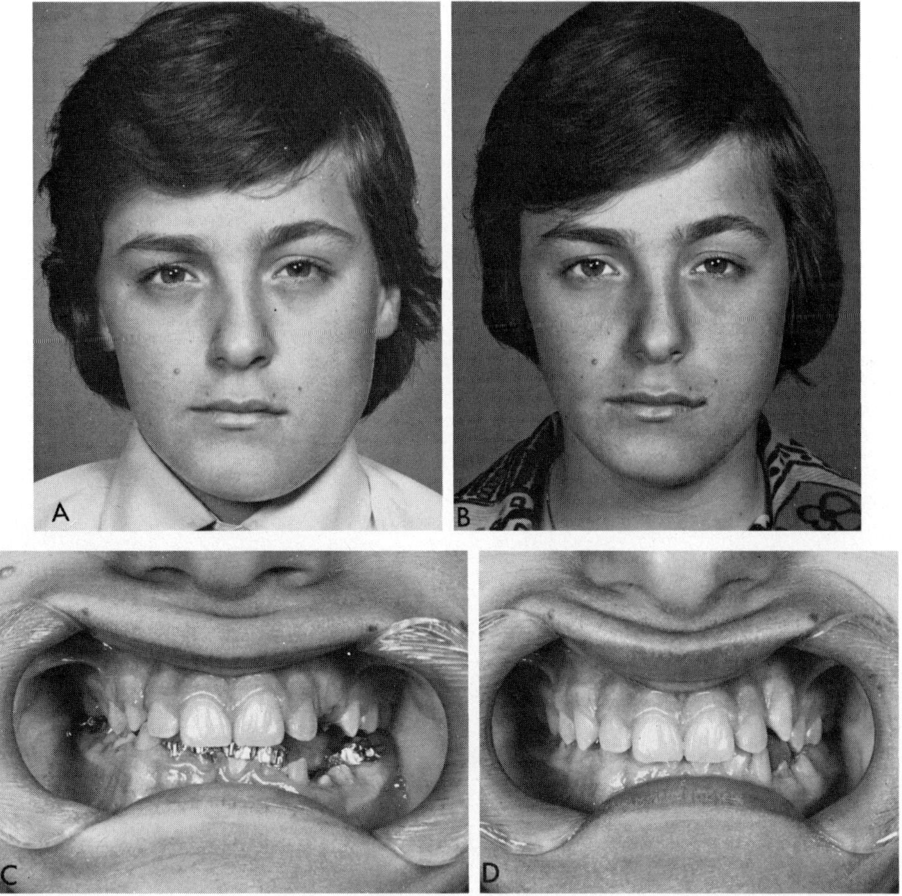

Figure 29–113. Lateral deviation of the mandible caused by elongation of the neck of the condyle. *A,* Patient with deviation of the chin to the right caused by an elongated condylar neck on the left side (see Fig. 29–114). *B,* After resection of a measured section of the neck of the left condyle. *C,* Occlusal relationships before the surgical correction. Note the deviation to the right. *D,* Dental occlusion after completion of the treatment. (Patient of Donald Wood-Smith, M.D.)

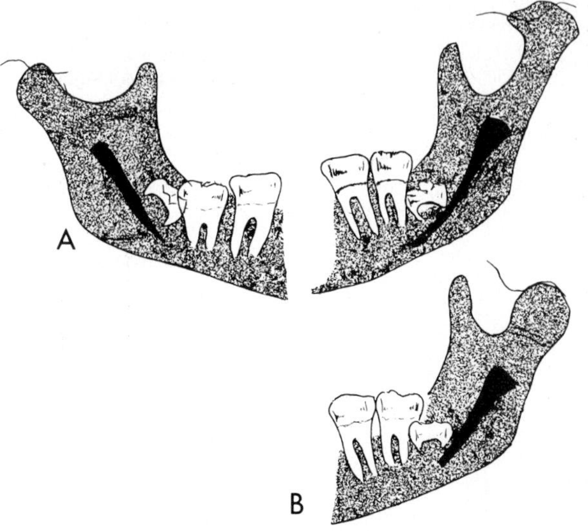

Figure 29–114. *A,* Tracings of a panoramic roentgenogram showing the elongation of the neck of the condyle on the left side. *B,* After resection of a measured segment from the condylar neck (see Fig. 29–113).

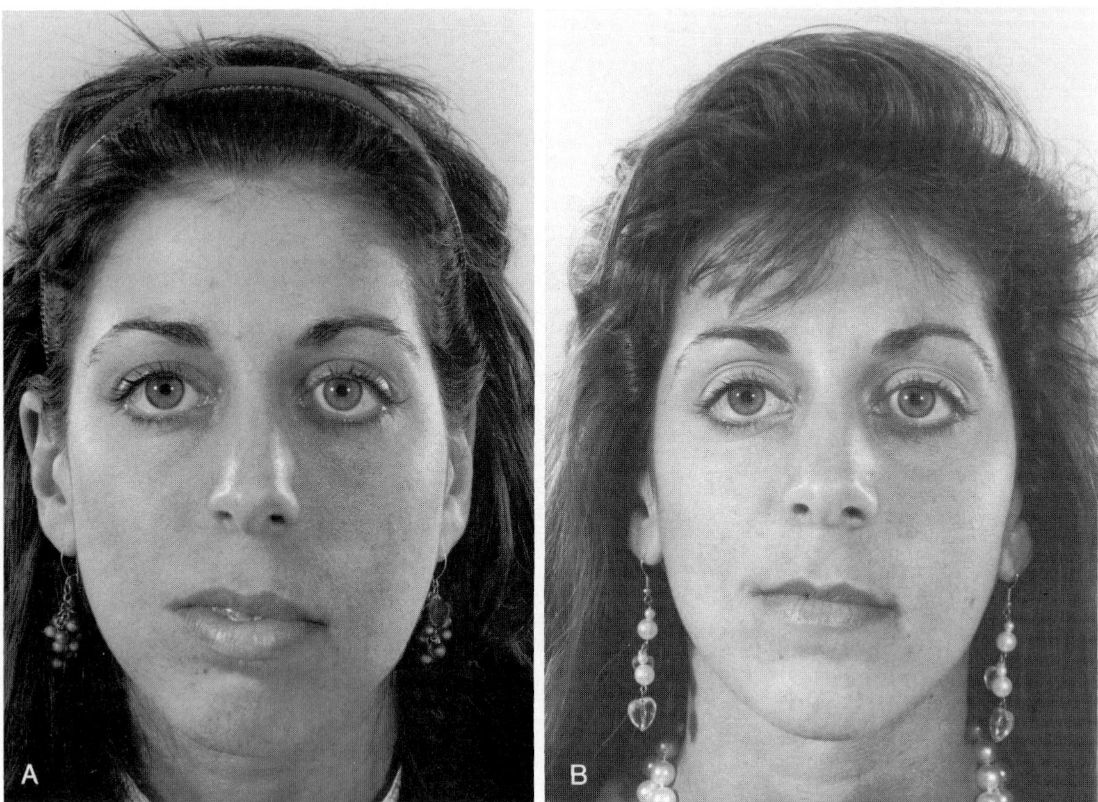

Figure 29–115. Hemifacial hyperplasia. *A, C, E,* Preoperative appearance of a female with hemifacial (corporal) hyperplasia including unilateral enlargement of the tongue. *B, D, F,* Appearance after debulking of the soft tissues of the left side of the face, in combination with Le Fort I osteotomy, mandibular rotation (sagittal splitting or ramisection), and genioplasty.

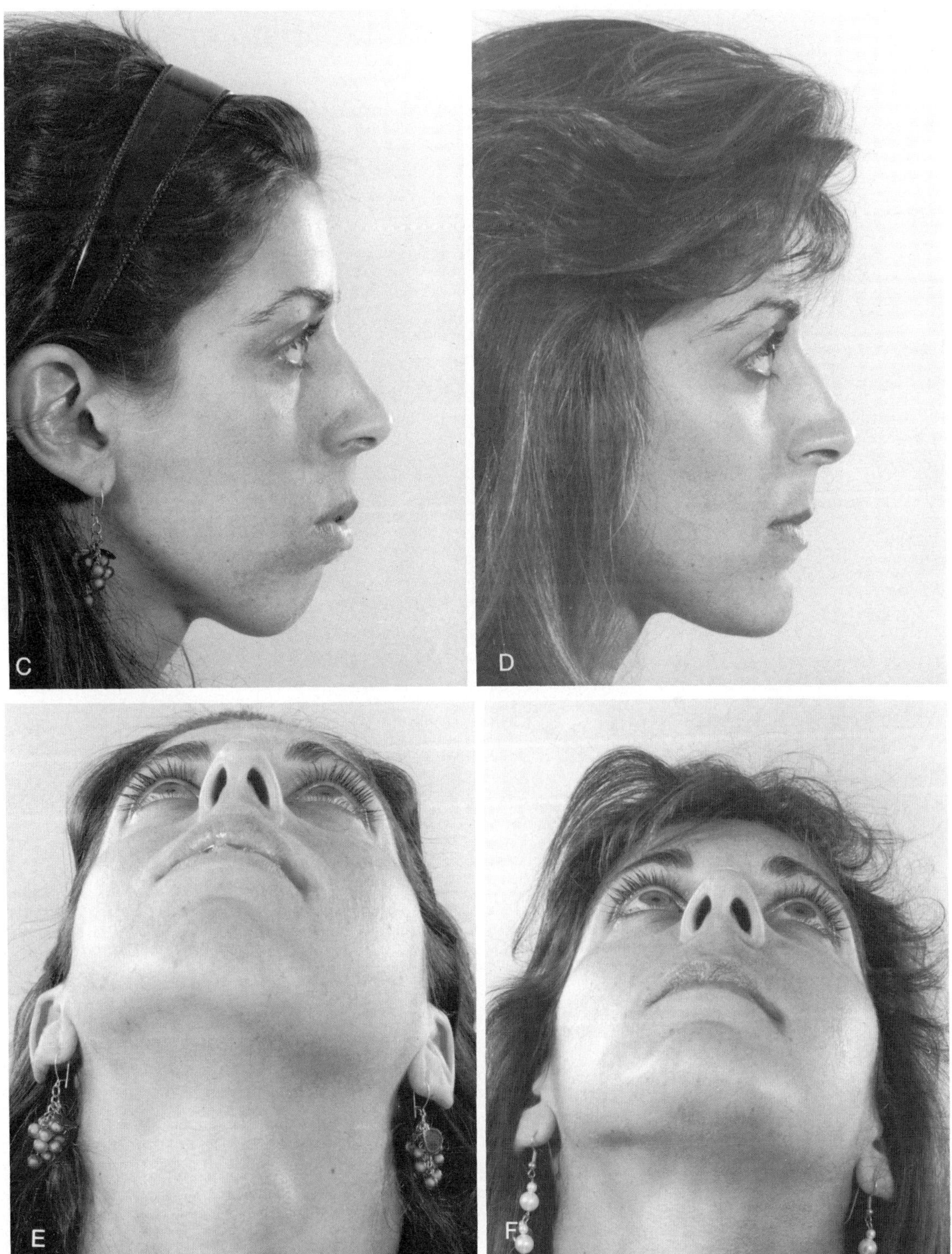

Figure 29–115 *Continued*

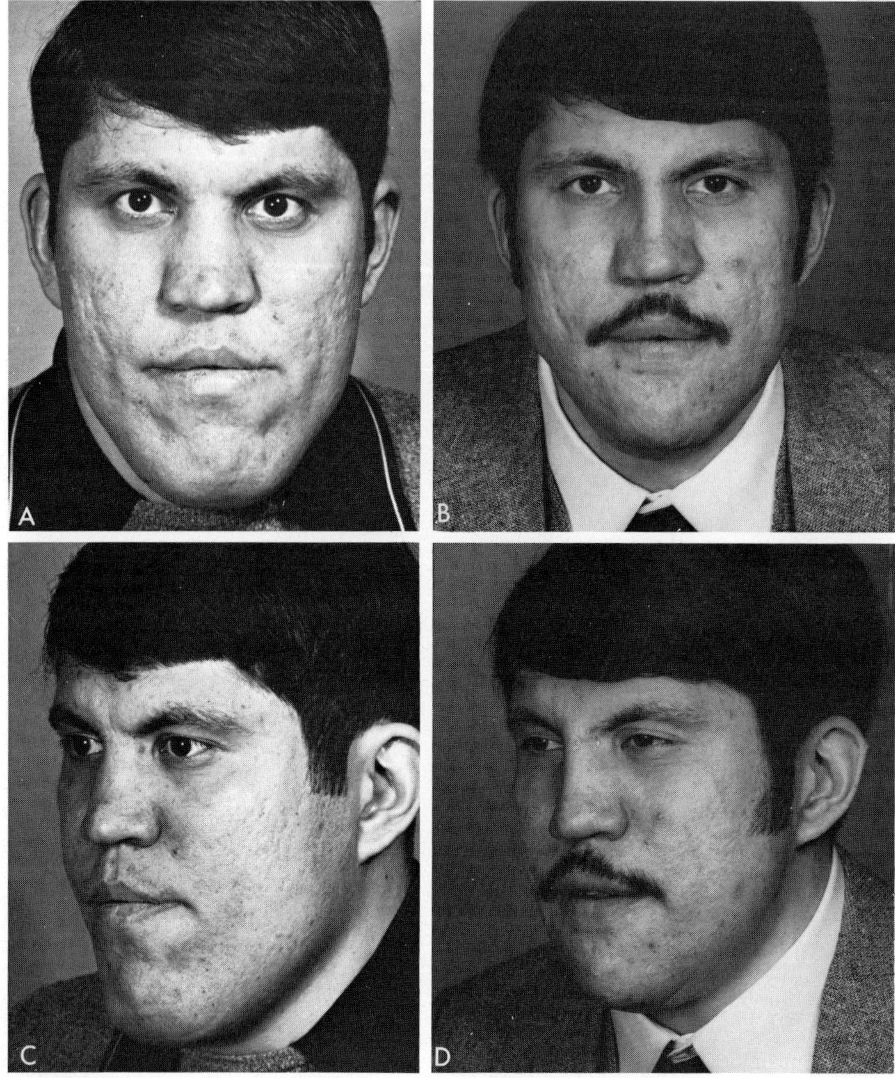

Figure 29–116. Patient with acromegalic features. *A, C,* Preoperative views. Note the elongated face and flat nose. *B, D,* Appearance after removal of a horseshoe segment from the inferior border of the mandible and transposition of some of the resected bone to a position anterior to the symphysis. In a separate stage a bone graft was placed over the nasal dorsum, and redundant submental soft tissue was resected.

HEMIFACIAL HYPERPLASIA

Hemifacial hyperplasia is a rare congenital deformity that affects the soft and bony tissues of the face (Fig. 29–115). The terms "hemifacial gigantism," "facial hemihypertrophy," and "hemifacial hypertrophy" have also been used. The latter two terms are obviously incorrect.

The etiology of the condition is unknown and no pattern of heredity is present. Rowe (1962), in reviewing the subject, found that the condition is more prevalent in males than in females and involves the right side more frequently than the left. The asymmetry is progressively accentuated through puberty. Abnormal enlargement generally ceases at the age of 17 or 18 years as skeletal maturation occurs.

Enlargement of the zygoma, maxilla, and mandible on the affected side is present (Fig. 29–115). The inferior alveolar canal is also increased in size. The cranium and extremities can be involved. Premature development and eruption of the teeth occur as well as macrodontia of varying degrees. Unilateral enlargement of the tongue and its papillae is also a feature. The overlying facial soft tissues are increased in bulk and the auricle may be enlarged. The entire ipsilateral side of the body, including the extremities, or in some cases the contralateral side, can be involved.

Treatment is difficult and consists of repositioning the jaws to a more normal location and reducing the bulk of the soft tissues (Fig. 29–115). Surgical procedures similar to those used to correct unilateral mandibular macrognathia and a Le Fort I osteotomy can be employed. Robinson, Shuken, and Dougherty (1969) recommended early condylectomy of the affected side to reduce the ongoing asymmetric growth.

LATERAL MANDIBULAR DEVIATION RESULTING FROM LOSS OF BONE

Acquired deformities due to bone loss usually require bone grafting and elongation osteotomies, procedures similar to those described in the section on mandibular hypoplasia (see p. 1260). Additional details about these deformities may be found later in this chapter (p. 1412).

FACIAL HYPERPLASIA

Pathologic states such as fibrous dysplasia, cherubism, and acromegaly result in an increase of facial skeletal size. Facial hyperplasia of unknown origin is rare.

Acromegaly, an endocrine disorder characterized by enlargement of the bones of the head and gigantism due to dysfunction of the pituitary gland, is one of the best-known examples of facial hyperplasia. A patient with acromegalic features is shown in Figure 29–116. A thorough evaluation, although it showed enlargement of the sella turcica, failed to demonstrate elevated growth hormone levels. A mandibular degloving procedure (see Fig. 29–46) was performed, and the mandibular angles were exposed through submandibular incisions. A horseshoe segment of the lower portion of the body of the mandible, including the mandibular angles, was resected through the combined approach. The symphyseal portion of the resected specimen was transplanted over the remaining mandibular symphysis to create adequate chin projection and a labiomental fold. The operation could presently be performed solely through the intraoral route. At a later session, an iliac bone graft was transplanted as part of the nasal reconstruction and an excision of the redundant submental soft tissue was required (Fig. 29–116*B,D*).

BENIGN MASSETERIC HYPERTROPHY

Benign masseteric hypertrophy is characterized by an asymptomatic unilateral or bilateral increase in size of the masseter muscle. Bilateral involvement is more common.

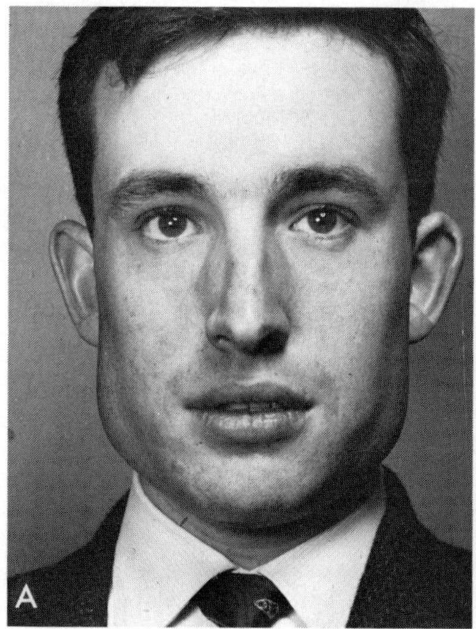

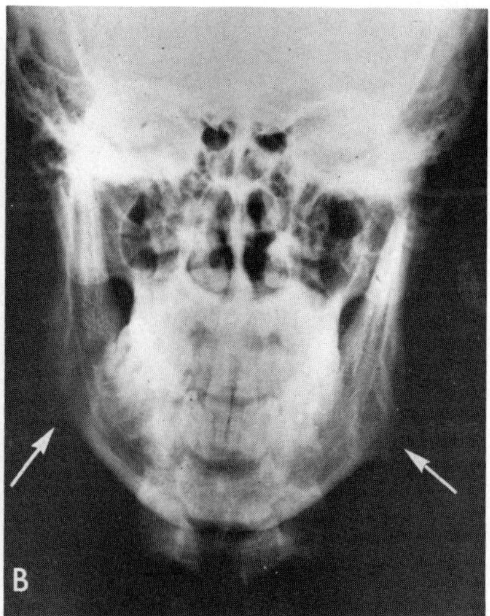

Figure 29–117. Bilateral masseteric muscle hypertrophy. *A*, Typical square jaw facial appearance. *B*, Roentgenogram showing hyperostosis in the region of the mandibular angles (*arrows*).

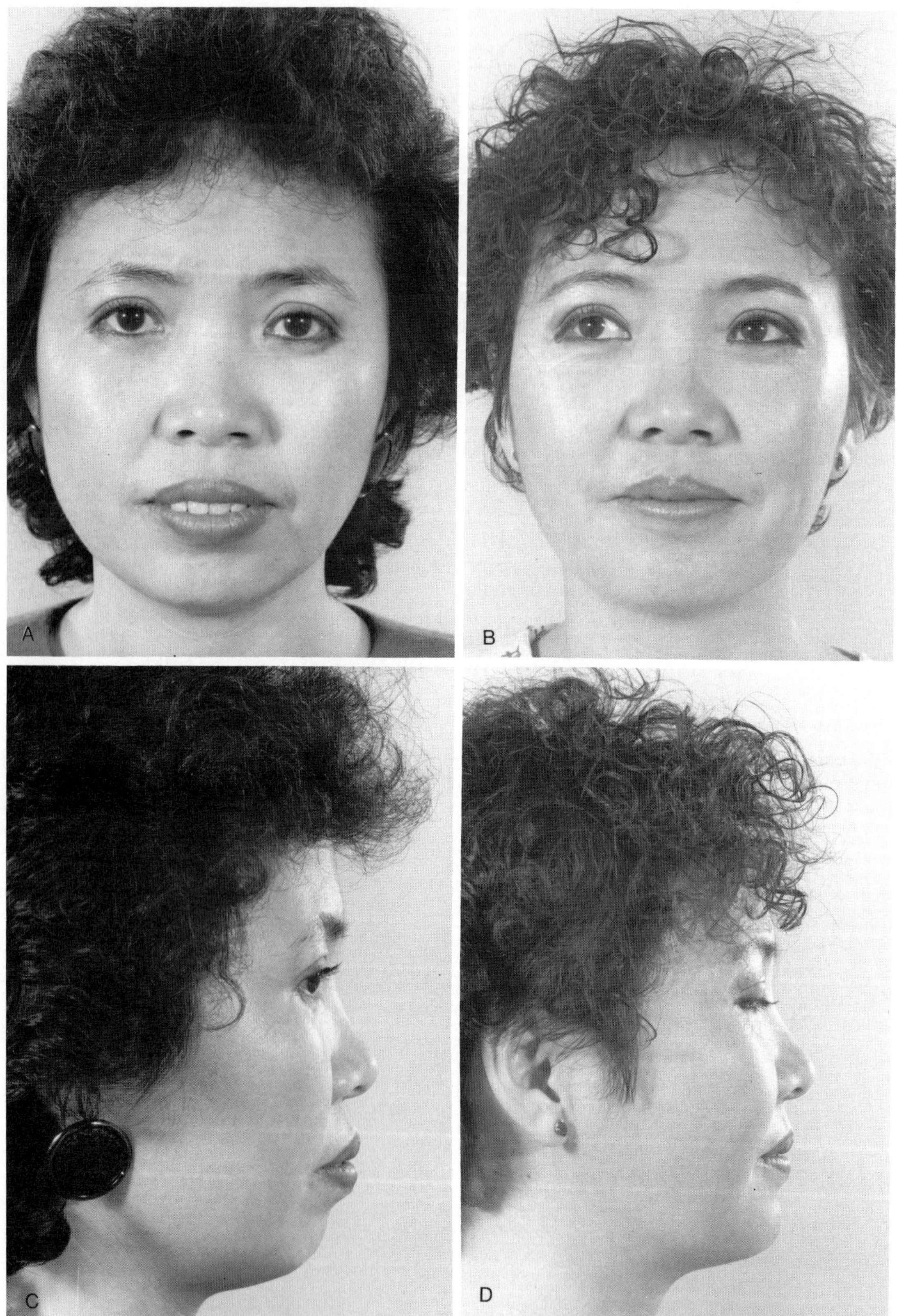

Figure 29–118. Masseteric hypertrophy. *A, C, E,* Preoperative appearance of an Oriental female with masseteric hypertrophy and mild anterior open bite. *B, D, F,* Appearance after combined maxillary and mandibular anterior segmental dentoalveolar setback osteotomies, partial masseter resections, recontouring of the mandibular angles, and removal of buccal fat pads.

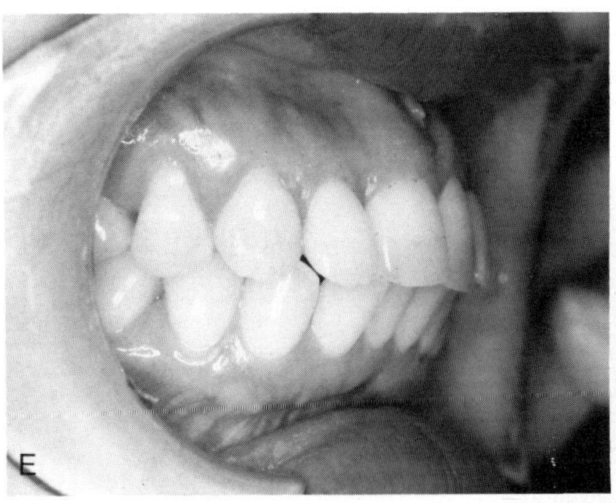

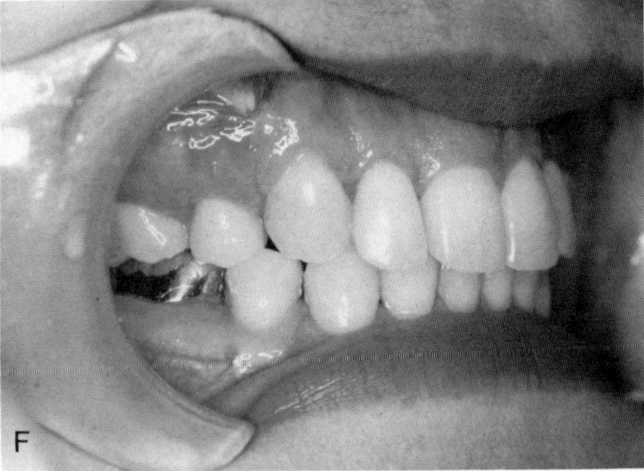

Figure 29–118 *Continued*

Legg (1880) first described the condition, and it was subsequently reported by Boldt (1930) and Coffey (1942). The surgical treatment of the abnormality was described by Gurney (1947) and Adams (1949).

The deformity occurs with equal frequency in both sexes and has its highest incidence in the third decade of life (Wolhynski, 1936; Oppenheim and Wing, 1959). There can be associated emotional instability (Guggenheim and Cohen, 1959, 1960, 1961). The patient may also have a "jaw clenching" habit, lending substance to Gurney's "work hypertrophy" theory. The etiology is unknown in most cases (Waldhart and Lynch, 1971).

Diagnosis

The face has a square contour with prominence of the preauricular and mandibular angle regions (Fig. 29–117*A*). The diagnosis is confirmed by palpating the masseter with the mandible at rest and during clenching. The condition has been mistaken for a parotid tumor or lymphangioma. Furthermore, a similar appearance without true hypertrophy of the masseter can be racial in origin, as frequently seen in Orientals (Fig. 29–118). Roentgenographic studies usually show hyperostosis with accentuation of the mandibular (gonial) angle (see Fig. 29–117*B*). The neurologic examination and electromyographic studies are usually inconclusive. Biopsy studies have reported "normal striated muscle" (Coffey, 1942).

Treatment

To convert the square facies to a more oval and tapering one, the bulk of the masseter and any hyperostosis of the mandibular angle must be reduced. Resection of the excess muscle is indicated to improve facial contour. Adams (1949) described the external inframandibular approach to remove the medial portion of the muscle and the hyperostotic areas under direct vision. Gurney (1947) excised only the lateral portion of the muscle, which is more hazardous because of the immediately superficial location of the facial nerve branches. Converse (1951) used the intraoral approach to resect the hypertrophied muscle and the protruding bone at the angle of the mandible (Fig. 29–119). Ginestet, Frezières, and Merville (1959) also recommended the intraoral approach, which avoids an external scar and the danger of damage to the marginal mandibular branch of the facial nerve.

The oral mucosa is incised over the anterior border of the ramus in a manner similar to that used for ramal osteotomies. The masseter is reflected in a subperiosteal manner from the lateral surface of the ramus. Using a scissor, the medial portion of the masseter is resected, a greater amount being removed inferiorly (Fig. 29–120). The protruding bone of the mandibular angle is reduced with a powered, large pear-shaped bur. A softer appearance can be achieved by converting the square mandibular angle to a slightly obtuse one, removing a section of bone that tapers superiorly from the posterior inferior border of the ramus with a right-angled saw.

The intraoral incision is closed with chromic sutures. Placement of an intraoral drain is optional. A compressive head dressing helps to minimize the postoperative edema. A full liquid diet is taken until the intraoral wounds have sealed.

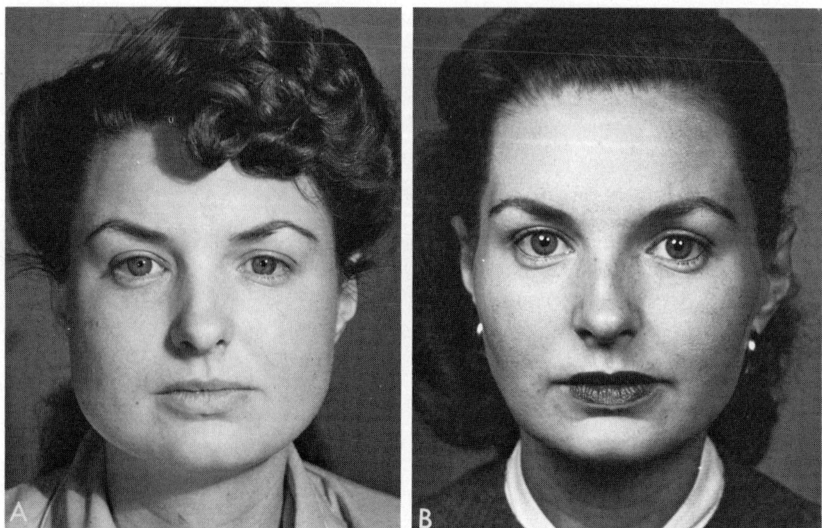

Figure 29–119. Bilateral masseteric muscle hypertrophy. *A,* Preoperative appearance. *B,* After resection of excess masseter muscle and removal of hyperostotic bone from the angle of the mandible by the intraoral approach.

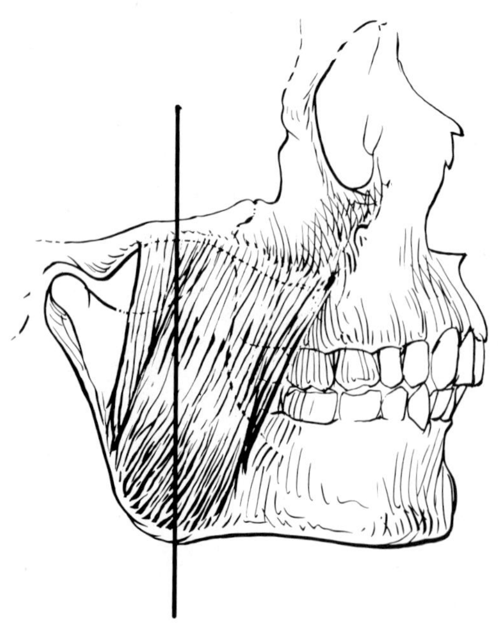

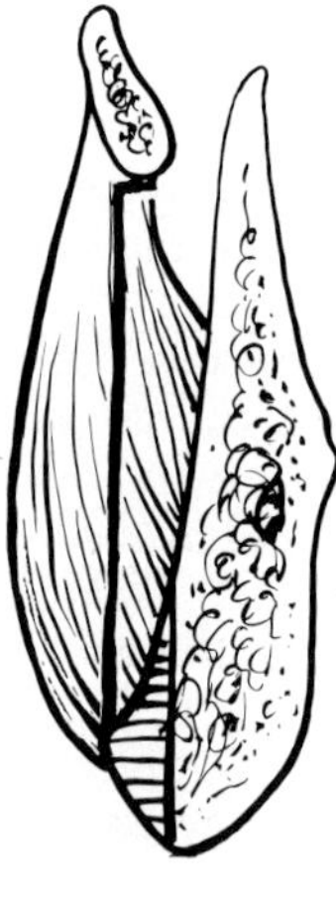

Figure 20–120. Combination resection of the masseter muscle and bony exostosis of the mandible through an intraoral route. The resection is illustrated on the cross section and the limits of the muscle and bony resection are designated by heavy lines.

Trismus and considerable swelling are to be expected after the operation. Active and passive exercises to open the mouth as wide as possible are to be encouraged, since jaw opening will be limited. Preoperatively, the patient should be warned not to expect a noticeable improvement in contour immediately after the operation. A change may not be evident for three to six months postoperatively. Furthermore, there may be residual asymmetry of the mandibular angles.

Chin Deformities

The position and contour of the chin are important components in facial harmony and balance. The chin also influences the posture and function of the lips. A deformity of the region may be an isolated problem, or may coexist with malformations of the jaws or other facial structures.

Anatomic Considerations. The mandible fuses in the midline during prenatal life. At the junction of the two halves, there is a ridge, the mental symphysis, which divides below and encloses a triangular eminence, the *mental protuberance* (Fig. 29–121). The base of the mental protuberance is depressed in its center. The raised portions on each side form the *mental tubercles.* On each side of the symphysis is a fossa, the *incisive fossa*, which gives origin to the mentalis and a small portion of the orbicularis oris muscle (Fig. 29–122). A faint ridge, the *oblique line*, extends posteriorly and upward from each mental tubercle and is continuous with the ridge that forms the anterior border of the ramus. This ridge passes below the mental foramen, which is situated below and usually slightly anterior to the second premolar tooth, and is an important surgical landmark. The quadratus labii inferioris and triangularis are attached to the oblique line immediately lateral to the origin of the mentalis. The platysma is attached to the lower portion of the lateral surface of the mandible below the oblique line.

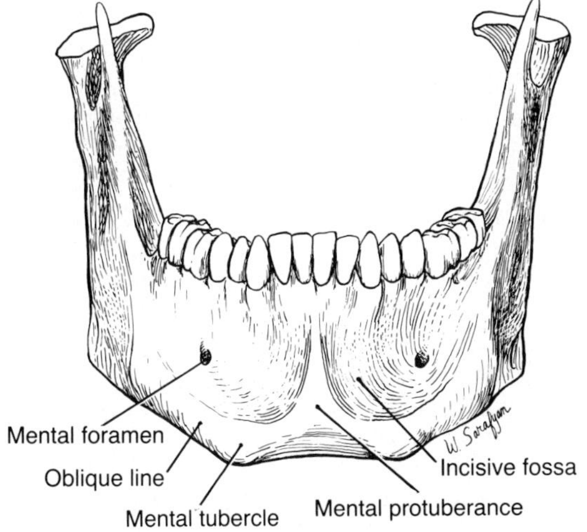

Figure 29–121. Skeletal anatomy of the chin.

On the lingual surface, near the lower part of the symphysis, are two pairs of small projections—the *mental spines.* The genioglossus muscles arise from the superior mental spines. The lower pair of spines serves as the origin of the geniohyoid muscles. An oval depression is present on each side below the level of the spines. The anterior bellies of the digastric muscles insert into these bony concavities. The mylohyoid muscle originates from the mylohyoid line, which extends posteriorly and upward from the lower part of the symphysis.

The function of the circumoral muscles is affected by the bone contour of the chin. Thus, alteration of the underlying skeleton changes the contour of the soft tissues and labial performance. For example, patients with a retruded chin may experience difficulty in occluding their lips and achieving lip seal. The muscles of the lower lip are placed under excessive tension as a result of their attachment to the abnormal backward and downward inclined bony chin. When the patient tries to occlude his lips, the chin pad (i.e., the mentalis muscles) rides upward to obliterate the labiomental fold, and stamps the chin with a puckered appearance (Zide and McCarthy, 1989). Increasing the projection of the chin helps to restore normal working relationships of the musculature of the lower lip (mentalis and depressor labii inferioris and triangularis). Thus, the muscular tension is relieved, labial competence is improved, and the contour of the chin is enhanced (see Fig. 29–138).

MICROGENIA

Microgenia, or "small chin," implies an underdevelopment of the region of the mental symphysis. The term should be neither confused nor interchanged with the word "micro-

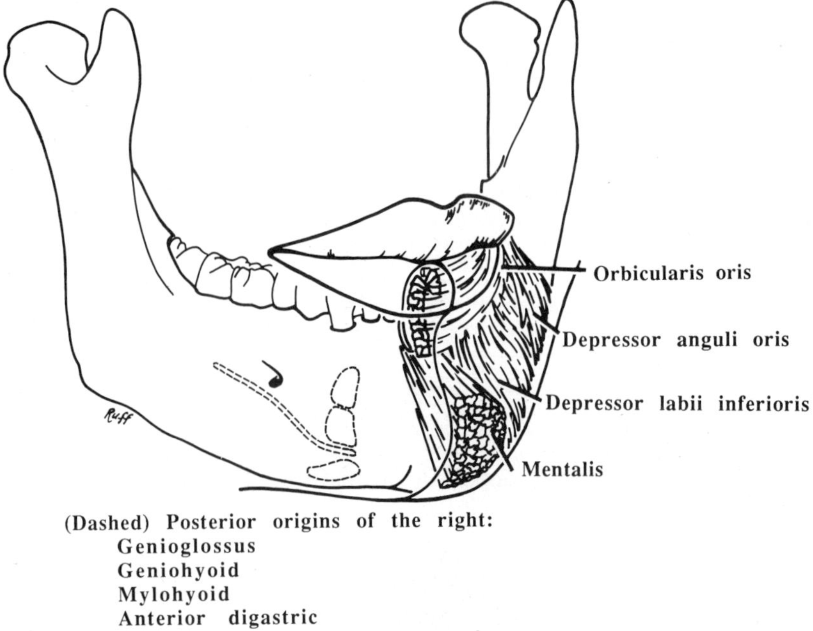

Figure 29–122. Soft tissue anatomy of the chin. (From McCarthy, J. G., and Ruff, G.: The chin. Clin. Plast. Surg., *15*:125, 1988.)

gnathia," in which all components of the jaw can be affected.

The small chin may be an isolated deformity, the remainder of the lower jaw being normal in size. It is also seen in patients with variable degrees of hypoplasia of the mandible (micrognathia) and, paradoxically, in mandibular prognathism. Thus, the associated occlusion and the dentoalveolar relationships may or may not be ideal. Frequently, the maxillary anterior dentoalveolar segment is protruded (Class II, division 1 malocclusion); bimaxillary protrusion may also be seen. Orthodontic therapy is helpful in deemphasizing the deformity of the tooth-bearing structures and thereby accentuating the appearance of the chin. However, in order to create a harmonious balance of the face, the symphyseal area requires augmentation.

Diagnosis and Preoperative Planning

Precisely oriented photographs and cephalometric roentgenograms help to confirm the clinical diagnosis. Various cephalometric measurements have been proposed to determine the ideal position of the chin (Ricketts, 1957; Hambleton, 1964; Merrifield, 1966; Zide, Grayson and McCarthy, 1981a,b, 1982). These measurements are limited by their two-dimensional nature and are useful only as guides; the final analysis depends more on the desires of the patient and the esthetic judgment of the surgeon.

The vertical dimension of the chin must be carefully noted. All too often the surgeon's attention is arrested by the retruded appearance of the chin, and an equally important vertical problem is overlooked. Soft tissue analysis of the chin is equally important: the quality (resilience, scar), labial muscular function, and the relationship of the chin pad (mentalis muscle) to the bony chin (McCarthy and Ruff, 1988).

The nose-chin relationship is an important aspect of vertical facial balance (see Fig. 29–3). The general appearance of the face is largely influenced by the size, shape, and position of the nose and chin. As stated earlier in the chapter, it has been proposed that a face divided into equal horizontal thirds represents the best artistic facial balance. The ratios of the divine proportions have also been used (Ricketts, 1982). However, many esthetically acceptable variations of the ideal ratio are found in nature.

Anteroposterior and vertical abnormalities can be accurately assessed by cephalometric studies and photographs. The amount of desired projection of the chin can be determined by tracing the new position of the chin and measuring the difference from the original contour (see Fig. 29–25). Not all cases require such an elaborate work-up, and in the average case of microgenia a reliable estimate of the amount of chin augmentation can be gained from a careful examination of the patient and the profile photograph.

Chin Augmentation

Nose-chin relationships to reestablish a balanced profile were emphasized by Aufricht (1934). His use of the dorsal excess of a large hump nose was one of the first means of increasing the projection of the chin. Stripped of mucoperiosteum and mucoperichondrium and shaped, the dorsal hump was introduced over the mental symphysis through a short submental incision.

Use of alloplastic implant materials in a wide range is the most popular method of augmenting the chin. A sliding advancement osteotomy of the lower border of the mental symphysis is favored by those who prefer the use of autogenous tissue. Bone and cartilage grafts are less frequently employed.

Surgical Approach. The surgical field should include the entire face and upper neck. A vertical ink line is traced on the skin to serve as a landmark for the proposed midline of the chin. An extraoral or an intraoral approach can be used for exposure.

Extraoral Approach. An incision is made under the mental symphysis. In this area, a superior scar is obtained when the incision is made along the inferior border of the mandible rather than in the submental fold. A subperiosteal pocket is developed by incising and raising the periosteum. If a supraperiosteal pocket is desired, the plane of dissection should be kept immediately on top of the periosteum. The pocket is only large enough to accommodate the implant or transplant, leaving no excess space.

Intraoral Approach. The amount of exposure desired dictates the choice of mucosal incision. Introduction of an implant calls for a limited pocket to minimize the risk of displacement of the material. A single midline incision or two vertical incisions placed laterally near the cuspid (Fig. 29–123) are made down to the underlying bone. A pocket is dissected, either immediately above or below

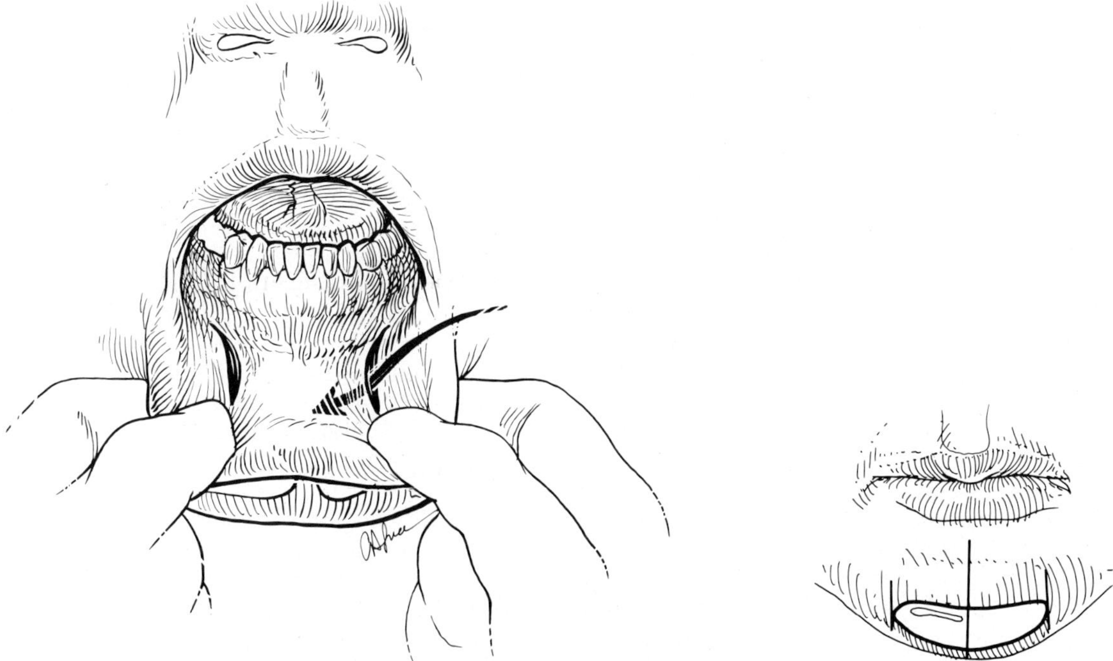

Figure 29–123. Technique of chin implant insertion. Surgical approach to the chin via parallel incisions at the cuspid level. The inset shows the proper position of the chin implant over the pogonion or basilar portion of the mandible.

the periosteum, over the most anteroinferior surface of the mental symphysis and directly over the thick, dense cortical bone. The dissection is continued laterally under the mental foramina to avoid injury to the mental nerves.

If a larger pocket is required, as when performing a horizontal (transverse) osteotomy of the symphysis, a horizontal intraoral incision is used (Converse, 1950). The incision should be made above the vestibular sulcus. Augmentation procedures, particularly in the mental symphyseal region, place tension on the tissue, which may cause separation of the wound edges and exposure of the material used to project the chin. Either the labiobuccal vestibular incision or the gingival incision (see Fig. 29–45) provides adequate exposure. Placement in the depth of the cul de sac should be avoided since the accumulation of saliva and food debris can interfere with the healing of the wound.

A horizontal incision is made through the mucosa below the labial frenulum. The mucosa alone is incised and raised from the underlying muscles, and the dissection is carried down to the bone. The periosteum is incised along a horizontal line. The extent of the subperiosteal dissection depends on the size of the implant or the needs of the osteotomy.

Technique of Contour Restoration in Microgenia

Four techniques are available to correct microgenia of the mandible. Contour restoration is made by (1) an alloplastic implant, (2) horizontal advancement osteotomy, (3) implantation of cartilage or bone, or (4) a skin graft inlay and prosthodontic support.

Contour Restoration by Alloplastic Implant. A variety of inorganic materials have been used to increase the prominence of the chin, most notable of which are polyethylene (Rubin and associates, 1948, 1971), methyl methacrylate (Gonzalez-Ulloa, 1957; Rish, 1960; Pitanguy, 1968), and Teflon (Brown and associates, 1960). However, solid or gel-filled silicone implants remain the most commonly used material (Rish, 1960; Safian, 1965; Bayne, 1966; Junghans, 1967; Snyder, 1975). These prefabricated implants are commercially available in various sizes and shapes, and can be used without modification of shape or trimmed to fit the individual deformity.

Because the operative procedure is simple, inorganic implants have become popular in the treatment of moderate degrees of microgenia and in conjunction with corrective rhinoplasty. The concomitant corrective procedures for the nose and the chin usually achieve a successfully balanced profile (Millard, 1965).

The use of alloplastic implants is best reserved for mild to moderate microgenic deformities that require projection of the chin point. They should not be used to camouflage a vertical discrepancy such as an excessively tall but retruded chin (retromacrogenia) or a short and retruded chin (McCarthy and Ruff, 1988).

The symphysis and the body of the mandible are formed of hard, dense bone in the lower basilar portion. The implant should be placed to rest on this thick cortical bone and not over the thin, weaker bone that surrounds the dentoalveolar structures. As a result of misplacement or upward displacement by the pressure of the overlying soft tissues, the implant may penetrate through the thin cortex into the softer cancellous bone and endanger the roots of the incisor teeth (see Fig. 29–234).

Technique. Depending on the surgeon's preference, the alloplastic implant can be introduced through an extraoral submental or intraoral approach (Fig. 29–123). Although it is difficult to detect, the patient may object to the placement of a cutaneous scar.

The operation is usually performed under local anesthesia with a 1:100,000 concentration of epinephrine to minimize bleeding. Regardless of the surgical route, two precautions should be observed in developing the pocket to receive the implant. The first is to place the pocket over the hard and resistant bone of the mental symphysis. Failure to heed this point can lead to malplacement of the implant over the thin cortical bone of the dentoalveolar region, which offers little resistance to bone erosion under the implant. The second is to make the pocket only large enough to accommodate the implant, to discourage its displacement, and to minimize redundant space and hematoma formation.

The pocket can be placed in a supraperiosteal or subperiosteal plane. A subperiosteal pocket is easier to create, but a supraperiosteal placement of the implant has been advocated to decrease underlying bone resorption (Parkes, 1973). Regardless of the plane of dissection, the important point is to position the implant over the dense bone of the lower portion of the symphysis.

To accommodate the flanges of the implant, especially the extended implants, the pocket must be extended in a posterior direction. Care should be exercised to avoid injury to the mental nerve by staying well below the mental foramen. With a small chin, less leeway space is present since the mental foramen can be located close to the inferior border.

After the implant is inserted, its midline should be checked to coincide with the ink reference mark on the skin. Many of the implants come with a midline marker; if not, a small notch can be made in the solid implants. The implant should be well adapted to the underlying bone contour to avoid instability and undesirable space. To minimize migration of the implant, some are manufactured with Dacron backing, or the surgeon may elect to fix the implant to the adjacent tissues with a nonabsorbable suture or an intraosseous wire.

The wound is closed in layers. Drains are infrequently needed. A small compressive dressing of 1 inch Microform or Elastoplast will discourage hematoma formation and help immobilize the implant (Fig. 29–124). The use of perioperative antibiotics is optional. If an intraoral incision is used, the patient should be maintained on food substances that are free of particulate matter for a few days until the wound has sealed over.

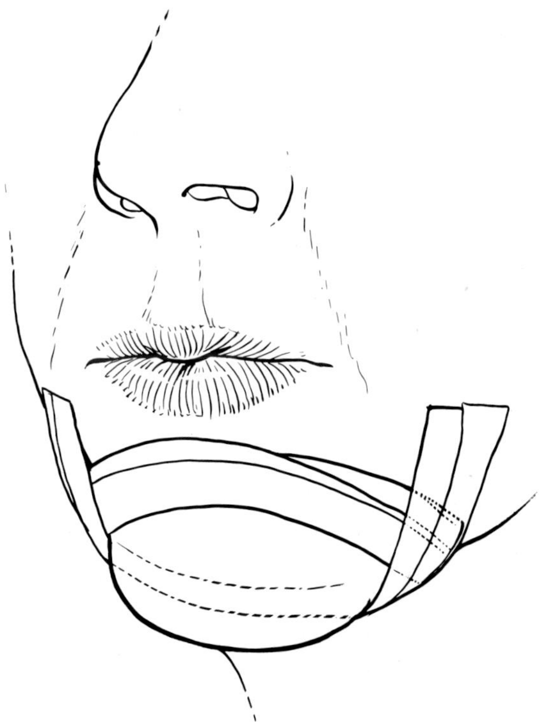

Figure 29–124. Type of chin dressing: Elastoplast strips applied to the skin after coating with an adhesive.

Complications. Of the various complications, the most worrisome is the upward displacement of the implant and resorption of the underlying bone with penetration of the mandible. A small amount of bone erosion and settling of the implant is to be expected, and patients should be informed preoperatively of this possibility. This is not altogether an unfavorable event since a small amount of settling in the bone prevents dislodgment of the implant.

However, when the implant migrates cephalad and penetrates the softer tooth-bearing portion of the mandible (see Fig. 29–235), it should be removed to prevent damage to the teeth.

As with any inorganic implant, capsule formation also occurs. If the contour of the implant is less than ideal, an esthetically objectionable outline of the implant will be seen as a lump on the chin. The implant should not be merely removed but replaced with one of more suitable contour or a horizontal osteotomy of the symphysis. If the implant is simply removed, the capsule will collapse toward its center, drawing in the origins of the overlying muscles. The resulting deformity is a disfiguring, balled-up, flabby, ptotic soft tissue mass that defies correction (Fig. 29–125).

Paresthesia of the lower lip can also occur. Since the distance between the lower border of the mandible and the mental foramen is often decreased in a microgenic mandible, the dissection of the pocket should be kept as close as possible to the lower border.

Infection is rare and usually results from a hematoma. In this event, removal of the implant is required. Extrusion as a result of excessive soft tissue pressure and closure of the wound under tension usually occurs through the newly healed oral wound. Migration of the implant is also seen (Fig. 29–126), as is its rotation in the soft tissues to produce an undesirable chin contour.

Results. The clinical application of the alloplastic implant should be limited to mild cases of microgenia (Fig. 29–127). When excessively large implants are placed, the pressure of the overlying tight tissues may cause

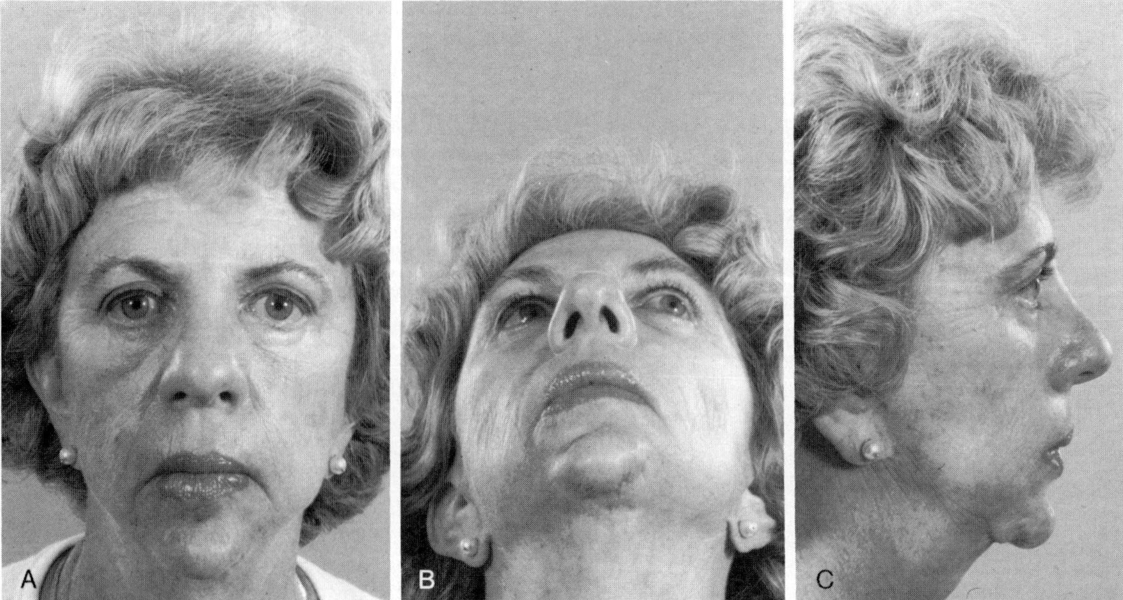

Figure 29–125. Chin appearance after removal of successively inserted implants. Note the ill-shaped and rolled-up soft tissue chin pad.

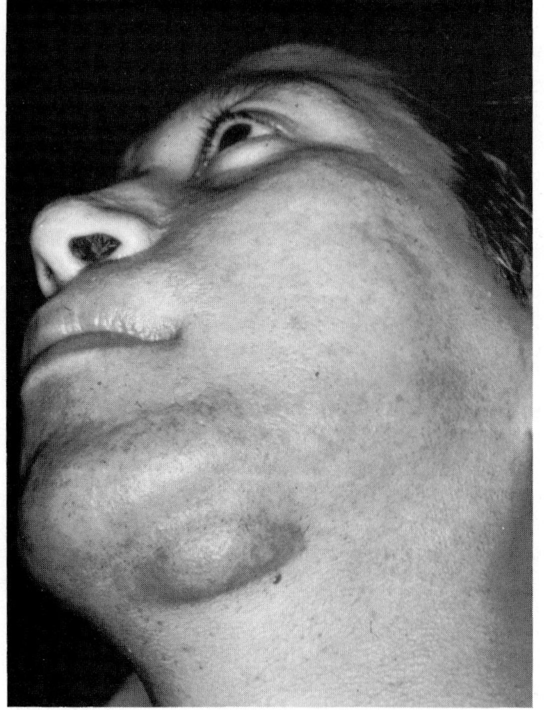

Figure 29–126. Migration of a chin implant into the neck. (Courtesy of Dr. Melvin Spira.)

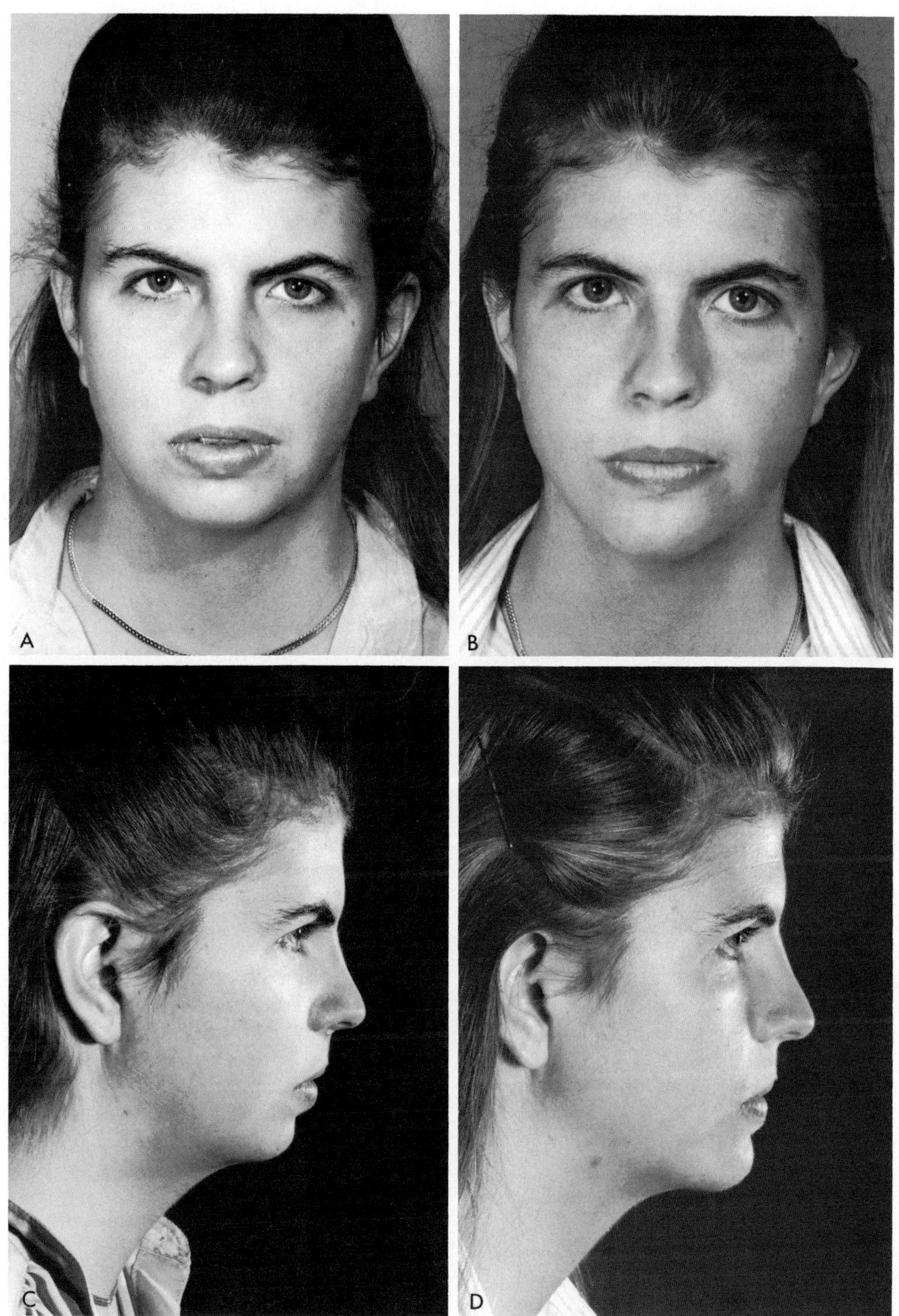

Figure 29–127. Microgenia corrected by chin implant. *A, C,* Preoperative views. *B, D,* Postoperative views.

bone erosion and resorption of the underlying mandible. Extrusion and migration of the implant are other problems that can follow injudicious use in such cases.

Erosion of the bone can be seen on the cephalometric roentgenogram within months after implantation. When the overlying tissues are tight, soft tissue pressure appears to be the principal factor in this process.

A cephalometric survey of 85 chin implants suggested that small and medium-sized implants are well tolerated in the absence of tight overlying soft tissues (Friedland, Coccaro, and Converse, 1976). Although some degree of erosion was noted, it did not appear to progress for more than a few months after implantation. The study also emphasized the advisability of placing the implant over the hard, resistant bone of the mental symphysis.

Contour Restoration by Horizontal (Transverse) Advancement Osteotomy (Genioplasty). The techniques of the horizontal osteotomy of the mandible (Hofer, 1942; Obwegeser, 1957; Converse and Wood-Smith, 1964; McCarthy and Ruff, 1988) consist of detaching the lower portion of the anterior mandibular body, usually moving it forward, occasionally laterally, and not infrequently transplanting it over the anterior aspect of the mandible (jumping genioplasty). It is a highly versatile technique capable of producing excellent results (Fig. 29–128).

The horizontal osteotomy was first proposed by Hofer (1942) using an external approach (Fig. 29–129). However, it is universally now performed through the intraoral degloving technique (see Fig. 29–45). Although general anesthesia is widely used, the procedure can be safely and comfortably performed under intravenous sedation and local anesthesia on an outpatient basis even in a properly equipped office setting (Spear, Mausner, and Kawamoto, 1987).

Technique. The symphyseal region is exposed through the degloving procedure. The horizontal incision can be placed on either the labial or dental side of the vestibule. A limited subperiosteal dissection is performed *preferably with preservation of the soft tissue attachment over the lower portion of the symphysis* and minimal dissection around the mental foramen (see Fig. 29–46).

A power oscillating and reciprocating saw is used to outline and complete the osteotomy (Fig. 29–130). A vertical midline score with a saw should be made initially as a reference line. The level and the angle of the line of osteotomy can be varied to suit the deformity. However, the osteotomy must always be situated below the apices of the teeth. It begins at the midline approximately 1 cm above the inferior border of the symphysis and extends posteriorly, according to the demands of the deformity, often reaching and continuing beyond the mental foramen below the level of the inferior alveolar canal. The position of the inferior alveolar canal and mental foramen is variable but can be identified on preoperative roentgenograms. The canal usually descends for a few millimeters before reaching the mental foramen. Failure to verify the position of the canal can result in its penetration by the line of osteotomy and severance of the inferior alveolar neurovascular bundle.

The entire osteotomy can be accomplished with powered saws. The use of a bur for the osteotomy is time consuming and creates a greater kerf. A conscious effort must be made in the posterior aspect to direct the saw blade around the inferior border of the mandible and through the lingual cortical plate. It is in this region that the osteotomy is apt to be incomplete, preventing the mobilization of the fragment. The blood supply to the mobilized symphysis is maintained through the remaining attached soft tissues. In effect, a pedicle flap of bone is created. The retained vascular supply promotes rapid consolidation of the segment. Furthermore, resistance to infection is increased even if there is a disruption of the incision. Vertical cuts through the reflected periosteum allow for greater expansion of the pocket to accommodate the advanced segment of bone.

The surgeon at this point can choose among various alternatives to satisfy the needs of the particular deformity (McCarthy and Ruff, 1988):

1. The inferior segment is simply advanced forward: a sliding osseous genioplasty (see Figs. 29–128*C*, 29–130, 29–131, 29–132) (Obwegeser, 1957).

2. The inferior segment is transposed as an onlay pedicled flap over the anterior mandibular cortex (Figs. 29–128*E*, 29–133, 29–134) (Converse and Shapiro, 1952; Converse, 1959). The technique ("jumping genioplasty," a term coined by Tessier) is indicated when the vertical dimension of the lower face is excessive and projection of the chin is also desirable. An intimate contact between the

Text continued on page 1318

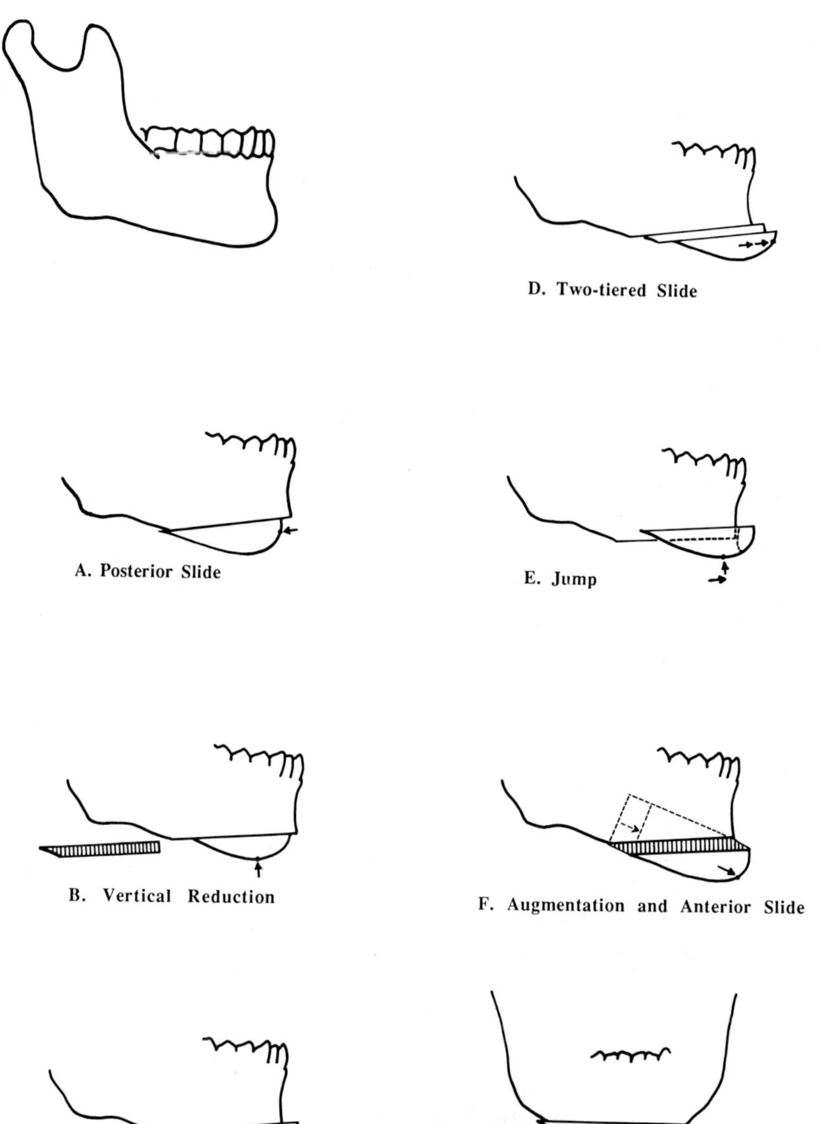

Figure 29–128. The horizontal osteotomy: variations. Note the net movement delineated by the vector (arrow). The dashed line in *F* effects the same movement as the horizontal osteotomy of the mandible but requires additional osteotomies and exposure. (From McCarthy, J. G., and Ruff, G.: The chin. Clin. Plast. Surg., *15*:125, 1988.)

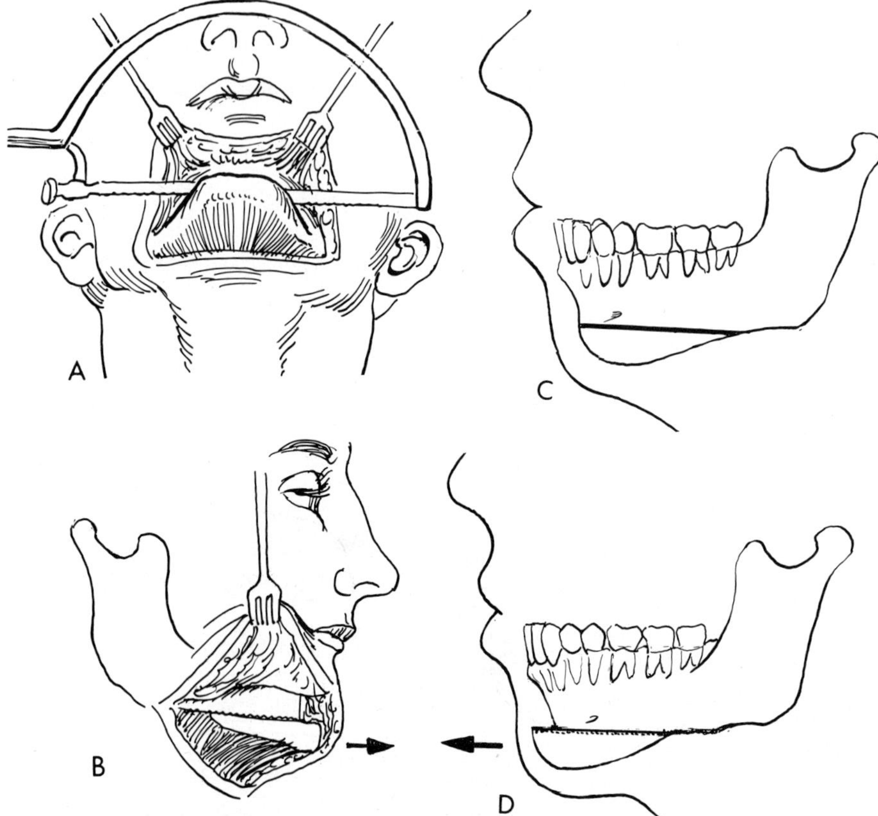

Figure 29–129. Horizontal osteotomy to advance the lower portion of the mandible. *A, B,* Hofer's technique (1942) of horizontal advancement osteotomy through an extraoral approach. *C,* Line of osteotomy passing below the mental foramen and inferior alveolar canal. *D,* A fragment is advanced to augment the contour of the chin.

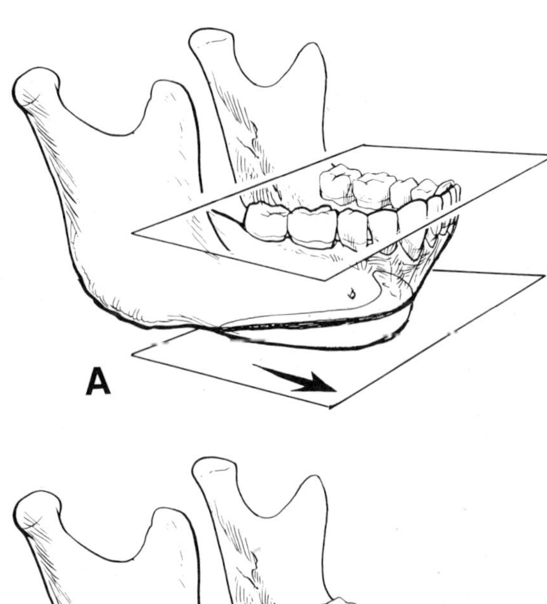

Figure 29–130. Sliding genioplasty. *A,* The osteotomy is made in a plane parallel to the occlusal surface. Consequently, there is no change in the vertical dimension. *B,* Lag screws provide fixation. The poles of the advanced segment have been contoured.

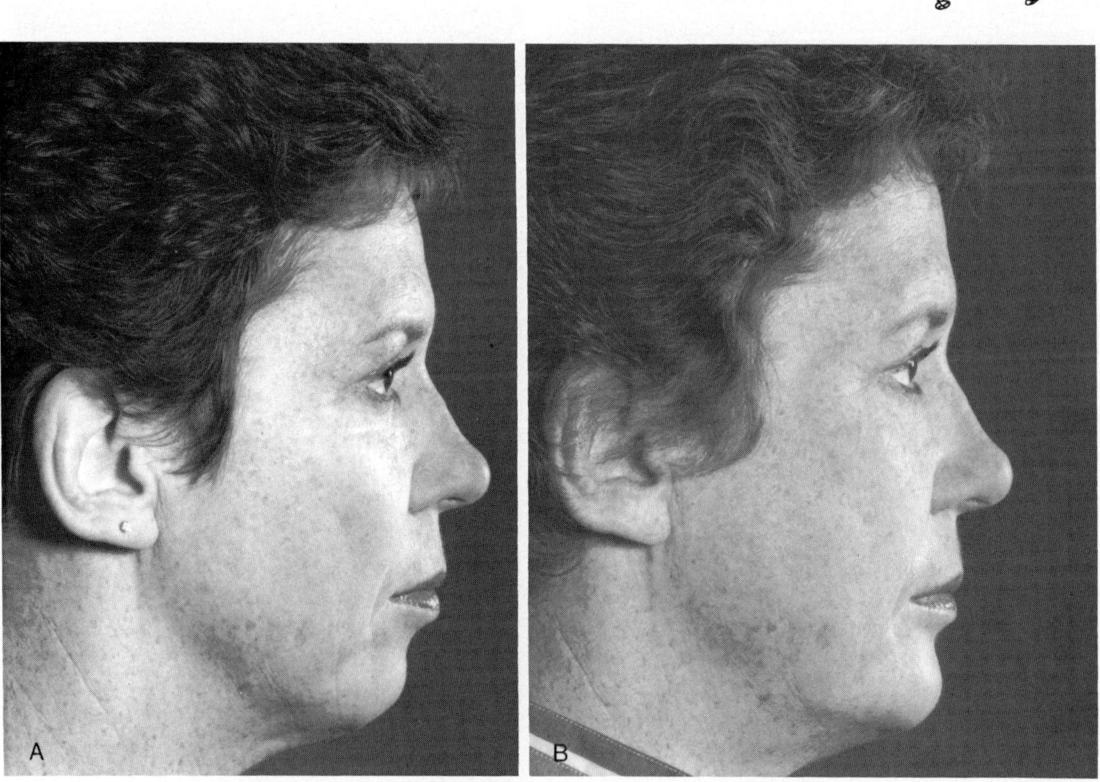

Figure 29–131. Sliding genioplasty. *A,* Preoperative profile. Note the disparity between the soft tissue and skeletal chin in a middle-aged woman. *B,* Profile after correction by the technique illustrated in Figure 29–130.

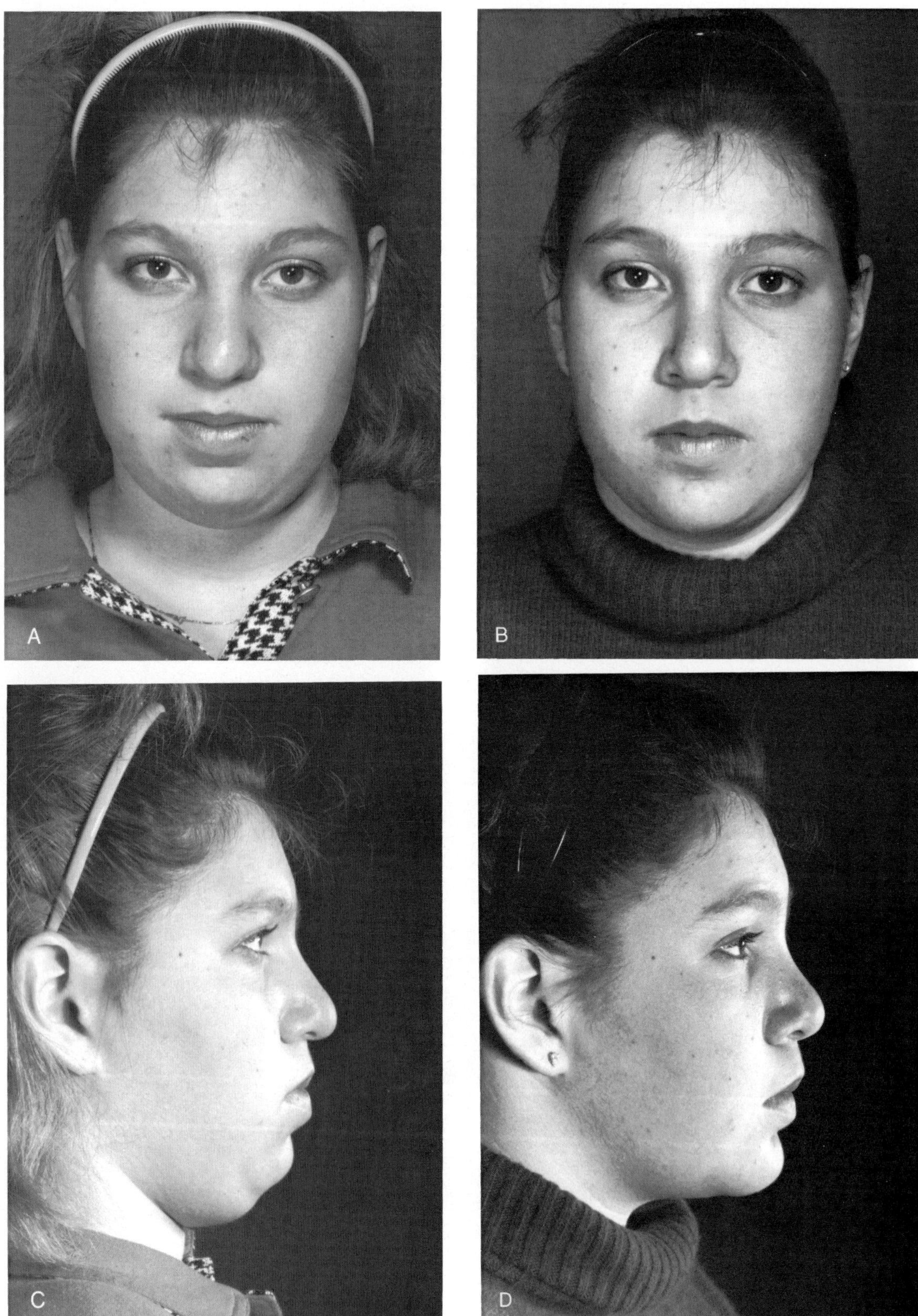

Figure 29–132. Sliding genioplasty. *A, C,* Preoperative views of an adolescent female with microgenia and submental excess. *B, D,* Postoperative views after a sliding genioplasty (see Fig. 29–130) and suction assisted lipectomy of the submental region.

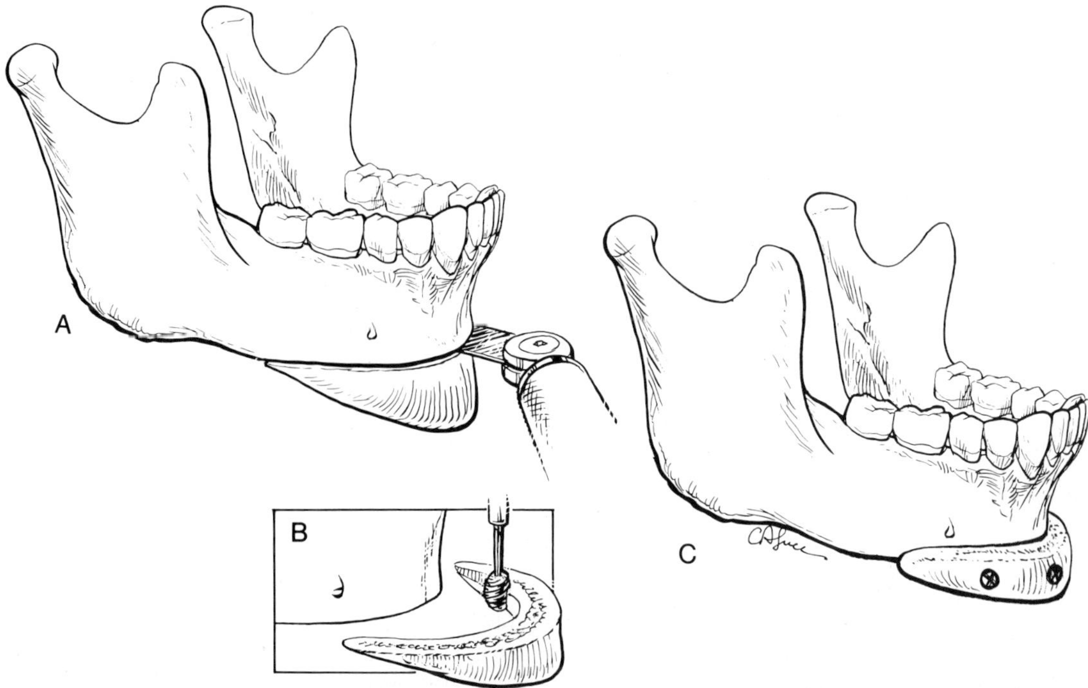

Figure 29–133. Jumping genioplasty. The segment is transposed as an onlay (muscle) flap over the anterior mandibular cortex. *A,* Lines of osteotomy. Note the anterior deficiency and vertical excess of the pogonion. *B,* After transposition of the osteotomized segment, contouring is done on the concave surface of the transplant to control the degree of advancement and achieve intimate bone to bone contact. Each pole of the segment may also require burring. *C,* Fixation with lag screws. The fragment pedicle has been preserved but is not illustrated.

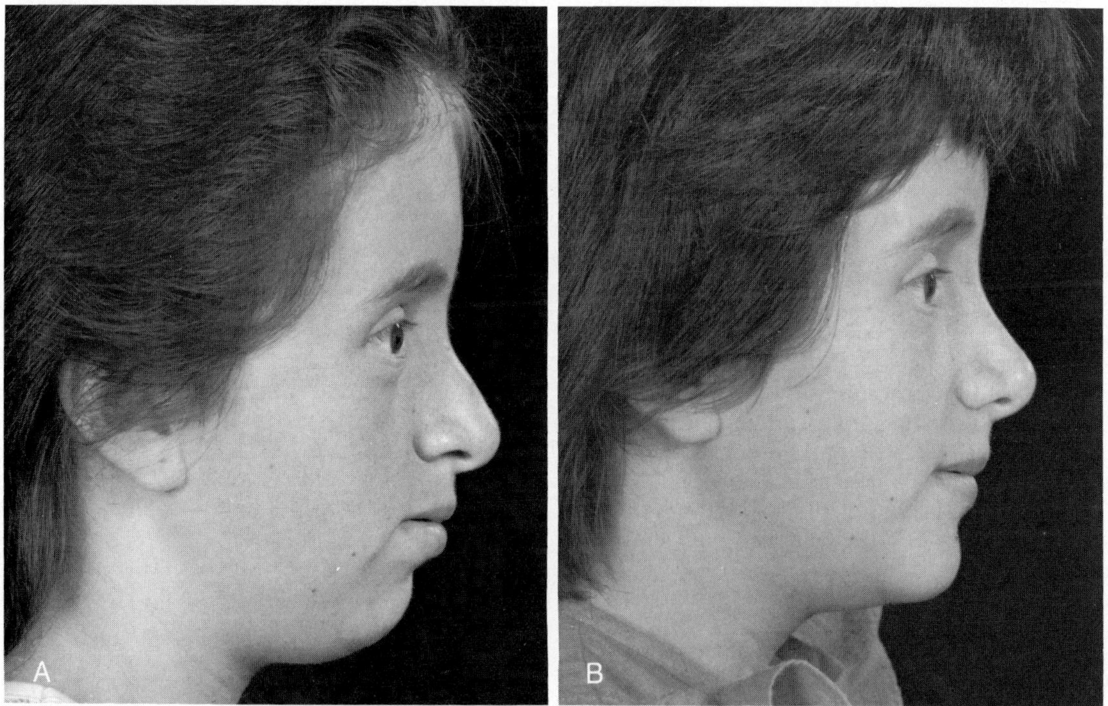

Figure 29–134. Jumping genioplasty (see Fig. 29–133) and nasalplasty. *A,* Preoperative profile. *B,* Postoperative view.

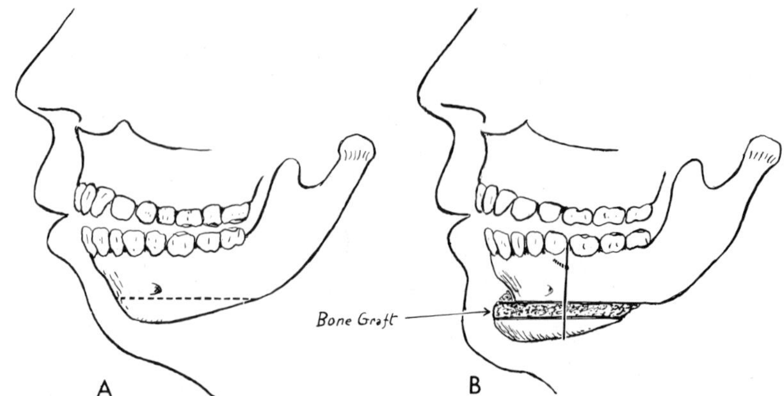

Figure 29–135. The sandwich procedure. The horizontal osteotomy is combined with an interposition bone graft or hydroxyapatite for vertical elongation of the anterior portion of the mandible and for increasing the prominence of the chin. *A,* The line of osteotomy. *B,* The bone graft has been interposed, in a sandwich fashion, between the lower segment and the body of the mandible. Circumferential wiring immobilizes the bone graft and the detached lower segment. Alternative fixation techniques include interosseous wires or lag screws. (From Converse, J. M., and Wood-Smith, D.: Horizontal osteotomy of the mandible. Plast. Reconstr. Surg., *34*:464, 1964. Copyright 1964, The Williams & Wilkins Company, Baltimore.)

mobilized segment and the host bone is obtained by adjusting the contour of the concave surface of the transplant with a power-driven, large, cutting bur.

3. When increased vertical dimension is required, a bone graft or hydroxyapatite is sandwiched between the mandibular body and the segment detached by the horizontal osteotomy (Figs. 29–135, 29–136) (Converse and Wood-Smith, 1964; Rosen, 1988).

4. In patients with an excessive vertical dimension of the symphyseal portion of the mandible, a horizontal wedge of bone is removed between the fragment that is to be advanced and the bone below the apices of the teeth (Figs. 29–128*B*, 29–137, 29–138). The inferior horizontal cut must be first. If in error the upper osteotomy is made first, the second horizontal cut must be made on the detached piece of bone. The vibration principle on which the saws operate will be defaulted and the second cut will be laboriously slow.

5. An oblique osteotomy (Fig. 29–139) permits simultaneous advancement and shortening of the vertical dimension of the symphyseal area (Fig. 29–140).

6. In lateral deviations of the mandible, when malocclusion of the teeth and shortening of the mandible on one side are relatively minor (Fig. 29–141), a horizontal osteotomy permits replacement of the chin in the midsagittal plane (Fig. 29–142) (Converse and Wood-Smith, 1964). In more severe lateral deviation, after mandibular body or ramus lengthening, the midline repositioning of the chin can also be used as a final-stage procedure.

7. The double-step osteotomy (Neuner, 1965) consists of a two-tier osteotomy, two osteotomies made one above the other (Fig. 29–143). The upper segment is advanced first and the fixation established; the lower segment is then advanced and secured to the upper segment. This is an excellent technique to use when the deformity requires considerable advancement (Fig. 29–144).

Fixation After Horizontal Advancement Osteotomy. Fixation of the advanced fragment to the mandible is efficiently maintained by interosseous wiring or miniplates and screws. Remodeling of the advanced symphyseal segment does occur. Therefore, if a miniplate is used, care must be exercised in its placement, otherwise the patient may complain of an irritating palpable mass.

Securing the mobilized fragment with No. 26 stainless steel wire works well, is universally available, and is less costly than the use of miniplates (Fig. 29–145). Generally, three interosseous wires are more than sufficient, one placed in the midline and the others in the cuspid region. The twisted ends of the stainless steel wire become incorporated into the bone and may remain permanently without causing local reaction, either in the soft tissue or in the bone. As with all well-tolerated, permanently buried, inert materials, the procedure is successful unless hematoma and local infection, fortunately rare complications, are superimposed. Nonunion is almost unheard of.

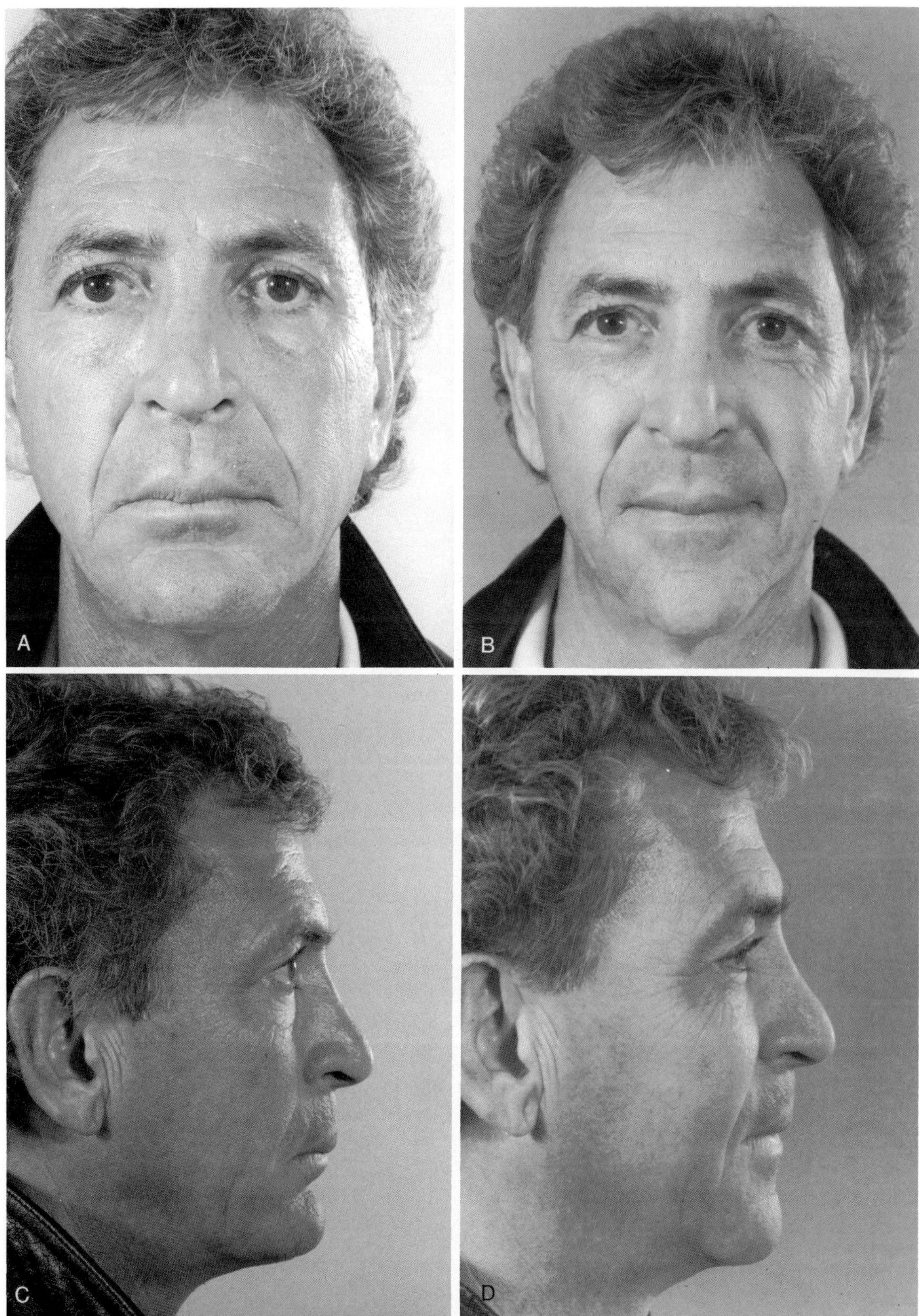

Figure 29–136. Sandwich genioplasty. *A, C,* Preoperative appearance after a previous unsuccessful chin implant. Note the deficiency of the chin in the sagittal and vertical dimensions. *B, D,* Appearance after genioplasty (see Fig. 29–135).

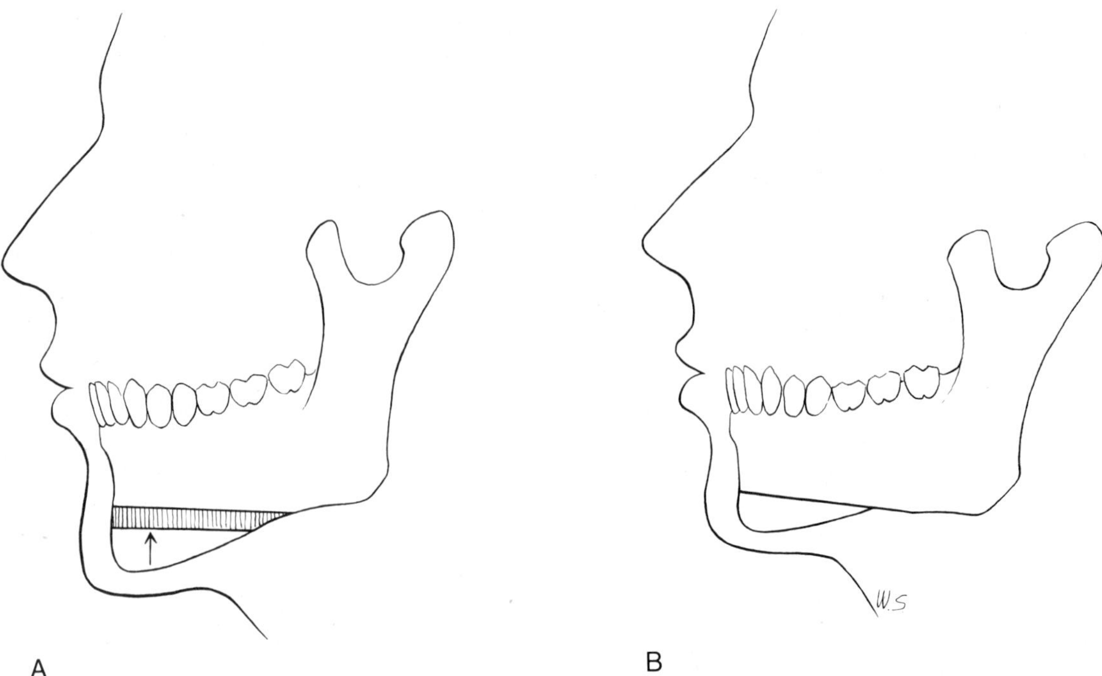

Figure 29–137. Vertical shortening of the chin by removal of a wedge of bone. *A,* Area of bone resection. *B,* The lower segment is wired into the desired position.

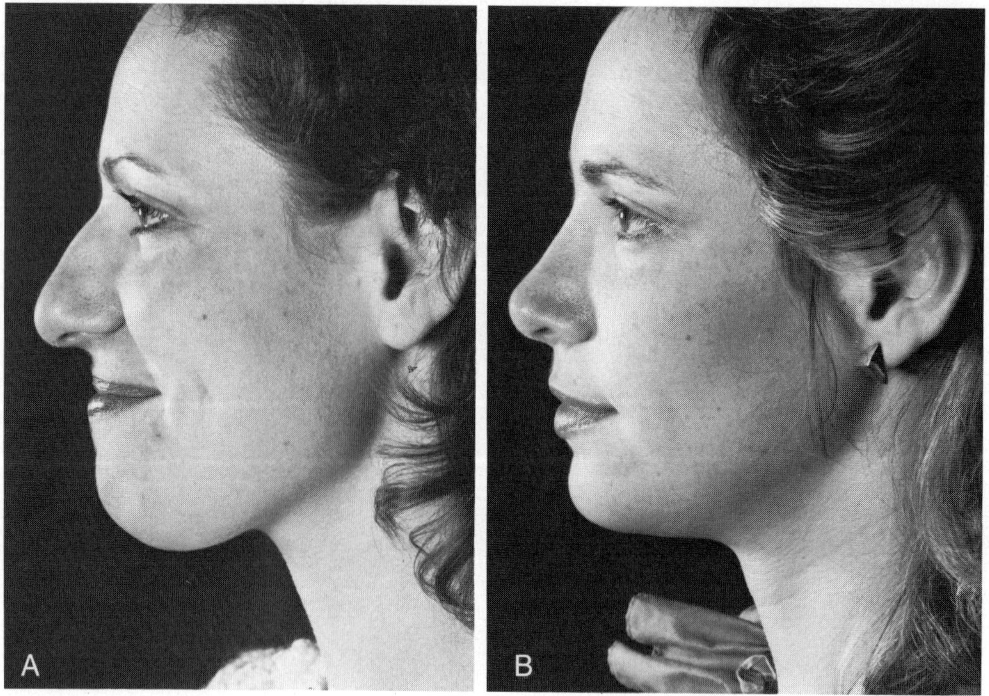

Figure 29–138. Vertical reduction of the chin (see Fig. 29–137). *A,* Preoperative view. *B,* Postoperative view. Note the improved contour. A nasalplasty was also performed.

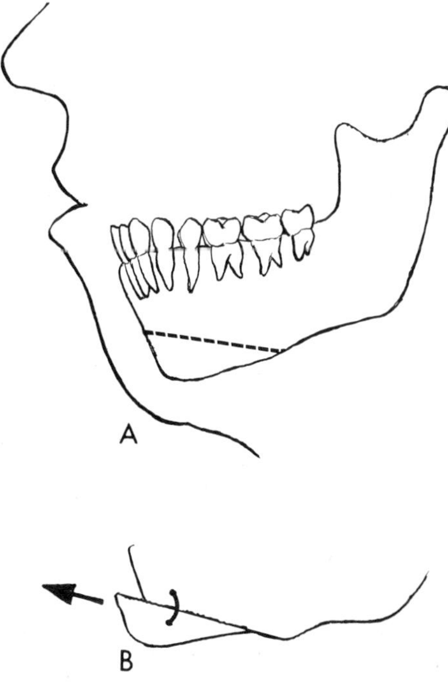

Figure 29–139. Oblique osteotomy for advancement and moderate shortening of the vertical dimension of the mandible. *A,* Design of the oblique osteotomy. *B,* The fragment is moved upward and forward and held in fixation by interosseous wiring (or rigid skeletal fixation). (From Converse, J. M., and Wood-Smith, D.: Horizontal osteotomy of the mandible. Plast. Reconstr. Surg., *34*:464, 1964. Copyright 1964, The Williams & Wilkins Company, Baltimore.)

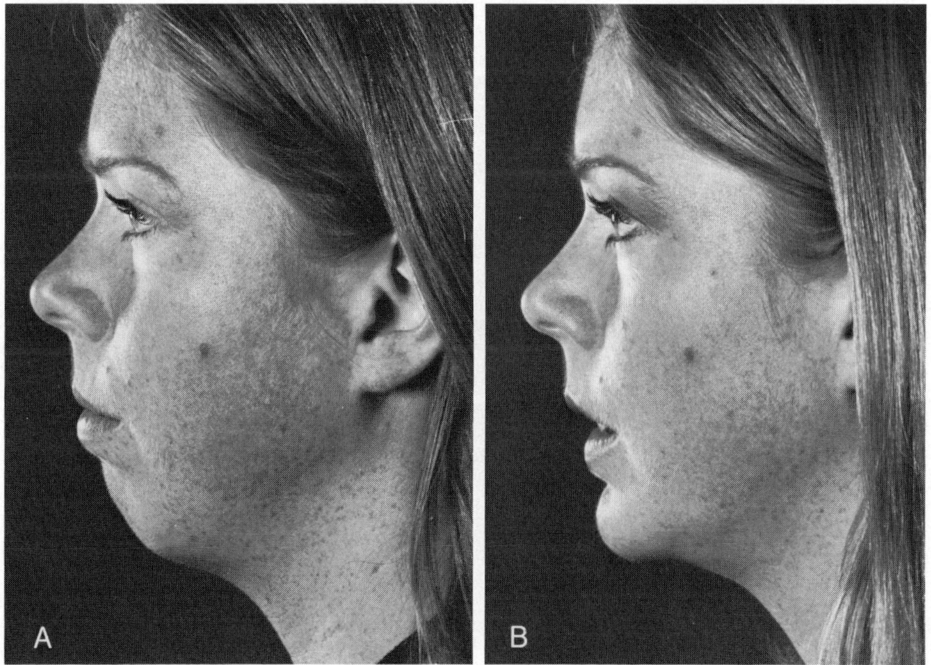

Figure 29–140. Microgenia corrected by an oblique osteotomy (see Fig. 29–139). *A,* Preoperative view. *B,* Postoperative profile.

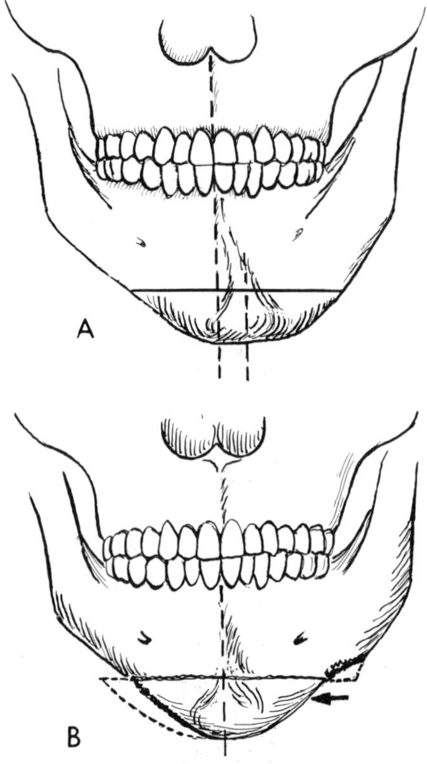

Figure 29–141. Correction of lateral deviation of the chin by horizontal osteotomy. *A,* Vertical (midsagittal) dotted line shows the amount of deviation of the chin to the left. *B,* After the horizontal osteotomy. The lower mandibular segment is displaced toward the right. The broken line outlines the protruding bone that is resected to obtain a smooth contour. (From Converse, J. M., and Wood-Smith, D.: Horizontal osteotomy of the mandible. Plast. Reconstr. Surg., *34*:464, 1974. Copyright 1964, The Williams & Wilkins Company, Baltimore.)

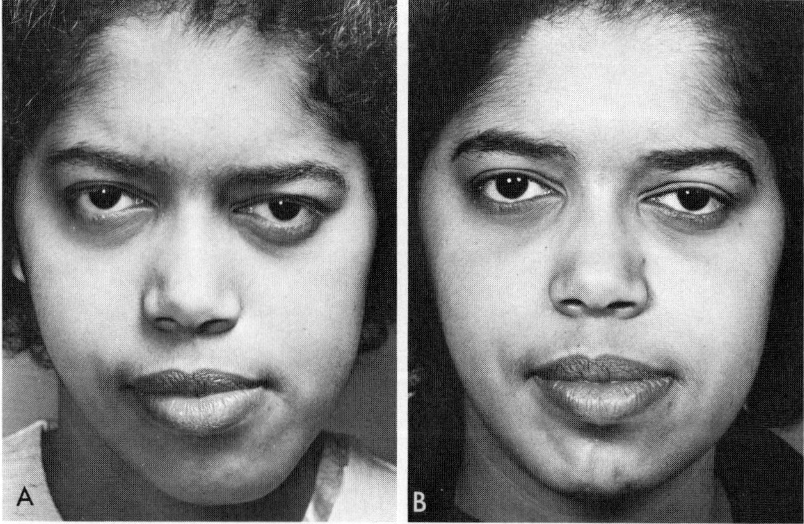

Figure 29–142. A patient with lateral deviation and retrusion of the chin corrected by the procedure shown in Figure 29–141. *A,* Preoperative full-face view showing the lateral deviation of the chin to the left. *B,* Facial symmetry restored by the horizontal osteotomy and displacement of the lower mandibular segment forward and to the right. (From Converse, J. M., and Wood-Smith, D.: Horizontal osteotomy of the mandible. Plast. Reconstr. Surg., *34*:464, 1964. Copyright 1964, The Williams & Wilkins Company, Baltimore.)

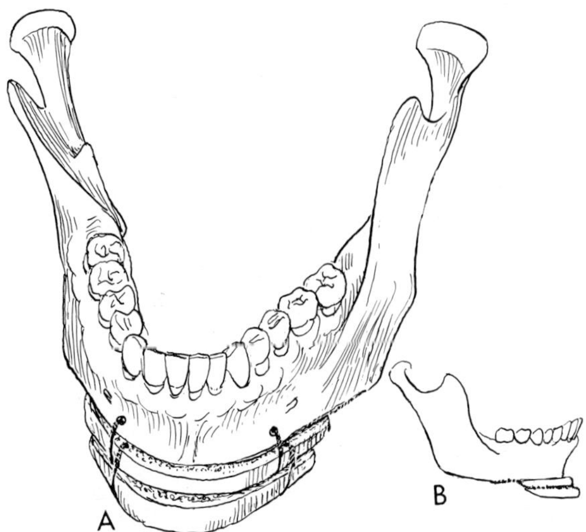

Figure 29–143. Double-step osteotomy. *A*, Advancement of the lower segment anterior to the upper segment by a two-tier osteotomy. Interosseous wire fixation is used to maintain the position of the fragments. *B*, Lateral view of the double-step osteotomy. Cancellous bone chips can be added to promote consolidation and to improve the contour. (After Neuner.)

When the symphyseal fragment is transposed forward and upward to rest on the mandible (jumping genioplasty), a rotational displacement force is imposed (Fig. 29–146). With a jumping genioplasty, bone contact is vertically oriented and cortical in nature, a combination that poorly resists the tipping action generated by the strong downward and backward pull of the suprahyoid musculature that remains attached to the symphyseal fragment. With a sliding genioplasty the situation is more favorable, since the apposition along the cut surfaces effectively counteracts the rotating forces, bone contact is more cancellous in amount, and the interosseous wires effectively prevent posterior slippage. Thus, with a jumping genioplasty, reinforcement with a miniplate (Fig. 29–147) or lag screws (Fig. 29–148, see Fig. 29–130) is recommended.

The sharp edge of the advancement segment needs no special attention since it will remodel during the period of osseous healing and remodeling.

Bone Grafting in Conjunction with Horizontal Advancement Osteotomy of Lower Portion of Mandible. When the symphyseal fragment is advanced to a point where contact is lost between the posterior surface of the segment and the body of the mandible (Fig. 29–149) or where bone contact is tenuous as in a tier (step) genioplasty, it is advisable to fill the intervening space with cancellous bone from the ilium, calvarial bone chips, or hydroxyapatite particles.

The careful application of a pressure dressing is an important final step. Elimination of unwanted space diminishes the risk of hematoma formation and the development of an infection. Antibiotic therapy is routine.

Results. The techniques of sliding genioplasty and jumping genioplasty have proved to be reliable and successful. The procedure not only increases the projection of the mental symphysis in the sagittal dimension but also can alter the vertical dimension of the chin. Furthermore, changes in the width (transverse dimension) of the chin are possible.

A cephalometric survey of cases of osseous genioplasty performed over a period of 30 years showed a high proportion of success with the procedure. During the first year, the edges of the advanced or transposed bone become rounded, with minimal change in the degree of projection of the pedicled bone. A small loss of volume of the mobilized fragment occurs; this is not clinically significant, since the facial contour is maintained with relatively little change. A final soft tissue projection can be confidently predicted to be approximately 80 per cent of the osseous change (Bell and Dann, 1973).

In the patient shown in Figure 29–150, the cephalometric roentgenograms taken before the operation, shortly afterward, and seven years later (Figs. 29–151, 29–152) show the remodeling process that has taken place. Loss of the projection of the advanced segment has not occurred.

The horizontal advancement osteotomy offers a distinct advantage over onlay bone grafts, since there is little resorption of the advanced bone. In mandibular micrognathia (as opposed to microgenia), it offers a particular advantage over inorganic implants, which are best suited for less severe deformities without vertical discrepancies. Moreover, the horizontal advancement osteotomy increases the horizontal dimension (width) of the chin more than an inorganic implant does (McCarthy and Ruff, 1988).

Contour Restoration by Cartilage or Bone Grafts. Although a *distinct third* choice after the previously described methods, two types of tissue are suitable for contour restoration of the symphysis: cartilage and bone. Allografts and xenografts of cartilage have

Text continued on page 1329

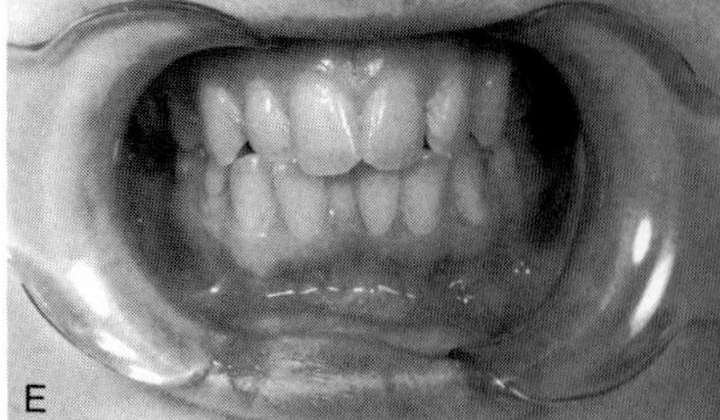

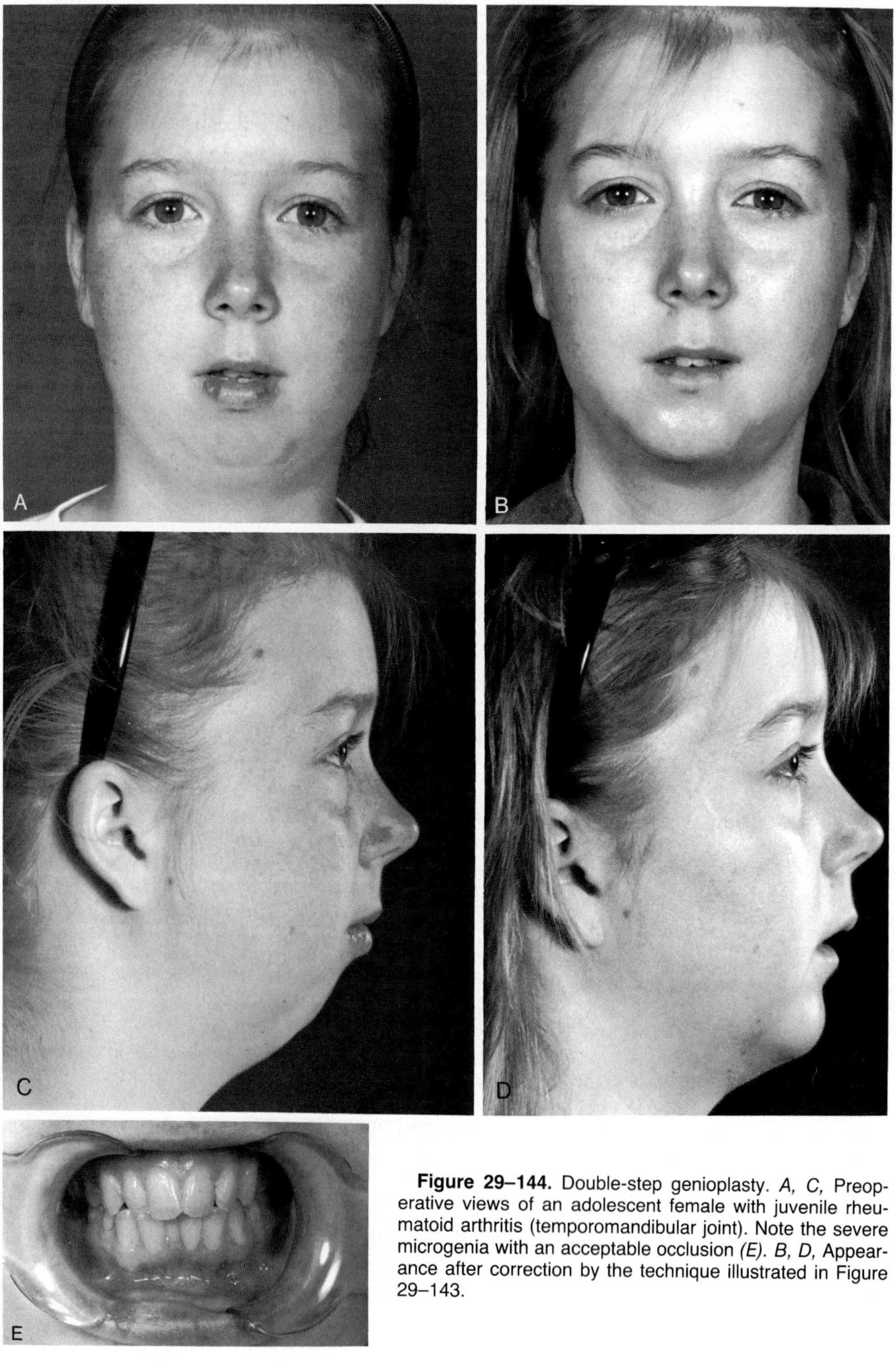

Figure 29–144. Double-step genioplasty. *A, C,* Preoperative views of an adolescent female with juvenile rheumatoid arthritis (temporomandibular joint). Note the severe microgenia with an acceptable occlusion *(E)*. *B, D,* Appearance after correction by the technique illustrated in Figure 29–143.

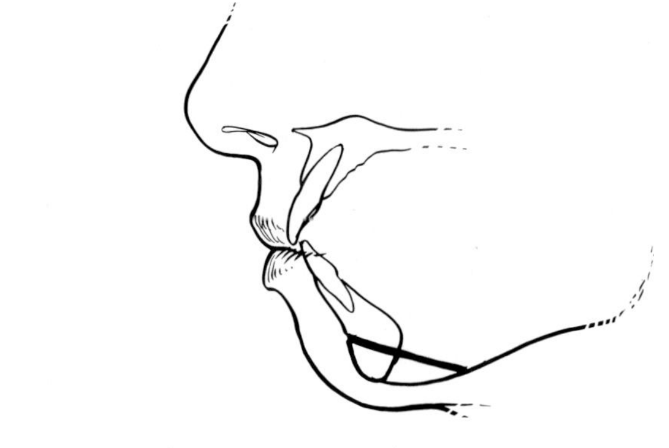

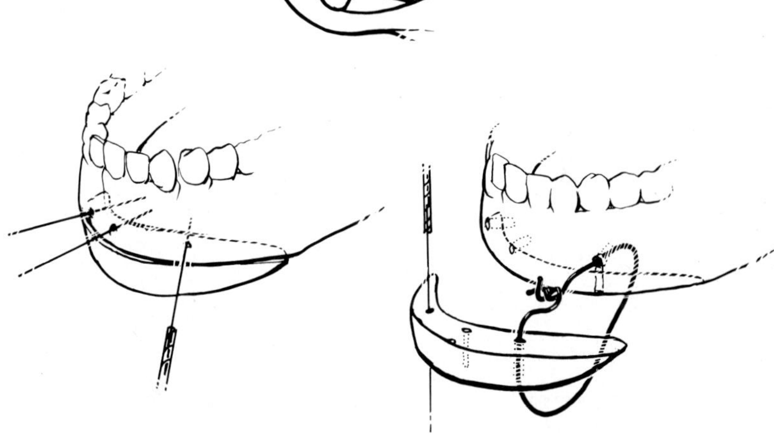

Figure 29–145. Interosseous wire (No. 26 stainless steel) fixation after a horizontal (oblique) advancement osteotomy. The holes are angulated at 45 degrees.

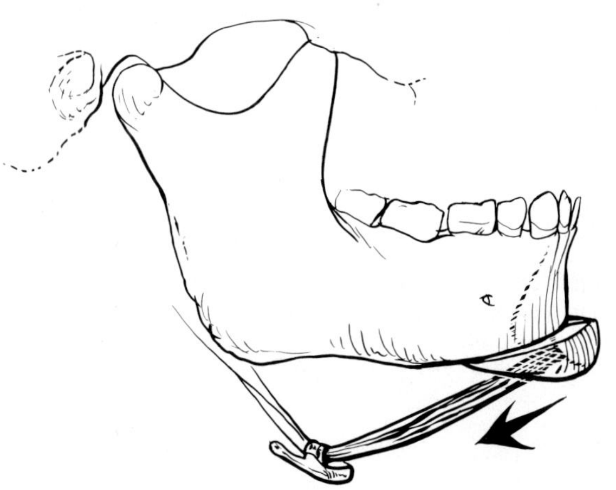

Figure 29–146. Rotational muscular displacement force (*arrow*) after a jumping genioplasty.

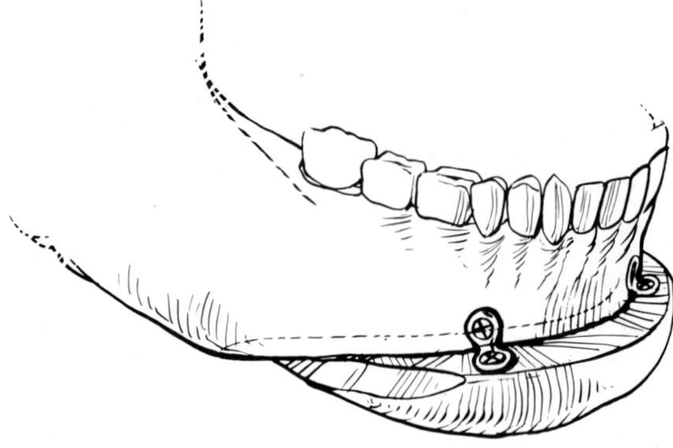

Figure 29–147. Miniplate fixation after a horizontal advancement osteotomy. The end of the advanced fragment has been contoured.

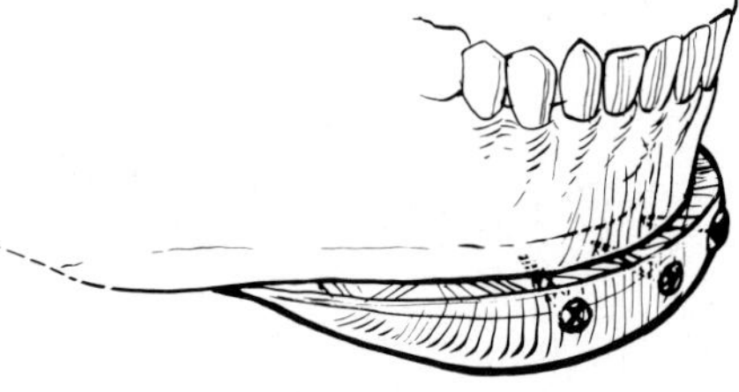

Figure 29–148. Lag screw fixation after a horizontal advancement osteotomy.

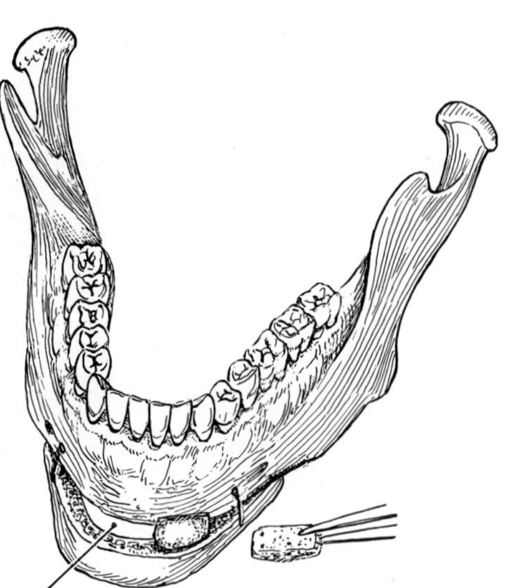

Figure 29–149. When contact is lost between the advanced segment and the body of the mandible, bone grafts are used to fill the void. The technique illustrated is recommended when such a degree of advancement is required.

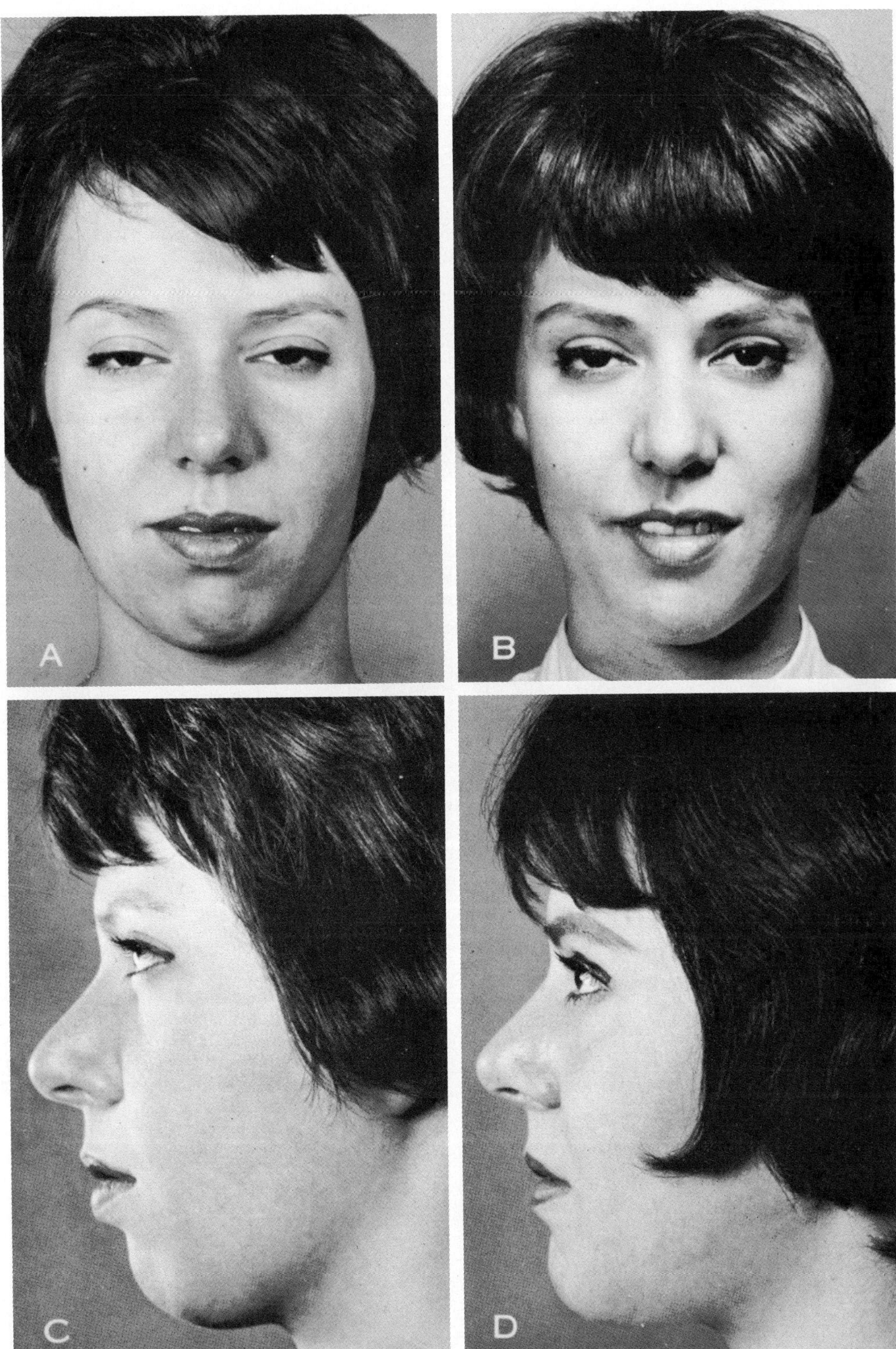

Figure 29–150. Correction of microgenia using a horizontal osteotomy. *A, C,* Preoperative views. *B, D,* After horizontal osteotomy and advancement of the lower mandibular segment. (From Converse, J. M., and Wood-Smith, D.: Horizontal osteotomy of the mandible. Plast. Reconstr. Surg., *34*:464, 1964. Copyright 1964, The Williams & Wilkins Company, Baltimore.)

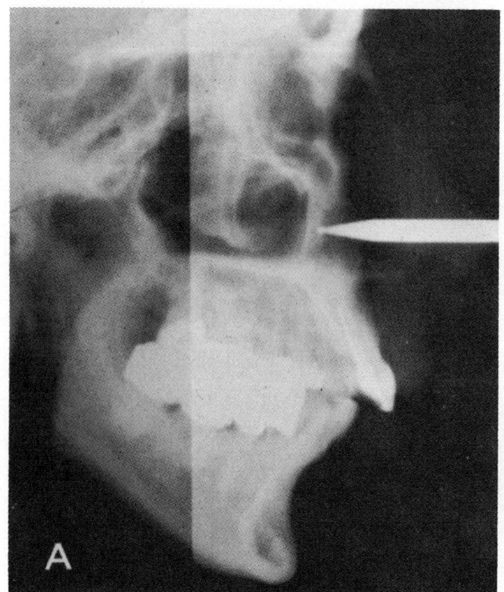

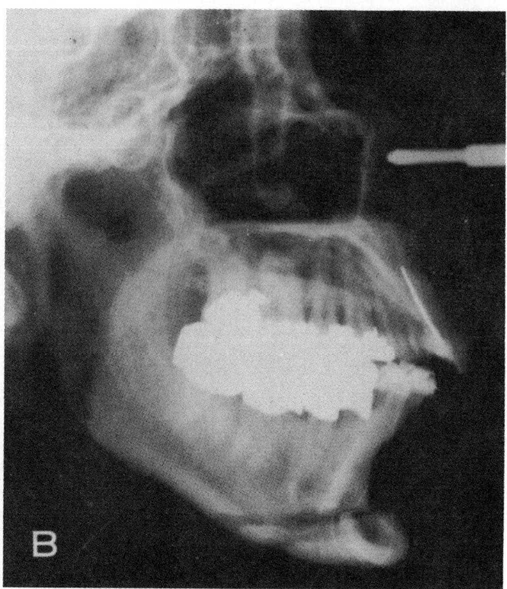

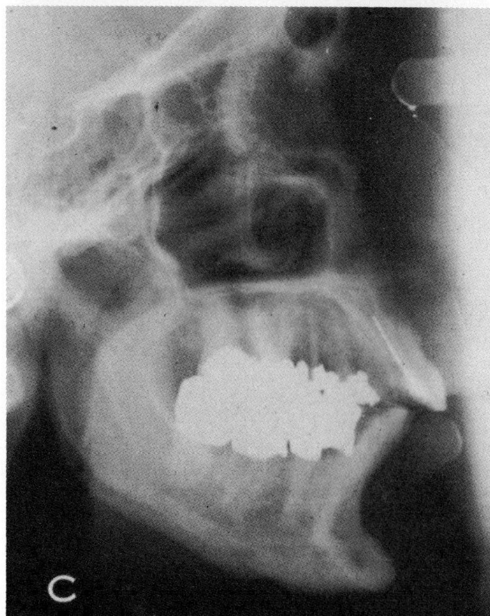

Figure 29–151. Cephalometric longitudinal study of the patient shown in Figure 29–150. *A,* Before surgery. *B,* During the postoperative period. *C,* Seven years after surgery. Note the rounding of the upper edge of the advanced bone as described in the text. (From Converse, J. M., and Wood-Smith, D.: Horizontal osteotomy of the mandible. Plast. Reconstr. Surg., *34*:464, 1964. Copyright 1964, The Williams & Wilkins Company, Baltimore.)

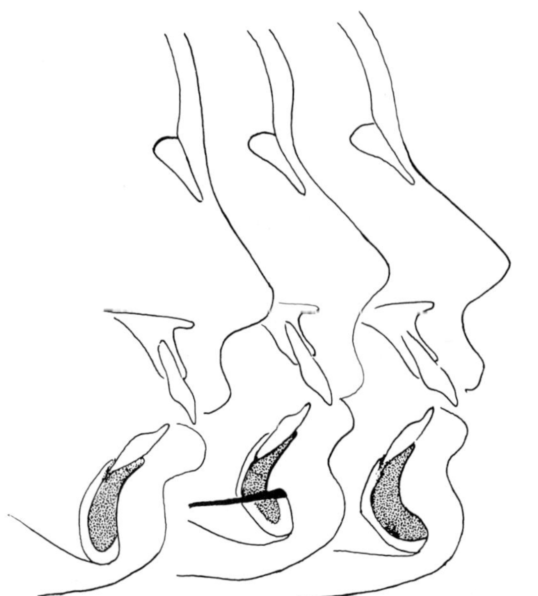

Figure 29–152. Tracings of the cephalometric longitudinal study of the patient shown in Figure 29–150.

been used but have their limitations, namely, progressive resorption (see Chap. 17). Autogenous cartilage grafts survive and maintain their contour but do not consolidate with the underlying bone. Although cartilaginous allografts have a tendency toward progressive resorption in patients with microgenia, the contour of the chin is preserved for a long time (Converse, 1964b).

Iliac bone grafts are generally preferred because they provide a greater proportion of cancellous bone than costal bone grafts. Calvarial bone undergoes less resorption but it is brittle, a property that makes it difficult to contour.

Technique. The amount of subperiosteal elevation is determined by the size of the graft. After intraoral exposure has been obtained (Fig. 29–153*A*,*B*), the bone graft is contoured and placed over the mental symphysis (Fig. 29–153*C*). When lengthening of the lower face is indicated, the graft is inserted under the mental symphysis (Fig. 29–153*D*). The bone graft is removed from the medial aspect and/or the iliac crest and shaped as shown in Figure 29–153*E*. A pressure dressing similar to that shown in Figure 29–124 is applied (Fig. 29–154).

If the surface of the mental symphysis is irregular and the mental tubercles are prominent, the recipient site is recontoured with a bur. Some of the cortex of the symphysis can be removed to achieve an intimate contact between the graft and host. The take of the bone graft is quicker when the cancellous surface is positioned against the host bone; this is especially so if an osteoperiosteal graft is employed. Contour adaptation is obtained by bending the graft and making a concavity in the cancellous surface.

Results. Onlay bone grafts are not uniformly successful, particularly when minor contour restoration is required. Progressive resorption has been observed in some of the grafts, and appears to be caused by the absence of functional stress. The best results from onlay bone grafts are obtained in the more severe types of micrognathic deformities; serial onlay bone grafts, placed one over the other, have yielded excellent permanent restoration of contour in these cases.

Contour Restoration by Skin Graft Inlay and Dental Prosthesis. The skin graft inlay technique, which is used for restoration of the buccal sulcus after reconstruction of the mandible, is discussed later in this chapter. It is rarely used in microgenia correction and is mainly of historical interest. It has been applied to achieve contour restoration in mandibular micrognathia when the mandible is edentulous. The labial flange of the denture is extended downward and has an anteriorly directed curvature in order to maintain the labiomental fold and adequate projection of the chin.

The technique (see Chap. 72) is not an entirely satisfactory method of restoring contour. It has its limitations, but is a justifiable compromise in older patients.

A skin graft inlay procedure was performed on the patient with mandibular micrognathia shown in Figure 29–155. Osteomyelitis had occurred after a fracture of the mandible resulting from the removal of a tooth early in childhood. The mandible had failed to develop beyond the childhood stage. The condyles were hypoplastic, and the mandible articulated with the base of the skull by way of the coronoid processes (Fig. 29–156*A*). Because of the posterior position of the micrognathic mandible, a base for a lower denture capable of articulating with the teeth of the maxilla could not be made. Insufficient bone was available to permit an elongation osteotomy. It was decided that bone should be added to the anterior mandible to provide bone support for a denture (Fig. 29–156*B*).

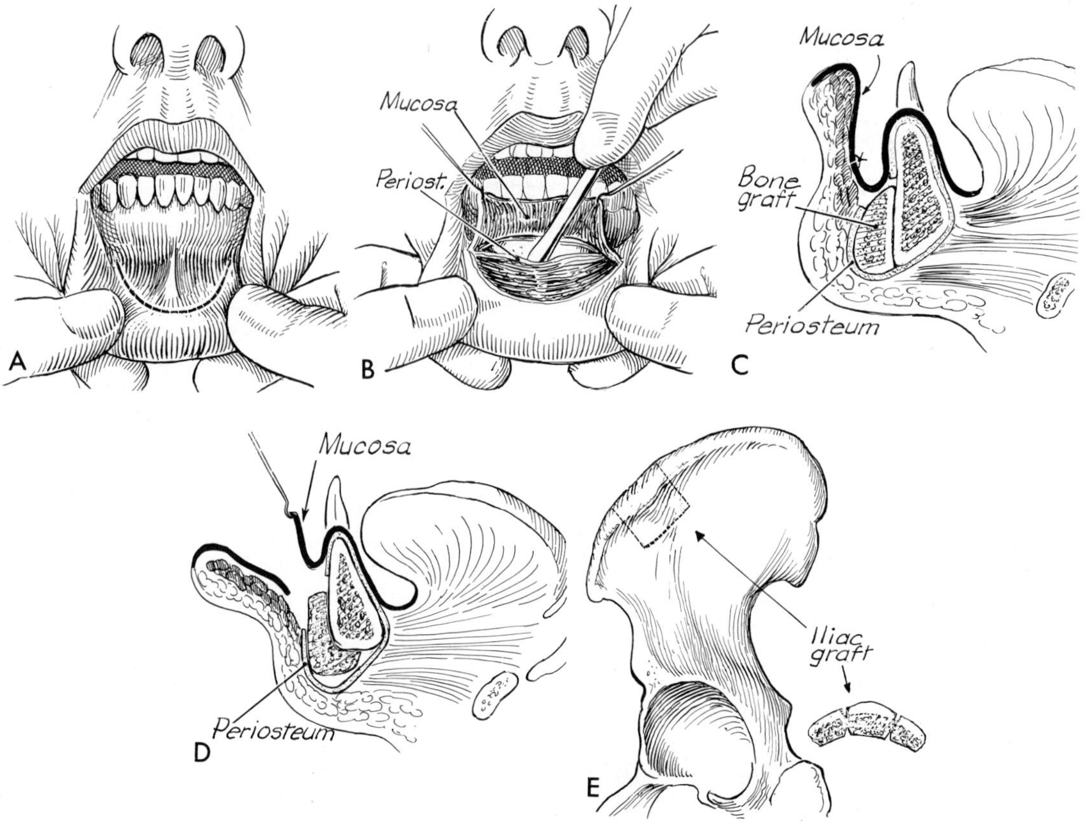

Figure 29–153. Iliac bone grafting through an intraoral approach for the correction of microgenia. *A,* Incision through the mucosa is made above the insertion of the frenulum. *B,* The periosteum is incised and raised after the mucosal flap is elevated. *C,* The bone graft is in position. *D,* When vertical increase as well as increased projection is indicated, the graft is hooked under the symphysis. *E,* Site of removal of the iliac bone graft from the medial aspect of the crest and inner aspect of the ilium.

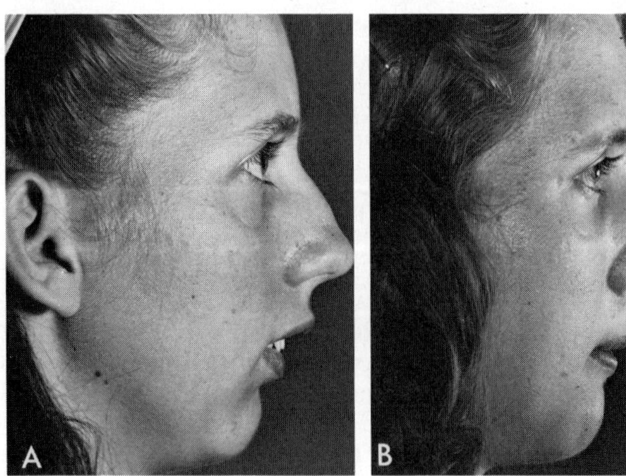

Figure 29–154. *A,* Microgenia with downward and backward slant of the lower lip. *B,* Improvement obtained by intraoral bone grafting over the mental symphysis and a corrective nasalplasty. (From Converse, J. M., and Campbell, R. M.: Bone grafts in surgery of the face. Surg. Clin. North Am., *34*:375, 1954.)

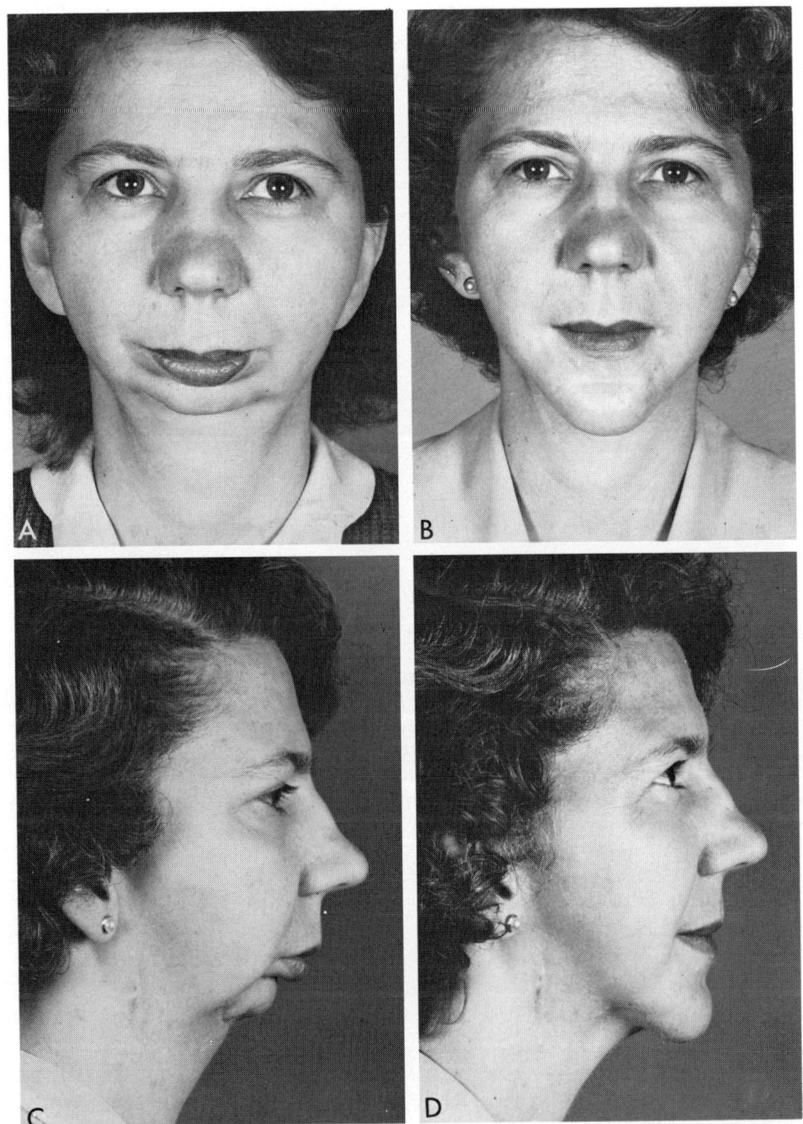

Figure 29–155. Contour restoration by bone grafting and prosthodontics in mandibular micrognathia. *A*, Preoperative chinless appearance. *B*, Restoration of contour obtained by bone grafting and a dental prosthesis. The labial sulcus was restored by the skin graft inlay technique to accommodate the overextended denture flange, which helped to restore the chin contour. *C*, Preoperative birdlike facial profile. *D*, Postoperative profile view. (From Converse, J. M., and Shapiro, H. H.: Treatment of developmental malformation of the jaws. Plast. Reconstr. Surg., *10*:473, 1952. Copyright 1952, The Williams & Wilkins Company, Baltimore.)

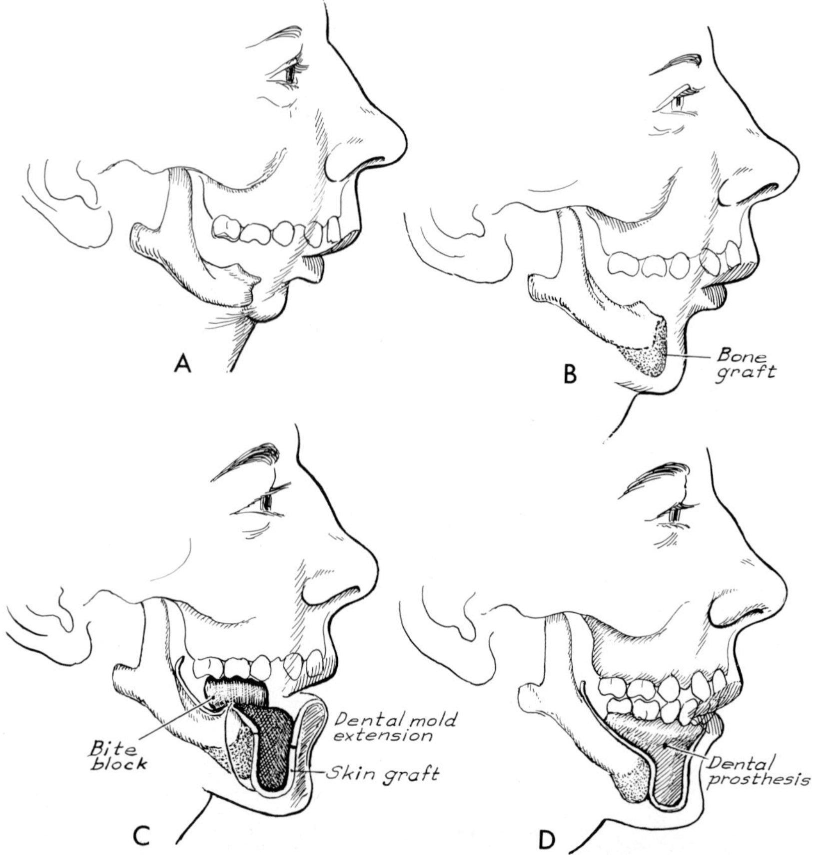

Figure 29–156. Correction of the mandibular micrognathia of the patient shown in Figure 29–155 by a combination of bone grafting, a skin graft inlay, and a dental prosthesis. *A,* Mandibular micrognathia with absence of the condyle. Note that the coronoid process of the mandible articulated with the infratemporal surface. *B,* An onlay bone graft was added to the anterior portion of the mandible in a preliminary operation. *C,* After healing of the bone graft, a skin graft inlay was done. The inlay is maintained by the downward extension of the biteblock into the newly formed sulcus. Circumferential wiring holds the prosthesis in position. *D,* Final denture with an enlarged labial flange that extends into the skin grafted labial sulcus to restore the contour of the lower portion of the face.

The inferior labial sulcus, anterior to the bone graft, was deepened with a skin graft inlay (Fig. 29–156*C*).

After the skin graft had healed, the compound mold was replaced by a denture constructed with an extended labial flange that filled the deepened sulcus. Denture retention was improved by the exaggerated sulcus, and the lower facial contour was also restored (Fig. 29–156*D*).

MACROGENIA

Macrogenia is the term used to describe the overdevelopment of the chin in all dimensions. This portion develops independently from the rest of the lower jaw and is strongly influenced by hereditary factors. A large chin is esthetically and socially acceptable in males, but a similar mental protuberance in females produces an unpleasing prognathic, aggressive appearance.

Macrogenia frequently occurs in conjunction with mandibular prognathism, but it is also seen as an independent malformation. The chief complaint of the patient usually centers on the lower facial imbalance and the prognathic appearance.

Surgical correction of macrogenia in the absence of true prognathism poses a difficult problem. Although the excess bone can technically be removed, the redraping and adaptation of the soft tissue to the reduced framework often are unsatisfactory (Kawamoto, 1982b). The chin pad takes on a flattened, uninteresting, and unnatural contour. Robbed of its concave platform, the muscles of the chin and the chin pad itself descend to produce a ptotic, unflattering appearance when the person smiles (Fig. 29–157). Furthermore, the relatively redundant soft tissue is also crowded posteriorly to create undesirable submental fullness and the suggestion of a double chin.

Cephalometric tracings can be used to determine the amount of excess mental projection. Unfortunately, the reduction (sagittal dimension) in the prominence of the soft tissue chin pad is disappointingly far less than that produced in the bone. The reduction in the vertical dimension is more predictable.

Three procedures are available to correct macrogenia. All have somber limitations.

Removal of Excess Bone. Removal of the bone from the symphyseal area by contour reduction of the cortical surface usually does not result in appreciable improvement in the soft tissue contour of the chin. The excess soft tissue more often than not drapes poorly over the newly contoured bone to produce undesirable side effects.

The thickness of the bone to be removed is always more than one would think. A one to one relationship between hard tissue reduction and the soft tissue change does not occur. The redundant bone can be removed with a saw, but it is safer to use a bur. A series of vertical grooves is cut with a bur to the depth of the desired amount of bone to be removed. The grooves are then filled with surgical ink. A large, pear-shaped cutting bur removes the excess bone until the depth of the grooves is reached as indicated by the presence of the ink stain. Care must be taken to avoid eliminating the labiomental fold by excess bone removal.

Horizontal Recession Osteotomy. A horizontal section and posterior displacement of the symphyseal fragment can also be employed. The basic technique is the same as that described for the treatment of microgenia (see Fig. 29–128*A*). It is best to leave as much as possible of the soft tissue attachments to the anterior surface of the recessed fragment (Fig. 29–158).

The horizontal osteotomy produces the most favorable results in patients whose macrogenia is mainly vertical in dimension. A wedge resection of the symphysis helps to restore better, if not perfect, facial harmony (see Figs. 29–137, 29–138).

Careful attention must be paid so that the soft tissue is repositioned by a carefully applied compressive dressing to minimize the danger of producing a postoperative flattened and double chin appearance.

Osteotomies Similar to Those Used to Correct Mandibular Prognathism. These procedures are rarely indicated for the treatment of macrogenia. Improved facial balance can be achieved but at the expense of incurring a dental malocclusion.

Maxillary and Mandibular Dentoalveolar Deformities

MAXILLARY DENTOALVEOLAR PROTRUSION

Maxillary dentoalveolar protrusion must be distinguished from *skeletal maxillary protrusion*. In the former there is labial inclination of the maxillary anterior teeth, and the facial convexity on profile examination is limited to the upper lip region (Fig. 29–159*A, B*). In the latter there is a convexity of the inferior orbital rims, anterior maxilla, and nose, in addition to that observed in the upper lip region (Fig. 29–159*C, D*).

In maxillary dentoalveolar protrusion, cephalometric anaylsis of several skeletal points and measurements confirms the clinical impression. Such measurements as PNS-ANS, Ba-ANS, PNS-UIE, and SNA are increased (see Fig. 29–7). As mentioned earlier in the chapter, no single cephalometric measurement is ever diagnostic.

Orthodontic therapy can often correct the inclined maxillary incisor teeth and result in competent lip posture and improved dentofacial balance. Orthodontic therapy is most commonly practiced during childhood or adolescence, and it has erroneously come to be regarded as a treatment available exclusively to the young. Age is not a limiting factor; treatment can be rendered at any time provided that the teeth and their supporting structures are in satisfactory physical condition.

Facial balance can be restored by surgical-orthodontic procedures when improvement in facial harmony cannot be achieved through orthodontic therapy alone, or when an adult patient is unwilling to accept the required appliance therapy. Such procedures consist of osteotomies that modify the occlusion of the teeth and the contour of the face. Two types of osteotomies are employed: the *segmental osteotomy*, in which a segment of the dental arch only is displaced, and a *complete hori-*

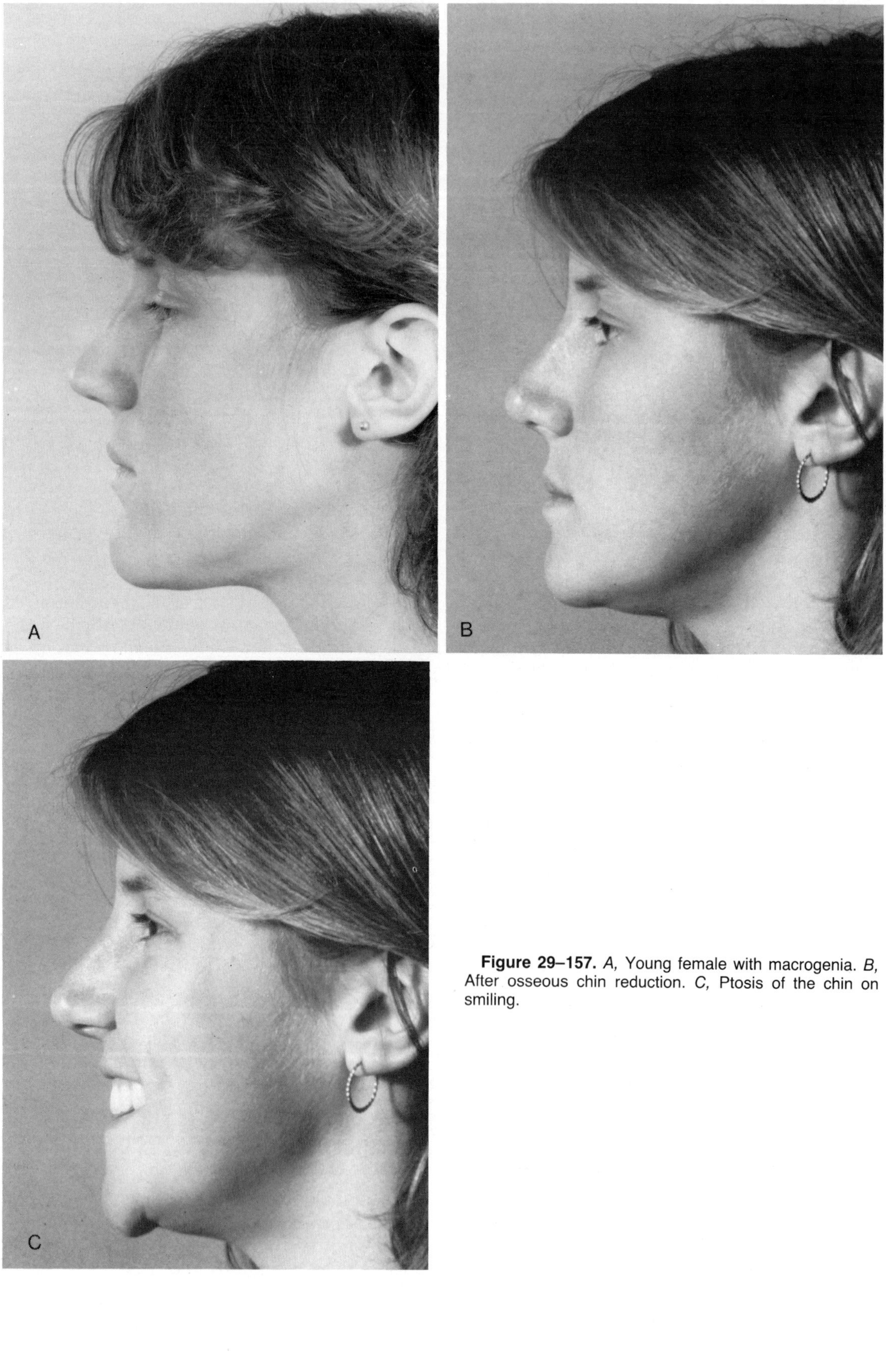

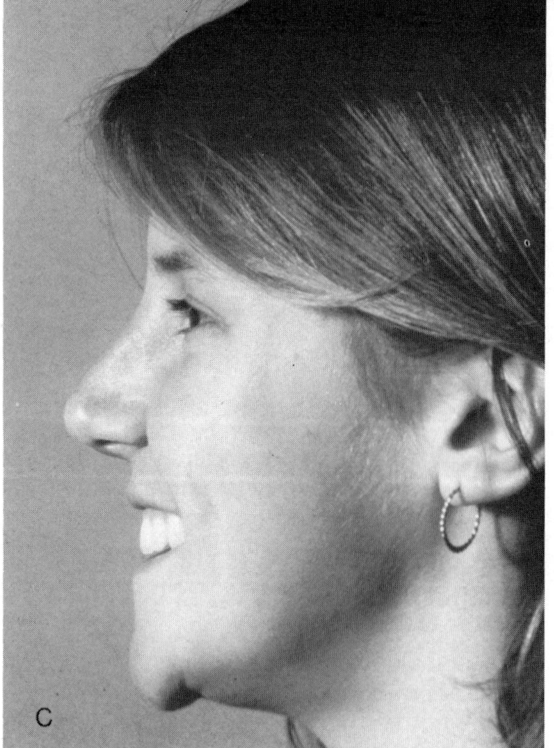

Figure 29–157. *A,* Young female with macrogenia. *B,* After osseous chin reduction. *C,* Ptosis of the chin on smiling.

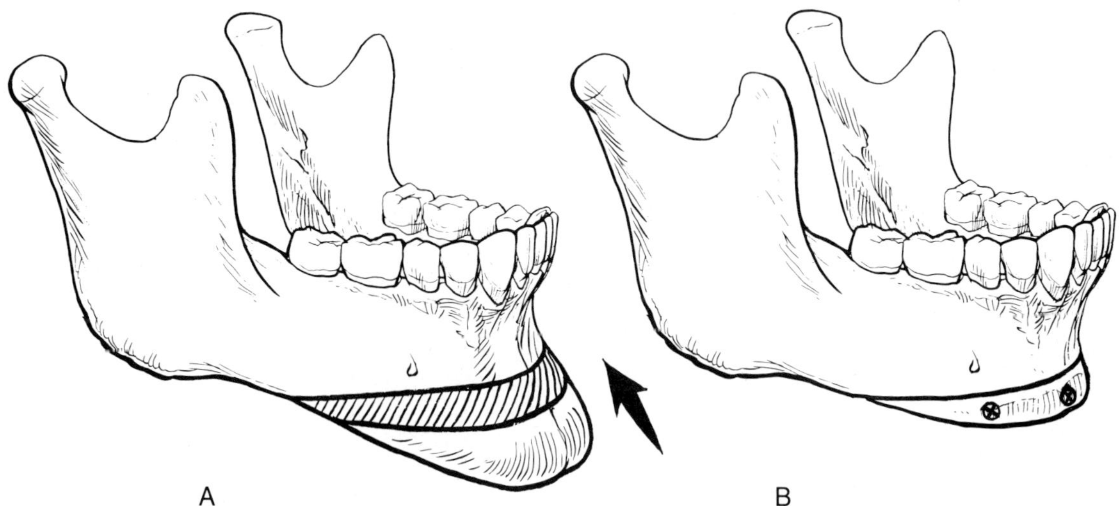

Figure 29–158. Horizontal resection and posterior displacement of the symphyseal fragment for the correction of macrogenia. The soft tissues of the pogonion are not disturbed. *A,* Area of resection and direction of recession of the symphyseal fragment. *B,* Lag screw fixation.

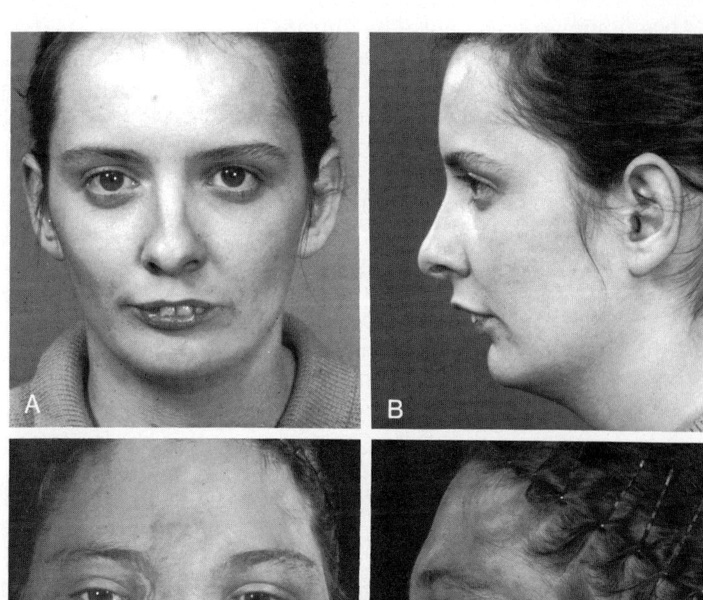

Figure 29–159. *A, B,* Maxillary dentoalveolar protrusion. *C, D,* Maxillary skeletal protrusion with an extensive arteriovenous malformation of the face.

zontal osteotomy, in which the entire dental arch is displaced (see Le Fort I osteotomy, p. 1369).

Segmental Osteotomies

Premolar Recession (Set-back) Osteotomy. Wilhelm (1954), who described the surgical technique, favored a two-stage procedure to correct maxillary protrusion. In the first stage the mucoperiosteum of the palate was raised, the second premolar teeth were extracted, and an osteotomy was performed through the palate and the alveolar arch. Three to four weeks later, the second stage completed the correction. Wilhelm considered the one-stage procedure dangerous. Wunderer (1962), however, disagreed and advocated a one-stage procedure (Fig. 29–160). He designed an anterior mucoperiosteal flap to maintain the blood supply. The operation is performed without risk provided that either a labial or a palatal mucoperiosteal flap remains attached to the repositioned segment, as previously mentioned. The abundant blood supply of the area explains the success of the single-stage operation.

Extraction of a premolar tooth on each side of the arch is usually required. The palatal mucoperiosteum is reflected subperiosteally from the anterior portion of the hard palate. The incision should be made posterior to the incisive papilla to avoid injury to the vascular supply originating from the incisive canal. Direct exposure for the palatal osteotomy site is thus obtained. The required amount of bone is resected from the alveolar process (Fig. 29–161*A*) and the hard palate (Fig. 29–161*B*).

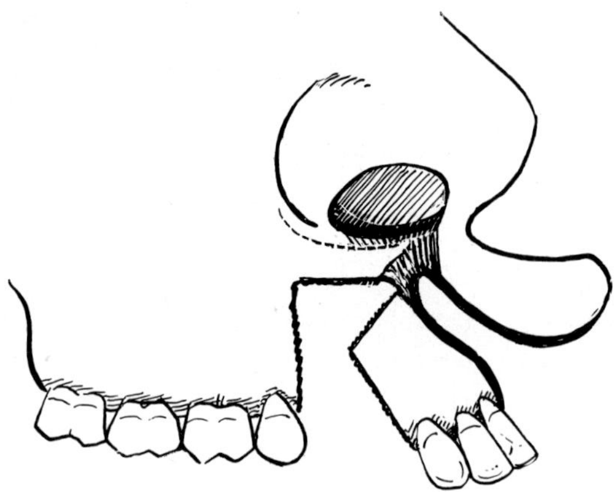

Figure 29–160. The labial mucoperiosteal flap. The blood supply to the mobilized maxillary segment is preserved by the anterior mucoperiosteal flap. (After Wunderer, 1962.)

The vertical buccal mucoperiosteal incisions in the premolar area should be placed posterior to the buccal osteotomy site. Designed in this manner, the incisions will not lie directly over the area where bone consolidation must take place. After the osteotomies are completed, the segment is outfractured (Fig. 29–161*C*) and recessed (Fig. 29–161*D*).

A more conservative technique is to raise a subperiosteal tunnel over the area of the proposed osteotomy for the resection of palatal bone and vomer. A short midline palatal mucosal incision aids in the exposure without jeopardizing the blood supply (Fig. 29–162). It is possible to incise the palatal mucoperiosteum at the site of the osteotomy without endangering the blood supply. The procedures illustrated in Figures 29–161 and 29–162 are obviously preferable.

Precaution should be taken to place the osteotomy in the recessed segment above the apices of the teeth so as to leave sufficient bone above the apices to ensure the blood supply to the teeth. Radiologic verification of the position of the teeth is helpful.

The palatal and alveolar osteotomies with resection of bone are illustrated in Figure 29–163. A curved (Fig. 29–163*B*) or V-shaped (Fig. 164*A*) segment of bone from the hard palate and vomer is resected. The septal cartilage may also require a limited resection to accommodate the maxillary recession and to permit repositioning of the anterior dentoalveolar segment. If a direct anteroposterior displacement is required, the V-shaped triangular resection of the palate prevents rotation of the anterior segment; if any degree of rotation is needed to achieve optimal occlusal relationships, a curved line of resection is preferable. The amount of maxillary recession is estimated by the double standard of reestablishment of correct occlusal relationships with the mandibular teeth and of attainment of a satisfactory facial contour (Fig. 29–165).

Occasionally, a midline palatal splitting osteotomy is required to realign the dental arch (see Fig. 29–164*C*). The dental arch increases in width posteriorly. When the anterior segment is displaced backward, the discrepancy of the arch width results in a poor buccopalatal alignment of the teeth adjacent to the osteotomy (see Fig. 29–164*B*). A midline palatal splitting osteotomy corrects the alignment (see Fig. 29–164*C*) (Heiss, 1934; Dautrey and Pepersack, 1971; Steinhauser, 1972). Alignment of segments is necessary to decrease the risk of periodontal pocket formation and disease (Hinds and Kent, 1972). The palatal flap is then reapplied.

Fixation of the detached fragment is maintained by an orthodontic appliance or arch bars to provide monomaxillary fixation. The molar teeth provide anchorage for the appliance. A continuous labial coating of quick-setting, tooth-colored acrylic assists in stabilization during the six week period of postoperative healing. Intermaxillary fixation usually is not necessary.

The maxillary set-back procedure is also combined with a mandibular dentoalveolar set-back operation in patients with bimaxillary protrusion (see Fig. 29–173).

Subnasal Dentoalveolar Segmental Osteotomy. In some cases, when it is not desirable to modify the position of the nasal spine and the anterior nasal floor, a more limited type of osteotomy may be indicated. In the subnasal premolar osteotomy technique, the edge of the piriform aperture is exposed subperiosteally, and the line of section extends below the nasal spine and the floor of the nose. The procedure is otherwise similar to the premolar set-back osteotomy described above. The osteotomy is directed posteriorly, transecting the bone above the apices of the teeth, then inferiorly in the region of the premolars (Fig. 29–166).

The technique can be used to close an anterior open bite. The subnasal dentoalveolar segment is detached and displaced downward to close the open bite, and bone chips are packed into the resultant subnasal defect. Conversely, the subnasal osteotomy can be used to correct a deep overbite. Resection of a segment of bone above the apices of the teeth permits the upward displacement of a maxillary anterior dentoalveolar segment that has drifted downward.

Advantages and Disadvantages of Segmental Dentoalveolar Osteotomies. Segmental osteotomy provides a means of selective surgical-orthodontic correction of a dentoalveolar malocclusion. Correction is achieved of only that part of the dental arch that is actually deformed. Body and ramus osteotomies can also be used, but they are more involved and may introduce a secondary malocclusion and an undesirable change in the facial contour. When the deformity is in the anterior portion of the dental arch, an additional advantage is that monomaxillary fixation need be only temporary and can be released after the desired occlusion is ensured. Intermaxillary fixation usually is not indicated.

Hogeman and Sarnäs (1967) studied patients for 14 months after a maxillary setback procedure. When the final result was achieved, no relapses were noted. Improvement in the lip relationship (contour, profile, and lip seal) was maintained. All the mobilized fragments were clinically stable despite roentgenographic evidence of incomplete healing in several patients who had undergone a premolar segmental osteotomy, and also in patients in whom a paramedian palatal splitting osteotomy had been performed.

The disadvantages are minimized by careful attention to technique. The survival of the mobilized segment depends on the preservation of either a lingual or a buccal mucoperiosteal flap. The flap should be protected throughout the operation. It should also be designed to provide coverage of the lines of osteotomy and bone graft sites. These precautions, and careful apposition of the alveolar bone adjacent to the interdental osteotomy, decrease the risks of excessive alveolar bone loss and subsequent periodontal problems (Kent and Hinds, 1971; Bell, 1971). Thin, tapered osteotomes must be used to complete the interdental aspect of the osteotomy, in order to prevent damage to the roots of the neighboring teeth. Injury to the apices of the teeth is always a possibility. Therefore, it is advisable to preserve at least 3 and preferably 5 mm of bone beyond the apices. The canine teeth have the longest roots and are the most apt to be injured. An estimate of their length can be obtained from intraoral dental roentgenograms. The teeth in the mobilized segment usually retain their vascularity and regain their sensibility if their apices are not directly damaged (Butcher and Taylor, 1951; Madritsch, 1968; Johnson and Hinds, 1969; Barton, 1973; Pepersack, 1973). In the study by Pepersack (1973), 94.5 per cent of the maxillary teeth and 75 per cent of the mandibular teeth responded to stimuli one year postoperatively. The incidence of damage to the mandibular teeth was higher—1.5 per cent compared with 0.3 per cent involving the maxillary teeth. The increased number of cases involving nonresponse and injury to the lower teeth is explained by the greater diffi-

Text continued on page 1342

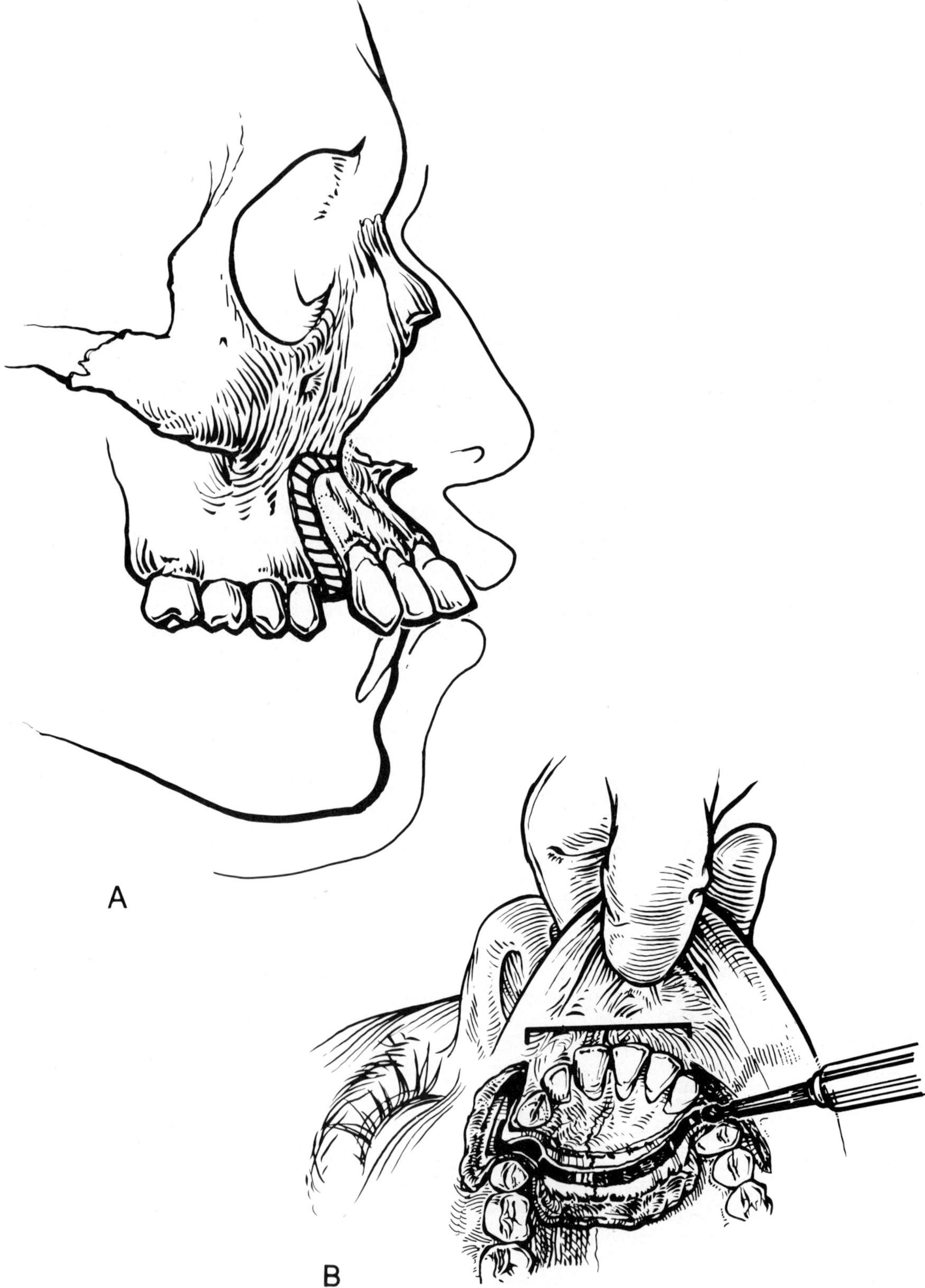

Figure 29–161. The premolar maxillary recession (set-back) osteotomy. *A,* Line of osteotomy and bone resection after removal of the premolar. *B,* Resection of the palatal segment with a bur. The bracket designates the width of the mucosal flap.

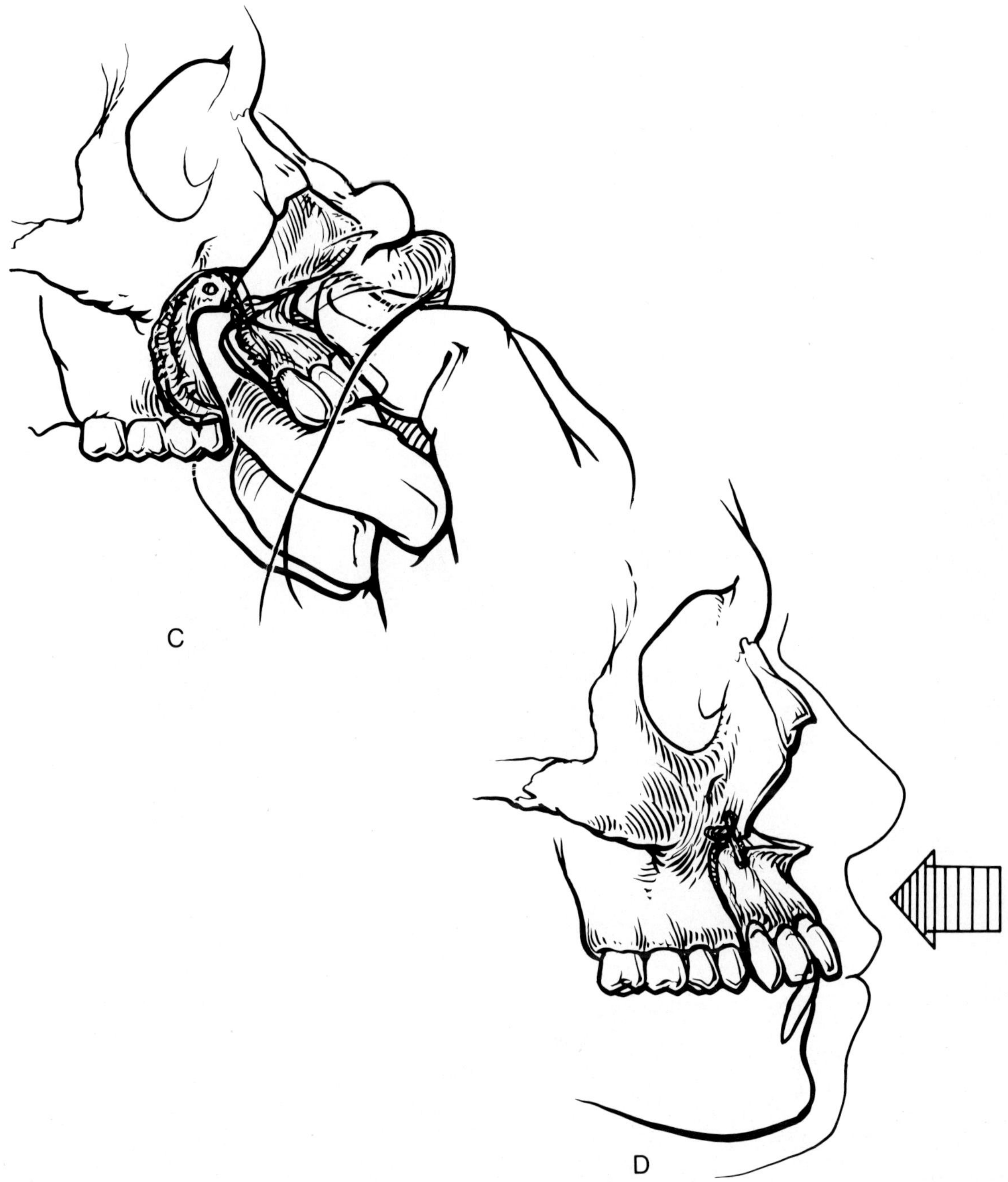

Figure 29–161 *Continued C,* Outfracturing maneuver. *D,* The segment has been recessed and secured with an interosseous wire.

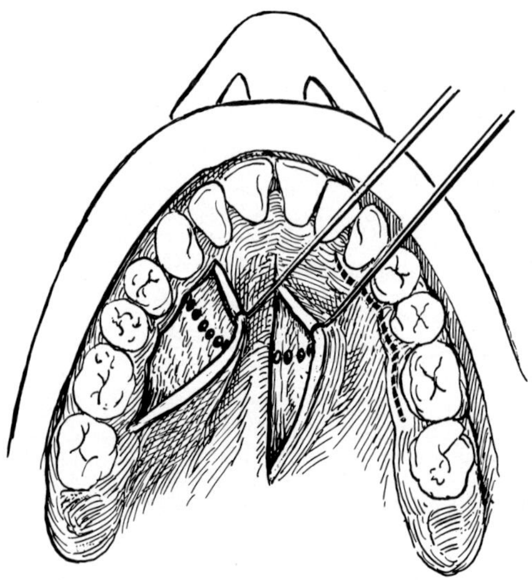

Figure 29–162. Tunneling technique to preserve the continuity of the blood supply of the palatal mucoperiosteal flap.

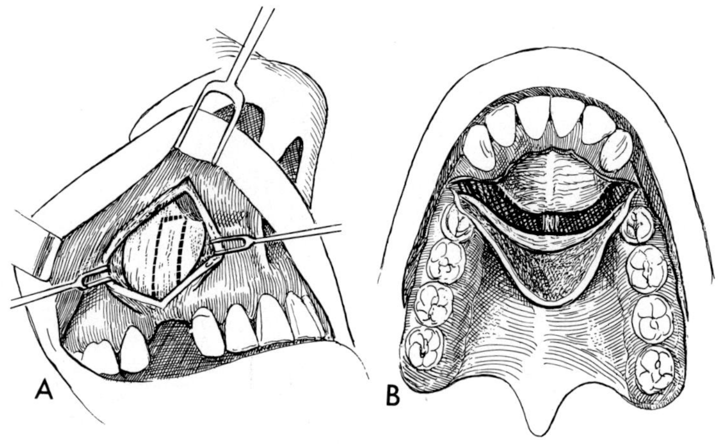

Figure 29–163. Premolar maxillary set-back osteotomy. *A,* Outline of the segment of bone to be resected when tilting of the dentoalveolar segment is not a problem and a straight set-back is desired. Resection of a triangular segment would be required to produce the tilting. *B,* The mucoperiosteal palatal flap has been elevated. The shaded area indicates the required resection of bone.

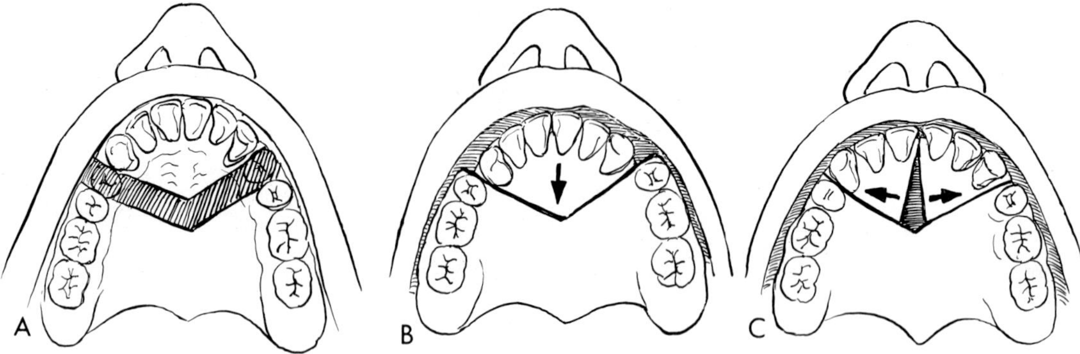

Figure 29–164. *A,* V-shaped osteotomy to prevent rotation of the recessed anterior maxillary segment. *B,* Loss of alignment of the dental arch after the set-back. *C,* A midline palatal osteotomy realigns the dental arch. A triangular bone graft fills the gap.

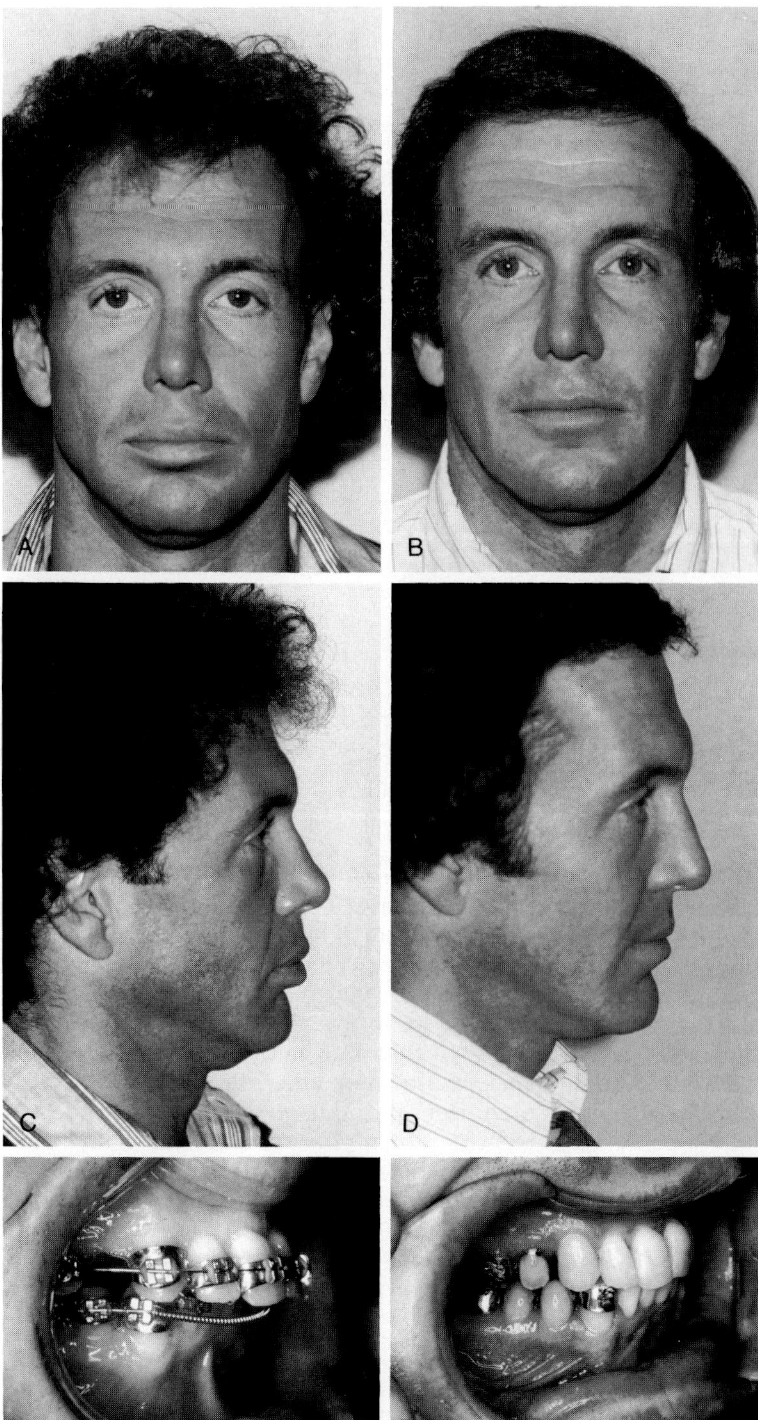

Figure 29–165. Anterior maxillary dentoalveolar protrusion corrected by a segmental dentoalveolar setback osteotomy and orthodontic therapy. *A, C, E,* Preoperative views. *B, D, F,* Postoperative views.

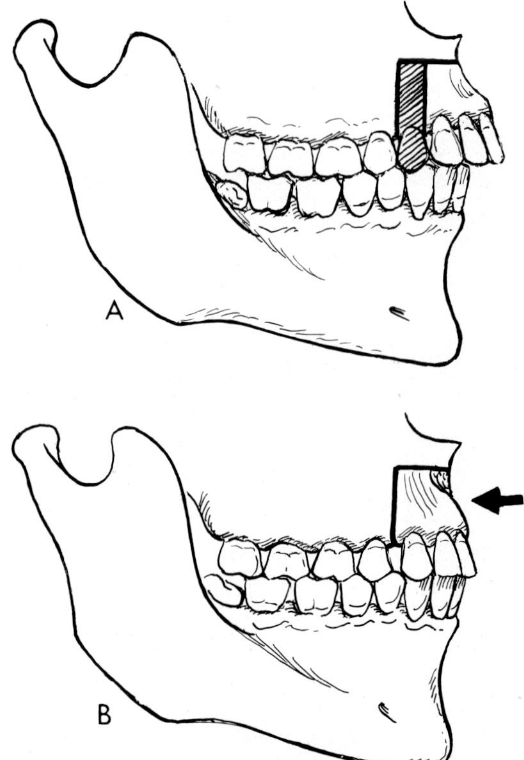

Figure 29–166. The subnasal premolar maxillary set-back osteotomy. *A*, The subnasal line of osteotomy. The bone to be resected is indicated by the shaded area. *B*, Relationships after completion of the procedure.

culty of the surgical approach and differences in the vascular and nerve supply. Teeth adjacent to the interdental osteotomy encounter the greatest risk. Poswillo (1972), in animal experiments, showed that progressive fibrosis and loss of odontoblasts occur in the pulp of the mobilized teeth. Nerve fibers do not regenerate, but the teeth retain their viability and vascularity. Hutchinson and MacGregor (1969) postulated that the return of sensibility is due to the perivascular nerve supply.

Relapse is always a possibility, especially if orofacial musculature dysfunction is overlooked. Detrimental habits and neuromuscular patterns are difficult to correct, but their control is crucial to the success of the operation.

Since the maxillary sinus is entered during the operation, alterations in sinus function theoretically may occur. Such problems have not been reported (Young and Epker, 1972). It is important to evaluate preoperatively any history of sinus disease and to eliminate any pathologic condition before the operation.

MAXILLARY DENTOALVEOLAR RETRUSION

On occasion the anterior maxillary dentoalveolar complex is retruded but the molar occlusal relationships are satisfactory. This type of malocclusion is frequently associated with the cleft lip-palate deformity.

The retruded appearance of the upper lip is apparent on frontal and especially on profile view (Figs. 29–167, 29–168). Usually the deficiency is limited to the upper lip region and does not extend to the zygomas and inferior orbital rims. The nasolabial angle may be acute and there is flattening of the piriform aperture region.

Cephalometric analysis confirms the clinical impression. The following measurements may be reduced: PNS-ANS, Ba-ANS, PNS-UIE, and SNA. As emphasized earlier in the chapter, no single cephalometric measurement is diagnostic.

Premolar Advancement Osteotomy. The outline of the premolar segmental advancement osteotomy (Converse and associates, 1964a) is similar to that of the premolar set-back osteotomy; the liberated anterior maxillary segment is advanced to correct the anterior maxillary retrusion (Fig. 29–169).

The degree of surgical advancement is planned preoperatively on the sectioned dental casts, using the dental occlusion and the cephalometric roentgenograms as guides.

The patient shown in Figure 29–167 is a typical example of a complex case in which the premolar segmental advancement osteotomy is specifically indicated. The bilateral cleft lip and palate had been repaired. The vermilion portion of the prolabial segment had been sacrificed in the repair of the bilateral cleft lip. When the patient was first seen at the age of 10 years (see Fig. 29–167*A*), the upper lip was tight, the anterior portion of the maxilla was hypoplastic, and the premaxilla was loose, lying lingually on a plane nearly horizontal with the palate (see Figs. 29–167*C* and 29–168*A,B*). In a first stage an Abbé flap from the lower lip was transposed to relieve the tight upper lip; the prolabial segment was used to lengthen the columella, and the tip of the nose was maintained in a forward projected position by a cantilever bone graft wired to the nasal bones. By orthodontic therapy, the premaxilla was realigned with the adjacent dentoalveolar segments. The premaxilla was then consolidated with the adjacent dentoalveolar segments by

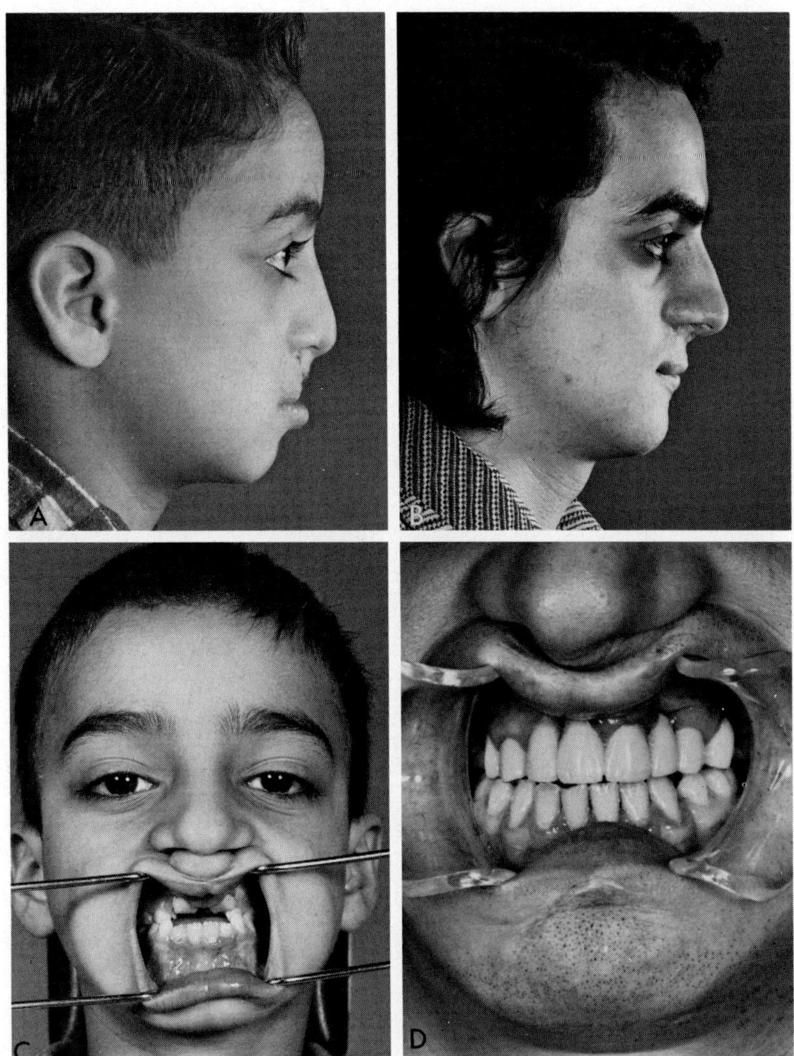

Figure 29–167. Premolar segmental maxillary advancement osteotomy. *A,* A 10 year old patient with a repaired bilateral cleft lip and palate. The vermilion portion of the prolabial segment of the lip has been sacrificed, resulting in a tight upper lip. The premaxilla is loose and lingually inclined against the hard palate (see *C*). The occlusal relationships between the molar teeth are adequate. *B,* Thirteen years after the following procedures: (1) an Abbé flap reconstruction to relieve the tight upper lip and to lengthen the columella at the expense of the prolabial segment and a cantilever bone graft wired to the nasal bones to maintain the projection of the nasal tip; (2) orthodontic therapy to realign the premaxilla; (3) consolidation of the premaxilla to the adjacent dentoalveolar segments by bone grafting; (4) premolar segmental advancement osteotomy (see Fig. 29–169) to correct the anterior maxillary hypoplasia. *C,* The dentition before treatment. Note the premaxilla lingually inclined against the palate. *D,* Final appearance of the dentition. Dental restorations were required and were completed after surgical-orthodontic treatment. (From Converse, J. M., Horowitz, S. L., Guy, C. L., and Wood-Smith, D.: Surgical and orthodontic procedures in bilateral cleft lip and cleft palate. Cleft Palate J., *1*:153, 1964.)

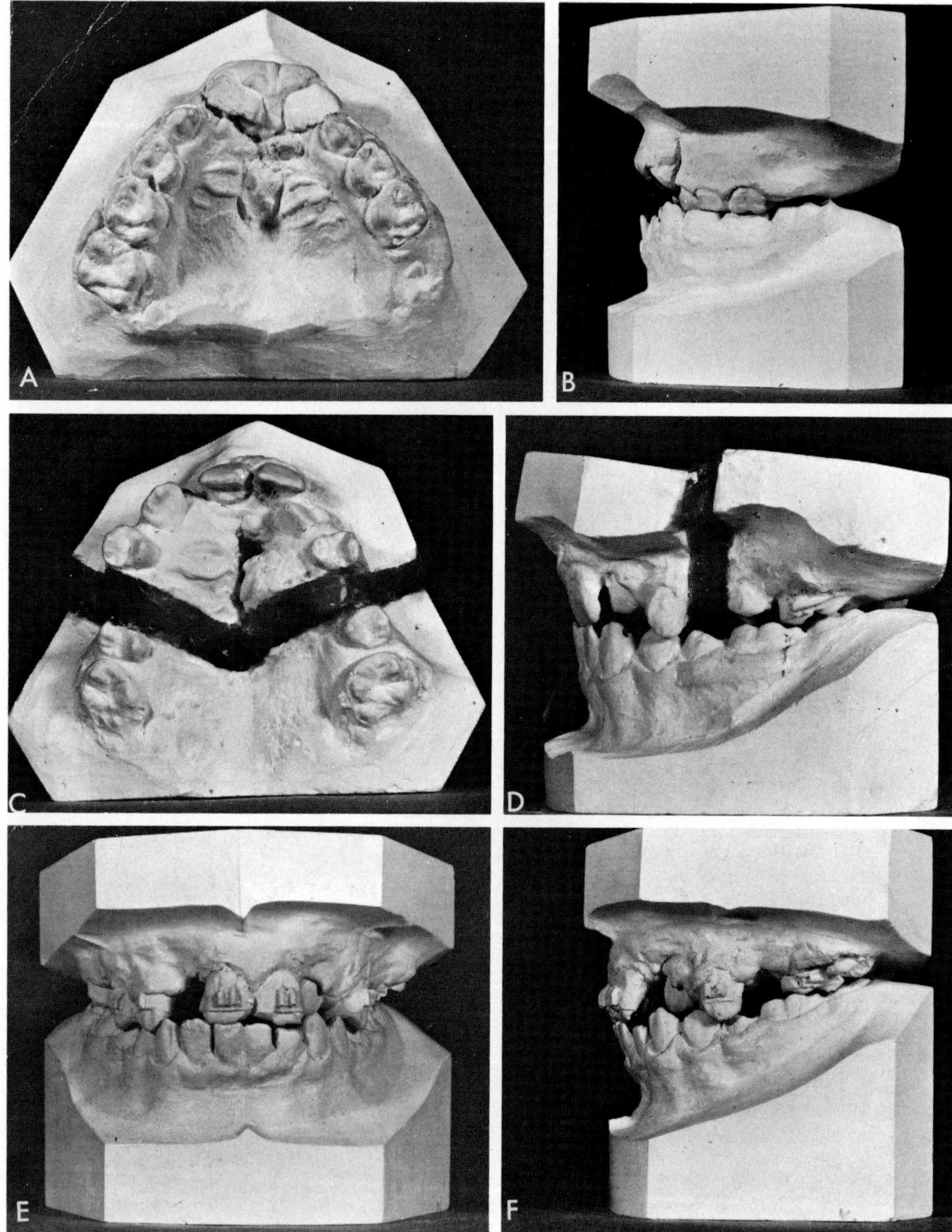

Figure 29–168. Use of dental casts in planning the combined orthodontic and surgical treatment to correct the malocclusion associated with bilateral cleft lip and palate (see Fig. 29–167). *A,* Preoperative view showing the lingual inclination of the mobile premaxilla. *B,* Preoperative profile view. *C,* After orthodontic repositioning of the premaxilla, the advancement of the anterior segment of the maxilla is planned by sectioning the study casts. *D,* Profile view of the planned advancement. *E, F,* Occlusal relationships after completion of surgical treatment. (From Converse, J. M., Horowitz, S. L., Guy, C. L., and Wood-Smith, D.: Surgical and orthodontic procedures in bilateral cleft lip and cleft palate. Cleft Palate J., *1*:153, 1964.)

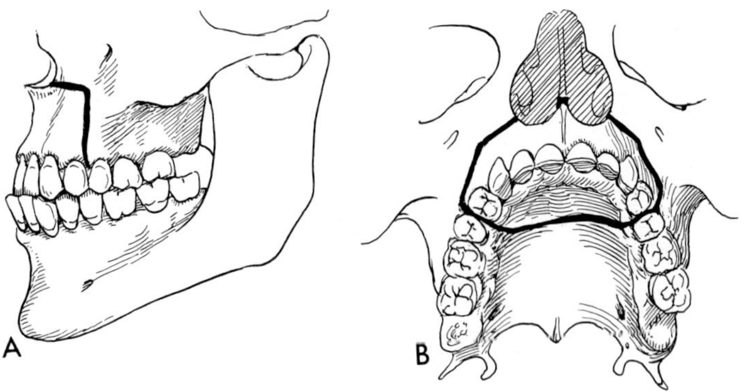

Figure 29–169. The premolar maxillary advancement osteotomy. *A,* Outline of the interdental osteotomy extending upward to the piriform aperture. *B,* The general outline of the osteotomy of the dentoalveolar region, hard palate, and septum.

bone grafting (see Chap. 55). At this point the patient still had a retruded and hypoplastic maxilla. However, the occlusal relationships between the maxillary and the mandibular molar teeth were adequate. Thus, a premaxillary segmental osteotomy was indicated rather than a Le Fort I advancement osteotomy, which would have disturbed the molar occlusal relationships. The planning of the premolar segmental osteotomy is shown in Figure 29–168*C,D*, and the result of the premolar segmental osteotomy is shown in Figure 29–168*E,F*.

The general outline of the osteotomy is similar to that of the set-back osteotomy (Fig. 29–169), except that the premolar teeth are retained, and bone is not removed from the hard palate. A labial mucoperiosteal tunnel is made over the proposed osteotomy site. With a small, round bur or an oscillating blade, the line of osteotomy is made from the edge of the piriform aperture to a line extending upward from the interdental space between the premolar teeth (Fig. 29–169*A*). A thin, tapered osteotome is used to make the interdental alveolar section, leaving sufficient bone on each side to protect the adjacent teeth. The palatal mucoperiosteum is raised and the osteotomy is continued across the hard palate, reaching the alveolar line of section of the contralateral side (Fig. 29–169*B*). In the midline of the palate, the osteotomy must be extended upward across and through the vomer.

The nasal septal framework is exposed by careful elevation of the mucoperiosteum and mucoperichondrium. The nasal septal cartilage is divided at its line of insertion in the vomer groove to a point that reaches the osteotomy through the vomer.

The mobilized anterior segment of the maxilla is advanced and rotated downward, upward, or laterally as needed. The anterior fragment is maintained in monomaxillary fixation in the corrected position by an orthodontic appliance or arch bar, using the teeth in the posterior fixed portion of the maxilla for anchorage (Fig. 29–170). A continuous thin coating of quick-curing acrylic is used to provide additional stabilization; intermaxillary fixation is not necessary but may be temporarily employed to ensure that the occlusion is achieved.

Small fragments of bone are wedged between the fragments to restore osseous continuity (Fig. 29–170). Interosseous wiring or miniplate fixation may be required for stabi-

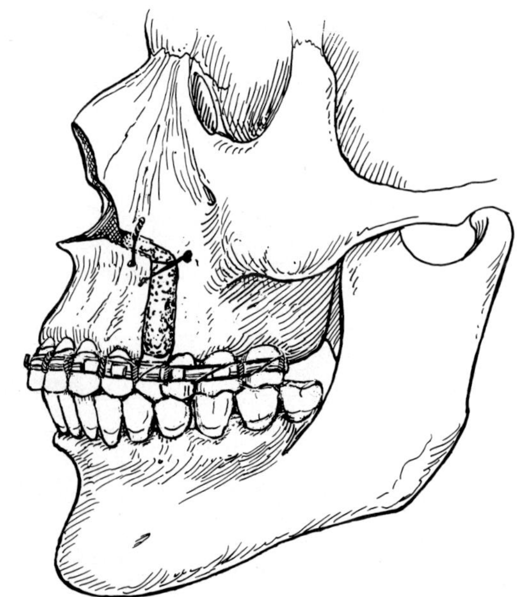

Figure 29–170. Monomaxillary fixation. Fixation is based on the stable posterior teeth. Intermaxillary fixation is not necessary except to adjust the occlusion. It can then be released. An arch bar is represented in the drawing but an orthodontic appliance or occlusal splint is preferred.

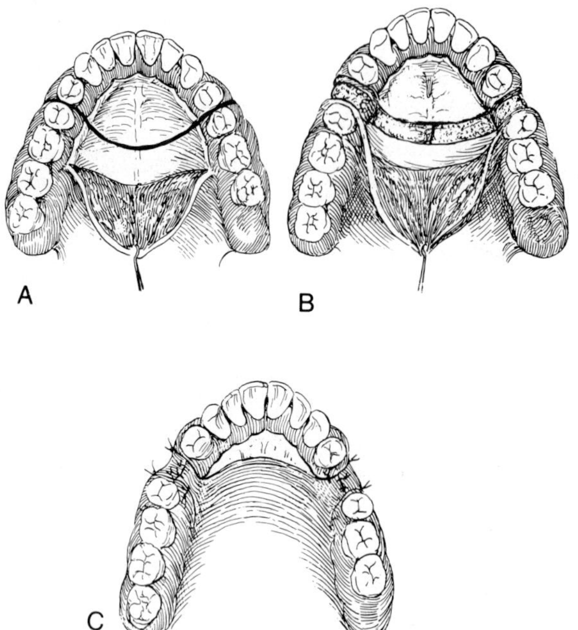

Figure 29–171. The premolar maxillary advancement osteotomy. *A,* A mucoperiosteal palatal flap has been raised, and the outline of the osteotomy is indicated. *B,* After the advancement, bone grafts are wedged into the line of osteotomy. *C,* The exposed portion of the anterior hard palate epithelizes spontaneously. The palatal flap is sutured to the buccal mucoperiosteum to cover the bone grafts in the alveolar area.

lization. Bone grafts may also be inserted around the edge of the piriform aperture and over the anterior surface of the maxilla if additional reinforcement of the bone continuity or contour restoration is required. The mucoperiosteal incision is closed (Fig. 29–171*C*).

The palatal mucoperiosteal flap serves to cover the bone grafts in the palatal defect (Fig. 29–171*C*). Depending on the amount of maxillary advancement, the palatal flap may not cover the anterior portion of the hard palate. The exposed bone, however, epithelizes secondarily. Usually there is sufficient vestibular and alveolar mucoperiosteum to cover the bone grafts in the alveolar defect. When the planned maxillary advancement exceeds 1 cm, an anteriorly based buccal

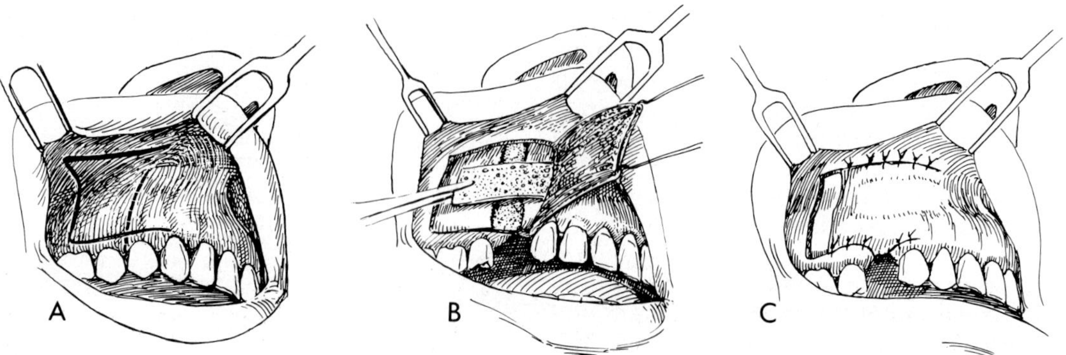

Figure 29–172. The premolar maxillary advancement osteotomy. *A,* When the advancement exceeds 1 cm, an anteriorly based mucoperiosteal flap is outlined to release the soft tissue tension and to cover the bone grafts. *B,* Bone grafts are wedged into the gap in the alveolar process. A thin cancellous bone onlay is placed over the area of the osteotomy. *C,* A mucoperiosteal flap is sutured over the bone grafts. The posterior raw surface epithelizes spontaneously. The drawing shows that a premolar tooth has been extracted; an interdental osteotomy usually obviates the need for the extraction.

mucoperiosteal flap should be employed to ensure coverage of the bone grafts (Fig. 29–172). Exposure to the open maxillary sinus does not complicate the healing of the bone grafts; the lining of the maxillary sinus rapidly covers the undersurface of the grafts.

MANDIBULAR DENTOALVEOLAR PROTRUSION

Isolated mandibular dentoalveolar protrusion is an uncommon deformity and must be distinguished from mandibular (skeletal) prognathism (see p. 1228).

In the former, the molar occlusal relationships are satisfactory and cephalometric analysis shows that the mandibular skeletal measurements are within normal limits.

The osteotomies employed to correct mandibular dentoalveolar protrusion are discussed under Anterior Open Bite (see p. 1351).

BIMAXILLARY DENTOALVEOLAR PROTRUSION

When the maxillary and mandibular incisors protrude so severely that lip seal cannot be achieved without severe straining, the condition is labeled *bimaxillary dentoalveolar protrusion* (Case, 1921).

Dental protrusion is generally more common in black and Oriental people than in whites and may even be considered a racial characteristic in the former groups.

In the typical patient, extreme protrusion of the maxillary and mandibular incisors is readily apparent on frontal and profile views (Fig. 29–173). Lip seal is never achieved involuntarily, and when the teeth are covered by the lips there is obvious straining of the lips, with contraction of the mentalis muscle and corrugation of the soft tissue chin (Fig. 29–173). The lips appear thick and the vermilion-cutaneous borders are everted. There is often an associated microgenia with loss of the labiomental crease.

Bimaxillary dentoalveolar protrusion must be distinguished from maxillary dentoalveolar protrusion or maxillary skeletal protrusion. Study of the molar occlusal relationships and cephalometric analysis both help to establish the diagnosis.

Classification of Treatment Modalities

The following is a classification of the available forms of treatment for bimaxillary dentoalveolar protrusion:

1. Extraction of first or second premolar teeth.
2. Preoperative orthodontic therapy to close the above extraction spaces by retraction of the incisors, and to level or correct an accentuated curve of Spee of the mandibular arch.
3. Anterior maxillary dentoalveolar segmental osteotomies to retract and (frequently) to intrude the protruding maxillary incisors. The osteotomies popularized by Cohn-Stock (1921), Wassmund (1927), and Wunderer (1962) are discussed on page 1336. The premolar set-back osteotomy of the maxilla (Wilhelm, 1954) is discussed on page 1336.
4. Anterior mandibular dentoalveolar segmental osteotomies to retract and (frequently) to intrude the protruding mandibular incisors. The Köle (1959b) procedure is discussed on page 1356.
5. Ancillary procedures, such as genioplasty and rhinoplasty, may also be indicated.

Surgical-Orthodontic Treatment of Bimaxillary Protrusion: Simianism. The face of modern man is distinguished from his early forebears and living primate relatives by a reduction in the forward projection of the jaws. Relative protrusion of the snout is seen in all simians but only rarely in humans (particularly whites); even when it does occur, it is usually confined to either the lower jaw (mandibular prognathism) or maxilla (skeletal Class II).

In the patient shown in Figure 29–174*A,C*, bimaxillary protrusion caused a severe and unusual facial deformity (Converse and Horowitz, 1973). The mandible and dentoalveolar arch are elongated, with contraction of the horizontal dimension (Fig. 29–175*A*), similar to the jaw of the primate (Fig. 29–175*B*).

Several factors were considered in planning the total corrective program for the patient: (1) the increased skeletal facial height, as shown in the cephalometric tracing (see Fig. 29–174*E*) and also demonstrated by the location of the chin pad above the mental symphysis (see Fig. 29–174*A*); (2) dental malocclusion (Class I) with severe crowding (Fig. 29–176*A*); and (3) protrusion of the upper and lower dentoalveolar processes in relation to other facial structures.

In planning the treatment, the principal objectives were to diminish facial height and reduce the bimaxillary dentoalveolar protrusion. Several staged procedures were used to accomplish these goals.

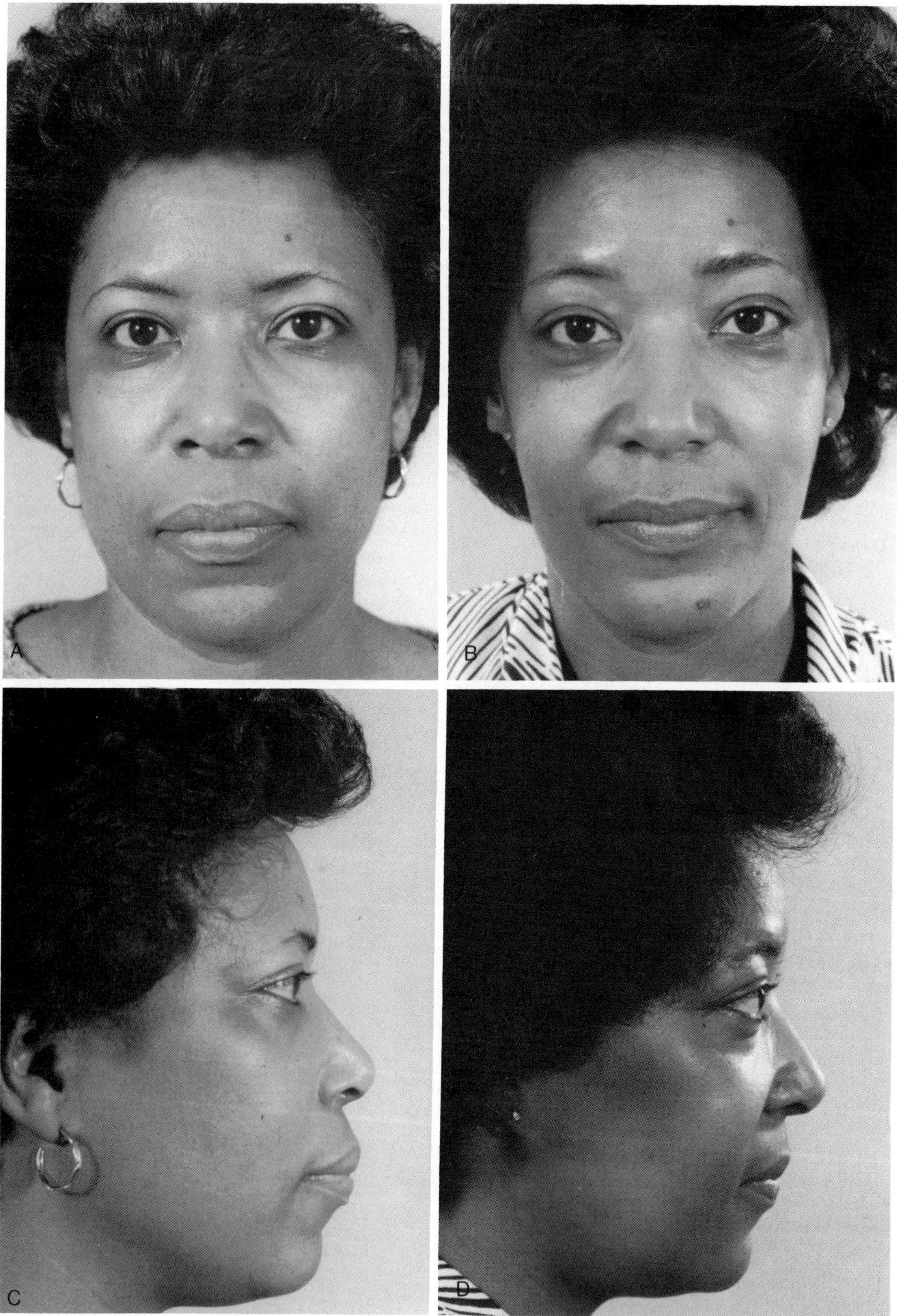

Figure 29–173. Bimaxillary protrusion. *A, C,* Preoperative appearance. *B, D,* After maxillary and mandibular anterior segmental dentoalveolar osteotomies.

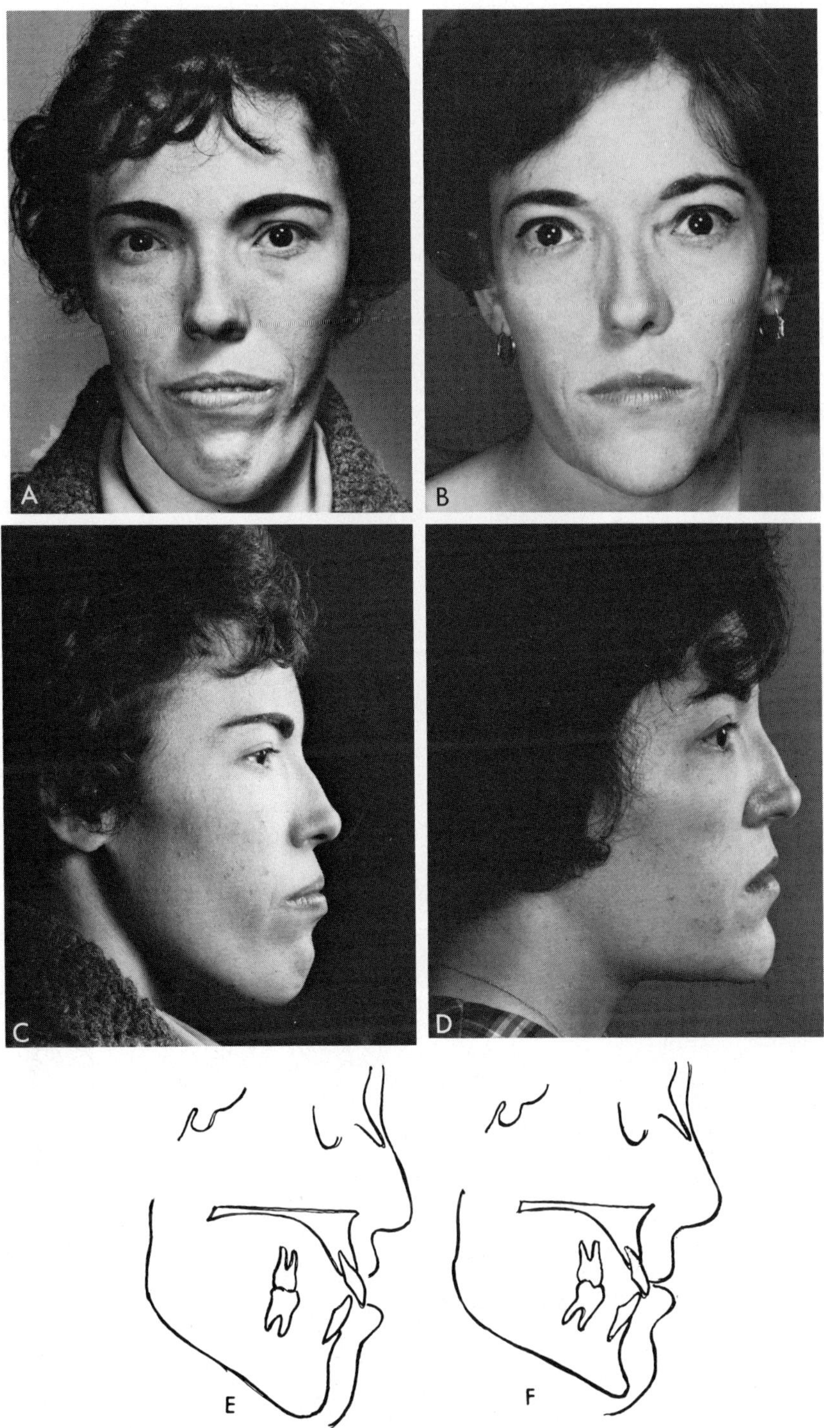

Figure 29–174. Bimaxillary protrusion. *A,* Appearance of a patient nicknamed "monkey face." Note the considerable increase in facial height. *B,* Postoperative photograph of the patient after completion of treatment. *C,* Profile view showing bimaxillary protrusion. *D,* Profile view of the patient after surgical-orthodontic treatment. *E,* A cephalometric tracing before treatment showing the increased skeletal facial height. *F,* Cephalometric tracing four years after completion of treatment showing changes in the dentoalveolar relationships, diminution in facial height, and adequate protrusion of the mental symphysis. (From Converse, J. M., and Horowitz, S. L.: Simianism: surgical-orthodontic correction of bimaxillary protrusion. J. Maxillofac. Surg., *1*:7, 1973. Georg Thieme Verlag, Stuttgart, Germany.)

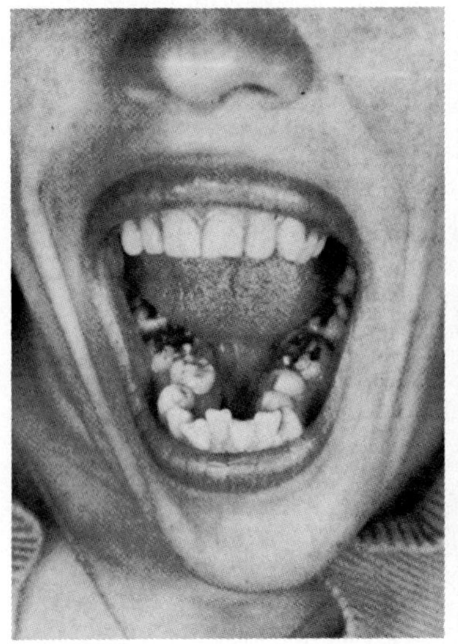

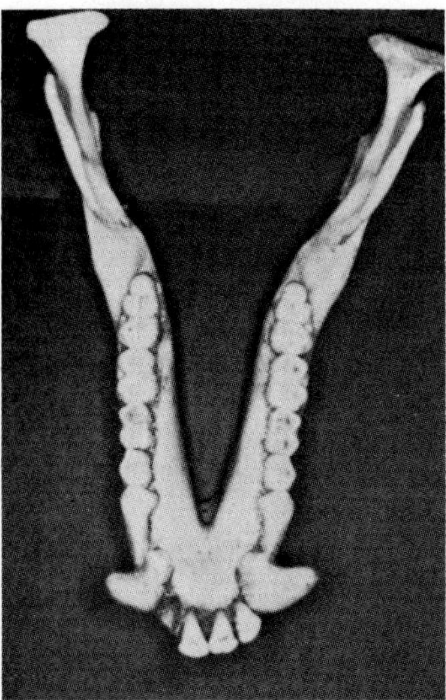

Figure 29–175. Comparison of the lower jaw of the patient shown in Fig. 29–174 with that of a primate. *A,* Note the elongated shape of the patient's mandible with restriction in the horizontal dimension reminiscent of the jaw of a primate (*B*). (From Converse, J. M., and Horowitz, S. L.: Simianism: surgical-orthodontic correction of bimaxillary protrusion. J. Maxillofac. Surg., *1*:7, 1973. Georg Thieme Verlag, Stuttgart, Germany.)

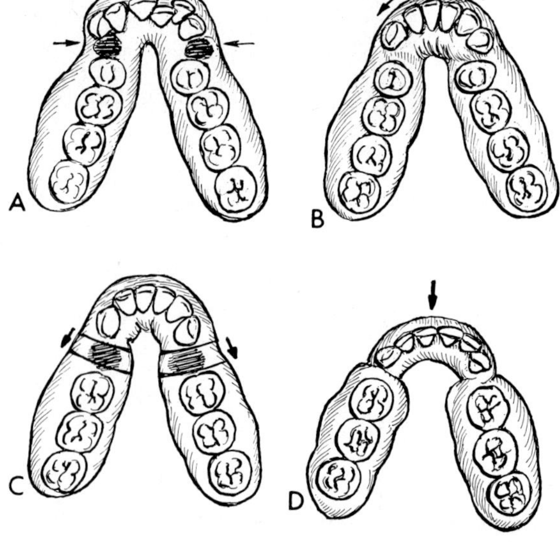

Figure 29–176. Drawing made from dental mandibular casts of the patient shown in Figure 29–174. *A,* Original dental malalignment of the mandibular teeth. The arrows indicate the extraction of the first premolars. *B,* Result obtained after orthodontic therapy. *C,* The arrows indicate the extraction of the second premolars before a dentoalveolar set-back procedure. *D,* Contour of the mandibular arch after the set-back osteotomy. (From Converse, J. M., and Horowitz, S. L.: Simianism: surgical-orthodontic correction of bimaxillary protrusion. J. Maxillofac. Surg., *1*:7, 1973. Georg Thieme Verlag, Stuttgart, Germany.)

Stage 1. The first operation consisted of a reduction in the vertical dimension of the mandibular body by resection of a predetermined segment of mandible along the inferior border, and transplantation of the resected segment anterior to the mental symphysis. The fragment was adapted to the contour of the mandible by buring the cortex of its posterior surface until the horseshoe-shaped graft was accurately fitted to the host bed (see Fig. 29–133). The procedure shortened the total face height and provided adequate protrusion of the mental symphysis. As can be observed on the cephalometric tracing of the patient four years after the procedure, a satisfactory contour was maintained (see Fig. 29–174*F*).

Stage 2. Orthodontic treatment to relieve the severe dental crowding and reduce the protrusion of the anterior maxillary and mandibular dentoalveolar areas made up the second stage of treatment. This required extraction of the maxillary and mandibular first premolar teeth. The spaces thus made available were used to realign the anterior teeth and retract them as much as possible, using upper and lower edgewise arch orthodontic appliances over a period of approximately one year (Fig. 29–177). Since much of the extraction space was required for tooth realignment (particularly in the mandibular dental arch), both the upper and lower dentoalveolar areas were still relatively protrusive after orthodontic therapy. In order to correct this disharmony, a combined surgical-orthodontic approach was planned to correct the remaining bimaxillary protrusion.

Stage 3. In the third phase the mandibular second premolars were extracted (see Fig. 29–176*C*); the dentoalveolar process was exposed subperiosteally, and an alveolar set-back osteotomy was performed below the level of the apices of the teeth (see Fig. 29–41). The dentoalveolar block was moved posteriorly almost the entire width of the extraction space, temporarily producing an overjet of nearly 1 cm between the upper and lower anterior teeth. The edgewise arch orthodontic appliance was used for fixation.

Stage 4. In order to harmonize the occlusion and complete the reduction of the bimaxillary protrusion, the upper second premolars were removed, and the anterior portion of the maxilla containing the six anterior maxillary teeth and dentoalveolar bone was moved posteriorly (Fig. 29–177*C,D*) by a maxillary premolar segmental set-back osteotomy.

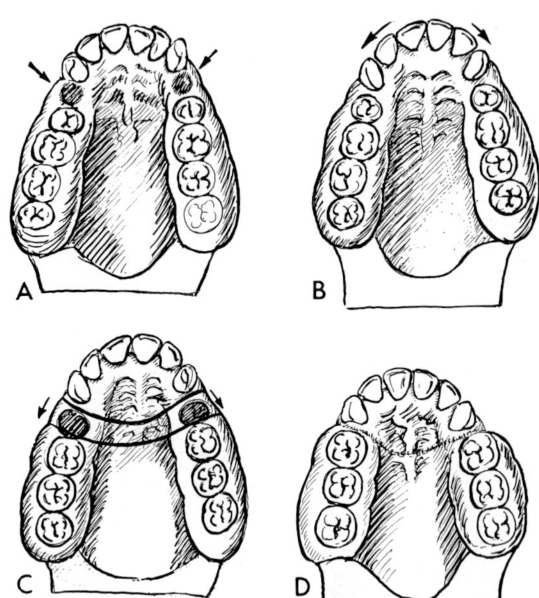

Figure 29–177. *A,* Drawing of the maxillary arch before treatment. The arrows indicate extraction of the first premolars. *B,* Contour of the arch after orthodontic therapy. *C,* The shaded areas indicate the extraction of the second premolars. *D,* Contour of the maxillary arch after the dentoalveolar set-back osteotomy. (From Converse, J. M., and Horowitz, S. L.: Simianism: surgical-orthodontic correction of bimaxillary protrusion. J. Maxillofac. Surg., *1*:7, 1973. Georg Thieme Verlag, Stuttgart, Germany.)

As seen from the drawings of the dental casts, the combination of orthodontic alignment and surgical set-back of the anterior dentoalveolar segments resulted in considerable improvement in the general contour of the dental arches, which assumed a parabolic rather than a simian form. Removal of the eight premolar teeth permitted foreshortening of the dental arches, without loss of dental arch continuity, and also provided reduction of the bimaxillary protrusion.

The period of treatment could have been shortened by combining Stages 3 and 4 through careful predetermination of the desired position of the dentoalveolar segments and simultaneous maxillary and mandibular dentoalveolar osteotomies.

OPEN BITE DEFORMITY

The term "open bite" (apertognathism) is applied to a condition in which the teeth fail to occlude when the jaws are brought together. An open bite can occur in the incisor segment (*anterior open bite*), in the premolar and molar segments (*posterior open bite*), or in both segments (*lateral open bite*) of the dentoalveolar arch. The deformity primarily affects the dentoalveolar complex, but both the dentoalveolar segment and the body of the jaw can be involved. Dysfunction of the orofacial musculature almost always accompanies the malocclusion. Because of the neuromuscular problem, the mandible is malpositioned relative to the maxilla. There is also differential eruption of the teeth and differential growth of various jaw segments—factors that accentuate the deformity.

Anterior open bite can be associated with a variety of functional and esthetic abnormalities. The functional disturbance is characterized by the absence of concerted and coordinated action of the tongue and teeth in pronouncing certain consonants; in addition to the speech impairment, many patients with anterior open bite have difficulty in mastication. Anterior open bite is also frequently characterized by an elongation of the lower third of the face, which may be sufficiently pronounced to constitute a conspicuous deformity.

Incidence

The true incidence of open bite deformity in the general population has never been established. Statistics supplied from the United States Public Health Survey reveal that 5.7 per cent of 8000 schoolchildren between the ages of 6 and 11 years demonstrated an open bite deformity (Kelly, Sanchez, and van Kirk, 1973).

Etiology

Most open bite deformities are caused either by imbalance of the orofacial musculature or by trauma. The etiologic factors can be listed as follows:

1. Thumb or other "non-nutritive" sucking patterns. In general, there is a direct association between the length of thumb sucking and the development and presence of an open bite deformity.
2. Disturbances of neuromuscular and tongue patterns that lead to tongue thrusting between the upper and lower teeth during the act of deglutition—the so-called *tongue thrust swallow*. Patients frequently have difficulty in obtaining lip seal, and hyperactivity and hypertrophy of the mentalis muscle represent a compensatory attempt to occlude the oral muscular sphincter.

   The open bite deformity in Down and Beckwith-Wiedemann syndromes is an example of the lip and tongue neuromuscular dysfunction observed in this syndrome.

   Approximately 50 per cent of 6 year old children demonstrate tongue thrust swallow, but by 15 years of age only 25 per cent show evidence of this phenomenon (Fletcher, Casteel, and Bradley, 1961). However, these figures greatly exceed the incidence of the open bite deformity in the population, and individuals with this type of neuromuscular dysfunction can also be observed without an open bite deformity. Consequently the cause and effect relationship between tongue thrust and open bite is not entirely clear.

   With the onset of puberty the incidence of open bite decreases significantly. This can be attributed to (1) the decrease in thumb sucking; (2) an increase in the vertical dimension of the mandible, which allows more intraoral space for the tongue; and (3) involution of the tonsils and adenoids with an associated increase in the airway.
3. Trauma.
   a. Bilateral fractures of the ramus, especially at the level of the condylar neck. These can be associated with posterior and superior displacement of the tooth-bearing mandibular segment and shortening of the vertical dimension of each ramus. Occlusal contact of the dentition occurs only in the region of the posterior molars.
   b. Malunited fractures of the mandibular body that interfere with masticatory efficiency.
   c. Fractures of the bones of the midface, the maxilla being displaced posteriorly and inferiorly, resulting in premature contact of the posterior teeth.
   d. Untreated jaw fractures in children.
   e. Distortion of the mandible by scar contractures after cervical burns.

Classification

Anterior open bite deformity was classified by Moyers (1963) as follows: *simple*, in which the interdental opening is anterior to the canines; *compound*, in which the opening extends back to the premolars; and *skeletal*, in which the open bite involves the molars. The occlusion should also be classified according to Angle (see p. 1193).

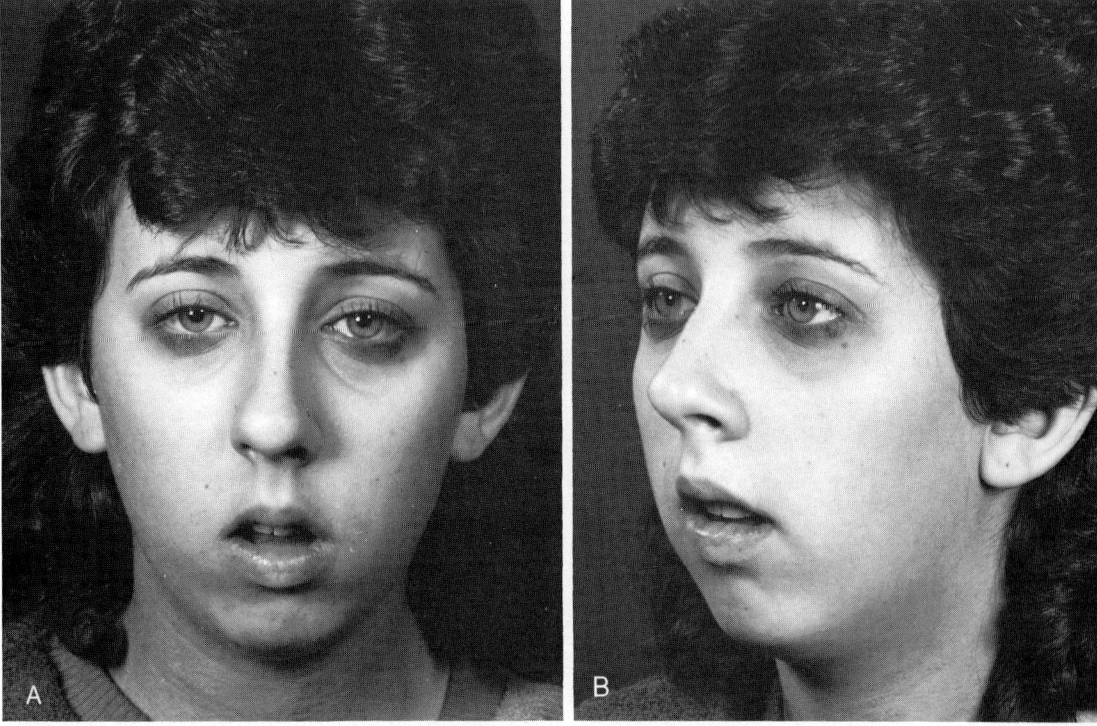

Figure 29–178. Anterior open bite. Note the elongation of the lower third of the face, microgenia, and lip incompetence.

Clinical Evaluation

The physician should ascertain whether there is a history of respiratory obstruction, thumb sucking, tongue thrust swallow, or craniofacial trauma.

The patient usually shows an obvious open bite and elongation of the lower third of the face (Fig. 29–178). There is lip incompetence at rest with hypertrophy of the mentalis muscle. It is not uncommon to observe maxillary incisor show at rest and gingival exposure on smiling. The nasolabial angle is usually obtuse and the nasal septum is deviated. There often is microgenia. Classes I, II, and III occlusion can be observed; Class II is most common because the mandible is rotated in an inferior and posterior direction.

An appreciation of the excess vertical dimension of the face should be obtained during the clinical examination. The height of the lower third of the face will influence the surgical treatment. The orofacial musculature pattern must also be carefully observed. Failure to recognize faulty muscular activity invites relapse and a poor final result.

Dental Examination. Examination of the occlusion (Fig. 29–179) can show protrusion (labial inclination) of the maxillary and mandibular incisors. There can also be disparity between maxillary and mandibular arch form. The maxillary arch can be significantly narrower than its mandibular counterpart.

Working dental casts are also sectioned to determine the optimal location for the osteotomies required to correct the deformity.

Cephalography. Cephalometric roentgenograms best define the skeletal component of the deformity. The anterior facial height (N-Me) is often elongated, and the mandibular plane (MP) is steep, as noted by the increased MP-SN angle (Fig. 29–180). Elongation of the lower third of the face is often caused by the downward tilt of the anterior portion of the mandibular body, which increases the distance between the anterior nasal spine (ANS) and menton (Me). The vertical dimension of the ramus (Ar-Go or posterior facial height) is often reduced. The gonial angle (Ba-Go-Po) is usually obtuse. The mandibular body is usually of normal length since the open bite deformity is usually a vertical problem. The palatal plane (ANS-PNS) can be tipped (higher posteriorly). The amount of eruption of the molar teeth and the inclina-

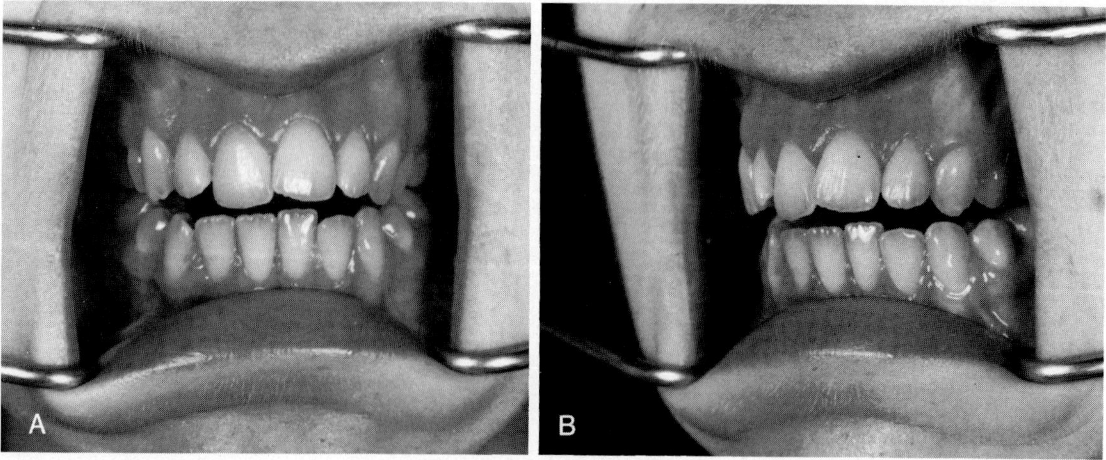

Figure 29–179. Occlusal views of the patient shown in Figure 29–178.

tion of the incisor teeth (L1-MP and U1-SN) should also be recorded, since they have a bearing on the type of treatment.

Treatment

Open bite deformities can be associated with vertical displacement in all or part of the upper or lower dentoalveolar segments, and with prognathism or retrognathism. In problems not amenable to orthodontic therapy alone, orthognathic surgery of the mandible, maxilla, or both is indicated. The choice of the corrective technique depends on whether the open bite is primarily due to a malformation of the mandible or maxilla, or both.

The differentiation between an anterior

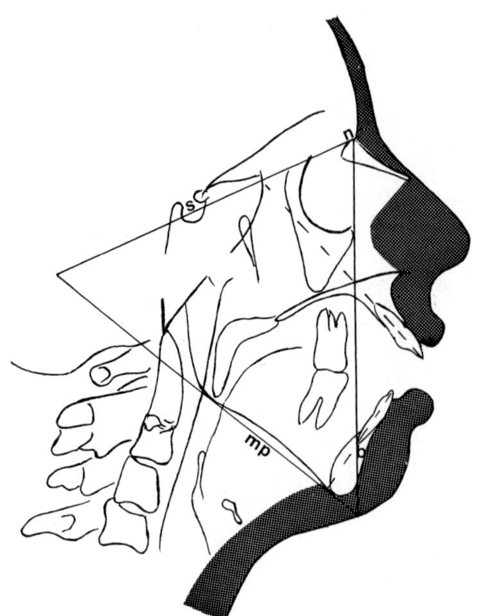

Figure 29–180. Cephalometric tracing of a patient with an anterior open bite. Note the increase in the facial height, the steep mandibular plane, and the downward tilt of the anterior aspect of the mandibular body. The angle mp–sn is increased. The hard palate shows an unusual downward tilt.

open bite of maxillary origin and a mandibular open bite is aided by study of the cephalogram. If the palatal plane (ANS-PNS) reflects an upward deflection anteriorly and a downward deflection posteriorly, the diagnosis of maxillary anterior open bite is confirmed. In mandibular open bite, the palatal plane is level, and the anterior portion of the mandible shows a downward cant.

Treatment also differs depending on whether or not there is an elongation of the lower third of the face. Vertical maxillary excess (see p. 1381) is another variable to be considered.

Thus, before surgery is attempted, the following questions must be answered: (1) is the basic defect (pathology) in the maxilla, in the mandible, or in both?; (2) is the deformity a dentoalveolar or a skeletal problem?; and (3) is there a vertical increase of the lower third of the face or of the maxilla?

In general, most open bite deformities caused by dentoalveolar malrelationships can be corrected by selective *segmental dentoalveolar osteotomies* of the jaws. *Skeletal open bite* caused by deformity of the main body of the jaw usually requires movement of a larger portion of the jaw.

The goals of treatment of the open bite deformity are the improvement of (1) occlusion, (2) appearance, (3) tongue function, and (4) speech.

Surgical-Orthodontic Treatment of Open Bite: Historical Background. The first operation in the United States to correct an open bite deformity and prognathism of the lower jaw was reported by Hullihen in 1849 (Fig. 29–181). The operation consisted of the resection of bilateral V-shaped segments of bone from the upper two-thirds of the mandible in the premolar region; a subapical horizontal osteotomy then connected the resected wedge-shaped areas. The anterior dentoalveolar segment was tilted backward and upward to close the open bite. Blair in 1897 (Angle, 1899) and von Eiselsberg (1906) performed similar operations. Lane (1905) and Pickrell (1912) corrected open bite deformities by the removal of a wedge-shaped segment of bone, which extended through the entire thickness of the mandible in the premolar area. Subsequently, osteotomies of the mandibular ramus and body to correct mandibular prognathism and micrognathism were adapted to close the open bite malocclusion. A reversed L vertical osteotomy of the ramus with resection of a V-shaped section of bone was described by Limberg (1925) for the treatment of micrognathia with an anterior open bite (Fig. 29–182). He later (1928) proposed the addition of a costal bone graft, a technique applied by Schuchardt (1958). Robinson (1957) used an iliac bone graft to fill the gap.

Selective movement of a segment of the dentoalveolar arch after osteotomy (segmental osteotomies) has also been used to correct an open bite. The principles for this type of operation were developed by Cohn-Stock (1921), Spanier (1932), Wassmund (1935), Schuchardt (1955), Köle (1959a), Wunderer (1962), and Kufner (1968).

Classification of Treatment Modalities. The following is a classification of the avail-

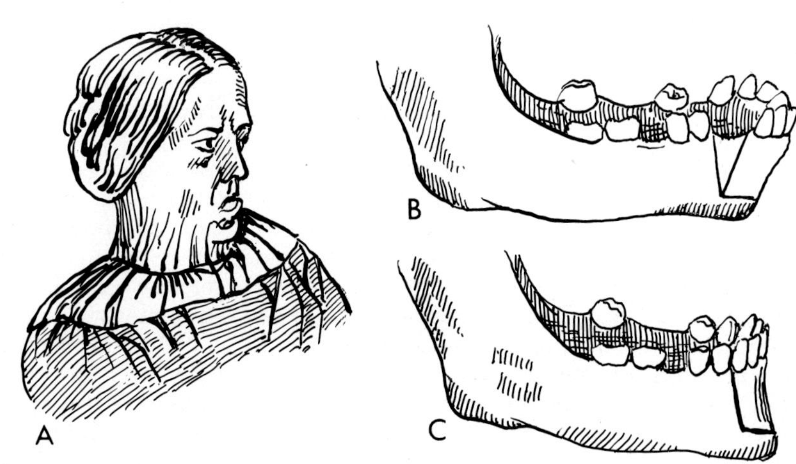

Figure 29–181. Hullihen's operation for the correction of an anterior open bite. *A,* The open bite was caused by contractures due to a third degree burn. *B,* Outline of the V-shaped segment to be resected and the dentoalveolar osteotomy. *C,* Result the operation.

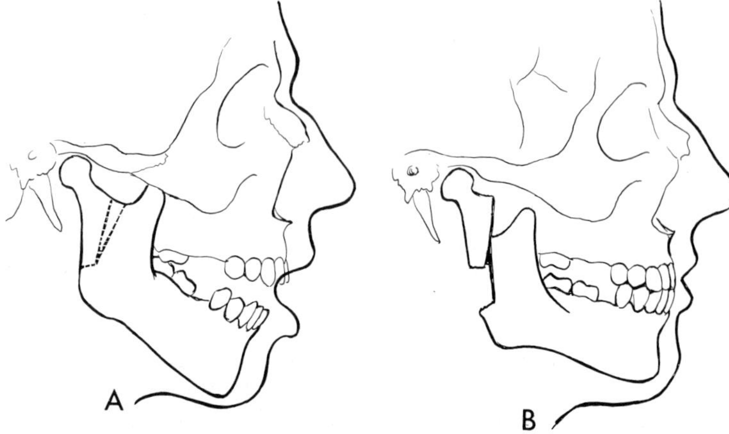

Figure 29–182. Limberg's operation for correction of an anterior open bite. *A*, Outline of osteotomy with V-resection of bone from the ramus. *B*, After closure of the open bite.

able treatment modalities for open bite deformity:

1. Orthodontic therapy.
2. Anterior segmental dentoalveolar osteotomy of the mandible.
3. Ramus osteotomy of the mandible.
4. Anterior segmental dentoalveolar osteotomy of the maxilla.
5. Posterior segmental dentoalveolar osteotomy of the maxilla.
6. Total maxillary (Le Fort I) osteotomy.
7. Tongue reduction.

Orthodontic Therapy. An open bite malocclusion that affects primarily the dentoalveolar segment responds well to orthodontic treatment if concomitant improvement is also achieved in the neuromuscular forces acting on the dentoalveolar structures. However, in patients with an open bite secondary to a developmental malformation of the jaw and craniofacial skeleton, the response to orthodontic therapy alone is often poor, and correction cannot be achieved without combined surgical-orthodontic treatment.

Orthodontic therapy is especially indicated in the preoperative and postoperative periods to correct any occlusal irregularities, as discussed previously (p. 1200).

Anterior Segmental Dentoalveolar Osteotomy of Mandible. Since Hullihen's original operation (1849), the mandibular anterior segmental dentoalveolar osteotomies have been refined by Köle (1959b) and Schuchardt (1963). A labial mucoperiosteal flap is raised, and vertical osteotomies are made at the selected interdental spaces (see Fig. 29–41). A transverse osteotomy below the apices of the teeth connects the lower limits of the vertical sections. A thin, tapered osteotome is used to complete the interdental vertical osteotomy. The blood supply is maintained by a lingual mucoperiosteal flap. The fragment is then elevated toward the occlusal plane to close the open bite deformity. Bone grafts are interposed into the resulting defect to support the transposed segment. Intermaxillary fixation is not required. The mobilized segment is secured by an orthodontic appliance or an arch bar, which is reinforced by quick-curing acrylic ("monomandibular fixation"). Fixation is maintained for six weeks.

The technique of Köle (1959b) consists of a mandibular dentoalveolar osteotomy to correct the anterior open bite malocclusion. The resected chin fragment is inserted into the space between the elevated dentoalveolar process and the remaining mandibular body (Fig. 29–183). Fixation of the anterior segment is established by the technique listed above and the fixation appliance is kept in place for six to eight weeks. The procedure can be used only when there is excessive vertical height of the mental symphysis; sufficient bone must be maintained in the remaining anterior portion of the mandible to preserve its strength and prevent accidental fracture.

A greater incidence of dental injuries (6.5 per cent) is associated with this technique (Pepersack, 1973). Because of the interposition of bone, the number of nonresponsive teeth is also increased (40 per cent). Kloosterman (1985), in a retrospective study of patients with anterior open bite corrected by the Köle procedure, noted a recurrence of the deformity in 32 per cent of patients in the series. Vitality of the teeth adjacent to the osteotomy was satisfactory if a tooth at the osteotomy site was extracted.

Segmental osteotomies require that the

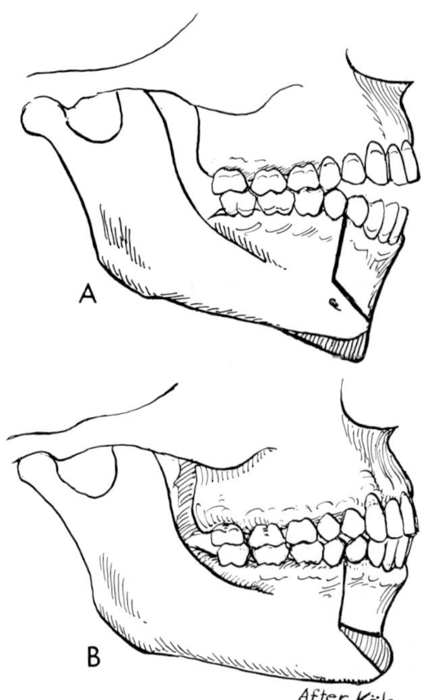

Figure 29–183. The Köle procedure to close an anterior open bite and reduce the vertical height of the symphysis. *A,* Outline of the osteotomies. Sufficient bone must be preserved between the anterior segmental dentoalveolar osteotomy and the horizontal osteotomy of the lower border of the mandible. The transverse cut of the dentoalveolar segmental osteotomy is made at least 5 mm below the apices of the teeth. *B,* The anterior open bite has been closed, and the resulting gap is filled with bone taken from the horizontal osteotomy. Monomaxillary fixation stabilizes the fragment; intermaxillary fixation is not required.

blood supply to the fragment be maintained through either a labial, buccal, or lingual mucoperiosteal flap. Elimination of the blood supply from both flaps leads to disastrous sequestration of the dentoalveolar segment. Parnes and Becker (1972) reported a case in which both the labial and palatal mucoperiosteum was elevated from the anterior maxillary segment; necrosis of the entire segment occurred. Revascularization studies in animals by Bell (1969), Bell and Levy (1970), and Brusati and Bottoli (1970) confirmed the long-standing clinical observation that preservation of a single mucoperiosteal flap is critical.

Ramus Osteotomy of Mandible. The sagittal split osteotomy of the ramus of the mandible has been employed to correct the anterior open bite deformity. As described on page 1280, the technique allows for counterclockwise rotation of the mandible to close the open bite and correct an associated micrognathia and Class II malocclusion. However, skeletal and dental relapse is common after this procedure for closure of Class II skeletal open bite deformity. It has been attributed to the required counterclockwise movement and the stretching of the suprahyoid and masticatory musculatures, as well as displacement of the condyle. Secondary procedures, such as an anterior mandibular dentoalveolar osteotomy, are required. *In general, it is preferable to correct open bite deformities with maxillary osteotomies.*

It has been reported that the inverted L-osteotomy of the mandibular ramus has more long-term stability in the horizontal and vertical dimensions when employed to correct a skeletal open bite deformity (Dattilo, Braun, and Sotereanos, 1985).

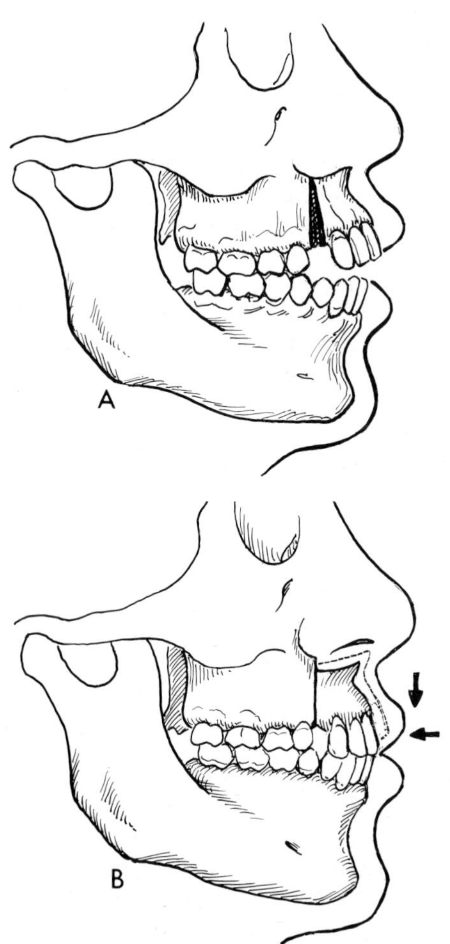

Figure 29–184. Anterior segmental dentoalveolar osteotomy for the closure of a maxillary open bite. *A,* An anterior dentoalveolar segment is outlined. *B,* The segment is mobilized; the open bite is closed.

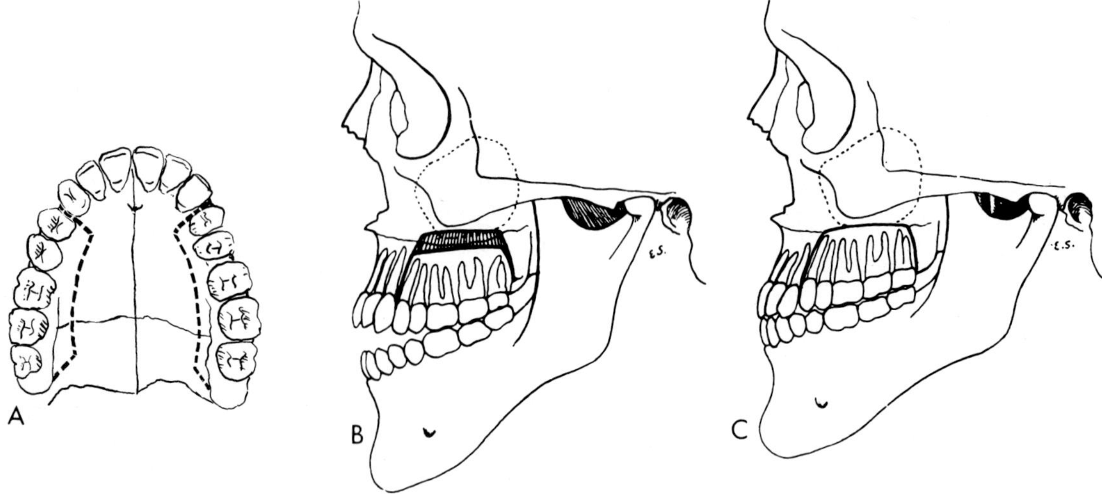

Figure 29–185. Schuchardt procedure for closure of an anterior open bite. *A,* In the first stage, bilateral osteotomies of the alveolar processes are performed as outlined. The palatal flap is reapplied, preserving the vascular supply. *B,* Six weeks later, a buccal mucoperiosteal flap is raised, and the lateral aspect of the maxilla is exposed. A segment of the maxilla above the apices of the teeth is resected as indicated by the shaded area. *C,* Correction achieved after vertical repositioning of the posterior maxillary segments; monomaxillary fixation is sufficient. (After Schuchardt.)

Anterior Segmental Dentoalveolar Osteotomy of Maxilla. This osteotomy was introduced by Cohn-Stock (1921) and modified by Wassmund (1927) and Wunderer (1962).

A transverse palatal mucosal incision provides exposure of the transverse osteotomy site (Fig. 29–184). Appropriately sized and shaped osteotomies can be performed through this incision. Vertical interdental osteotomies are then made between selected teeth. The anterior maxillary segment is repositioned with posterior and inferior pressure applied by the surgeon's fingers. Monomaxillary fixation is established with the posterior maxillary teeth.

Posterior Segmental Dentoalveolar Osteotomy of Maxilla. Schuchardt (1955) described a two-stage method applicable to the closure of a posterior open bite and also to the closure of an anterior open bite resulting from premature contact of overerupted posterior teeth (Fig. 29–185). In a first stage, after a palatal flap is raised, an anteroposterior osteotomy of the hard palate is performed along the base of the alveolar process on each side (Fig. 29–185*A*). In a second stage six weeks later, a buccal mucoperiosteal flap is raised, and anterior and interdental osteotomies are performed in a vertical direction to a level above the apices of the teeth; the two vertical osteotomies are joined by a horizontal osteotomy. Bone is resected above the apices of the teeth (Fig. 29–185*B*), and the anterior open bite is closed (Fig. 29–185*C*).

In the case of an anterior open bite, a segment of bone is resected superiorly, and the premolar-molar segment is elevated into the maxillary sinus to close the anterior open bite. Care must be taken when the hard palate osteotomy is being performed to direct the line of section into the maxillary sinus and not into the floor of the nose. If the osteotomy is made into the floor of the nose, the lateral nasal wall must be comminuted, or partly resected, when the mobilized dentoalveolar segment is impacted into the maxillary sinus.

When a posterior open bite is present, the mobilized fragment is lowered toward the occlusal plane to close the bite, and a bone graft is inserted in the resulting bony gap.

Kufner (1968) modified the Schuchardt procedure by performing the posterior maxillary segmental dentoalveolar osteotomy in one stage. A horizontal incision is made through the buccal mucosa, and the mucoperiosteal flap is raised. After the buccal osteotomy is performed and a predetermined segment of bone is resected (Fig. 29–186), a narrow, thin, tapered osteotome is introduced through the buccal osteotomy line, traversing the maxilary sinus to perform the osteotomy without injuring the palatal mucoperiosteum (Fig.

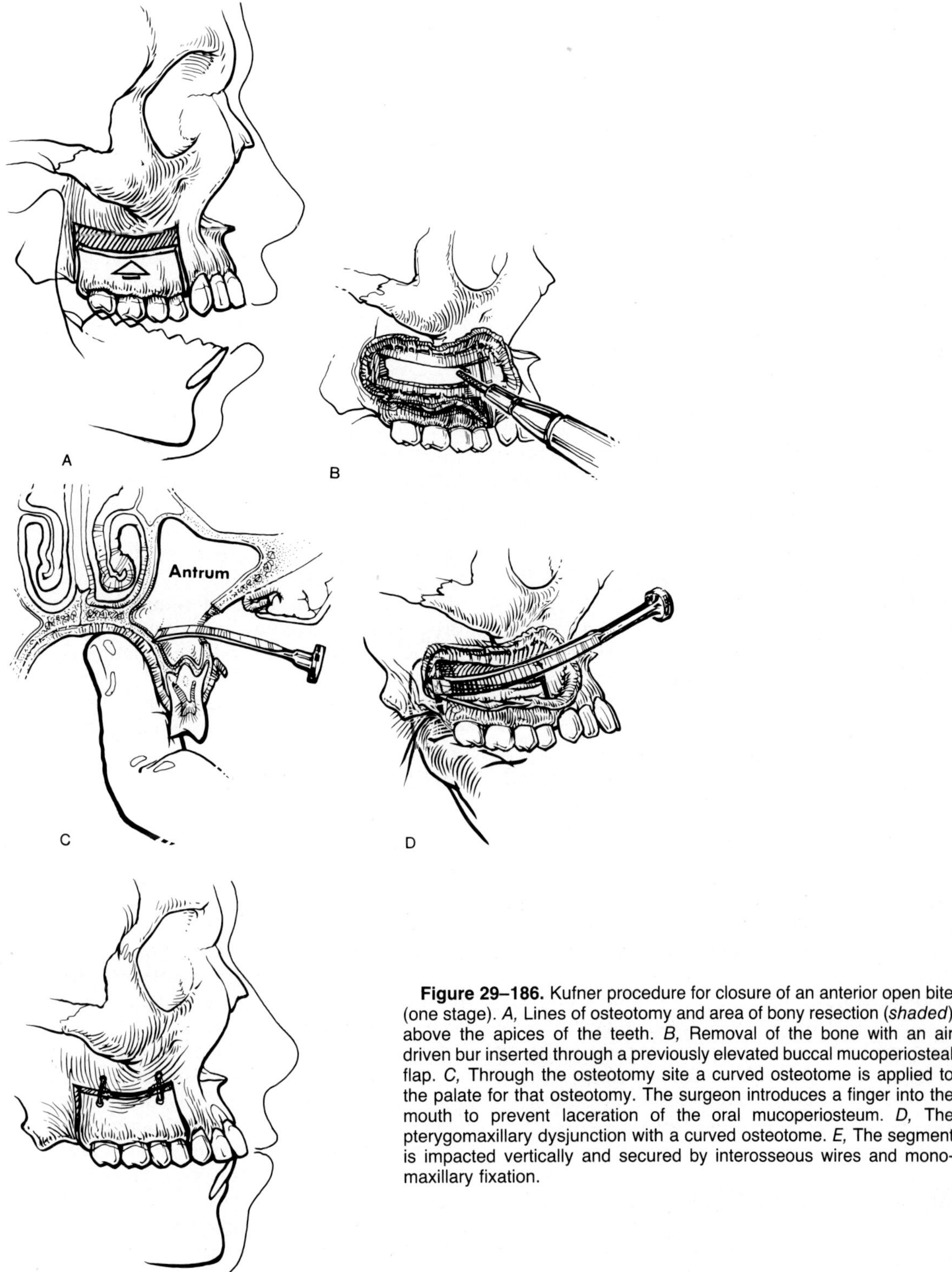

Figure 29–186. Kufner procedure for closure of an anterior open bite (one stage). *A,* Lines of osteotomy and area of bony resection (*shaded*) above the apices of the teeth. *B,* Removal of the bone with an air driven bur inserted through a previously elevated buccal mucoperiosteal flap. *C,* Through the osteotomy site a curved osteotome is applied to the palate for that osteotomy. The surgeon introduces a finger into the mouth to prevent laceration of the oral mucoperiosteum. *D,* The pterygomaxillary dysjunction with a curved osteotome. *E,* The segment is impacted vertically and secured by interosseous wires and monomaxillary fixation.

29–186*C*). The operator's finger inserted through the mouth and resting on the palatal mucosa ensures that the latter is not transected. Intermaxillary fixation is initially established to ensure the occlusion, but the patient is quickly placed in monomaxillary fixation for six to eight weeks (Fig. 29–186*E*). A patient who underwent the procedure is illustrated in Figure 29–187.

West and Epker (1972) applied a similar technique to correct unilateral or bilateral posterior maxillary crossbite, and to reposition the posterior maxillary alveolus distally when there is insufficient space for an unerupting canine or premolar tooth.

The posterior maxillary segmental osteotomy was criticized by surgeons because of the high incidence of relapse. However, Kufner (1968) and West and Epker (1972) showed that this is not the case if the mobilization is complete and the segment can be repositioned with ease. The transverse posterior palatal osteotomy (see Fig. 29–202), when indicated, is another technique that ensures complete mobilization and eliminates recurrence.

Total Maxillary Osteotomy. The Le Fort I osteotomy (see Fig. 29–196) can be employed to correct the sagittal, vertical, and horizontal aspects of the open bite deformity. In order to achieve satisfactory esthetic and occlusal relationships, it may be necessary to segmentalize, in addition to intruding, the posterior aspect of the Le Fort I segment.

Tongue Reduction. There are relatively few indications for tongue reduction in the correction of anterior open bite. In contemporary practice it is performed most commonly in patients with Down syndrome or other types of macroglossia in which the tongue is grossly enlarged by a pathologic process such as a lymphangioma (Maisels, 1979).

In a study of patients who underwent surgical correction of an anterior open bite deformity, all demonstrated improvement in tongue function (interdental lisp, tongue thrust) in the period of postoperative follow-up (Turvey, Journot, and Epker, 1976).

Maxillary Deformities

Deformities of the maxilla are often more complex than those of the mandible. Although the actual defect may be confined to the maxilla, other portions of the midfacial skeleton frequently are involved because of the intimate relationships among the maxilla, the nasal skeleton, the orbit, and the zygoma. Maxillary deficiencies are often part of a clefting syndrome such as a cleft lip-palate or an orbitofacial cleft (see Chap. 59). It should also be noted that there is often an element of maxillary hypoplasia in patients with mandibular prognathism and Class III malocclusion. The most severe maxillary deformities are observed in the craniosynostosis syndromes.

The growth and development of the nasomaxillary complex are discussed in Chapter 47.

CLASSIFICATION

Because of the intimate interrelationship of the bones of the midfacial skeleton, maxillary deformities should be considered in terms of the *dentoalveolar* and *skeletal* components. Dentoalveolar malocclusions occur alone or in combination with a skeletal jaw deformity, which in turn can be associated with malformations of the adjacent bony structures. By dividing a complex deformity into its dentoalveolar and skeletal parts, the analysis, diagnosis, and treatment are simplified.

When the maxillary anterior *dentoalveolar* segment is projected more labially than normal, the term *maxillary protrusion* (see p. 1333) is used; when the teeth are inclined more lingually than normal, *maxillary retrusion* (see p. 1342) is present. A similar buccolingual dentoalveolar segment malrelationship can be found between the posterior teeth. When the posterior maxillary arch width is excessive, a *unilateral* or *bilateral buccal crossbite* is produced. Transverse maxillary arch collapse, as seen in a patient with cleft palate, leads to a *lingual crossbite* malocclusion of the posterior teeth.

Some maxillary deformities exist mainly in the *anteroposterior* dimension of the skeletal maxilla. *Maxillary hypoplasia* or *micrognathia* designates underdevelopment or reduction of the skeletal component. This type of malformation is often seen in the patient with cleft palate or craniofacial synostosis (Crouzon's disease and Apert's syndrome). The maxilla is of normal size but in a retruded position in *maxillary retrognathia* (or retropositioned maxilla or retromaxillism). A common example is the retropositioned max-

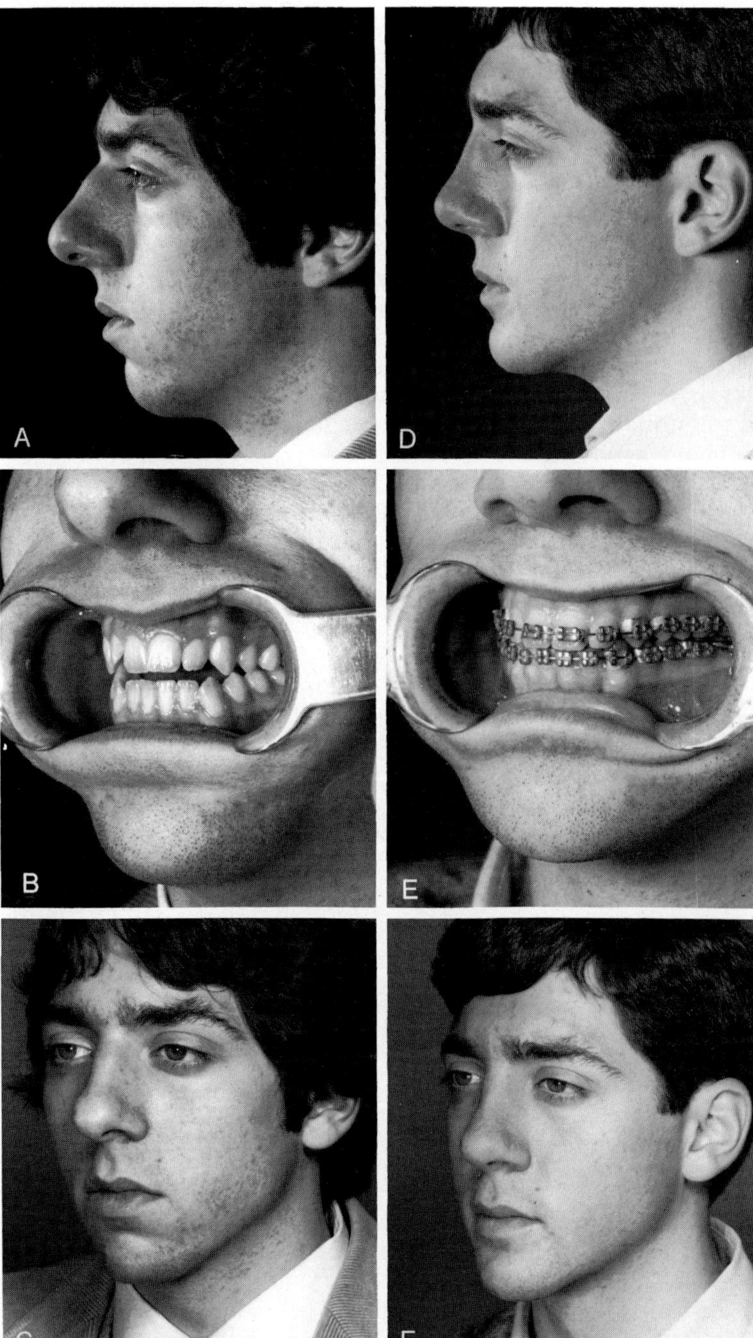

Figure 29–187. Correction of an anterior open bite by the Kufner procedure (see Fig. 29–186). *A* to *C*, Preoperative views. *D* to *F*, Postoperative appearance. A corrective rhinoplasty and genioplasty were also performed. The patient had undergone minor orthodontic adjustments in the postoperative period.

illa that is found after a malunited midfacial fracture. In all the above examples, the mandible, though normal in size, appears to be prognathic (mandibular pseudoprognathism).

Idiopathic *maxillary prognathism*, in which the entire maxilla is anteriorly positioned, is a rare condition. Usually the protrusion is localized in the anterior dentoalveolar segment, and the maxillary dentoalveolar segment drifts forward and downward. This type of maxillary deformity is seen in patients with mandibular micrognathia. With associated hemangiomas or lymphangiomas, as well as tumors such as fibrous dysplasia, the maxilla is often severely protruded.

The "dish-face" deformity is an example of a nasomaxillary skeletal deformity. The entire nasomaxillary complex is displaced posteriorly. This type of deformity results from a malunited midfacial fracture, or is seen in Binder's syndrome.

Other maxillary deformities are apparent in the *transverse* dimension (decrease in maxillary arch width) and *vertical* dimension (vertical maxillary excess or long face syndrome, and vertical maxillary deficiency or short face syndrome).

PREOPERATIVE PLANNING

The diagnosis made from the clinical examination of the patient is correlated with analysis of the photographs, the dental study models, and the cephalometric roentgenogram.

It is critical to assess lip posture and relationships. The amount of maxillary incisor show at rest should not exceed 3 mm and there should not be more than 1 mm of gingival exposure on smiling. The nasolabial angle is usually obtuse in vertical maxillary excess.

Dental casts are invaluable aids in studying dentoalveolar malformations. A duplicate cast is sectioned and the fragments repositioned to simulate the maxillary osteotomies in a manner similar to the planning employed in the correction of mandibular deformities (see Fig. 29–21).

Cephalometric measurements of primary concern are the SN length, SNA and SNB angles, midfacial height (N-ANS, ANS-SD, ANS-UIE) and U1-SN angles (see Figs. 29–8, 29–10). The U1-SN cephalometric measurement is used to assess the amount of protrusion or retrusion of the anterior maxillary dentoalveolar segment. Cephalometric analysis provides a means of distinguishing the respective anatomic characteristics of nasomaxillary hypoplasia and craniofacial dysostosis (Firmin, Coccaro, and Converse, 1974; Zide, Grayson, and McCarthy, 1981a,b, 1982). When the midfacial advancement procedures are planned, it is helpful to record the SN length and the vertical midfacial dimension. The SNA and SNB angular measurements can be misinterpreted if the SN length is not taken into consideration. Smaller SN measurements contribute toward a larger SNB angle, indicating mandibular prognathism in the presence of an average-sized mandible (Fig. 29–188). SNA angles are similarly affected by the decreased SN length.

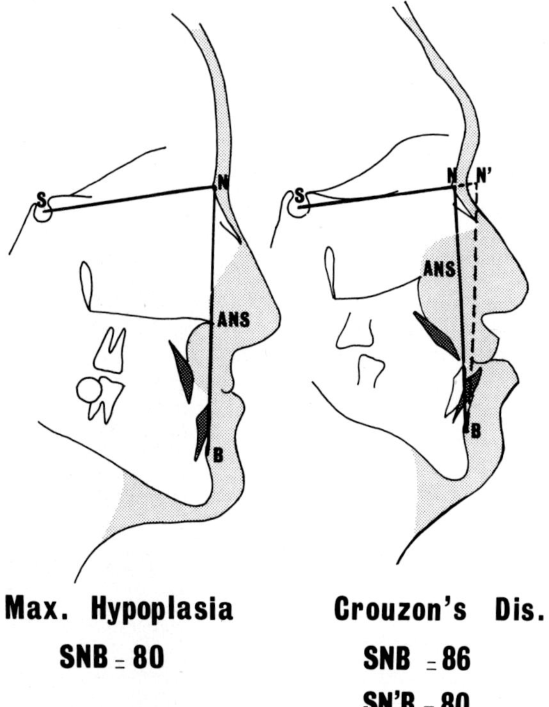

Figure 29–188. Relationship between sella-nasion (SN) and facial profile angles. Although the patient with maxillary hypoplasia and the patient with Crouzon's disease appear to have mandibular prognathism, neither has an abnormal lower jaw. The pseudoprognathic appearance is caused by hypoplasia of the maxilla. In the patient with maxillary hypoplasia, SNB = 80 degrees (which measures the projection of the mandible), within the average range. In the patient with Crouzon's disease, SNB = 86 degrees; however, if SN were extended to a normal length (SN′), the SN′B angle would fall within the normal range. (From Firmin, F., Coccaro, P. J., and Converse, J. M.: Cephalometric analysis in diagnosis and treatment planning of craniofacial dysostoses. Plast. Reconstr. Surg., *54*:300, 1974. Copyright 1974, The Williams & Wilkins Company, Baltimore.)

The hypoplastic maxillary region may require an advancement as well as a downward rotation to provide the necessary forward projection and increase in vertical facial dimension. The amount of midfacial elongation needed is estimated from the vertical midfacial measurements. In addition to assessing the amount of displacement required, the cephalogram aids in indicating the size and volume of the bone grafts required to fill the voids in the skeletal framework.

Henderson (1974) described a technique that combines the use of transparent cephalometric and photographic cut-outs to help predict the final facial profile. Photographs are enlarged to the dimensions of the cephalogram and are sectioned along the lines of the osteotomies. The parts of the photograph are recomposed to conform to the movement of the skeleton (see Fig. 29–25).

SURGICAL APPROACH TO MIDFACE

The maxilla and midface can be exposed through an intraoral incision, the midface degloving procedure, an extraoral incision through the lower eyelid, a conjunctival approach, a coronal scalp flap, or a combination of these incisions.

Intraoral Approach. The oral cavity offers a direct approach to the craniofacial skeleton. Incisions in the oral vestibule, extended through the periosteum, permit subperiosteal exposure of the bones. Through this approach the maxilla and zygoma are exposed up to the level of the infraorbital rims.

The two basic types of intraoral incisions previously described for the exposure of the mandible are also applicable to the maxilla. These are the *labiobuccal vestibular incision* and the *mucogingival incision* (see Fig. 29–45). The mucogingival incision has limitations, since it is more difficult to suture without tension if the maxillary skeleton is advanced or augmented with onlay bone grafts.

Midface Degloving Procedure. Converse described the intraoral approach to the maxilla and the mandible in 1950 and the mandibular degloving procedure in 1959 (see Fig. 29–46). Casson, Bonanno, and Converse (1974) described a midfacial degloving procedure that is performed in a similar fashion.

Bilateral intercartilaginous incisions are made between the alar and lateral cartilages (Fig. 29–189*A*). The soft tissues over the lateral cartilages and the nasal bones are elevated (Fig. 29–189*B*). A transfixion incision is extended down along the dorsal and caudal portions of the septal cartilage to the nasal spine (Fig. 29–189*C*). An intraoral incision is made through the mucosa on the labial aspect of the upper vestibule (Fig. 29–189*D*); the periosteum is raised, and the nasal spine and the piriform aperture are exposed. The attachments of the nasal tissues to the piriform aperture are exposed and severed. The premaxillary dissection is joined to the transfixion incision. Retractors are inserted and the subperiosteal elevation is continued upward to the inferior orbital rim, exposing and preserving the infraorbital nerve. Complete exposure of the midfacial skeleton can thus be obtained (Fig. 29–189*E*). After the skeletal procedures are completed, the nasal tissues are carefully redraped and the transfixion incision is sutured; the intranasal and labial incisions are also sutured.

Lower Eyelid Approach. The lower eyelid incision is an excellent approach to the upper portion of the maxilla. The preferred incision is one made along the lower border of the tarsus; the septum orbitale is readily exposed, after a horizontal incision is made through the orbicularis oculi muscle, and is followed down to the orbital rim. This approach avoids penetration of the septum orbitale and extrusion of orbital fat (see Chap. 33).

Conjunctival Approach. An alternative approach is through an incision in the conjunctiva of the lower eyelid (see Chap. 33). Because this approach may result in extrusion of orbital fat and vertical shortening of the lower lid, the cutaneous incision below the tarsus is preferred. The lower eyelid incision, combined with the midfacial degloving incision and other supplementary incisions, provides adequate exposure of the midface skeleton.

Exposure of Midface Skeleton Through Coronal Scalp Flap. The coronal scalp flap extends behind the hairline from preauricular area to preauricular area. It is wise to place the incision sufficiently posterior to the hairline in male patients to allow for a receding hairline. The flap is raised through the areolar tissue between the galea aponeurotica and the pericranium. The pericranium is then raised from the bone with a periosteal elevator.

The subperiosteal elevation is extended to the supraorbital rims, along the lateral or-

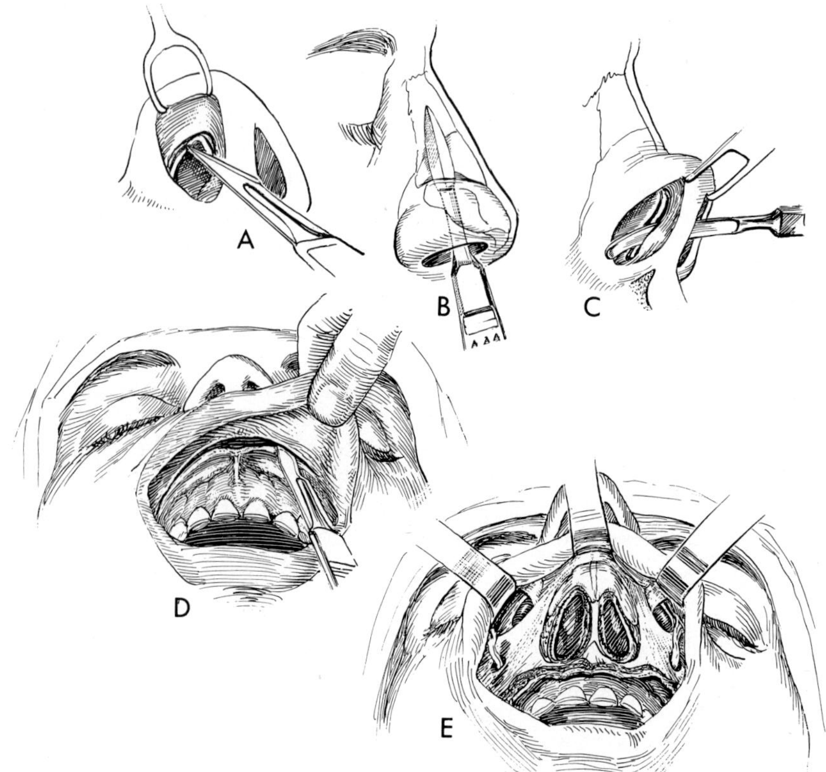

Figure 29–189. The midface degloving procedure. *A,* Bilateral intercartilaginous incisions are made as in a rhinoplasty. *B,* The soft tissues are dissected over the lateral nasal cartilages bilaterally. *C,* The transfixation incision is illustrated. *D,* An incision is made through the mucosa on the labial aspect of the sulcus. *E,* The midfacial skeleton is exposed subperiosteally, respecting the infraorbital nerves. (From Casson, P. R., Bonanno, P. C., and Converse, J. M.: The midface degloving procedure. Plast. Reconstr. Surg., *53*:102, 1974. Copyright 1974, The Williams & Wilkins Company, Baltimore.)

bital rims down to the zygomatic arch, and over the zygoma on each side. If additional exposure is required, the periorbita is raised from the roof, from the medial and lateral walls of the orbits, and along the bony dorsum of the nose. The scalp flap is thus loosened, providing exposure of a major portion of the midface skeleton (see also Chap. 33).

Blood Supply. Preservation of the blood supply to the mobilized skeletal segment is of paramount importance. The blood supply of the anterior maxillary teeth is derived from branches of the internal maxillary artery (Fig. 29–190). The anterosuperior alveolar branches originate from the infraorbital artery within the infraorbital canal, and descend through the anterior alveolar canals to supply the upper incisors and canine teeth and the mucous membrane. The posterosuperior alveolar artery originates from the internal maxillary artery in the pterygopalatine fossa. As it descends over the tuberosity of the maxilla, it divides into numerous branches to supply the molars and premolars. Other branches continue forward on the alveolar process to supply the gingiva. All these vessels anastomose with various branches of the ophthalmic and external maxillary arteries that supply the face.

The descending palatine artery, a branch of the internal maxillary artery, descends through the pterygopalatine canal and emerges at the greater palatine foramen. It courses forward toward the incisive canal in a groove on the hard palate on the medial aspect of the alveolar border. The artery then anastomoses with branches of the posterior septal arteries, which pass through the canal.

The sphenopalatine artery, another branch of the internal maxillary artery, enters the nasal cavity through the sphenopalatine foramen and terminates on the nasal septum.

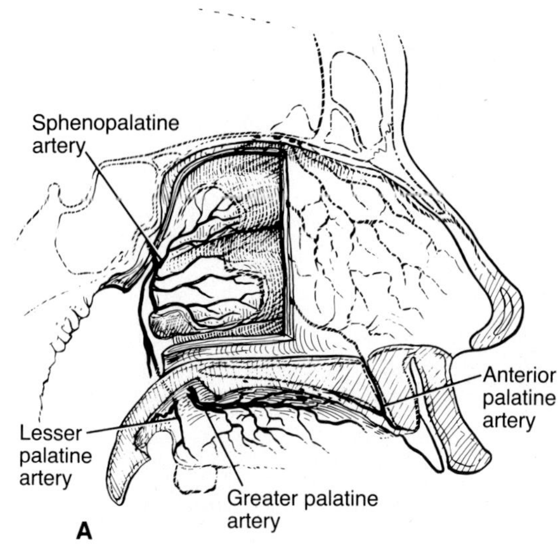

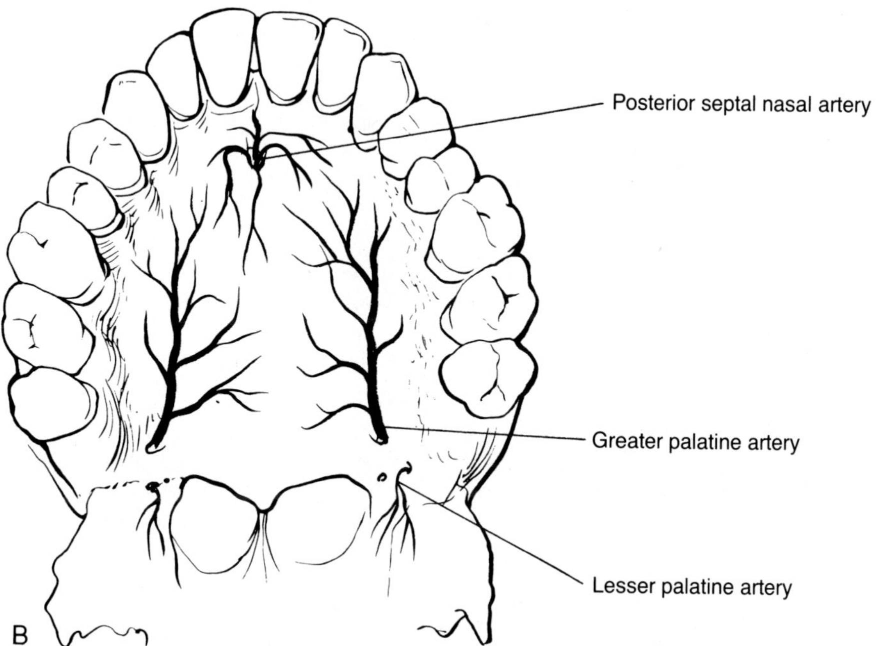

Figure 29–190. Blood supply of the maxilla. *A,* The vascular supply of the maxilla originates from the pterygopalatine portion of the internal maxillary artery. The *posterosuperior alveolar artery* passes over the maxillary tuberosity. The *infraorbital artery,* which also originates from the internal maxillary artery in similar fashion, gives the *anterosuperior alveolar* branches. The *descending palatine artery,* passing through the pterygopalatine canal, supplies a major portion of the palate and forms anastomoses with branches of the *anterior palatine artery,* which passes through the incisive foramen. *B,* Palatal view.

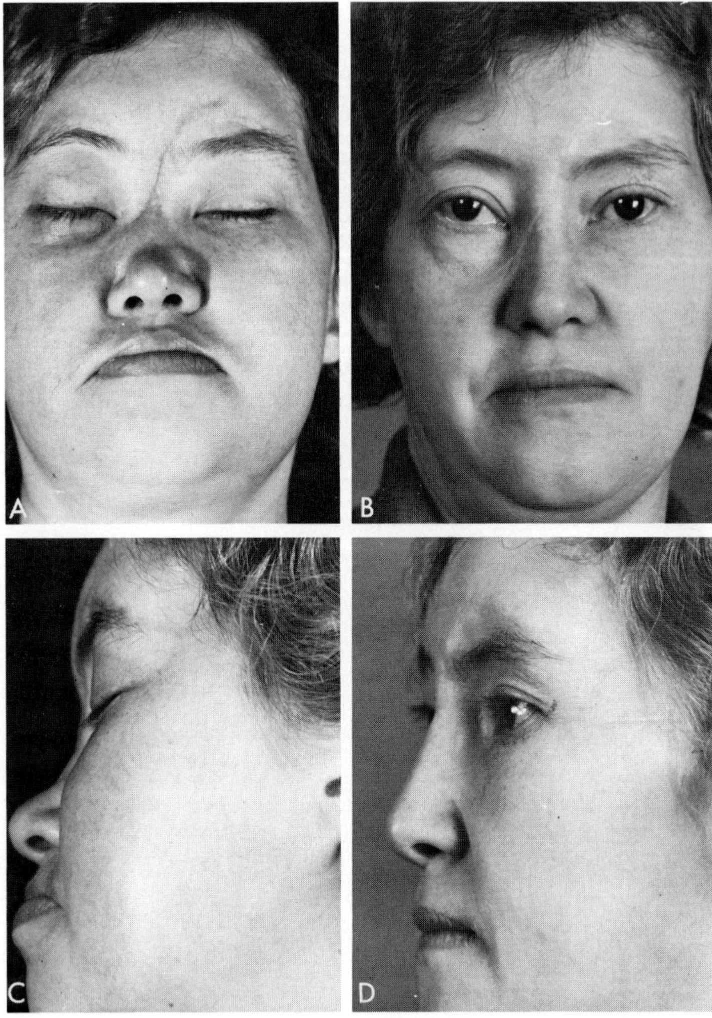

Figure 29–191. Contour improvement in an edentulous patient by a denture. *A, C,* Preoperative appearance. The deformity resulted from an automobile accident. Note the saddle nose deformity and the retrusion of the nasomaxillary area. *B, D,* Appearance after iliac bone graft reconstruction of the nose and a denture with an upward extension into the labiobuccal sulcus deepened by a skin graft inlay.

It forms anastomoses with branches of the descending (greater) palatine artery and the septal branch of the superior labial artery.

The vascularity of the area permits a mucoperiosteal flap to maintain the blood supply to a mobilized maxillary segment.

MICROGNATHIA-RETROGNATHIA

Three types of treatment are available to correct maxillary micrognathia-retrognathia: prosthodontic treatment, onlay bone grafts, and osteotomy of the maxilla.

Prosthodontic Treatment

This is the oldest method and it was originally used in edentulous or partially edentulous patients. A denture that protrudes under the upper lip increases the projection and thus improves contour. To obtain further projection, the sulcus is deepened and lined with a skin graft inlay (Fig. 29–191). The denture can then be extended upward as far as the piriform aperture or even along the sides of the piriform aperture. In the past the prosthodontic appliance was more extensively applied in patients with a normal complement of teeth; an overlay denture was made over the patient's teeth to improve contour. The nasomaxillary skin graft inlay technique (see p. 1389) involves an even more extensive application of prosthodontic techniques to obtain contour restoration.

Prosthodontic restoration can be combined with bone grafting of the alveolar process in edentulous patients to obtain improved retention and contour.

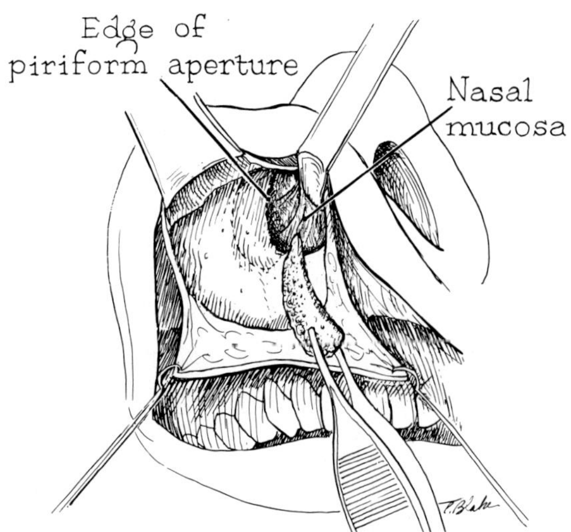

Figure 29–192. Crescent-shaped bone grafts are placed around the piriform aperture and are combined with a graft to the nose to correct a saddle nose deformity with naso-maxillary depression. Costal cartilage grafts can also be employed. (From Converse, J. M.: Technique of bone grafting for contour restoration of the face. Plast. Reconstr. Surg., *14*:332, 1954. Copyright 1954, The Williams & Wilkins Company, Baltimore.)

Onlay Bone Grafts

Restoration of contour can be achieved by bone grafts applied through either the intraoral or extraoral route (Converse, 1950; Schmid, 1952; Converse and Shapiro, 1954).

In nasomaxillary deformities with depression not only of the nose but also of the adjacent maxillary portion of the face, bone grafts are placed over the dorsum of the nose and over the maxilla around the edge of the nose and around the edge of the piriform aperture. The exposure is obtained subperiosteally through the intraoral approach. Crescent-shaped, pyramidal pieces of cancellous bone are placed on each side to correct the nasomaxillary depression (Fig. 29–192). Large, depressed areas of the maxilla are repaired by a bone graft, which consists of a shell-like segment that is shaped from the calvaria or the medial aspect of the ilium (Fig. 29–193). The onlay bone graft is applied as a bridge over the defect. Small chips of cancellous bone are placed in the intervening crevices beneath the onlay bone to improve contact with the host bone and to increase the projection of the graft. An overcorrection is necessary to compensate for some degree of bone absorption, particularly if a large quantity of bone is employed. After the vestibular incision is sutured, an external pressure dressing immobilizes the graft and prevents hematoma formation. A contour restoration obtained by this technique is shown in Figure 29–194. Other techniques of contour restoration by bone grafting are discussed later in this chapter. It should be noted that cartilage grafts and alloplastic implants are alternative techniques.

Onlay bone grafts are not as reliable in maintaining contour as the actual modification of the facial skeleton by advancement osteotomy combined with bone grafting. Much progress has been made in the treatment of skeletal deformities of the maxilla by the development of selective osteotomies.

Maxillary Osteotomies to Correct Skeletal Deformities

When the maxillary deformity is skeletal and extends beyond the dentoalveolar complex, major osteotomies must often be performed. The choice of type of osteotomy depends on (1) the extent of the maxillary deformity, (2) the portion of the maxilla that is affected, (3) the type of malocclusion, and (4) the degree of involvement of the neighboring structures, such as the nose, zygoma, and orbits.

Maxillary osteotomies are generally performed along the classic lines of fracture as described by Le Fort (1901): the lower maxillary osteotomy (Le Fort I), the pyramidal naso-orbitomaxillary osteotomy (Le Fort II), and the high maxillary osteotomy (Le Fort III), in which the midfacial skeleton is detached from the cranium. Variations and combinations of these osteotomies are indicated for a wide variety of malformations, such as maxillary micrognathia and retrognathia, open bite deformities, and craniofacial malformations.

Complete Horizontal Low Maxillary Osteotomy (Le Fort I). The complete horizontal low maxillary osteotomy transects the maxilla at the level of a Le Fort I maxillary fracture, above the dentoalveolar segment of the jaw and the floor of the nose. Wassmund performed this type of procedure in 1927 to close an open bite malocclusion. Axhausen (1934) was the first to advance the lower portion of the maxilla using this technique. Schuchardt (1942) applied forward traction by means of a pulley and weight system to produce an advancement of the sectioned

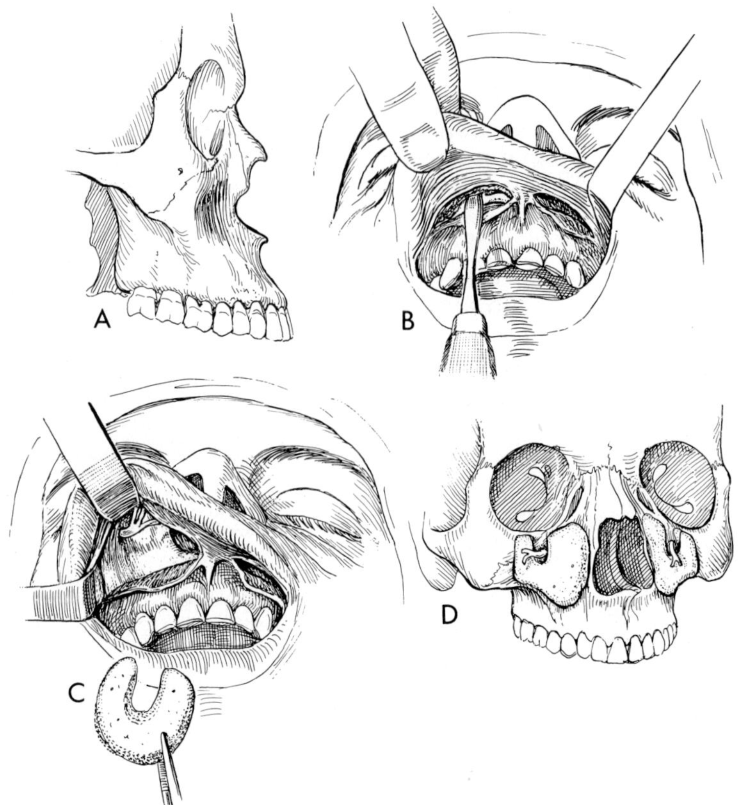

Figure 29–193. Contour restoration by onlay bone grafts through the intraoral route. *A,* Profile view of the depression of the anterior maxillary wall. *B,* After an incision is made through the mucosa on the labial aspect of the sulcus, the periosteum is raised from the bone. *C,* The exposed piriform aperture and infraorbital nerve. *D,* Onlay bone grafts in position filling the depressed areas of the maxilla.

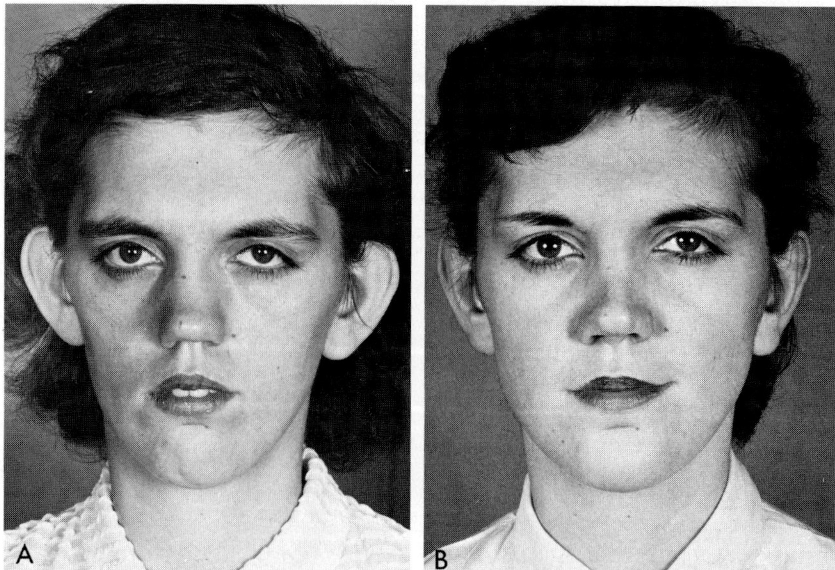

Figure 29–194. Contour restoration of the maxilla by bone grafting. *A,* Preoperative appearance showing retrusion of the nasomaxillary area. *B,* Restoration of contour obtained by bone grafts applied over the maxilla through the intraoral approach, as illustrated in Figure 29–193. Additional corrective measures included orthodontic treatment, a corrective rhinoplasty, and corrective surgery for protruding ears.

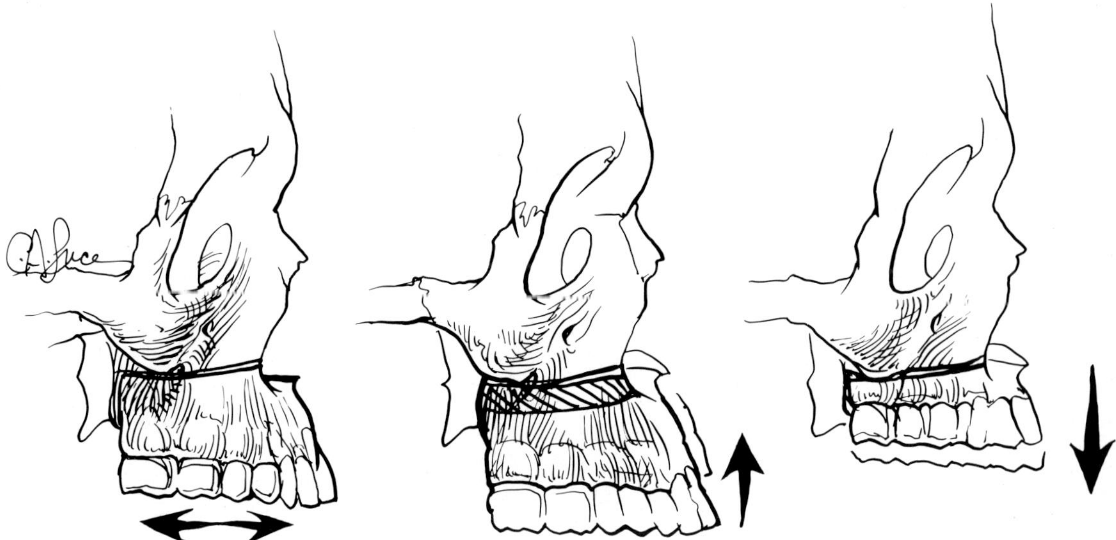

Figure 29–195. The versatility of the Le Fort I osteotomy. Note the multiple dimensions in which the segment can be mobilized.

maxillary segment. Transection of the pterygoid processes in the Le Fort I osteotomy was described by Moore and Ward (1949), and was recommended by Ullik (1970) in adult patients who had been operated on for cleft lip and palate. Hogeman and Willmar (1967) reported a series of 49 cases of maxillary retrusion treated by a complete low maxillary osteotomy, which included the pterygoid processes in the transection. Colantino and Dudley (1970) used a similar complete horizontal osteotomy, including the pterygoid plates, to retroposition the maxilla in the correction of maxillary prognathism.

Willmar (1974), in reviewing the historical aspects of the Le Fort I osteotomy, noted that Dingman and Harding (1951) were the first to separate the maxillary tuberosities from the pterygoid processes in performing the operation. Converse and Shapiro (1952), in a different type of operation, also separated the tuberosities from the pterygoid processes but preserved the posterior portion of the hard palate. Dupont, Ciaburro, and Prévost (1974) advocated sectioning through the tuberosity rather than at the pterygomaxillary interface.

The use of bone grafts over the osteotomy sites was reported by Gillies and Rowe (1954), Cupar (1954), Cernéa and associates (1955), and Lévignac (1958). In 1969 Obwegeser introduced the technique of wedging a bone graft between the pterygoid process and the tuberosity of the maxilla for stabilization and the bony consolidation of the advanced maxillary segment. In recent years, rigid skeletal fixation has been employed more frequently for stabilization of the mobilized segment and has decreased the need for bone grafting this gap.

The Le Fort I osteotomy is an extremely versatile technique since it allows multidimensional movement of the maxilla (Fig. 29–195).

Technique of Le Fort I Osteotomy. The procedure (Fig. 29–196) is performed under general hypotensive anesthesia administered through a nasotracheal tube that is sutured to the membranous septum. An incision is made through the mucoperiosteum approximately 7 mm above the mucogingival junction; the mucoperiosteum is undermined backward to and around the maxillary tuberosity. The procedure is repeated on the contralateral side. The mucosa is then elevated from the lateral wall and floor of the nasal cavity as well as the lower aspect of the septum.

The maxilla is sectioned transversely from the edge of the piriform aperture back to the maxillary tuberosity (Fig. 29–196*A*) with a mechanical saw. The level of the osteotomy should be sufficiently high to leave 3 to 5 mm of bone above the apices of the teeth. An additional 2 to 3 mm should be preserved if miniplate fixation is to be used.

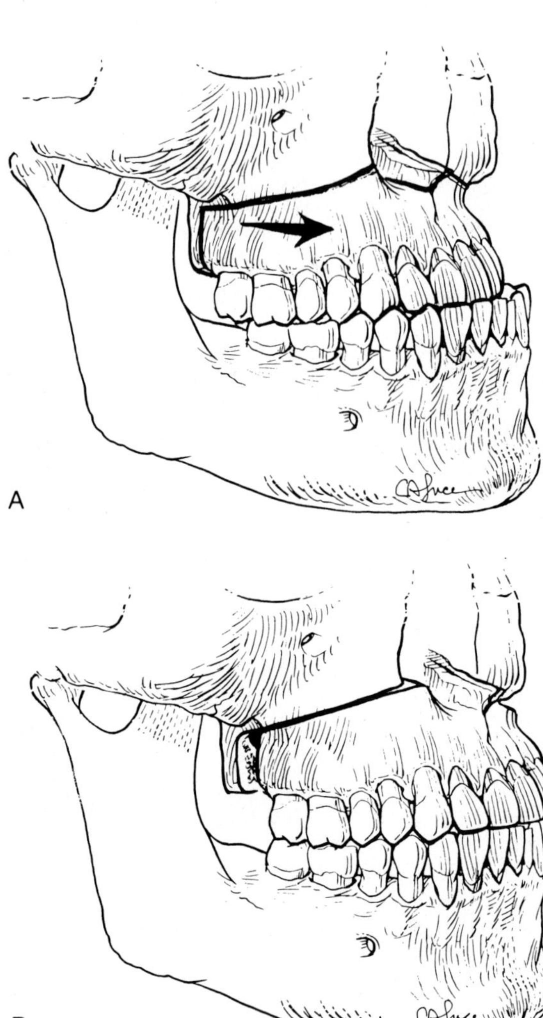

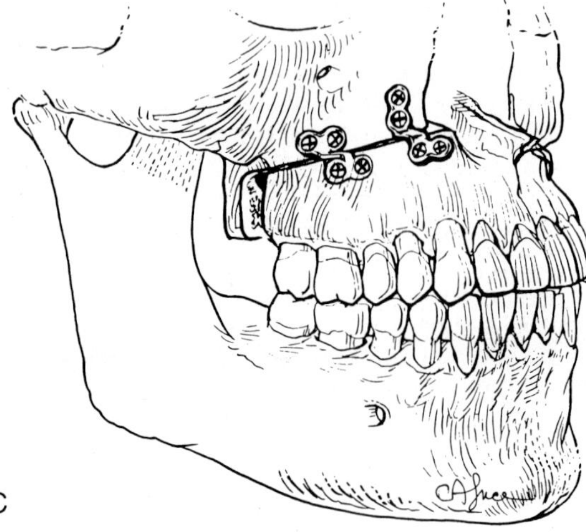

Figure 29–196. The Le Fort I advancement osteotomy. *A,* Lines of osteotomy. *B,* Anterior mobilization of the maxillary segment. *C,* Miniplate fixation of the buttresses.

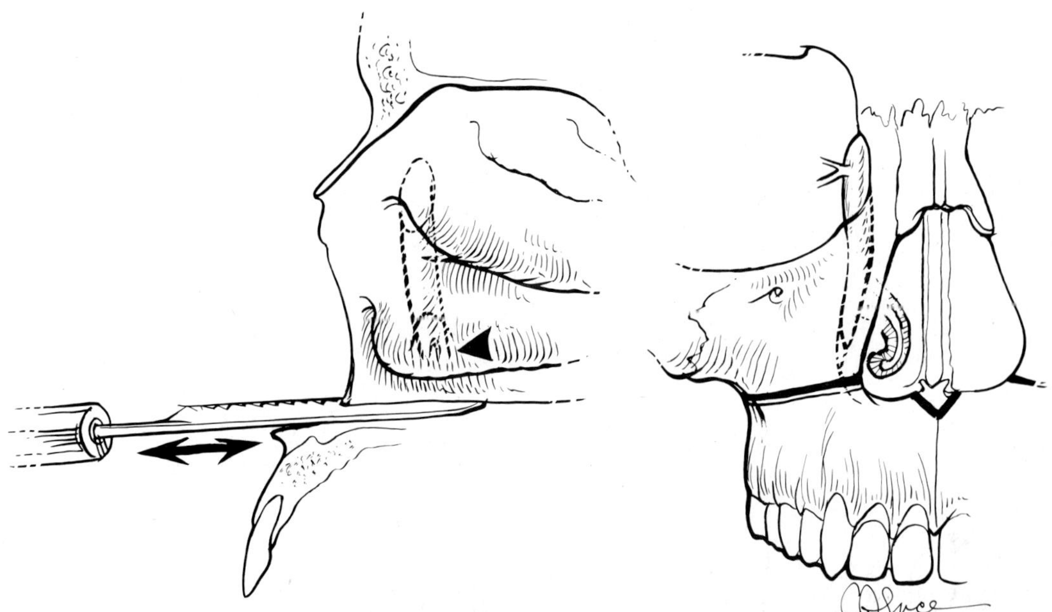

Figure 29–197. Le Fort I osteotomy: reciprocating saw to section the septum in a V-like fashion without disrupting the anterior nasal spine. Note the position of the nasolacrimal duct.

The septum is sectioned at the base of the vomer along the entire length of the nasal floor (Fig. 29–197). Despite the presence of the nasotracheal tube, the septal procedure is performed without difficulty. The nasotracheal tube must be protected. The safest methods of sectioning the septum are to use a double-guarded osteotome or a reciprocating saw placed alongside the tube and directed away from it during the sawing movement.

The lateral walls of the nasal cavity are sectioned with an osteotome or a reciprocating saw. The approach is through the nasal cavity or across the maxillary sinus through the previously made osteotomy along the anterior surface of the maxilla. The line of osteotomy is kept at the level of the nasal floor to avoid injury to the orifice of the nasolacrimal duct (Fig. 29–197).

The maxillary segment is separated posteriorly from its attachment at the pterygopalatine suture (see Fig. 29–196*B*). A curved periosteal elevator is placed beneath the mucoperiosteum to and around the maxillary tuberosity as far back as the pterygomaxillary junction. A thin, sharp, curved osteotome (Kawamoto-Tessier) *gently* severs the connection between the tuberosity and the pterygoid processes (Fig. 29–198). Undue force applied during the disjunction can fracture the pterygoid plates. If the pterygoid plates are fractured, the bone graft placed in the area will be deprived of a posterior buttress.

The osteotomized maxillary segment can be "downfractured" (Fig. 29–199). At this point there is usually a remaining portion of skeletal attachment at the posterior aspect of

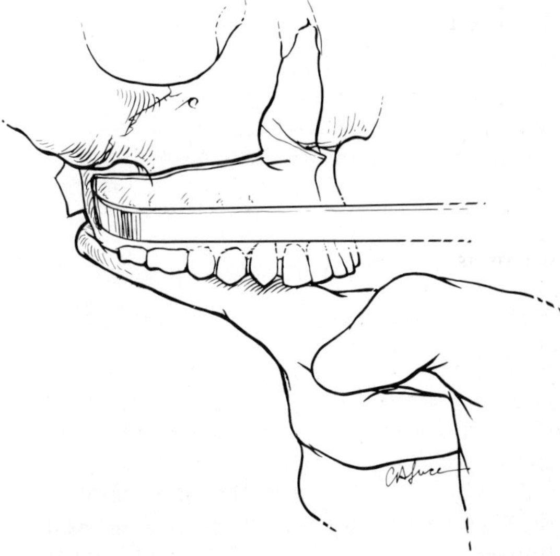

Figure 29–198. Pterygomaxillary disimpaction with a curved osteotome. Note that the operator's index finger, placed along the maxillary occlusal surface, ensures proper placement of the osteotome.

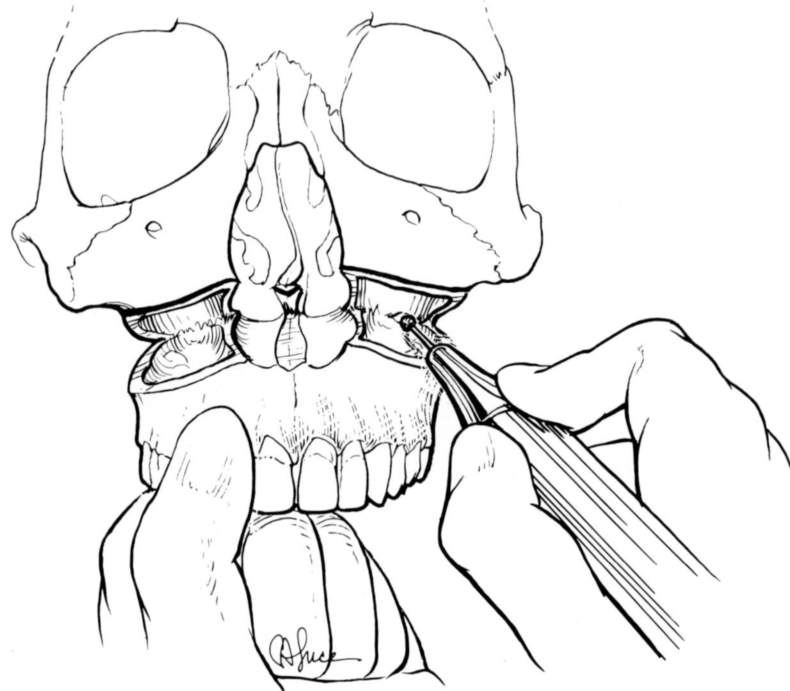

Figure 29–199. Downfracture of the Le Fort I segment with the surgeon's fingers allows completion of the osteotomy of the posterior maxillary sinus under direct vision.

the maxillary sinus. This can be divided with an air-driven bur under direct vision.

The remaining resistance to advancement is encountered from the soft tissues, and is overcome by side to side distal pressure or by slow and careful manipulation with a pair of Rowe disimpaction forceps. One branch of the forceps is placed on the floor of the nose and the other on the hard palate. Forward traction and rocking are exerted in a circular motion until the desired position is attained. The lower maxillary segment, once "rocked" loose, can be advanced into position. The new occlusal relationships are maintained by intermaxillary fixation using an orthodontic appliance or by miniplate fixation (see Figs. 29–38, 29–196).

Before the establishment of osseous fixation, the mandible is recessed so as to place the condyles into the glenoid fossae. *Failure to seat the condyles properly will result in a posterior and upward movement of the mandible and a malocclusion when the intermaxillary fixation is released.* If miniplates are used, they are placed in the thick bone of the piriform rim and the zygomaticomaxillary buttress. The plates must be perfectly adapted to the bone, and the compression mode should not be used or a shift in the occlusion will occur; the bone will move toward the plate and not vice versa. If stainless steel wire (26 gauge) is employed for the osteosynthesis, 1 mm drill holes are placed in the same thick bony regions. Internal suspension wires can be passed through the upper set of drill holes and secured through an intermediary loop of wire to the maxillary arch wire. This secondary loop of wire can be adjusted, if necessary, during the postoperative period without jeopardizing the main suspension loop.

Bone grafts are not required if the maxilla is advanced less than 6 to 7 mm. Their presence is required whenever the vertical dimensions of the maxilla are concomitantly increased or when the osteotomy is performed in patients with cleft palate. A measured bone graft can be wedged into the pterygopalatine space to help maintain the forward projection of the detached maxilla, or can be placed along the osteotomy lines to assist bone consolidation.

The advancement of the maxillary segment produces a step between the repositioned segment and the intact portion of the maxilla; bone grafts placed over this area improve contour and facilitate bone consolidation.

The mucoperiosteal incision is sutured. If miniplate fixation is not employed, intermaxillary fixation and internal wires are usually left in position for six to eight weeks. After removal of the intermaxillary wires, orthodontic surveillance is continued to verify the maintenance of the corrected occlusal relationships (Fig. 29–200).

Maxillary Advancement in Cleft Palate Patients. Maxillary hypoplasia is commonly associated with unilateral and bilateral clefts. When the molar relationships are adequate and there are maxillary dental spaces, a premolar segmental maxillary advancement osteotomy may be indicated (see Fig. 29–169). When the maxillary dental arch is in a Class III malocclusion, the Le Fort I advancement osteotomy is the operation of choice (Fig. 29–201). After the osteotomy, the advancement is more difficult than in idiopathic maxillary hypoplasia, and requires considerable force and forward and downward traction with the Rowe disimpaction forceps.

Retromolar Segmental Advancement of Maxilla. This operation was designed to preserve the posterior potion of the hard palate and to avoid advancement of the soft palate and consequent velopharyngeal incompetence. It is indicated in patients in whom velopharyngeal competence is threatened by a Le Fort I advancement osteotomy (see p. 1376).

The operation (Converse and Shapiro, 1952) was devised to advance the lower portion of the maxilla with the dentoalveolar component, to reestablish dental occlusion, and to restore facial contour.

Exposure of the maxilla is similar to that employed in the Le Fort I advancement osteotomy; the incision is extended backward toward the maxillary tuberosity on each side. The osteotomy is performed on both sides beyond and around the maxillary tuberosities (Fig. 29–202*A*, *B*). The osteotomy around the maxillary tuberosity extends through the pterygopalatine interface to a point above the level of the roots of the molar teeth; it extends around the tuberosity and in a forward direction on the palatal aspect of the alveolar process to a point situated anterior to the greater palatine foramen on each side (Fig. 29–202*C*). The palatine process of the maxilla is sectioned transversely, including the vomer, leaving intact the attachment of the greater portion of the vomer to the floor of the nose. The septal cartilage is exposed by raising a mucoperichondrial flap and is severed along its insertion into the vomer groove; the incision through the cartilage joins the transverse palatal osteotomy. The severed portion of the maxilla is mobilized, loosened, and advanced to the planned intermaxillary relationships (Fig. 29–202*D*). Bone grafts are wedged into the line of osteotomy through the hard palate. Sutures are placed to reapply the mucoperiosteal flap to the gingival tissues. Fixation is maintained by intermaxillary wiring or miniplate fixation, as previously described.

Results. The results of the Le Fort I advancement osteotomy are usually satisfactory when the operative steps outlined above are followed. An example of such a result is shown in Figure 29–203. The intraoral views before and after the surgical advancement are shown in Figure 29–204. The preoperative and postoperative cephalograms illustrate the degree of advancement obtained (Fig. 29–205).

Willmar (1974) reported the long-term dentoalveolar and skeletal changes observed after Le Fort I osteotomies in 106 patients. Metallic implants accurately recorded the positional changes of the maxilla relative to the anterior cranial base. It was noted that the dentoalveolar relationships remained stable throughout the observation period of up to three years; small changes were insignificant. The posterior portion of the maxillary skeleton in patients with cleft lip and palate shifted by upward of 1.0 mm during the first postoperative year and remained stable thereafter. In patients with idiopathic and post-traumatic anterior crossbites, the entire maxilla had a tendency to move upward during the period of intermaxillary fixation. The anterior portion of the maxilla was displaced superiorly 1.8 to 2.3 mm and the posterior portion 0.8 to 1.1 mm. The upward shift was greater in males. Changes in maxillary position did not occur after removal of the intermaxillary fixation. Since the occlusal relationships remained fairly constant, one must assume that the dentoalveolar segment compensated for the skeletal changes.

Similar findings were reported by Teuscher and Sailer (1982) in their long-term follow-up of patients who had undergone Le Fort I advancement osteotomy for correction of a retropositioned maxilla. The osteotomized maxilla remained stable, but the upper lip lost 44 per cent of its advanced position within the first year of surgery. Long-term stability of the Le Fort I segment was also documented by Carlotti and Schendel (1987).

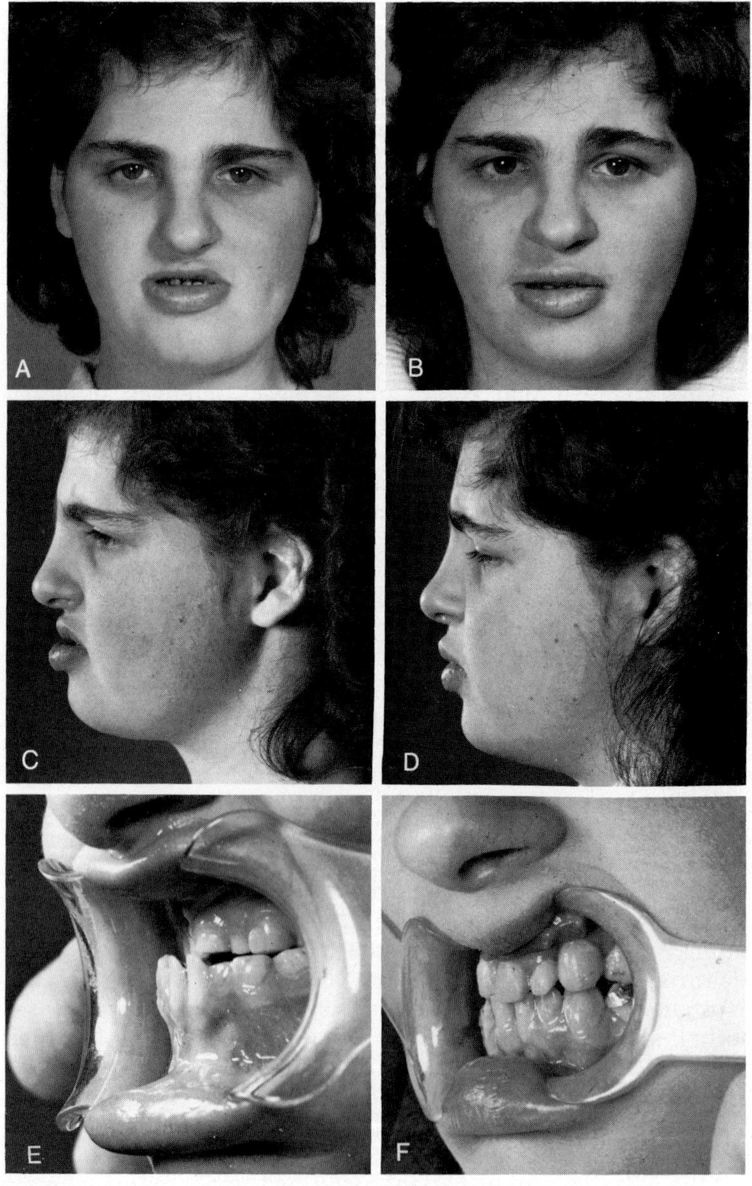

Figure 29–200. Le Fort I osteotomy. *A, C, E,* Preoperative views demonstrating maxillary hypoplasia and anterior crossbite after surgical correction of choanal atresia in childhood. *B, D, F,* Appearance after Le Fort I advancement. Note the improvement in the nasal tip and labial relationships.

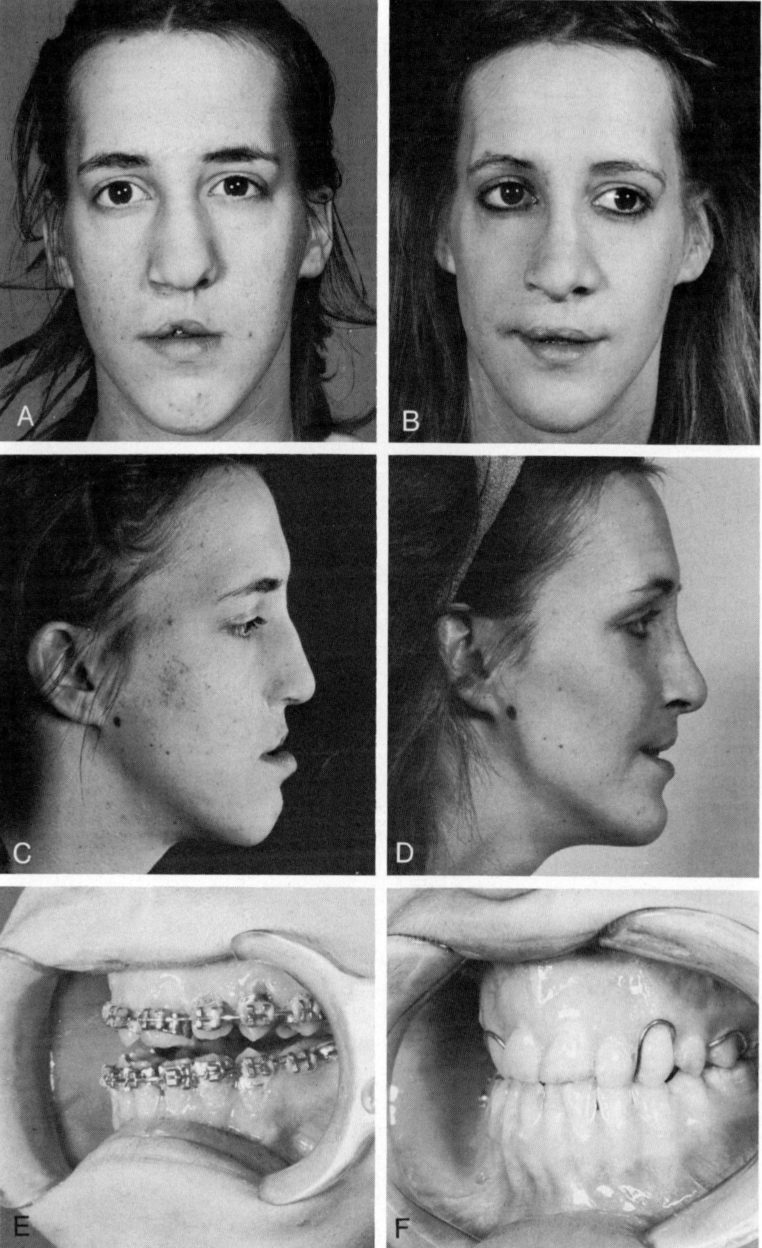

Figure 29–201. Le Fort I advancement osteotomy in a patient with cleft palate. *A, C,* Preoperative views. Note the associated nose and lip deformities. *B, D,* After Le Fort I advancement, reduction genioplasty, corrective rhinoplasty, and lip revision. *E,* Preoperative occlusion. *F,* Occlusion after combined orthodontic-prosthodontic-surgical rehabilitation.

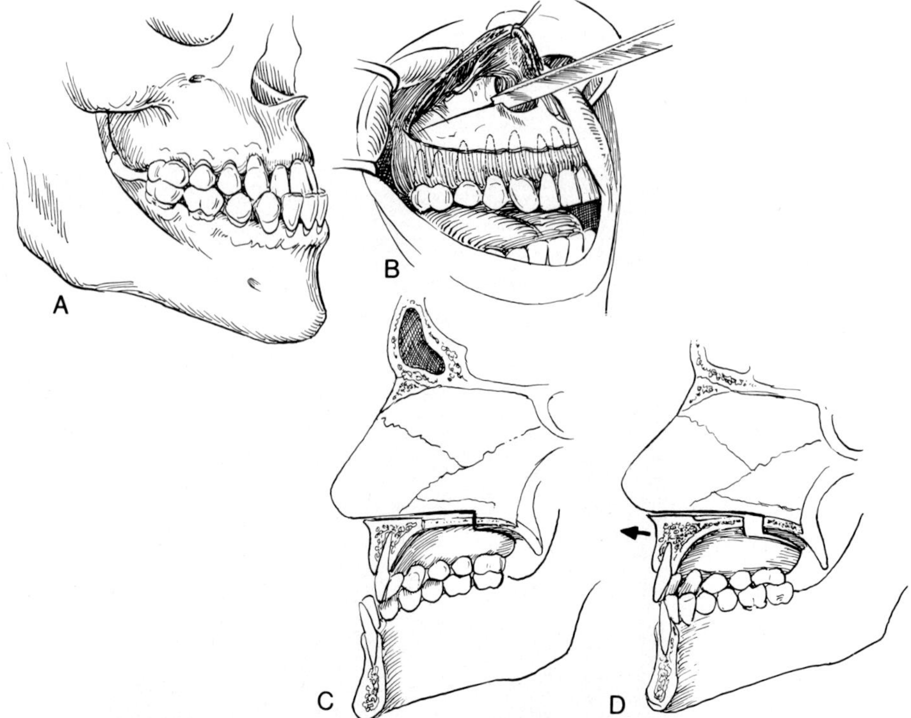

Figure 29–202. Technique of the retromolar segmental advancement osteotomy. *A,* Drawing illustrating the skeletal deformity. *B,* The mucoperiosteum is reflected to demonstrate the line of osteotomy. *C,* Sagittal section illustrating the line of section of the vomer and hard palate. *D,* The maxillary segment is advanced.

The postoperative skeletal stability reported in the above studies could be accounted for by the long-term study of Compton, Jacobs, and Dunsworth (1984), which documented healing of the Le Fort I osteotomy sites by mature compact bone on biopsy and histologic study.

In a study of lip-nose esthetics after Le Fort I osteotomy, Rosen (1988) noted that the width of the alar base increases with anterior (and superior) repositioning of the maxilla. Nasal tip projection is increased only with advancement of the maxillary segment. Horizontal displacement of the upper lip was approximately 0.82 mm for every 1.0 mm of advancement (sagittal) at the incisal edge, and approximately 0.51 mm at the subnasale for every 1.0 mm advancement at the cephalometric point A. With vertical impaction of the maxilla, lip shortening ranged from 20 to 50 per cent of the skeletal intrusion.

Velopharyngeal Incompetence After Maxillary Advancement. The incidence of velopharyngeal incompetence after maxillary advancement procedures is not known. It is suspected that patients with a repaired cleft palate incur a greater risk of this postoperative complication than those undergoing maxillary advancements for other reasons.

Since these procedures involve forward movement of the palate for distances often ranging between 10 and 20 mm, it is thought that such advancement, carrying as it does the soft palate, might be responsible for the development of postoperative velopharyngeal incompetence.

Witzel and Munro (1977) reported an adolescent male with a repaired cleft lip and palate who developed velopharyngeal incompetence after a Le Fort I advancement. In a subsequent study, Witzel and associates (1983) reported a series of 70 patients who underwent a Le Fort I advancement and who were examined for velopharyngeal function before and six to 12 months after surgery. Patients with a repaired cleft palate were at risk for the development of velopharyngeal incompetence postoperatively, especially the cleft palate patients with preoperative evidence of nasal air emission, nasal resonance, borderline velopharyngeal competence, or some combination of these. The latter group,

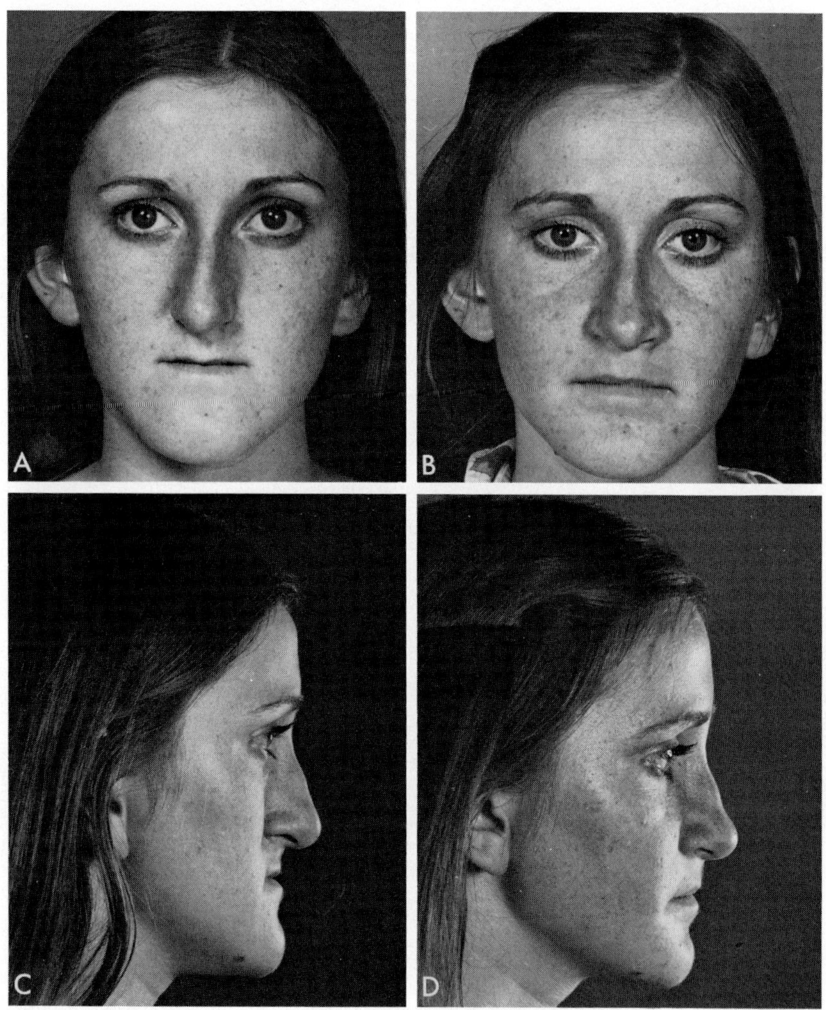

Figure 29–203. Le Fort I advancement osteotomy. *A,* Preoperative view of a patient with idiopathic maxillary hypoplasia. *B,* Appearance after advancement of the maxilla. *C,* Lateral preoperative view showing pseudoprognathism of the mandible. *D,* Change in the appearance after maxillary advancement. Note the additional projection of the nasal tip. (Patient of Dr. Donald Wood-Smith.)

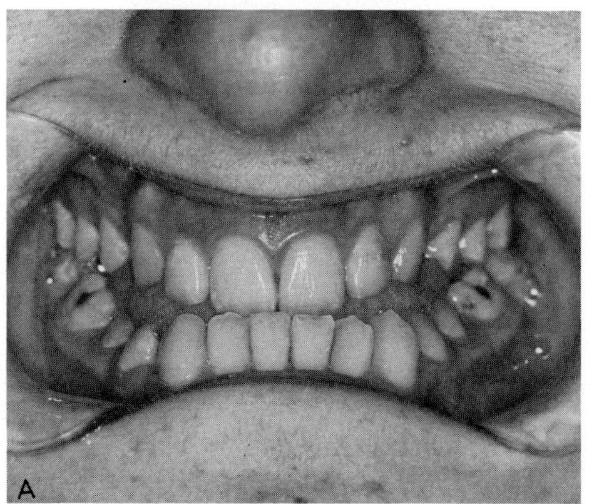

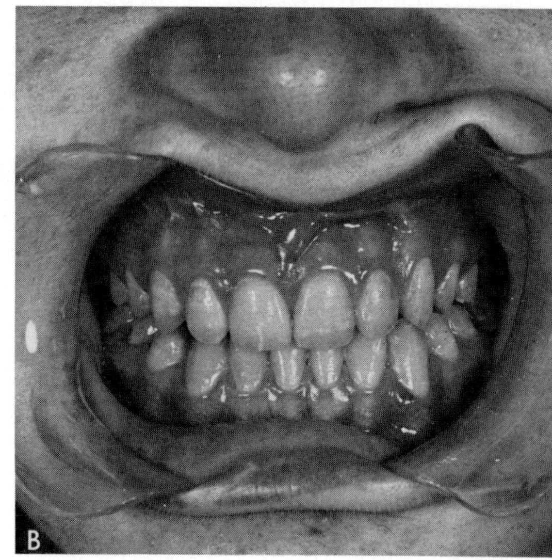

Figure 29–204. Intraoral views of the patient shown in Figure 29–203. *A,* Before surgery. *B,* After completion of treatment.

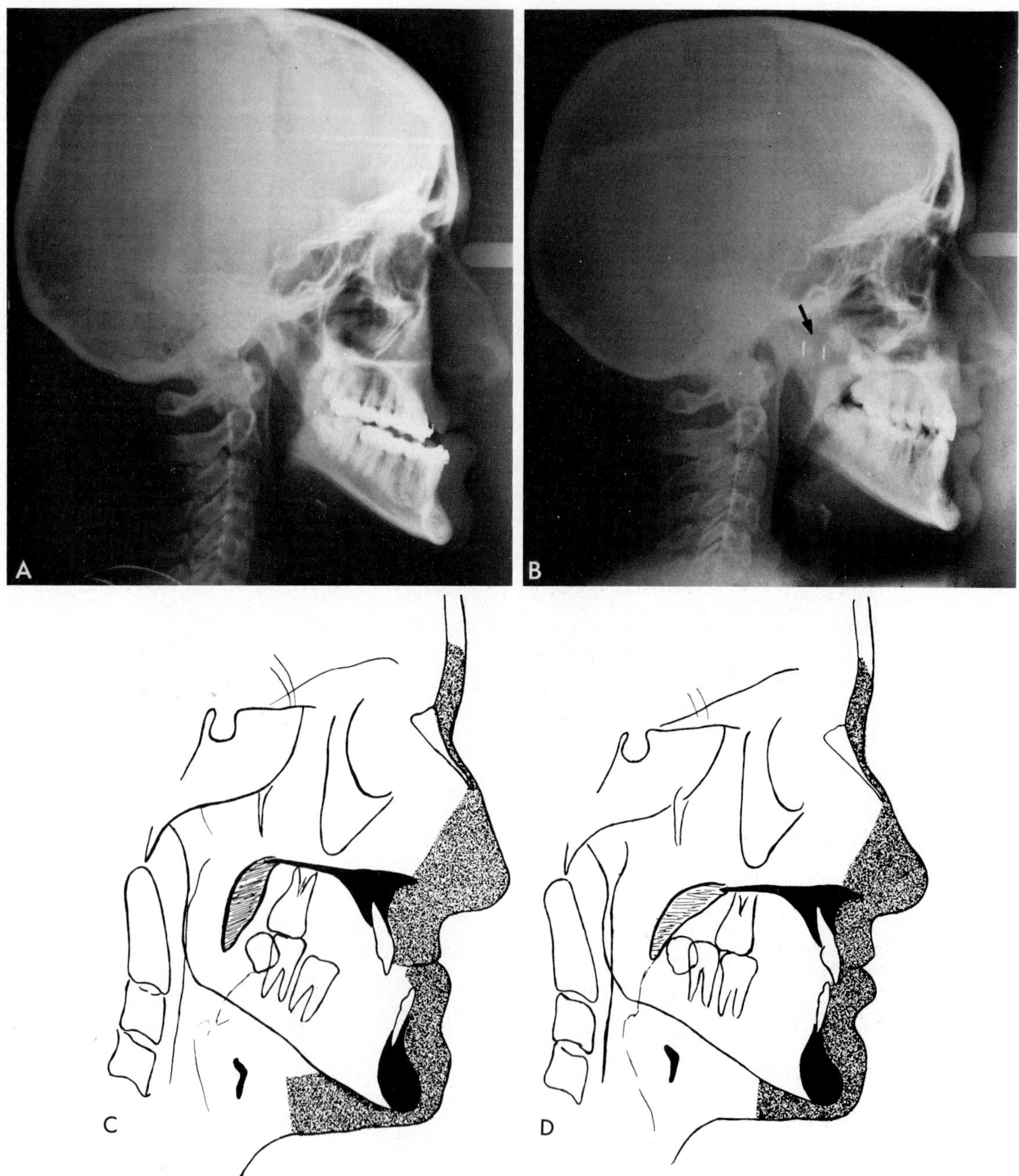

Figure 29–205. Cephalograms and tracing of patient shown in Figure 29–203. *A,* Preoperative cephalogram. *B,* Six months after the operation. The bone graft placed at the pterygomaxillary junction is indicated by the arrow. *C,* Preoperative tracing. *D,* Postoperative tracing.

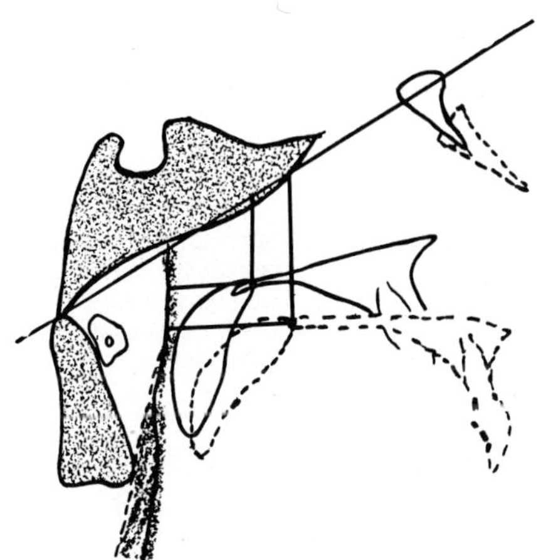

Figure 29–206. Lateral preoperative (*solid line*) and postoperative (*dotted line*) cephalometric tracings of a patient with Crouzon's disease. Note the anterior and inferior displacement of the maxilla following the maxillary advancement. There is a concomitant change in the position of the velum and its relationship to the posterior pharyngeal wall; the nasopharyngeal volume has also been increased.

as well as any patient with preoperative velopharyngeal incompetence, were considered by the authors as candidates for a pharyngoplasty at the time of Le Fort I advancement.

In a longitudinal postoperative study of 40 patients with craniosynostosis who had undergone Le Fort III advancement of the maxilla-midface, none developed velopharyngeal incompetence when studied by clinical and aerodynamic examination (McCarthy, Coccaro, and Schwartz, 1979). Serial cephalometric studies documented a short, tethered velum in the cleft palate subgroup (14 of 40). Postoperatively there was a slight increase in velar length as well as in the depth, height, and volume of the nasopharyngeal space. In the craniofacial synostosis group without a cleft palate, there was an elongated velum with a decreased anteroposterior nasopharyngeal dimension on the preoperative lateral cephalogram (Fig. 29–206). Consequently, this type of patient has the nasopharyngeal spatial anatomy that can accommodate a maxillary advancement without the development of velopharyngeal incompetence. In fact, in five patients with craniofacial synostosis, speech was improved because hyponasality was eliminated by the maxillary advancement, which significantly lengthened the velum and enlarged the nasopharyngeal volume (McCarthy, Coccaro, and Schwartz, 1979).

It should be stressed that patients with a repaired cleft palate are at risk of developing velopharyngeal incompetence, particularly if they have undergone a maxillary advancement in excess of 10 mm.

Pharyngeal Flaps and Maxillary Advancement Procedures. In planning a maxillary advancement in a patient who has undergone a pharyngeal flap procedure for the correction of velopharyngeal incompetence, the surgeon is faced with several possibilities:

1. If the pharyngeal flap is narrow and tethered and there is evidence of velopharyngeal incompetence, the flap is divided and inhalation anesthesia can be administered by a nasotracheal route. At a later stage the velopharyngeal incompetence can be corrected by some type of pharyngoplasty (see Chap. 58). However, Witzel and associates (1983) recommended that a pharyngoplasty be performed at the same time as maxillary advancement.

2. If the pharyngeal flap is functional and sufficiently large, with only slitlike nasopharyngeal ports, and intubation is not possible or it is feared that the proposed operation will jeopardize the airway, a temporary tracheotomy is the procedure of choice. Endotracheal intubation is accomplished through an oral route, and the tracheotomy is performed over the endotracheal tube. The latter is withdrawn as the tracheostomy tube is inserted, and an alternative inhalation anesthetic route is provided.

3. If the pharyngeal flap is inferiorly based and is tethered, and it is thought that advancement of the maxillary complex will result in velopharyngeal incompetence, the length of the flap can be augmented by dividing the inferior pedicle, raising a new superiorly based pharyngeal flap, and inserting it into the nasal surface of the velum or the divided flap (Weber, Chase, and Jobe, 1970; McEvitt, 1971; Owsley, Creech, and Dedo, 1972).

Correction of Transverse Maxillary Deformity. Palatal expansion may be required for the correction of transverse maxillary deficiency and lingual crossbite of the posterior teeth in nonsurgical cases as well as in preparation for sagittal or vertical movement of the maxilla by osteotomy techniques. The lingual crossbite malocclusion is usually bilateral.

Palatal expansion appliances are effective

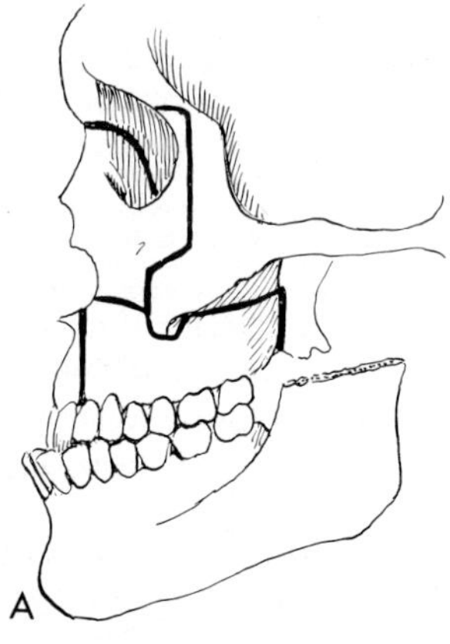

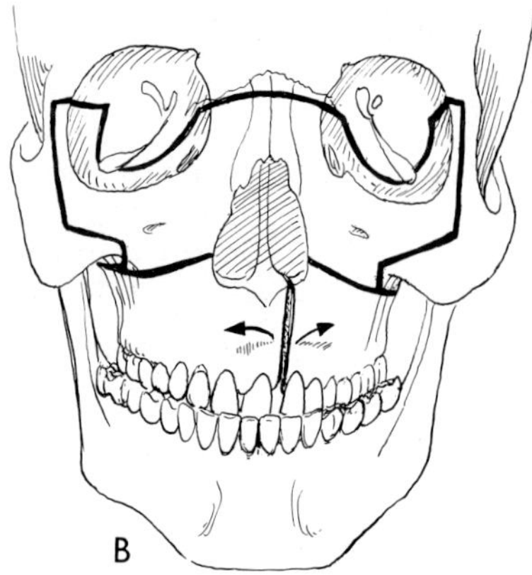

Figure 29–207. Maxillary expansion osteotomy combined with the Le Fort I and III osteotomies. *A,* Lateral view of the osteotomies. *B,* Frontal view illustrating parasagittal splitting of the alveolar bone and palate. The arrows designate the maxillary expansion. (After Obwegeser.)

in children and adolescents but such attempts in adults are frequently unsuccessful. The failure to open the midpalatal suture in adults has been attributed to fusion of the suture or the resistance offered by the remaining maxillary articulations (Isaacson and Ingram, 1964).

In the adult patient with transverse maxillary deficiency a variety of osteotomies, combined with orthodontic treatment, can be employed.

Axhausen (1934) described the "midline" palatal split to correct a malunited fracture. The sagittal osteotomy of the hard palate was made through the bone immediately lateral to the vomer. In cleft palate cases the maxillary osteotomy is facilitated by the cleft, but expansion may be hindered when the palatal mucosa is excessively scarred.

Obwegeser (1969) combined the maxillary expansion osteotomy with the Le Fort I and III osteotomies (Fig. 29–207). The maxillary fragments were immobilized by fixation appliances. The gaps in the bone skeleton resulting from the expansion were filled with bone grafts for further stabilization. West and Epker (1972) demonstrated the feasibility of independent repositioning of various portions of the maxilla.

Turvey (1985) reported expansion of the maxillary-palatal segments by two paramidline osteotomies performed through a Le Fort I downfracture osteotomy (Fig. 29–208). The osseous defects can be filled with bone grafts. In a more conservative technique, Lehman and associates (1984) confined the osteotomies to the pterygomaxillary buttress and the anterior aspect of the lateral nasal wall. A rigid palatal expansion appliance, cemented to the maxillary premolar and molar teeth, was activated in the postoperative period.

Preoperative model surgery is a key element of success. The maxillary cast is sectioned and the fragments are repositioned to align properly with the mandibular dental arch. The fragments are temporarily held together with dental wax and are then rigidly

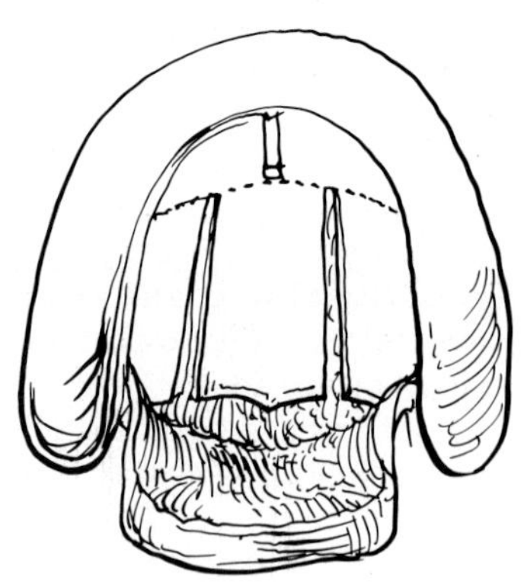

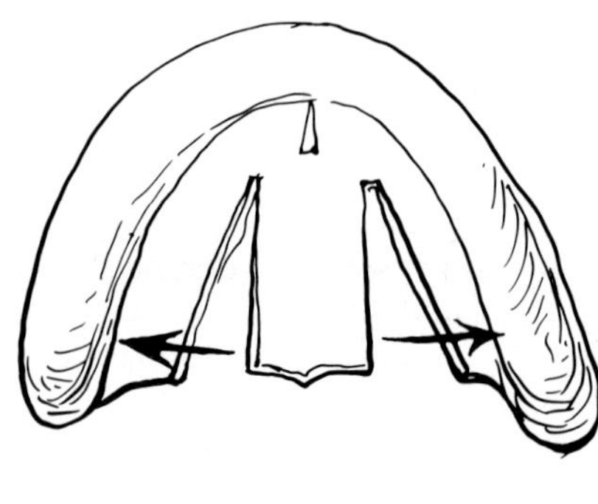

Figure 29–208. Transverse expansion of the palatal-maxillary segment by two paramedian osteotomies (after Turvey, 1985). The osteotomies (*right*) can be done after elevation of a palatal flap (*left*) or through the Le Fort I downfracture osteotomy.

maintained with a slab of plaster applied to the base of the divided cast. An occlusal, acrylic, horseshoe-shaped splint is fabricated on the articulated casts. The splint should not encroach more than a few millimeters onto the palatal mucosa to prevent compromise by compression of the vascular supply.

VERTICAL EXCESS

Maxillary Intrusion to Correct Long Face Deformity

One of the most common uses of the Le Fort I osteotomy is to shorten the face. Willmar (1974) used the term "long face" (vertical maxillary excess) to describe the consortium of traits associated with the long face deformity.

The principal physical finding of the deformity is an exaggerated anterior facial height due to maxillary vertical hyperplasia. The nose is frequently narrowed in the alar base region and the nasolabial angle is open or obtuse. The so-called adenoid facies is seen with a propensity toward breathing through the mouth. The palate is often high-arched and narrow. The mandible is forced into a clockwise rotation, and a Class II malocclusion may be present. The chin may be excessively tall as well as retruded. With the lips in repose, the interlabial gap is inordinate. The incisal edges of the maxillary incisors exceed the commonly accepted esthetically pleasing 2 to 3 mm of show (Burstone, 1967). On smiling, the gingival display is lavish and unflattering: the so-called "gummy smile." The upper lip normally reaches the crown-gingival junction or may reveal 1 mm of gingiva when a person smiles. Because of the physical distance that must be spanned, the lips must strain to achieve a seal. The resulting hyperactivity of the mentalis muscles bunches up the chin pad and bestows a puckered appearance upon the overlying soft tissues. The presence of an anterior open bite malocclusion may further exaggerate the facial distortion. However, in this situation the maxillary vertical excess is usually in the posterior region, and the relationship between the upper lip and the underlying incisors falls within an acceptable range.

To restore function and facial harmony, the long face deformity is corrected by a Le Fort I osteotomy (see Fig. 29–195) with minor modifications. Cephalometric analysis is used as a *guide* to the amount of desired maxillary reduction; however, the most important parameter is the *clinical* assessment. The amount of incisal disclosure with the lips in repose and the magnitude of gingival exhibition on smiling are recorded. The final goal for incisal display is usually 2 to 3 mm. Subtracting this count from the amount of dental show with the lip in a tranquil pose will equal the amount of maxillary shortening. More likely than not, this figure will closely agree with the previous measurement

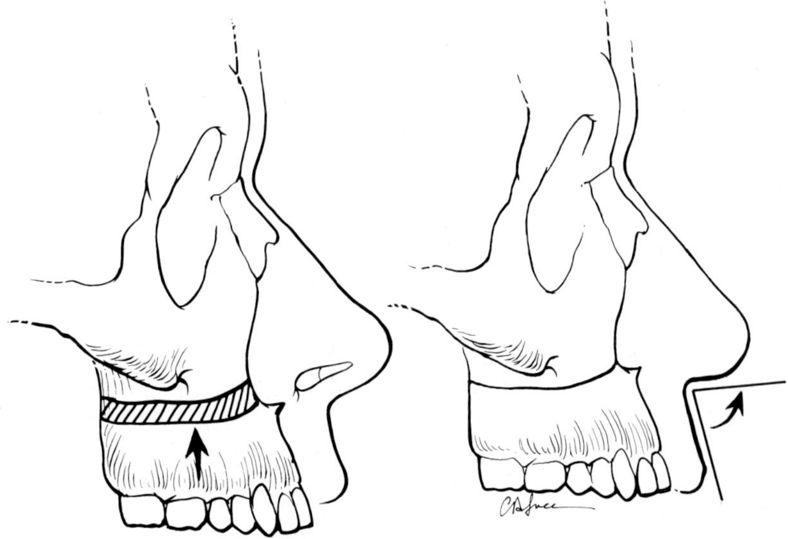

Figure 29–209. Vertical impaction of the maxilla (Le Fort I) with the anterior nasal spine left attached to the mobilized segment. Note that the nasolabial angle is decreased.

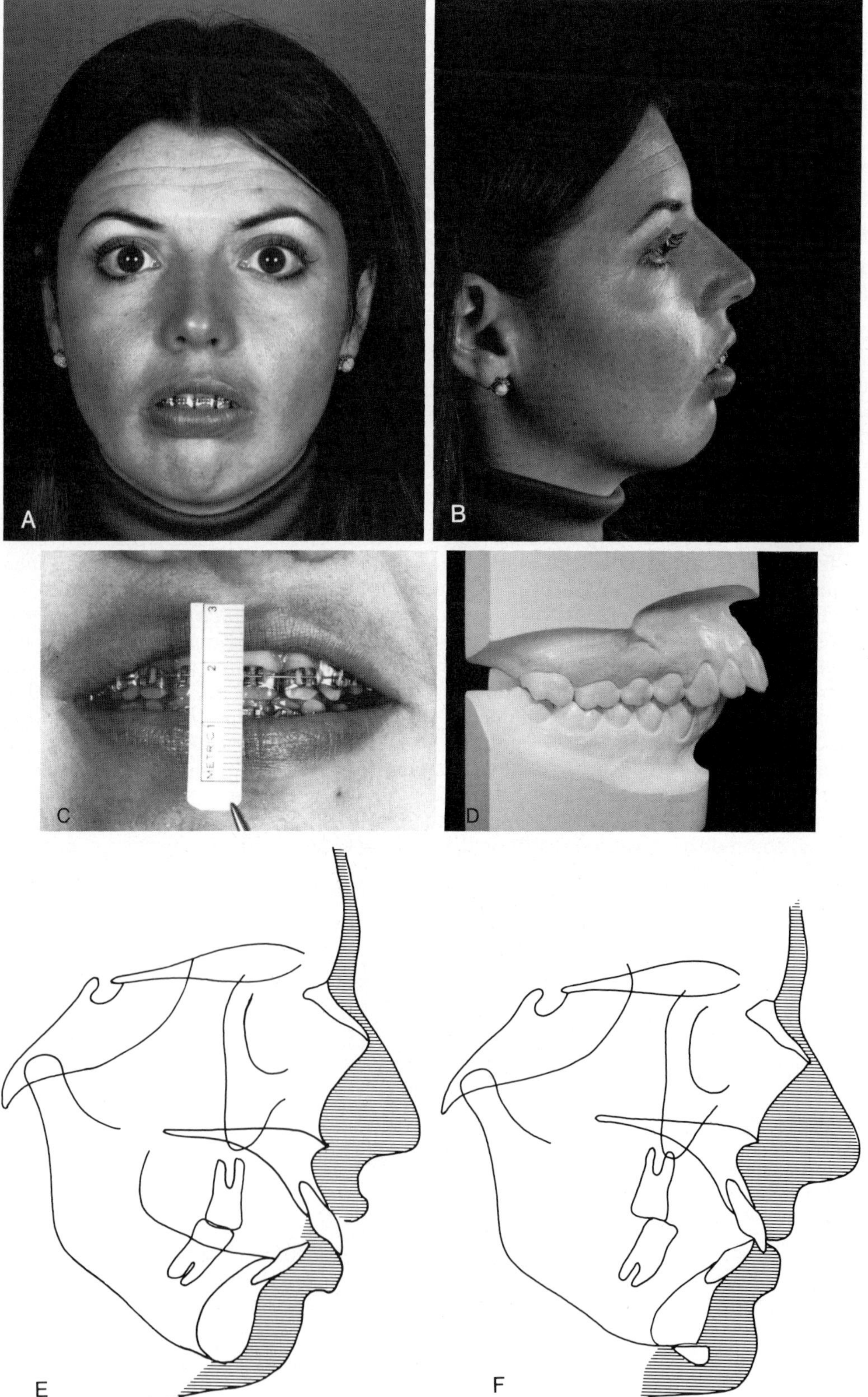

Figure 29–210 *See legend on opposite page*

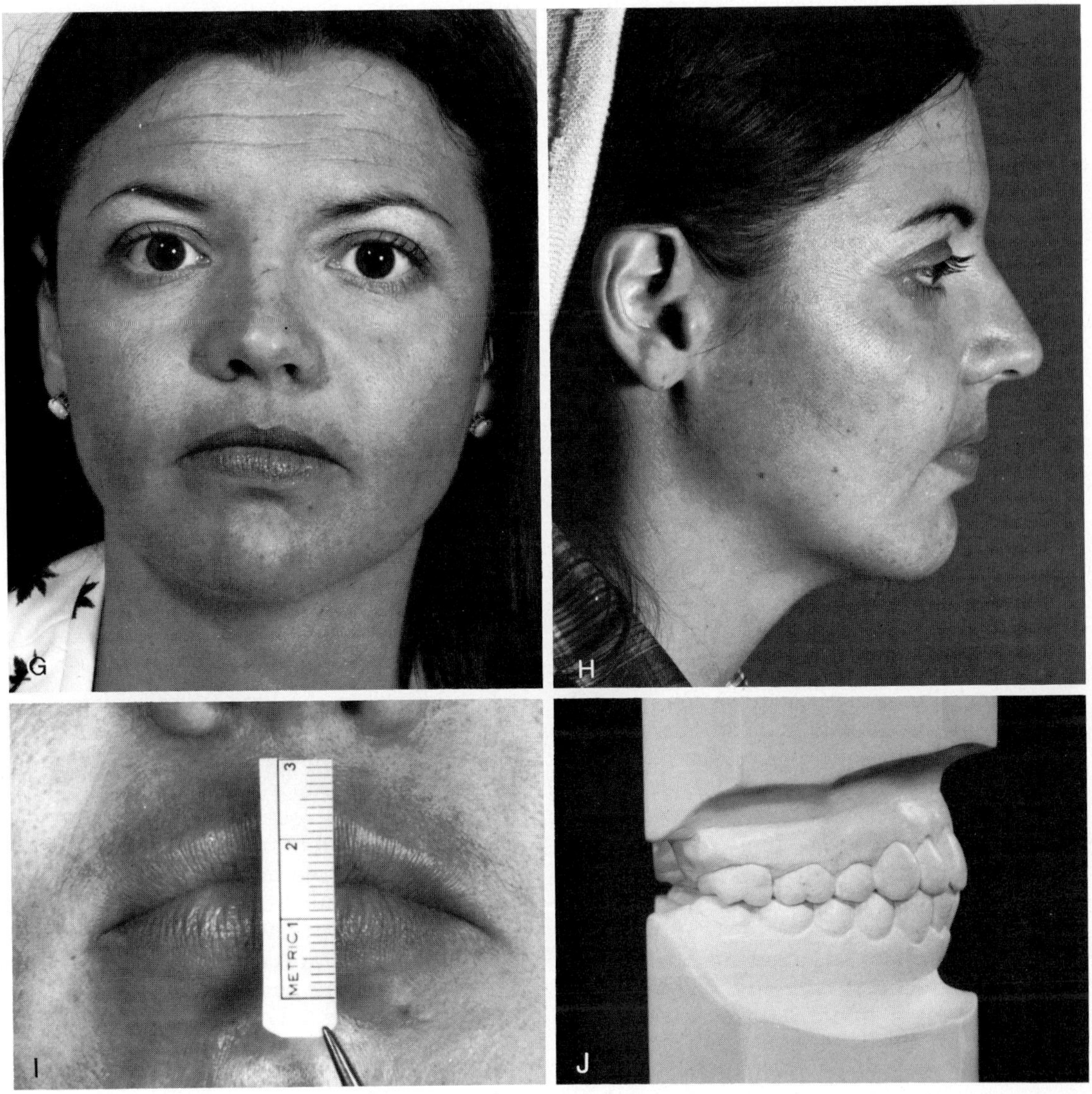

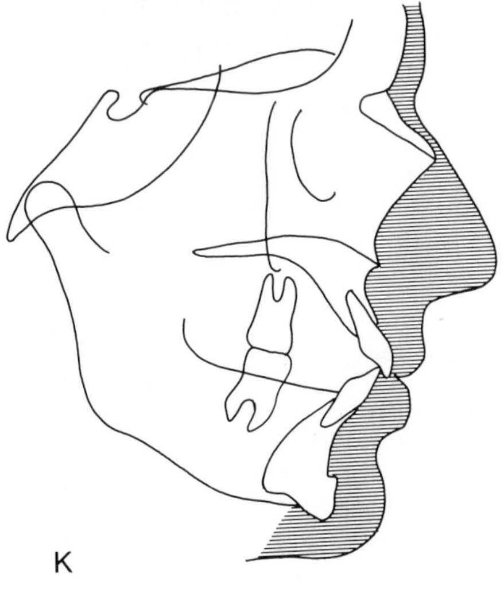

Figure 29–210. Vertical maxillary excess, overjet, and microgenia in an adult female treated by vertical impaction of the maxilla and genioplasty in combination with preoperative and postoperative orthodontic therapy. *A, B,* Preoperative views. *C,* Preoperative lip seal. *D,* Preoperative dental model. *E,* Preoperative lateral cephalogram. Note the skeletal and soft tissue (shading) profile. There is evidence of excessive incisor show at rest, lip incompetence, overjet, vertical maxillary excess, and mandibular deficiency. *F,* Surgical plan: vertical impaction and slight setback of maxilla, and mandibular advancement secondary to autorotation and genioplasty. *G, H,* Postoperative views. *I,* Postoperative lip seal. *J,* Postoperative dental model. *K,* Lateral cephalogram four years postoperatively.

of gingival exposure during smiling. When the maxilla is surgically elevated, the upper lip is correspondingly shortened by approximately 20 per cent (Bell, Creekmore, and Alexander, 1977). This ascent of the lip should be taken into account, especially in cases in which the amount of intrusion is great. However, the amount of shortening of the upper lip varies with the individual case (Bell and Dann, 1973; Schendel and associates, 1976) and may shorten even when the vertical position of the maxilla is unaltered (Radney and Jacobs, 1981).

At the beginning of the operation, the position of the maxillary incisors should be registered. A simple method is to place a tattoo mark with a needle and surgical ink in the region of the medial canthus (Kawamoto, 1982a). The distance between the mark and the incisal edge is recorded. At the end of the procedure, this measurement should equal the original observation minus the amount of desired shortening.

The general outline of the Le Fort I osteotomy is followed. A modification may be required in the management of the anterior nasal spine. Close attention should be directed preoperatively to the nasolabial angle. If the angle is acceptable, it is advisable to alter the line of the osteotomy by creating a "V" cut below the anterior nasal spine and allowing it to remain attached to the nasal septum. If the anterior nasal spine were left with the maxillary segment, as in the conventional Le Fort I (see Fig. 29–195), the nasolabial angle would be decreased as the maxilla is intruded (Fig. 29–209).

After the Le Fort I osteotomy, the maxilla is placed in intermaxillary or rigid skeletal fixation (see Fig. 29–213). With the condyles properly seated in the glenoid fossa, the maxillomandibular complex is rotated cephalad. The maxillary bony interferences are removed with a rongeur or a bur until the planned shortening is achieved. The nasal septum must be reduced to prevent its buckling as the maxilla is elevated. If it was elected to preserve the attachment of the anterior nasal spine to the septum, the maxilla should be relieved in the area to avoid a deflection of the caudal septal border.

Osteosynthesis is established in the usual manner after the planned superior repositioning of the maxilla and the incision is closed (see Fig. 29–196). The alar width of the nose widens as the maxilla is superiorly positioned (Rosen, 1988); this may be welcomed when the alar width is narrow before the operation. In addition, there is a tendency for the upper lip to flatten and the vermilion to thin. To counteract these postoperative findings and to produce a pleasing nasal appearance and a pouting lip, a horizontal mattress suture can be placed between the alar bases, and a V-Y advancement is used to close the oral incision (Schendel and Williamson, 1983).

Because of the frequently associated retromacrogenia, an osseous advancement and vertical reduction genioplasty are often necessary (Fig. 29–210). However, it should be noted that vertical impaction of the maxilla is associated with an autorotation (anterior) of the mandible and thus a sagittal projection of the bony chin.

VERTICAL DEFICIENCY

Maxillary Elongation to Correct Short Face Deformity

In addition to the long face problem, Willmar (1974) described the idiopathic maxillary deformity of the short face. The lower half of the face is disproportionately short and in full view it has a square-shaped outline with prominent mandibular angles. During speaking and smiling the maxillary anterior teeth are hidden behind the upper lip, resulting in an edentulous appearance. The ends of the interlabial line are depressed at the oral commissures, and this inverted design imparts a sad visage. The lips, crowded by the decreased anterior facial height, are folded outward to accentuate the labiomental fold.

Intraoral examinations show an adequate or Class II dental occlusion and teeth of normal size. The maxillary alveolar process is unusually diminished in its vertical dimension. With the mandible in a rest position, Willmar (1974) found the average distance between the maxillary and mandibular teeth (freeway space) to be more than 10 mm (three to four times the expected range).

Cephalometric Examination

Reference points and lines used by Willmar (1976) are illustrated in Figure 29–211. The most significant differences noted in the profile of patients with the short face deformity are the decreased height of the alveolar process (*sp′-is′*), the concealed incisors by the

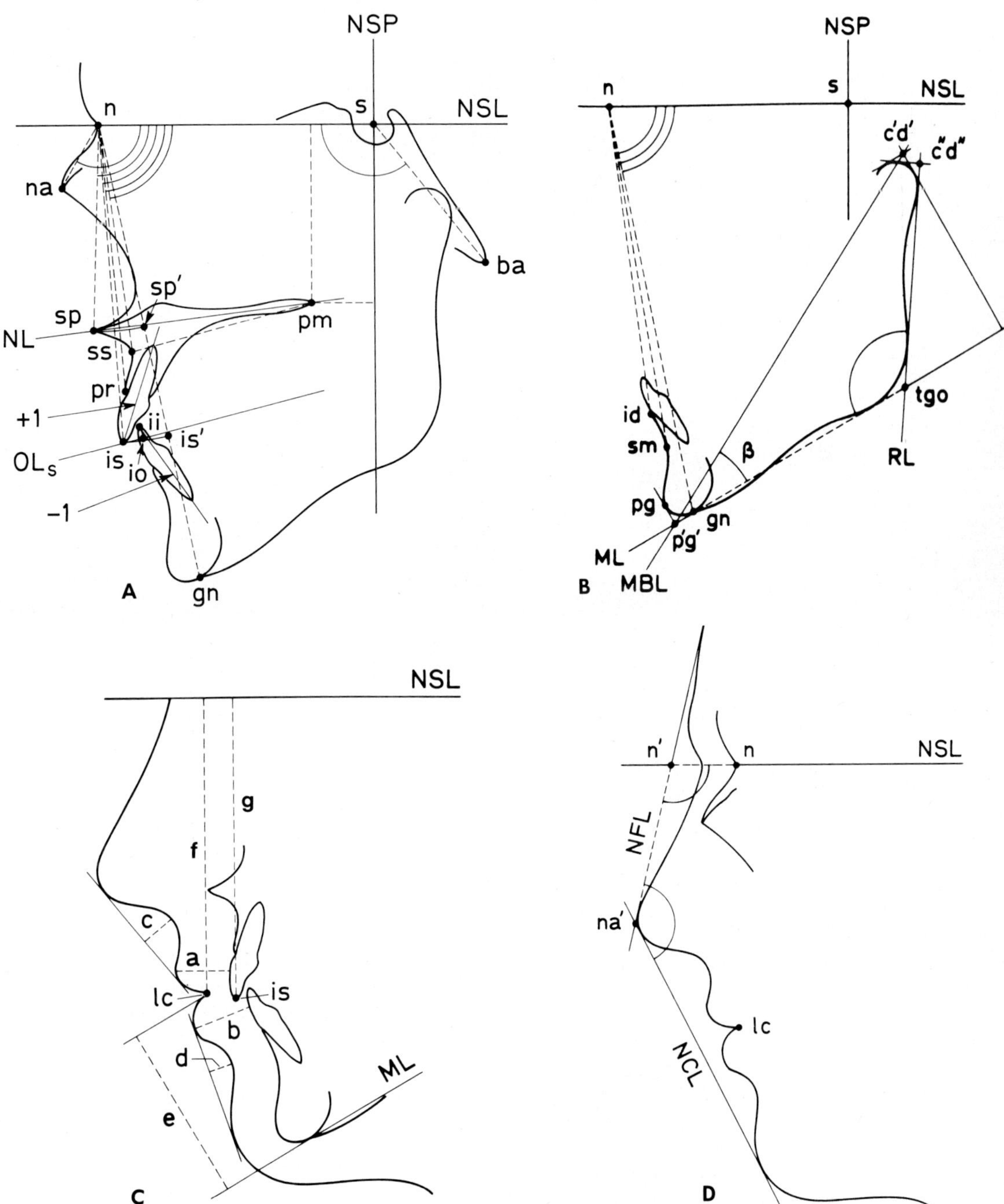

Figure 29–211. *A,* Reference points and lines. *B,* Reference points and lines related to the mandible. *C,* Lines NSL and ML. *D,* Construction of the soft tissue lines NFL and NCL. (Courtesy of Dr. K. Willmar.)

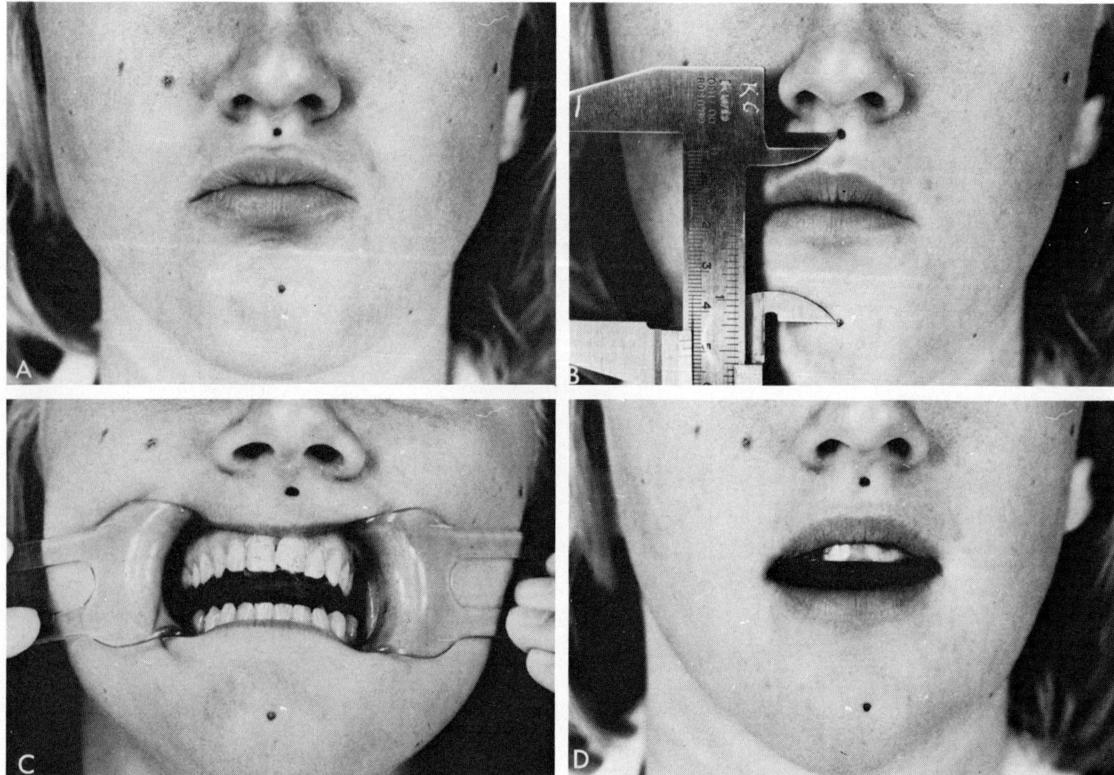

Figure 29–212. Determination of freeway space. *A,* Midline inkmarks on the upper lip and chin serve as reference points. The jaws are held with the teeth in centric occlusion. The distance between the ink marks is measured. *B,* The mandible is in its rest position. The distance between the skin marks is again recorded. *C,* The jaws are closed on the wax wafer to within 3 mm of the distance between the skin marks in *B. D,* The wafer is trimmed to a level corresponding to the border of the upper lip. (Courtesy of Dr. K. Willmar.)

upper lip (the difference between *s-lc vert* and *s-is vert*), and the reduced anterior lower facial height (*sp-gn*). The total facial height (*n-gn*) and *NSL/ML angle* are less than normal. The gonial angle is more square. In the soft tissues the lower vermilion is thicker, the lower lip height shorter, and the facial angle (NFL/NCL) more obtuse.

Clinical and radiographic studies confirm the underdevelopment of the maxillary alveolar process, particularly in its anterior portion. To increase the vertical dimension and to reestablish the relations between the maxillary incisor and the upper lip, it is necessary to perform a Le Fort I osteotomy, with lowering of the mobilized maxillary segment and filling of the defect along the osteotomy sites with bone grafts or hydroxyapatite.

Preoperative Planning

The distance between the relaxed upper lip and the buried incisor edge is measured. To this measurement, 2 to 3 mm is added, which represents the ideal position of the free vermilion border to the incisal edge. Although firm figures have yet to be established, vertical relapse does occur; therefore, an additional 20 to 30 per cent of lengthening should be provided (Fig. 29–212).

As the maxilla is elongated, the mandible undergoes a clockwise (posterior) rotation. Thus, the prominence of the chin is decreased. Accommodation for this change should be made when planning the profile correction.

Surgical Technique

Because of the reduced height of the alveolar process, the roots extend further into the sinus than normal. Therefore, a higher Le Fort I than one might expect is required in order to avoid injury to the apices of the teeth (Fig. 29–213). Reference points, as mentioned in the maxillary intrusion technique, are used as measurement guides. The mobilized

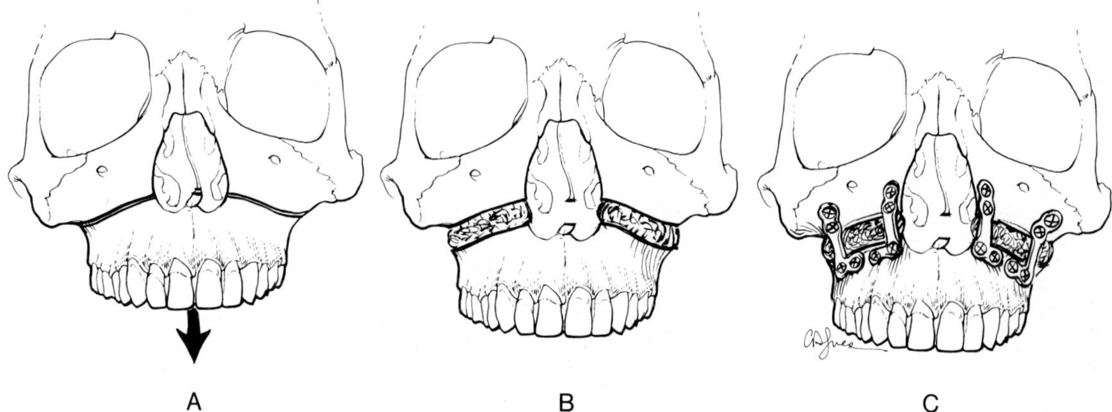

Figure 29–213. Le Fort I osteotomy to correct vertical maxillary deficiency or the short face syndrome. *A,* Note that the lines of osteotomy are made high to avoid injury to the teeth apices. *B,* Either autogenous bone or hydroxyapatite is placed in the resulting void. *C,* Miniplates are inserted across the osteotomy site at the buttresses.

maxilla is placed in intermaxillary fixation and inferiorly repositioned by the calculated amount. Miniplates are used for the osteosynthesis, and autogenous bone grafts or hydroxyapatite are used to fill the resulting gaps (Fig. 29–214).

Nasomaxillary Hypoplasia

Nasomaxillary hypoplasia is a generic term coined by Converse and associates (1970) for a variety of clinical states characterized by underdevelopment of the nasomaxillary complex. A clinical classification was further provided by Henderson and Jackson (1973) and was based on the presence or absence of involvement of the dentoalveolar segment.

In recent years Binder's syndrome has been defined; it covers a major portion of patients with the diagnosis of nasomaxillary hypoplasia. The syndrome was originally described by Binder (1962) and there is an occasional hereditary component. The facies has a characteristic appearance: retruded or pressed-in nose with a low-set, flat nasal tip; crescent-shaped nostrils; a short, retracted columella without the usual triangular base; an acute nasolabial angle; a minimal or missing nostril sill; and a wide, shallow philtrum (Fig. 29–215). There are two types of nasal deformities: a flattened nose of normal length and a significantly foreshortened nose (Rintala and Ranta, 1985). The columella and upper lip are drawn into the nostril floor, and the nasal spine and floor of the piriform fossa cannot be palpated (Jackson, Moos, and Sharpe, 1981). Holmstrom (1986a,b), in a study of 50 patients with Binder's syndrome, noted that the salient skeletal features were a palpable depression in the anterior nasal floor (prenasal fossa) and a localized maxillary hypoplasia in the alar base region. The piriform aperture region and infraorbital rims may be retruded with exposure of the sclera. There can be elements of orbital hypotelorism and other evidence of problems of forebrain differentiation in some patients with nasomaxillary hypoplasia (see Chap. 60). If the dentoalveolar segment is involved, there is an anterior crossbite.

Cephalometric evaluation usually confirms the nasomaxillary hypoplasia and there is a pathognomonic absence of the anterior nasal spine.

TREATMENT

Preoperative assessment includes a clinical examination and radiographic evaluation. On orthodontic study maxillary crowding is frequently observed, usually associated with maxillary labial protrusion and mandibular incisor retrusion. An anterior crossbite reflects involvement of the maxillary dentoalveolar segment.

A variety of treatment courses are available depending on the clinical findings (Table 29–3).

Nasal Lengthening

The dorsum of the nose can be augmented with an onlay bone graft (Fig. 29–216) (Con-

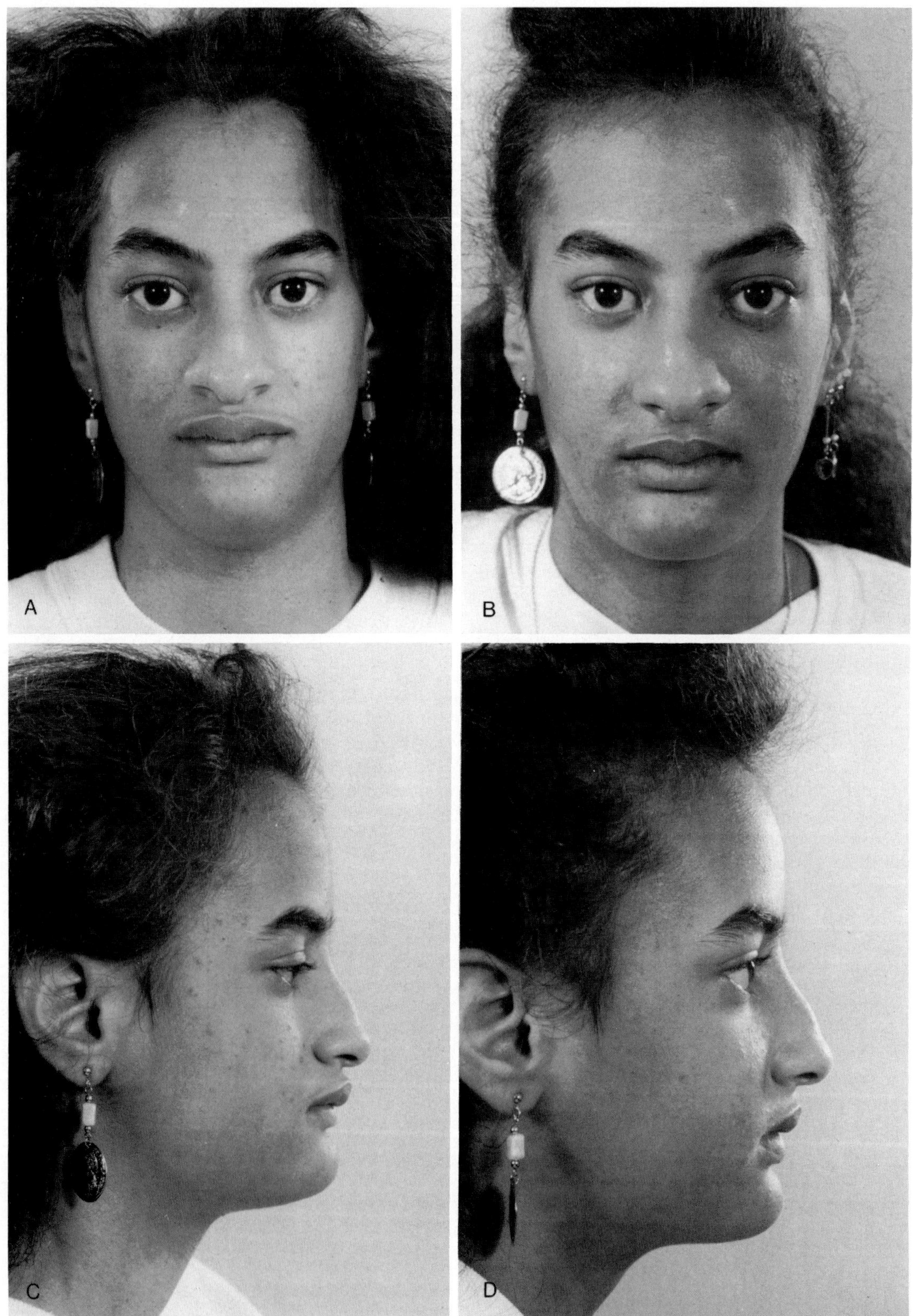

Figure 29–214. Correction of short face syndrome (vertical maxillary deficiency). *A, C,* Preoperative appearance. Note the camouflage of the maxillary teeth by the upper lip and vertical facial deficiency. *B, D,* Appearance after Le Fort I osteotomy and interposition bone grafting (see Fig. 29–213).

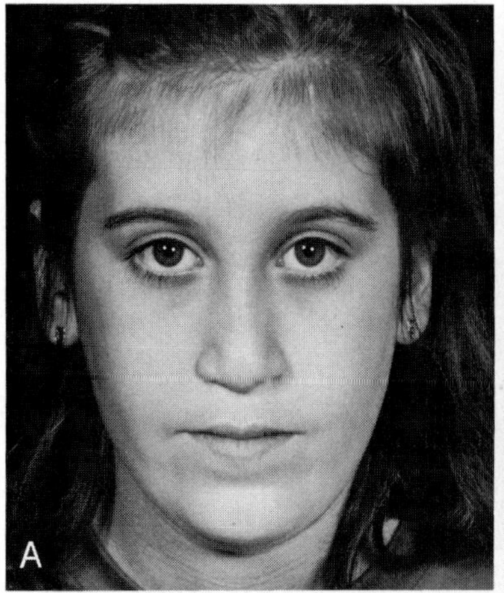

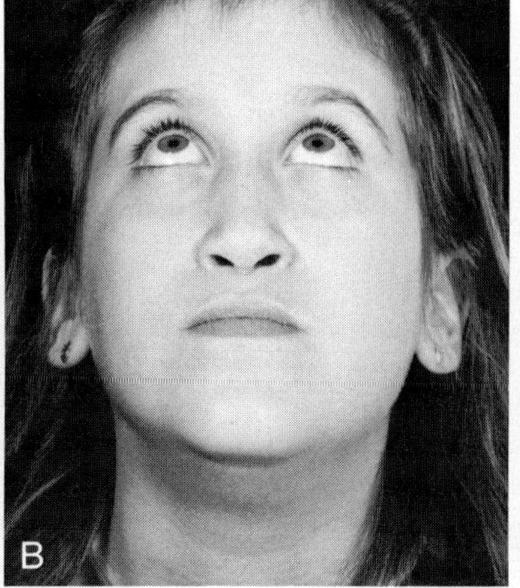

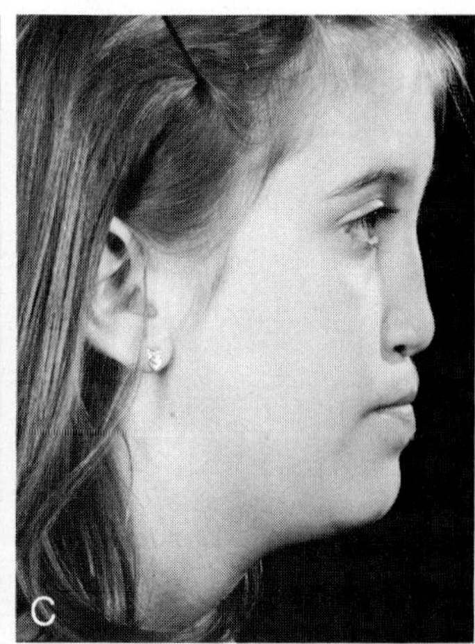

Figure 29–215. Nasomaxillary hypoplasia (Binder's syndrome). Note the retruded nose, flat nasal tip, retracted columella, crescent-shaped nostrils, acute nasolabial angle, and absent nostril sills. *A,* Frontal view. *B,* Basilar view. *C,* Profile.

verse and associates, 1970; Munro, Sinclair, and Rudd, 1979; Jackson, Moos, and Sharpe, 1981; and Tessier, 1981) (see Chap. 35). However, the nasal tip remains depressed because of the short columella. Consequently, L-shaped bone grafts (dorsum and columella) are prepared (Holmstrom, 1986b). Through an intraoral vestibular incision the columella and nasal dorsum are undermined, the nasal bones are exposed in a subperiosteal plane, and the soft tissue dissection extends widely over the maxilla. The L-shaped graft can be secured with a K-wire or simple stainless steel wire. The vestibular incision is closed in a V-Y fashion to lengthen the mucosal lining of the upper lip. Bone grafting of the piriform aperture area can be accomplished at the same time.

An alternative technique proposed by Holmstrom (1986b) is an advancement of the septum after it has been exposed in a submucoperichondrial plane (Fig. 29–217). Bone grafting of the nasal floor and maxilla can be done concomitantly. This technique gives a more natural appearance to the nasal tip.

Nasomaxillary Skin Graft Inlay

Gillies (1923) described the nasomaxillary skin graft inlay technique, which can be employed in patients who have lost a major portion of the nasal bones or central maxilla. In these patients, construction of a permanent dental appliance is essential and the latter can be incorporated into the surgical reconstruction. The technique has been used on occasion by the authors in patients who have sustained trauma or undergone radical premaxillectomies. Antia (1974) reported excellent results in correcting the saddle nose deformity of leprosy by this technique.

The technique, which involves the inconvenience that the patient must continuously wear, cleanse, and replace the appliance, is best suited for the edentulous patient, since the prosthetic support for the nose is an extension of the denture.

The nasal skin graft inlay technique is illustrated in Figure 29–218. A patient requiring such reconstruction is shown in Figure 29–219.

A description of the operative procedure follows. Under oroendotracheal anesthesia, an incision is made in the upper buccal sulcus (Fig. 29–218*A*), the nasal fossa is entered

Table 29–3. Nasomaxillary Hypoplasia: Surgical Techniques

Nasal lengthening procedures
Onlay bone grafting: anterior maxilla, piriform aperture, nostril sill, columella, nasal dorsum
Cartilage grafting: anterior maxilla, piriform aperture, nostril sill, columella, nasal tip, and dorsum
Nasomaxillary skin graft inlay
Osteotomies:
Perinasal osteotomy
Naso-orbitomaxillary osteotomy ± advancement of dentoalveolar segment
Le Fort II osteotomy ± advancement of dentoalveolar segment
Other: Le Fort I, premolar

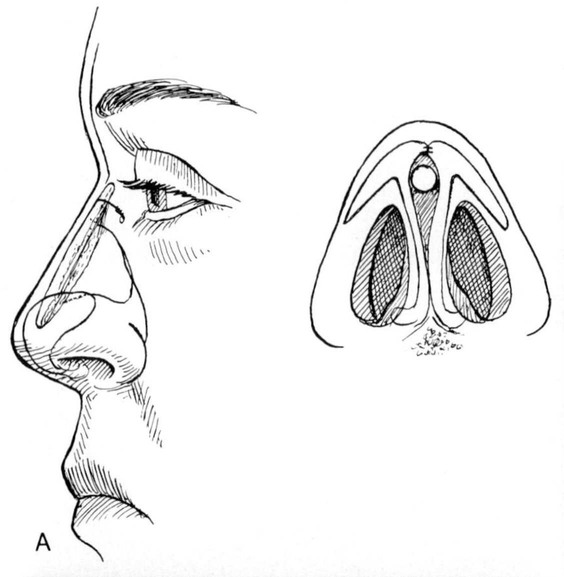

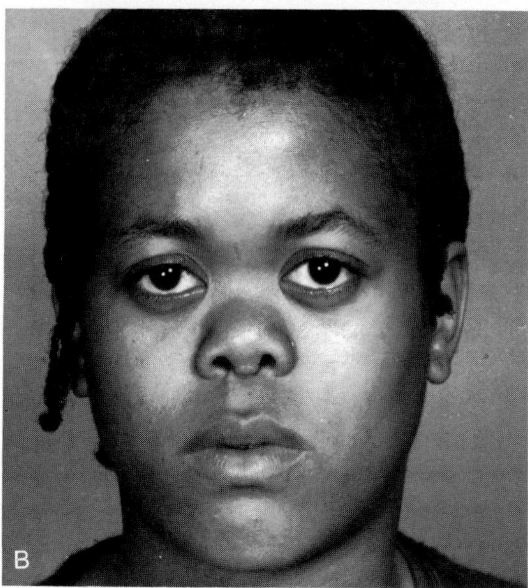

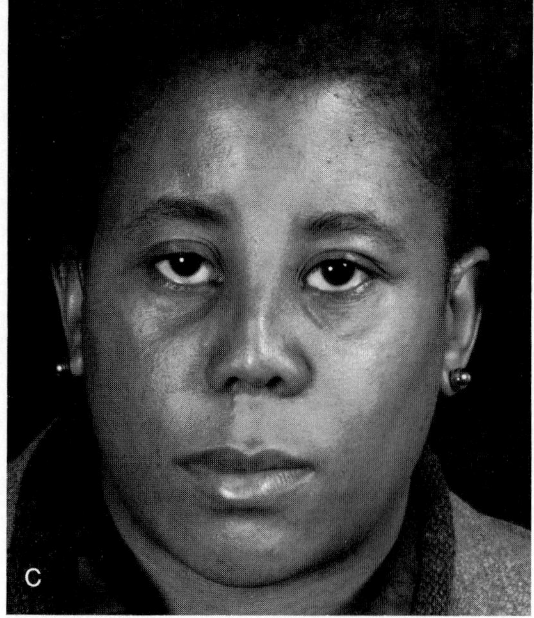

Figure 29–216. Nasal augmentation and lengthening with an onlay iliac bone graft in a 20 year old female with Binder's syndrome. *A,* Technique. *B,* Preoperative view. *C,* Postoperative view.

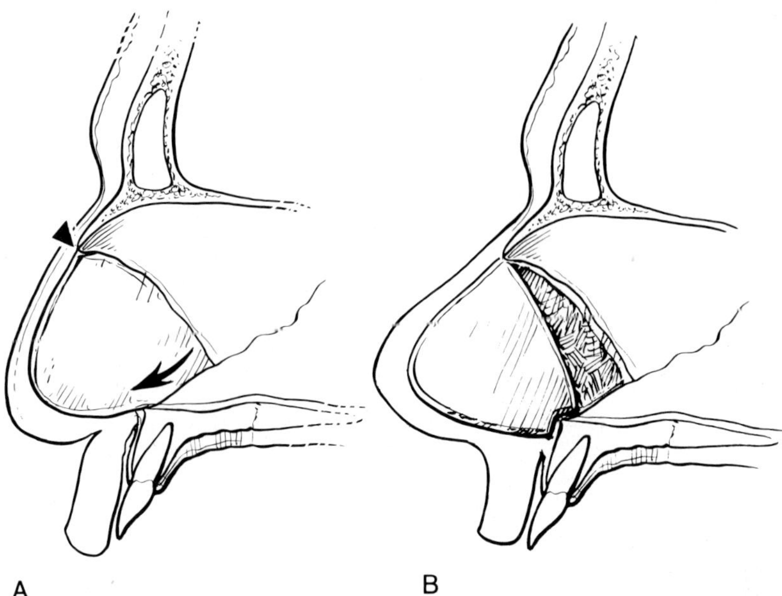

Figure 29–217. Septal lengthening by the method of Holmstrom (1986b). *A,* Line of septal sectioning. Note the pivot point on the dorsal border and direction of the advancement *(arrow)*. *B,* After advancement the septum is secured to the site of the deficient nasal spine.

from within the sulcus (Fig. 29–218*B*), and the nasal structures are freed of adhesions; an extensive raw area results. The nasal spine is removed (Fig. 29–218*C*). A dental compound mold is constructed to fit the resulting pyramidal cavity (Fig. 29–218*D*) with the apex pointing upward so that the mold can be inserted and removed easily. The mold is duplicated to construct a permanent acrylic prosthesis. The permanent prosthesis may be prepared in the operating room using quick-curing acrylic. A split-thickness skin graft from a nonhairy donor site is spread over the mold, raw surface outward, and inserted into the nasal cavity (Fig. 29–218*E* to *G*). The skin graft–carrying mold is maintained by a splint attached to the molar teeth (Fig. 29–218*H*). The preoperative contour of the patient is shown in Figure 29–218*I*. The tissues should be distended by the compound mold in order to ensure close coaptation of the graft with the soft tissues and to counteract possible subsequent contraction of the graft (Fig. 29–218*J*); the mold is removed after two weeks and the cavity examined and cleansed. At intervals during subsequent weeks, the size of the mold is diminished. After a period of many weeks, a permanent acrylic prosthesis maintains the contour of the final nose (Figs. 29–218*K*, 29–219). When the patient is edentulous, the prosthesis is an upper extension of the denture.

The nasomaxillary skin graft inlay technique has also been employed in patients who received radiation early in life and in whom the nose failed to develop (Fig. 29–219).

Perinasal Osteotomy

The perinasal osteotomy (Fig. 29–220) can be employed to lengthen the cartilaginous and bony skeletal framework.

Exposure is obtained preferably through a coronal incision. The area of junction of the nasal bones with the frontal bone is exposed subperiosteally, and the dissection is extended backward to the lacrimal groove, the lacrimal sac being raised from the groove. The lamina papyracea situated posterior to the posterior lacrimal crest is also exposed. The attachment of the medial canthal tendon is not disturbed. An incision made in the nasal vestibule immediately lateral to the base of the piriform aperture allows the passage of a periosteal elevator, which raises the periosteum from the base of the lateral wall until the elevator rejoins the medial orbital area; exposure can also be obtained by an intraoral incision.

Exposure having been obtained, the perinasal osteotomy is performed. A transverse osteotomy is carried out at the junction of the nasal bone with the frontal bone. The osteotomy is extended posteriorly above the lac-

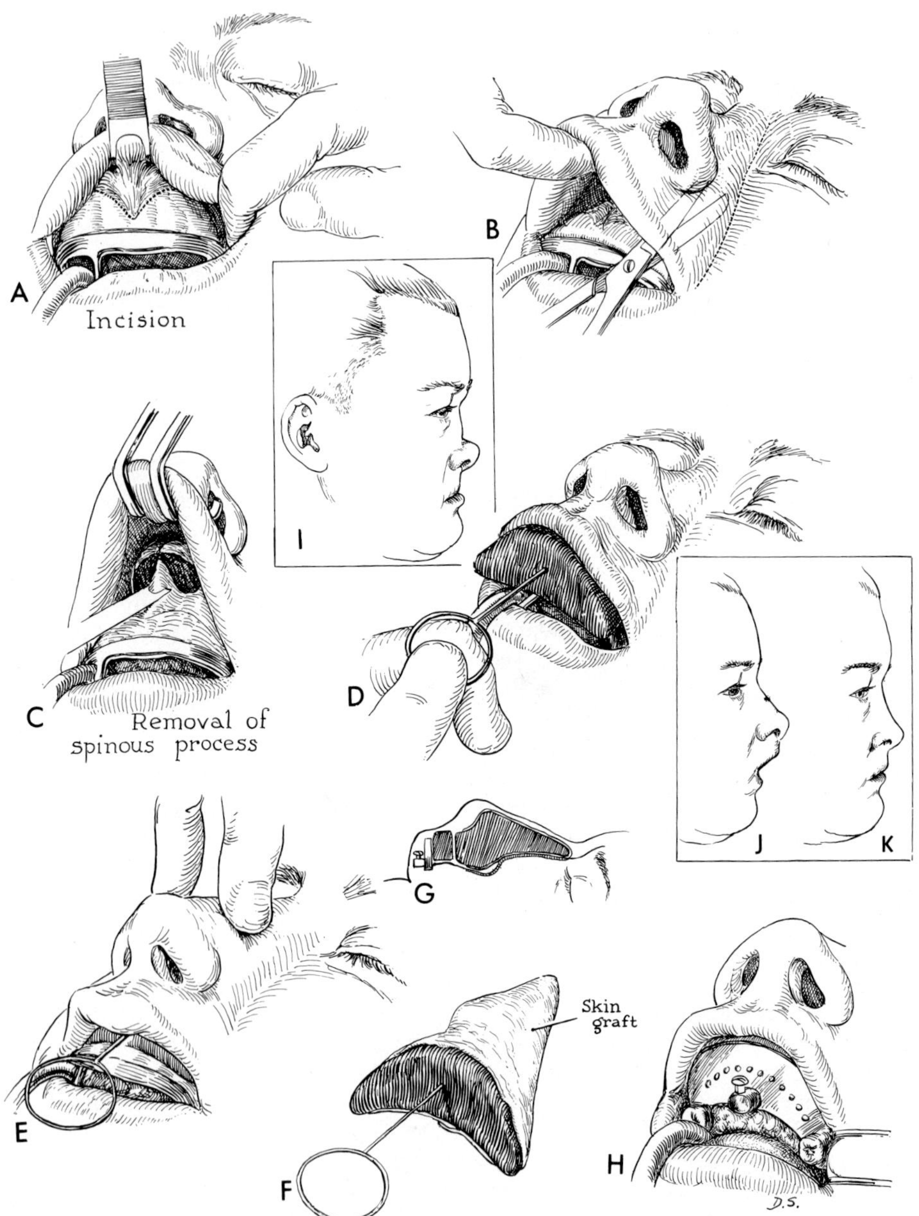

Figure 29–218. Technique of the nasomaxillary skin graft inlay (Gillies, 1923). *A,* Outline of the intraoral incision. *B,* The nasal cavity is entered through the mouth. *C,* The nasal spine is resected. *D,* A dental compound mold is fitted to the nasomaxillary cavity. *E,* The softened dental compound is molded to the nasomaxillary cavity by external digital pressure. *F,* The mold is covered with a split-thickness skin graft, raw surface outward. *G,* The mold carrying the skin graft is placed inside the maxillary cavity. It is held in position by a splint anchored to the upper molar teeth. In this patient, the remainder of the maxillary teeth are absent. *H,* The dental appliance maintaining the mold in the nasomaxillary cavity. *I* to *K,* Appearance of the patient before, during, and after the skin graft inlay procedure.

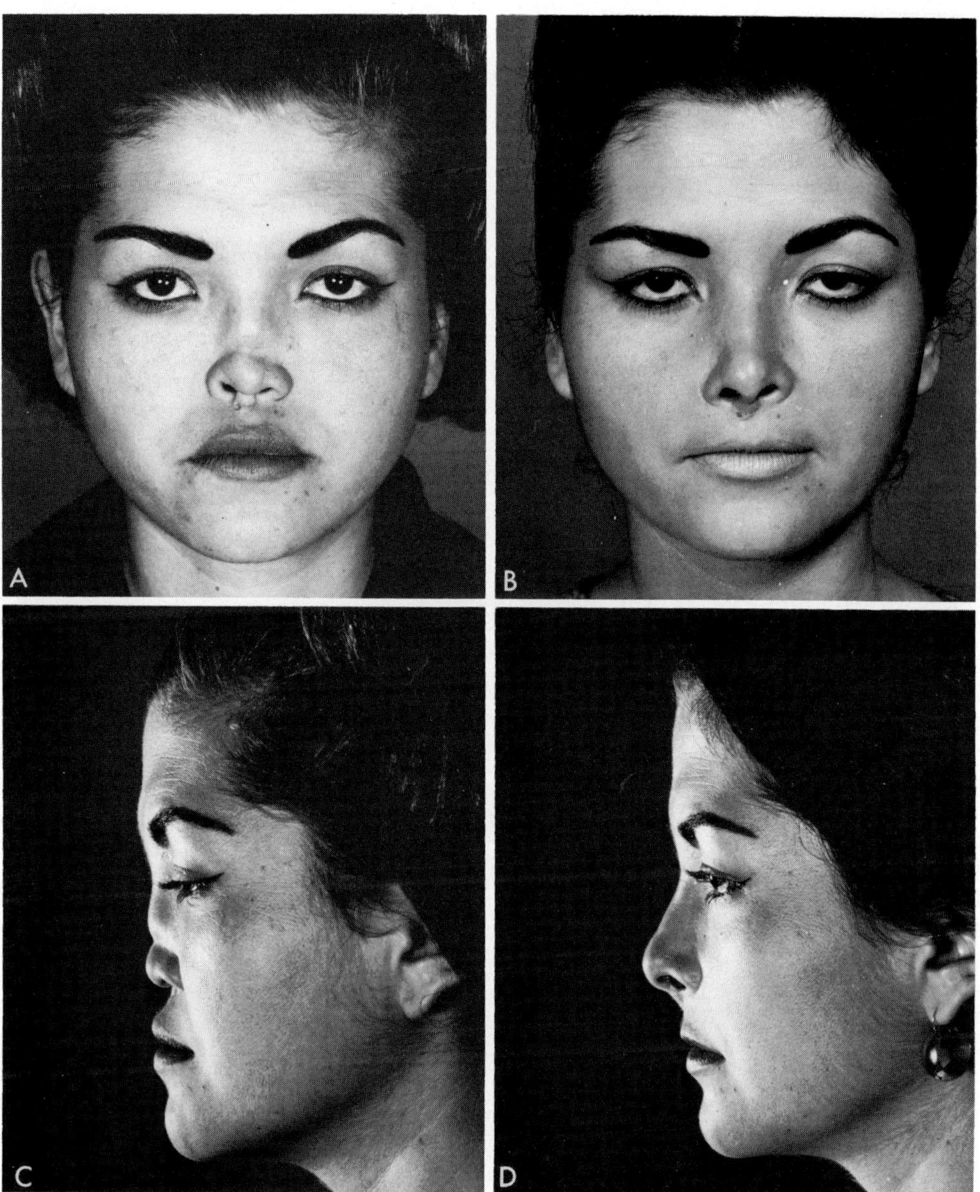

Figure 29–219. Contour restoration by the nasomaxillary skin graft technique. *A,* Appearance of the patient with complete loss of nasal lining and nasal obstruction resulting from the application of radon seeds at the age of 8 years for the treatment of epistaxis. *B,* Result obtained by the nasomaxillary skin graft inlay technique. *C,* Preoperative profile view showing nasomaxillary retrusion. *D,* Postoperative result.

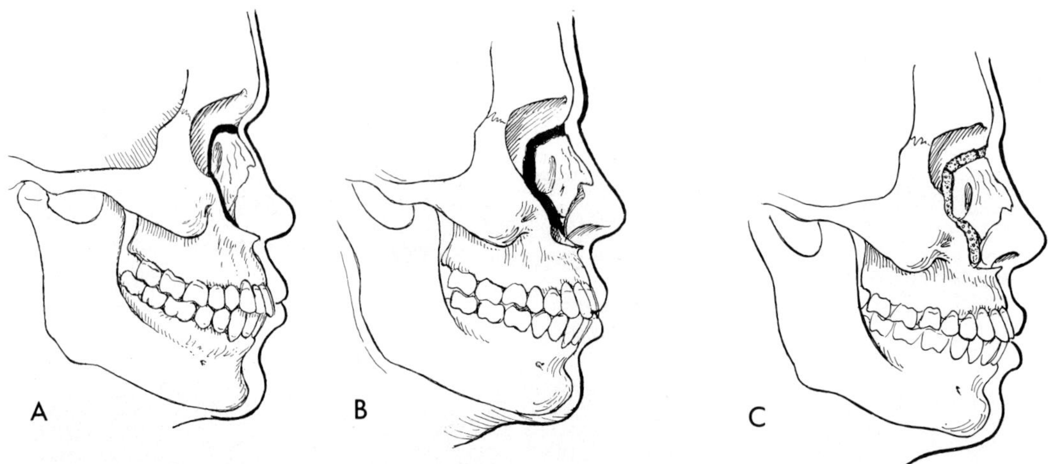

Figure 29–220. The perinasal osteotomy. Further lengthening and increase in the projection of the nose is obtained by the perinasal osteotomy. *A,* Nasomaxillary hypoplasia and a foreshortened nose. *B,* The osteotomy begins at the nasofrontal junction and extends posteriorly to the lacrimal groove, descending along the medial orbital wall and rim and joining a line of osteotomy extending through the base of the frontal process of the maxilla. The nasal skeleton can then be lifted to increase its forward projection. *C,* Small bone grafts are placed in the interstices left by the forward mobilization of the nasal structures.

rimal sac to an area situated posterior to the posterior lacrimal crest. The osteotomy extends downward, posterior to the lacrimal groove through the medial portion of the orbital floor and rim, and downward along the base of the lateral wall of the nose. This latter portion of the osteotomy can be performed with a nasal saw or osteotome. The separation of the nasal bones from the frontal bone can be completed with a small osteotome, which is levered downward. The area of the root of the nose then opens up. If resistance to downward displacement of the bones is noted, scissors are introduced into the nasal cavity, and the posterior portion of the septum is divided. Wedges of bone graft are placed between the frontal bone and the nasal bones, thus providing the desired lengthening of the bony portion of the nose. Thin plates of cancellous bone can be placed over the areas of osteotomy along the medial wall of the orbit. Wedges of bone are placed between, and thin plates of bone over, the edges of the line of osteotomy in the lateral wall of the nose. The detelescoping procedures required to lengthen the cartilaginous nasal skeletal framework (Fig. 29–221) are carried out when indicated. A bone graft placed along the dorsum of the nose is usually necessary to restore adequate contour and projection of the dorsum. The main criticism of this technique is that the mobilized segment is small and stabilization is difficult. However, microplates and screws have helped in this regard.

Naso-orbitomaxillary Osteotomy

Converse and associates (1970) designed a pyramidal naso-orbitomaxillary osteotomy to correct both the nasal and maxillary components of the deformity. The patient shown in Figure 29–222 had a history of a nasal septal hematoma-abscess following injury at the age of 4 years. An abscess and subsequent necrosis of the septal cartilage resulted in failure of growth and development of the nasomaxillary area.

The principles of the procedure include the following: (1) the foreshortened nasoseptal framework must be advanced, as it will oppose nasal lengthening; (2) a forward and downward repositioning of the underdeveloped nasomaxillary complex is required to correct the maxillary retrusion and to elongate the nose; (3) the nasolacrimal apparatus must not be disrupted; (4) bone grafts are used to restore the nasal contour and to fill the defects resulting from the advancement of the nasomaxillary complex; and (5) skin coverage and nasal lining must be provided to accommodate the nasal elongation.

Exposure of Nasal Framework. The nasal framework and medial orbital wall are exposed through a coronal or trapdoor inci-

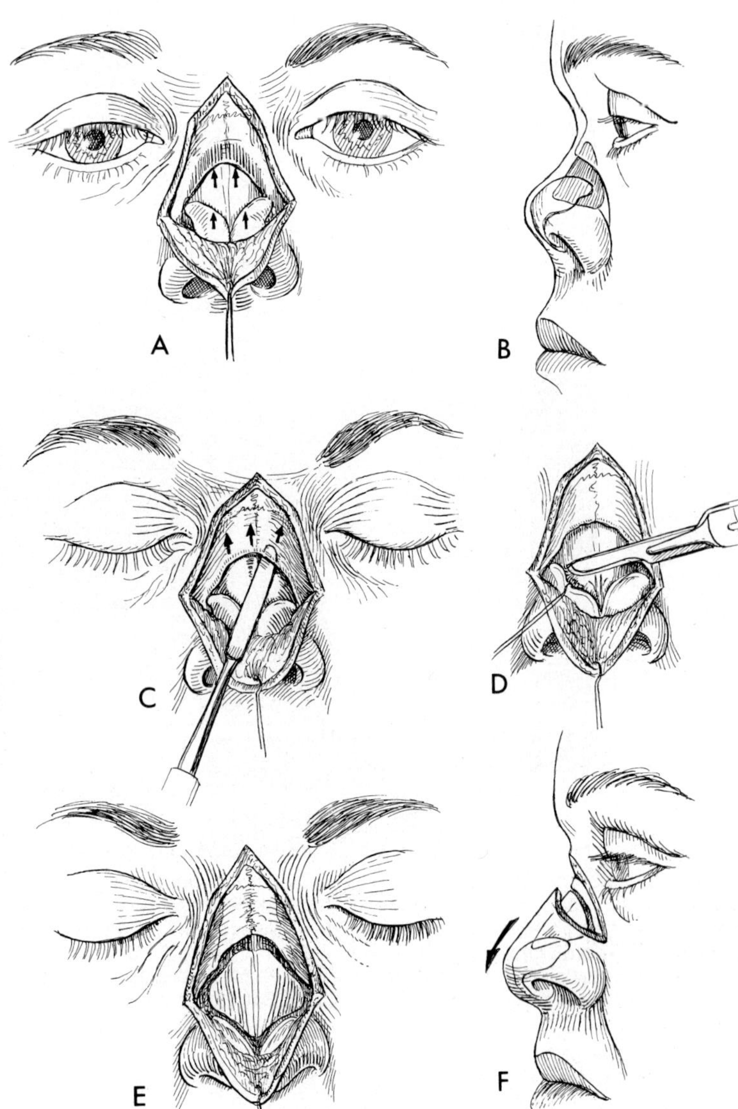

Figure 29–221. Elongation of the cartilaginous framework. *A, B,* The arrows indicate the usual direction of the overlapping of the nasal bones and the alar cartilages over the lateral cartilages. *C,* Detaching the lateral cartilages and the mucoperiosteum from under the nasal bones. After the lining tissues have been severed transversely under the nasal bones, they can be drawn downward to elongate the lining of the nose. *D,* Further elongation is obtained by separating the alar from the lateral cartilages and advancing the alar cartilages caudad. *E, F,* Elongation obtained.

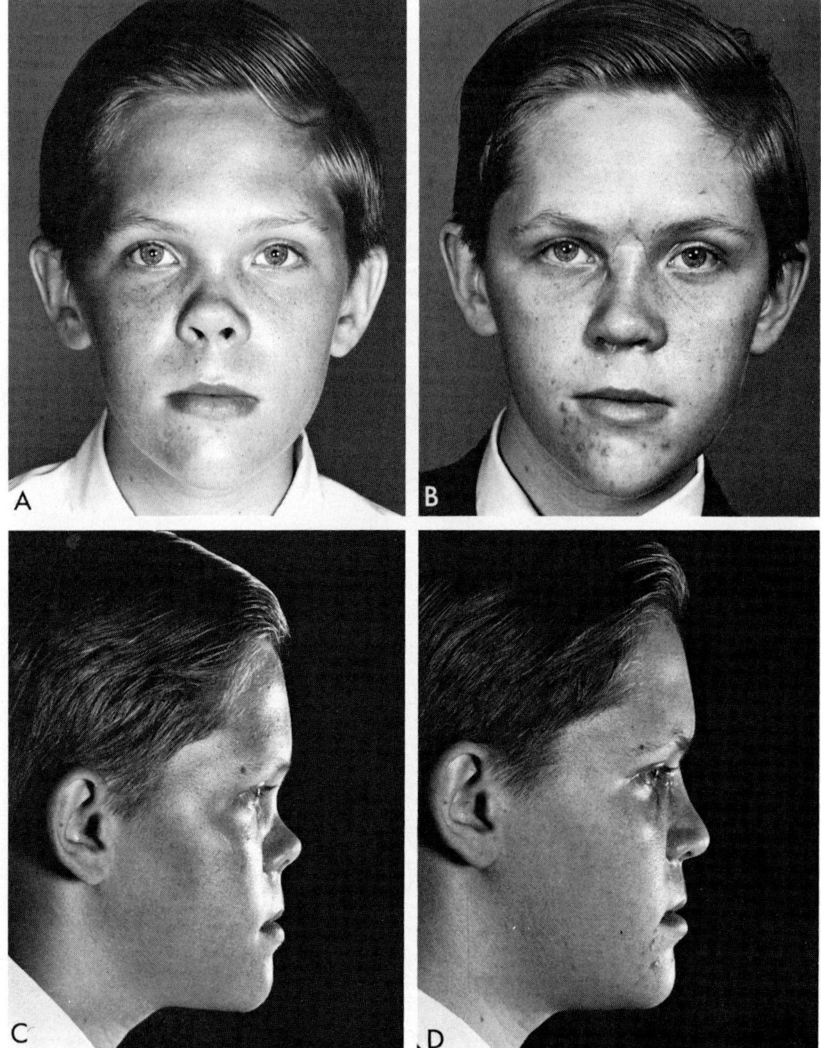

Figure 29–222. Correction of nasomaxillary hypoplasia by naso-orbitomaxillary advancement osteotomy. *A,* Preoperative appearance showing the retrusion of the midfacial skeleton. *B,* Appearance after advancement. *C, D,* Preoperative and postoperative profile views. Note the elongation of the nose and the increased nasomaxillary forward projection. A coronal scalp incision is preferred. (From Converse, J. M., Horowitz, S. L., Valauri, A. J., and Montandon, D.: The treatment of nasomaxillary hypoplasia. A new pyramidal naso-orbital maxillary osteotomy. Plast. Reconstr. Surg., *45*:527, 1970. Copyright 1970, The Williams & Wilkins Company, Baltimore.)

sion, triangular in shape with its apex at the glabella (Fig. 29–223); the incision also provides additional skin coverage by means of a V-Y advancement. Retraction of the flap provides exposure and permits subperiosteal elevation of the soft tissues from the bone framework of the nose and the nasal cartilages. The dissection is extended to the base of the piriform aperture. The periosteum is reflected from the lacrimal groove, and the medial wall of the orbit is exposed. The medial canthal tendon and the lacrimal sac are left attached.

The first phase of the skeletal surgery involves lengthening the cartilaginous nose. A submucous exposure of the residual septal framework is effected. Released from the restrictive influence of the septum, the cartilaginous portion of the nose becomes more extensible. By reflecting the trapdoor flap downward, the area of junction of the lateral cartilages with the nasal bones is exposed. The lateral cartilages are separated from the undersurface of the nasal bones. The mucoperiosteum underlying the nasal bones is undermined as far upward as possible and

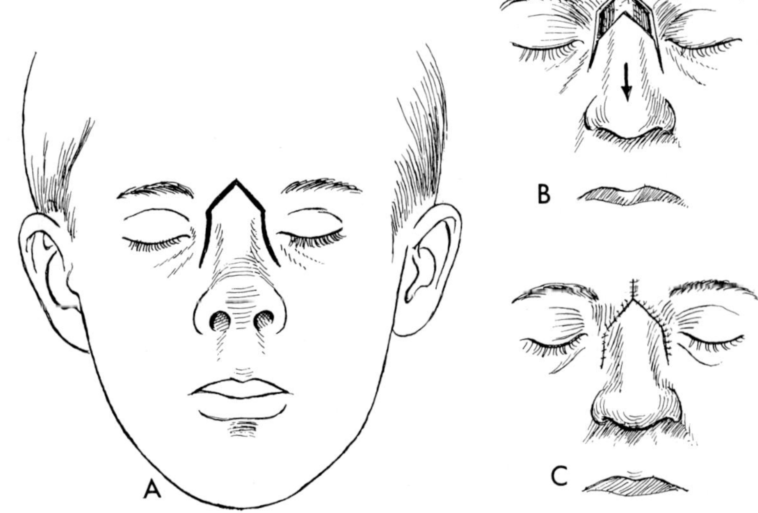

Figure 29–223. Exposure of the nasal framework and elongation of the nose. *A,* Incision, outlining the trapdoor flap. *B, C,* V-Y advancement to elongate the skin of the nose. (From Converse, J. M., Horowitz, S. L., Valauri, A. J., and Montandon, D.: The treatment of nasomaxillary hypoplasia. A new pyramidal naso-orbital maxillary osteotomy. Plast. Reconstr. Surg., *45*:527, 1970. Copyright 1970, The Williams & Wilkins Company, Baltimore.)

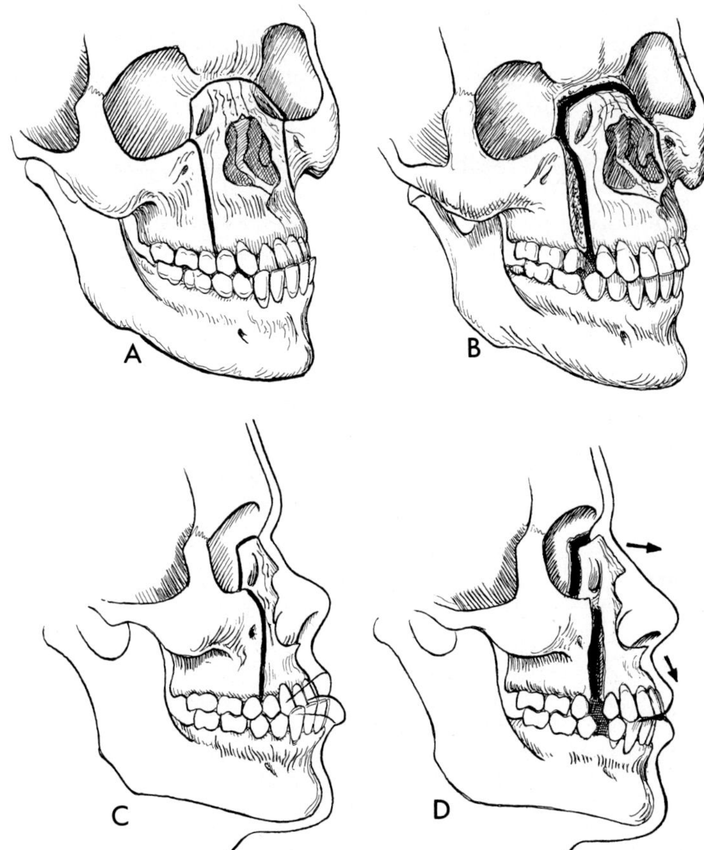

Figure 29–224. Naso-orbitomaxillary osteotomy for forward and downward displacement of the nasomaxillary complex. *A,* The line of osteotomy extends across the nasofrontal junction, posterior to the lacrimal groove, through the rim of the orbit, downward through the maxilla into the premolar area, and across the hard palate. *B,* After the posterior portion of the nasal septum is severed, the nasomaxillary block is mobilized. *C,* Lateral view of the line of osteotomy. *D,* Forward and downward displacement made possible by the osteotomy. Bone grafts are wedged into the gaps to maintain the position of the nasomaxillary complex and to ensure consolidation. When the molar relationships are in a Class III malocclusion, the osteotomy can be modified and is extended posteriorly as far as the pterygomaxillary junction. (From Converse, J. M., Horowitz, S. L., Valauri, A. J., and Montandon, D.: The treatment of nasomaxillary hypoplasia. A new pyramidal naso-orbital maxillary osteotomy. Plast. Reconstr. Surg., *45*:527, 1970. Copyright 1970, The Williams & Wilkins Company, Baltimore.)

incised transversely. At this point, by placing the thumb and index finger on each side of the columella near the tip of the nose, it is possible to draw the nasal structures downward. Further elongation is also obtained by dividing the loose connective tissue joining the alar and lateral nasal cartilages.

A transverse osteotomy separates the nasal bones from the frontal bone (Fig. 29–224). The line of osteotomy is extended along the medial orbital wall and is then directed vertically downward to the medial portion of the floor of the orbit, anterolaterally to the lacrimal groove but medial to the infraorbital foramen to preserve the lacrimal apparatus and the infraorbital nerve. It is continued downward through the anterior wall of the maxillary sinus and through the alveolar process between the first and second premolar teeth.

A posteriorly based mucoperiosteal flap is raised from the palatal vault, exposing the hard palate. The osteotomy is completed by cutting transversely across the palate into the floor of the nose and through the vomer if it has not been resected during the submucous resection of the septum (Fig. 29–225). The posterior portion of the maxilla provides a strong abutment and the molar teeth can be used as stable posterior points of fixation. The entire nasomaxillary segment is advanced the desired distance and the position is maintained by the orthodontic appliance anchored on the posterior maxillary teeth. Intermaxillary fixation is not necessary. The forward movement of the mobilized segment is also accompanied by a downward movement to lengthen the nose.

The gaps in the facial skeleton are filled with fragments of autogenous bone. Wedges of bone are placed into the bony defect in the nasofrontal area and over the perinasal and anterior maxillary portions of the skeleton. The open spaces in the hard palate and the alveolar process are also packed with bone grafts. A carved iliac or cranial bone graft is introduced over the dorsum of the nose (see Fig. 29–216). The upper portion of the bone graft is maintained by transosseous wire fixation or lag screws near the nasofrontal osteotomy, and the distal tip of the bone graft is placed between the domes of the alar cartilages, which are sutured to each other over the graft.

A V-Y advancement of the skin in the glabellar area provides the necessary additional cutaneous coverage. The operation is completed by placing over the nose a carefully applied splint, which is left in position for five days.

Psillakis, Lapa, and Spina (1973) employed a modification of the naso-orbitomaxillary osteotomy in patients whose dental occlusion was adequate. The osteotomy does not include the dentoalveolar segment of the maxilla and is similar to the perinasal osteotomy previously described. The disadvantage of creating a gap in the dental arch is thus avoided.

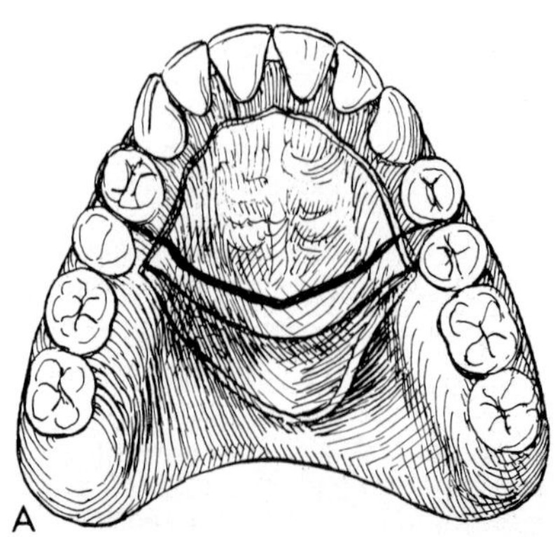

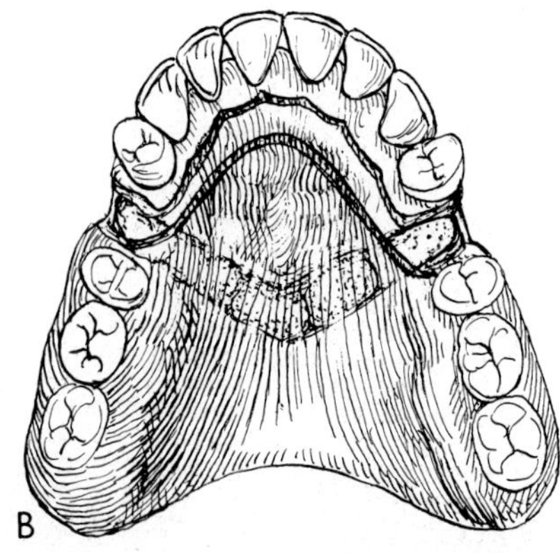

Figure 29–225. Line of section through the hard palate in the naso-orbitomaxillary osteotomy. *A,* After the mucoperiosteal palatal flap has been raised, the palatal osteotomy is made as outlined. After the naso-orbitomaxillary segment has been advanced, bone grafts are wedged into the defect in the hard palate, and the palatal flap is returned to cover the bone grafted area. The denuded anterior portion of the hard palate is left to epithelize spontaneously. (From Converse, J. M., Horowitz, S. L., Valauri, A. J., and Montandon, D.: The treatment of nasomaxillary hypoplasia. A new pyramidal naso-orbital maxillary osteotomy. Plast. Reconstr. Surg., *45*:527, 1970. Copyright 1970, The Williams & Wilkins Company, Baltimore.)

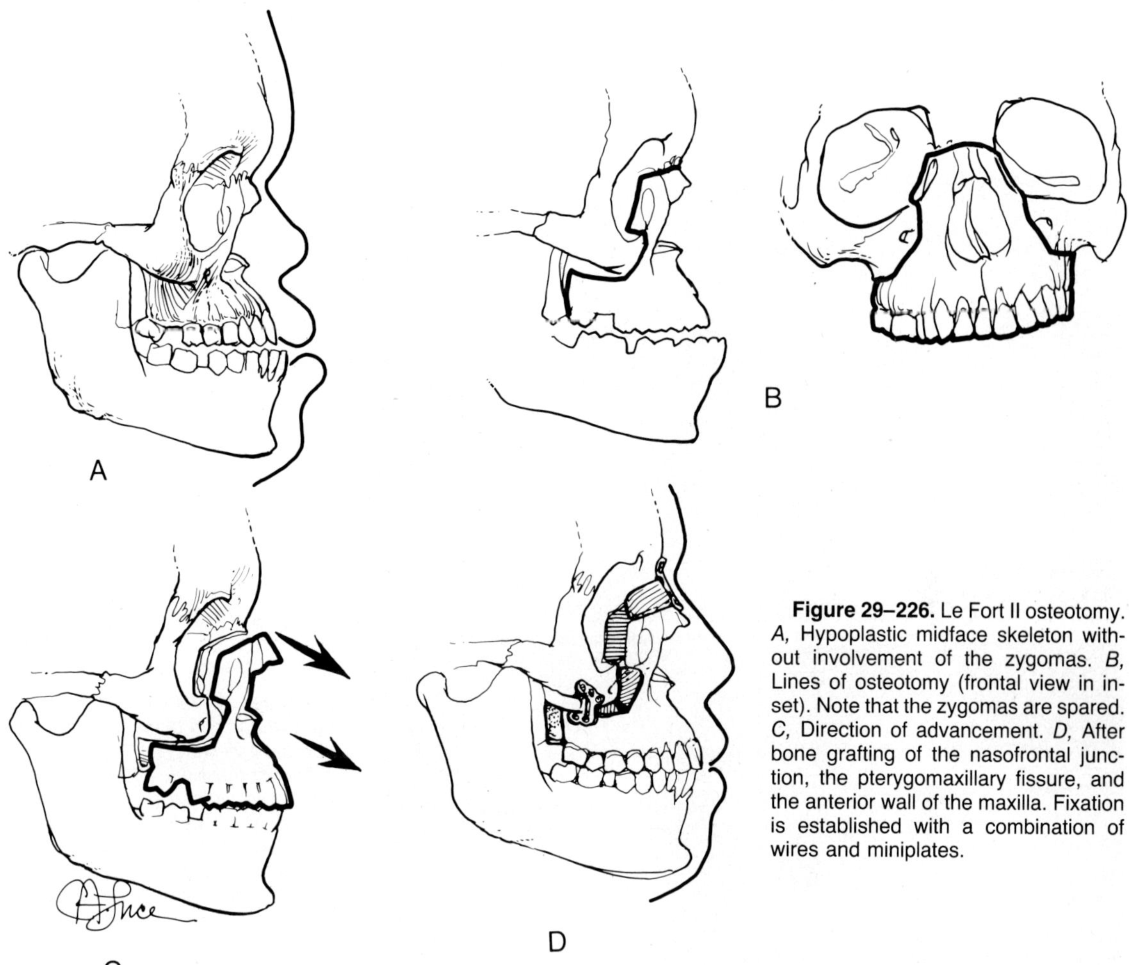

Figure 29–226. Le Fort II osteotomy. *A,* Hypoplastic midface skeleton without involvement of the zygomas. *B,* Lines of osteotomy (frontal view in inset). Note that the zygomas are spared. *C,* Direction of advancement. *D,* After bone grafting of the nasofrontal junction, the pterygomaxillary fissure, and the anterior wall of the maxilla. Fixation is established with a combination of wires and miniplates.

Le Fort II Osteotomy

This osteotomy (Henderson and Jackson, 1973) is indicated when the patient has nasomaxillary hypoplasia in addition to recession of the lower maxillary segment and Class III malocclusion. The zygomas are not involved and consequently a Le Fort III osteotomy is not indicated. The lines of osteotomy follow the classic Le Fort II fracture lines (Fig. 29–226). Through a coronal incision or incisions made over the frontal process of the maxilla on each side of the nose (Henderson and Jackson, 1973), a subperiosteal dissection exposes the medial wall of the orbit. The medial canthus is left attached and the lacrimal sac is raised from the lacrimal groove on each side.

Through an intraoral vestibular approach the maxilla is exposed subperiosteally, and the infraorbital nerves are identified. Laterally, the junction of the zygoma with the maxilla on each side is exposed.

The osteotomy across the nasofrontal junction is made with a power-driven mechanical saw and is continued posteriorly along each medial orbital wall until it reaches the lamina papyracea of the ethmoid, posterior to the lacrimal groove. The osteotomy then changes direction, extending vertically downward to the floor of the orbit and lateral to the lacrimal groove (medial to the infraorbital foramen); it curves laterally along the area of junction of the maxilla and zygoma and backward to the pterygomaxillary junction. Pterygomaxillary dysjunction is accomplished with a curved osteotome.

The ethmoid plate of the septum is divided with scissors after the midface has been rocked forward and downward.

The nasomaxillary segment is then advanced with Rowe forceps into the planned

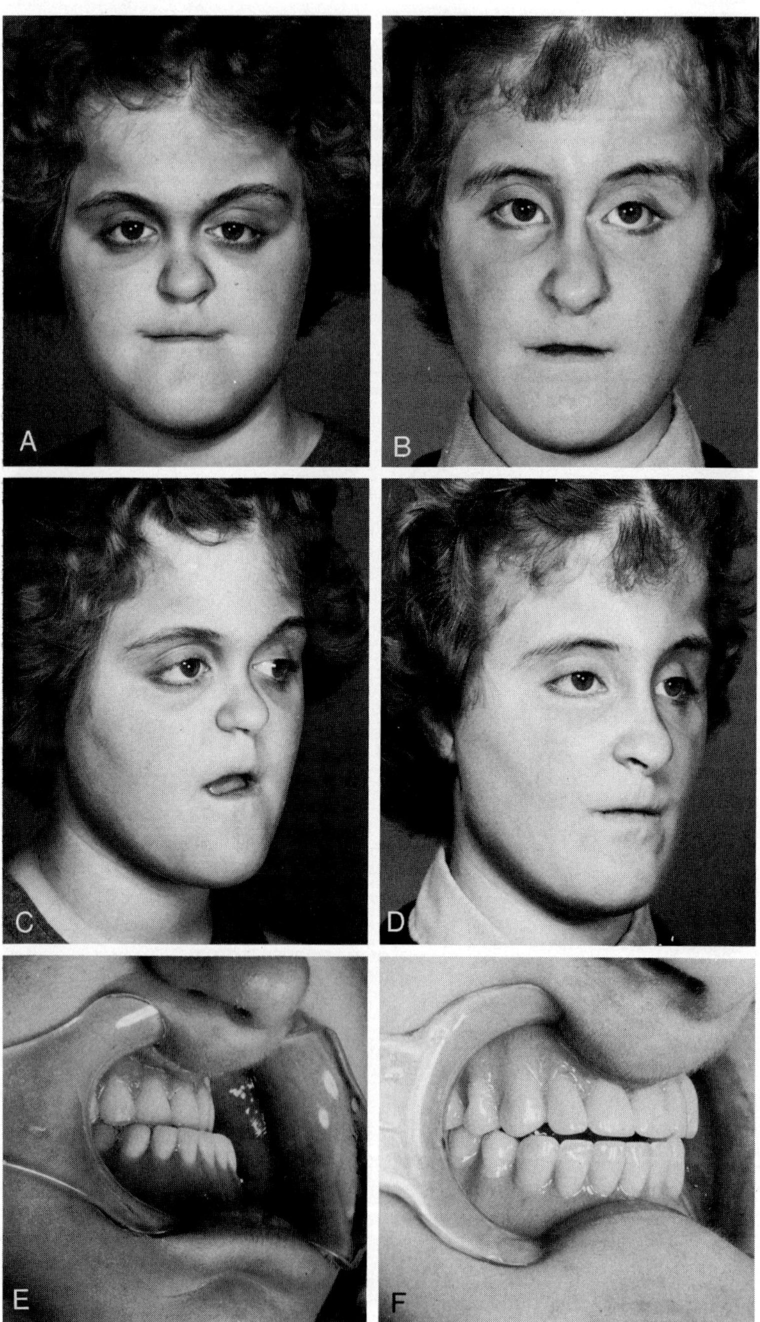

Figure 29–227. Le Fort II advancement osteotomy. *A, C,* Preoperative views of a 17 year old girl with nasomaxillary hypoplasia secondary to vitamin D resistant rickets. *B, D,* Appearance after a Le Fort II osteotomy. *E,* Preoperative occlusion. The patient wore a complete set of dentures. *F,* Postoperative view after prosthodontic replacement.

position and secured by intermaxillary fixation techniques. Bone grafts are wedged into the nasofrontal, medial orbital, and pterygomaxillary defects. Craniofacial suspension wiring or miniplate fixation at the nasofrontal osteotomy site provides additional fixation. Direct interosseous wiring or miniplate fixation at the osteotomy sites on the inferior orbital rims is usually practiced (Fig. 29–227).

Munro, Sinclair, and Rudd (1979) recommended a Le Fort II advancement combined with a Le Fort I osteotomy in those patients with Binder's syndrome in whom the occlusion is acceptable but in whom projection of the nasomaxillary area above the dentoalveolar level is desired.

A modification of the Le Fort II osteotomy was introduced by Kufner (1971) and subsequently termed the *quadrangular* osteotomy by Steinhauser (1980). It differs from the classical Le Fort II osteotomy in that the nasal root is not mobilized (Fig. 29–228). It is particularly suited to patients in whom additional elongation of the nose is not desired.

For the Le Fort II osteotomy, relapse is also a concern. Ward-Booth, Bhatia, and Moos (1984), in a sample of patients with cleft palate, showed a reversal of more than 30 per cent in approximately one-third of their patients. In patients without cleft palate undergoing the operation at the same institution, there was stability of the advanced fragment with little evidence of relapse (Stirrups, Patton, and Moos, 1986).

Other Osteotomy Techniques

Other techniques that can be employed include the Le Fort I osteotomy (see Fig. 29–196) and the premolar segmental osteotomy (see Fig. 29–169). Both procedures advance the maxillary dentoalveolar segment, but neither gives sufficient projection of the nasomaxillary segment. One of the principal advantages of the Le Fort I osteotomy is that the dental arch continuity remains intact; edentulous spaces are not produced by the operation.

The advantage of the premolar segmental osteotomy is that molar relationships are not disturbed when they are satisfactory, a not infrequent condition in patients with cleft palate. The premolar osteotomy also offers the advantage of maintaining a stable posterior segment for monomaxillary fixation. Intermaxillary fixation is not necessary and velopharyngeal competence is not jeopardized.

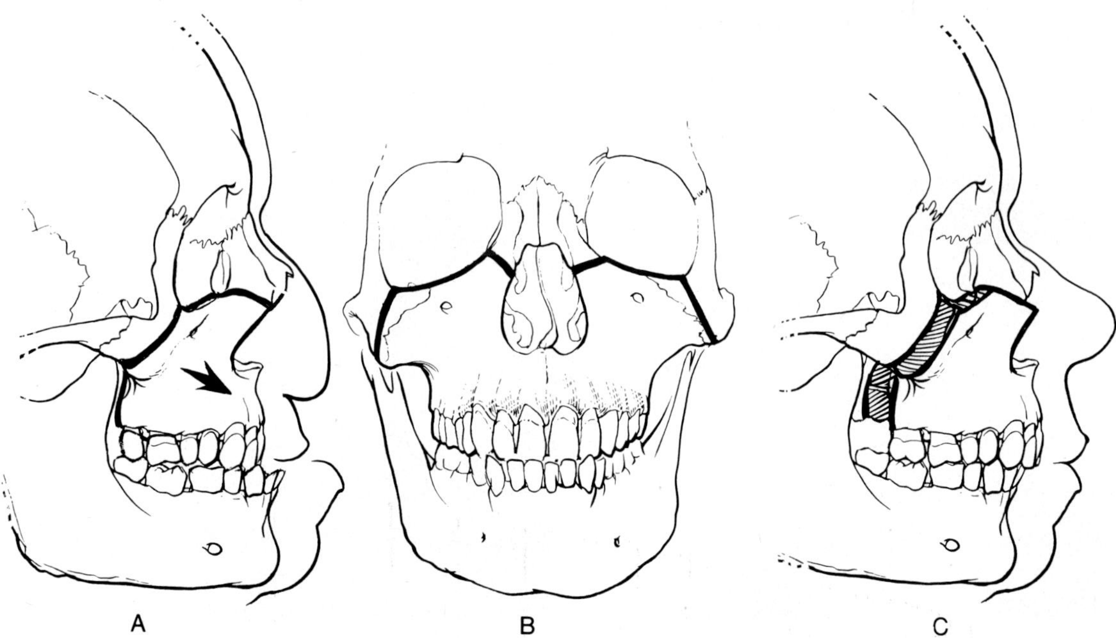

Figure 29–228. Modification of the Le Fort II osteotomy or the quadrangular osteotomy (Kufner, 1971; Steinhauser, 1980). *A, B,* Lines of osteotomy and the direction *(arrow)* of the midface advancement. *C,* After advancement.

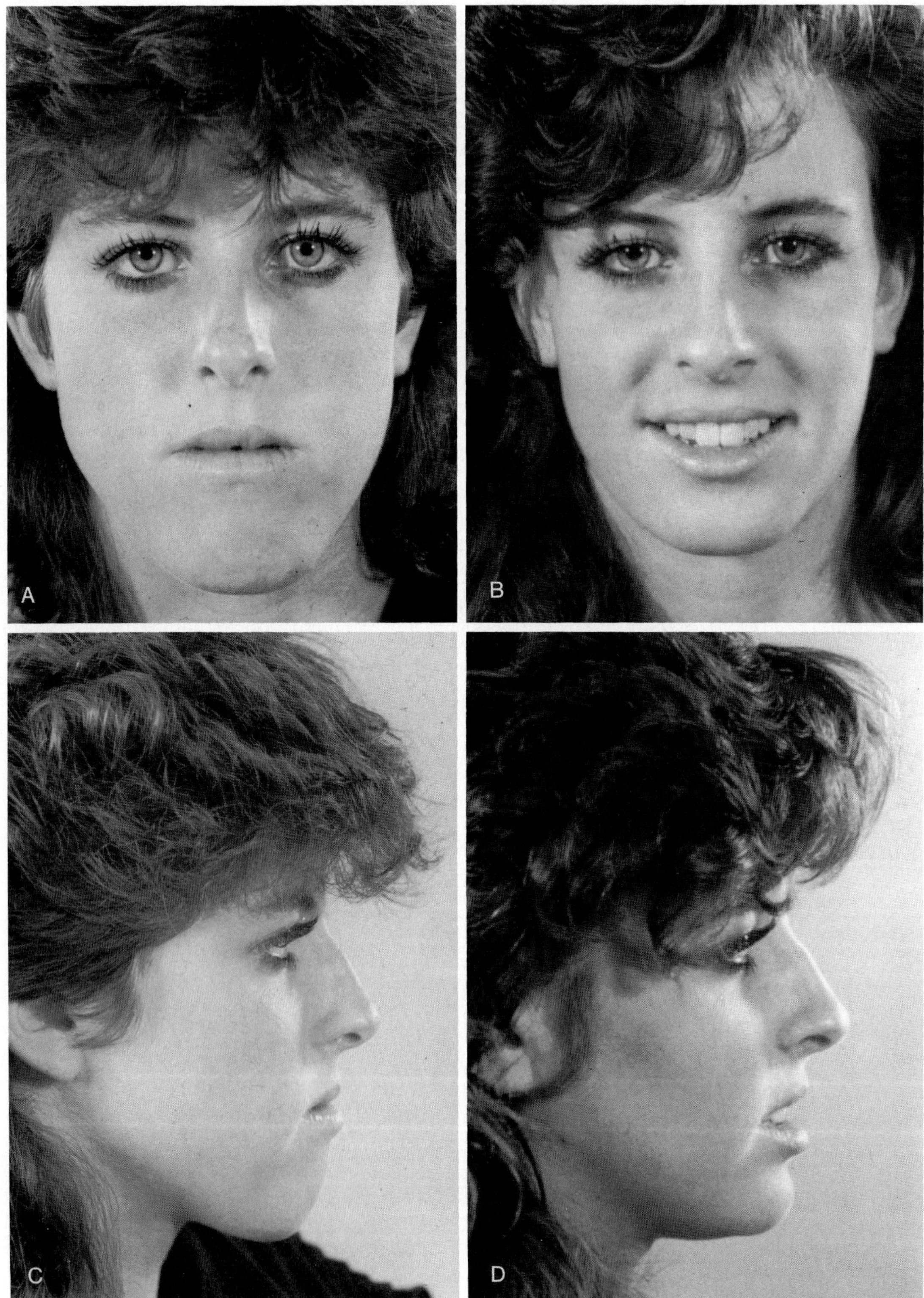

Figure 29–229 *See legend on opposite page*

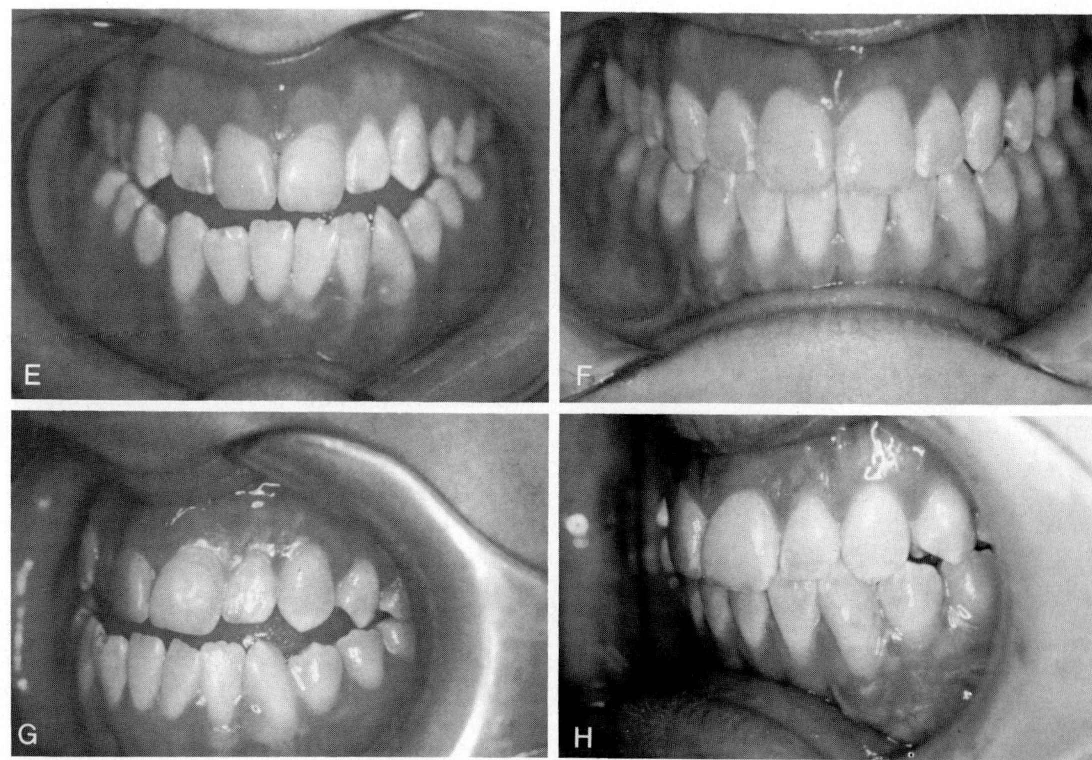

Figure 29–229. Maxillomandibular dysharmony. *A, C, E, G,* Preoperative appearance of an adolescent female with anterior open bite, maxillary deficiency, mandibular prognathism, and vertical excess of the chin. *B, D, F, H,* Appearance after one-stage Le Fort I osteotomy, bilateral oblique osteotomies of the mandibular rami (intraoral), and genioplasty.

Maxillomandibular Disharmonies

Disparities in size and position can exist between the maxilla (midface) and mandible. The most common example is a maxillary micrognathia and mandibular prognathism.

There are three indications for simultaneous surgical mobilization of the maxilla and mandible (Moser and Freihofer, 1980). The first is evidence of skeletal pathology in each jaw. Second, if the desired mobilization of either jaw exceeds 10 mm, the likelihood of relapse is greater with a single jaw mobilization of 11 mm than with a combined maxillary advancement of 6 mm and mandibular recession of 5 mm. The third indication is improved facial esthetics.

In the preoperative assessment the clinical examination must consider the relationship of the maxillary incisors to the lip, the amount of incisor show, the degree of the nasolabial angle, the contour of the infraorbital region and mandible, and the steepness of the mandibular plane.

Cephalometric analysis should confirm the clinical impression and document the skeletal pathology in each jaw.

From the study models two occlusal wafers are fabricated: an *intermediate* and a *definitive* occlusal splint (see Fig. 29–23) (Lindorf and Steinhauser, 1978; Turvey, 1982).

The most common combination of osteotomies in two-jaw surgery is a sagittal split recession of the mandible and a Le Fort I advancement of the maxilla.

The surgical sequence is as described. Initially the mandibular rami are exposed and the sagittal split osteotomies are made bilaterally. However, the sectioning of the rami is not completed (only 90 per cent) in order to preserve mandibular stability.

Attention is then turned to the maxilla; the osteotomies are made and the upper jaw is mobilized. The *intermediate* splint is used to relate the mobilized maxilla to the nonmobilized mandible. Intermaxillary fixation is established and miniplate fixation of the advanced maxillary segment is achieved (see Fig. 29–196).

This maneuver is followed by completion of the osteotomy and repositioning of the mandible. The *intermediate* splint is removed and replaced by the *definitive* splint. In this way the mandible can be oriented to the surgically corrected maxilla by intermaxillary fixation. A genioplasty often completes the procedure.

A patient who underwent operative procedures on both jaws is shown in Figure 29–229. The preoperative cephalogram documented the fact that the maxilla required advancement and the mandible recession. A high Le Fort I osteotomy was performed (see Fig. 29–196) concomitantly with bilateral sagittal osteotomy of the ramus to recess the mandible. A case study is illustrated in Figure 29–230.

Complications of Orthognathic Surgery

Complications after corrective jaw surgery are usually secondary to inadequate preoperative planning and faulty surgical technique (McCarthy, 1977). Many of the reported complications are common to any surgical procedure; others are unique to jaw surgery. The more common complications following maxillary and mandibular surgery will be discussed.

HEMATOMA

Hematoma is a major complication and serves as a culture medium for bacterial organisms, often with the development of a wound infection. A hematoma can also jeopardize the viability of a skin or mucosal flap. Hematoma can be minimized by meticulous surgical technique, dissection in a subperiosteal plane, and careful attention to hemostasis. Dependent suction drainage should be used if there is any question of inadequate hemostasis or residual dead space.

In jaw surgery, hemorrhage and hematoma formation are usually more common after sagittal split osteotomy of the ramus of the mandible. The internal maxillary vessels can be damaged while performing the osteotomy on the medial side of the mandible, and the facial (external maxillary) vessels can be damaged in the course of sectioning the lateral aspect of the ramus (Behrman, 1972). In the vertical osteotomy of the ramus the internal maxillary vessels can also be inadvertently lacerated. Oscillating saws tend not to lacerate soft tissues, and malleable retractors placed between the ramus and the vessels protect the latter during the ramisection. Hemorrhage can also be encountered at the time of pterygomaxillary disimpaction. This osteotomy is best accomplished with a curved, tapered osteotome that is kept close to the maxillary tuberosity to avoid damage to the pterygoid plexus.

The descending palatine vessels can be lacerated in the course of a Le Fort I osteotomy. With downfracture of the maxillary segment, hemostasis can be obtained by applying clips to the bleeding vessels.

Hemorrhage can usually be controlled by inserting well wrung-out epinephrine packs into the bleeding site for several minutes. Vessel ligation often is not required.

INFECTION

In terms of infection the head and neck area is a relatively privileged site because of the rich regional blood supply and local immunologic factors. Fragmentation of the bone segments and hematoma formation are principal factors promoting the development of a local wound infection.

Although the nonhemolytic streptococci are the predominating organisms, it is the anaerobic streptococci in association with fusiform bacilli and spirochetes that can be extremely destructive of local tissue. Since the flora of the oral cavity are multiple in number and the possibility of contamination of the operative field is often unavoidable, the routine use of prophylactic antibiotics has been questioned (Converse and McCarthy, 1972). However, their clinical use is widespread, and the absolute indications for the use of prophylactic antibiotics, which should be administered preoperatively and again during the surgical procedure, include the following:

1. An intraoral surgical approach.
2. Previous irradiation of the operative site.
3. Use of a bone graft.
4. Use of an alloplastic implant.
5. Poor dental hygiene.
6. Patients prone to infection, i.e., those with impoverished local blood supply, carrier state, malnutrition, remote preexisting infection, or therapy that alters the host defense mechanisms.

Once an infection is established, treatment consists of surgical drainage of the infected area, curettement of any areas of osteitis, and removal of infected grafts or alloplastic materials. In addition, it is essential to remove any interosseous wire at the site of infection. A chronically draining sinus tract (Fig. 29–231) should be completely excised and the underlying infected bone resected. The wound should be closed loosely with only a few sutures, and a catheter placed for continuous irrigation of the wound with an antiobiotic solution (Fig. 29–232). Parenteral antibiotics, chosen according to individual sensitivities determined on bacteriologic study, should be administered. Treatment, in general, should be aggressive, because relapse of the osseous deformity is an almost inevitable consequence of infection after corrective jaw surgery.

PAROTID FISTULA

Parotid fistula has been reported as a rare complication after bilateral oblique osteotomies of the mandibular rami (Goldberg, Marco, and Googel, 1973). In the reported case, drainage ceased spontaneously on the 19th postoperative day, but incision and drainage of a cyst were required earlier in the postoperative period.

BONE NECROSIS

Areas of exposed bone within the oral cavity result either from local infection or failure to provide sufficient soft tissue coverage of the osteotomy or bone graft sites. Behrman (1972), in a survey of a group of surgeons, reported this complication in eight of 64 patients undergoing sagittal split osteotomy of the mandibular ramus. The protective role of the periosteum was also emphasized because the blood supply to the lateral mandibular fragment comes from the condyle. Consequently, the lateral segment should be only conservatively skeletonized.

The best prophylaxis against this complication is the provision of soft tissue coverage. Mucosal flaps can be transferred over the osteotomy sites and bone graft recipient areas from the adjacent buccal and lingual areas.

When an area of exposed bone is detected, curettement of the involved area is indicated until bleeding from viable bone is observed. *The procedure can often be salvaged.* If there is careful attention to local wound care, bone grafts, as they acquire an independent blood supply, show remarkable vitality and ability to survive, especially after they are covered by granulation tissue and mucosa from the periphery of the defect.

MALUNION AND NONUNION

Malunion and nonunion are caused by faulty surgical planning and inadequate postoperative fixation. Other contributing factors include inaccurate intraoperative bone alignment and apposition, failure to impact the ends of the bone segments at the osteotomy site, inadequate blood supply and soft tissue coverage, and wound sepsis. Bone grafts should be used to fill any residual defects at the osteotomy sites if there is absence of apposition of the osteotomized fragments.

Guernsey and DeChamplain (1971) reported five cases of intraoperative fracture of the mandible during the sagittal split procedure; this is another factor that interferes with bone healing and favors the development of malunion.

Postoperative fixation must be secure, particularly in view of the pull of the powerful muscles of mastication on the individual bone fragments. The elevator muscles can displace the ramus fragments after a sagittal split osteotomy, and in addition the suprahyoid musculature can cause recurrence of an open bite deformity because of the pull on the mandibular symphysis. Secure postoperative fixation employed for a sufficient length of time ensures stabilization of the mobilized fragments. The newer rigid (miniplate) fixation systems provide additional means of obtaining optimal skeletal stabilization.

Treatment of malunion or nonunion consists of redoing the osteotomy with resection of any intervening fibrous tissue between the bone fragments. The resulting defect should be filled with autogenous bone grafts, and an appropriate period of fixation is indicated.

LOSS OF TEETH AND VITALITY

The loss of individual teeth or teeth vitality is a problem usually associated with segmental dentoalveolar osteotomies. One must distinguish between *tooth sensibility*, which is a parameter of nerve function, and *tooth vitality*, which depends on the pulp blood supply. Nerve function (sensibility) is best tested by carbon dioxide snow, thermography, and liquid crystal methods. Problems in vitality are manifested by color changes and loosening of

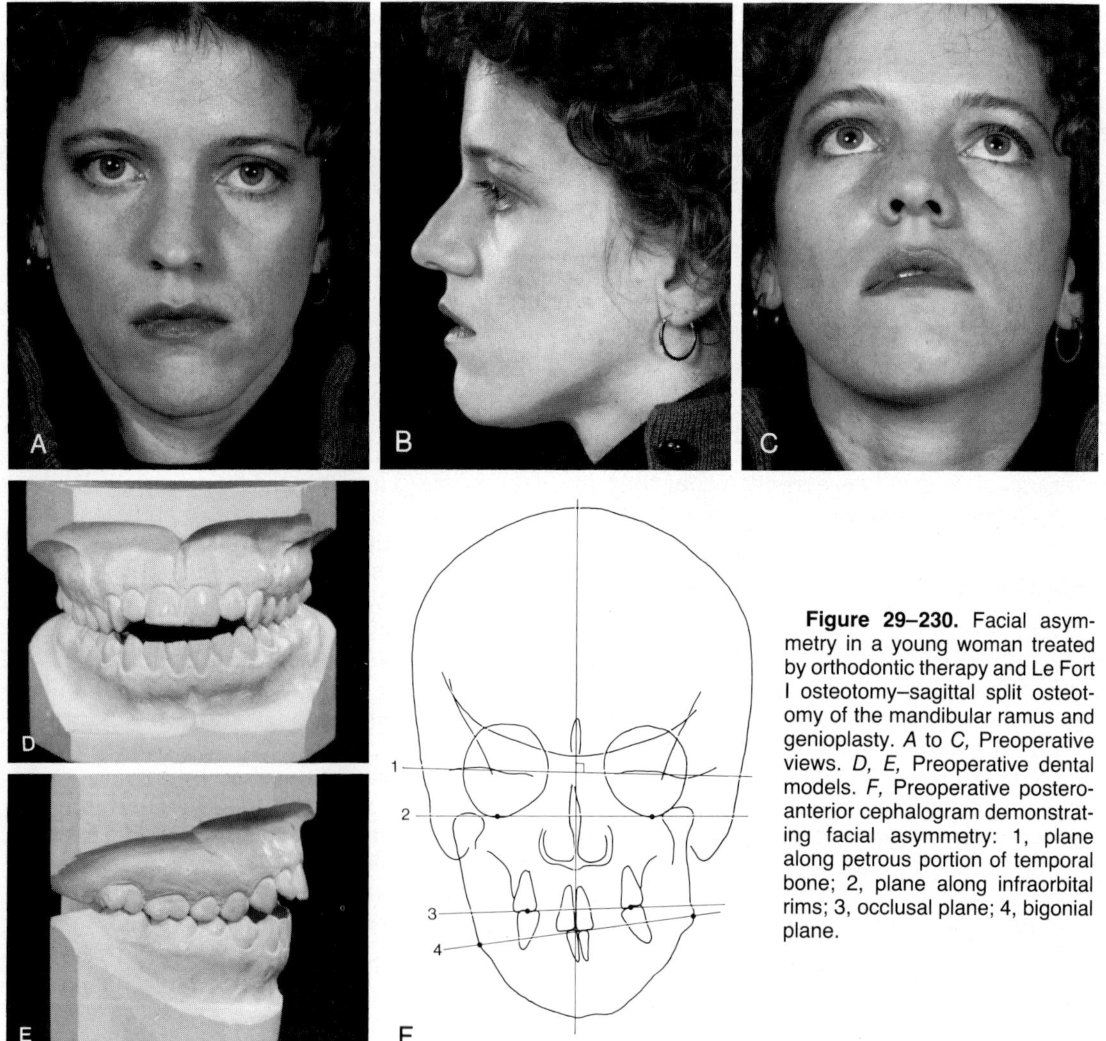

Figure 29–230. Facial asymmetry in a young woman treated by orthodontic therapy and Le Fort I osteotomy–sagittal split osteotomy of the mandibular ramus and genioplasty. *A* to *C,* Preoperative views. *D, E,* Preoperative dental models. *F,* Preoperative posteroanterior cephalogram demonstrating facial asymmetry: 1, plane along petrous portion of temporal bone; 2, plane along infraorbital rims; 3, occlusal plane; 4, bigonial plane.

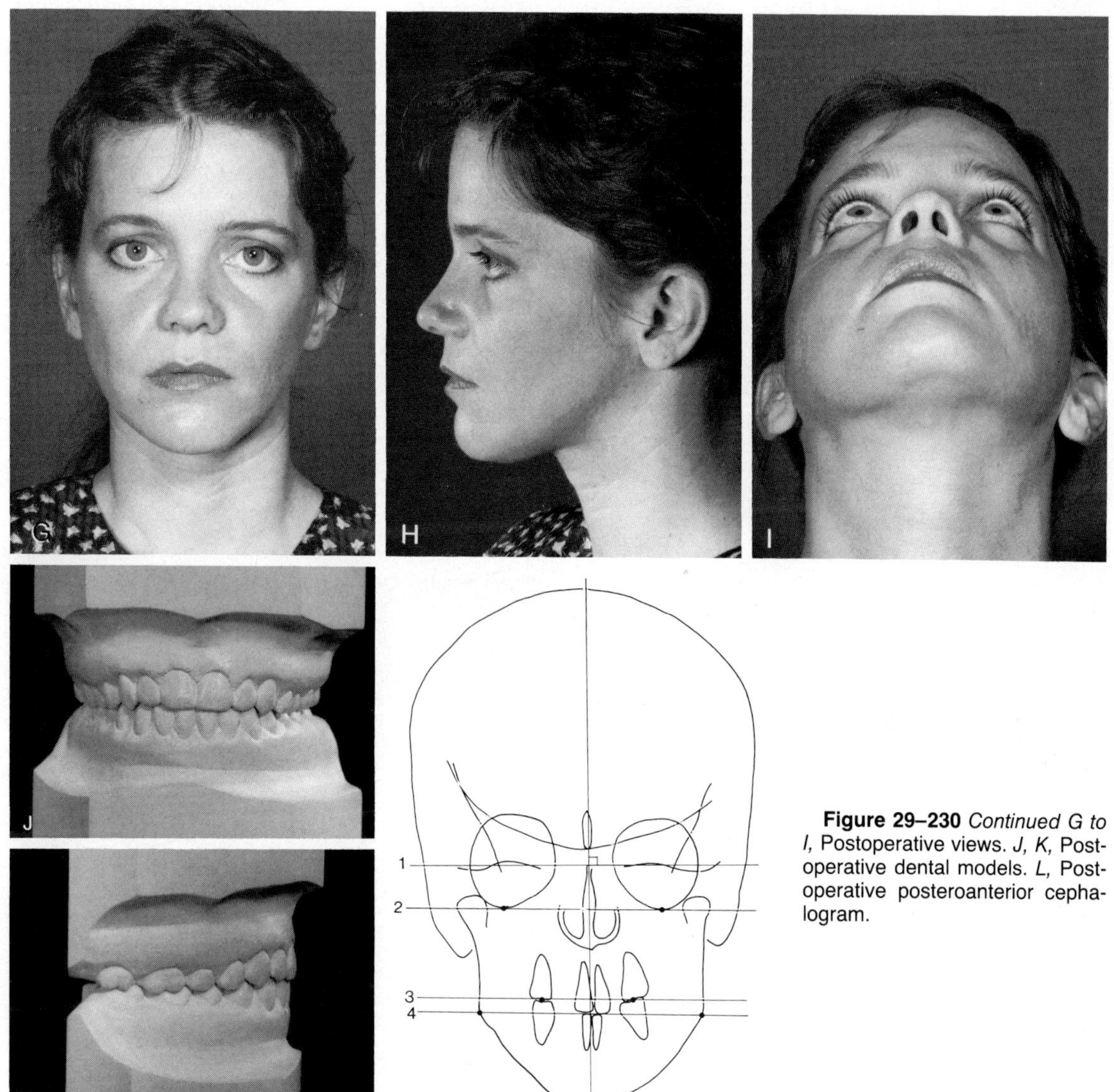

Figure 29–230 *Continued G to I,* Postoperative views. *J, K,* Postoperative dental models. *L,* Postoperative posteroanterior cephalogram.

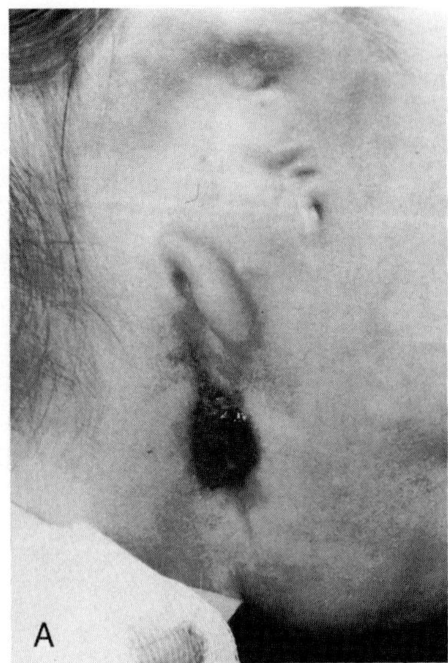

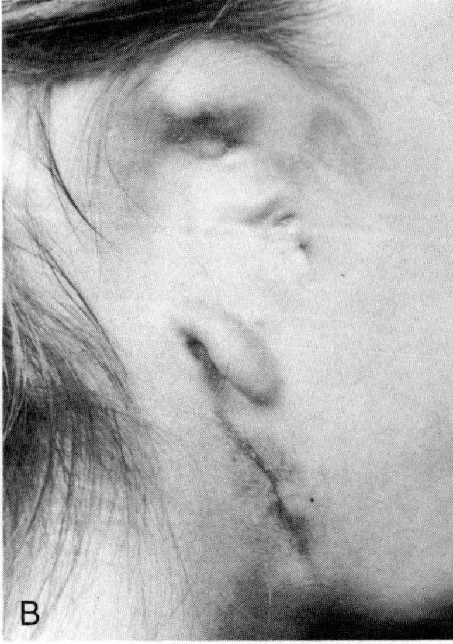

Figure 29–231. Chronic draining sinus at an osteotomy site. *A,* Appearance after ramus reconstruction in unilateral craniofacial microsomia. *B,* Several months after removal of an interosseous wire, curettement of the bone, and antibiotic therapy. (From McCarthy, J. G.: Complications of Jaw Surgery. St. Louis, C. V. Mosby Company, 1977.)

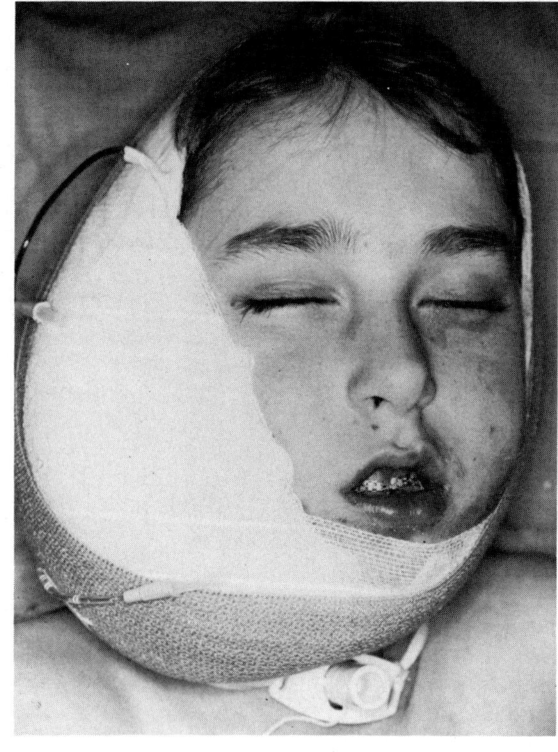

Figure 29–232. Continuous antibiotic irrigation system. The fluffed gauze absorbs the fluid escaping from the wound. (From McCarthy, J. G.: Complications of Jaw Surgery. St. Louis, C. V. Mosby Company, 1977.)

the affected teeth; there often is accompanying periodontal disease.

Several technical factors must be considered in order to preserve an adequate blood and nerve supply to the mobilized alveolar segments. At least one mucosal, i.e., a labial, buccal, or lingual, flap must be left attached to the alveolar fragment (see Fig. 29–160), and thin tapered osteotomes must be used for the individual interdental osteotomies. Bell (1969), in a primate study, demonstrated the presence of vascular anastomoses that permit maintenance of the osseous and pulpal vascularity in segmental maxillary alveolar osteotomies, provided that a single mucoperiosteal flap is preserved. It was also noted that if the horizontal osteotomy component was made 0.5 cm or more from the apices of the teeth, there was no interruption of the pulpal circulation. The fragments healed by osseous union within six weeks without the need for intermaxillary fixation. Poswillo (1972) demonstrated that after segmental alveolar osteotomies the development of progressive fibrosis in the pulp of the mobilized teeth occurred with total loss of odontoblasts. Although no nerve fibers persisted, vascularity was preserved and the teeth remained viable. Teeth were extracted serially from the osteotomized segment eight to 52 weeks after an anterior mandibular subapical osteotomy in a primate model (Banks, 1977). No normal pulps were found on histologic study; progressive fibrosis and calcification were observed in all teeth.

Kent and Hinds (1971) reported a one- to 3-year evaluation of patients undergoing anterior alveolar segmental osteotomies. With electric pulp testing, they noted that only one of 25 patients who had undergone 65 vertical alveolar osteotomies showed either poor bone healing or severe tooth injury. In addition, radiographs of 45 osteotomy sites demonstrated interdental bone loss of 1 to 5 mm one year after surgery. Cratering with invagination of gingiva was also observed, but there was less periodontal damage in the younger patient. These authors also emphasized the role of proper mucosal flap design.

Pepersack (1973) studied a larger number of patients who had undergone segmental alveolar osteotomies. It was noted that in most cases sensibility returned between the third and sixth postoperative months. At the end of the 12th postoperative month, 94.5 per cent of all injured teeth reacted positively after maxillary alveolar osteotomies. However, after mandibular alveolar osteotomy only 72.5 per cent of the teeth reacted positively at the end of 12 months. After the 12th postoperative month, few of the nonreacting teeth subsequently demonstrated a positive reaction. After maxillary alveolar osteotomy, the apices of only two of the 588 surgically endangered teeth were damaged, and one tooth required endodontic treatment. Damage to the apices of the teeth, however, was five times more frequent after mandibular alveolar osteotomy. In general the actual rate of tooth loss was small.

Egyedi and Visser (1973) demonstrated in a canine study that one root can be damaged without jeopardizing the vitality of the affected tooth.

NERVE DAMAGE

In the course of jaw operations the marginal mandibular, inferior alveolar, facial, and lingual nerves can be damaged. The auriculotemporal (Frey) syndrome represents another manifestation of intraoperative nerve damage. Every effort should be made to avoid nerve injury. The nerves should be identified and protected; retraction should not be excessive, otherwise neuropraxia, although reversible, results.

The marginal mandibular branch of the facial nerve can be damaged in the course of a submandibular (Risdon) incision as part of the exposure of the body and ramus of the mandible. Dingman and Grabb (1962), in an anatomic study, noted that the position of the nerve posterior to the facial artery was above the inferior border of the mandible in 81 per cent of the specimens; anterior to the facial artery the nerve was found to lie above the inferior border of the mandible in 100 per cent of the specimens. Over the mandible the nerve tends to have multiple branches. It was therefore recommended that in the area of the mandibular body the incision should be in the skin lines approximately a fingersbreadth, or 2 cm, below the inferior border of the mandible. Blunt dissection should then be carefully extended in a superior direction beneath the platysma muscle. Hinds and Kent (1972) modified the Risdon incision by placing it posterior to the posterior border of the ramus; the location of the incision obviated the need for careful dissection and identification of the facial nerve branches.

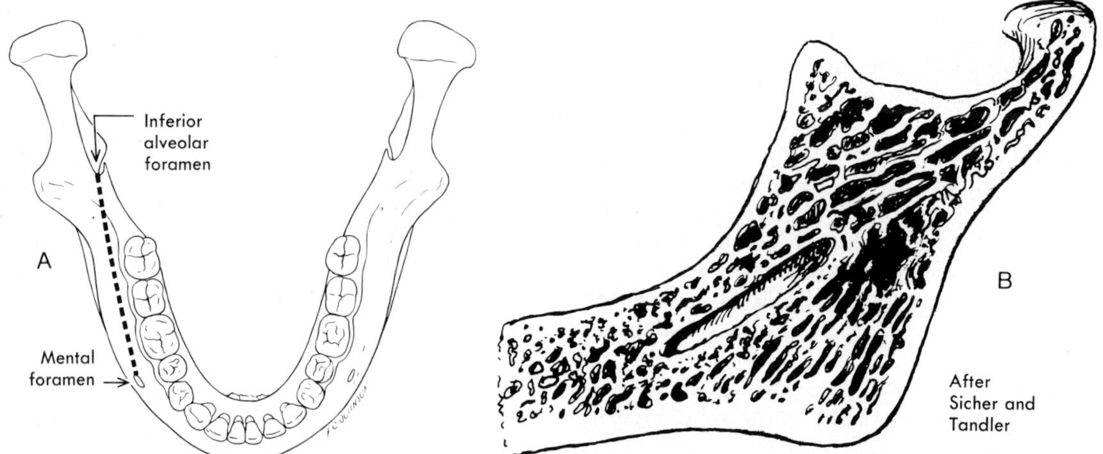

Figure 29–233. Interosseous pathway of the inferior alveolar nerve. Note that the nerve courses in an oblique direction and bows out toward the outer cortex.

The most annoying, and not infrequent, complication following osteotomies on the ramus of the mandible, especially in the sagittal split procedure, has been the development of hypoesthesia in the distribution of the inferior alveolar nerve. It must be emphasized that the nerve courses in an oblique direction as it continues into the body of the mandible (Fig. 29–233); thus, the bundle lies closer to the anterior border (outer table) of the mandible as it descends through the ramus.

Guernsey and DeChamplain (1971) reported bilateral inferior alveolar neuropathy in 19 of 22 patients who had undergone the sagittal split procedure; neuropathy was defined as either hypoesthesia or anesthesia. Return of sensation was observed in 12 patients; in six the ultimate nerve function was not known; and in three varying degrees of residual hypoesthesia persisted for 18 months postoperatively. Pepersack and Chausse (1974) examined a large number of patients from the Zürich clinic who had undergone the sagittal split procedure; 45 per cent had some degree of decrease in sensibility of the lower lip for at least five years after the operation.

The possible mechanisms of the injury include pinching of the nerve between the mobilized bone fragments (Fig. 29–234), direct injury by the osteotome, or stretching of the nerve. Dautrey (1986) modified the Obwegeser–Dal Pont procedure by sectioning the ramus through the lateral cortex of the mandibular ramus and body with an extremely thin (5 to 7 mm wide) osteotome (Fig. 29–70). The osteotome must be directed along the plane that is parallel to the lateral cortex, and rotation of the osteotome should be avoided for fear of causing a fracture and comminution of the bone fragments. The introduction of the C-osteotomy (Hayes, 1973) represented an attempt to obtain the advantages of the Obwegeser–Dal Pont procedure, i.e., a wide area of bone apposition, without the distinct disadvantage of injury to the inferior alveolar nerve.

Turvey (1985) reported a 7.0 per cent incidence of nerve injury after sagittal split osteotomy of the mandibular ramus. Consequently he recommended restricting the osteotomy posterior to the third molar to minimize the length of nerve exposed and to avoid injury to the inferior alveolar neurovascular bundle. The Dal Pont extension should be reserved for patients with a mandibular advancement in excess of 10 mm.

Injury to the main trunk of the facial nerve was reported by Behrman (1972) in four of 64 patients in a national survey who had undergone sagittal osteotomy of the mandibular ramus. All injuries resolved with time and were probably secondary to impingement of the facial nerve with retrodisplacement of the mandible. This survey, however, represented the early experience with this osteotomy.

In the same series (Behrman, 1972), injury of the lingual nerve was reported in a small number of patients. Guernsey and

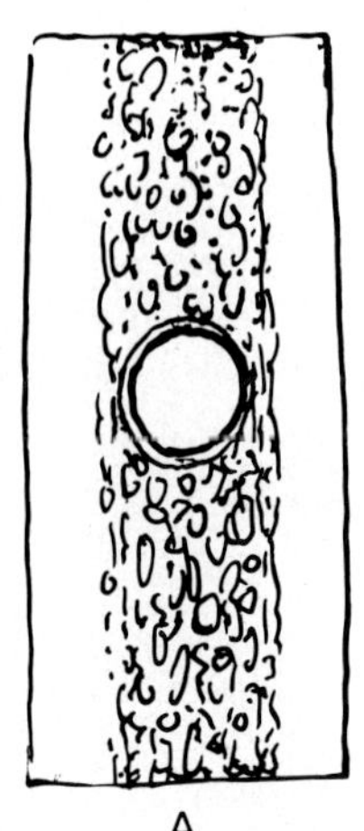

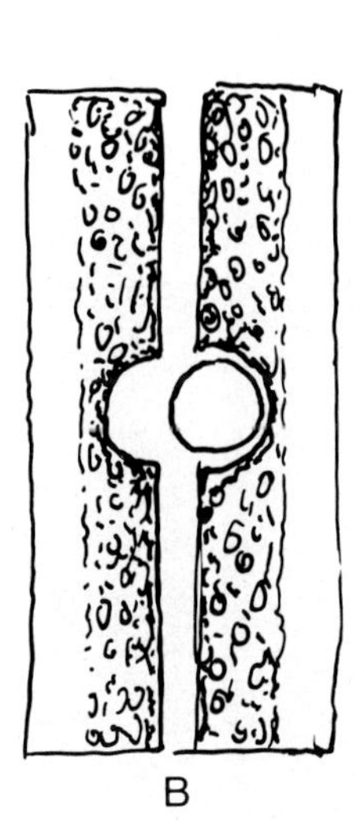

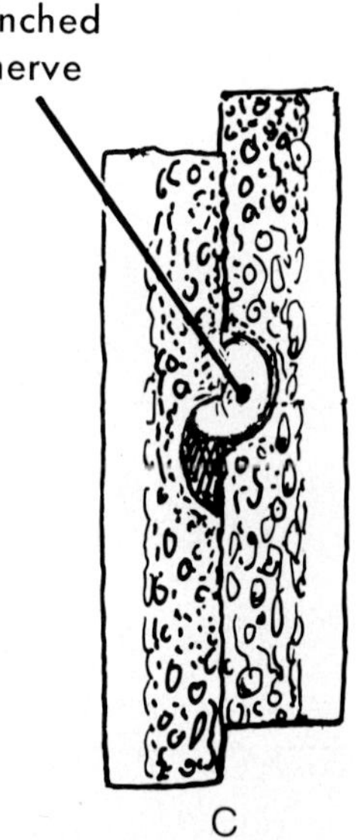

Figure 29–234. Mechanism of intraosseous compression of the inferior alveolar nerve in the course of a sagittal split ramisection.

DeChamplain (1971) reported two cases of transient lingual nerve paresthesia following intraoral sagittal split of the mandible. These complications can be avoided by precise osteotomies with fine, tapered osteotomes while the mandible is immobilized by specially designed retractors.

KELOIDS AND HYPERTROPHIC SCARS

After the submandibular or Risdon incision, keloids or hypertrophic scars can develop. Black patients are especially at risk, and the surgeon should consider an intraoral approach.

SPEECH CHANGES

The patient with a repaired cleft palate is at risk for the development of velopharyngeal incompetence after a Le Fort maxillary advancement (see p. 1376).

MISCELLANEOUS

Bone resorption has been reported after the insertion of alloplastic chin implants. Robinson and Shuken (1969) recalled 14 patients after chin augmentation and demonstrated radiographic evidence of bone resorption in 12. Friedland, Coccaro, and Converse (1976) reported a retrospective study of 85 patients who had undergone chin augmentation, and demonstrated radiographic evidence of bone resorption in 47 (Fig. 29–235). Less bone resorption was observed when the implant was placed over the hard bone of the lower part of the mandible (pogonion) rather than in a higher position over the alveolar bone.

If the degree of bone resorption is only minimal and the apices of the teeth are not involved, the implant can be safely left in place. However, removal of the implant is imperative when the apices of the teeth are threatened.

If, after removal of the implant, there is a resultant bone defect with lack of projection of the chin, the anteroinferior border of the mandible can be advanced by a horizontal osteotomy and any osseous defect filled with autogenous bone grafts or hydroxyapatite.

Airway Obstruction. Compromise of the airway produces great anxiety and a life-threatening event. If the jaws are wired together, the patient will experience some resistance to air exchange. During the postoperative night, monitoring of the patient in the intensive care unit is advised.

In mandibular procedures the nasal airways remain open. However, osteotomies of the maxilla that encroach upon the nasal cavity pose a peril. The nasal passages are quickly jeopardized by swelling of the nasal mucosa and blood clots.

The insertion of a nasopharyngeal tube is recommended immediately after the removal of the nasotracheal tube. Frequent suctioning of the tubes is required since they tend to clog quickly. It is a safe practice to have additional nasopharyngeal tubes at the bed-

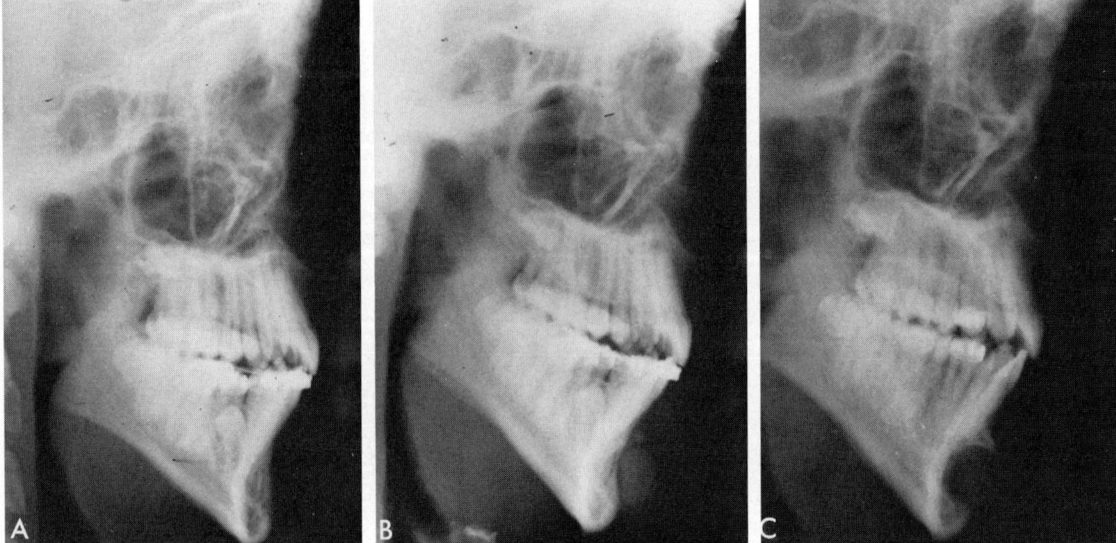

Figure 29–235. Penetrating silicone implant. *A,* Preoperative cephalogram. *B,* Four months after placement of the silicone implant. Note the erosion of the bone. *C,* Two years after surgery, the implant has penetrated the bone, endangering the roots of the teeth.

side so that they can be changed as needed. In addition, administration of humidified air is helpful. As the facial edema subsides, the nasopharyngeal tube can be removed and vasoconstricting nasal drops can be used to maintain the nasal air passages.

With Le Fort I intrusion procedures, it can be reasoned that diminution of the nasal cavity may cause restriction of nasal air flow. The opposite occurs (Gotzfried and Masing, 1984; Turvey, Hall, and Warren, 1984). As the maxilla is raised, the alar base of the nose and the internal nasal valve are widened. Nasal air exchange is thus improved.

Maxillary Sinus Infections. With the maxillary osteotomies the maxillary sinuses are routinely transgressed. The collection of blood in these cavities would theoretically favor the promotion of sinusitis. In practice, however, such infection is surprisingly rare (Stoker and Epker, 1974; Bell, 1975). Possible explanations for this include the use of prophylactic antibiotics and drainage of the sinus through the osteotomy site along the floor of the nose.

ACQUIRED DEFORMITIES

An acquired jaw deformity with associated loss of bone and soft tissue is one of the greatest challenges faced by the plastic surgeon. The achievement of form, function, and esthetics is the surgeon's combined goal. The functions of speech, swallowing, mastication, and respiration are dependent on the successful restoration of a bony arch, properly oriented to the opposing maxilla, lined by a thin soft tissue layer, and capable of functional temporomandibular joint motion. Perhaps in no other area of reconstruction are the demands for precision in planning and technical execution so important if one is to consider the result successful.

The size of the bone segment requiring replacement, and more important the quality of the soft tissue bed into which the bone reconstruction is to be performed, are the two factors that ultimately determine whether the technique chosen will be a success or failure. The spectrum of clinical problems is illustrated when one compares the young patient undergoing a subperiosteal and limited resection for a benign tumor with the elderly patient undergoing a composite resection of oral lining, external coverage, and a large, full-thickness anterior segment of mandible in which postoperative radiation will be used. The goals and principles of the reconstruction are the same for both patients, but the types of techniques required to achieve these goals are vastly different in complexity.

Mandibular Defects

HISTORICAL REVIEW

It is informative to review the history of man's attempt to replace a missing portion of the mandible. The imagination and the ingenuity of the reconstructive surgeon are reflected in the wide variety of techniques and materials used since Martin described the immediate restoration of a resected segment of the mandible with a prosthetic appliance in 1889. Partsch (1897) used a metal band to restore the continuity of the jaw. A pessary made of celluloid material was recommended by Berndt (1898). White (1909) favored a silver wire. Scudder (1912) reported that Ollier and Martin were replacing segments of the mandible with hard rubber, while Konig bridged the gap with ivory. Well-tolerated metals, such as vitallium (Castigliano, 1941), stainless steel mesh (Attie, Cantania, and Ripstein, 1953), and ticonium (Walsh, 1954), have also been used. With the introduction of alloplastic materials, surgeons have looked toward this type of material to reconstruct the jaw. Acrylic was used by Aubry and Pillet (1950) and Edgerton, Ward, and Sikes (1950). Despite the appeal of the alloplastic materials, the complications and extrusions that followed their use led to their abandonment except as temporary prostheses. *The method of choice in treating skeletal defects of the jaws remains replacement by autogenous bone.*

The pioneer work in bone grafting jaw defects is found in the German literature. Autogenous bone grafts from either rib or tibia were transferred in a delayed fashion to the jaw by Bardenheuer (1892) and Sykoff (1900). World War I gave rise to the need for, and spurred interest in, the bone grafting of jaw defects.

Bone Grafts. On the basis of the early experimental work of Ollier (1860, 1867) and the clinical experience of Delagénière (1916), tibial osteoperiosteal grafts were favored to bridge bone defects of the jaws during World War I (Imbert and Réal, 1916; DuBouchet, 1917; Lemaitre and Ponroy, 1920). The Germans continued to use ribs and tibia as sources of bone grafts during the early part of the war.

Around 1915 the superiority of cancellous bone was recognized by Lindemann (1916) and Klapp and Schroeder (1917). According to Ivy (1951), the British surgeons adopted the ilium as the osseous donor site when word reached plastic surgery centers via Dolamore from Holland of the success of the Germans. After an exchange of wounded prisoners, in British soldiers returning to the Plastic Surgery Hospital at Sidcup excellent results were found after iliac bone grafting by the German surgeons. Waldron and Risdon (1919), Gillies (1920), and Chubb (1920) soon reported the British experience with iliac bone grafts. Chubb (1920) was also one of the first to report the use of composite skin-clavicular bone flaps for mandibular reconstruction.

Ivy (1921) reported a case of resection of a part of the mandible with immediate grafting using iliac bone. The bone graft remained in place and functioned well, as noted in a 38-year follow-up report (Ivy and Eby, 1958).

During World War II, Mowlem (1944) reemphasized the importance of cancellous bone. Realizing that cortical bone grafts are almost noncellular, are slowly revascularized, and are a poor source of osteoblasts, he reconstructed the jaw with cancellous bone chips from the ilium. Fragmentation of the cancellous bone increases the surface of contact with the soft tissue and enhances the opportunity for rapid revascularization of the grafts.

Use of Trays Combined with Cancellous Bone Chips. During World War II, Converse (1945) used a fenestrated metal tray with bone chips to reconstruct the entire body of the mandible that was destroyed by a gunshot wound. The fenestrated tantalum tray served as an internal splint and as a means of carrying the bone chips (see Fig. 29–253). The tantalum tray was later removed and iliac bone grafts were added to reinforce the reconstructed mandibular body. Soderberg, Jennings, and McNelly (1952) employed a perforated vitallium tray and blocks of iliac bone graft to reconstruct the mandible. After consolidation was obtained, the metallic tray was removed.

Renewed interest in this concept was stimulated by Boyne's report (1969) of the use of a chromium-cobalt alloy crib, and his later report (1973) of a titanium tray to support particulate cancellous bone grafts and to act as an internal splint. A cellulose acetate micropore filter was recommended to line the crib to prevent connective tissue invasion. The impediment to revascularization of the bone grafts due to the presence of the millipore filters appears to defy the concept that rapid revascularization of a bone graft is as essential as it is for a skin graft (see Chap. 18). Morgan and Thompson (1975) reported that, on the removal of such trays, a layer of fibrous tissue of varying thickness was found between the graft and the filter.

Swanson and associates (1973) reported the use of a wire-reinforced silicone tray with windows to hold chips of bone. Repeated aspirations of serous fluid that collected around the silicone trays were required. In a subsequent report, Murray (1976) stated that the method had been abandoned because of a high failure rate.

Boyne and Zarem (1976) reported their experience using cancellous bone chips in a titanium mesh tray in 53 patients after tumor resections. Reconstruction was performed six months to one year after tumor resection, and the reconstructions were delayed 12 to 18 months if radiation therapy had been given. The authors described an 88 per cent success rate.

Leake and Rappaport (1972) developed the dacron-urethane prosthesis as an alternative to the metallic tray as a method to support cancellous bone chips. Schwartz (1984) reported his experience utilizing this prosthesis in 32 patients with only one failure. Albert and associates (1986) reported their experience with the dacron-urethane mesh prosthesis in 17 patients; 15 developed solid, functional mandibles.

Bone Allografts. Early encouraging results were reported with the use of lyophilized, decalcified allograft mandibles carved into the shape of a trough into which cancellous bone chips are packed (Pike and Boyne, 1973, 1974). Orthopedic surgeons were the first to use banked allografts of bone (Inclan, 1942; Bush, 1947; Wilson, 1948). Converse and Campbell (1950) described their experience with banked bone allografts as onlay grafts to restore facial contour. Reidy (1956) and Markowitz (1958) reported the successful application of bone allografts for the restoration of mandibular continuity.

Replacement of Resected Mandible. It is occasionally possible to use the resected mandible after sterilization as a scaffold for new bone growth. Freeze-dried autogenous mandible replacement in humans was reported by Cummings and Leipzig (1980). Mandibles invaded by tumor have also been sterilized by repeated freezing (Leipzig and Cummings, 1984). However, on careful follow-up of the clinical experience, the procedure was abandoned because of consistent failure.

Hamaker and Singer (1986) reported long-term follow-up of 19 patients who underwent sterilization of the mandibles with 10,000 rads of radiation, and reported a success rate of only 53 per cent. Autopsy histologic studies of the replaced irradiated mandibles showed no evidence of residual tumor. There was uniform failure when postoperative radiation therapy was utilized.

Despite interest over the years in alloplastic materials, metal trays, allografts, and sterilized autografts of the mandible, the success rates have been inconsistent. Autogenous bone remains the mainstay when mandibular replacement is required.

Cardinal Prerequisites of Successful Bone Grafting. Kazanjian (1952) listed the cardinal prerequisities of successful bone grafting of mandibular defects: (1) bone transplantation into healthy tissues, (2) a recipient area with adequate blood supply, (3) wide contact between the adjacent bone and graft, and (4) positive fixation. Currently available techniques for autogenous bone replacement include nonvascularized bone grafts, bone flaps, and microsurgical bone flaps. The appropriate technique for the specific clinical situation is determined by several factors. Foremost is the quality of the soft tissue environment into which the bone reconstruction is to be performed. A history of radiation, scarring from previous bone graft failures, or previous infection lessens the probability that vascularization of a nonvascularized bone graft will occur. In a compromised soft tissue environment, the ability to transfer bone with an inherent blood supply offers considerable advantage, making either pedicled bone flaps or microvascular bone flaps the procedures of choice.

Another consideration is whether adequate soft tissue exists to provide both internal (mucosal) lining and external soft tissue coverage to the bone segment requiring reconstruction. Adequate soft tissue must always be provided at a previous operation if a nonvascularized bone transfer is to be used. The ability of bone flaps, either pedicled or microsurgical, to provide both bone and soft tissues in a one-stage procedure makes these reconstructive options preferable when both bone and soft tissue replacement is required. The larger the bone segment requiring reconstruction, the more critical is the quality of the soft tissue bed if nonvascularized bone is to be used. Immobilization and fixation techniques are also more difficult with large-segment reconstruction. In these situations bone flaps have the advantage of their intrinsic blood supply, making early bone healing more likely. However, in the ideal soft tissue environment, successful reconstruction of large bone segments with nonvascularized grafts has been reported.

In summary, although nonvascularized bone grafts are frequently the procedure of choice and can provide successful results, bone flaps, either pedicled or microvascular, are indicated when the soft tissue bed is compromised, when both bone and soft tissue replacement is required, and when large segments of the mandible require reconstruction. Furthermore, it is clear that vascularized bone flaps heal more rapidly, require shorter periods of immobilization, and have less chance of nonunion. There is less risk of bone resorption, and vascularized bone transfers have demonstrated a greater resistance to infection.

The immediate reconstruction of the mandible at the time of tumor resection has several advantages. The requirements of size, contour, and bone orientation to the opposing maxilla can be evaluated and achieved more precisely when done at the time of tumor resection. The secondary deformities of the remaining mandibular segment and surrounding soft tissues after tumor resection and radiotherapy are exceedingly difficult to correct. When adequate soft tissues are present after the resection of a benign tumor, immediate mandibular reconstruction can be successfully performed using nonvascularized bone grafting techniques. When complex postablative defects exist, vascularized bone flaps are essential if an immediate reconstruction is to be performed successfully. The requirements of internal lining, bone, and external coverage, capable of withstanding postoperative radiotherapy, can be satisfied in a single stage by use of microvascular bone flaps.

The discussion of mandibular reconstruction will be divided into two main sections: traditional (nonvascularized) bone grafting techniques, when adequate soft tissues are available that are capable of revascularizing the bone graft, and bone flap techniques, both pedicled and microsurgical, when either poor quality soft tissues are present or the reconstruction requires both bone and soft tissues in a single stage. Special consideration and discussion will be given to the specific problems encountered in cases of immediate reconstruction.

METHODS OF FIXATION

A wide variety of methods of fixation of the fragments of the mandible is available to provide immobilization during the period of healing of bone grafts. Depending on the size of the defect, these vary from relatively simple techniques, such as intermaxillary fixation, monomaxillary fixation with a splint, and rigid skeletal (miniplate) fixation, to more complex methods providing cranial fixation by specially constructed external fixation appliances.

Intraoral Fixation

Teeth are Present on Both Sides of Defect. When teeth are present on both sides of the defect, a splint is made (monomaxillary fixation) and applied before the bone grafting procedure. Intermaxillary wiring is advisable to relieve some of the stress placed on the appliance and to prevent breaking or slippage during the operation. In the early postoperative period, the intermaxillary fixation is released and the monomaxillary splint is retained for stabilization. Early movement of the mandible is thus permitted.

In defects of the symphysis, each lateral fragment is provided with a splint; the two splints are joined by a lock-bar. The lock-bar is removed before the operation and each mandibular fragment is wired to the teeth of the maxilla. The lock-bar is replaced after completion of the operation. The intermaxillary wires are removed a few days later and fixation of the mandibular fragments is maintained by the splint and lock-bar appliance.

Ramus Fragment is Loose. In patients who have no teeth on the posterior fragments, the residual fragment is usually displaced forward and medially by the muscles of mastication after resection of the mandibular body when provision has not been made to prevent the displacement of the ramus. The masseter and medial pterygoid muscles should be detached subperiosteally from the ramus; the procedure frees the posterior fragment and allows its repositioning. The control of the posterior fragment can be accomplished by a number of methods: (1) the graft is

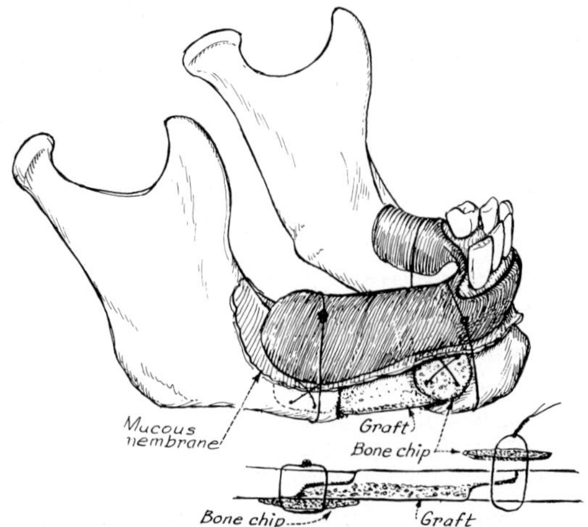

Figure 29–236. The loose ramus fragment. Control and fixation of the ramus by a prosthodontic appliance. The patient's denture was relined (in the operating room) and was maintained by circumferential wiring after placing of the bone graft. This type of fixation appliance requires the services of a maxillofacial prosthodontist. Excessive pressure over the mucoperiosteum should be avoided to prevent necrosis.

wedged into position between the anterior and posterior fragments to prevent forward displacement of the posterior fragment; (2) an intraoral appliance with a forked wire extension is used to maintain the retroposition of the edentulous posterior fragment until the bone graft is in place; (3) an acrylic splint maintained by circumferential wire around the mandible (Fig. 29–236) controls the posterior fragment as well as the anterior portion of the mandible during consolidation of the bone graft; (4) an external fixation appliance is used (see Figs. 29–238 to 29–243).

Mandible is Edentulous: Maxillary Dentition is Present. A biteblock is fitted over the remaining portion of the mandible and is maintained in position by circumferential wires around the mandible (see Fig. 29–236). Holes are drilled through the acrylic biteblock for the passage of the circumferential wires. Hooks are imbedded into the biteblock to establish intermaxillary fixation with the maxillary teeth.

Maxilla is Edentulous. A biteblock or the patient's denture is maintained in cranial fixation by wires passed around each zygomatic arch or anchored to the frontal bone. The mandibular fragments are held in intermaxillary fixation with the upper denture either by wiring the teeth or by means of the biteblock described above if the mandible is edentulous.

Maxilla and Mandible are Edentulous. The maxillary biteblock is maintained in cranial fixation by internal wire fixation as described above; intermaxillary fixation is established between the mandibular biteblock, fixed to the mandible by circumferential wiring, and the maxillary biteblock (Fig. 29–237).

Rigid skeletal (miniplate) fixation techniques have also become popular in recent years in mandibular bone grafting procedures (see p. 1216).

The collaboration of an expert prosthodontist is essential in order that the appliances be made with precision, thus avoiding excessive compression and necrosis of the mucoperiosteum, loosening of the fixation appliances, and loss of the bone graft.

External Fixation. External fixation is indicated when insufficient dentition is present to secure an interdental fixation appliance and when fixation cannot be obtained by means of prosthodontic appliances. An external fixation appliance is particularly useful when the posterior fragment is edentulous and there is a large anterior defect of the mandible.

The external fixation device has also been useful when immediate reconstruction at the time of tumor resection is planned. The device is placed prior to tumor resection to maintain proper relationships of the rami to each other in order to allow proper placement of the

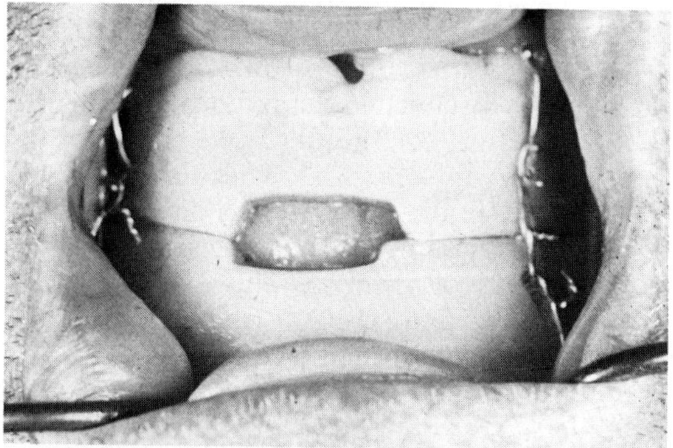

Figure 29–237. When both jaws are edentulous, biteblocks are fabricated. The maxillary biteblock is maintained by cranial fixation. The mandibular biteblock is adjusted and relined in the operating room after the bone grafting. Intermaxillary fixation is established after the mandibular biteblock has been attached to the mandible by circumferential wiring. Note the anterior opening to provide an airway and space for feeding.

bone graft in its anatomic position. The external hardware can be placed out of the field for the tumor surgeon, thus facilitating the resection.

Anderson (1936) reported the use of an external appliance to treat fractures of the shaft of the femur. The converging pins technique of the Roger Anderson appliance was applied by Converse and Waknitz (1942) to fractures of the mandibular angle. Two pins are placed in each remaining mandibular fragment, each pin converging with its twin at an angle of approximately 70 degrees. The pins are usually inserted side by side along a line parallel with the lower border of the mandible, or one above the other in the region of the angle of the ramus. Each pin is carefully passed through the skin and soft tissues and is drilled into the bone, penetrating both the outer and inner cortical plates. After the fragments are returned to their normal position, the connecting portion of the appliance is adjusted and the joints are locked to secure fixation.

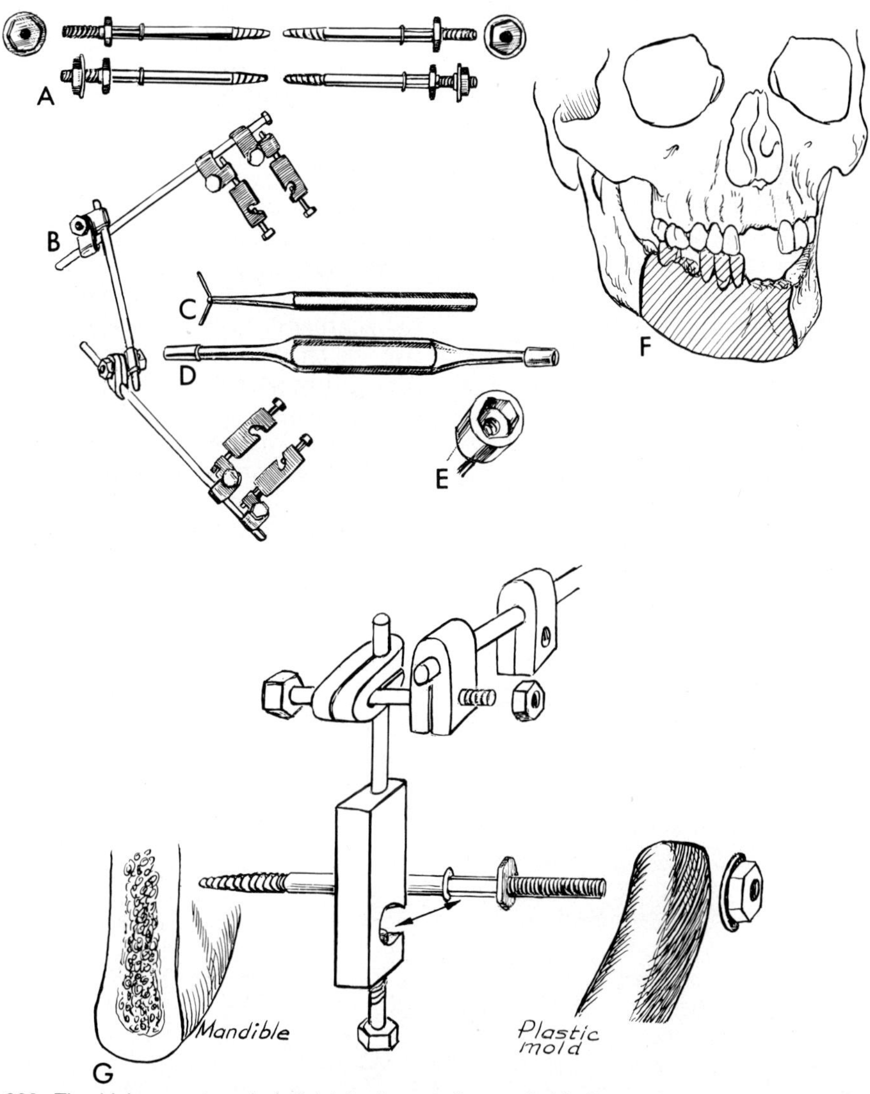

Figure 29–238. The biphase external skeletal fixation appliance. *A,* Vitallium bone screws with special heads and washer-faced lock nuts. *B,* Primary assembly of the splint fixation appliance with rods and screw clamps in position for adjustment. *C,* Antitorque wrench. *D,* The wrench. *E,* The end of the wrench, which accepts hexagonal nuts. *F,* The shaded area represents the mandibular bone defect that is to be repaired. *G,* Details of the vitallium bone screw and screw clamp. The hexagonal surface of the screw facilitates positive no-skid fixation. Rod clamps are shown above as they maintain the primary splint rods in position. (From Kazanjian and Converse; drawings according to Dr. A. J. Valauri.)

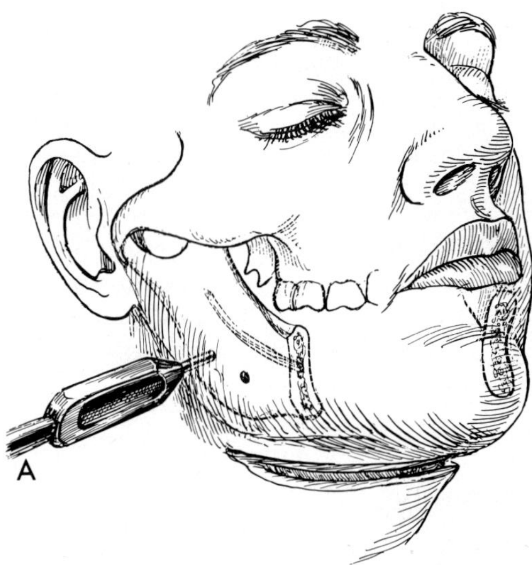

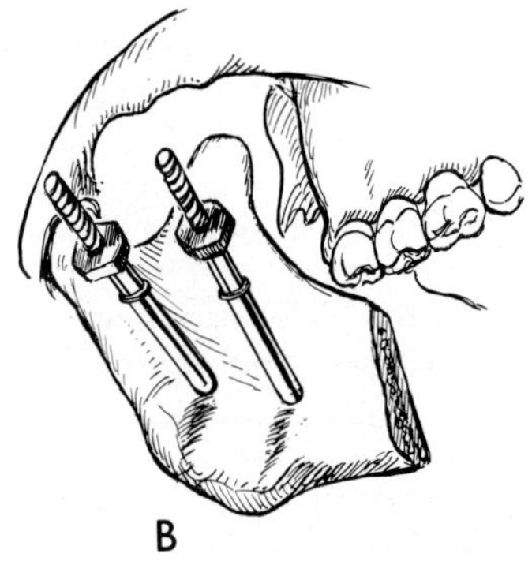

Figure 29–239. The biphase external skeletal fixation appliance. *A,* Drill holes are made with a drill to receive the bone screws. *B,* The bone screws are threaded into position. (From Kazanjian and Converse.)

Twin-Screw Morris Biphase Appliance. The twin-screw Morris biphase appliance (Morris, 1949; Fleming and Morris, 1969) is highly versatile (see also Chap. 72). The Morris external fixation splint (Figs. 29–238 to 29–243) employs vitallium bone screws ⅛-inch in diameter. The screws are threaded at both ends; one end is inserted into bone, and the other receives a washer-faced nut that secures an acrylic bar to join the two units of parallel screws (Fig. 29–238). A stablike soft tissue incision is made over the proposed site of insertion of the screw, and a hole is drilled into the bone with a 3/32-inch twist drill (Fig. 29–239). A drill of smaller dimension is preferred to place holes into the ramus. The screws are inserted with a distance of at least 2 cm between each screw of the pair. After realignment of the fragments is achieved, the two units of parallel screws are joined by a connecting portion of the apparatus (the first phase), which is designed to maintain the position of the two units (Fig. 29–240) until an acrylic bar (the second phase) ensures permanent fixation (Fig. 29–241). The term "biphase" defines the double maneuver.

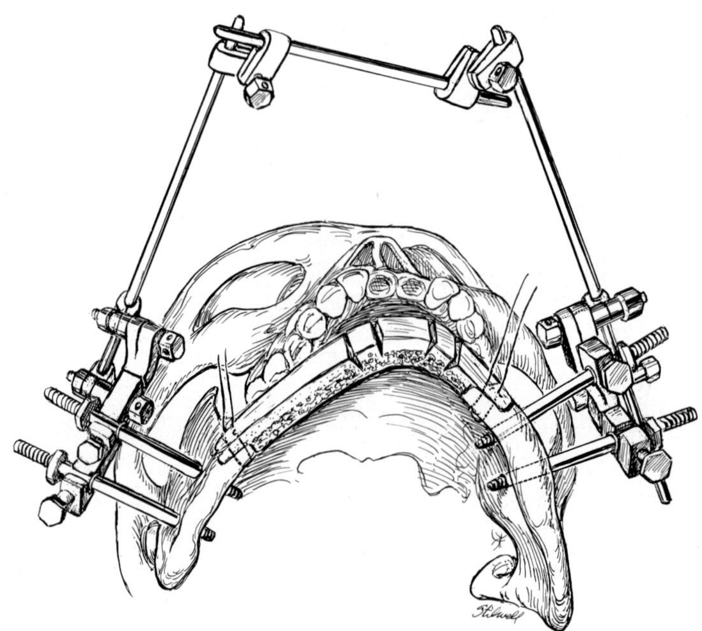

Figure 29–240. Biphase external skeletal fixation appliance. The primary splint appliance and the bone graft in position before the fixation wires are twisted. (From Kazanjian and Converse.)

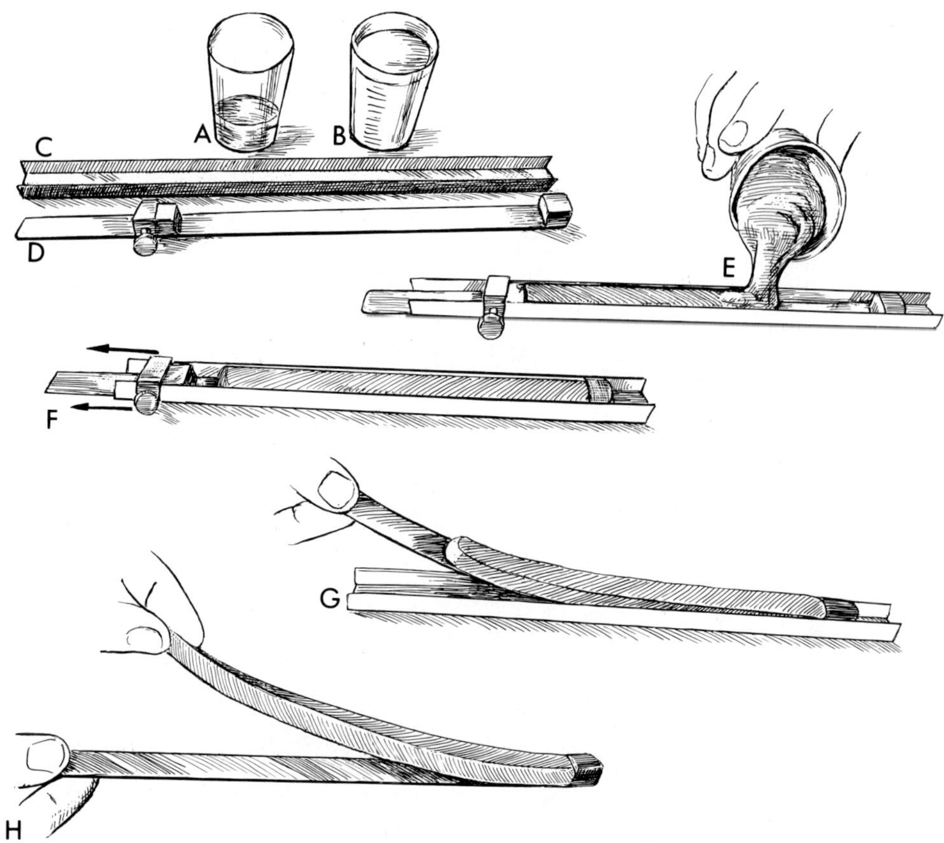

Figure 29–241. Fabrication of an acrylic resin bar. *A,* Acrylic liquid monomer. *B,* Acrylic resin polymer powder. The liquid monomer and powdered polymer are mixed in a 1:3 ratio. *C, D,* The metallic tray and rod that make up the take-apart mold. *E,* Acrylic mixture being poured into the take-apart mold. *F,* Mold being separated from the "room temperature curing" acrylic splint. *G, H,* The still pliable acrylic bar is carefully removed from the mold without deforming its shape. (From Kazanjian and Converse.)

Quick-curing acrylic, while it is in its rubber-like, pliable state (Fig. 29–241), is molded and adapted over the ends of the screws of each unit (Fig. 29–242). After the acrylic bar has hardened, a washer-faced nut is secured to the exposed thread of each screw. The temporary connecting splint is removed. The Morris apparatus is strong, although light in weight. The vitallium screws are well tolerated and can be left in position for long periods (Fig. 29–243).

The external splint controls the remaining mandibular fragments during the consolidation of the bone grafts. Before bone grafting, the external fixation appliance is used to retain the edentulous fragments in position. After the bone is transplanted and fastened with interosseous wires to the remaining mandibular segments, additional fixation methods are not required.

The Morris external fixation device has been especially useful in cases in which an immediate mandibular reconstruction is being performed at the time of tumor resection. Before the resection the device is placed to control the relationship of the mandibular rami. The acrylic bar is positioned superiorly over the forehead and scalp so as to be out of the way of the tumor resection. After the resection of a large anterior segment, the technique allows maintenance of the normal relationships of the mandibular rami, and facilitates proper placement of the mandibular reconstruction. The device, when used in conjunction with prefabricated biteblocks (when there are no remaining teeth) and intermaxillary fixation, allows control of both the vertical and horizontal dimensions of the mandibular reconstruction. Fixation of the bone graft to the remaining mandibular seg-

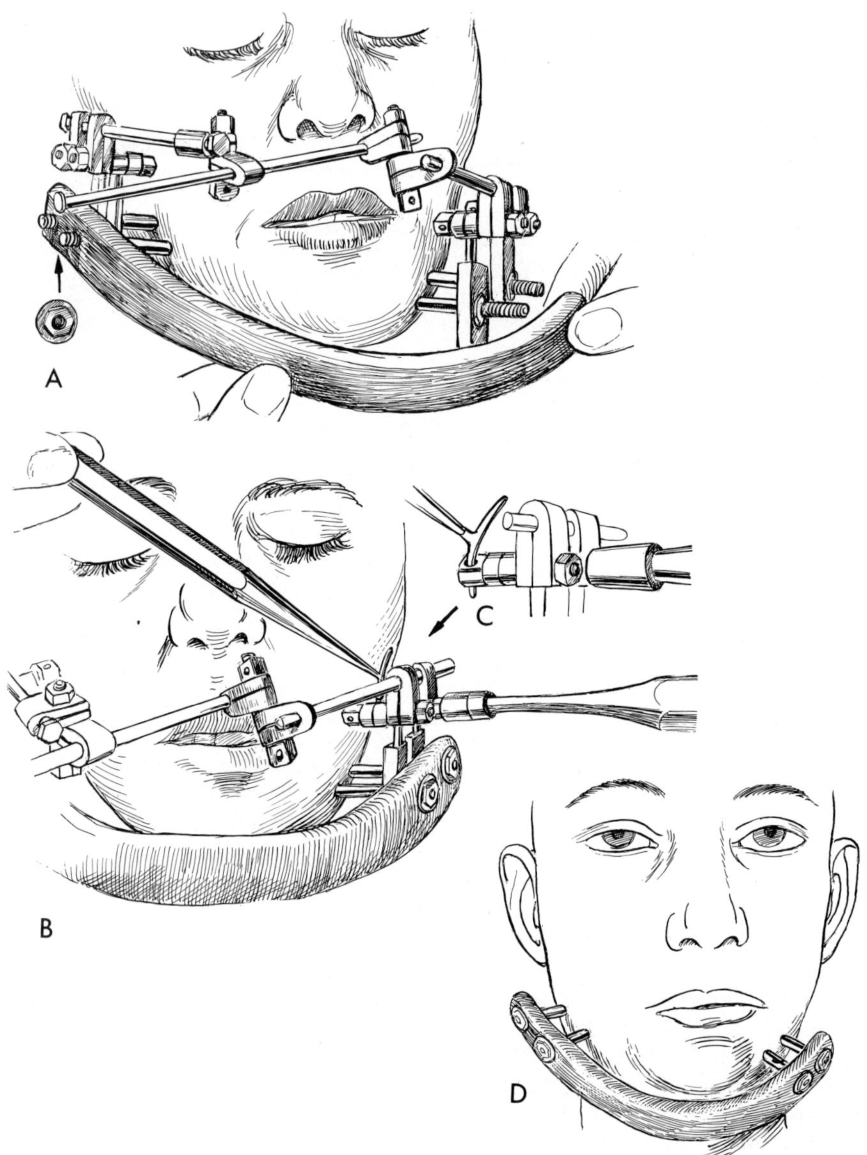

Figure 29–242. Adapting the acrylic resin splint. *A,* While still in a semiputty condition, the acrylic bar is gently pressed onto the machined threads of the bone screws. Washer-faced lock nuts are initially twisted to a position just short of being flush with the end of the screw. *B, C,* After the heat of polymerization has dissipated three to five minutes later and the acrylic bar has hardened, final tightening of the lock nuts is performed. To overtighten the lock nut while the acrylic is soft invites weakness in the splint due to excessive thinning of the bar at this site. The primary mechanical splint is removed in the reverse order of its application—that is, first unlock the rod clamps, then release the screw clamp, and finally remove the screw clamp from the bone screw. *D,* The secondary rigid, resilient, light acrylic bar (biphase splint) is relatively unobtrusive as the bone graft heals. (From Kazanjian and Converse.)

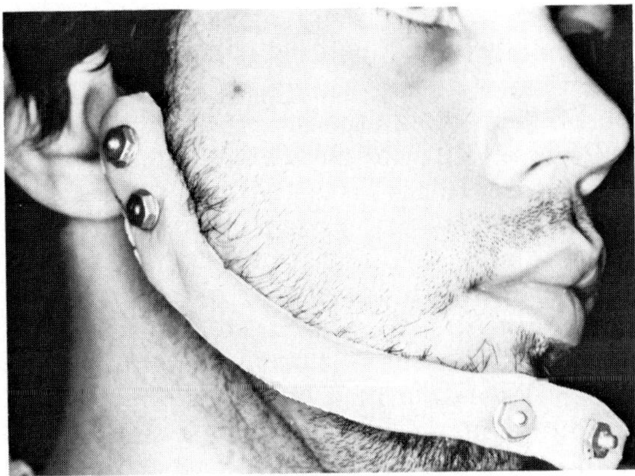

Figure 29–243. Morris appliance in position controlling the posterior edentulous fragment. A large portion of the body of the mandible has been reconstructed by a bone graft. (From Kazanjian and Converse.)

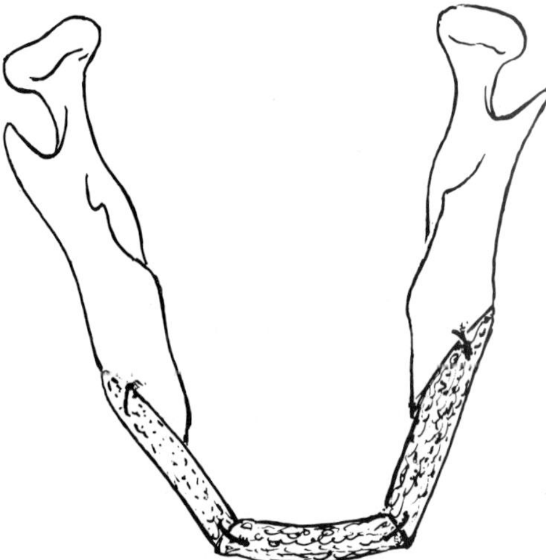

Figure 29–244. Reconstruction of the missing portion of the mandibular arch by three bone grafts wired to each other and to the posterior mandibular fragments.

ments can be achieved with interosseous wiring, screws, or bone plates.

Internal Fixation. Fixation of the remaining fragments is provided by the bone graft (or grafts), which bridge(s) the gap between the mandibular fragments. In moderate-sized defects, the main bone graft, containing cortical bone, is sufficiently strong to maintain the position of the fragments in the edentulous mandible. Successful results have been obtained in patients in whom bone grafts were wired to each other and to the mandibular stumps (Figs. 29–244, 29–245). Some type of internal fixation splint (stainless steel, tantalum, ticonium, a dacron mesh) holding the fragments may be required in larger defects (see Fig. 29–253). Such internal splints are usually removed after the consol-

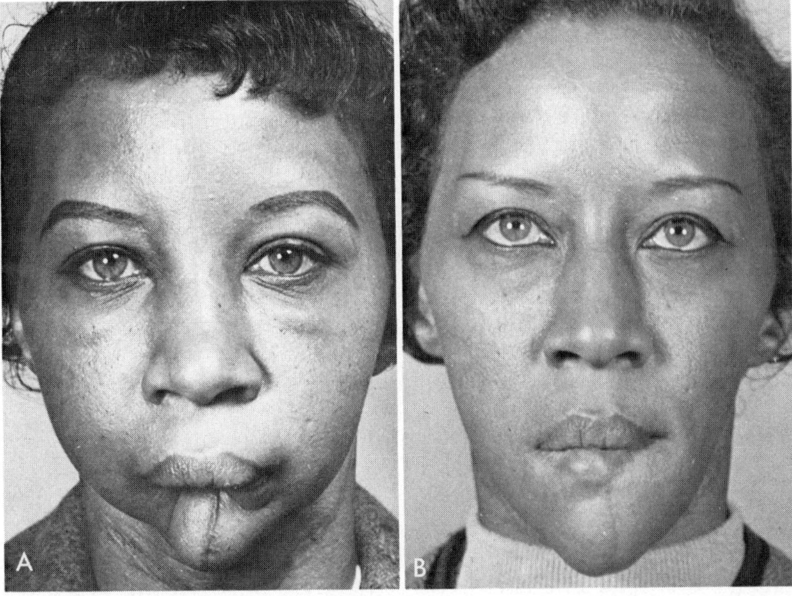

Figure 29–245. Reconstruction of the mandibular arch by three bone grafts wired to each other as illustrated in Figure 29–244. *A*, Appearance after resection of the major portion of the mandibular arch and floor of the mouth for the eradication of carcinoma. *B*, After reconstruction by bone grafts and skin graft inlay procedure (see Figs. 29–275 and 29–276).

idation of the fragments, as they may interfere with the subsequent restoration of a functional buccal sulcus.

The use of screws and miniplates securing the bone graft or flap to remaining mandibular segments has greatly facilitated the achievement of rigid internal fixation.

NONVASCULARIZED BONE GRAFTING TECHNIQUES

Conditions are favorable for nonvascularized bone reconstruction if there has been little or no loss of soft tissue and the bone graft is placed in a well-vascularized bed. The bone graft is placed in contact with the adjacent bone fragments, which have been stripped of periosteum; thus, a bone to bone contact is obtained. Chips of cancellous bone are packed in any interstices between the ends of the fragments and also over the junction line; the additional grafts promote bone consolidation as they are revascularized rapidly.

If adequate fixation of the mandibular fragments is provided and the defect is not too large, the consolidation of the graft is usually uneventful. Careful hemostasis to avoid hematoma formation (suction drainage when there is any doubt concerning the hemostasis), intermaxillary fixation (which is maintained for a variable period if monomaxillary fixation has been established), and a pressure dressing complete the operation. The following factors must also be considered: (1) as much cancellous bone as possible must be included in the graft for rapid revascularization; (2) cortical bone is required to provide strength to the graft; and (3) periosteum, if preserved over the cortex, is a vascular structure that will assist in the revascularization of the graft through the cortical layer (see Chap. 18).

Iliac Bone Grafts Versus Split Rib Grafts. Corticocancellous bone grafts removed from the crest of the ilium, as initiated by Lindemann (1916) during World War I, were successful in a high proportion of patients during World War II. This procedure remains the favorite technique of reconstruction of the mandible with average-sized defects.

Whole rib grafts have been less successful because of the absence of exposed cancellous bone and the slow rate of revascularization. Split rib grafts, however, have been highly successful in some extensive defects when their cancellous surfaces are exposed to the soft tissues to encourage rapid revascularization (see Fig. 29–255).

Primary Bone Grafting After Tumor Resection. In nonmetastasizing tumors, such as ameloblastomas, primary bone grafting is feasible and has been successful in treating large defects. In the 7 year old child shown in Figure 29–246, the resection of a giant tumor diagnosed as fibrous dysplasia (Fig. 29–247) resulted in a defect extending from the premolar region on the left side of the mandible to the subcondylar area on the right side. The defect was successfully bone grafted after the mandible had been "degloved" (see Fig. 29–46) and the tumor exposed and resected (Fig. 29–246). Intermaxillary fixation had been established between the remaining mandibular teeth and the maxillary teeth. A guide plane was placed on the left side to prevent the tendency toward deviation to the right after intermaxillary fixation was released. Healing was uneventful except for the extrusion of some bone chips at the area of junction of the bone grafts and the remaining mandibular body (Fig. 29–248). The success of such a procedure can be attributed to the fact that adequate soft tissue was available to ensure coverage of the transplanted bone.

Primary Bone Grafting of Post-traumatic Defects. In defects caused by trauma, when the soft tissues are intact or can be sutured primarily, primary bone grafting is successful provided that adequate fixation of the fragments is established. Unthinkable before the advent of antibiotics, the intraoral approach is employed for exposure of the mandibular fragments, bone grafting, and soft tissue coverage; the tissues are sutured without tension so as to ensure primary healing.

Technique of Bone Grafting Small and Medium-Sized Defects. When the gap between the two fragments of bone is narrow, as in nonunited fractures, the ends of the fragments are exposed through either a short incision made below the lower border of the mandible or an intraoral approach. The interposed fibrous tissue is removed and the bone stumps are trimmed with a rongeur or an osteotome. A bone graft (cancellous) from the crest of the ilium is packed between the fragments; an additional bone graft onlay over the fragments bridges the gap.

A larger defect requires a solid piece of

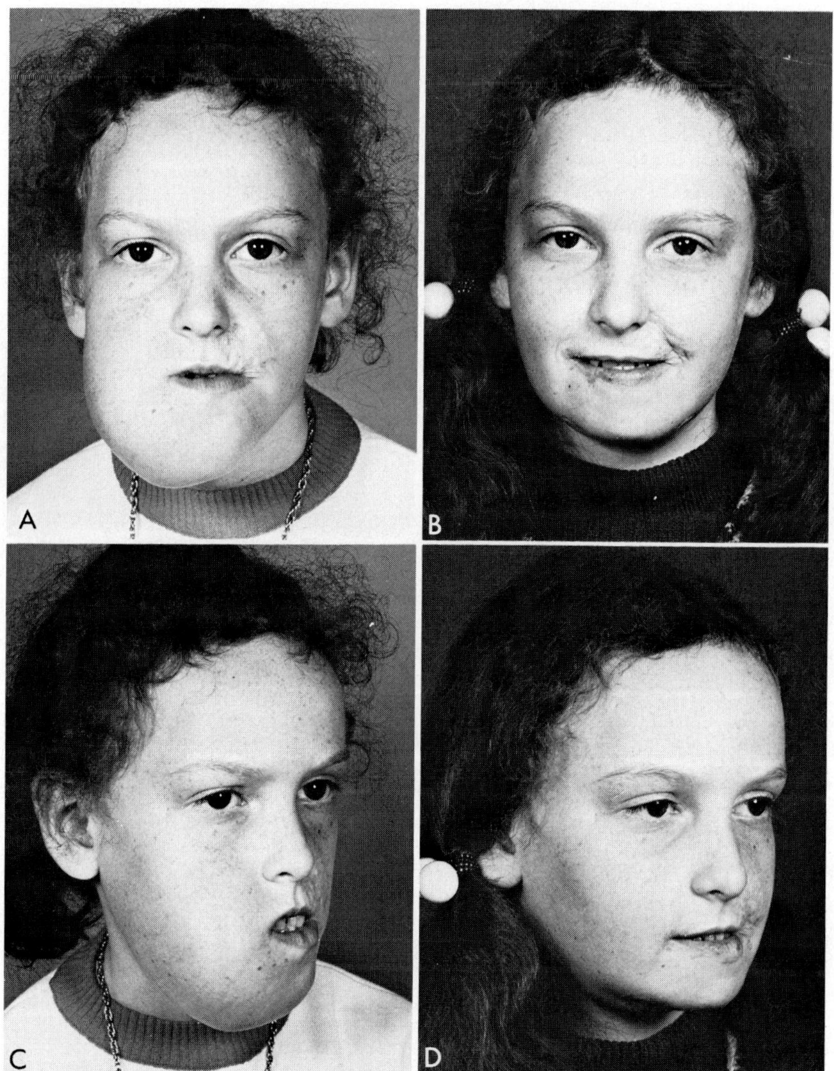

Figure 29–246. Primary reconstruction of the mandible after resection of a large area of fibrous dysplasia. *A,* Appearance of a 7 year old child with a giant tumor. Note the radiation scarring in the region of the left nasolabial fold. *B,* After resection and primary bone grafting through the intraoral approach. *C,* Preoperative view. *D,* Postoperative view. (Surgery in conjunction with Dr. A. J. Valauri.)

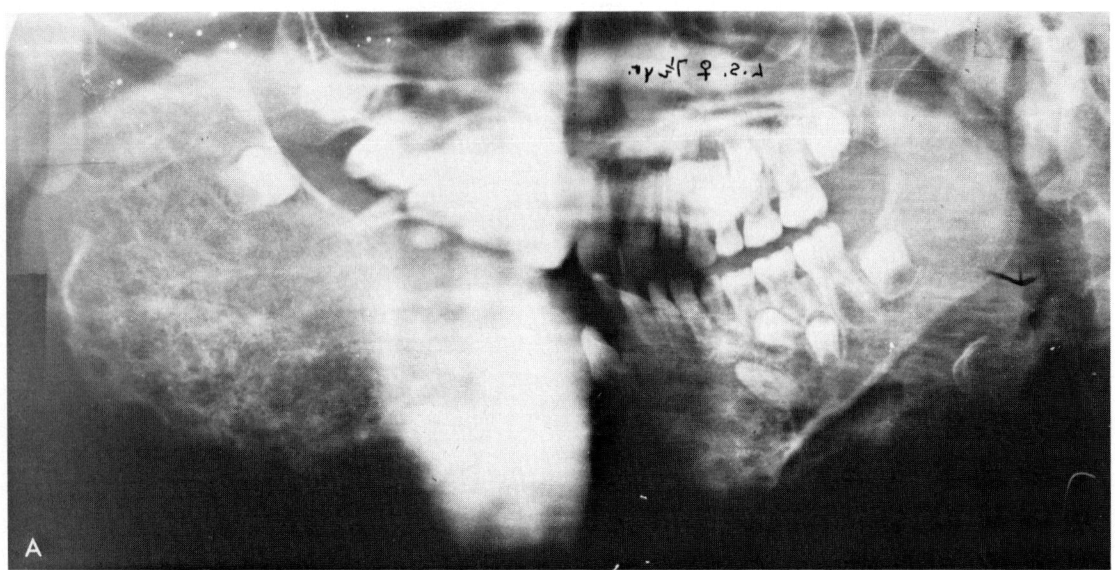

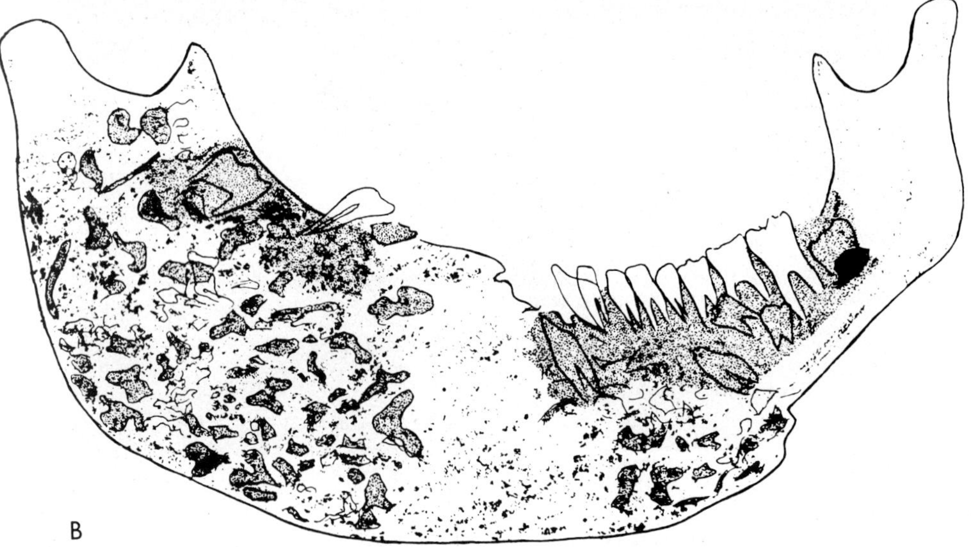

Figure 29–247. *A,* Panoramic roentgenogram of the mandible showing the large area of involvement extending from the neck of the right condyle to the premolar area on the left side. *B,* Diagram outlining the extent of the tumor.

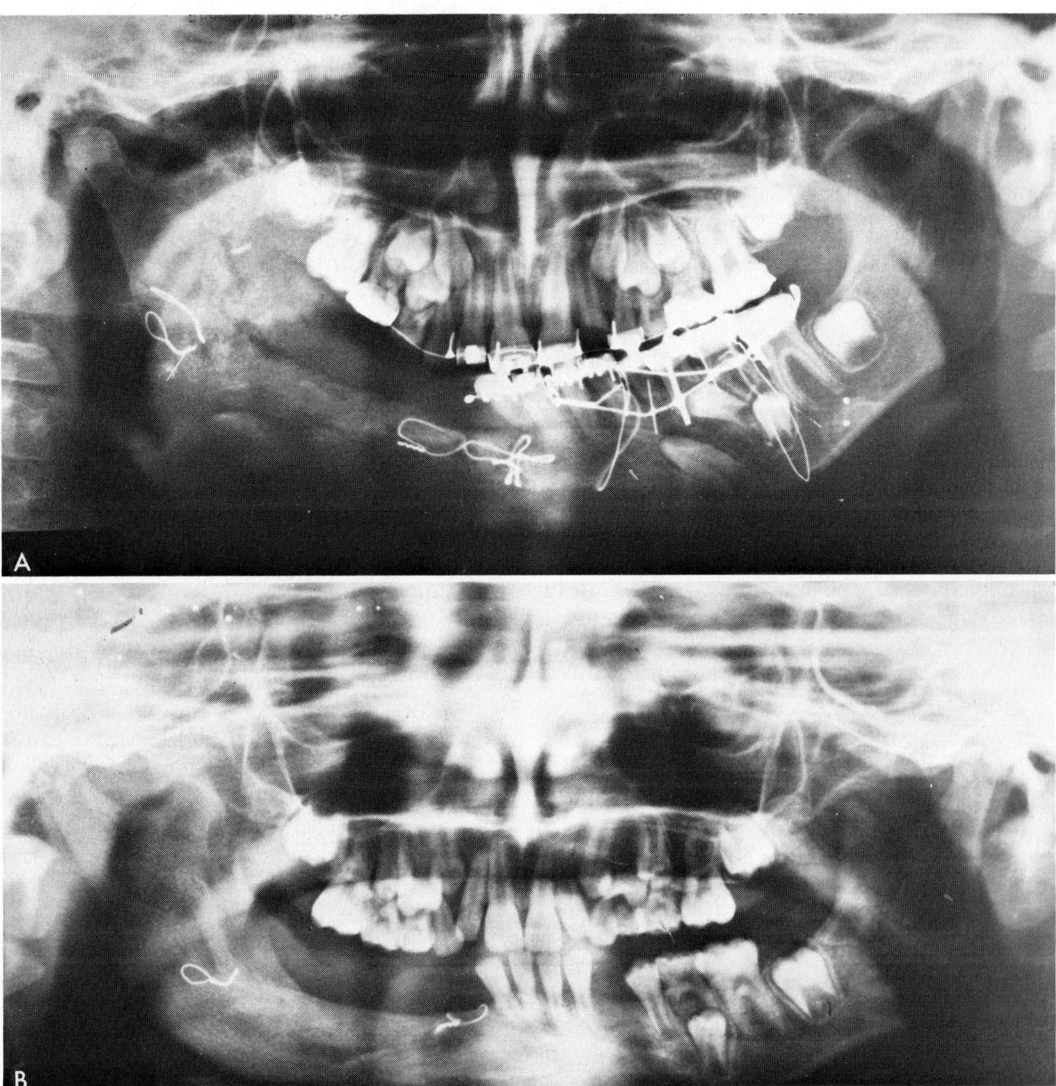

Figure 29–248. Radiographic follow-up of the patient shown in Figure 29–246. *A,* Panoramic roentgenogram taken a few days after bone grafting. *B,* One year after the operation, the mandible has been reconstructed with adequate symmetry with the contralateral hemimandible.

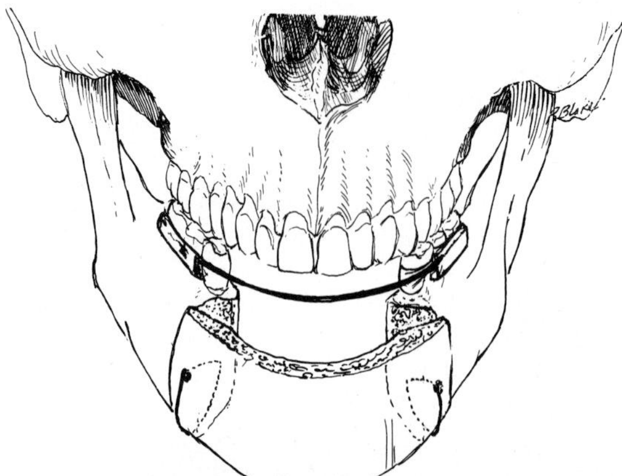

Figure 29–249. Large block of iliac bone carved, fitted, and wired to the remaining mandibular fragments. Two molars were present on each posterior fragment and served as a means of anchorage by bands placed around the teeth and an arch bar joining the two mandibular fragments.

bone shaped to overlap the ends of the fragments (Figs. 29–249, 29–250). The graft is held in place by direct interosseous wiring or miniplates supplemented by intraoral or external fixation. The surface of contact between the graft and the host bone should be as wide as possible. The interstices between the transplant and the mandible are filled with bone chips. The curvature of the iliac crest supplies a suitable graft, since it simulates the curvature of the mandibular arch.

Iliac bone grafts are successful for the repair of small, medium-sized, and even large defects in a high percentage of patients with mandibular defects. Split rib grafts are rapidly revascularized and can also be used successfully in extensive defects (see Fig. 29–255).

Bone Grafting to Reconstruct Major Portion of, or Entire Body of, Mandible. As stated earlier, a defect involving the symphysis and part of the body of the mandible can be reconstructed by the use of three large iliac bone grafts: one median graft in the area of the symphysis, and one on each side (see Fig. 29–244). The bone grafts are wired to each other and to the posterior mandibular fragments. Rigid fixation of the remaining mandibular fragments by intermaxillary fixation is of critical importance for success. Gillies and Millard (1957) used lengths of rib that were notched on the inner aspect and bent to a suitable shape by means of making a series of greenstick fractures. The degree of success of this technique has not been reported.

When the entire or major portion of the mandibular arch is absent and no teeth are present for intermaxillary fixation, one method of treatment is to use an internal splint filled with chips of iliac bone consisting mostly of cancellous bone. The patient shown in Figures 29–251 and 29–252 lost the body of the mandible after severe comminution by a shell fragment. Reconstruction was achieved using a fenestrated tantalum splint filled with bone grafts (Fig. 29–253) (Converse, 1945). Six months after the bone grafts had become consolidated, the splint was removed and onlay bone grafts were added to increase the bulk of the reconstructed mandibular body. At a later stage the buccal sulcus was deepened by the skin graft inlay technique (see Fig. 29–275).

Albee (1919) advocated using a U-shaped piece of bone removed from the ilium. A similar U-shaped piece of bone cut from the ilium was used by Seward (1974) to reconstruct the mandibular body after resection of an ameloblastoma. To obtain a pattern of the proposed U-shaped bone graft, Seward used a tracing of the outline of the lower border of the mandible from angle to angle as recorded from a submental vertex radiograph, in conjunction with a dental model cast from an impression of the lower arch. A roll of wax was bent to the shape of the mandible and tested against the lower border of the patient's jaw. Care must be taken that the shape of the jaw is precisely followed and that the posterior portion of the U has adequate width to fit over the angle of the jaw on each side. The latter precaution is of particular importance, as the ramus normally lies lateral to the occlusal line of the molar dental arch.

Fry (1975) employed a technique using split ribs. Two symmetric rib grafts are removed from the region of the posterior axillary line where the curvature is greatest. The length of each graft is 13 cm. The ninth or tenth ribs are usually satisfactory. The grafts are removed, care being taken to preserve the periosteum, even at the expense of penetrating the pleura (Figs. 29–254, 29–255*A*).

Muscle tissue is dissected from the rib grafts, the periosteum being preserved. The ribs are split with an osteotome. Each rib therefore provides two sections of cortical bone, curved top and bottom, covered by periosteum and enclosing an inner layer of cancellous bone. The sections are light but sufficiently strong because of the shape of the

Text continued on page 1432

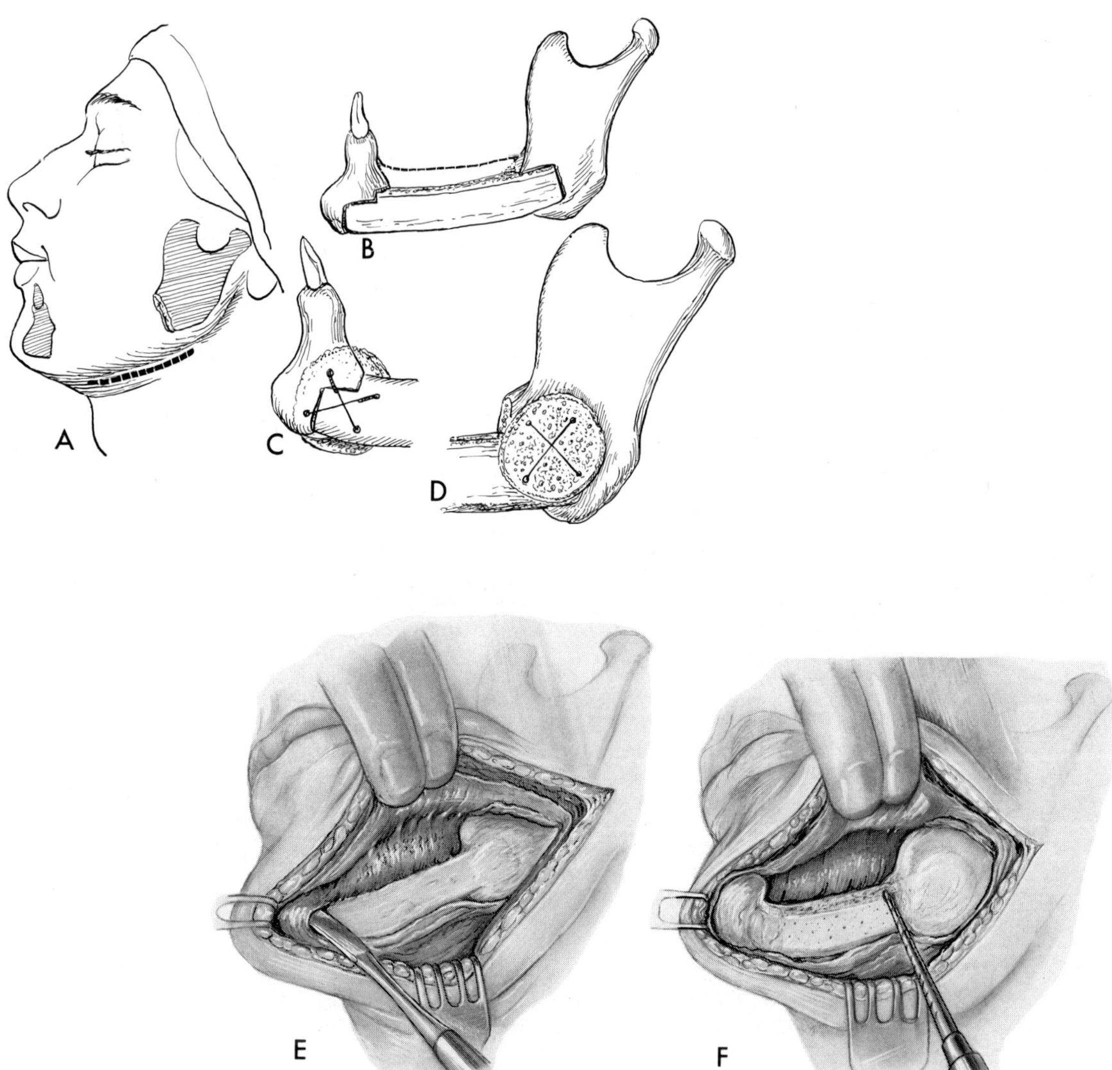

Figure 29–250. Reconstruction of the body of the mandible by bone grafting and subsequent addition of bone to increase the vertical dimension of the alveolar ridge. *A,* Extensive defect involving the body of the mandible. *B,* The iliac bone graft in position. Note the overlap between the bone graft and the mandibular fragments. *C,* A piece of cancellous bone has been crosswired into place on the lingual aspect of the junction between the graft and the anterior mandibular fragment. *D,* Cancellous bone has been placed over the junction of the posterior end of the bone graft and the ramus fragment. *E,* In a second stage, after consolidation of the bone graft, the height of the alveolar ridge was increased to improve retention of the denture. Subperiosteal exposure of the grafted area is shown. *F,* The cortex is removed from the upper portion of the bone graft.

Illustration continued on following page

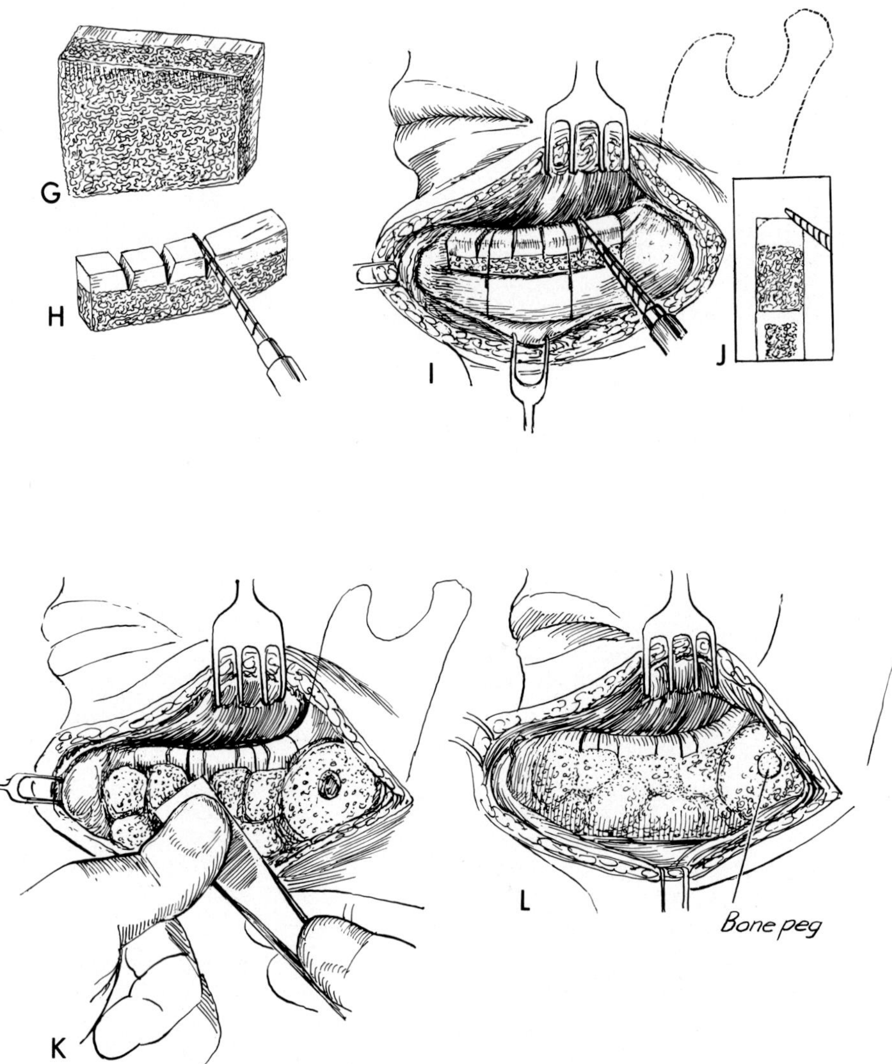

Figure 29–250 *Continued G,* A block of iliac bone. *H,* The cortex is cut as shown to permit contouring of the graft to form the new alveolar ridge. *I,* Circumferential wiring is used to secure the added bone graft. *J,* The sharp edges of the upper portion of the bone graft are contoured. *K,* Cancellous bone is added to the buccal surface of the new alveolar arch to increase the bulk of the mandible. *L,* Note the use of a bone peg for fixation of a piece of cancellous bone.

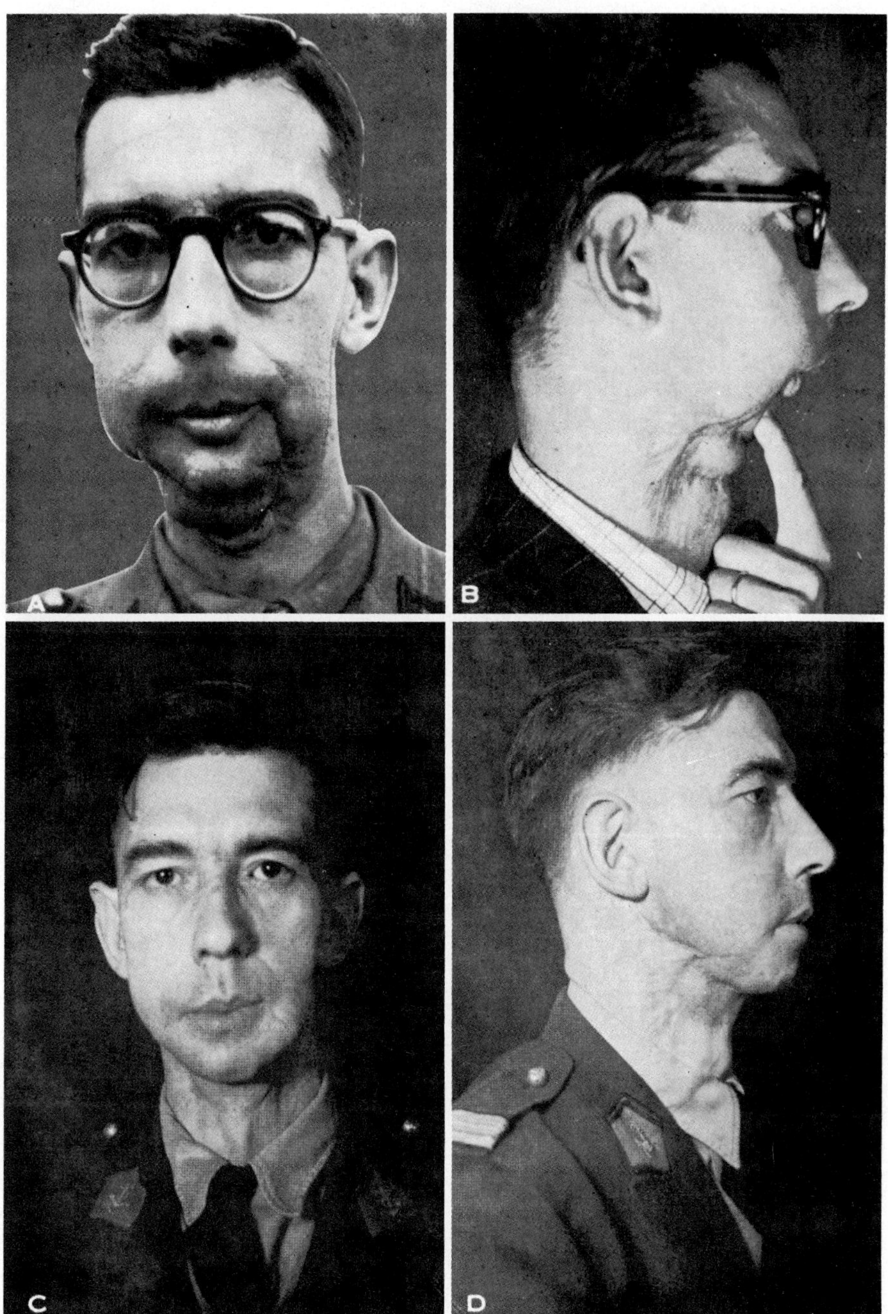

Figure 29–251. Reconstruction of the body and symphyseal region of the mandible. *A,* Appearance after loss of a major portion of the mandible as a result of injury by a shell fragment. Although the defect was large, little loss of the soft tissues occurred. *B,* The patient demonstrates the loss of the bone support by pressing the soft tissue backward. *C, D,* After completion of the mandibular reconstruction according to the technique illustrated in Figure 29–253. The patient is wearing a full denture. (From Converse, J. M.: Early and late treatment of gunshot wounds of the jaws in French battle casualties in North Africa and Italy. J. Oral Surg., *3*:112, 1945.)

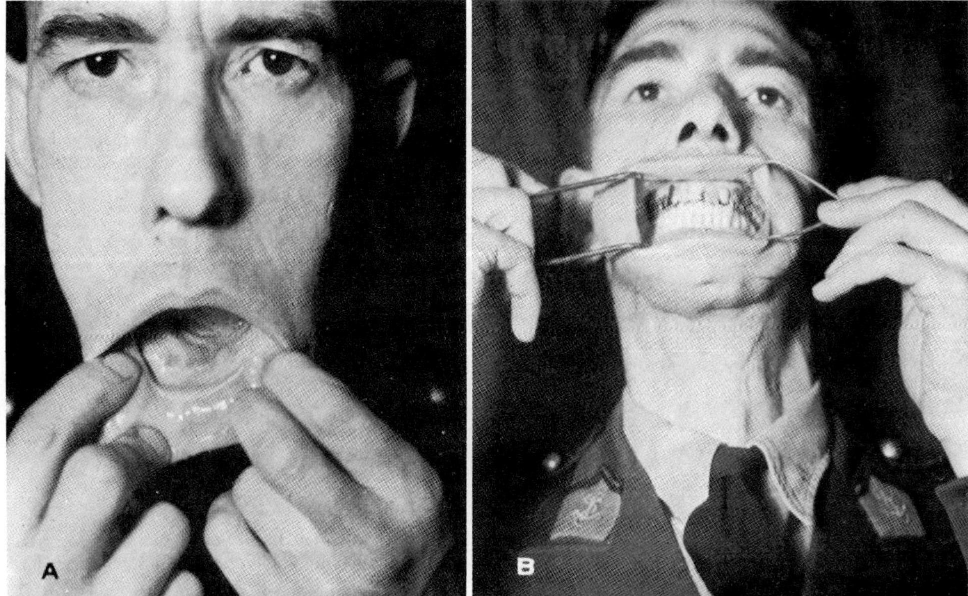

Figure 29–252. Intraoral views of the patient shown in Figure 29–251. The body of the mandible has been restored. The tantalum splint (see Fig. 29–253) has been removed. *A,* The sulcus was deepened by the skin graft inlay technique (see Figs. 29–275 and 29–276). *B,* Full denture in position. (From Converse, J. M.: Early and late treatment of gunshot wounds of the jaws in French battle casualties in North Africa and Italy. J. Oral Surg., *3*:112, 1945.)

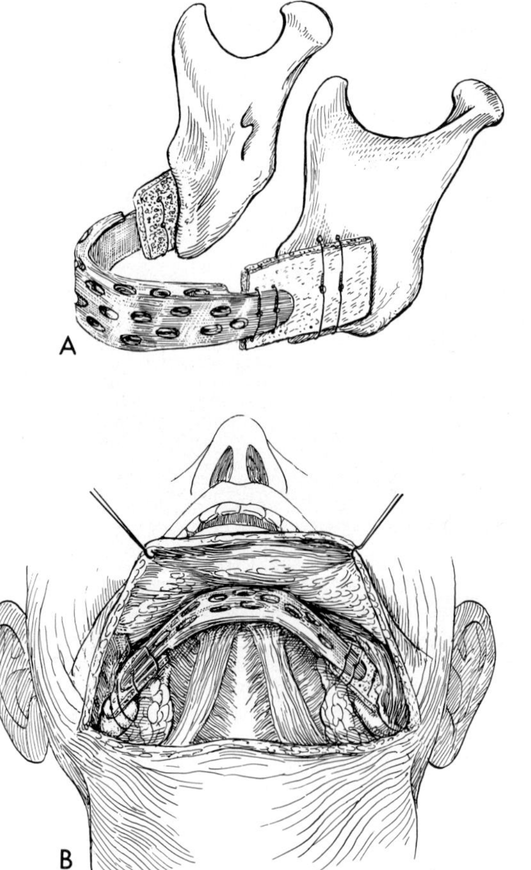

Figure 29–253. Internal fixation by a metallic splint. *A,* The fenestrated tantalum splint is wired to a bone graft, which in turn is wired to the ramus stump. Greater stability can be achieved by direct fixation of the metallic splint to the ramus stump. The splint maintains the alignment of the bone grafts, not represented in the drawings, which consist mostly of cancellous bone. *B,* The metallic splint in position. The metallic splint can be removed and additional onlay bone grafts placed to increase the bulk of the reconstructed mandibular arch.

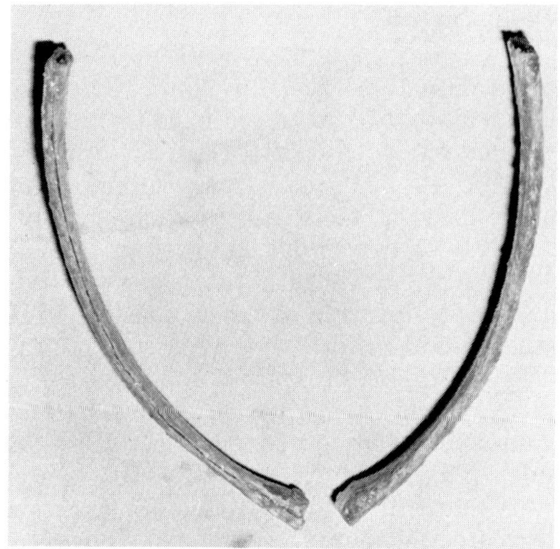

Figure 29–254. Fry's technique. Two ribs are removed from the region of the posterior axillary line (ninth and tenth ribs). Each graft is 13 cm in length.

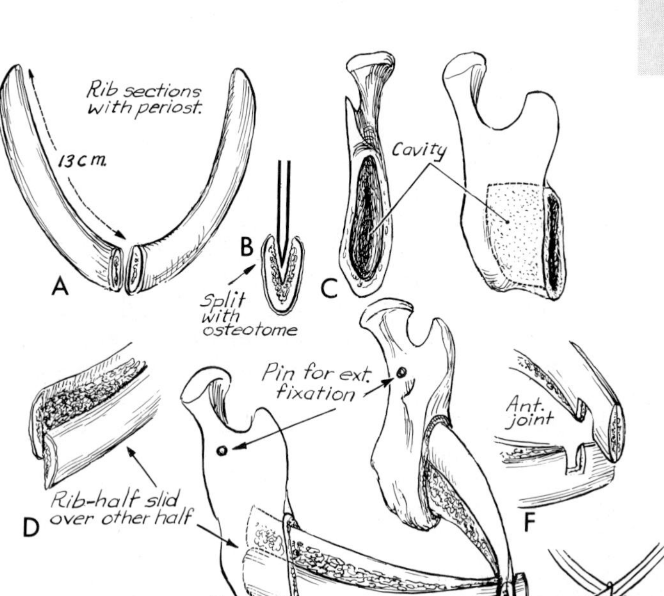

Figure 29–255. Osteoperiosteal split rib grafts for mandibular construction. *A,* Two ribs (ninth and tenth) are removed with attached periosteum from the region of the posterior axillary line. *B,* The rib is split. *C,* The medullary cavity of the ramus remnant is reamed out. *D,* The split ribs are joined by a halving technique. Note that a wide surface of cancellous bone is exposed, thus accelerating the revascularization of the grafts. *E,* The grafts have been inserted into the reamed-out cavity of the ramus, and fixation is obtained by transosseous wiring. *F,* Technique of joining the grafts anteriorly. *G,* A suture secures the joint and also attaches it to the tissues of the floor of the mouth. (After Fry, 1975.)

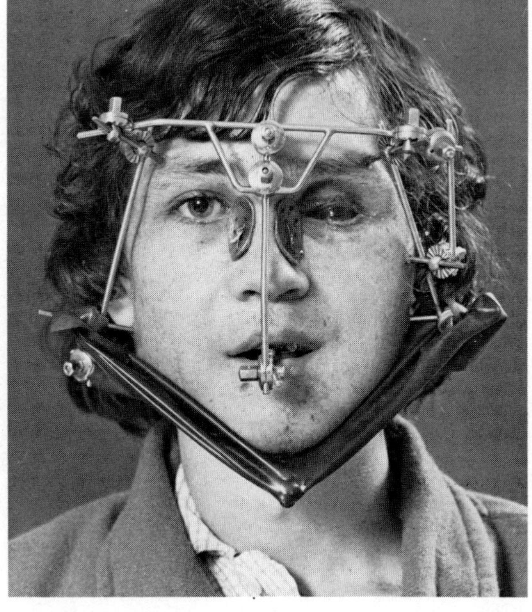

Figure 29–256. Technique of fixation of the ramus on each side by the Levant frame. (From Fry, 1975.)

cortical section (Fig. 29–255*B*). The medullary cavity of the mandibular remnants is reamed out with a drill (Fig. 29–255*C*). The two halves of a split rib are joined together by a halving technique, which entails the removal of cancellous bone (Fig. 29–255*D*), and are pressed together; the ends of the two halves are inserted as far as possible into the reamed-out medullary cavity of the ramus (Fig. 29–255*E*). Fixation is secured with a through and through wire suture. The same manuever is repeated on the contralateral side, and it is found that the split ribs cross over naturally in a satisfactory position to recreate the mental symphsis. The anterior joint is made by slotting one rib unit into the other, as shown in Figure 29–255*F*. At the anterior joint there is little if any sliding of one rib half over the other, and the joint is secured by a suture, which also attaches it to the tissue of the floor of the mouth (Fig. 29–255*G*).

The grafts are carefully covered by soft tissues. The reconstructed jaw is immobilized by pins inserted into the mandibular remnants above the grafts and fixed by a Levant frame (Fig. 29–256). The patients treated with this method are usually immobilized for eight weeks.

Fry (1975) achieved successful reconstruction of the mandibular body in two patients who required angle to angle reconstruction. The first patient had sustained severe injuries, including multiple facial fractures with loss of the mandible from angle to angle, in a traffic accident. The result of the reconstruction 15 months after the reconstruction is shown in Figure 29–257*A*. There has been no bone resorption. There was evidence of bone union both clinically and radiologically at the posterior and anterior joints (Fig. 29–257*B*).

Reconstruction of Ramus, Angle, and Posterior Portion of Mandibular Body. A defect involving the ramus and a major portion of the mandible requires an angular bone graft. Such a graft is obtained from the medial aspect of the anterosuperior iliac spine and the iliac table, including the medial portion of the iliac crest (Fig. 29–258). The bone graft is obtained from the iliac bone on the same side as the defect. The vertical portion of the graft serves as the ramus, and the horizontal portion restores the body; the angle between the two portions of the graft forms the new mandibular angle. The cancellous surface of the graft is placed inward for optimal revascularization. The graft is out-

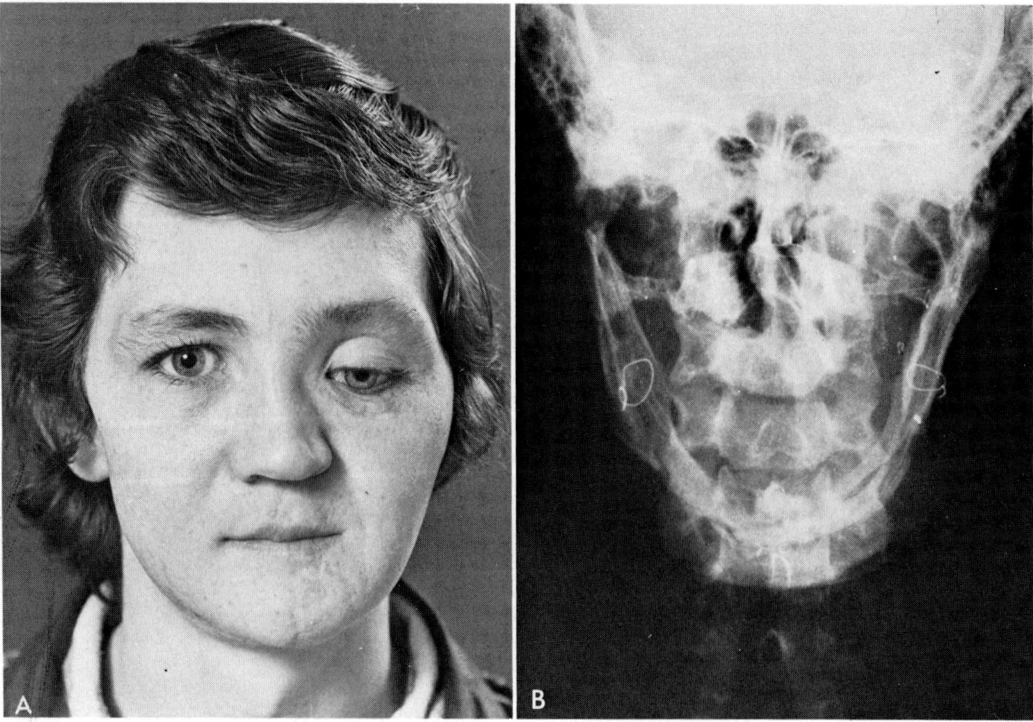

Figure 29–257. *A*, Appearance of the patient after reconstruction of the mandibular arch. *B*, Roentgenogram showing the consolidated bone grafts. (From Fry, 1975.)

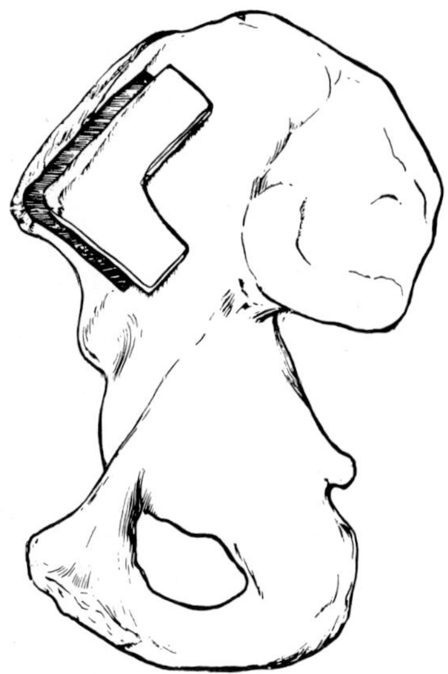

Figure 29–258. Angular bone graft removed from the medial aspect of the anterosuperior spine of the ilium for reconstruction of the ramus and body of the mandible.

lined at its donor site from a template cut from a piece of Asch metal and applied over the bone. The template is prepared after the exposure of the mandibular defect. The outline on the iliac bone is marked with an osteotome.

A dual approach provides adequate access: (1) a preauricular incision that extends upward into the temporal area and exposes the remaining condylar or ramus fragment; and (2) a submandibular (Risdon) incision that exposes the posterior portion of the mandibular body. A cleavage plane, deep to the masseter muscle, the parotid gland, and the facial nerve branches, is sought. The absence of the ramus results in an intimate relationship between the masseter and medial pterygoid muscle. The plane of cleavage for the insertion of the bone graft lies between these two muscles and must be carefully dissected. The bone graft is securely wired to the posterior portion of the mandibular body and overlies the stump of the ramus, which has been denuded of periosteum. Cancellous bone chips are added around the junction of the graft and the body of the mandible, and thin, flat pieces are placed between the graft and the remaining portion of the ramus. The soft tissues are sutured. The lower borders of the masseter and the medial pterygoid muscles are sutured to each other. Immobilization must be maintained for six to eight weeks to ensure consolidation. Figure 29–259 shows photographs and roentgenograms of a patient who was treated in this manner to reconstruct the major portion of the right side of the mandible.

Reconstruction of Hemimandible. Manchester (1965) reproduced the anatomy of the hemimandible for immediate reconstruction after resection for tumors that are slow-growing and not aggressively malignant (Fig. 29–260*A*). In one patient the resection was performed for the eradication of fibrous dysplasia; in two patients the tumor was a myxoma; and in a fourth patient the jaw was resected because of a melanoma of the cheek that had invaded the mental foramen and the inferior alveolar canal.

It is important to preserve the meniscus of the temporomandibular joint when the mandible is being resected in order to obtain a satisfactory functioning joint.

A template (Fig. 29–260*B*) of the resected hemimandible is prepared after intermaxillary fixation is established by silver cap splints. The template is applied over the lateral surface of the ilium on the same side as the defect (Fig. 29–261). The outline of the graft is marked with a chisel, and the graft is partly shaped before it is finally harvested. The graft includes the full thickness of the ilium. Final shaping of the graft is completed, precaution being taken to avoid making the condyle excessively large, as this would interfere with the hinge action of the temporomandibular joint. The graft is placed against the meniscus. A stainless steel (Kirschner) wire is used to fix the anterior end of the graft to the uninvolved hemimandible, which is maintained in position by the cast cap splint. An excellent result was obtained by Manchester (Fig. 29–262). Radiographic studies documented survival of the graft.

At the autopsy of the patient with melanoma performed 11 months after the operation, the graft was grossly normal in appearance. The radiographic examination of the graft, particularly the condyle, showed that morphologic changes had begun to occur under the influence of functional stress.

Bilateral Reconstruction of Ramus. Reconstruction of both rami is required in bilateral and unilateral craniofacial microsomia (see Chap. 62). Kazanjian (1956) reconstructed both rami in a patient with this type of deformity.

The patient shown in Figure 29–263 had a retracted chin and a conspicuous depression on each side of the face. The ramus on the left side was represented by a tenuous, stem-

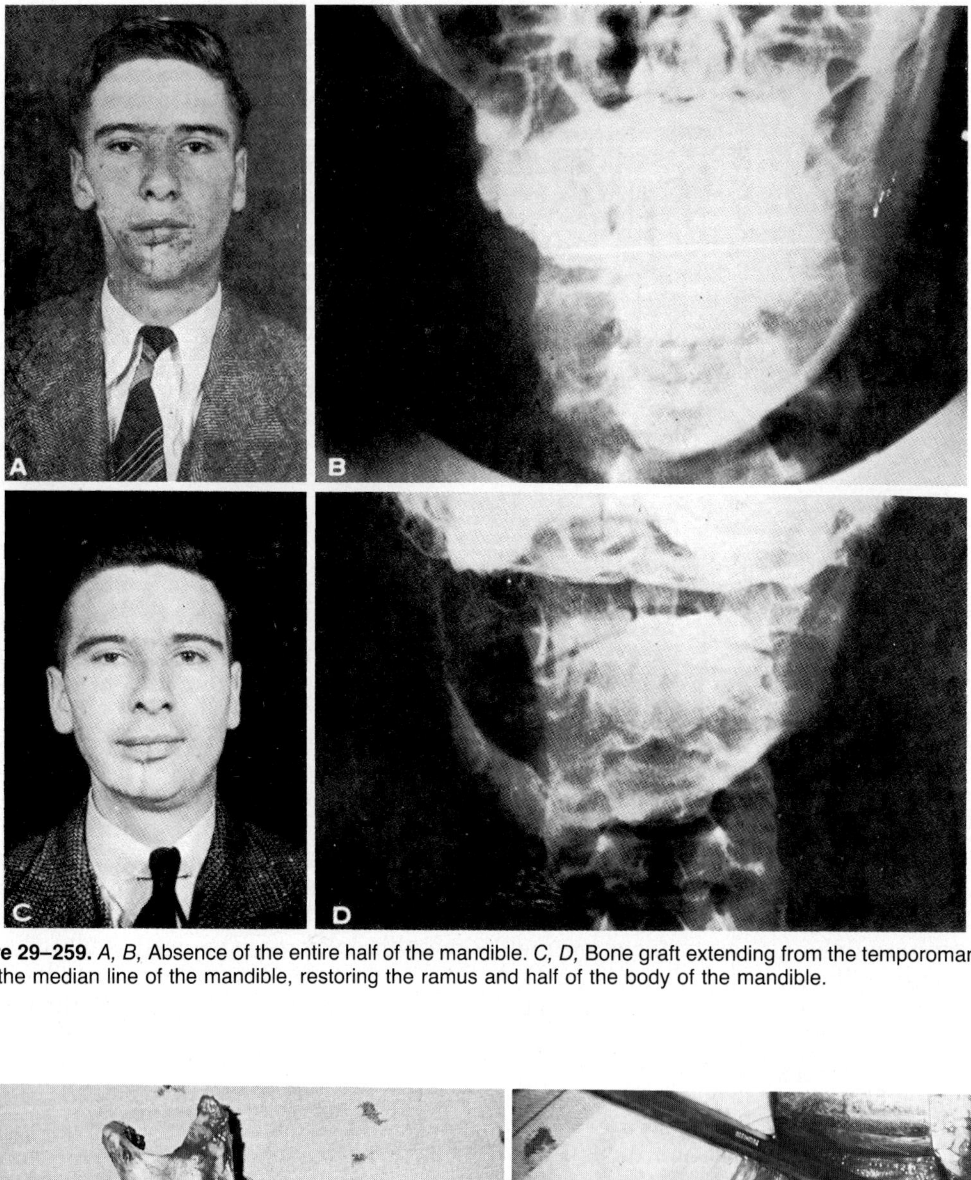

Figure 29–259. *A, B,* Absence of the entire half of the mandible. *C, D,* Bone graft extending from the temporomandibular joint to the median line of the mandible, restoring the ramus and half of the body of the mandible.

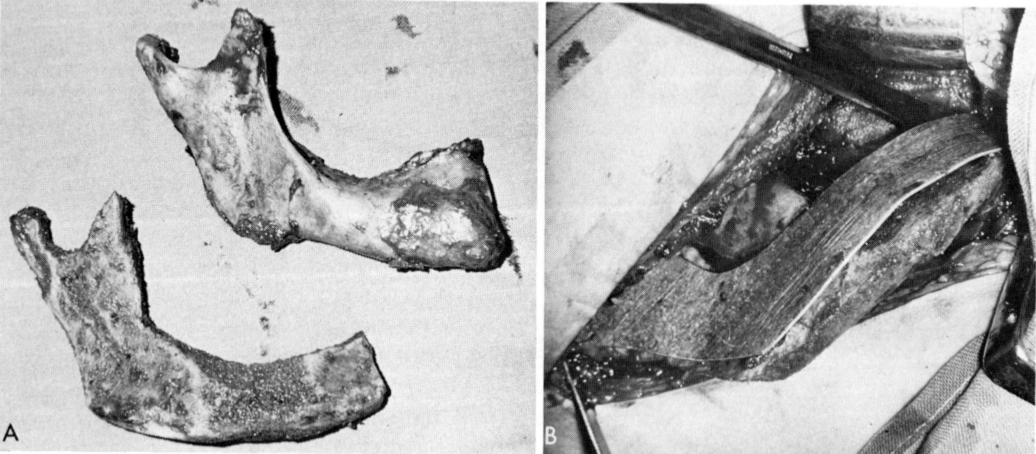

Figure 29–260. Immediate reconstruction of the hemimandible. *A,* The resected hemimandible (*above*) and the sculptured iliac bone (*below*). *B,* An aluminum template is resting on the hemimandible prior to the resection. It will serve as the pattern for the graft. (From Manchester, W. M.: Immediate reconstruction of the mandible and temporomandibular joint. Br. J. Plast. Surg., *18*:291, 1965.)

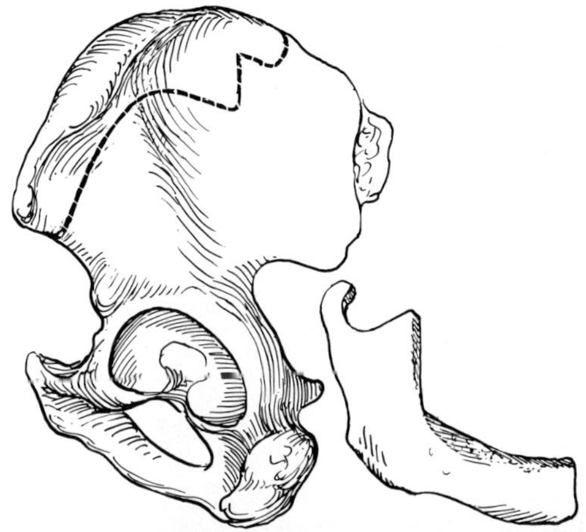

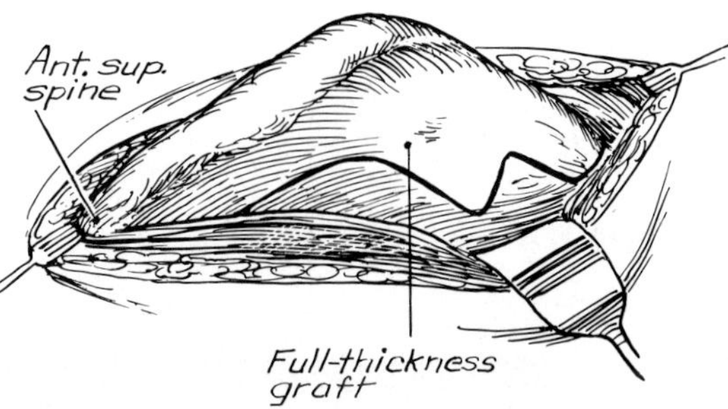

Figure 29–261. Removal of the iliac bone graft. The pattern is applied over the lateral portion of the ilium and iliac crest, and a full-thickness bone graft is removed as illustrated. (Drawn after Manchester, W. M.: Immediate reconstruction of the mandible and temporomandibular joint. Br. J. Plast. Surg., *18*:291, 1965.)

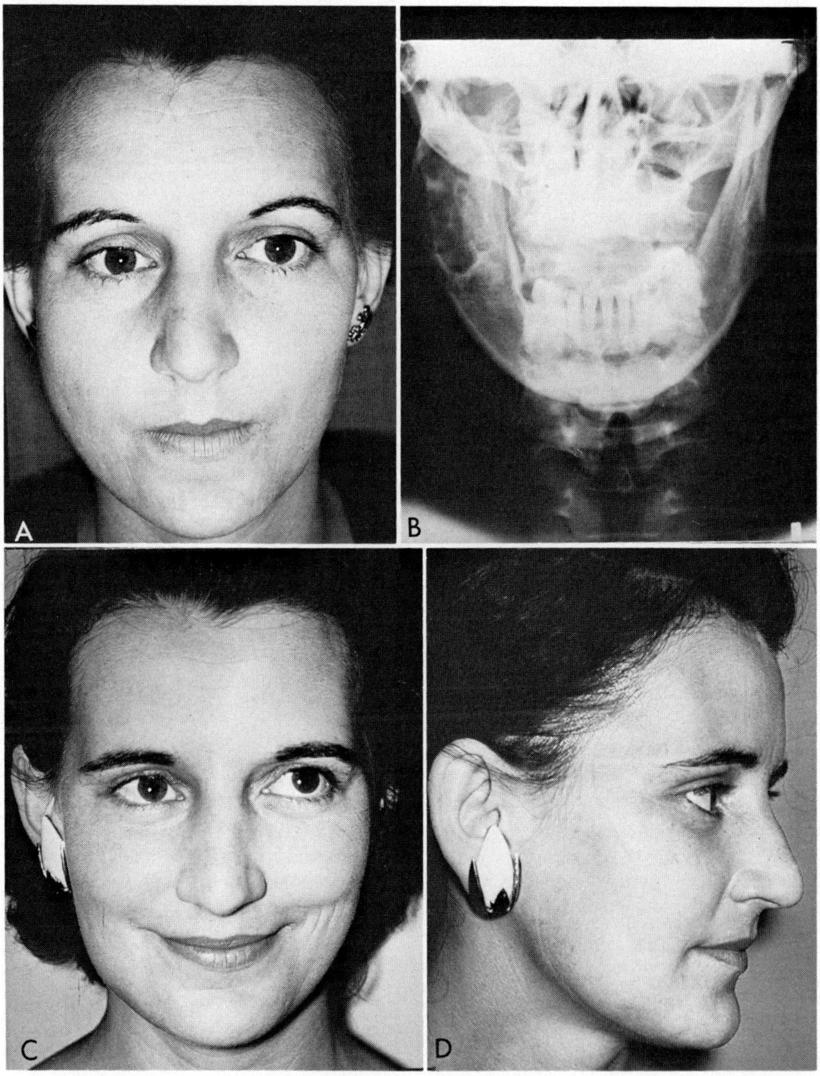

Figure 29–262. *A,* Patient, age 27 years, showing a swelling of the right cheek caused by fibrous dysplasia. *B,* The roentgenogram shows the pathologic process extending to the base of the condyle. *C, D,* Postoperative result two years later. (From Manchester, W. M.: Immediate reconstruction of the mandible and temporomandibular joint. Br. J. Plast. Surg., *18*:291, 1965.)

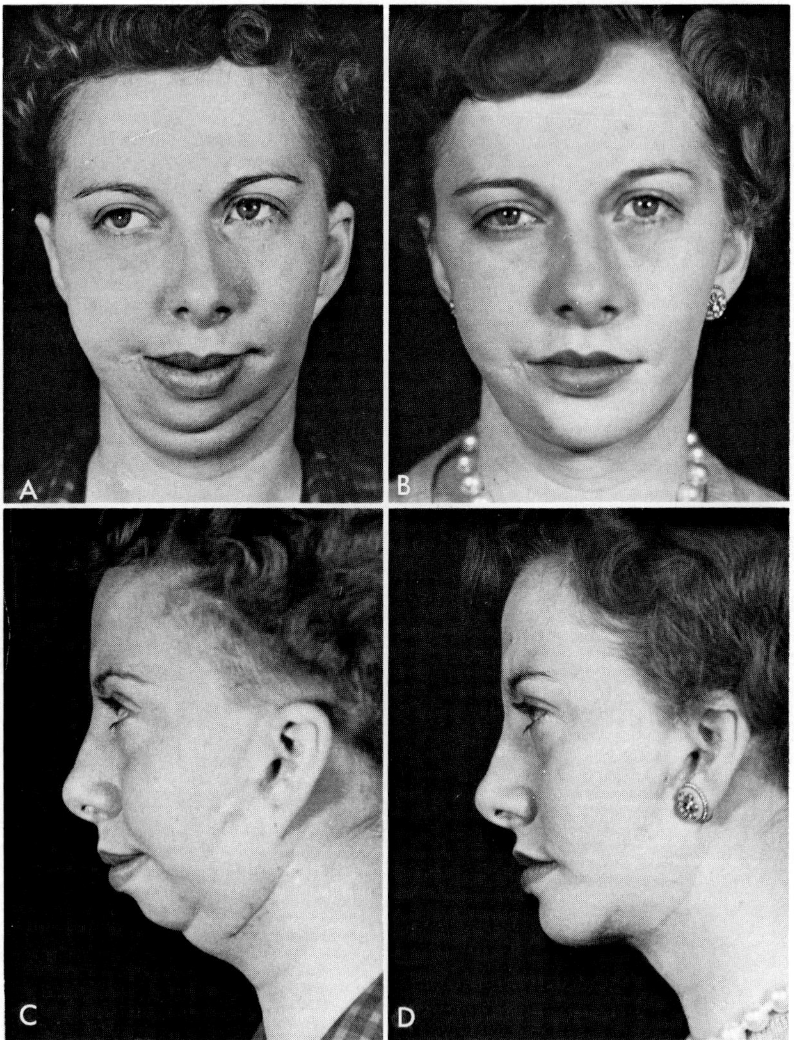

Figure 29–263. Congenital absence of the right mandibular ramus and near-complete absence of the left ramus. *A, C,* Preoperative views showing pronounced retraction of the chin and retrusion of the mandible. The transverse ridge of soft tissue below the chin is caused by the downward retraction of the mental symphysis. *B, D,* Postoperative appearance. (From Kazanjian, V. H.: Bilateral absence of the ascending rami of the mandible. Br. J. Plast. Surg., *9*:77, 1956.)

like structure; the ramus and the angle of the mandible were absent on the right side (Fig. 29–263*A,C*). The body of the mandible was "floating" and could easily be manipulated in any direction. The symphyseal region was increased considerably in its vertical dimension, and the cortical border was greatly thickened, giving the external appearance of a transverse shelf across the front of the neck, above the thyroid cartilage. This type of hypertrophy may have resulted from the overuse of the suprahyoid muscles in achieving opening of the mouth, since the lateral pterygoid muscles appeared to be absent. To construct the ramus, combined preauricular and submandibular (Risdon) incisions were used to introduce iliac bone grafts. Each graft extended from the rudimentary glenoid fossa to the posterior portion of the mandibular body.

The right iliac crest was exposed, and two large sections of bone and several smaller sections were removed from the crest to be used as "fill." A section of bone was transplanted into the prepared tunnel, the graft extending from the rudimentary glenoid fossa to the posterior portion of the right body of the mandible, where the bone graft was wired firmly to the body with two stainless steel wires. Several small chips of cancellous bone were placed in strategic areas to reconstruct the angle of the jaw and to add fullness where required.

The anomalous conditions found on the right side were also present on the left. A similar reconstructive operation was performed on the left side. The lower end of the bone graft was wired directly to the posterior portion of the body as on the contralateral side, and cancellous bone chips were also

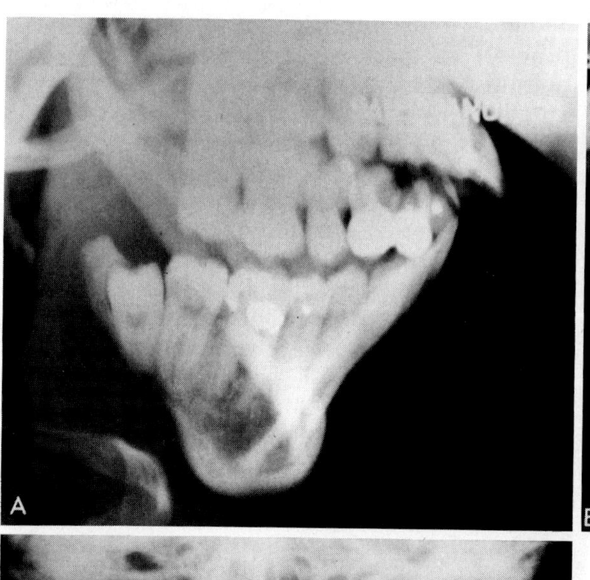

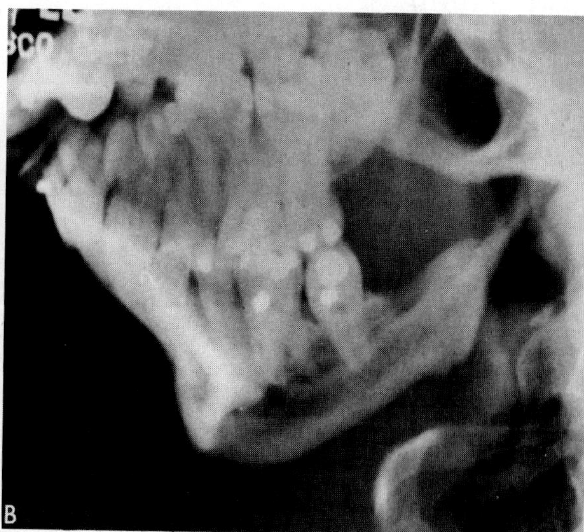

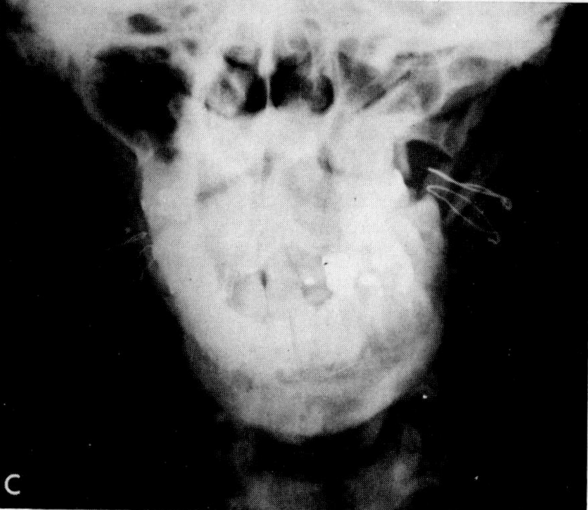

Figure 29–264. Roentgenograms of the patient shown in Figure 29–263. *A,* Absence of the right ramus. *B,* Stemlike ramus on the left side. Note the hypertrophy of the bone of the mental symphysis. *C,* Bone grafts articulating with the base of the skull. (From Kazanjian, V. H.: Bilateral absence of the ascending rami of the mandible. Br. J. Plast. Surg., 9:77, 1956.)

placed where indicated. Both wounds were closed in layers. The intermaxillary wires were removed, and the teeth were retained in satisfactory temporary occlusion by elastic bands (maintained for approximately six weeks). Radiographs (Fig. 29–264) showed that the bone grafts reconstructing each ramus articulated with the base of the skull and that there was satisfactory bone union at the points of contact of the bone grafts with the mandibular body (Fig. 29–264*C*).

Five months after the initial surgical procedures, the dental occlusion remained satisfactory and the patient could chew food without difficulty. Although a slight grinding action of the teeth could be detected during mastication, the patient could control mandibular motions effectively.

Satisfactory function of the mandible was achieved and the depression on each side of the face was corrected; the retracted appearance of the chin, however, had not been appreciably altered. Two subsequent operations were performed to restore facial contour, additional onlay iliac bone grafts being transplanted to the region of the chin and to the lateral aspect of the mandible.

An additional operation was performed to obtain further improvement in contour. Bone was again removed from the ilium; some of this bone was transplanted to the chin to accentuate the mental prominence. Other portions of bone were added to the lateral aspect of the body of the mandible on the left side to achieve symmetry with the contour of the right side (Fig. 29–263*B,D*).

NERVE GRAFTING AFTER RESECTION OF MANDIBULAR BODY AND BONE GRAFT RECONSTRUCTION

After resection of a segment of the mandible, the proximal and distal nerve stumps are tagged with a suture. After the reconstruction of the mandible by a bone graft or flap, a sural nerve graft is placed without tension between the stumps of the inferior alveolar nerve. Hausamen, Samii, and Schmidseder (1973) placed the nerve graft at a distance from the healing bone below the mandibular angle in the midst of well-vascularized soft tissue.

VASCULARIZED BONE TRANSFERS

In the clinical situation in which an adequate soft tissue bed to support a traditional bone graft is not present and when the reconstruction is to be done at the time of malignant tumor resection, vascularized bone transfers and composite bone and soft tissue flaps are the techniques of choice. The bone and soft tissue may be transferred as either a pedicle flap or a microvascular flap.

Much discussion has focused on whether living bone can be reliably transferred on its periosteal blood supply or whether the nutrient medullary vessels must be maintained. Before various bone flap techniques are discussed, this issue must first be examined.

The conclusions of Östrup and Fredrickson (1975) concerning the transfer of a free living bone can be summarized as follows: (1) survival of the isolated bone is predicated on maintaining the nutrient vessels; (2) both arteries and veins must be anastomosed; (3) linear bone formation within the transferred bone remains comparable with the rest of the skeleton and is unaffected by limited ischemia; (4) the quality of the recipient bed does not influence survival, thus permitting placement of the bone in heavily irradiated sites; (5) the union between the graft and recipient bone is a process similar to that of fracture healing, with bone of the transferred bone and recipient bone contributing to callus formation; and (6) the bone transfer is not replaced by creeping substitution. These conclusions were based on numerous experimental free rib transfers with long-term follow-up and use of multiple radioactive labeling techniques.

An understanding of the prime significance of the nutrient artery, as opposed to the periosteal vessels, has evolved as more experience is gained both clinically and experimentally. Experimental data by Berggren and associates (1982) found no difference in bone union when comparing vascularized posterior (nutrient artery) rib transfers and posterolateral (periosteal vessels) rib transfers in dogs. Extensive communication between the haversian canals within bone to both periosteal and endosteal lamellae has been demonstrated by Cohen and Harris (1958). Studies by Gothman (1960) on the rabbit tibia suggested that the inner two-thirds of the cortex was supplied by medullary arteries and the outer one-third by periosteal arteries. He used microangiographic techniques to show extensive communications between the two systems. Rhinelander (1968) suggested that when the medullary circulation becomes blocked, the periosteal circulation has the capacity to nourish that segment of cortex previously dependent on the endosteal vessels. In 1978 Ariyan and Finseth reported their first case of an anterior rib osteocutaneous free flap based on the periosteally supplied internal mammary artery. In 1980 Ariyan reported two additional cases with documentation of bone viability using fluorochrome markers and histologic examinations. In 1980 Cuono and Ariyan performed an anterior rib osteomusculocutaneous flap, clearly periosteally perfused, and documented viable bone following transfer using tetracycline labeling. Numerous reports in the literature now agree that the periosteal blood supply is capable of fulfilling the initial conclusion of Östrup and Fredrickson (1975), which previously had been thought to be solely dependent on a nutrient medullary blood supply. One must remember that different osseous segments rely on either periosteal or nutrient vessels in different ways. It is now apparent that the choice of flap must not be based solely on nutrient versus periosteal blood supply but rather on the specific requirements of the reconstruction.

Pedicled Vascularized Bone. A large number of cutaneous muscle and musculocutaneous flaps incorporating a segment of bone with its periosteal blood supply have been described. The clavicle, rib, sternum, calvarium, and scapular spine have all been used in this fashion.

In 1918 Blair described the transfer of a segment of rib or clavicle in a compound flap to jaw defects. This work was confirmed by Snyder and associates in 1970. Conley (1972a) reconstructed a series of mandibular defects utilizing the clavicle pedicled on the sternocleidomastoid muscle. A success rate of 78 per cent was reported in a mixed group of patients. The transfer of a rib as an island flap on the internal mammary vessels alone was described by Strauch, Bloomberg, and Lewin (1971). They isolated the seventh rib on the skeletonized internal mammary vessels for mandibular defects in dogs. This concept was carried out clinically by Ketchum, Masters, and Robinson (1974). Siemssen, Kirby, and O'Connor (1978) reported the use of the medial one-half of the clavicle transferred on the sternocleidomastoid muscle. In 1980 Cuono and Ariyan reported a single case of successful mandibular reconstruction using rib pedicled on the pectoralis major muscle (Fig. 29–265). In 1981 Bell and Baron used a similar flap in 14 cases, and in 1983 they published their experience with 22 rib and pectoralis major pedicled flaps. They had seven cases of rib exposure and complete loss of five ribs. In 1982 Baek, Lawson, and Biller reported five cases with one partial and two complete failures. Robertson (1986) detailed his experience with 24 cases of osteomyocutaneous pedicled mandibular reconstructions, all carried on the pectoralis major muscle. Six ribs and 18 outer tables of the sternum were used. Two cases required bilateral sternal flaps. Five of six of the rib cases had problems with bone survival. Only two sternal bone reconstructions had associated problems. Modifications by Little, McCullough, and Lyons in 1983 to include the pectoralis minor and lateral thoracic artery, and by Richards, Poole, and Godfrey (1985) using the serratus anterior muscle, have been reported. The latissmus dorsi muscle (Schmidt and Robson, 1982; Maruyama, Vrita, and Ohnishi, 1985) has been used as a pedicle to transfer rib segments for mandibular reconstruction as well. Ariyan (1980) demonstrated that rib remains viable when transferred on its periosteal blood supply, but such transfers involve many problems in clinical practice. The thin cortex and small caliber make the rib less than ideal as a replacement for the mandible. As a pedicled osteomyocutaneous flap, proper contouring and positioning are severely limited by the vascular pedicle. Complex three-dimensional reconstructions requiring precise orientation of skin and bone are often impossible to achieve.

Demergasso and Piazza (1979) were the first to describe the use of the scapular spine pedicled on the trapezius muscle. Panje and Cutting (1980) reported a successful case using an osteomyocutaneous trapezius-scapular spine flap. Panje in 1985 reported his follow-up of 24 cases: 85 per cent involved reconstruction of anterior mandibular segments secondary to osteoradionecrosis. He reported an 87 per cent success rate. Bone viability was confirmed by bone biopsy in five cases and tetracycline labeling in one. Early and late bone scans were suggestive of bone viability in eight of the 24 cases. An area of bone measuring approximately 12 × 2.5 cm is available if one does not disturb the acromion. Two of three of Panje's failures occurred when more than 10 cm of bone was used. He stated that contouring and fixation may dis-

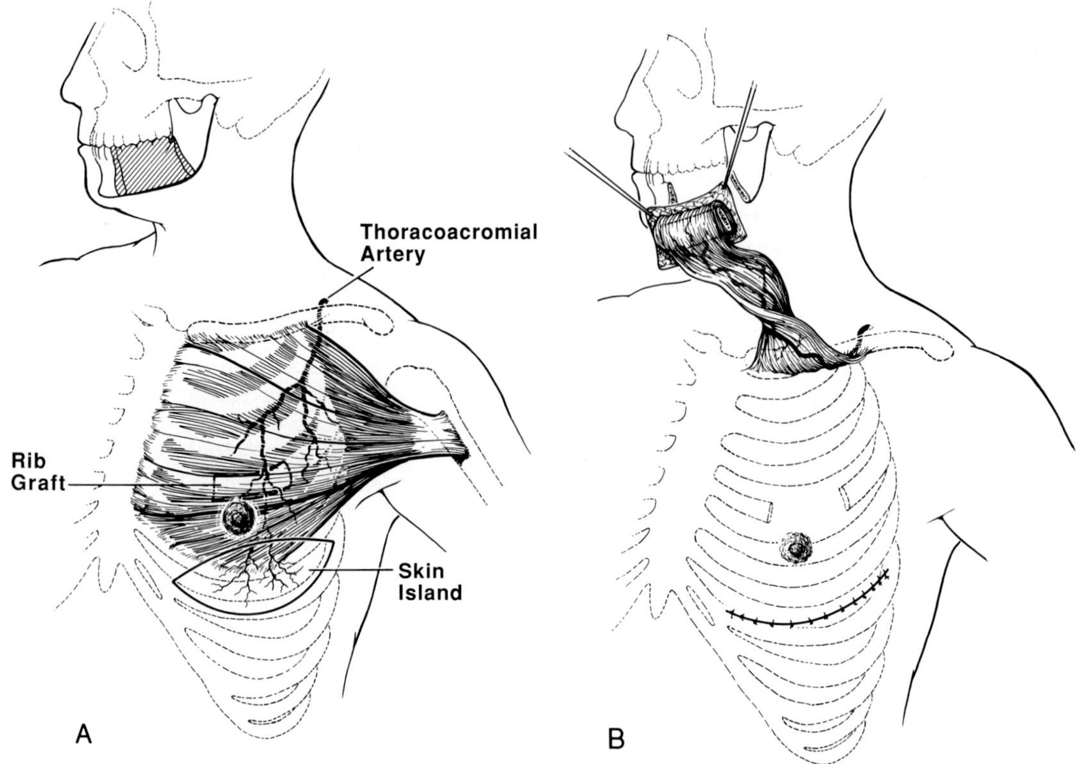

Figure 29–265. Pectoralis major osteomusculocutaneous flap. *A,* Design of the flap. Note the rib and skin island components and the thoracoacromial pedicle. *B,* Transfer of the flap.

turb the pedicle and he warned against loss of shoulder mobility postoperatively.

Dufresne and associates (1987) reported their experience with eight clinical cases utilizing the trapezius osteomyocutaneous flap for mandibular reconstruction. Tetracycline labeling and bone biopsies confirmed viable bone transfer. The paper reviewed the anatomy of the transverse cervical pedicle and its anatomic variations (Fig. 29–266). Approximately 10 cm of bone can be harvested without disturbing the acromion. Gregor and Davidge-Pitts (1985) included the acromion with negligible instability of the shoulder in 18 cases.

While various osteomyocutaneous flaps are capable of delivering vascularized bone and soft tissues to the oral cavity, the procedures should probably be reserved for small-segment bone replacement when orientation of the skin and bone is not a problem. Most failures have occurred when large segments of bone needing osteotomies for contour and complex soft tissue replacements have been required. In the later cases microvascular flaps are preferred.

Microvascular Osseous and Osteocutaneous Flaps. McCullough and Fredrickson first described the experimental use of microvascular bone flaps in dogs in 1973, and their experiments were followed by Östrup and Fredrickson (1974, 1975) and Östrup and Tam in 1975. They transferred the posterior ninth rib on its posterior intercostal nutrient vessels to irradiated mandibular beds in dogs. Similar experiments were made by Adelaar, Soucacos, and Urbaniak (1974), Fujimaki (1977), and Doi, Tominaga, and Shibata (1977).

The first clinical report of a microvascular free bone transfer was published by Taylor, Miller, and Ham (1975), who reconstructed tibial defects by transferring the contralateral vascularized fibula. In 1977 Buncke and associates reconstructed a missing segment of both bone and soft tissue in the tibia with a free osteocutaneous flap composed of the posterior ninth rib and its overlying skin. Harashina, Nakajima, and Imai (1978) reported two successful mandibular reconstructions using posterior rib segments based solely on the periosteal blood supply. Bone

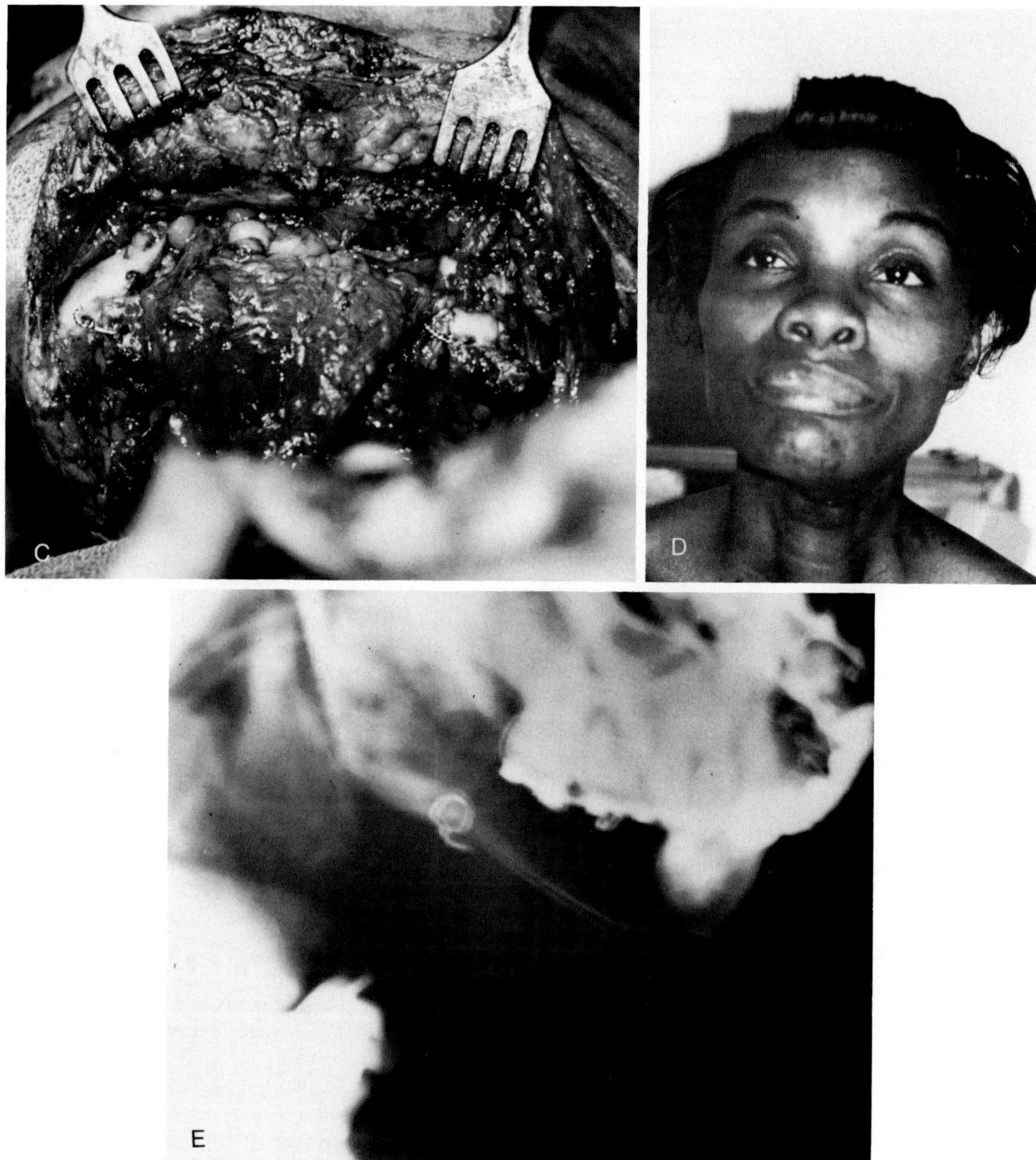

Figure 29–265 *Continued C,* Bone wired in place. *D,* Appearance at six months. *E,* Radiograph at six months. (Courtesy of Dr. S. Ariyan.)

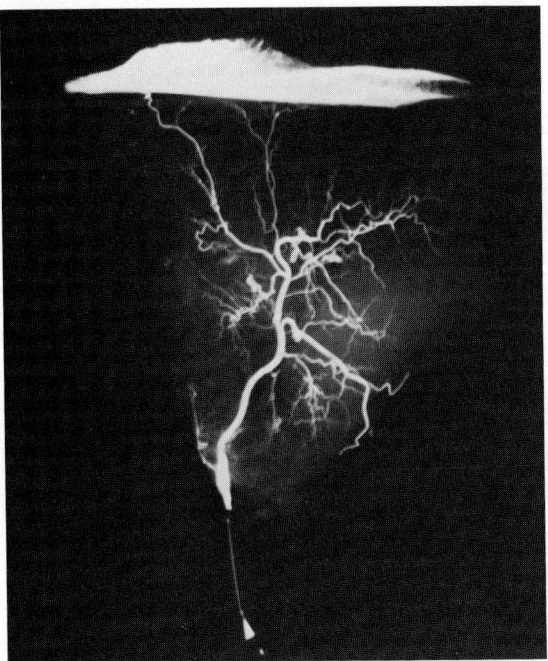

Figure 29–266. Injection of the transverse cervical artery demonstrating vessels supplying the periosteum of the scapular spine.

viability was confirmed by bone scans and biopsies.

Complex mandibular reconstructions requiring large bone replacements and multiple osteotomies in a compromised soft tissue environment are the prime indications for microsurgical reconstruction, especially when both soft tissue and bone require replacement. Successful reconstructions have been widely reported with either nutrient supplied bone flaps or periosteally supplied bone flaps. Currently available nutrient supplied flaps include (1) rib, (2) second metatarsal, and (3) iliac crest. Periosteally supplied segments of scapular, rib, radius, and fibula have been successfully used (Fig. 29–267). The choice of flap is based on several factors: (1) the size and contour of the bone defect, (2) the associated intraoral lining and/or external soft tissue coverage requirements, (3) the availability and orientation of the recipient vessels, and (4) the experience of the surgeon.

The normal adult mandible measures approximately 17 to 18 cm from angle to angle. The reconstruction of an anterior segment requires osteotomies in the bone flap while the vascularity of the bone transfer is maintained. The attached skin paddles of certain flaps are more appropriate for intraoral lining, while others provide excellent external coverage. Some pedicles are long and large; others are short and small. All factors are important considerations in flap choice.

Presently available microvascular flaps used in mandibular reconstruction that incorporate the nutrient blood supply are the rib, the second metatarsal, and the iliac crest. The posterior segment of the rib receives its nutrient vessel from the posterior intercostal artery slightly after its origin from the aorta. Its dissection requires a formal thoracotomy. The overlying soft tissue territory is bulky and frequently unreliable. The morbidity associated with the dissection, as well as the availability of other flaps, has made the posterior segment rib flap obsolete for clinical practice.

The second metatarsal, based on the dorsalis pedis artery and first dorsal metatarsal branch, was first described by O'Brien, Morrison, and Dooley (1979). It is capable of providing a well-vascularized segment of bone up to 7 cm in length. The skin island incorporated with this flap is thin, pliable, and hairless and it can be designed for up to 6 × 10 cm in area. The skin provides excellent internal lining when required.

Mandibular reconstruction from midbody to midbody is easily achieved with this flap. Experience with this technique has been reported by multiple authors (MacLeod and Robinson, 1982; Rosen and associates, 1985). Duncan and associates (1985) described its use in 26 osteocutaneous mandibular reconstructions with only three failures. The disadvantages of the flap are based on the variability in the course of the first dorsal metatarsal artery (Fig. 29–268), the potential for atherosclerotic disease, and the consistent donor site problems with incomplete skin graft vascularization. It also provides poor external soft tissue coverage. Despite these disadvantages, Duncan and associates (1985) considered it the flap of choice when a 7 cm segment of bone in association with intraoral lining is required.

When a larger bone segment requires reconstruction, the flap of choice is the iliac crest based on the deep circumflex iliac vessels, as described by Taylor, Townsend, and Corlett (1979). Up to 18 cm of vascularized bone is available (Fig. 29–269). Multiple osteotomies on the outer table of the ilium allow complex contour requirements to be achieved while still maintaining bone perfusion (Fig.

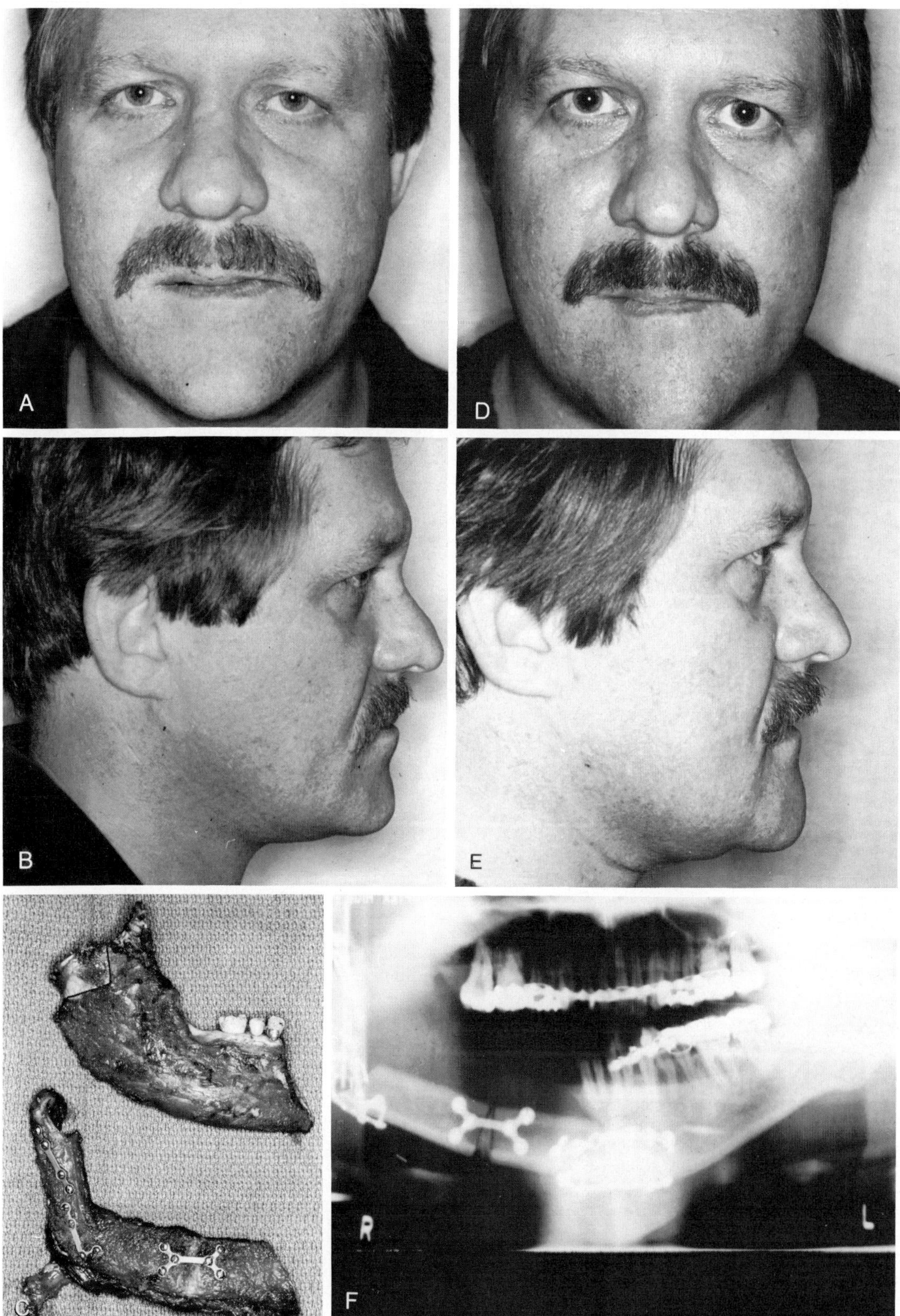

Figure 29–267. Primary reconstruction after partial mandibulectomy for an ossifying fibroma. *A, B,* Preoperative views. *D, E,* Postoperative views. *C,* The resected hemimandible is shown above the contoured fibula flap. Note the pedicle at the angle. *F,* Postoperative roentgenogram. (Courtesy of Dr. David Hidalgo.)

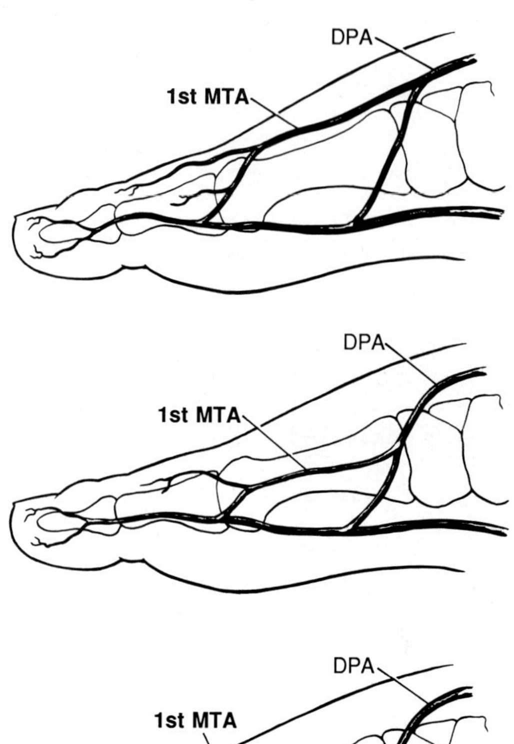

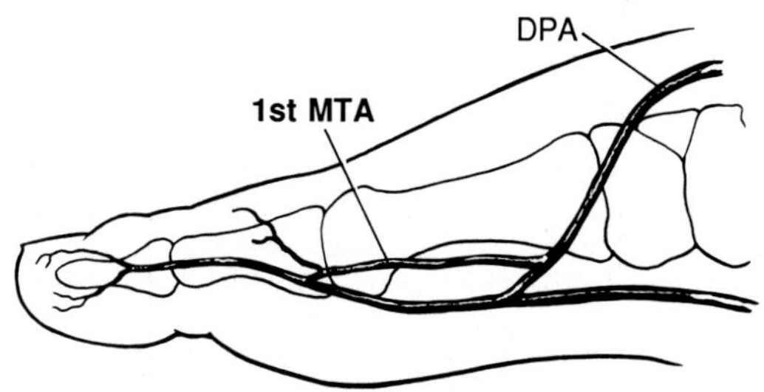

Figure 29–268. Variability in the course of the first metatarsal artery (MTA). *Upper,* The first MTA passes superficially from the dorsalis pedis artery (DPA). *Middle,* The MTA runs within the intermetatarsal space. *Lower,* The MTA has a plantar course. (From Gilbert.)

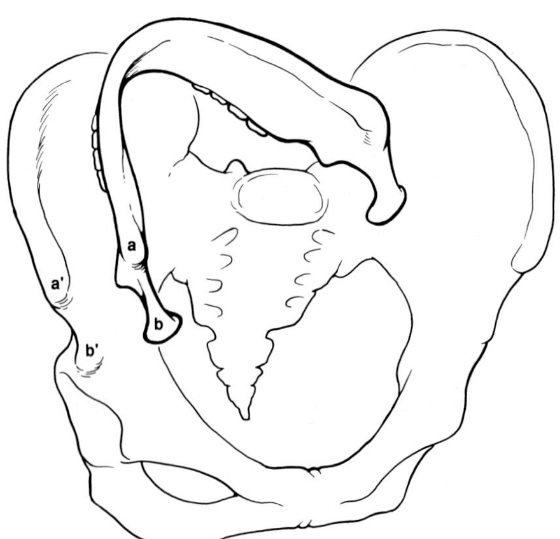

Figure 29–269. Bone harvested from the ilium on a pedicle simulates mandibular size and shape. a' = anterior superior iliac spine; b' = anterior inferior iliac spine; a = mandibular angle; b = condyle. (After Taylor.)

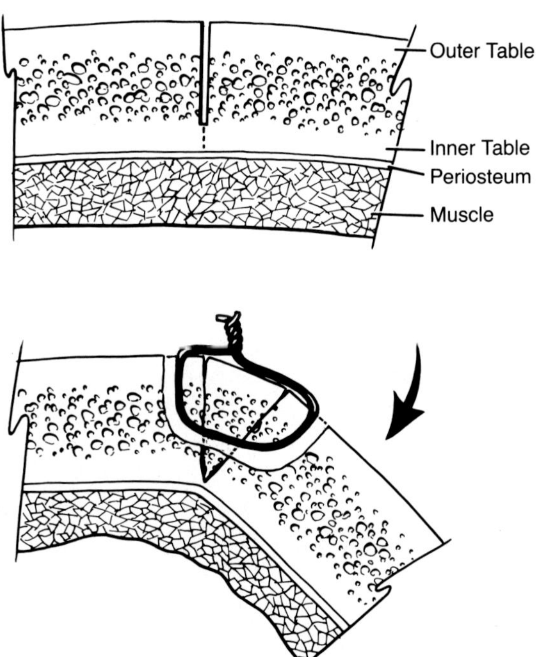

Figure 29–270. Partial osteotomy for contouring of the bony component of the flap. The blood supply is maintained by preserving the inner table and periosteum. (After Taylor.)

29–270). Taylor, Townsend, and Corlett (1979) demonstrated the versatility of this bone flap, allowing either ilium to be used, thus facilitating pedicle orientation on either side of the neck (Fig. 29–271). Furthermore, the inherent anatomy of the ilium simulates mandibular contour (see Fig. 29–269). The excellent quality of the bone transferred has facilitated the use of osteointegrated implants for denture construction (Fig. 29–272). The major disadvantage of the flap is its cutaneous portion. The skin island is generally bulky and is not suited for intraoral lining replacements, except in the situation when total glossectomy has been performed and the bulkiness of the skin flap is useful to achieve an oral seal to assist in swallowing. The perfusion of large skin islands is frequently inconsistent and it is often advisable to anastomose the superficial circumflex iliac vessels as well when a large skin component is required (Fig. 29–273). After the initial report by Taylor and associates (1979), Rosen and associates (1985) noted satisfactory results in 31 of 33 cases (Fig. 29–274).

Donor site closure must be precisely performed if complications are to be avoided. Colen, Shaw, and McCarthy (1986) reported four complications in ten patients, including hernia and transient femoral nerve palsy.

The periosteally supplied rib, as either an anterior, lateral, or posterior segment based on the intercostal vessels, presents the same difficulties with osteotomies and proper contour establishment as those previously described. Furthermore, its cutaneous component is bulky because of the necessity of

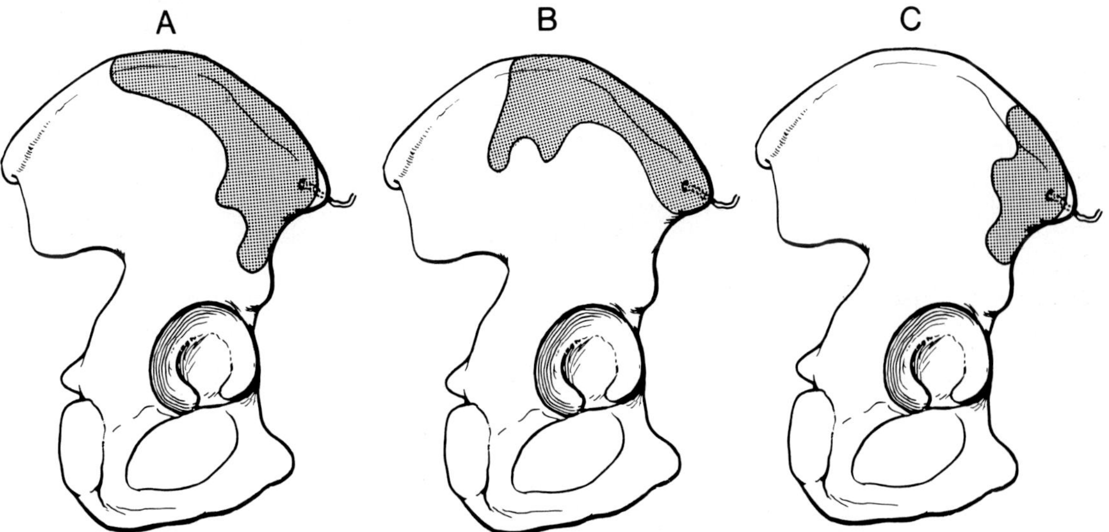

Figure 29–271. The ilium as a donor site for vascularized osseous reconstruction of the mandible. *A*, Flap design for hemimandibular reconstruction with the ipsilateral pelvis. Note that the recipient vessels are on the same side as the mandibular defect. *B*, Contralateral pelvic donor site with the recipient vessels on the contralateral side of the mandibular reconstruction. *C*, Contralateral pelvic donor site with the recipient vessels on the ipsilateral side of the mandibular reconstruction. (After Taylor.)

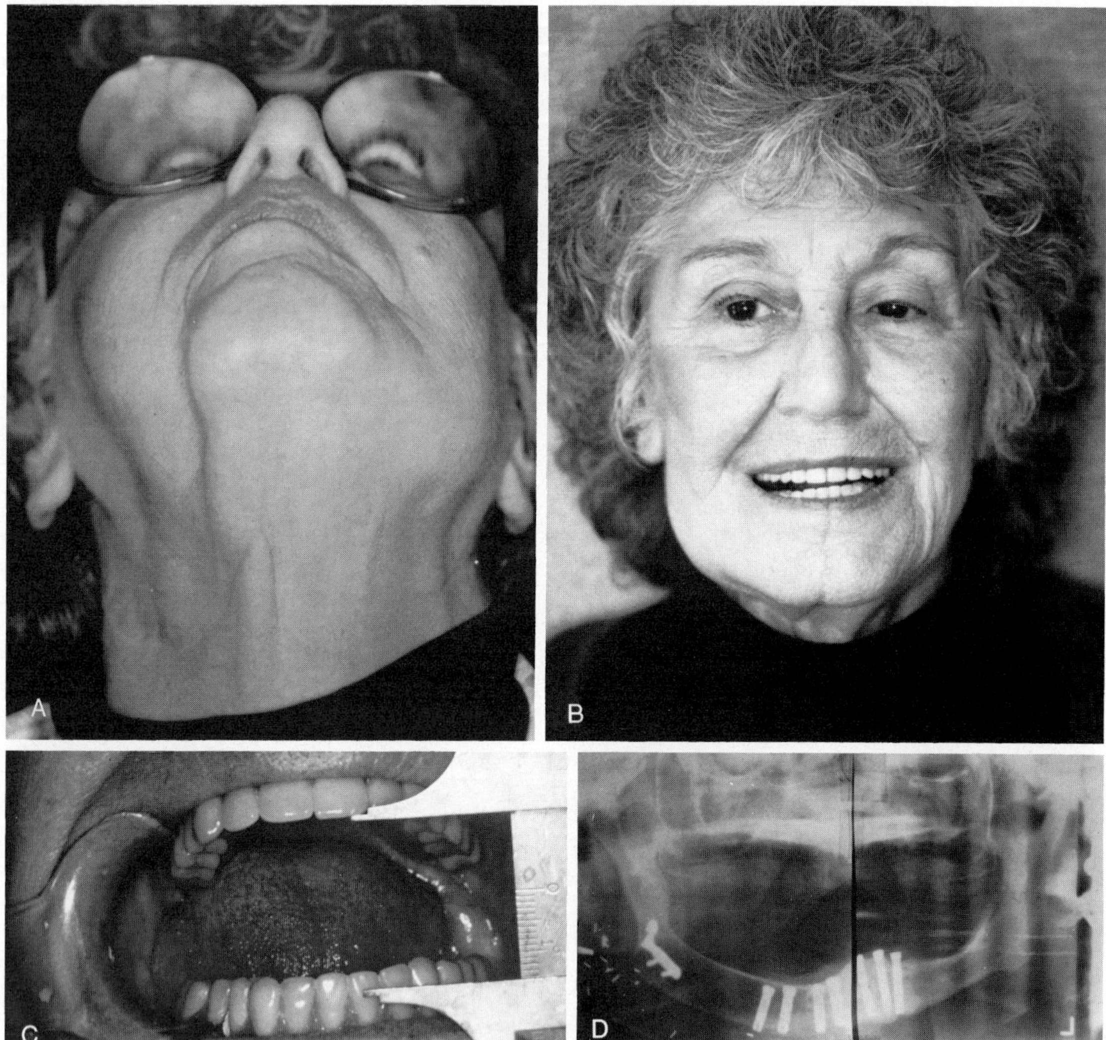

Figure 29–272. Vascularized iliac transfer reconstruction and osteointegration denture. *A,* Deformity after hemimandibulectomy. *B,* Postoperative view. *C,* Postoperative opening to greater than 32 mm with the osteointegrated denture in place. *D,* Postoperative radiograph. (Courtesy of Dr. Frederick N. Lukash.)

including muscle in the soft tissue attachments. Its clinical applications at the present time are limited.

The lateral border of the scapular receives a rich network of periosteal vessels from the circumflex scapular artery as it ascends from the omotricipital space. Approximately 10 to 14 cm of bone is available for harvesting.

Swartz and associates (1986) reported 21 mandibular reconstructions utilizing this flap; 14 of these required osteotomies for contour, with consistently satisfactory results. The major advantage of this flap is its independent cutaneous component based on the cutaneous branches of the circumflex scapular artery. Complex geometric soft tissue and bone reconstructions are more easily accomplished. Its long and large vascular pedicle also facilitates proper flap orientation, independent of recipient vessel availability. Its primary limitation is the quality of the bone and the difficulty in maintaining osseous perfusion when multiple osteotomies are required. Donor site morbidity is reported as minimal, only two patients having limited shoulder mobility (Swartz and associates, 1986).

Several authors (Sauter and McGregor, 1986; Sauter and Widdowson, 1986) recommended the use of segments of radius periosteally supplied by the radial artery, in conjunction with a forearm skin flap. Sauter and Widdowson (1986) reported 14 consecutive cases with one failure and one postoperative death.

A successful oromandibular reconstruction must not only restore the continuity of the missing bone segment but also provide soft tissues for external coverage and internal lining. It must also improve the functions of speech, swallowing, mastication, and respiration if it is to be considered successful. This is particularly important when patients have undergone large anterior composite resections. Opinions have differed with regard to the surgical management of patients requiring total or subtotal glossectomies with anterior arch resections. Some surgeons (Razack and associates, 1983; Krespi and Sisson, 1983) emphasized the need for laryngectomy in these patients to prevent aspiration, whereas others thought laryngectomy unnecessary if adequate palatal seal can be achieved with an intraoral flap (Myers, 1972; Effron and associates, 1981). Salibian, Rappaport, and Allison (1985) reported their experience in ten patients in whom oromandibular reconstruction was performed using the iliac crest osteocutaneous flap. Two patients had resections of major portions of the tongue. The authors specifically evaluated the functions of speech and swallowing and the prevention of aspiration. They noted excellent results; all patients had intelligible speech and were capable of eating a soft diet without aspiration. The authors made the following recommendations for patients undergoing simultaneous subtotal glossectomy: (1) the bone should be placed in the horizontal position to support the intraoral soft tissue and (2) the skin flap should be contoured to simulate the shape of the tongue without displacing the base of the tongue. They also emphasized the frequent need to anastomose the superficial circumflex iliac arterial system as well to support the large skin paddle. Duncan and associates (1985) evaluated 19 patients after oromandibular reconstructions by microvascular flaps and studied the functions of speech, swallowing, and oral continence. All patients reported that their speech was adequate for daily needs. Oral continence was dependent on several factors: lower lip sensation and contour, lower lip muscular function, the extent of tongue resection, the presence of an intraoral sulcus, and the degree of postradiation xerostomia.

None of the 19 patients had significant drooling. The adequacy of swallowing appeared to be most related to the extent of the tongue resection. Two patients remained gastrostomy dependent.

It became apparent from reviewing the previous reports as well as evaluating the authors' experience with 28 oromandibular microsurgical reconstructions that the planning of these reconstructions must not only address bone and soft tissue contour but lip sensation, tongue function, and denture construction. Flap selection and positioning, as well as restoration of a sensate functioning lower lip with an adequate buccal sulcus, are critical to a truly successful functional and cosmetic end result.

In summary, despite numerous reports in the literature of successful mandibular reconstructions using osteomusculocutaneous flaps, these procedures all have inherent limitations based on pedicle length, the quality and quantity of bone available, and the difficulty in achieving proper bone contour and orientation. Most oromandibular reconstruc-

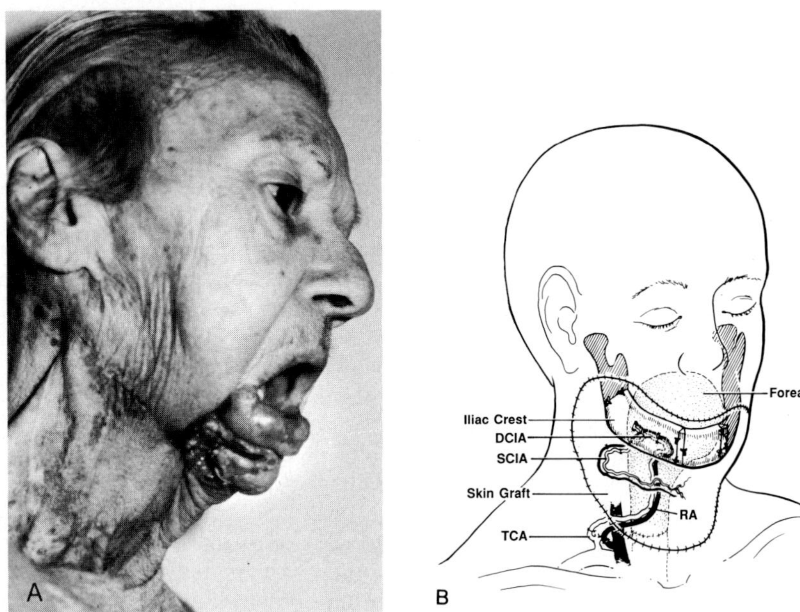

Figure 29–273. Combined deep circumflex iliac and forearm microvascular free flaps. *A*, Patient with a T4 recurrent squamous cell carcinoma of the floor of the mouth. *B*, Reconstruction of the anterior wall of the cervical esophagus, hypopharynx, and floor of the mouth with a forearm microsurgical flap. Reconstruction of an 18 cm segment of mandible and external soft tissues with an osteocutaneous iliac crest flap. Both the deep circumflex iliac artery (DCIA) and the superficial circumflex iliac artery (SCIA) are included in the flap pedicle. The radial artery (RA) was anastomosed to the transverse cervical recipient vessels (TCA).

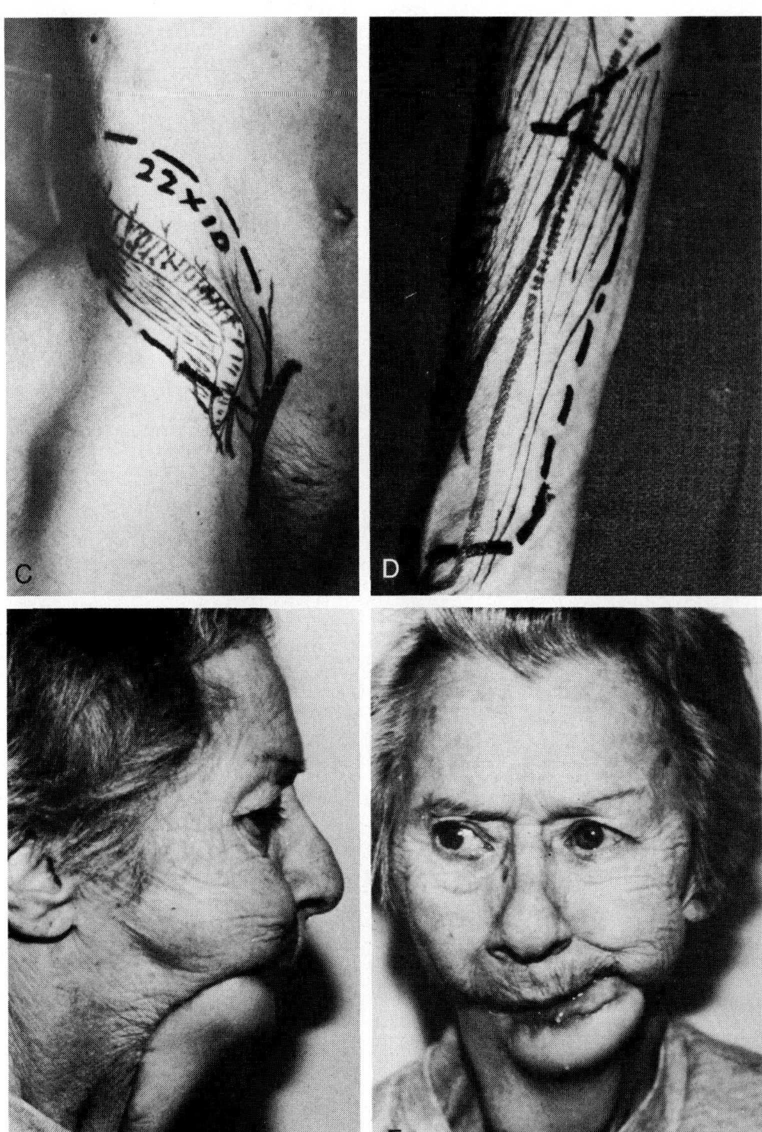

Figure 29–273 *Continued C,* Iliac donor site. *D,* Forearm donor site. *E, F,* Final result.

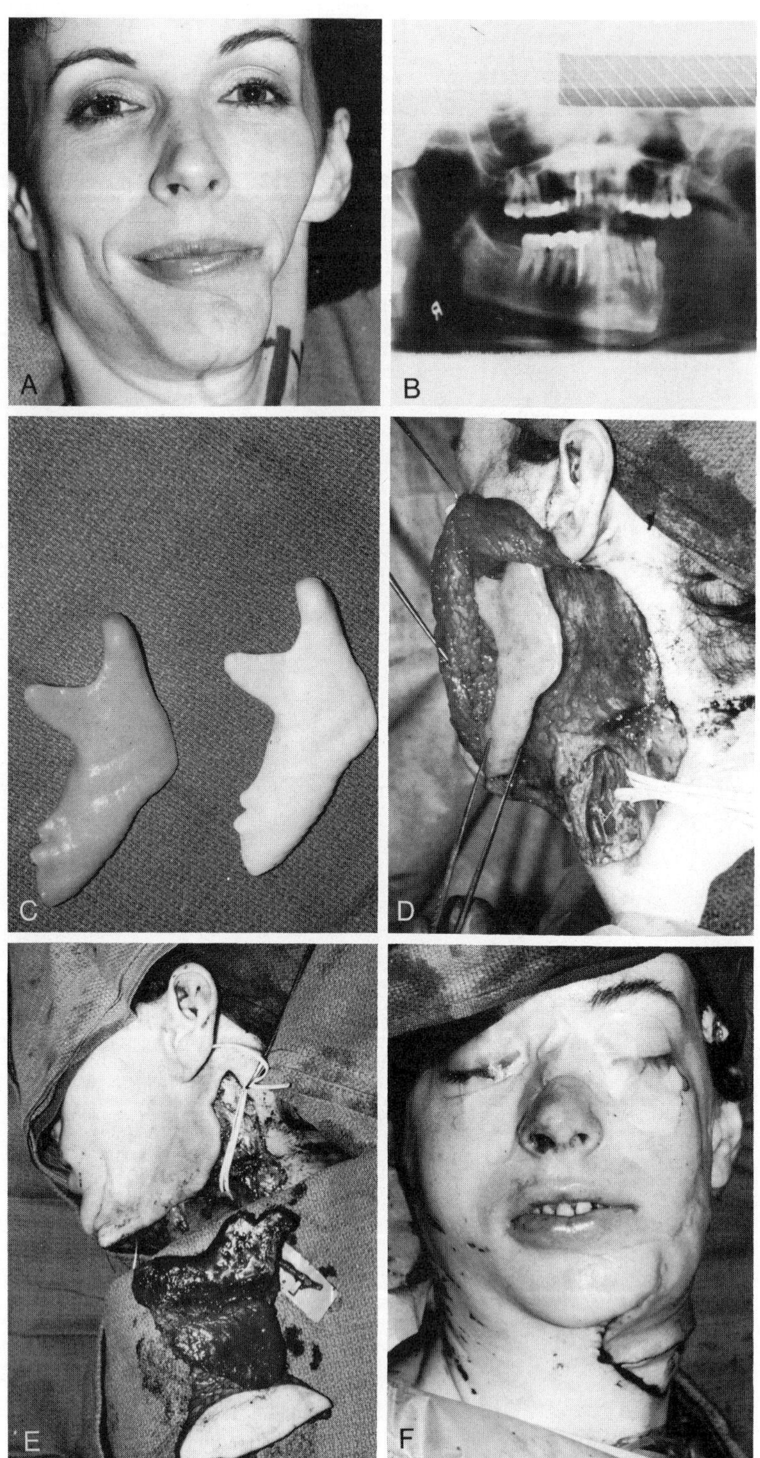

Figure 29–274. *A,* A patient who had undergone previous resection of an osteogenic sarcoma of the mandible. *B,* Preoperative radiograph demonstrating the bone defect. *C,* Prefabricated, CT scan-generated, acrylic model of mandibular segment to be reconstructed. *D,* Acrylic model being fitted into defect. *E,* The iliac crest flap is carved to the proper contour using the acrylic model as a guide. *F,* Immediate result of the operating room. (This procedure was performed by Mr. Ian Taylor.)

tions require precise placement of both the bone component and the soft tissues. When flaps are used, care must be taken to prevent pedicle kinking, often at the sacrifice of proper flap orientation. Composite flaps should most appropriately be reserved for cases in which the geometry is simple and the bone reconstruction limited. Microvascular osseous and osteocutaneous flaps allow more precise placement of both the bone and soft tissue components. The large number of microvascular flaps now available allow the exact requirements of the reconstruction to be more easily achieved. Recipient vessels are numerous in the head and neck region and their orientation can be modified with vein grafts when required. Large, well-vascularized bone reconstructions requiring multiple osteotomies for contour are best accomplished with microsurgical flaps. Simultaneous oral lining and external soft tissue coverage are also more easily accomplished with microvascular flaps.

RESTORATION OF BUCCAL SULCUS AND FUNCTIONAL ALVEOLAR RIDGE: SKIN OR MUCOSAL GRAFT INLAY TECHNIQUE

Operative procedures that restore the external contour of the face and reestablish the bone continuity of the mandible should be supplemented by artificial dentures to restore masticatory function. Skin or mucosal grafting is often a necessary procedure to provide an adequate sulcus and a retentive alveolar ridge after bone graft reconstruction of the mandible. The recent development of osteointegrated implants (see Chap. 72) placed into the mandibular reconstruction has greatly facilitated denture construction in these patients (see Fig. 29–272).

The term "epithelial" inlay was used by Esser (1917), who devised the technique of intraoral skin grafting. The term is a misnomer, since the graft, which includes both epidermis and dermis, is composed of more than epithelium alone, as the original term employed by Esser implies. It is preferable to use the term "skin graft" inlay. Esser (1917) conceived the technique for the purpose of establishing a buccal sulcus in patients in whom the mandible had been reconstructed by means of bone grafts. The purpose of restoring a vestibule is to facilitate the retention of a denture. Esser made an incision through the skin in the submandibular area, extending the incision to the lower border of the reconstructed mandible, upward along the buccal aspect of the mandible as far as the mucosa of the floor of the mouth. Into this cavity he molded a piece of softened dental impression compound. Around the mold, a split-thickness skin graft, raw surface outward, was wrapped and the compound mold was placed into the cavity; the submandibular incision was sutured.

In a second-stage operation several weeks later, Esser incised through the mucosa of the floor of the mouth into the skin grafted cavity, removed the dental compound mold, and extended the buccal flange of the patient's denture into the restored sulcus.

Waldron, an American surgeon during World War I, modified the technique by placing the skin graft directly into the new sulcus through an intraoral incision (Waldron and Risdon, 1919). Since World War I, the skin graft inlay technique has been used extensively to restore an adequate lining in the oral cavity. The typical skin graft inlay technique consists of three parts: the incision, the prosthesis, and the graft (Fig. 29–275).

The Incision. The incision is made through the mucosa on the labiobuccal aspect of the alveolar ridge down to the periosteum. The reason for leaving the periosteum intact over the bone is that skin grafting is more successful over the vascular bed provided by the periosteum. The incision is extended downward along the buccal surface of the mandible, and the mucosal flap thus formed is reflected inferiorly to line partially the labiobuccal aspects of the new sulcus (Fig. 29–275*A,B*). This type of incision has the advantage that the cut edges of the oral mucosa are not situated at the same level; thus, a constrictive scar band is not formed at the junction of the skin and the mucosa after the skin graft has healed. Careful hemostasis is obtained by pinching the bleeding vessels with fine forceps and occluding them by electrocoagulation. Complete hemostasis is essential to prevent hematoma, which would interfere with the revascularization of the skin graft.

In order that the revascularization of the graft may occur without interference, two conditions must be met. First, the contact between the graft and host must be as intimate as possible and there must be no interposition of blood or serum, which would act as a barrier to the ingrowth of host vessels.

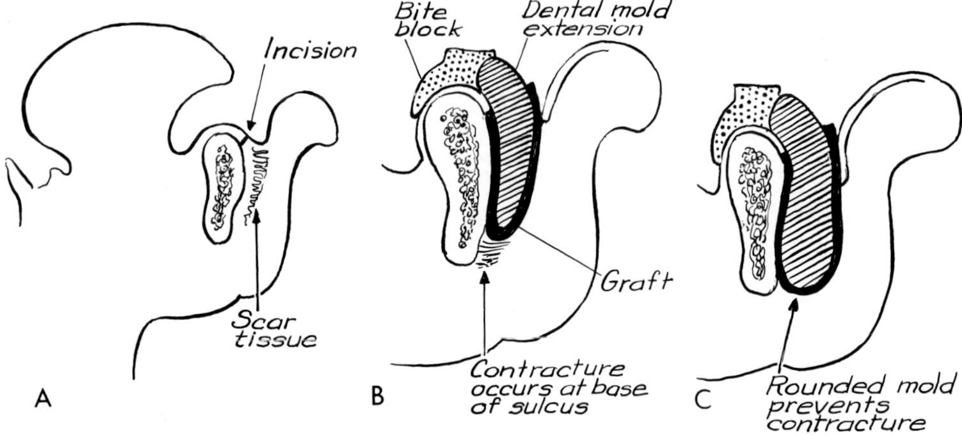

Figure 29–275. The skin graft inlay for restoration of a labiobuccal sulcus. *A,* The incision is made through the mucosa but does not extend through the periosteum. A flap is raised and reflected forward to line the lower lip (see *B*). *B,* The sulcus has been deepened: an impression has been taken with soft dental compound and hardened in situ with cold water. A split-thickness skin graft covers the dental compound mold. Note that the pointed shape of the tip of the mold results in contracture of the grafted tissues postoperatively. *C,* Correct shape of the mold to maintain the depth of the sulcus. Fixation of the biteblock or denture that maintains the skin grafted mold is often best obtained by circumferential wiring around the mandible.

Second, satisfactory fixation and immobilization (Fig. 29–276) must be provided so that the vessels are not torn during the period of vessel penetration into the graft.

In large skin graft inlays, considerable distention of the soft tissues in the region of the symphysis is necessary to permit the introduction of a compound mold of sufficient size. In such cases, it may be necessary to sever the lower attachments of the musculature of the lower lip and the platysma to permit adequate stretching of the soft tissues.

The Prosthesis. Three features are essential to the construction of the dental compound mold: (1) it must provide an accurate impression of the new surgical cavity, (2) it must be considerably larger than the cavity in order to distend the tissues in every direction, and (3) it must be free of sharp edges that would cut into the tissues. One cannot overemphasize the need for considerable distention of the soft tissues, and the construction of a grossly oversized mold, which can be reduced progressively during subsequent weeks. An oversized mold is important for two reasons. First, all skin grafts tend to contract during the healing period; thus, if the skin graft is placed over a mold that is oversized, an excess of skin graft will be transplanted, thus counteracting the eventual contraction of the graft. Second, hematoma formation, which would interfere with the revascularization of the graft, is prevented.

Newly developed synthetic materials have made possible the fabrication of a definitive prosthesis while the patient is in the operating room. However, this procedure causes considerable delay despite the rapidity of curing of some of the resins. In most complicated cases, it is more practical to prepare two appliances. The first is a temporary biteblock (occlusal wafer), which serves to anchor the compound mold for the primary skin grafting procedure, the second is a definitive denture with an oversized flange that fills the reconstructed sulcus. The flange is gradually reduced during the weeks after the operation. The shaping of the flange is important: it should fill the entire cavity and be of a shape that will ensure its retention (see Fig. 29–275*C*).

The Graft. Grafts of split-thickness skin are the most frequently used tissue to reline the raw surface of the surgically prepared cavity.

Skin grafts have the disadvantages of lacking pliability, of having a keratin surface that is difficult to "wet," of being malodorous, and of occasionally transferring hair to the oral cavity. The "wetness" is an especially desirable feature when maxillary vestibuloplasties are performed (Steinhauser, 1971).

To provide a more physiologic vestibular lining, a split-thickness graft of oral mucosa can be removed from the inner aspect of the lower lip by a Castroviejo mucotome (a small electric dermatome) (Converse, 1964c; Stein-

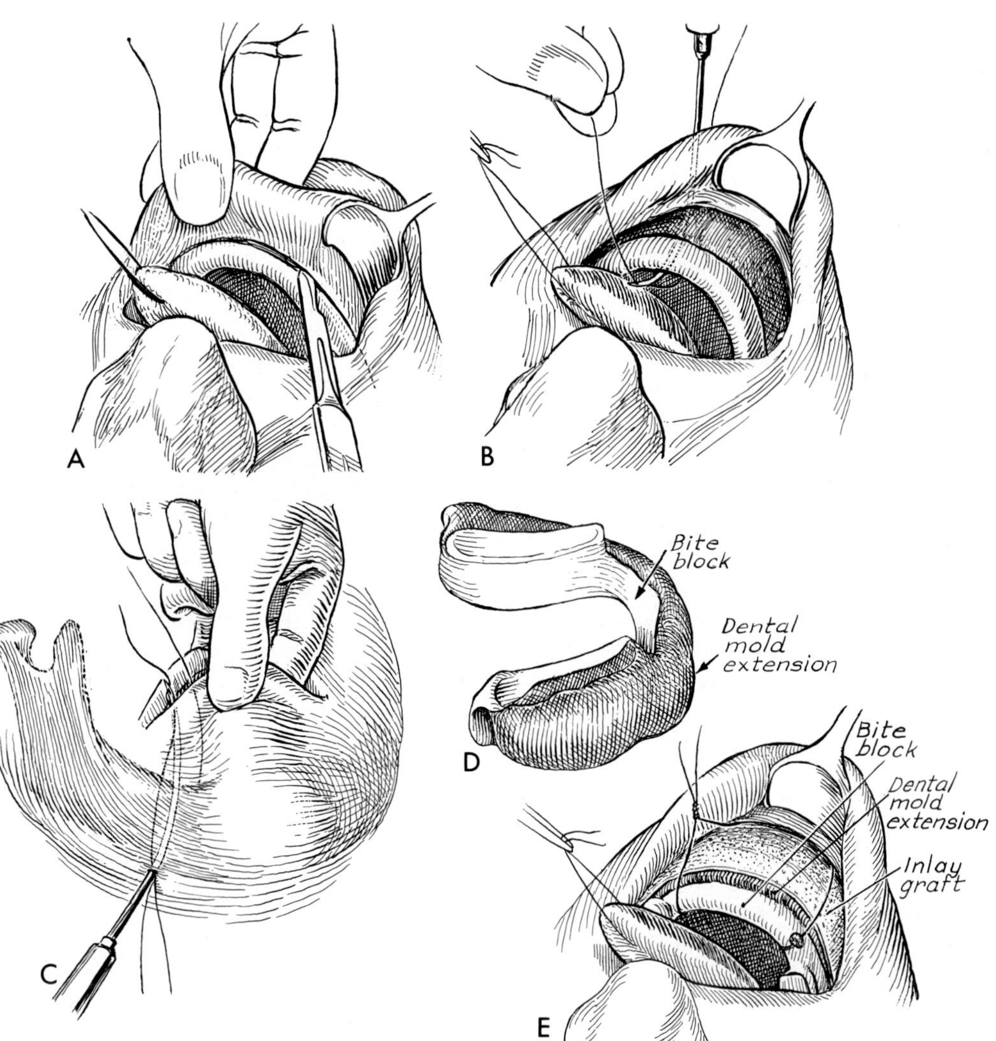

Figure 29–276. The skin graft inlay for the restoration of the labiobuccal sulcus in the edentulous patient. *A,* Incision through the mucosa. *B, C,* Passing a circumferential wire. *D,* The biteblock with the skin graft–carrying mold. *E,* Circumferential wires hold the skin graft inlay in position.

hauser, 1969). The cheeks and the undersurface of the tongue can also serve as donor sites. The entire hard palatal mucoperiosteum has also been used (Hall and O'Steen, 1970). In an effort to increase the area of coverage, Morgan, Gallegos, and Frileck (1973), using the mucoperiosteum of the hard palate, placed the graft through a skin mesher to expand the graft. Thus, a greater surface area could be covered by the limited amount of graft. The denuded hard palate reepithelized spontaneously.

The skin graft inlay was originally made with thick split-thickness grafts. The thin graft, although it becomes vascularized rapidly, has the disadvantage of contraction during the postoperative healing period. For this reason, thicker varieties of split-thickness grafts are preferred. The usual thickness is 0.014 inches (0.035 cm), as calibrated on American dermatomes. The skin graft should be removed from a hairless area of the body to prevent subsequent growth of hair within the oral cavity.

Fixation of Skin Graft–Carrying Prosthesis. The fixation of the appliance that maintains the skin graft in the newly made sulcus varies according to the status of the dentition. When the patient has teeth, it is possible to provide fixation of the partial denture by fixed band and arch appliances. When the patient is edentulous, a complete denture or biteblock (occlusion rim) is maintained by circumferential wiring around the body of the mandible (Fig. 29–276). In patients who have teeth a denture can be made on portions of the adjacent mandible. Clamps stabilize the denture to the teeth, and circumferential wires ensure completion of the fixation. Softened dental compound is added to the denture and extended into the deepened sulcus; a definitive appliance can be made immediately in the operating room with quick-curing methylmethacrylate.

Postoperative Care. The skin graft is immobilized for seven days, after which the compound mold is removed under sedation. Any excess skin graft overlapping the edges of the sulcus and any points where granulation tissue is seen are trimmed and cauterized with a silver nitrate stick. The appliance is *immediately replaced* to prevent contraction of the graft and diminution of the sulcus. At no time during the subsequent months should the prosthesis be left out of the skin grafted cavity, because contraction of the skin graft will prevent replacement of the prosthesis. The duplicate acrylic resin mold is used to replace the primary mold. This prosthesis is left undisturbed for another four or five days, when it is removed for cleansing. After this, it is removed every few days. As previously emphasized, the prosthetic mold should be oversized for all large skin graft inlays. After a period varying between three and five weeks, the size of the acrylic resin prosthesis is reduced by progressively grinding it down to the desired size and shape. All skin grafts contract; the period of maximal contraction spans several months, and the reduction in size should be slow and progressive. The best results are obtained if a period of approximately eight to ten weeks is spent in developing the final size and shape of the prosthesis. The patient should be told to avoid removing the appliance for any length of time, to prevent contraction in the skin grafted area.

PROCEDURES TO INCREASE AREA OF PURCHASE FOR DENTURE IN EDENTULOUS MANDIBLE

Recession of Muscular Attachments on Lingual Aspect of Mandible and Lowering Floor of Mouth. In the edentulous jaws, the attachments of the muscles are closer to the alveolar ridges, thus limiting the depth of the labiobuccal sulcus and the lingual sulcus.

In certain cases, it may be advantageous to increase the purchase surface of the denture by increasing the vertical height of the alveolar ridge on the lingual aspect of the transplanted bone. This is accomplished by recessing the attachments of the muscles of the floor of the mouth, thus lowering the floor. This technique was first demonstrated by Trauner in 1950 and published in 1952; it was later modified by Rehrmann (1953) and Obwegeser (1964). In such cases, deepening the buccal sulcus is not enough; it is also necessary to recess the structures on the lingual aspect of the mandible to establish an adequate ridge (Fig. 29–277).

The procedure consists of detaching the muscles attached to the lingual surface of the mandible, principally the mylohyoid muscle, and recessing the muscular attachment more inferiorly on the bone so as to gain additional vertical dimension for the alveolar ridge, and thus extra purchase for the prosthesis. The procedure is carried out without disturbing the periosteum over the alveolar bone. After

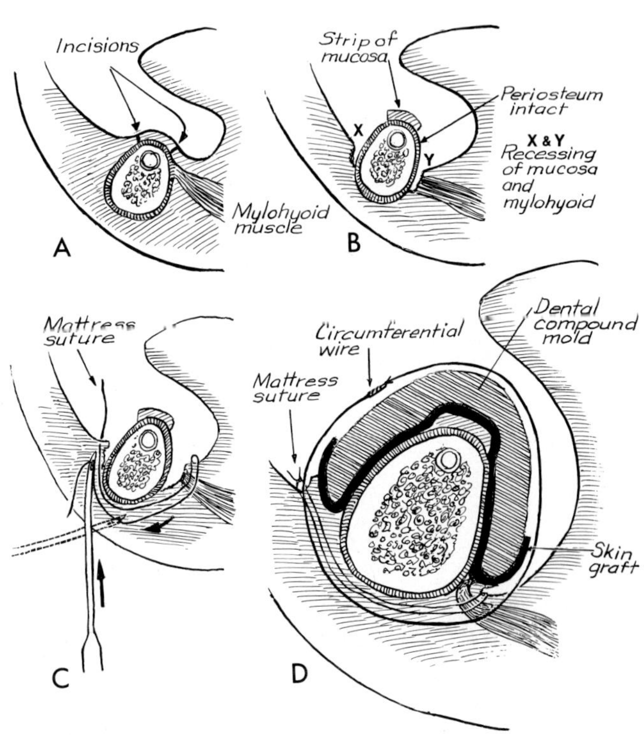

Figure 29–277. Technique for increasing the depth of the sulcus on the labiobuccal and lingual aspect of the mandible by muscle recession. *A,* Cross sectional appearance of the atrophied alveolar process. The buccal sulcus is shallow, and the floor of the mouth is close to the alveolar crest. Incisions are placed below the crest of the alveolar process, and a strip of mucosa is allowed to remain and cover the ridge. *B,* The buccal and lingual mucosa is dissected from the periosteum, as is the attachment of the mylohyoid muscle. The periosteum is left intact. *C,* The buccal and lingual mucosa and the mylohyoid muscle are displaced inferiorly and held by a catgut mattress suture passed below the border of the mandible. *D,* An acrylic splint maintains the molded dental compound and a split-thickness skin graft in position. The appliance is maintained in position by circumferential mandibular wires. (After Trauner.)

infiltration with a local anesthetic vasoconstrictor solution, an incision is made from the retromolar region to the retromolar region on the contralateral side, the incision being placed immediately lingual to the crest of the ridge. The entire periosteal surface on the lingual side of the mandible is exposed to a point immediately above the lower border of the mandible. In the most posterior portion of the wound, it is necessary to divide the superior fibers of the superior constrictor muscle. Blunt dissection avoids injury to the lingual nerve. In the anterior aspect, the lateral and superior fibers of the genioglossus muscle are resected. However, one should avoid complete section of the genioglossus muscle to prevent a backward displacement of the tongue and difficulty in control of eating and swallowing. The edge of the mucous membrane of the recessed floor of the mouth is then displaced downward, and catgut sutures are passed under the lower border of the mandible, rejoining the depth of the newly constructed vestibule on the buccal surface of the mandible. Fibrous tissue that may have accumulated over the lingual aspect of the mandible is resected down to the periosteum. At this point in the operation, it will be noted that a portion of the crest and the lingual aspect of the mandible are denuded of mucous membrane. A split-thickness skin graft is used to resurface the area. An impression is taken using the patient's own denture or a preoperatively prepared acrylic biteblock as a tray. Softened dental compound is molded over the area and hardened with ice water. A split-thickness skin graft, raw surface outward, is placed over the dental compound, and the skin graft–carrying denture or splint is immobilized by circumferential wires. After the skin graft has healed, a definitive denture with fully extended flanges is inserted.

Increasing Vertical Projection of Edentulous Mandibular Arch. Exposure of the alveolar process is obtained preferably through an intraoral or an extraoral approach. A bone graft is fashioned and fitted over the bone and maintained by circumferential wires laid into grooves on the upper surface of the graft (Fig. 29–278). There is usually sufficient mucosa to redrape it over the bone graft and deepen the sulcus.

There is considerable resorption of the graft bone, but usually enough bone remains to protect the inferior alveolar nerve and furnish a retentive alveolar process. Although bone resected from the lower border of the mandible is less prone to resorption, the edentulous mandible is often so tenuous that

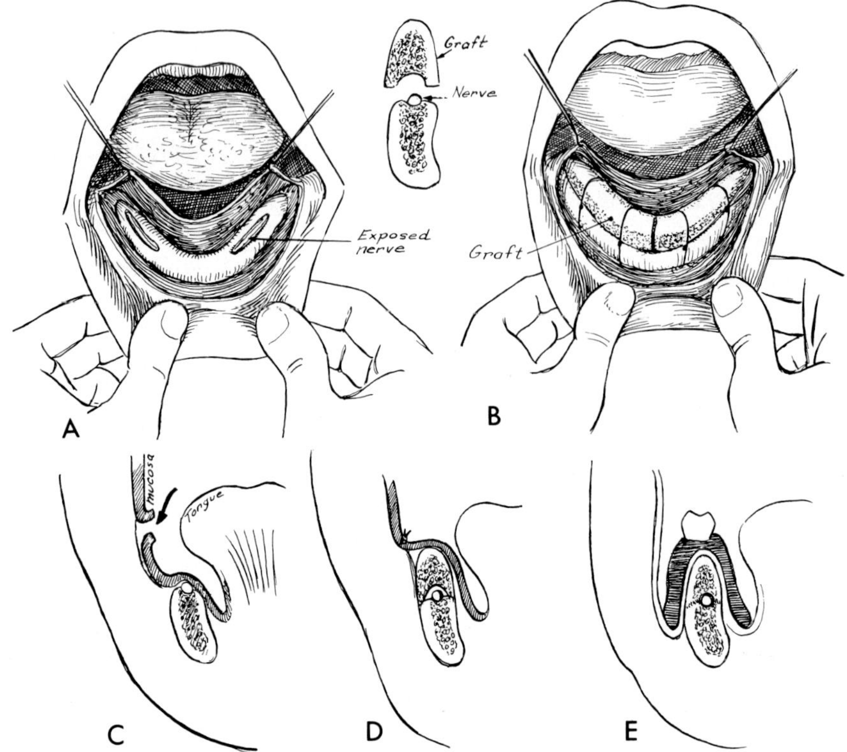

Figure 29–278. Increasing the vertical projection of the mandibular arch. *A,* Exposure of the mandible through a labiobuccal incision. The inferior alveolar nerves are exposed. *B,* The bone graft or hydroxyapatite segment is shaped to fit over the nerves and is secured by circumferential wires. *C,* The labiobuccal incision is made. *D,* Suture completed. *E,* The denture now has better retention as a result of the increased height of the alveolar process. Often the labiobuccal sulcus must be reconstructed as a secondary procedure.

little bone is available for this purpose. Autogenous cartilage grafts have also been successfully employed.

Encouraging results have been reported by several authors (Kent and associates, 1982, 1983; Rothstein, Paris, and Zacek, 1984; Block and Kent, 1984) from the use of particulate ceramic hydroxyapatite either alone or in combination with cancellous bone, placed subperiosteally for alveolar ridge augmentation. No significant advantages are obtained when cancellous bone is incorporated. Secondary vestibular surgery is frequently unnecessary. Ridge height resorption has been less than 10 per cent at four-year follow-up of 74 patients reported by Block and Kent (1984).

OSTEOINTEGRATED IMPLANTS

Osteointegrated implants have also found recent application for retention of a denture in the reconstructed mandible (Riediger, 1988); the subject is discussed in Chapter 72.

Maxillary Defects

In contrast to the many references in the literature to reconstructive surgery of the mandible, little has been written about reconstruction of the maxilla. Upper jaw defects have been treated by closing the palatal defect with an obturator connected with a denture, which is retained by the maxillary teeth on the contralateral side (see Chap. 72). By deepening the buccal sulcus, an upward extension of the denture improves the contour of the middle third of the face.

The forces applied to a prosthodontic appliance have an adverse effect on the remaining teeth that serve as anchoring points. Design of the appliance is critical. Obtaining support and retention of the prosthesis may be difficult. The problem of retention is compounded in the patient with an edentulous maxilla. Nevertheless, a skilled maxillofacial prosthodontist can overcome many of these problems and provide a valuable service to the facially crippled patient.

Bone grafts are employed in the reconstruction of the maxilla, either as onlay grafts to restore contour or as framework grafts to replace the missing maxillary skeleton.

In 1938 Figi used iliac bone to reconstruct the maxilla after removal of a malignant tumor of the maxillary sinus. Campbell (1948), borrowing from the principles of Figi, reported the successful restoration of half the midfacial skeleton after a resection of the maxilla and the malar bone. In a first stage, the void left by the resection was filled by a flap consisting of the anterior third of the temporalis muscle (Gillies, 1920). Lining was obtained from the remaining half of the palate. Iliac bone grafts were used, according to the technique described by Figi (1938), in a second stage to reconstruct the skeletal defect and restore contour. The buccal sulcus was restored in a third stage by the skin graft inlay technique (see Figs. 29–275 and 29–276).

When the floor of the orbit has been removed along with the remainder of the maxilla, the perioribita and the orbital fascia, including the suspensory ligament of Lockwood, are undisturbed. A progressive sagging of the orbital contents results in the ocular globe being situated at a lower level than the unaffected eye. Since the extraocular musculature is not appreciably disturbed, diplopia does not usually follow. These patients, however, complain of transient diplopia when fatigued.

Destructive injuries, such as a gunshot wound, or disruption of the floor of the orbit followed by sequestration of bone fragments after wound sepsis can cause extensive loss of the orbital floor. As a result, direct injury of the periorbita and the inferior oblique and inferior rectus muscles can occur. Scar tissue contraction compounds the problem: it may cause downward displacement and rotation of the ocular globe, and interfere with the ocular rotary movements. The bone defect can include a major segment of the orbital floor in its maxillary and zygomatic portions and also a large portion of the body of the zygoma.

In 1950 Converse and Smith (1950b) reported the reconstruction of the upper portion of the maxilla, the zygoma, and the orbital floor with bone grafts. The palatal defect was closed with an obturator, and an upward extension of the appliance restored the contour of the lower portion of the cheek (Fig. 29–279).

Reconstruction of the hard palate is contraindicated after resection of the maxilla for malignant disease, since the palatal defect permits direct observation of the affected area. Reconstruction of the hard palate and alveolar process is indicated, however, after resection of benign or nonmetastasizing tumors.

RECONSTRUCTION OF HARD PALATE AND ALVEOLAR PROCESS

The reconstruction is achieved in two stages (Obwegeser, 1973). In a first stage, a two-layer soft tissue closure is obtained by local flaps; in a second stage, bone grafts restore the bony continuity of the palate and reconstruct the alveolar process.

The nasal lining is obtained by making a circumferential incision around the rim of the defect and freeing the mucoperiosteum from the nasal septum and from the lateral wall of the defect (Fig. 29–280*A*). The turnover flaps are approximated with inverting sutures that are left long (Fig. 29–280*B*). Bone grafts are used to reconstruct the hard palate and the alveolar process (Fig. 29–280*C*). Direct interosseous wiring stabilizes the alveolar bone graft to the remaining alveolar process anteriorly and to the pterygoid process posteriorly. The sutures that had been left long during the closure of the nasal cavity are passed through the bone grafts used to restore the hard palate and the alveolar ridge (Fig. 29–280*C*). The oral lining and coverage of the grafts are provided by a large rotation flap from the remaining hard palate mucoperiosteum and the labiobuccal mucosa (Fig. 29–280*D*). The long sutures are passed through the flaps and tied to eliminate dead space. Three weeks after the bone grafting, a temporary denture is placed over the reconstructed structures. A skin graft inlay is performed three months later to reform a sulcus that aids in the retention of the maxillary denture (Fig. 29–281).

Costal grafts have also been used to correct bone defects produced by resection of half of the maxilla and the infraorbital region (Obwegeser, 1973). The palatal defect is closed, and the alveolar process is reconstructed as shown in Figures 29–282 and 29–283. The Weber-Ferguson incision is reopened to obtain exposure. The exposure facilitates reconstruction of the alveolar process with a section of undivided rib, which is maintained by wire fixation to the alveolar process on the

Text continued on page 1463

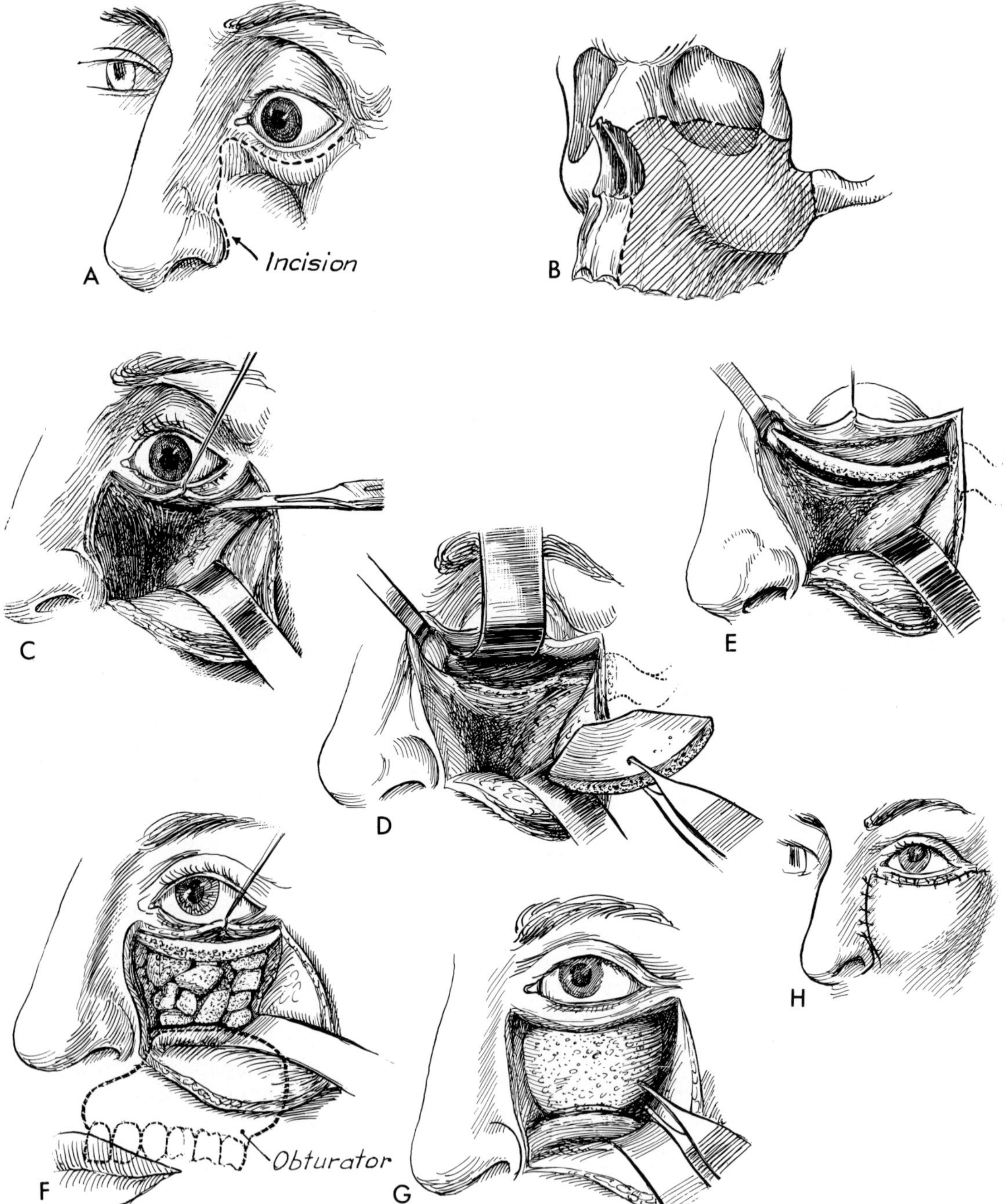

Figure 29–279. Technique of reconstruction of the upper portion of the maxilla, the floor of the orbit, and the zygoma by bone grafts. *A,* Line of incision outlining the cheek flap. *B,* The shaded area shows the extent of bone resected. *C,* The cheek flap has been elevated. The orbital contents are freed from the binding scar tissue. *D,* The orbital contents are raised. After subperiosteal exposure of the frontal process, the maxilla, and the zygomatic arch, a bone graft is prepared for insertion. *E,* Bone graft in position, restoring the floor of the orbit. *F,* The depressed area is filled with cancellous bone chips. *G,* An overlay contour restoring bone graft is placed over the bone chips. *H,* Suture of the edges of the skin flap to the edges of the defect has been completed. In the older patient and in the patient reconstructed following resection for a malignant tumor, closure of the palate is usually contraindicated, since the palatal defect allows clinical observation of the affected area. (From Converse, J. M., and Smith, B.: Case of reconstruction of the maxilla following resection for carcinoma of the antrum. Plast. Reconstr. Surg., *5*:426, 1950. Copyright 1950, The Williams & Wilkins Company, Baltimore.)

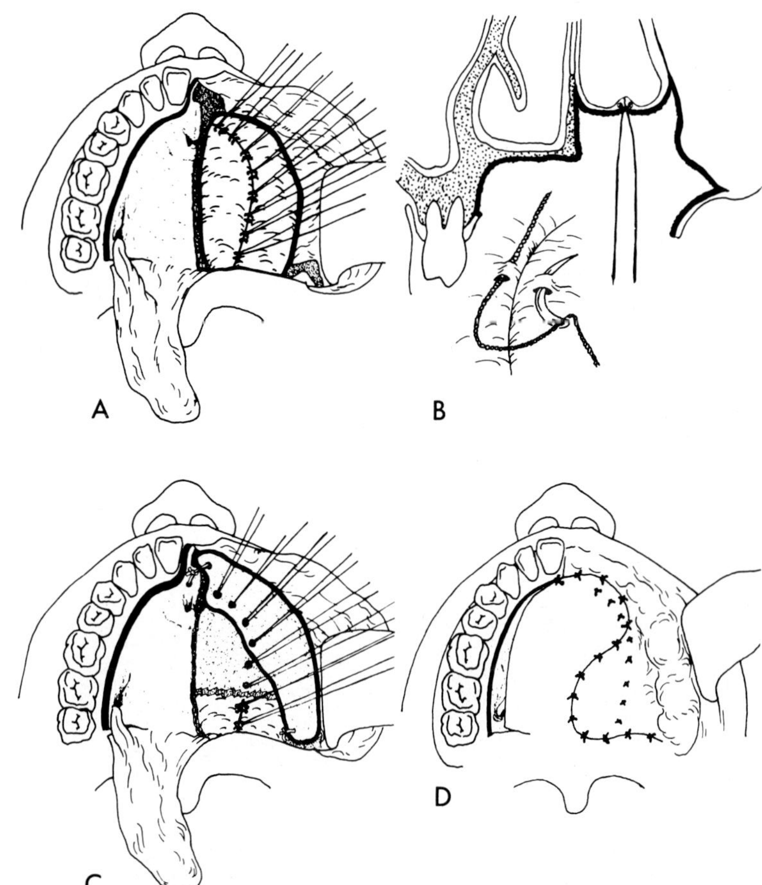

Figure 29–280. Technique of reconstruction of the hemimaxilla and alveolar process. *A,* Closure of the nasal cavity is obtained by turned-in flaps of mucoperiosteum from the lateral rim of the defect and the nasal septum. *B,* Frontal section showing the closure of the nasal layer. Mattress sutures are used to invert the mucosal edges into the nasal cavity. The ends of the sutures are left long. *C,* The hard palate and the alveolar process are restored by bone grafts, which are fixed by interosseous wiring to the remaining hard palate, the anterior portion of the alveolar process, and the pterygoid processes. The long ends of the sutures are passed through the bone grafts and the oral mucosal covering. *D,* Rotation flaps from the remaining hard palate and the buccal mucosa provide the oral lining. The sutures are tied to eliminate dead space. (From Obwegeser, H. L.: Late reconstruction of large maxillary defects after tumor resection. J. Maxillofac. Surg., *1*:19, 1973. Georg Thieme Verlag. Stuttgart, Germany.)

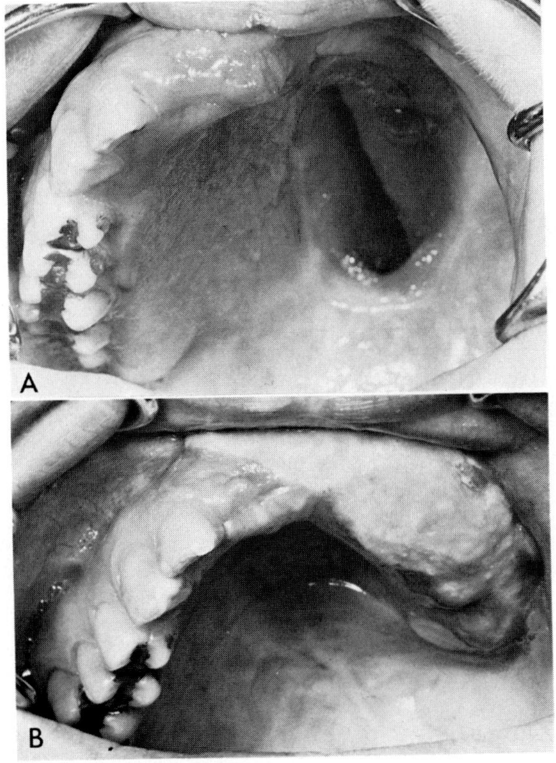

Figure 29–281. Reconstruction of a hemimaxillary defect and the alveolar process using the technique shown in Figure 29–280. *A,* A defect of the maxilla and alveolar process 30 years after resection of a malignant tumor. *B,* Postoperative appearance showing restoration of the maxilla and the alveolar ridge. In a first stage the soft tissue defect was closed and the bony support was restored. In a second operation the buccal sulcus was reestablished by the skin graft inlay technique. (From Obwegeser, H. L.: Late reconstruction of large maxillary defects after tumor resection. J. Maxillofac. Surg., *1*:19, 1973. Georg Thieme Verlag, Stuttgart, Germany.)

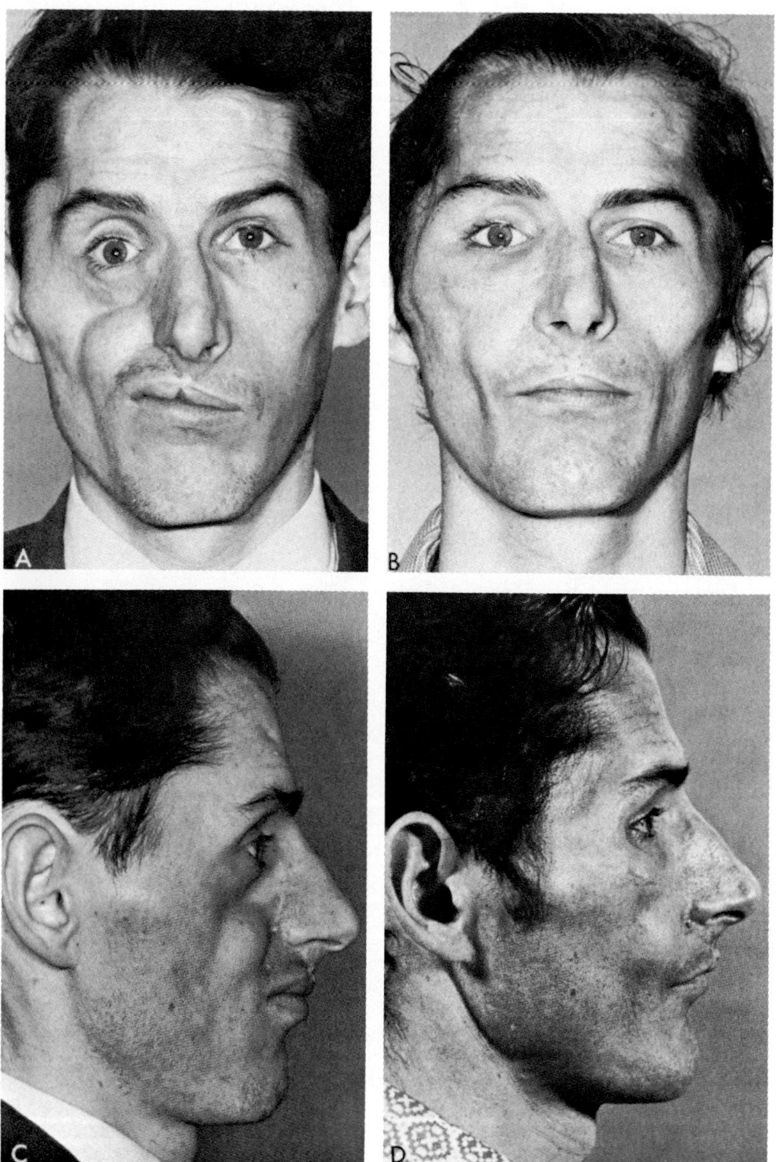

Figure 29–282. *A,* Facial deformity caused by a defect of the major portion of the maxilla resulting from the resection of a tumor in childhood. *B,* Appearance after reconstruction of the hard palate by a skin flap, followed by reconstruction of the alveolar process, floor of the orbit, and infraorbital area by iliac bone grafts; and posterior recession of the prognathic mandible by a bilateral sagittal split of the mandibular rami. *C,* Preoperative profile appearance. *D,* Postoperative profile appearance. (From Obwegeser, H. L.: Late reconstruction of large maxillary defects after tumor resection. J. Maxillofac. Surg., *1*:19, 1973. Georg Thieme Verlag, Stuttgart, Germany.)

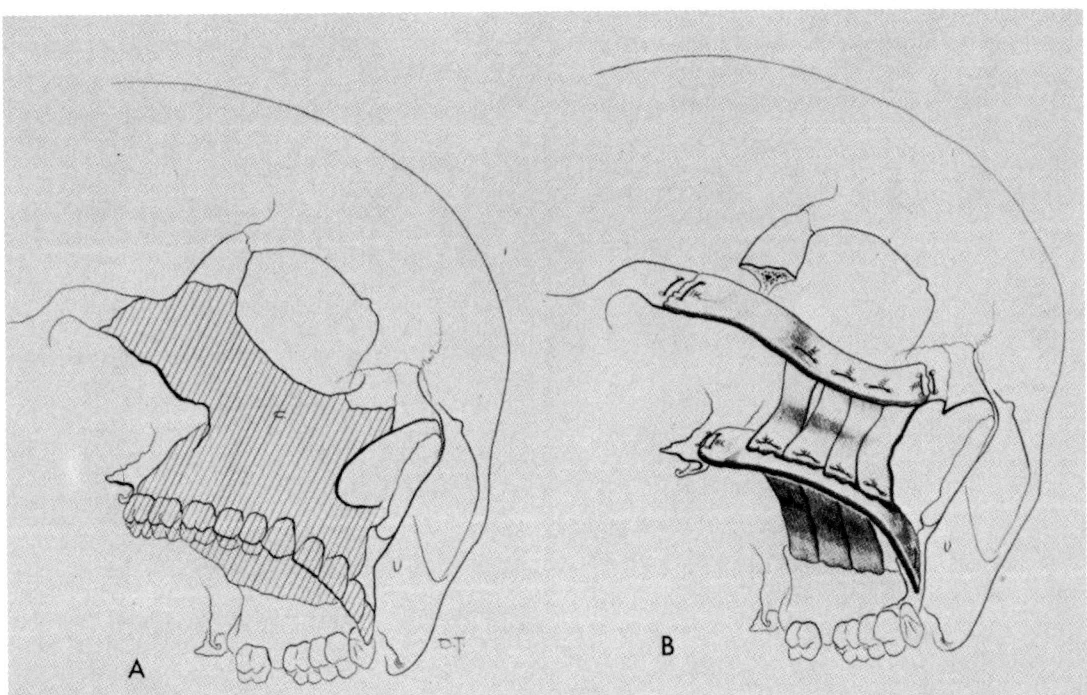

Figure 29–283. Reconstruction of the maxilla, orbital floor, zygoma, hard palate, and alveolar process. *A,* The shaded area represents the extent of the defect. *B,* Placement of costal bone grafts. Undivided rib grafts are used to reconstruct the zygoma, inferior orbital rim, and alveolar process. The hard palate and the lateral wall of the maxilla are restored with split rib grafts. (From Obwegeser, H. L.: Late reconstruction of large maxillary defects after tumor resection. J. Maxillofac. Surg., *1*:19, 1973. Georg Thieme Verlag, Stuttgart, Germany.)

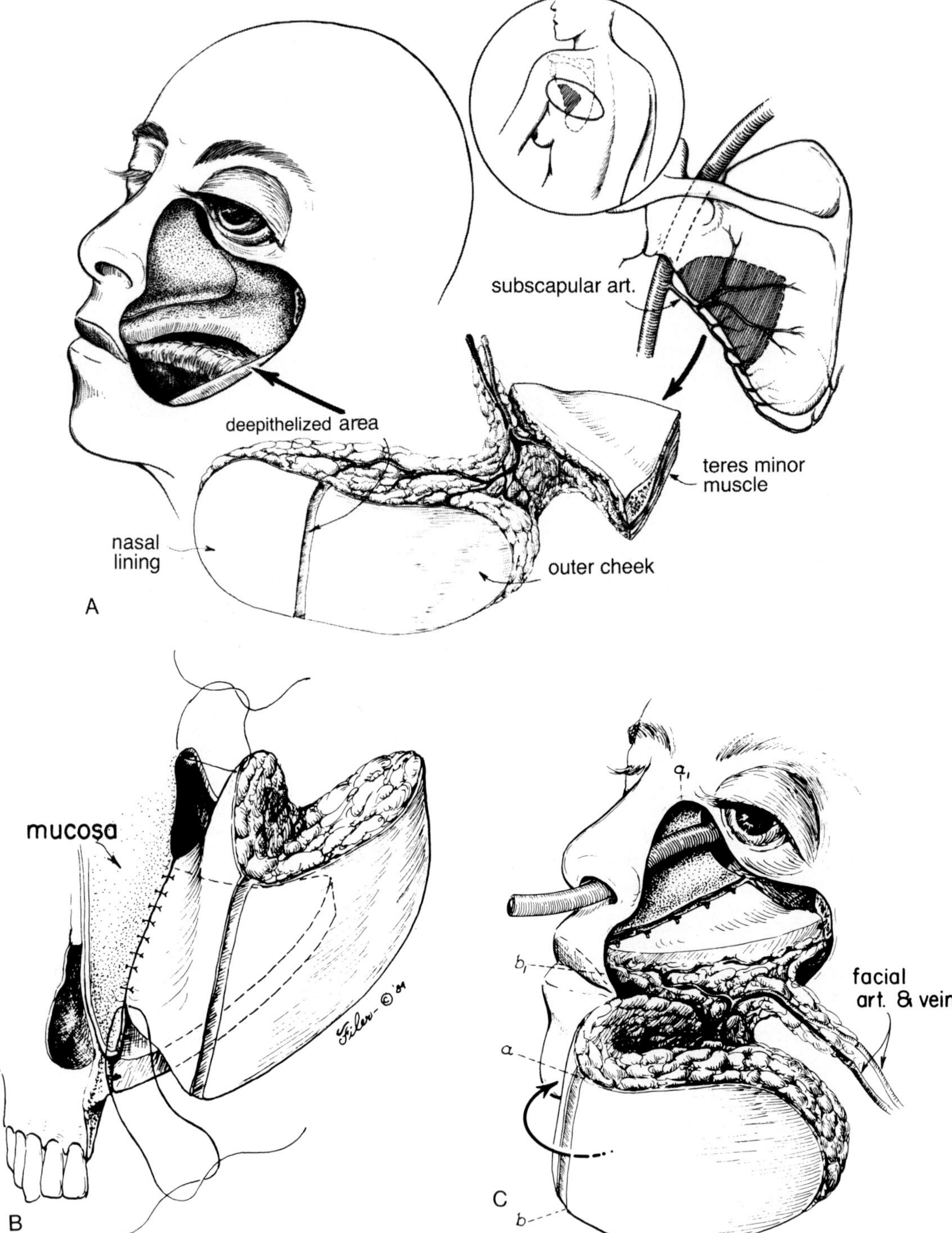

Figure 29–284. *A,* Total maxillectomy defect including the palate, nasal and oral lining, and exterior cheek several years after resection of a squamous cell carcinoma. *B,* Reconstruction of the nasal lining, outer cheek, and bony palate accomplished in one stage by using a scapular osteocutaneous free flap. *C,* Nasal lining and outer cheek contour accomplished by folding the cutaneous portion of the scapular flap. The bony palate is reconstructed utilizing the blade of the scapula wired to the vomer. Oral lining was provided by skin grafting the muscle layer to the underside of the scapula. Anastomosis of the circumflex scapular vessels to the facial artery and vein was carried out to revascularize the flap.

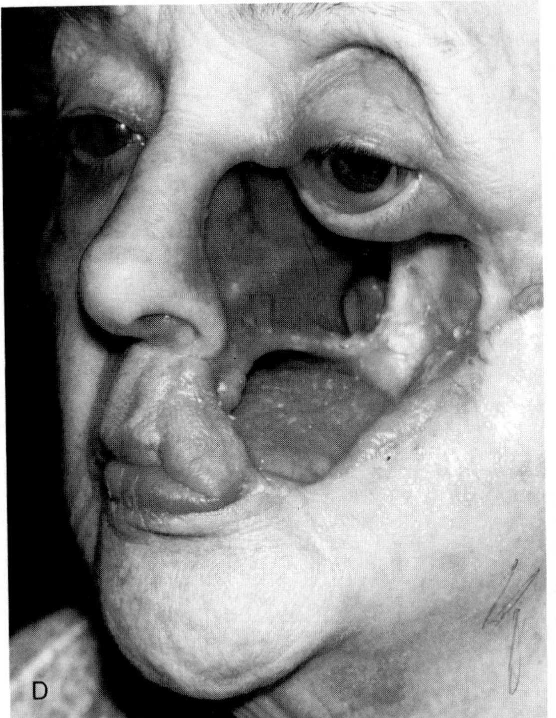

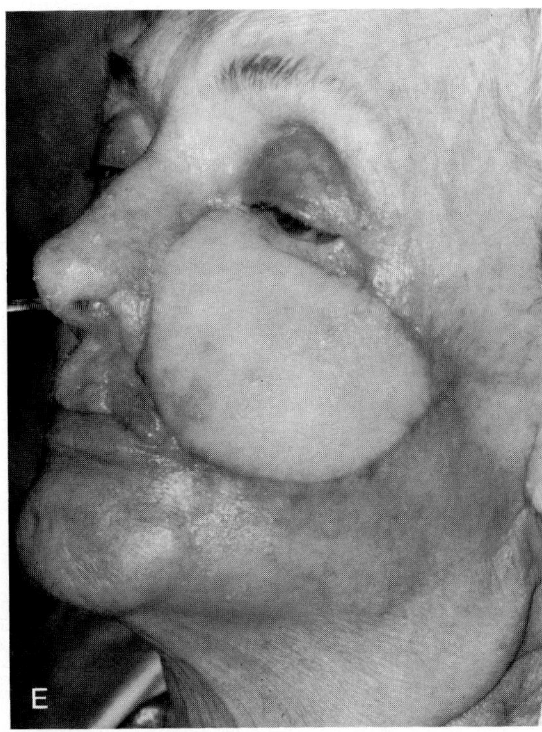

Figure 29–284 *Continued D,* Preoperative appearance. *E,* Result at one month. (Courtesy of Dr. William Swartz.)

contralateral side and the remainder of the pterygoid processes on the same side.

In 1986 Swartz and associates reported their experience with maxillary reconstruction in five patients, using the scapular osteocutaneous microvascular flap. They were able to reconstruct the bone defects in the orbital floor, maxilla, zygoma, and palate as well as providing soft tissue contour restoration (Fig. 29–284). The ability to satisfy complex bony and soft tissue requirements in a single surgical stage with a vascularized flap has revolutionized maxillary reconstruction. It is apparent from this report that the microvascular osteocutaneous flap has assumed a prime role in complex maxillary reconstructions.

REFERENCES

Aaronson, S. A.: A cephalometric investigation of the surgical correction of mandibular prognathism. Angle Orthod., *37*:251, 1967.

Abbott, L. C.: The operative lengthening of the tibia and fibula. J. Bone Joint Surg., *9*:128, 1927.

Adams, W. M.: Bilateral hypertrophy of the masseter muscle. An operation for the correction. Br. J. Plast. Surg., *2*:78, 1949.

Adelaar, R. S., Soucacos, P. N., and Urbaniak, J. R.: Autologous cortical bone grafts with microsurgical anastomosis of periosteal vessels. Surg. Forum, *25*:487, 1974.

Albee, F. H.: Orthopedic and Reconstructive Surgery. Philadelphia, W. B. Saunders Company, 1919.

Albert, T. W., Smith, J. D., Everts, E. C., and Cook, T. A.: Dacron mesh tray and cancellous bone in reconstruction of mandibular defects. Arch. Otolaryngol. Head Neck Surg., *112*:53, 1986.

Aller, T. G.: Operative treatment of prognathism. Dent. Cosmos, *59*:394, 1917.

Anderson, R.: An ambulatory method of treating fractures of the shaft of the femur. Surg. Gynecol. Obstet., *62*:865, 1936.

Angle, E. H.: Double resection of the lower maxilla. Dent. Cosmos, *40*:635, 1898.

Angle, E. H.: Classification of malocclusion. Dent. Cosmos, *41*:240, 1899.

Antia, N. H.: The scope of plastic surgery in leprosy: a ten-year progress report. Clin. Plast. Surg., *1*:69, 1974.

Ariyan, S.: The viability of rib grafts transplanted with the periosteal blood supply. Plast. Reconstr. Surg., *65*:140, 1980.

Ariyan, S., and Finseth, F. J.: The anterior chest approach for obtaining free osteocutaneous rib grafts. Plast. Reconstr. Surg., *62*:676, 1978.

Åstrand, P., Eckerdal, O., and Sund, G: Intraosseous wiring in ramus osteotomy. J. Oral Surg., *41*:789, 1983.

Attie, J. N., Catania, A., and Ripstein, C. B.: Stainless steel mesh prosthesis for immediate replacement of hemimandible. Surgery, *33*:712, 1953.

Aubry, M., and Pillet, P.: Sur les implants d'acrylique dans la résection du maxillaire inférieur. Ann. Otol. (Paris), *67*:553, 1950.

Aufricht, G.: Combined nasal plastic and chin plastic; correction of microgenia by osteocartilaginous transplant from large hump nose. Am. J. Surg., *25*:292, 1934.

Axhausen, G.: Zur Behandlung veralteter disloziert geheilter Oberkieferbrüche. Dtsch. Zahn. Mund. Kieferheilkd., *1*:334, 1934.

Babcock, W. W.: Surgical treatment of certain deformities of the jaw associated with malocclusion of the teeth. J.A.M.A., *53*:178, 1909.

Babcock, W. W.: The field of osteoplastic operations for the correction of deformities of the jaws. Items of interest, *32*:439, 1910.

Babcock, W. W.: Advancement of the receding chin. Ann. Surg., *105*:115, 1937.

Baek, S. M., Lawson, W., and Biller, H. F.: An analysis of 133 pectoralis major myocutaneous flaps. Plast. Reconstr. Surg., *69*:460, 1982.

Banks, P.: Pulp changes after anterior mandibular subapical osteotomy in a primate model. J. Maxillofac. Surg., *5*:39, 1977.

Bardenheuer, P.: Ueber Unterkiefer- und Oberkiefer-Resection. Arch. Klin. Chir., *44*:604, 1892.

Barton, P. R.: Segmental surgery. Br. J. Oral Surg., *10*:265, 1973.

Bayne, H. R.: Pseudoretrognathia: evaluation and treatment. Dent. Dig., *762*:112, 1966.

Behrman, S. J.: Complications of sagittal osteotomy of the mandibular ramus. J. Oral Surg., *30*:554, 1972.

Bell, H. B.: Biologic basis for maxillary osteotomies. Am. J. Phys. Anthropol., *38*:279, 1973.

Bell, M. S., and Baron, P. T.: The rib–pectoralis major osteomyocutaneous flap. Ann. Plast. Surg., *6*:347, 1981.

Bell, W. H.: Revascularization and bone healing after anterior maxillary osteotomy: a study using adult Rhesus monkeys. J. Oral Surg., *27*:249, 1969.

Bell, W. H.: Correction of skeletal type of anterior open bite. J. Oral Surg., *29*:706, 1971.

Bell, W. H.: Le Fort I osteotomy for correction of maxillary deformities. J. Oral Surg., *33*:412, 1975.

Bell, W. H., and Creekmore, T. D.: Surgical-orthodontic correction of mandibular prognathism. Am. J. Orthod., *63*:256, 1973.

Bell, W. H., Creekmore, T. D., and Alexander, R. G.: Surgical correction of the long face syndrome. Am. J. Orthod., *71*:40, 1977.

Bell, W. H., and Dann J. J., III: Correction of dentofacial deformities by surgery in the anterior part of the jaws. Am. J. Orthod., *64*:162, 1973.

Bell, W. H., and Levy, B. M.: Revascularization and bone healing after anterior mandibular osteotomy. J. Oral Surg., *28*:196, 1970.

Bell, W. H., and Levy, B. M.: Revascularization and bone healing after posterior maxillary osteotomy. J. Oral Surg., *29*:313, 1971.

Berggren, A., Weiland, A. J., Östrup, L. T., and Dorfman, H.: Microvascular free bone transfer with revascularization of the medullary and periosteal circulation or the periosteal circulation alone. A comparative experimental study. J. Bone Joint Surg., *64A*:73, 1982.

Berndt: Prosthesis after jaw resection. Arch. Klin. Chir., *52*:210, 1898.

Binder, K. H. von: Dysostosis maxillo-nasalis, ein arhinencephaler Missbildungskomplex. Dtsch. Zahnaerztl. Z., *17*:438, 1962.

Björk, A.: The Face in Profile: An Anthropological X-ray Investigation of Swedish Children and Conscripts. Lund. Berlingska Boktryckerret, 1947.

Björk, A.: Facial growth in man, studied with the aid of metallic implants. Acta Odontol. Scand., *13*:9, 1955.

Björk, A.: The relationship of the jaws to the cranium. *In* Lundström, A. (Ed.): Introduction to Orthodontics. New York, McGraw-Hill Book Company, 1960.

Björk, A.: Variations in the growth pattern of the human mandible: a longitudinal radiographic study by the implant method. J. Dent. Res., *42*:400, 1963.

Björk, N., Eliasson, S., and Sörensen, S.: Relative rotation of fragments during the time of intermaxillary fixation after transverse osteotomy bilaterally in the ascending ramus of the mandible. Sven. Tandlak. Tidskr., *63*:111, 1970.

Blair, V. P.: Operations on the jaw-bone and face; a study of the etiology and pathological anatomy of developmental malrelations of the maxilla and mandible to each other and to the facial outline, and of their operative treatment when beyond the scope of the orthodontist. Surg. Gynecol. Obstet., *4*:67, 1907.

Blair, V. P.: Instances of operative correction of malrelation of the jaws. Int. J. Orthod., *1*:395, 1915.

Blair, V. P.: Surgery and Diseases of the Mouth and Jaws. St. Louis, MO. C. V. Mosby Company, 1918.

Block, M. S., and Kent, J. N.: Long-term radiographic evaluation of hydroxyapatite-augmented mandibular alveolar ridges. J. Oral Maxillofac. Surg., *42*:793, 1984.

Boldt, H.: Ein Beitrag zur Kenntnis der einfachen Masseter Hypertrophy. Thesis No. 31, Berlin, 1930.

Booth, D. F.: Control of the proximal segment by lower border wiring in the sagittal split osteotomy. J. Maxillofac. Surg., *9*:125, 1981.

Bosworth, F. H.: A Treatise on Diseases of the Nose and Throat. Vol. 1. New York, William Wood & Company, 1889.

Boyne, P. J.: Restoration of osseous defects in maxillofacial casualties. J. Am. Dent. Assoc., *78*:767, 1969.

Boyne, P. J.: Implants and transplants. Review of recent research in the area of oral surgery. J. Am. Dent. Assoc., *87*:1074, 1973.

Boyne, P. J., and Zarem, H.: Osseous reconstruction of the resected mandible. Am. J. Surg., *132*:49, 1976.

Broadbent, B. H., Broadbent, B. H., and Golden, W.: Bolton Standards of Developmental Growth. St. Louis, C. V. Mosby Company, 1975.

Bromberg, B. E., Walden, R. H., and Rubin, L. R.: Mandibular bone grafts, a technique in fixation. Plast. Reconstr. Surg., *32*:589, 1963.

Brown, J. B., Fryer, M. P., and Ohlwiler, D. A.: Study and use of synthetic materials, such as silicones and Teflon, as subcutaneous prostheses. Plast. Reconstr. Surg., *26*:264, 1960.

Brusati, R., and Bottoli, V.: L'osteotomia mascellare segmentaria anteriore: ricerche sperimentali sulla vascolarizzazione del settore osseo osteotomizzato. Riv. Ital. Stomatol., *25*:446, 1970.

Buncke, H. J., Furnas, D. W., Gordon, L., and Achauer, B. M.: Free osteocutaneous flap from rib to the tibia. Plast. Reconstr. Surg., *59*:799, 1977.

Burstone, C. J.: The integumental profile. Am. J. Orthod., *44*:1, 1958.

Burstone, C. J.: Lip posture and its significance in treatment planning. Am. J. Orthod., *53*:262, 1967.

Bush, L. F.: Use of homogenous grafts. Preliminary report on bone bank. J. Bone Joint Surg., *29*:620, 1947.

Butcher, E. O., and Taylor, A. C.: The effects of denervation and ischemia upon the teeth of a monkey. J. Dent. Res., *30*:265, 1951.

Caldwell, J. B.: Developmental deformities of the jaws.

In Kruger, G. O. (Ed.): Textbook of Oral Surgery. 2nd ed. St. Louis, MO., C. V. Mosby Company, 1964, p. 461.

Caldwell, J. B., and Amaral, W. J.: Mandibular micrognathia corrected by vertical osteotomy of the rami and iliac bone graft. J. Oral Surg., *18*:3, 1960.

Caldwell, J. B., Hayward, J. R., and Lister, R. L.: Correction of mandibular retrognathia by vertical "L" osteotomy: a new technic. J. Oral Surg., *26*:259, 1968.

Caldwell, J. B., and Letterman, G. S.: Vertical osteotomy in the mandibular rami for correction of prognathism. J. Oral Surg., *12*:185, 1954.

Campbell, H. H.: Reconstruction of left maxilla. Plast. Reconstr. Surg., *3*:66, 1948.

Carlotti, A. E., Jr., and Schendel, S. A.: An analysis of factors influencing stability of surgical advancement of the maxilla by the Le Fort I Osteotomy. J. Oral Maxillofac. Surg., *45*:924, 1987.

Case, C. S.: A Practical Treatise on the Techniques and Principles of Dental Orthopedia. Chicago, C. S. Case Company, 1921.

Casson, P. R., Bonanno, P. C., and Converse, J. M.: The midface degloving procedure. Plast. Reconstr. Surg., *53*:102, 1974.

Castigliano, S.: Massive metallic implant in situ five years after resection of mandible. Am. J. Surg., *88*:490, 1941.

Cernéa, P.: Déviations mandibulaires par hypertrophie condylienne unilatérale et leur traitement chirurgical. *In* Deuxième Congrès International d'Odontostomatologie. Paris. Julien Prélat. 1954.

Cernéa, P., Grignon, J. L., Crépy, C., and Benoist, M.: Les ostéotomies totales des maxillaires superieurs. Rev. Stomatol., *56*:700, 1955.

Champy, M., Lodde, J. P., Wilk, A., and Grasset, D. Plattenosteosynthesen bei Mittelgesichts-Frakturen end-osteotomien. Dtsch. Z. Mund-Kiefer-Gesichts-Chir., *2*:26, 1978.

Cheever, D. W.: Displacement of the upper jaw. Med. Surg. Rep. Bost. City Hosp., 1870, p. 154.

Chubb, G.: Bone grafting of the fractured mandible, with an account of 60 cases. Lancet, *2*:9, 1920.

Coccaro, P. J.: Restitution of mandibular form after condylar injury in infancy (a 7-year study of a child). Am. J. Orthod., *55*:32, 1969.

Coffey, R. J.: Unilateral hypertrophy of the masseter muscle. Surgery, *11*:815, 1942.

Cohen, J., and Harris, W. H.: The three-dimensional anatomy of haversian systems. J. Bone Joint Surg., *40A*:419, 1958.

Cohn-Stock, H.: Die chirurgische Immediatreguherung der Kiefer, speziell die chirurgische Behandlung der Prognathie. Vjschr. Zahnheild., *37*:320, 1921.

Colantino, R. A., and Dudley, T.: Correction of maxillary prognathism by complete alveolar osteotomy. J. Oral Surg., *28*:543, 1970.

Colen, S. R., Shaw, W. W., and McCarthy, J. G.: Review of the morbidity of 300 free flap donor sites. Plast. Reconstr. Surg., *76*:948, 1986.

Compton, J. E., Jacobs, J. D., and Dunsworth, A. R.: Healing of the bone incision following Le Fort I osteotomy. J. Oral Maxillofac. Surg., *42*:665, 1984.

Conley, J. J.: Use of composite flaps containing bone for major repairs in the head and neck. Plast. Reconstr. Surg., *49*:522, 1972a.

Conley, J. J.: Regional bone-muscle-skin pedicle flaps in surgery of the head and neck. Trans. Am. Acad. Ophthalmol. Otolaryngol., *76*:946, 1972b.

Converse, J. M.: Early and late treatment of gunshot wounds of the jaw in French battle casualties in North Africa and Italy. J. Oral Surg., *3*:112, 1945.

Converse, J. M.: Restoration of facial contour by bone grafts introduced through the oral cavity. Plast. Reconstr. Surg., *6*:295, 1950.

Converse, J. M.: Masseter muscle hypertrophy. Unpublished case, 1951.

Converse, J. M.: Technique of bone grafting for contour restoration of the face. Plast. Reconstr. Surg., *14*:332, 1954.

Converse, J. M.: Transplantation of the inferior mandibular segment after horizontal osteotomy. *In* Kazanjian, V. H., and Converse, J. M.: The Surgical Treatment of Facial Injuries. Baltimore. Williams & Wilkins Company, 1959, p. 867.

Converse, J. M.: Micrognathia. Br. J. Plast. Surg., *16*:197, 1963.

Converse, J. M.: Surgical elongation of the traumatically foreshortened nose: the perinasal osteotomy. Plast. Reconstr. Surg., *47*:539, 1971.

Converse, J. M.: The degloving procedure. *In* Kazanjian, V. H., and Converse, J. M.: Surgical Treatment of Facial Injuries, 3rd ed. Baltimore, Williams & Wilkins Company, 1974a, p. 1022.

Converse, J. M.: Elongation by sagittal splitting of the body of the mandible. *In* Kazanjian, V. H., and Converse, J. M.: Surgical Treatment of Facial Injuries. 3rd ed. Baltimore. Williams & Wilkins Company, 1974b, p. 1061.

Converse, J. M., and Campbell, R. M.: Experiences with a bone bank in plastic surgery. Plast. Reconstr. Surg., *5*:258, 1950.

Converse, J. M., and Campbell, R. M.: Bone grafts in surgery of the face. Surg. Clin. North Am., *34*:375, 1954.

Converse, J. M., Horowitz, S. L., Guy, C. L., and Wood-Smith, D.: Surgical and orthodontic procedures in bilateral cleft lip and cleft palate. Cleft Palate J., *1*:153, 1964a.

Converse, J. M., Horowitz, S. L., and Wood-Smith, D.: Deformities of the jaws. *In* Converse, J. M. (Ed.): Reconstructive Plastic Surgery. Philadelphia, W. B. Saunders Company, 1964b, p. 869.

Converse, J. M., Horowitz, S. L., Valauri, A. J., and Montandon, D.: The treatment of nasomaxillary hypoplasia. A new pyramidal naso-orbito-maxillary osteotomy. Plast. Reconstr. Surg., *45*:527, 1970.

Converse, J. M., Horowitz, S. L., Coccaro, P. I., and Wood-Smith, D.: The corrective treatment of the skeletal asymmetry in hemifacial microsomia. Plast. Reconstr. Surg., *52*:221, 1973.

Converse, J. M., and Horowitz, S. L.: The surgical-orthodontic approach to the treatment of dentofacial deformities. Am. J. Orthod., *55*:217, 1969.

Converse, J. M., and Horowitz, S. L.: Simianism: surgical-orthodontic correction of bimaxillary protrusion. J. Maxillofac. Surg., *1*:7, 1973.

Converse, J. M., and McCarthy, J. G.: Infections in plastic surgery. Surg. Clin. North Am., *52*:1459, 1972.

Converse, J. M., and Shapiro, H. H.: Treatment of developmental malformations of the jaws. Plast. Reconstr. Surg., *10*:473, 1952.

Converse, J. M., and Shapiro, H. H.: Bone grafting malformations of the jaws; cephalographic diagnosis in the surgical treatment of malformations of the face. Am. J. Surg., *8*:858, 1954.

Converse, J. M., and Smith, B.: Reconstruction of the floor of the orbit by bone grafts. Arch. Ophthalmol., *44*:1, 1950a.

Converse, J. M., and Smith, B.: Case of reconstruction of the maxilla following resection for carcinoma of the antrum. Plast. Reconstr. Surg., *5*:426, 1950b.
Converse, J. M., and Waknitz, F. W.: External skeletal fixation in fractures of the mandibular angle. J. Bone Joint Surg., *24*:154, 1942.
Converse, J. M., and Wood-Smith, D.: Horizontal osteotomy of the mandible. Plast. Reconstr. Surg., *34*:464, 1964.
Cotton, W. A., Takano, W. S., and Wong, W. M. W.: The Downs analysis applied to other ethnic groups. Angle Orthodont., *21*:213, 1951.
Crockford, D. A., and Converse, J. M.: The ilium as a source of bone grafts in children. Plast. Reconstr. Surg., *50*:270, 1972.
Cryer, M. H.: Studies of anterior and posterior occlusion. Dent. Cosmos, *55*:683, 1913.
Cummings, C. W., and Leipzig, B.: Replacement of tumor-involved mandible by cryosurgically devitalized autograft. Human experience. Arch. Otolaryngol., *106*:252, 1980.
Cunat, J. J., and Gargiulo, E. A.: Changes in mandibular morphology after surgical correction of prognathism: report of case. J. Oral Surg., *31*:694, 1973.
Cuono, C. B., and Ariyan, S.: Immediate reconstruction of a composite mandibular defect with a regional osteomusculocutaneous flap. Plast. Reconstr. Surg., *65*:477, 1980.
Cupar, I.: Die chirurgische Behandlung der Formund Stellungs-Veränderung des Oberkiefers. Österr, Z. Stomatol., *51*:565, 1954.
Cutting, C., Grayson, B., Bookstein, F., Fellingham, L., and McCarthy, J. G.: Computer-aided planning and evaluation of facial and orthognathic surgery. Clin. Plast. Surg., *13*:449, 1986.
Cutting, C. B., McCarthy, J. G., and Karron, D. B.: Three-dimensional input of body surface data using a laser light scanner. Ann. Plast. Surg., *21*:38, 1988.
Dal Pont, G.: L'osteotomie retromolare per la correzione della progenia. Minerva Chir., *14*:1138, 1959.
Dal Pont, G.: Retromolar osteotomy for correction of prognathism. J. Oral Surg., *19*:42, 1961.
Dann, J. J., Fonseca, R. J., and Bell, W. H.: Soft-tissue changes associated with total maxillary advancement: a preliminary study. J. Oral Surg., *34*:19, 1976.
Dattilo, D. J., Braun, T. W., and Sotereanos, G. C.: The inverted L osteotomy for treatment of skeletal openbite deformities. J. Oral Maxillofac. Surg., *43*:440, 1985.
Dautrey, J.: Personal communication, 1974.
Dautrey, J.: Personal communication, 1975.
Dautrey, J.: Personal communication, 1986.
Dautrey, J., and Pepersack, W.: Le traitement chirurgical de la proalvéolie supérieure. Acta Stomatol. Belg., *68*:335, 1971.
Delagénière, H.: Les greffes ostéoperiostiques prises au tibia. Bull. Mém. Soc. Chir. Paris, *42*:1048, 1916.
Demergasso, F., and Piazza, M. V.: Trapezius myocutaneous flap in reconstructive surgery for head and neck cancer. An original technique. Am. J. Surg., *138*:533, 1979.
Dingman, R. O.: Surgical correction of mandibular prognathism; an improved method. Am. J. Orthod. Oral Surg., *30*:683, 1944.
Dingman, R. O., and Grabb, W. C.: Surgical anatomy of mandibular ramus of the facial nerve based on the dissection of 100 facial halves. Plast. Reconstr. Surg., *29*:266, 1962.
Dingman, R. O., and Grabb, W. C.: Reconstruction of both mandibular condyles with metatarsal bone grafts. Plast. Reconstr. Surg., *34*:441, 1964.
Dingman, R. O., and Harding, R. L.: Treatment of malunion fractures of facial bones. Plast. Reconstr. Surg., *7*:505, 1951.
Doi, K., Tominaga, S., and Shibata, T.: Bone grafts with microvascular anastomosis of vascular pedicles. An experimental study in dogs. J. Bone Joint Surg., *59A*:809, 1977.
Downs, W. B.: Variations in facial relationships; their significance in treatment and prognosis. Am. J. Orthod., *34*:812, 1948.
Drommer, R., and Luhr, H. G.: The stabilization of osteotomized maxillary segments with Luhr miniplates in secondary cleft surgery. J. Maxillofac. Surg., *9*:166, 1981.
DuBouchet, C. W.: New method of bone grafting for pseudoarthrosis of the mandible. Bull. Mém. Soc. Chir. Paris, *43*:1328, 1917.
Dufourmentel, L.: Essai de reconstitution totale du massif maxillaire inférieur, Restaur. Maxillofac., *3*:141, 1919.
Dufourmentel, L.: Le traitement chirurgical du prognathisme. Presse Méd., *29*:235, 1921.
Dufresne, C., Cutting, C., Valauri, F., Klein, M., Colen, S., and McCarthy, J. G.: Reconstruction of mandibular and floor of mouth defects using the trapezius osteomyocutaneous flap. Plast. Reconstr. Surg., *79*:687, 1987.
Duncan, M. J., Manktelow, R. T., Zuker, R. M., and Rosen, J. B.: Mandibular reconstruction in the radiated patient: the role of osteocutaneous free tissue transfers. Plast. Reconstr. Surg., *76*:829, 1985.
Dupont, C., Ciaburro, H., and Prévost, Y.: Simplifying the Le Fort I type of maxillary osteotomy. Plast. Reconstr. Surg., *54*:142, 1974.
Edgerton, M. T., Ward, A. E., and Sikes, T. E.: Fixation and plastic repair after partial mandibular resection. Plast. Reconstr. Surg., *5*:231, 1950.
Edlund, J., Hansson, T., Petersson, A., and Willmar, K.: Sagittal splitting of the mandibular ramus. Scand. J. Plast. Reconstr. Surg., *13*:437, 1979.
Effron, M. Z., Johnson, J. T., Myers, E. N., Curtis, H., Berry, Q., and Sigler, B.: Advanced carcinoma of the tongue. Arch. Otolaryngol., *107*:694, 1981.
Egyedi, P.: Evaluation of operations for mandibular protrusion. Oral Surg., *19*:451, 1965.
Egyedi, P., Houwing, M., and Juten, E.: The oblique subcondylar osteotomy; report of results of 100 cases. J. Oral Surg., *39*:871, 1981.
Egyedi, P., and Visser, W. J.: Pulp vitality of multirooted teeth after injury to one root. J. Maxillofac. Surg., *1*:207, 1973.
Ellis, E., and Gallo, J.: Relapse following mandibular advancement with dental plus skeletal maxillomandibular fixation. J. Oral Surg., *44*:509, 1986.
Entin, M. A.: Reconstruction in congenital deformity of temporomandibular component. Plast. Reconstr. Surg., *21*:461, 1958.
Epker, B. N.: Modifications in the sagittal osteotomy of the mandible. J. Oral Surg. *35*:157, 1977.
Esser, J. F.: Studies in plastic surgery of the face. Ann. Surg., *65*:297, 1917.
Figi, F. A.: Plastic repair after removal of extensive malignancy of the antrum. Arch. Otolaryngol., *28*:29, 1938.
Firmin, F., Coccaro, P. J., and Converse, J. M.: Cepha-

lometric analysis in diagnosis and treatment planning of craniofacial dysostoses. Plast. Reconstr. Surg., *54*:300, 1974.

Fish, L. C., and Epker, B. N.: Prevention of relapse in surgical-orthodontic treatment. J. Clin. Orthodont., *20*:826, 1986.

Fleming, I. D., and Morris, J. H.: Use of acrylic external splint after mandibular resection. Am. J. Surg., *118*:708, 1969.

Fletcher, S. G., Casteel, R. L., and Bradley, D. P.: Tongue-thrust swallow, speech articulation, and age. J. Speech Hearing Dis., *26*:201, 1961.

Foley, J., and Van Dam, A.: Fundamentals of Interactive Computer Graphics. Reading, PA, Addison-Wesley, 1982.

Freihofer, H. P.: Probleme der Behandlung der Progenie durch sagittale Spaltung der aufsteigenden Unterkieferäste. Schweiz. Mschr. Zahnheilk., *86*:679, 1976.

Freihofer, H. P.: Modellversuch zur Lageveränderung des Kieferköpfchens nach sagittaler Spaltung des Unterkiefers. Schweiz. Mschr. Zahnheilk., *87*:12, 1977.

Freihofer, H. P. Jr., and Petresevic, D.: Late results after advancing the mandible by sagittal splitting of the rami. J. Maxillofac. Surg., *3*:250, 1975.

Friedland, J. A., Coccaro, P. J., and Converse, J. M.: Retrospective cephalometric analysis of mandibular bone absorption under silicone rubber chin implants. Plast. Reconstr. Surg., *57*:144, 1976.

Fromm, B., and Lundberg, M.: Postural behaviour of the hyoid bone in normal occlusion and before and after surgical correction of mandibular protrusion. Svensk Tandlak. T. *63*:425, 1970.

Fry, H. J. H.: Reconstruction of the mandible from angle to angle. Paper read at the Sixth International Congress of Plastic and Reconstructive Surgery, Paris, France, August, 1975.

Fujimaki, A.: Free vascularized bone graft to fill up bone defect. Saigai Igaku, *20*:537, 1977.

Georgiade, N. G., and Quinn, G. W.: Newer concepts in surgical correction of mandibular prognathism. Plast. Reconstr. Surg., *27*:185, 1961.

Gillies, H. D.: Plastic Surgery of the Face. London, Oxford University Press, 1920.

Gillies, H. D.: Deformities of the syphilitic nose. Br. Med. J., *29*:977, 1923.

Gillies, H. D., and Millard, D. R., Jr.: Principles and Art of Plastic Surgery. Boston, Little, Brown & Company, 1957.

Gillies, H. D., and Rowe, N. L.: L'ostéotomie du maxillaire supérieur envisagée essentiellement dans les cas de bec-de-lièvre total. Rev. Stomatol., *55*:545, 1954.

Ginestet, G., Frezières, H., and Merville, L.: La correction chirurgicale de l'hypertrophie du masseter. Ann. Chir. Plast., *4*:187, 1959.

Glahn, M., and Winther, J. E.: Correction of unilateral mandibular hypoplasia due to early loss of mandibular condyle. Acta Chir. Scand., *129*:312, 1965.

Goldberg, M. H., Marco, W., and Googel, F.: Parotid fistula: a complication of mandibular osteotomy. J. Oral Surg., *31*:207, 1973.

Gonzalez-Ulloa, M.: Temporomandibular arthroplasty in the treatment of prognathism. Plast. Reconstr. Surg., *8*:136, 1951.

Gonzalez-Ulloa, M.: Mentoplasty with acrylic implants. Rev. Lat. Am. Cir. Plast., *3*:13, 1957.

Gonzalez-Ulloa, M., and Stevens, E.: The role of chin correction in profileplasty. Plast. Reconstr. Surg., *41*:477, 1968.

Gothman, L.: The arterial pattern of the rabbit's tibia after the application of an intramedullary nail. A microangiographic study. Acta Chir. Scand., *120*:211, 1960.

Gotzfried, H. F., and Masing, H.: On the improvement of nasal breathing following mid-face osteotomies, and possible reasons for the phenomenon. J. Maxillofac. Surg., *12*:29, 1984.

Grabb, W. C.: The Habsburg jaw. Plast. Reconstr. Surg., *42*:442, 1968.

Grant, J. C. B.: An Atlas of Anatomy. Baltimore, Williams & Wilkins Company, 1951.

Grayson, B., Cutting, C., Bookstein, F. L., Kim, H., and McCarthy, J. G.: The three dimensional cephalogram: theory, technique and clinical application. Am. J. Orthod., *94*:327, 1988.

Gregor, R. T., and Davidge-Pitts, K. J.: Trapezius osteomyocutaneous flap for mandibular reconstruction. Arch. Otolaryngol., *111*:198, 1985.

Gruca, A., and Meiselles, F.: Asymmetry of the mandible from unilateral hypertrophy. Ann. Surg., *83*:755, 1926.

Guernsey, L. H., and DeChamplain, R. W.: Sequelae and complications of the intraoral sagittal osteotomy in the mandibular rami. Oral Surg., *32*:176, 1971.

Guggenheim, P., and Cohen, L. B.: External hyperostosis of the mandible angle associated with masseteric hypertrophy. Arch. Ortolaryngol., *70*:674, 1959.

Guggenheim, P., and Cohen, L. B.: The histopathology of masseteric hypertrophy. Arch. Orolaryngol., *71*:906, 1960.

Guggenheim, P., and Cohen, L. B.: The nature of masseteric hypertrophy. Arch. Otolaryngol., *73*:15, 1961.

Guilford, J. P.: Psychometric Methods. New York, McGraw-Hill Book Company, 1954.

Gurney, C. E.: Chronic bilateral benign hypertrophy of the masseter muscles. Am. J. Surg., *73*:137, 1947.

Hall, H. D., Chase, D. C., Payor, L. G.: Evaluation and refinement of the intraoral vertical subcondylar osteotomy. J. Oral Surg., *33*:333, 1975.

Hall, H. D., and O'Steen, A. N.: Free grafts of palatal mucosa in mandibular vestibuloplasty. J. Oral Surg., *28*:565, 1970.

Hamaker, R. C., and Singer, M. I.: Irradiated mandibular autografts update. Arch. Otolaryngol. Head Neck Surg., *112*:277, 1986.

Hambleton, R. S.: The soft-tissue covering of the skeletal face as related to orthodontic problems. Am. J. Orthod., *50*:405, 1964.

Harashina, T., Nakajima, H., and Imai, T.: Reconstruction of mandibular defects with revascularized free rib grafts. Plast. Reconstr. Surg., *62*:514, 1978.

Harii, K., Ohmori, K., and Ohmori, S.: Successful clinical transfer of ten free flaps by microvascular anastomoses. Plast. Reconstr. Surg., *53*:259, 1974.

Harsha, W. M.: Prognathism with operative treatment. J.A.M.A., *59*:2035, 1912.

Hausamen, J. E., Samii, M., and Schmidseder, R.: Repair of the mandibular nerve by means of nerve grafting after resection of the lower jaw. J. Maxillofac. Surg., *1*:74, 1973.

Hayes, P. A.: Correction of retrognathia by modified "C" osteotomy of the ramus and sagittal osteotomy of the mandibular body. J. Oral Surg., *31*:682, 1973.

Heiss, J.: Ueber die chirurgische Unterstuetzung der Dehnung im comprimierten Oberkiefer. Dtsch. Zahnärztebl., *8*:560, 1934.

Hellman, M.: An introduction to growth of the human face from infancy to adulthood. Int. J. Orthod., *18*:777, 1932.

Henderson, D.: The assessment and management of bony

deformities of the middle and lower face. Br. J. Plast. Surg., *27*:287, 1974.

Henderson, D., and Jackson, I. T.: Naso-maxillary hypoplasia—the Le Fort II osteotomy. Br. J. Oral Surg., *11*:77, 1973.

Herbert, J. M., Kent, J. N., and Hinds, E. C.: Correction of prognathism by an intraoral vertical subcondylar osteotomy. J. Oral Surg., *28*:651, 1970.

Hilbert, D., and Cohn-Vossen, S.: Geometry and the Imagination. New York, Chelsea Publishing Company, 1952.

Hinds, E. C.: Surgical correction of acquired mandibular deformities. Am. J. Orthod., *43*:161, 1957.

Hinds, E. C., and Girotti, W.: Vertical subcondylar osteotomy: a reappraisal. Oral Surg., *24*:164, 1967.

Hinds, E. C., and Kent, J. N.: Surgical Treatment of Developmental Jaw Deformities. St. Louis, MO., C. V. Mosby Company, 1972.

Hofer, O.: Operation der Prognathie und Microgenie. Dtsch. Zahn. Mund. Kieferheilkd., *9*:121, 1942.

Hogeman, K. E.: Surgical-orthopaedic correction of mandibular protrusion. Acta Chir. Scand., Suppl. 159, 1951.

Hogeman, K. E., and Sarnäs, K. V.: Surgical and dental-orthopedic correction of maxillary protrusion or Angle Class II, division 1 malocclusion. Scand. J. Plast. Surg., *1*:101, 1967.

Hogeman, K. E., and Willmar, K.: Die Vorveriagerund des Oberkiefers zur Korrektur von Gebissanomalien. Fortschr, Kiefer. Gesichtschir., *12*:275, 1967.

Holmstrom, H.: Clinical and pathologic features of maxillonasal dysplasia (Binder's syndrome): significance of the prenasal fossa in etiology. Plast. Reconstr. Surg., *78*:559, 1986a.

Holmstrom, H.: Surgical correction of the nose and midface in maxillonasal dysplasia (Binder's syndrome). Plast. Reconstr. Surg., *78*:568, 1986b.

Horowitz, S. L., Gerstman, L. J., and Converse, J. M.: Craniofacial relationships in mandibular prognathism. Arch. Oral Biol., *14*:121, 1969.

Hovell, J. H.: Surgical correction of facial deformities. Ann. R. Coll. Surg. Engl., *46*:92, 1970.

Hullihen, S. P.: Case of elongation of the under jaw and distortion of the face and neck, caused by a burn, successfully treated. Am. J. Dent. Soc., *9*:157, 1849.

Hunsuck, E. E.: A modified intraoral sagittal technic for correction of mandibular prognathism. Oral Surg., *26*:249, 1968.

Hunter, J.: Works of John Hunter (with notes by James F. Palmer). London, Longman, Rees, Orme, Brown, Breen and Longman, 1835–1837.

Hutchinson, D., and MacGregor, A.: Tooth survival following various methods of sub-apical osteotomy. Int. J. Oral Surg., *29*:256, 1969.

Imbert, L., and Réal, P.: Le traitement chirurgical des pseudoarthroses du maxillaire inférieur. Marseille Med., *53*:193, 1916.

Inclan, A.: Use of preserved bone grafts in orthopedic surgery. J. Bone Joint Surg., *24*:81, 1942.

Indresano, A. T.: Simplified technique for wiring the condyloid process after intraoral vertical subcondylar osteotomy. J. Oral Surg., *33*:384, 1975.

Isaacson, R. J., and Ingram, A. H.: Forces produced by rapid maxillary expansion. II. Forces present during treatment. Angle Orthod., *34*:261, 1964.

Isaacson, R. J., Kopytov, O. S., Bevis, R. R., and Waite, D. E.: Movement of the proximal and distal segments after mandibular ramus osteotomies. J. Oral Surg., *36*:263, 1978.

Ive, J., McNeill, R. W., and West, R. A.: Mandibular advancement: skeletal and dental changes during fixation. J. Oral Surg., *35*:881, 1977.

Ivy, R. H.: Extensive loss of substance of mandible due to removal of sarcoma, replaced by bone graft from crest of ilium. Int. J. Orthod., *7*:483, 1921.

Ivy, R. H.: Benign bony enlargement of the condyloid process of the mandible. Ann. Surg., *85*:27, 1927.

Ivy, R. H.: Bone grafting for restoration of defects of mandible, collective review. Plast. Reconstr. Surg., *7*:333, 1951.

Ivy, R. H.: Iliac bone graft to bridge a mandibular defect. 49-year clinical and radiological follow-up. Plast. Reconstr. Surg., *50*:483, 1972.

Ivy, R. H., and Eby, J. D.: Thirty-nine and 38 year follow-ups of mandibular bone grafts in three cases. Plast. Reconstr. Surg., *22*:548, 1958.

Jaboulay, M.: Les effets de la resection des condyles du maxillaire inférieur sur la situation de la rangée dentaire et la forme du mention. Lyon Med., *75*:519, 1895.

Jackson, D.: Lip positions and incisor relationships. Br. Dent. J., *112*:147, 1962.

Jackson, I. T., Moos, K. F., and Sharpe, D. T.: Total surgical management of Binder's syndrome. Ann. Plast. Surg., *7*:25, 1981.

Jacobsen, P. U., and Lund, K.: Unilateral overgrowth and remodeling processes after fracture of the mandibular condyle: a longitudinal radiographic study. Scand. J. Dent. Res., *80*:68, 1972.

Johanson, B., Kahnberg, K. -E., Lilja, J., and Ridell, A.: Surgical correction of mandibular prognathism by the oblique sliding osteotomy: a clinical and radiological follow-up study of 112 consecutive cases. Scand. J. Plast. Reconstr. Surg., *13*:453, 1979.

Johnson, J. V., and Hinds, E. C.: Evaluation of teeth vitality after subapical osteotomy. J. Oral Surg., *27*:256, 1969.

Joy, E. D., and Cronan, J. C., Jr.: Pin fixation of the proximal segment in intraoral oblique subcondylar osteotomy of the mandible. J. Oral Maxillofac. Surg., *41*:206, 1983.

Junghans, J. A.: Profile reconstruction with Silastic chin implants. Am. J. Orthod., *53*:217, 1967.

Karabouta, I., and Martis, C.: The TMJ dysfunction syndrome before and after sagittal split osteotomy of the rami. J. Maxillofac. Surg., *13*:185, 1985.

Kawamoto, H. K.: Treatment of the elongated lower face and the gummy smile. Clin. Plast. Surg., *9*:479, 1982a.

Kawamoto, H. K.: Discussion of reduction mentoplasty. Plast. Reconstr. Surg., *70*:151, 1982b.

Kazanjian, V. H.: The treatment of gunshot wounds of the face accompanied by extensive destruction of the lower lip and mandible. Br. J. Surg., *5*:74, 1918.

Kazanjian, V. H.: Jaw reconstruction. Am. J. Surg., *43*:249, 1939.

Kazanjian, V. H.: *In* Kazanjian, V. H., and Converse, J. M.: The Surgical Treatment of Facial Injuries. 1st ed. Baltimore, Williams & Wilkins Company, 1949.

Kazanjian, V. H.: Bone transplanting of the mandible. Am. J. Surg., *83*:633, 1952.

Kazanjian, V. H.: The surgical treatment of prognathism: an analysis of 65 cases. Am. J. Surg., *87*:691, 1954.

Kazanjian, V. H.: Bilateral absence of the ascending rami of the mandible. Br. J. Plast. Surg., *9*:77, 1956.

Kazanjian, V. H., and Burrows, H.: Treatment of maxillary fractures. Br. Dent. J., *37*:126, 1917–1918.

Kazanjian, V. H., and Converse, J. M.: Intraoral approach. *In* Kazanjian, V. H., and Converse, J. M.: The

Surgical Treatment of Facial Injuries. 2nd ed. Baltimore, Williams & Wilkins Company. 1959, pp. 838–866.

Kazanjian, V. H., and Converse, J. M.: Open-bite deformities of the jaw. *In* Kazanjian, V. H., and Converse, J. M.: Surgical Treatment of Facial Injuries. 3rd ed. Baltimore, Williams & Wilkins Company. 1974a. p. 1118.

Kazanjian, V. H., and Converse, J. M.: Intraoral approach. *In* Kazanjian, V. H., and Converse, J. M.: Surgical Treatment of Facial Injuries. 3rd ed. Baltimore, Williams & Wilkins Company, 1974b, p. 1022.

Kelly, J. E., Sanchez, M., and van Kirk, L. E.: An assessment of the occlusion of the teeth of children. National Center for Health Statistics, U. S. Public Health Service, 1973, DHEW Publ. HRA 74–1612.

Kelsey, C. C.: Radiographic cephalometric study of surgically corrected mandibular prognathism. J. Oral Surg., *26*:239, 1968.

Kent, J. N., and Hinds, E. C.: Management of dental facial deformities by anterior alveolar surgery. J. Oral Surg., *29*:13, 1971.

Kent, J. N., Quinn, J. H., Zide, M. F., Finger, I. M., Jarcho, M., and Rothstein, S. S.: Correction of alveolar ridge deficiencies with nonresorbable hydroxyapatite. J. Am. Dent. Assoc., *105*:993, 1982.

Kent, J. N., Quinn, J. H., Zide, M. F., Guerra, L. R., and Boyne, P. J.: Alveolar ridge augmentation using nonresorbable hydroxyapatite with or without autogenous cancellous bone. J. Oral Maxillofac. Surg., *41*:629, 1983.

Ketchum, L. D., Masters, F. W., and Robinson, D. W.: Mandibular reconstruction using a composite island rib flap. Plast. Reconstr. Surg., *53*:471, 1974.

Klapp, R., and Schroeder, H.: Die Unterkieferschussbruche. Berlin. Hermann Meusser, 1917.

Kloosterman, J.: Köle's osteotomy, a follow-up study. J. Maxillofac. Surg., *13*:59, 1985.

Knize, D. M.: The influence of periosteum and calcitonin on onlay bone graft survival. Plast. Reconstr. Surg., *53*:190, 1974.

Knowles, C. D.: Changes in the profile following surgical reduction of mandibular prognathism. Br. J. Plast. Surg., *18*:432, 1965.

Koblin, I., and Reil, B.: Die Sensibilität der Unterlippe nach Schonung bzw. Durchtrennung des Nervus alveolar mandibularis bei Progenie Operationen. Vortag auf der XII Jahrestagung der Deutschen Gesellschaft für Kiefer-und Gesichtschirurgie in Berlin, *24*:27, 1972.

Köle, H.: Surgical operations on the alveolar ridge to correct occlusal abnormalities. Oral Surg., *12*:277, 413, 515, 1959a.

Köle, H.: Nouvelles interventions chirurgicales à la hauteur du processus alveolaire en vue de la correction des malformations de l'arcade et des malpositions dentaires. Rev. Belg. Stomatol., *56*:247, 1959b.

Kopp, W. K.: Auriculotemporal syndrome secondary to vertical sliding osteotomy of the mandibular rami: report of case. J. Oral Surg., *26*:295, 1968.

Kostečka, F.: Surgical correction of protrusion of the lower and upper jaws. J. Am. Dent. Assoc., *15*:362, 1928.

Krause, F.: Unterfiefer Plastik. Zentralbl. Chir., *34*:1045, 1907.

Krespi, P. Y., and Sisson, A. G.: Reconstruction after total or subtotal glossectomy. Am. J. Surg., *146*:488, 1983.

Krevszig, E.: Introduction to Differential Geometry and Riemannian Geometry. Toronto, University of Toronto Press, 1968.

Kufner, J.: Experience with a modified procedure for correction of open bite. Transaction of the Third International Conference of Oral Surgery. London, E. & S. Livingstone, 1968.

Kufner, J.: Four-year experience with major maxillary osteotomy for retrusion. J. Oral Surg., *29*:549, 1971.

Lane, W. A.: Cleft Palate and Hare Lip. London, London Medical Publishing Company, 1905.

Lanigan, D. T., Wray, J. D., and Chasmar, L. R.: Reconstruction of the atrophic mandible. Ann. Plast Surg., *16*:333, 1986.

Leake, D. L.: Mandibular reconstruction with a new type of alloplastic tray: a preliminary report. J. Oral Surg., *32*:23, 1974.

Leake, D. L., and Rappaport, M.: Mandibular reconstruction: bone induction in an alloplastic tray. Surgery, *72*:332, 1972.

Le Fort, P.: Etude expérimentale sur les fractures de la machoire supérieure. Rev. Chir., *23*:208, 360, 479, 1901.

Legg, W.: Enlargement of the temporal and masseter muscles on both sides. Trans. Pathol. Soc. London, *31*:361, 1880.

Lehman, J. A., Haas, A. J., and Haas, D. G.: Surgical orthodontic correction of transverse maxillary deficiency: a simplified approach. Plast. Reconstr. Surg., *73*:62, 1984.

Leibold, D. G., Tilson, H. B., and Rask, K. R.: A subjective evaluation of the re-establishment of the neurovascular supply of teeth involved in anterior maxillary osteotomy procedures. J. Oral Surg., *32*:531, 1971.

Leipzig, B., and Cummings, C. W.: The current status of mandibular reconstruction using autogenous frozen mandibular grafts. Head Neck Surg., *6*:992, 1984.

Lemaitre, F., and Ponroy, J.: Greffes du maxillaire inférieur. Rev. Stomatol., *18*:260, 1920.

Lévignac, J.: Traitement d'un enforcement consolidé du tiers moyen de la face par osteotomies et greffes d'os. Rev. Stomatol., *59*:551, 1958.

Limberg, A. A.: Treatment of open-bite by means of plastic oblique osteotomy of the ascending rami of the mandible. Dent. Cosmos, *67*:1191, 1925.

Limberg, A. A.: A new method of plastic lengthening of the mandible in unilateral microgenia and asymmetry of the face. J. Am. Dent. Assoc., *15*:851, 1928.

Lindegård, B.: Variations in human body-build. Acta Psychiatr. Neurol. Scand., Suppl. 86, 1953.

Lindemann, A.: Bruhn's Ergebnisse aus dem Dusseldorfer Lazarett, Behandlungen der Kieferschussverletzungen. Weisbaden, 1916, p. 243.

Lindorf, H. H., and Steinhauser, E. W.: Correction of jaw deformities involving simultaneous osteotomy of the mandible and maxilla. J. Maxillofac. Surg., *6*:239, 1978.

Little, J. W., III, McCulloch, D. T., and Lyons, J. R.: The lateral pectoral composite flap in one-stage reconstruction of the irradiated mandible. Plast. Reconstr. Surg., *71*:326, 1983.

Longacre, J. J.: Surgical correction of extensive defects of scalp and cranium with autogenous tissues. Internatl. Soc. Plastic Surgeons, 1st Congress, Stockholm, 1955. Baltimore, Williams & Wilkins Company, 1957.

Longacre, J. J., and DeStefano, G. A.: Further observations of the behavior of autogenous split-rib grafts in reconstruction of extensive defects of the cranium and face. Plast. Reconstr. Surg., *20*:281, 1957.

Luhr, H. G.: Skelettverlagernde Operationen zur Harmonisierung des Gesichtsprofils—Probleme der stabilen Fixation von Osteotomiesegmenten. *In* Pfeifer, G. (Ed.): Die Ästhetik von Form und Funktion in Plastischen u. Wiederherstellungschirurgie. Berlin, Heidelberg, Springer-Verlag, 1985, pp. 87–92.

Luhr, H. G.: A micro-system for cranio-maxillofacial skeletal fixation; preliminary report. J. Craniomaxillofac. Surg., *16*:312, 1988.

Luhr, H. G., Schauer, W., Jager, A., and Kubein-Meesenburg, D.: Formveränderung des Unterkiefers durch kieferorthopädisch-chirurĝische Massnahmen mit stabiler Fixation der Segmentê. Forstschr. Kieferorthop., *47*:39, 1986.

Lund, K., and Jacobsen, P. U.: Overgrowth of a hypoplastic mandibular ramus after autoplastic bone grafting: an 18-year longitudinal radiographic study, using metallic implants. Tandlaegebladet, *75*:1279, 1971.

MacLeod, A. M., and Robinson, D. W.: Reconstruction of defects involving the mandible and floor of mouth by free osteocutaneous flaps derived from the foot. Br. J. Plast. Surg., *35*:239, 1982.

Madritsch, E.: Spätergebnisse nach Korrektur von Dysgnathien und Zahnstellungsanomalien durch Alveolarfortsatzbewegungen und Kortikotomien. Dissertation, University of Zürich, 1968.

Maisels, D. O.: Spontaneous regression of anterior open bite following treatment of macroglossia. Br. J. Plast. Surg., *32*:309, 1979.

Manchester, W. M.: Immediate reconstruction of the mandible and temporomandibular joint. Br. J. Plast. Surg., *18*:291, 1965.

Markowitz, A.: The use of homogenous bone grafts in mandibular reconstruction. Am. J. Surg., *96*:755, 1958.

Marsh, J. L., and Vannier, M. W.: The "third" dimension in craniofacial surgery. Plast. Reconstr. Surg., *71*:759, 1983.

Marsh, J. L., Vannier, M. W., Stevens, W. G., Warren, J. O., Gayou, D., and Dye, D. M.: Computerized imaging for soft tissue and osseous reconstruction in the head and neck. Clin. Plast. Surg., *12*:279, 1983.

Mårtensson, G.: Dental injuries following radical surgery on the maxillary sinus. Acta Otolaryngol., Suppl. 84, 1950.

Martin, C.: De la prothèse immédiate, appliquée à la résection des maxillaires: rhinoplastie sur appareil prothétique permanent; restauration de la face, lèvres, nez, langue, voûte et voile du palais. Paris, Masson et Cie, 1889.

Maruyama, Y., Urita, Y., and Ohnishi, K.: Rib–latissimus dorsi osteomyocutaneous flap in reconstruction of a mandibular defect. Br. J. Plast. Surg., *38*:234, 1985.

Massey, G. B., Chase, D. C., Thomas, P. M., and Kohn, M. W.: Intraoral oblique osteotomy of the mandibular ramus. J. Oral Surg., *32*:755, 1974.

Mayer, R.: Le traitement chirurgical de la prognathie mandibulaire. Acta Stomatol. Belg., *68*:383, 1971.

McCarthy, J. G.: Complications of Jaw Surgery. St. Louis, C. V. Mosby Company, 1977.

McCarthy, J. G., Coccaro, P. J., and Schwartz, M. D.: Velopharyngeal function following maxillary advancement. Plast. Reconstr. Surg., *64*:180, 1979.

McCarthy, J. G., Grayson, B., and Zide, B.: The relationship between the surgeon and orthodontist in orthognathic surgery. Clin. Plast. Surg., *9*:423, 1982.

McCarthy, J. G., and Ruff, G. L.: The chin. Clin. Plast. Surg., *15*:125, 1988.

McCullough, D. W., and Fredrickson, J. M.: Neovascularized rib grafts to reconstruct mandibular defects. Can. J. Otolaryngol., *2*:96, 1973.

McEvitt, W. G.: Conversion of an inferiorly based pharyngeal flap to a superiorly based position. Plast. Reconstr. Surg., *48*:36, 1971.

McKee, D.: Microvascular rib transposition for reconstruction of the mandible. Presented at the Annual Meeting of the American Society of Plastic and Reconstructive Surgeons, Montreal, Canada, 1971.

McNeill, R. W., Hooley, J. R., and Sundberg, R. J.: Skeletal relapse during intermaxillary fixation. J. Oral Surg., *31*:212, 1973.

McNichol, J. W., and Rogers, A. T.: An original method of correction of hyperplastic asymmetry of the mandible. Plast. Reconstr. Surg., *1*:288, 1945.

Meredith, H. V.: Changes in the profile of the osseous chin during childhood. Am. J. Phys. Anthrop., *15*:247, 1957.

Merrifield, L. L.: Profile line as an aid in critically evaluating facial esthetics. Am. J. Orthod., *52*:804, 1966.

Merville, L. C.: The choice of the procedure in surgical correction of mandibular prognathia. *In* Walker, R. V. (Ed.): Transactions of the 3rd International Conference on Oral Surgery. London, E. & S. Livingstone, 1970.

Merz, B.: Computer guides facial reconstruction [news]. J.A.M.A., *249*:1409, 1983.

Michelet, F. X., Deymes, J., and Desus, B.: Osteosynthesis with miniaturized screwed plates in maxillofacial surgery. J. Maxillofac. Surg., *1*:79, 1973.

Millard, R.: Adjuncts in augmentation mentoplasty and corrective rhinoplasty. Plast. Reconstr. Surg., *3*:48, 1965.

Moore, F. F., and Ward, F. G.: Complications and sequelae of untreated fractures of the facial bones and their treatment. Br. J. Plast. Surg., *1*:262, 1949.

Moose, S. M.: Correction of abnormal mandibular protrusion by intraoral operation. J. Oral Surg., *3*:304, 1945.

Morgan, L. R., Gallegos, L. T., and Frileck, S. P.: Mandibular vestibuloplasty with a free graft of the mucoperiosteal layer from the hard palate. Plast. Reconstr. Surg., *51*:359, 1973.

Morgan, L. R., and Thompson, C. W.: Mandibular reconstruction. Clin. Plast. Surg., *2*:561, 1975.

Morris, J. H.: Biphase connector, external skeletal splint for reduction and fixation of mandibular fractures. Oral Surg., *2*:1382, 1949.

Moser, K., and Freihofer, H. P. M.: Long-term experience with simultaneous movement of the upper and lower jaw. J. Maxillofac. Surg., *8*:271, 1980.

Moss, M. L.: Functional analysis of human mandibular growth. J. Prosthet. Dent., *10*:1149, 1960.

Mowlem, R.: Cancellous chip bone grafts; report of 75 cases. Lancet, *2*:746, 1944.

Moyers, R.: Handbook of Orthodontics. 2nd ed. Chicago, Year Book Medical Publishers, 1963.

Munro, I. R.: Personal communication, 1988.

Munro, I. R., Boyd, J. B., and Wainwright, D. J.: Effect of steroids in maxillofacial surgery. Ann. Plast. Surg., *17*:440, 1986.

Munro, I. R., Chen, Y. U., and Park, B. Y.: Simultaneous total correction of temporomandibular ankylosis and facial asymmetry. Plast. Reconstr. Surg., *77*:517, 1986.

Munro, I. R., Sinclair, W. J., and Rudd, N. L.: Maxillonasal dysplasia (Binder's syndrome). Plast. Reconstr. Surg., *63*:657, 1979.

Murray, J.: Personal communication, 1976.

Myers, E. N.: The role of total glossectomy in the management of cancer of the oral cavity. Otolaryngol. Clin. North Am., *5*:343, 1972.

Neuner, O.: Chirurgische Orthodontie. Schweiz. Monatsschr. Zahnkeilkd., *75*:940, 1965.

Neuner, O.: Surgical correction of mandibular prognathism. Oral Surg., *42*:415, 1976.

New, G. B., and Erich, J. B.: The surgical correction of mandibular prognathism. Am. J. Surg., *53*:2, 1941.

Niebergall, C. F., and Mercuri, L. G.: Intraoral vertical subcondylar osteotomy: a national survey. J. Oral Maxillofac. Surg., *43*:450, 1985.

Niederdellmann, H., and Dieckmann, J.: Neurologiache Storungen nach Chirurgischer Korrektur der Progenie und Mikrogenie. Fortschr. Kiefer. Gesichtschir., *18*:186, 1974.

Nordendram, Å.: and Waller, Å.: Oral-surgical correction of mandibular protrusion. Br. J. Oral Surg., *6*:64, 1968.

O'Brien, B. McC., Morrison, W. A., and Dooley, B. J.: Microvascular osteocutaneous transfer using the groin flap and iliac crest, the dorsalis pedis flap and second metatarsal. Br. J. Plast. Surg., *32*:188, 1979.

Obwegeser, H. L.: *In* Trauner, R., and Obwegeser, H. L.: The surgical correction of mandibular prognathism and retrognathia with consideration of genioplasty. I. Surgical procedures to correct mandibular prognathism and reshaping of the chin. Oral Surg., *10*:677, 1957.

Obwegeser, H. L.: Surgical preparation of the maxilla for prosthesis. J. Oral Surg., *22*:127, 1964.

Obwegeser, H. L.: Surgical correction of small or retrodisplaced maxilla; the "dish-face" deformity. Plast. Reconstr. Surg., *43*:351, 1969.

Obwegeser, H. L.: Late reconstruction of large maxillary defects after tumor resection. J. Maxillofac. Surg., *1*:19, 1973.

Ollier, L.: Récherches éxperimentales sur les greffes osseuses. J. Physio., *3*:88, 1860.

Ollier, L.: Traité experimental et clinique de la regénération des os et de la production artificielle du tissue osseux. Paris, V. Masson & Fils, 1867.

Oppenheim, H., and Wing, M.: Benign hypertrophy of the masseter muscle. Arch. Otolaryngol., *70*:207, 1959.

Ortiz-Monasterio, F., Fuente del Campo, A., and Carrillo, A.: Advancement of the orbits and the midface in one piece, combined with frontal repositioning, for the correction of Crouzon's deformities. Plast. Reconstr. Surg., *61*:507, 1978.

Osborne, R.: The treatment of the underdeveloped ascending ramus. Br. J. Plast. Surg., *17*376, 1964.

Östrup, L. T.: The Free Living Bone Graft. Stockholm, Linkoping University, 1975.

Östrup, L. T., and Fredrickson, J. M.: Distant transfer of free living bone graft by microvascular anastomoses. An experimental study. Plast. Reconstr. Surg., *54*:274, 1974.

Östrup, L. T., and Fredrickson, J. M.: Reconstruction of mandibular defects after radiation, using a free living bone graft transferred by microvascular anastomoses. An experimental study. Plast. Reconstr. Surg., *55*:563, 1975.

Östrup, L. T., and Tam, C. S.: Bone formation in a free living bone graft transferred by microvascular anastomosis. A quantitative microscopic study using fluorochrome markers. Scand. J. Plast. Reconstr. Surg., *9*:101, 1975.

Owsley, J. Q., Creech, B. J., and Dedo, H. H.: Poor speech following the pharyngeal flap operation; etiology and treatment. Cleft Palate J., *9*:312, 1972.

Panje, W. R.: Mandible reconstruction with the trapezius osteomusculocutaneous flap. Arch. Otolaryngol., *111*:223, 1985.

Panje, W. R., and Cutting, C.: Trapezius osteomyocutaneous island flap for reconstruction of the anterior floor of mouth and mandible. Head Neck Surg., *3*:66, 1980.

Parkes, M.: Avoiding bone absorption under plastic chin implants. Arch. Orolaryngol., *98*:100, 1973.

Parnes, E. T., and Becker, M. L.: Necrosis of the anterior maxilla following osteotomy. Oral Surg., *33*:326, 1972.

Partsch: Prosthesis of lower jaw after resection. Arch. Klin. Chir., *55*:746, 1897.

Peck, H., and Peck, S.: A concept of facial esthetics. Angle Orthod., *40*:284, 1970.

Pepersack, W. J.: Tooth vitality after alveolar segmental osteotomy. J. Maxillofac. Surg., *1*:85, 1973.

Pepersack, W. J., and Chausse, J. M.: Long term follow up for the correction of prognathism by sagittal split osteotomy. Second Congress. European Association for Maxillofacial Surgery, Zurich. Sept. 16–21, 1974.

Pichler, H.: Unterkieferresektion wegen Progenie. Z. Stomatol., *16*:190, 1918.

Pichler, H., and Trauner, R.: Lehrbuch der Mund- und Kiefer-chirurgie. Wien. Urban & Schwarzenberg, 1948.

Pickrell, H. P.: Double resection of the mandible. Dent. Cosmos. *54*:1114, 1912.

Pike, R. L., and Boyne, P. J.: Composite autogenous marrow and surface decalcified implants in mandibular defects. J. Oral Surg., *31*:905, 1973.

Pike, R. L., and Boyne, P. J.: Use of surface decalcified allogeneic bone and autogenous marrow in extensive mandibular defects. J. Oral Surg., *32*:177, 1974.

Pitanguy, I.: Augmentation mentoplasty. Plast. Reconstr. Surg., *42*:460, 1968.

Poswillo, D. E.: Early pulp changes following reduction of open bite by segmental surgery. Int. J. Oral Surg., *1*:87, 1972.

Poulton, D. R., Taylor, R. C., and Ware, W. H.: Cephalometric x-ray evaluation of the vertical osteotomy correction of mandibular prognathism. Oral Surg., *16*:807, 1963.

Poulton, D. R., and Ware, W. H.: Surgical-orthodontic treatment of severe mandibular retrusion (part II). Am. J. Orthod., *63*:237, 1973.

Psillakis, J. M., Lapa, F., and Spina, V.: Surgical correction of midfacial retrusion (nasomaxillary hypoplasia) in the presence of normal dental occlusion. Plast. Reconstr. Surg., *51*:67, 1973.

Radney, L. J., and Jacobs, J. D.: Soft tissue changes associated with surgical total maxillary intrusion. Am. J. Orthod., *80*:191, 1981.

Ragnell, A.: Der Moderna Plastikkirurgien inklusive den Kosmetiska Kirurgien, dess verksamhetsfalt och arbetsmethoder. Nord. Med. Tidskr., *15*:361, 1938.

Razack, S. M., Sako, K., Bakamjian, Y. V., and Shedd, P. D.: Total glossectomy. Am. J. Surg., *146*:509, 1983.

Rehrmann, A.: Beitrag zur Alveolarkammplastik am Unterkiefer. Zahnaerztl. Rdsch., *62*:505, 1953.

Reidy, J. B.: Homogenous bone grafts. Br. J. Plast. Surg., *9*:89, 1956.

Rhinelander, F. W.: The normal microcirculation of a diaphyseal cortex and its response to fracture. J. Bone Joint Surg., *50A*:784, 1968.

Rice, J.: Numerical methods, software, and analysis: IMSL reference edition. *In* Finite Element Methods. New York, McGraw-Hill Book Company, 1983, pp. 320–324.

Richards, M. A., Poole, M. D., and Godfrey, A. M.: The serratus anterior/rib composite flap in mandibular reconstruction. Br. J. Plast. Surg., *38*:466, 1985.

Ricketts, R.: Planning treatment on the basis of the facial pattern and on estimate of its growth. Angle Orthod., *27*:14, 1957.
Ricketts, R. M.: Esthetics, environment and the law of lip relation. Am. J. Orthod., *54*:272, 1968.
Ricketts, R. M.: Divine proportions in facial esthetics. Clin. Plast. Surg., *9*:401, 1982.
Ricketts, R. M., and Kawamoto, H. K., Jr.: Personal communication, 1980.
Riedel, R. A.: An analysis of dentofacial relationships. Am. J. Orthod., *43*:103, 1957.
Riediger, D: Restoration of masticatory function by microsurgically revascularized iliac crest bone grafts using enosseous implants. Plast. Reconstr. Surg., *81*:861, 1988.
Rintala, A., and Ranta, A.: Nasomaxillary hypoplasia—Binder's syndrome. Morphology and treatment of two separate varieties. Scand. J. Plast. Reconstr. Surg., *19*:127, 1985.
Riolo, M. L., Moyers, R. E., McNamara, J. A., and Hunter, S. W.: An Atlas of Craniofacial Growth. Monograph 2. Ann Arbor, Center for Human Growth and Development, University of Michigan, 1974.
Rish, B. B.: Alloplastic materials in the creation of facial contour. Arch. Otolaryngol., *72*:212, 1960.
Rittersma, J., Van der Veld, R. G. M., van Gool, A. V., and Koppendraaier, J.: Stable fragment fixation in orthognathic surgery: review of 30 cases. J. Oral Surg., *39*:671, 1981.
Robertson, G. A.: A comparison between sternum and rib in osteomyocutaneous reconstruction of major mandibular defects. Ann. Plast. Surg., *17*:421, 1986.
Robinson, M.: Prognathism corrected by open vertical condylotomy. J. South. Calif. Dent. Assoc., *24*:22, 1956.
Robinson, M.: Micrognathism corrected by vertical osteotomy of ascending ramus and iliac bone graft. Oral Surg., *10*:1125, 1957.
Robinson, M., and Lytle, J. J.: Micrognathism corrected by vertical osteotomies of the rami without bone grafts. Oral Surg., *15*:641, 1962.
Robinson, M., and Shuken, R.: Bone resorption under plastic chin implants. J. Oral Surg., *27*:116, 1969.
Robinson, M., Shuken, R., and Dougherty, H.: Surgical orthodontic treatment of hemigigantism; report of case. Oral Surg., *27*:744, 1969.
Rockey, K., Evans, H., Griffiths, D., and Nethercot, D.: The Finite Element Method. New York, John Wiley & Sons, 1983.
Rogers, D., and Adams, J. A.: Three-dimensional transformations and projections. *In* Mathematical Elements for Computer Graphics. New York, McGraw-Hill Book Company, 1976.
Rontal, E., and Hohmann, A.: Lateral alveolomaxillary osteotomies. Arch. Otolaryngol., *95*:18, 1972.
Rosen, H. M.: Miniplate fixation of Le Fort I osteotomies. Plast. Reconstr. Surg., *78*:748, 1986.
Rosen, H. M.: Lip-nasal aesthetics following Le Fort I osteotomy. Plast. Reconstr. Surg., *81*:171, 1988.
Rosen, H. M.: Surgical correction of the vertically deficient chin. Plast. Reconstr. Surg., *82*:247, 1988.
Rosen, I. B., Manktelow, R. T., Zuker, R. M., and Boyd, B.: Application of microvascular free osteocutaneous flaps in the management of post-radiation recurrent oral cancer. Am. J. Surg., *150*:474, 1985.
Rothstein, S. S., Paris, D. A., and Zacek, M.: Use of hydroxyapatite for augmentation of deficient alveolar ridges. J. Oral Maxillofac. Surg., *42*:224, 1984.
Rougier, J., Tessier, P., Hervouet, F., Woillez, M., Lekieffre, M., and Derome, P.: Chirurgie Plastique Orbito-Palpebrale. Paris, Masson et Cie, 1977, p. 292.
Rowe, N. H.: Hemifacial hypertrophy. Oral Surg., *15*:572, 1962.
Ruberg, R. L., Randall, P., and Whitaker, L. A.: Preservation of a posterior pharyngeal flap during maxillary advancement. Plast. Reconstr. Surg., *57*:335, 1976.
Rubin, L. R., Bromberg, B. E., and Walden, R. H.: Long term human reaction to synthetic plastic. Surg. Gynecol. Obstet., *132*:603, 1971.
Rubin, L. R., Robinson, G. W., and Shapiro, R. N.: Polyethylene in reconstructive surgery. Plast. Reconstr. Surg., *3*:586, 1948.
Rusconi, L., Brusati, R., and Bottoli, V.: Indagini elettromiografiche sull'equilibrio muscolare post operatorionel trattamento chirurgico del progenismo secondo la techica di Obwegeser-Dal Pont. Riv. Ital. Stomatol., *25*:9, 1970.
Rushton, M. A.: Malformation of the mandibular ramus treated by bone graft. Dent. Rec., *62*:272, 1942.
Rushton, M. A.: Growth of mandibular condyle in relation to some deformities. Br. Dent. J., *76*:57, 1944.
Rydigier, L. R.: Zum osteoplastistischen Ersatz nach Unterkieferresektion. Zentralbl. Chir., *35*:1321, 1908.
Safian, J.: Silastic chin implant. The Bulletin 14–085, Medical Products Division, Dow Corning Corp., 1965.
Salibian, A. H., Rappaport, I., and Allison, G.: Functional oromandibular reconstruction with the microvascular composite groin flap. Plast. Reconstr. Surg., *76*:819, 1985.
Salzmann, J. A.: Practice of Orthodontics. Philadelphia, J. B. Lippincott Company, 1966.
Sanborn, R. T.: Differences between the facial skeletal patterns of class III malocclusion and normal occlusion. Angle Orthod., *25*:208, 1955.
Sarnäs, K. V.: Inter- and intra-family variations in the facial profile. Odontol. Rev. *10*(Suppl. 4), 1959.
Sarnäs, K. V.: The adult facial profile. A radiographic study of 317 male and female students aged 19–23 years. Unpublished data, 1973.
Sassouni, V.: A classification of skeletal facial types. Am. J. Orthod., *55*:109, 1969.
Sauter, D. S., and McGregor, I. A.: The radial forearm flap in intraoral reconstruction: the experience of 60 consecutive cases. Plast. Reconstr. Surg., *78*:1, 1986.
Sauter, D. S., and Widdowson, W. P.: Immediate reconstruction of the mandible using a vascularized segment of radius. Head Neck Surg., *8*:232, 1986.
Schendel, S. A., Eisenfeld, J. H., Bell, W. H., and Epker, B. N.: Superior repositions of the maxilla: stability and soft tissue osseous relations. Am. J. Orthod., *70*:663, 1976.
Schendel, S. A., and Epker, B. N.: Results after mandibular advancement surgery: an analysis of 87 cases. J. Oral Surg., *38*:265, 1980.
Schendel, S. A., and Williamson, L. W.: Muscle reorientation following superior repositioning of the maxilla. J. Oral Maxillofac. Surg., *41*:235, 1983.
Schmid, E.: Ueber neue Wege in der plastichen Chirurgie der Nase. Beitr. Klin. Chir., *184*:385, 1952.
Schmidt, D. R., and Robson, M. C.: One-stage composite reconstruction using the latissimus myo-osteocutaneous free flap. Am. J. Surg., *144*:470, 1982.
Schuchardt, K.: Ein Beitrag zur chirurgischen Kieferorthopädie unter Berücksichtigung ihrer Bedeutung für die Behandlung angeborener und erworbener Kieferdeformitäten bei Soldaten. Dtsch. Zahn. Mund. Kieferheilk., *9*:73, 1942.
Schuchardt, K.: *In* Bier, Braun, and Kümmel (Eds.): Chirurgisch Operationslehre, Leipzig, 1954. Johann Ambrosius Barth, Bd. II. Operationen im Gesicht-Kieferbereich, 1954a.

Schuchardt, K.: Die Chirurgie als Helferin der Kieferorthopädie. Fortschr. Kieferorthop., *15*:1, 1954b.

Schuchardt, K.: Formen des offen Bisses und ihre Operativen. Behandlungsmoglichkeiten. Fortschr. Kiefer. Gesichtschir., *1*:22, 1955.

Schuchardt, K.: Erfahrungen bei der Behandlung der Mikrogenie. Langenbecks Arch. Klin. Chir., *289*:651, 1958.

Schuchardt, K.: Personal communication, 1963.

Schwartz, H. C.: Mandibular reconstruction using the dacron-methane prosthesis and autogenic cancellous bone: review of 32 cases. Plast. Reconstr. Surg., *73*:387, 1984.

Schwartz, M. F.: The acoustics of normal and nasal vowel production. Cleft Palate J., *5*:125, 1968.

Schwartz, M. F.: Personal communication, 1976.

Scudder, C. L.: Tumors of the Jaws. Philadelphia, W. B. Saunders Company, 1912.

Seward, G. J.: Replacement of the anterior part of the mandible by bone graft. J. Maxillofac. Surg., *2*:168, 1974.

Siemssen, S. O., Kirby, B., and O'Connor, T. P. F.: Immediate reconstruction of a resected segment of the lower jaw, using a compound flap of clavicle and sternocleidomastoid muscle. Plast. Reconstr. Surg., *61*:724, 1978.

Smith, A. E., and Chambers, F. W.: Mandibular prognathism corrected by newly divised osteotomy of the ramus. J. Am. Dent. Assoc., *64*:328, 1962.

Smith, A. E., and Robinson, M.: Surgical correction of mandibular prognathism by subsigmoid notch ostectomy with sliding condylotomy: a new technic. J. Am. Dent. Assoc., *49*:46, 1954.

Snyder, C. C., Bateman, J. M., Davis, C. W., and Warden, G. D.: Mandibulo-facial restoration with live osteocutaneous flaps. Plast. Reconstr. Surg., *45*:14, 1970.

Snyder, C. C., Levine, G. A., Swanson, H. M., and Browne, E. Z.: Mandibular lengthening by gradual distraction. A preliminary report. Plast. Reconstr. Surg., *51*:506, 1973.

Snyder, G.: Personal communication, 1975.

Soderberg, B. N., Jennings, H. B., and McNelly, J. E.: Restoration of the jaw. U.S. Armed Forces Med. J., *3*:1423, 1952.

Solow, B.: The pattern of craniofacial associations. Acta Odontol. Scand., *24*(Suppl. 46), 1966.

Spanier, F.: Prognathie-Operationen. Z. Zahnärztl. Orthop. (München), *24*:76, 1932.

Spear, S. L., Mausner, M. E., and Kawamoto, H. K., Jr.: Sliding genioplasty as a local anesthetic outpatient procedure: a prospective two-center trial. Plast. Reconstr. Surg., *80*:55, 1987.

Spiessl, B.: Osteosynthese bei sagittaler Osteotomie nach Obwegeser/Dal Pont. *In* Schuchardt, K. (Ed.): Fortschritte der Kiefer- und Gesichtsschirugie. Stuttgart, Thieme/Verlag, 1974.

Spiessl, B.: The sagittal splitting osteotomy for correction of mandibular prognathism. Clin. Plast. Surg., *9*:491, 1982.

Steiner, C. C.: Cephalometrics for you and me. Am. J. Orthod., *39*:729, 1953.

Steiner, C. C.: Cephalometrics in clinical practice. Angle Orthod., *29*:8, 1959.

Steinhauser, E. W.: Free transportation of oral mucosa for improvement of denture retention. J. Oral Surg., *27*:955, 1969.

Steinhauser, E. W.: Vestibuloplasty-skin grafts. J. Oral Surg., *29*:777, 1971.

Steinhauser, E. W.: Midline splitting of the maxilla for correction of malocclusion. J. Oral Surg., *30*:413, 1972.

Steinhauser, E. W.: Advancement of the mandible by sagittal ramus split and suprahyoid myotomy. J. Oral Surg., *31*:516, 1973.

Steinhauser, E. W.: Variations of Le Fort II osteotomies for correction of midfacial deformities. J. Maxillofac. Surg., *8*:258, 1980.

Steinhauser, E. W. Bone screws and plates in orthognathic surgery. Int. J. Oral Surg., *11*:209, 1982.

Stirrups, D. R., Patton, D. W., and Moos, K. F.: A cephalometric analysis of the Le Fort II osteotomy in the non-cleft patient. J. Maxillofac. Surg., *14*:260, 1986.

Stoker, N. G., and Epker, B. N.: The posterior maxillary osteotomy: a retrospective study of treatment results. Int. J. Oral Surg., *3*:153, 1974.

Strauch, B., Bloomberg, A., and Lewin, M. L.: Artery island composite rib grafts for mandibular replacement. Surg. Forum, *20*:516, 1969.

Strauch, B., Bloomberg, A. E., and Lewin, M. L.: An experimental approach to mandibular replacement. Island vascular composite rib grafts. Br. J. Plast. Surg., *24*:334, 1971.

Stuteville, O. H.: Surgical reconstruction of the mandible. Plast. Reconstr. Surg., *19*:229, 1957.

Stuteville, O. H., and Lanfranchi, R. P.: Surgical reconstruction of the temporomandibular joint. Am. J. Surg., *90*:940, 1955.

Swanson, L. T., Habal, M. B., Leake, D. L., and Murray, J. E.: Compound silicone-bone implants for mandibular reconstruction: development and application. Plast. Reconstr. Surg., *51*:402, 1973.

Swartz, W. M., Banis, J. C., Newton, E. D., Ramasastry, S. S., Jones, N. F., and Acland, R.: The osteocutaneous scapular flap for mandibular and maxillary reconstruction. Plast. Reconstr. Surg., *77*:530, 1986.

Sykoff, V.: Zur Frage der Knocken-Plastic am Unterkiefer. Zentralbl. Chir., *27*:881, 1900.

Takagi, Y., Gamble, J. W., Proffit, W. R., and Christiansen, R. L.: Postural change of the hyoid bone following osteotomy of the mandible. Oral Surg., *23*:687, 1967.

Taylor, G. I., Miller, G. D., and Ham, F. J.: The free vascularized bone graft. A clinical extension of microvascular techniques. Plast. Reconstr. Surg., *55*:533, 1975.

Taylor, G. I., Townsend, P., and Corlett, R.: Superiority of the deep circumflex iliac vessels as the supply for free groin flaps. Clinical work. Plast. Reconstr. Surg., *64*:745, 1979.

Tessier, P.: Aesthetic aspects of bone grafting to the face. Clin. Plast. Surg., *8*:279, 1981.

Teuscher, U., and Sailer, H.: Stability of Le Fort I osteotomy in Class III cases with retropositioned maxillae. J. Maxillofac. Surg., *10*:80, 1982.

Thoma, K. H.: Oral Surgery, Vol. 2. St. Louis, MO., C. V. Mosby Company, 1948, p. 1438.

Thoma, K. H.: Oblique osteotomy of the mandibular ramus. Oral Surg., *14*:23, 1961.

Thompson, N., and Casson, J. A.: Experimental onlay bone grafts to the jaw—a preliminary study in dogs. Plast. Reconstr. Surg., *46*:341, 1970.

Toman, J.: Le traitement chirurgical de la progénie par la méthode d'inlay ostectomie. Rev. Stomatol., *67*:551, 1966.

Trauner, R.: Alveoloplasty with ridge extensions on the lingual side of the lower jaw to solve the problem of a lower dental prosthesis. J. Oral Surg., *5*:340, 1952.

Trauner, R.: The surgical correction of mandibular prognathism and retrognathia with consideration of genioplasty. Part II. Operating methods for microgenia and distoclusion. B. Distoclusion. Oral Surg., *10*:899, 1957.

Turvey, T. A.: Simultaneous mobilization of the maxilla and mandible: surgical technique and results. J. Oral Maxillofac. Surg., *40*:96, 1982.

Turvey, T. A.: Intraoperative complications of sagittal osteotomy of the mandibular ramus: incidence and management. J. Oral Maxillofac. Surg., *43*:509, 1985.

Turvey, T. A., Hall, D. J., and Warren, D. W.: Alterations in nasal airway resistance following superior repositioning of the maxilla. Am. J. Orthod., *85*:109, 1984.

Turvey, T. A., Journot, V., and Epker, B. N.: Correction of anterior open bite deformity: a study of tongue function, speech changes, and stability. J. Maxillofac. Surg., *4*:93, 1976.

Tweed, C. H.: The Frankfort-mandibular plane angle in orthodontic diagnosis, classification, treatment planning and prognosis. Am. J. Orthod., *32*:175, 1946.

Ullik, R.: Erweiterte Osteotomi des Oberkiefers. Osterr. Z. Stomatol., *4*:122, 1970.

Urist, M. R.: Surface decalcified allogenic implants. Clin. Orthrop., *56*:37, 1968.

Vannier, M., Marsh, J., and Warren, J.: Three-dimensional CT reconstruction images for craniofacial surgical planning and evaluation. Radiology, *150*:179, 1984.

Van Zile, W. N.: Triangular ostectomy of the vertical rami, another technique for correction of prognathism. Oral Surg., *21*:3, 1963.

von Eiselsberg, A.: Ueber Plastic bei Ectropium des Unterkiefers (Progenie). Wien. Klin. Wochenschr., *19*:1505, 1906.

Waldhart, E., and Lynch, J. B.: Benign hypertrophy of the masseter muscles and mandibular angles. Arch. Surg., *102*:115, 1971.

Waldron, C. W., and Risdon, R.: Mandibular bone grafts. Proc. R. Soc. Med., *12*:11, 1919.

Walsh, T. S., Jr.: Buried metallic prosthesis for mandibular defects. Cancer, *7*:1002, 1954.

Ward-Booth, R. P., Bhatia, S. N., and Moos, K. F.: A cephalometric analysis of the Le Fort II osteotomy in the adult cleft patient. J. Maxillofac. Surg., *12*:208, 1984.

Ware, W. A., and Taylor, R. C.: Condylar repositioning following osteotomies for correction of mandibular prognathism. Am. J. Orthod., *54*:50, 1968.

Ware, W. H., and Ashamalla, M.: Pulpal response following anterior maxillary osteotomy. Am. J. Orthod., *60*:156, 1971.

Warren, D. W.: Velopharyngeal orifice size and upper pharyngeal pressure-flow patterns in normal speech. Plast. Reconstr. Surg., *33*:148, 1964.

Warren, D. W., and Ryan, V. E.: Oral port constriction, nasal resistance, and respiratory aspects of cleft palate speech: an analog study. Cleft Palate J., *4*:38, 1967.

Wassmund, M.: Fracturen und Luxationen des Gesichtschadels unter Beruksichtigung der Komplikationen des Hirnschadesl. *In* Klinik und Therapie. Praktischen Lehrbuch. Vol. 20. Berlin, Hermann Meusser, 1927, p. 384.

Wassmund, M.: Lehrbuch der praktischen Chirurgie des Mundes und der Kiefer. Berlin, Hermann Meusser, 1935.

Weber, J., Jr., Chase, R. A., and Jobe, R. P.: The restrictive pharyngeal flap. Br. J. Plast. Surg., *23*:347, 1970.

West, R. A., and Epker, B. N.: Posterior maxillary surgery; its place in the treatment of dentofacial deformities. J. Oral Surg., *30*:562, 1972.

West, R. A., and McNeill, R. W.: Diagnosis and treatment planning: a coordinated effort between oral and maxillofacial surgery and orthodontics. J. Oral Surg., *39*:809, 1981.

White, R. P., Peters, P. B., Costich, E. R., and Page, H. L.: Evaluation of sagittal split-ramus osteotomy in 17 patients. J. Oral Surg., *27*:851, 1969.

White, S.: The employment of silver wire to bridge the gap after resection of a portion of the lower jaw. Br. Med. J., *2*:1525, 1909.

Wilbanks, J. L.: Correction of mandibular prognathism by double-oblique intraoral osteotomy: a new technique. Oral Surg., *31*:321, 1971.

Wildt: Über partielle Unterkieferresektion und Bildung einer natürlichen Prothese durch Knochentransplantion. Zentralbl. Chir., *23*:1177, 1896.

Wilhelm, W.: The surgical treatment of prognathism of the maxilla. Bol. Odontol., *20*:146, 1954.

Willmar, K.: On Le Fort I osteotomy. A follow-up study of 106 operated patients with maxillo-facial deformity. Scand. J. Plast. Reconstr. Surg., Suppl. 12, 1974.

Willmar, K.: Personal communication, 1976.

Willmar, K., Hogeman, K.-E., and Thiésus, S.: Sagittal split osteotomy in our experience: a follow-up study of 100 operated patients. Scand. J. Plast. Reconstr. Surg., *13*:445, 1979.

Wilmott, D. R.: Soft tissue profile changes following correction of class III malocclusions by mandibular surgery. Br. J. Orthod., *8*:175, 1981.

Wilson, P. D.: Experiences with a bone bank. Ann. Surg., *210*:932, 1948.

Winstanley, R. P.: Subcondylar osteotomy of the mandible and the intra-oral approach. Br. J. Oral Surg., *6*:134, 1968.

Witzel, M. A., and Munro, I. R.: Velopharyngeal insufficiency after maxillary advancement. Cleft Palate J., *14*:176, 1977.

Witzel, M. A., Munro, I. R., Ross, R. B., and Huang, S.: The effect of maxillary advancement on velopharyngeal function. Transactions of the Seventh International Congress of Plastic and Reconstructive Surgeons, Montreal, 1983.

Wolhynski, F. A.: Qualitative und quantitative Struklurveranderung de M. masseter des Menschen. Anat. Anz., *82*:260, 1936.

Wunderer, S.: Die Prognathieoperation mittels frontal gestieltem Maxilla Fragment. Osterr. Z. Stomatol., *39*:98, 1962.

Young, R. A., and Epker, B.: The anterior maxillary ostectomy: a retrospective evaluation of sinus health, patient acceptance, and relapses. J. Oral Surg., *30*:69, 1972.

Zallen, R. D., and Strader, R. J.: The use of prophylactic antibiotics in extraoral procedures of mandibular prognathism. J. Oral Surg., *29*:178, 1971.

Zide, B. M., Grayson, B., and McCarthy, J. G.: Cephalometric analysis: Part I. Plast. Reconstr. Surg., *68*:816, 1981a.

Zide, B. M., Grayson, B., and McCarthy, J. G.: Cephalometric analysis for upper and lower midface surgery: Part II. Plast. Reconstr. Surg., *68*:961, 1981b.

Zide, B. M., Grayson, B., and McCarthy, J. G.: Cephalometric analysis for mandibular surgery: Part III. Plast. Reconstr. Surg., *69*:155, 1982.

Zide, B. M., and McCarthy, J.: The mentalis muscle: an essential component of chin and lower lip position. Plast. Reconstr. Surg., *83*:413, 1989.

30

Barry M. Zide

The Temporomandibular Joint

ANATOMY

TEMPOROMANDIBULAR JOINT DYSFUNCTION
- Muscular Problems
- Capsular and Ligamentous Problems
- Internal Derangement
- Condylar Dislocations

DEVELOPMENTAL ABNORMALITIES

ANKYLOSIS

FRACTURES OF THE CONDYLE

ARTHRITIS

RADIOGRAPHIC STUDY

SURGICAL APPROACH

The temporomandibular joint (TMJ) afflictions fall within the province of numerous specialists, each with his own special interest. When pain is involved, the dilemma of making the correct diagnosis arises. Although some clinicians propose emotional stress as a key etiologic factor in causing muscle imbalance, others point to dental occlusion or intrinsic joint dysfunction. The tendency is to try to give one simple explanation for all the symptoms. The signs and symptoms vary greatly among the patients. This chapter aims to provide the clinician with a basic understanding of TMJ problems that will allow him to deal with these patients in a knowledgeable way. The management of fractures, ankylosis, arthritis, and hyperplasia is also presented.

ANATOMY

The condyle of the mandible articulates with the squamous portion of the temporal bone at the TMJ (Fig. 30–1).

This freely mobile synovial joint has certain functionally adapted anatomic features that distinguish it from other bodily joints. The bone surfaces are covered by fibrocartilage, i.e., an avascular fibrous connective tissue that contains cartilage cells. Moreover, certain movements of this joint are determined by the teeth, which are firmly imbedded within the bone of the two articulating complexes. The right and left articulations must function together. The meniscus, or articular disc, is interposed between the condyle and the temporal bone, separating the joint spaces into upper and lower divisions. As the jaw opens, the condyle first rotates as a hinge and then translates or glides forward and down the articular eminence (Fig. 30–2).

The condyle has a relatively elliptic shape, and each side is not exactly the same. In the mediolateral dimension the condyle measures almost 2 cm, but only about 1 cm in the anteroposterior plane. The concave articular fossa, i.e., the articulating surface of the temporal bone, has the following relations. The anterior wall of the glenoid fossa is formed by the posterior slope of the articular eminence. During translation, the condyle rides down this path. Posteriorly the tympanic bone and superiorly the thin squamous temporal bone form most of the fossa. This thin temporal bone is occasionally fractured, allowing displacement of the condyle superiorly into the middle cranial fossa (Zecha, 1977; Ihalainen and Tasanen, 1983).

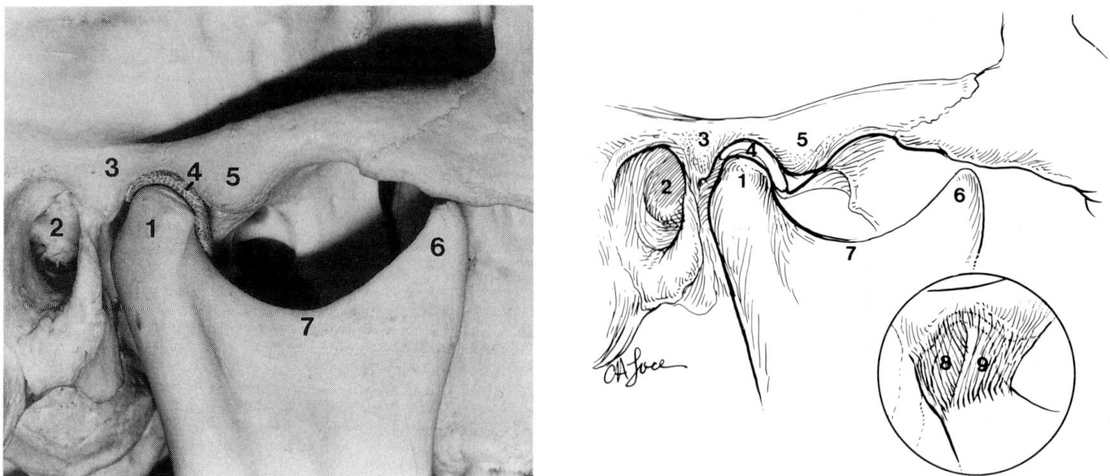

Figure 30–1. Temporomandibular joint anatomy. *1,* Mandibular condyle. *2,* External auditory canal. *3,* Zygomatic portion of temporal bone. *4,* Meniscus (artificial). *5,* Articular eminence. *6,* Coronoid process. *7,* Sigmoid notch. *8,* (Posterior) capsule. *9,* (Anterior) TM ligament.

On the lateral aspect the TMJ structures are protected by a capsule that is attached superiorly to the lower edge of the posterior zygomatic process of the temporal bone. This capsule tapers prior to its attachment on the condylar neck. Posteriorly the capsule extends from the tympanic plate to the posterior condyle. The capsule fuses with the meniscus along the entire lateral edge close to the condylar attachment. The portion of the capsule that thickens laterally and anteriorly has been termed the TMJ ligament (see Fig. 30–1). It is clinically important that after the usual condylar fracture, the condylar head is displaced medially. Therapeutic early movement and limited intermaxillary fixation time may allow the condylar head to upright itself. If the condylar head is displaced laterally (a rare finding), the head may be forced through the TMJ capsule, in which case the

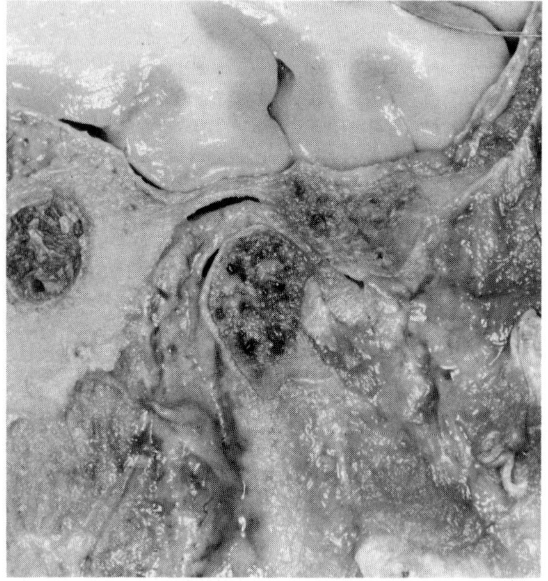

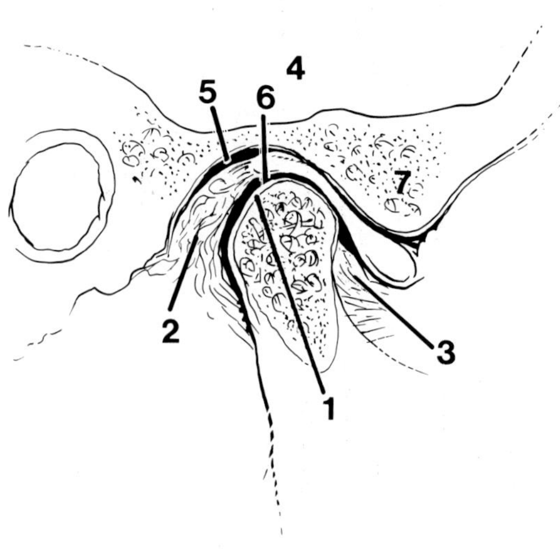

Figure 30–2. Temporomandibular joint anatomy. *1,* Fibrocartilaginous condylar cap. *2,* Highly innervated and vascular bilaminar zone. *3,* Inferior head of lateral pterygoid muscle. *4,* Middle cranial fossa. *5,* Superior joint space. *6,* Inferior joint space. *7,* Articular eminence.

head cannot right itself. The situation is demonstrable by CT scan and requires open reduction.

Between the head of the condyle and the temporal bone, the firm but flexible meniscus or articular disc acts as a shock absorber. This avascular, noninnervated fibrous sheet with a few cartilage cells consists of a thinner central zone, the pars gracilis, with thickening posteriorly and anteriorly. The anterior projection, the pes meniscus or anterior band, is attached superiorly to the articular eminence and to the superior belly of the lateral pterygoid. Inferiorly this structure attaches to the condyle via a synovial membrane along the superior margin of attachment of the inferior head of the lateral pterygoid muscle.

As the upper surface of the disc is uniquely contoured to the shape of the fossa and posterior slope of the articular eminence, the lower surface contours itself to the shape of the mandibular condyle.

In the posterior aspect the thickened disc or posterior band is confluent with highly innervated and vascularized tissue, which has been termed the bilaminar zone or retromeniscal pad (Fig. 30–2). The bilaminar zone consists of two layers of fibers separated by loose connective tissue. The upper layer attaches to the tympanic plate of the temporal bone, while the lower stratum proceeds from the posterior meniscus to the neck of the condyle. Although this posterior attachment provides considerable *anterior* freedom of movement for the meniscus, it cannot tolerate any pressure itself.

In the anteromedial direction the superior head of the external pterygoid muscle is attached to the disc. The lateral pterygoid muscle consists of two heads that function independently (Grant, 1973; McNamara, 1973; Juniper, 1981). The larger inferior head inserts into the anterior aspect of the condyle and assists in mouth opening in conjunction with the suprahyoid muscles. The muscle pull of the inferior head is obliquely downward to move the chin to the opposite side. The belly of the lateral pterygoid is inactive during closing.

The smaller superior head, which pulls obliquely upward, is active only during closing. It attaches to the joint capsule and disc along the medial two-thirds of the anterior border. The superior head contributes to joint stability by directing the condylar head against the back slope of the eminence during closing. During mastication and swallowing, the superior head braces the meniscus and condylar head against the posterior slope. Anterolaterally and laterally the disc is attached to the joint capsule. Medially the discal attachment occurs firmly on the condyle.

The meniscus and its attachments divide the TMJ into the upper and lower joint spaces (Dolwick and associates, 1983) (Fig. 30–3). The upper joint space spans the glenoid fossa to the articular eminence and extends farther anteriorly than the lower joint space. The lower joint space proceeds from just above the insertion of the lateral pterygoid muscle anteriorly and then spreads over the condyle. The volume of each space is small, approximately 1 ml for the upper and 0.50 ml for the lower space.

The blood supply arises both from the superficial temporal vessels and from branches of the masseteric artery, a derivative of the internal maxillary (Boyer, Williams, and Stevens, 1964). The masseteric branches pass through the sigmoid notch of the mandible. The nerve supply is derived from the mandibular division of the trigeminal, specifically, the auriculotemporal, masseteric, and deep temporal branches.

Condylar Action

The motion of the condyle combines an initial rotation (hinge) movement followed by a translation (glide). During opening, a pure *rotation* occurs around a horizontal axis through the condylar heads. The meniscus and condyle then function together in the second gliding or *translational* movement.

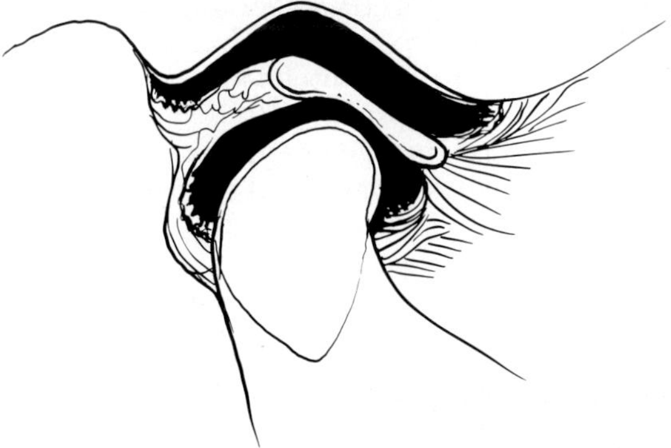

Figure 30–3. The meniscus and its attachments separate the joint into upper and lower joint spaces. Dye is usually injected into the lower joint space in performing an arthrogram.

When the teeth are in occlusion, the thicker, more vascular posterior band of the meniscus covers the superior portions of the condyle. During rotation, the posterior band becomes slightly more posterior. As the condyles begin the translational movement, the midzone of the meniscus articulates between the articular eminence and the condylar head. The condyle slides down the articular eminence during the full translation. The head may rotate under the anterior band of the meniscus.

The posterior attachment of the meniscus, i.e., the bilaminar zone, fills with blood to increase in size when the condyles move anteriorly within the fossa. Thus, the space left by the condylar repositioning becomes occupied. The blood empties during closure or retrusive movement of the condyle.

TEMPOROMANDIBULAR JOINT DYSFUNCTION

A pathologist in medical school once told the author, "You cannot diagnose beyond your realm of thought." By this statement he meant that many diagnostic errors are caused not by making the wrong diagnosis but by not knowing the possible diagnoses. For this reason, this section is included to describe certain unusual conditions that are neither developmental nor indicative of a disease state. They are acquired dysfunctions that may present as pain in and around the TMJ.

1. Muscular problems.
   a. Myalgia from grinding (bruxism) or malocclusion.
   b. Muscular incoordination.
   c. Masseter parotid hypertrophy.
   d. Intramuscular pathology.
2. Capsular or ligamentous problems.
   a. Posterior capsulitis.
   b. Loose or sprained capsular ligaments.
   c. Traumatized external capsular ligaments.
3. Internal derangement.
4. Condylar dislocations: acute and chronic.

Muscular Problems

MYALGIA FROM GRINDING OR MALOCCLUSION

Patients who grind their teeth tend to do so in a lateral or protrusive position. This motion causes wear facets on the teeth, frequently associated with muscle spasm of the lateral pterygoid or posterior deep fibers of the masseter. Night grinders wake up with pain primarily in the muscles used for bruxing. As a rule, pain from eccentric bruxism occurs in the muscle that causes the jaw to move toward the position of the facet. For example, a wear facet on the right cuspid (canine) might require movement by the left lateral pterygoid, which would be tender by intraoral palpation. Treatment involves occlusal equilibration to round off and reduce the wear facets to produce equal contacts of other teeth during the same excursive movement.

As stated, the lateral pterygoids are frequently in spasm or are hypertonic as they attempt to hold the disc properly. When the mandible is thrust backward, the patient will complain of pain in front of the condyle. The maneuver may assist evaluation.

For years, excessive emphasis was placed on malocclusion as the prime cause of TMJ problems. Dentists tried to equilibrate the occlusion of people whose teeth just did not fit properly. Repeated adjustments were frustrating and patients became neurotic about their "bite." In most cases, failure to adjust properly was due to the fact that the disc was displaced anteriorly, but this finding went unnoticed for years. Dentists aimed to make centric occlusion (maximal intercuspation of teeth) coincident with centric relation (the most posterior position of the condyle). Undoubtedly this type of occlusal adjustment merely aggravated the problem by pushing the condyle even more posteriorly. The symptoms were therefore perpetuated.

MUSCULAR INCOORDINATION

A small group of patients protrude the jaw during speech and opening. Pain may be a presenting symptom and the clinician should note any evidence of excessive anterior movement during the interview and examination. Simple exercises to keep the mandible in the hinge position may help.

MASSETER PAROTID HYPERTROPHY

Patients occasionally present with bilateral masseter pain from overuse. They may be gum chewers or have an idiopathic hypertrophy on one or both sides. Such hypertrophy can be caused by excessive bruxism; the muscle excess may at times block salivary flow through the parotid duct, leading to swelling and even infection of the parotid gland. Associated with the masseteric hypertrophy, the gonial angle may be flared outward. Surgical correction may be performed by an intraoral route to reduce the bony excess and debulk some of the masseter muscle.

INTRAMUSCULAR PATHOLOGY

Acute trismus may be caused by injury to any of the masticatory muscles. Anesthetic block injections through the internal (medial) pterygoid muscle may cause acute bleeding within the muscle. The patient will have pain during opening, which subsides over a week or two with a simple jaw exercise regimen. This represents an acute myositis.

On occasion the elevator muscles can suffer an injury that does not subside rapidly. This type of chronic problem is due to a localized or diffuse fibrosis within one or more muscles. If marked fibrosis occurs within the muscle, *opening is severely limited, usually 8 to 20 mm.* With disc dislocations the opening is usually 22 to 28 mm. In addition, with elevator muscle "myofibrositis," *lateral movements are usually unaffected.* The joint spaces also appear normal on transcranial or tomographic x-rays.

Treatment consists of heating pad, progressive exercises, and occasionally injections of a lidocaine/steroid solution directly into the area of pain. The injections create more pain for several days, which then subsides. Some patients may in fact require muscle release, which is done by an intraoral approach (Minami, 1981). The jaw may appear osteoporotic from nonuse.

Occasionally a single traumatic episode or multiple minor injuries result in pain and trismus. In these cases one may palpate a firm mass, usually in the masseter muscle. The diagnosis of myositis ossificans may be made by radiographic study. The lesion should be removed (Arima, Shiba, and Hayashi, 1984).

Capsular and Ligamentous Problems

POSTERIOR CAPSULITIS

Posterior capsulitis has also been called intracapsular edema or retrodiscitis. The tissues posterior to the disc are comprised of the posterior superior and posterior inferior disc attachments, i.e., the bilaminar zone, and the posterior capsular ligament (see Figs. 30–2 and 30–3). These tissues are well innervated with considerable vascularity and lymphatic drainage. Acute injury, inflammation, or infection causes the retrodiscal structures to become inflamed and edematous. The signs and symptoms relative to this are directly proportional to the edema, which proportionately causes anterior displacement of the condyle (Fig. 30–4) and a posterior open bite.

The lateral pterygoid muscle that equilibrates the position of the disc and condyle may become spastic or hypertonic as a result of the constant traction required to prevent this pressure against the inflamed posterior tissues. This aggravates the problem.

The problem represents a common early complaint of patients who later present with definite joint derangements. Many of these patients may receive either intrinsic or extrinsic jaw trauma (e.g., occlusal trauma vs. a fall on the chin) or suffer inflammation from any of the arthritides or infection as the inciting cause. Owing to the swelling in the posterior joint structures, the mandibular midline is deviated away from the affected side even at rest. This may not be very noticeable. However, as the jaw opens, the mandible tends to deviate toward the affected side, which becomes quite obvious at maximal opening. This occurs because the condyle cannot glide and stretch the inflamed bilaminar zone. A similar type of opening is observed in acute dislocation of the disc, i.e., deviation toward the affected side with opening. With disc dislocation the cause is the disc lying anterior to the condyle.

Two simple physical tests may be used to make the diagnosis of posterior capsulitis (Fig. 30–4*B*, *C*).

Test 1: The examiner grasps the patient's chin and, with the patient's help, moves the jaw from side to side. When he has moved the jaw slightly toward the affected side, the clinician suddenly pushes the chin backward, forcing the condyle posteriorly also. The patient is asked to point to the area of maximal pain. Pain in front of the ear or over the joint helps the diagnosis. However, if the pain is anterior to the joint, the clinician should consider myalgia of the spastic lateral pterygoid, most often caused by irregular dental contacts.

Test 2: A cotton roll or tongue blades are

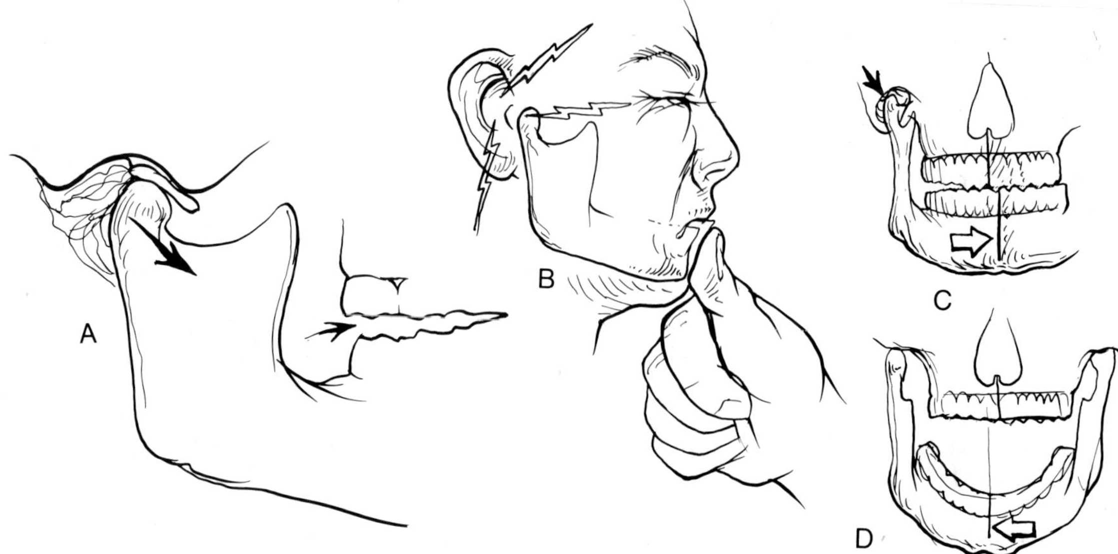

Figure 30–4. Posterior capsulitis. *A,* When the retromeniscal pad becomes inflamed, the swelling displaces the jaw downward, giving the patient a posterior open bite. The patient may state that his teeth do not meet. *B,* Anterior pressure applied toward the affected side produces pain. *C,* The midline is slightly shifted on closing. *D,* On opening, the jaw's motion is restricted on the affected side owing to pain, and thus it deviates off the midline.

placed in the canine-bicuspid region on the opposite side. The patient is asked to bite quickly and firmly on the object. The opposite side biting thrust will torque the condyle backward on the affected side, causing considerable pain. The patient is asked to point to the area of discomfort. *Note:* Do not attempt this test more than once in the presence of pain. The patient will not appreciate it.

Transcranial or tomographic radiographs demonstrate an anteriorly displaced condyle at closed position. The space behind the condyle is increased. During maximal opening, translation of the condylar head is limited slightly on the affected side and the difference is easily noted in comparing sides.

If there is a history of arthritis or infection, the appropriate tests should be arranged, such as complete blood count, uric acid, sedimentation rate, and rheumatoid arthritis factor. These should be ordered after fabrication of a repositioning appliance that allows for mandibular closure in a more anterior position. If the pain persists even after insertion of the appliance and there is suspicion of infection or arthritis, one should embark on the laboratory work-up.

LOOSE OR SPRAINED CAPSULAR LIGAMENTS

Sprained capsular ligaments heal after two to three weeks. The causes may be intrinsic (e.g., malocclusion) or extrinsic trauma. The key diagnostic test is the presence of pain provoked by light pressure over the lateral aspect of the joint. Since the situation is self-limiting, a splint is not provided. The patient is provided with analgesics and a soft food regimen, and a reappointment in two to three weeks is scheduled.

If the same severe occlusal irregularities that cause the signs of acute sprain become chronic, stretching of the capsular ligaments may occur. With *loose capsular ligaments* the patient may be able to open excessively, i.e., more than 54 mm, with predisposition to disc displacement and its associated clicking or locking. The patient requires slow occlusal equilibration, preceded by the fabrication of a bite plate to reduce the pain.

TRAUMATIZED EXTERNAL CAPSULAR LIGAMENTS

The patient usually provides the history of some event, such as surgical dissection of the facial nerve. The transcranial radiograph shows a normal joint with limited motion during the opening phase. Tests for posterior capsulitis and sprained lateral ligaments are negative. The mandible deviates toward the affected side.

For therapy, bite opening regimens, along with analgesics, are required. Commonly used regimens for increasing opening in such

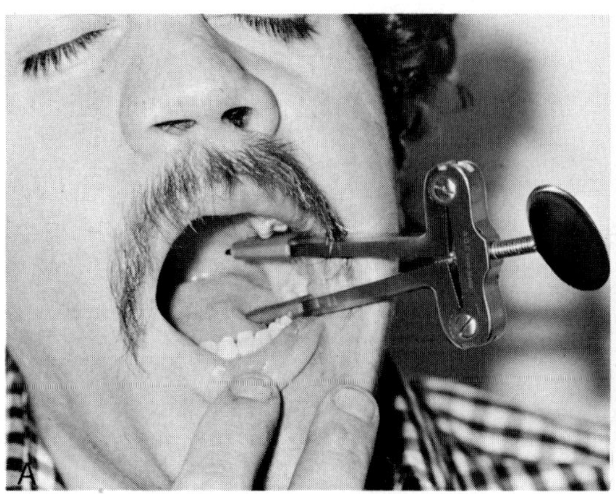

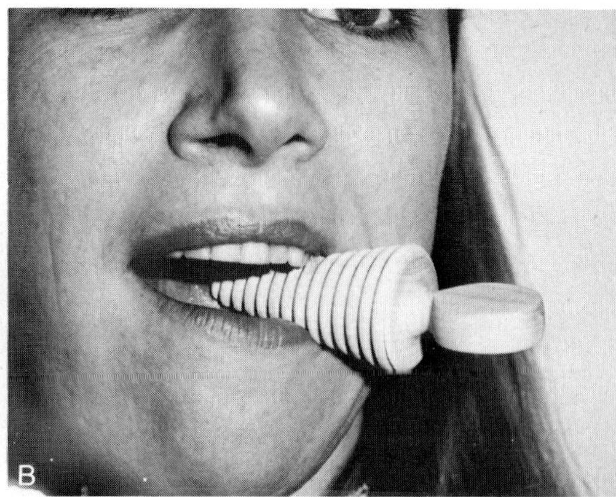

Figure 30–5. Trismus assistance. *A,* The Heister mouth prop is straight bladed or curved. The ends must be taped or covered with rubber tubing. This device works well after removal of intermaxillary fixation or after ankylosis surgery. *B,* The oral screw comes small or large in wood or plastic. This device works well in the earlier phases of treatment.

types of trismus are the oral screw, tongue blades, and the Heister mouth prop (Fig. 30–5). These devices may be required for many months.

Internal Derangement

The usual (98 per cent) internal derangement consists of an anterior disc displacement associated with a posterior-superior displacement of the condyle in the closed jaw position (Isbert-Holm and Westesson, 1980). However, in about 2 per cent of cases, the disc may be anteriorly displaced, but the condyle is undisplaced even while in occlusion. In all cases, therefore, an abnormal relationship exists between the disc and the condyle, fossa, and articular eminence.

ABNORMAL ANATOMY

Autopsy studies have noted a common finding (Blackwood, 1964; Dolwick and associates, 1983), namely, anterior displacement of the meniscus with attenuation of the posterior attachment tissues, and occasional tearing of the posterior attachment. Meniscus thickness varies considerably. Owing to the anterior disc displacement, the lower joint space extends farther anteriorly than normal. This finding may be noted on an arthrogram when dye is injected into the space. In fact, the anterior extent of the lower joint space is directly proportional to the amount of meniscus displacement. The lower border of the posterior band of the meniscus may present as a concavity into the lower joint space in front of the condyle.

When the disc is improperly positioned, the mandible functions improperly. Usually the first sign of mandibular dysfunction is the *reciprocal click* (Helms, Katzberg and Dolwick, 1983) (Fig. 30–6). This term refers to an opening click followed by a closing click. During opening in these cases, the condyle is not seated properly below the disc. The thickened posterior band, seated anterior to the condyle, is pushed first. Normally the head of the condyle would be rotating under the thin intermediate zone of the disc. The opening click occurs when the condyle quickly shifts under the posterior band into the intermediate area. The tightness or laxity of the posterior attachment determines when the click will sound. A looser bilaminar zone allows more anterior disc displacement, and this would provide a later opening click. Similarly the closing click occurs as the condyle slips behind the posterior band, allowing the meniscus to displace anteriorly again.

If the meniscus never slips over the condyle and remains anterior to it throughout the opening and closing cycle, the condition is called a *closed lock.* The dislocated meniscus is not *captured* or *reduced* by the condyle and acts to obstruct the opening of the mandible. The mandible deviates toward the impeded side during opening.

Chronic mandibular function against the highly vascularized and innervated posterior attachment tissue may result in severe pain. If these tissues are finally perforated, *crepitus* may occur within the joint because of bone rubbing against bone. When the disc is nonreducible or if a bone to bone situation develops, the condyle may begin to undergo the changes associated with degenerative joint

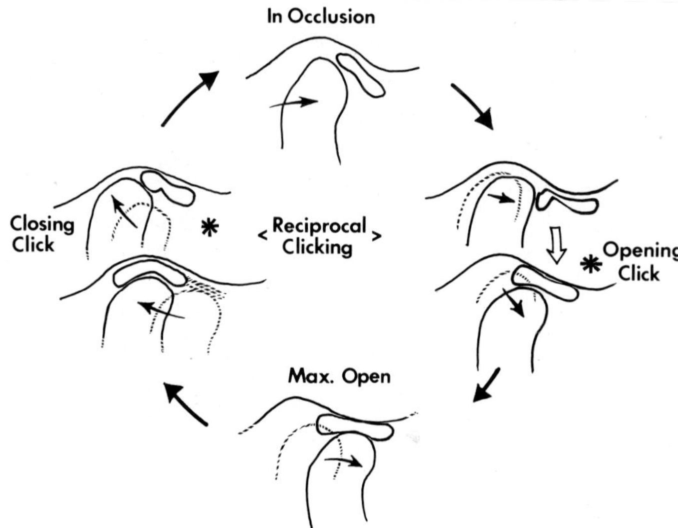

Figure 30–6. Anterior disc displacement predisposes the patient to reciprocal clicking, i.e., an opening *and* closing click. This is never innocuous and predisposes the patient to degenerative joint disease.

disease (see p. 1498). Since painful clicking is an important sign of early joint disease, crepitus distinctly points to evidence of advanced degenerative arthritis. Incidentally, an occasional transmission of sound from one side to another may occur and cause confusion in the more common clinical setting.

Clinical Presentation and Patient Evaluation. The surgeon who evaluates TMJ problems must be willing not to operate much more frequently than to operate. In fact, the conservative approach is more rewarding 90 per cent or more of the time (Bessette and associates, 1985; Farrar and McCarty, 1982). The key to proper diagnosis rests with the clinician, who must become part anatomist, radiologist, psychologist, neurologist, otolaryngologist, and full-time friend or teacher to a patient with a problem. Many questions remain to be answered. The plight of the patient is often to be misdiagnosed and mistreated by those who are unwilling to take the necessary step to unravel the true problem. The following protocol offers a rational approach to diagnosis and treatment of internal derangements.

Although a verbal interchange is critical with the patients, a questionnaire is also very helpful. The patient is given enough time and space to answer questions briefly and quietly in an unstressed environment (Table 30–1). Of course, a complete medical history is *always* taken.

History. The presence of pain and dysfunction in or around the TMJ does not de facto pinpoint the problem. The more common complaints of patients with internal derangements are: "My jaw locks," "I can't chew or eat," or "I have painful clicking." These statements can be associated with neuromuscular (myofascial) disorders alone or also with an internal derangement. The clinician must keep an open mind. The only pathognomonic sign of internal derangement is *reciprocal clicking,* i.e., an opening (protrusive) click followed by a closing (retrusive) click that *does not occur at exactly the same time.* This is due to the variance in stretch between the anterior and posterior disc retaining structures.

The patient may report a headache of some type and describe its onset, duration, and intensity. Farrar and McCarty (1979b) reported that retro-orbital headaches represent the most common sign in internal derangement. Although no specific diagnostic pattern of headache pain exists, the clinician should ask the patient to localize the areas of discomfort before the physical examination. This can be helpful, especially if a definite relationship exists between the headache and jaw use. The patient, for example, may point to the temporal area. An anteriorly displaced disc with malposition of the condyle (and thus the ramus) may place abnormal stress on the more horizontal fibers of the temporal muscle when the patient attempts to position his jaw properly (Fig. 30–7).

An earache is never diagnostic either, although vertigo, tinnitus, and even decreased hearing acuity have been reported (Myrhaug, 1969).

The patient should be asked about associated psychologic stresses or emotional factors

Table 30–1. TMJ Questionnaire

1. Do you have headaches? ________ Temple? ________ Neck pain? ________ Jaw pain? ________ Ear pain? ____
   Eye pain? ________ Other? ________
2. Exactly where is the pain? ________
   Right? ________ Left? ________ Both? ________
3. How long have you had these symptoms? ________
4. Do you recall any associated event(s) that may have brought on this problem? ________
5. Describe the pain (e.g., constant, aching, shooting, burning, etc.). ________
6. When is the pain worse? Morning? ________ Evening? ________ After chewing? ________ On opening? ________
   During chewing? ________
7. What major dental work or problems have you had? ________
   Extractions? ________ Orthodontic retainer? ________ Bridgework? ________ Bite off? ________
8. Does your jaw make any noise (or did it)? ________
   Clicking? ________ Grinding? ________ Other? ________
9. Does your jaw ever "lock" or slip out? ________
10. Do you clench or grind your teeth? ________ When? ________
11. Do you have any problems with your ears? ________ Hearing? ________ Dizziness? ________
12. Any pain or difficulty swallowing? ________
13. Note all previous therapy (including splinting, medicine, x-rays, etc.) and names of doctors. ________
14. Describe this problem in your own words (use back of sheet if required). ________

that might be contributing to the problem. The referring physician or dentist often comments that the patient is tense or "high strung," a common finding in those with myofascial pain dysfunction (MPD). The patient may be clenching his teeth at night in response to emotional trauma, which makes him awaken in pain in the morning. The masticatory muscles are the focus of discomfort in such a situation, and the surgeon must palpate the muscles individually (pterygoids, masseters, and temporal muscles). Diagnostic injections of local anesthetic solution may be made directly into the painful area. Muscle complaints, however, need not be localized to the face. Patients frequently complain of neck, shoulder, arm, or even chest muscle spasm. Antispastic medication and physical therapy may be required, and in fact some therapists actually specialize in "craniomandibular" treatment.

Direct questioning to determine the exact mode of onset is helpful in pinpointing the original traumatic episode. Often the cause seems relatively mild, i.e., a dental appointment during which the mouth was held open for a long time, biting on an unexpected piece of bone or fish claw, or even a forced yawn. Third molar extraction, tonsillectomy, and endoscopy performed with jaw hyperextension have been implicated. Some patients have forcefully bumped their chins in accidents three to six months before the onset of pain. Since all the radiographs were negative for fracture and the occlusion was normal, such patients were released. Pain began to

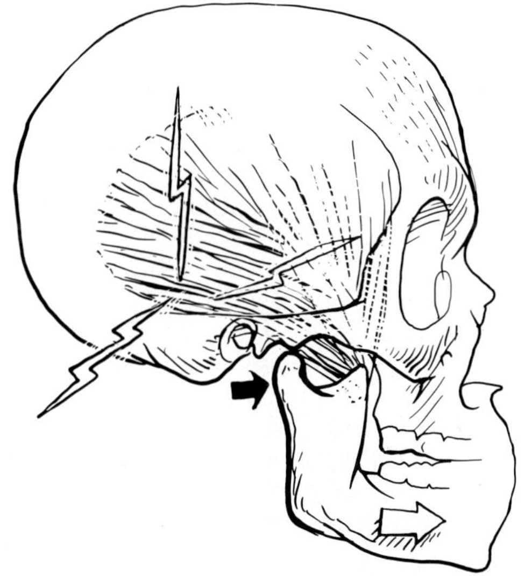

Figure 30–7. The patient whose disc is displaced anteriorly may attempt to reposition his condyle appropriately under the disc. This minor change may stretch the more horizontal temporalis muscle fibers. The patient thus complains of supra-auricular or postauricular headache.

occur in the joint region, with obvious clicking three to six months *after* injury.

Although the examiner must ask whether "the bite is off," malocclusion rarely aids the specific diagnosis of internal derangement. The examiner should enquire about and examine for the absence of posterior teeth or a posterior bite collapse, since such conditions allow the condyle to retroposition, a precondition for internal derangement. The presence of prognathism, long face syndrome, and especially open bite conditions are often found in conjunction with TMJ problems. These should preferably be corrected before or immediately after any arthroplastic surgery to maintain a stable joint.

The patient often may have recently concluded orthodontic banding and may be wearing an anterior retainer. As the posterior teeth settle, the lower anterior teeth may occlude heavily on the lingual of the upper anterior teeth. This may cause condylar retropositioning, and thus initiate disc displacement (McCarty, 1980). Thus, the orthodontic history is important. The author frequently sees patients who have worn braces for inordinately long periods in an attempt to correct obvious major orthognathic problems. The parents may have tried to "save" their children from surgery, but just as often the orthodontist was reluctant to refer the case to the surgeon. The patient presents with an unstable occlusion and joint pain.

Pain and tenderness associated with internal derangements are usually located in front of the ear or over the joint region. Such pain is relatively constant, occurring primarily with jaw use and thus joint motion. The joint is often tender to palpation or to placement of a finger into the external acoustic canal. The muscles of mastication, masseter and temporalis, can also be tender as a result of coincident spasm. The clinician should understand that, since jaw motion is precise and occurs in synchrony with the opposite side, muscle dysfunction and thus pain may also occur on the opposite side.

Clinical Examination. In many cases the patient accurately describes his problem and the diagnosis seems relatively obvious. The clinical examination may corroborate the clinician's initial impression. More than one-third of patients referred for "TMJ problems" require only one office visit and leave with mild analgesics, a jaw exercise regimen, or even reassurance that the condition is not cancer related. Nevertheless, the clinician must always be dubious of his own diagnoses. He must be wary of patients who blame another clinician who may have caused a ligamentous strain when previous symptoms may have existed. There is also the tendency to overinterpret mild malocclusions. More tests cannot replace sound clinical judgment. The following is a list of critical *clinical* data required to study such patients.

1. Joint noise.
   a. Click.
   b. Crepitus.
2. Limited range of motion.
   a. Diminished opening.
   b. Diminished lateral movement.

The *click* may act as a dubious diagnostic element in TMJ evaluation. Farrar and McCarty (1982) suggested that 70 per cent of all patients with TMJ symptoms have some form of disc displacement. The mere presence of a click provides little information. Consider two situations. In the first, the superior belly of the lateral pterygoid muscle could be holding the disc anteriorly owing to spasm. Treatment directed at spasm reduction, such as splinting, may eliminate the clicking. In the second case, the disc may be displaced as a result of injury to the retrodiscal pad. This could be irreversible, unlike the former case. Forty per cent of the normal population may have some evidence of clicking during function (Agerberg and Carlsson, 1975). No one knows what happens to those joints in ten years. No one knows whether painless clicks require treatment or whether they will cause further deterioration in the TMJ apparatus, in the form of degenerative arthritis. However, we know that some clicks are worse than others and that painful reciprocal clicking should be treated.

If a patient clicks, one should ask about associated pain with clicking, the number of clicks, their loudness, and the consistency of timing. During reciprocal clicking, the disc is anteriorly positioned. As opening begins and the condyle translates forward, the posterior band of the articular disc bunches up (Fig. 30–8) in front of the condyle until the click occurs. The condyle moves forward under the thick posterior band, which snaps back. The rest of the translation proceeds in a normal fashion. During the closing phase, disc and condyle position are normal until the end of the retrusive movement. As the closing click occurs, the condyle is suddenly displaced pos-

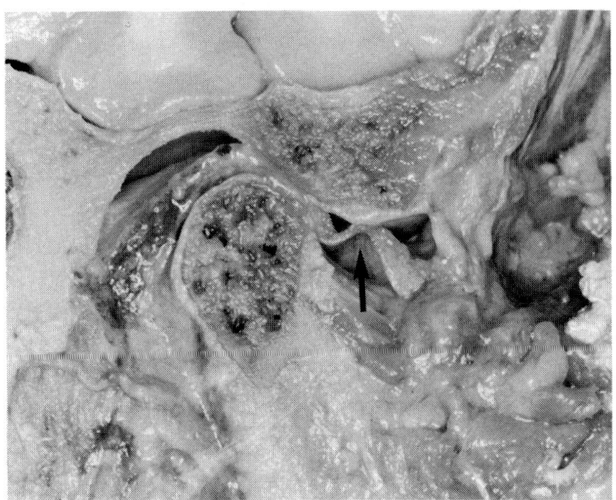

Figure 30–8. When the disc is displaced, the condyle must click and "capture" to achieve proper position. Note the folded disc. Dye injected into the lower joint space would demonstrate this "beaking" (*arrow*), a finding pathognomonic of internal derangement of this type.

terosuperiorly and the disc is displaced anteriorly. Opening clicks are usually more pronounced than the closing click. As previously stated, with internal derangements the opening and closing clicks never occur at the same time (see Fig. 30–6). As the derangement becomes more severe, i.e., with continued stretching of the retromeniscal pad, the opening click occurs later and later. Finally, as the disc becomes lodged in front of the condyle, the click stops completely.

The normal mandibular opening is measured from incisal edge to incisal edge, and the overbite (approximately 2 mm) is included. This measures 40 to 56 mm in the normal individual. If one draws a thin vertical line or dot at midchin and another in the mid–upper lip, deviation off the midline can be noted during opening. As an aid, a clear millimeter ruler can be held between the dots (Fig. 30–9) during the opening. Mandibular deviation off the midline may be noted. Usually the jaw deviates toward the side of the click until the sound occurs, whereupon it shifts back to the midline.

The opening click (anterior dislocation with reduction) may be defined generally as early, intermediate, or late, depending on the amount of dislocation. Closing clicks almost always occur at the terminus of the closing movement, but never at the same time as the opening sound. Clicks occurring at the same time would suggest the presence of a solid obstacle within the joint itself.

As the reciprocal click becomes chronic, the opening click occurs later in the cycle, as measured from the retruded condylar position. Eventually the disc remains dislocated throughout condylar translation and is *never captured,* except perhaps during very wide opening, eating, or yawning. In this situation the patient "locks" intermittently. He may report that his jaw catches or becomes immobile. At this phase the patient may actually be able to unlock himself by moving his jaw or pressing laterally on the condyle with his thumb. Finally, as the disc remains in an anterior position, *locked* during opening, no click occurs. The opening becomes

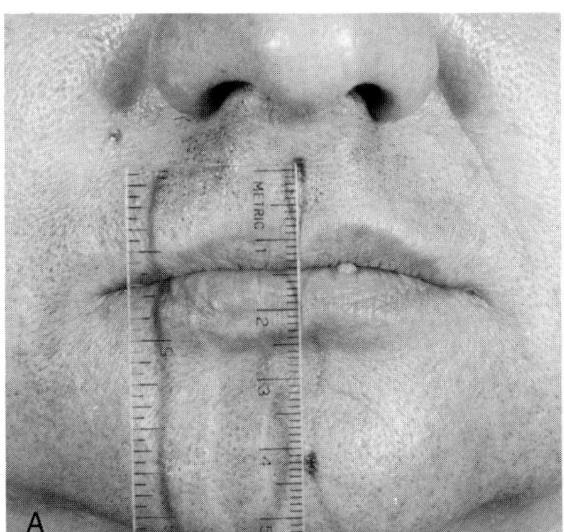

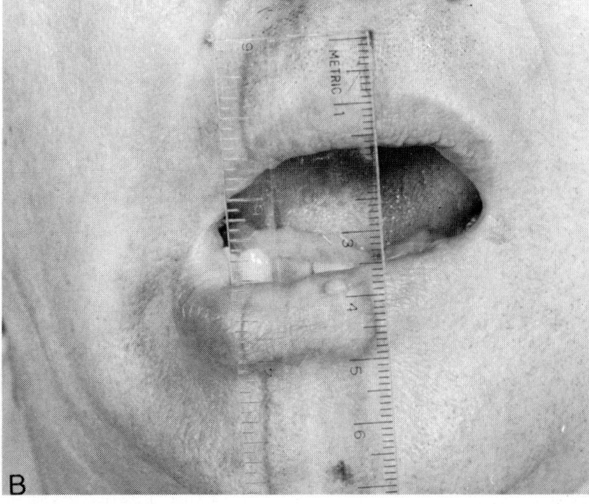

Figure 30–9. Deviation on opening. Although deviated opening may be obvious to the examiner, it may be subtle. A dot is placed on the midphiltrum and the central point of the chin. During opening the jaw may shift toward one side. *A,* Closed. *B,* Open.

limited owing to the jamming of the disc anterior to the condyle. This is called complete anterior dislocation with locking, or without reduction, or without disc capture.

Note: Displacement implies that the range of jaw movement is not limited. *Dislocation* of the disc or disc lodging creates a blocking action to jaw movement.

This phase of disc dislocation may progress as the lateral and posterior attachments of the disc are stretched. During the early locking period, mandibular opening may be limited to 25 to 30 mm, but with stretching the opening increases gradually as the disc becomes more entrapped anteriorly. Mandibular opening motions show deviation toward the affected side. As the disc becomes more and more compacted anteriorly, mandibular motion may show no deviation at all and, of course, no clicking. The condyle, however, is riding on the stretched retrodiscal pad. This state represents a precondition for later degenerative joint disease, because no shock absorber or substance remains between the condyle and fossa.

Since lateral jaw movement as well as opening may be restricted, it should also be checked and recorded. The normal range of maximal lateral movement at 1 cm opening is 9 to 13 mm (Fig. 30–10). The normal ratio of maximal lateral to maximal vertical movement is approximately 1:4 or 1:5. The lateral ranges may not be affected greatly in the earlier pathologic states, but once locking or more reduction of the disc occurs the lateral movements from one side to another vary greatly. A simple chart drawing is helpful (Fig. 30–10).

The vertical line represents the mandibular opening with the marks at every centimeter. Lateral motion is noted by the lateral wings. For example, Figure 30–10*B* denotes an opening of 50 mm. The mandible begins to shift to the right; at 10 mm a click occurs. Lateral motion is unrestricted on each side; this represents an early click. The patient instinctively positions the disc in proper relationship with the condyle very early. During rest, his mouth may be slightly open. This characteristic of jaw movement has a favorable prognosis. A therapeutic bite opening or protrusive splint will allow the disc to be seated properly over the condyle.

In the schema illustrated in Figure 30–10*C*, the click occurs very late. The disc is out of place for a long time and the jaw finally shifts back toward the midline at almost maximal opening. Lateral motion is slightly retracted to the opposite side. This situation is unfavorable for conservative treatment.

When there is complete anterior disc dislocation without capture or reduction, lateral motion to the opposite side is limited. The condyle jams against the disc; the translational motion is limited, and the opening is limited. The ratio of lateral movement (e.g., 5 mm) to maximal opening (28 mm) is approximately 1:6. As the locking becomes more

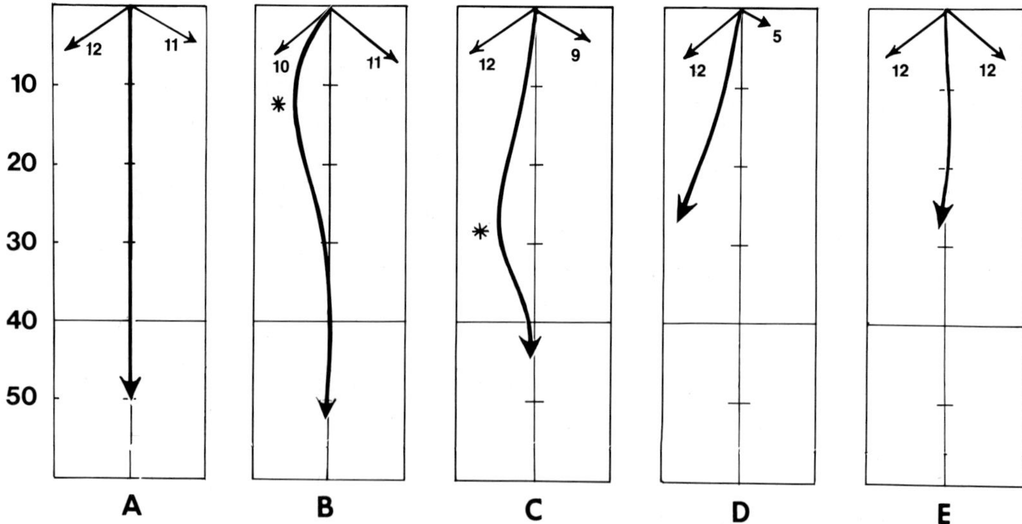

Figure 30–10. *A,* Normal opening. Normal lateral excursions. *B,* Early deviation and click (*). No restrictions. *C,* Late opening click. Mild lateral restriction to opposite side. *D,* Opening and excursion limited. Disc is dislocated and not captured. *E,* Extracapsular problem usually; limited opening. No lateral restriction.

chronic, the range of motion increases since the disc becomes less of a hindrance (Fig. 30–10*D*). The opening increases but is definitely deviated. The midline and lateral motions are still limited. In the later stages of locking the range of motion may be normal.

Note: If a patient presents with limited jaw opening even with some deviation and *the lateral movements are almost normal,* it may be assumed that the trismus is due to an extracapsular problem, such as a myofibrositis, rather than an internal derangement.

The timing of clicks has important clinical implications. Occlusal therapy with splints aims primarily to capture the disc by repositioning the mandibular occlusal table. If one grades the clicks in some way, an inexact cut-off point can be made beyond which occlusal therapy may not be helpful. The opening clicks are usually graded on a scale of 1 to 5; i.e., if the click occurs at a jaw opening (interincisal distance) of 1 cm, the grade is 1, at 2 cm the grade is 2, and so on. Although the closing click may be graded by a tracing curve, the simplest way is as follows. Instruct the patient to close maximally, and mark the teeth to record the position of the vertical alignment. Tell him to open widely and past the opening click, then to close in a protrusive (bulldog) position. The patient then glides backward slowly to make his teeth fit together. During retrusion, the mandible hesitates when the posterior band of the disc jams against the posterior aspect of the condyle prior to the closing click. That point is recorded several times to determine precisely how many millimeters of posterior condylar displacement occur coincident with the closing click. For each millimeter the closing click is graded, grade 2 for 2 mm, 3 for 3 mm, and so on. The opening and closing clicks are averaged. Thus, if a person has a grade 3 opening click (sound at 3 cm opening) and a grade 2 closing click (2 mm of posterior condylar displacement with closure), these are averaged to *2.5* as a composite grade. This grade may be used only adjunctively. If the patient is uncooperative or refuses to wear the splint consistently, the grading may be meaningless. For the purpose of occlusal therapy, however, the chances of capturing a dislocated disc and stabilizing it are practically nil if the composite grade is 3 or more.

Some patients report a grating or grinding sound in the joint. *Crepitus* is indicative of far-advanced disease and is caused by movement across irregular surfaces. This sound often signifies the presence of a perforation of the posterior disc or supporting ligaments. Although all patients with perforation have crepitus, the presence of crepitus is not necessarily pathognomonic for perforation. Dye studies further elucidate the situation. Furthermore, some patients with grinding may not have pain and may present primarily because of their concern about the noise. The surgeon must ask whether he should violate the joint in such situations, especially if motion is not severely limited.

Condylar Dislocations

The condylar head(s) may be dislocated with or without fracture in any direction. When forces sufficient for fracture occur, the head may be dislocated backward into the ear canal, upward into the middle cranial fossa (Zecha, 1977), laterally through the capsule (Sanger and Greer, 1979; Zide and Kent, 1983), or, more commonly, medially. Dislocation may also occur anteriorly, and in these situations previous or coincident fracture need not be present. The condylar head slips so far forward that the posterior articulating surface of the condyle advances ahead of the articular eminence (Fig. 30–11) and may become entrapped. The condyle thus moves from the glenoid fossa into the temporal fossa. When this type of condylar displacement occurs, repositioning techniques

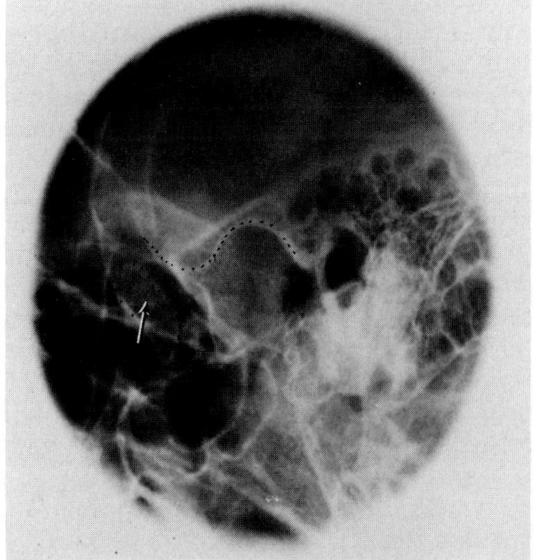

Figure 30–11. The condyle (*arrow*) hypertranslates forward in front of the articular eminence.

may be effective. When such dislocation occurs frequently, the ligaments around the joint stretch concomitantly. Severe concurrent lateral pterygoid muscle spasm and joint pain tend to keep the patient in the dislocated position. In some cases the condylar heads may be malposed anteriorly for long periods, as in chronic dislocation, and surgical intervention may be required to reposition the heads. The methods of treatment for both chronic and acute dislocation are discussed below.

In an acute dislocation, manual reduction may be possible. In one method the operator seats the patient in front of him, places both his index fingers on the mandibular external oblique ridges, and pushes downward. The thumbs are used simultaneously to push the mandible backward (Georgiade, 1977). The author's preferred technique, which provides more force (Lewis, 1981), uses the thumbs to push downward. This can be done from either in front of or behind the patient. By standing behind the patient the operator may exert sufficient thumb forces at the retromolar areas to reduce first one side, then the other. The thumbtips exert downward pressure at the base of the coronoid processes, with one hand under the chin.

If this initial maneuver is unsuccessful, one should reduce spasm in the lateral pterygoid muscle and reduce pain in the pericapsular area of the joint. This may be required only on one side. A 25 or 27 gauged 1½″ needle with 1 per cent lidocaine (Xylocaine) is passed preauricularly to the joint capsule. The needle puncture should be made anterior to the intertragal notch, aiming toward the neck of the condyle and capsular ligaments. After aspiration and injection, remanipulation should be attempted. If this is still unsuccessful, extraoral block of the mandibular branch of the trigeminal nerve should be performed, or *this can be done as the sole injection* (Eriksson, 1979). After the skin has been infiltrated directly over the sigmoid notch, a spinal needle is passed through the notch until the surgeon detects the lateral pterygoid plate. By redirection posteriorly for approximately 1 cm, injection should provide excellent muscle relaxation and analgesia. The surgeon may find the administration of intravenous diazepam and meperidine helpful at this time. Use of such drugs, however, may result in the patient being supine during manipulation. If the above measures fail, the patient should be scheduled for a general anesthetic with muscle relaxation. Following reduction, the motion of the mandible must be restricted for two to three weeks to allow the capsule to heal. Bonded brackets with four to eight orthodontic rubber bands, sufficient to reduce opening to 20 to 35 mm, may be helpful.

Surgery for dislocation is performed to reduce a chronic dislocation or to prevent redislocation in patients who frequently require relocation. When the patient is dislocated at the time of surgery, a Gillies approach is used to provide passage for an elevator to approach the temporal space (Lewis, 1981). The elevator is passed behind the zygomatic arch. The elevator is directed to the neck of the condyle (Fig. 30–12), where downward and posterior force can be placed along the posterior arc of the sigmoid notch. Laskin (1973) has suggested an intraoral temporal muscle myotomy as an adjunctive step. If the surgeon decides to approach the joint at this time for further work, the Gillies temporal incision may be extended for preauricular access to the joint.

Many methods have been proposed to alleviate the dislocation problem permanently. The eminectomy technique of Hale (1972) or Irby (1974) works well. Whereas the articular

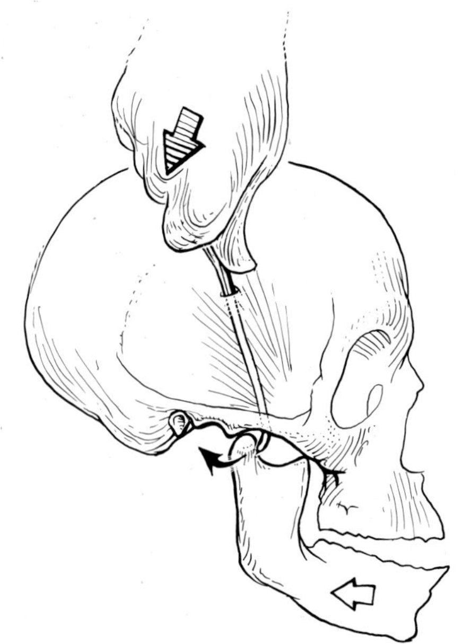

Figure 30–12. Chronic dislocation (after Lewis, 1981). The Gillies approach provides access to the front of the condyle and posterior notch. Downward and posteriorly directed force may help to reduce the dislocation.

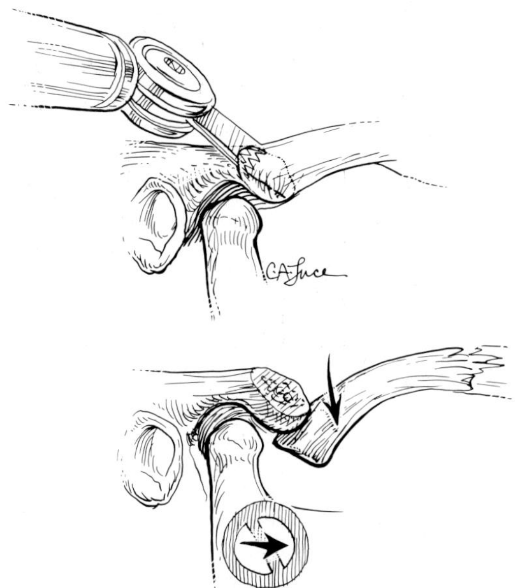

Figure 30–13. Blocking hypertranslation of the condyle (after Dautrey and Pepersack, 1982). The zygomatic arch may be osteotomized and displaced downward to block condylar dislocation.

eminence formerly blocked the repositioning of the dislocated condylar head back into the glenoid fossa, its absence provides free anteroposterior movement. Plication or reefing of the joint capsule (Morris, 1930) may temporarily work, but will not prevent recurrence if the ligaments stretch. In addition, ligamentous reefing alone does not address the meniscal problem that may need to be assessed. It has been suggested that an autogenous or demineralized bone wedge be inserted into an osteotomized niche in the posterior articular eminence, thus blocking the translational movement of the condylar head. Dautrey and Pepersack (1982) recommended an osteotomy at the root of the zygomatic arch (Fig. 30–13). After the arch is divided at 45 degrees, the bony arch is gently rocked on its temporozygomatic articulation until it can be replaced inferiorly. The height of the articular eminence is thus doubled, and dislocation is prevented.

DEVELOPMENTAL ABNORMALITIES

Condylar Hypoplasia

See Chapter 62, which discusses craniofacial microsomia.

Coronoid Impingement (Shira and Lister, 1958; Fitzpatrick, 1970; Sperling, 1973; van Hoof and Besling, 1973; Monks, 1978; Shuken and Girard, 1979; Hecker and Corwin, 1980).

The coronoid processes may be responsible for limitation of protrusive or lateral mandibular motion. They may be enlarged, restricted by local bony trauma or disease, or relatively malposed. The patient has pain and demonstrates grinding joint sounds. In reality the noise is located anterior to the joints.

When the condyle is shortened for any reason, the coronoid process is positioned more superiorly relative to it. In some cases, however, the relative increase in coronoid height may far exceed that of the opposite side regardless of the state of the condyle. An enlarged coronoid may also be part of an overall enlarged prognathic mandible (Fig. 30–14).

It is this hypertrophic state that is frequently associated with tendinitis or myositis of the temporal muscle, an obvious contributing factor to temporal headache. Pain or headache arising at the attachment of the temporal tendon may be diagnosed by intraoral block into the area. Most of the temporalis insertion is *medial.* However, in these cases 0.5 per cent bupivacaine hydrochloride (Marcaine) may be injected within the infratemporal fossa on both sides of the coronoid to verify the diagnosis.

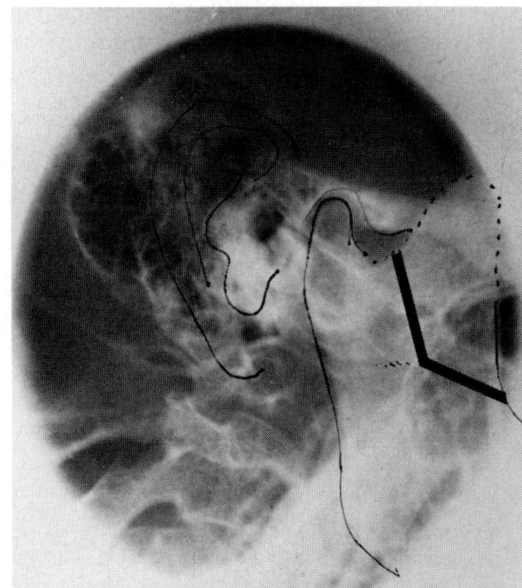

Figure 30–14. Enlarged coronoid process. This patient had grating bilaterally at 22 mm opening. Lateral excursions were equal bilaterally. The mandible was prognathic and the joints were normal. The dark line denotes the extent of the bilateral coronoidectomy.

When the coronoid process is enlarged, it may impinge on the zygomatic arch or maxillary tuberosity, causing pain and trismus. Rib grafts placed for zygomatic reconstruction may cause the obstruction, and depressed zygomatic arch fractures may act the same way. During rapid palatal expansion the tuberosity may also be displaced laterally, promoting obstruction. Similarly, acquired causes of reduced mandibular posterior height, e.g., condylar neck fractures, condylectomy, and degenerative joint disease, may effectively allow for vertical repositioning of the coronoid process with resulting impingement.

When severe incapacitating headache arises from the temporalis-coronoid attachment, or when obstruction is considerable, coronoidectomy can be performed by an intraoral approach (Fig. 30–14). The temporalis tendon, whose primary attachment is medial, must be stripped from the bone. The coronoid process should be removed from the sigmoid notch obliquely to the anterior notch of the mandible. Transoral suction drainage in these wounds is helpful, since postoperative hematoma formation promotes fibrosis and neoformation of bone. Regeneration of a smaller coronoid and reattachment of the temporal muscle is usually noted after one to two years.

Multiple Chondromas

Single chondromas are occasionally noted in the region of the condyle, coronoid, zygoma, or articular eminence. Limitation of movement and pain may occur. Radiographs are nonspecific. Surgical resection, when required, provides the definitive histologic diagnosis. This topic is also discussed under Condylar Hyperplasia below.

In certain cases, multiple loose bodies of ossifying cartilage ("joint mice") may be noted. The chondromatosis is similar to that seen in other joints. Such loose bodies may be positioned anywhere within the joint, and in fact removal may affect the occlusion.

Eagle's Syndrome

The presence of throat, ear, and jaw pain should alert the clinician to the possibility of Eagle's syndrome. The patient may complain of a feeling of something stuck in his throat. Radiographs may reveal a calcified or elongated stylohyoid ligament that is painful on intraoral examination; this should be removed surgically (Marano, Fenster, and Gosselin, 1972; Messer and Abramson, 1975).

Condylar Hyperplasia and Osteochondroma

When the condyle is hyperplastic, the facial skeleton elongates vertically on that side. The oversized condylar neck-ramus may be associated with unilateral posterior open bite, a bowing of the inferior border of the mandible, and occasionally an elongated maxilla. When the hyperplastic condyle grows, it maintains an almost normal shape, a distinguishing feature since condylar hyperplasia must be differentiated from osteochondroma, which is much more irregular in shape. The chondromas may grow on the condyle, coronoid, articular eminence, or zygoma and must be removed surgically, since they cause limitation of movement (Eller and associates, 1977; Keen and Callahan, 1977; Sanders and McKelvy, 1977; Simon, Kendrick and Whitlock, 1977; Pool and associates, 1979; Kaneda and associates, 1982).

Condylar hyperplasia does not stop growing after cessation of generalized development. Patients in their 30's and 50's may present with overgrowth for unknown reasons. Often an unsuspecting orthodontist will have been using vertical elastic bands to correct the posterior open bite, which is relentless as the growth continues. Some patients present with severe TMJ pain on the opposite side (Farrar and McCarty, 1982). This type of one-sided overgrowth causes the opposite, unaffected condylar head to become malposed in the fossa, leading to degenerative joint disease on the opposite side. The dentition may shift to compensate for the overgrowth in certain cases (Fig. 30–15). In short, when an unexplainable unilateral posterior open bite occurs in a patient, one should consider condylar hyperplasia and obtain a panoramic radiograph.

Treatment of this problem depends on: (1) evaluation of the condylar growth and (2) the severity of the resultant or concomitant maxillomandibular deformity. Since condylar hyperplasia is not limited to the growing individual, the disease does not necessarily stop spontaneously. The surgeon may evaluate the

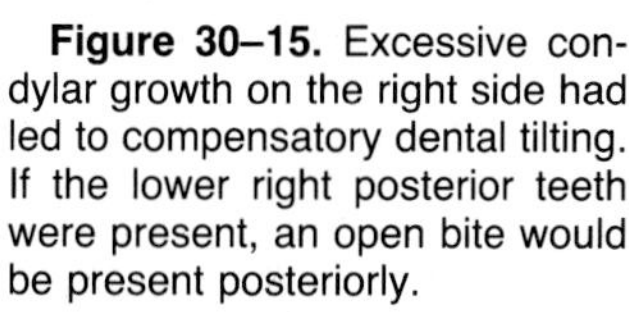

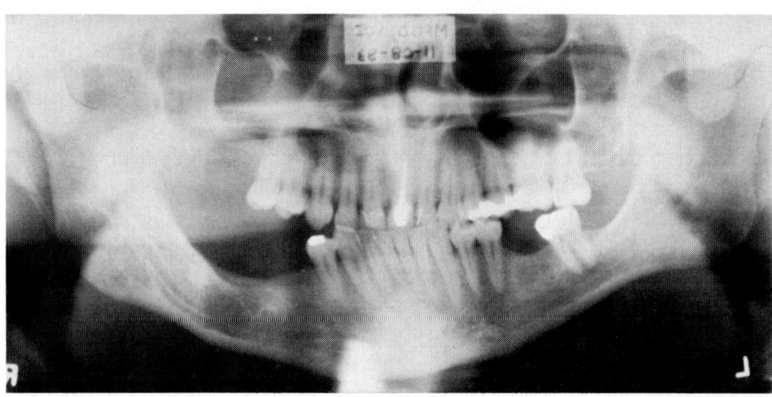

Figure 30–15. Excessive condylar growth on the right side had led to compensatory dental tilting. If the lower right posterior teeth were present, an open bite would be present posteriorly.

size of the condyle by comparing panoramic radiographs taken six to 12 months apart. This method tends to be inexact and difficult because of variations in radiographic technique, beam direction, or head position. More definitive evaluation may be performed by technetium scanning (Beirne and Leake, 1980; Murray and Ford, 1982). An affected condyle shows increased uptake, unlike the normal side (Fig. 30–16). The severity of the associated dentofacial deformity depends on how long the condyle has been growing, on whether the patient had preexisting malocclusion, and on the patient's age.

One should optimally prefer to make the diagnosis of condylar hyperplasia early, and thus treat early (Jonck, 1981). If the patient has no preexisting dentofacial deformity, the disease may be eradicated by a high condylectomy. High condylectomy is effective since the hyperplastic cartilage cells almost never penetrate more than 4 mm from the head of the hyperplastic condyle, and most are within the first 2 to 3 mm.

If the condylar hyperplasia becomes active in a young patient, the ultimate dentofacial deformity, i.e., bowing canted occlusal plane and hyperplastic maxilla, is more severe than if the disease starts in an adult. Treatment must, therefore, be aimed at eradicating the pathologic condylar process as early as possible. The surgeon must always be mindful that the diagnosis of condylar hyperplasia may be incorrect and osteochondroma may actually be present. Both processes may present with a vertical lengthening and a posterior unilateral open bite.

Proper correction of the patient with condylar hyperplasia may take four possible paths as well as combinations:

1. Orthodontic therapy plus. . . .
2. Condylar surgery.
3. Mandibular with or without maxillary surgery.
4. Inferior border and chin surgery.

Preoperative orthodontic therapy should not aim at correcting the vertical problem since it will only be exaggerated. In addition, vertical elastics tip the maxillary occlusal plane adversely. Rather, the dental arches should be leveled. Crossbites should be corrected to avoid postoperative discrepancies in

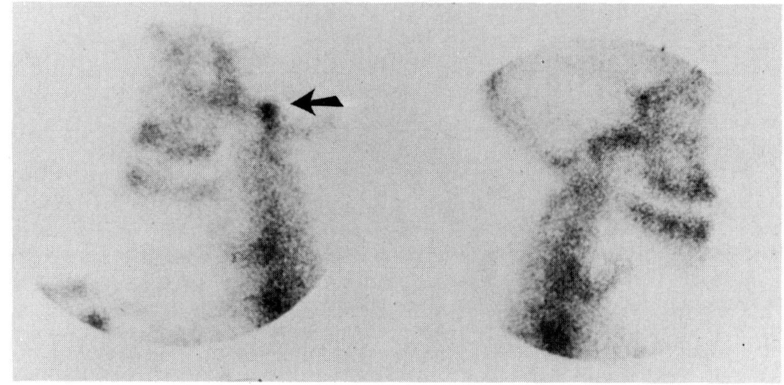

Figure 30–16. Technetium scanning in condylar hyperplasia. Note that one condyle (*arrow*) picks up dye more than the opposite side, evidence of continued growth.

transverse arch width. The required extractions for proper equilibration of tooth mass should be performed preoperatively.

If it is determined by bone scan or serial panoramic radiography that the condyle is still active, the condyle must be approached surgically. Since the meniscus should *not* be affected by a condylar shave, orthognathic surgery may be performed at the same time, although such combined procedures tend to be very time-consuming. If orthodontic preparation is required, the condyle may be approached during that time of preparation. A preauricular approach (Kreutziger, 1984) is performed using loupe magnification, and at least 4 mm of the condylar head is shaved and rounded from lateral to medial side.

If the cant of the maxillary occlusal plane is severe (Fig. 30–17), surgery is required in both jaws. These cases often have excessive gingival show and tooth exposure on the affected side: in effect, a unilateral long face. Such skeletal adaptations occur in response to the untreated growing condyle. The maxilla requires leveling, and bilateral sagittal or vertical ramus osteotomies of the mandible are needed. The surgeon must be aware of the rotational movement of the mandible toward the affected side. The contralateral ramus may be pushed outward and require intraoperative correction. The patient is maintained in intermaxillary fixation for six to eight weeks, depending on the expected stability and on his age, or plated.

The bowing of the inferior border of the mandible on the affected side requires special attention (Blair and Schneider, 1977). The inferior alveolar nerve often skirts the lower border of the mandible and must be protected after decortication (Fig. 30–18). The soft tissue incision made for the ramus osteotomies must be carried forward to the midsymphysis in the midbuccal sulcus. The mental nerve should be liberated for a short distance to provide adequate exposure of the inferior border. By comparing the panoramic radiographs of each side, the amount to be removed can be determined. After careful removal of the lateral cortex by sequentially fracturing small segments, the nerve can be teased out. The redundant periosteum must be adapted well to the new inferior border by suture or by postoperative compression dressing, otherwise regrowth of bone will occur.

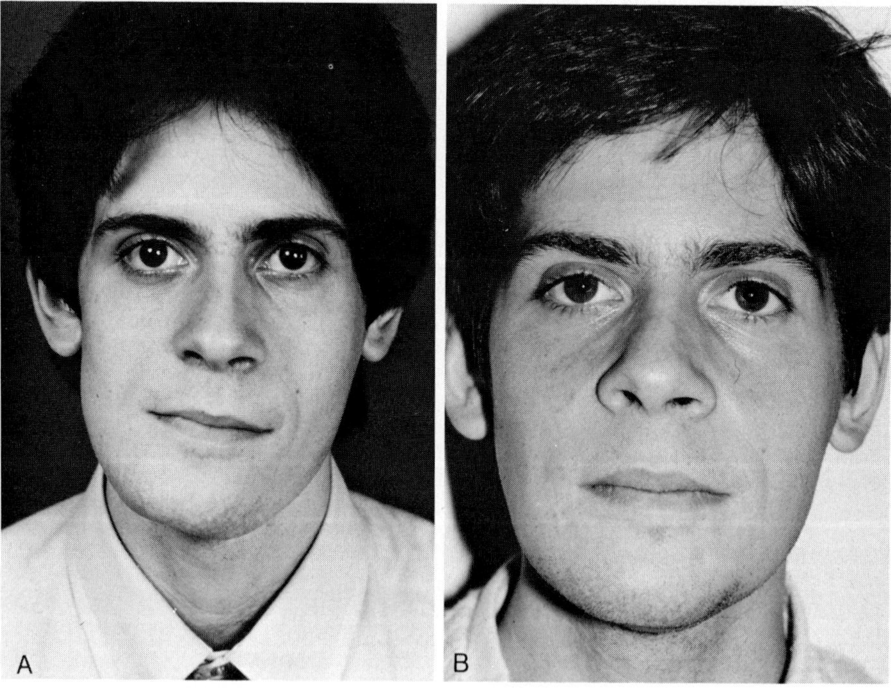

Figure 30–17. Condylar hyperplasia—surgical correction. First stage: Condylar shave to remove the activity of the overactive condylar cartilage. Second stage: Asymmetric Le Fort I maxillary impaction and downfracture on the unaffected side with interposition graft and inferior mandibular border reduction with ramisection. Asymmetric genioplasty, i.e., symphyseal osteotomy, was done for final contour correction. *A*, Preoperative. *B*, Postoperative.

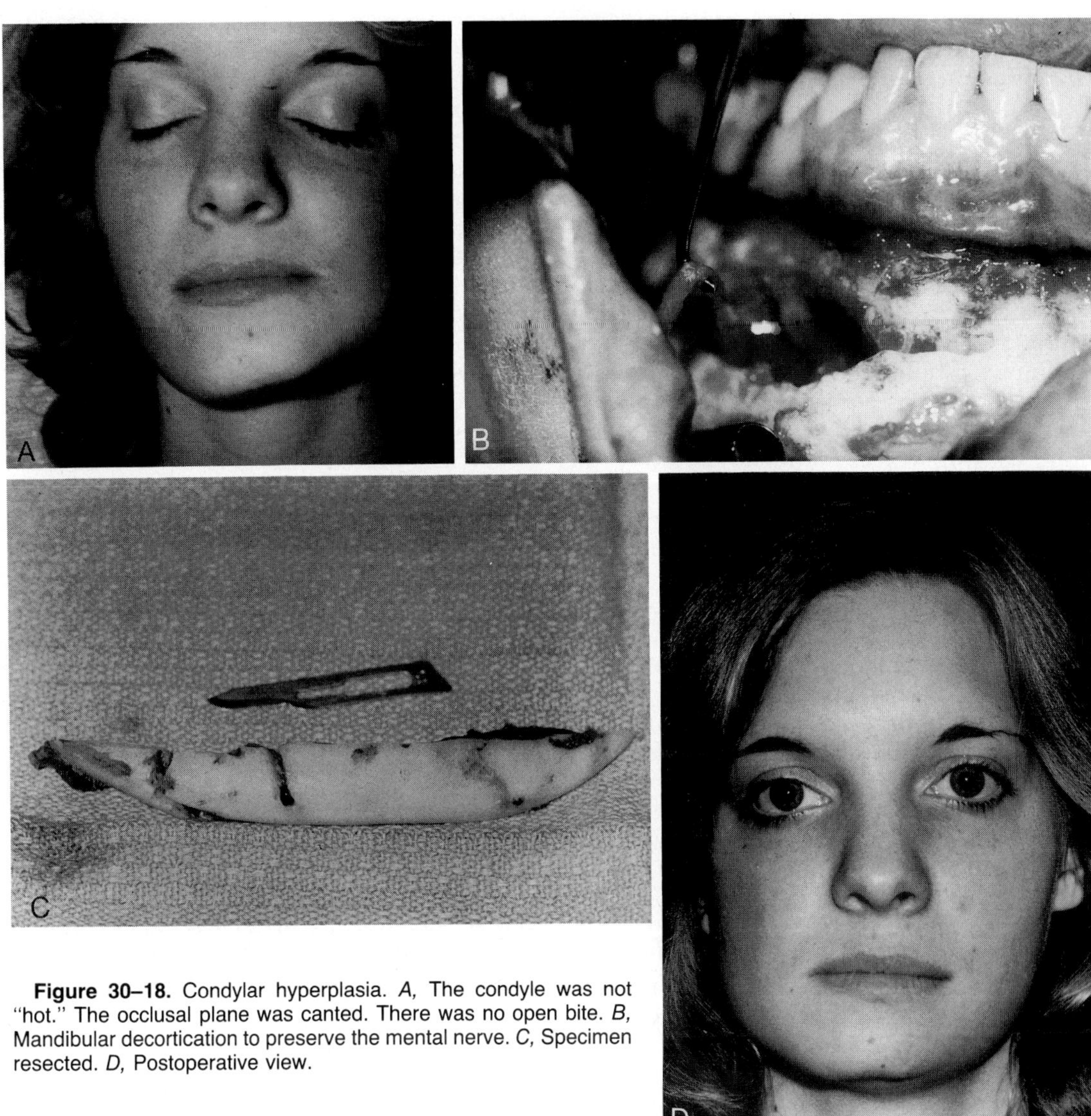

Figure 30–18. Condylar hyperplasia. *A,* The condyle was not "hot." The occlusal plane was canted. There was no open bite. *B,* Mandibular decortication to preserve the mental nerve. *C,* Specimen resected. *D,* Postoperative view.

If the vertical disparity in growth was caused by an osteochondroma as opposed to hyperplasia, the entire tumor must be removed and replaced by costochondral rib grafts (MacIntosh, 1985). Since the grafts vascularize slowly, excessive forces on them must be prevented for up to 12 weeks. The technique for removal of the affected condyle and subsequent reconstruction must use two incisions: a preauricular and a retromandibular or inframandibular approach. The retromandibular approach (preferred) involves an incision approximately 1.5 cm behind the posterior ramal border from just under the lobule of the ear and downward for 3 cm. The dissection may course through or behind the parotid gland and fascia. The mandibular branch of VII is anterior to this plane of dissection. After exposure of the posterior border, the masseter is elevated by subperiosteal dissection carried to the sigmoid notch. Gentle medial subperiosteal dissection allows placement of the malleable retractor before removal of the pathologic condylar process. The rib graft is contoured, leaving approximately 5 mm of cartilage on the graft to simulate the condylar head. It should be fixed so that the maximal width of cartilage is mediolateral, as is usually found in the normal articulation. After graft placement, the patient must be maintained *solidly* in intermaxillary fixation for eight weeks. The next four to eight weeks should provide gentle mobilization with minimal vertical compressive forces on the graft.

ANKYLOSIS

The causes of ankylosis or hypomobility of the mandibular ramus may be within the TMJ or external to the joint. Cases of *true* or *intra-articular* ankylosis usually occur unilaterally and are most frequently secondary to trauma. The fusion at the articular level may be fibrous or bony in nature. When the fusion occurs during the growth of the mandible, varying degrees of facial deformity result, and the maxilla may also become deformed. Since the attachment of the lateral pterygoid muscle to the condyle and meniscus may also be altered, the patient presents with limited protrusion and diminished lateral excursions as well as trismus. These movements may not be restored coincident with surgical correction of the hypomobility.

Of 185 cases of temporomandibular ankylosis (Topazian, 1964), trauma was involved in 29 per cent, infection in 48.7 per cent, congenital factors such as forceps delivery in 2.6 per cent, and unknown causes in 19 per cent. Younger patients have a greater tendency toward post-traumatic ankylosis, mostly before the age of 10 years (Laskin, 1978). Considering the fact that only 6 per cent of all condylar fractures occur in the first decade, this statement takes on greater significance (Miller, Page, and Griffith, 1975). Perhaps the articular capsule, not as well developed in children, permits easier displacement of the condyle out of the fossa. The inability of the more trabecular condyle of the child to withstand trauma may predispose toward a crushing type of intracapsular fracture. The comminution and hemarthrosis in a highly osteogenic environs may produce grave consequences. However, such injury in animals does not uniformly produce ankylosis (Beekler and Walker, 1969). The length of postfracture immobilization may be surgeon or patient induced and surely contributes to the incidence of hypomobility. A critical factor, according to Laskin (1978), in determining whether post-traumatic ankylosis develops is the position of the meniscus. When meniscal displacement or comminution (tearing) occurs, allowing bone to bone contact either directly or via blood clot, the potential for osteogenesis and resultant fusion is extensive. According to Kent and Zide (1984), "In all cases of hypomobility (intra-articular) displacement or destruction of the meniscus is universal."

False ankylosis from extra-articular causes may be due to a variety of conditions affecting the muscles of mastication, the facial nerve, and coronoid process. Post-traumatic fibrosis resulting from infection, injection, or hematoma often causes trismus. Patients with neurogenic disorders such as epilepsy and cerebrovascular accidents often present with limited mouth opening. An enlarged coronoid process or one obstructed by local fracture or surgically placed bone grafts prevents proper translational movement of the mandible. Concomitant hematoma and fracture in the temporalis muscle-zygoma-coronoid zone often confuses the surgeon (Rankow and Mignogna, 1978). Of prime importance, therefore, is the differentiation between ankylosis from intra-articular causes and that from extra-articular causes. Tomography, CT scan, and clinical examination allow the physician to solve the dilemma and choose the optimal therapeutic approach.

Intra-articular ankylosis is usually fibrous, but often the fibrous tissue ossifies. The ossification process may extend beyond the joint area to involve the cranial base, sigmoid notch, zygoma, external ear canal, and beyond. The surgical approach for release of such an extensive area of ankylosis may be submandibular, preauricular (Kreutziger, 1984), or occasionally temporal (Obwegeser, 1985) in very severe cases. Treatment of the more usual ankyloses may be broadly classified into three main groups (Moorthy and Finch, 1983):

1. Condylectomy (rare).
2. Gap arthroplasty.
3. Interpositional arthroplasty (alloplastic or biologic).

In a sense, condylectomy is similar to gap arthroplasty, since it involves the creation of a gap at or below the site of ankylosis and has been described as an operation for the relief of ankylosis. The technique has been rejected because it is technically difficult to release the fused remnants of the condylar head exactly at the joint space.

Gap arthroplasty, which is actually a more extensive condylectomy or ostectomy below the prior joint level, involves the removal of at least 1 cm of bone *without* the interposition of any material. The 1 cm zone of excision should be sufficiently wide to prevent reankylosis but should produce little change in vertical height of the mandible. Since prevention of reankylosis is difficult, Rajgopal and associates (1983) have suggested radical condyle and neck removal as well as coronoidectomy. Of course, the vertical ramus height becomes greatly reduced.

Most surgeons tend to agree, however, that recurrent ankylosis is less likely if material is interposed between the divided bone ends. Controversy arises over whether to place alloplastic material (Proplast, Teflon, Silastic, methyl methacrylate, etc.) or autogenous tissue (fascia lata, muscle, full-thickness skin or cartilage) into the defect.

The most commonly used alloplastic material has been silicone rubber. In addition to producing a pseudoarticulation, the vertical dimension of the ramus is maintained (Hartwell and Hall, 1974; Gallagher and Wolford, 1982). In adults, carved Silastic blocks, split silicone tubing, ulnar head prostheses (Lewin and Wright, 1978), and modified chin implants have been used with success for years. When appropriately placed and stabilized to the temporal bone or condylar neck (the latter is less preferable), long-term functional restoration usually occurs. In an effort to reduce the incidence of implant displacement, or extrusion, Gallagher and Wolford (1982) suggest using Proplast in the TMJ. Owing to the porous structure and potential for tissue ingrowth, postoperative stabilization is more secure. In ten cases the Proplast implants were wired to the condylar neck and no postoperative slippage occurred. In children it is less desirable to perform a large ostectomy since function is compromised and deviation occurs. It is preferable to use Silastic sheets or split tubing secured to the articulating mandibular stump (Caldwell, 1978).

The use of biologic materials such as skin, fascia lata, or muscle may not preserve the vertical dimension of the mandibular ramus. In these cases, retrognathia and apertognathia (open bite) develop. Biologic transplants of metacarpal or costochondral bone and cartilage may provide a new growing unit within the existing "functional matrix" (MacIntosh and Henny, 1977; MacIntosh, 1985; Munro, Chen, and Park, 1986). In growing individuals these grafts may cause an increase in mandibular ramal height (Murray, Kaban, and Mulliken, 1984) but cannot shift a deviated midline back to normal. Formal, long-term studies using such autogenous implants are still pending. Biologic materials present many drawbacks. Vertical dimension of the mandible is not maintained if the graft becomes displaced. Resorption may occur, and certainly the necessary postoperative immobilization may limit function. In addition, donor site morbidity from rib or metatarsal harvest may occur, but in spite of the problems, autogenous grafting may represent the optimal approach.

Kent and associates (1983) have described a chromium cobalt molybdenum alloy prosthesis to reduce vertical height loss. This prosthesis has a shank coated with Proplast to improve stabilization (Fig. 30–19). This type of implant is also advocated for cases such as:

1. Severe degenerative joint disease with condylar collapse.
2. Advanced rheumatoid arthritis with condylar collapse and open bite.
3. Condylar and meniscus loss secondary to trauma and tumor ablation.

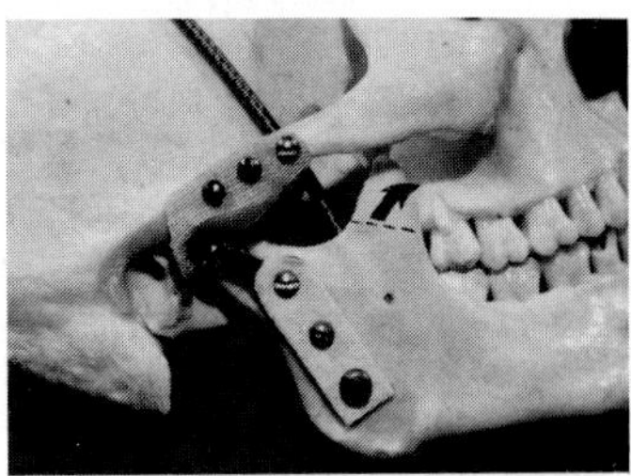

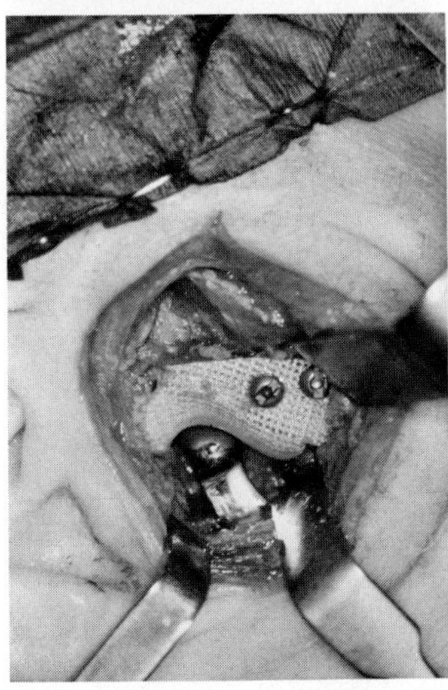

Figure 30–19. The Kent prosthesis demonstrated on a skull (*above*) and in situ (*below*). Coronoidectomy (*arrow*) is usually done as part of the procedure. (Courtesy of Jack Kent, D.D.S.)

4. Severe idiopathic condylysis.

Such prostheses correct the facial asymmetry, retrognathia, and open bite. Furthermore, immediate postoperative function is possible.

FRACTURES OF THE CONDYLE

The mandibular condyle appears to be well protected from direct trauma owing to its posterior position. However, it becomes indirectly fractured in 30 per cent of all mandibular fractures (Olson and associates, 1982). The most commonly seen associated mandibular fractures are parasymphyseal and the contralateral condyle (James, Fredrickson, and Kent, 1981). Thus, direct trauma to the anterior mandible should always arouse suspicion of condylar fracture.

Classification

Condylar fractures have been classified with respect to the level of fracture, e.g., the head of the condyle versus the neck, the position of the condylar head, and the amount of overriding of the fracture segments (Rees and Weinberg, 1983). The radiographically based classifications do not provide the surgeon with any therapeutic guidelines. In addition, CT examination of the condyles (Horowitz, Abrahami, and Mintz, 1982), which now provides excellent views, has never been included in previous classifications. Age is also a key factor, since considerable evidence exists that children below the age of 12 years can heal and remodel after condylar injury far better than teenagers or adults (Lund, 1974; Spence, 1982). In fact, Keizer and Tuinzing (1985) reported spontaneous regeneration of a totally absent condyle in a 5 year old child, and Nagase and associates (1985) reported regeneration in a 12 year old after hemimandibulectomy. According to Lund (1974), the condyle may even be resorbed and replaced, depending on the age and amount of displacement (Fig. 30–20).

Diagnosis

Patients may present at the time of injury or well after the traumatic event complaining of pain or limitation of movement. The patient or examiner may note an anterior open bite. One should seek the following information: (1) intra- or extraoral evidence of trauma to the symphyseal region; (2) localized discomfort or edema in the preauricular region; (3) limitation or deviation of opening; (4) occlusal interferences, crossbites, and the presence or absence of posterior tooth support; (5) blood or soft tissue swelling in the external ear canal; (6) pain or step defect by palpation at the condylar fracture site; and (7) no palpable movement in the condylar area on opening.

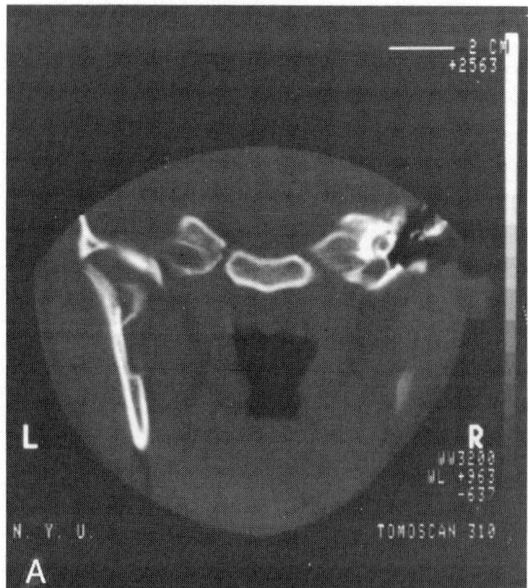

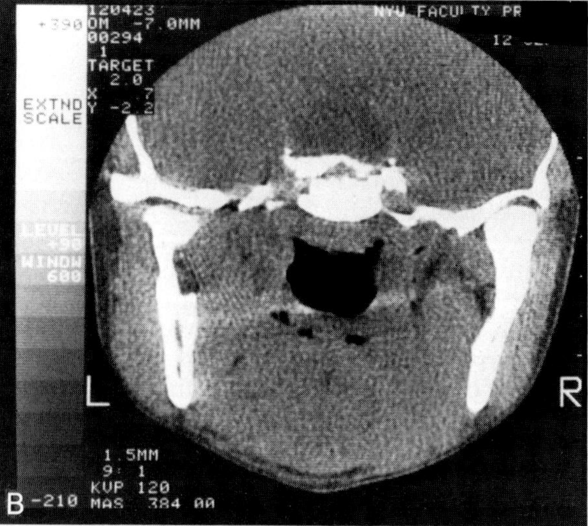

Figure 30–20. *A*, CT scan demonstrates medial displacement of the fractured condyle in a 7 year old child. *B*, At six months the condylar fragment is reconstituted.

Roentgenography

The usual facial radiographs obtained in most emergency rooms do not include panoramic roentgenograms, CT scans, or tomograms. These are the best methods to visualize the condylar region. Only CT scans or tomograms demonstrate intracapsular fractures, and these have the tendency to give rise to late complications, such as disc problems and ankylosis. In summary, if a doubt exists, the CT scan provides the best source of information (Horowitz, Abrahami, and Mintz, 1982).

Closed or Conservative Management

Nonoperative management of condylar fractures consists of immobilization of the mandible by intermaxillary fixation. In the adult or adolescent, arch bars are placed as the initial step. This may be done under local anesthesia without difficulty in most cases. The author keeps the patient in fixation for approximately seven to ten days to allow for edema and spasm reduction. By varying the number and strength of the orthodontic rubber bands, opening and closing are allowed to occur after the initial fixation period. The *key* is to keep the mandible in the midline during opening. After initial release of fixation, three or four vertically or obliquely directed elastics on each side allow for mild opening. These should be attached to the arch bar; brackets should not be placed on individual teeth. The rubber bands are subsequently reduced in number, but may be directed obliquely to prevent the mandible from retruding (in bilateral cases) or shifting to one side (in unilateral cases). Finally, the patient is able to open in the midline with only one or two elastics to direct motion (Fig. 30–21). These adjustments may take six to 14 weeks. The patient is seen weekly and, of course, the arch bars are maintained until he can open and close unassisted in the midline. If the surgeon chooses to keep the patient in intermaxillary fixation for longer periods (e.g., because of other fractures), he must release the fixation at least weekly after one to two weeks to exercise the mandible, otherwise ankylosis may occur. In addition, the surgeon must follow the patient for at least six months, since late disc displacements or discal problems may become more obvious.

For children, splints (not arch bars) may require placement in the operating room owing to the presence of a mixed dentition. Usually the splints are held in position by circum-mandibular wires for the lower splint and drop wires from the pyriform aperture and zygomatic arch to the upper splint. Fixation may be short term (one to two weeks), but the patient must be able to resume wearing the splint easily. If the mandible tends to return to a deviated or retruded position, the maxillary teeth may require *temporary* interconnected orthodontic brackets or bands for obliquely directed rubber band traction to direct mandibular opening.

If the condylar displacement is minimal and the patient, either adult or child, can obtain a proper occlusal relationship, fixation may not be necessary. In such cases, the author sees the patient frequently (two to three times a week) during the first two weeks to check for deviation. During this period the patient may consume a soft diet.

Open Reduction

Open reduction for fractures of the mandibular condyle is rarely performed since the procedure may be complicated, and closed reduction usually is sufficient. However, as noted by Rees and Weinberg (1983) as well as by Zide and Kent (1983), there are late and acute requirements for open reduction.

Rees and Weinberg (1983) reported five

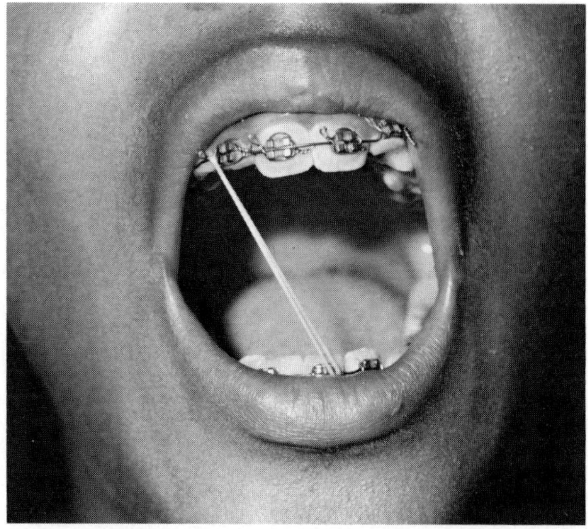

Figure 30–21. Midline maintenance. By varying the number, direction, and strength of the intermaxillary elastics, the surgeon directs the patient to open maximally in the *midline*.

cases presenting with varying degree of nonunion, disrupted occlusion, and limitation of movement after weeks to months of conservative treatment of condylar fractures. The surgical technique to reestablish proper occlusion varied, depending on the problem, but all were directed at proper reestablishment of posterior ramal height.

Zide and Kent (1983) have criticized some of the data on closed reduction. Specifically they suggested more long-term follow-up, since late arthritic changes may occur in joints that were not corrected into the appropriate anatomic position.

Some of the indications for open reduction were considered absolute, while others were considered relative.

ABSOLUTE INDICATIONS

1. Displacement into the middle cranial fossa (Zecha, 1977; Ihalainen and Tasanen, 1983).
2. Impossibility of obtaining adequate occlusion by closed reduction.
3. Lateral extracapsular displacement of the condyle (Sanger and Greer, 1979).
4. Invasion by foreign body (e.g., gunshot wound).

RELATIVE INDICATIONS

1. Bilateral condylar fractures in an edentulous patient when splinting is unavailable or impossible owing to severe alveolar ridge atrophy.
2. Unilateral or bilateral condylar fractures when splinting is not recommended (e.g., seizure disorders, severe alcoholism, refractory behavior).
3. Bilateral condylar fractures associated with comminuted midface fractures.
4. Bilateral condylar fractures and associated gnathologic problems (e.g., multiple tooth loss, open bite with severe periodontal problems, retrognathia, prognathism).

TECHNIQUES FOR OPEN REDUCTION

The European surgeon seems more disposed toward open reduction for condylar fractures, as evidenced by the literature (Tasanen and Lamberg, 1976; Petzel and Bulles, 1982; Cadenat and associates, 1983; Brown and Obeid, 1984). Before any reduction, however, proper methods must be used to maintain solid intermaxillary fixation postoperatively. New prostheses or old dentures must often be constructed or adjusted to obtain the correct vertical dimension. Posterior edentulous molar regions cannot be left unattended.

The surgical correction for such fractures often requires both a preauricular approach and the routine Risdon or retromandibular type of incision. Alternatively a face lift incision, after which the facial nerve is identified (Zide and Kent, 1983), also provides adequate exposure. The preauricular approach (see Surgical Approach, p. 1505) is relatively simple once the anatomy is well understood (Al-Kayat and Bramley, 1979; Kreutziger, 1984).

Multiple direct wiring techniques may be used, but these all require some postoperative time in intermaxillary fixation. The use of small compression plates with two screws on each side of the fracture (Koberg and Momma, 1978) allows immediate mobilization. As noted by Brown and Obeid (1984) and Wennogle and Delo (1985) (Fig. 30–22), the preauricular approach is required to retrieve the displaced condylar head. The standard submandibular exposure (Risdon) allows access for traction on the ramus. A large Kocher clamp, lion's jaw clamp, or towel clip may be used to grasp the large distal segment inferiorly to position the condylar head.

The transfacial puncture method for fixation of condylar head displacement (Georgiade, 1977) should be discarded, since proper preauricular exposure techniques provide adequate visualization. If the dissection is properly performed (Kreutziger, 1984), the seventh cranial nerve frontal branch may often be avoided and one need not spend time identifying these branches.

ARTHRITIS

The temporomandibular joint is subject to the same afflictions as all the other joints: arthritis, infection, tumors, fractures, and so forth. The surgeon should know how to differentiate and treat the more common arthritic conditions discussed below. The pain and disease may often be palliated by antiinflammatory drugs, but when discal displacement is severe and marked bony changes have occurred, surgery may be required for unrelenting pain.

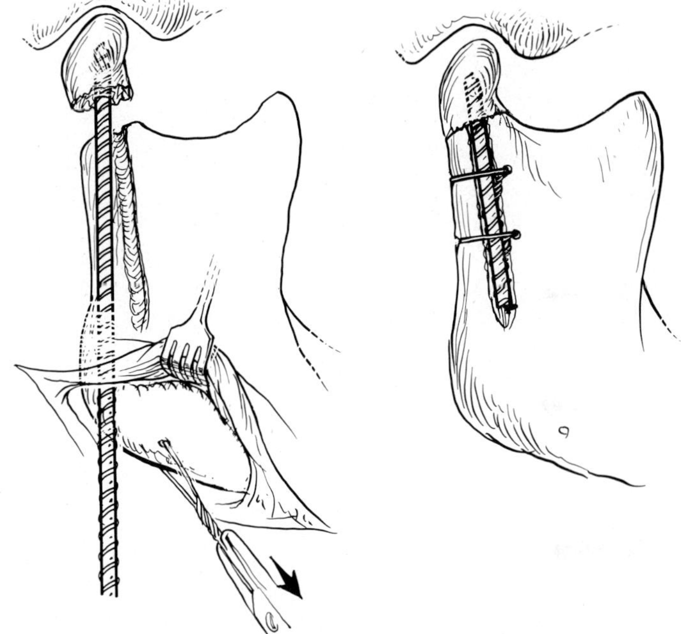

Figure 30–22. Open reduction of a condylar fracture (after Wennogle and Delo, 1985). The preauricular approach is required to stabilize the displaced head, while the submandibular (Risdon) approach is required for ramal traction and placement of the pin. Note the groove in the outer cortex of the ramus to accommodate the threaded pin.

Degenerative Arthritis

Degenerative joint disease (DJD), often unilateral, is first manifest by reduction of joint space, typically caused by disc displacement. Although the pain may vary, the symptoms of reciprocal clicking and locking should never be considered innocuous even if pain is minimal. Disc problems must be distinguished from the muscle pain of bruxism, malocclusion, and myofascial pain dysfunction. *Documented* disc displacement results in decreased joint spacing, which ultimately produces some type of degenerative arthritis. No bony changes are noted at this early stage. To reiterate, the superior joint space *should be no less than 2.0 mm, the posterior space no less than 2.2 mm, and the anterior joint space no less than 1.8 mm on transcranial radiographic study* (Fig. 30–23). Surgical treatment should be rendered if splint therapy and medical management fail to diminish the pain. Only *7 per cent* of patients with painful clicking diagnosed by arthrography as having displacement *with* reduction show evidence of arthritis (Stanson and Baker, 1976).

In the early stage of DJD the anterior displacement of the disc allows the condylar head to appear closer to the glenoid fossa posteriorly (Fig. 30–24). Splint therapy is designed to open the bite slightly and allow the condyle to *recapture* the disc in its more anterior position. If the opening click occurs early in the opening phase (less than 2.5 cm interincisal distance), disc capture may be possible, but the splint must be worn 24 hours a day. If the disc is irreducible by splint therapy and the patient experiences persistent pain, surgery is usually required. Arthrography documents the pathologic condi-

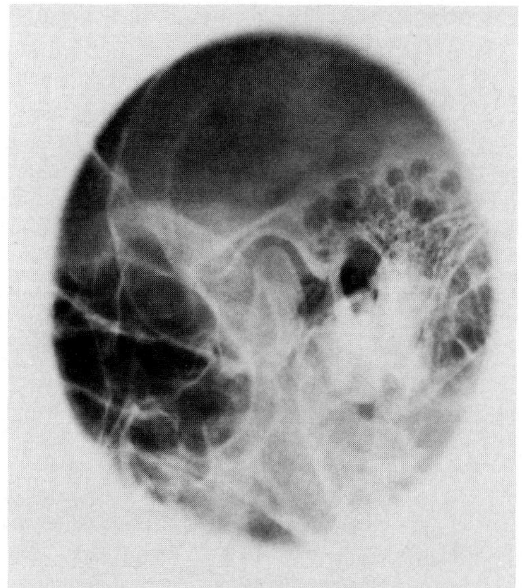

Figure 30–23. Normal joint space and condylar contour (left side). Note the smooth guide plane of the articular eminence. The eminence may be pneumatized in certain patients.

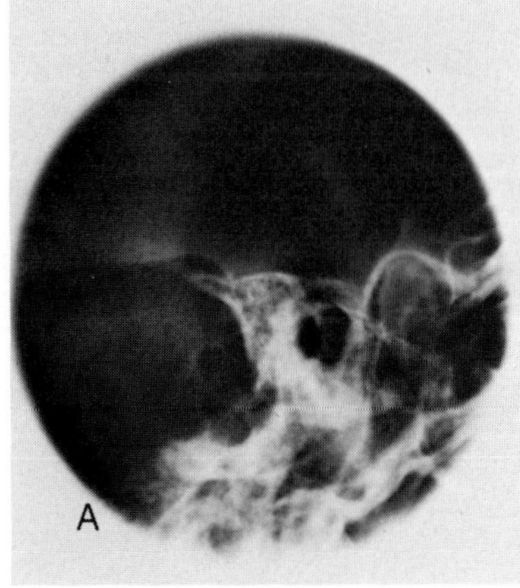

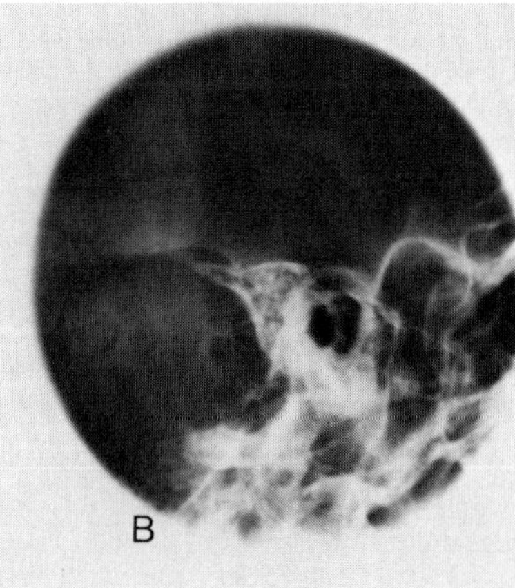

Figure 30–24. Degenerative arthritis. *A,* The joint space is reduced posterosuperiorly when the disc slips forward (right side closed). *B,* On opening, the disc is captured late.

tion. Such surgery aims to displace the disc posteriorly by removing a small wedge from the anterior bilaminar zone or suture fixation to the condylar head (Walker and Kalamchi, 1987). Sutures used to return the disc to proper position are checked by opening and closing movements in the operating room. Sutures placed totally within the posterior disc will not heal, as the disc is avascular.

Bony changes are next seen in the progression of the disease and the disc becomes more displaced. Thirty-six per cent of patients with unilateral pain and limitation of opening who cannot capture the disc have arthritis, i.e., obvious bony changes (Helms, Katzberg, and Dolwick, 1983). In this, the regressive phase of DJD, the articular surfaces of the condylar head and the articular eminence begin to flatten and erode, with sclerotic changes noted below the articular surfaces (Fig. 30–

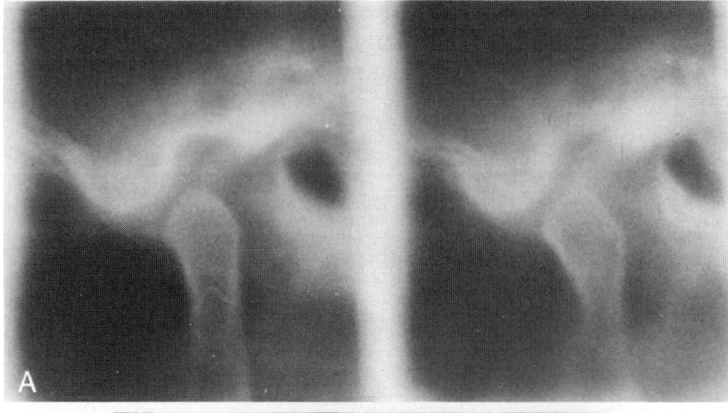

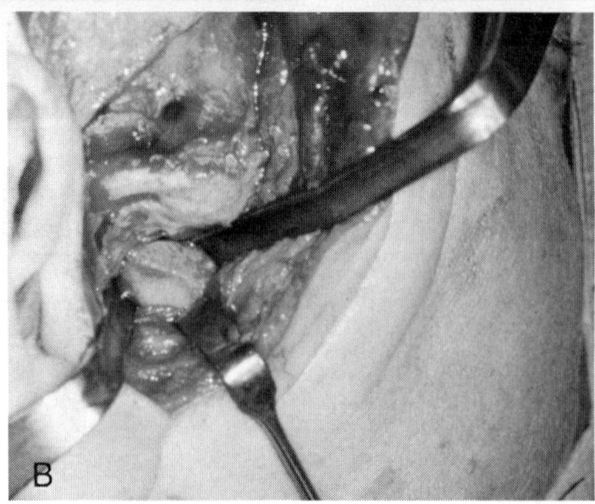

Figure 30–25. Degenerative arthritis. *A,* Tomograms show the flattening of the articular surface, an early bony change found in degenerative joint disease (left side). *B,* Clinical example (right side).

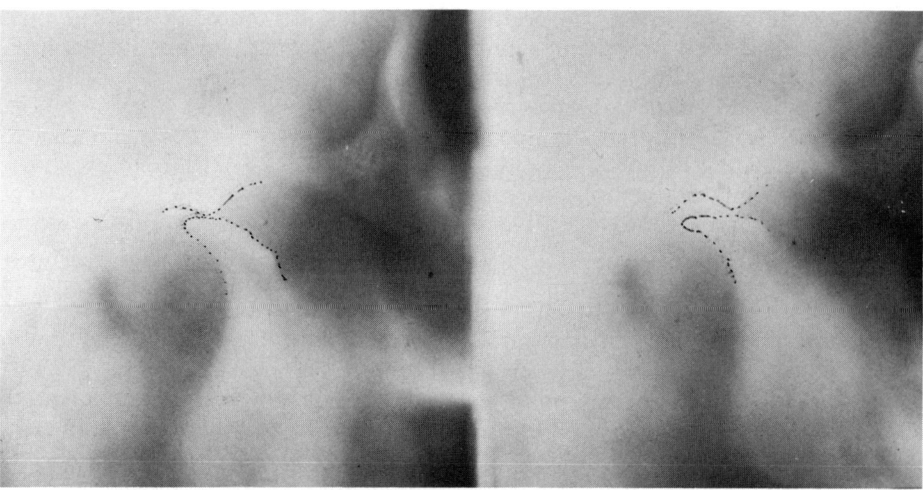

Figure 30–26. Degenerative joint disease. Osteophytic remodeling phase. Note the lipping of the condyle.

25). As the joint space decreases and the disease continues, peripheral changes occur and may be noted on the anteroposterior radiographs, the tomograms, or the transcranial studies (Fig. 30–26). This lipping or mushroom phenomenon represents an arthritic, osteophytic remodeling phase in the bone since the disc has shifted in position. Small radiographic lucencies, termed Ely's cysts, may be noted in the cortical bone at the time, evidence of resorption within the condyle (Murphy and Adams, 1981).

When the disc is totally dislocated, the condyle remodels progressively, usually with associated pain and crepitus (Fig. 30–27). As the condyle shortens, the molar teeth alone contact and an anterior open bite occurs. The head of the condyle is obviously irregular, with thickening of the cortical bone both in the fossa and the condyle. Sclerosis may be noted in the condyle, neck, or fossa. Osteophytic changes are common in these cases. The spurring may be observed on the condylar surface and is associated with more pain than the lateral lipping seen previously.

As the condylar height decreases during

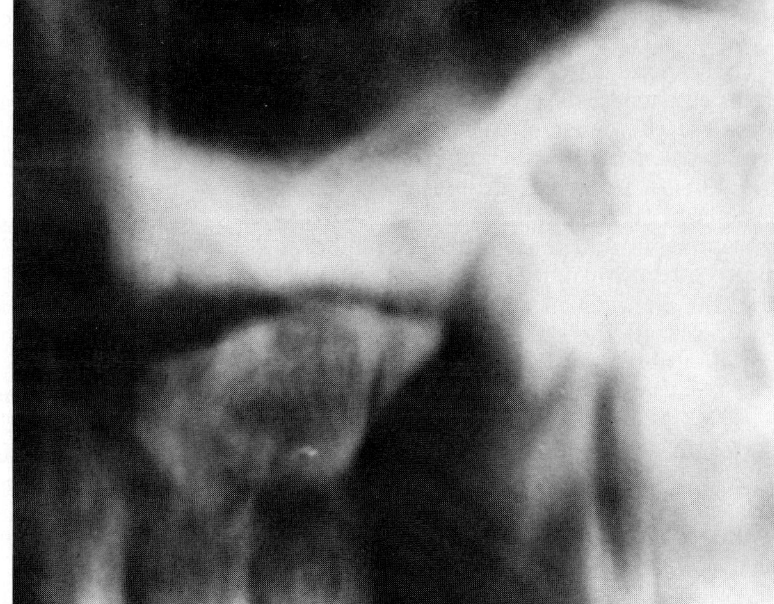

Figure 30–27. Advanced degenerative joint disease. A 57 year old patient who presented with pain and crepitus. The tomogram demonstrates condylar shortening and irregularity as well as posterior lipping.

the arthritic remodeling process, the occlusion changes progressively. With one-sided disease, the mandibular midline shifts toward the affected joint. As the midline shifts, the open bite becomes more lateral on the opposite side as well as in the anterior position. The disc gradually displaces medially owing to the lateral thrust of the condyle. Regressive unilateral DJD eventually causes internal derangement on the opposite side.

When bony changes become obvious by radiographic study and the patient has pain, surgical intervention is probably necessary and splinting usually fails. In spite of this, short-term conservative splinting is still performed. Surgery consists of disc repositioning or meniscal replacement with alloplastic sheeting after removal. A diamond bur is used to reshape the condylar head and remove the osteophytes when required (Kraut, 1981). If more than 2 to 3 mm of the articulating surface is removed, maintenance of the vertical dimension is accomplished with reinforced sheets of silicone rubber or Teflon-Proplast laminate (Kent and Zide, 1984). The benefit of the latter laminate is that the Teflon wears well as a meniscus substitute and the Proplast adheres to the glenoid surface. The problem of implant slippage seen with silicone is thus reduced. However, the author personally has removed numerous Proplast laminates, which in some cases produce a severe inflammatory reaction.

Osteochondritis

Osteochondritis, also called idiopathic condylar osteonecrosis, occurs primarily in young females. The cause of this usually seronegative type of arthritis is unknown. The condyles begin to resorb, dramatically reducing the joint space. The disease may progress to retrognathia and open bite. The amounts of pain and limitation vary. Radiology may reveal the changes of a severe erosive arthritis with associated crepitus in one or both joints. Fortunately, this does not occur frequently. The disease is often self-limiting. If minimal pain exists, orthognathic surgery should be performed to correct the retrognathia and open bite. If pain or persistent dysfunction arises, one might wait for the resolution of pain and condylysis which may occur. Alternatively the use of a condylar implant has been suggested (Kent and associates, 1983); however, total condylar replacement in young women has not been evaluated over the long term.

Rheumatoid Arthritis

The patient with rheumatoid arthritis (RA) rarely presents with TMJ disease as the original manifestation. Laboratory data, namely ESR (erythrocyte sedimentation rate), rheumatoid factor, and SLE tests should be obtained if there is any doubt. More likely the patient is already under medical treatment for *bilateral* proliferative inflammatory arthritis of some other synovial joints. The radiographs show evidence of varying destructive patterns in both joints, similar to those seen in later DJD. As the articular cartilage becomes eroded, the vertical length of the ramus decreases, with a resulting anterior open bite and retrognathia (Seymour, Crouse, and Irby, 1975). In patients with long-standing rheumatoid arthritis of the TMJ, the condyle may appear "penciled" or eroded (Fig. 30–28). Patients with psoriatic arthritis (Lowry, 1975) may show the same bony changes as patients with rheumatoid disease. Although the RA factor is negative, the ESR is increased and the patient has psoriatic lesions. Condylar bony changes tend to occur rapidly (within four to six weeks) and may even progress to necrosis and severe ankylosis. The treatment of other seronegative arthritides, e.g., ankylosing spondylitis, Reiter's syndrome, collagen vascular diseases (Lanigan and associates, 1979), and enteropathic arthritides, is similar to that of rheumatoid joint disease, both medically and surgically.

These patients usually have the clinical stigmata of deep auricular pain, stiffness, and vague ear problems (Ogus, 1975; Trenwith and Beale, 1977). Tenderness, crepitus, and hypomobility may also be present (Morgan, 1975). In advanced cases and in juvenile rheumatoid arthritis, Class II malocclusions may occur with or without open bite (Morgan, 1975; Turpin and West, 1978). The arthrogram clearly distinguishes the synovial changes of inflammatory arthritis from the meniscal dysfunction of an internal derangement. The surgeon must realize that the more usual, straightforward internal derangements (DJD) may also occur in patients with rheumatoid arthritis.

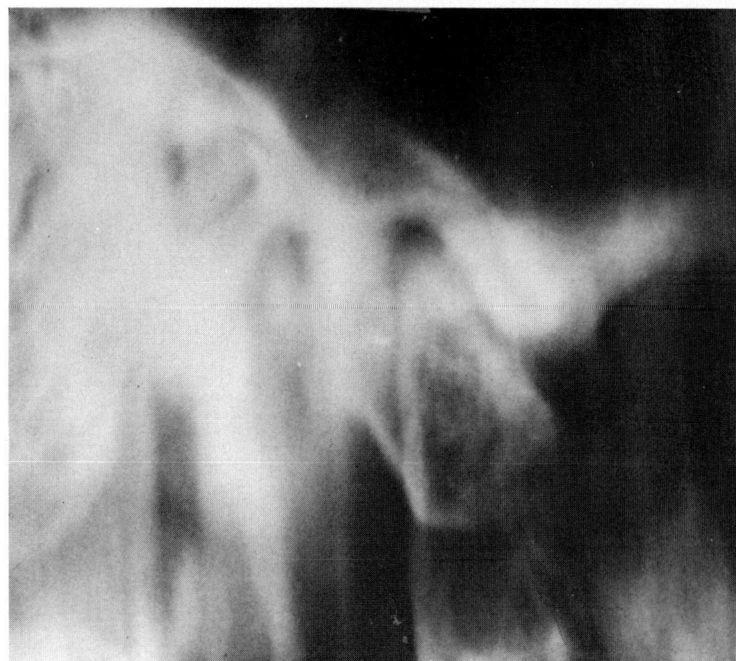

Figure 30 28. Rheumatoid arthritis: the penciled erosive late phase.

Surgery for rheumatoid or seronegative joint disease may be required to reduce pain that does not respond to medical management. Surgery may also be indicated for improved function or the correction of secondary deformity. Intra-articular steroid injections may lead to erosive articular changes (Irby, 1980). For patients with severe pain and bony changes but normal occlusion, the joint alone should be explored. The condylar head requires recontouring and an interpositional implant should be placed between the condyle and fossa. If the vertical dimension is decreased as a result of bone loss, patients show evidence of an open bite and retrognathic malocclusion. Such individuals require total TMJ reconstruction. The Kent prosthesis is designed for these problems (Kent and associates, 1983; Kent and Zide, 1984). Alternatively, costochondral reconstruction allows biologic, nonalloplastic reconstruction in these patients (MacIntosh, 1985). Such surgery may be required in addition to the usual orthognathic techniques for advancement of the jaw. If the malocclusion exists with minimal pain, minimal progression of joint disease, and little functional impairment, orthognathic surgery may be performed to provide optimal occlusion and cosmetic rehabilitation.

Juvenile rheumatoid arthritis (Still's disease) may cause hypoplasia of the entire mandible, i.e., condyle, body, and ramus. Early treatment should be aimed at maximizing jaw opening, to prevent trismus. Later jaw surgery (sagittal split and advancement genioplasty) may be necessary (Turpin and West, 1978).

RADIOGRAPHIC STUDY

Four radiographic methods, each with its own drawbacks, may be used to study the joint (Helms, Katzberg, and Dolwick, 1983):

1. Transcranial radiography/panoramic radiography.
2. Arthrography.
3. Tomography.
4. Computerized tomography.

Transcranial radiography allows excellent visualization of condylar size, profile, and position without the disc being seen (Farrar and McCarty, 1982). Open and closed mouth views should be obtained. The patient's head must be inclined approximately 15 degrees off the vertical to view the joint structures properly (Helms, Katzberg, and Dolwick, 1983). In closed mouth position, the condylar head should be centered within the glenoid fossa and the joint space should be uniform. With open mouth views, the condylar head

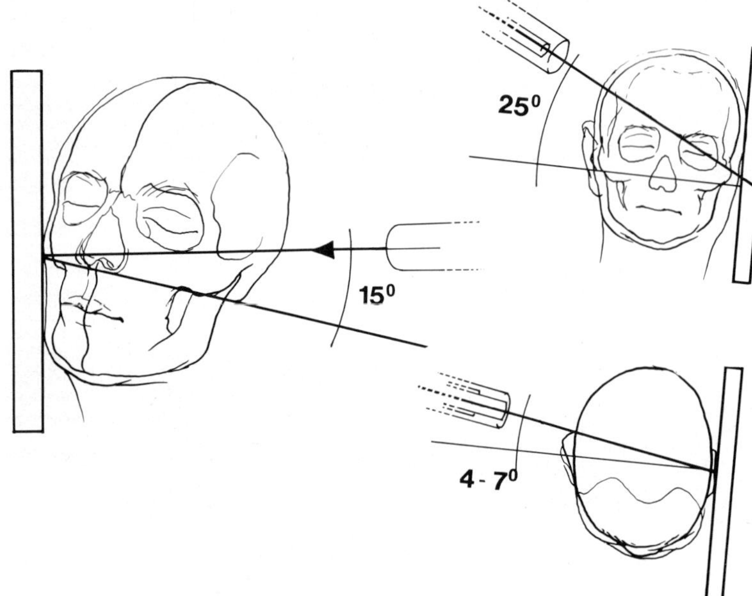

Figure 30–29. Transcranial radiographs (see normal control in Fig. 30–23) provide an excellent baseline view for joint study. Unfortunately, they must be taken at exact angles as noted to provide an accurate picture. Thus, some type of head-holding device is often required.

moves to a position within 5 mm in front of or behind the apex of the articular eminence. Although early internal derangements may be noted as a decrease in joint space, these radiographs are subject to great variability unless a head positioning device is used or the technician is extremely adept at proper positioning in every case (Fig. 30–29).

The panoramic radiograph, although helpful for comparison of right and left size and evaluation of fractures, does not provide satisfactory visualization of joint spaces.

Arthrography is the single most important diagnostic study for internal derangement (Wilkes, 1978; Katzberg and associates, 1980a, 1981; Bronstein, Tomasetti, and Ryan, 1981; Murphy, 1981). Patients who have painful clicking or locking, or those whose joints never respond to symptomatic or splint therapy, should be studied. Table 30–2 lists the indications for arthrography.

The aim of the arthrography is to detail meniscal position, movement, and integrity. It is performed by injecting dye into the lower joint space and asking the patient to open and close. The jaw dynamics are fluoroscoped until a definitive diagnosis can be made. The lower joint space is widest anteriorly with a smooth contour. During opening, the dye changes its configuration to allow study of the disc above (Fig. 30–30). In general, patients who have severe arthritic symptoms before arthrography have more pain during and after the study, but even patients with normal joints have temporary trismus or discomfort. Postinjection anti-inflammatory medicine is often helpful.

Linear (or multidirectional) tomography may also help to assess osseous detail and allow comparison between both sides (Delfino and Eppley, 1986). True lateral projections often provide excellent evaluation for ankylosis cases in that the surgeon may view the exact area of bony or fibrous fusion. Tomograms also display the early flattening and erosive changes of degenerative arthritis, often not well visualized in conventional radiographic studies. In addition, the progression or healing of the head of the condyle

Table 30–2. Indications for Arthrography of the Temporomandibular Joint*

Pain
Tenderness
Clicking with pain
Locking ("closed-lock")
Persistent complaints or vague symptoms not responding to symptomatic therapy
Evaluation of splint therapy
Arthrographically assisted splint therapy
Postoperative evaluation
Acute injury
Loose bodies
Diagnostic aspiration

*From Helms, C. A., Katzberg, R. W., and Dolwick, M. F.: Internal Derangements of the Temporomandibular Joint. San Francisco Radiology Research and Education Foundation, 1983.

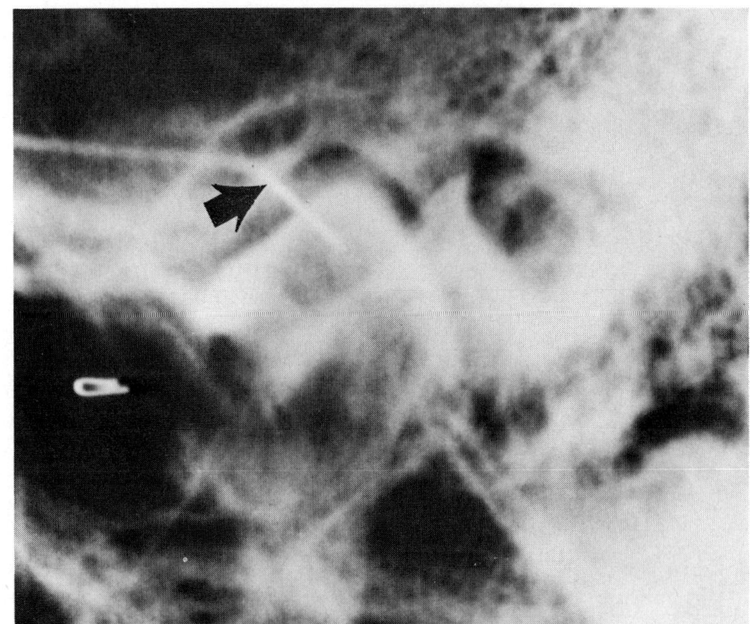

Figure 30–30. Arthrography. A needle (*arrow*) is placed into the lower joint space into which dye is injected. The pattern of movement of the dye allows accurate diagnosis of discal problems. Advanced techniques, in which dye and air are injected into both joint spaces, are available. The disc becomes outlined by this method.

in arthritic situations may be followed by tomography.

Computerized tomography (CT) scanners may also be used to evaluate DJD. Joint narrowing and osteophytic and sclerotic changes are well seen by the CT mode. The meniscus can occasionally be seen on routine CT, but this diagnostic approach is not highly reliable unless special techniques are used. Reformatting of CT slices for highlighting of the disc with a special identity mode provides a satisfactory picture of the disc. This is exactly what the arthrogram provides and it is noninvasive.

Unfortunately, CT scans are at least twice as expensive as arthrograms. Kursunoglu and associates (1986) recently demonstrated the use of three-dimensional CT analyses of the normal joint. They reported that meniscal problems may be observable with this mode in the near future. At this time, however, the dynamics of disc function and perforations cannot be seen as well as in the arthrogram. However, for fractures and ankylosis, the CT is an excellent diagnostic tool. The use of nuclear magnetic imaging (NMR) may be helpful in reducing x-ray exposure, but the expense and inability to view the disc dynamically are drawbacks.

SURGICAL APPROACH

The preauricular approach to the joint is probably used most commonly, although an endaural or a postauricular technique may also provide access. The usual incision resembles the preauricular face lift incision except for a shorter, 45 degree extension into the hair with the inferior limit above the lobule. After injecting the area and placing a cotton pledget in the ear canal, the surgeon dissects in the scalp, directly down to the *temporalis fascia,* i.e., the thickened white layer of fascia that lies directly on the temporal muscle (Fig. 30–31). The deep layer lies *below* the superficial fascia and superficial temporal vessels, some of which may require ligation. Staying slightly anterior to the vessels may reduce the chance of transecting the auriculotemporal branch of V_3 (mandibular trigeminal branch), which provides sensation to the supra-auricular temporal scalp.

The surgeon must stay *exactly* on and *bare* the white temporalis fascia, which splits approximately 1 inch above the zygomatic arch before enveloping it (Fig. 30–32). The temporal muscle lies behind the fascia. The space between the layers contains fat incompletely separated by irregular tracts of dense fibrous tissue, and often large veins are present. This thick layer continues inferiorly to join the periosteum that covers the zygomatic arch. The fascia is continuous inferiorly with the fascia lying directly on the masseter muscle and is connected to the parotid, the so-called parotid-masseteric fascia.

The key structure at risk during surgery is the frontal branch of the seventh cranial

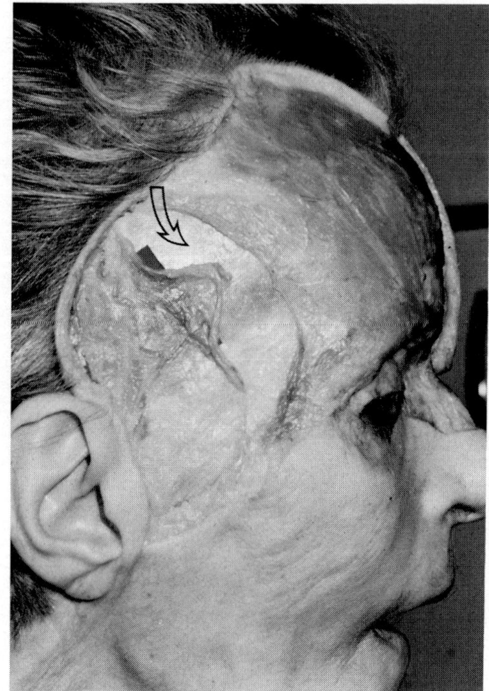

Figure 30–31. The arrow points to the deep temporalis fascia. Lying on this layer is the superficial temporalis fascia, which contains the superficial temporal vessels. A piece of plastic (dark color) is noted below the superficial layer.

nerve. In fact, Hall, Brown, and Lebowitz (1985) reported a *25 per cent* incidence of postoperative frontal nerve *loss* in 88 joints operated on between 1976 and 1981. Dolwick and Kretzschmar (1982) reported a *32 per cent* incidence of frontal nerve "weakness" until they altered their approach. Al-Kayat and Bramley (1979) recorded the distance from the most anterior concavity of the bony ear canal to the most posterior significant branch of the frontal nerve along the midzygomatic arch. This distance measured 2 cm $\pm$ 0.5 cm with a low of $\pm$ 0.28 cm from the lowest concavity of the external canal with a range of 1.5 to 2.8 cm. Topographically, the frontal branches, usually two, lie over the region of the articular eminence.

The preauricular incision provides the maximal anterior and lateral exposure. The submandibular, Risdon, or retromandibular approaches are reserved for subcondylar procedures or patients in whom the coronoid notch might require exposure. The preauricular incision risks injury to the frontal branch unless the above basic dissection methods are followed. The postauricular incision (Alexander and James, 1975), although cosmetically superior and less likely to cause nerve injury, provides access only to the posterior joint structures.

Two preauricular dissection techniques are possible and, when properly done, injury to the facial nerve branches should be minimal.

Method 1: Subfascial Technique

(Al-Kayat and Bramley, 1979;
Kreutziger, 1984)

After the glistening deep temporalis fascia is exposed (*bared*) to the upper zygomatic arch, an incision is made from the root of the arch anteriorly at a 45 degree angle (Fig. 30–33*A*). The incision is carried superiorly until a few muscle fibers are noted below the fascia. Hooks are placed along the thick anterior edge, and dissection is extended inferiorly until the splitting of the temporalis fascia occurs. Fat and veins will be noted between the split layers. The temporal muscle will lie behind the deeper layer. A knife is used to cut vertically across the root of the zygomatic arch to bone and approximately 2 cm beyond into the parotid fascia. An additional cut is made between the split fascial layer, 2 cm forward and directly along the upper bony edge of the arch. An elevator is placed between the fat and anterior thick fascial

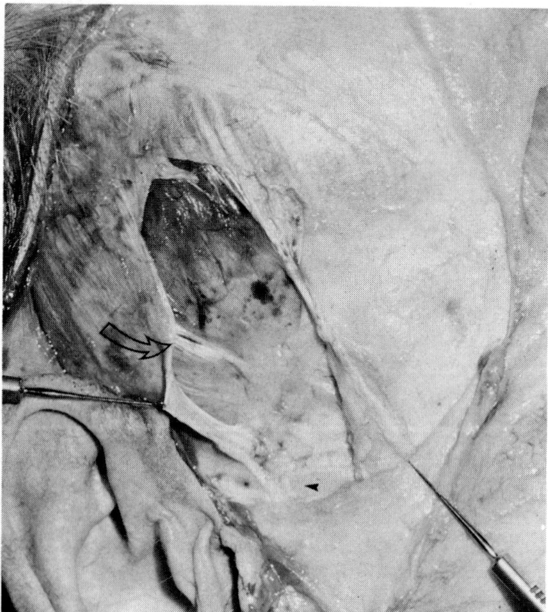

Figure 30–32. The deep temporalis fascia splits (*arrow*) to envelop the zygomatic arch. Within this split may be found fat and the middle temporal vessels.

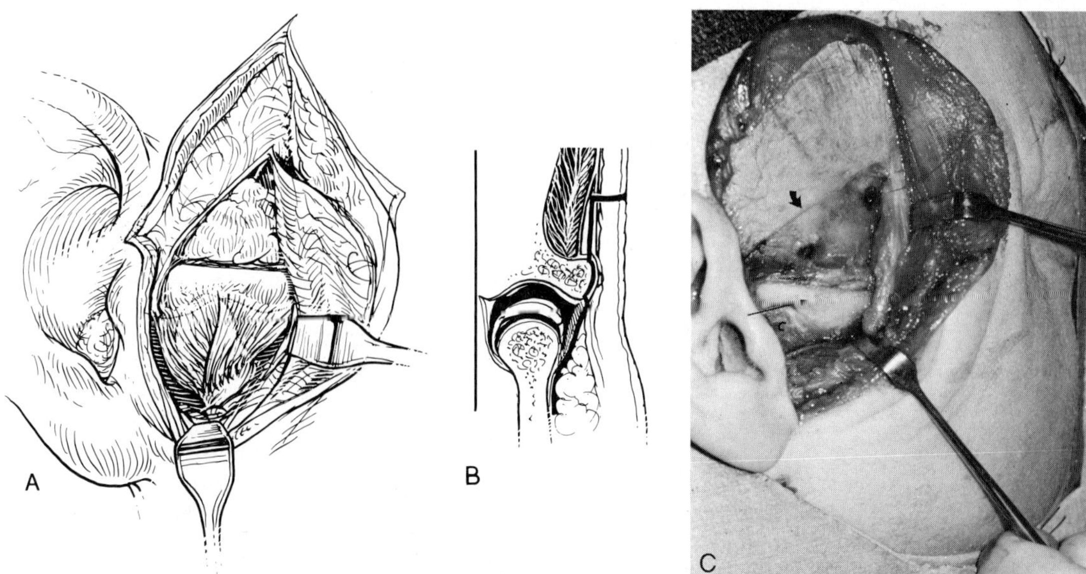

Figure 30–33. Subfascial technique. The skin incision is carried down to the deep temporalis fascia. The fascial cut is perpendicular to the root of the arch and is extended superiorly at a 45 degree angle. A cut between the fascial split on the upper arch allows subperiosteal exposure in a forward direction. *A,* Lateral drawing. *B,* Sagittal drawing. Note that the incision goes deep to the temporalis fascia on to the arch to expose the TMJ capsule after forward retraction. (Modified from Kreutziger, 1984.) *C,* Clinical views. The fascia has been reflected. c = capsule; broad arrow = fascial cut; arrow = arch. (Courtesy of M. F. Zide.)

sheath and the entire flap is lifted off the zygomatic arch, exposing the bare bone (Fig. 30–33*B*). The frontal branch is totally protected and cannot be injured when the dissection is made in the subperiosteal plane. The dissection progresses anteriorly, elevating the tissue off the arch. The vertical extension of the fascial incision allows sufficient anterior mobilization of this flap to expose the articular eminence, the temporomandibular ligament and capsule. A self-retaining retractor is then placed. The capsule may be opened by a T-shaped incision, a transverse incision with a posterior vertical extension, or a U-shaped flap based posteriorly. The incisions must leave some capsule for closure. Sutures are placed for retraction of the capsule and later identification and closure (Fig. 30–34*C, D*). Manipulation of the mandible at this time allows the surgeon to view the meniscus and its attachments during function. The superior joint space, meniscus, and glenoid fossa are visible. A lateral meniscus incision is made to explore the inferior joint space. The incision actually curves downward posteriorly, as does the bilaminar zone, and downward slightly anteriorly, as does the anterior meniscus. The condylar head is inspected at rest as well as during function. By distracting the mandible inferiorly with a towel clip at the gonial angle, the condylar head, joint spaces, and glenoid fossa should be inspected.

Method 2: Suprafascial Technique

In the above *subfascial* method the glistening deep temporalis fascia is exposed and incised to gain access to the joint. In the previous technique, the dissection is carried downward to the arch below the fascial plane to avoid damage to the frontal branch of the facial nerve. At variance with the former technique, the surgeon may continue dissection downward exactly on top of this fascia and avoid injury to the nerve (Fig. 30–34*A, B*). The periosteal elevator, not the knife, is used to clear the tissues from this layer, which continues inferiorly over the arch to the parotid-masseteric fascia. Any deviation from this plane in the region of the eminence or below places the frontal branch at risk, as evidenced by clinical studies (Dolwick and Kretzschmar, 1982; Hall, Brown, and Lebowitz, 1985). After the fascioperiosteal layer is bared over the arch to the level of the artic-

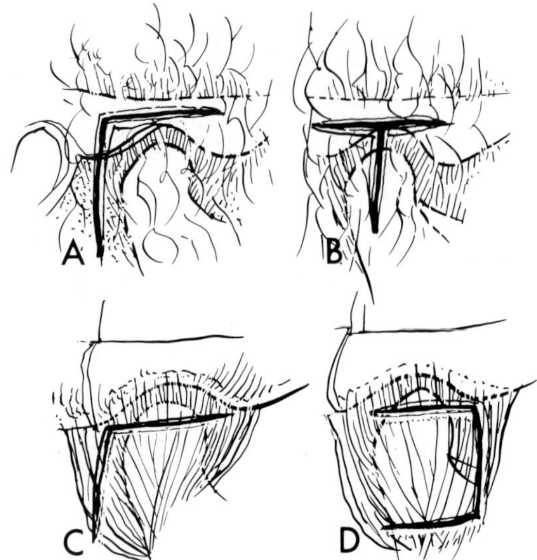

Figure 30–34. Suprafascial technique. *A, B,* When a suprafascial approach is used, the incidence of damage to the frontal branch of the facial nerve is higher. In addition the deep temporal fascia overlying the zygoma must be opened to expose the capsule. The usual incision into the upper level of the fascia is illustrated.

Subfascial capsular incisions. *C, D,* The inverted L incision provides excellent joint exposure. However, when the meniscus may need excision and/or replacement, the horizontal component is released from the lower arch directly so as not to interfere with wiring of a prosthesis. *D,* An alternative capsular incision for joint exposure.

ular eminence, a transverse incision is made at midarch with a posterior vertical extension inferiorly. The tissues are reflected subperiosteally in an inferior direction until the underside of the arch is reached. The mandible is moved and the upper joint space is entered and cleared. Meniscus position is checked. The lower joint space is entered by making an incision along the lateral attachment of the meniscus to the condyle. The meniscus is grasped and checked as the jaw is manipulated through a range of motion. This technique allows easier closure of the capsule, but it places the facial nerve more at risk.

What to Do Once the Joint Is Exposed

1. The surgeon should evaluate the fossa, articular eminence, meniscus, and condylar head, then
2. Reposition the meniscus *or*
3. Remove the meniscus (all or part) *or*
4. Replace the meniscus (all or part) *in conjunction with*
5. Shaving the condylar head and reducing the articular eminence, if necessary.

After the joint is exposed, the surgeon should distract the ipsilateral ramus downward by traction at the angle with a towel clip. Joint work may be simplified, however, with the Wilkes distractor (Fig. 30–35), which holds the joint open while the surgeon appropriately deals with the distorted or displaced structures.

If there are no degenerative bone changes and the meniscus is merely displaced anteriorly and not perforated, disc repositioning may be successful. A small wedge of posterior disc but preferably bilaminar zone will require removal and repair (McCarty and Farrar, 1979; Helms, Katzberg, and Dolwick, 1983). Following wedge excision or bilaminar zone plication the disc is repositioned more posteriorly by closure (Fig. 30–36). More lateral and secure positioning of the disc may also be helpful, a maneuver that can be accomplished by suturing or attaching the disc to the lateral condylar head (Walker and Kalamchi, 1987). Function is checked by putting the mandible through range of motion.

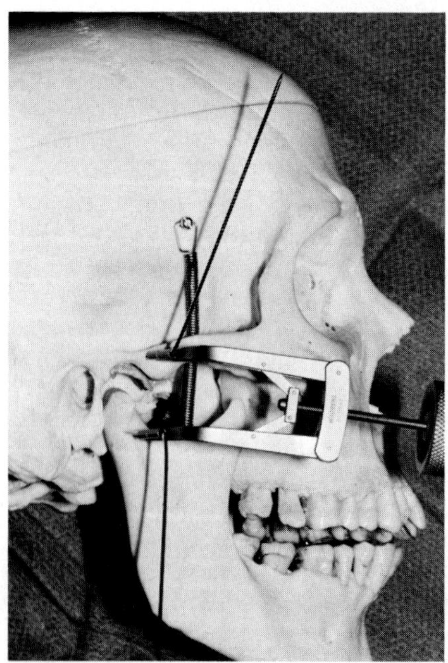

Figure 30–35. The Wilkes retractor may be used in lieu of gonial traction to provide sufficient exposure. K-wires are placed into the condylar neck and zygomatic arch and passed through the tube in the instrument. The wires are bent and the instrument screwed down to open the joint.

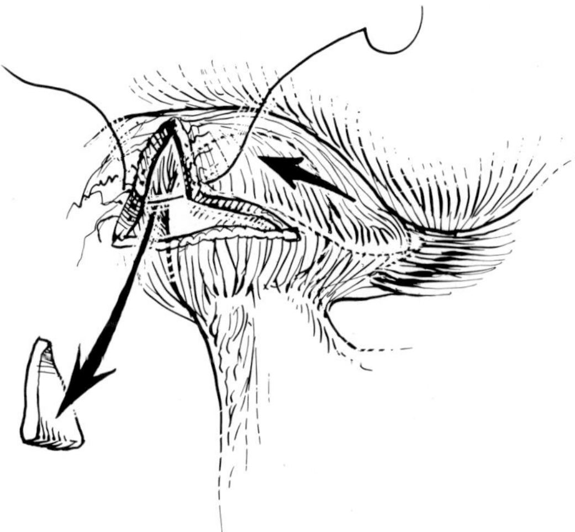

Figure 30–36. A posterior wedge may be excised from the bilaminar zone to place the disc in proper position. Alternatively, the upper condyle may be shaved and the disc repositioned by suture fixation to a hole in the lateral aspect of the condyle.

The author has found that discal repositioning works approximately 75 per cent of the time. The avascular disc probably does not "heal" to the bilaminar zone, and thus permanent sutures alone are required to hold disc position. In addition the joint must be "stabilized" postoperatively: i.e., the proper vertical dimension should be maintained. Thus, if the patient is missing posterior tooth support, this must be corrected either preoperatively by splinting or immediately postoperatively, otherwise the condyle tends to position itself posteriorly in the glenoid fossa.

If the meniscus is dislocated far anteriorly or crushed, the surgeon must decide to save some of the disc (Bessette and associates, 1985) or discard it totally. Meniscectomy, i.e., total disc removal (Kiehn, 1952; Eriksson and Westesson, 1985), has had more limited success when an intermediate substance was not placed in the joint space to prevent postoperative bone to bone contact. However, the presence of grating, joint noise, and loss of joint space due to lack of spacing material does not necessarily mean that the patient will experience postoperative pain in spite of the presence of documented DJD. Silastic sheeting or some other alloplastic material is wired to the zygomatic arch (Fig. 30–37). Eminectomy may be helpful when this technique is used for disc replacement, since translation motion may be impeded. Eminectomy will rapidly and effectively "decompress the intracapsular compartment by creating a large anterior recess in the superior joint space" (Weinberg, 1984). Just as eminectomy increases joint space, so too does condylar shave. These adjustments are especially helpful in patients who have pain at rest or a history of swelling. They tend to compensate for the joint space narrowing found in the earlier stages. Bessette and associates (1985) suggested salvage of part of the disc and suturing the Silastic sheeting between the bilaminar zone and the retained anterior disc.

The head of the condyle should then be reshaped with diamond bur and irrigation. Osteophytic spurring and roughened areas should be eliminated. When severe DJD is

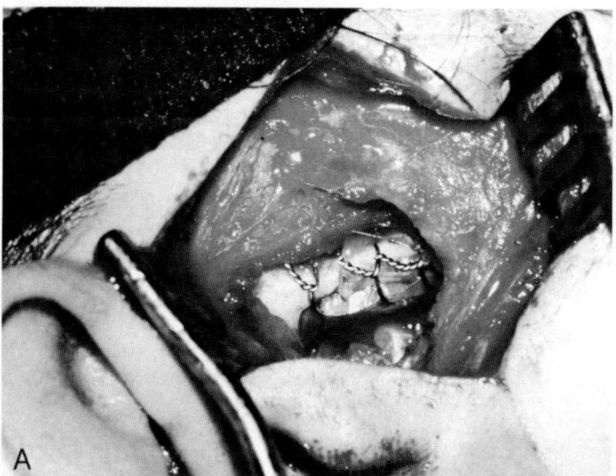

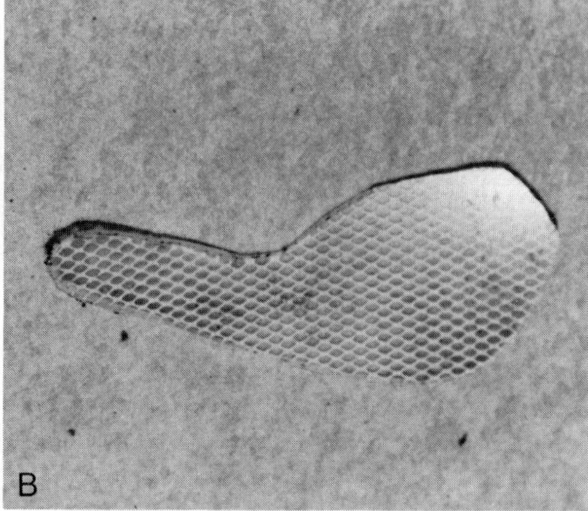

Figure 30–37. When the disc is destroyed or nonsalvageable, it is replaced. The implant is placed in the fossa. The implant tongue is wrapped around the arch by going through the space medial to the arch. This method prevents implant dislodgement (after Rippert and associates, 1986). *A*, Implant wired in position. *B*, Implant.

present, the entire articular surface may need recontouring. If the vertical dimension is lost, an implant is required to restore vertical height. The joint is irrigated clean and the capsule closed. Postoperative physiotherapy is aggressive (Helms, Katzberg, and Dolwick, 1983). Nonsteroidal anti-inflammatory drugs (e.g., ibuprofen) are often required for up to one month postoperatively. The patient should begin opening exercises with protrusive movement within two days. Attention toward midline opening is encouraged so that an interocclusal distance of 10 to 15 mm is possible by the end of the first week, 25 to 35 mm by the end of the second week, and at least 40 mm by one month. Before exercising (at least five minutes four times a day), the patient should place a warm pack over the joint. If the meniscus is removed and sheeting wired to the arch, a 35 mm opening is all that is expected. The patient should be instructed to avoid hard foods and very wide opening for at least six weeks. The bite may need adjustment after surgery, and the patient should be informed of this preoperatively.

REFERENCES

Agerberg, G., and Carlsson, G. E.: Symptoms of functional disturbances of the masticatory system: a comparison of frequencies in a population sample and in a group of patients. Acta Odontol. Scand., *33*:183, 1975.

Akers, J. O., Narang, R., and DeChamplain, R. W.: Posterior dislocation of the mandibular condyle into the external ear canal. J. Oral Maxillofac. Surg., *40*:369, 1982.

Alexander, R. W., and James, R. B.: Postauricular approach for surgery of the temporomandibular articulation. J. Oral Surg., *33*:346, 1975.

Al-Kayat, A., and Bramley, P.: A modified pre-auricular approach to the temporomandibular joint and malar arch. Br. J. Oral Surg., *17*:91, 1979.

Anderson, J., and Blair, G.: Screening in a dental clinic for adult rheumatoid arthritis involving the temporomandibular joint, using a statistical discriminant function. J. Oral Rehabil., *2*:187, 1975.

Arima, R., Shiba, R., and Hayashi, T. L.: Traumatic myositis ossificans in the masseter muscle. J. Oral Maxillofac. Surg., *42*:521, 1984.

Beekler, D. M., and Walker, R. V.: Condyle fractures. J. Oral Surg., *27*:563, 1969.

Beirne, O. R., and Leake, D. L.: Technetium 99m pyrophosphate uptake in a case of unilateral condylar hyperplasia. J. Oral Surg., *38*:385, 1980.

Bell, W. H.: Surgical Correction of Dentofacial Deformities: New Concepts. Philadelphia, W.B. Saunders Company, 1985.

Bessette, R. W., Katzberg, R., Natiella, J. R., and Rose, M. J.: Diagnosis and reconstruction of the human temporomandibular joint after trauma or internal derangement. Plast. Reconstr. Surg., *75*:192, 1985.

Blackwood, H. J. J.: Pathology of the temporomandibular joint. J. Am. Dent. Assoc., *79*:118, 1964.

Blair, A. E., and Schneider, E. K.: Intraoral inferior border osteotomy for correction of mandibular asymmetry. J. Oral Surg., *35*:493, 1977.

Blaschke, D. D., Solberg, W. K., and Sanders, B.: Arthrography of the temporomandibular joint: review of current status. J. Am. Dent. Assoc., *100*:388, 1980.

Boyer, C. C., Williams, T. W., and Stevens, F. H.: Blood supply of the temporomandibular joint. J. Dent. Res., *43*:224, 1964.

Bronstein, S. L., Tomasetti, B. J., and Ryan, D. E.: Internal derangements of the temporomandibular joint: correlation of arthrography with surgical findings. J. Oral Surg., *39*:572, 1981.

Brown, A. E., and Obeid, G.: A simplified method for the internal fixation of fractures of the mandibular condyle. Br. J. Oral Maxillofac. Surg., *22*:145, 1984.

Cadenat, H., Combelles, R., Boutault, F., and Hemous, J. D. Osteosynthesis of subcondylar fractures in the adult. Central medullary "up and down" pinning via a temporal approach. J. Maxillofac. Surg., *11*:20, 1983.

Caldwell, J. B.: Surgical management of temporomandibular ankylosis in children. Int. J. Oral Surg., *7*:354, 1978.

Dautrey, J., and Pepersack, J.: Functional surgery of the temporomandibular joint. Clin. Plast. Surg., *9*:591, 1982.

Delfino, J. J., and Eppley, B. L.: Radiographic and surgical evaluation of internal derangements of the temporomandibular joint. J. Oral Maxillofac. Surg., *44*:260, 1986.

Dolwick, M. F., Katzberg, R. W., Helms, C. A., and Bales, D. J.: Arthrotomographic evaluation of the temporomandibular joint. J. Oral Surg., *37*:793, 1979.

Dolwick, M. F., and Kretzschmar, D. P.: Morbidity associated with the preauricular and perimeatal approaches to the temporomandibular joint. J. Oral Maxillofac. Surg., *40*:699, 1982.

Dolwick, M. F., Lipton, J. S., Warner, M. R., and Williams, V. F.: Sagittal anatomy of the human temporomandibular joint spaces: normal and abnormal findings. J. Oral Maxillofac. Surg., *41*:86, 1983.

Eller, D. J., Blakemore, J. R., Stein, M., and Byers, S.: Transoral resection of a condylar osteochondroma: report of case. J. Oral Surg., *35*:409, 1977.

Eriksson, E. K. G.: Illustrated Handbook in Local Anesthesia. 2nd Ed. Chicago, Year Book Medical Publishers, 1979.

Eriksson, L., and Westesson, P. L.: Long-term evaluation of meniscectomy of the temporomandibular joint. J. Oral Maxillofac. Surg., *43*:263, 1985.

Eyanson, S., Hutton, C., and Brandt, K. D.: Erosive temporomandibular joint disease as a feature of the spondyloarthropathy of ulcerative colitis. Oral Surg. Oral Med. Oral Pathol., *53*:136, 1982.

Farrar, W. B.: Diagnosis and treatment of painful temporomandibular joints. J. Prosthet. Dent., *20*:494, 1968.

Farrar, W. B., and McCarty, W. L., Jr.: Inferior joint space arthrography and characteristics of condylar paths in internal derangements of the TMJ. J. Prosthet. Dent., *41*:548, 1979a.

Farrar, W. B., and McCarty, W. L., Jr.: The TMJ dilemma. J. Ala. Dent. Assoc., *63*:19, 1979b.

Farrar, W. B., and McCarty, W. L., Jr.: A Clinical Outline of Temporomandibular Joint Diagnosis and Treatment. 7th Ed. Montgomery, Normandie Publications, 1982.

Farrar, W. B., and McCarty, W. L., Jr.: TMJ Course in New York City, 1983.

Fitzpatrick, B. N.: Bilateral hyperplasia of the mandibular coronoid process. Oral Surg. Oral Med. Oral Pathol., *29*:184, 1970.

Gallagher, D. M., and Wolford, L. M.: Comparison of Silastic and Proplast implants in the temporomandibular joint after condylectomy for osteoarthritis. J. Oral Maxillofac. Surg., *40*:627, 1982.

Georgiade, N.: Disturbances of the temporomandibular joint. *In* Converse, J. M. (Ed.): Reconstructive Plastic Surgery. Vol. 3. Philadelphia, W. B. Saunders Company, 1977, p. 1521.

Grant, P. G.: Lateral pterygoid: 2 muscles? Am. J. Anat., *138*:1, 1973.

Hale, R. H.: Treatment of recurrent dislocation of the mandible: review of the literature and report of cases. J. Oral Surg., *30*:527, 1972.

Hall, M. B., Brown, R. W., and Lebowitz, M. S.: Facial nerve injury during surgery of the temporomandibular joint: a comparison of two dissection techniques. J. Oral Maxillofac. Surg., *43*:20, 1985.

Hartwell, S. W., and Hall, M. D.: Mandibular condylectomy with silicone rubber replacement. Plast. Reconstr. Surg., *53*:440, 1974.

Hecker, R., and Corwin, J. O.: Bilateral coronoid hyperplasia: review of the literature and report of case. J. Oral. Surg., *38*:606, 1980.

Helms, C. A., Katzberg, R. W., and Dolwick, M. F.: Internal Derangements of the Temporomandibular Joint. San Francisco Radiology Research and Education Foundation, 1983.

Helms, C. A., Katzberg, R. W., Dolwick, M. F., and Bales, D. J.: Arthrotomographic diagnosis of meniscus perforations in the temporomandibular joint. Br. J. Radiol., *53*:283, 1980.

Helms, C. A., Morrish, R. B., Jr., Kircos, L. T., Katzberg, R. W., and Dolwick, M. F.: Computed tomography of the meniscus of the temporomandibular joint: preliminary observations. Radiology, *145*:719, 1982.

Horowitz, I., Abrahami, E., and Mintz, S. S.: Demonstration of condylar fractures of the mandible by computed tomography. Oral Surg. Oral Med. Oral Pathol., *54*:263, 1982.

Ihalainen, U., and Tasanen, A.: Central luxation or dislocation of the mandibular condyle into the middle cranial fossa. A case report and review of the literature. Int. J. Oral Surg., *12*:39, 1983.

Irby, W. B.: Surgery of the temporomandibular joint. *In* Irby, W. B. (Ed.): Current Advances in Oral Surgery. Vol. 1. St. Louis, C. V. Mosby Company, 1974.

Irby, W. B. (Ed.): Current Advances in Oral Surgery. Vol. 3. St. Louis, C. V. Mosby Company, 1980, p. 313.

Isbert-Holm, A., and Westesson, P. L.: Temporomandibular joint clicking (thesis). Malmo, 1980.

James, B. R., Fredrickson, C., and Kent, J. N.: Prospective study of mandibular fractures. J. Oral Surg., *39*:275, 1981.

Jonck, L. M.: Condylar hyperplasia. A case for early treatment. Int. J. Oral Surg., *10*:154, 1981.

Juniper, R. P.: The superior pterygoid muscle? Br. J. Oral Surg., *19*:121, 1981.

Kaneda, T., Torii, S., Yamashita, T., Inoue, N., and Shimizu, K. Giant osteochondroma of the mandibular condyle. J. Oral Maxillofac. Surg., *40*:818, 1982.

Katzberg, R. W., Dolwick, M. F., Bales, D. J., and Helms, C. A.: Arthrotomography of the temporomandibular joint: New technique and preliminary observations. AJR, *132*:949, 1979.

Katzberg, R. W., Dolwick, M. F., Helms, C. A., and Bales, D. J.: Arthrotomography of the temporomandibular joint. *In* Dalinka, M. K. (Ed.): Arthrography. New York, Springer, 1980a.

Katzberg, R. W., Dolwick, M. F., Helms, C. A., Hopens, T., Bales, D. J., and Coggs, G. C.: Arthrotomography of the temporomandibular joint. AJR, *134*:995, 1980b.

Katzberg, R. W., Dolwick, M. F., Keith, D. A., Helms, C. A., and Guralnick, W. C.: New observations with routine and CT-assisted arthrography in suspected internal derangements of the temporomandibular joint. Oral Surg. Oral Med. Oral Pathol., *51*:569, 1981.

Keen, R. R., and Callahan, G. R.: Osteochondroma of the mandibular condyle: report of a case. J. Oral Surg., *35*:140, 1977.

Keizer, S., and Tuinzing, D. B.: Spontaneous regeneration of a unilaterally absent mandibular condyle. J. Oral Maxillofac. Surg., *43*:130, 1985.

Kent, J. N., Misiek, D. J., Akin, R. K., Hinds, E. C., and Homsy, C. A.: Temporomandibular joint condylar prosthesis: a ten year report. J. Oral Maxillofac. Surg., *41*:245, 1983.

Kent, J. N., and Zide, M. F.: Wound healing: bone and biomaterials. Otolaryngol. Clin. North Am., *17*:273, 1984.

Kiehn, C. L.: Meniscectomy for internal derangement of the temporomandibular joint. Am. J. Surg., *83*:364, 1952.

Koberg, W. R., and Momma, W. G.: Treatment of fractures of the articular process by functional stable osteosynthesis using miniaturized dynamic compression plates. Int. J. Oral Surg., *7*:256, 1978.

Koehl, G. L., and Tilson, H. B.: Osteochondromas associated with facial asymmetry and masticatory dysfunction: report of two cases. J. Oral Surg., *35*:934, 1977.

Kraut, R. A.: Treatment of osteoarthritis of the temporomandibular joint. Oral Surg. Oral Med. Oral Pathol., *51*:355, 1981.

Kreutziger, K. L.: Surgery of the temporomandibular joint. I. Surgical anatomy and surgical incisions. Oral Surg. Oral Med. Oral Pathol., *58*:637, 1984.

Kursunoglu, S., Kaplan, P., Resnick, D., and Sartoris, D. J.: Three-dimensional computed tomographic analysis of the normal temporomandibular joint. J. Oral Maxillofac. Surg., *44*:257, 1986.

Lanigan, D. T., Myall, R. W., West, R. A., and McNeill, R. W.: Condylysis in a patient with a mixed collagen vascular disease. Oral Surg. Oral Med. Oral Pathol., *48*:198, 1979.

Laskin, D.: Myotomy for the management of recurrent and protracted mandibular dislocation. Trans. 4th Internatl. Conf. on Oral Surg. Copenhagen, Munksgaard, 1973, p. 254.

Laskin, D. M.: Role of the meniscus in the etiology of post-traumatic temporomandibular joint ankylosis. Int. J. Oral Surg., 7:340, 1978.

Lewin, R. W., and Wright, J. A.: Silastic ulnar head prostheses for use in surgery of the temporomandibular joint. J. Oral Surg., *36*:906, 1978.

Lewis, J. E. S.: A simple technique for reduction of long-standing dislocation of the mandible. Br. J. Oral Surg. *18*:52, 1981.

Lowry, J.: Psoriatic arthritis involving the temporomandibular joint. J. Oral Surg., *33*:206, 1975.

Lund, K.: Mandibular growth and remodelling processes after condylar fractures. Acta Odontol. Scand. [Suppl.], *32*:3, 1974.

MacIntosh, R. B.: Current spectrum of costochondral

grafting. *In* Bell, W. H. (Ed.): Surgical Correction of Dentofacial Deformities: New Concepts. Philadelphia, W. B. Saunders Company, 1985.

MacIntosh, R. B., and Henny, F. A.: A spectrum of application of autogenous costochondral grafts. J. Maxillofac. Surg., *5*:257, 1977.

Marano, P. D., Fenster, G. F., and Gosselin, C. F.: Eagle's syndrome necessitating bilateral styloid amputation. Oral Surg. Oral Med. Oral Pathol., *33*:874, 1972.

McCarty, W. L.: Diagnosis and treatment of internal derangements of the articular disc and mandibular condyle. *In* Solberg, W. K., and Clark, G. T. (Eds.): Temporomandibular Joint Problems: Biologic Diagnosis and Treatment. Chicago, Quintessence, 1980.

McNamara, J. A., Jr.: The independent functions of the two heads of the lateral pterygoid muscle. Am. J. Anat., *138*:197, 1973.

Messer, E. J., and Abramson, A. M.: The stylohyoid syndrome. J. Oral Surg., *33*:664, 1975.

Miller, G. A., Page, H. L., Jr., and Griffith, C. R.: Temporomandibular joint ankylosis: review of the literature and report of 2 cases of bilateral involvement. J. Oral Surg., *33*:792, 1975.

Minami, R. T.: Temporomandibular joint ankylosis—experience with a case of 20 years' duration. Ann. Plast. Surg., *7*:228, 1981.

Monks, F. T.: Bilateral hyperplasia of the mandibular coronoid processes: a case report. Br. J. Oral Surg., *16*:31, 1978.

Moorthy, A. P., and Finch, L. D.: Interpositional arthroplasty for ankylosis of the temporomandibular joint. Oral Surg. Oral Med. Oral Pathol., *55*:545, 1983.

Morgan, D. H.: Surgical correction of temporomandibular joint arthritis. J. Oral Surg., *33*:766, 1975.

Morris, J.: Chronic recurring temporomaxillary subluxation. Surg. Gynecol. Obstet., *50*:483, 1930.

Munro, I. R., Chen, Y. R., and Park, B. Y.: Simultaneous total correction of temporomandibular ankylosis and facial asymmetry. Plast. Reconstr. Surg., *77*:517, 1986.

Murphy, W. A.: Arthrography of the temporomandibular joint. Radiol. Clin. North Am., *19*:365, 1981.

Murphy, W. A., and Adams, R. J.: The temporomandibular joint. *In* Resnick, D. (Ed.): Diagnosis of Bone and Joint Disorders with Emphasis on Articular Abnormalities. Philadelphia, W. B. Saunders Company, 1981, pp. 3061–3101.

Murray, I. P., and Ford, J. C.: TC-99m medronate scintigraphy in mandibular condylar hyperplasia. Clin. Nucl. Med., *7*:474, 1982.

Murray, J. E., Kaban, L. B., and Mulliken, J. B.: Analysis and treatment of hemifacial microsomia. Plast. Reconstr. Surg., *74*:186, 1984.

Myrhaug, H.: The incidence of ear symptoms in cases of malocclusion and temporomandibular joint disturbances. Br. J. Oral Surg., *2*:28, 1969.

Nagase, M., Ueda, K., Suzuki, I., and Nakajima, T.: Spontaneous regeneration of the condyle following hemimandibulectomy by disarticulation. J. Oral Maxillofac. Surg., *43*:218, 1985.

Obwegeser, H. L.: Temporal approach to the TMJ, the orbit, and the retromaxillary-infracranial region. Head Neck Surg., *7*:185, 1985.

Ogus, H.: Rheumatoid arthritis of the temporomandibular joint. Br. J. Oral Surg., *12*:275, 1975.

Olson, R. A., Fonseca, R. J., Zeitler, D. L., and Osbon, D. B.: Fractures of the mandible: a review of 580 cases. J. Oral Maxillofac. Surg., *40*:23, 1982.

Oster, C., Katzberg, R. W., Tallents, R. H., Morris, T. W., Bartholomew, J., et al.: Characterization of temporomandibular joint sounds. A preliminary investigation with arthrographic correlation. Oral Surg. Oral Med. Oral Pathol., *58*:10, 1984.

Petzel, J. R.: Instrumentarium and technique for screw-pin osteosynthesis of condylar fractures. J. Maxillofac. Surg., *10*:8, 1982.

Petzel, J. R., and Bulles, G.: Stability of the mandibular condylar process after functionally stable traction screw osteosynthesis (T.S.O.) with a self tapping screw pin. J. Maxillofac. Surg., *10*:149, 1982.

Pool, J. W., Tilson, H. B., Thornton, W. E., and Steed, D. L.: Osteochondroma of the zygomatic arch: report of case. J. Oral Surg., *37*:673, 1979.

Rajgopal, A., Banerji, P. K., Batura, V., and Sural, A.: Temporomandibular ankylosis. A report of 15 cases. J. Maxillofac. Surg., *11*:37, 1983.

Rankow, R. M., and Mignogna, F. V.: Ankylosis of the temporalis-coronoid complex of the mandible. Ann. Plast. Surg., *1*:280, 1978.

Rees, A. M., and Weinberg, S.: Fractures of the mandibular condyle: review of the literature and presentation of five cases with late complications. Oral Health, *73*:37, 1983.

Rippert, E. T., Flanigan, T. J., and Middlebrooks, M. L.: New design for Silastic implants in temporomandibular joint surgery. J. Oral Maxillofac. Surg., *44*:163, 1986.

Sanders, B.: Temporomandibular joint ankylosis secondary to Marie-Strümpell disease. J. Oral Surg., *33*:784, 1975.

Sanders, B., and McKelvy, B.: Osteochondromatous exostosis of the condyle. J. Am. Dent. Assoc., *95*:1151, 1977.

Sanger, R., and Greer, R.: Facially displaced condylar fractures. Oral Surg. Oral Med. Oral Pathol., *47*:492, 1979.

Seymour, R., Crouse, V., and Irby, W.: Temporomandibular ankylosis secondary to rheumatoid arthritis. Oral Surg. Oral Med. Oral Pathol., *40*:584, 1975.

Shira, R. B., and Lister, R. L.: Limited mandibular movement due to enlargement of the coronoid process. J. Oral Surg., *16*:183, 1958.

Shuken, R. A., and Girard, K. R.: Bilateral mandibular coronoid hyperplasia. J. Oral Surg., *37*:744, 1979.

Simon, G. T., Kendrick, R. W., and Whitlock, R. I.: Osteochondroma of the mandibular condyle. Case report and its management. Oral Surg. Oral Med. Oral Pathol., *43*:18, 1977.

Spence, D. R.: Post-injury condylar remodeling in children. Oral Surg. Oral Med. Oral Pathol., *53*:340, 1982.

Sperling, A.: Limitation of mandibular movement secondary to coronoid impingement. J. Oral Surg., *31*:780, 1973.

Stakesby-Lewis, J. E.: A simple technique for reduction of long-standing dislocation of the mandible. Br. J. Oral Surg., *19*:52, 1981.

Stanson, A. W., and Baker, H. L., Jr.: Routine tomography of the temporomandibular joint. Radiol. Clin. North Am., *14*:105, 1976.

Tasanen, A., and Lamberg, M. A.: Transosseous wiring in the treatment of condylar fractures of the mandible. J. Maxillofac. Surg., *4*:200, 1976.

Topazian, R. G.: Etiology of ankylosis of the temporomandibular joint. Analysis of 44 cases. J. Oral Surg., *22*:227, 1964.

Trenwith, J. A., and Beale, G.: Rheumatoid arthritis in the temporomandibular joint. N.Z. Dent. J., *73*:195, 1977.

Turpin, D. L., and West, R. A.: Juvenile rheumatoid arthritis: a case report of surgical/orthodontic treatment. Am. J. Orthod., *73*:312, 1978.

van Hoof, R. F., and Besling, W. F. J.: Coronoid process enlargement. Br. J. Oral Surg., *10*:339, 1973.

Walker, R. V., and Kalamchi, S.: A surgical technique for management of internal derangement of the temporomandibular joint. J. Oral Maxillofac. Surg., *45*:299, 1987.

Weinberg, S.: Eminectomy and meniscorrhaphy for internal derangements of the temporomandibular joint. Rationale and operative technique. Oral Surg. Oral Med. Oral Pathol., *57*:241, 1984.

Wennogle, C. F., and Delo, R. I.: A pin-in-groove technique for reduction of displaced subcondylar fractures of the mandible. J. Oral Maxillofac. Surg., *43*:659, 1985.

Wilkes, C. H.: Arthrography of the temporomandibular joint in patients with TMJ pain-dysfunction syndrome. Minn. Med., *61*:645, 1978.

Worthington, P.: Dislocation of the mandibular condyle into the temporal fossa. J. Maxillofac. Surg., *10*:24, 1982.

Zecha, J. J.: Mandibular condyle dislocation into the middle cranial fossa. Int. J. Oral Surg., *6*:141, 1977.

Zide, M. F., and Kent, J. N.: Indications for open reduction of mandibular condyle fractures. J. Oral Maxillofac. Surg., *41*:89, 1983.

31

Charles P. Vallis

Hair Replacement Surgery

HISTORY

ANATOMY OF HAIR AND SCALP

GROWTH CYCLE

HAIR TYPES

FACTORS INFLUENCING HAIR GROWTH

SURGICAL TREATMENT OF ALOPECIA
- Composite Scalp Grafts
- Scalp Flaps
- Scalp Reduction

The surgical replacement of hair has progressively become an important part of the practice of plastic surgery. The ever-increasing success of hair transplantation for the treatment of male pattern baldness has made it the most common cosmetic procedure in the male. For many years nonvascularized hair-bearing grafts were the sole means of transferring hair follicles to correct male pattern baldness. During the past 15 years various types of flap and scalp reduction procedures have proved their usefulness. The surgeon should be well versed in several methods of hair replacement. Versatility in the various surgical techniques is essential to achieving a suitable growth of hair.

Anthropologic studies have shown that man's early ancestors had a heavy covering of body hair, and this was obviously useful in protecting him from the elements. Actually, hair has practically no functional significance in our present-day life. Berg (1951) states: "Although hair has ceased to be the over-coat provided by nature against the elements, it has not ceased to be of psychological, as distinct from physical, significance."

Since his early beginnings, man has always devoted a considerable portion of his daily existence to some form of interference with his hair. There has always been a normal concern, and occasionally even an intense anxiety, about the general condition of the hair, whether it is becoming thin, shedding, or becoming gray.

In every civilization some special meaning has been attributed to the presence or absence of hair. Some examples of the symbolic nature of hair are pertinent to the understanding of present-day man's concern in losing his hair and his desire to restore it. Among primitive and civilized people, hair has always had a symbolic significance. Hair has been regarded as the seat of strength, as a symbol of royalty and social status, as a fetish and index of sensuality, and more often as the emblem of juvenescence itself. The absence or presence of hair was also symbolically significant as a form of punishment, religious sacrifice, or mourning. In every civilization, the length of hair, the presence or absence of hair, and the hair styling also played an important role in revealing an individual's occupation and professional status, moral conduct, age, sex, and marital status.

HISTORY

Since the dawn of history, man has been searching for a method to correct or at least retard male pattern baldness (Byron, 1931). Repair of scalp defects due to trauma or disease has been practiced by surgeons for many years using skin grafts and flaps (Kazanjian and Webster, 1946; Straith and Beers, 1950; Vallis and Humphreys, 1956). However, consideration was rarely given to the esthetic correction of the simple loss of scalp hair. Until recently the attitude of plastic surgeons toward the treatment of baldness was one of indifference. Padgett and Stephenson (1948) wrote: "We were consulted several times by patients for relief of alopecia. The patients have our sympathy but so far, we have turned a cold shoulder to the petitioner."

Before 1959 only sporadic reports appeared in the literature relative to the surgical treatment of baldness. Hunt (1926) was one of the first to propose surgical procedures for correction of alopecia and alopecia areata. He reasoned that, if baldness was not too extensive, it could be entirely corrected by a series of excisions of the balding scalp, and by advancing the hair-bearing scalp to close the defects.

Passot, in his classic text published in 1931, described the use of long, narrowly based, hair-bearing transposition flaps to treat alopecia (Fig. 31–1). His method was revolutionary and imaginative, and is the precursor of many flap techniques used today.

In 1939 Tauber, applying Passot's technique, described the use of local flaps elevated from the lateral and posterior scalp for replacement of hair in the denuded frontal areas in 50 cases of male pattern baldness.

In 1939, a paper by Okuda first described the use of punch grafts for transplanting hair in 200 cases of cicatricial alopecia. Okuda also advocated this technique for alopecia of the eyebrows and mustache areas.

In 1950, Barsky reported a case of cicatricial alopecia in the occipital scalp improved by implanting small grafts of hair-bearing scalp skin.

Nothing further of any significance appeared in the literature relative to the surgical approach to baldness until 1957, when Lamont described lateral scalp flaps for the treatment of frontotemporal baldness. Correa-Iturraspe and Arufe (1957) attempted several different methods to correct partial alopecia. They reduced the bald area by excising full-thickness segments of hairless skin and by closing the wound margins primarily. In addition, they used bipedicle and unipedicle flaps to transfer hair-bearing segments to the bald areas.

The modern age of hair transplantation for the treatment of male pattern baldness was launched in 1959 by the classic publication of Orentreich entitled "Autografts in alopecias and other selected dermatological conditions." Orentreich described the results of transplanting hair-bearing scalp punch grafts in areas of alopecia and other skin sites with dermatologic disorders. After this work was published, many surgically oriented dermatologists used the punch graft technique to treat male pattern baldness. Within a short time the operation became the most commonly used method of hair transplantation.

In 1964, Vallis described the combination of the strip graft and the punch graft method. In 1965, Fleming reported a case of bilateral frontotemporal alopecia corrected by the excision of the two triangular bald areas and the immediate reconstruction of the defects with rotation flaps. In 1971, Coiffman introduced the use of the free square scalp graft.

Harii, Ohmori, and Ohmori (1974) made use of recently developed microsurgical techniques to transplant hair to heavily scarred areas with free scalp flaps. In 1975, Juri reported several hundred cases of male pattern baldness treated with large, narrowly based, temporo-parieto-occipital flaps. In 1976, Blanchard and Blanchard described the technique of scalp reduction, which they called "obliteration of alopecia by hair lifting."

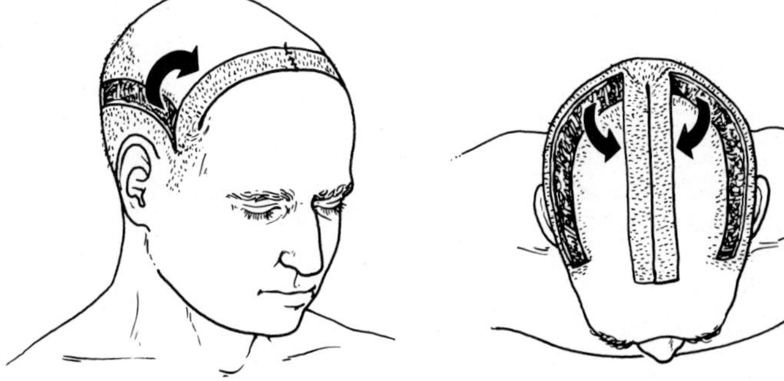

Figure 31–1. Passot's technique of scalp transposition flaps for the treatment of alopecia.

Radovan (1976) was the first to describe the use of tissue expansion in reconstructive surgery. In 1977, Elliott described the use of a smaller, temporo-parietal scalp flap. Manders and associates (1984) reported the use of tissue expanders to reconstruct large scalp defects.

ANATOMY OF HAIR AND SCALP

The hair shaft is composed of keratin and is essentially a collection of dead cells cemented together in the form of threads. It is a protein end product of a living structure, the hair follicle (Flesch, 1945).

The hair follicle is a pouchlike depression or invagination of the epidermis into the dermis (Montagna, 1956). At the base, the follicles have an onion-shaped dilatation called the bulb. The bulb is hollowed out at its base, forming an envelope around a small remnant of dermis known as the dermal papilla. When the hair is of considerable length, the follicle extends into the subcutaneous tissue. The hair follicle commences on the surface of the skin and passes inward in an oblique or angulated direction. The direction may also be curved and angulated when the hair is curly.

The hair follicle consists of two coats, a dermal or outer coat and an epidermal or inner coat. The dermal coat is continuous with the corium and is composed of fibrous tissue. It is highly vascular and has numerous minute nerve filaments (Gray, 1942).

The arrectores pilorum is a single muscle. There is one for every hair follicle in the scalp. These muscles, which have several points of origin in the corium, are inserted into the hair follicle just below its neck and below the duct entrance of the sebaceous gland. The action of this muscle is to elevate the hair and express the sebaceous secretion from the duct of the gland.

The scalp is composed of five layers (Fig. 31–2).

Skin. The skin of the scalp is very thick and is attached by dense fibrous septa to the underlying aponeurosis and muscle. Movements of the underlying muscle move the skin. The skin contains much hair, densely set together, and numerous sweat and sebaceous glands.

Subcutaneous Tissue. The subcutaneous layer is a firm, dense, fibrofatty layer. It has several fibrous septa intimately attached to the skin and underlying epicranius. The blood vessels are contained in the deeper aspect of this layer. Since the fibrous septa are tough and inelastic, the blood vessels imbedded in this unyielding tissue bleed profusely when incised because of their inability to contract. The nerves are also contained in this layer. Sepsis in the scalp usually remains localized because of the fibrous septa. However, purulent collections are associated with pain because the nerves are compressed within closed compartments.

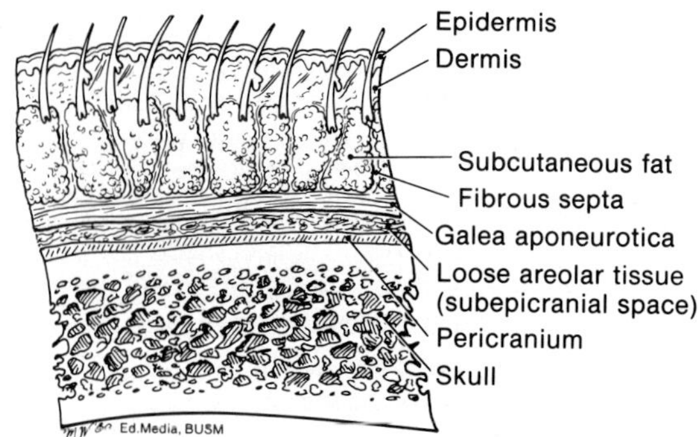

Figure 31–2. The layers of the scalp.

Epicranius. This is a broad, musculofibrous layer that covers the top of the scalp (Fig. 31–3). It is attached posteriorly to the superior nuchal line of the occipital bone, laterally to the temporal fascia, and anteriorly it intermingles with the orbicularis oculi fibers. It consists of two parts, the occipitalis muscle and the frontalis muscle, connected by an intervening aponeurosis, the galea aponeurotica. The latter covers the vertex of the skull.

Subepicranial Space. This is a layer of loose, areolar connective tissue between the galea and the periosteum or pericranium. The looseness of this layer allows for easy dissection and elevation of scalp flaps at this level. This space contains small blood vessels, which supply the pericranium and emissary veins. The latter connect the intracranial venous sinuses with the superficial veins of the scalp.

Pericranium. The pericranium is the periosteum overlying the skull. It is a thin, yet strong, membrane that strips easily from the bone except at the suture line, where it dips to merge with the dura.

The scalp is a unique structure. Its outer three layers are independent of the skull. They are intimately fused together and move

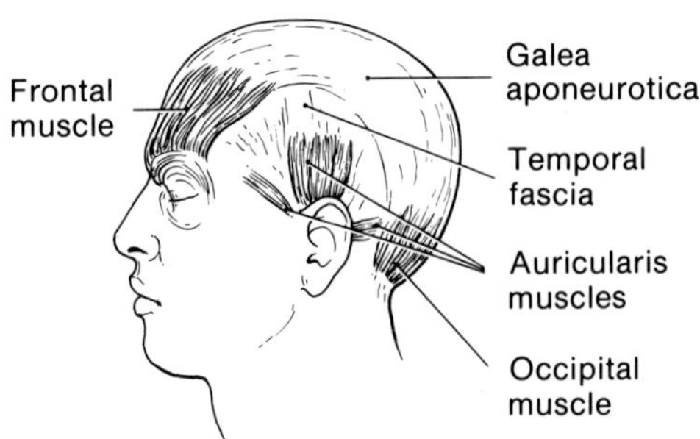

Figure 31–3. The epicranius.

over the skull as a unit with contraction of the associated frontalis and occipitalis muscles. The major blood supply and nerves enter the scalp from the periphery. These vessels traverse through the subcutaneous tissue and interconnect freely throughout the scalp. The vascular anastomosis is such that one set of intact vessels could nourish the entire scalp. This type of vascular network is unlike any other in the body and makes it possible to construct a wide range of flaps. Long, narrow flaps that would never survive elsewhere in the body can be constructed on the scalp, and often are transposed without delay.

The main blood supply to the scalp is derived from the external carotid artery through four branches (Cutting, McCarthy, and Berenstein, 1984; Casanova and associates, 1986) (Fig. 31–4):

1. Superficial temporal artery.
2. Occipital artery.
3. Internal maxillary artery.
4. Posterior auricular artery.

Two branches from the internal carotid by way of the ophthalmic artery also supply the frontal scalp:

1. Supratrochlear artery.
2. Supraorbital artery.

Preserving and respecting the blood supply to the scalp is the most important factor in ensuring a successful result in any type of hair transplantation. Transplanting too many grafts in the recipient site or inserting the grafts too close together, with short intervals between operations, diminishes the blood supply.

The veins accompany the arteries and empty into the external jugular, with the exception of the emissary veins, which drain into the superior sagittal sinus. The frontal and supraorbital veins empty first into the ophthalmic veins and then into the cavernous sinus. These last two venous systems are of particular importance, since infection may be conveyed from the scalp and upper part of the face directly into the interior of the skull.

The sensory innervation to the frontal part of the scalp is supplied by the supratrochlear nerve and the two branches of the supraorbital nerve (Fig. 31–5). Both nerves are branches of the frontal nerve, which is the middle branch of the ophthalmic, a branch of the trigeminal. The zygomatic nerve innervates the temporal region through its zygomaticotemporal branch. The zygomatic nerve is a lateral branch of the maxillary nerve, the second branch of the trigeminal nerve. The auriculotemporal nerve, a lateral branch of the mandibular nerve, innervates the parietal area of the scalp. The mandibular nerve is the third branch of the trigeminal nerve.

The greater auricular and lesser occipital nerves innervate the scalp behind the ear. The greater occipital nerve supplies sensation to the occiput and crown of the scalp. These nerves arise from the second and third branches of the cervical plexus.

The motor branch of the occipitalis muscle is the posterior auricular branch of the facial

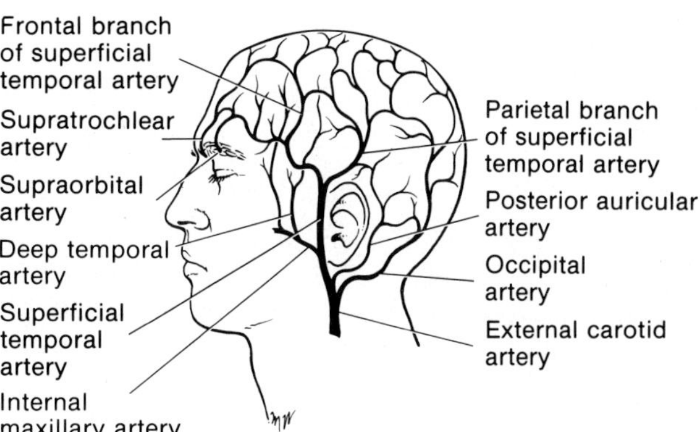

Figure 31–4. The arterial supply of the scalp.

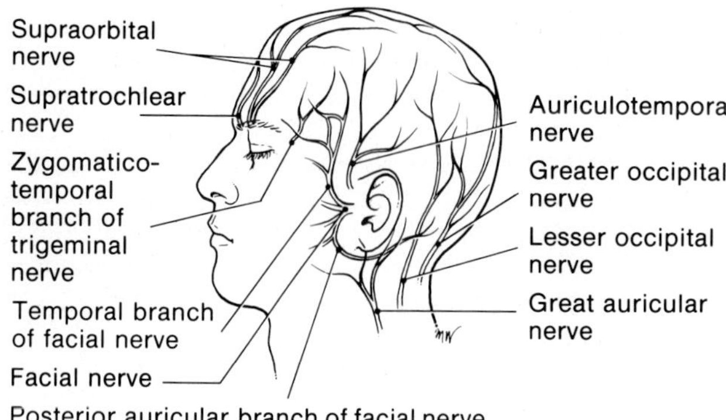

Figure 31–5. The nerve (motor and sensory) supply of the scalp.

nerve. The frontalis muscle is supplied by the temporal branch of the facial nerve.

All the nerves of the scalp traverse the dense superficial fascia between the galea and the overlying integument. Injection with local anesthesia can cause intense pain if the anesthetic solution is given rapidly, owing to compression of the nerves that results from the inability of this space to expand. The distribution of the nerves also allows for block anesthesia, especially in the frontal and occipital areas of the scalp.

GROWTH CYCLE

The living cells at the base of the hair follicle show active mitotic growth. They eventually form a compact column, which extends toward the surface of the skin. A zone of keratinization forms directly above the actively dividing cells. The living cells become dehydrated, eventually die, and are converted into a mass of keratin. The keratin filaments are cemented together by a matrix rich in cystine.

An average of 100,000 hairs make up the scalp hair of adults. The ratio of hair growth in man was measured by two groups of investigators, and their results are in close agreement (Myers and Hamilton, 1951; Saitoh, Uzuka, and Sakamoto, 1969). The average rate of growth of scalp hair is about 0.35 mm per day, or about 1 cm per month.

The dermal papilla, situated just under the actively dividing cells of the follicle, actually plays a vital role in the regulatory control of the hair's growth cycle. The hair follicle passes through a life cycle (Fig. 31–6), which is divided into three phases.

Anagen Phase. The anagen phase is the actively growing period of the hair. The follicular cells are actively multiplying and keratinizing. Approximately 90 per cent of the hairs on the scalp are in the anagen phase, which in man lasts approximately three years.

Catagen Phase. When a hair is approaching the catagen phase, the base of the hair becomes keratinized to form a club, and the melanocytes change and cease producing melanin. A constricted epidermal strand remains, joining the dermal papilla with the hair club, which moves toward the surface, completing catagen. The follicular bulb is largely destroyed, leaving the follicle much

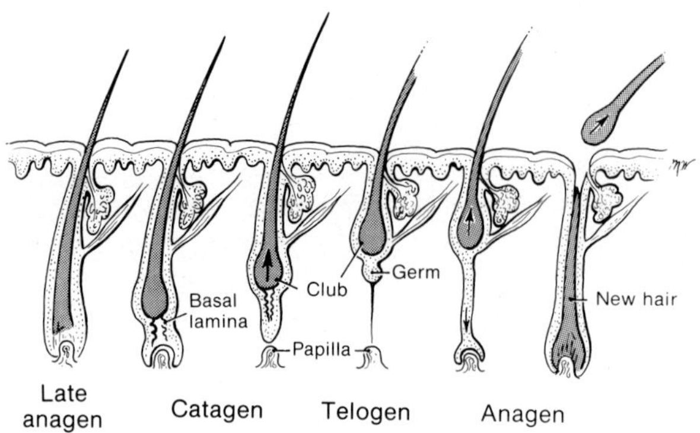

Figure 31–6. The growth cycle of the hair.

shorter. Catagen lasts about one to two weeks.

Telogen Phase. The dermal papilla becomes released from its epidermal investment as the follicle passes into the telogen or resting phase. A small nipple of undifferentiated tissue known as the secondary germ is left. Telogen lasts about three to four months. During this period the follicle is inactive and hair growth ceases. When the attachment of the hair to the base of the follicle is weakened, the hair is shed. Approximately 10 per cent of the hairs are in telogen. The average daily loss of scalp hair is about 100 hairs. When the rate of hair loss is greater than the rate of regeneration, thinning of the scalp occurs, with eventual alopecia.

Anagen begins again when the secondary germ lengthens and becomes invaginated by the dermal papilla.

Hair has a characteristic histologic appearance during anagen and telogen, which makes it possible to determine the *anagen:telogen ratio* in the scalp at any time. Determining the ratio can be accomplished by plucking several hairs and examining them microscopically. A high telogen count could indicate an abnormal amount of hair loss.

HAIR TYPES

There are three types of hair.

Lanugo Hair. Lanugo hair is soft and fine, usually unpigmented and without a medulla. This hair is found on the fetus and is usually shed about the eighth month of gestation.

Vellus Hair. Vellus hair is also soft and unmedullated. It is short, rarely exceeding 2 cm in length, and may be pigmented. It replaces lanugo hair in the postnatal period, and it is spread over the entire body surface.

Terminal Hair. Terminal hair is longer, coarser, pigmented, and medullated. It replaces vellus hair at specific sites on the body. In areas of the scalp that are destined by age and heredity to become bald, the vellus hairs that first fall out are replaced by those of less vigorous growth, and these in turn are shed to make way for still weaker ones until a short vellus-type hair of static growth becomes evident. The process continues until complete baldness results. Biopsies of bald sites show persistent hair follicles that are much smaller than normal. There is no apparent decrease in the number of follicles. The fact that the hair follicles are still present, albeit in miniaturized form, has led some investigators to believe that these may regain their function of hair growth if the androgenic effect on the hair follicle is eliminated. Hamilton (1958) showed that once the hair follicle is affected by androgens, it does not necessarily revert to its prestimulated state after androgen deprivation.

FACTORS INFLUENCING HAIR GROWTH

Male pattern baldness, or androgenic alopecia, is the most common type of hair loss in both sexes. Androgenic alopecia is controlled by a single, dominant, sex-limited autosomal gene. Regardless of how strong is the inherited predisposition to baldness, alopecia does not result if inciting agents such as androgens are missing. Conversely, the androgenetic inciting agents are not able to induce baldness in individuals not genetically predisposed to baldness.

Alopecia occurs only in those scalp follicles that have the genetic potential to be inhibited by androgens over a period of time. The capacity for development of baldness appears to be controlled by factors resident in localized areas of the scalp. The hair follicles most typically subjected to androgenic alopecia are in the frontal and crown regions of the scalp. Each hair follicle carries the genetic capability to produce hair associated with the area from which it is obtained. The follicle is not affected by the area in which it is placed. Consequently, it is important when transplanting hair, especially in male pattern baldness, whether it be nonvascularized grafts or flaps, that the donor site be in an area of the scalp containing follicles of high longevity. The transplanted hair in the recipient site will continue to grow and remain viable for as long as it would have remained viable in the donor area.

Orentreich (1959) suggested the terms *donor dominant* and *recipient dominant* to describe the results in transplanting grafts in areas of alopecia and other sites possessing certain dermatologic disorders. When the transposed graft of skin maintains its integrity and characteristics independent of the recipient site, it is donor dominant. When the transposed graft of skin takes on the characteristics of the recipient site, it is recipient dominant. Donor dominance is observed in all cases of alopecia of the scalp. Grafts containing hair continue to grow in the area of alopecia and the hair continues to have the same texture and color and to grow at the same period of anagen that governs the nature of the hair in the donor site.

The nonsurgical treatment of male pattern alopecia has a long history of association with quackery. In 1979 the United States Food and Drug Administration (FDA) approved the marketing of minoxidil as an effective oral antihypertensive agent. A side effect of the drug was the development of generalized body hair. Dermatologists prepared hydroalcoholic solutions of minoxidil for topical application to the balding scalp with sporadic success. In 1983 double-blind and placebo-controlled multi-institutional clinical trials were initiated to assess the safety and efficiency of a 2 and 3 per cent minoxidil solution for male pattern alopecia. These studies have been completed, and chronic use studies continue (Savin, 1987).

Current knowledge suggests that twice daily application of a 2 per cent minoxidil solution gives optimal results. Almost all patients experience a diminution in the rate of hair loss, often perceptible after only a few weeks of use. Approximately two-thirds of patients note an improvement in the texture of existing hair, a finding attributed to enlargement of the hair follicle with the production of a thicker hair shaft. Approximately one-third of patients have visible new hair growth, but only about one-third of these (10 per cent of all users) show profuse growth. The best responses were observed in individuals just beginning to bald (the nonsurgical group). Extensive safety testing failed to reveal any systemic toxicity. There were occasional instances of irritation of the scalp, especially in individuals with underlying scalp dermatoses.

A commercial preparation is being marketed in Canada, and approval by the U.S. FDA is imminent. The product has several drawbacks. It is expensive. Chronic use is necessary since discontinuance results in rapid reversal of all benefits. The optimal dosing frequency for chronic use has yet to be determined. Many patients are unwilling to comply with chronic use, being reluctant to expend the effort necessary for regular applications. Finally, the long-term side effects of chronic topical application, either locally or systemically, are unknown, although animal studies suggest safety.

The advent of the first drug demonstrably capable of influencing male pattern alopecia has opened the door to new clinical studies searching for more effective agents. Trials are now in progress using prostaglandin analogues, topical vasodilators, and topical angiogenesis factors.

Topical minoxidil is not capable of replacing surgical methods, but it is useful in early male pattern alopecia where it may prevent or delay progression. The ability of minoxidil to stimulate the hair follicle may make it a suitable adjunct to surgical hair replacement techniques where postoperative application may help to maximize the cosmetic result.

SURGICAL TREATMENT OF ALOPECIA

There are essentially three major methods of transplanting hair to bald areas of the scalp:

1. Composite hair-bearing scalp grafts.
   a. Punch grafts.
      (1) Round.
      (2) Square.
   b. Strip grafts.
2. Scalp flaps.
   a. Rotation flaps.
   b. Transposition flaps.
      (1) Temporo-parieto-occipital flaps.
      (2) Lateral scalp flaps.
      (3) Temporal vertical flaps.
   c. Bipedicle flaps.
   d. Multiple flaps.
   e. Microvascular free flaps.
3. Scalp reduction.
   a. Fractional excision of alopecia.
   b. Excision of alopecia with the aid of scalp expanders.

Composite Scalp Grafts

ROUND PUNCH GRAFTS

Healthy, highly motivated patients with moderate hairline recession and with dense hair of good quality in the donor areas are considered candidates for this procedure. These patients are even better candidates if

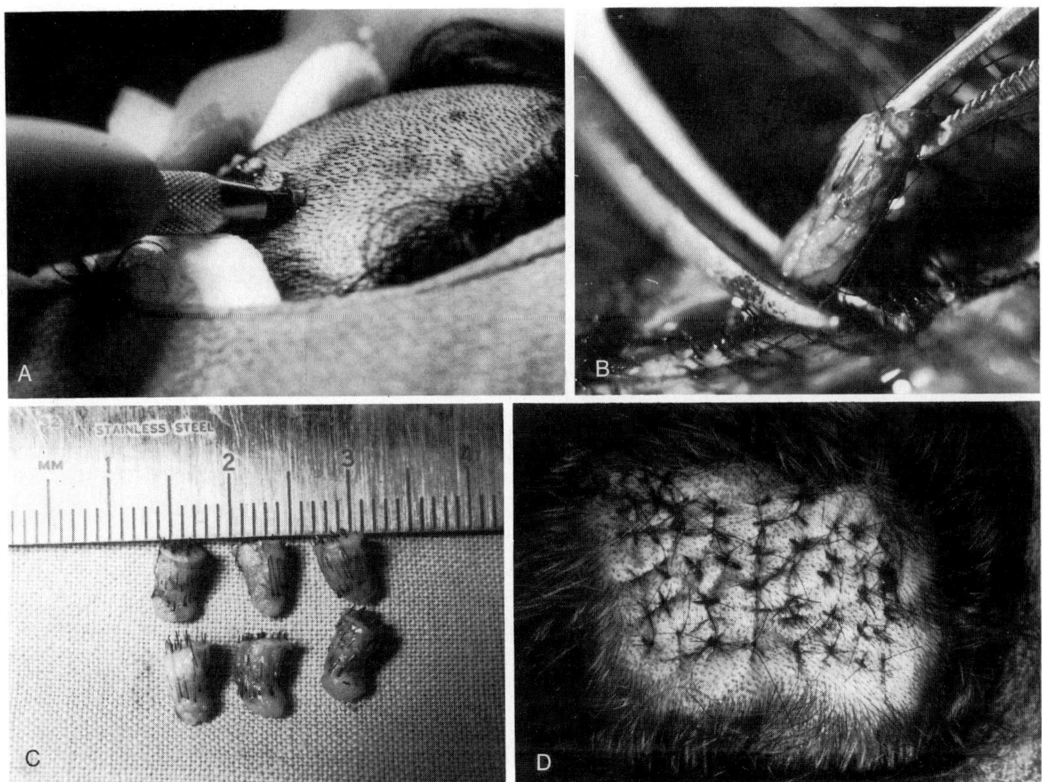

Figure 31–7. *A,* Sharp angulation of the instrument in the direction of the hair shafts. *B,* Severance of the basal attachment of the graft below the base of the hair follicles. *C,* Several 4.5 mm grafts. *D,* Sutured donor sites.

they are over 30 years of age and the pattern of their baldness has been more or less established. Younger patients between 20 and 30 years of age are also good candidates. However, they should be forewarned that their hairline recession will probably continue and that they will likely require additional operations in the future.

The punch graft has proved an ingenious procedure to both surgeon and patient because of its simplicity and versatility. It is the most common procedure used for the surgical correction of male pattern baldness. Punch scalp grafts have also been useful in transplanting hair in patients with other forms of alopecia of the scalp, such as cicatricial alopecia.

The operation is done as an office or outpatient procedure under local anesthesia. The lower occipital and parietal areas of the scalp are used for the donor sites. Punch grafts measuring 4 to 4.5 mm in diameter are most frequently used. The razor-sharp punch graft instrument fits into a larger holder, a feature that allows for easier manipulation. The graft is taken with a gentle rotary motion of the instrument. The instrument should penetrate the skin easily with only minimal pressure and rotation. A dull instrument requires increased pressure and may actually damage the graft, resulting in less hair growth. A dull instrument also causes coning of the grafts. Many surgeons use a revolving hand piece powered by an electric motor or battery.

The hair in the donor site is shaved. A few millimeters of hair are left intact so that the exact angulation of the hair shaft is easily determined during the cutting of the graft and its placement in the recipient site.

In the taking of the graft (Fig. 31–7), the instrument is placed on the scalp perpendicular to the surface of the skin. The instrument is then angulated sharply to a position parallel to the direction of the hair shaft for penetration of the skin and subcutaneous tissue. Sharp, curved scissors sever the underlying attachment of the graft beneath the base of the hair follicle. It should be noted that the hair follicles in each plug are of varying length and the graft should be inspected on all sides before it is cut from its base. A small amount of fatty tissue left

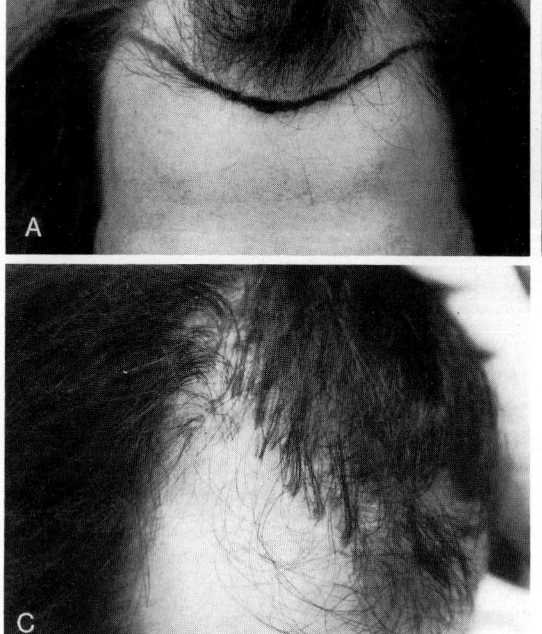

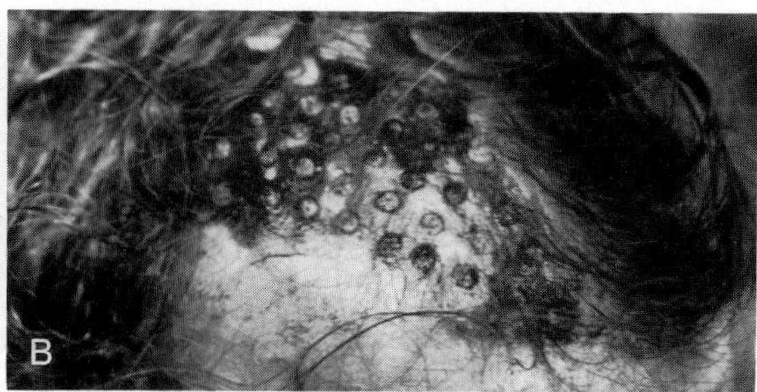

Figure 31–8. *A,* Proposed site of the frontal hairline outlined. *B,* Placement of grafts at the first operative session. *C,* Hair growth from the first set of grafts five months postoperatively.

under the follicles does not jeopardize the viability of the graft.

The number of grafts taken from the donor site in one procedure varies with the size of the recipient site to be grafted. In the average case a total of 50 to 75 punch grafts are taken during each stage. When the punch grafts are removed, each donor wound is closed with a single 4–0 nylon suture. Suturing is important to control bleeding and to lessen the amount of scarring. A space at least as wide as the graft is left between each graft site in order to facilitate closure and to ensure adequate growth of hair to camouflage the donor site scars.

Regardless of which technique is used for the reconstruction of the frontal hairline, it is important that its position be carefully planned and designed preoperatively with the patient in a sitting position. After local anesthesia is achieved along the proposed frontal hairline, a hand-operated punch graft instrument that is 0.25 mm smaller in size is used to remove the bald plugs from the recipient site. In some cases in which the donor plugs appear more shallow and the follicles are finer and less distinct, a punch graft measuring 0.5 mm smaller in size is taken from the recipient site. The difference in size is important because the grafts contract slightly and the recipient sites expand slightly. The instrument is carried through the skin and the entire thickness of the subcutaneous layer to the level of the galea. The grafts should fit snugly and smoothly in each recipient opening to avoid the disfiguring "cobblestone" effect. The direction of the instrument in the recipient site is perpendicular to the skin surface.

Positioning of the grafts in the scalp is important (Fig. 31–8). A good rule to follow is to separate the grafts by a width of skin at least equal to the diameter of the graft. When the donor plugs are placed into the recipient sites, an attempt is made to arrange the grafts so that the hair shafts angulate in the natural direction of the hair in all areas of the scalp.

At least four months or more should elapse before a new crop of grafts is placed between previously implanted grafts. After four months the surgeon can make a judgment relative to the adequacy of hair growth. Despite the abundant blood supply, the circulation can easily be abused during hair transplantation. The harvesting of an excess number of grafts from a donor site and their insertion over a large recipient area can cause injury to the vessels, with untoward results. Preserving and respecting the blood supply of the scalp are the most important factors in ensuring a successful result in any type of

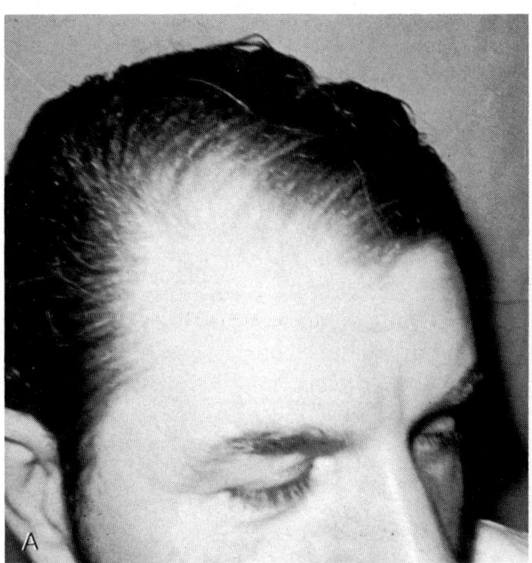

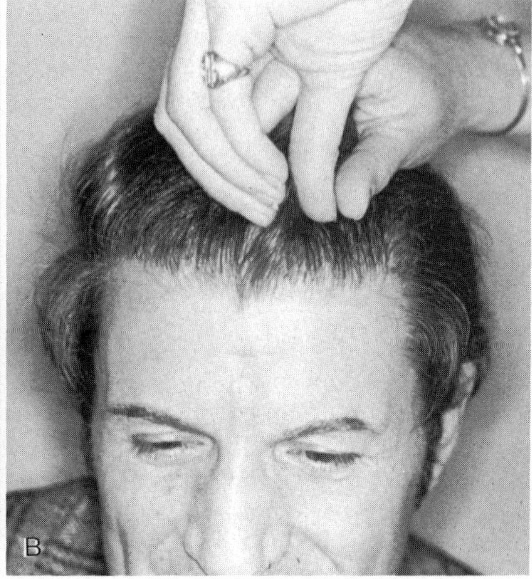

Figure 31–9. *A,* A 38 year old man with moderate frontotemporal recession. *B,* Frontal hairline enhanced by insertion of multiple small grafts.

hair transplantation. Friederich and Gloor (1970) reported that, following hair transplantation with punch grafts in humans, the blood supply in the recipient site showed optimal recovery after only three months. Periodic skin temperature and heat loss measurements were taken to document the gradual recovery of the circulation.

If proper spacing of the grafts is ensured with each procedure, a total of four separate operations is necessary to cover any bald segment significantly. Additional small grafts may be required to fill in residual hairless areas. Miniplugs measuring 3 mm or less in diameter can be inserted between or near the grafts in the most anterior row to create a more natural frontal hairline (Fig. 31–9). Deepithelized micrografts (Nordström, 1981) containing two to three hairs apiece and inserted in small stab wounds can also be used to enhance the frontal hairline.

Punch grafts are often used for restoration of hair in areas of cicatricial alopecia of the scalp. The surgical technique for inserting the punch grafts in the scarred recipient area is crucial for their survival. Insertion of the punch graft in the scarred scalp may be difficult since the graft is usually thicker than the depth of the recipient hole. Some form of fixation is necessary to maintain the grafts in place. If the graft projects, a continuous suture over the top of each graft and inserted through opposite sides of the recipient site is used to keep it level with the surrounding skin.

When the recipient site is shallow, as in atrophic scarring of the scalp, interrupted anchoring sutures may be necessary. The recipient opening is undermined circumferentially, the graft is inserted, and four interrupted sutures are placed in opposing poles.

Another method of anchoring the grafts in areas covered with a split-thickness skin graft or thin scar was proposed by Nordström (1979). After the recipient hole is made with the punch instrument, the adjacent skin is undermined to form a pocket for insertion of the graft. Local fixation is attained with strips of microporous surgical tape.

The introduction of scalp expansion techniques (see p. 1535) has obviated the need for punch grafts in most cases of cicatricial alopecia of the scalp.

In the postoperative period the hair follicles in all scalp grafts behave similarly. There is an initial false growth of hair for approximately three to four weeks. This hair is shed as the hair follicles pass into a telogen phase, which lasts two to three months after surgery. A new, permanent growth then begins. Since hair growth proceeds at approximately 1 cm per month, a period of six months or more is required before significant hair growth is noted.

SQUARE SCALP GRAFTS

Coiffman (1971) proposed the use of a square or hexahedral graft in place of a round graft. In the recipient site the square perforations are made with a square trephine. After the perforations are completed, the extraction of each square segment is accomplished with a circular punch whose diameter is 0.5 mm greater than the width of the square punch. The orifices are counted and the area of the segment to be removed from the donor site is calculated.

Parallel strips are traced in the donor area with a double-bladed scalpel. The strips are removed using a single-bladed scalpel under direct vision. Magnification ensures that the path of the scalpel passes between the hair follicles without damaging them. The donor site is sutured in a linear fashion.

Under magnification the strips are divided into squares of the correct size. The end result is the formation of hexahedral plugs with a square base. The plugs are placed in the prepared sites of the recipient area, particular care being given to orient the hair in its natural direction. Coiffman (1971) listed the advantages of the hexahedral grafts:

1. Each graft is handled under direct magnification using microsurgical techniques that minimize damage to the hair follicles.
2. The donor site is sutured leaving only a straight line of scar. This permits extension of the technique to patients with large areas of alopecia.
3. A square graft produces an average of 25 per cent more hair than a circular graft by virtue of the greater area for the equivalent diameter.

Devine (1982) used the square graft technique combined with strip grafts with considerable success for the treatment of male pattern baldness.

In the author's opinion the ease in performing the highly successful round punch graft technique far outweighs any slight advantage that the more intricate square graft method may have.

STRIP SCALP GRAFTS

The strip graft is essentially a long composite segment of hair-bearing skin and subcutaneous tissue (Vallis, 1969, 1982). The graft is primarily used to reconstruct a frontal hairline in patients with male pattern baldness, although it can be grafted successfully in any area of the scalp.

Most patients are first treated with a series of punch graft procedures. In some cases the frontal hairline created by the punch grafts may be rather spotty and sparse. In these patients the strip graft enhances the appearance of the frontal hairline (Fig. 31–10).

The length of the strip graft is variable and limited only by the existing donor site and the length of the frontal area to be reconstructed. The width of the graft is important relative to the ultimate take of the graft. The width is limited and ranges from 3 to 8 mm. A graft as wide as 7 to 8 mm can be successfully placed in areas of normal scalp previously untouched by surgery. If a strip graft is to be placed near a row of previously implanted punch grafts, a narrower strip (5 to 6 mm) has a better chance of survival.

The strip graft operation is done as an office or outpatient procedure under local anesthesia. The graft is taken in a horizontal direction from the parieto-occipital area of the scalp with a simple instrument called the parallel double-bladed holder. This instrument was designed to allow the surgeon to take a strip graft with a predetermined and uniform width (Fig. 31–11). The instrument is used to make the initial incision through the epidermis in the donor site. A single-bladed knife is then used to make a deeper incision on either side of the graft. It is important that the deeper incisions are made parallel to the angulation of the hair follicles. The incisions are carried down to the galea. The graft is lifted off its bed with a sharp, curved scissors or scalpel. The donor wound is closed with a continuous 3–0 nylon suture. The graft is carefully pared of excess fascia and fat. The paring of the fat should not be excessive. Care should be taken not to expose the underlying hair follicles.

A simple linear incision is made through the skin in the recipient site, slightly angulated superiorly and extending through the subcutaneous tissue and underlying fascia. Incising the fascia or galea allows the wound to expand to receive the graft. Bleeding is controlled and the graft is placed in the recipient site with the hair follicles directed forward, consistent with the normal angulation of the hair growth in the frontal scalp. The strip graft is sutured to the skin superiorly and inferiorly with a continuous 6–0 nylon suture, and a nonadherent pressure dressing is placed over the graft.

Some surgeons proposed modification in the size of the strip graft (Nataf, 1979). These grafts are given names such as navicular, spindle, or fusiform. Their average size is 3 mm in width and up to 35 mm in length.

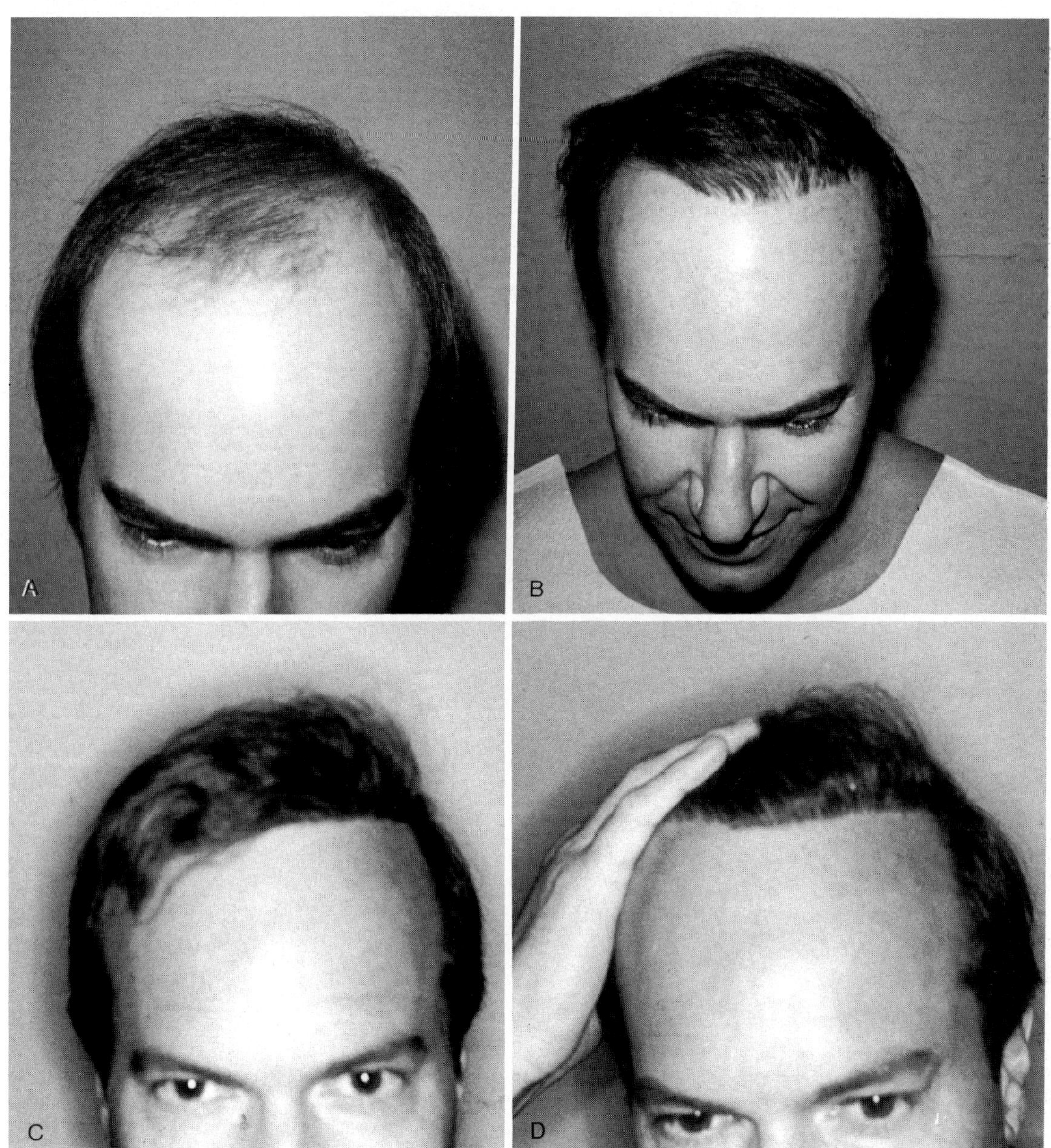

Figure 31–10. *A,* Preoperative appearance of a 43 year old man. *B,* Appearance after insertion of 200 punch grafts. *C, D,* Appearance following enhancement with a strip graft.

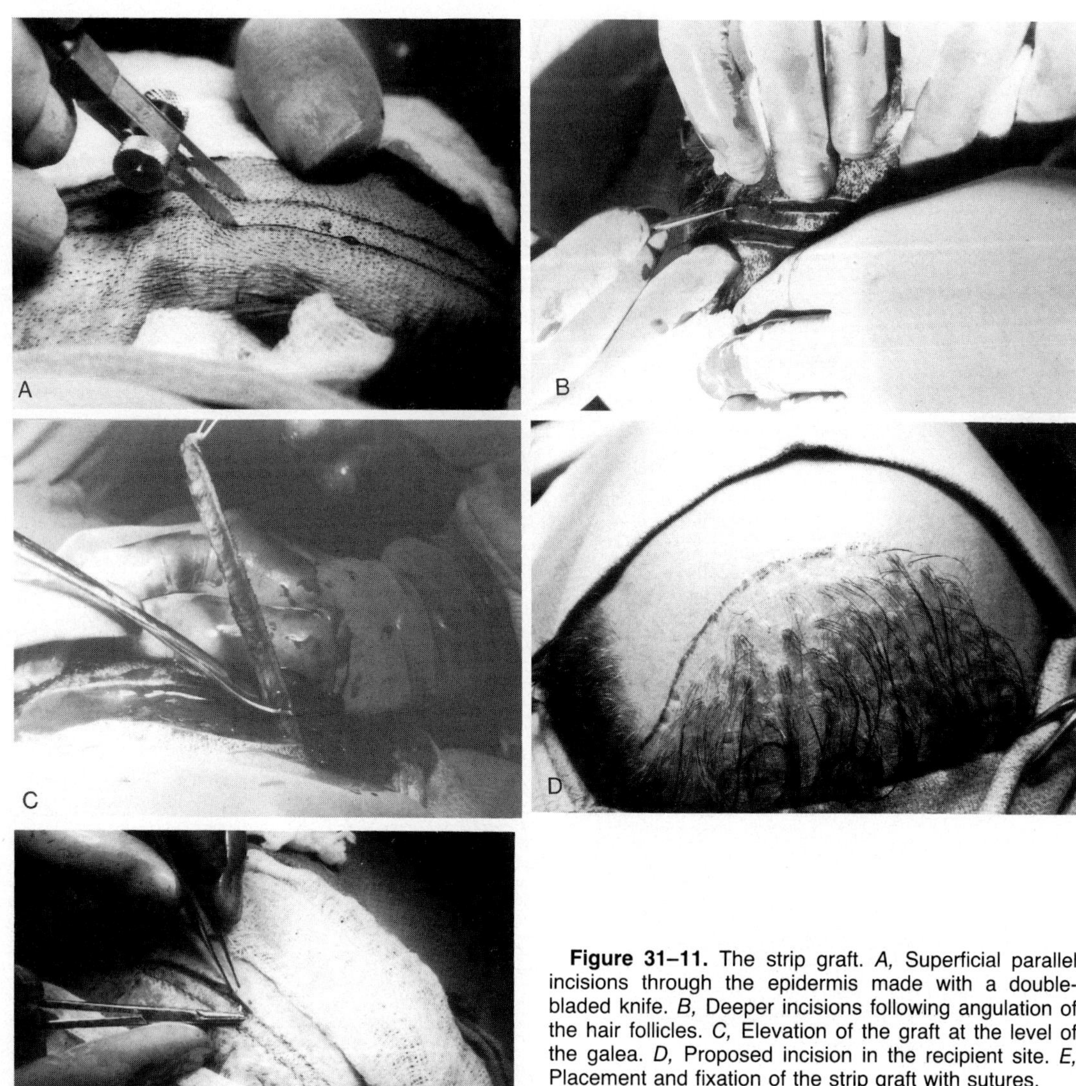

Figure 31–11. The strip graft. *A,* Superficial parallel incisions through the epidermis made with a double-bladed knife. *B,* Deeper incisions following angulation of the hair follicles. *C,* Elevation of the graft at the level of the galea. *D,* Proposed incision in the recipient site. *E,* Placement and fixation of the strip graft with sutures.

The wide strip graft has not been used frequently in cicatricial alopecia since it does not survive in scar tissue in which the circulation has been severely compromised. Thin strip grafts measuring 3 to 4 mm in width can be successfully employed in some cases of cicatricial alopecia (Coiffman, 1982).

If patients are carefully selected and if the procedure is performed properly, there should be few complications following scalp grafting. Early in the author's experience two strip grafts were lost because of infection. All patients are given prophylactic antibiotics. Another graft failed to survive when the patient accidentally struck his forehead against a firm object several days after the operation. In a small percentage of strip grafts there may not be a complete growth of hair in certain spots, although the graft may have taken completely. These areas of alopecia in the graft may be small or may involve as much as 50 per cent or more of the total area of the graft. The smaller area can be easily corrected by implanting punch grafts. The larger area can be corrected by excising the segment of alopecia and replacing it with a small strip graft.

Scalp Flaps

Scalp flaps were initially used in patients with cicatricial alopecia to transfer hair-bearing skin from inconspicuous areas of the scalp to the more obvious critical areas. One of the prime objectives in treating any form of alopecia (prematura or cicatricial) is to reestablish a frontal hairline. All scalp flaps should be planned with care. Knowledge of the arterial supply is critical in designing the proper flap. If a particular vessel is difficult to identify, a Doppler apparatus can be used to define its course and integrity. Because of the extensive collateral circulation of the scalp, delay of most scalp flaps is often unnecessary. Delay procedures are done by simply incising the lateral margins of the flap down to the periosteum. Elevation of the flap is deferred until it is ready for transposition.

Kazanjian (1953) observed that the areas of scalp loss following burns are usually frontal, temporal, and parietal. The occiput is more often spared. Figure 31–12 illustrates the replacement of an area of cicatricial alopecia on the frontal aspect of the scalp with two rectangular flaps of hair-bearing skin from the occipitoparietal regions. The total scarred area of the scalp is not diminished but is repositioned to a less conspicuous location.

The type of flap used for transplanting hair in areas of alopecia depends on the area and location of the alopecia. This principle holds true whether the alopecia is due to scarring following trauma or whether it is the result of male pattern baldness.

ROTATION FLAPS

Small areas of cicatricial alopecia can often be excised and replaced with hair-bearing rotation flaps. The rotation flap is usually large in comparison with the excised area of alopecia. According to Dingman and Argenta (1982), the flap margin that represents the axis of rotation over which the flap will travel should be at least five times the length of the defect to be covered, to avoid undue tension. If the flap is properly planned, the donor defect can usually be closed primarily.

TRANSPOSITION FLAPS

If the area of alopecia is extensive, the method of hair restoration becomes more complex. If the destruction of hair has been in a conspicuous area such as the frontal region of the scalp, it is often wise to transpose a hair-bearing flap from a location that can be more easily camouflaged. The defect that remains after transposition of the flap can be closed primarily, if small, or covered with a split-thickness skin graft, if large.

In the past, most transposition flaps were wide based and were used primarily to repair traumatic defects of the scalp. They were also used to restore hair in areas of cicatricial alopecia of the frontal scalp. During the past decade, however, long, narrow flaps for transplanting hair in areas of alopecia have become popular.

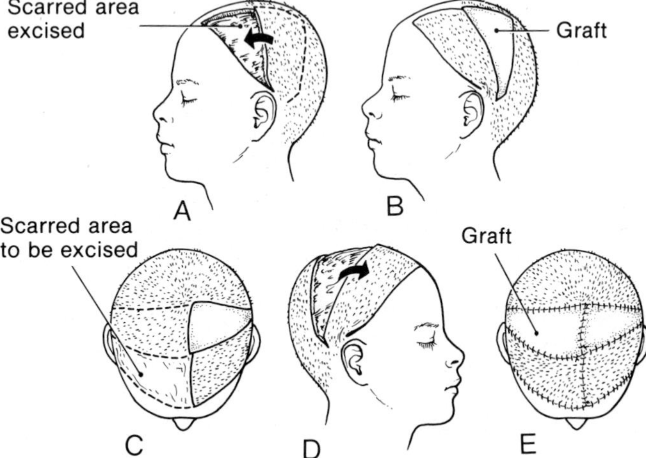

Figure 31–12. Replacement of cicatricial alopecia in the frontal scalp with rectangular hair-bearing flaps. The base of the flap is ideally wider.

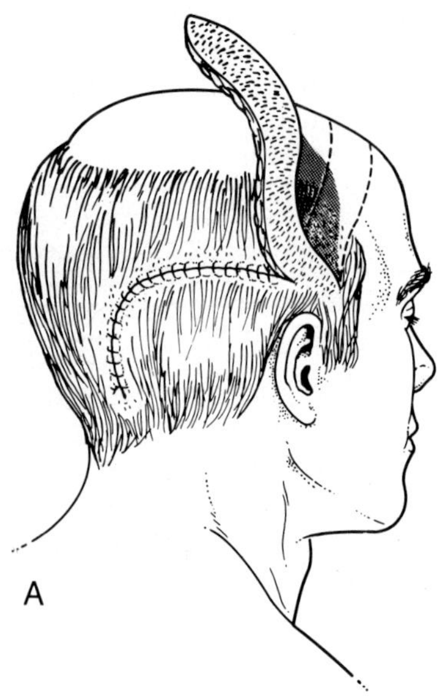

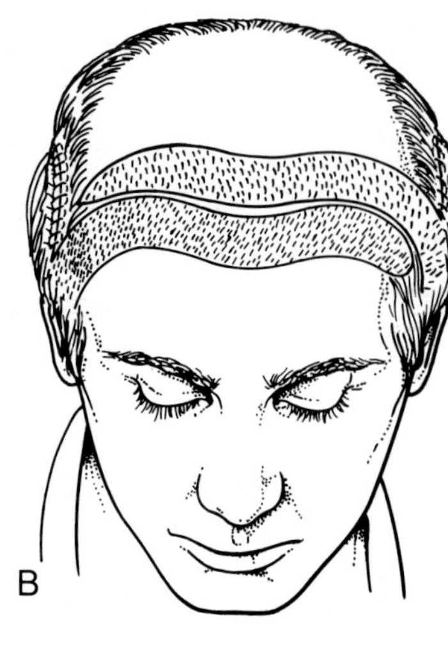

Figure 31–13. *A,* The parieto-occipital flap (after Juri). *B,* Position of the second flap from the contralateral side.

The benefits of a long, narrow flap are many. Transfer of the flap is facilitated, and a large redundant fold at the base of the pedicle is not usually evident, resulting in less wastage of hair-bearing scalp. In most situations, the donor site can be closed primarily with less possibility of a secondary defect.

A very important consideration in designing flaps, especially in males with a genetic background of baldness, is to select a donor site containing hair follicles of high longevity. The parietal and occipital areas of the scalp retain their hairs indefinitely and in most cases are the best donor sites, provided they are not damaged by the original injury.

There are many types of narrow-based pedicle flaps, varying in length, width, and location.

Temporo-Parieto-Occipital Flaps

Temporo-parieto-occipital flaps have been used with effectiveness by Juri, Juri, and Arufe (1978) and Juri and Juri (1981). These flaps are used in varying numbers and designs according to the distribution and extent of baldness (Fig. 31–13). Juri flaps were designed primarily to treat male pattern baldness. They were constructed so that each flap would extend across the entire width of alopecia of the scalp. The flaps measured 4 cm in width, and each had the necessary length (approximately 25 cm) to reach across the scalp to the opposite hair area. The base of the flaps is located on the temporal scalp at the site of the superficial temporal artery. Two flap delays are made at one week intervals. The first delay includes both longitudinal margins of the flap, and the second delay severs the occipital attachment. Two delays are not always necessary. The author has handled many of these flaps with a single delay, following which the entire flap was transposed in one week.

In transposition of the flap, the donor site can usually be closed primarily with some difficulty. Extensive undermining in the retroauricular area in an inferior direction toward the neck is necessary in order to allow primary closure of the donor site. The width of the Juri flap can actually be as small as 3.5 cm and still be transposed successfully. This dimension makes closure of the donor site much easier.

Careful management of the anterior margin of the flap is essential to avoid an ugly scar. Juri deepithelizes a 2 mm width of the anterior margin of the flap and sutures the frontal skin on top of the deepithelized margin with 6-0 nylon sutures, to avoid damaging the underlying follicular bulbs.

Juri also designed a parieto-occipital flap based in the retroauricular area to treat occipital baldness.

The Juri flap has been especially useful in cases of cicatricial alopecia (Fig. 31–14). Because of the extensive surgery involved in

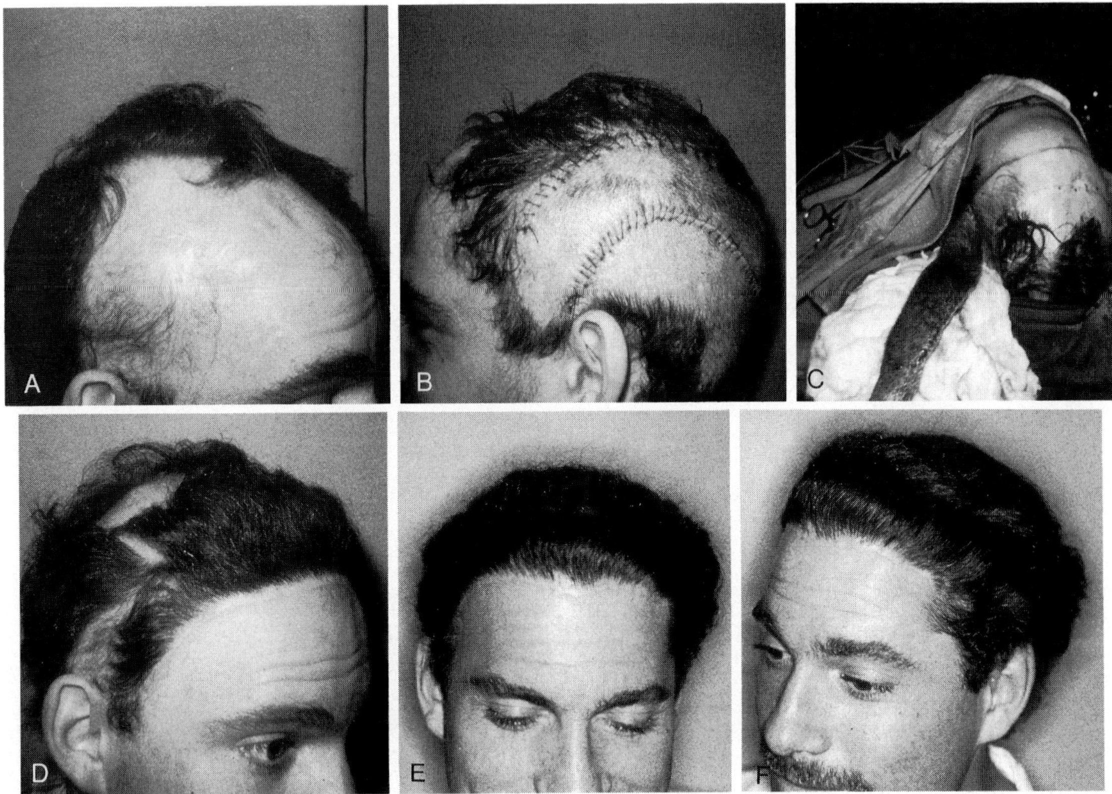

Figure 31–14. *A,* A 19 year old man with cicatrical alopecia resulting from radiation therapy. *B,* Delay of Juri flap on the left side of the scalp. *C,* Elevation of the flap. Note the length. *D,* Reconstructed frontal and right temporal scalp. *E, F,* Final appearance.

the transposition of these flaps, there has been no general acceptance of Juri's method for the treatment of ordinary male pattern baldness.

A slightly shorter temporo-parieto-occipital flap with a narrow base has been used successfully by Stough, Cates, and Dean (1982) and Mayer and Fleming (1982). The former flap has a width at the base of 2 cm and gradually widens to a maximum of 3 cm. The flap is delayed once for ten days. This flap reaches at least two-thirds across the forehead when transposed. The narrow base of the flap facilitates transposition without a dog ear. Closure of the donor site is accomplished without extensive undermining.

Lateral Scalp Flaps

Elliott (1982,a,b) developed a simplified technique for transposing undelayed lateral scalp flaps or temporoparietal flaps to the frontal scalp for treatment of male pattern baldness (Fig. 31–15). The use of shorter, narrower flaps eliminates the necessity of delay procedures and allows for relatively simple closure of the donor sites. The technique is easily performed as an office or outpatient procedure. The lateral scalp flap is based on the anterior hairline in the temporal region. The flap, averaging 2.5 cm in width, is directed posteriorly above the ear and curved across the parietal scalp.

The flap is elevated in the areolar plane deep to the galea. The donor defect is sutured as far anteriorly as possible without tension. The small triangular defect remaining near the base of the pedicle is closed with a flap from the recipient site.

Elliott (1982a,b) reported that the lateral flap is safe and reliable and does not require a delay before transfer. Bilateral one-stage flap reconstruction can be done safely but closure of the donor site is much easier when the opposite flap is transposed two to four months later. Patients with extensive baldness require free grafts posterior to the flaps. The scar along the anterior hairline and the

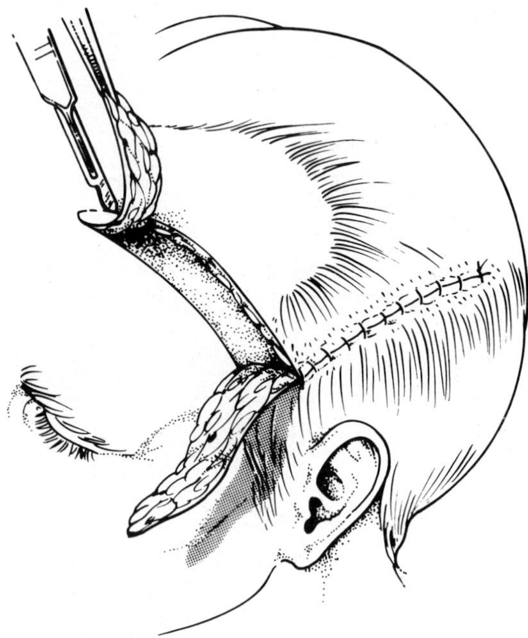

Figure 31–15. The lateral scalp flap with primary closure of the donor site (after Elliott).

faulty direction of the hair on the flap are disadvantages that can be masked by styling the hair. The lateral scalp flap has been useful in many cases of cicatricial alopecia involving the frontal areas of the scalp (Fig. 31–16).

Temporal Vertical Flaps

The temporal vertical flap, as designed by Nataf (1984), is based superiorly in the parietal scalp and extends inferiorly and vertically along either the pre- or retroauricular areas. This flap has been used exclusively in cases of male pattern baldness. It was designed primarily to orient the hair in a natural, forward direction in the frontal scalp. Because of its retrograde circulation, there are flap survival problems. The wide rotation angle of the flap often results in a redundant fold at the base. Nataf (1984) claimed that flaps measuring 2 to 3 cm in width by 20 cm in length could be designed. By delaying the flaps twice over a period of up to three months, Nataf was able to transpose them successfully.

Shorter temporal vertical flaps may be used to cover a remaining area of frontal alopecia not reached by a temporo-parieto-occipital flap from the opposite side.

BIPEDICLE FLAPS

Bipedicle flaps can be used in selected cases of cicatricial alopecia of the scalp. The "visor" flap was used for many years to transfer hair-bearing skin from the occipital scalp to the critical frontal area of the scalp. Small bipedicle flaps based on both temporal areas can be used to replace hair in localized areas of cicatricial alopecia in the frontal scalp (Fig. 31–17). The donor defect following transposition of the flap can be closed primarily by extensive undermining of the scalp posteriorly.

MULTIPLE FLAPS

Orticochea (1971) developed a rather radical method for repairing scalp defects by completely dividing the remaining intact

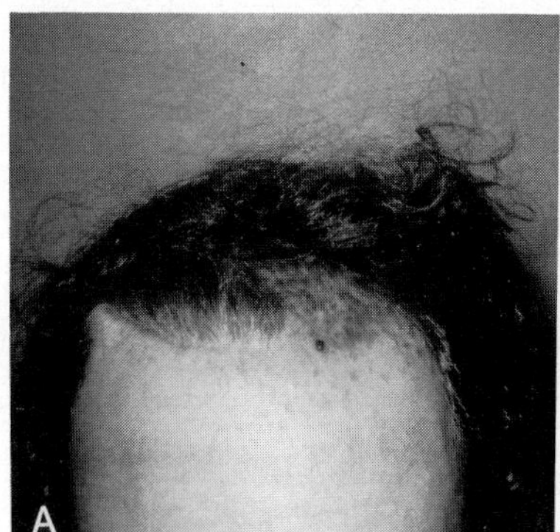

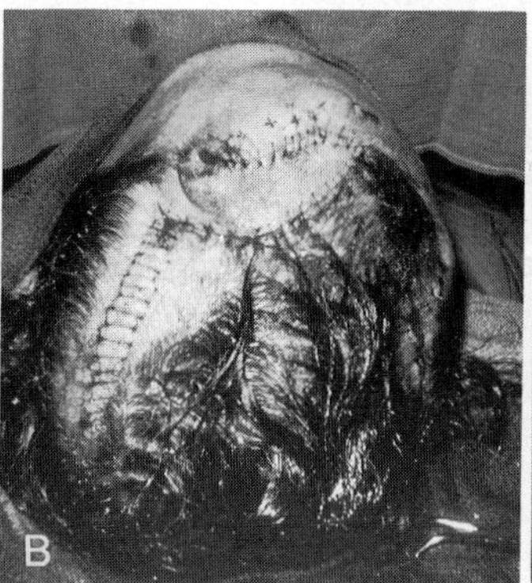

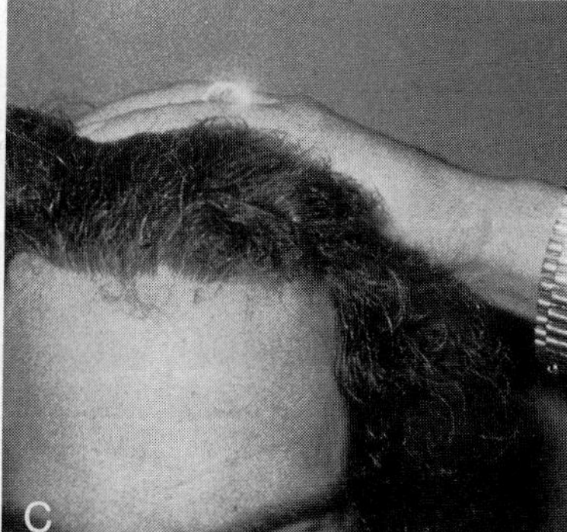

Figure 31–16. *A,* A 28 year old man. Chronic inflammation and scarring of the frontal scalp. The right side had been repaired with a lateral flap. *B,* Replacement of the scarred scalp on the left side with a scalp flap. *C,* Completion of the scalp reconstruction.

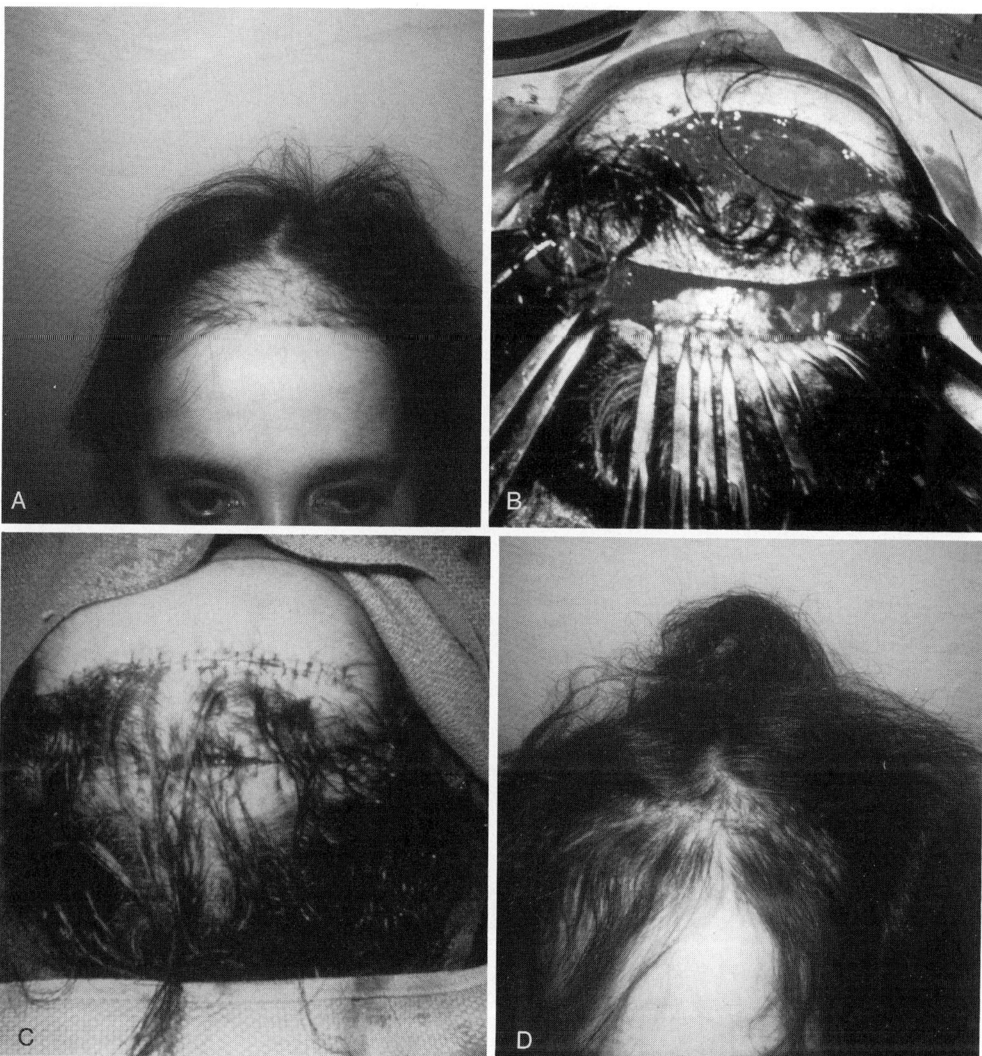

Figure 31–17. *A,* A 48 year old woman with cicatricial alopecia of the frontal scalp resulting from infection during infancy. Note the sparse hair growth from 50 punch grafts. *B,* Excision of alopecia and transposition of the bipedicle scalp flap. *C,* Closure of the donor site after extensive posterior undermining of the scalp. *D,* Final appearance.

scalp into three large flaps, each having its own pedicle. He transposed them geometrically to cover the defect, often in its entirety. The flexibility of the scalp is increased by making parallel incisions through the galea transversely relative to the longitudinal axis of the skull, great care being taken not to injure the underlying vessels. Orticochea (1971) stated that with this technique the whole scalp can be expanded to cover large defects at the frontal and occipital regions. The scalp is subjected to a distribution of even tensions throughout its full extent and in all directions.

MICROVASCULAR FREE SCALP FLAPS

Traditional scalp flaps have certain disadvantages. Because of the fixed attachment of the pedicle, positional adjustment of the flap in the recipient site is somewhat limited. The surgeon may have difficulty in controlling the direction of the hair, and a redundant fold of skin may often occur at the base of the pedicle. The latter becomes more pronounced as the rotation angle becomes wider.

Harii, Ohmori, and Ohmori (1974) made use of microsurgical techniques to transplant hair by free scalp flaps. They reported a one-stage

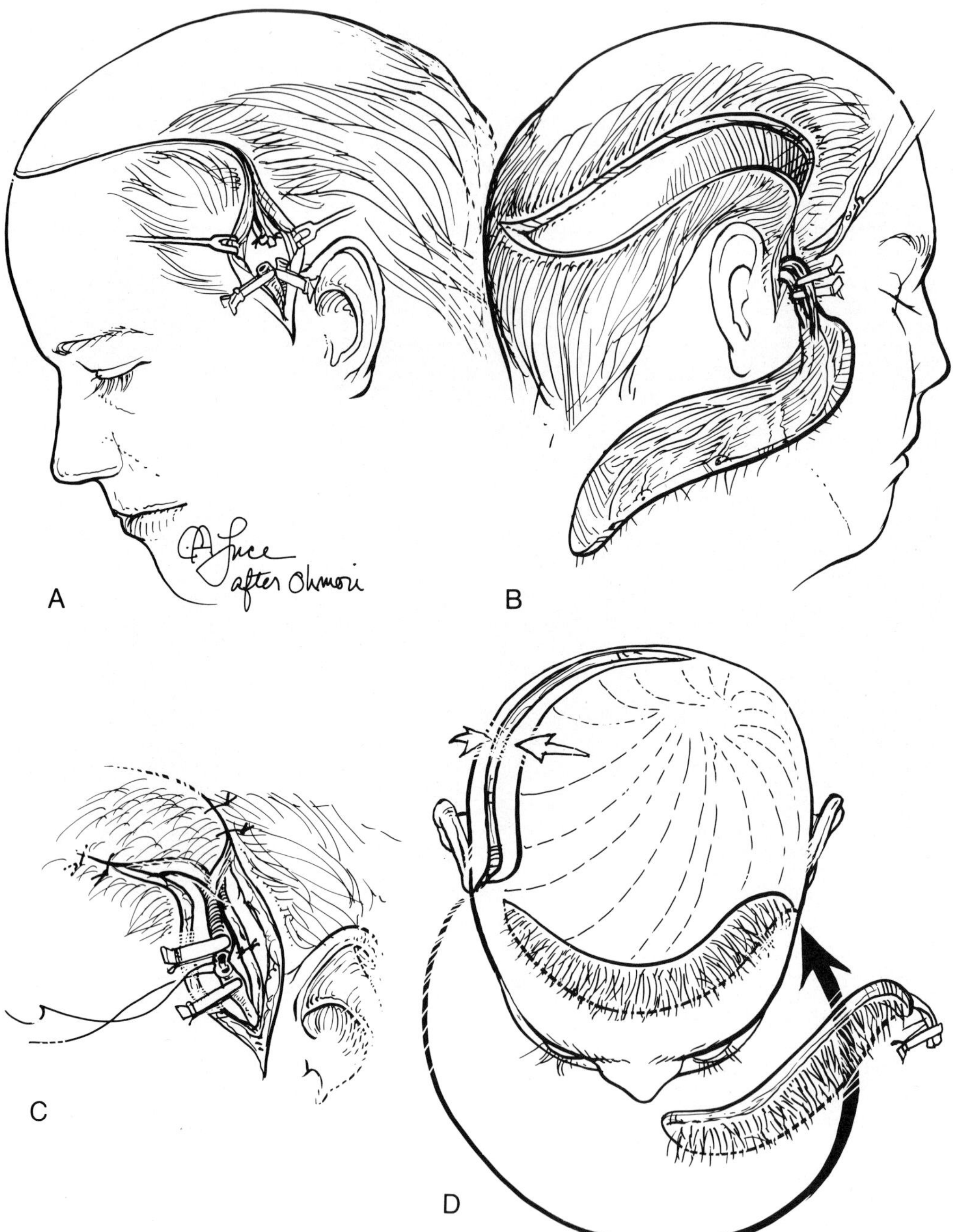

Figure 31–18. Microvascular free scalp flap (Ohmori). *A,* Preparation of the recipient site superficial temporal artery and vein. *B,* Design of a large free scalp flap based on the superficial temporal vessels. *C,* Microvascular repair of the artery and vein. *D,* Flap transferred and sutured to recreate the anterior hairline. The donor site is closed primarily after extensive undermining. Note the direction of the scalp hair. The flap technique optimizes hair position in the flap to recreate the hairline.

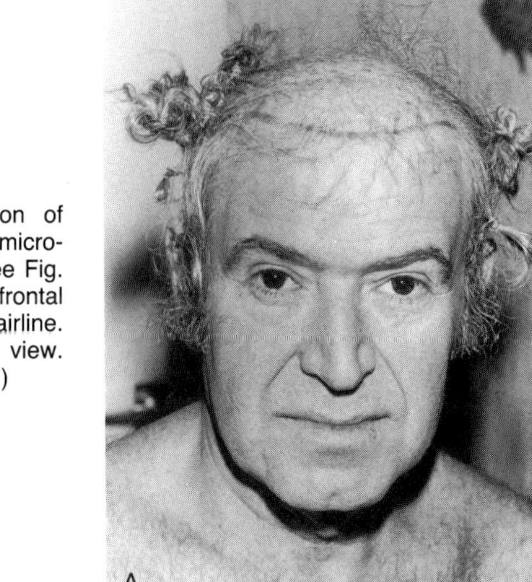

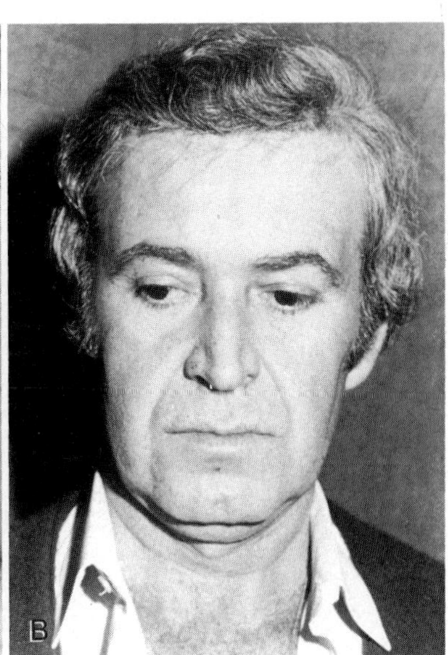

Figure 31–19. Correction of male pattern alopecia by a microvascular free scalp flap (see Fig. 31–18). *A,* Preoperative frontal view showing projected hairline. *B,* Postoperative frontal view. (Courtesy of Dr. K. Ohmori.)

reconstruction of the frontal temporal hairline in cases of cicatricial alopecia that used a large, hair-bearing free scalp flap. The flaps averaged 12 by 2.5 cm. In most cases the free scalp flap was taken from the occipital area and transplanted by microsurgical anastomosis of the occipital vessels to the superficial temporal vessels to reconstruct the hairline. The donor sites were closed primarily.

Ohmori (1980) designed a large Juri flap in the temporo-parieto-occipital area and transformed it into a free scalp flap for treatment of postburn alopecia in the frontal temporal region. The flap is elevated from the intact side of the scalp and transplanted to the opposite temporal vessels (Fig. 31–18). A total of 43 free scalp flap transfers were reported with only one failure. The advantage of this technique, which can also be used to treat male pattern baldness, is the ability to transplant a large amount of hair in one stage and to position the flaps so that the hair is oriented in a natural direction (Figs. 31–19, 31–20).

Scalp Reduction

Scalp reduction has gained considerable popularity during the past decade for the treatment of male pattern baldness (Bell, 1982). It is indicated for complete or partial elimination of alopecia on the vertex of the scalp. The bald frontal areas of the scalp are best covered with scalp grafts or flaps. Scalp reduction can be very useful in decreasing the number of hair transplants needed for any given patient.

Scalp flexibility is different in every patient and is the limiting factor relative to the amount of bald scalp that can be excised. Flexibility is usually more marked in the older patient.

The bald scalp is excised in an anteroposteriorly directed ellipse, beginning approximately 2 cm behind the proposed frontal hairline and extending to the occipital scalp (Fig. 31–21). The ellipse has a maximal width of 3.5 to 4 cm and extends up to 12 to 15 cm in length. If there is scalp flexibility in the occipital area, a fishtail excision may be added to the posterior end of the ellipse. The size and design of the excised scalp often depend on the shape and extent of the alopecia. Undermining is done below the galea, and is extensive laterally and less so posteriorly. The mobility and abundant arterial supply of the scalp make possible primary closure of comparatively large defects by this method. The scalp is not as elastic as the skin of the face and neck but, after the surrounding scalp has been widely undermined, longitudinal incisions can be made in the galea to increase the elasticity. After a series of partial excisions have been completed, the residual scar can be further improved with multiple Z-plasties or replaced with punch grafts. In selected cases, replacement of the

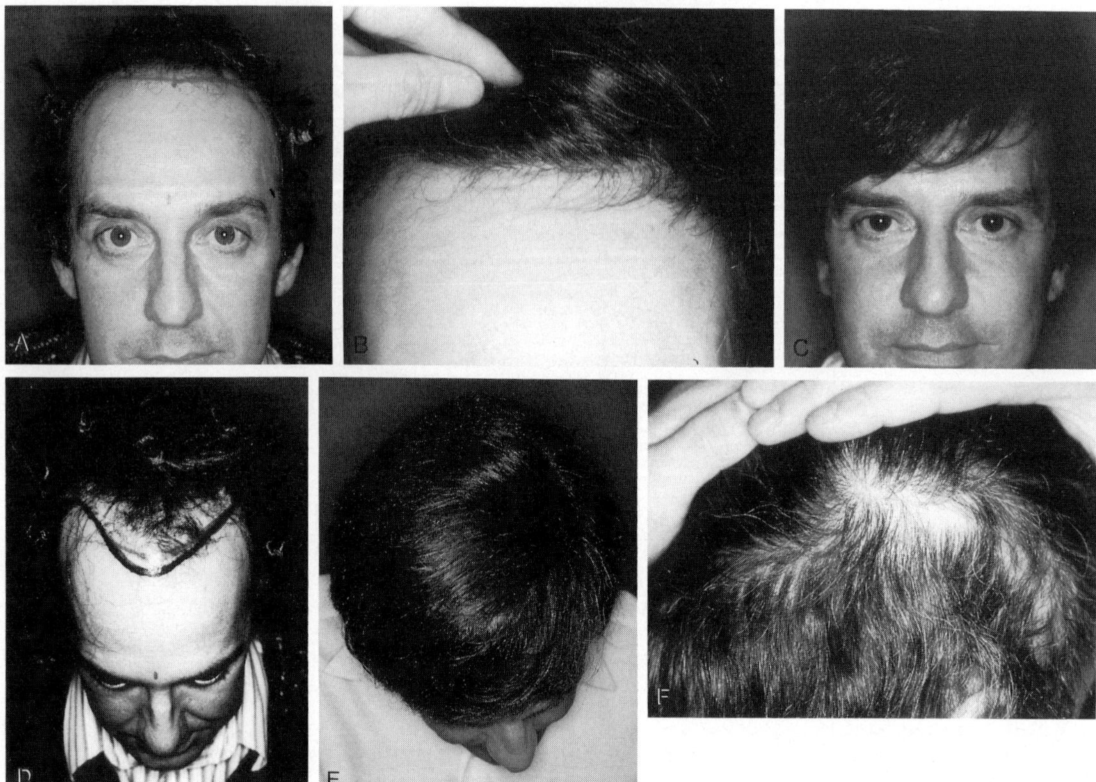

Figure 31–20. Correction of male pattern alopecia by microvascular free scalp flap (see Fig. 31–18). *A,* Preoperative view outlining the proposed recipient site of the flap. *B,* Reconstructed anterior hairline (postoperatively). *C,* Postoperative view. *D,* Preoperative superior view outlining the proposed recipient site. *E,* Postoperative superior view. *F,* Healed donor site with minimal scar. (Courtesy of Dr. K. Ohmori.)

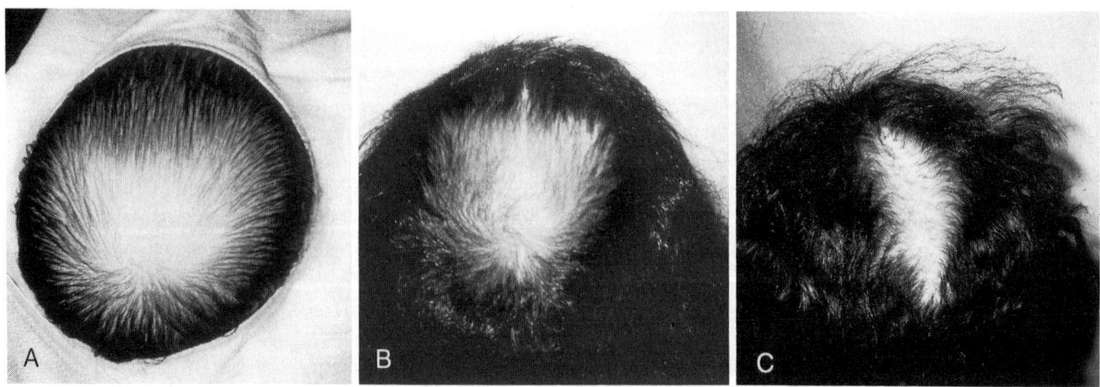

Figure 31–21. *A,* A 33 year old man with severe alopecia of the crown. *B,* Appearance after the first scalp reduction. *C,* Appearance after two additional reductions over a period of one year.

scar with a narrow, posteriorly based scalp flap is preferable.

Areas of burn scar of the scalp can often be diminished in size by serial excisions. If the scar is atrophic and avascular, it should be excised along its periphery, gradually advancing the hair-bearing scalp on both sides until the surgeon considers that further partial excision is not feasible.

SCALP REDUCTION WITH THE AID OF EXPANDERS

The use of temporary silicone expanders to increase the surface of the skin is one of the recent advances in plastic surgery (see Chap. 13). The technique of expanding the scalp will probably replace many of the surgical methods now used for transplantation of hair in large areas of cicatricial alopecia (Manders and associates, 1984; Nordström and Devine, 1985; Leonard and Small, 1986). Although scalp expansion has been used for scalp reduction in cases of male pattern baldness, it probably will not be accepted by many patients because of the head distortion that necessarily accompanies the period of scalp expansion.

Skin expanders are composed of silicone elastomer and are designed in various shapes and sizes. They are usually round or rectangular in shape and vary from 200 to 700 ml in size.

The expander is placed in a subgaleal location, usually through an incision at the junction of the normal scalp and the defect that is to be replaced. The size of the defect dictates the size of the expander. Placement of the expander depends on the location of the scarred area. For example, expanders can be placed in both parietal areas of the scalp if the defect is in the crown. They can be placed singly in any area of healthy scalp or paired in any combination.

The preferred position for the scalp expander is adjacent to the defect being reconstructed (Fig. 31–22). This allows simple advancement of the scalp. Placement of the incision at the edge of the defect avoids additional scars. The adjacent normal scalp is

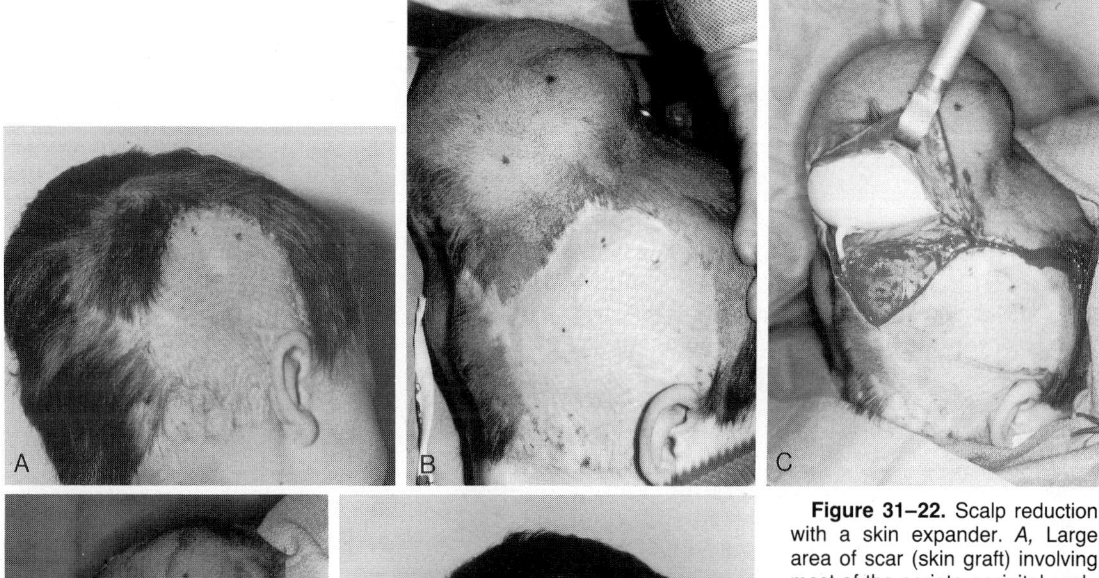
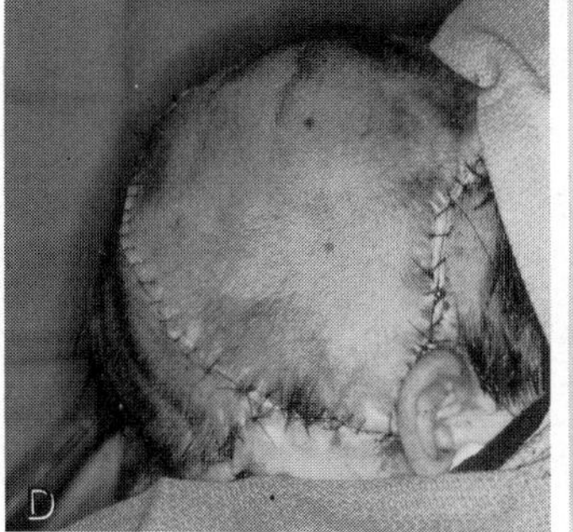
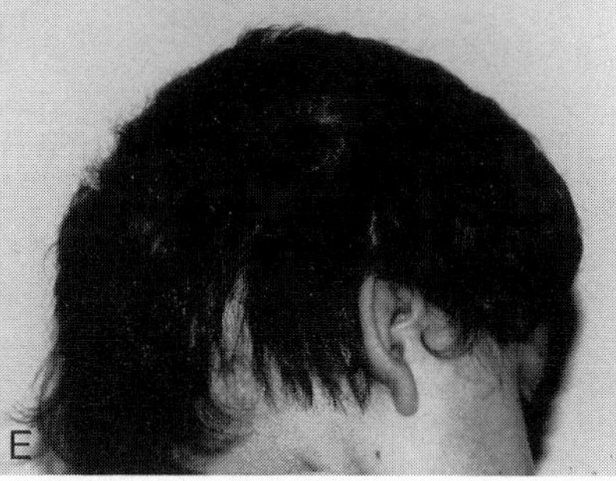

Figure 31–22. Scalp reduction with a skin expander. *A,* Large area of scar (skin graft) involving most of the parieto-occipital scalp (right side). *B,* After serial expansion of the adjacent scalp. *C,* Intraoperative view at the time of removal of the expander. *D,* After removal of the expander, excision of the scar and advancement of the adjacent scalp. *E,* One year later showing luxuriant hair growth in the advancement flap. (Courtesy of Dr. Barry Zide.)

elevated in a subgaleal plane by blunt dissection. The subgaleal pocket should be made large enough to accommodate the entire dimension of the expander. The reservoir dome is placed at some distance from the inflatable bag in an area accessible for injecting the saline solution. A suitable location is the upper postauricular area. Possible leakage in the inflatable bag and the integrity of the reservoir dome should be checked before insertion.

Inflation of the expander is commenced two weeks after its insertion. The sutures in the scalp are left in place for at least two to three weeks. Expansion of the scalp is done weekly, depending on scalp flexibility. The amount of saline injected into the expander each time is limited by the tenseness of the scalp during the injection. When the scalp becomes tense, the injection should stop. As much as 20 to 50 ml can be injected at one time. A period of six to eight weeks may be necessary before satisfactory expansion is achieved. The patient may experience some discomfort during the expansion. The scalp becomes soft and readily compressible approximately 24 hours after each fluid injection.

After expansion has been completed, the original incision is reopened, and the expander is deflated and removed. The expanded scalp is advanced over the defect. Lateral incisions may be necessary to facilitate advancement of the flap. If there is incomplete removal of the defect, another expander can be inserted in the same pocket and the process repeated.

The major advantage of the expander technique is that large areas of alopecia of the scalp are replaced with normal hair-bearing scalp. In patients in whom a large expansion is necessary, there may be some decrease in density of the hair; however, the decrease is slight and does not present a problem. Radiographic studies (Manders and associates, 1984) showed that the underlying cranial vault was not affected after scalp expansion. However, the cranial sutures should be closed, limiting the approach to children 3 years of age and older.

Adson, Anderson and Argenta (1987) reported three cases of male pattern baldness treated by the expansion technique. By expanding the temporo-parieto-occipital areas they were able to design Juri flaps measuring 5 cm in width and up to 23 cm in length. Transposition of bilateral flaps with easy closure of the donor site was carried out in two cases. In one patient the flaps were based in the occipital scalp, and transposition of the flaps in the anterior scalp created a hairline with natural orientation of the hair.

REFERENCES

Adson, M. H., Anderson, R. D., and Argenta, L. C.: Scalp expansion in treatment of male pattern baldness. Plast. Reconstr. Surg., *79*:906, 1987.

Barsky, A. J.: Principles and Practice of Plastic Surgery. Baltimore, Williams & Wilkins Company, 1950.

Bell, M. C.: Scalp reduction. Clin. Plast. Surg., *9*:269, 1982.

Berg, C.: The Unconscious Significance of Hair. London, Allen & Unwin. 1951.

Blanchard, G., and Blanchard, B.: La reduction tonsurale: concept nouveau dans le traitement chirurgical de la calvitie. Rev. Chir. Esth. L. Fr., *4*:5, 1976.

Byron, C. P. (Trans.): The Papyrus Ebers. New York, D. Appleton & Company, 1931.

Casanova, R., Cavalcante, D., Grotting, J. C., Vasconez, L. O., and Psillakis, J. M.: Anatomic basis for vascularized outer-table calvarial bone flaps. Plast. Reconstr. Surg., *78*:300, 1986.

Coiffman, F.: Injertos de cuero cabelludo. Trib. Med. (Bogota), March, 1971.

Coiffman, F.: Square scalp grafts. Clin. Plast. Surg., *9*:221, 1982.

Correa-Iturraspe, M., and Arufe, H. N.: La cirugía plastica en las alopecias parciales definitivas del cuero cabelludo. Bol. Trab. Soc. Cir. Buenos Aires, *41*:10, 1957.

Cutting, C. B., McCarthy, J. G., and Berenstein, A.: Blood supply of the upper craniofacial skeleton: the search for composite calvarial bone flaps. Plast. Reconstr. Surg., *74*:603, 1984.

Devine, J. W., Jr.: Square scalp grafts combined with strip grafts for treatment of male pattern baldness. *In* Vallis, C. P. (Ed.): Hair Transplantation for the Treatment of Male Pattern Baldness. Springfield, IL, Charles C Thomas, 1982.

Dingman, R. O., and Argenta, L. C.: The surgical repair of traumatic defects of the scalp. Clin. Plast. Surg., *9*:131, 1982.

Elliott, R. A., Jr.: Lateral scalp flaps for instant results in male pattern baldness. Plast. Reconstr. Surg., *60*:699, 1977.

Elliott, R. A., Jr.: Lateral scalp flaps. *In* Vallis, C. P. (Ed.): Hair Transplantation for the Treatment of Male Pattern Baldness. Springfield, IL, Charles C Thomas, 1982a.

Elliott, R. A., Jr.: The lateral scalp flap for anterior hairline reconstruction. Clin. Plast. Surg., *9*:241, 1982b.

Fleming, J. P.: Surgery for baldness: a case report. Canad. J. Surg., *8*:400, 1965.

Flesch, P.: Hair growth. *In* Rothman, S.: Physiology and Biochemistry of the Skin. Chicago, University of Chicago Press, 1945.

Friederich, H. C., and Gloor, M. E.: Experimentelle Untersuchungen über die Bedeutung der Durchblutung für das Angehen behaarter Vollhautransplantate beim Menschen. Arch. Klin. Exp. Dermatol., *237*:625, 1970.

Gray, H.: Anatomy of the Human Body. W. H. Lewis, Ed. 24th Ed. Philadelphia, Lea & Febiger, 1942.

Hamilton, J. B.: Age, sex and genetic factors in the regulation of hair growth in man. *In* Montagna, W., and Ellis, R. (Eds.): The Biology of Hair Growth. New York, Academic Press, 1958.
Harii, K., Ohmori, K., and Ohmori, S.: Hair transplantation with free scalp flaps. Plast. Reconstr. Surg., *53*:410, 1974.
Hunt, H. L.: Plastic Surgery of the Head, Face and Neck. Philadelphia, Lea & Febiger, 1926.
Juri, J.: Use of parieto-occipital flaps in the surgical treatment of baldness. Plast. Reconstr. Surg., *55*:456, 1975.
Juri, J., and Juri, C.: Two new methods for treating baldness: temporo-parieto-occipito-parietal pedicled flap and temporo-parieto-occipital free flap. Ann. Plast. Surg., *6*:38, 1981.
Juri, J., Juri, C., and Arufe, H. N.: Use of rotation scalp flaps for treatment of occipital baldness. Plast. Reconstr. Surg., *61*:23, 1978.
Kazanjian, V. H.: Repair of partial losses of the scalp. Plast. Reconstr. Surg., *12*:325, 1953.
Kazanjian, V. H., and Webster, R. C.: The treatment of extensive losses of the scalp. Plast. Reconstr. Surg., *1*:360, 1946.
Lamont, E. S.: A plastic surgical transformation; report of a case. West. J. Surg. Obstet. Gynecol., *65*:164, 1957.
Leonard, A. G., and Small, J. O.: Tissue expansion in the treatment of alopecia. Br. J. Plast. Surg., *39*:42, 1986.
Manders, E. K., Graham, W. P., III, Schenden, M. J., and Davis, T. S.: Skin expansion to eliminate large scalp defects. Ann. Plast. Surg., *12*:305, 1984.
Mayer, T. G., and Fleming, R. W.: Short flaps—their use and abuse in the treatment of male pattern baldness. Ann. Plast. Surg., *8*:296, 1982.
Montagna, W.: The Structure and Function of Skin. New York, Academic Press, 1956.
Myers, R. J., and Hamilton, J. B.: Regeneration and rate of growth of hairs in man. Ann. N.Y. Acad. Sci., *53*:562, 1951.
Nataf, J.: Special techniques of hair transplantation by fusiform grafts and flaps of many types. J. Dermatol. Surg. Oncol., *5*:620, 1979.
Nataf, J.: Surgical treatment for frontal baldness: the long temporal vertical flap. Plast. Reconstr. Surg., *74*:628, 1984.
Nordström, R. E. A.: Punch hair grafting under split-skin grafts on scalps. Plast. Reconstr. Surg., *64*:9, 1979.
Nordström, R. E. A.: "Micrografts" for improvement of the frontal hairline after hair transplantation. Aesth. Plast. Surg., *5*:97, 1981.
Nordström, R. E. A., and Devine, J. W.: Scalp stretching with a tissue expander for closure of scalp defects. Plast. Reconstr. Surg., *75*:578, 1985.
Ohmori, K.: Free scalp flap. Plast. Reconstr. Surg., *65*:42, 1980.
Okuda, S.: Clinical and experimental studies of transplantation of living hairs. Jpn. J. Dermatol. Urol., *46*:135, 1939.
Orentreich, N.: Autografts in alopecias and other selected dermatological conditions. Ann. N.Y. Acad. Sci., *83*:463, 1959.
Orticochea, M.: New three-flap scalp reconstruction technique. Br. J. Plast. Surg., *24*:184, 1971.
Padgett, E. C., and Stephenson, K. L.: Plastic and Reconstructive Surgery. Springfield, IL, Charles C Thomas, 1948.
Passot, R.: Chirurgie Esthétique Pure: Techniques et Résultats. Paris, G. Doin et Cie., 1931.
Radovan, C.: Adjacent flap development using expandible Silastic implant. Presented at the annual meeting of the ASPRS, Boston, MA, Sept. 1976.
Saitoh, M., Uzuka, M., and Sakamoto, M.: Rate of hair growth. *In* Montagna, W., and Dobson, R. L. (Eds.): Hair Growth. New York, Pergamon Press, 1969.
Savin, R. C.: Use of topical minoxidil in the treatment of male pattern baldness. J. Am. Acad. Dermatol., *16*:696, 1987.
Stough, D. B. III, Cates, J. A., and Dean, A. J., Jr.: Updating reduction and flap procedures for baldness. Ann. Plast. Surg., *8*:287, 1982.
Straith, C. L., and Beers, M. D.: Scalp avulsions. Plast. Reconstr. Surg., *6*:319, 1950.
Tauber, H.: Alopecia prematura and its surgical treatment (flap method of plastic surgery). J. Ceylon Br., Br. MA, *36*:237, 1939.
Vallis, C. P.: Surgical treatment of the receding hairline. Plast. Reconstr. Surg., *33*:247, 1964.
Vallis, C. P.: Surgical treatment of the receding hairline. Plast. Reconstr. Surg., *44*:271, 1969.
Vallis, C. P.: The strip scalp graft. Clin. Plast. Surg., *9*:229, 1982.
Vallis, C. P., and Humphreys, S. P.: Treatment of extensive defect of scalp and skull. Report of a case. J. Int. Coll. Surg., *26*:249, 1956.

32

Daniel Marchac

Deformities of the Forehead, Scalp, and Cranial Vault

ANATOMY OF THE SCALP
PHYLOGENY AND GROWTH OF THE CRANIAL BONES
CONGENITAL SCALP AND SKULL DEFECTS
Aplasia Cutis Congenita
Craniopagus
Premature Craniosynostosis
TRAUMATIC DEFECTS OF THE SCALP
Total Scalp Avulsion
Partial Scalp Defects
Scalp Expansion
Cicatricial Alopecia of the Scalp
CRANIOPLASTY
Historical Review
Cranial Vault Defects
Splitting the Remaining Calvaria
Split Rib Cranioplasty
Methylmethacrylate Implants
FRONTAL BONE REPAIR AND CONTOURING
Repair of Full-Thickness Defects
Iliac or Cranial Vault Bone Graft
Frontal Bone Contouring
Frontal Bone Repositioning

ANATOMY OF THE SCALP

The soft tissue over the cranium consists of four layers (Fig. 32–1): skin; subcutaneous tissue; the occipitofrontalis muscle (epicranius) or the galea aponeurotica (a lax layer of subaponeurotic fibroareolar tissue); and the pericranium. From a surgical standpoint the first three strata are considered as forming the scalp proper, since they are intimately connected and are not easily separated.

The *skin* of the scalp is thick and is attached by firm, fibrous septa to the underlying galea. It has an abundant blood and lymphatic supply and numerous sweat and sebaceous glands.

The *subcutaneous tissue*, because of its fibrous septa, forms an inelastic but firm layer containing the blood vessels. The blood vessels embedded in the unyielding tissue bleed freely when divided because they cannot contract. Because of the abundant anastomoses of the temporal, supraorbital, supratrochlear, posterior auricular, and occipital vessels, scalp flaps with only a small pedicle usually survive and large flaps heal uneventfully. Infection is prone to remain localized because of the fibrous septa, but purulent collections are painful since the nerves are compressed within enclosed compartments.

The paired *occipitofrontalis muscles* (epicranius) and their galeal aponeuroses, which join them across the vertex of the cranium, are attached posteriorly to the external occipital protuberance and the superior nuchal line of the occipital bone. They fuse laterally with the temporal fascia, and attach through the substance of the frontalis muscle to the

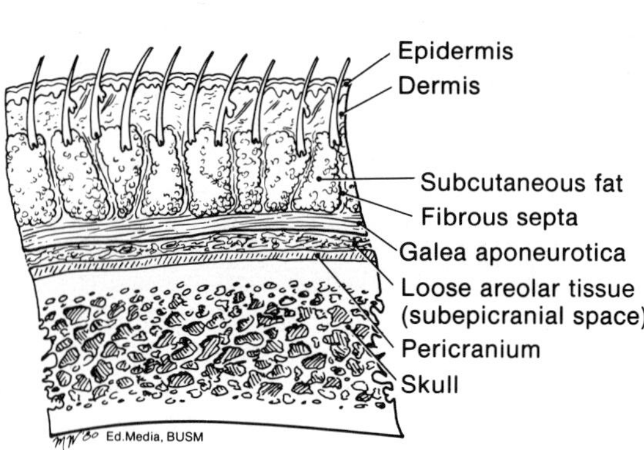

Figure 32–1. The layers of the scalp.

supraorbital ridges and adjacent soft tissue (orbicularis oculi).

The *subepicranial space* lies between the epicranius muscle and the pericranium (see below). This potential space is traversed by small arteries that supply the pericranium, and by the emissary veins connecting the intracranial venous sinuses with the superficial veins of the scalp. This space is considered the danger zone of the scalp because hematoma and infection can spread easily through it, and thrombosis of the emissary veins may extend to the dural sinuses. Purulent material trapped in this space may destroy the pericranium and cause necrosis of the skull, and can even spread intracranially.

The periosteum overlying the cranium is known as the *pericranium*. In the neonatal skull, the fontanels are bridged by pericranium externally and dura mater internally. When the fontanels are obliterated, the dura mater and pericranium are bound closely to the suture line. Spreading infection and hematoma thus are usually limited to the confines of a single bone. The blood vessels that traverse the pericranium and the small vessels in the outer table of the cranium may afford pathways along which infection extends to the diploë and causes osteomyelitis. When the sutures are obliterated, the pericranium extends from one bone to another without deep sutural attachment.

PHYLOGENY AND GROWTH OF THE CRANIAL BONES

In describing the development of the cranium it is well to consider first its basic neural and visceral (branchial) components. The neural portion supports and protects the brain and sense organs. Phylogenetically, this part of the skull is a composite consisting of an old cranial base with which are associated the capsular investments of the sense organs. To this has been added more recently the facial skeleton plus a vaulted cranial roof. Thus, the skull eventually consists of two components: cranial and facial. Phylogenetically, man inherited only two of the original five bones that protect the eye: the lacrimal and the malar bones. The decrease in the number of bones accompanying the movement forward of the orbits from their more lateral position allows for binocular vision. The progressive decrease in the number of bones in the skull as one passes from fish to man is known as "Williston's law." In general the older basal portion is preformed in cartilage, whereas the new facial and roofing bones are formed in membrane (*membranous bone*). There is, however, so much fusion and overlapping that it is unwise to try to draw too sharp a line of distinction.

The visceral (branchial) portion of the skull consists of reduced and modified remains of the gill arches, which played such an important role in food seizure (jaws) and respiration (gill arches) in our aquatic ancestors. It is of interest that most of the parts retained are still concerned with the same functions, although they have been utilized under different conditions since lung respiration replaced the gill mechanism.

Under air living conditions, the sound receiving mechanism evolves into a more elaborate form with the conversion of the obsolescent proximal ends of the first two visceral arches into the auditory ossicles. The inner aspect of the first branchial pouch becomes the eustachian tube, while the external portion forms the external auditory canal. Around the external auditory orifice, budlike proliferations form as the anlagen of the external ear. The remaining portion of the first branchial arch (Meckel's cartilage) continues forward and becomes the anlage around which two membrane bones are later laid down to form the mandible. The second branchial arch is represented by the stylohyoid ligament and the upper portion of the hyoid bone. The third arch is represented by the lower portion of the hyoid bone, and the thyroid cartilage is formed by the fourth. In the developing embryo the muscles of the face and neck are formed by mesenchymal migration carrying along the original nerve innervation and blood supply from each visceral arch.

The cranial base is first laid down in cartilage, and this model is gradually replaced with chondral bone in the developing infant. In contrast, the calvaria is formed by the ossification of the preexisting condensed mesenchyma (desmocranium) and by the periosteum, respectively. The preexisting fibrous structures are incorporated with a large number of newly formed fibers in the new bone matrix. Likewise with the maxilla and mandible, the first bone appears in an area of

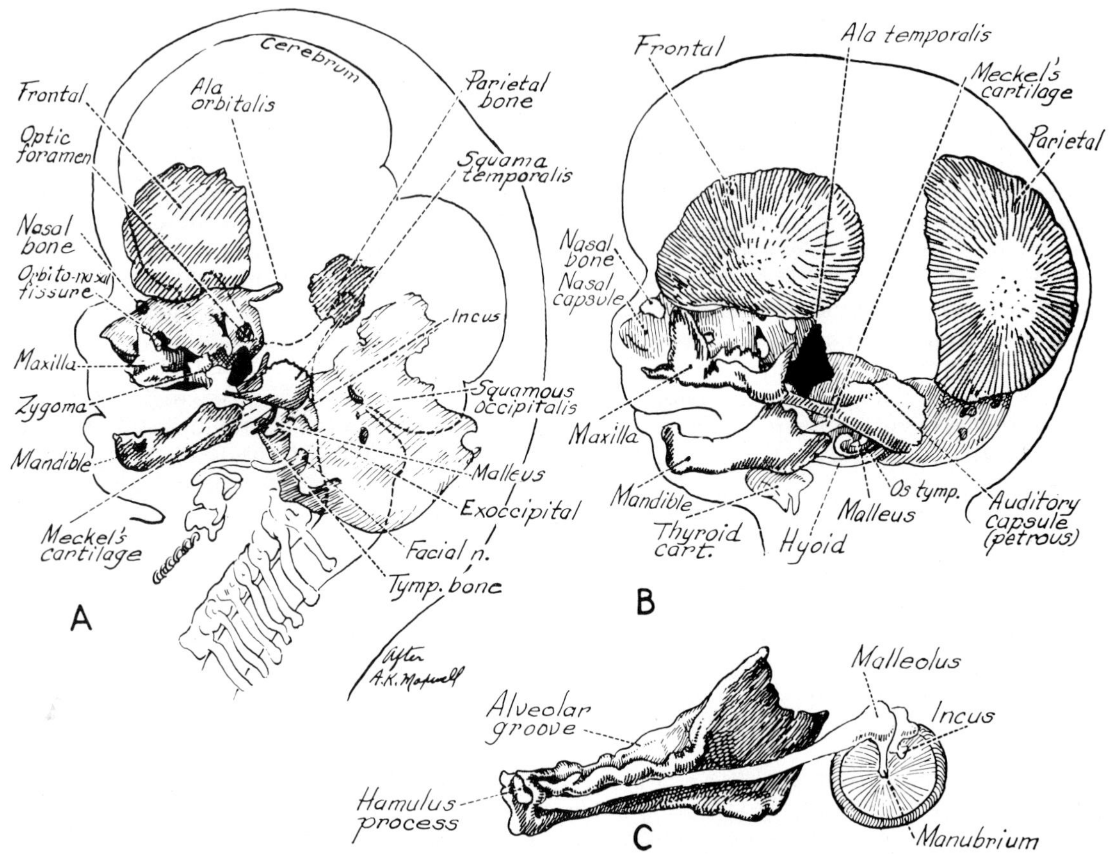

Figure 32–2. *A,* Lateral aspect of the skull of a human embryo of approximately 40 mm (based on Macklin, 1914, 1921). *B,* Lateral aspect of the skull of an 80 mm human embryo (based on Hartwig's model from Kollman's Handatlas, 1907). (*A* and *B* redrawn from Hamilton, W. J., Boyd, J. D., and Mossman, H. W.: Human Embryology. 3rd Ed. Baltimore, Williams & Wilkins Company, 1962.) *C,* Meckel's cartilage, malleus, and incus of a human fetus 80 mm long. (Redrawn from Kollmann, J., Kiebel, F., and Mall, F. R.: Human Embryology. Philadelphia, J. B. Lippincott Company.)

mesenchyme in which definitive collagen fibers are not present until immediately before ossification. In a third type of formation, bone appears among the dense fibers of preexisting fascia, aponeurosis, tendon, ligament, or cartilage, e.g., Meckel's cartilage (Fig. 32–2).

As is well known, the brain grows rapidly; consequently, the cranium triples in volume in the first two years of life, except in premature cranial synostosis (craniostenosis). Growth of the cranium continues but at a slower rate until the seventh year, at which time it has attained 90 per cent of its adult size. Thereafter, the annual increment in growth is almost negligible.

The facial bones do not keep up with the rapid pace of the cranium. After the first year the facial skeleton grows faster and continues to grow over a much longer period.

Craniofacial growth is discussed in more detail in Chapters 46 and 47.

CONGENITAL SCALP AND SKULL DEFECTS

Aplasia Cutis Congenita

Aplasia cutis congenita was first described by Campbell (1826), whose patient died of hemorrhage from the superior sagittal sinus. Since then approximately 500 cases have been reported, but the questions remain the same: (1) how to prevent early bleeding or infection and (2) how to ensure proper skull and scalp repair.

There is no agreement as to the etiology of congenital scalp and skull defects. A genetic cause is supported by many familial cases, with chromosomal abnormalities (trisomy D), but placental infarcts and intrauterine amniotic adhesions have also been implicated.

The scalp or skull defects occur most frequently in the first-born female children, and

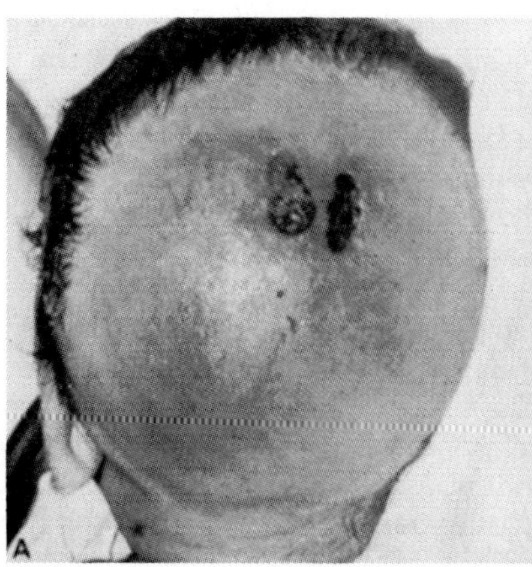

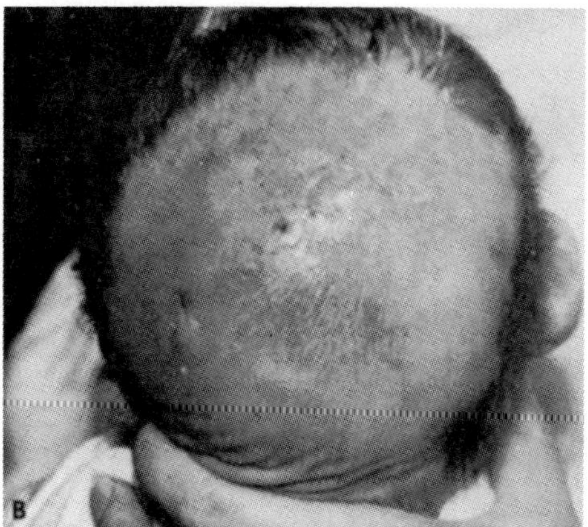

Figure 32–3. *A,* Congenital absence of an area of the scalp with beginning necrosis of the dura in a newborn infant. *B,* One month after excision of the necrotic areas and reconstruction by double rotation flaps.

most often are on the midline in the region of the posterior fontanel. Two or more lesions have been reported in 25 per cent of the cases, and associated trunk defects have been observed as well as hydrocephalus, myelomeningoceles, cleft lip and palate, and deformities of the fingers and cranium (Spear and Mickle, 1983).

The size and depth of the defect is variable. In most cases it is less than 2 cm in diameter, is symmetric or stellate in configuration, involves only the scalp and not the underlying bone, and heals spontaneously. These cases are, of course, simple to manage and require only careful dressings during the healing period. The small area of residual alopecia can be corrected later by a local scalp flap.

A difficult problem exists when the bone is missing and the dura is left unprotected (Fig. 32–3). A local flap is used for coverage. The scalp in these infants is especially fragile and should be manipulated with great care (Fig. 32–4).

The defect can be even larger and make up the full thickness of scalp, vault, and dura (Fig. 32–5). The sagittal sinus is apparent under a fine membrane, which is the thin pia covering the brain. When the defect can be closed easily by local flaps, they are recommended (Irons and Olson, 1980; Schneider, Berg, and Kaplan, 1980) to prevent hemorrhage and infection. There are, however, large defects beyond the scope of local rotation flaps. In these cases, conservative management has been advocated by several authors (Muakkassa, King, and Stark, 1982; Handa, Nakasu, and Matsuda, 1982). Muakkassa, King, and Stark (1982) reported a child presenting with an 11 × 7 cm full-thickness defect that healed spontaneously in six weeks. The defect was kept moist with sterile normal saline and topical antibiotic dressings. Reverse isolation was employed for four weeks. The surface of the scalp defect gradually epithelized from the margins. When the child was 1 year of age a soft, mobile skin with scattered hair was present over a 7 × 6 cm pulsatile defect. The bone grew from the edges of the skull defect toward the vertex, and at 3 years of age there was a normal skull contour.

In contrast to this case, there have been many case reports of dramatic hemorrhage and infection (Schneider, Berg, and Kaplan, 1980; Irons and Olson, 1980; Glasson and Duncan, 1985), especially if an eschar was allowed to form. It is essential to keep the defect moist immediately after birth.

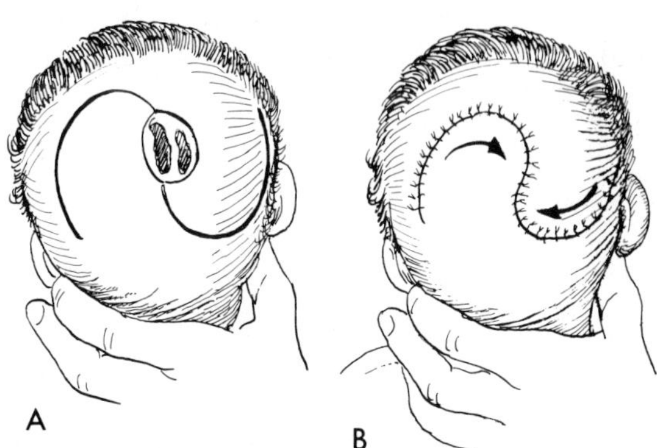

Figure 32–4. *A,* Outline of the proposed rotation flaps for the closure of the occipital defect of the scalp and skull in the infant shown in Figure 32–3. *B,* The rotation flaps have been interpolated, providing adequate coverage of the cranial defect.

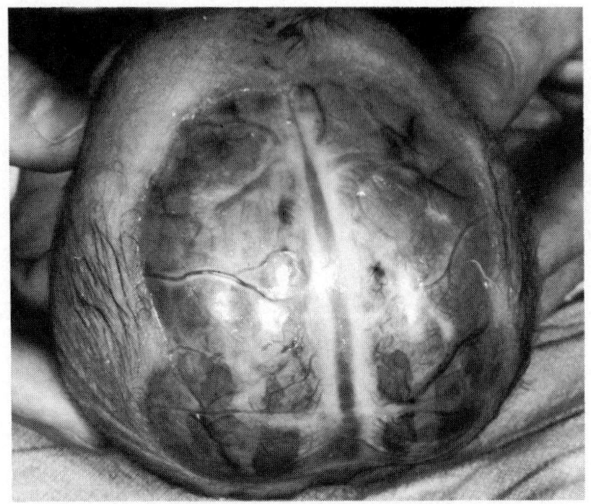

Figure 32–5. Appearance of a congenital defect of the scalp, cranium, and dura 11 days after birth.

An important point is to define the exact depth of the defect, and this is a difficult problem. Montgomery (1967) reported that the brain is covered by a thin, flattened layer of cuboidal cells arranged in a regular manner in a simple layer. Dingman, Weintraub, and Wilensky (1977) noted only a thin pia covering the brain, whereas Muakkassa, King, and Stark (1982) reported a thin, parchment-like membrane covering an opaque vascularized tissue. They thought the latter represented the dura—the cerebral cortex and sagittal sinus being not visible. These differing descriptions of the deformity suggest that the thickness of the defect can be variable.

Surgical treatment of these large defects is difficult. The case reported by Dingman, Weintraub, and Wilensky in 1977 is illustrative of these problems. The infant presented with a 7.5 × 5 cm defect of the skull, scalp, and dura. An associated omcephalocele had to be treated first, and the skull defect was kept moist and covered with cadaver allografts (Fig. 32–6).

Flap coverage was undertaken at 11 days of life, but fluorescein tests showed nonperfusion of the distal ends of the scalp flaps; the flaps were consequently delayed. Another delay was done eight days later until finally the flaps were transposed and the donor areas covered with split-thickness skin autografts (Fig. 32–7). The child did well postoperatively but had grand mal seizures. Seizures did not reappear after completion of scalp coverage. At 12 months of age, there was no evidence of spontaneous closure of the bony defect.

The technique of skin expansion offers a possible solution to facilitate the closure, but it requires a wait of at least a few weeks before flap coverage is begun (Argenta, Watanabe, and Grabb, 1983). Skull repair should not be undertaken immediately, to allow for spontaneous reossification (Muakkassa, King, and Stark, 1982; Handa, Nakasu, and Matsuda, 1982). If this does not occur, a variety of cranioplasty techniques can be considered according to the size of the defect. A residual alopecia is treated by scalp reduction (McCray and Roenigk, 1981) or skin expansion and local flaps (Argenta and Dingman, 1986) (Fig. 32–8) (see also Chap. 31).

Craniopagus

This dramatic anomaly, first described by Münster in 1556, is extremely rare and affects only one out of 600 twin births (Edmonds

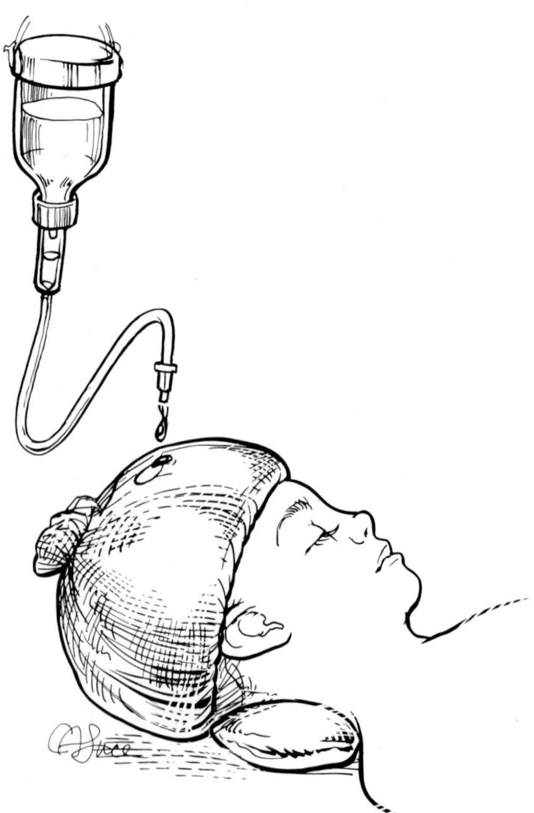

Figure 32–6. The patient was fitted with a tube gauze head dressing kept moist by a continuous drip of normal saline solution.

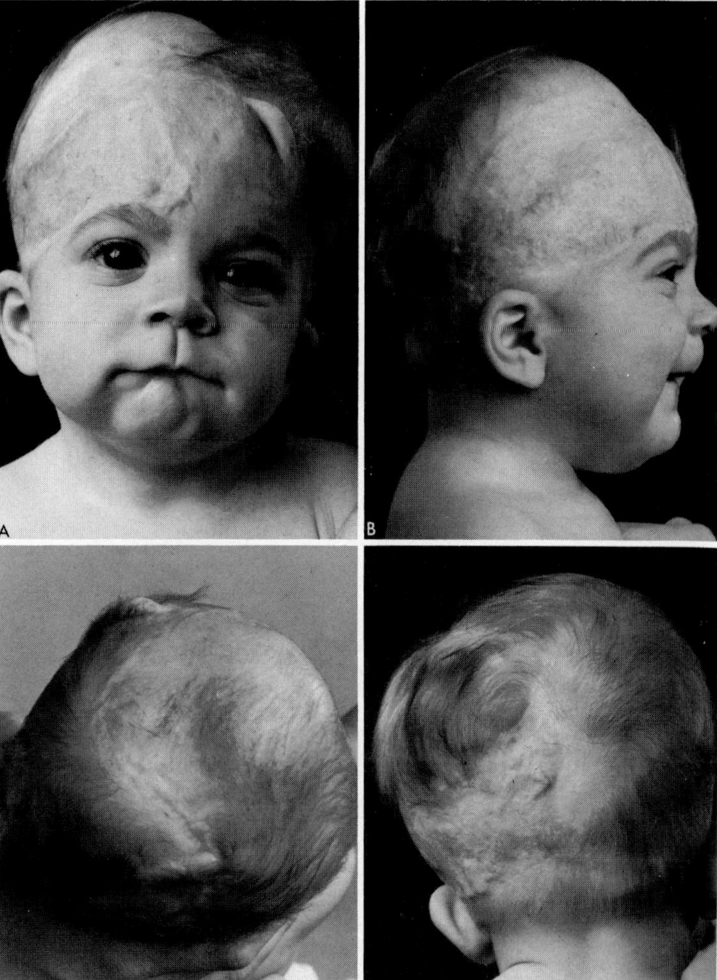

Figure 32–7. Appearance of the patient at the age of 10 months. *A, B,* The skin grafted area of the donor site of the right scalp flap, which covers half of the original defect. *C,* The left scalp flap covers the other half of the defect. *D,* View of the vertex.

and Layde, 1982) or one in 2.5 million births (O'Connell, 1976), despite the fact that the potential for double monsters exists in all fertilized eggs, and more specifically in twins.

The surgical separation is obviously much more difficult in total craniopagus, in which the brains are connected, than in partial craniopagus (O'Connell, 1976), in which the union of both heads involves only the skull and the skin and/or the scalp. The dura can generally be separated in these cases. Successful cases of separation of partial craniopagus were reported by Voris and associates (1957), Baldwin and Debakan (1958), and Wolfowitz and associates (1968).

In total craniopagus the brains are connected, a finding that presents a most difficult problem for the neurosurgeon. Three-dimensional CT scans and angiography are helpful to an understanding of the anatomic relationship between the two brains (Fig. 32–9).

The problems associated with dural repair, cerebrospinal fluid circulation, and skull and skin repair can be solved, but reestablishment of the cerebral venous drainage is the major problem. In the case reported by Grossman and coworkers (1953), only one longitudinal sinus was found. All the veins in one twin had to be clipped and divided; he never recovered consciousness and died 34 days later. O'Connell (1976), who performed three total craniopagus separations with one survivor each time, suggested that venous drainage should be modified before separation.

In partial or total craniopagus separation, the coverage of the scalp defects was previ-

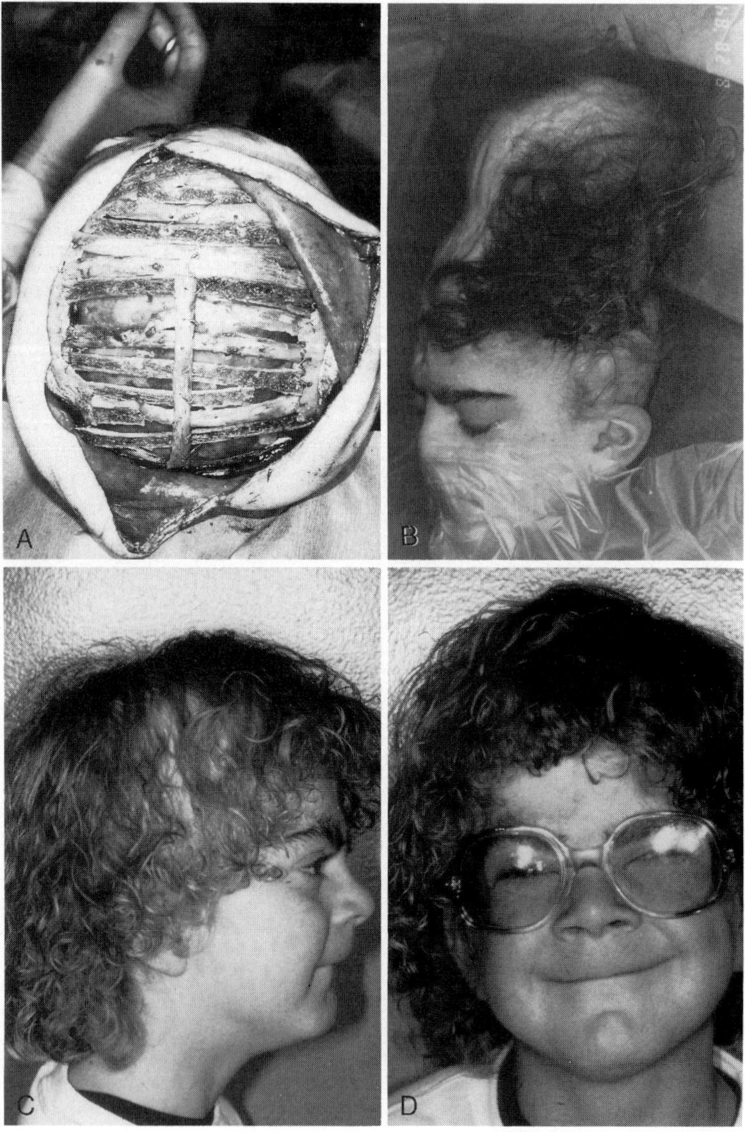

Figure 32–8. Calvarial reossification did not occur in the patient illustrated in Figures 32–5, 32–6, and 32–7. *A,* At 7 years of age, a cranial vault reconstruction was performed with split rib grafts, after previous skin expansion with a steel-reinforced silicone sheet placed over the brain. *B,* One year later a second skin expansion (1100 ml) permitted removal of the skin graft and correction of the alopecia. *C, D,* Final result. Note the luxuriant hair coverage. (From Argenta, L. C., and Dingman, R. O.: Total reconstruction of aplasia cutis congenita involving scalp, skull, and dura. Plast. Reconstr. Surg., *77*:650, 1986.)

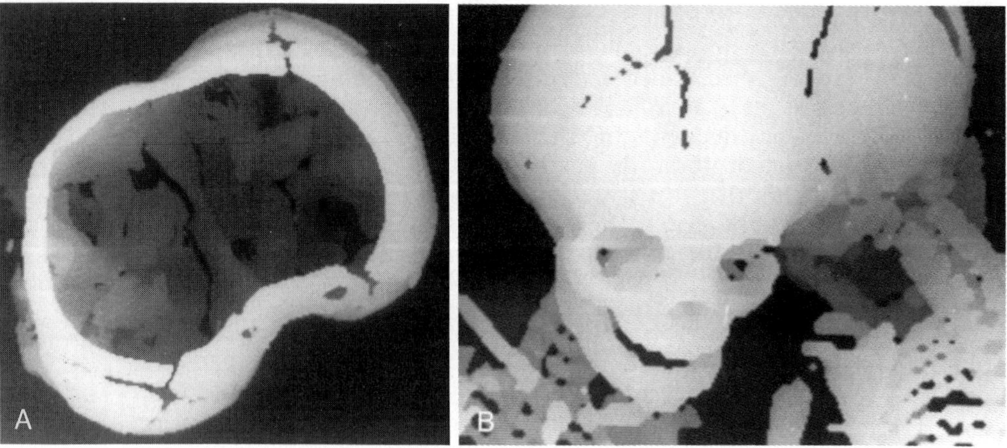

Figure 32–9. *A, B,* Three-dimensional CT imaging shows the connection between the two skulls (see Fig. 32–10). (Courtesy of Dr. R. E. Shively.)

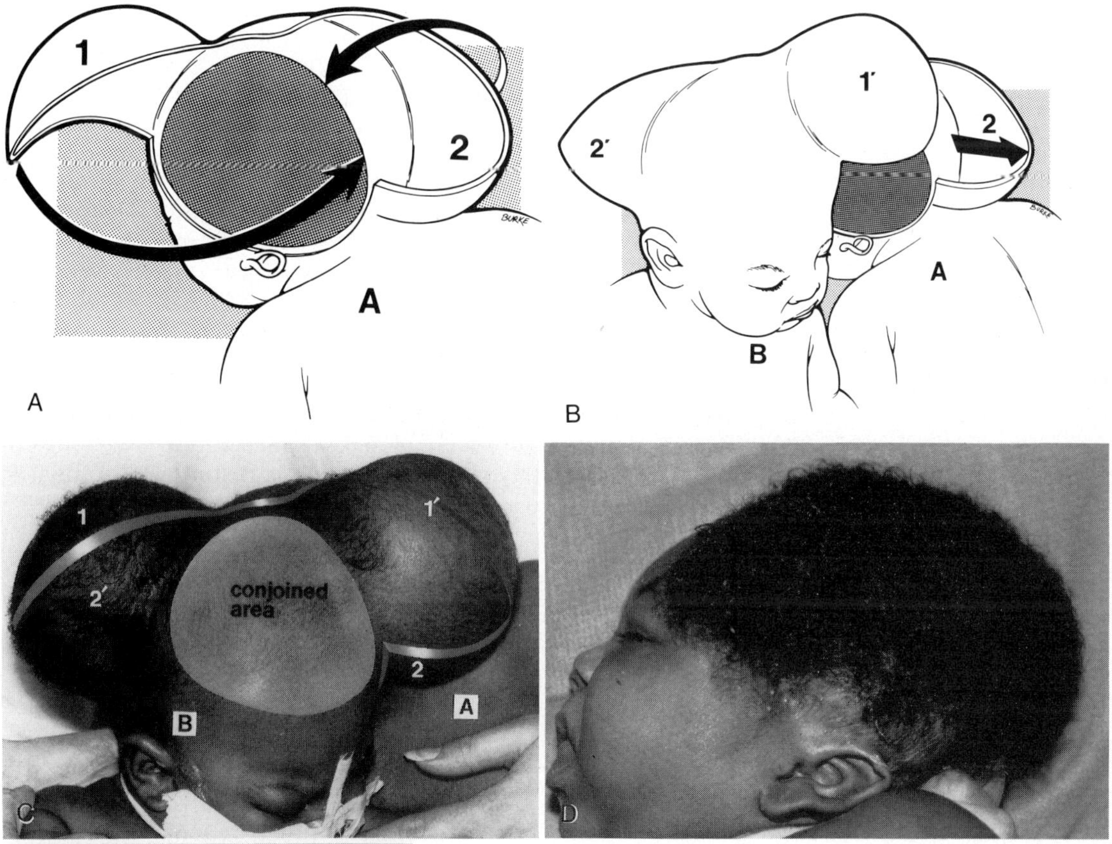

1
2
A
A

1′
2′
2
A
B
B

1
1′
2′
conjoined area
2
B
A
C

D

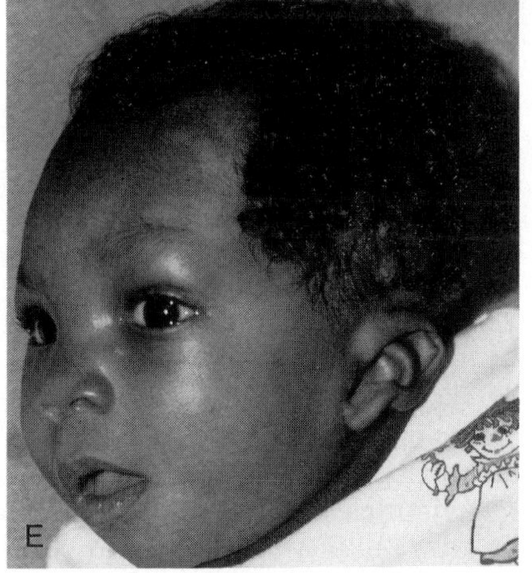

Figure 32–10. Skin expansion permitted complete coverage of the two heads after separation of the craniopagus twins (see Fig. 32–9). *A, B, C,* Planning of the repair with two large tissue expanders. *D, E,* Appearance of the two twins without evidence of alopecia. (From Shively, R. E., Bermant, M. A., and Bucholz, R. D.: Separation of craniopagus twins utilizing tissue expanders. Plast. Reconstr. Surg., *76*:765, 1985.)

ously obtained with skin grafts and flaps. Shively, Bermant, and Bucholz (1985) reported the first case of successful separation of craniopagus with utilization of skin expanders for the scalp repair. The twins were connected in the parietal area, on a surface of 90 sq cm. The brains were also connected. Neurosurgical separation was performed in two stages, at 9 and 46 days respectively. The parietal brain was separated as well as an ectopic dural sinus connecting the two existing sagittal sinuses. During the second operation, two 200 ml expanders were placed in a subgaleal location over the occiput in each child. Expansion was achieved in six weeks. When the twins were 106 days of age, final separation was accomplished. Expanded skin flaps permitted an easy closure, but an episode of severe bleeding due to venous abnormalities affected one of the twins, who demonstrated a significant developmental delay. The careful planning of the flaps allowed a complete coverage of the scalp defects and considerably simplified the scalp repair (Fig. 32–10).

Premature Craniosynostosis

The shape of the head may be severely altered by premature closure of one or more of the cranial sutures (see also Chap. 61). Familial history is present in 39 per cent of the cases, and a search for associated anomalies should also be made (Marchac and Renier, 1982).

When an abnormal shape of the head is observed at birth, a radiograph rules out the frequent positional distortions. In the case of craniosynostosis, the affected sutures are not visible or are less visible, and in most cases the orbital shape is modified on frontal view.

The shape of the head depends on the sutures involved, the limitation of growth being at right angles to the line of the involved sutures. Synostosis of the metopic midline suture produces a triangular forehead with hypotelorism (*trigonocephaly*). Involvement of the sagittal suture creates *scaphocephaly*, with an elongated and narrow head. Synostosis of one coronal suture causes *plagiocephaly*, with flattening of the forehead, elevation of the orbit, and nasal deviation toward the affected side. Bilateral coronal synostosis creates *brachycephaly*, the skull being shortened sagittally and widened transversally, with a recession of the supraorbital rim. *Cloverleaf skull* due to synostosis of the temporoparietal suture, or various associations, can also be observed.

All the craniosynostoses are detectable at birth. Early craniofacial surgery (Marchac, 1978; Marchac and Renier, 1982) has improved the prognosis, allowing functional brain decompression and resolution of the morphologic problem in one operation, in most cases.

There is also a late-appearing craniosynostosis (at 2 to 4 years of age), which affects the coronal suture and creates a pointed head, or *oxycephaly*. Increased intracranial pressure is especially frequent (Renier and associates, 1987).

All these syndromes and their early and late treatment are discussed extensively in Chapter 61. Later correction of the recessed forehead of oxycephaly is discussed in this chapter under contour restoration of the frontal bone (see p. 1565).

TRAUMATIC DEFECTS OF THE SCALP

Total Scalp Avulsion

This dramatic injury is generally caused by long hair being caught in a machine. Partial avulsions are rare because the strong galea resists the traction, the tearing occurs at the periphery, and the scalp is removed in a single piece. The forehead, eyebrows, upper lids, and part of the ear are often avulsed with the scalp, the plane of cleavage being between the galea and the periosteum. Nevertheless, the fragile periosteum is occasionally torn away with the scalp.

For decades, plastic surgeons considered it futile to try to replace the scalp, as reported by Davis in 1911 and McWilliams in 1924. Despite the unique case of successful replacement reported by Lu (1969), it even seemed useless to try to defat and replace the avulsed scalp (Robinson, 1952). The treatment of choice was split-thickness grafting when the periosteum was present (Kazanjian and Webster, 1946; Converse, 1955).

Miller, Anstee, and Snell (1976) opened a new era in the treatment of scalp avulsion by reporting successful total scalp replantation by microvascular anastomosis (Fig. 32–11). Subsequently, Buncke and associates (1978)

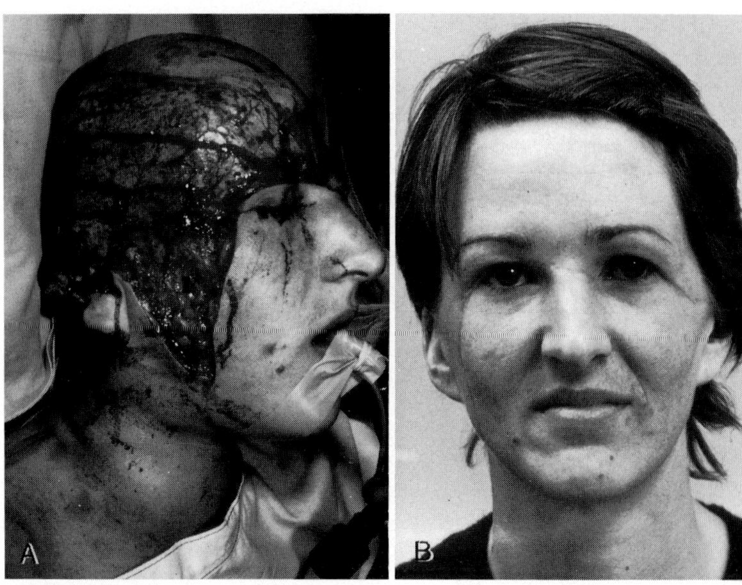

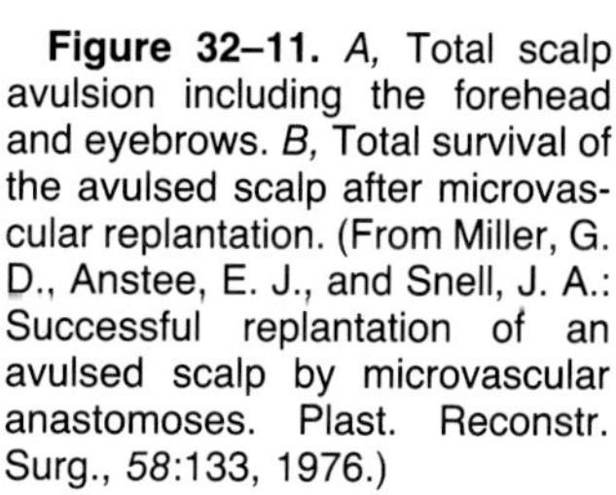

Figure 32–11. *A,* Total scalp avulsion including the forehead and eyebrows. *B,* Total survival of the avulsed scalp after microvascular replantation. (From Miller, G. D., Anstee, E. J., and Snell, J. A.: Successful replantation of an avulsed scalp by microvascular anastomoses. Plast. Reconstr. Surg., *58*:133, 1976.)

and others reported similar cases that had remarkable success. *Replantation of the avulsed scalp* is now, therefore, the treatment of choice provided that the scalp has not been damaged and has been kept moist and refrigerated. The patient reported by Miller, Anstee, and Snell (1976) was admitted to the hospital 45 minutes after the accident, and the scalp was revascularized four and one-half hours later. Successful replantations have been reported with as long as 17 hours' delay (Nahai, Hurteau, and Vasconez, 1978). Even if the vessels have been damaged at the periphery, vein grafts can be used to bridge the vascular defects.

When the scalp is not usable, the surgeon is faced with the problem of repairing an enormous scalp defect. When the periosteum is present, it should be carefully moistened to prevent drying, and coverage can be accomplished with split-thickness skin grafts harvested from the buttocks or the thighs.

When the periosteum is absent, the outer table of the calvaria is in jeopardy because it receives its blood supply from the scalp through the periosteum. Microsurgical techniques can be utilized to provide coverage. Greater omentum or groin flaps are useful; latissimus dorsi flaps are preferred by Alpert, Buncke, and Mathes (1982), including the dorsal skin when the defect is smaller than 9 cm in diameter. In larger defects the muscle alone, covered with a split-thickness graft, is the preferred technique.

When microsurgical techniques cannot be utilized, multiple perforations of an exposed calvaria, as advocated by Celsus, can provide granulation tissue coming from the diploë. Chiseling of the outer table, with immediate skin grafting, is recommended by Feierabend and Bindra (1985), after their experience with 46 cases. However, thin, tethered skin graft on calvaria does not represent optimal scalp coverage.

For cases in which the outer table has desiccated or has sequestrated, Shanoff and Tsur (1981) have reported success with perforation of the inner table of calvaria, the granulation tissue rising from the dura. These perforations obviously must be made very carefully, preferably with a small trephine. Skin grafting is possible after the granulation tissue has covered the exposed bone, because otherwise "it skins remarkably slow, generally taking two years," as stated by Patrick Vance in 1776. The skin graft is adherent, tight, and unstable and carries a risk of late malignancy.

Partial Scalp Defects

The scalp is a privileged area for tissue expansion (Radovan, 1976), and most partial scalp defects can be reconstructed from the residual hair-bearing areas after expansion (see Chaps. 13 and 31).

Expanded scalp is transferred in the same manner as a large flap, success depending on (1) absence of infection and (2) absence of scars around the planned flaps.

For management of acute trauma of the scalp, the surgeon should immediately consider the possible use of expanders, but must be conservative. If the periosteum is intact, a split-thickness skin graft from the buttocks or thigh is the best solution (Dingman and Argenta, 1982).

If the periosteum is absent, several solutions can be considered, depending on the size and bacterial status of the wound: (1) perforation of the calvaria and moist dressings for subsequent grafting and (2) coverage of the exposed bone with a periosteal (pericranial) flap, which is covered with a split-thickness skin graft (Fonseca, 1983). Preferably the periosteal flap should be dissected without additional incisions in the scalp.

The classic solution of a large scalp flap to cover the denuded area, and skin grafting of the donor defect, can still be used, as long as sufficient expandable scalp is kept adjacent to the donor area to enable the skin graft to be removed later after tissue expansion.

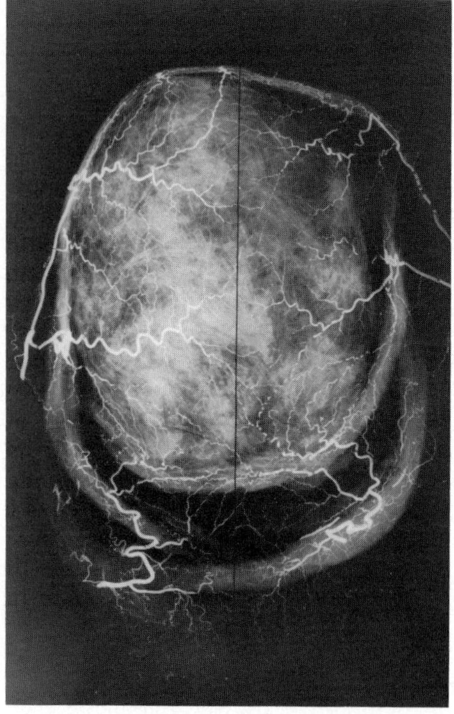

Figure 32–12. Cast study demonstrating that the vascularization of the scalp originates from the periphery and has a rich anastomotic network (Courtesy of Dr. Ricbourg).

Local scalp flaps are numerous. They should take into consideration the blood supply of the scalp (Fig. 32–12), which originates from the periphery but has numerous anastomoses forming a rich network.

A description of the scalp flaps has been given by Converse (1955). All medium-sized defects can be covered by a variety of local flaps (Fig. 32–13). Multiple incisions in the galea, according to the technique of Kazanjian and Converse (1959), facilitate stretching of the scalp flaps. The flaps are undermined in the plane between the galea and periosteum, and elevated, and transverse or crisscrossed incisions are made across the galea, taking care not to injure the blood vessels that lie on the latter.

Orticochea (1971) devised an ingenious three-flap technique for the closure of moderate-sized and large defects with variations (Figs. 32–14, 32–15). A four-flap technique is also feasible (Fig. 32–16) (Orticochea, 1967). All the available scalp is lifted, as one peels a banana, and defects up to 20 cm can be resurfaced with hair-bearing skin (Jurkiewicz and Hill, 1981). The Orticochea principle of mobilizing large scalp flaps pedicled at the periphery is also utilized after tissue expansion.

Large defects of scalp and cranium secondary to burns cannot be repaired with local scalp flaps if the surrounding or potential donor tissue is subject to circulatory and dystrophic alterations. Such a condition is often seen in recurrent carcinoma treated by irradiation. In this situation, tissue must be transferred from a distance. Classic tube flaps have been replaced by microvascular free flaps. Two types of free flaps can be used: the omentum covered with a skin graft (McLean and Buncke, 1972), or a microvascular free flap, such as the scapular flap (Fig. 32–17). With time such flaps shrink and a suitable scalp thickness results. Free flaps including skin tend to be more bulky, with the exception of free flaps from the dorsum of the foot or the forearm, both of which, however, leave objectionable donor sites.

Scalp Expansion

When one has manipulated a scalp flap with its galea, it would seem unlikely that expansion of this strong tissue can be obtained, but clinical experience (Argenta, Wa-

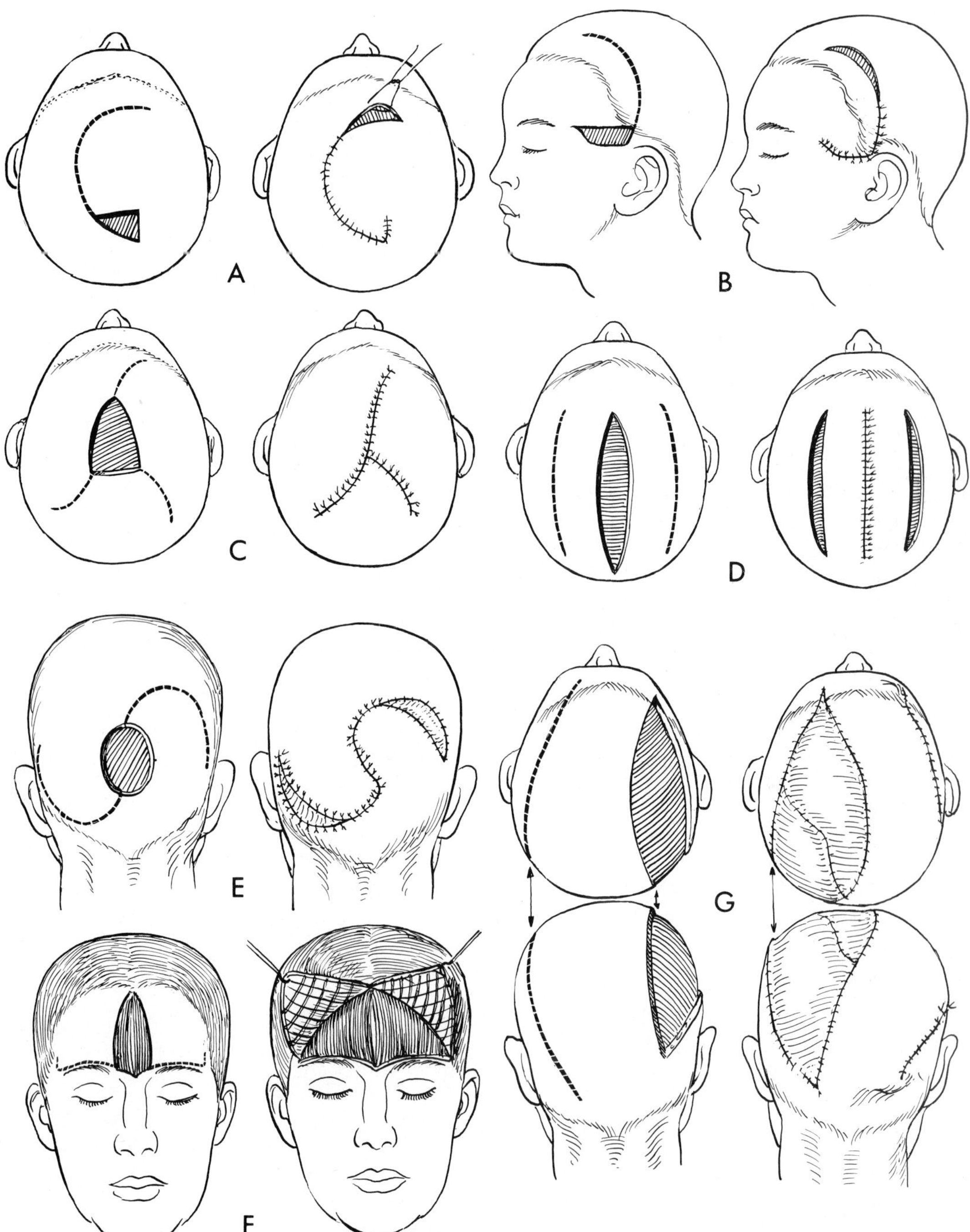

Figure 32–13. Some techniques for the closure of scalp defects. *A, B,* Rotation flaps. *C,* Gillies' tripod technique (1944). *D,* Bipedicle flaps. *E,* Double opposing rotation flaps. If complete closure cannot be obtained, split-thickness skin grafts are applied over the pericranium to cover the remaining exposed areas. *F,* Kazanjian and Converse's crisscross incisions through the frontalis muscle and/or the galea aponeurotica to distend the flaps and achieve closure of the defect. *G,* A large flap transposed over a lateral scalp defect. The residual defect is covered with a split-thickness skin graft over the pericranium.

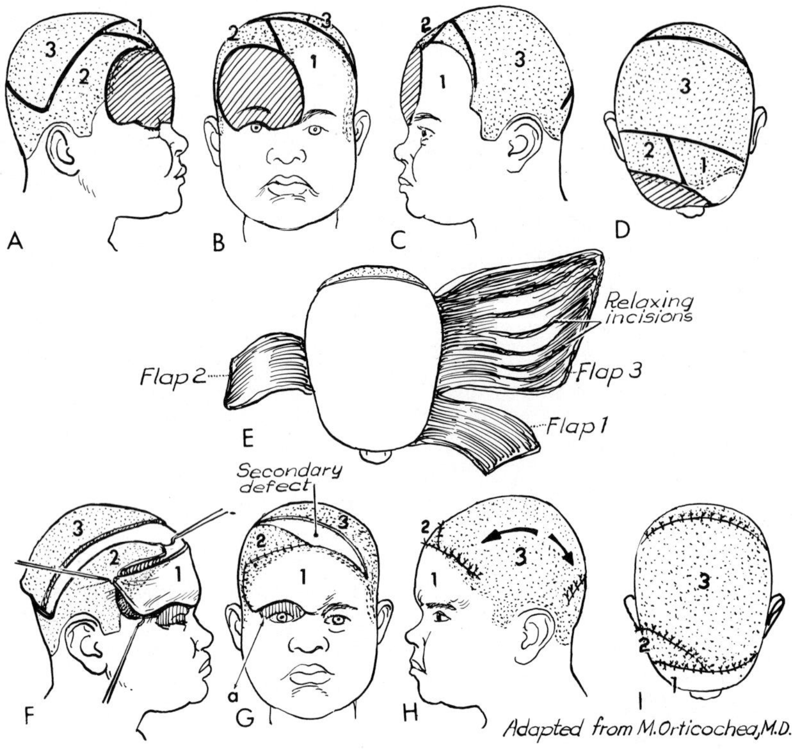

Figure 32–14. Development of the three-flap technique. It is preferable to cut flaps 1 and 2 at an angle as shown. The secondary defect that results after juxtaposing flaps 1 and 2 is smaller than the primary one. (Modified from Orticochea, M.: New three-flap scalp reconstruction technique. Br. J. Plast Surg., *24*:184, 1971.)

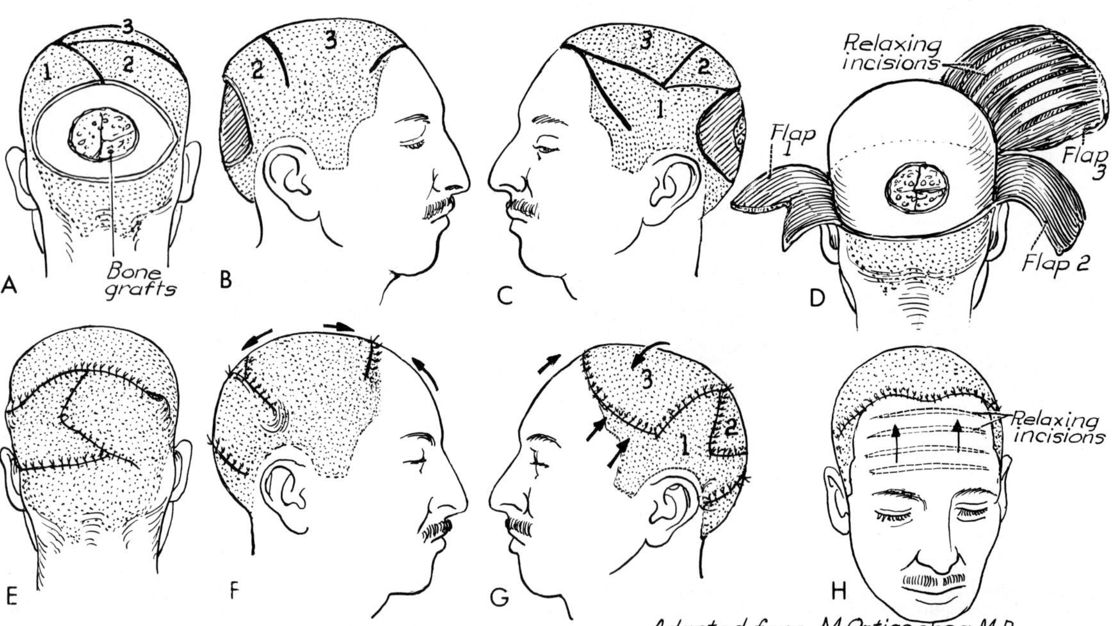

Figure 32–15. The three flaps have been mobilized. Parallel incisions have been made in the aponeurosis of the large flap (*3*) transverse to the longitudinal axis of the skull. Flaps 1 and 2 are sutured in juxtaposition but without tension because their pedicles are narrow. (Modified from Orticochea, M.: New three-flap scalp reconstruction technique. Br. J. Plast. Surg., *24*:184, 1971.)

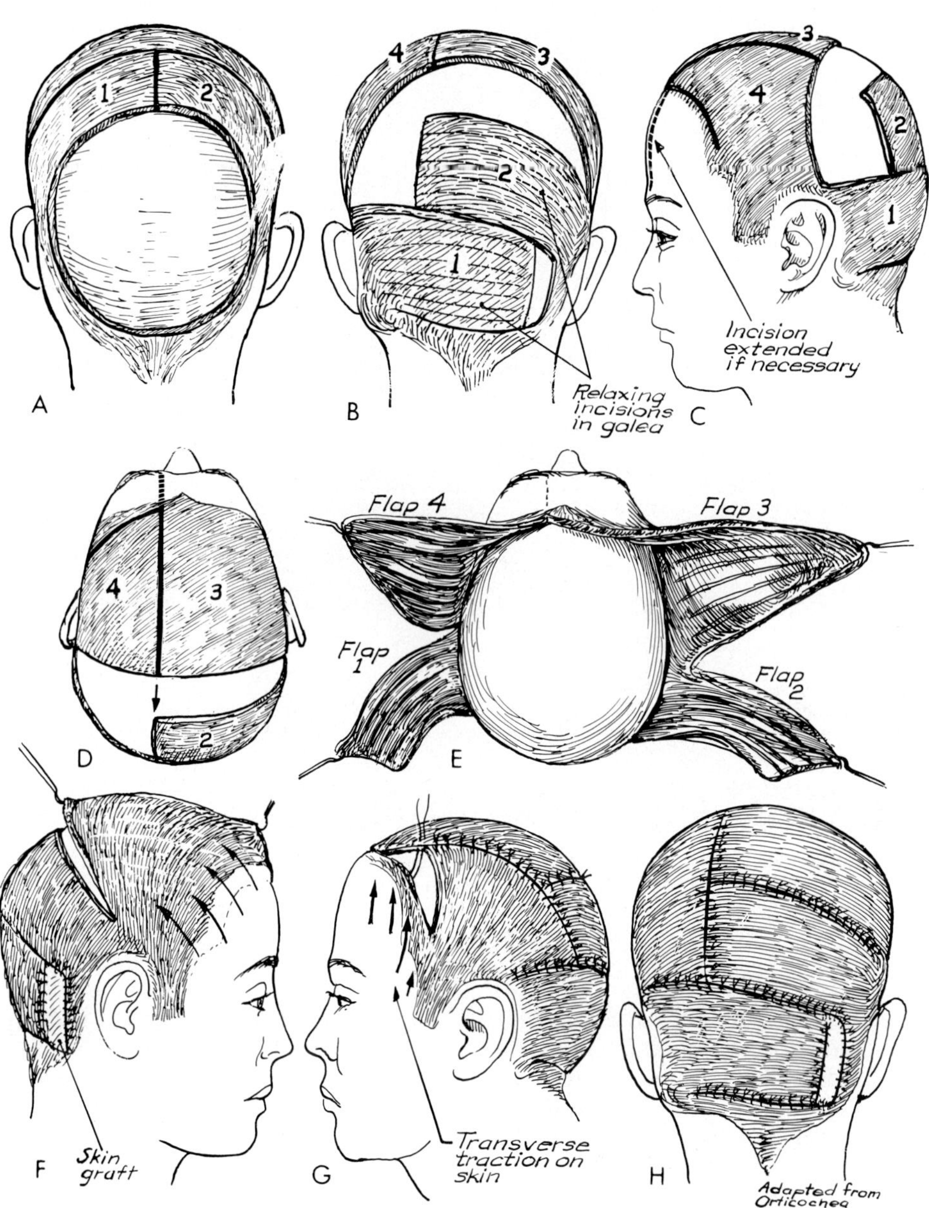

d. (Modified from Orticochea,

Figure 32–16. Four-flap technique, which is particularly applicable in a child. (Modified from Orticochea, M.: Four-flap scalp reconstruction technique. Br. J. Plast. Surg., *20*:159, 1967.)

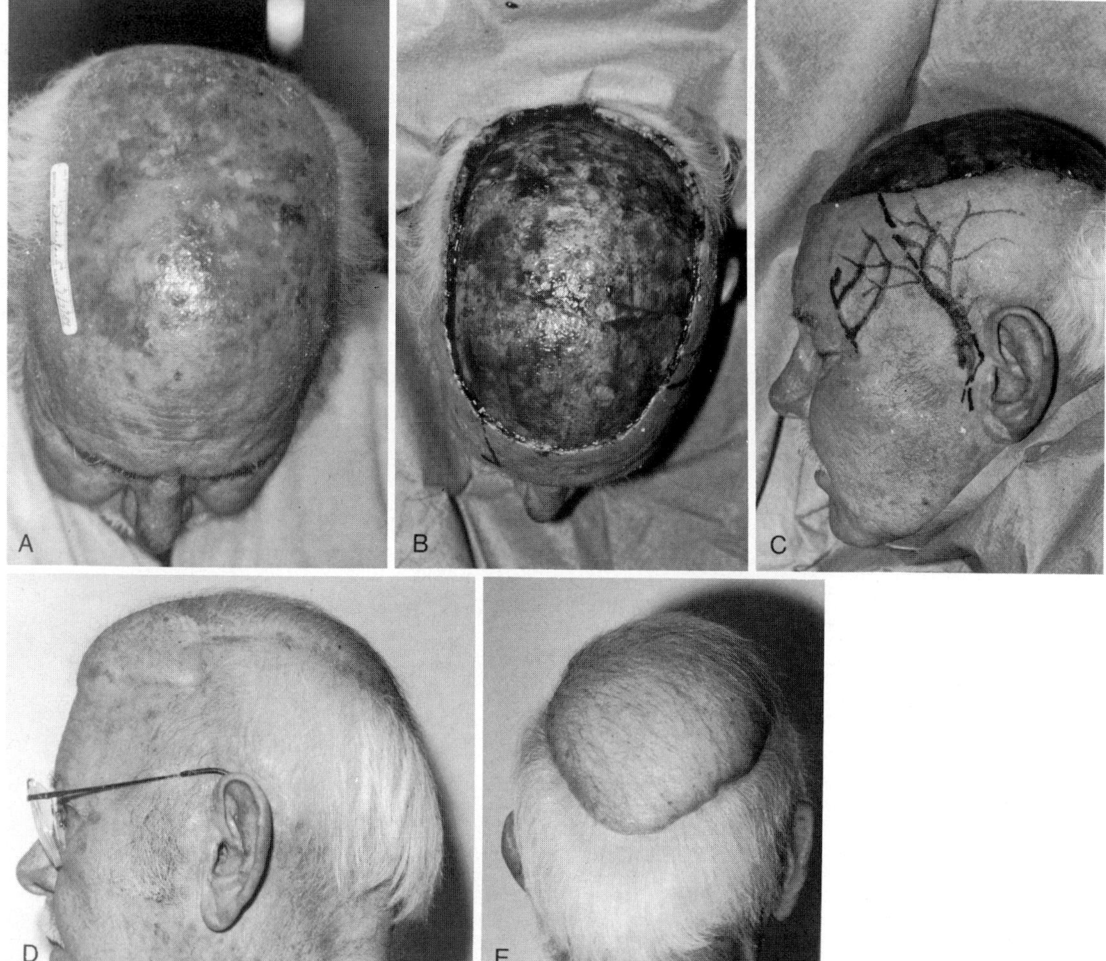

Figure 32–17. Reconstruction of a scalp defect with a microvascular scapular free flap. *A,* Multifocal superficial squamous cell cancer of the scalp in a 65 year old male. *B,* Excisional defect. *C,* Outline of recipient superficial temporal vessels. *D, E,* Appearance several months later. (Courtesy of Dr. William Shaw, Institute of Reconstructive Plastic Surgery.)

tanabe, and Grabb, 1983; Manders and associates, 1984) has shown that the scalp is, on the contrary, expandable, without visible changes in hair thickness. The technique represents perhaps the best indication for tissue expansion.

Large scalp flaps can therefore be obtained, the excess tissue created being mobilized as a rotation flap, an advancement flap, or a random flap (see Figs. 32–8, 32–10, and 32–18).

The technique of skin expansion is discussed in detail in Chapter 13. However, a few points are of particular importance in scalp expansion:

1. Large expanders must be used, 400 ml usually being the minimum, and often it is useful to employ two expanders.

2. The incision for placement of the expander should be small and should not interfere with the design of the planned scalp flap. Suction drainage is also advisable (Manders and associates, 1984).

3. The sutures should be retained for three weeks (Manders and associates, 1984).

4. Inflation should proceed slowly at first and later progress rapidly, the total time of expansion being approximately three to four months.

5. Two successive expansions can be performed.

The pressure exerted by the expander has no adverse effect on the underlying cranium. Manders and associates (1984) recommended, however, that scalp expansion should not be

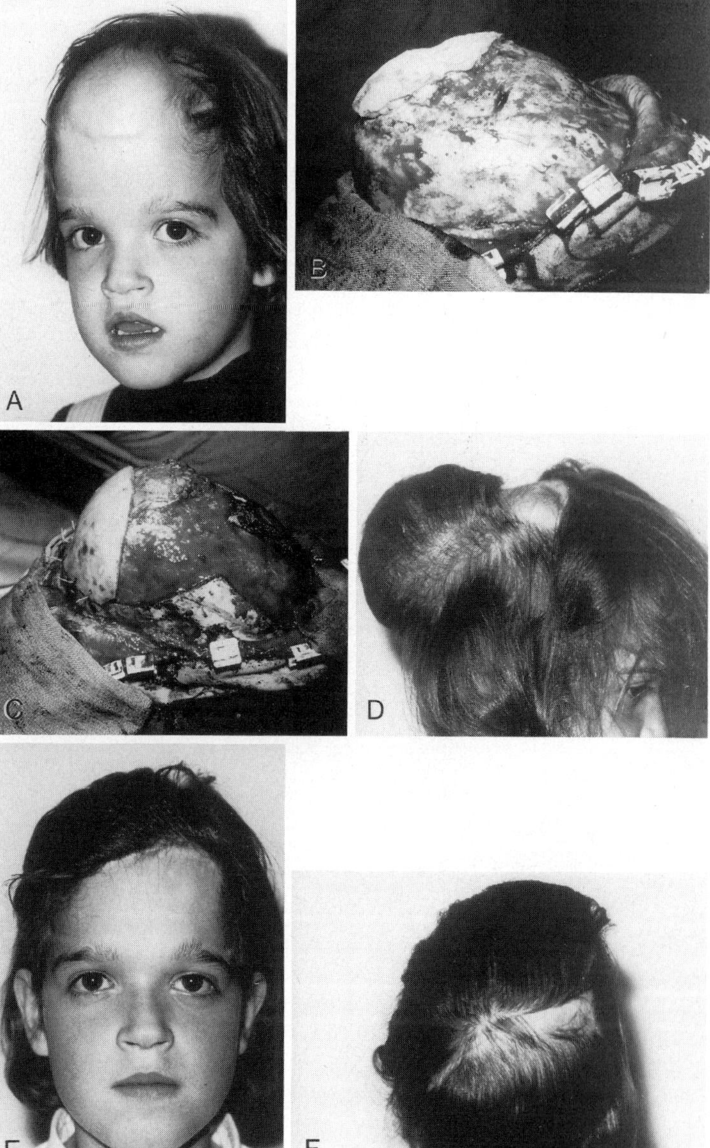

Figure 32–18. *A, B,* A lipoma of the corpus callosum has been removed in this 6 year old girl and the high frontal bony defect repaired with a poorly fitting methylmethacrylate implant. *C,* During frontocranial repair, the frontal bone was replaced by a calvarial bone graft harvested posteriorly, and the remainder of the vault is to be repaired by split calvarial and rib bone grafts. *D,* The anterior bald area was covered with a rotation scalp flap and, in a second stage, an occipital scalp expansion was performed in anticipation of excising the skin graft placed in the original flap donor area. *E, F,* Final appearance with evidence of only minimal alopecia.

performed before the patient reaches the age of 3 years.

Cicatricial Alopecia of the Scalp

One of the most frequently encountered problems is postburn alopecia with partial absence of the frontal hairline (see also Chap. 31). Since the cicatricial alopecia represents a contraction of the initial wound, its correction is usually beyond local flap's repair. Moreover, the temporofrontal area is not favorable for the Orticochea (1967) type of procedure. The Juri (1975) temporo-occipital flap can provide only limited cover (Fig. 32–19) but can be helpful (see Chap. 31). It is best delayed and can be used in association with rotation flaps or anteriorly based midline flaps (Fig. 32–20) (Mitz, Dabos, and Vilain, 1984).

The direction of hair growth is an important variable in the reconstruction of a normal hairline. This is the great advantage of the free flap harvested on the opposite side in a vertical direction (Harii, Ohmori, and

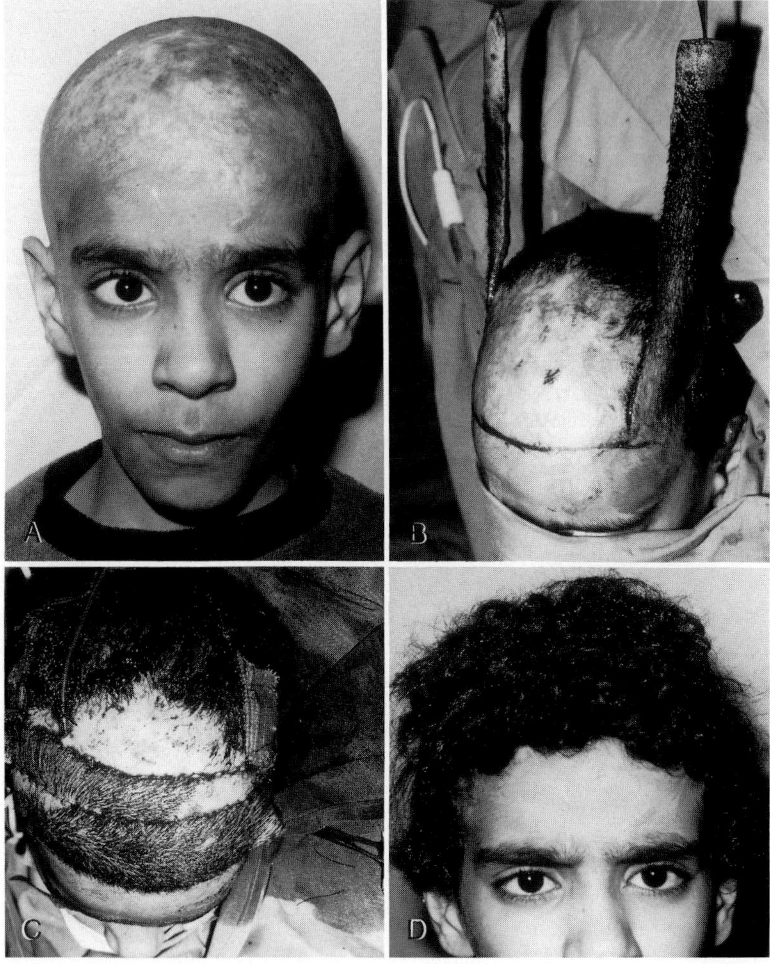

Figure 32–19. The temporo-occipital flap (Juri, 1975). *A,* Postburn alopecia. *B, C,* Two long temporo-occipital flaps are elevated and inset after delay. *D,* Satisfactory hair growth camouflages the residual central alopecic area.

Ohmori, 1974) or horizontally in the temporo-occipital region (Ohmori, 1980). Nevertheless, the free flap must be narrow in order to close the donor site primarily. This flap usually does not resurface all areas of alopecia (see Chap. 31).

Scalp expansion is often the procedure of choice. It allows complete correction of large areas of alopecia and is eventually used with a free flap to obtain the most optimal hair growth direction.

CRANIOPLASTY

Historical Review

In 1889, Seydel used an osteoperiosteal graft from the tibia, reduced in small pieces, to repair a cranial defect. Müller (1890) and König (1890) used a flap of scalp with a portion of the outer calvarial table attached. Von Hacker (1903) transplanted a single osteoperiosteal graft from the tibia for reconstruction of a cranial defect. Keen (1909) filled calvarial defects with calvarial grafts removed by drilling the outer table of the skull, anticipating the chip-bone grafting technique of Mowlem (1944). During a six year period Delagénière and Lewin (1920) reported 104 cases of cranial reconstruction with tibial osteoperiosteal grafts in which there were only two failures. Kazanjian and Converse (1940) reported 18 successful cranioplasties using tibial osteoperiosteal grafts.

In 1915, Kappis employed the full thickness of the 12th rib with periosteum to cover a dural and skull defect. Weber (1916) and Schmidt (1916) reported their experience with rib grafts. In 1917 Brown suggested splitting the rib, leaving the inner half as a protection for the thoracic cavity. In 1921,

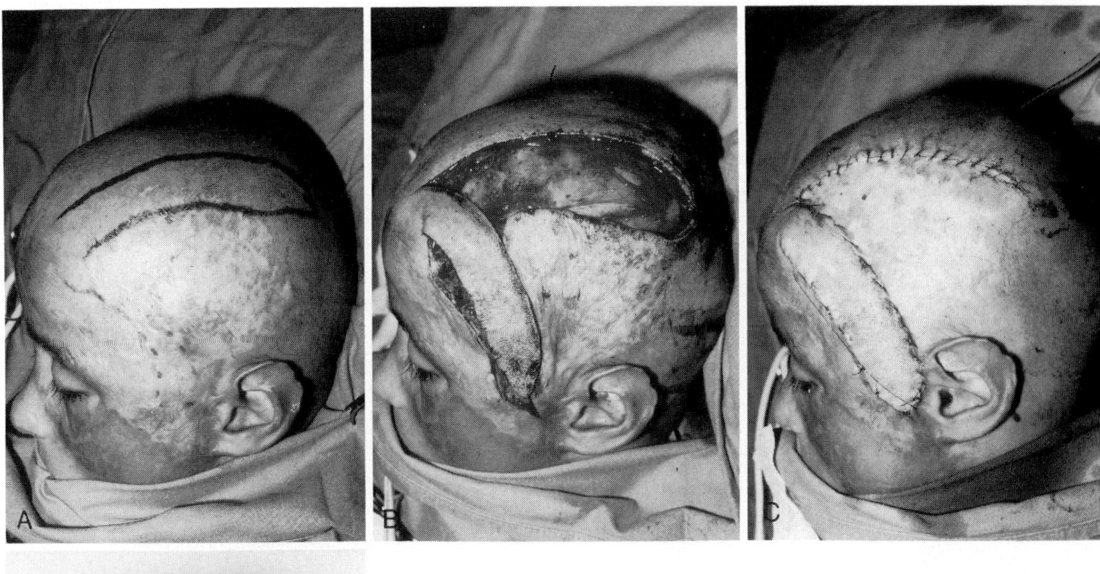

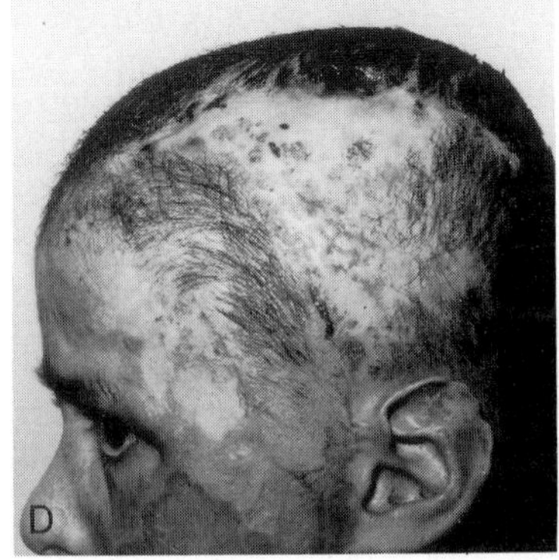

Figure 32–20. Anteriorly based midline scalp flap. *A,* Postburn temporoparietal alopecia. A midline flap along the edge of the bald area is designed with an anteriorly based pedicle. *B,* The flap is elevated and placed without delay in its new location. *C,* The donor defect can be closed primarily after wide undermining. *D,* Early result shows that the flap hair has a satisfactory direction of growth.

Ballin suggested repairing a dural defect with fascia and laying the split ribs "cut" face down on the fascia. Fagarasanu (1937) split the rib in order to gain more bony substance.

Morestin in 1915 recommended costal cartilage. Westermann (1916) transplanted a graft from the sternum, and in 1920 MacLennan used scapula. Mauclaire (1908) and Phemister (1914) advocated the iliac crest as a donor site. Pickerill (1931) employed the inner table of the ilium for reconstruction of cranial defects and later in 1946, in a long-range follow-up, concluded that autogenous tissues provide the best means of reconstruction.

In 1928, Brown presented a ten year follow-up of patients who underwent split rib graft reconstruction. Mowlem (1944) emphasized the merits of autogenous cancellous bone grafts. Macomber (1949) used cancellous iliac bone for reconstruction of defects of the forehead, nose, and chin. Soderberg and Mulvey (1947) also claimed that cancellous bone had superior osteogenic properties. McClintock and Dingman (1951) reported the successful use of autogenous iliac bone in 14 cranioplasties. Kiehn and Grino (1953) described three cases in which tantalum plates were removed and the calvarial defects reconstructed with iliac bone grafts and skin flaps.

In a monograph on cranioplasty, Woolf and Walker (1945) stated that for defects up to 8 cm in diameter, autogenous bone graft was the preferred choice; for larger defects, alloplasts should be used. It is of interest that a hammered gold plate was used before the dawn of history, to repair a frontal defect of the skull in a Neolithic Peruvian chieftain (Fig. 32–21). The same type of gold plate was suggested by Fallopio, but later decried by Paré. Gold was utilized by the French (Estor, 1917) during World War I, but it was found to be too soft and expensive. Lead plates were used by Mauclaire (1908), but produced symp-

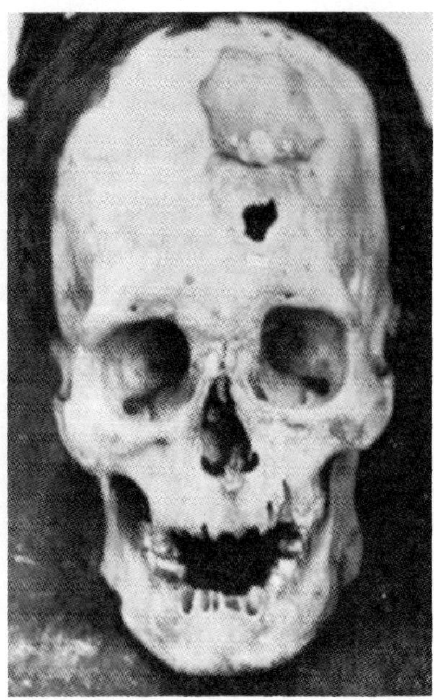

Figure 32–21. Prehistoric Peruvian skull with frontal defect repaired with hammered gold plate.

toms of lead poisoning. Silver was utilized by Savariaud (1912), and resulted in localized argyria.

Subsequently, tantalum (Pudenz and Odom, 1942), vitallium (Geib, 1941), and stainless steel (Scott and Wycis, 1946) have been extensively utilized, but all these materials have the following disadvantages: (1) they are radiopaque, (2) they conduct heat and cold, (3) they produce varying degrees of local reaction at the time of implantation, and (4) the incidence of infection and subsequent extrusion is fairly high. White (1948), in an extensive follow-up of patients operated on during the period between 1943 and 1946, reported that complications occurred in 10.6 per cent of 66 cranioplasties performed with lucite, and in 12.3 per cent of 130 after plating with tantalum. It was noted that the scarred scalp is likely to break down over a plate and that plates over the mastoid, frontal, and supraorbital areas tend to loosen and perforate the soft tissues.

Pastoriza, Tessier, and Delbet (1973) stressed the advantages of autologous bone. Wilflingseder (1983) also reported satisfactory experience with 83 patients in whom split rib and diced cartilage grafts were used. Utilization of the cranial vault as a donor site by removal of the outer table (Santoni-Rugiu, 1969) or splitting of a mobilized cranial bone flap (Marchac and associates, 1973; Psillakis, Nocchi, and Zanini, 1979; McCarthy and Zide, 1984; Wolfe, 1986) is gaining wide acceptance and is an elegant technique when feasible. This bone splitting can often be performed on children with fine chisels. The inner table can even be taken from the edges of the cranial defects, as performed by Lovaas (1985).

Banked bone can be used with success, either as reimplanted bone flaps (Steinhauser and Hardt, 1977) or as cadaver bone (Merville, Brunet, and Derome, 1982). Poole and associates (1987) used irradiation for sterilization. Shehadi (1970) advocated bone paste; Habal, Leake, and Maniscalco (1978) combined the bone paste with a mesh of polyurethane to ensure proper contour; and Anderl, Muhlbauer, and Marchac (1987) mixed the bony paste with fibrin glue to obtain a solid mass.

Among alloplastic implants, methylmethacrylate is the most widely used, even in acute trauma, by Subczynski (1977), who reported 25 cases with only one infection. Preformed plates are advocated by several authors (Van Gool, 1985) to ensure optimal contour and to avoid the heat and possible release of monomer associated with the use of cold cured in situ implants. A porous acrylic cement is recommended by Vandraager, Van Mullen, and Wijn (1983), whereas Manson, Crawley, and Hoopes (1986) advocated acrylic on a wire mesh, even in patients who had had a previous infection.

Mulliken and Glowacki (1980) induced osteogenesis from a powder of demineralized cadaver bone, whereas hydroxyapatite is used as a matrix for bone formation in powder form by Haasner, Krokowski, and Rach (1967) or in blocks of prepared devitalized corals by Salyer, Ubinas, and Snively (1985).

At the present time, when faced with a cranial defect, the surgeon must still decide between autogenous bone grafts, which give security for the future but are of limited size and have donor site morbidity, and implants, mainly methylmethacrylate, which are easier to use but provide no security for the future.

Cranial Vault Defects

Reconstruction of cranial vault defects, except for forehead deformities, is here discussed. They can be observed after (1) a

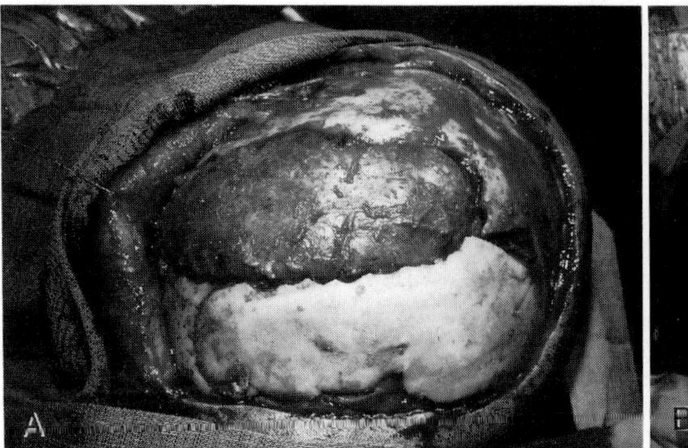

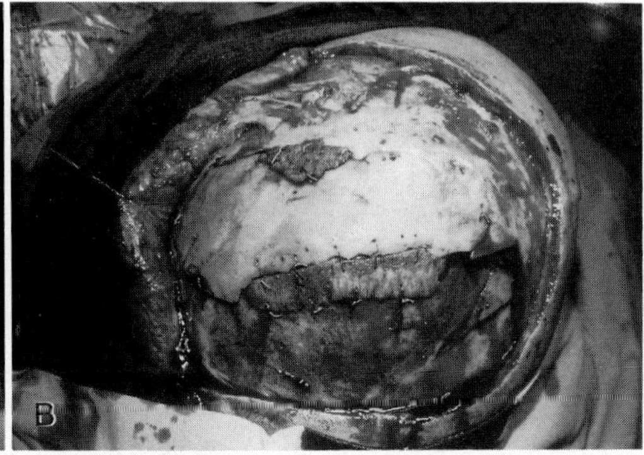

Figure 32–22. Splitting of the adjacent calvaria. *A,* A post-traumatic temporoparietal left-sided defect in a 6 year old boy. The outer table adjacent and posterior to the defect is split with oscillating saws and chisels. *B,* The posterior outer table has been wired into the defect. Additional pieces of split calvaria are utilized to complete the reconstruction. The inner table has been left in place posteriorly.

neurosurgical procedure in which the neurosurgical bone flap was discarded for intracranial decompression or became infected; (2) tumor resection, mostly epitheliomas of the skin that involved the calvaria; and (3) calvariectomies for treatment of craniosynostosis with insufficient secondary reossification.

Scalp reconstruction has been discussed previously, and it is obvious that no cranial vault reconstruction can be undertaken before adequate soft tissue coverage is provided. Since the undermining of a flap or skin graft adherent to the dura is difficult, it is advisable to provide scalp coverage, if necessary, at the time of the cranial vault reconstruction. Preliminary scalp expansion with inflatable prostheses provides the necessary surface and quality of scalp coverage when difficulties of closure are expected.

The coronal incision provides complete exposure to all of the cranial vault, and allows comparison with the contralateral side in unilateral defects. When there is an existing scar it can be partially used, extending the coronal incision.

The undermining between the scalp and the dura is generally not difficult, if one proceeds with care. Walton and Krizek (1980) confirmed in the laboratory a clinical observation that a dural defect regenerates under a periosteal or lyophilized dural patch. They consequently advocated direct application of the galea of scalp flaps directly over the brain without repair of the dura after full-thickness losses.

After the cranial vault defect has been exposed and the surgeon is faced with the bone repair, several solutions can be utilized. The author's first choice is the splitting of the remaining cranial vault, which has the advantage of (1) the security of autologous bone graft, (2) minimal donor site problems, and (3) optimal curvature and form (Fig. 32–22).

If cranial vault splitting is not possible because of (1) the poor quality of the cranial vault bone, (2) the unwillingness of the neurosurgeons to extensively undermine the dura, or (3) the size of the defect, it is necessary to choose between a split rib cranioplasty and a methylmethacrylate implant.

In cases of previous infection or exposure to the nasal cavity or paranasal sinuses, only autogenous bone can be considered. It is also a satisfactory solution in cases of young, active individuals. Implants can be considered for large defects, when the taking of many ribs can be a problem for elderly or debilitated patients.

Splitting the Remaining Calvaria

The use of the outer table of the calvaria was apparently first described by Müller (1890), who employed a periosteal flap attached to the split outer table. He was followed by many surgeons, as stated by Santoni-Rugiu (1969), who advocated a large outer table graft. The development of craniofacial surgery in the last 20 years has familiarized plastic surgeons with cranial vault anatomy, and the use of thin motorized blades and fine chisels has permitted a variety of cranial (calvarial) splitting techniques. The inner table is the preferred donor site in order to avoid residual irregularities. It is much

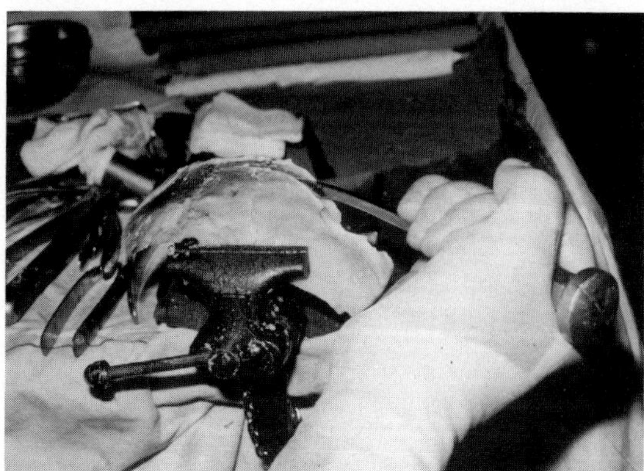

Figure 32–23. A bench vise is useful in splitting the full-thickness cranial vault flaps.

easier to harvest after the bone flaps have been removed by the neurosurgeon, as recommended by Psillakis, Nocchi, and Zanini (1979), Marchac and associates (1973, 1982), and McCarthy and Zide (1984). It can be split in situ, as performed by McCarthy and Zide (1984) and Lovaas (1985), but is potentially more hazardous.

After the cranial defect is exposed and the dura is undermined from its edges, a pattern is made with a piece of metal or any other material and a suitable cranial (calvarial) donor site is sought. When found, the bone flap is cut in a full-thickness fashion with an oscillating saw, the dura being protected. The author prefers not to use a Gigli saw because of the width of its bony cut. After removal, the bony flap is split by utilizing long oscillating saws and curved, thin chisels. A bench vise (Fig. 32–23) is useful for this maneuver. The outer table is used for the repair of the defect if the latter is anterior in location or is more visible than the donor site. The split calvarial bone graft is intimately adjusted to the bony edges of the cranial defect after they have been freshened with a rongeur. Wires are utilized for immobilization. The inner table is replaced and wired to the donor site. The wound is closed in two layers over suction drainage. Another possibility is to use strips of calvarial bone as recommended by Tessier (1982), the strip being split by osteotomes.

The in situ elevation of the outer table alone should be done with care, the danger being inadvertent perforation of the inner table. A 19 year old patient who had an outer table graft harvested for supraorbital rim remodeling developed an extradural hematoma after surgery. At operation, only a thinning of the inner table was noted. The cranial vault is a remarkable donor site, but the presence of the underlying dura and brain should always be remembered. During cranial defect repairs, protection of the underlying dura is recommended even if the outer table is only lifted, and it is safer to elevate the full thickness of the cranial vault, split it, and return the inner table. Details of harvesting of cranial or calvarial bone grafts are also discussed in Chapter 18.

In situ techniques are used by many (McCarthy and Zide, 1984; Wolfe and Berkowitz, 1988). Elevation of the outer table is carried out after a groove has been drilled around the proposed bone plate. A bur flattens the ridge around the groove, so that a chisel can be introduced at a proper angle between the outer and inner tables. It also softens the ridges of the depression after the graft has been taken. The chisel is gently tapped as it finds its way between the two tables (see also Chap. 18).

It is essential to avoid the sutures area, and the parietal area is the donor site of choice (Fig. 32–24). A study by Pensler and McCarthy (1985) demonstrated that the thickest portion for calvarial bone grafts is that region of the parietal bone posterior to the coronal suture.

Vibrations produced by the hammering on the cranium can be a potential problem. Hendel and Nadell (1987) have devised a special chisel and also a motor-driven instrument to facilitate these maneuvers.

Split Rib Cranioplasty

If it is Brown (1928) who described the splitting of ribs, it is Longacre who popularized their clinical application with experience of over 500 cases (Longacre, 1955; Longacre and de Stefano, 1957a, b, c; Longacre and coworkers, 1959). These authors showed that the ribs can regenerate as long as the periosteum is left intact (Fig. 32–25). However, the reformed ribs are often irregular and are rarely suitable for another grafting procedure.

There are no respiratory problems as long as one does not take more than two ribs in continuity. When several ribs must be harvested, an alternative intact rib should be left between removed ribs. Accidental puncture of the pleura is easily managed by lung expansion; closure of the defect is accom-

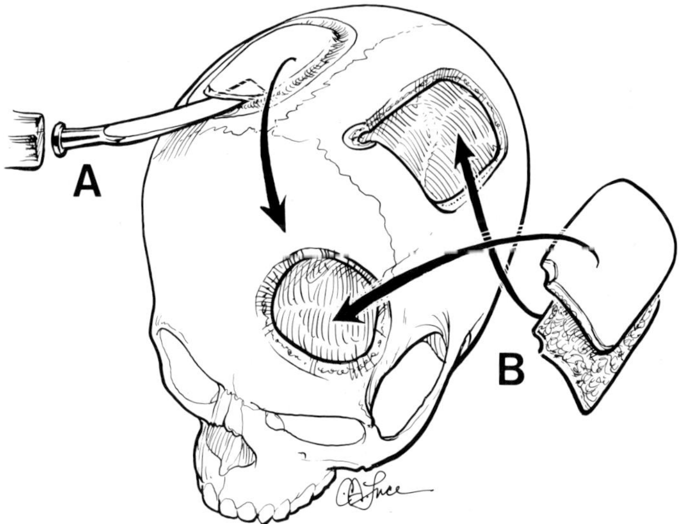

Figure 32–24. Harvesting of cranial grafts. It is best to avoid the sutures when selecting the donor area. *A,* On the right side of the skull, the in situ technique with splitting of the outer table is illustrated. A groove has been drilled around the future graft, and the outer edge beveled to allow the chisel to follow the loose plane between the inner and outer table. On the left (*B*), after a trephine hole has been drilled, the full thickness of the vault is elevated. The bone flap is split and the inner table wired back in the donor site. The outer table is placed in the forehead defect.

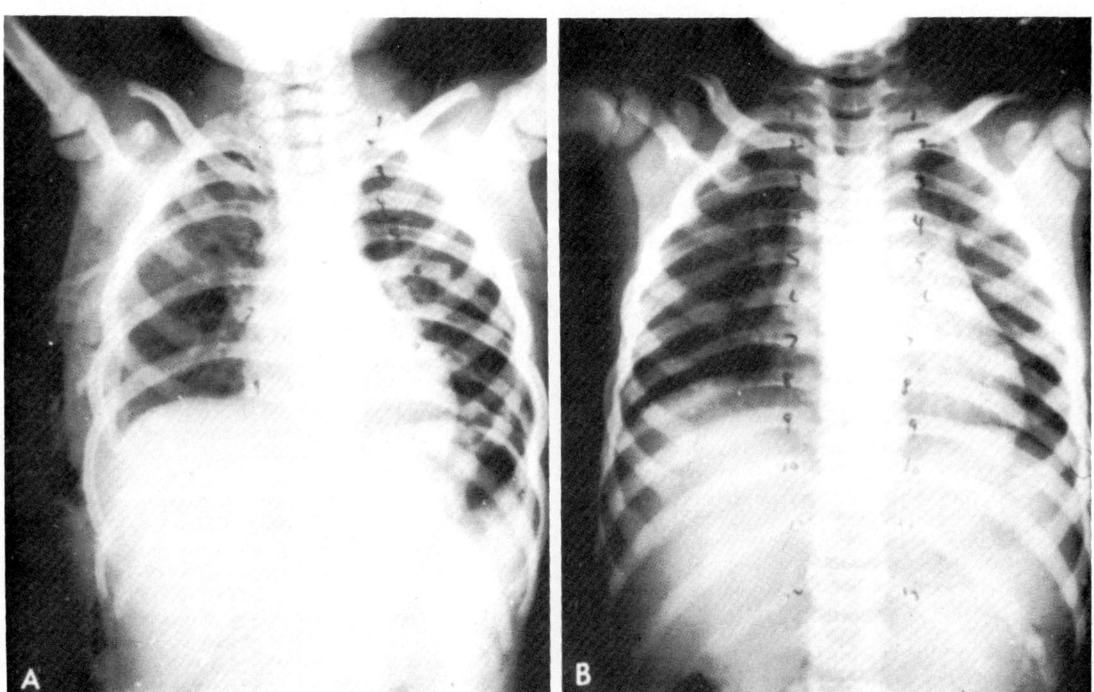

Figure 32–25. *A,* Roentgenogram shows regeneration of the left sixth, eighth, and tenth ribs, removed three weeks before resection of the right fifth, seventh, ninth, and 11th ribs. *B,* Completed regeneration and growth one year after resection.

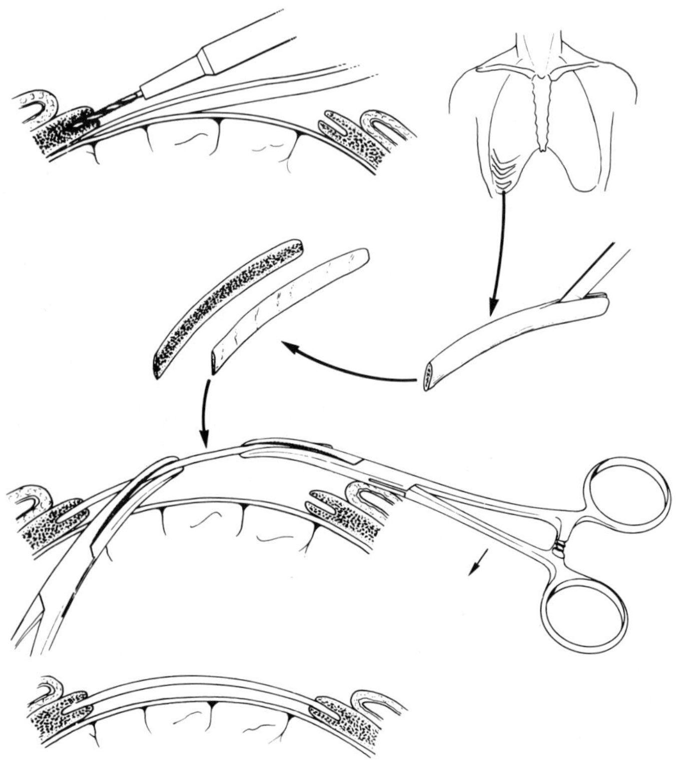

Figure 32–26. Imbedding of split ribs. The ribs are split with a chisel or a strong knife, and introduced in a groove drilled between the outer and inner tables of the calvaria, after the edges have been freshened with a rongeur. Force bent, they hold by themselves at the desired curvature. (From Marchac, D., and Cophignon, J.: Technique for imbedding split-ribs in a cranioplasty. Plast. Reconstr. Surg., *55*:237, 1975.)

plished by watertight pleural suture, if possible, and tight muscle and skin suture. Any pain associated with pneumothorax usually subsides in a few days.

The ribs must be cut as long as possible, and special angled bony cutters are useful. The splitting of the ribs is easily done with a fine chisel or a strong knife.

Various ways of fitting the split ribs to the cranial defect have been described: under the inner table of the cranium (Pastoriza, Tessier and Delbet, 1973), over the outer table, interposed with wires, or wedged between the edges (Korlof, Nylen, and Rietz, 1973).

The imbedding of split ribs in a groove drilled at the periphery of the defect (Marchac and Cophignon, 1975) (Fig. 32–26) has several advantages:

1. It allows easy maintenance of the desired curvature, the rib being introduced under forced bending and released afterward.
2. It increases the contact between the ribs and the calvaria.
3. It gives great stability without wire fixation.

To perform the imbedding, the edges of the calvarial-cranial defect must be freshened with rongeurs, and the groove drilled at 1 cm of depth in the diploë. The end of the ribs, thin at the anterior end, is easily flattened at the posterior end so that it can be introduced into a rather narrow groove (Fig. 32–27). The ribs must be bent over the defect before they are cut, and 1 cm should be added on each side for the imbedding. The elasticity of the ribs allows them to be easily introduced on one side first, and after exaggerating the bending, on the other (Fig. 32–28). They are alternatively cortex out and diploë out, and

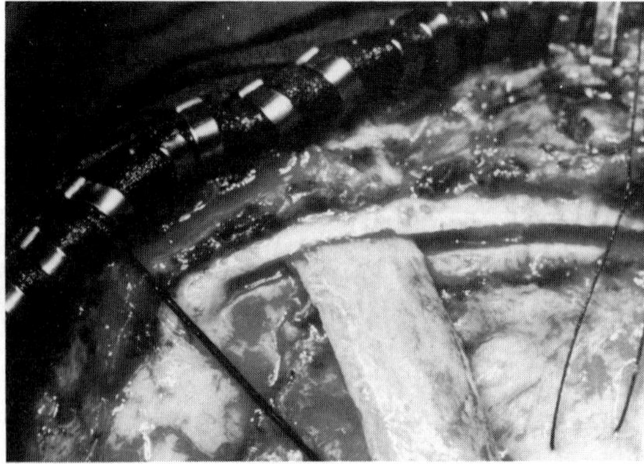

Figure 32–27. The groove is drilled with a high speed bur 1 cm deep, and the rib is snugly introduced.

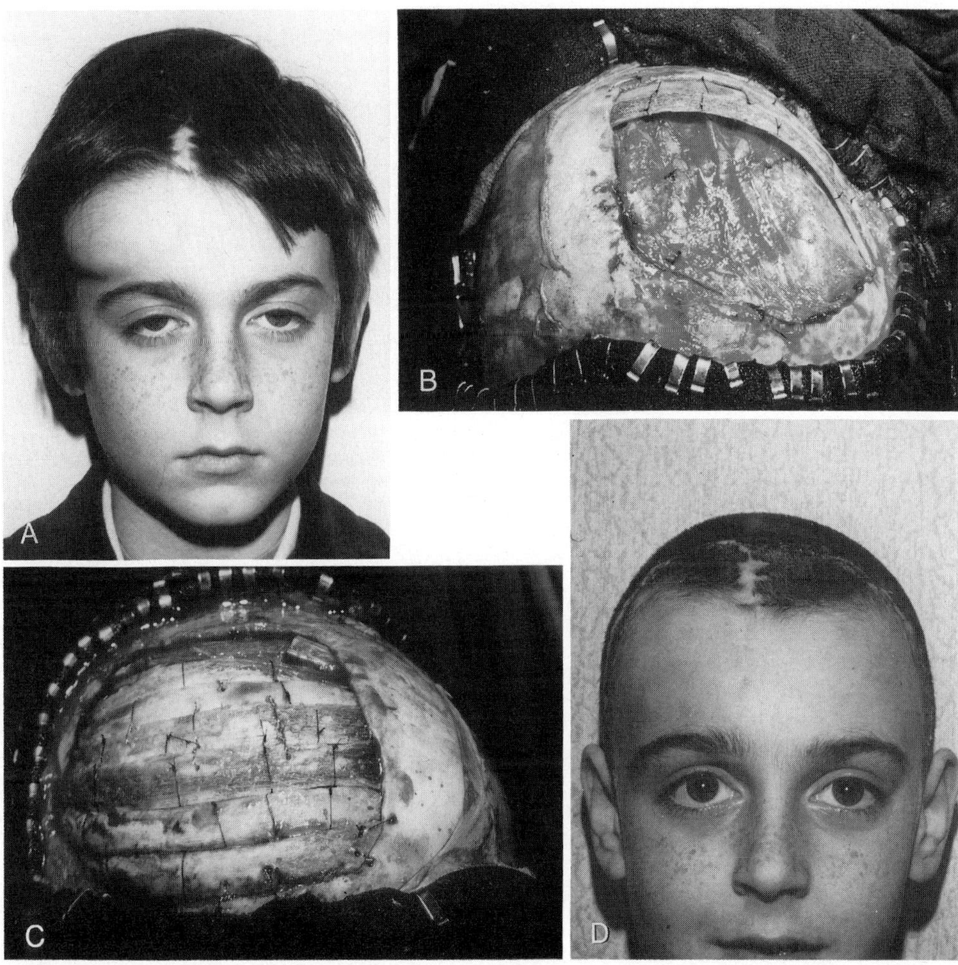

Figure 32–28. Post-traumatic frontoparietal split rib cranioplasty in a 13 year old boy. *A,* The bulge in the right forehead is caused by a dural cyst. *B,* The large frontoparietal defect and the curvature obtained. The imbedded ribs are clearly visible. *C,* The repair is completed with the use of several wires. The dura is suspended to the ribs by silk sutures. Anterior view. *D,* Postoperative appearance.

the dura is suspended to the ribs. Two to three ribs are the usual amount of graft, and these can cover a surface of 100 to 150 sq cm without problems. One can also combine bone harvesting techniques, e.g., split calvaria plus ribs.

In the author's series of 38 split rib cranioplasties, there was only one case of resorption (following a postoperative hematoma) and no infections. On the negative side, the surface usually becomes irregular with time (Fig. 32–29) and this technique might not produce an esthetically acceptable result. It can be improved by an onlay if this irregularity becomes visible, but it is preferable to avoid the split rib in favor of a calvarial graft in the nonhairy area of the scalp.

Munro and Guyuron (1981) further strengthened the imbedded split ribs by the use of chain link fence wiring. This technique may be useful when mobility persists between the ribs, since absolute immobilization is fundamental to vascularization of all bone grafts. The technique suffers the disadvantage of using an inordinate amount of wires, which can be subsequently palpated by the patient.

Methylmethacrylate Implants

Alloplastic implants have enjoyed a bad reputation in plastic surgery, especially among craniofacial surgeons who have seen many patients referred after implant removal. Munro and Guyuron (1981) stated that "in reconstructive craniofacial surgery,

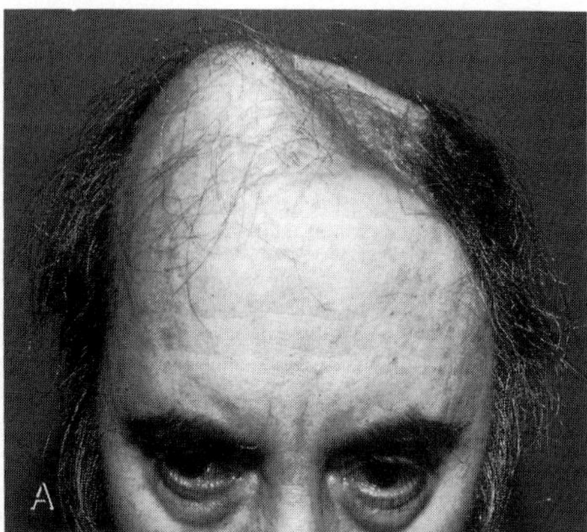

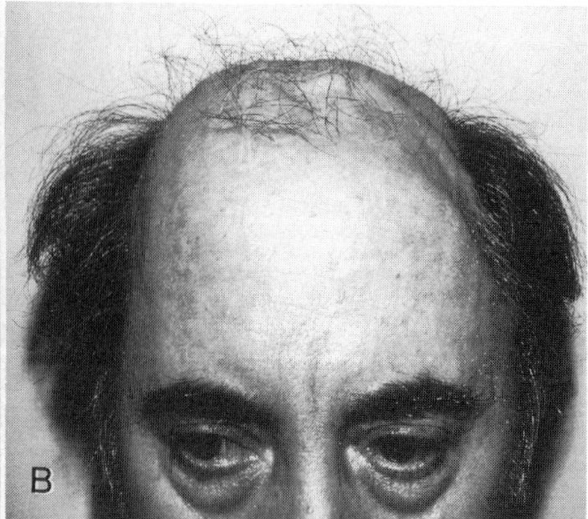

Figure 32–29. Split rib cranioplasty. *A,* Large defect of the cranial vault following removal of an acrylic implant. *B,* One and one-half years after repair with imbedded split rib grafts. Note the surface irregularities. (From Marchac, D., and Cophignon, J.: Technique for imbedding split-ribs in a cranioplasty. Plast. Reconstr. Surg., *55*:237, 1975.)

there is no place for alloplastic materials." It is true that the first choice should always be autogenous bone, and that the use of alloplastic material is definitely contraindicated if (1) the defect is adjacent to or involves the nose or paranasal sinuses, (2) there is a history of infection, or (3) the overlying soft tissue coverage is deficient.

However, it is the author's opinion that alloplastic material can be considered in two circumstances: (1) for an onlay on a deformed frontal bone and (2) for cranial vault cranioplasties (in carefully selected cases). In these situations, utilizing a careful technique, the surgeon can achieve satisfactory results.

Methylmethacrylate has been used extensively for 30 years by neurosurgeons, and the number of problems encountered is limited compared with the total number of cases (Cabanela and associates, 1972; Schultz, 1979; Richaud, Lazorthes, and Caraoué, 1985; Argenta and Newman, 1986). The main problem associated with an alloplastic implant is late exposure and infection leading to removal. Even though Thomson, Munro, and Birch (1977) reported that they were able to salvage exposed implants by flap coverage, it is an unpleasant situation for the patient.

The author has performed 24 methylmethacrylate cranioplasties since 1976 and has removed only one. Nevertheless, at the time of consultation the patient is always warned of the possibility of a problem leading to implant removal in the future.

Prefabricated implants utilized by Van Gool (1985) and Richaud, Lazorthes, and Caraoué (1985) have the advantage of satisfactory contour and avoidance of heat. The author prefers cold cure technology.

Technique of Methylmethacrylate Implants. After the cranial defect is exposed and the periosteum reflected around the edges, wires are passed at the periphery and left long. Methylmethacrylate monomers (powder and liquid) are mixed in a bowl, and after a few minutes a paste is obtained. It is usable when it is still malleable and keeps its shape. It is applied on the recipient area and contoured by hand and with spatulas. The surgeon passes wires through the paste, being especially careful to soften the edges. Water is poured abundantly while the implant is cooling, to avoid heating the brain. When the implant is cooler and hard, it is leveled with a sharp polishing bur, and the wires are twisted (Fig. 32-30).

FRONTAL BONE REPAIR AND CONTOURING

Repair of Full-Thickness Defects

Attention to the presence of a frontal sinus and to a history of a previous infection of the frontonasal area is the first concern when a patient requiring a repair of a frontal bone defect is examined. The best reconstruction is ruined if infection results from a mucosal cul-de-sac that has not been removed.

If there is residual frontal sinus, the preferred technique is to open the sinus as completely as possible to remove all of the mucosa

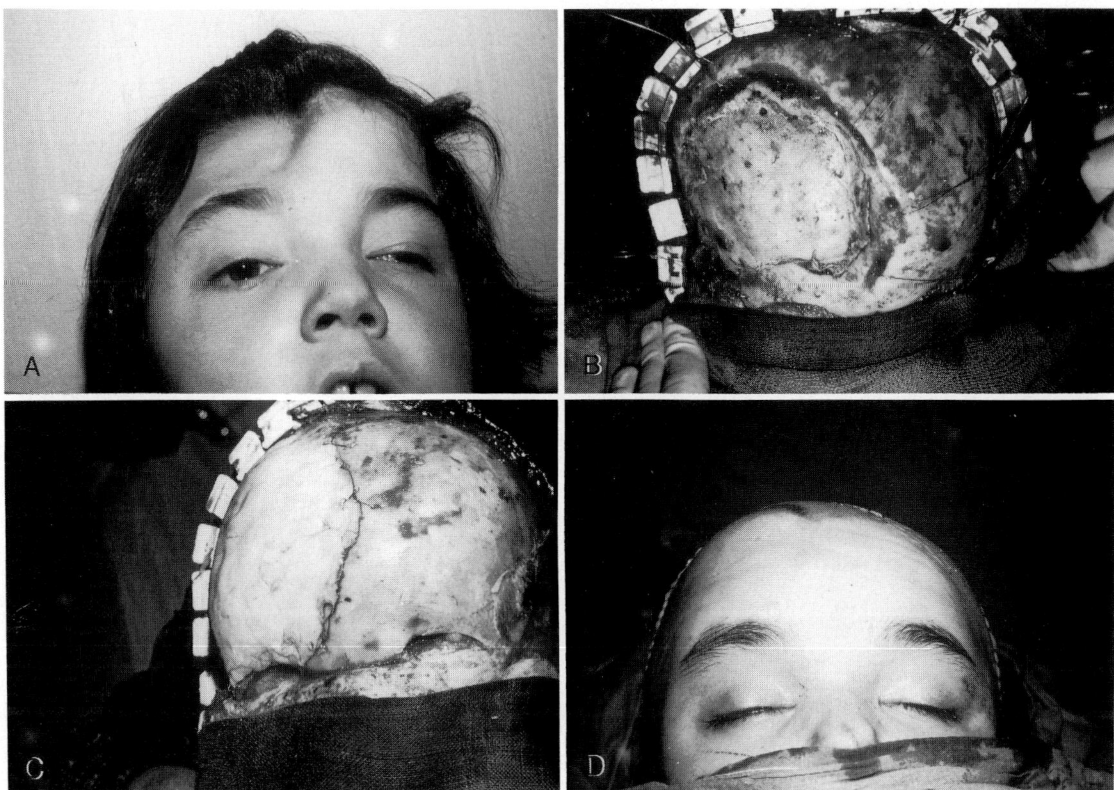

Figure 32–30. *A,* A 7 year old boy had sustained severe frontal trauma with a depressed frontal bone on the right side. The neurosurgeons were opposed to an intracranial procedure because of dural and brain damage. *B,* The edges of the defect are exposed. Wires are passed and left long. *C,* The paste is laid over the defect, the edges feathered, and the wires tied. *D,* Camouflaging of the depression was accomplished with methylmethacrylate, but cranial bone grafting would have been preferable, especially in a young boy.

with a bur, to resect the posterior bony wall, and to elevate and advance the mucosal remnants into the frontonasal canal, which is plugged with bone chips. This technique can be done when the cranial cavity is open, either through a defect of the posterior wall of the sinus or through removal of the frontal bone as in a formal craniotomy. If the cranial cavity is not open and one is faced with only a defect of the anterior wall of the frontal sinus, it is better to rebuild a normal sinus by draining the cavity in the nose and reconstructing only the missing anterior wall with an autogenous bone graft (Fig. 32–31).

The preferred material to reconstruct an opened frontal sinus, and to build a barrier between the frontal area and the nasal cavities, is cancellous bone, harvested from the calvaria, the ilium, or another site.

In cases with a history of extensive infection and loss of frontal bone, Merville, Brunet, and Derome (1982) recommended a two-stage procedure: (1) careful reconstruction of the supraorbital rim area, after removal of all sinusal remnants and isolation of the nasal cavity with iliac cancellous bone grafts; and (2) later reconstruction of the frontal bone with an irradiated bank bone graft.

The preference for autogenous bone in frontal reconstruction has been criticized by Manson, Crawley, and Hoopes (1986), who reported that acrylic repair produced an equally good and often better result, even in cases of previous infection. They emphasized that the late repair (at least one year after eradication of the infection) and careful treatment of the sinus is more important than the type of reconstructive material used. In a series of 42 frontal cranioplasties, 25 were performed after previous infection. Fifteen had an acrylic implant with no recurrence of infection, and ten underwent bone reconstruction with four patients showing recurrence of infection.

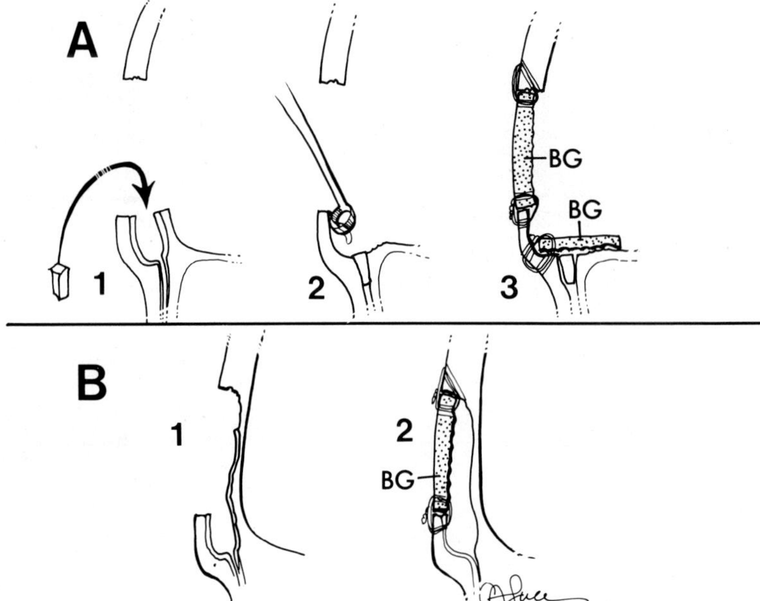

Figure 32–31. Treatment of an open frontal sinus. *A,* When the cranial cavity is open, it is preferable to perform a cranialization and to resect the frontal sinus (*1*). The posterior wall is removed, the sinus mucosa carefully curetted (*2*), the frontonasal duct plugged with bone, and a cancellous bone graft (BG) placed over it (*3*). *B,* When only the anterior wall is open (*1*) and the sinus clean, it is possible to reconstruct only the anterior wall with a bone graft (*2*), leaving the frontonasal canal open for natural drainage.

The data are completely opposite to the experience of Wolfe (1986), who had no infections in a series of 73 bone cranioplasties. An analysis of the series of Manson, Crawley, and Hoopes (1986) reveals that bone was employed only in severe cases with simulataneous repair of the nose and orbits, and that all cases of recurrence of infection were among this group. However, in isolated frontal defect repair, acrylic and bone did equally well.

For most craniofacial surgeons, autogenous bone graft is the first choice for frontal reconstruction. Postoperative irregularities can nevertheless be visible, and it is not always easy to recreate a smooth, gently curved natural surface. Splitting of the calvaria or iliac bone graft is the preferred choice for small and medium-sized defects. For very large defects, transposition of a segment of the cranial vault (see under Frontal Bone Contouring) gives the best contour. Split rib grafts can be used for large defects, but suffer the disadvantage of possibly showing contour irregularities. Converse (1955) suggested covering them with slivers of cancellous bone graft, and Korlof, Nylen, and Rietz (1973) recommended placing a second layer of rib grafts later.

Iliac or Cranial Vault Bone Graft

In this procedure, wide exposure is obtained through a coronal incision, placed well behind the hairline. This type of exposure is preferable to exposure through residual scars, unless they are conspicuous, require repair, and provide adequate surgical exposure. The coronal approach allows complete visualization of all the frontal bone, comparison with the unaffected side in unilateral cases, and access to the cranial-calvarial donor sites. Elevation of the flap is done usually in the loose plane between the pericranium and the galea aponeurotica.

As the raising of the flap reaches the bony defect, careful dissection is required because of the adherence of the dura to the overlying tissues, and dense scar tissue may be present. The extent of the bony defect is outlined and the periosteum is incised at its periphery. A periosteal elevator raises the periosteal cuff thus formed around the defect, and the cuff is folded into the defect.

In defects involving the lower portion of the frontal bone, the periosteum is incised and elevated, the supraorbital nerve is liberated from its canal, and the periorbita is raised from the anterior portion of the roof of the orbit when the defect involves the supraorbital rim.

With the bicoronal approach, it is advisable to elevate a large frontal periosteal flap, pedicled on the side opposite to the defect. It allows exposure of all the frontal bone for better comparison of contours, and coverage of the complete reconstruction with a periosteal flap. After checking that there is no problem with the frontal sinuses, the bony

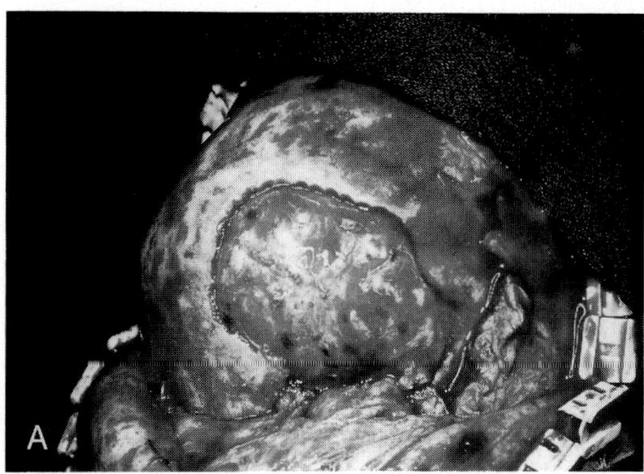

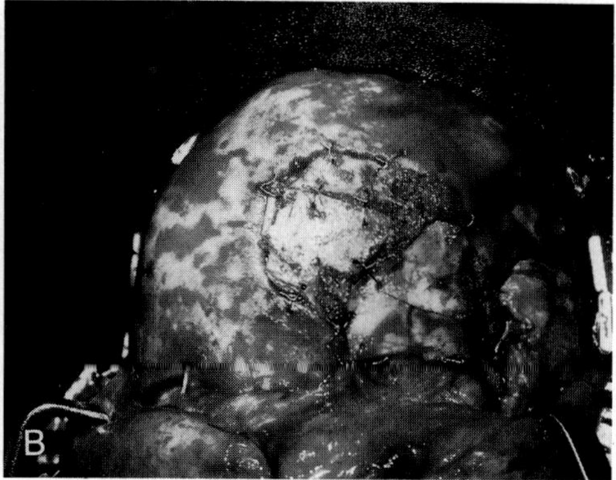

Figure 32–32. Frontal reconstruction with an iliac bone graft. *A,* A post-traumatic defect of the left frontal area, including the supraorbital rim, has been exposed through a bicoronal incision in an 8 year old girl. The edges of the defect have been freshened with rongeurs. The frontal sinus was not opened. *B,* Iliac bone grafts have been adjusted to the defect, with incomplete bony cuts (cortical) for contouring. Cancellous bone is used to eradicate irregularities.

defect is measured and a pattern taken. The bone graft is harvested. The first choice is the split calvarial bone graft (see p. 1557); if this is not feasible, the iliac bone graft is chosen.

The iliac bone graft is taken after the crest is split with its attached muscles and the iliac wing exposed (see also Chap. 18). If one table is sufficient, the inner table usually has the best curvature for restoring forehead contour. Both inner and outer tables can be taken, if necessary, without secondary problems. The iliac crest is carefully reconstructed in its original location. The curvature of the graft can be modified by bending the graft, after weakening the cortex by a number of parallel cuts through the partial thickness of the cortex. This maneuver is easier to perform in younger patients.

The edges of the defect are freshened with rongeurs to open the diploë. A few wires are passed through the outer table and the graft is strongly fitted and immobilized with the wires, any residual gap between the graft and the edges of the defect being filled with cancellous bone (Fig. 32–32). When the dura tends to fall backward, it is advisable to suspend it by a few stitches passed through holes made in the bone graft. The symmetry is checked against the contralateral side if the defect is unilateral. The surface is smoothed with a bur, and the periosteal flap is placed over the bone graft if a coronal approach is utilized.

When the defect is larger, it can exceed the possibilities of an iliac bone graft. If a large split cranial or transposition (see the discussion of forehead contouring below) is not feasible or not advised by the neurosurgeon because of a previous pathologic condition, rib grafts can be utilized (see p. 1558). Converse (1955) suggested that layers of cancellous bone be immediately added, whereas Korlof, Nylen, and Rietz (1973) recommended serial layers of costal grafts. An alloplastic onlay can also be added on the rib graft in a second surgical stage if the surface is not sufficiently smooth. An allograft of irradiated bone was utilized by Brunet and Visot (1982) and Poole and associates (1987).

Frontal Bone Contouring

In congenital or post-traumatic cases in which there is no skin or bony defect, but only a contour problem, two approaches are possible: (1) the addition of material (onlay) in front of the malpositioned bone, which is left in place; or (2) mobilization of the frontal bone by osteotomies.

The use of autogenous onlay bone grafts has been disappointing because they tend to resorb a great deal. Utilization of alloplastic material is also suspect in the frontal area and is reserved only for a few cases in which there are contraindications to frontal bone repositioning.

Frontal Bone Repositioning

In post-traumatic cases, the displaced bones are mobilized to restore normal skeletal anatomy. Neurosurgeons are reluctant to perform a formal craniotomy in cases of severe dural and brain damage incurred at the time of injury or "primary repair."

A coronal approach is used for exposure,

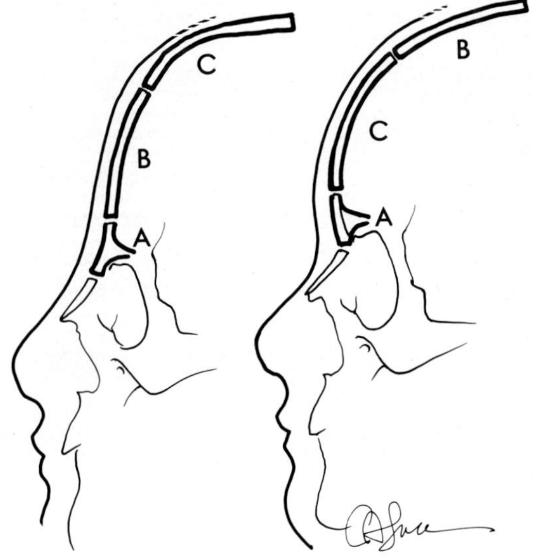

Figure 32–33. The two components of the forehead: the supraorbital bar (*A*) is responsible for definition of the nasofrontal angle, projection of the eyebrows, and the supratarsal fold. The upper forehead (*B*) ideally should be made of one piece of bone of the proper curvature, which can often be obtained from *C*. *Left,* Oxycephaly. *Right,* Normal contour. (From Marchac, D., and Renier, D.: Craniofacial Surgery for Craniosynostosis. Boston, Little, Brown & Company, 1982.)

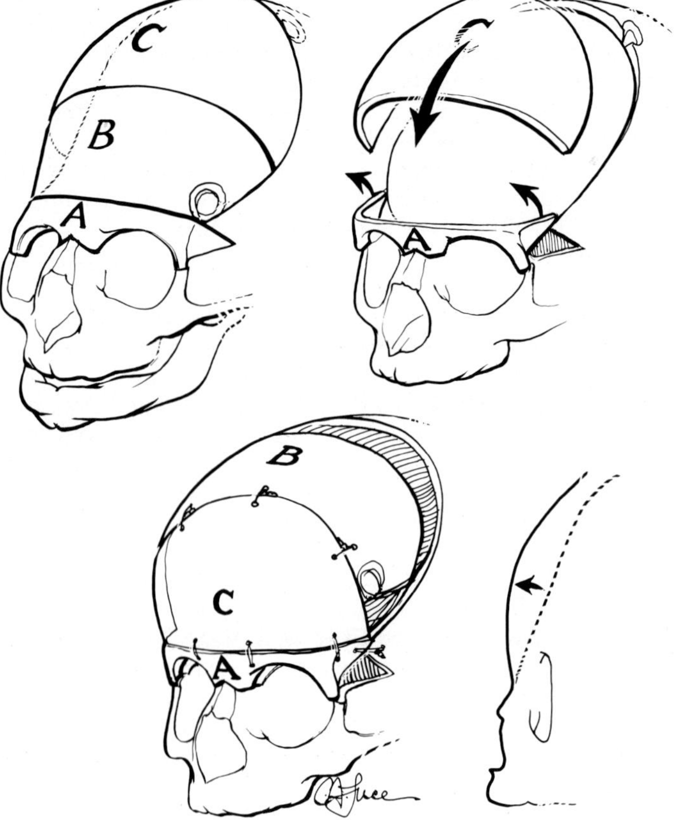

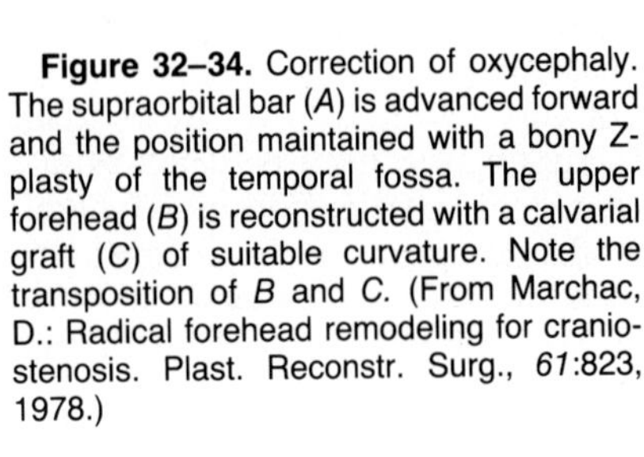

Figure 32–34. Correction of oxycephaly. The supraorbital bar (*A*) is advanced forward and the position maintained with a bony Z-plasty of the temporal fossa. The upper forehead (*B*) is reconstructed with a calvarial graft (*C*) of suitable curvature. Note the transposition of *B* and *C*. (From Marchac, D.: Radical forehead remodeling for craniostenosis. Plast. Reconstr. Surg., *61*:823, 1978.)

but shaving of the hair is not necessary; several shampoos and hair draping are sufficient.

If there are no bone defects, bur holes are drilled around the deformed area, the dura is retracted and displaced, and the bone is elevated with an oscillating saw or an osteotome.

An open sinus is carefully obliterated and the bony pieces are wired in normal position. If bone is missing, adjacent calvaria is split and used for repair.

In *congenital anomalies*, all the structures of the forehead and of the cranial vault should be considered in relation to the face. The forehead can be distorted or recessed in many congenital anomalies, especially in craniosynostosis (discussed in Chap. 61). This section discusses only the problem of adolescents or adults who seek esthetic improvement without functional problems.

The typical problem is that of a recessed forehead, which lies in a plane in continuity with the nasal dorsum. The cranial vertex is usually pointed.

The forehead can be considered as made up of two parts (Fig. 32–33):

1. The *supraorbital bar*, which is responsible for the definition of the frontonasal angle, the projection of the eyebrows, and the supratarsal fold of the upper eyelid.

2. The *upper forehead*, which should be curved in the transverse dimension to meet with the temporal fossae and in the vertical dimension to continue with the cranial vault.

Frontal repositioning usually requires forward rocking of the supraorbital bar, and the transposition of cranial grafts of suitable shape with the existing upper forehead (Fig. 32–34) (Marchac and associates, 1974). Figure 32–35 illustrates a girl, age 15 years, who had been operated on for a craniosynostosis at the age of 4 years. A total craniectomy was performed followed by spontaneous reossification. Brain decompression was obtained but the shape of the cranial vault was defective. The technique illustrated in Figure 32–34 was used and a favorable result was maintained seven years later.

The 23 year old man illustrated in Figure 32–36 has the typical features of oxycephaly. This type of craniosynostosis, observed predominantly in North Africa, is characterized by a late-appearing coronal synostosis and increased intracranial pressure. Some untreated patients manage to compensate for the frontal recession by elevation of the height of the cranial vault, and have no functional problems. Irregularities of the undersurface of the calvaria are frequent, and dural undermining must consequently be carefully performed and the dura protected during the osteotomies, which are made with an oscillating saw.

If the frontal sinus is open during elevation of the supraorbital bar, the posterior wall is resected and the frontonasal canal occluded (see Fig. 32–31).

Special care must be taken at the junction of the frontal bone with the temporal fossae. The bony contour should be carefully reconstructed and the temporal muscle reattached to the temporal crest.

In a series of 51 frontal remodelings for oxycephaly, there have been no major complications; no patient developed osteitis or bone resorption.

The recessed forehead can also be recontoured with alloplastic materials. Prefabricated prostheses are recommended in Silastic by Nataf, Elbaz, and Pollet (1976) and in methylmethacrylate by Ousterhout, Baker, and Zlotolow (1980) and Argenta and Newman (1986). The immediate result is usually favorable if the implant is well placed but the future remains uncertain in such cases, since the implant may have to be removed years later, e.g., as a result of a direct blow. The other disadvantage is that the associated anomaly of the cranial vault is also uncorrected. Massive forehead implants should be considered only if the neurosurgeons are of the opinion that the craniotomy is dangerous. However, the patient must be warned that extrusion of the implant could occur at any time.

In the author's opinion (Marchac and Renier, 1982), implants for forehead contour can be considered only as a limited onlay on a moderate bony irregularity to restore symmetry. Methylmethacrylate is utilized with careful fixation to ensure perfect immobilization of the implant on the bone.

A hydroxyapatite type of bone substitute may provide a solution for limited forehead contour anomalies in the future (Salyer, Ubinas, and Snively, 1985), but in major forehead recessions the only complete long-term correction is provided by frontocranial remodeling.

Simple forehead contouring, by removing the excess pathologic bone, can be considered in cases of fibrous dysplasia or frontometapla-

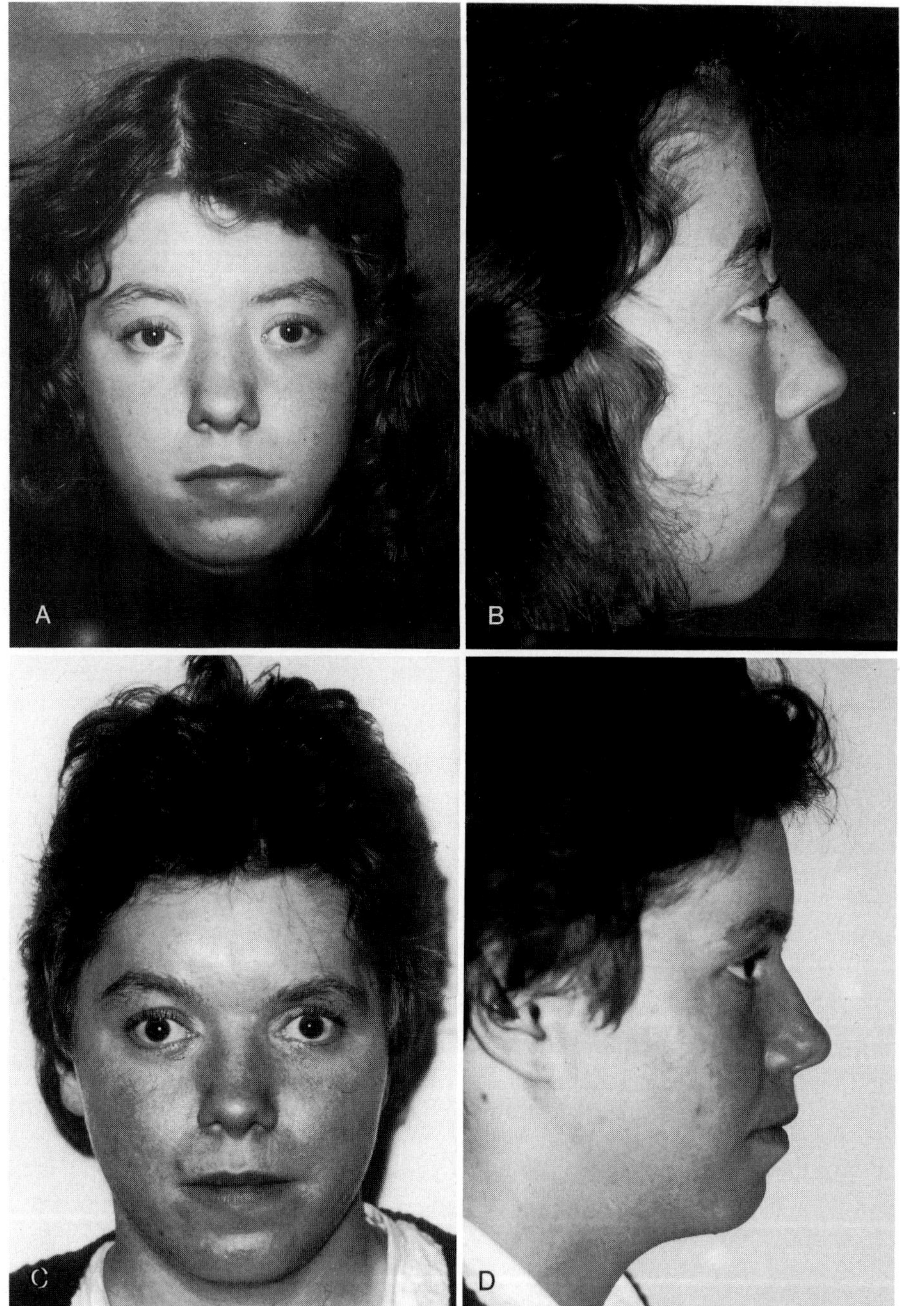

Figure 32–35. *A, B,* Female patient, age 15, requested a forehead reshaping because of a recessed and vertically elongated forehead. A total craniectomy had been done at age 4 for craniosynostosis. *C, D,* Seven years after frontocranial remodeling performed as illustrated in Figure 32–34.

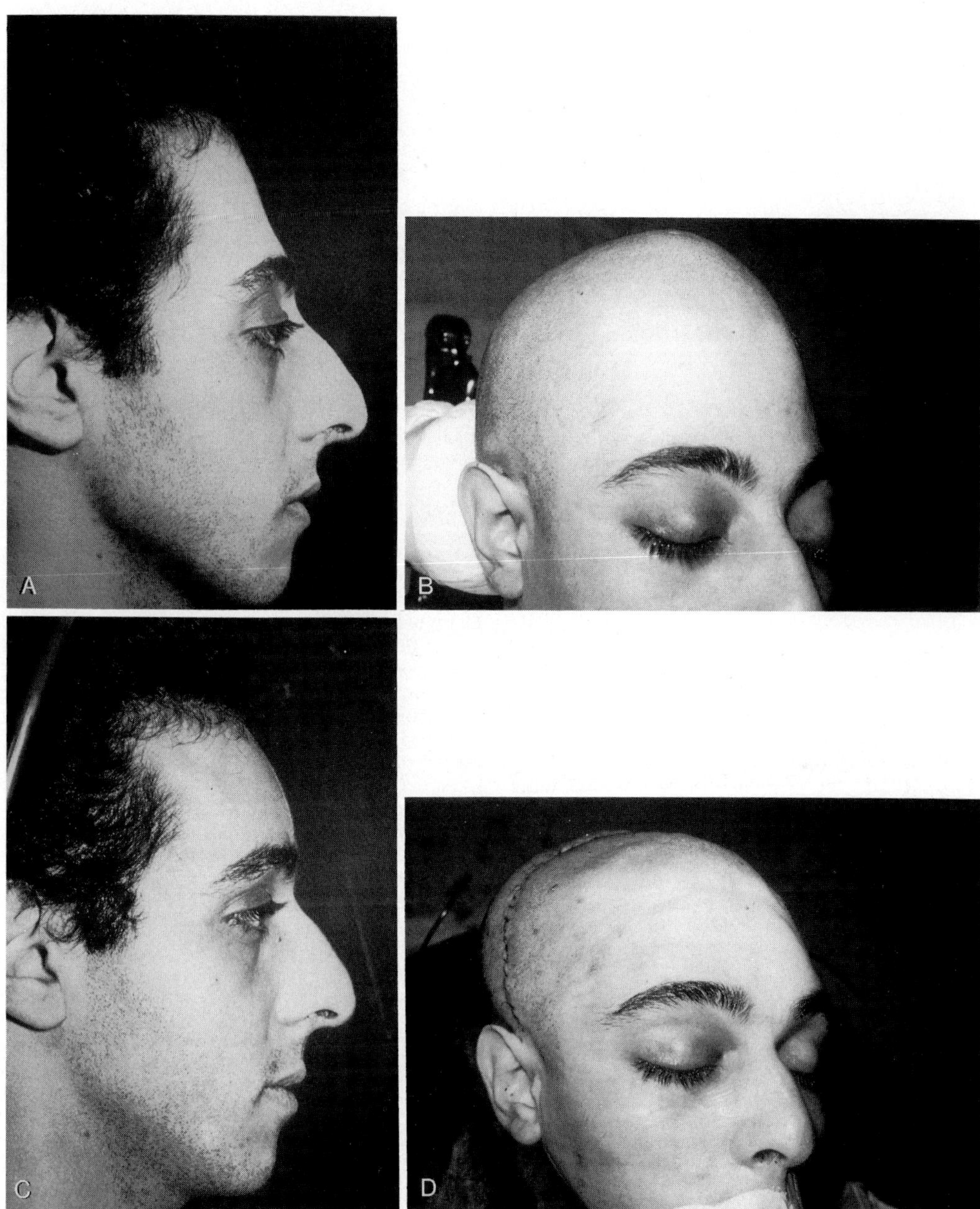

Figure 32–36. Oxycephaly correction. *A, B,* A male, aged 23, requested a frontal bone correction. He had an untreated oxycephaly without functional problems. *C, D,* Frontal remodeling according to the technique illustrated in Figure 32–34 allowed simultaneous correction of the forehead and the cranial vault. Note that the profile is improved and the nose, which seemed prominent previously, appears normal in countour.

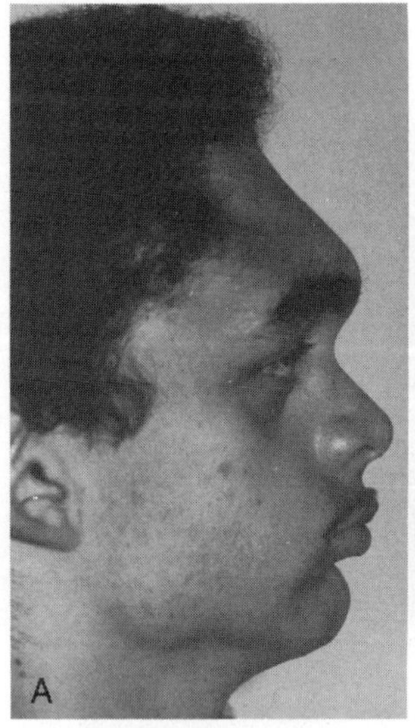

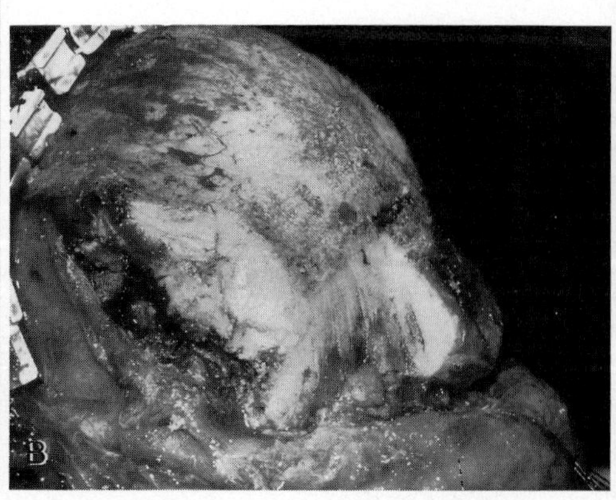

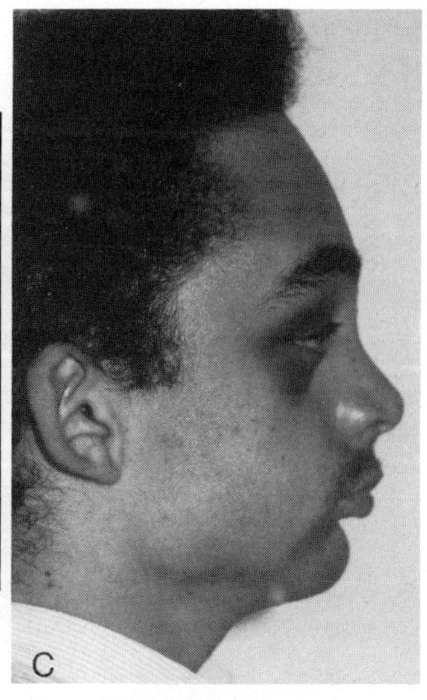

Figure 32–37. Simple forehead recontouring. *A,* A male, aged 20, requested contour improvement of his forehead distorted by frontometaplasia. *B,* Bone carving was performed through a thickened supraorbital rim and frontal bone. *C,* Resulting contour.

sia, as in the patient illustrated in Figure 32–37.

REFERENCES

Alpert, B. S., Buncke, H. J., and Mathes, S. J.: Surgical treatment of the toally avulsed scalp. Clin. Plast. Surg., *9*:145, 1982.

Anderl, H., Muhlbauer, W., and Marchac, D.: Moulding the craniofacial skeleton with a paste of concentrated fibrin and bone dust. *In* Marchac, D. (Ed.): Craniofacial Surgery. Transactions of the 1st Congress of the International Society of Craniomaxillofacial Surgery. Heidelberg, Springer Verlag, 1987, p. 274.

Argenta, L. C., and Dingman, R. O.: Total reconstruction of aplasia cutis congenita involving scalp, skull, and dura. Plast. Reconstr. Surg., *77*:650, 1986.

Argenta, L. C., and Newman, M. H.: The use of methylmethacrylate cranioplasty in forehead reconstruction. Eur. J. Plast. Surg., *9*:94, 1986.

Argenta, L. C., Watanabe, M. J., and Grabb, W. C.: The use of tissue expansion in head and neck reconstruction. Ann. Plast. Surg., *11*:31, 1983.

Baldwin, M., and Debakan, A.: The surgical separation of Siamese twins conjoined by the heads (cephalopagus frontalis) followed by normal development. J. Neurol. Neurosurg. Psychiatr., *21*:195, 1958.

Ballin, M.: A method of cranioplasty using as a graft one-half the thickness of bony part of rib. Surg. Gynecol. Obstet., *33*:79, 1921.

Brown, R. C.: Cranioplasty by split-rib method. J. Coll. Surg. Aust., *1*:238, 1928.

Brunet, C., and Visot, A.: Stérilisation des os de banque. Crânioplasties par homogreffes. Ann. Chir. Plast., *27*:211, 1982.

Buncke, H. J., Rose, E. H., Brownstein, M. J., et al.: Successful replantation of two avulsed scalps by microvascular anastomoses. Plast. Reconstr. Surg., *61*:666, 1978.

Cabanela, M. E., Coventry, M. B., MacCarthy, C. S., and Miller, W. E.: The fate of patients with methylmethacrylate cranioplasty. J. Bone Joint Surg., *54*:278, 1972.

Campbell, W.: Case of congenital ulcer on the cranium of a fetus. Edinburgh J. Med. Sci., *2*:82, 1826.

Converse, J. M.: Surgical closure of scalp defects. *In* Kahn, E. A., Bassett, R. C., Schneider, R. C., and Crosby, E. C. (Eds.): Correlative Neurosurgery. Springfield, IL, Charles C Thomas, 1955.

Davis, J. S.: Scalping accidents. Johns Hopkins Hosp. Rep., *16*:257, 1911.

Delagénière, H., and Lewin, P.: A general method of repairing loss of bony substance and of reconstructing bones by osteoperiosteal grafts taken from the tibia. Surg. Gynecol. Obstet., *30*:441, 1920.

Demmel, V.: Clinical aspects of congenital skin defects. Congenital skin defects on the head of the newborn. Eur. J. Pediatr., *121*:21, 1975.

Dingman, R. O., and Argenta, L. C.: The surgical repair of traumatic defects of the scalp. Clin. Plast. Surg., *9*:131, 1982.

Dingman, R. O., Weintraub, W. H., and Wilensky, R. J: Congenital absence of the scalp, cranial vault, and dura. *In* Converse, J. M. (Ed.): Plastic and Reconstructive Surgery. 2nd Ed. Philadelphia, W. B. Saunders, 1977, p. 828.

Dufourmentel, L.: Plastic operations on the skull. Paris Med., *8*:503, 1918.

Edmonds, L. D., and Layde, P. M.: Conjoined twins in the United States, 1970–1977. Teratology, *24*:301, 1982.

Estor, E.: Cent cas de prosthèse cranienne par plaque d'or. Bull. et Mem. Soc. Chir. Paris, *43*:463, 1917.

Fagarasanu, I.: Procédé de cranioplastie par des greffons costaux redoublés; procédé du "grillage protecteur." Tech. Chir., *29*:57, 1937.

Feierabend, T. C., and Bindra, R. N.: Injuries causing major loss of scalp. Plast. Reconstr. Surg., *76*:189, 1985.

Fonseca, J. L.: Use of pericranial flap in scalp wounds with exposed bone. Plast. Reconstr. Surg., *72*:786, 1983.

Geib, F. W.: Vitallium skull plates. J.A.M.A., *117*:306, 1941.

Glasson, D. W., and Duncan, G. M.: Aplasia cutis congenita of the scalp. Delayed closure complicated by massive hemorrhage. Plast. Reconstr. Surg., *75*:423, 1985.

Grossman, H. J., Sugar, O., Greeley, P. W., and Sadove, M. S.: Surgical separation in craniopagus. J.A.M.A., *153*:201, 1953.

Haasner, E., Krokowski, E., and Rach, K.: Normal values of hydroxyapatite content in the skeleton dependent upon localization, age, and sex. Klin. Wochenschr., *45*:575, 1967.

Habal, M. B., Leake, D. L., and Maniscalco, J. E.: Repair of major cranio-orbital defects with an elastomer-coated mesh and autogenous bone paste. Plast. Reconstr. Surg., *61*:394, 1978.

Handa, J., Nakasu, Y., and Matsuda, M.: Conservative management of congenital defect of skull and scalp. Surg. Neurol., *17*:152, 1982.

Harii, K., Ohmori, K., and Ohmori, S.: Hair transplantation with free scalp flaps. Plast. Reconstr. Surg., *53*:410, 1974.

Hendel, P. M., and Nadell, J. M.: A new approach for harvesting cranial bone grafts: the guided osteotome. *In* Marchac, D. (Ed.): Craniofacial Surgery. Transactions of the 1st Congress of the International Society of Craniomaxillofacial Surgery. Heidelberg, Springer Verlag, 1987.

Irons, G. B., and Olson, R. M.: Aplasia cutis congenita. Plast. Reconstr. Surg., *66*:199, 1980.

Juri, J.: Use of parieto-occipital flaps in the surgical treatment of baldness. Plast. Reconstr. Surg., *55*:456, 1975.

Jurkiewicz, M. J., and Hill, H. L.: Open wounds of the scalp: an account of methods of repair. J. Trauma, *21*:769, 1981.

Kappis, A.: Zur Deckung von Schädeldefekten. Zentralbl. Chir., *42*:897, 1915.

Kazanjian, V. H., and Converse, J. M.: Reconstruction after radical operation for osteomyelitis of frontal bone. Arch. Otolaryngol., *31*:94, 1940.

Kazanjian, V. H., and Converse, J. M.: The Surgical Treatment of Facial Injuries. 2nd Ed. Baltimore, Williams & Wilkins Company, 1959.

Kazanjian, V. H., and Webster, R. C.: The treatment of extensive losses of the scalp. Plast. Reconstr. Surg., *1*:360, 1946.

Keen, W. W.: Surgery, Its Principles and Practice. Philadelphia, W. B. Saunders Company, 1909.

Kiehn, C. L., and Grino, A.: Iliac bone grafts replacing tantalum plates for gunshot wounds of the skull. Am. J. Surg., *85*:395, 1953.

König, F.: Der knocherne Ersatz grosser Schädeldefekte. Zentralbl. Chir., *17*:467, 1890.

Korlof, B., Nylen, B., and Rietz, K. A.: Bone grafting of skull defects. A report of 55 cases. Plast. Reconstr. Surg., *52*:378, 1973.

Longacre, J. J.: Surgical correction of extensive defects of scalp and skull with autogenous tissues. Transactions of 1st International Congress of Plastic Surgeons, Stockholm, 1955, p. 346.

Longacre, J. J., and de Stefano, G. A.: Reconstruction of extensive defects of the skull with split-rib grafts. Plast. Reconstr. Surg., *19*:186, 1957a.

Longacre, J. J., and de Stefano, G. A.: Further observations of the behavior of autogenous split-rib grafts in reconstruction of extensive defects of the cranium and face. Plast. Reconstr. Surg., *20*:281, 1957b.

Longacre, J. J., and de Stefano, G. A.: Repair of extensive defects of the scalp and skull with autogenous tissues. J. Int. Coll. Surg., *27*:324, 1957c.

Longacre, J. J., de Stefano, G. A., Davidson, D. A., and Holmstrand, K.: Observations on the behavior of split-rib grafts in the reconstruction of extensive defects of the calvarium and facial skeleton. Transactions of 2nd International Congress of Plastic Surgeons, London, 1959, p. 290.

Lovaas, G.: Personal communication, 1985.

Lu, M. M.: Successful replacement of avulsed scalp. Plast. Reconstr. Surg., *43*:231, 1969.

MacLennan, A.: The repair, by bone graft, of gaps in the skull due to congenital deficiency, injury, or operation. Glasgow Med. J., *93*:251, 1920.

Macomber, D. W.: Cancellous iliac bone in depressions of forehead, nose and chin. Plast. Reconstr. Surg., *4*:157, 1949.

Manders, E. K., Graham, W. P., III, Schenden, M. J., and Davis, T. S.: Skin expansion to eliminate large scalp defects. Ann. Plast. Surg., *12*:305, 1984.

Manson, P. N., Crawley, W. A., and Hoopes, J. E.: Frontal cranioplasty; risk factors and choice of cranial vault reconstructive material. Plast. Reconstr. Surg., *77*:888, 1986.

Marchac, D.: Radical forehead remodeling for craniostenosis. Plast. Reconstr. Surg., *61*:823, 1978.

Marchac, D., and Cophignon, J.: Technique for embedding split-ribs in a cranioplasty. Plast. Reconstr. Surg., *55*:237, 1975.

Marchac, D., Cophignon, J., Clay, C., and Rey, A.: La réfection du toit de l'orbite par dédoublement du volet frontal. Nouv. Presse Med., *2*:2413, 1973.

Marchac, D., Cophignon, J., Rey, A., Chai and Clay, C.: Réparation des fracas fronto-orbitaires par reposition ou ostéotomie et greffes osseuses. Ann. Chir. Plast., *19*:41, 1974.

Marchac, D., and Renier, D.: Craniofacial Surgery for Craniosynostosis. Boston, Little, Brown & Company, 1982.

Mauclaire, P.: Breche cranienne restaurée par la prothèse métallique. Comments on article by Rouvillois. Bull. Mem. Soc. Chir. Paris, *34*:232, 1908.

McCarthy, J. G., and Zide, B. M.: The spectrum of calvarial bone grafting: introduction of the vascularized calvarial bone flap. Plast. Reconstr. Surg., *74*:10, 1984.

McClintock, H. G., and Dingman, R. O.: The repair of cranial defects with iliac bone. Surgery, *30*:955, 1951.

McCray, M. K., and Roenigk, H. H.: Scalp reduction for correction of cutis aplasia congenita. J. Dermatol. Surg. Oncol., *7*:655, 1981.

McLean, D. H., and Buncke, H. J., Jr.: Autotransplant of omentum to a large scalp defect, with microsurgical revascularization. Plast. Reconstr. Surg., *49*:268, 1972.

McWilliams, C. A.: Principles of the four types of skin grafting; with an improved method of treating total avulsion of scalp. J.A.M.A., *83*:183, 1924.

Merville, L., Brunet, C., and Derome, P.: Reconstruction frontale et des sinus frontaux. Ann. Chir. Plast., *27*:205, 1982.

Miller, G. D., Anstee, E. J., and Snell, J. A.: Successful replantation of an avulsed scalp by microvascular anastomoses. Plast. Reconstr. Surg., *58*:133, 1976.

Mitz, V., Dabos, N., and Vilain, R.: Stratégie thérapeutique dans la réparation des alopécies temporo-pariétales: intérêt du lambeau sagittal médian ou paramédian. Ann. Chir. Plast., *29*:48, 1984.

Montgomery, H.: Congenital aplasia. *In* Montgomery, H.

(Ed.): Dermatopathology. Vol. 1. New York, Harper & Row, 1967.

Morestin, H.: Les transplantations cartilagineuses dans la chirurgie réparatrice. Bull. Mem. Soc. Chir. Paris, *41*:1994, 1915.

Mowlem, R.: Cancellous chip bone grafts; report on 75 cases. Lancet, *2*:746, 1944.

Muakkassa, K. F., King, R. B., and Stark, D. B.: Nonsurgical approach to congenital scalp and skull defects. J. Neurosurg., *56*:711, 1982.

Müller, W.: Zur Frage der temporären Schädelresektion an Stelle der Trepanation. Zentralbl. Chir., *17*:65, 1890.

Mulliken, J. B., and Glowacki, J.: Induced osteogenesis for repair and construction in the craniofacial region. Plast. Reconstr. Surg., *65*:553, 1980.

Munro, I. R., and Guyuron, B.: Split-rib cranioplasty. Ann. Plast. Surg., *7*:341, 1981.

Münster, S.: La Cosmographie Universelle. Basle, H. Pierre, 1556.

Nahai, F., Hurteau, J., and Vasconez, L. O.: Replantation of an entire scalp and ear by microvascular anastomoses of only one artery and one vein. Br. J. Plast. Surg., *31*:339, 1978.

Nataf, J., Elbaz, J. S., and Pollet, J.: Critical study of scalp transplantations and proposal of an approach. Ann. Chir. Plast., *21*:CP199, 1976.

O'Connell, J. E.: Craniopagus twins: surgical anatomy and embryology and their implications. J. Neurol. Neurosurg. Psychiatry, *39*:1, 1976.

Ohmori, K.: Free scalp flap. Plast. Reconstr. Surg., *65*:42, 1980.

Orticochea, M.: Four-flap scalp reconstruction technique. Br. J. Plast. Surg., *20*:159, 1967.

Orticochea, M.: New three-flap scalp reconstruction technqiue. Br. J. Plast. Surg., *24*:184, 1971.

Ousterhout, D. K., Baker, S., and Zlotolow, I.: Methylmethacrylate onlay implants in the treatment of forehead deformities secondary to craniosynostosis. J. Maxillofac. Surg., *8*:228, 1980.

Paré, A.: Of wounds made by gunshot, other fierie engeines and all sorts of weapons. In the Workes of that Famous Chirurgion Ambrose Parey. Translated from the Latin and compared with the French by T. Johnson. London, T. Cotes & R. Young, 1634.

Pastoriza, J., Tessier, P., and Delbet, J. P.: Cranioplasties de la voûte. Ann. Chir. Plast., *18*:261, 1973.

Pensler, J., and McCarthy, J. G.: The calvarial donor site: an anatomic study in cadavers. Plast. Reconstr. Surg., *75*:648, 1985.

Phemister, D. B.: The fate of transplanted bone and regenerative power of its various constituents. Surg. Gynecol. Obstet., *19*:303, 1914.

Pickerill, H. P.: New method of osteoplastic restoration of the skull. Med. J. Aust., *2*:228, 1931.

Pickerill, H. P.: Advantages of early skin grafting. N.Z. Med. J., *45*:45, 1946.

Poole, M., Briggs, M., Ashworth, G., and Timmons, M.: Use of prepared cadaver bone in cranial reconstruction. A preliminary report. *In* Marchac, D. (Ed.): Craniofacial Surgery. Transactions of the 1st Congress of the International Society of Craniomaxillofacial Surgery. Heidelberg, Springer Verlag, 1987.

Psillakis, J. M., Nocchi, V. L., and Zanini, S. A.: Repair of large defect of frontal bone with free grafts of outer table of parietal bones. Plast. Reconstr. Surg., *64*:827, 1979.

Pudenz, R. H., and Odom, G. L.: Meningocerebral adhesions: experimental study of effect of human amniotic membrane, amnioplastin, beef allantoic membrane, cargile membrane, tantalum foil and polyvinyl alcohol films. Surgery, *12*:318, 1942.

Radovan, C.: Adjacent flap development using expandable Silastic implants. American Society of Plastic and Reconstructive Surgeons Forum, Boston, MA, Sept. 30, 1976.

Renier, D., Sainte-Rose, D., and Marchac, D.: Intracranial pressure in craniostenosis: 302 recordings. *In* Marchac, D. (Ed.): Craniofacial Surgery. Transactions of the 1st Congress of the International Society of Craniomaxillofacial Surgery. Heidelberg, Springer Verlag, 1987.

Richaud, J., Lazorthes, Y., and Caraoué, F.: Cranioplasties acryliques thermopolymérisables. Technique et résultat à propos de 37 cas. Ann. Chir. Plast., *30*:133, 1985.

Robinson, F.: Complete avulsion of the scalp. Br. J. Plast. Surg., *5*:37, 1952.

Salyer, K. E., Ubinas, E. E., and Snively, S. L.: Growth following craniofacial remodeling in craniosynostosis. Prog. Clin. Biol. Res., *187*:161, 1985.

Santoni-Rugiu, P.: Repair of skull defects by outer table osteoperiosteal free grafts. Plast. Reconstr. Surg., *43*:157, 1969.

Savariaud, M.: Prothèse du crâne avec plaque d'argent extensible. Bull. Mem. Soc. Chir. Paris, 38:238, 1912.

Schmidt, G. B.: Schädelplastik: Besprechung. Beitr. Klin. Chir., *98*:604, 1916.

Schneider, B. M., Berg, R. A., and Kaplan, A. M.: Aplasia cutis congenita complicated by sagittal sinus hemorrhage. Pediatrics, *66*:948, 1980.

Schultz, R. C.: Restoration of frontal contour with methylmethacrylate. Ann. Plast.Surg., *3*:295, 1979.

Scott, M., and Wycis, H. T.: Experimental observations on the use of stainless steel for cranioplasty; comparison with tantalum. J. Neurosurg., *3*:310, 1946.

Seydel, H.: Eine neue Methode, grosse Knochendefekten, des Schädels zu Keckung. Zentralbl. Chir., *16*:209, 1889.

Shanoff, E., and Tsur, H.: Fenestration and delayed skin grafting for the cover of the exposed inner table of the skull. Br. J. Plast. Surg., *34*:331, 1981.

Shehadi, S. I.: Skull reconstruction with bone dust. Br. J. Plast. Surg., *23*:227, 1970.

Shively, R. E., Bermant, M. A., and Bucholz, R. D.: Separation of craniopagus twins utilizing tissue expanders. Plast. Reconstr. Surg., *76*:765, 1985.

Soderberg, B., and Mulvey, J. M.: Mandibular reconstruction in jaw deformities. Plast. Reconstr. Surg., *2*:191, 1947.

Spear, S. L., and Mickle, J. P.: Simultaneous cutis aplasia congenita of the scalp and cranial stenosis. Plast. Reconstr. Surg., *71*:413, 1983.

Steinhauser, E. W., and Hardt, N.: Secondary reconstruction of cranial defects. J. Maxillofac. Surg., *5*:192, 1977.

Subczynski, J. A.: One-stage debridement and plastic repair of compound comminuted depressed skull fractures with methylmethacrylate. J. Trauma, *17*:467, 1977.

Tessier, P.: Autogenous bone grafts taken from the calvarium for facial and cranial applications. Clin. Plast. Surg., *9*:531, 1982.

Thomson, H. G., Munro, I. R., and Birch, J. R.: Exposed cranial implants—a salvage operation. Plast. Reconstr. Surg., *59*:395, 1977.

Tysvaer, A. T., and Hovind, K. H.: Stainless steel mesh-acrylic cranioplasty. J. Trauma, *17*:231, 1977.

Vandraager, J. M., Van Mullen, P. J., and Wijn, J. R.:

Porous acrylic cement for the correction of craniofacial deformities and repair of defects, animal experimentation and two years of clinical application. Biomaterials, *4*:128, 1983.
Van Gool, A.: Preformed polymethylmethacrylate cranioplasties: report of 45 cases. J. Maxillofac. Surg., *13*:2, 1985.
Von Hacker, V.: Ersatz von Schädeldefekten durch unter der Kopfschwartz verschobener oder ein gelappte Periostknochen. Beitr. Klin. Chir., *37*:499, 1903.
Voris, H. C., Slaughter, W. B., Christian, J. R., and Cayia, E. R.: Successful separation of craniopagus twins. J. Neurosurg., *14*:548, 1957.
Walton, R. L., and Krizek, T. J.: The scalp flap only onlay: a method for managing large dural defects. Plast. Reconstr. Surg., *66*:684, 1980.
Weber, H.: Schädelplastik. Berl. Klin. Wochenschr., *53*:1115, 1916.
Westermann, C. W. J.: Zur Methodik der Deckung von Schädeldefekten. Zentralbl. Chir., *43*:113, 1916.
White, J. C.: Late complications following cranioplasty with alloplastic plates. Ann. Surg., *128*:743, 1948.
Wilflingseder, P.: Cranioplasties by means of diced cartilage and split rib grafts. Minerva Chir., *38*:837, 1983.
Wolfe, S. A.: Discussion of Manson et al. paper. Plast. Reconstr. Surg., *77*:901, 1986.
Wolfe, S. A., and Berkowitz, S.: Cranioplasty. *In* Wolfe, S. A. (Ed.): Plastic Surgery of the Facial Skeleton. Boston, Little, Brown and Company, 1988.
Wolfowitz, J., Kerr, E. M., Levin, S. E., Walker, D. H., and Vetten, K. B.: Separation of craniopagus twins. S. Afr. Med. J., *42*:412, 1968.
Woolf, J. I., and Walker, A. E.: Cranioplasty: a collective review. Int. Abstr. Surg., *81*:2, 1945.
Zins, J. E., and Whitaker, L. A.: Membranous vs. endochondral bone autografts: implications for craniofacial reconstruction. Surg. Forum, *30*:521, 1979.

33

Joseph G. McCarthy
Glenn W. Jelks
Augustus J. Valauri
Donald Wood-Smith
Byron Smith

The Orbit and Zygoma

EMBRYOLOGY
ANATOMY
CLINICAL EVALUATION
RADIOGRAPHIC TECHNIQUES
SURGICAL PRINCIPLES
MALUNITED FRACTURES OF THE ORBIT AND ZYGOMA
- Roof (Fronto-orbital)
- Floor and Medial and Lateral Walls
- Nasoethmoido-orbital Fractures
- Dislocation

ORBITAL DYSTOPIA
ORBITAL DECOMPRESSION
- Orbital Pathology in Graves' Disease (Hyperthyroidism)
- Thyrotoxic Exophthalmos

ANOPHTHALMOS AND MICROPHTHALMOS
RECONSTRUCTION OF THE ANOPTHTHALMIC ORBIT
MISCELLANEOUS ORBITAL PATHOLOGY
- Fibrous Dysplasia
- Neurofibroma
- Hemangioma
- Lymphangioma

RECONSTRUCTION OF THE ZYGOMA

In man, as with lower animals, the face is the seat of the principal sensory organs. In evolutionary progression, as man assumed the upright position, olfaction was destined to partial retrogression and vision attained greater importance. Consequently, comparative anatomic studies disclose enlargement of the brain, visual cortical centers and cranial vault (forehead and roof of the orbit), and the development of a protective circumferential bony orbit with a zygomatic arch.

EMBRYOLOGY

By the 22nd day (*fourth week*) of embryonic life there is a distinct cephalic end of the C-shaped embryo, containing the brain, the frontonasal prominence, the maxillary and mandibular processes, and the beginning of the second branchial arch. The *optic sulcus* appears on approximately the 22nd day; it evaginates as the *optic placode* (Fig. 33–1) and becomes the *optic vesicle*. The latter eventually projects through the ectoderm in the 28-day embryo (Rogers, 1977).

In the *fifth embryonic* week the optic vesicle enlarges and becomes attached to the brain by the *optic stalk*. The posterior aspect of the optic vesicle is transformed into the *optic cup*,

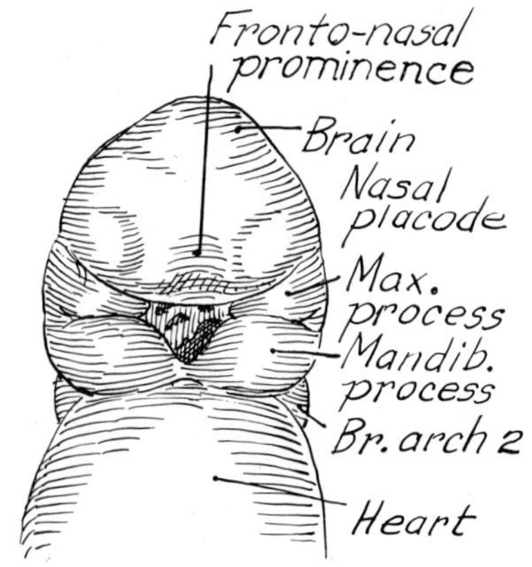

Figure 33–1. Human embryo, estimated age 26 days (2.5 mm). (After Hamilton, W. J., Boyd, J. D., and Mossman, H. W.: Human Embryology. 3rd Ed. Baltimore, Williams & Wilkins Company, 1962.)

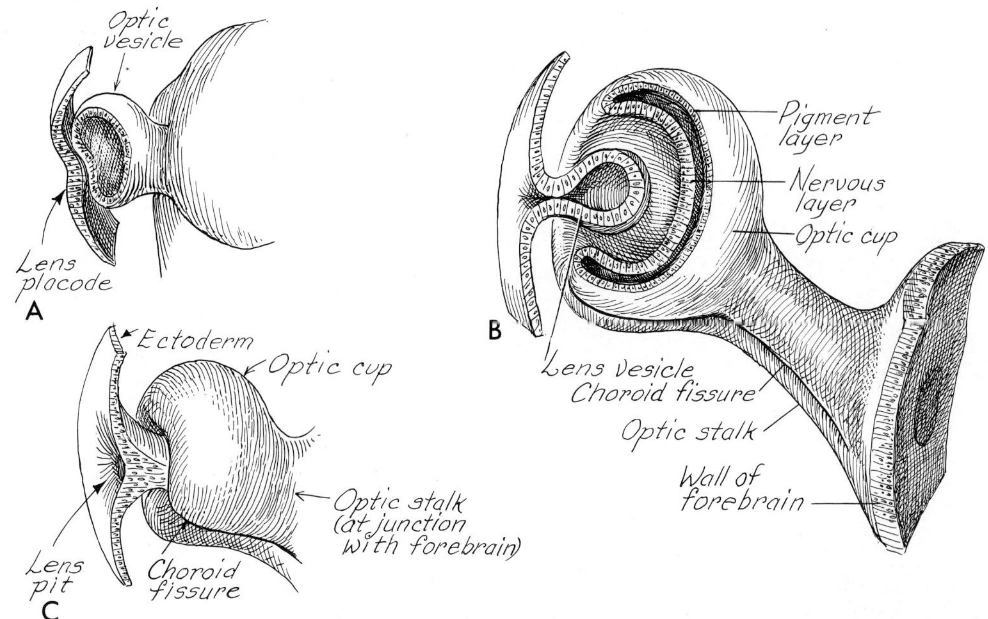

Figure 33–2. Embryonic development of the optic system. *A,* At 4.5 mm, 30 to 31 days. *B,* At 5.5 mm, 32 to 33 days. *C,* At 7.5 mm, 34 to 35 days. (After Hamilton, W. J., Boyd, J. D., and Mossman, H. W.: Human Embryology. 3rd Ed. Baltimore, Williams & Wilkins Company, 1962.)

which eventually becomes the retina (Fig. 33–2). The lens placodes, lens vesicles, and choroidal fissures have also made their appearance by this time.

The axes of the primitive eye region are initially located at an angle of approximately 180 degrees to each other. Between the third fetal month and term the angle is reduced from 105 to approximately 71 degrees (Fig. 33–3).

By the *sixth week* there is pigment in the optic vesicles and the choroidal fissures have fused in the inferior portion of the optic cup.

During the *seventh week* the eyelids, composed of ectoderm and mesoderm, are first noted above and below the developing lens and optic cup. The eyelids remain fused until the seventh fetal month (Fig. 33–4).

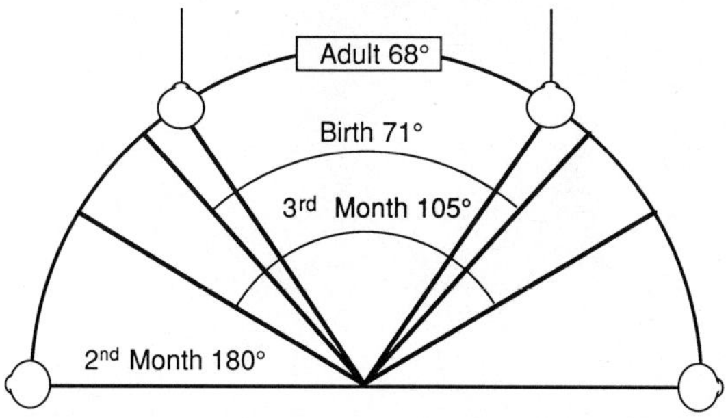

Figure 33–3. Changes in the orbital axes beginning at the second fetal month and continuing until adulthood.

By the *eighth week* the globular eye and eyelid region have differentiated into the oval-almond shape of the human. There is also progressive medial translation of the developing eye areas toward the midline of the head.

ANATOMY

The orbits are paired cavities separated in the midline by the interorbital space (nasal cavity and ethmoid and sphenoid sinuses) (Fig. 33–5), which is delimited superiorly by the anterior cranial fossa, cribriform plates, and crista galli. The superior aspect of the orbit is bounded by the frontal sinus (variable) and anterior cranial fossa. The orbits sit above the maxillary sinuses and medial to the temporal fossae.

The orbital contents are protected by strong skeletal abutments: the nasal bones, the nasal process of the frontal bone, and the frontal process of the maxilla medially; the supraorbital arch of the frontal bone superiorly; the frontal process of the zygoma and the zygomatic process of the frontal bone laterally and inferiorly the thick infraorbital rims formed by the zygoma and maxilla (Fig. 33–6).

Seven bones of the craniofacial skeleton

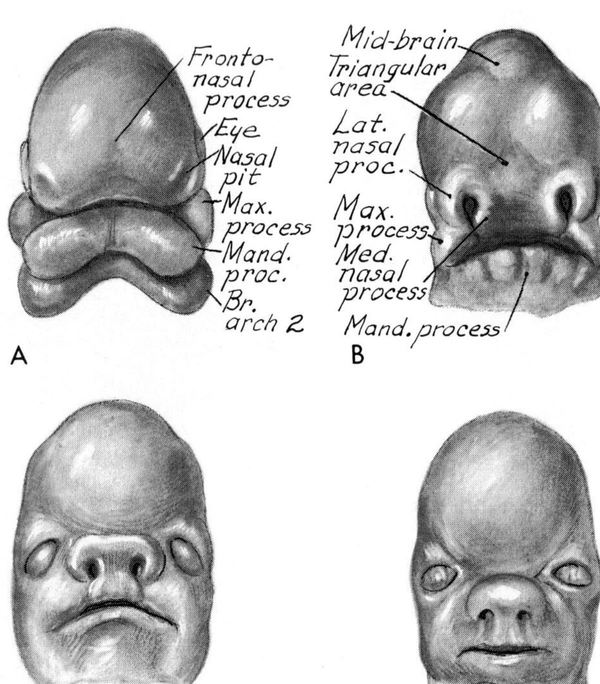

Figure 33–4. Embryonic development of the human face. *A,* Embryo approximately 33 days old. *B,* Embryo approximately 37 days old. *C,* Embryo approximately 42 days old. *D,* Embryo approximately 47 days old. (After Peter. *In* Arey, L. B.: Developmental Anatomy. 6th Ed. Philadelphia, W. B. Saunders Company, 1970.)

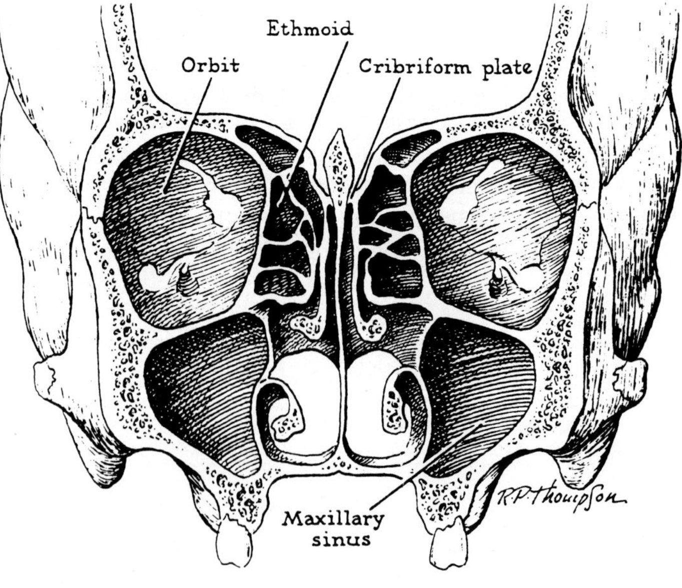

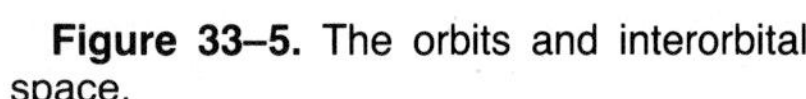

Figure 33–5. The orbits and interorbital space.

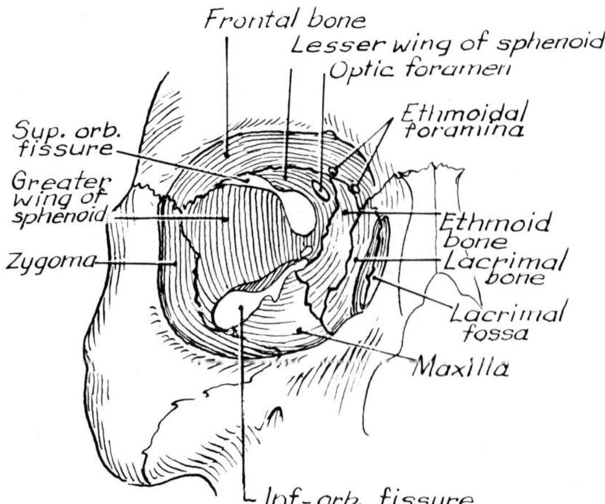

Figure 33–6. Frontal view of the right orbit. The contribution of the palatine bone is not illustrated.

contribute to the form of the orbit: the frontal, ethmoidal, sphenoidal, maxillary, zygomatic, lacrimal, and palatine bones.

The bony orbits have been described as pyramidal in shape (Fig. 33–6), but there are some inaccuracies in this analogy. The widest orbital diameter is not at the orbital rim but approximately 1.5 cm within the orbital cavity. The medial wall of the orbit has a quadrilateral rather than a triangular configuration. The optic foramen does not lie posterior to the middle point of the base but lies on a more medial and slightly superiorly situated axis. In children the floor of the orbit is situated at an even lower level in relation to the orbital rim because the maxillary sinus has not reached full development. The adult orbit is usually slightly wider than it is high. The angle between the lateral orbital walls of the orbits is 90 degrees and the angle between the lateral and medial wall of each orbit is 45 degrees.

Although the division is artificial, it is helpful in studying the bony orbit to divide it into four component parts: the roof, lateral wall, medial wall, and floor (Fig. 33–6). The *roof of the orbit* is composed mainly of the orbital plate of the frontal bone, but posteriorly it receives a minor contribution from the lesser wing of the sphenoid. The fossa lodging the lacrimal gland is a depression situated along the anterior and lateral aspect under the shelter of the zygomatic process of the frontal bone. The anterior portion of the roof can be invaded by the supraorbital extension of the frontal sinus (Fig. 33–7). The thin roof separates the orbit from the anterior cranial fossa and from the middle cranial fossa in its posterolateral aspect (Fig. 33–8).

The *lateral wall*, which is relatively stout, is formed by the orbital plate of the greater wing of the sphenoid, the frontal process of the zygomatic bone, and the lesser wing of the sphenoid lateral to the optic foramen. The superior orbital fissure is a cleft that runs forward and upward from the apex between the roof and lateral wall. The fissure, which

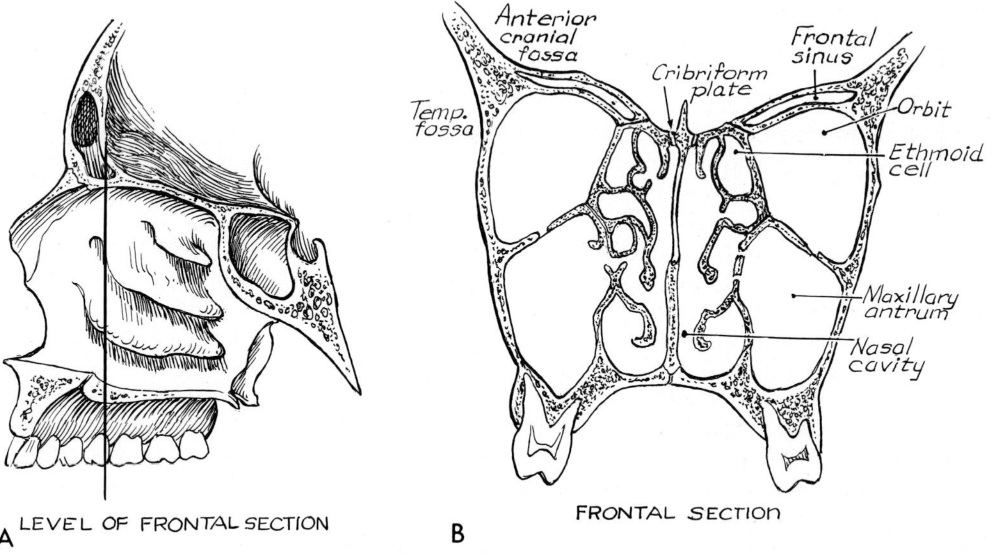

Figure 33–7. Frontal section showing relationship of the bony orbits and the interorbital space to the anterior cranial fossa, frontal sinus, temporal fossa, maxillary sinus, and ethmoidal sinus.

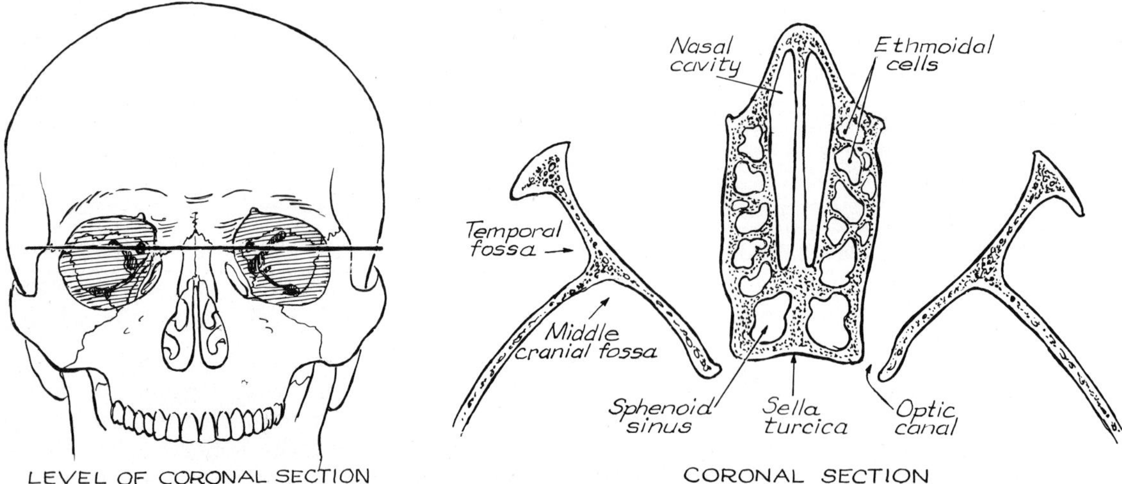

Figure 33–8. Horizontal section showing relationship of the orbit to the temporal fossa and middle cranial fossa.

separates the greater and lesser wings of the sphenoid, gives passage to the three motor nerves to the extraocular muscles and branches of the ophthalmic division of the trigeminal nerve. The superior orbital fissure communicates with the middle cranial fossa. The lateral wall of the orbit is related to the temporal fossa, and posteriorly a small part of the wall lies between the orbit and the middle cranial fossa and temporal lobe of the brain–hence the ease and danger of entering the middle cranial fossa in performing an osteotomy through the posterior portion of the lateral orbital wall (Fig. 33–8). Between the floor and the lateral wall of the orbit is the inferior orbital fissure, which communicates with the infratemporal fossa. The maxillary division of the trigeminal nerve, the infraorbital artery, the zygomatic nerve, the branches of the sphenopalatine ganglion, and the branches from the ophthalmic vein pass through the inferior orbital fissure.

The *medial wall*, reinforced anteriorly by the frontal process of the maxilla, is relatively fragile and is formed from the frontal bone, the lacrimal bone, the lamina papyracea of the ethmoid, and part of the lesser wing of the sphenoid around the optic foramen (see Fig. 33–6). The lamina papyracea is the largest component and accounts for the structural weakness of the medial wall. The groove for the lacrimal sac is a broad vertical fossa lying partly on the anterior aspect of the lacrimal bone and partly in the frontal process of the maxilla: the anterior and posterior margins of the lacrimal groove form the respective lacrimal crests. The groove is continuous with the nasolacrimal duct at the junction of the floor and the medial wall of the orbit, passing down into the inferior meatus of the nose. Between the roof and the medial wall of the orbit are the anterior and posterior ethmoidal foramina, which lead into canals communicating with the medial part of the anterior cranial fossa. The anterior ethmoidal artery and the anterior ethmoidal branch of the nasociliary nerve pass through the former, and the posterior ethmoidal artery and the sphenoethmoidal branch of the nasociliary nerve through the posterior foramen.

The *floor of the orbit*, a frequent site of fracture, has no sharp line of demarcation with the medial wall because the orbital floor tilts upward in its medial aspect, while the medial wall has a progressively lateral inclination. It is separated from the lateral wall by the inferior orbital (sphenomaxillary) fissure. The floor of the orbit (the roof of the maxillary sinus) is composed mainly of the orbital plate of the maxilla, a paper-thin structure medial to the infraorbital groove, and partly of the zygomatic bone anterior to the inferior orbital fissure. The infraorbital groove extends across the floor of the orbit beginning at about the middle of the inferior orbital fissure. Anteriorly it penetrates the thick inferior orbital rim as the infraorbital canal, which opens on the anterior surface of the maxilla as the infraorbital foramen. The middle superior alveolar nerves descend from the posterior aspect of the infraorbital canal; the anterosuperior alveolar branches of V_2 pass from the anterior aspect of the canal.

The periosteum of the orbit is designated

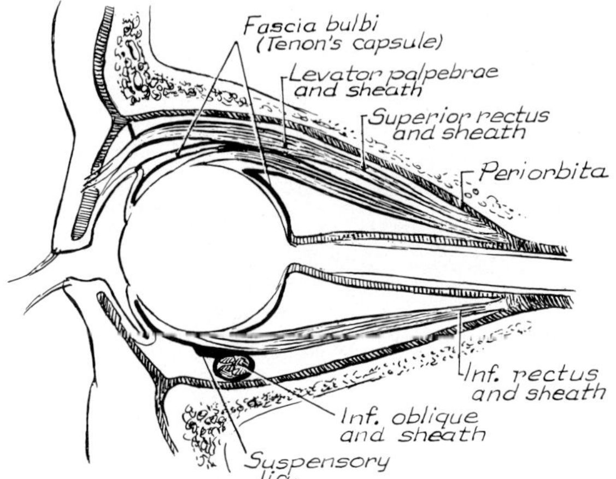

Figure 33–9. Sagittal section through the orbit showing the periorbita and intraorbital contents.

as the periorbita and is continuous with the dura at those sites where the orbit communicates with the cranial cavity, e.g., the optic foramen, the superior orbital fissure, and the anterior and posterior ethmoidal canals (Fig. 33–9). The optic canal, 4 to 10 mm in length, is the passage through which the optic nerve and ophthalmic artery pass from an intracranial to an intraorbital position. The canal is framed medially by the body of the sphenoid and laterally by the lesser wing, and is thus in close approximation to the sphenoid sinus and the posterior ethmoidal cells.

The *superior orbital rim* is formed by the frontal bone and is variable in its anterior projection, often depending on the degree of pneumatization of the enclosed frontal sinus. The supraorbital notch (a true foramen in 25 per cent of individuals) is approximately 25 mm lateral to the midline of the glabella. The supraorbital notch (foramen) lies on the same vertical plane with the infraorbital and mental foramina. The supraorbital artery and nerves pass through the notch; the supratrochlear vessels and nerves cross over the rim in a more medial location. The cartilaginous pulley for the superior oblique muscle attaches to the trochlear fossa approximately 8 mm within the orbit behind the junction of the medial and superior orbital rims.

The *lateral orbital rim*, composed of components from the frontal and zygomatic bones, is well defined. The lateral orbital tubercle of Whitnall, 10 mm inferior to the frontozygomatic suture and 3 mm within the orbit, is the attachment for the lateral canthal tendon, the check ligament of the lateral rectus muscle, the suspensory ligament of Lockwood, and the lateral extension of the aponeurosis of the levator muscle (Zide and Jelks, 1985).

The *medial orbital rim* is made up of the frontal process of the maxilla and the anterior lacrimal crest. The medial orbital rim is the main component of the "naso-orbital valley," a key topographic cosmetic feature of the face.

The *inferior orbital rim* includes the zygomaticomaxillary suture, which unites the two components: the maxilla and the zygoma. The infraorbital foramen, through which the infraorbital nerve and vessels exit, lies approximately 10 mm inferior to the suture.

The *anterior cranial fossa* supports the frontal lobes of the brain (Fig. 33–10). The floor of the anterior cranial fossa is composed largely of the orbital process of the frontal bone and, to a lesser extent, the cribriform plates of the ethmoid and the sphenoid bone (body and lesser wing). The lesser wing or sphenoid ridge forms a distinct margin between the anterior and middle cranial fossae.

The *middle cranial fossa* is thicker than the anterior cranial fossa. It is formed anteriorly by the greater wing of the sphenoid and posteriorly by the squama and upper surface of the petrous portions of the temporal bone. The sella turcica in the body of the sphenoid serves to connect the two sides. Posteromedially, the posterior and middle cranial fossae are separated by the petrous ridges or edges of the petrous pyramids.

The *maxilla*, formed of paired halves, is relatively cuboidal in shape. It is situated anterior to the pterygoid processes, inferior to the ocular globes, and lateral to the nasal cavities. The maxilla, along with the zygoma, accounts for the prominence of the cheeks and also encloses the maxillary sinuses. The

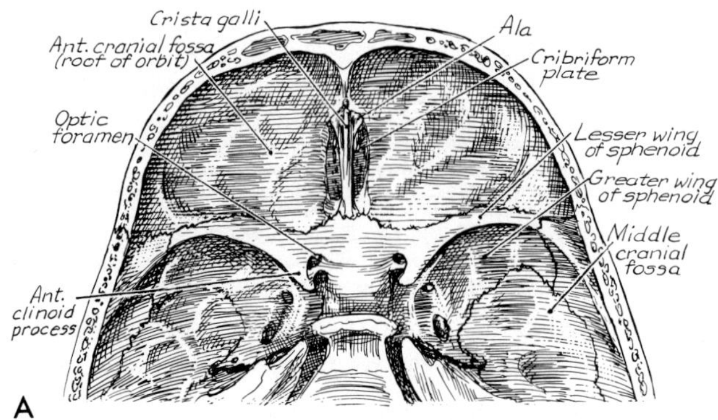

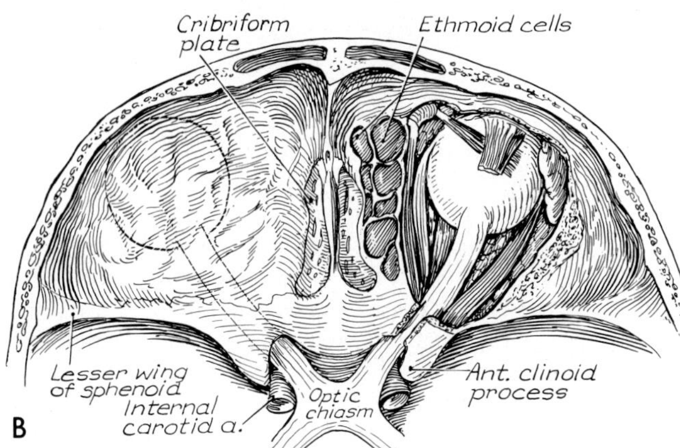

Figure 33–10. *A,* Superior view of the anterior and middle cranial fossae. *B,* Close-up view of *A* with the roof of the orbit and ethmoidal sinus removed.

medial wall of the maxillary sinus is completed by the palatine plate, the ethmoidal and maxillary processes of the inferior nasal concha, and the uncinate process of the ethmoid.

The maxilla joins with the orbital, nasal, zygomatic, and palatine structures to form the midfacial skeleton. The anterior (approximately) three-fourths of the palate is formed by the palatine processes of the maxilla and the palatine bones. The piriform aperture of the nose is bounded above by the lower margin of the nasal bones, and laterally and below by the strong frontal processes of the maxilla.

The *zygoma* (see Fig. 33–6) consists of a body that accounts for cheek prominence. It articulates with the maxilla at the zygomaticomaxillary suture, with the frontal bone at the zygomaticofrontal suture and the temporal bone at the zygomaticotemporal suture. The zygomatic arch is formed from the temporal process of the zygoma and the zygomatic process of the temporal bone. The zygomaticofacial nerve exits the foramen of the same name located in the midportion of the body of the zygoma; it innervates the overlying skin and fascia.

The reader is referred to Chapter 34 for additional details of soft tissue orbital anatomy and to Chapter 60 for craniofacial skeletal anatomy.

CLINICAL EVALUATION*

Clinical evaluation of the orbit must include a complete history and detailed physical examination of the eye and its associated structures (Jelks, Jelks, and Ruff, 1988). Whether the evaluation is for a traumatic, infectious, inflammatory, or neoplastic condition, the main concern is to determine the visual status and to preserve vision. The initial ocular examination can be easily performed with a few basic tools (Fig. 33–11). When there is associated intracranial pathology, a multidisciplinary approach to management may be necessary. In order to establish proper priorities, the ocular status must be documented so that there is a reduced risk of further damage during subsequent surgical

*Taken in part from Jelks, G. W., Jelks, E. B., and Ruff, G.: Clinical and radiographic evaluation of the orbit. Otolaryngol. Clin. North Am., *21*:13, 1988.

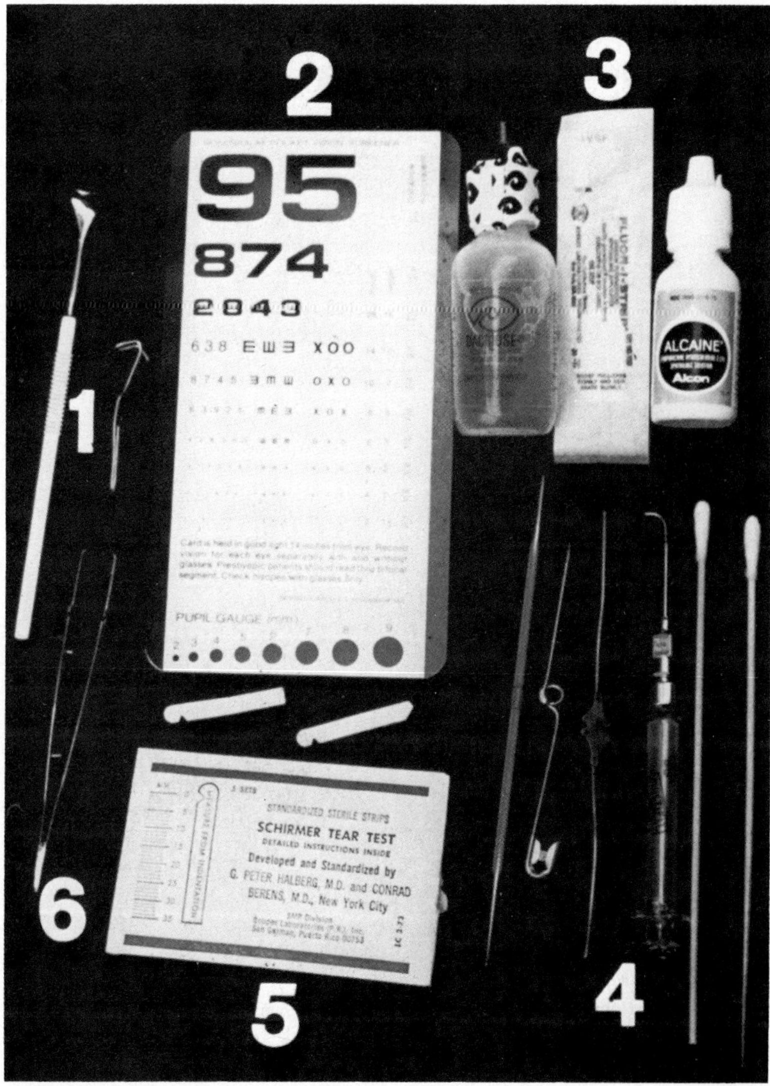

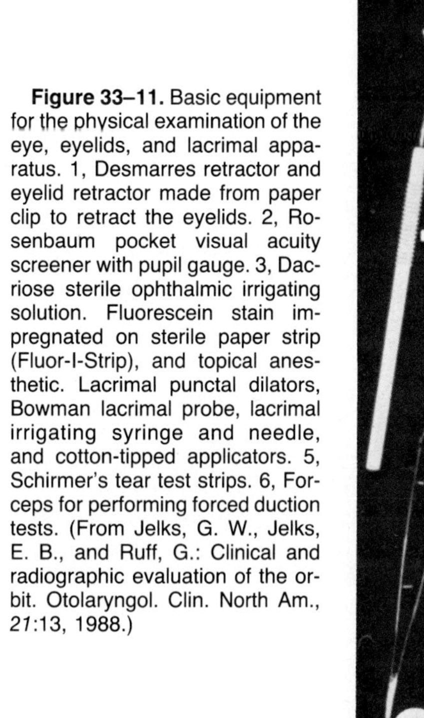

Figure 33–11. Basic equipment for the physical examination of the eye, eyelids, and lacrimal apparatus. 1, Desmarres retractor and eyelid retractor made from paper clip to retract the eyelids. 2, Rosenbaum pocket visual acuity screener with pupil gauge. 3, Dacriose sterile ophthalmic irrigating solution. Fluorescein stain impregnated on sterile paper strip (Fluor-I-Strip), and topical anesthetic. Lacrimal punctal dilators, Bowman lacrimal probe, lacrimal irrigating syringe and needle, and cotton-tipped applicators. 5, Schirmer's tear test strips. 6, Forceps for performing forced duction tests. (From Jelks, G. W., Jelks, E. B., and Ruff, G.: Clinical and radiographic evaluation of the orbit. Otolaryngol. Clin. North Am., *21*:13, 1988.)

Table 33–1. Evaluation of the Orbit

Clinical Evaluation	Radiographic Evaluation
History	Plain roentgenograms
Visual acuity	Computed tomography
Inspection and palpation	Ultrasound
Pupils	Angiography
Motility	Magnetic resonance imaging
Slit lamp examination	
Intraocular tension	
Dilated funduscopic examination	

From Jelks, G. W., Jelks, E. B., and Ruff, G.: Clinical and radiographic evaluation of the orbit. Otolaryngol. Clin. North Am., *21*:13, 1988.

intervention. The essential components of a complete evaluation of the orbit are summarized in Table 33–1.

History

It is essential to establish any history of ocular or orbital trauma or decreased vision, and the need for correction for distant and/or near visual acuity. If the patient is not mentally alert, family members or other persons knowledgeable of pertinent information should be questioned. For the obtunded patient, it is important to determine whether contact lenses are in place, and if so to remove them to prevent possible corneal damage. The subjective change in visual acuity and any associated history of pain, tearing, discharge, photophobia, periorbital swelling, proptosis, or double vision should be documented. Delineation of the temporal sequence of the patient's complaints as an acute, subacute, or chronic process is important in directing priorities to the remainder of the clinical evaluation. Examination of old photographs can be useful in determining the duration of an eyelid, ocular, or orbital deformity.

Visual Acuity

It is important to determine the patient's best possible visual acuity. This requires the patient to read the smallest letter possible from a standard Snellen wall chart at 20 feet while wearing distance corrective lenses if needed. When a Snellen chart is unavailable or impractical, a determination of near vision with a Rosenbaum pocket chart (Fig. 33–11) may be used. It is important to test each eye individually and to record the right and left eye separately. Both Snellen and pocket charts are available with numbers and the letter "E" in various orientations to allow testing of illiterate patients or of children unfamiliar with the alphabet. When the "E" chart is used, the patient describes the correct orientation of the "E." If the patient's spectacles are not available, a pinhole device may be substituted. When a patient looks through a pinhole, the light rays entering the eye are maintained parallel and are therefore less subject to alteration by any ocular refractive error (Fig. 33–12). The pinhole determination of visual acuity should be used when the degree of impaired vision is not compatible with the findings of the ocular examination. The best vision is recorded as the distance equivalent, which is printed to the right of each line of the visual acuity chart, i.e., 20/400 to 20/20 (see Fig. 33–11). If the patient is unable to read the largest distance equivalent figure (20/400), one should determine the farthest distance for counting fingers (CF), e.g., "counts fingers at 2 feet." If fingers cannot be counted, one should determine the ability to detect a waving hand in front of the eye, i.e., hand motion (HM). If hand motion vision is not present, determine light perception (LP) with or without knowledge of its direction (LP c̄ or s̄ projection). The inability to perceive light is designated as "no light perception" (NLP).

Other visual tests that may be employed include color perception, visual fields, electroretinography (ERG), visual evoked response (VER), and fluorescein angiography.

Inspection and Palpation

The bony orbital rims are palpated to detect masses, irregularities, and tenderness.

Lid movement and position in primary, downward, and upward gaze must be assessed to determine the status of the levator mechanism. Probing and irrigation can be performed to assess the patency of the lacrimal system.

Exophthalmos, globe proptosis, or enophthalmos can be evaluated by observing the level of the globes looking down across the forehead or up across the chin (Fig. 33–13). If available, an exophthalmometer can be used for more exact documentation and for future comparison (Fig. 33–14). The same anatomic baseline (e.g., the lateral orbital bone rims) should be used each time a measurement is made.

Pupils

The pupils are best examined in a semidarkened room to enhance slight inequalities that may not be observed under bright light.

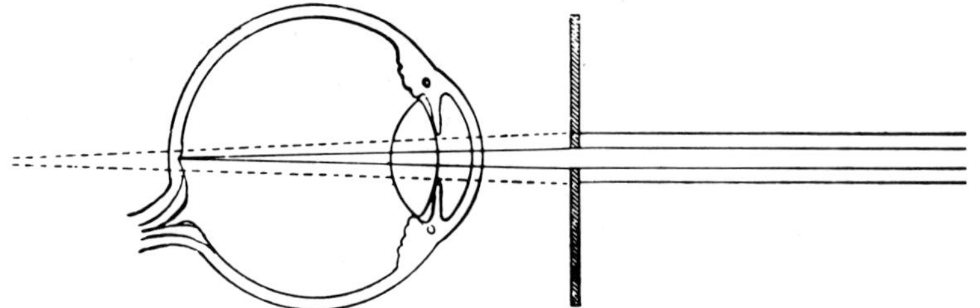

Figure 33–12. Effect of a pinhole device placed in front of the eye to assist in focusing light rays, thus eliminating the need for corrective lenses. (From Jelks, G. W., Jelks, E. B., and Ruff, G.: Clinical and radiographic evaluation of the orbit. Otolaryngol. Clin. North Am., *21*:13, 1988.)

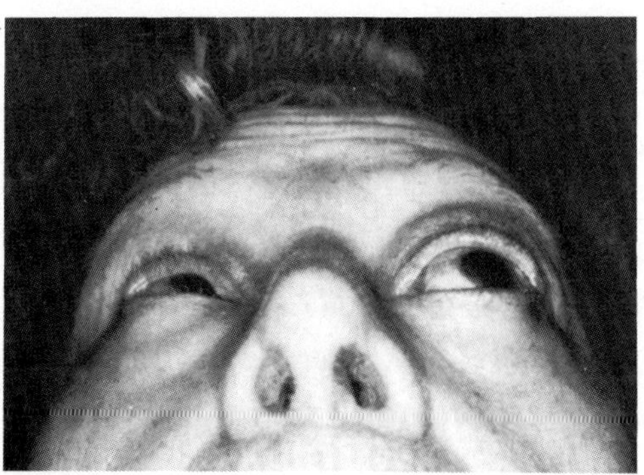

Figure 33–13. Patient with 8 mm of left ocular globe proptosis best visualized by the "worm's eye" view. (From Jelks, G. W., Jelks, E. B., and Ruff, G.: Clinical and radiographic evaluation of the orbit. Otolaryngol. Clin. North Am., *21*:13, 1988.)

The size and shape should be documented by measuring the pupillary diameter in millimeters with the patient fixating at a distant object. Most pocket vision charts have pupil gauge charts for this purpose (see Fig. 33–11). Anisocoria (unequal pupil size) may be an indication of intracranial, orbital, or ocular pathology. An eccentrically located oval or slitlike pupil may be the result of a perforating injury to the globe.

The reactivity of each pupil to bright light should also be carefully evaluated. Note whether they react sluggishly or briskly. The swinging flashlight test is performed in looking for a relative afferent pupillary defect (RAPD), also known as a Marcus Gunn pupil. When one eye is stimulated by a bright light, there is an equal constricting response in both eyes owing to the direct and consensual light reflexes. There is decreased or no stimulation of the afferent visual system if there is a lesion interrupting the optic nerve, chiasm, or tract carrying the pupillary light fibers. Thus, when light is changed from a normal to an affected eye (impaired afferent visual pathway), there is a dilation of both pupils. When the light is moved back to the unaffected eye, both pupils constrict again. An RAPD usually is not caused by a cataract, but can be present with a dense vitreous hemorrhage or severe amblyopia.

Motility

The ability of the eyes to move in all directions is tested by having the patient follow the examiner's finger or a penlight held at a 45-degree angle to avoid glare. If the patient complains of diplopia, it is necessary to document the position of gaze in which it occurs and to determine whether it is associated with visual disturbances, pain, or systemic complaints. One should examine for diplopia in the primary (straight-ahead position) and in the cardinal positions of gaze: up and right, up and left, right, left, down and right, and down and left (see subsequent discussion).

When there is a question of mechanical restriction in a field of gaze, a forced duction test is performed to differentiate this from an extraocular muscle paresis. Several drops of a topical anesthetic are placed in the eye. A

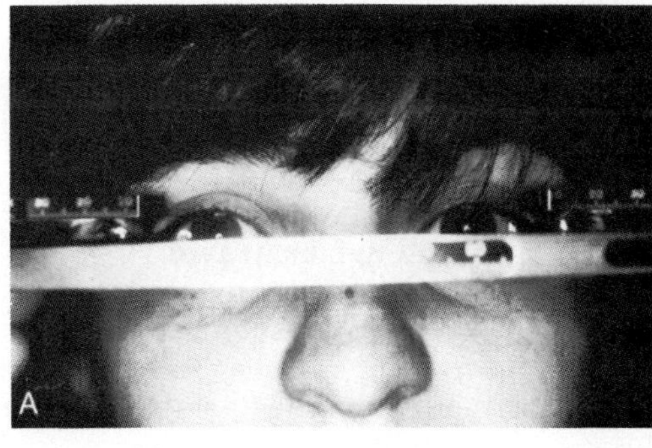

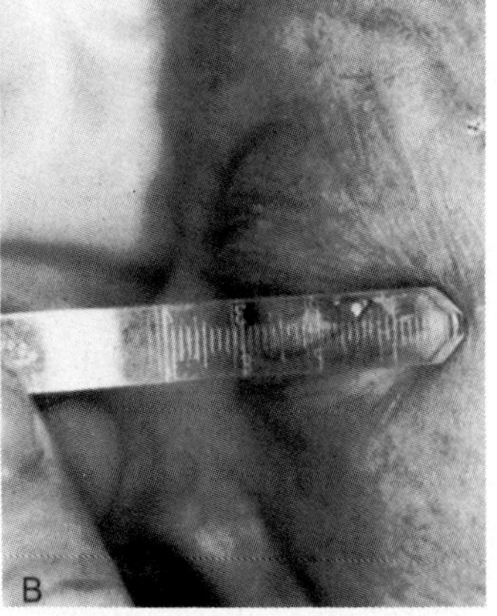

Figure 33–14. *A,* Determination of relative anterior projection of the globe by use of a Hertel exophthalmometer. *B,* Ludde exophthalmometer used to measure the anterior position of the ocular globe relative to the lateral orbital rim. (From Jelks, G. W., Jelks, E. B., and Ruff, G.: Clinical and radiographic evaluation of the orbit. Otolaryngol. Clin. North Am., *21*:13, 1988.)

small cotton pledget soaked in 10 per cent cocaine is placed over the muscle to be grasped for 1 minute. The patient is instructed to look in the field of decreased muscle function, the muscle is grasped through the conjunctiva with a fine-toothed forceps, and the globe is gently forced into the field of suspected restriction. If there is a notable resistance, the restriction is mechanical in etiology. Often the test must be performed on the fellow eye to determine the significance and magnitude of the restriction (see also Chap. 27).

Slit Lamp Examination

A slit lamp examination is used to evaluate the conjunctiva, cornea, anterior chamber, iris, and lens. If the anterior chamber is deepened, a ruptured globe with vitreous loss may have occurred. A tonometer on the slit lamp may be used to check the intraocular pressure.

Dilated Funduscopic Examination

Dilation is usually accomplished with 1 per cent tropicamide and 2.5 per cent phenylephrine solution instilled into the conjunctival sac. The direct ophthalmoscope provides 15 × magnification and should be used to study the clarity of the ocular media and the status of the optic nerve, and to determine any visible ocular pathology. The ophthalmologist will want to use the indirect ophthalmoscope for a complete view of the retina, looking for edema, hemorrhage, or other evidence of a pathologic condition.

RADIOGRAPHIC TECHNIQUES

Diagnostic strategies should keep pace with the latest technologic innovations. Improved imaging with diagnostic thin-slice computed tomography (CT), ultrasound (US), and magnetic resonance imaging (MRI) has modified existing diagnostic approaches for problem solving in orbital pathology. However, the selection of the appropriate modality and consideration of its utility and availability and the possibility of redundancy must be made with a firm grasp of the normal anatomy and the spectrum of potential pathology.

The diagnostic modalities considered below are plain roentgenograms, CT, US, angiography, and MRI; reformation of CT has supplanted multidirectional tomography and has achieved enhanced definition with less radiation exposure.

Plain Roentgenograms

The standard views of the orbit best delineate structures located tangential to the x-ray. To minimize distortion, the area of interest is placed closest to the film. The most useful radiographs for routine evaluation of the orbit are the Caldwell and Waters views (Fig. 33–15). When indicated, direct lateral, optic foramen, and submentovertex views may also be employed.

The Caldwell projection superimposes the petrous ridges on the maxilla, thereby depicting the medial, superior, and lateral aspects of the orbit and the crista galli. The orbital roof, as the floor of the anterior cranial fossa, is convoluted by the frontal lobes and is more clearly evaluated on CT. The greater wing of the sphenoid is readily visible as the temporal boundary of the superior orbital fissure, and creates the oblique or innominate line.

The Waters view (Fig. 33–15) is tangential to the orbital floor, projecting its posterior aspects below the inferior rim. The infraorbital canal can occasionally be seen, and because the petrous pyramids lie below the maxillary sinus, the foramen rotundum is often visible along the medial wall of the antrum.

The lateral radiographic view obscures orbital detail owing to the interposed ethmoid air cells; however, the sella turcica, clivus, sphenoid sinus, and cribriform plate are usually well demonstrated.

By virtue of their reliability, the relatively low cost, and the low radiation exposure, plain radiographs are recommended for screening a wide variety of orbital conditions (Rao and Gonzalez, 1986).

Computed Tomography

Computed tomography (CT) exploits the differential x-ray absorption of the orbital

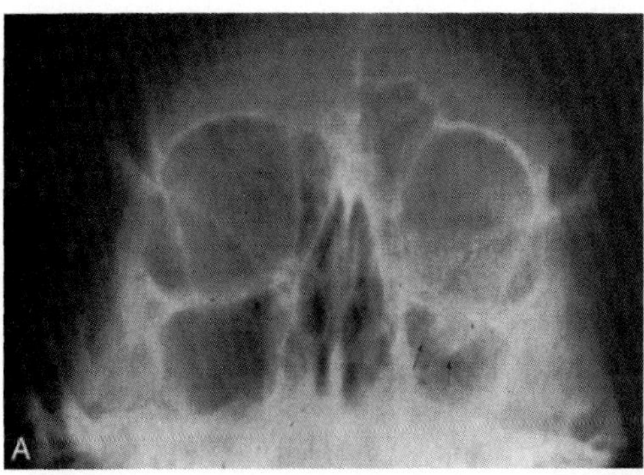

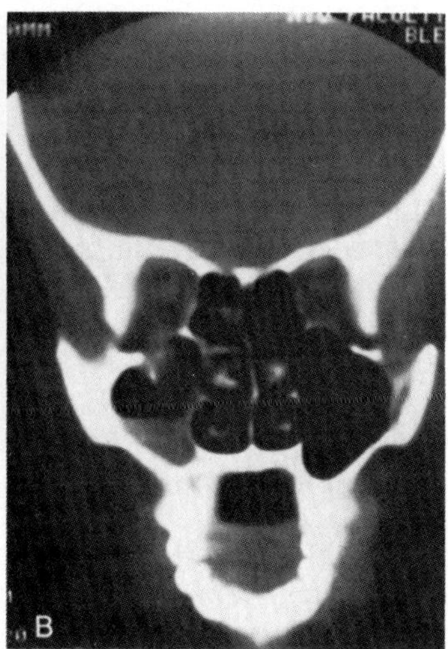

Figure 33–15. *A,* Waters view demonstrating the foramen rotundum (*asterisk*) on the right side along the medial wall of the maxillary antrum. Prolapse of orbital tissues into the left maxillary antrum is seen (*arrows*) owing to a pure orbital floor fracture. *B,* Coronal CT scan demonstrates a dehiscence in the left orbital floor, prolapse of the orbital contents, and fluid in the maxillary sinus. (From Jelks, G. W., Jelks, E. B., and Ruff, G.: Clinical and radiographic evaluation of the orbit. Otolaryngol. Clin. North Am., *21*:13, 1988.)

muscle and neurovascular tissues, which register a radiographic density of approximately 35 Hounsfield units, and the surrounding fat, which has a value of −100 Hounsfield units. The disparity in density permits clear demonstration of the orbital structures. With thin-slice CT imaging and computer software programs, reformatting in multiple planes and three-dimensional reconstruction is possible (Weinstein and associates, 1981). Intravenous contrast material may also be used to delinate vascular lesions (Hammerschlag, Hesselink, and Weber, 1983) (Fig. 33–16).

Computed tomography can define the ex-

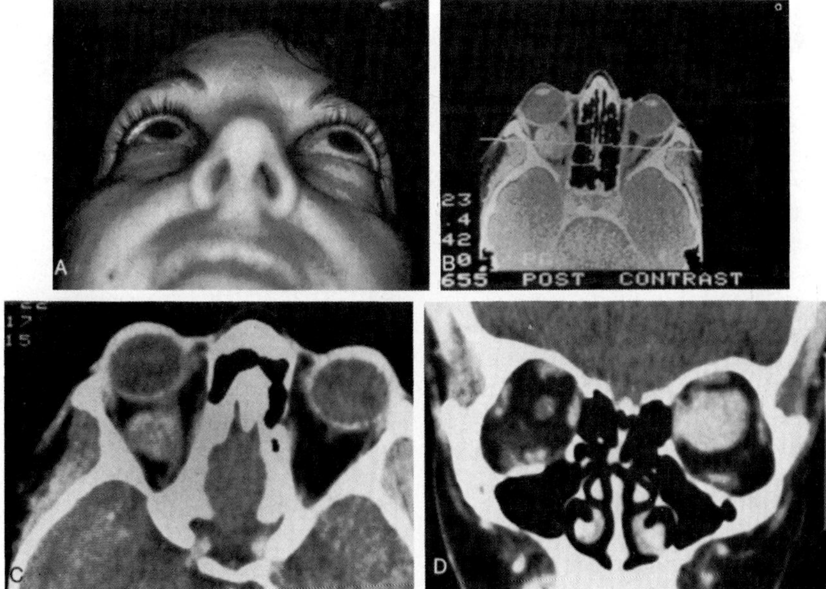

Figure 33–16. *A,* "Worm's eye" view of a patient with 6 mm of left ocular globe proptosis. *B* to *D,* CT scans demonstrating (contrast enhancing) a well-defined mass in the superolateral muscle cone without apical involvement. The optic nerve is displaced medially and there is minimal involvement of the optic nerve with the mass. The findings are typical of a cavernous hemangioma of the orbit. (From Jelks, G. W., Jelks, E. B., and Ruff, G.: Clinical and radiographic evaluation of the orbit. Otolaryngol. Clin. North Am., *21*:13, 1988.)

tent of a neoplastic process and characterize its tissue type. The clinical differentiation of an optic nerve sheath meningioma from optic nerve gliomas has been radiographically corroborated. A glioma causes fusiform enlargement with the isodense nerve indistinguishable from its sheath, whereas a meningioma is cylindrically hyperdense, creating a "railroad track" sign when visualized parallel to the optic nerve.

Computed tomography can diagnostically delineate variants of the idiopathic inflammation known as orbital pseudotumor. Dacryoadenitis, perineuritis, lymphoid hyperplasia, scleritis, and orbital myositis each manifest an increased density of the involved tissue owing to inflammatory edema. Distinct from this form of inflammatory edema, Graves' ophthalmopathy spares the tendinous extraocular muscle insertion and is bilateral in 90 per cent of cases (Enzmann, Donaldson, and Kriss, 1979).

Ultrasonography

Ultrasound (US) confers unique diagnostic capabilities in the heterogeneous milieu of the orbit. High frequency sound penetrates the various soft tissues of the orbit, and that portion reflected by the tissue is recorded, providing an accurate measure of the distance and consistency of the tissues. The A and B modes depict one and two dimensions, respectively. Both plot time as an index of distance along the path of the ultrasound beam. The second parameter is the distance perpendicular to the beam for the B-scan, and the amplitude for the echo of the A mode.

With this noninvasive modality, four patterns of internal reflectivity can be distinguished: (1) cysts exhibit large amplitudes corresponding to their walls; (2) solid masses show an exponential time decay; (3) hemangiomas display consistently high, regularly spaced, internal echoes or reflectivity; and (4) hemorrhage elicits much lower ultrasonic amplitudes.

Ultrasonic resolution increases from 1.0 mm at 5 MHz to 0.07 mm at 20 MHz, sacrificing the depth of penetration for sensitivity of resolution (Dallow, 1986). The eye contains recognizable interfaces at the cornea, iris, lens, and retina. Like the aqueous humor of the anterior chamber and the vitreous gel posteriorly, the crystalline structure of the lens is anechoic unless a cataract is present. The orbital fat exhibits a solid pattern on the A-scan, whereas the muscles and optic nerve are relatively homogeneous and generate few A-scan reflections. The differentiation in each pattern allows evaluation of subtle differences at the interface of these tissues.

Ultrasonography is unsurpassed for intraocular evaluation when opacification of the lens is present and precludes direct observation of the posterior globe. Vitreous membrane formation and retinal or choroidal detachment are routinely well delineated as causes of visual loss. Foreign bodies of high density are readily seen if they project one side perpendicular to the beam. Each of the four most common intraocular tumors presents a characteristic pattern. Melanomas and metastases show rapid attenuation of closely spaced echoes on A-scan. On B-scan the former typically indent the posterior globe and grow in a polypoid configuration, and the latter remain flat and may be multicentric. Hemangiomas are benign and indolent, and project little above the choroid from which they arise. The A-scan echoes are of a regular texture and high amplitude. Retinoblastomas undergo necrosis and hemorrhage, with associated retinal detachment and calcification contributing to a heterogeneous signal with high amplitude echoes. US clearly distinguishes neoplastic invasion from inflammation largely because of the reliability with which it can characterize edematous fat with its characteristic ultrasonic features.

The ability to discriminate cystic, solid, angiomatous, and infiltrative tissues commends US as an adjunct in the diagnosis of orbital pathology (Fig. 33–17).

Angiography

Angiography (Fig. 33–18) utilizes intraluminal visualization by the injection of contrast material to illustrate the vascular arborizations. Well-perfused regions are assessed directly, and interferences in perfusion are demonstrated by displacement of the normal vascular architecture.

The ophthalmic artery arises as the first branch of the internal carotid artery and courses through the optic canal inferior to the nerve. Upon entering the orbit, it crosses the optic nerve superiorly to supply the eye and ocular adnexa (Zide and Jelks, 1985). Its

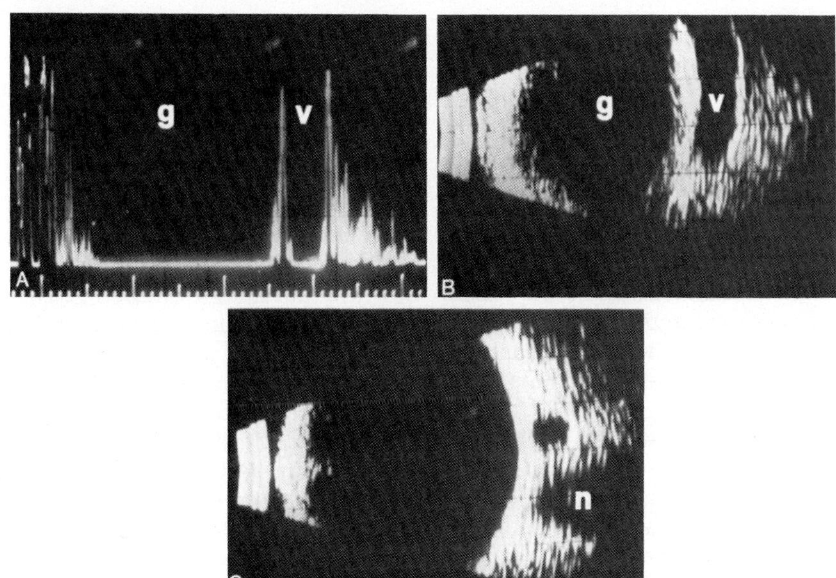

Figure 33–17. Transocular A- and B-scans of a dilated superior ophthalmic vein. *A,* A-scan revealing an echoic intraocular globe (g) followed by medium range echo of the posterior aspect of the globe, and very high peaks of the anterior and posterior walls of the dilated ophthalmic vein (v). *B, C,* B-scans of a dilated vessel (v) in longitudinal (*B*) and cross-sectional (*C*) views. The optic nerve echo shadow (n) is seen in *C.* (Courtesy of Richard Koplin, M.D.) (From Jelks, G. W., Jelks, E. B., and Ruff, G.: Clinical and radiographic evaluation of the orbit. Otolaryngol. Clin. North Am., *21*:13, 1988.)

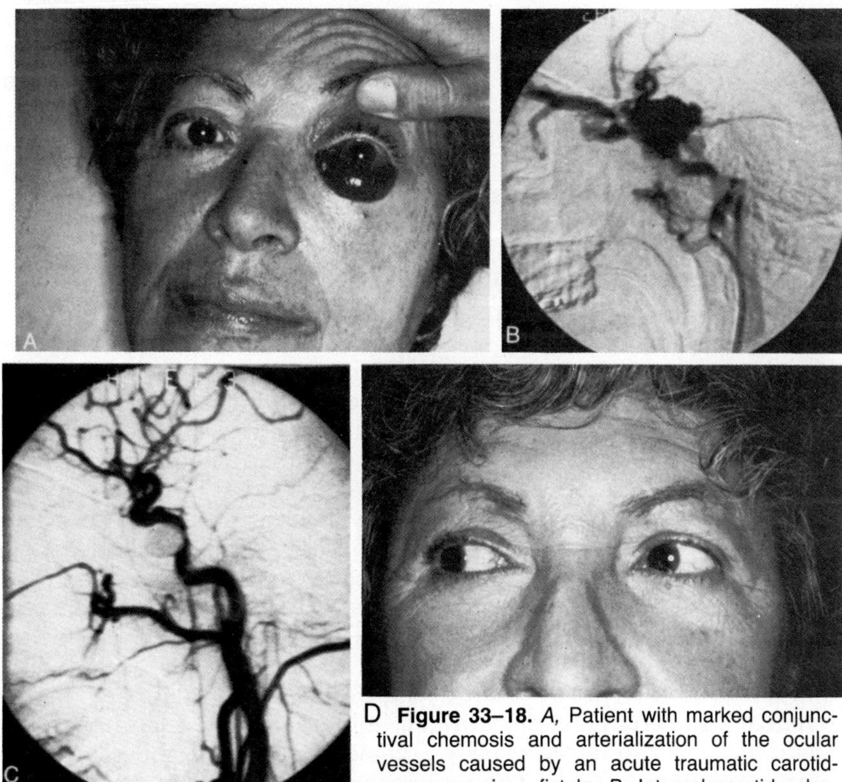

Figure 33–18. *A,* Patient with marked conjunctival chemosis and arterialization of the ocular vessels caused by an acute traumatic carotid-cavernous sinus fistula. *B,* Internal carotid selective, subtraction angiography demonstrating a high flow carotid-cavernous sinus fistula and associated dilation of the superior ophthalmic veins. *C,* Balloon occlusion of the fistula and normalization of the vascular patterns. *D,* Patient six weeks after angiographic balloon occlusion of the carotid-cavernous sinus fistula, showing resolution of the vascular ocular and orbital congestion. (Courtesy of Alejandro Berenstein, M.D., N.Y.U. Medical Center. From Jelks, G. W., Jelks, E. B., and Ruff, G.: Clinical and radiographic evaluation of the orbit. Otolaryngol. Clin. North Am., *21*:13, 1988.)

first branch is the lacrimal artery, which forms an anastomosis with the recurrent middle meningeal artery within the superior orbital fissure. This anatomic finding is angiographically important, because the meningeal artery may be the main arterial source to the eye and orbit in a small, albeit significant number of individuals (Handle and associates, 1973). Therefore, angiography may be necessary before the sacrifice of the lacrimal arterial connections to the orbit during an extirpation procedure.

The most common suprasellar masses are (1) pituitary adenoma, (2) cerebral arterial aneurysm, (3) meningioma, and (4) craniopharyngioma, which present with similar CT characteristics but different angiographic findings. The surgical approach may possibly be altered by the preoperative angiographic evaluation. Because a pituitary adenoma can readily be resected by a transsphenoidal approach, arteriographic diagnosis may obviate the need for a craniotomy (Zimmerman and Russell, 1986).

Magnetic Resonance Imaging

Magnetic resonance imaging (MRI) promises greater discrimination than other modalities because it characterizes tissues using a four-parameter analysis, whereas CT recognizes only electron density, and US distinguishes only attenuation and velocity of sound waves. The lack of ionizing radiation, the potential for spectroscopic analysis, and three-dimensional and real-time imaging promote the use of this format for orbital examination.

Elemental nuclei with odd numbers of protons or neutrons generate a magnetic moment as they spin, a process similar to a wobbling top about a randomly oriented axis. The hydrogen atom is the most biologically abundant when compared with the other elements contained in the human body, namely, C^{13}, N^{14}, F^{19}, Na^{23}, and P^{31}. Quantum mechanics dictate that nuclei equilibrate in two energy states, the excited and the ground state, with a slight preponderance for the latter at body temperature. MRI exploits the fact that those nuclei in the ground state align their axes with a magnetic field, whereas excited nuclei oppose it (arbitrarily designated as 0 degrees and 180 degrees, respectively, in the Z axis). Their procession projects a component vector in the X-Y plane perpendicular to the Z axis. Ground-state nuclei are excited by electromagnetic radiation delivered at a frequency equal to their rate of procession. The Larmor relation states that the resonant frequency equals the field strength divided by a constant for any particular element. During resonance the individual magnetic moments progress in phase and thus acquire a net X-Y component. Upon cessation of the radiofrequency (RF) pulse, the acquired energy is emitted, providing an MRI signal.

The portion dispersed as heat is known as spin-lattice relaxation. This restores the Z-axis component in the direction of the ground state over time, conventionally known as T1. The energy is transferred magnetically to unexcited protons and generates heat in dissimilar elements. Magnetic exchange between protons or spin-spin relaxation results in loss of phase coherence and hence reduction of the X-Y component over time (T2). The resultant MRI signal, therefore, represents the effects on the proton density and tissue T1 and T2 characteristics. These variables are manipulated to enhance the disparity between normal and pathologic tissues when the resultant signal is displayed on a black-to-white or "gray" scale (Pavlicek, Modik, and Weinstein, 1984). Tissues differ in spin-lattice and spin-spin relaxation, which increase and decrease, respectively, in an exponential fashion when measured along their corresponding axes.

The duration and amplitude of the RF pulse can be varied to induce resonance and excite sufficient protons to deflect and thus be recorded. Proton density can be assessed when tissue relaxation differences are small and signal strengths large. The normal MRI contrast of periorbital structures ranges from the most intense (fat) to the least (the sinuses), which (like bone) have a relative paucity of protons. The soft tissues of the orbit, however, have a spectrum of proton densities that vary only 10 per cent, and thus relaxation differences offer the greatest degree of tissue discrimination. Water manifests long relaxation times under MRI, reflecting a high rate of molecular collisions. As protein content increases, the relaxation times are attenuated.

The degree of tissue organization is helpful in allowing differentiation at the MRI level by emphasizing the T1 or T2 image. The lens contains 35 per cent protein and the vitreous only 1 per cent. Electronic emphasizing of T1 generates a greater signal and hence a brighter image for the lens. By accentuating the more rapid T2 relaxation of the lens, it appears correspondingly darker than the vitreous on T2-weighted scans. Even the liquid cerebrospinal fluid (CSF) can be distinguished from the vitreous gel on the basis of T2 differences despite similar protein content. Fat exhibits a short T1 and moderate T2, whereas more solid tissues such as sclera and cornea have a longer T1 and short T2. The latter two structures have a low water content and, thus, low protein density, a property that renders them relatively dark with any pulse sequence.

Pathologic processes are readily discerned amid the strong MRI contrasts normally present within the orbit. MRI is superior to CT in demonstrating intracranial extensions of mass lesions (Fig. 33–19) (Haik, Saint-Louis, and Smith, 1985). As a group, neoplasms generate a brighter T1-weighted image than does vitreous. The ability of MRI to distinguish intraocular melanomas with amazing accuracy demonstrates the capability of MRI to detect subtle changes in chemical composition. The loosely bound electrons in the melanin pigment are paramagnetic, which promotes relaxation. Thus, densely pigmented tumors present dark images with T2 weighting. However, MRI may fail to distinguish retinoblastomas when their only ab-

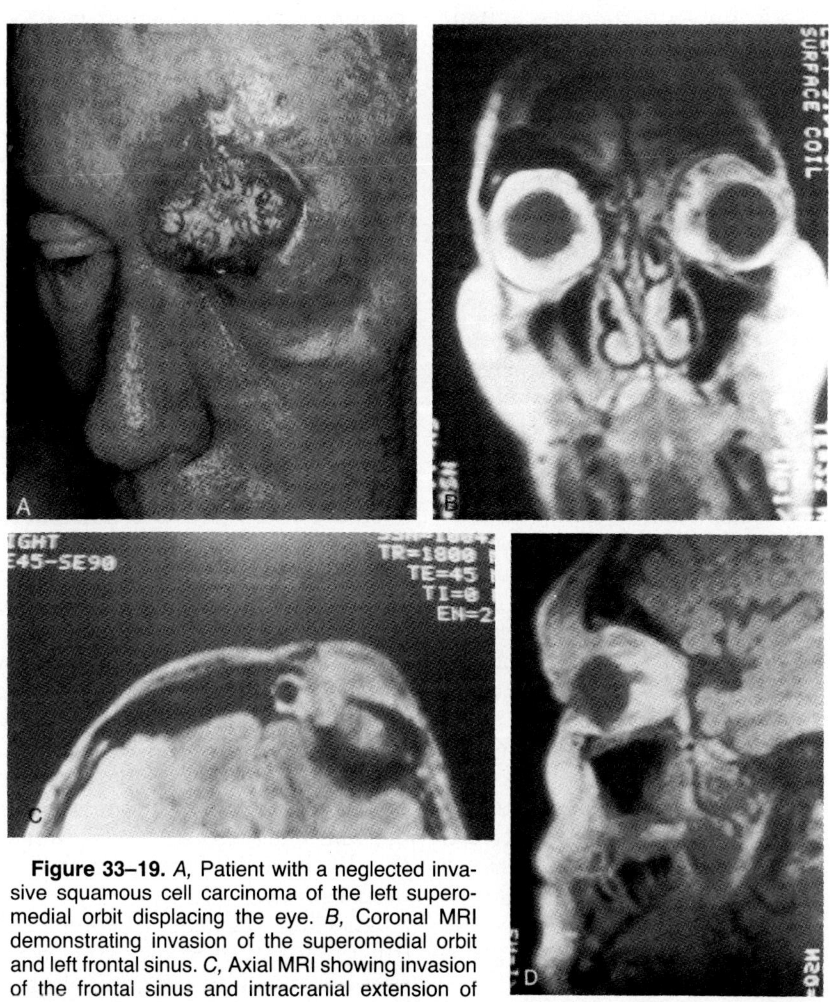

Figure 33–19. *A,* Patient with a neglected invasive squamous cell carcinoma of the left superomedial orbit displacing the eye. *B,* Coronal MRI demonstrating invasion of the superomedial orbit and left frontal sinus. *C,* Axial MRI showing invasion of the frontal sinus and intracranial extension of the tumor. *D,* Lateral MRI showing tumor filling the frontal sinus and invading the orbital tissues. (From Jelks, G. W., Jelks, E. B., and Ruff, G.: Clinical and radiographic evaluation of the orbit. Otolaryngol. Clin. North Am., *21*:13, 1988.)

normality is punctate calcification. Neoplastic erosion of bone and even the sclera is well visualized because of the contrast their low MRI signal affords (Fig. 33–19).

Inflammatory changes accompanied by edema substantially alter relaxation times. In orbital pseudotumor the image intensity of the retrobulbar fat is reduced on both T1- and T2-weighted studies. Demyelination is a process in which loss of intraneural lipid occurs, and this is reflected on the MRI as prolonged relaxation. The unique ability of MRI to detect demyelinated plaques recommends it for the diagnosis of optic neuritis and other demyelinating processes (Brant-Zawadski and associates, 1983). Low flow or acutely clotted blood exhibits a long T2 compared with CSF but a slightly shorter T1. The paramagnetic effect of methemoglobin alters the MRI so that acute and subacute hemorrhages produce bright images on both T1- and T2-accentuated scans. With resorption of the blood components, the remaining fluid resembles the MRI signal of CSF. These MRI characteristics allow detection of bleeding into a lymphangioma or other structure. Furthermore, accurate differentiation of a hemorrhagic from an exudative retinal detachment can be made.

Nuclear magnetic resonance (NMR) signals are produced by placing patients in a strong magnetic field and preexciting their nuclei by passing a strong RF and electromagnetic field through them. Virtually all MRI uses excitation of the hydrogen atom, because of its presence in such large quantities in the body (65 per cent water). Soft tissue contrast is higher in MRI than in CT scans. The intensity and/or diagnostic contrasts of MRI scans may be varied, depending on the method of signal generation (T1- or T2-weighted images). Another advantage of the MRI scan is the ability to obtain coronal views by electronic manipulation without the need for radiation or awkward positioning. Furthermore, the visualization of blood-containing systems can be imaged without the injection of contrast material. In addition, because bone produces virtually no NMR signal, areas of the body surrounded by bone, e.g., the orbital contents, can be examined in great detail.

The disadvantages of MRI are that it currently requires a great deal of time per examination and the patient must remain motionless during the study. MRI is also contraindicated in the evaluation of the orbit for metallic foreign bodies (Lagouros and associates, 1987; Zheutlin, Thompson, and Shofner, 1987). CT has scan times of approximately five to ten seconds per slice; MRI requires three to eight minutes per slice. In addition, the resolution of CT scanning is currently at 1 to 1.5 mm per computed slice. MRI, with its increased time, currently has a resolution of 5 to 12 mm per slice. However, the use of surface magnetic coils may help to overcome this gap in technology.

SURGICAL PRINCIPLES

The first concern in orbital surgery is protection of the cornea from desiccation and trauma during the operative procedure. Plastic contact protective shells should be used to protect the corneas on both sides (Fig. 33–20).

In like fashion the corneas should also be protected in the postoperative period. At the conclusion of the operation the conjunctival sac should be liberally irrigated with a balanced salt solution to clear any foreign body. An ophthalmic ointment should also be instilled to lubricate the cornea.

An *occlusive suture* (Fig. 33–21) provides corneal protection, and if secured by tape to the forehead it supports the lower eyelid. The latter function is especially important since repeated incisions in the lower eyelid tend to result in lid retraction.

A double-armed 4–0 silk suture is passed sequentially through the gray line of the upper lid, in a horizontal mattress suture fashion through the gray line of the lower lid, and finally through the upper lid (Fig. 33–21). The suture is tied and can be secured to the forehead, as previously mentioned, to provide vertical support to the lower eyelid.

A *tarsorrhaphy* (formation of a lid adhesion), although extensively used in the past to ensure occlusion of the eyelids, should be condemned because it permanently deforms the lid margins and carries a high rate of dehiscence.

Another method of occlusive suture is a continuous, buried suture between the upper and lower eyelid margins (Fig. 33–22). The suture may be left in place for many weeks and is as effective as the tarsorrhaphy in maintaining lid occlusion without causing damage to the lid margins.

Figure 33–20. Protective lens being inserted into the conjunctival sac. A transparent lens is shown in the photograph in order to allow the sclera and the cornea to be seen through the lens. Colored lenses are preferable, since there is less risk of forgetting to remove them postoperatively and thus risking corneal abrasion.

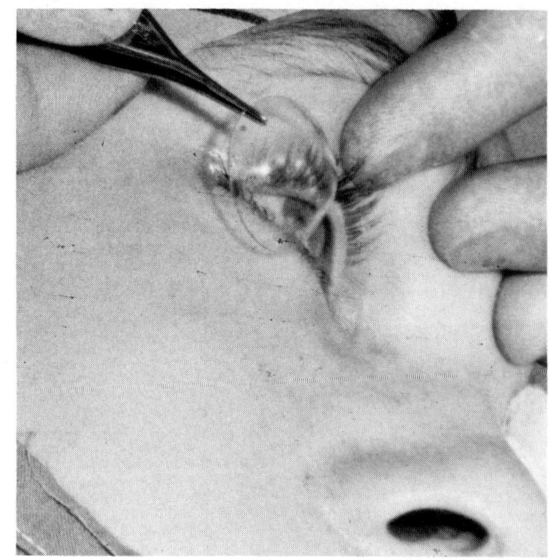

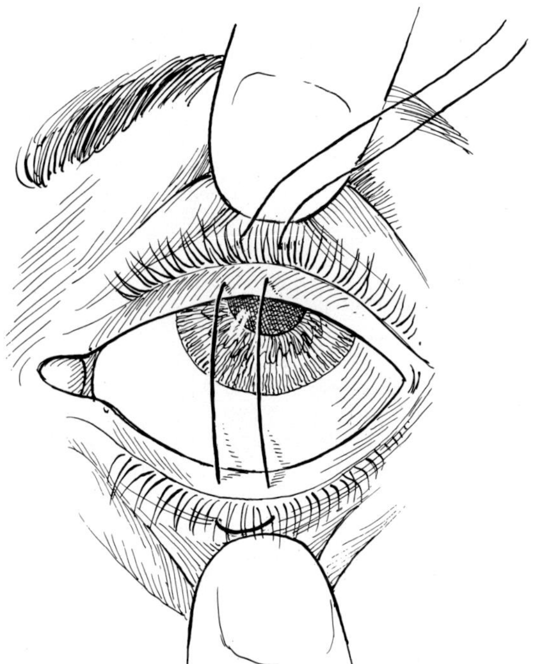

Figure 33–21. Occlusive suture used to prevent opening of the palpebral fissure and corneal abrasion. It can be suspended to the forehead to support the lower eyelid.

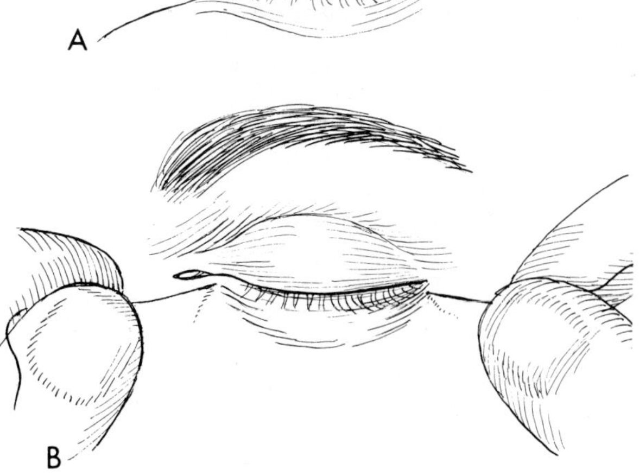

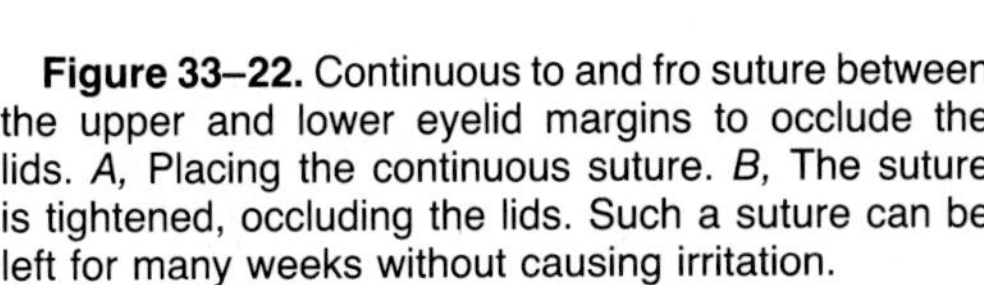

Figure 33–22. Continuous to and fro suture between the upper and lower eyelid margins to occlude the lids. *A,* Placing the continuous suture. *B,* The suture is tightened, occluding the lids. Such a suture can be left for many weeks without causing irritation.

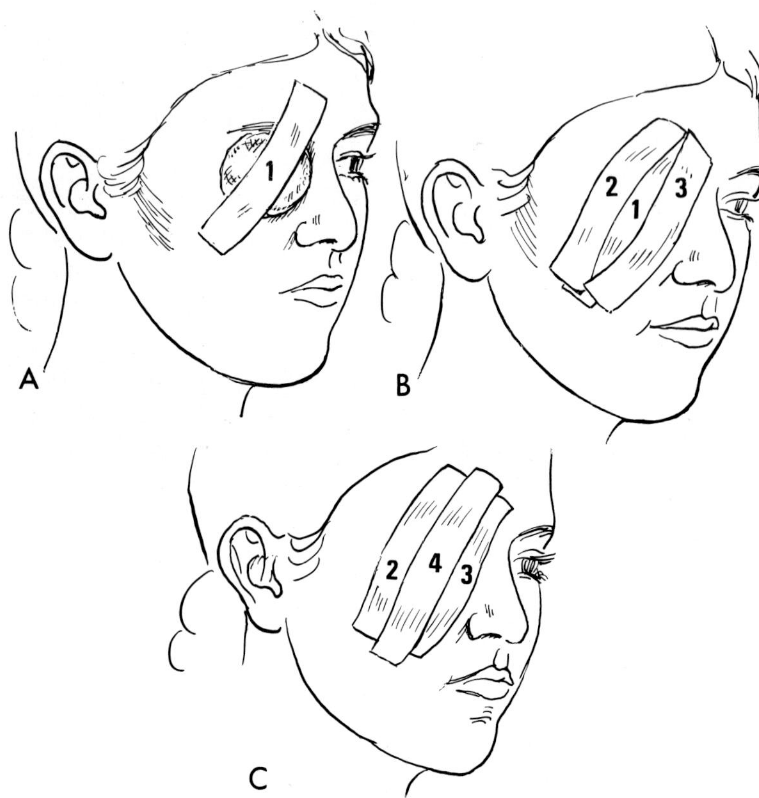

Figure 33–23. The eye dressing. *A,* An eye pad has been placed over the orbital region and is maintained in place with a strip of paper tape. *B, C,* The dressing is reinforced with additional tape. A moderately compressive pressure dressing may be placed over the eye pad and maintained by a head bandage when required.

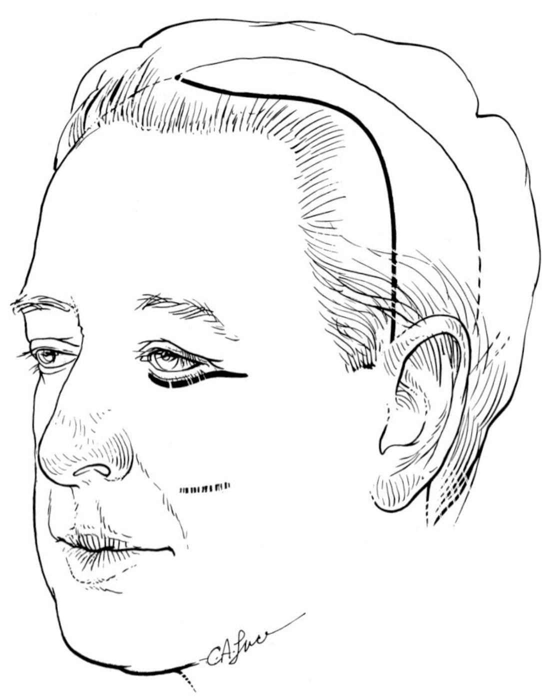

Figure 33–24. Various incisions for exposure of the orbit and zygoma: bicoronal, transcutaneous eyelid, and buccovestibular (*interrupted line*). The transconjunctival-lateral canthal incision is not illustrated.

It should be emphasized that, as a principle, sutures should be inserted in the eyelids, conjunctiva, and lid margins so that the knots and suture ends do not cause corneal abrasion. Skin grafts should not be placed in the conjunctival sac if they are in contact with the cornea; only conjunctiva or other mucosal tissue is tolerated by the cornea.

If a dressing is employed, it should be meticulously applied (Fig. 33–23). If a pressure dressing is used, a lid occlusive suture should first be inserted.

Surgical Approaches

There are multiple surgical approaches to the orbit. The *bicoronal incision* (Fig. 33–24), popularized by Tessier, provides wide access to the orbits, nose, and zygomas as well as the cranium. It is the preferred incision for extensive orbital surgery, especially when the roof of the orbit must be visualized and the orbital contents must be mobilized 360 degrees. It has obvious disadvantages in patients with male pattern baldness and in black patients with short curly hair.

There are multiple *eyelid incisions*. Converse, Cole, and Smith (1961) popularized a steplike *transcutaneous* lower eyelid incision (Fig. 33–25*A*). The incision, extending from the punctum to the lateral canthus, is made approximately 3 mm below the lid margin and is carried only through the skin. The dissection is made in an inferior direction over the orbicularis muscle. Below the tarsus the orbicularis is incised along the width of the incision until the septum orbitale is clearly identified (Fig. 33–25*B,C*). The dissection is carried on the septum orbitale in an inferior direction until a point is reached approximately 2 mm below the inferior orbital rim. The periosteum is incised and elevated from the rim and floor of the orbit (Fig. 33–25*D*). Through this incision one can gain access to the lateral and medial walls and floor of the orbit as well as the anterior wall of the maxilla and zygoma (Fig. 33–26).

The *transconjunctival* incision was advocated by Tessier (1973) for the correction of

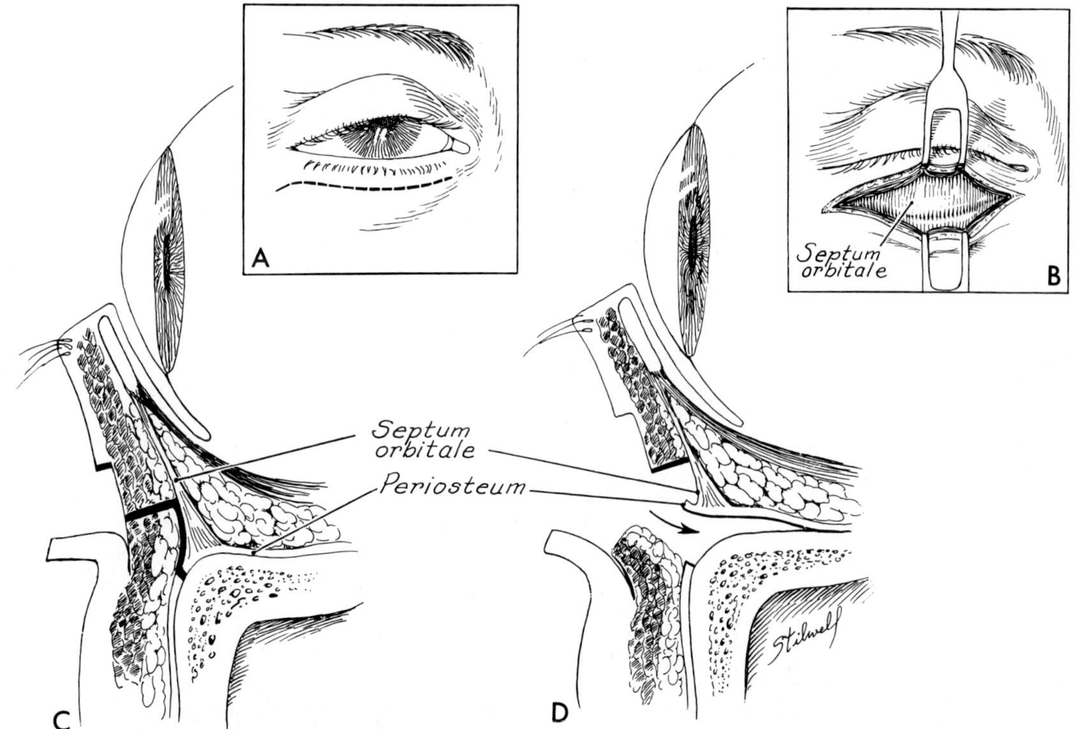

Figure 33–25. Technique of the transcutaneous eyelid incision and exposure of the orbital floor. *A,* Outline of the eyelid incision. *B,* Septum orbitale exposed. *C,* Sagittal section showing the skin incision through the orbicularis oculi muscle and the path of dissection over the septum orbitale to the orbital rim. *D,* Periosteum of the orbit (periorbita) is raised from the orbital floor. (From Converse, J. M., Cole, J. G., and Smith, B.: Late treatment of blowout fracture of the floor of the orbit. A case report. Plast. Reconstr. Surg., *28*:183, 1961.)

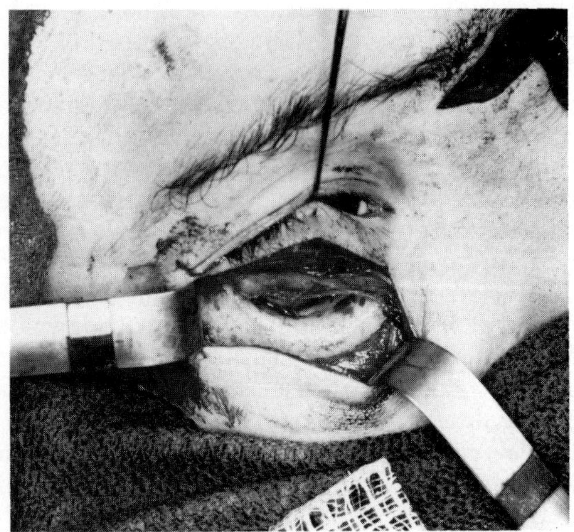

Figure 33–26. Exposure obtained through a transcutaneous eyelid incision.

congenital orbital deformities and by Converse and associates (1973) for post-traumatic deformities. The incision can take either a *preseptal* or a *retroseptal* route as illustrated in Figure 33–27.

A simplified technique employed by Tenzel and Miller (1971) consists of a direct incision in the fornix that reaches the orbital rim and a retroseptal approach that exposes the orbital fat. A Desmarres retractor is used to retract the lower eyelid away from the globe. A malleable retractor placed posterior to the orbital rim gives adequate exposure (Fig. 33–28). The incision is made through the conjunctiva, capsulopalpebral fascia (lid retractors), and periosteum of the orbital rim. This incision directly exposes the orbital fat without incising the septum orbitale. Tenzel and Miller employed this type of incision in patients who had small blow-out fractures without restriction of ocular rotary movements of the globe. They did not employ the incision in patients with massive fractures and herniation of the orbital contents into the maxillary sinus.

The conjunctival incision avoids an external scar, albeit an inconspicuous one, and claims have been made that it prevents postoperative lower lid lagophthalmos in the upward gaze.

Because of the need to preserve the orbital fat and recover fat that has extruded into the maxillary sinus, it is preferable to avoid extrusion of fat through the septum orbitale, whenever possible.

McCord and Moses (1979) described a combined lateral canthal (cutaneous) and inferior fornix (conjunctival) incision that can give exposure of all four walls of the orbit (Fig. 33–29).

The *lateral brow* incision (Fig. 33–30) provides exposure of the frontozygomatic suture and part of the lateral wall and roof of the orbit. If it is carefully placed, an inconspicuous scar results. *Medial canthal* incisions (Fig. 33–30) are usually made in a curvilinear direction. They give excellent exposure of the medial canthus, the medial wall of the orbit, and the nasal bones. The quality of the resulting scar is unpredictable and the need for this type of incision is often obviated when a bicoronal incision is used. The *intraoral ap-*

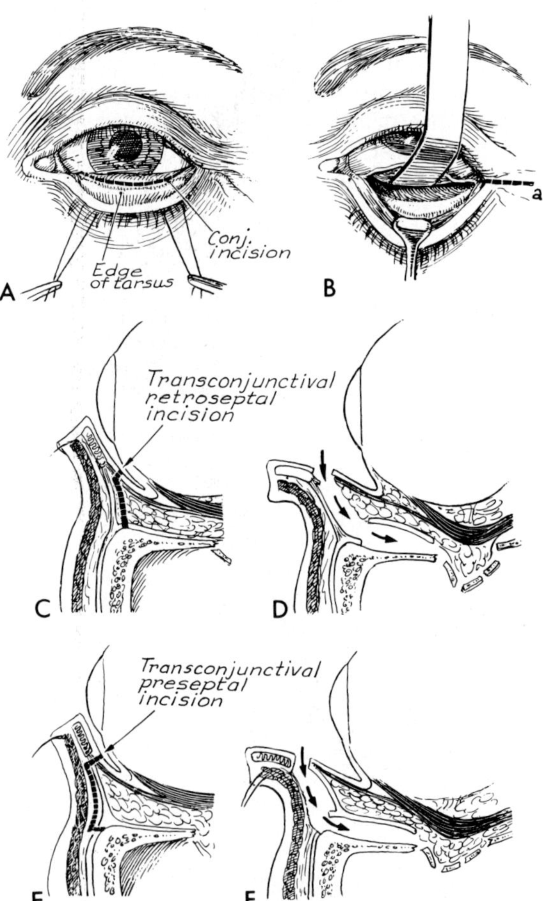

Figure 33–27. Transconjunctival approach. *A,* Conjunctival incision below the lower border of the tarsus. *B,* Subperiosteal exposure of the orbital floor. Dotted line shows the lateral canthal extension for additional exposure. *C,* Retroseptal approach. *D,* Sagittal view of the retroseptal approach to the fracture. *E,* Preseptal incision. *F,* Sagittal view of the preseptal approach to the fracture.

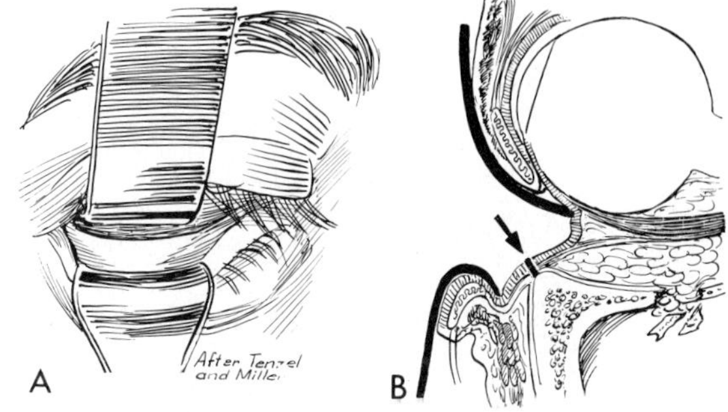

Figure 33–28. The direct conjunctival approach to the orbital floor. *A,* One retractor displaces the globe; another depresses the lower lid. The infraorbital rim protrudes under the conjunctiva. *B,* The conjunctiva is incised, exposing the orbital rim.

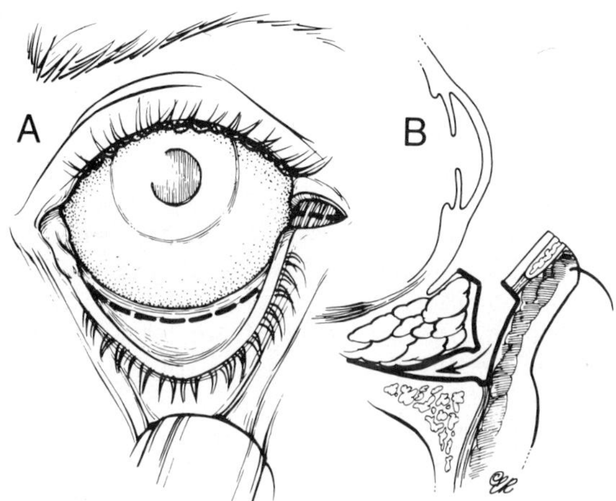

Figure 33–29. *A,* Schematic representation of lateral canthotomy, lateral cantholysis, and subtarsal transconjunctival incisions. *B,* Sagittal view demonstrating the preseptal approach to the inferior orbital rim. (From Jelks, J. W., and La Trenta, G.: Orbital fractures. *In* Foster, C. A., and Sherman, J. E. (Eds.): Surgery of Facial Bone Fractures. New York, Churchill Livingstone, 1987, p. 80.)

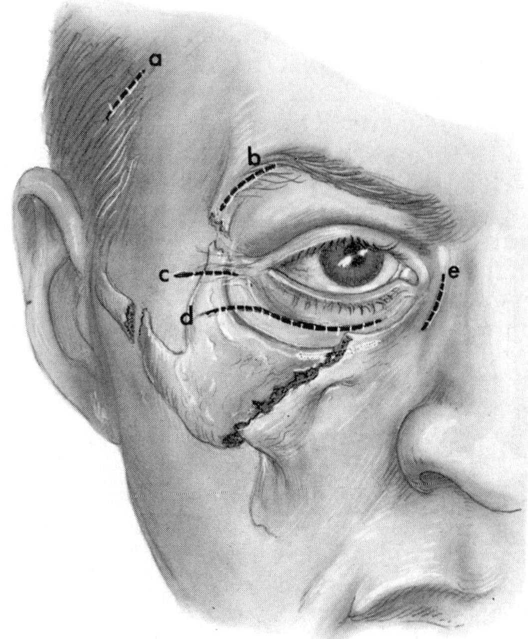

Figure 33–30. Various incisions for orbital exposure. a = Gillies; b = lateral brow; c = lateral canthal; d = transcutaneous eyelid; e = medial canthal. A coronal scalp flap may also be indicated for extensive defects.

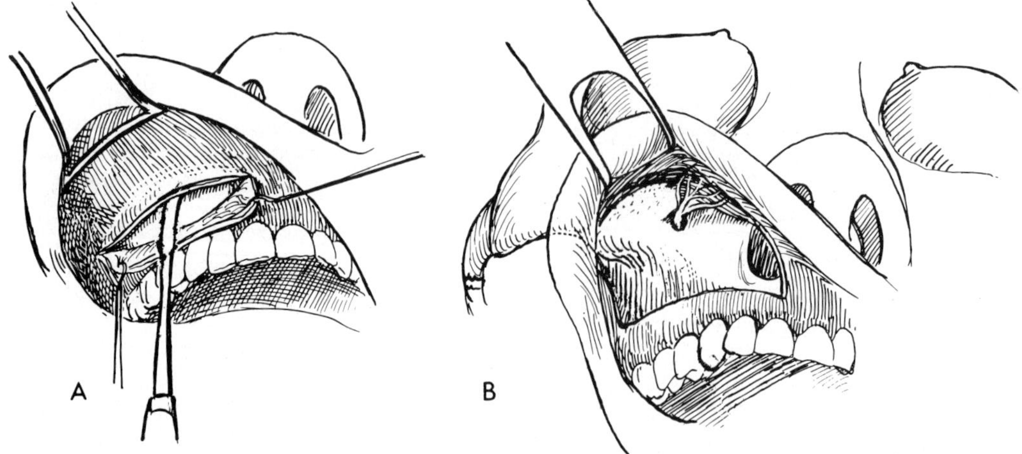

Figure 33–31. Intraoral approach to the inferior orbital rim, maxilla, and zygoma. *A,* The incision through the mucosa has been made on the labial aspect of the oral vestibule. *B,* The periosteum has been incised and elevated. The subperiosteal exposure has been extended to the inferior orbital rim. The subperiosteal exposure is also extended medially to the edge of the piriform aperture and laterally over the zygoma.

proach (Fig. 33–31) gives excellent exposure of the zygoma, maxilla, and inferior orbital rim.

MALUNITED FRACTURES OF THE ORBIT AND ZYGOMA

High speed motor vehicle collisions are the most common cause of severe comminuted fractures involving the upper portion of the midface, the orbits, and the intervening structures. Because this area of the face contains important functional structures, patients who have not received expert early treatment may be left with a gross deformity. Inadequate primary treatment (see Chap. 27) of an orbital fracture, including failure to restore the skeletal anatomy, can contribute to a residual orbital deformity and disorganization of the intraorbital contents. Disruption of the lacrimal apparatus, diplopia, and enophthalmos are frequent sequelae of malunited orbital fractures.

Roof (Fronto-orbital)

Fractures of the roof of the orbit usually involve the prominent supraorbital ridge, frontal bone, and frontal sinus. Traumatic defects are seen particularly in the thin portion of the orbital plate of the frontal bone situated in the medial aspect of the orbital roof. Enophthalmos and the transmission of brain pulsations to the ocular globe are signs of such a defect when it is of moderate size. Exophthalmos may result from massive herniation of the brain into the orbit in large defects of the roof.

Large orbital roof defects are repaired through an intracranial approach similar to that employed for the treatment of orbital hypertelorism (Merville and associates, 1983). The anatomic details of the defect can be assessed preoperatively by three-dimensional CT scan.

An area of frontal bone sufficient to provide exposure is resected. The frontal lobe is raised, the area of elevation remaining lateral to the cribriform plate. A plane of cleavage usually is readily found between the dura and periorbita. A thin bone graft (calvaria or ilium) is carefully wired within the defect. The frontal bone segment is replaced into the frontal defect.

A small defect can be repaired through an orbital approach. An incision is made immediately below the supraorbital rim. The periorbita is raised until the defect is reached, and the periorbita is separated from the dura over the extent of the defect. The dura is also separated over the intracranial surface of the bone along the edge of the defect by an angulated elevator. A thin bone graft is placed into the defect, bridging over the defect and resting on the anterior cranial fossa. In general the intracranial approach is preferred because of the exposure and safety associated with the technique.

The trochlea of the superior oblique muscle is often damaged owing to its proximity with the surface of the roof and contact with the bone fragment. Transitory diplopia usually results from this specific injury.

The sixth cranial nerve may also be traumatized in orbital injuries, resulting in paralysis of the lateral rectus muscle and limitation of ocular abduction. A period of at least six months should elapse to allow for recovery before corrective muscle surgery is undertaken.

Floor and Medial and Lateral Walls

Deformities and functional impairment are late complications that can be prevented by early diagnosis and treatment; however, primary treatment is often inadequate and the skeletal anatomy is not restored. Modern surgical principles of orbital fracture treatment have been established by Merville and associates (1983), Gruss (1985), and Manson (1986a,b) (see Chap. 27). Occasionally, despite early treatment of the orbital fracture, progressive ocular muscle imbalance and enophthalmos ensue.

These patients show a variety of deformities and functional disturbances: impairment of oculorotary action with resultant diplopia, enophthalmos (Fig. 33–32), depression of the zygomatic prominence, ptosis of the upper eyelid, downward displacement of the orbital contents, medial canthal deformities, reduction of the horizontal dimensions of the palpebral fissure, shortening of the vertical dimension of the lower eyelid, saddle nose deformity, widening of the nasal bone bridge, and occasionally deformities of the supraorbital arch.

Functional disturbances may include diminution of vision and blindness or loss of the eye. Blindness or eye loss is remarkably infrequent, in view of the severity of some of the injuries sustained. Epiphora resulting from interruption of the continuity of the lacrimal apparatus and cystic dilatation of the lacrimal sac (mucocele) require treatment. Lacerations through the eyelids may result in severe structural disorganization and may sever the canaliculi, the medial canthal tendon, or the levator palpebrae superioris.

True ptosis of the upper eyelid is to be differentiated from pseudoptosis resulting from the downward displacement of the globe and enophthalmos. True ptosis results from loss of function of the levator palpebrae superioris muscle after transection of the muscle or the aponeurosis, intramuscular hematoma causing subsequent fibrosis, or an injury to the third cranial nerve.

The most frequent and severe sequelae of inadequately treated fractures of the orbital floor are *diplopia* and *enophthalmos*.

DIPLOPIA

Permanent diplopia is usually produced by interference with the oculorotary mechanism as a result of entrapment of orbital structures in orbital fractures. The patient has diplopia because he is unable to rotate the affected eye in various directions. The degree of diplopia is dependent on the degree of oculorotary disturbance. Thus, in the patient shown in Figure 33–32, inability to rotate the ocular globe resulted in diplopia except when the patient compensated by tilting her head backward and looking toward the left. Relief of this type of diplopia is obtained by releasing the orbital contents from the area of entrapment and repairing the orbital defect.

Many fractures of the orbital floor occur without blow-out fracture. In most zygomatic fractures and fractures involving the rim of the orbit without blow-out fracture, diplopia is transitory and is attributed to hematoma causing muscular imbalance by elevating the ocular globe, or to injury of the extraocular musculature temporarily affecting the oculorotary mechanism. In patients with malunited fracture of the zygoma that involves separation of the frontozygomatic suture and downward displacement of the orbital floor, a period of transitory diplopia occurs. A remarkable degree of binocular fusion can compensate for the displacement of the ocular globe, permitting single vision. Most of these patients complain of diplopia only when fatigued.

Malunited depressed fractures of the orbital floor are frequently accompanied by restriction of upward gaze (Fig. 33–32). The eye cannot be rotated upward with the forced duction test. Trauma and fracture affect the extraocular muscles by causing edema, ecchy-

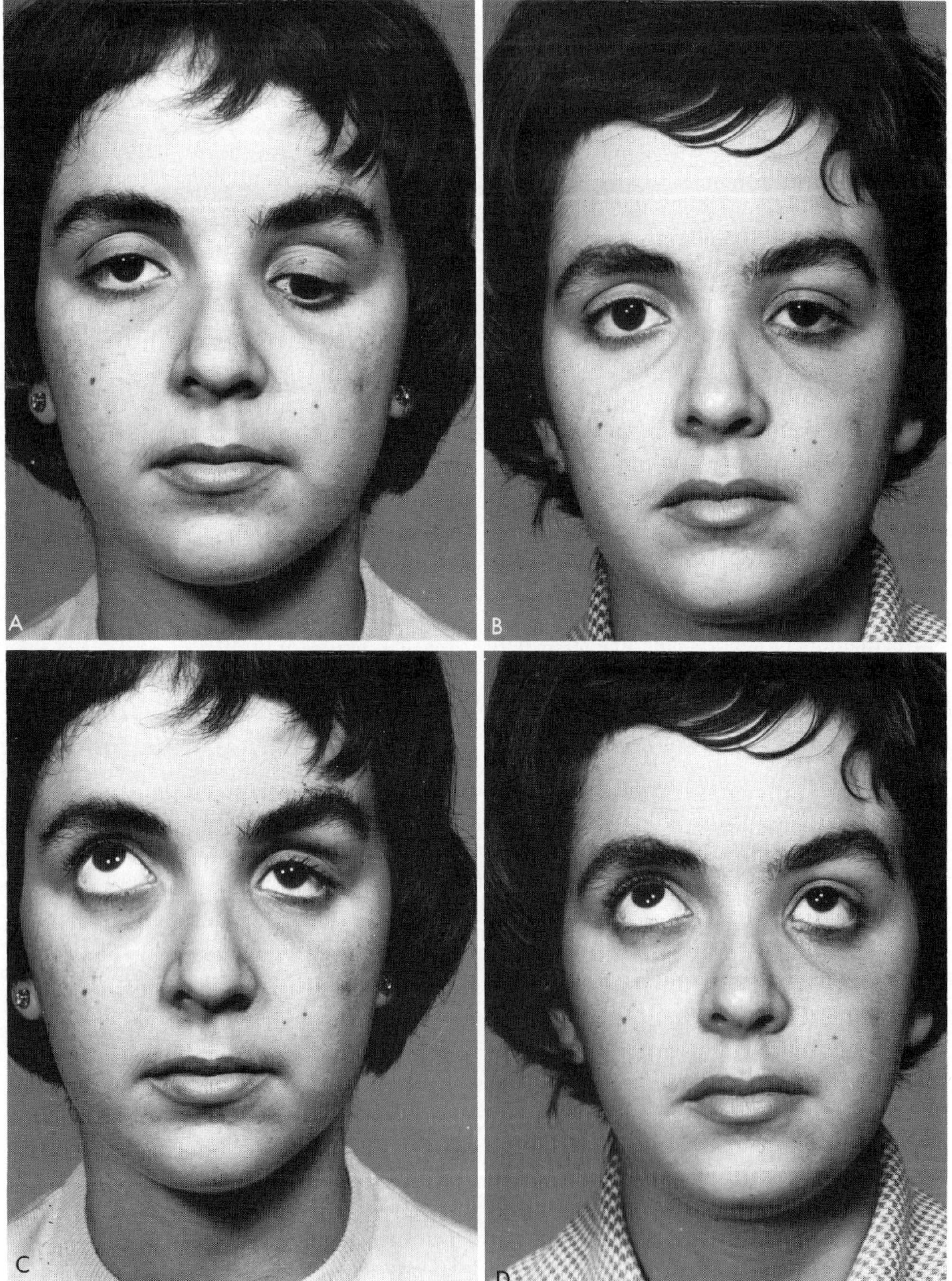

Figure 33–32. *A,* Patient four months after blow-out fracture of the left orbit. Note the deepened supratarsal fold and the downward rotation of the left ocular globe. *B,* Two months after operation. Note the improved position of the left ocular globe and the restored supratarsal fold. *C,* The left eye shows limited oculorotary movement in the upward gaze. *D,* Improved oculorotary movement of the left eye in the upward gaze after surgery. (From Converse, J. M., Cole, J. C., and Smith, B.: Late treatment of blow-out fracture of the floor of the orbit. A case report. Plast. Reconstr. Surg., *28*:183, 1961.)

mosis, hematoma, displacement, and entrapment. The intimate anatomic relationship of the inferior rectus and inferior oblique muscles to the common fracture site is one of the reasons for their vulnerability. The inferior oblique muscle arises from the orbital floor near the temporal margin in the lacrimal groove. It passes inferior to the belly of the inferior rectus muscle, and inserts into the sclera behind the equator of the globe deep to the belly of the lateral rectus. The sheath of the inferior rectus muscle is loosely attached to that of the inferior oblique. While the muscles themselves may not be entrapped, the fascial expansions, the capsulopalpebral fascia, may be tethered to the fracture site.

Tests for Diplopia. Inasmuch as diplopia is a subjective condition, the tests for its analysis depend on the cooperation of the patient. Subjective results from tests for diplopia must therefore be correlated with objective findings for proper diagnosis and treatment.

Occlusion Test. Alternating a small cover in front of the eyes permits the patient to tell the examiner what happens to the double image. Persistence of the double image when one eye is occluded means that the diplopia is monocular rather than binocular; disappearance of one image indicates binocular diplopia. The image seems to move when the occluding apparatus is rapidly alternated from one eye to the other. The apparent motion of the image is opposite to the direction of movement of the eyeball. This test enables the examiner to observe the motion of the eye and to decide whether the deviation is horizontal, vertical, or a combination of each. The amount of ocular deviation in the various fields of gaze may be estimated by testing with prisms (Fig. 33–33). Interpretation of the findings leads to a presumptive diagnosis as to the specific muscles involved. The occlusion test is reliable because it offers both a subjective and an objective analysis.

Red Glass Test. A simple red filter placed in front of one eye helps the patient to describe the displacement of images. Although a diplopia field may be plotted by means of this test, it is not as accurate as the cover or occlusion test. The red glass may be modified so that its image is perceived as a linc rather than a point. This modification is known as the Maddox rod test and has the advantage of separating the horizontal from the vertical displacement by observation of the line in the vertical and horizontal meridians, respectively.

Monocular Diplopia. Monocular diplopia is a one-eyed phenomenon and consequently represents a visual rather than an oculorotary disturbance. If functional, the condition is managed as any other psychosomatic disorder. Organic monocular diplopia is caused by any alteration or obstruction along the visual axis that is conducive to duplication or multiplicity of monocular retinal images. Abrasions of the cornea; opacities in the cornea, lens, or transparent media; aberrations in the iris diaphragm; displacement of the lens; disturbance of the retina and choroid; and other similar conditions may contribute to monocular diplopia. Organic monocular diplopia is purely an ophthalmologic problem.

Binocular Diplopia. Binocular double vision is caused by images upon noncorresponding retinal points in both eyes. These images, transmitted to consciousness under normal circumstances, are the fused images from corresponding points of the retina. The sharply focused, fused images received by the cerebral cortex from the macular areas are those registered in the area of consciousness.

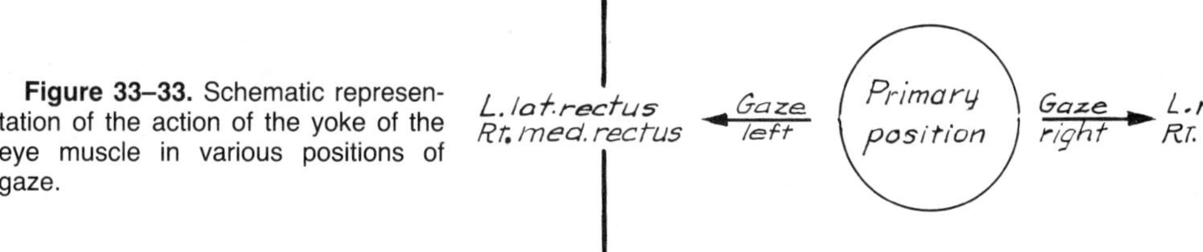

Figure 33–33. Schematic representation of the action of the yoke of the eye muscle in various positions of gaze.

Images received from noncorresponding points on the peripheral retina are poorly perceived in consciousness and are used as a means of orientation rather than attentive fixation.

A normal person can observe the diplopia arising as a result of peripheral images being focused on noncorresponding retinal points. Most people are not plagued with this type of diplopia (physiologic diplopia) because they have learned to suppress the peripheral images. Ordinarily, one sees but a single image; if one tries, however, physiologic diplopia may occur. This simple experiment is conducted by holding a pencil in a central position approximately 2 feet in front of the eyes and focusing across the room. The pencil is seen double. Likewise, focusing on the pencil and observing objects across the room produces a double image of the distant objects.

Occasionally, patients discover physiologic diplopia and suffer from its symptoms until explanations and reassurances lead them back to normal peripheral visual suppression.

Suppression is a psychologic mechanism by which the individual learns to ignore ocular images. Suppression may be central, peripheral, or both. Suppression is one means by which a person may learn to overcome double vision caused by extraocular muscle imbalance.

Binocular diplopia due to deviation of the visual axes, secondary to extraocular muscle imbalance, is the diplopia usually encountered after orbital fracture. Ocular deviation and diplopia resulting from organic muscle changes are caused by edema, hemorrhage, laceration, fibrosis and disturbances in the nerve supply, and displacement of the eyeball. Deviation may also follow diminution of visual acuity because the normal mechanism is not sufficiently stimulated to bring about binocular vision. Ocular deviation may also occur in the presence of satisfactory vision in each eye as a result of a defect in the fusion mechanism.

Individuals with normal vision and a normal fusion mechanism become conscious of double vision when the visual axes are carried beyond the range of normal fusion. Even slight restriction of extraocular muscular activity in orbital fractures may result in diplopia. Individuals with defective vision or poor fusion tolerate extreme limitations of ocular motility without diplopia. Because the range of vertical fusion is much less than that of horizontal fusion, the binocular mechanism is less tolerant of vertical imbalance.

Horizontal deviations frequently develop secondarily to the vertical deviation; this is partly the result of direct involvement of the horizontally acting muscles. Secondary actions of the vertically acting muscles are also influential in the superimposed horizontal deviation.

ENOPHTHALMOS

Enophthalmos in excess of 5 mm is disfiguring. The deformity seen in the malunited orbital fracture is characteristic (see Fig. 33–32*A*). The ocular globe appears depressed and recessed, the horizontal dimension of the palpebral fissure is diminished, the superior tarsal fold is deepened, and the upper lid droops. The latter finding has been mistakenly interpreted as ptosis caused by severance of the levator palpebrae superioris aponeurosis or by a nerve injury.

Etiopathogenesis. Converse and Smith (1957) attributed enophthalmos to the effect of gravity on the intraorbital soft tissues in an *enlarged bony orbital volume.* However, this theory failed to explain the absence of enophthalmos in cases in which the orbital floor had been resected, as in a radical maxillectomy. Such findings prompted the theory of intraorbital *fat atrophy,* since Lockwood's ligament and the intraorbital musculofibrous ligament system described by Koornneef (1982) prevent inferior displacement of the globe when the orbital floor is removed. Converse, Smith, and Wood-Smith (1977) also speculated that *entrapped intraorbital soft tissue structures* (the inferior rectus muscle) and *post-traumatic scar* could pull the globe posteriorly and inferiorly and give the appearance of enophthalmos.

In a series of classic papers, Manson and associates (1986a,b) described the etiopathogenic factors involved in enophthalmos. In fresh cadaver studies they demonstrated that removal of *intra*muscular fat (contained within the muscle cone) produced globe displacement similar to that observed in clinical enophthalmos. In patients undergoing bilateral cosmetic blepharoplasty, removal of anterior *extra*muscular fat did not significantly affect globe position. In fresh cadavers there was no displacement of the globe when the orbital floor was removed, provided that there was neither disruption of the periosteum (periorbita) or distortion of the supporting musculofibrous ligament system (Koornneef, 1982).

Quantitative CT scans (Manson and associates, 1986a,b) were performed on 16 patients with post-traumatic orbital deformity. The orbits were evaluated according to component parts: soft tissue orbital volume (STOV), bony orbital volume (BV), retrobulbar volume (RV), globe volume (GV), and fat volume (FV) (Fig. 33–34). These studies demonstrated that, in patients with enophthalmos, (1) BV was enlarged (up to 18 per cent) by expansion into the maxillary and ethmoid sinuses (rarely adjacent to the inferior orbital fissure or by displacement of the sphenoid) (Figs. 33–35, 33–36); (2) STOV showed a slight increase (approximately 5 per cent), and this was attributed to edema and fibrosis; (3) FV was increased only slightly (approximately 5 per cent); and (4) GV was slightly lower (approximately 1 per cent). These findings are also illustrated in Figure 33–37. In summary, the data indicate that the principal mechanism in the development of post-traumatic enophthalmos is a displacement of a relatively constant volume of orbital soft tissue into an enlarged bony orbit. Loss of musculofibrous ligament support permits posterior displacement of the intraorbital soft tissue and a change in orbital soft tissue shape (under the influence of gravity and scar contracture) from a "conal" to a "spherical" configuration (see Fig. 33–35). Fat atrophy does not appear to play an etiopathogenic role.

Measurement of Enophthalmos. Determination of the degree of enophthalmos is based on the relative position of a line projected from the lateral orbital margin to the profile of the zenith of the cornea. When there is bone loss and displacement, fixed points on the affected and unaffected sides cannot be used in diagnosis. In such cases, the degree of ocular protrusion or recession is determined by differences in the number of millimeters required to focus an instrument on each cornea.

Roentgenographic Studies. Roentgenographic examination offers additional orbital information and employs five projections: the Caldwell, Waters, lateral, optic canals, and base views. However, optimal visualization of orbital pathology is provided by quantitative CT scans (see Figs. 33–34 to 33–37) (Manson and associates, 1986a,b).

Surgical Treatment

Restoration of Orbital Architecture and Release of Entrapped Structures. The object of treatment is the release of the entrapped orbital tissues and the restoration of the bone architecture of the orbit.

In the late treatment of malunited orbital fractures, the authors prefer an eyelid incision combined, if necessary, with a bicoronal scalp incision.

Surgical exploration through fibrosed tissues may be laborious. Subperiosteal elevation from the orbital rim backward to the area of fracture is followed by elevation over the nonfractured medial and lateral aspects of the orbital floor. The bicoronal incision facilitates subperiosteal dissection of the orbital roof and lateral and medial walls. Painstaking elevation of the periorbita from the fracture area is performed. The orbital contents that have prolapsed into the maxillary and ethmoid sinuses are extracted from the skeletal defect. Preservation of the infraorbital nerve is necessary to avoid permanent anesthesia of the upper lip and cheek.

Tessier (1982a) described the *marginal orbitotomy* (Fig. 33–38). By removing the inferior orbital rim and that portion of the orbit anterior to the bone defect, the surgeon has better exposure of the pathologic condition, and the surgical maneuver facilitates the extraction of the orbital contents from the maxillary and ethmoid sinuses.

Correction of Diplopia. After separation of the entrapped orbital contents from the infraorbital nerve, it is essential to verify that they have been freed and that oculorotary movement has been restored. The *forced duction test* should be performed to verify that free oculorotary movements are fully restored. The periorbita should be raised from the orbit circumferentially (360 degrees). Because an associated fracture of the medial wall is common, an adhesion in this area may be responsible for persistent impairment of oculorotary movements after the floor is freed. The exposure of the floor must often be extended into the posterior reaches of the orbital cavity. The most frequent cause of surgical failure is fear of freeing posteriorly entrapped tissues.

Restoration of free oculorotary movements to the ocular globe is the first and most important step toward rehabilitation of the patient with a malunited orbital fracture. The

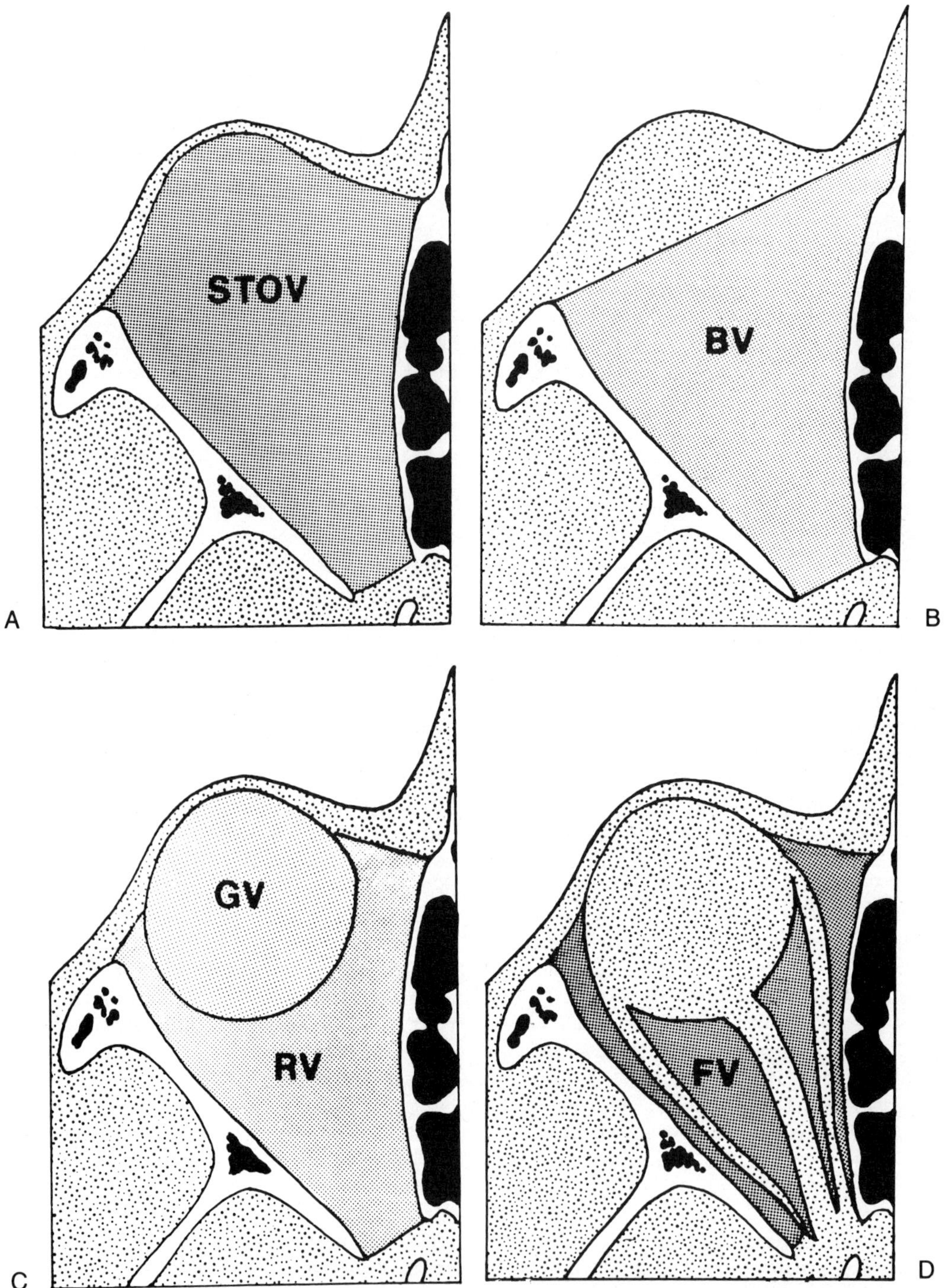

Figure 33–34. *A,* Soft tissue orbital volume (STOV). *B,* Bony orbital volume (BV). *C,* Retrobulbar volume (RV) and globe volume (GV). *D,* Fat volume (FV). (From Manson, P. N., Grivas, A., Rosenbaum, A., Vannier, M., Zinreich, J., and Iliff, N.: Studies on enophthalmos. II. The measurement of orbital injuries and their treatment by quantitative computed tomography. Plast. Reconstr. Surg., 77:203, 1986.)

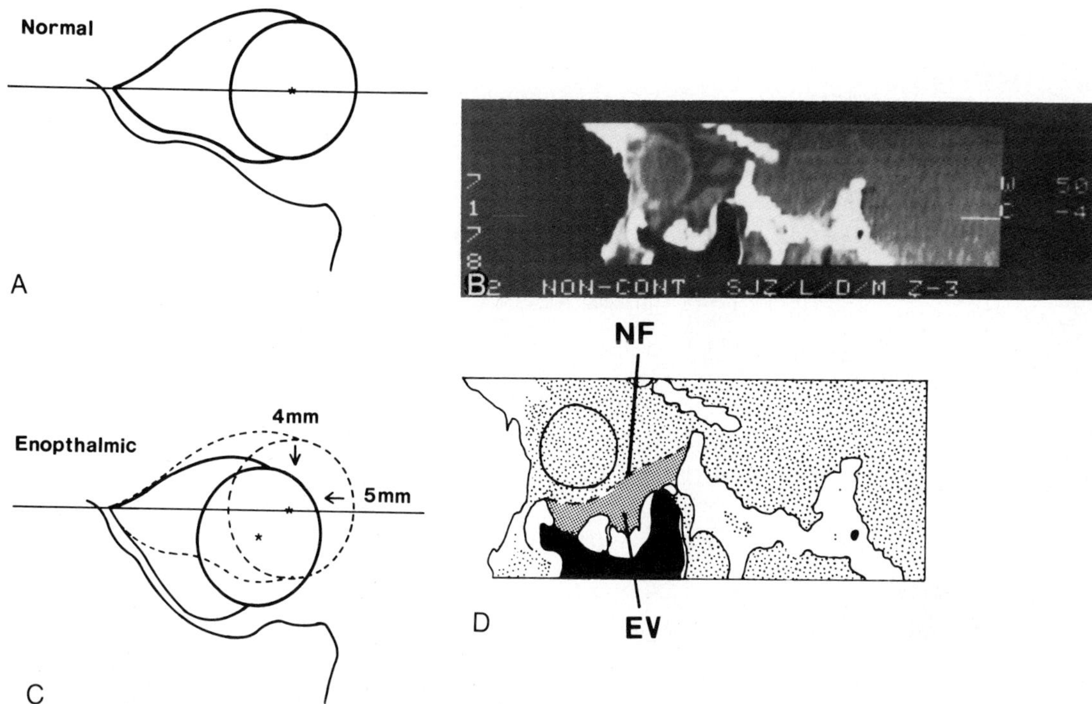

Figure 33–35. *A,* Normal orbital shape in the longitudinal axis of the orbit. The maxillary sinus bulges upward behind the globe (and the ethmoid bulges inward). *C,* Post-traumatic orbital shape. The orbital floor bulges inferiorly and there is a "spherical" configuration to the shape of the orbital soft tissue. *B, D,* Representative CT scan and drawing showing post-traumatic orbital deformity of enophthalmos, globe ptosis, and enlargement of the retrobulbar orbit. NF = normal floor position; EV = extra volume created by floor displacement. (From Manson, P. N., Clifford, C. M., Su, C. T., Iliff, N. T., and Morgan, R.: Mechanisms of global support and posttraumatic enophthalmos. I. The anatomy of the ligament sling and its relation to intramuscular cone orbital fat. Plast. Reconstr. Surg., *77*:193, 1986.)

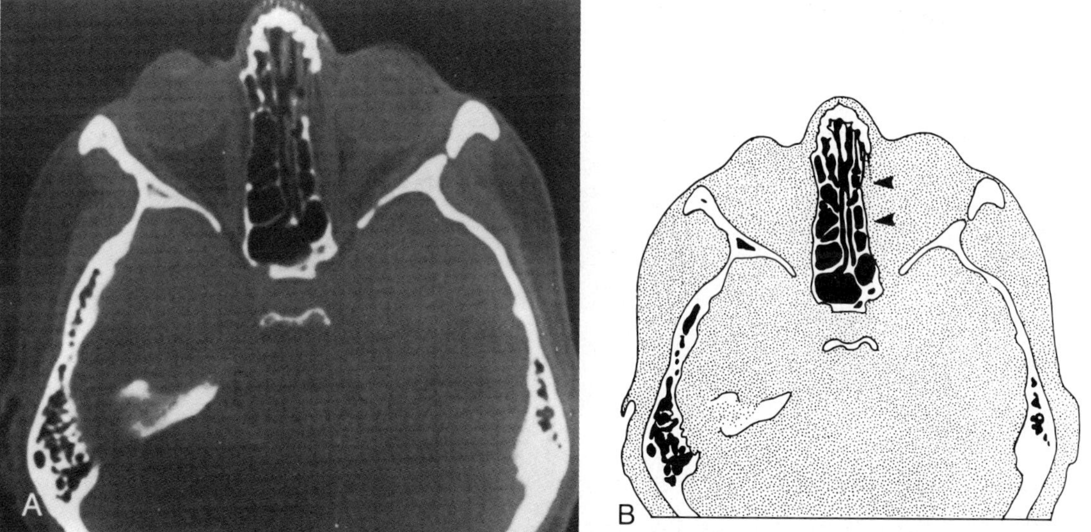

Figure 33–36. Medial compression of the ethmoid air cells produced by orbital fractures resulting in enophthalmos. These fractures are usually continuous with the floor fracture and the maxillary sinus compression seen in Figure 33–35*B, D.* Compression of the ethmoid air cells without actual bone defects is a frequent cause of orbital enlargement. *A,* CT scan. *B,* Drawing. (From Manson, P. N., Grivas, A., Rosenbaum, A., Vannier, M., Zinreich, J., and Iliff, N.: Studies on enophthalmos. II. The measurement of orbital injuries and their treatment by quantitative computed tomography. Plast. Reconstr. Surg., *77*:203, 1986.)

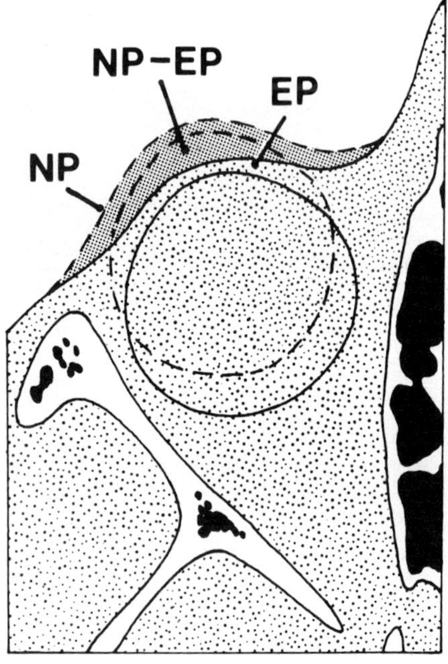

Figure 33–37. Change in orbital volume observed on axial CT scan with displacement of the globe 4 mm posteriorly. NP = normal globe position; EP = enophthalmic globe position; NP-EP = volume difference in axial mid-globe section to produce enophthalmos of 4 mm. (From Manson, P. N., Grivas, A., Rosenbaum, A., Vannier, M., Zinreich, J., and Iliff, N.: Studies on enophthalmos. II. The measurement of orbital injuries and their treatment by quantitative computed tomography. Plast. Reconstr. Surg., *77*:203, 1986.)

next step is to restore the bone continuity of the orbit and relieve the enophthalmos.

Correction of Enophthalmos. The orbital skeletal defect causing the enophthalmos must be defined by appropriate CT studies.

The bone architecture of the orbit can be restored by means of bone grafts, inorganic implants, or osteotomies.

Late correction of enophthalmos is difficult to achieve. Some information concerning the prognosis for the surgical correction of enophthalmos may be obtained by the *forward*

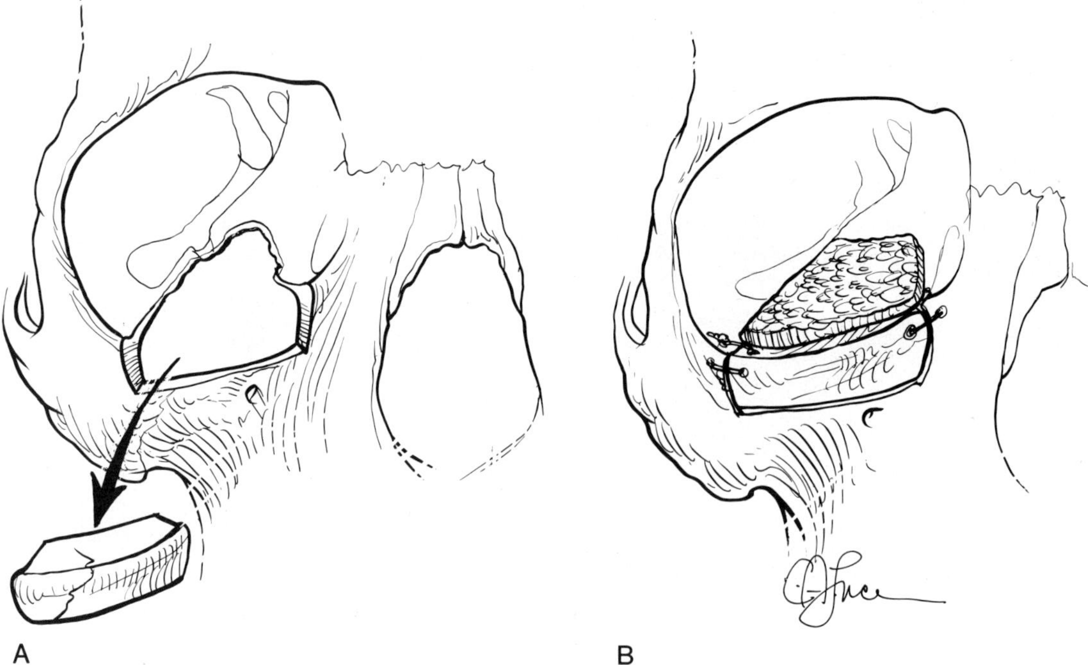

Figure 33–38. Marginal orbitotomy (Tessier). *A,* With a combination of a mechanical saw and osteotome, a segment of the right inferior orbital rim is removed to facilitate exposure of the orbital defect and extraction of the orbital tissues from the maxillary sinus. *B,* After restoration of the orbital architecture the segment is wired into position and the orbital defect is covered with an autogenous bone graft.

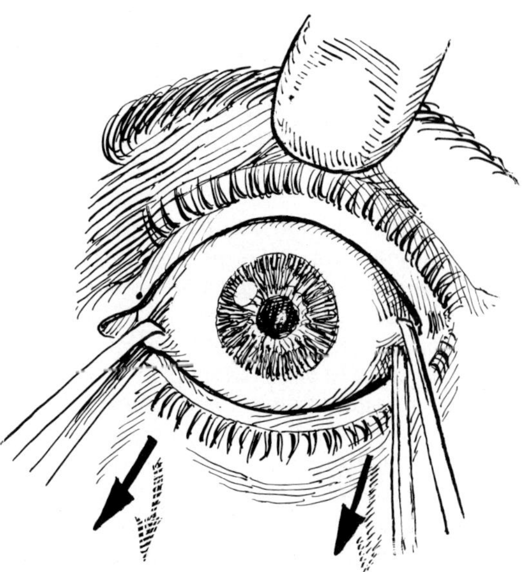

Figure 33–39. The forward traction test. Two forceps grasp the medial and lateral rectus muscles and exert a forward traction on the eyeball. Freedom of forward displacement of the orbital contents is a favorable prognostic sign for the correction of enophthalmos by orbital implants; resistance to forward traction is a relatively poor prognostic sign. (From Converse, J. M., Smith, B., Obear, M., and Wood-Smith, D.: Orbital blow-out fracture: a ten-year survey. Plast. Reconstr. Surg., *39*:20, 1967.)

traction test (Fig. 33–39), which consists of application of two forceps to the eyeball, one to the lateral rectus and the other to the medial rectus muscle. Forward traction is then exerted. If the ocular globe cannot be advanced readily, the prognosis for surgical correction of the enophthalmos is less favorable. The musculature and other soft tissue structures have become fibrosed and shortened, thus opposing surgical correction.

In assessing the patient with enophthalmos, the surgeon must distinguish between a *displaced* and a *normally positioned* lateral orbital rim-zygoma. Kawamoto (1982) emphasized that the position of the lateral orbital wall influences the anteroposterior position of the globe, and described a technique for correction of enophthalmos in the patient with lateral displacement of the orbitozygomatic complex (Fig. 33–40). Through a hemicoronal and lower eyelid incision, subperiosteal dissection is accomplished in the orbit in 360 degrees (but the apex is spared) and the anterior wall of the maxilla and the zygoma are exposed. The temporalis muscle is reflected from the lateral wall of the orbit. The malpositioned orbitozygomatic fracture frag-

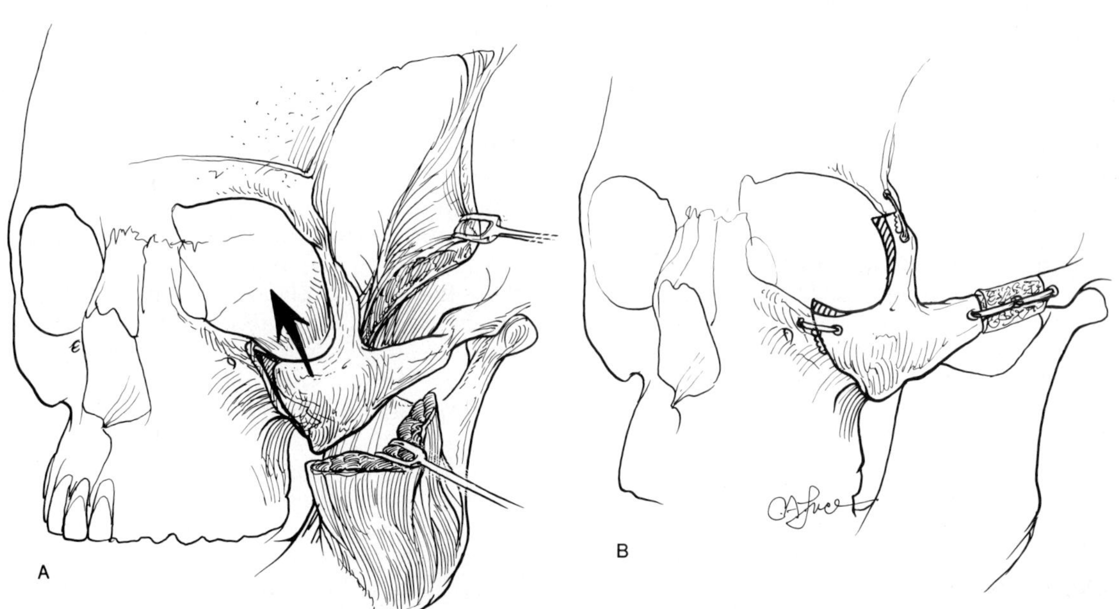

Figure 33–40. Correction of enophthalmos and a displaced orbitozygomatic complex (Kawamoto). *A,* The orbitozygomatic complex is exposed through a hemicoronal and lower eyelid incision. Note the direction (*arrow*) of the planned mobilization of the bony segment. The masseter muscle has been detached. *B,* After skeletal mobilization, interosseous wiring (or miniplate fixation) is established. Note the bone graft in the zygomatic arch and the recontouring (*diagonal lines*).

ment is liberated with a power saw and is freed of all soft tissue attachments. The segment is then placed in its anatomic position under direct vision (in an overcorrected superior and medial direction). The orbital volume is thus reduced; the enophthalmos is corrected and the zygomatic projection is restored. Orbital rim irregularities are recontoured with a power-driven bur and skeletal defects of the orbital floor, medial wall, or zygomatic arch are reconstructed with autogenous bone grafts (Fig. 33–41).

If the increase in bony orbital volume can be attributed to orbital defects only (without displacement of the orbitozygomatic complex), restoration of the bone orbit (and reduction of bony orbital volume) is indicated. The authors prefer a combined coronal-eyelid approach (see Fig. 33–24) with circumferential subperiosteal dissection of the intraorbital contents. The orbital apex is spared. The marginal orbitotomy of Tessier (see Fig. 33–38) facilitates dissection of the herniated soft tissue and its repositioning in the orbit.

All defects are carefully reconstructed with autogenous bone grafts carefully contoured to size and wired in position. Through the bicoronal incision, calvarial bone grafts are easily harvested (McCarthy and Zide, 1984). Alternative donor sites include the ilium and ribs. Alternative materials have included costal cartilage (LaGrange, 1918) and irradiated cartilage allografts (Dingman and Grabb, 1974). It should be emphasized that resorption or loss of volume is still a disadvantage of autogenous bone grafts. Consequently at the conclusion of the procedure the globe on the operated side should be in a slightly overcorrected position. The patient illustrated in Fig. 33–42 underwent such a surgical correction for enophthalmos.

In the patient with a nonseeing or prosthetic eye, the posterior reaches of the orbit may be approached by raising the periorbita along the lateral wall of the orbit, because the danger of causing blindness, ever present in the seeing eye, is nonexistent. Alloplastic implants (Spira, Gerow, and Hardy, 1974) may be placed in the posterior aspect of the orbital cone medially and laterally after raising the periorbita from the orbital wall (Fig. 33–43). A technique used by Smith, Obear, and Leone (1967) consisted of placing Pyrex glass beads in the apex of the orbit, but this has been abandoned because of migration of the beads.

To correct enophthalmos in the anophthalmic orbit, Iverson, Vistnes, and Siegel (1973) advocated the subperiosteal injection of RTV (room temperature vulcanizing) Silastic along the superior, lateral, and inferior aspects of the orbit (see Fig. 33–90).

In most patients, complete correction of the enophthalmos is not achieved. In most patients the enophthalmos is best corrected by the placement of implants over the orbital floor, the lateral orbital wall, and the lamina papyracea behind the lacrimal sac. It is essential to recall that the optic foramen is situated at the apex of the medial orbital wall; implants placed far posteriorly along this wall risk injuring the nerve. The lateral orbital wall, because it is situated in an anterolateral-posteromedial plane, is the most favorable site for implant placement, since it is at a distance from the optic foramen. In patients with residual enophthalmos, contour restoration of a malunited depressed zygoma with onlay grafts should be carried out with prudence. It must be emphasized that an increased projection of the zygoma causes the enophthalmic eye to appear relatively more enophthalmic.

Quantitative CT studies on patients who underwent surgical reconstruction for enophthalmos have demonstrated a postoperative reduction of orbital volume, an improvement in soft tissue position, and a slight decrease in soft tissue volume (Manson and associates, 1986b).

Correction of Other Deformities and Functional Impairment

Extraocular Muscle Imbalance. Extraocular muscle imbalance is a frequent sequela of orbital fracture. Secondary muscle imbalance occurs in the ptotic ocular globe only when the eye is enophthalmic. Muscle surgery is planned only after the muscle pattern has been established as a permanent deviation. The time of the first muscle surgery in late repairs is usually a minimum of six months after the treatment of the orbital fracture. Second and third muscle operative procedures are often necessary. The aim of these procedures is to obtain fusion in the primary and eyes-down positions, which are the most functional positions for speaking, eating, and reading. To achieve this result, it may be necessary to sacrifice fusion in the eyes-up position, an unphysiologic one at best.

Extraocular muscle surgery is not infre-

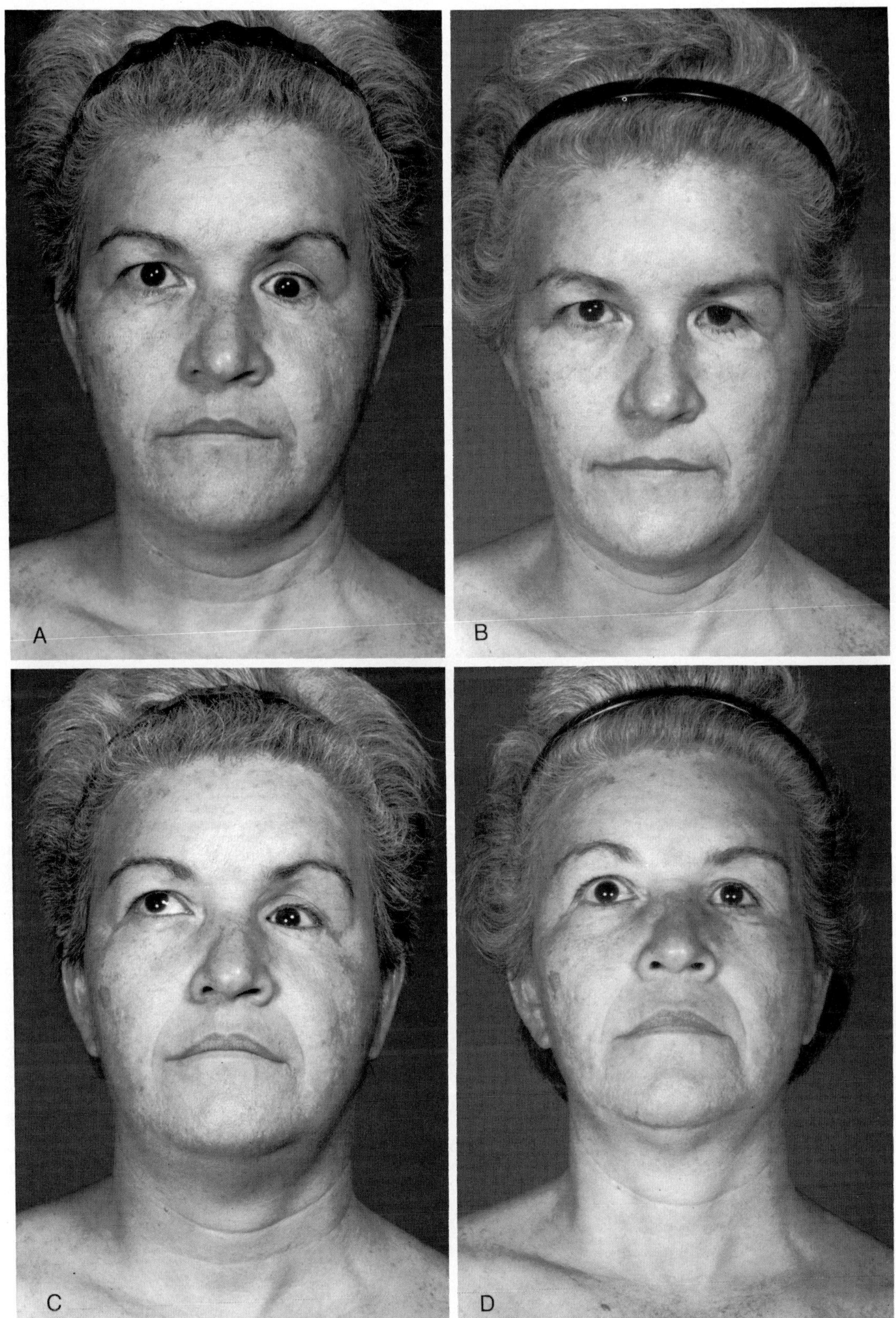

Figure 33–41. Correction of enophthalmos and a displaced orbitozygomatic complex. *A, C,* Preoperative views of a middle-aged woman with a displaced orbitozygomatic complex, enophthalmos, pseudoptosis, deepened supratarsal fold, and inferior displacement of the globe. *B, D,* Appearance after surgical correction (see Fig. 33–40).

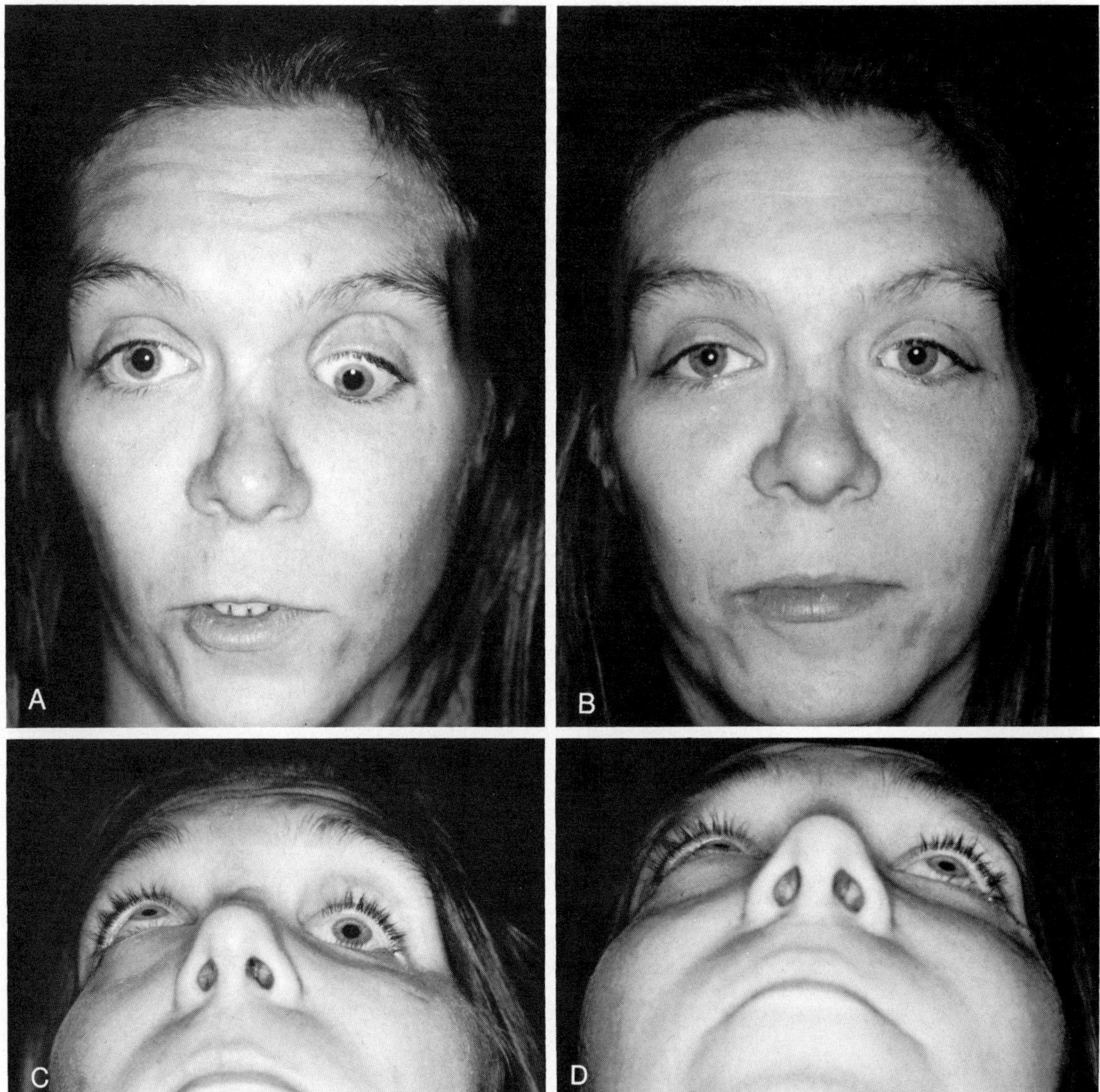

Figure 33–42. Late correction of enophthalmos. *A,* Patient with blow-out fracture of the left orbit of many months' duration, showing enophthalmos and inferior globe displacement with pseudoptosis of the upper eyelid. *B,* Correction after release of the entrapped orbital contents in the area of the blow-out site and bone grafting of the floor of the orbit. *C,* Preoperative basilar view. *D,* Improvement obtained after bone grafting and release of the structures entrapped in the orbital floor. (From Converse, J. M.: *In* Georgiade, N. G. (Ed.): Plastic and Maxillofacial Trauma Symposium. Vol. 1. St. Louis, C. V. Mosby Company, 1969.)

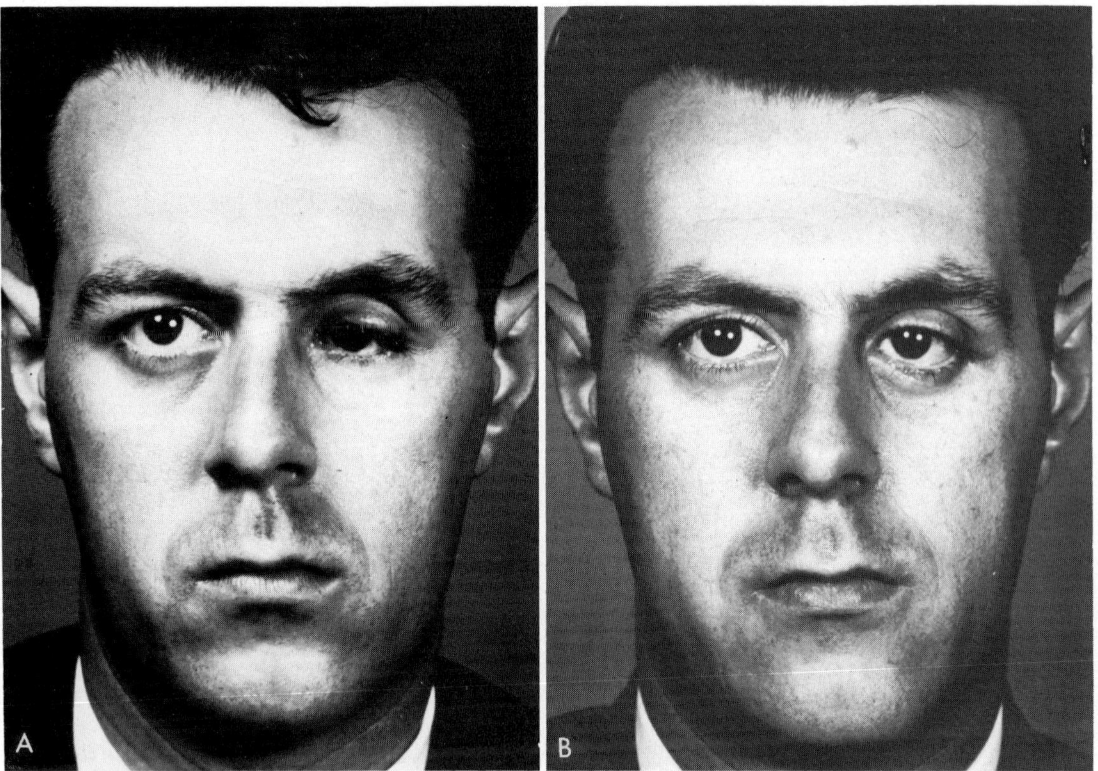

Figure 33–43. Treatment of enophthalmos in a patient with a nonseeing eye. *A,* The patient has suffered a blow-out fracture of the left orbit producing enophthalmos. Note the esotropia of the blind left eye. *B,* Correction of the enophthalmos by insertion of an alloplastic implant. Subsequent extraocular muscle surgery corrected the esotropia.

quently indicated in the unaffected eye in order to obtain binocular fusion.

Medial and Lateral Canthal Deformities. These are sequelae of orbital fractures more frequently found in association with multiple midfacial bone fractures and nasoethmoido-orbital fractures. Medial canthal deformities are usually seen after malunited nasoethmoido-orbital fractures. Zygomatic fractures and dislocations dislodge the lateral raphé and lateral canthal tendon, and an antimongoloid slant of the lid may result. Complete detachment of the lateral canthal tendon and raphé produces a rounded lateral canthus and decreased intercanthal distance. The techniques of lateral and medial canthopexy are discussed in Chapter 34.

Superior Sulcus Deformity. Even after bone graft restoration of the orbital bone contour and volume, some degree of deepening of the supratarsal fold may persist. Several "camouflaging" surgical techniques can be used, including the insertion of banked scleral allograft under the orbicularis muscle along the supratarsal fold (Smith and Lisman, 1983).

Vertical Shortening of Lower Eyelid. Exposure of the sclera below the limbus of the globe in the primary position (the "scleral show" or "white eye" syndrome) may result from scar contracture (vertical shortening of the lower eyelid) because of downward and backward displacement of the fractured inferior orbital rim, or because the periorbita has been sutured to the septum orbitale after placement of the implant. Release of the scar tissue and replacement of the orbital rim into the corrected position usually restore the lid to normal position. If the fractured rim is malunited, release of the septum orbitale attachment from the orbital rim and restoration of the orbital rim by a bone graft are procedures that can elevate the lid margin. If primary operative procedures fail, a lateral canthoplasty with release of the lid retractor system (see Chap. 34) is indicated to increase the vertical dimension of the lower lid and raise the lid margin up to 4 mm. A skin graft may be necessary for surgical correction of a deficiency of lower eyelid skin.

Infraorbital Nerve Anesthesia. Infraorbital nerve anesthesia may be disconcerting

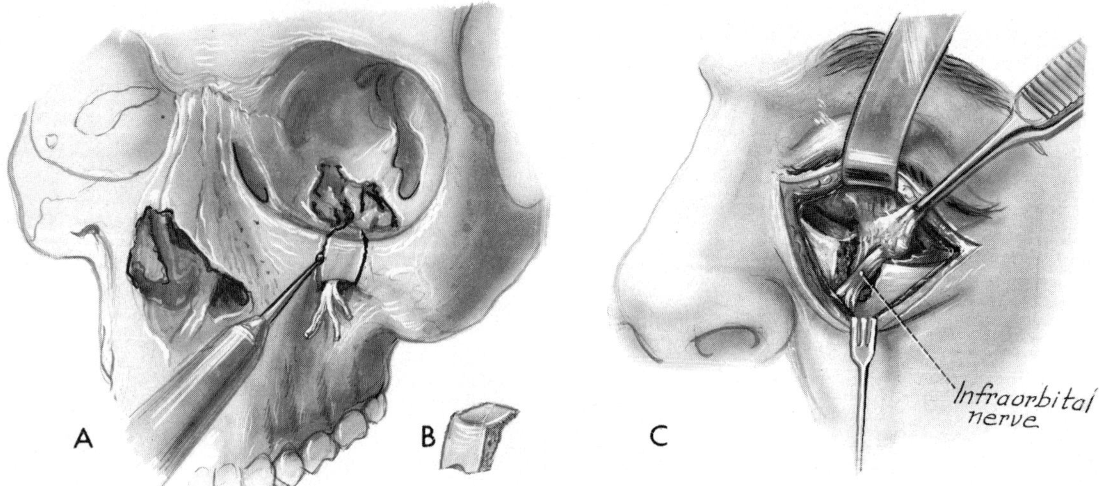

Figure 33–44. Decompression and identification of the infraorbital nerve. *A,* When difficulty is encountered in the orbital fracture area, the nerve is exposed at the infraorbital foramen, and a section of bone is outlined for removal to uncover the infraorbital canal. *B,* A block of bone is removed and set aside for later replacement. *C,* The infraorbital nerve is traced back to the blow-out fracture area and dissected from the orbital contents. The block of bone illustrated in *B* is replaced. (From Converse, J. M., Smith, B., Obear, M. R., and Wood-Smith, D.: Orbital blow-out fracture: a ten-year study. Plast. Reconstr. Surg., *39*:20, 1967.)

to some patients. The area of sensory loss usually extends from the lower lid over the cheek and lateral ala to the upper lip. Release of the infraorbital nerve from the pressure of bone fragments within the canal may be performed (Fig. 33–44). Sensation may recur spontaneously as late as one year after fracture but the results of surgery are unpredictable.

Nasoethmoido-orbital Fractures

Medial orbital wall fractures often accompany orbital floor fractures and are a hidden cause of residual postoperative enophthalmos. In their more severe form, they are usually associated with naso-orbital fractures, hence the preferred term *nasoethmoido-orbital* fractures (Gruss, 1985).

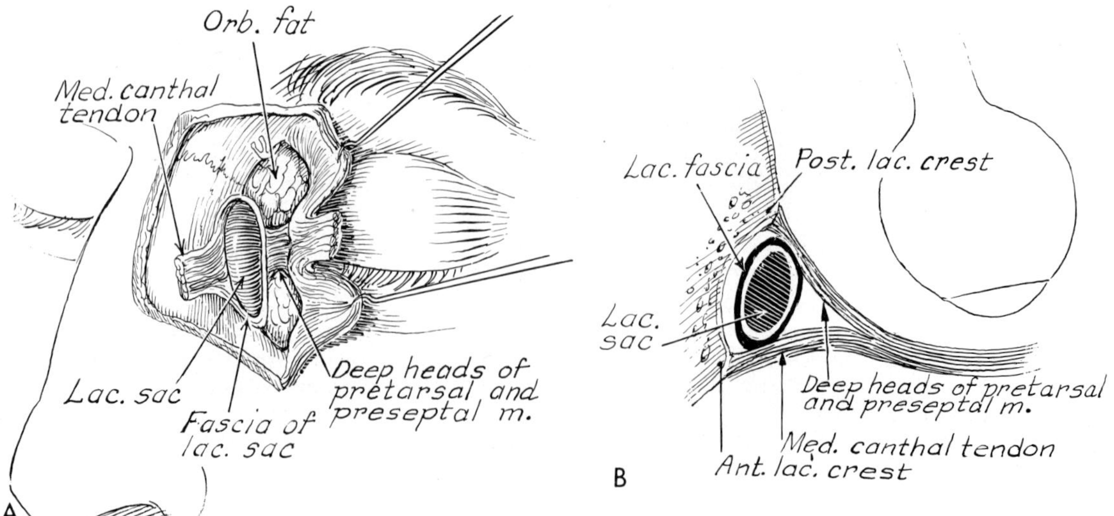

Figure 33–45. The left medial canthal region. The medial canthal tendon and the deep heads of the pretarsal and preseptal muscle embrace the lacrimal sac. *A,* Oblique view. *B,* Cross sectional view.

Because of the presence of the lacrimal system in the medial canthal area (Fig. 33–45), the treatment of malunited fractures involving the medial wall may be complex. The proximity of the anterior cranial fossa may also complicate the treatment.

The most vulnerable structures, however, are the anatomic complex formed by the lacrimal sac lodged in the lacrimal groove, and the nasolacrimal duct and the tendinous structures that surround the sac (Fig. 33–46).

Malunited fracture of the medial orbital wall may result from posterior displacement of comminuted fragments of the nasal bones and frontal processes of the maxilla. The fragments may enter the orbital cavity, injuring the lacrimal sac (Fig. 33–46*B*), or they may be forced into the ethmoidal labyrinth, outfracturing the medial orbital wall and reducing the horizontal dimension of the orbit (Fig. 33–46*C*).

In untreated or maltreated nasoethmoido-orbital fractures, the patient has a characteristic appearance; the bony bridge of the nose is depressed and widened, and the eyes appear far apart (Fig. 33–47). In severe midfacial fractures associated with nasoethmoido-orbital fractures, the degree of deformity is such that the patient is unrecognizable (Fig. 33–48). Post-traumatic telecanthus is caused by an increase in the distance between the medial canthi (intercanthal distance), resulting from fracture displacement of the bone forming the skeletal framework of the nose and medial orbital walls. In contrast to orbital hypertelorism, the circumferential (360 degree) orbit is not displaced laterally. The medial canthi are deformed, cutaneous scars and epicanthal folds may be present, and the function of the lacrimal apparatus is disturbed. The deformity may be unilateral or bilateral. The pseudohyperteloric appearance of the orbits is increased by the flattening of the bony dorsum of the nose (see Fig. 33–47).

Roentgenographic studies and CT scans at the axial plane extending through the lacrimal groove are of assistance in diagnosing and defining the extent of the pathology (Fig. 33–49).

Post-traumatic telecanthus is produced by various types of backward displacement of the bone structures and injury to the medial canthal tendon, the lacrimal sac, and the posterior heads of the pretarsal (tensor tarsi) and preseptal muscles (see Fig. 33–45).

In a first type of fracture, the nasal bones

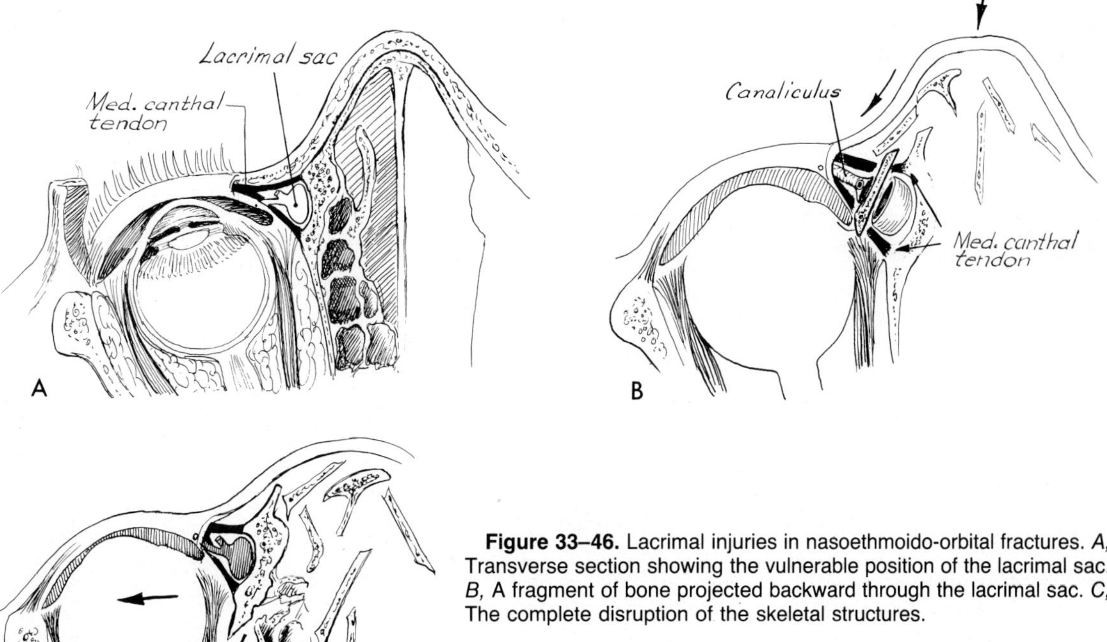

Figure 33–46. Lacrimal injuries in nasoethmoido-orbital fractures. *A,* Transverse section showing the vulnerable position of the lacrimal sac. *B,* A fragment of bone projected backward through the lacrimal sac. *C,* The complete disruption of the skeletal structures.

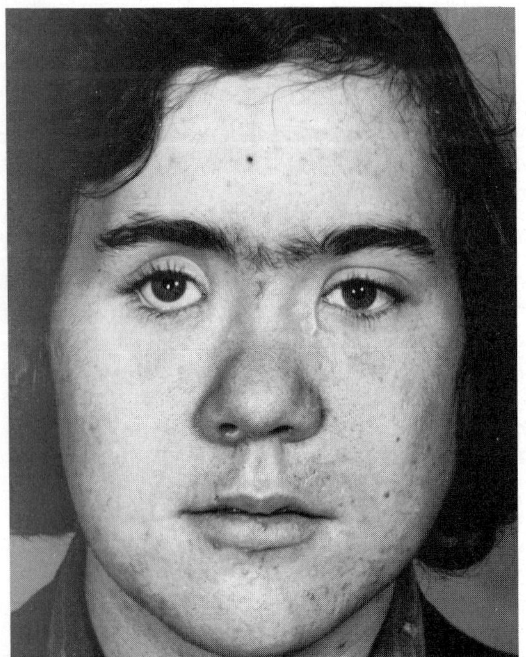

Figure 33–47. The typical deformity of nasoethmoido-orbital fracture. The nose is flattened, and the eyes appear far apart because of the telecanthus. The caruncles are covered. The epicanthal fold is the result of the penetration of a piece of glass in a head-on automobile crash. Note also the reduction in the horizontal dimension of the right palpebral fissure and vertical shortening of the lower eyelid.

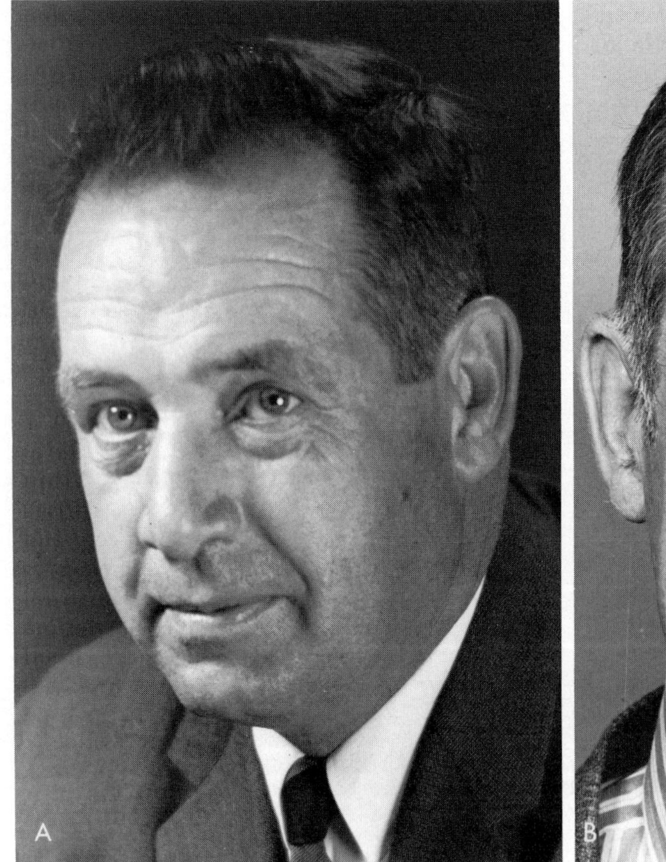

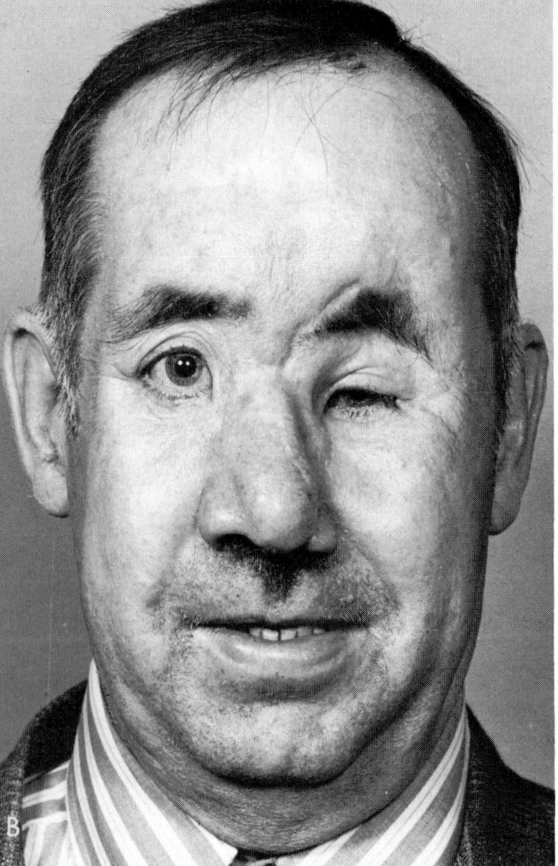

Figure 33–48. *A,* Portrait of a patient before an automobile crash. *B,* Photograph when the patient was first seen with malunited nasoethmoido-orbital and bilateral orbital fractures. Note the total disorganization of the upper and midfacial skeletal framework, the severity of the deformities, and the tragic change in the patient's appearance.

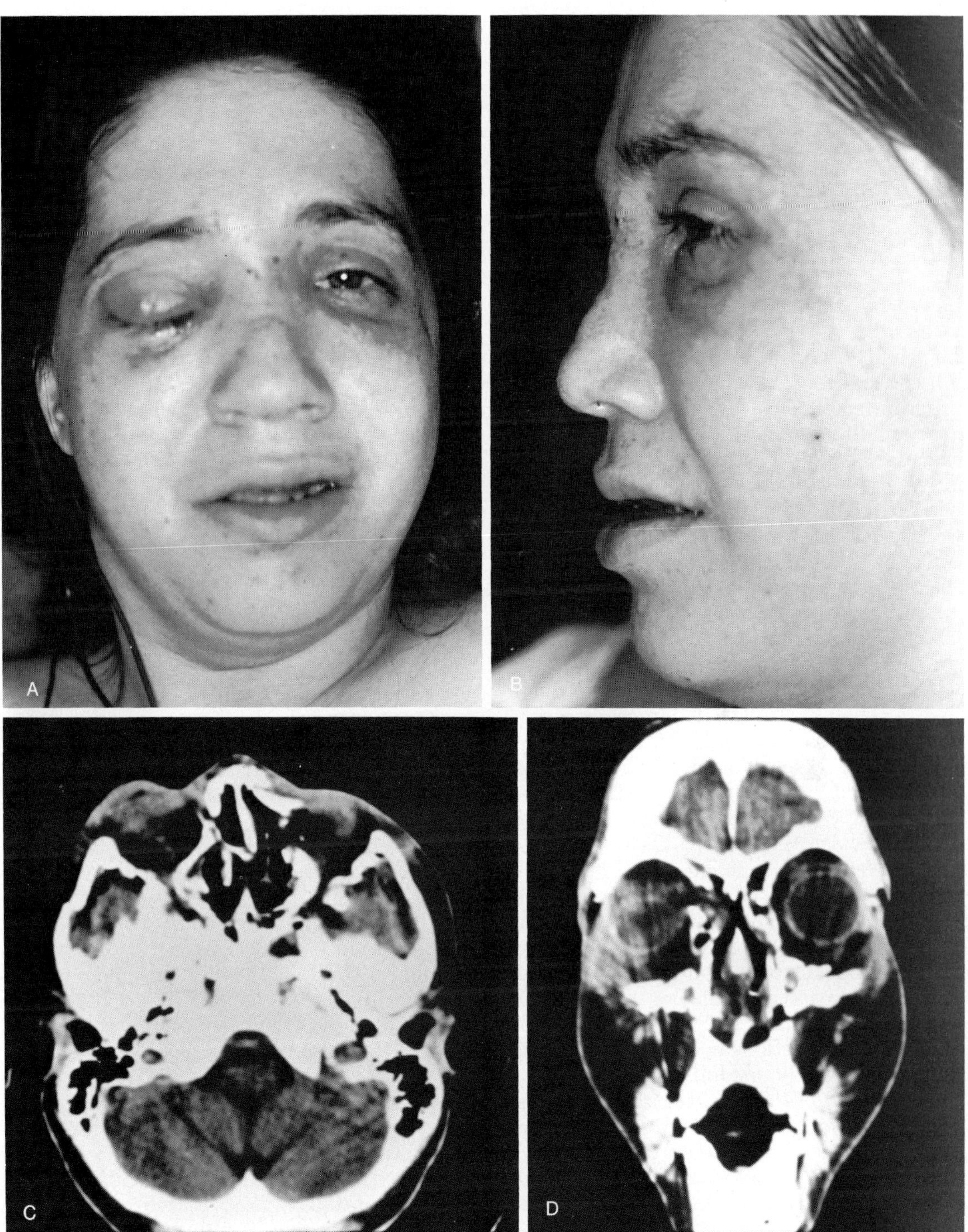

Figure 33–49. Nasoethmoido-orbital fracture. *A, B,* Appearance of the patient. There is ocular globe disruption with telecanthus and flattening of the nasal dorsum. *C,* Axial cut CT scan demonstrating telescoping of the nasoethmoido-orbital complex posteriorly. *D,* Coronal CT scan showing the extent of the bilateral medial orbital wall fracture.

and frontal process of the maxilla are splayed outward. The bones fill the medial portion of the orbital cavity, being pushed backward along the outer aspect of the medial orbital wall, severing the medial canthal tendon and traversing the lacrimal sac or severing the canaliculi (see Fig. 33–46). Considerable increase in the thickness of the medial orbital wall may result from overlapping of the bone fragments. Injury to the medial rectus muscle has been noted in this type of fracture (see Fig. 33–46*C*).

In a second type of fracture, the bones enter the interorbital space, comminuting the ethmoid cells and outfracturing the medial wall of the orbit. The medial canthal deformity is the result of lateral displacement of the medial canthal tendon with a loose fragment of comminuted bone to which the tendon is still attached; the unopposed contraction of the orbicularis muscle pulls the structures laterally (Fig. 33–50).

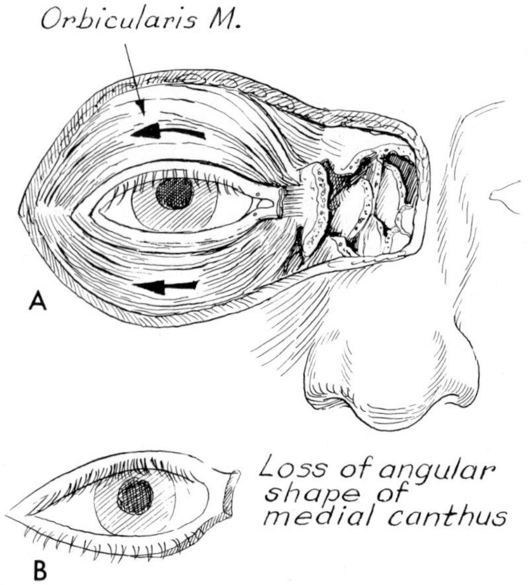

In the medial canthal deformity, the *medial canthus* loses its angular shape and the caruncle is often no longer visible (Fig. 33–50), being covered by an epicanthal fold of skin and subcutaneous tissue. This results in a reduction of the horizontal dimension of the palpebral fissure, a laxity of the eyelids, and a tendency to eversion of the lower eyelid margin. The punctum is no longer in contact with the ocular globe and epiphora results.

Downward displacement of the fractured bone fragment on which the medial canthal tendon is inserted can result in a *canthus inversus* deformity (see Fig. 33–59).

When the nasoethmoido-orbital fracture is unilateral, comparison of the post-traumatic telecanthus with the unaffected side demonstrates the lateral displacement of the medial canthus (Fig. 33–51). In bilateral fractures, the telecanthus is obvious.

Epicanthal folds (see Fig. 33–47) usually result from lacerations or poorly planned incisions through the medial canthal region.

Malfunction of the lacrimal apparatus may be present even in the absence of severance or interruption of any portion of the lacrimal system. Relaxation of the medial canthal soft tissue structures, and the inability of the orbicularis oculi muscle to maintain normal muscle tone cause relaxation of the lower eyelid, eversion of the lacrimal punctum, and inadequate evacuation of tears from the lacrimal lake. Interference with the function of the orbicularis oculi muscle also hampers the

Orbicularis M.

A

Loss of angular shape of medial canthus

B

Figure 33–50. *A,* Traction exerted by the orbicularis oculi muscle on the medial canthus when the medial canthal tendon is severed or detached. *B,* This results in a characteristic deformity of the medial canthus and a diminution of the horizontal dimension of the palpebral fissure. (From Converse, J. M., and Smith, B.: Naso-orbital fractures and traumatic deformities of the medial canthal region. Plast. Reconstr. Surg., *38*:147, 1966. Copyright © 1966, The Williams & Wilkins Company, Baltimore.)

evacuation of tears from the lacrimal sac into the nasolacrimal duct, the evacuation being largely dependent on the contraction of the orbicularis oculi fibers over the lacrimal sac (the “lacrimal pump”).

Interruption of the continuity of any portion of the lacrimal system may occur: the canaliculi, the common canaliculus, the lacrimal sac, or the nasolacrimal duct. The canaliculi are usually severed by a sharp object, such as a piece of glass lacerating the medial portion of the lids and the lacrimal sac. The nasolacrimal duct may be obstructed or lacerated along its course through the lateral wall of the nose or at its point of exit below the inferior turbinate.

The lacrimal sac becomes distended and filled with mucoid material when the nasolacrimal duct is obstructed. This is readily expressed when pressure is exerted over the medial canthal region. A mucocele of the lacrimal sac is manifest by a swelling at the medial canthus, which adds to the distortion of the area resulting from the fractures and the detachment or severance of the medial canthal tendon. The lacrimal sac may be dilated and displaced (Fig. 33–52). There may

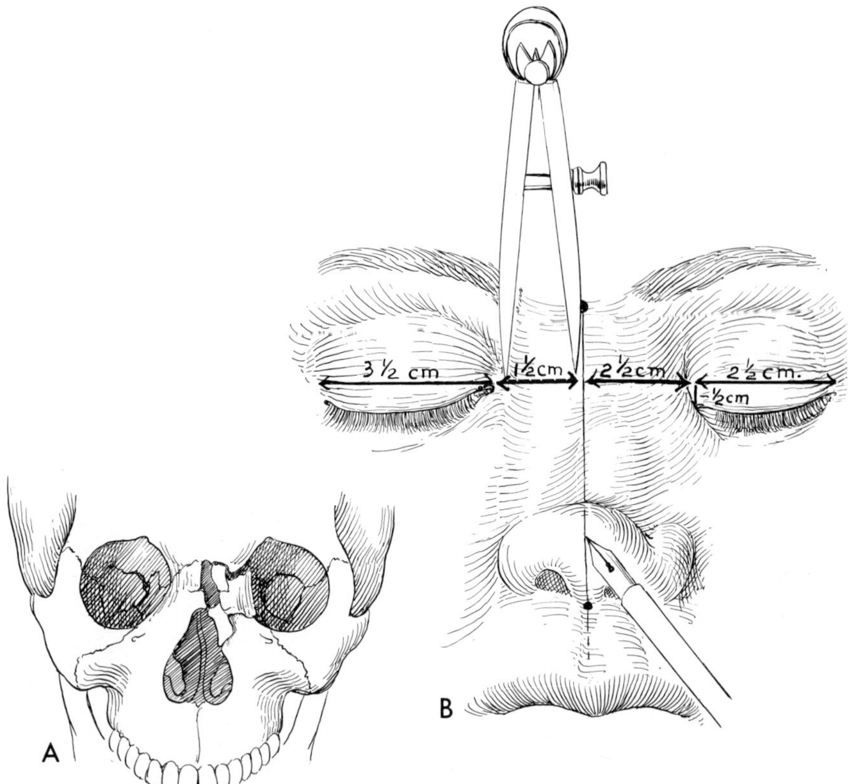

Figure 33–51. Traumatic telecanthus. *A,* Deformity resulting from fracture of the left nasal bone and frontal process of the maxilla. Bone fragments fill the medial portion of the orbital cavity. *B,* The left medial canthus is displaced laterally. (From Converse, J. M.: Two plastic operations for the repair of orbit following severe trauma and extensive comminuted fracture. Arch. Ophthalmol., *31*:323, 1944.)

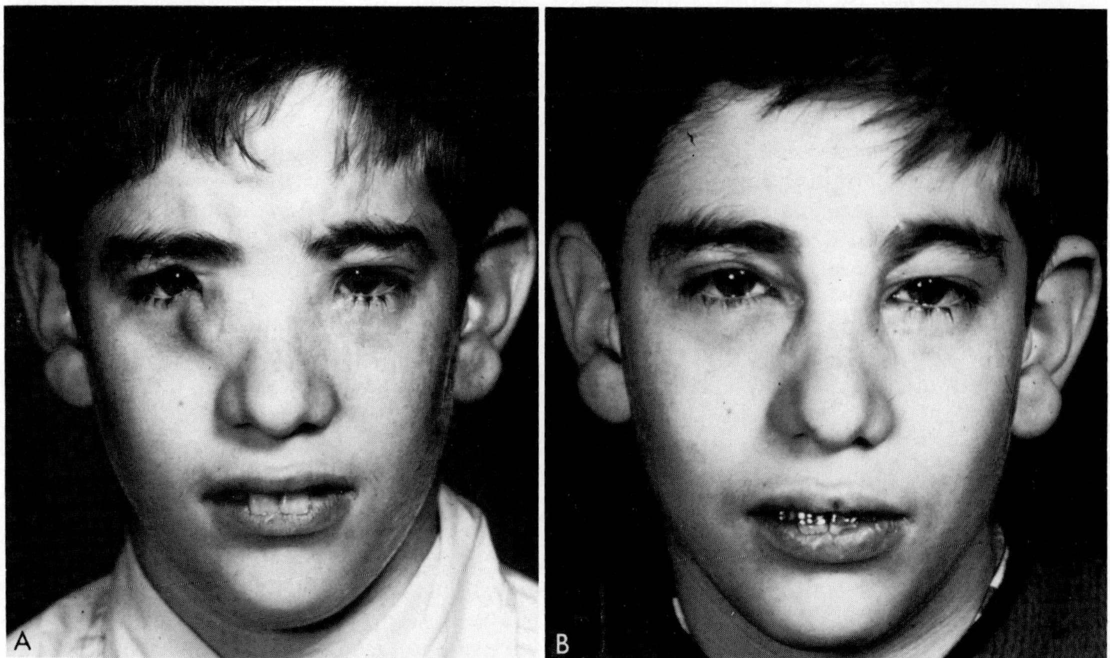

Figure 33–52. *A,* Nasoethmoido-orbital fracture that has caused obstruction of the nasolacrimal ducts. The patient has dilated lacrimal sacs (mucoceles) in addition to the telecanthus. *B,* Result obtained after bilateral dacryocystorhinostomy and restoration of the bony contour of the nasal bones and medial orbital walls.

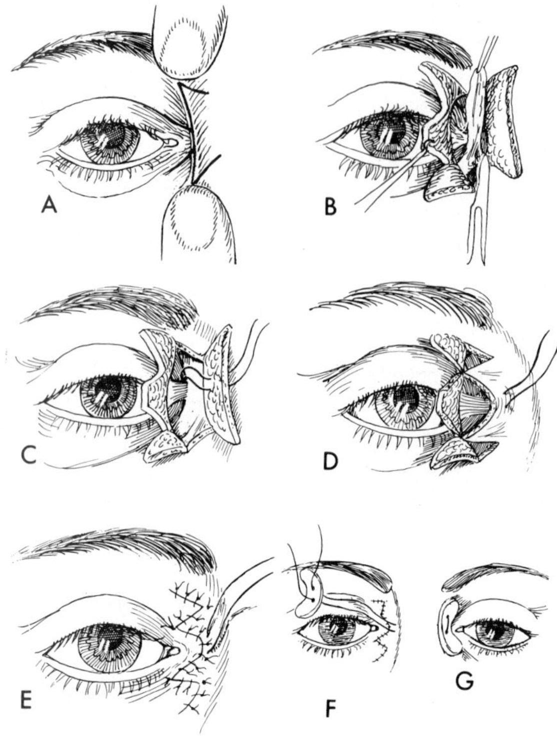

Figure 33–53. Double-opposing Z-plasties. Two Z-plasties done in opposing directions constitute a technique for relaxing tension and releasing contracture of a linear scar. It is of particular usefulness in areas where only small flaps may be designed. A limited amount of tissue in the confined nasoorbital valley limits the size of the Z-flaps. *A*, Design of the opposing Z-plasties. *B*, Flaps are raised, and the deep scar tissue is excised. *C*, Transosseous wires have been placed through the bony skeleton of the nose for fixation of the canthal buttons (see *F* and *G*). *D*, The flaps have been transposed. *E*, Double opposing Z-plasties completed. *F*, *G*, The canthal buttons are maintained by through and through wiring, ensuring the coaptation of the flaps to the underlying skeleton and preventing hematoma. The buttons should not be tightened excessively (Converse, 1964.)

also be dacryocystitis, which usually responds to antibiotic therapy.

Extraocular muscle injury may also be noted, the insertion of the inferior oblique being disrupted, since the medial portion of the floor of the orbit is frequently involved in the fracture. The inferior rectus or its check ligament is also vulnerable.

Some patients with malunited nasoethmoido-orbital fractures also have true *ptosis of the upper lid* from injury, hematoma, or a severance of the levator palpebrae superioris muscle or its aponeurosis (Converse and Smith, 1966).

TREATMENT

Treatment of a malunited nasoethmoido-orbital fracture should not be undertaken until progressive softening of the tissues has occurred and the general health of the patient has improved.

Lacrimal probes introduced through the lower or upper punctum and canaliculus are employed to test the continuity of the canaliculi. The lacrimal sac is usually dilated and forms a mucocele. Contrast media may also be injected through the punctum, and roentgenograms obtained show the outline of the lacrimal apparatus (see Chap. 34).

Surgical correction involves four different types of surgical procedures, which are best performed in the same operating session whenever possible. Staged procedures carry the inconvenience that each is made more difficult by the scar tissue resulting from the previous operation; however, staged procedures may be necessary for severe injuries.

Correction of Epicanthal Fold. The double-opposing Z-plasty technique (Converse, 1964) (Fig. 33–53) is most effective in correcting the epicanthal fold associated with nasoethmoido-orbital fractures. Mustardé's (1959) rectangular flap technique for the correction of the congenital type of epicanthal fold may also be employed. It is critical in correcting the epicanthal fold deformity that the medial canthal tendons are anatomically inserted into the craniofacial skeleton. In general, the medial epicanthal folds tend to disappear with restoration of nasal height (bone grafting), obviating the need for local incisions and flaps.

Restoration of Bone Contour of the Area. This component requires osteotomy (Fig. 33–54), replacement with bone graft,

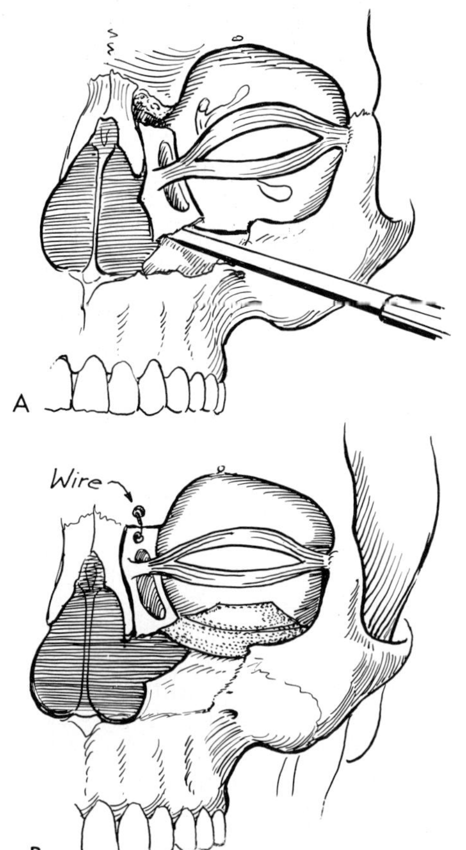

Figure 33–54. Osteotomy for malunited nasoethmoido-orbital fracture. *A*, An osteotome frees and elevates the malunited fragment. *B*, Wire fixation maintains the fragment. A bone graft is placed to reconstruct the floor of the orbit.

and reduction of the thickness of the medial orbital wall that results from overlapping fractured fragments. Occasionally the medial orbital wall may require reconstruction by a bone graft if it has been severely comminuted or destroyed. Restoration of contour of the bone bridge of the nose by bone grafting is usually required. Realignment of the bony portion of the nasal pyramid after osteotomy may be necessary. *The bone anatomy must be restored.*

Reestablishment of Continuity of Lacrimal System. The reestablishment of nasolacrimal apparatus function is an integral and essential aspect of the treatment of malunited nasoethmoido-orbital fractures when the lacrimal system is damaged (see Fig. 33–56 and Chap. 34).

Medial Canthoplasty and Canthopexy. This is achieved through reattachment of the medial canthal tendon by means of wire fixation of the tissues of the medial canthus to the bone of the medial orbital wall, after the removal of all scar tissue and realignment of displaced bone fragments. The details are discussed in Chapter 34.

Correction of Epicanthal Folds, Canthopexy, Dacryocystorhinostomy, Bone Grafting: A One-Stage Procedure

The preferred surgical approach is through a bicoronal incision (see Fig. 33–24), which gives excellent exposure of the nasoethmoido-orbital area, medial orbital walls, nasal dorsum, and frontal bone. It also affords the opportunity to harvest calvarial bone grafts (see Chap. 18). Additional exposure can be provided by lower eyelid incisions (see Fig. 33–25). If a Z-plasty procedure is required to correct an epicanthal fold, the Z-plasty incisions can also be employed.

The periosteum is raised posteriorly over the anterior lacrimal crest, the lacrimal groove, and the lamina papyracea of the ethmoid bone. Identification of the lacrimal apparatus may be extremely tedious when the area is filled with scar tissue left in the wake of penetrating lacerated wounds. Staining the lacrimal sac by injecting a solution of methylene blue through the lower or upper punctum and canaliculus, and placing a lacrimal probe through the same route, may help to identify the structures during the surgical exploration of the area.

The protruding and overlapping bone fragments are exposed. When severe comminution has resulted in destruction of a section of the medial orbital wall or when the bone has been reduced to mere pulp, a relatively thin bone graft (usually calvarial) is maintained in position by transosseous transnasal wires (Fig. 33–55). The dissection should be extended across the orbital floor. If there is extensive herniation of orbital soft tissues into the maxillary antrum, the marginal orbitotomy (Tessier, 1982a) facilitates exposure and reduction of the herniated tissue (see Fig. 33–38). Replacement of the medial canthus into its corrected position is achieved by reattaching the remnants of the medial canthal tendon to the medial orbital wall. The stump of the tendon can usually be identified and traction exerted upon it to mobilize the canthus in a medial direction (Zide and McCarthy, 1983).

Often, in long-standing deformities, dense

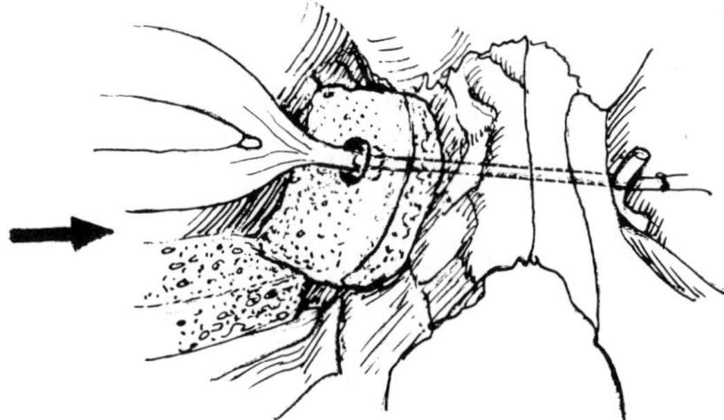

Figure 33–55. The use of a bone graft to reconstruct the medial wall of the orbit, thus furnishing an area of purchase for the medial canthal tendon. The bone graft and the medial canthal tendon are maintained in fixation by transosseous wiring. A batten of stout wire provides fixation on the contralateral side. The wire can be inset into the bone to avoid excessive protrusion under the skin. The bone graft must be relatively thin.

scar tissue lies between the medial canthus and the medial orbital wall. Resection of this tissue is essential if the canthus is to be reapproximated to the orbital wall and the depth of the nasoorbital valley regained. Traction is exerted to approximate the tissues to the bone, and the tip of a curved hemostat placed into the conjunctival sac in the medial canthal area assists in the approximation. Difficulty may be experienced in mobilizing the canthus toward the medial orbital wall. The scar tissue is the result of fractures of the orbital rim, penetrating lacerations, or previous unsuccessful attempts at surgical correction, and must be resected.

If difficulty is experienced in moving the canthus in a medial direction, the septum orbitale should be incised as widely as possible. In severe deformities the periorbita should be raised circumferentially (360 degrees) from the periphery of the orbital cavity, with the exception of the apex, as described earlier in the text under treatment of enophthalmos. This procedure is effective in releasing the canthus, thus permitting its replacement into the corrected position. The details of the medial canthopexy are discussed in Chapter 34.

Before reattaching the medial canthal tendon to the medial orbital wall, dacryocystorhinostomy should be performed, if required (Fig. 33–56). This procedure (see Chap. 34) restores the continuity of the lacrimal system by short-circuiting the tears into the nasal cavity. This operation, as well as other operations on the lacrimal system, is best done concomitantly with procedures to restore the medial canthal region; dacryocystorhinostomy is not performed until the wires for the canthopexy are in position (see Fig. 33–57).

When the lacrimal sac is destroyed, badly damaged, or grossly displaced, the sac should be resected. The common canaliculus, the point of juncture of the superior and inferior canaliculi, may be introduced into the nasal cavity through an opening made in the lateral wall of the nose in an attempt to reestablish lacrimal continuity. Techniques for the restoration of the continuity of the lacrimal system are discussed in Chapter 34.

Transosseous Wiring for Medial Canthopexy. If the bone landmarks (the anterior and posterior lacrimal crests) have been preserved, which usually is not the case, a drill hole is made well posterior to the lacrimal groove (Zide and McCarthy, 1983) (Fig. 33–57*A*). The hole must be wide enough to permit the entry of the wires and tendon. The posterior position of the bone fenestration through the medial orbital walls and the perpendicular plate of the ethmoid assists in maintaining the position of the medial canthi. This is the most important principle in the medial canthopexy. With a passageway thus established through the interorbital space, five wires are passed with a large curved needle or an instrument such as an awl. The needle should be passed in such a way that it curves backward to penetrate through the hole in the perpendicular plate of the ethmoid. The wires are twisted around each other after one of them has been threaded through the stump of the medial canthal tendon by means of a curved cutting needle (Fig. 33–57*B*); the cut ends of the wires are bent flat against the bone. On the contralateral side a similar procedure is executed, tightening the wires and snugging the medial canthal tendon into the bone opening. This maneuver is carefully performed under direct vision to ensure proper placement of the tendon in the bone fenestration.

One of the transnasal wires may be used to aid in the fixation of a dorsal nasal bone graft (Fig. 33–57*E*). The bone graft serves to reestablish the projection of the dorsum and to help improve the appearance of the nasoorbital valley. The remaining wires are brought through the skin to secure the canthal buttons (acrylic), which are optional.

The operation is completed by closing the skin incisions.

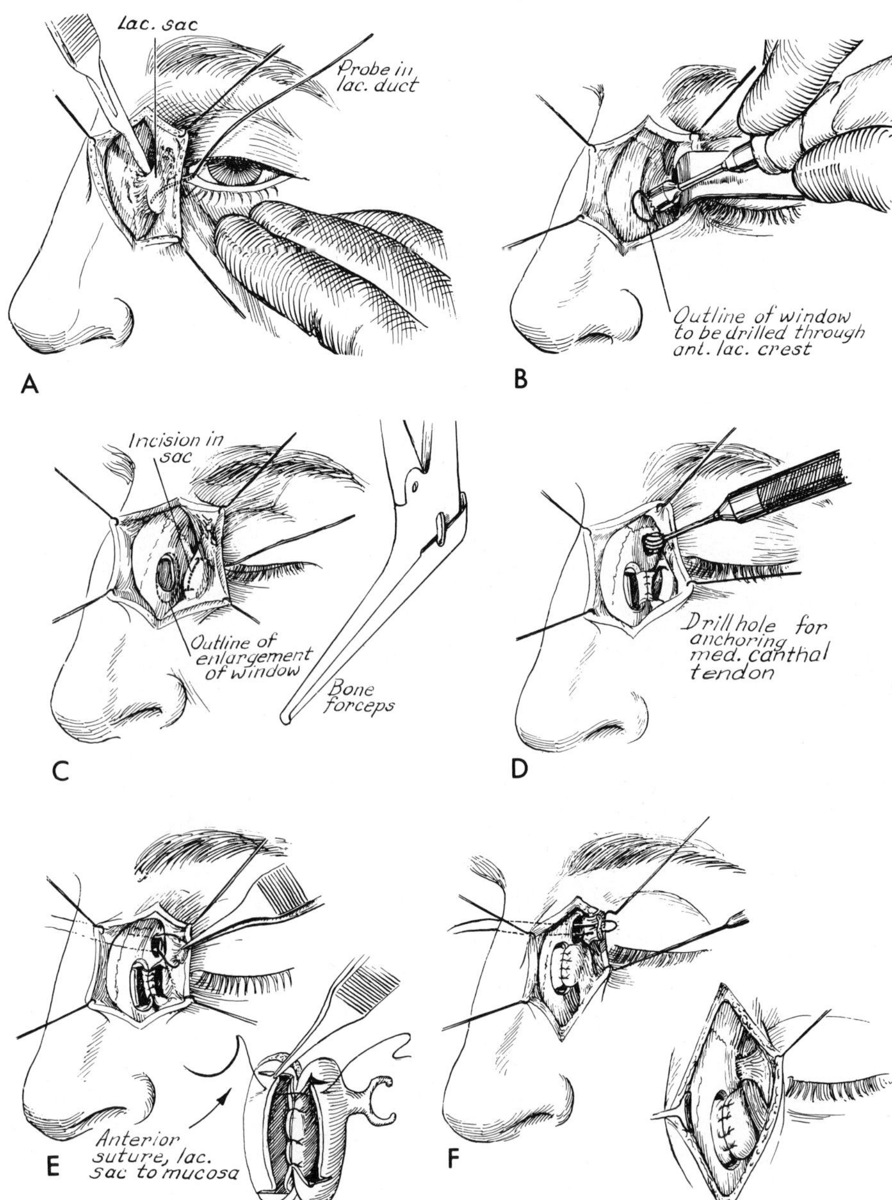

Figure 33–56. Technique of dacryocystorhinostomy combined with medial canthoplasty and canthopexy. *A,* Exposure of the medial orbital wall. The lacrimal probe placed into the lower lacrimal punctum (or an injection of methylene blue into the sac) helps to identify the lacrimal sac. The sac is dissected from the scar tissue resulting from the fracture. The sac is being raised from the lacrimal groove. *B,* A circular section of bone approximately 10 mm in diameter is removed from an area situated slightly below and anterior to the lacrimal groove without perforating the nasal mucoperiosteum. *C,* The bone opening is enlarged to a diameter of 15 to 20 mm, the diameter of the sac, which is usually dilated by the accumulation of secretion as a result of the obstruction of the nasolacrimal duct (mucocele). A vertical I-shaped incision is made through the sac and the nasal mucoperiosteum. *D,* The posterior nasal flap is sutured to the posterior flap of the lacrimal sac. A drill hole posterior and superior to the lacrimal groove is prepared for the attachment of the medial canthal tendon. *E,* The suture of the anterior flaps is begun. The transosseous wires have been passed through the medial canthal tendon. *F,* Suture is completed. The wires are twisted, and traction is exerted from the contralateral medial wall to maintain the fixation of the medial canthal tendon and canthus.

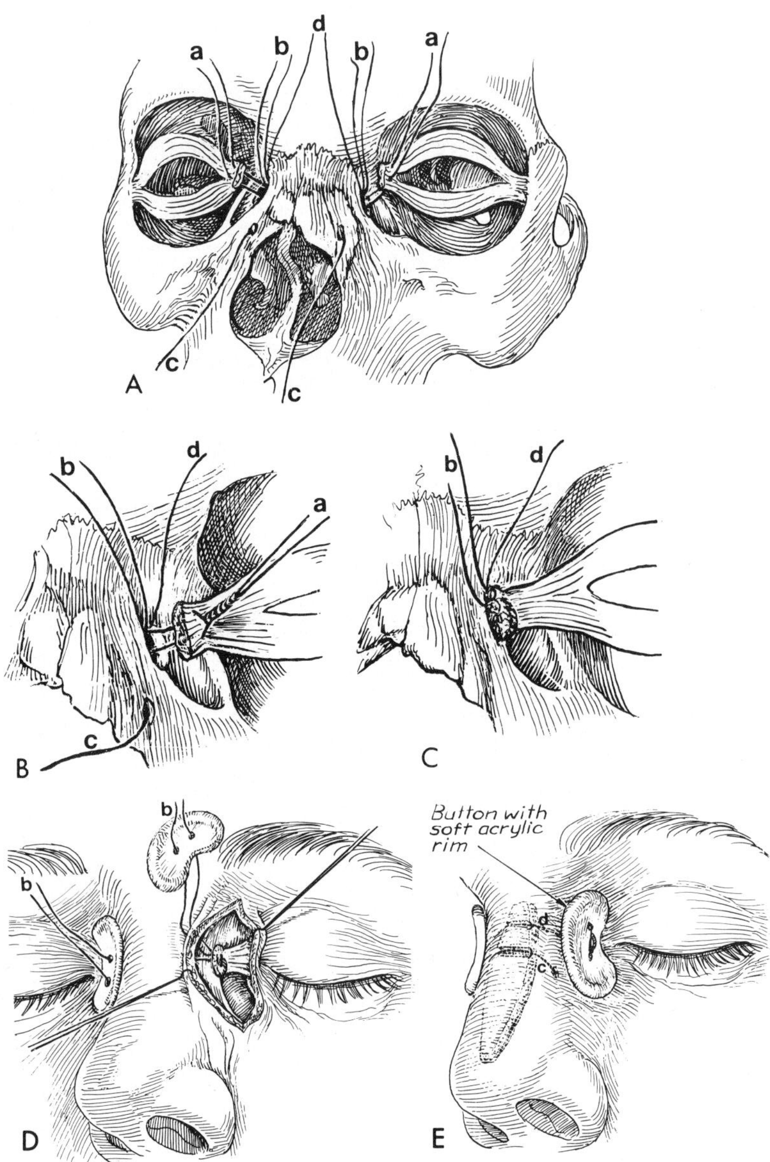

Figure 33–57. Respective positions of the transosseous wires (canthoplasty). The five wires placed posterior and superior to the posterior lacrimal crest are used as follows: two wires (a) for fixation of the medial canthal tendons (high to correct the canthus inversus deformity), and two others (b) for the canthal buttons. The other wire (d) will be looped around a bone graft (along with wire c). The drawing represents a medial orbital wall with well-preserved anatomic landmarks. In malunited nasoethmoido-orbital fractures, the landmarks are not present, because the bones are telescoped and overlapped. The point of reattachment in these cases should be high and posterior in order to reestablish the naso-orbital valley. The bone graft can also be secured by rigid skeletal fixation and the buttons are optional.

Contour Restoration of Nasal Dorsum. In malunited nasoethmoido-orbital fractures, it is usually necessary to increase the projection of the nasal dorsum of the nose by a bone graft at the same stage, because the scars resulting from the canthoplasties render a subsequent bone grafting procedure more difficult. Iliac bone is preferred because it lends itself to better shaping; however, calvarial and rib bone grafts have also been successfully used. The fixation of the graft is maintained by a circumferential wire (see Fig. 33–57*E*). The periosteum over the nasal bridge is elevated, and all deep scar tissue should be resected until bare bone is exposed before placing the bone graft (Fig. 33–58).

When scars overlying the bony bridge of the nose require resection and repair, it is relatively easy to restore the contour of the depressed nasal dorsum by a bone graft inserted under direct vision. If there is a deficiency of soft tissue, a forehead flap can provide extra tissue.

A *canthus inversus*, or downward tilt of the medial canthus, can result from a nasoethmoido-orbital fracture. When the displaced bone can be replaced by osteotomy, as shown in Figure 33–54, the canthus may return to

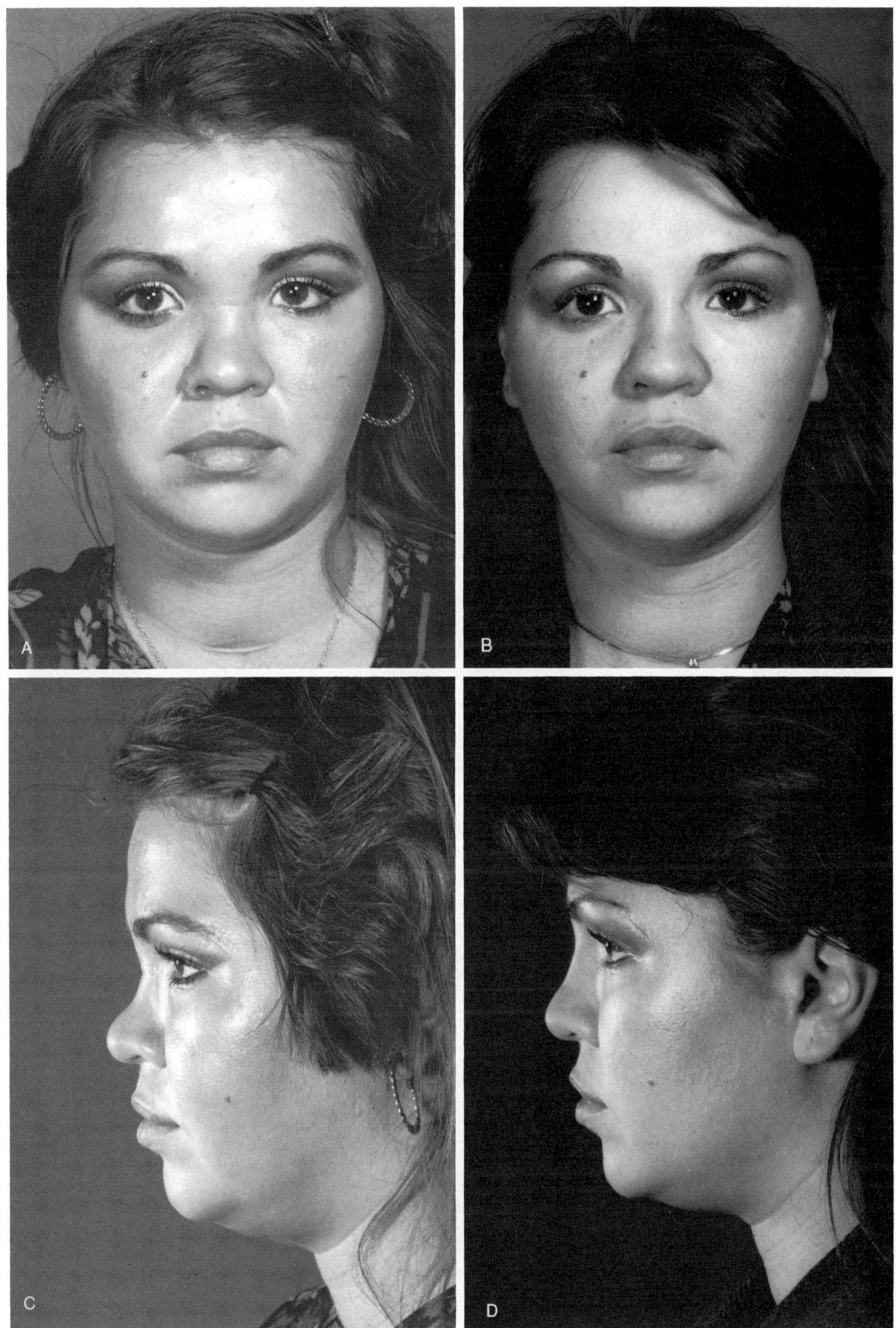

Figure 33–58. Contour restoration of the nose in conjunction with medial canthopexies. *A, C,* Nasoethmoido-orbital fracture with a depressed frontal bone fracture after a motor vehicle accident. *B, D,* After bone graft restoration of the nose and frontal bone and medial canthopexy.

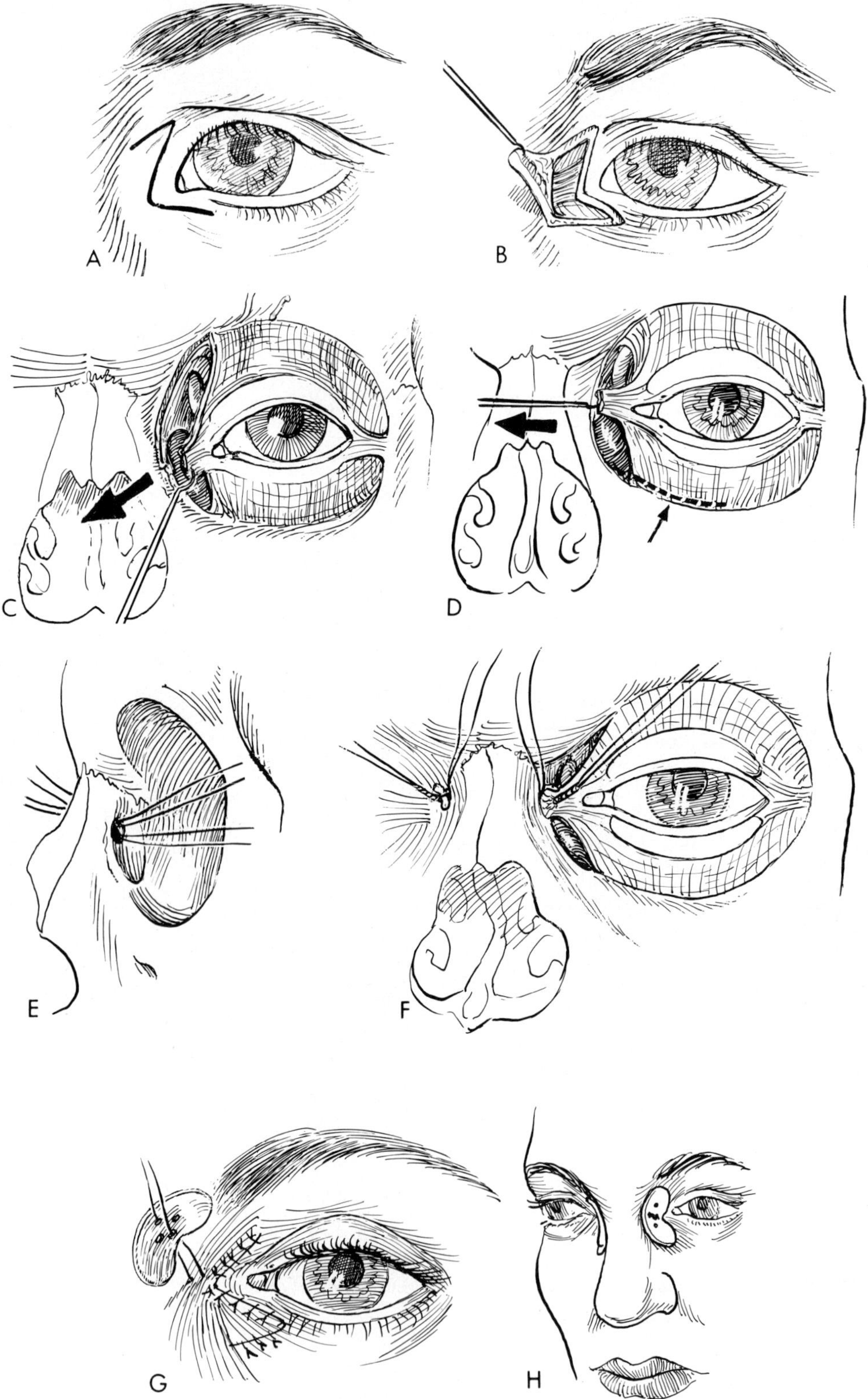

Figure 33–59. Correction of canthus inversus. *A,* Z-plasty incision. *B,* Elevation of the skin flaps. *C,* Note the inferiorly displaced insertion of the medial canthal tendon. *D,* Repositioning of the medial canthal tendon. Dotted line indicates release of the septum orbitale. *E, F,* Transnasal wiring to secure the tendon in the new position. *G,* Approximation of the wound edges. *H,* Appearance with canthal buttons in position.

its anatomic position. More often a cantilever bone graft over the dorsum of the nose, combined with Z-plasties of the medial canthal skin and medial canthopexies (Fig. 33–59), is required in a single operative stage.

Complicated Malunited Nasoethmoido-orbital Fracture: A Case Report

Some cases are complicated not only by the presence of associated orbital and midface fractures but also by loss of the ocular globe, loss of soft tissue of the nose, a depressed fracture or loss of the frontal bone, or fracture-dislocation of the entire orbit.

The patient shown in Figure 33–60 was injured in an automobile accident; after striking the dashboard she was projected through the windshield, suffering a nasoethmoido-orbital fracture, multiple lacerations, and loss of the right eye. She also sustained a laceration through the levator aponeurosis, with resulting ptosis of the left upper lid, as well as loss of the nasal bones and an appreciable amount of nasal soft tissue, with consequent foreshortening of the nose. The medial orbital walls had been splayed outward as a result of the severe trauma, causing telecanthus.

After treatment in a local hospital, the patient was referred with the residual deformity shown in Figure 33–61*A,C*). The telecanthus was severe, the right ocular globe had been enucleated, the left upper lid was ptotic, and the nose was grossly foreshortened.

In a *first stage*, skin was raised through a trapdoor flap, exposing the interorbital space over the depressed nasal dorsum (Fig. 33–62). The medial orbital walls were exposed. After a transverse osteotomy at the nasofrontal junction and resection of a central segment of bone, an osteotomy of the medial orbital walls was performed, and they were moved medially. The floor of the right orbit was repaired by a bone graft.

The telecanthus and the increased distance

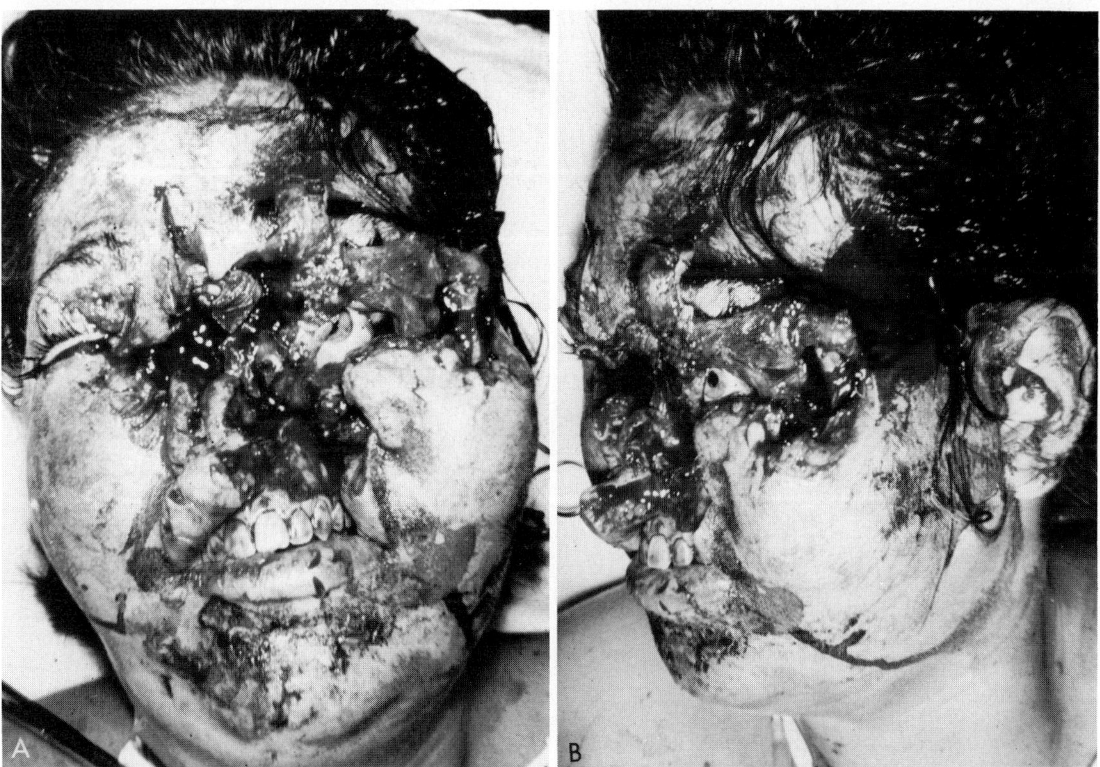

Figure 33–60. *A, B,* Severe facial injuries incurred by an 18 year old girl who was projected against the dashboard of the automobile and through the windshield in a head-on collision. The nasal bones were pulverized and projected into the interorbital space; the right eye required enucleation; the levator palpebrae superioris aponeurosis of the left upper eyelid was severed; the maxilla suffered multiple fractures; and the right lacrimal system was obstructed. (From Converse, J. M.: Surgical elongation of the traumatically foreshortened nose: the perinasal osteotomy. Plast. Reconstr. Surg., *47*:539, 1971. Copyright © 1971, The Williams & Wilkins Company, Baltimore.)

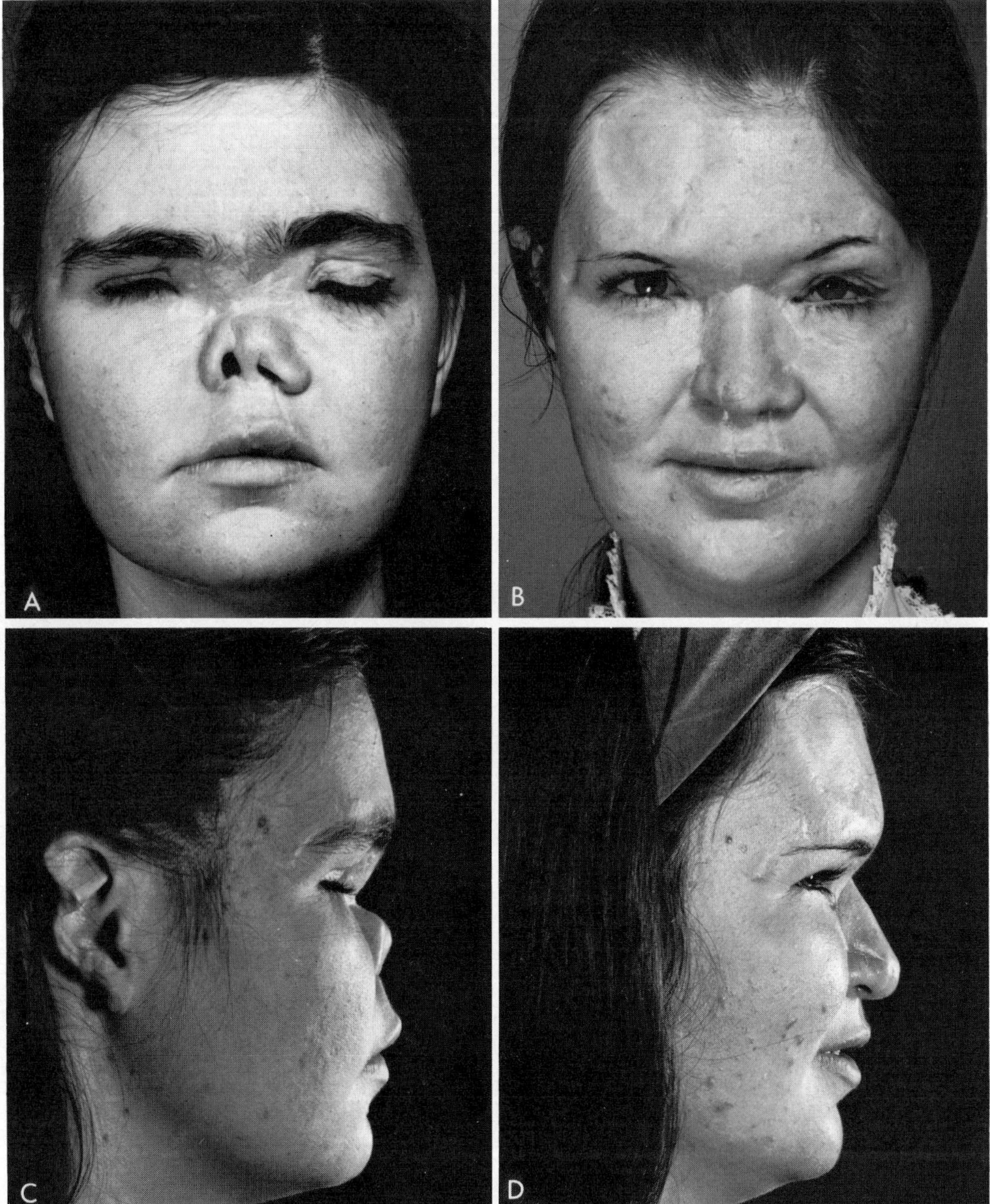

Figure 33–61. *A,* The patient shown in Figure 33–60 after primary surgery in a local hospital. Note the severe foreshortening of the nose, the telecanthus, the loss of the right eye, and the ptosis of the left upper eyelid. *B,* Early result after the procedures shown in Figures 33–62 to 33–64. A dacryocystorhinostomy was done on the right side, and a shortening of the levator aponeurosis remedied the ptosis of the left upper eyelid. *C,* Preoperative and *D,* postoperative profile views. (From Converse, J. M.: Surgical elongation of the traumatically foreshortened nose: the perinasal osteotomy. Plast. Reconstr. Surg., *47*:539, 1971. Copyright © 1971, The Williams & Wilkins Company, Baltimore.)

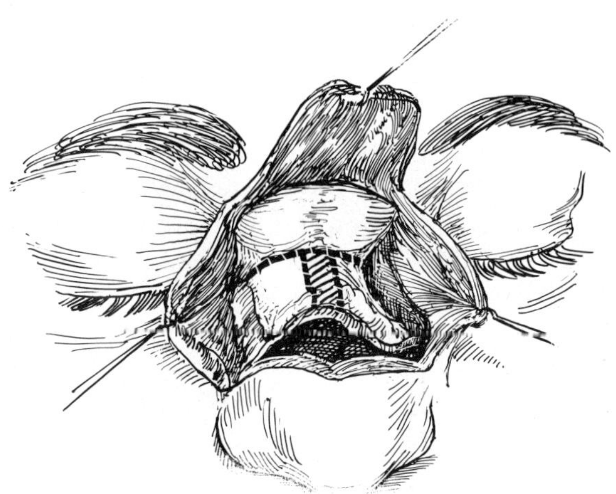

Figure 33–62. Stage 1. In a first procedure, the telecanthus was corrected by raising a skin flap to expose the interorbital area. Both medial orbital walls were exposed. A transverse osteotomy, resection of bone from the midline, and medial mobilization of the medial orbital walls reduced the telecanthus. A dacryocystorhinostomy was performed on the right side, and the medial canthal tendons were reattached after freeing the periorbita. The nose was divided by a transverse incision, and the tip of the nose was displaced into its anatomic position. (From Converse, J. M.: Surgical elongation of the traumatically foreshortened nose: the perinasal osteotomy. Plast. Reconstr. Surg., *47*:539, 1971. Copyright © 1971, The Williams and Wilkins Company, Baltimore.)

between the medial orbital walls were manifest. Subperiosteal elevation along the medial orbital walls showed multiple fractures and loss of the anatomic bone landmarks (the anterior and posterior lacrimal crests and lacrimal groove).

Projecting fragments of bone along the medial orbital walls were removed; a section of bone was removed from the small amount of bone remaining between the medial orbital walls (Fig. 33–62), and a submucous resection was made of what remained of the greatly thickened septum. An osteotomy of the medial walls was performed, followed by their mobilization toward the midline to correct the telecanthus. Drill holes were made through each medial wall, and four transosseous wires were passed from side to side for the triple purpose of (1) maintaining the medial translocation of the medial orbital walls, (2) reattaching the medial canthal tendons, and (3) placing canthal buttons. A dacryocystorhinostomy was performed on the right side (see Figs. 33–56, 33–57).

The first stage in the reconstruction was completed by passage of the wires through the skin of the medial canthus on each side, suturing the skin incision, and tightening the transosseous wires over the acrylic canthal buttons (see Fig. 33–57).

The lower portion of the nose was displaced inferiorly, drawbridge fashion, so that the tip of the nose assumed a position slightly overcorrecting the above foreshortening (Fig. 33–63). Mucous membrane was sutured to the skin along the edges of the defect. The downward position of the lower portion of the nose was maintained by dental compound. A second mold was duplicated in acrylic and was worn by the patient for three months (Fig. 33–63*C*).

During the subsequent three months, an eye prosthesis was fitted on the right side, and a levator shortening operation corrected the ptosis of the upper lid on the left side.

The *second stage* of the nasal reconstruction was started by raising a trapdoor flap from the tip of the nose, hinged on the edge of the defect (Fig. 33–64). The cartilages being thus exposed, the nasal tip was remodeled under direct vision; cartilage was excised and sutured with catgut sutures. The trapdoor flap was reflected to serve as lining for the defect, and was sutured to a similar trapdoor flap from the upper portion of the nose and to smaller flaps on each side of the defect. A scalping forehead flap (see Chap. 37) furnished the covering skin.

In a *third stage* of the reconstruction, a costal cartilage graft was removed, shaped, and introduced between the flaps to provide shape and support for the nasal dorsum. The patient's final appearance one year later is shown in Figure 33–65*B*.

Dislocation

In unusual cases, the circumferential orbit (360 degrees) is displaced by fracture. Such fracture-dislocations are seen after comminuted midfacial fractures combined with fracture of the frontal bone. The orbit is downwardly displaced and occasionally rotated upon itself. In such cases, a craniofacial approach similar to that employed for the treat-

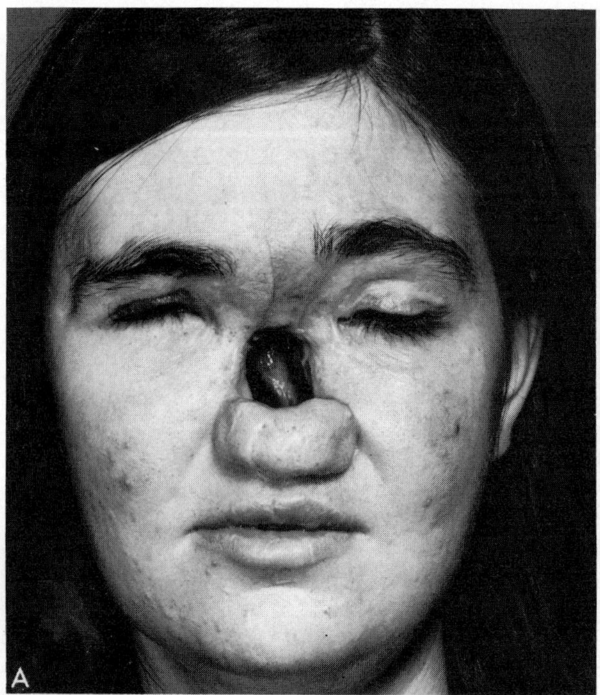

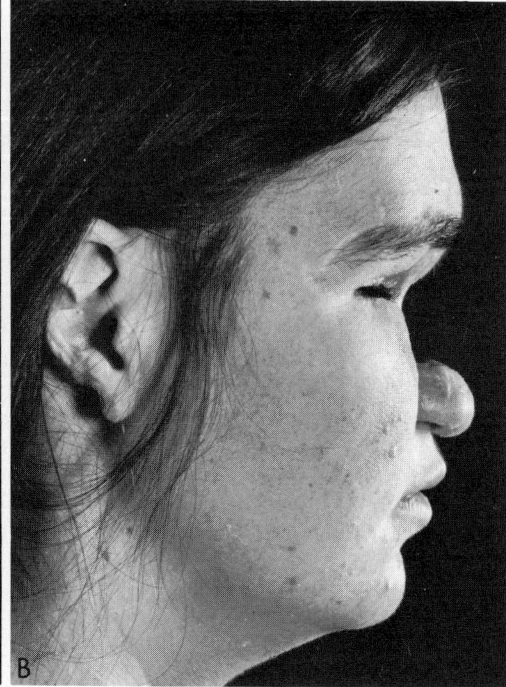

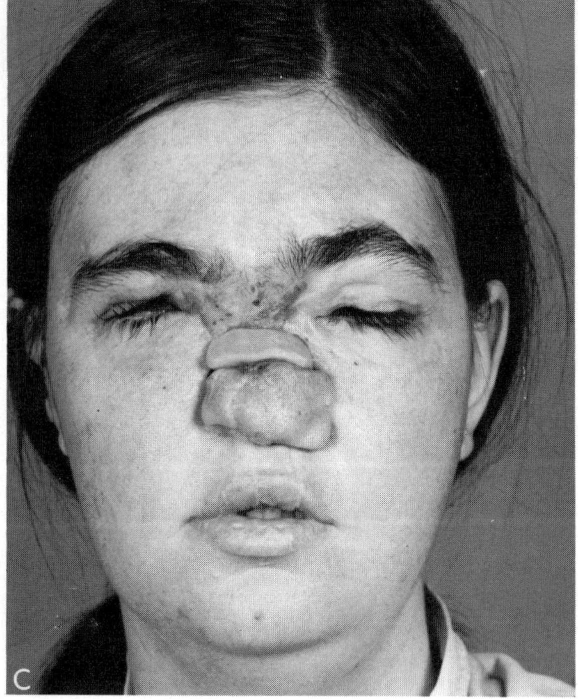

Figure 33–63. *A, B,* The patient shown in Figures 33–60 and 33–61 after the procedures illustrated in Figure 33–62. An acrylic mold was placed in the nasal opening to prevent superior retraction of the tip and was maintained for three months before additional reconstructive surgery. *C,* Note the acrylic mold placed in the defect to prevent the recurrence of nasal foreshortening. (From Converse, J. M.: Surgical elongation of the traumatically foreshortened nose: the perinasal osteotomy. Plast. Reconstr. Surg., *47*:539, 1971. Copyright © 1971, The Williams & Wilkins Company, Baltimore.)

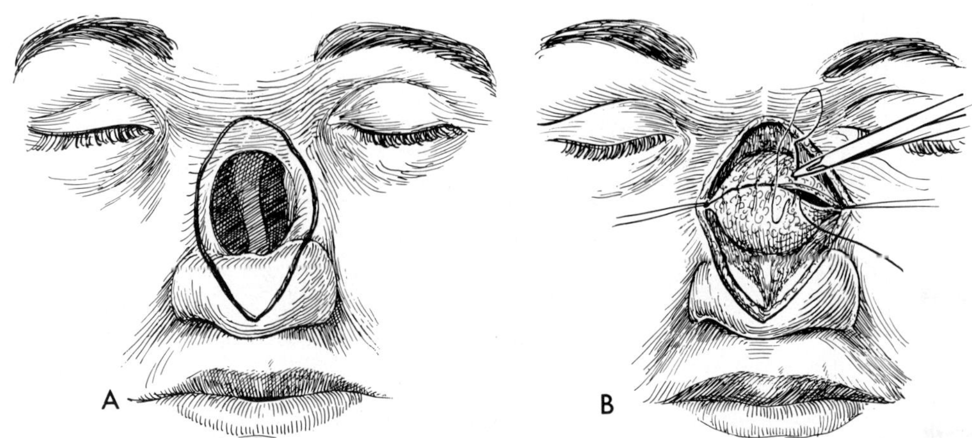

Figure 33–64. *A,* An ellipse of skin was outlined and used to provide adequate nasal lining four months after the procedure shown in Figure 33–62. *B,* The flaps are hinged on the edge of the defect and sutured. The nasal tip was remodeled under direct vision, and a scalping forehead flap provided the cutaneous cover. (From Converse, J. M.: Surgical elongation of the traumatically foreshortened nose: the perinasal osteotomy. Plast. Reconstr. Surg., *47*:539, 1971. Copyright © 1971, The Williams & Wilkins Company, Baltimore.)

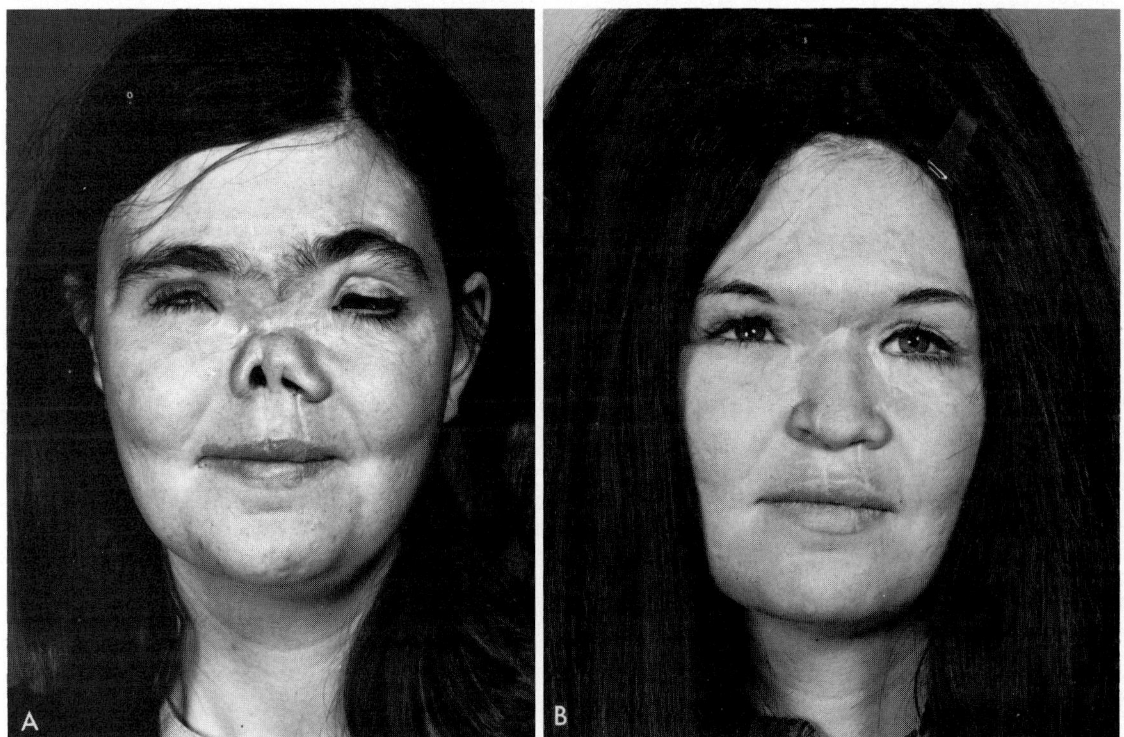

Figure 33–65. Comparative views of the patient before (*A*) and after (*B*) the reconstructive procedures. A costal cartilage graft furnished the skeletal framework of the nose. (From Converse, J. M.: Surgical elongation of the traumatically foreshortened nose: the perinasal osteotomy. Plast. Reconstr. Surg., *47*:539, 1971. Copyright © 1971, The Williams & Wilkins Company, Baltimore.)

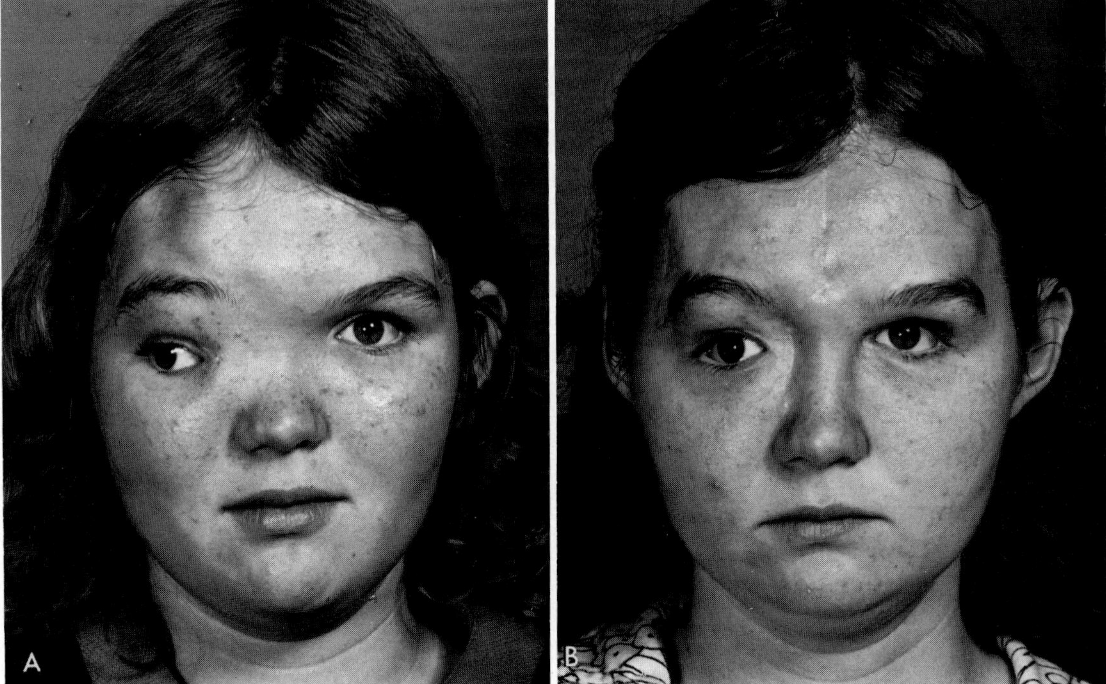

Figure 33–66. *A,* Patient with post-traumatic orbital hypertelorism (dislocation). In this unusual case the orbits were splayed apart in an automobile accident at the age of 1 year. Note the wide interorbital space and the exotropia of the right ocular globe. *B,* Postoperative result before extraocular surgery to correct the residual exotropia of the right ocular globe and a medial canthoplasty.

ment of orbital dystopia provides the only means of obtaining a satisfactory correction (see below under Orbital Dystopia).

Post-traumatic orbital hypertelorism is rare. However, the aftermath of untreated nasoethmoido-orbital fractures is usually telecanthus, an increased distance between the medial canthi and medial orbital walls.

The patient shown in Figure 33–66 is believed to represent one of the rare cases of post-traumatic orbital hypertelorism. Orbital hypertelorism occurred as a result of an automobile accident at the age of 1 year. At this age, the patient's nasofrontal area was splayed apart in the region of the metopic suture and the orbits were displaced laterally. Neurosurgical care was provided and a bone graft was placed in the median defect. No other treatment was provided and the patient was seen at the age of 14 years with post-traumatic orbital hypertelorism.

The technique for the correction of post-traumatic orbital hypertelorism is similar to that employed for congenital orbital hypertelorism (see Chap. 60). An improvement in the patient's appearance was obtained after this procedure (Fig. 33–66*B*).

ORBITAL DYSTOPIA

Vertical orbital dystopia can be defined as a condition in which one globe is higher or lower than the other in the vertical plane.

The skeletal pathology can vary from an inferior displacement of the orbital floor and zygoma (see Fig. 33–41) to a circumferential (360-degree) lowering of the entire orbit (see Fig. 33–69).

In the series of patients with vertical orbital dystopia reported by Edgerton and Jane (1981), the etiology was as follows: 62 per cent congenital (craniosynostosis, craniofacial microsomia, orbitofacial clefts, hypoplasia of the sphenoid); 26 per cent post-traumatic (fractures and irradiation therapy in children); and 12 per cent neoplastic (fibrous dysplasia, carcinoma of the maxillary antrum, intracranial lesions, neurofibromatoses) and miscellaneous (Romberg's disease).

In vertical orbital dystopia the surgeon must ask the following questions (Edgerton and Jane, 1981):

1. Are both eyes displaced? Or only one?
2. What vertical shifts of the orbits would produce (a) the best esthetic effect? (b) the

optimal retention of identity? or (c) the best chance of obtaining binocular fusion in all positions of gaze?

3. Exactly how many millimeters of shift up or down will be needed for each eye?

4. Will the palpebral fissures and canthi need the same amount of shift as the globes?

5. If the eye must be elevated, must the orbital roof also be raised, or must the supraorbital rim also be raised (or lowered) as a unit along with the orbital roof?

6. May some lesser operation be undertaken to give the illusion of correcting the eye levels? Or will complete translocation of one or both bony orbits be required?

It should be emphasized that some patients can tolerate a severe degree of vertical dystopia and be free of diplopia. However, diplopia may become apparent only after surgical transposition of the orbit. In general, surgical repositioning of the globe in the *vertical* dimension produces visual disturbances (diplopia) much more commonly than in the *horizontal* dimension (correction of orbital hypertelorism).

Preoperative Evaluation

A complete ophthalmologic assessment should be made, including complete strabismus testing. Three-dimensional CT provides the best definition of the skeletal pathology (Fig. 33–67). The scan is especially helpful in determining whether a *partial* or *subtotal* osteotomy-mobilization of the orbit is indicated.

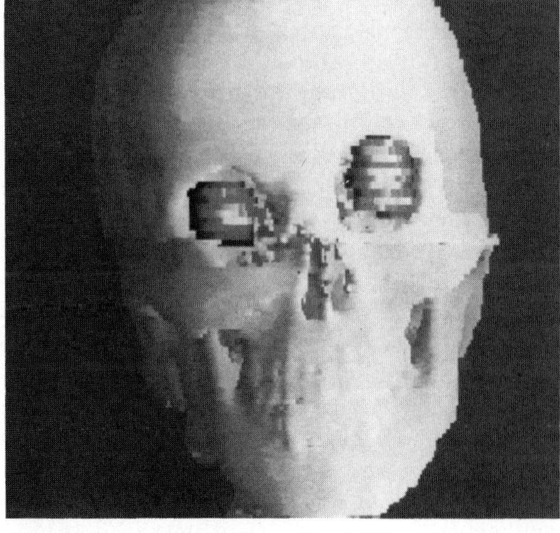

Figure 33–67. Three-dimensional CT scan of post-traumatic orbital dystopia.

Surgical Treatment

The *partial* osteotomy-mobilization of the orbit was previously described for the treatment of the malunited orbitozygomatic complex and enophthalmos (see Fig. 33–40) (Kawamoto, 1982). Similar techniques have been described by Edgerton and Jane (1981) and Furnas and Achauer (1981).

Subtotal osteotomy-mobilization of the orbit was described by Tessier (1967) and involves movement of the circumferential orbit (360 degrees); the orbital apex and optic stalk are spared. In this technique (Fig. 33–68) a limited anterior or frontal craniotomy provides exposure of the anterior cranial fossa

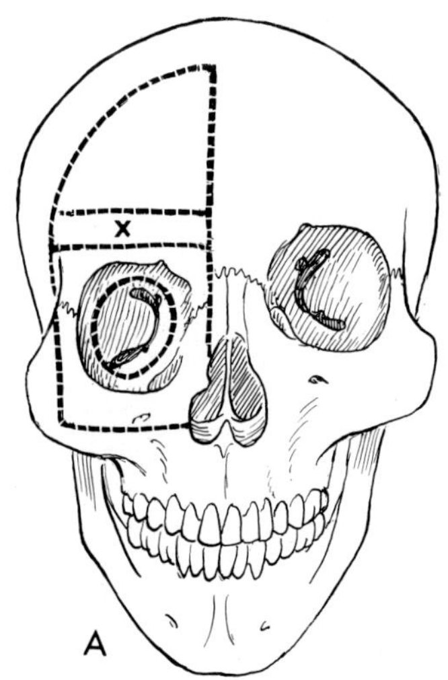

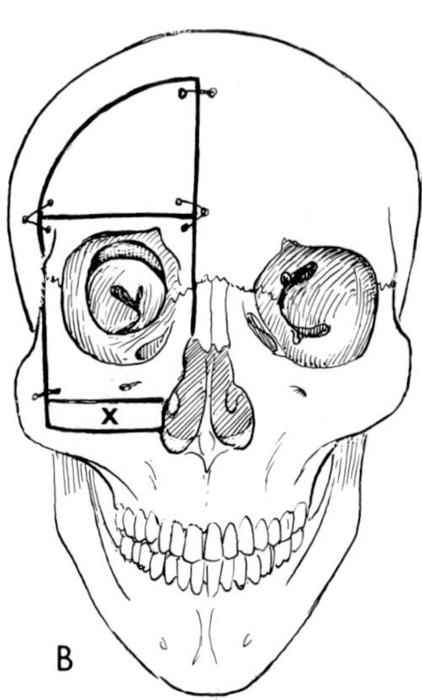

Figure 33–68. Rectangular orbital osteotomy to correct vertical orbital dystopia. *A,* Outline of the osteotomy lines and the area of the frontal bone resection (x). *B,* The orbit is displaced upward; the resected segment of frontal bone (x) is placed in the resulting maxillozygomatic defect. (Courtesy of Dr. Paul Tessier.)

to allow osteotomies of the orbital roof. A segment of bone (marked x) is removed from the frontal bone, and the height (in millimeters) of this resection determines the amount of superior mobilization of the orbit. The locations of the remaining osteotomies are similar to those employed to correct orbital hypertelorism: the medial and lateral walls and floor and roof of the orbit, the zygoma, and the anterior wall of the maxilla. The osteotomized orbital segment is translocated superiorly and segment x is placed in the resulting bone void in the anterior wall of the maxilla. The frontal bone flap is replaced and all segments are secured with interosseous wires. Patients who underwent subtotal orbital mobilization for the correction of vertical orbital dystopia are illustrated in Figures 33–69 and 33–70.

ORBITAL DECOMPRESSION*

Exophthalmos may be defined as a volume increase of the orbital contents with protrusion of the eye from the orbital cavity. *Exorbitism* (Tessier) is a volume reduction of the bony orbit with protrusion of the orbital contents.

Exophthalmos can occur in the following condition:

Increase of the orbital contents, such as occurs in thyrotoxic ophthalmopathy (Fig. 33–71), intraorbital tumors, or arteriovenous aneurysm.

Exorbitism can occur in the following conditions:

1. Reduction of the bone volume of the orbit by fractured fragments, osteomas, mucocele of the frontal sinus, meningioma, and fibrous dysplasia.

2. Decrease in the size of the orbit in patients with developmental skeletal disorders such as craniofacial synostosis. In such cases, frontal bone advancement and Le Fort III osteotomy effectively increase bony orbital volume.

Orbital Pathology in Graves' Disease (Hyperthyroidism)

According to Mayo (1914), Morgagni and Parry in the late 18th century had already mentioned a connection between hyperthyroidism and exophthalmos. However, the credit belongs to Graves (1840) and Basedow (1840) for having recognized the clinical entity of thyrotoxic exophthalmos.

Later it was realized that the exophthalmos persists and may even occur or progress after hyperthyroidism has been controlled by thyroidectomy (Dollinger, 1911; Kuhnt, 1912; Böhm, 1929; Andersson, 1932; Guyton, 1946; Wood, 1936; Craig and Dodge, 1952a,b; Heydenreich, Morczek, and Kurrals, 1966; Kuehn, Newell, and Reed, 1966; Long and Ellis, 1966; Long, 1967). Additional endocrine factors from the pituitary gland were studied, such as TSH (thyroid stimulating hormone) (Smelser, 1943; Pochin, 1944; Albert, 1945; Dobyns and Steelman, 1953; Canadell, 1959; Sonnenberg and Money, 1960; Sedan and Harter, 1966; Valenti and Cordella, 1967a,b); EPS (exophthalmos producing substance) and LATS (long-acting thyroid stimulator) (McKenzie, 1961; Adams, 1961); and other steroids (Alterman, 1954; Slansky, Kolbeit, and Gartner, 1967). A combination of hormones (Smelser, Ozanics, and Zugibe, 1958) was found to participate in malignant exophthalmos. It has also been suggested that Graves' disease may be one of the autoimmune disorders, with possible links to rheumatoid arthritis and systemic lupus erythematosus (Eversman, Skillern, and Senhauser, 1966; Werner, 1967).

The orbital pathology in Graves' disease and the tissue alterations that result in exophthalmos have been reviewed by Wybar (1957), Smelser (1961), and Riley (1972). It has been reported that mast cells, mucopolysaccharides, and water content are increased in orbital tissues. An inflammatory infiltration, consisting predominantly of lymphocytes and plasma cells, is found in all orbital tissues. An etiologic role has been ascribed to mast cells in the production of mucopolysaccharides and the resultant exophthalmos. The extraocular muscles are usually involved, and the extraocular muscle imbalance is another complicating factor. The final stage is fibrous replacement of the extraocular muscles with a fixed gaze.

At present, Graves' disease is universally considered a multisystem disease of unknown cause (Chopra and Solomon, 1970), characterized by (1) hyperthyroidism associated with diffuse hyperplasia of the thyroid gland, (2) infiltrative ophthalmopathy, and (3) infiltrative dermopathy (pretibial myxedema) (Odell and associates, 1970).

---

*Some of this material was prepared for the previous edition by Serge Krupp, M.D.

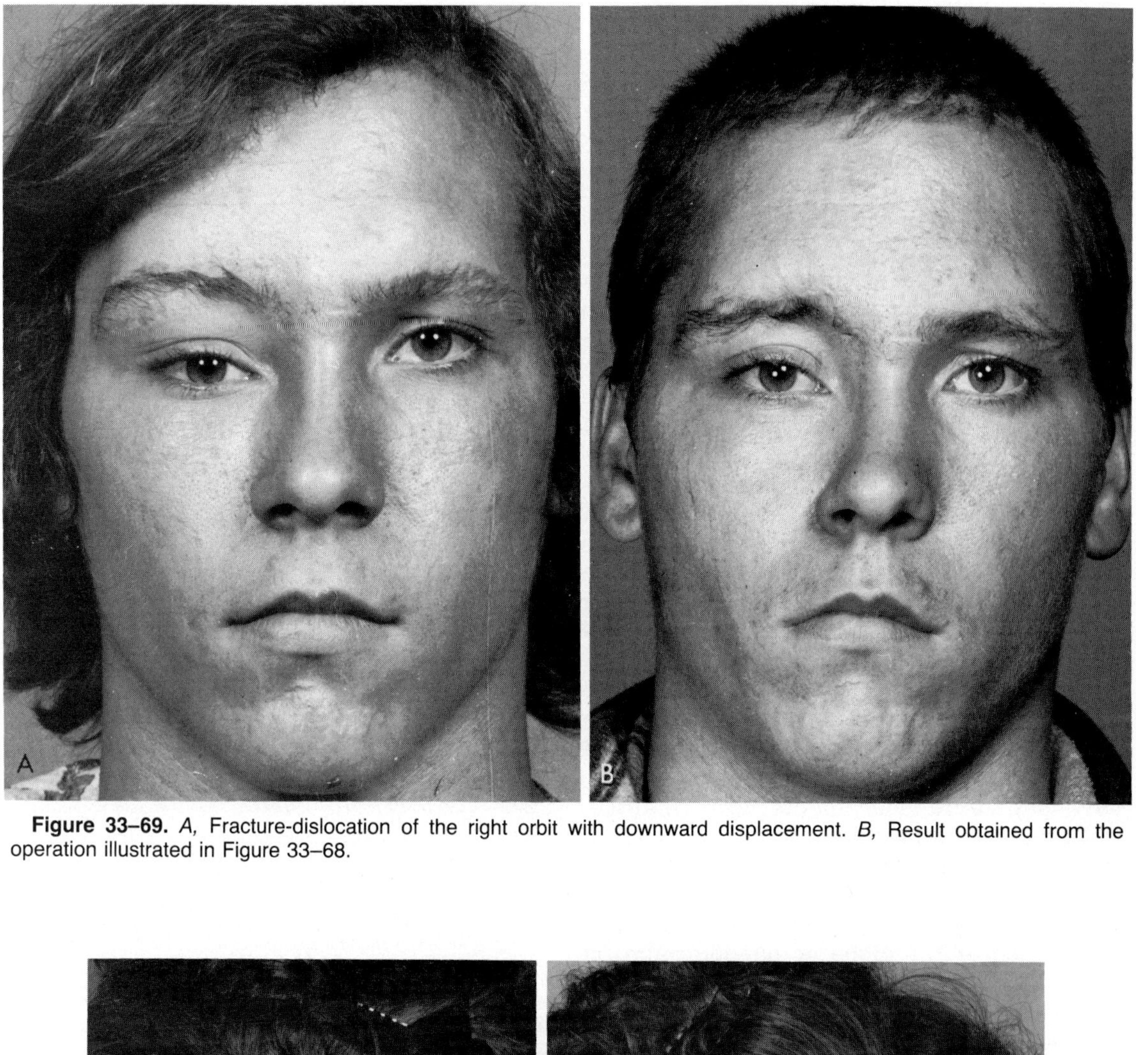

Figure 33–69. *A,* Fracture-dislocation of the right orbit with downward displacement. *B,* Result obtained from the operation illustrated in Figure 33–68.

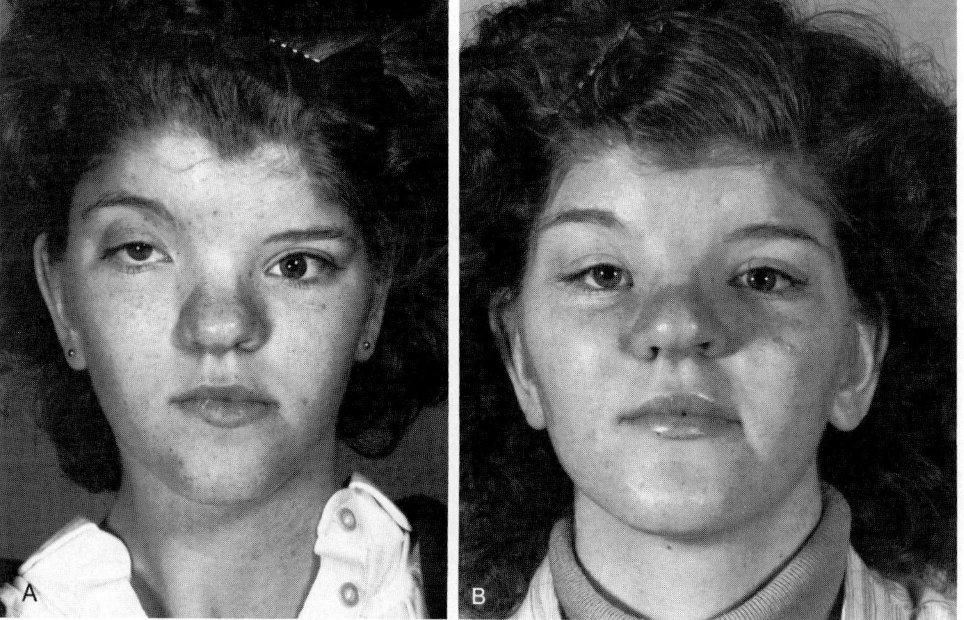

Figure 33–70. Orbital dystopia of the congenital type (craniofacial clefting) corrected by lowering the right orbit (the opposite of the procedure shown in Fig. 33–68). *A,* Preoperative and *B,* postoperative views.

Thyrotoxic Exophthalmos

The exophthalmos in Graves' disease is usually bilateral (Fig. 33–71), but in some patients it may be unilateral (Fig. 33–72) (Andersson, 1932; Rintoul, 1968). It is more common in females than in males, the ratio being about 6:1, but in males it usually leads to more complications (Graefe, 1867).

According to Means (1941), the severe form of thyrotoxic exophthalmos is observed in about 4.5 per cent of cases of hyperthyroidism. Craig and Dodge (1952b) and Poppen (1950) reported that only 1 per cent of the patients develop *malignant exophthalmos*. If the increasing proptosis in malignant thyrotoxic exophthalmos is not arrested, a progressive fullness of the eyelids occurs, followed by lacrimation and epiphora. With increasing proptosis, the lids are unable to cover the globe (lid retraction and lid lag), resulting in exposure and potential ulceration of the cornea. The scleral conjunctiva appears watery, and later chemosis of the conjunctiva of the lower eyelid develops. Diplopia due to muscular imbalance is followed by increasing limitation of globe movements; ultimately, only downward movements are retained. With increasing proptosis, edema can lead to optic nerve compression with varying degrees of retinal hemorrhage, papillitis, and loss of vision. There is always the danger of either perforation of the globe or panophthalmitis and death caused by infection (Würdemann and Becker, 1906; Merrill and Oaks, 1933; Naffziger, 1933).

The American Thyroid Association has adopted a system of classification of exophthalmos. Class I is termed mild; Class 2 represents the earlier involvement of soft tissue; Class 3 indicates proptosis; Class 4 has extraocular muscle involvement; in Class 5 the cornea is involved; and in Class 6 the optic nerve is threatened.

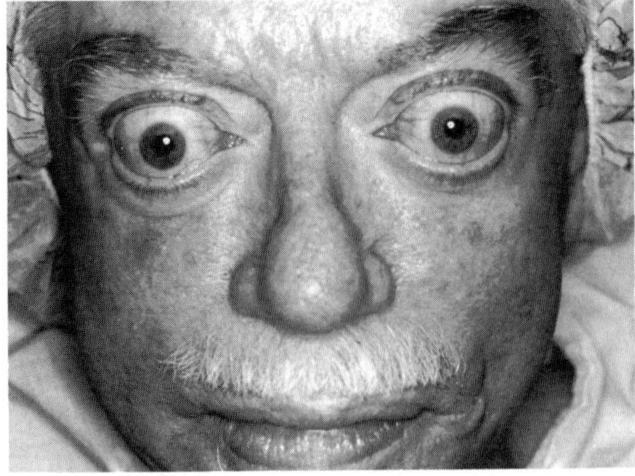

Figure 33–71. Patient with bilateral exophthalmos (thyrotoxic).

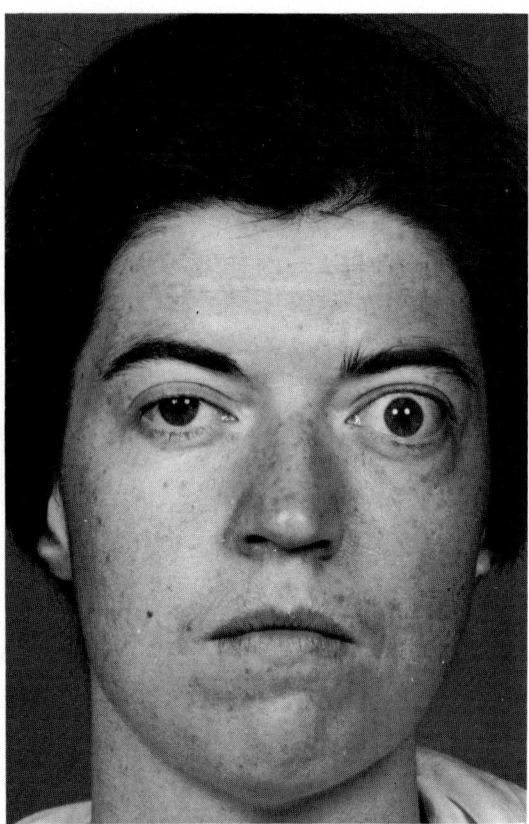

Figure 33–72. Patient with unilateral exophthalmos due to thyroid ophthalmopathy.

The diagnosis is confirmed by CT scan of the orbits that shows diffuse enlargement of one or more extraocular muscles (Fig. 33–73).

DEVELOPMENT OF ORBITAL DECOMPRESSION OPERATIONS

The various techniques employed for the decompression of the orbit in Graves' disease are summarized in Figure 33–74.

In 1888 Krönlein advocated a *temporal* approach to enter the orbital cavity for removing a dermoid cyst. In 1911 Dollinger performed the first recorded orbital decompression in a case of severe thyrotoxic exophthalmos, using the Krönlein-type approach (*one-wall decompression*). Tinker (1912) suggested removal of the floor, in ad-

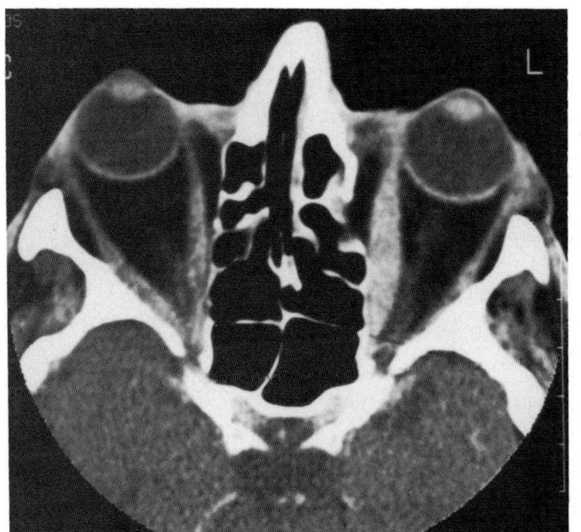

Figure 33–73. CT axial scan showing a diffusely enlarged medial rectus muscle in a patient with thyroid ophthalmopathy.

dition to temporal decompression, to obtain further enlargement of the orbit, but did not perform such an operation.

The temporal access to the orbital cavity for decompression in severe cases of exophthalmos in Graves' disease was popularized by Moran (1937) and Swift (1935), who approached the lateral orbital wall through a T-type incision. The technique was later standardized by Berke (1954) (Fig. 33–75) as an approach for the resection of intraorbital tumors.

In 1942 Welti and Offret reported another modification of the temporal decompression of the orbital cavity in Graves' disease. A curved incision exposed not only the lateral wall of the orbit but also part of the floor of the orbit, which could be resected, as well as the floor of the frontal sinus and even part of the orbital roof, without entering the cranial cavity. Schimek (1972) also advocated additional resection of the floor of the orbit to obtain a satisfactory decompression.

Hirsch and Urbanek in 1930 described a different technique for decompression of the orbital cavity. By a Caldwell-Luc type of approach (*transantral*), they removed the orbital floor, preserving the infraorbital nerve (see Fig. 33–74). In 1936 Sewall enlarged the orbit by removing the ethmoid cells through a curved incision over the frontal process of the maxilla to obtain access to the lamina papyracea (see Fig. 33–74). This method was also used by Kistner (1939), Schall and Regan (1945), and Boyden (1956). However, the technique was popularized by Walsh and

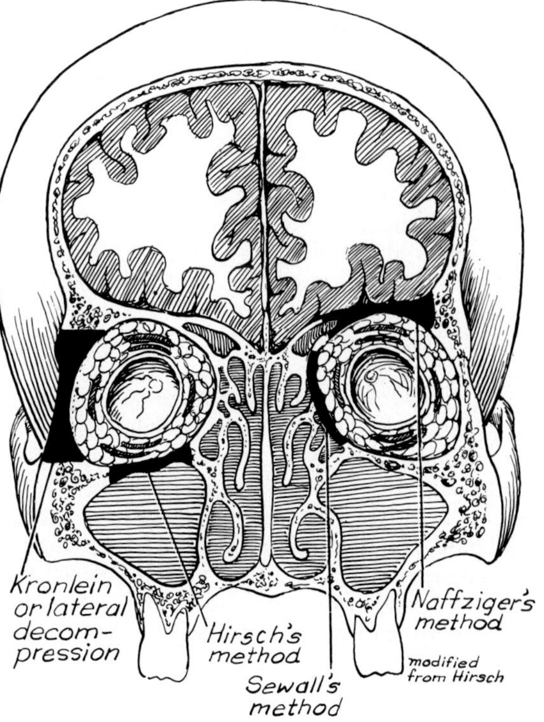

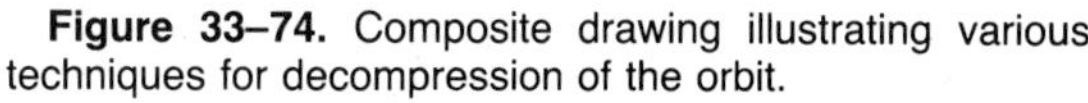
Figure 33–74. Composite drawing illustrating various techniques for decompression of the orbit.

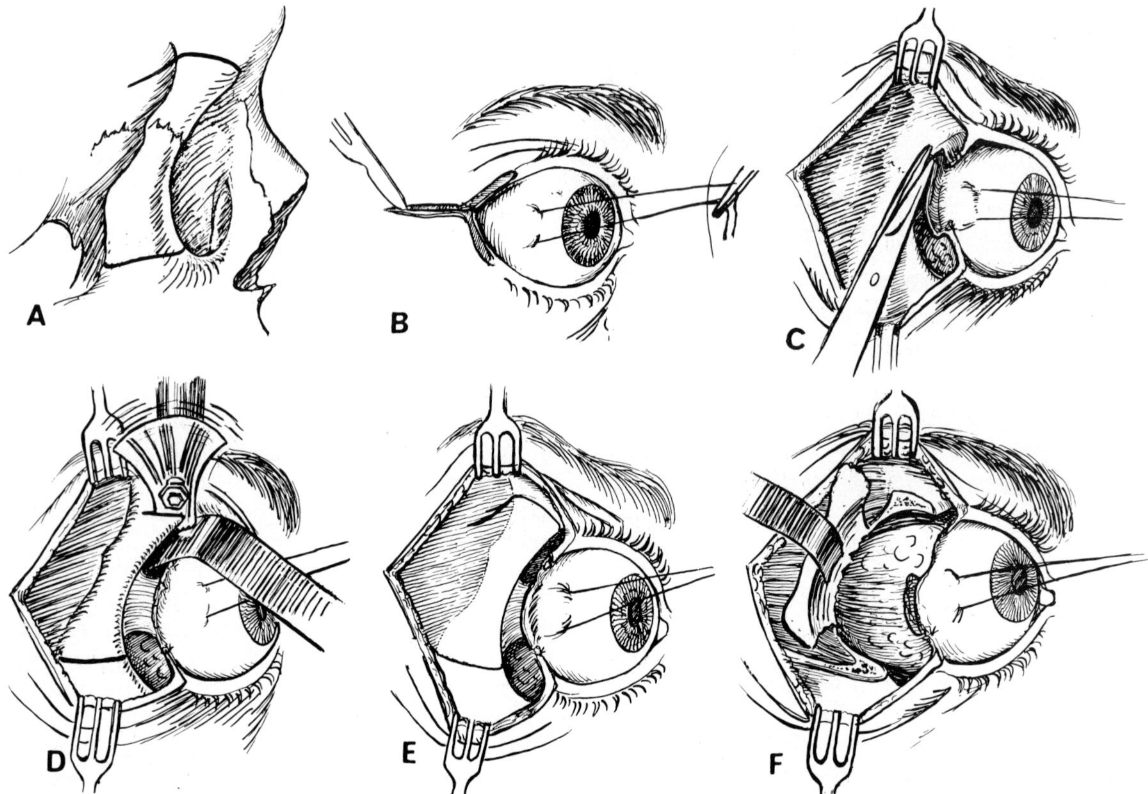

Figure 33–75. Lateral decompression: the Krönlein-Berke operation. *A,* The lines of osteotomy. *B,* T incision for exposure. *C,* The lateral canthal raphé is raised from the bone, and the check ligament of the lateral rectus muscle is severed. *D* to *F,* The section of the lateral wall, the outfracture, and removal of the bone.

Ogura (1957) and Ogura and Walsh (1962) in a large series of patients. These authors resected the orbital floor as well as the ethmoids and the lamina papyracea (*two-wall decompression*).

Naffziger in 1931 decompressed the orbits in severe thyrotoxic exophthalmos by an intracranial approach to the orbital roof, which was resected (see Fig. 33–74). Later, this type of operation was modified by Poppen (1944), who approached the orbital roof in a similar fashion but extended the resection of the orbital roof into the ethmoids and the frontal sinus. The Poppen modification was adopted by Craig and Dodge (1952a), who extended the decompression to include the sphenoid ridge (Fig. 33–76).

The disadvantage of the Naffziger operation and the Poppen modification is the resultant contact of the brain with the orbital contents, which receive the pulsations of the brain; this can cause a pulsating exophthalmos.

On the basis of his craniofacial surgical experience, Tessier (1969) described an orbital expansion technique in which the medial orbital wall was fractured into the ethmoid sinus. The orbital floor was lowered and a valgus osteotomy of the lateral orbital wall was performed (*three-wall decompression*). This procedure was modified by Wolfe (1979) to achieve a greater degree of orbital volume expansion.

Maroon and Kennerdell (1982) described a *four-wall decompression*. Through a combined lateral canthal-transconjuctival incision (McCord and Moses, 1979), all four walls of the orbit are partially resected.

INDICATIONS FOR SURGICAL DECOMPRESSION OF ORBIT

Surgical decompression in the severe type of exophthalmos in Graves' disease is performed if other forms of treatment have failed to control the exophthalmos. These include radioactive isotopes (^{131}I); thyroidectomy (Andersson, 1932; Naffziger, 1954; Sedan and

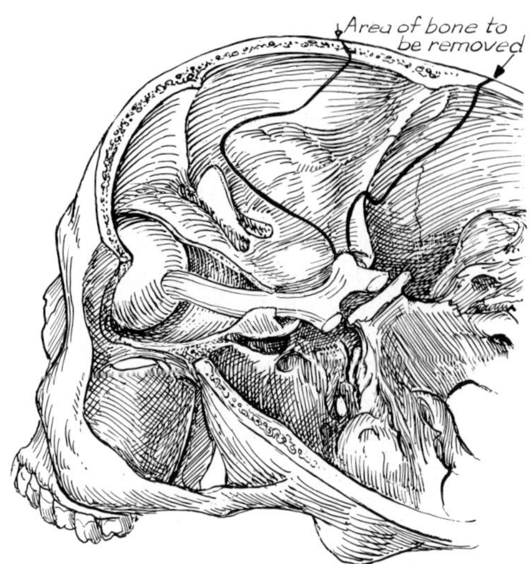

Figure 33–76. Decompression of the orbit by removal of the orbital roof: the Naffziger operation modified by Craig and Dodge. As outlined, the operation involves intracranial-extradural removal of the roof of the orbit, the sphenoid ridge, and the lateral orbital wall.

Harter, 1966; Mueller and associates, 1967); radiation treatment of the pituitary gland (Ljungren and Walander, 1959; Heydenreich, Morczek, and Kurrals, 1966; Kuehn and coworkers, 1966; Sedan and Harter, 1966); and hormonal or other forms of treatment (Ljungren and Walander, 1959; Slansky, Kolbeit, and Gartner, 1967; Werner, 1967). Although Graves' disease may be controlled by these various forms of therapy, the proptosis of the orbital contents may persist.

A survey of 75 surgeons by McCord (1985) demonstrated that over 60 per cent of orbital decompression procedures were performed to correct mild to severe proptosis with true or threatened corneal exposure or orbital disfigurement. Almost 40 per cent of the patients had been threatened with visual loss or compressive neuropathy.

The objectives of surgical decompression of the orbit are (1) to restore or preserve the threatened vision, the function of the extraocular muscles, and the ability to occlude the eyelids; (2) to relieve the increased orbital tension by allowing the periocular tissues to herniate into an enlarged orbital space; and (3) to attain a satisfactory cosmetic result (Welti and Offret, 1942; Naffziger, 1948, 1954; Craig and Dodge, 1952a,b; Walsh and Ogura, 1957; Kroll and Casten, 1966; Long, 1967; Low, 1967; Tessier, 1969; Maroon and Kennerdell, 1982).

The primary indications (functional) for the operation are increasing exposure of the cornea with impending ulcerative keratitis, increasing loss of visual acuity by papillitis and hemorrhages into the fundus, and loss of extraocular muscle function (Naffziger, 1948; Ogura and Walsh, 1962; Ogura, 1968). Secondary considerations (cosmetic) for operative decompression are relief of increasing exophthalmos, chemosis of the conjunctiva, and orbital edema (Naffziger, 1948, 1954; Ogura and Walsh, 1962; Ogura, 1968; Wolfe, 1979).

CHOICE OF SURGICAL PROCEDURE FOR ORBITAL DECOMPRESSION

The *Naffziger-Poppen-Craig intracranial approach* is indicated for malignant exophthalmos, a condition less often seen than formerly; the possibility of ocular pulsations and the greater risk involved in the intracranial approach are responsible for its decreased popularity. The *Krönlein-Berke approach (one-wall decompression)* and its modifications provide adequate access for decompression of the orbital contents provided that the lateral orbital rim is also resected as far posterolaterally as the inferior orbital fissure. The procedure also provides access to the orbital floor and the frontal sinus. The *transantral (two-wall) decompression* leaves no visible scar, does not alter the nasal physiology, and provides ample space for herniation of the orbital contents into the ethmoids and the maxillary sinus. In the hands of experienced surgeons, it is recognized as an effective procedure without serious complications, especially when combined with resection of the lateral wall (*three-wall decompression*) through a combined conjunctival-lateral canthal incision. The *four-wall decompression* is an extension of the latter combining subcranial partial resection of the orbital roof (Maroon and Kennerdell, 1982).

Medial Decompression Through an External Incision: Sewall Operation. The external approach through an incision extending through the skin and subcutaneous tissues over the frontal process of the maxilla, and curving upward below the eyebrow and supraorbital rim, leaves an inconspicuous scar. The ethmoid cells can be removed under direct vision; control of hemorrhage is assured, and the approach allows a direct inspection of the orbital cavity and the cribriform plate. The technique suffers the disadvantage of leaving a residual scar.

Lateral Decompression: Krönlein-Berke Operation or One-wall Decompression. Under general anesthesia with the cornea protected by occlusive sutures through the lids over a scleral lens, a horizontal incision is made through the skin for a distance of 3 cm or more in length from the lateral canthus to the temporalis fascia (see Fig. 33–75*A,B*). The tissues are widely undermined. The temporalis muscle is retracted, and the entire temporal aspect of the lateral wall of the orbit is exposed. The soft tissues are widely retracted, exposing the rim of the orbit in its supraorbital, lateral, and inferior aspects. An incision through the periosteum is made immediately medial to the edge of the orbital rim. The periorbita is elevated, the lateral canthal mechanism is freed from the bone, and the check ligament of the lateral rectus muscle is severed (Fig. 33–75*C*). The orbital contents are thus separated from the lateral orbital wall and retracted; the lateral orbital wall is sectioned with a mechanical saw and fractured outward through the thinner bone at the base (Fig. 33–75*D* to *F*).

As mentioned earlier in the text, additional orbital decompression can be obtained by removing the floor of the frontal sinus and also by resecting the floor of the orbit, as advocated by Schimek (1972).

Medial Decompression Through a Maxillary Sinus Approach: Walsh-Ogura Operation or Two-wall Decompression. The operation uses a Caldwell-Luc approach (Walsh and Ogura, 1957). A large opening is made through the anterior wall of the maxillary sinus. The operation is usually performed under general anesthesia with an endotracheal tube. The location of the ethmoidal sinus is indicated by the point at which the superoposterior and medial walls of the maxillary sinus come together. A line is drawn anteriorly along the junction of the superior medial wall to the point where the superior medial and anterior walls join. At the midpoint along this line an opening is made into the ethmoid labyrinth, and ethmoidal cells are opened until the point of junction of the superomedial and posterior walls is reached. At this point a transverse bone ridge is seen, under which are located the second division of the fifth nerve and the terminal branch of the internal maxillary artery (Fig. 33–77*A*). The bone ridge obstructs further exposure of the remaining ethmoid cells. The ridge is removed with a chisel, thus permitting complete exposure of the whole ethmoid labyrinth. The lamina papyracea is used as a landmark, and all the posterior ethmoidal cells are removed as far as the anterior face of the sphenoid. It is essential to remain medial to the lamina papyracea in performing the exenteration, because of the close relationship of the optic foramen with the posterior portion of the lamina papyracea. The other precaution is to avoid perforating the roof of the ethmoid, thus entering the anterior cranial fossa; another

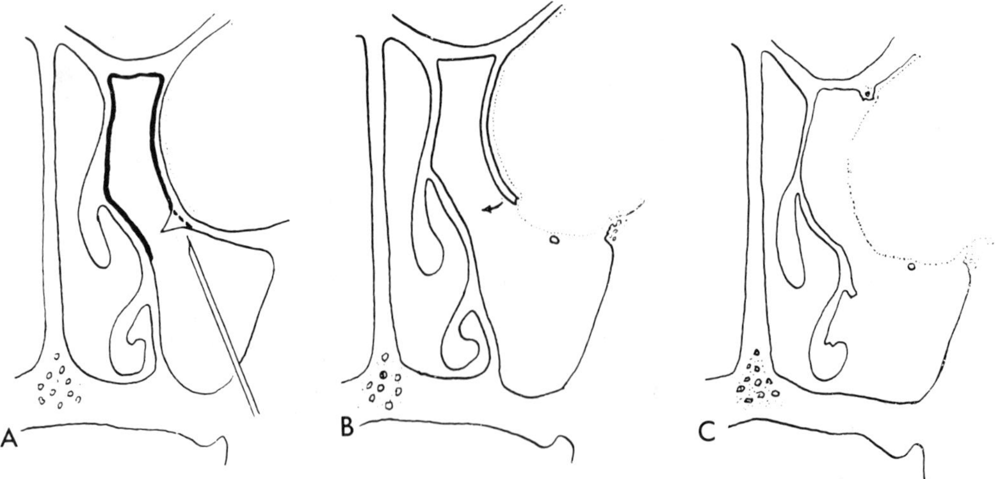

Figure 33–77. Medial decompression through a maxillary sinus approach: the Walsh-Ogura operation. *A,* The maxillary sinus is entered through a Caldwell-Luc approach. The ethmoid sinus is entered and the ethmoid cells are exenterated. A bony ridge obstructs further exposure of the remaining ethmoid cells and must be resected (see text). *B,* The floor of the orbit is removed; the arrow indicates the infracture of the lamina papyracea. *C,* Extent of the decompression. In this drawing the lamina papyracea has been resected rather than infractured. (Courtesy of Dr. Joseph H. Ogura.)

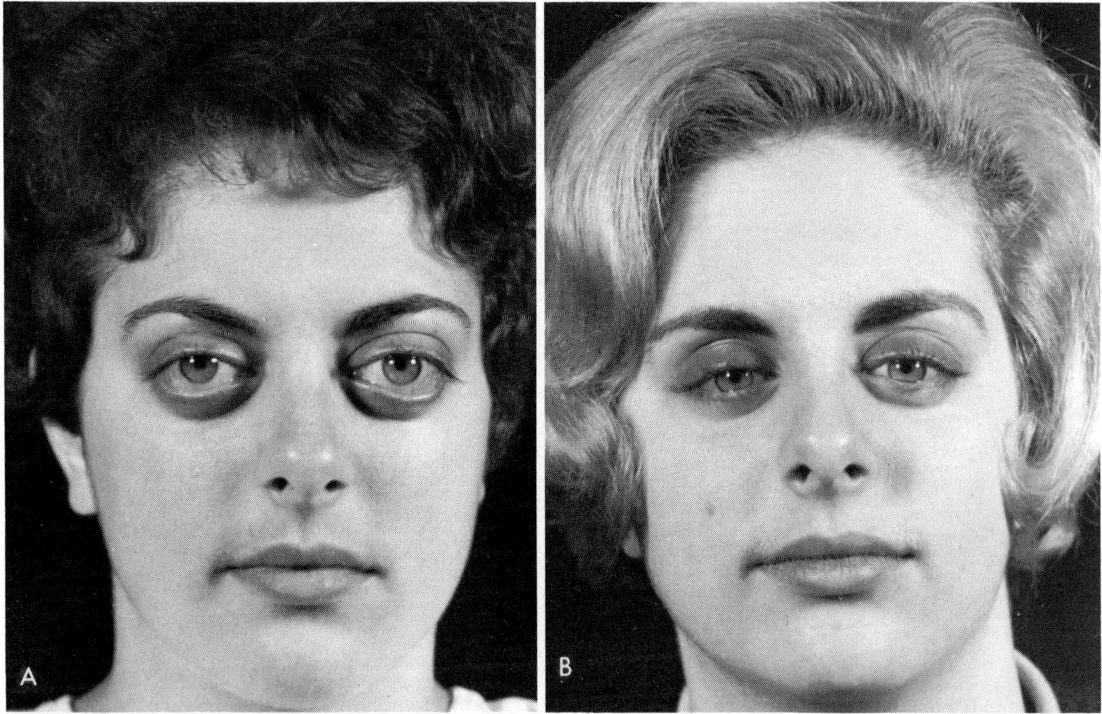

Figure 33–78. *A,* Moderate exophthalmos. *B,* Result obtained by medial orbital decompression (see Fig. 33–77). (Courtesy of Dr. Joseph H. Ogura.)

precaution is to remain medial to the cribriform plate in order to avoid cerebrospinal rhinorrhea. The floor of the orbit is removed after raising the periorbita and also the lining of the maxillary sinus (Fig. 33–77*B*); both of these structures are preserved, as well as the infraorbital nerve. The fragile lamina papyracea is fractured medially (Fig. 33–77*B*) or resected (Fig. 33–77*C*) except for its posterior portion, which is in close proximity to the optic nerve.

Several posteroanterior incisions are made through the periorbita, care being taken to avoid injury to the medial and inferior rectus muscles and the inferior oblique muscle; the orbital fat is seen to herniate into the maxillary and ethmoid sinuses. A window into the maxillary sinus is made under the inferior turbinate, and the mucoperiosteal incision line over the maxillary sinus is closed (Fig. 33–78).

Lateral Canthal or Three-wall Decompression. The three-wall orbital decompression is performed through a lateral canthal-conjunctival incision (see Fig. 33–29) (McCord and Moses, 1979; McCord, 1981). It includes a partial antral-ethmoidal-lateral orbital wall decompression.

Tessier-Wolfe Three-wall Orbital Expansion. In this technique (Fig. 33–79) the medial orbital wall (lamina papyracea) is displaced toward the midline, and the floor is lowered into the maxillary sinus. An osteotomy through the inferior orbital rim, lateral orbital wall, and superior orbital rim permits lateral displacement of the lateral wall. The periorbita is widely opened to allow the intraorbital contents to fill the expanded bony orbital volume.

Maroon-Kennerdell Four-wall Decompression. The Maroon-Kennerdell four-wall orbital decompression (1982) should be reserved for patients with bilateral proptosis measuring at least 30 mm or unilateral proptosis measuring at least 10 mm.

A 35 mm lateral canthal skin incision permits a T-shaped incision of the temporalis fascia with reflection of the underlying muscle and the intraorbital contents (Fig. 33–80). A major portion of the lateral orbital wall is resected. A fenestration is made in the orbital roof to expose the dura that is reflected. The orbital roof is resected posteriorly with rongeurs medially to the cribriform plate and lateral margin of the ethmoid, and posteriorly to the lesser wing of the sphenoid.

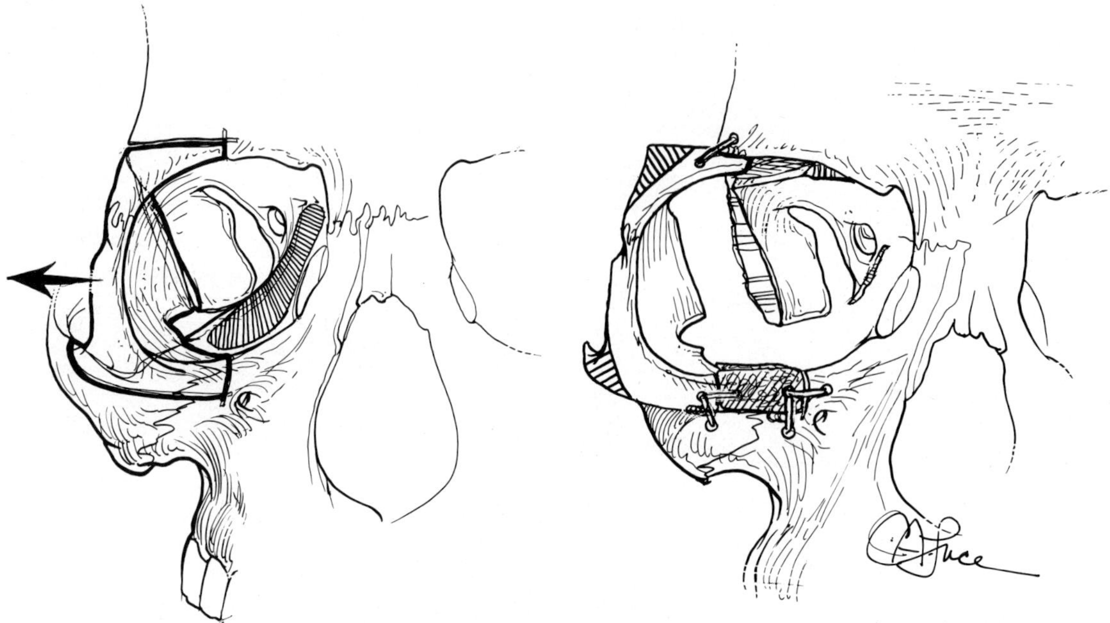

Figure 33–79. The Tessier-Wolfe three-wall orbital expansion. Note the outfracture of the medial wall into the ethmoid sinus, and of the floor into the maxillary sinus, as well as the osteotomy displacement of the lateral wall. The latter is contoured *(diagonal lines)* and secured with interosseous wires (or miniplates). A bone graft is placed in the inferior orbital rim defect.

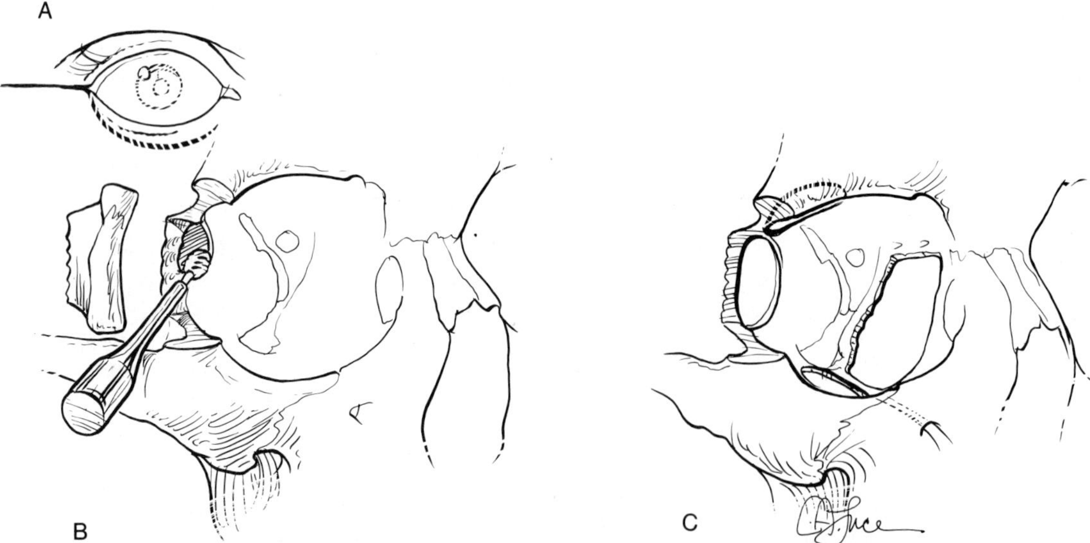

Figure 33–80. The Maroon-Kennerdell four-wall orbital decompression. *A,* Straight line 35 mm skin incision. It is extended with a conjunctival incision as far as the punctum *(dotted line)*. *B,* Removal of the posterior aspect of the lateral orbital wall with a bur. *C,* Orbital expansion after resection of the orbital floor and medial wall. Note also the excised portion of the posterolateral orbital roof. The periorbita must be incised to allow expansion of the soft tissue into the expanded orbit.

Through the conjunctival incision, exposure of the floor and medial orbital wall is obtained by subperiosteal dissection. The floor and medial wall are resected in a subtotal fashion with the aid of rongeurs (Fig. 33–80*C*). The periorbita and mucosa are widely excised to permit full extrusion of the intraorbital contents.

Major complications in the subcranial types of operations are unusual. In nearly all cases, transient diplopia occurs. If this condition become persistent, corrective extraocular muscle surgery is required. Extraocular muscle imbalance is more frequent in advanced cases, in which intrinsic degenerative changes have occurred in the musculature (Naffziger, 1948, 1954; Walsh and Ogura, 1957; Low, 1967).

Upper Lid Retraction. Although congestion and edema of the lids, conjunctiva, and orbit are partly responsive to systemic or repository steroid therapy, extraocular imbalance, restriction of upward gaze, lid retraction and puffy swelling of the lids, as well as varying degrees of exophthalmos, may persist.

The exact mechanism responsible for eyelid retraction is not fully understood; spasm or overactivity of the eyelid musculature has been presumed to cause the deformity, consisting of an altered position of the eyelid. The disorder is almost always bilateral, rarely unilateral, frequently symmetric, and rarely asymmetric.

Upper eyelid retraction may be caused by overactivity or spasm of Müller's muscle and/or the levator palpebrae superioris muscle. Aside from the undesirable appearance, corneal and conjunctival exposure mandates surgical correction.

Surgical Correction. Lid retraction alone is not an indication for orbital decompression, although the latter may make the lid retraction less obvious. Retraction of the upper eyelid has been treated by weakening of the levator, as advocated by Moran (1956) and Berke (1965). The surgical approach to the two muscles, Müller's muscle and the levator palpebrae superioris muscle, has also been undertaken by Henderson (1965, 1967).

Müller's muscle is composed of smooth muscle fibers innervated by the sympathetic nervous system; the levator muscle is a striated type of muscle, innervated by the third cranial nerve.

Putterman and Urist (1972) described a technique for distinguishing between the eyelid retraction due to overaction of Müller's muscle alone, and that secondary to the combined overaction of both Müller's muscle and the levator muscles. This is determined first by completely excising Müller's muscle and observing the height of the lid. If the lid is insufficiently lowered, additional lowering is obtained by partial tenotomy of the levator aponeurosis.

In order to obtain a block anesthesia of the upper eyelid, Putterman and Urist (1972) employed the sensory nerve block described by Hildreth and Silver (1967). A 25 gauge needle is inserted 4 cm into the orbit, the needle penetrating immediately below the midsuperior orbital rim and hugging the roof of the orbit. Lidocaine (Xylocaine), 2 per cent, is injected in a dosage of 0.5 ml. Anesthesia of the upper eyelid is obtained while the motility of the lid is preserved.

The patient is placed in a sitting position, and the levels of the upper eyelids are compared with each other in the primary position of gaze and looking up and down. The upper lid is everted over a Desmarres retractor, exposing the superior tarsal border. The important structures above the tarsus are the conjunctiva, Müller's muscle, and the levator aponeurosis. Müller's muscle attaches to the superior tarsal border, whereas the levator aponeurosis extends over the anterior surface of the tarsus and inserts into the inferior border of the tarsus as well as into the skin.

The lid being everted, an incision is made 2 mm above the superior tarsal border at its lateral aspect. Scissors are inserted between the plane of the conjunctiva and layer by layer along the central part of the lid. This procedure gradually lengthens the tendon and allows the lid to come down slowly. The patient is again checked in a sitting position several times during the levator stripping procedure to evaluate the position of the lid. If the lid level continues to be high, additional levator fibers are stripped. If the lid level is higher temporally than nasally, additional stripping can be done on the temporal half of the levator aponeurosis.

ANOPHTHALMOS AND MICROPHTHALMOS

Anophthalmos

Anophthalmos (anophthalmia) is defined as a condition in which no ocular globe, however small, can be found in the orbit. It is difficult to distinguish between true anophthalmos and an extreme degree of microphthalmos, in which there is an ocular globe remnant. The answer lies in microscopic examination of serial sections of the orbital contents, a procedure that is impractical in the living.

In *primary anophthalmos*, the single originating fault is a failure of the optic pit to deepen and form an optic outgrowth from the forebrain (see Embryology). In *secondary anophthalmos*, there is complete suppression or abnormal development of the entire forebrain; absence of the eye is merely the consequence of the lack of development of the entire region, and is one of a host of concomitant abnormalities. A third type of anophthalmos may be recognized, in which an optic vesicle forms but subsequently degenerates and disappears. This type is linked with extreme degrees of microphthalmos and is designated *consecutive* or *degenerative anophthalmos*.

In *primary anophthalmos*, the cause is probably germinal, since in a typical case no other defect is present. Moreover, there are clinical and experimental records of an occasional familial and hereditary character in which the *ectodermal* elements alone are missing. The orbit, eyelids, lacrimal apparatus, conjunctival sac, and extrinsic ocular muscles and their nerves are all self-determining and can develop without any stimulus from the optic vesicle. The lens, not being self-determining but arising from the surface ectoderm only, in response to a stimulus received from the optic vesicle, is absent. The cornea and sclera, on the other hand, form normally as condensations around an optic cup, but even in its absence there usually appears to be some attempt at a mesodermal condensation. The relationships of parts and the balance of growth between them are obviously interfered with by the absence of an optic cup, around which the subsidiary mesodermal structures should group themselves. As a result, the orbit is present but usually smaller than normal. The upper and lower eyelids are present, but the palpebral aperture is small. The lids are often adherent at their margins but can be separated without the need for cutting them; eyelashes and meibomian glands are usually present, although the puncta may be absent; there is a small conjunctival sac; the lids appear concave and are usually closed (Fig. 33–81); the lacrimal gland is present; and tears issue from the conjunctival sac when the child cries. The brain in primary anophthalmos shows no abnormality other than atrophy of the central optic paths from disuse.

The clinical appearance of primary anophthalmos in man corresponds closely with the findings of experimental embryologists (Fig. 33–82).

Secondary anophthalmos due to complete suppression or gross abnormality of the anterior end of the medullary tube is better known to experimental teratologists than to clinicians, since the fetuses are not usually viable.

Degenerative or *consecutive anophthalmos* is a term used to include cases in which an optic outgrowth appears to have formed and to have degenerated subsequently. Embryos are occasionally found in which a great disparity of size is observed between the two optic cups, one being normal and the other stunted and not in contact with the surface ectoderm. Such an eye might be expected either to attain an extreme degree of microphthalmos or to become overwhelmed by the growth of surrounding parts and to disappear almost completely.

If the fate of the ectodermal optic outgrowth is followed a stage further (after invagination), there is a group of abnormalities arising in man between the 7 mm and 14 mm stages. This growth period includes the time between invagination of the optic vesicle and complete closure of the embryonic cleft. These abnormalities lead to gross defects of the entire ocular globe, known clinically as microphthalmos with orbital clefts, and typical coloboma of the retina, choroid, and iris.

Microphthalmos

Microphthalmos has been described as a uniocular congenital deformity in which lack of development of one eye is in striking contrast to the development of the other. In some cases it may be said that the eye is not present at all, although a firm cystic tumor occupying the normal site of the globe in the orbit has sometimes been mistaken for an eye. Fuchs (1924) described such a cyst as being attached to the lower lid, where it is seen glimmering with a bluish luster. When opened, the cyst contains a rudimentary retina floating in a serous fluid. In cases of less severe deformity,

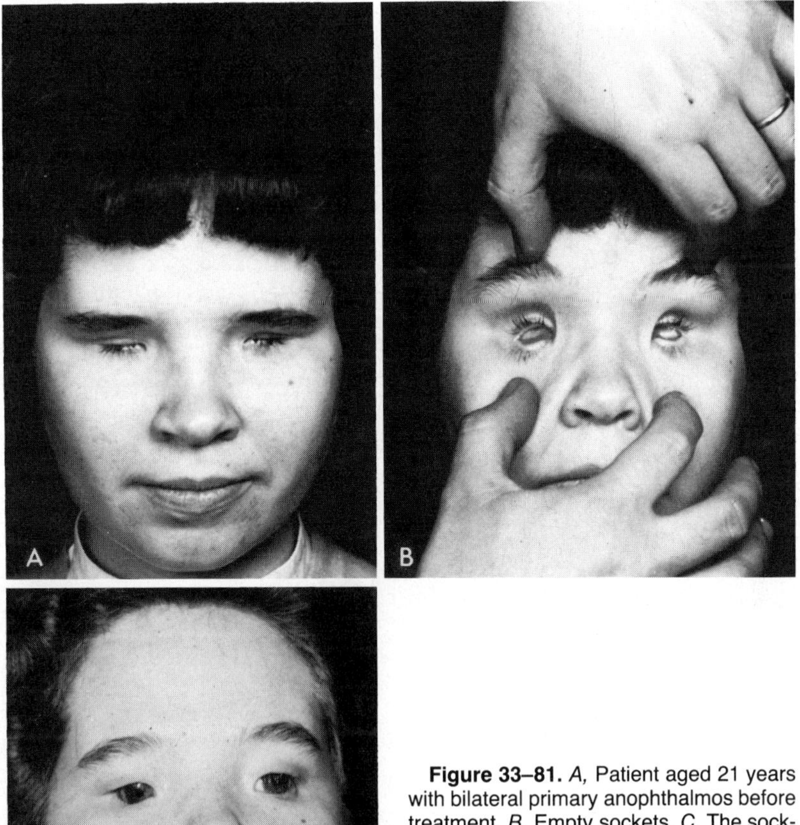

Figure 33–81. *A,* Patient aged 21 years with bilateral primary anophthalmos before treatment. *B,* Empty sockets. *C,* The sockets have been enlarged and prosthetic globes inserted.

coloboma or congenital fissure of the iris and of the optic nerve is usually present. Some observers claim that associated deformities are less frequent in patients with anophthalmos. In microphthalmos, a cyst of the lower eyelid that contains a rudimentary eye is nearly always found. In almost all patients, other congenital stigmata are seen, of which a hypoplastic orbit is the most common. Other defects in the order in which they may occur are cleft lip, cleft palate, orbitofacial cleft (see Chap. 59), supernumerary auricle, and supernumerary digits.

Etiology. In 1903 Hippel laid the foundation for the modern view that the defect is due to an inherent abnormality of growth in the optic cup. He pointed out the hereditary nature of the condition but still considered that persistence of mesoderm played a large part in failure of closure. He was the earliest observer to realize that, since coloboma is hereditary in rabbits, specimens at various stages of embryonic development can be obtained for examination. He disproved the inflammatory theory and laid the foundation for the work of Koyanagi (1921) and Szily (1913), who concluded that

1. The fault is primarily ectodermal, the persistence of mesoderm being secondary and not present in every case.

2. The affected individual shows transmission of the typical coloboma of choroid, retina,

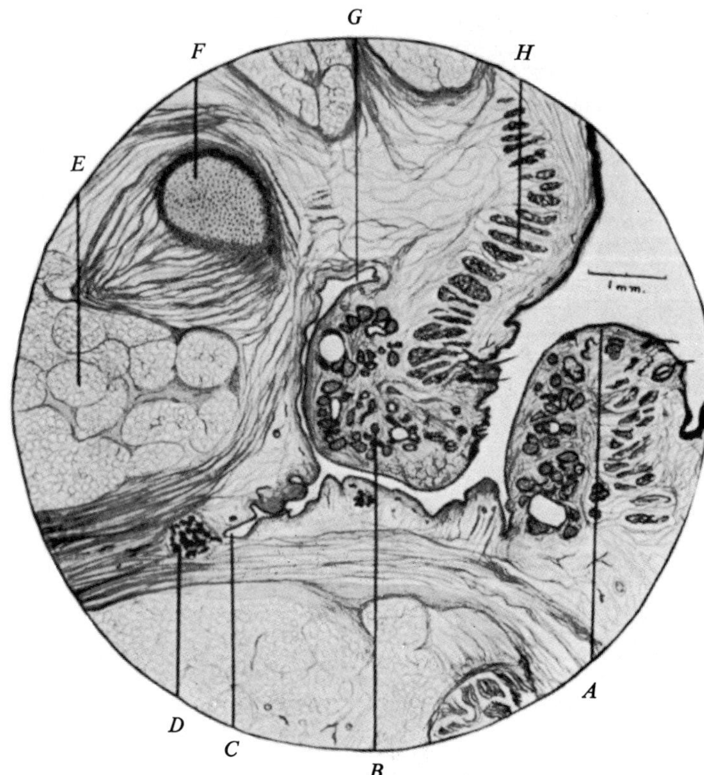

Figure 33–82. Section through the lids and orbital contents in a case of anophthalmos. *A,* Lower lid; *B,* upper lid; *C,* lower conjunctival fornix; *D,* accessory lacrimal gland; *E,* orbital fat; *F,* nodule of cartilage; *G,* upper conjunctival fornix; *H,* fibers of the orbicularis oculi muscle. (From Mann, I.: Developmental Abnormalities of the Eye. Philadelphia, J. B. Lippincott Company, 1957.)

and iris, coloboma of optic nerve, and orbital cysts interchangeably, but never of cyclopia and anophthalmos.

3. The condition is mendelian recessive.

Incidence. Congenital anophthalmos is rare, but microphthalmos occurs frequently in degrees varying from only a vestige to a complete miniature ocular globe. The deformity is usually unilateral (Fig. 33–83), occasionally bilateral.

Treatment. Microphthalmos and anophthalmos are deformities that are distressing to the parents and affect the psychologic development of the afflicted child. Correction of the deformity is difficult.

In the favorable case with *microphthalmos,* treatment consists of placing a small, plastic, concave-convex conformer in the conjunctival socket within the first four weeks of life. The conformer must be changed to one of a larger size approximately every two weeks. The sequence is continued with increasing intervals until the patient is past puberty. A peg can be attached to the anterior surface of the prosthesis as an aid in its manipulation (Fig. 33–84). Pressure can also be transmitted to the conformer through this attachment.

Depending on the degree of microphthalmos, expansion of the cul-de-sac with graduated prostheses may be of prime importance. In the average case of microphthalmos, a sufficient cul-de-sac is present to accommodate an adequate prosthesis without the need for an expansion technique. The orbit and the palpebral fissure are usually near normal size.

A shell prosthesis can be fashioned. Before prosthetic fittings are begun, the position of the cornea should be established to prevent irritation from the posterior surface of the shell. It is important to stain the cornea after fitting to be certain that it was not abraded by the prosthesis. Usually two or three fittings are necessary before a satisfactory prosthesis is achieved. The size and motility of the microphthalmic eye determine the motility of the prosthesis. Extraocular muscle surgery is required in some cases. In unilateral microphthalmos, the motility can be expected only to approach that of the uninvolved eye. There is usually an associated ptosis. The procedure used to correct the ptosis is determined by the type of ptosis involved (see Chap. 34).

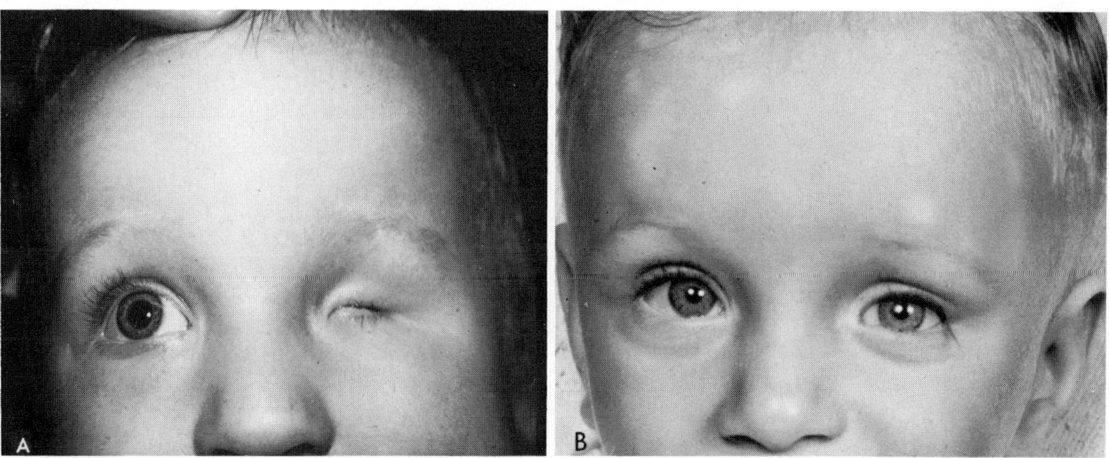

Figure 33–83. *A,* Child aged 2½ years with congenital microphthmos of the left eye, concave and closed lids, and a small palpebral fissure. *B,* Patient with an ocular prosthesis after five months of treatment, showing the growth of the lids and an almost normal palpebral fissure.

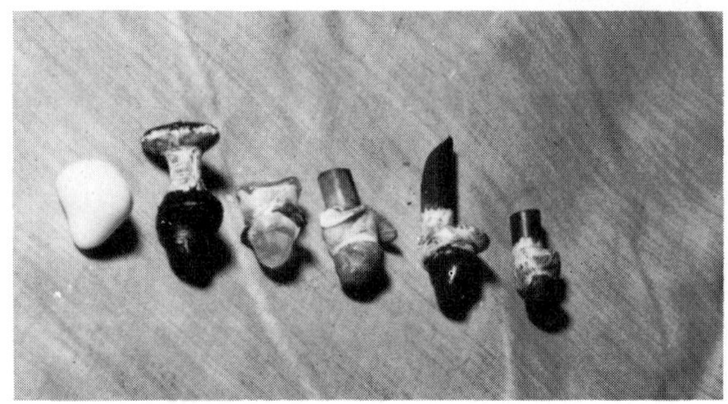

Figure 33–84. *A,* Graduated expanders employed during treatment of the patient shown in Figure 33–83. Note the size and the form of the cul-de-sac during pressure expansion. *B,* Prostheses used for expansion treatment. Note the progressive change of size from 9 mm wide and 6 mm vertically to 16 mm wide and 11 mm vertically in a period of five months.

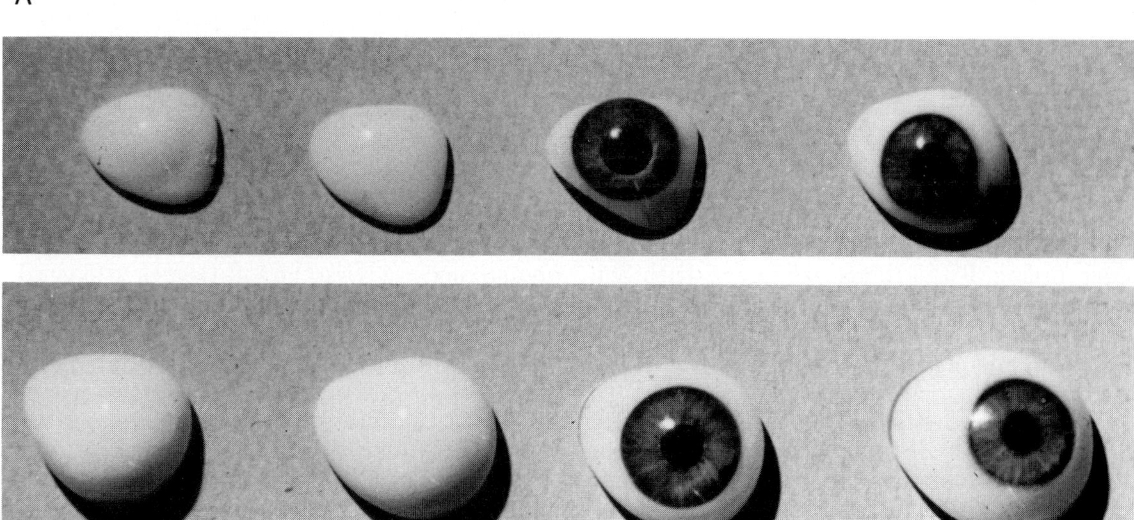

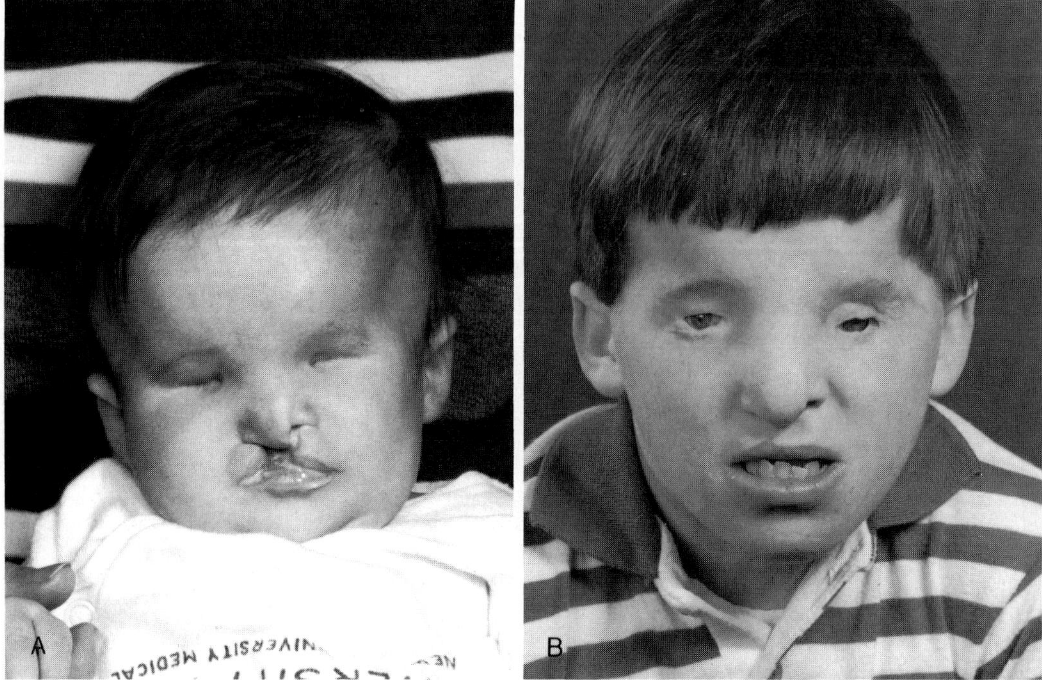

Figure 33–85. Bilateral microphthalmos and severe orbitofacial clefting. *A,* Infant with associated unilateral cleft lip and nose deformity. *B,* Appearance at age 12 years after multiple procedures: cleft lip repair, rhinoplasty, orbital expansion (see Fig. 33–87), and conjunctival dilatation.

In *congenital anophthalmos* the problem is much more involved. A hypoplastic bone orbit is usually associated with the anophthalmos, with a small palpebral aperture, scant eyelashes, miniaturized eyelid, and ptosis. The first corrective measure should be the enlargement of the socket. Forcing dental molding compound into the contracted socket produces a progressive enlargement, and the dental compound provides a pattern from which an acrylic prosthesis can be made. The prosthesis is placed in the socket and initially held in place with a moderately compressive dressing. A stem on the prosthesis protruding through the palpebral opening facilitates secure fitting. The orbital expansion with the compound implant is repeated at suitable intervals over a period of months until a socket of adequate size is obtained (Figs. 33–85, 33–86).

In some patients an impasse is reached. The conjunctival socket cannot accept a larger conformer than can be passed through the narrow palpebral aperture, and a lateral canthoplasty must be done to elongate the palpebral aperture. If a simple canthoplasty is not sufficient, a more expansive lateral canthoplasty extending lateral to the bone margin of the orbit is performed. The raw area is lined with a split-thickness buccal mucous membrane graft. The expansion of the palpebral fissure permits the fitting of a prosthesis of more suitable size.

During treatment a number of complications may arise, the most frequent and troublesome being lack of retention of the conformer. In order to overcome this obstacle, various devices have been tried, the simplest being that of taping the eyelids in order to maintain the prosthesis within the socket. In the early stages, under general anesthesia, positive pressure can be exerted by means of a dental compound stick, softened, yet with enough body to force the soft tissues to expand inside the cul-de-sac. This phase of the expansion is rapid. The dental compound is often self-retentive; it may be maintained by means of a tight bandage with pressure applied to a peg left on the stick and extending outward through the palpebral aperture.

When the socket has attained a relatively satisfactory size, impressions are taken with a rubber base material or a plastic base using a hand syringe and a shell conformer as a carrier tray. The shell conformer is fitted inside the lids; through an opening in its

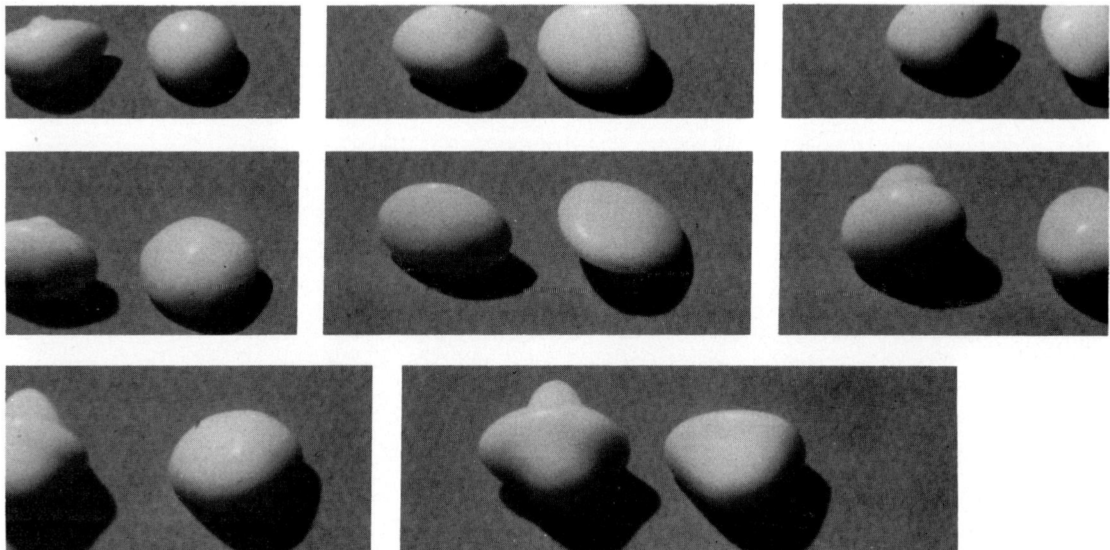

Figure 33–86. Prostheses used for expansion treatment of a patient with bilateral anophthalmos.

stem, a hypodermic syringe needle is inserted, and impression material is injected into the socket in a manner similar to the way in which an impression is taken for a contact lens. From this impression a wax pattern is made and fitted in the orbital socket; proper adjustments are made to the shape and contour by adding or shaping wax. The pattern is invested and "cured" into scleral material with a peg or handle attached to the anterior surface; the "cured" sclera is highly polished and fitted into the socket. This operation is repeated a number of times until the desired size and maximal expansion are attained.

The complication of entropion occurs frequently and may be caused by too large a conformer. The eyelashes begin to point toward the palpebral fissure rather than away from it.

When the entropion is allowed to progress, the cilia become adherent to the anterior face of the prosthesis with dried secretion, causing discomfort and an undesirable appearance. This complication is an indication either to proceed with caution in enlarging the size of the conformer or to enlarge the conjunctival fornices with mucosal grafts.

When mechanical expansion is not possible, more radical surgery may be required. The periosteum along the orbital margins may be incised and as much bone as possible recontoured to enlarge the bony orbit. The raw areas are covered with buccal mucosal grafts to enlarge the cavity in order that an artificial eye more comparable in size with the opposite eye may be fitted. Hartman (1962) stated that Strampelli enlarged the entire conjunctival sac by cutting through the conjunctiva along the tarsal edge of both upper and lower eyelids, undermining and cutting free the conjunctiva around the entire 360 degrees, working toward the center and allowing it to bunch up as a central stump. Both eyelids were completely everted and held in this extended position until a large, thin, labial mucous membrane graft that was applied over the raw area had healed. An orbital socket large enough to contain a satisfactory artificial prosthesis with some possibility of motion was obtained. In the authors' experience such techniques are usually unsuccessful since there is a severely hypoplastic bony orbit that prevents retention of the prosthesis.

Surgical expansion of the anophthalmic orbit has been achieved through an intracranial approach.

Tessier (1969) proposed enlargement of the bony orbit by a lateral displacement of the lateral orbital wall and an inferior movement of the zygoma. Marchac and associates (1977) described a multidirectional orbital expansion by osteotomies done in a steplike fashion. The three orbital rim segments are wired into their expanded position. A similar combined craniofacial procedure had been earlier described by Converse and associates (1974).

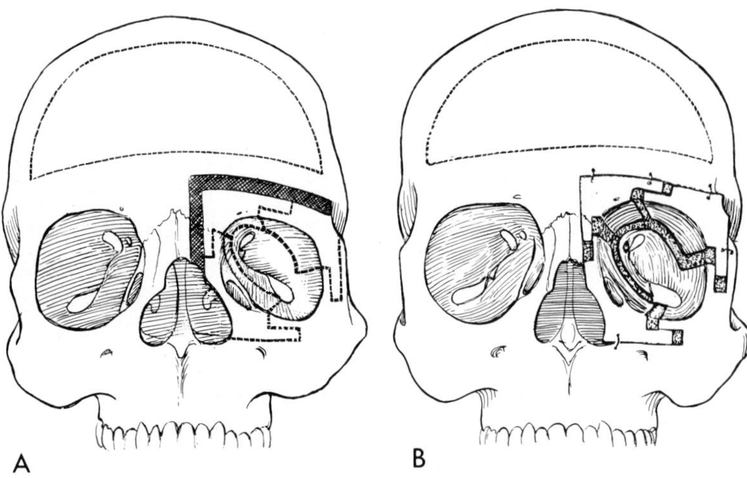

Figure 33–87. *A,* The osteotomies and bone resection (ostectomy) used in the expansion of the micro-orbit. *B,* The bone gaps are filled with autogenous grafts.

After exposure of the anterior cranial fossa (for osteotomy of the orbital roof) and dissection of the orbital contents via an eyelid incision, an ostectomy is accomplished in the nasofrontal and supraorbital region (Fig. 33–87). The resulting bone voids allow for expansion of the orbital segments. Steplike osteotomies are made as indicated in Figure 33–87. The three orbital segments are expanded and wired into position; bone grafts can be placed in the bone defects (this is optional) (Fig. 33–88). The skeletal expansion of the orbit must usually be associated with surgical reconstruction of the conjunctival sac, eyelids, and canthi (see Fig. 33–85).

RECONSTRUCTION OF ANOPHTHALMIC ORBIT

Successful reconstruction of the anophthalmic socket for the maintenance of an

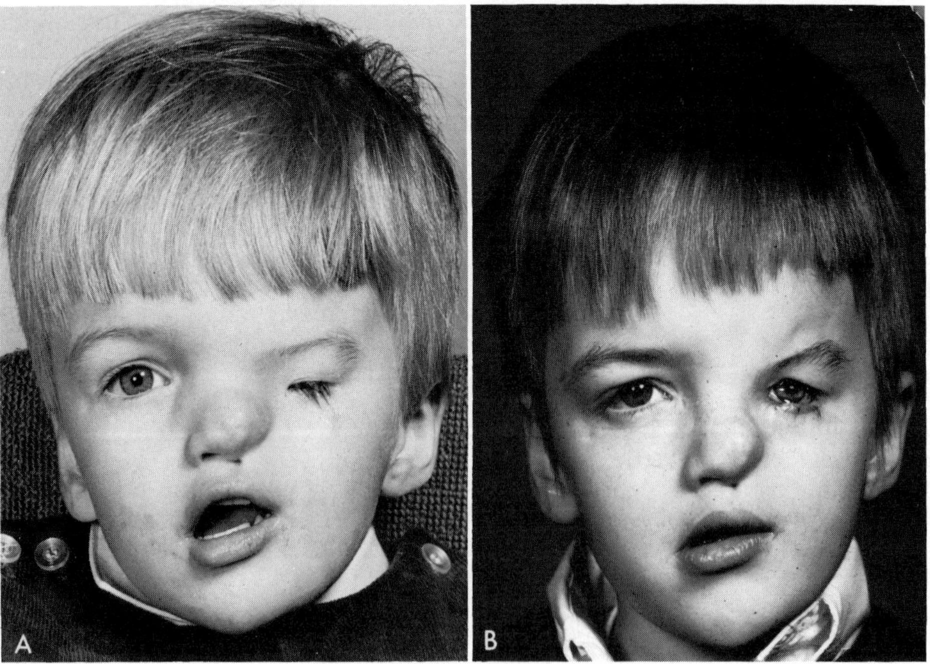

Figure 33–88. Child with orbital cleft and microphthalmos. *A,* Preoperative appearance. Note that the cleft involves the left alar base, the inferior and superior orbital rims, and the frontal bone. *B,* Postoperative appearance after expansion of the bony orbit (see Fig. 33–87) and subsequent expansion of the conjunctival sac to permit the wearing of a prosthetic eye. Additional nasal and jaw surgery is planned.

artificial eye depends on a cavity of sufficient size and shape. This necessitates the presence of eyelids and fornices deep enough to keep the prosthesis within the socket. A socket may be lined with a graft of skin or mucous membrane; the best socket has a mucous membrane lining. A skin socket is dry and has a tendency to accumulate desquamated epidermis, producing a foul odor. In addition, the bone orbit must be of sufficient volume not to impinge on the prosthesis.

Surgical Management. The surgical technique in socket reconstruction is contingent upon whether total or partial socket reconstruction is required. The simplest type of socket revision is the type in which there is sufficient socket lining but the lining is malpositioned or scarred. The surgical revision of such a socket is done by undermining the socket lining and thinning it and dissecting the fornices into the proper shape, repositioning the mucous membrane or conjunctiva by placing a conformer within the socket and maintaining its position until healing has taken place. The assurance of the proper positioning of the conformer during the healing process necessitates careful fixation.

The technique is relatively simple (Fig. 33–89). After the socket has been dissected and designed in proper configuration, an incision is made through the lower lid overlying the inferior orbital rim (Fig. 33–89*A,B*). In the middle third of the inferior orbital rim, a drill hole is placed through the rim from the outside to the inside (Fig. 33–89*B,C*). A stainless steel wire is passed through the hole and into the socket, and the other end of the wire is passed over the inferior orbital rim into the socket. The prepared conformer is perforated, and the wire is passed from behind forward through the hole in the conformer and twisted with the other end of the wire (Fig. 33–89*D,E*). This maneuver pulls the conformer down toward the orbital rim and maintains it in an upright position. The wire knot is tied within the socket and tucked into the hole in the conformer. The best type of conformer is made of gutta-percha and is prepared at the time of surgery. The graft may be sutured to itself after it has been wrapped around the conformer raw surface outward (Fig. 33–89*F*).

If the upper half of the socket is normal and the lower half deficient, the dissection consists of making an incision along the lower eyelid margin, thinning the lower lid, and extending the dissection to the inferior orbital rim. The partially covered conformer is placed in the socket and wired. Because some lids tend to contract in a vertical fashion during the healing process, it is advisable to insert a lid occlusal suture over the central third of the lid during the healing process. After the socket has healed and softened, the wire is divided and the conformer removed. The socket should not be left without some type of a prosthetic device during the postoperative phases.

When the lining is deficient in the upper fornix, the surgery required to reconstruct the fornix is somewhat more difficult. The dissection in the upper lid is extended upward (Fig. 33–89*C* to *F*), and attempts are made to preserve the levator if at all possible. After the dissection has been completed, a conformer is fashioned with a drill hole for fixation to the lower orbital rim. The upper part of the conformer is covered with a graft and inserted and wired into proper position.

Complete restoration of the socket combines the two previously described techniques, and the conformer is completely covered with a graft rather than partially covered. If the Castroviejo mucotome is used to obtain the graft from the oral cavity, a graft of 0.3 mm thickness is obtained. Ordinarily the membrane must be 0.3 mm thick or more, otherwise it does not handle with ease. A moderate pressure dressing is applied, and changed after 48 hours.

The anophthalmic orbit syndrome (Nolan and Vistnes, 1983) consists of (1) enophthalmos, (2) superior sulcus depression, (3) lower eyelid ptosis, and (4) upper eyelid ptosis.

Lower eyelid ptosis was observed in 40 per cent of anophthalmic orbits in the series presented by Nolan and Vistnes (1983). These authors reported that fascia lata suspension is a satisfactory reconstructive technique to correct lower eyelid ptosis. A strip of fascia 2.0 mm in width is passed through the lower eyelid and secured to the lateral orbital rim and medial canthal tendon. Mustardé (1975) advocated transplantation of septal cartilage in the lower lid to prevent the fold that forms under the prosthesis in the lower eyelid.

Room temperature vulcanizing silicone has been employed to correct anophthalmic enophthalmos (Fig. 33–90) (Iverson, Vistnes, and Siegel, 1973; Neuhaus and Shorr, 1982).

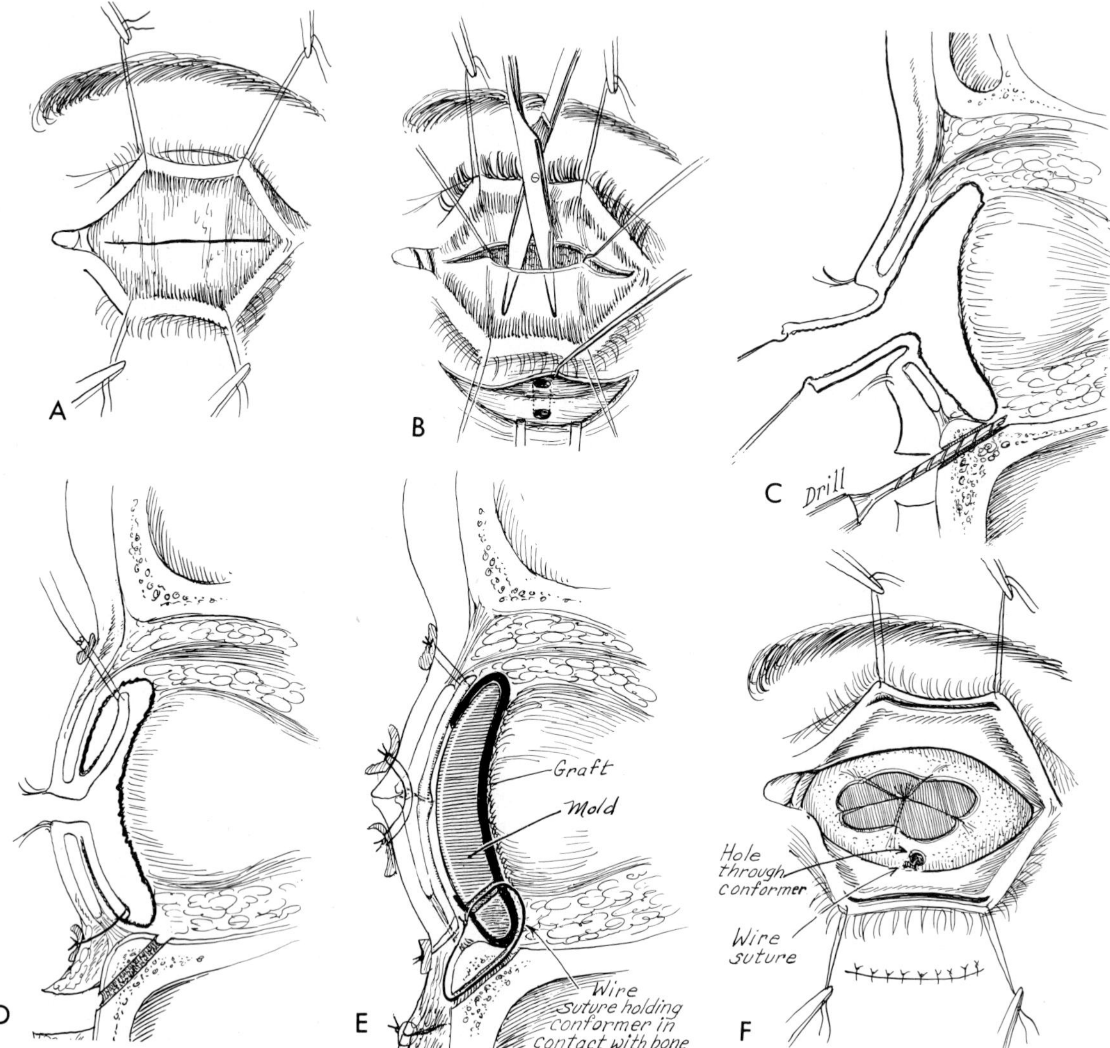

Figure 33–89. Anophthalmic orbit. *A,* Contracted socket showing obliteration of the fornices. The horizontal line across the center represents the line of incision across the dome of the socket. Traction sutures are placed in the lid to exert traction on the mucous membrane lining the socket during dissection. *B,* The wound edges are retracted with hooks, and the membrane is undermined from the incision toward the lid margin. The socket is dissected downward toward the orbital rim and upward and outward in all directions to prepare a cavity to receive the conformer. A horizontal incision is made over the orbital margin approximately 10 mm below the lid edge, after the margin has been cleared of periosteum. The drill hole is placed in the position shown by the dotted lines. *C,* A cross section of the orbit and lids, showing the dissection of the new socket cavity and the retracted conjunctiva between the lid margins. The drill hole is shown in its position across the angle of the orbital margin near its midpoint. *D,* The dissected conjunctiva is retracted and sutured as shown by interrupted sutures tied over rubber tubes on the outer surface of the lid margin. A cross section of the drill hole and its relationship to the lower socket margin are shown. *E,* The conformer in place surrounded by a graft of skin or mucous membrane. The drill hole in the bone is connected to a drill hole through the lower portion of the conformer by a wire suture; the knot of the suture is tied and tucked into the hole within the conformer in order to avoid irritation of the soft tissues. The suture across the inner palpebral fissure maintains the central lid adhesion until healing has taken place. *F,* The conformer is shown in place with the wire suture maintaining the lower margin of the conformer in approximation to the lower orbital rim. The skin wound is closed with interrupted 6-0 silk sutures. The incisions for the lid adhesion are shown along the lid margin. At the end of two months the lid adhesion is severed; the wire is removed; and the conformer is replaced by an artificial eye.

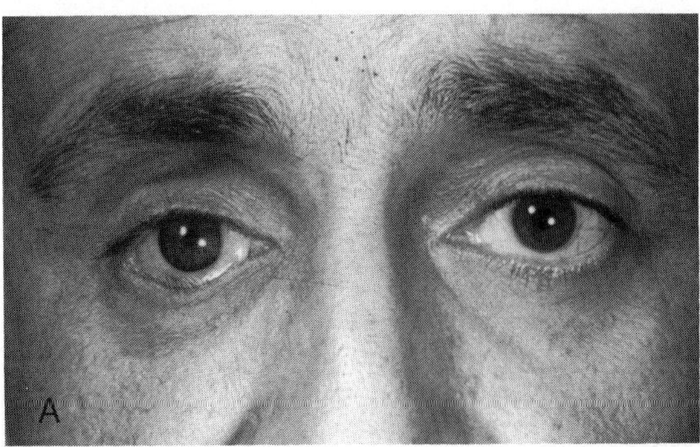

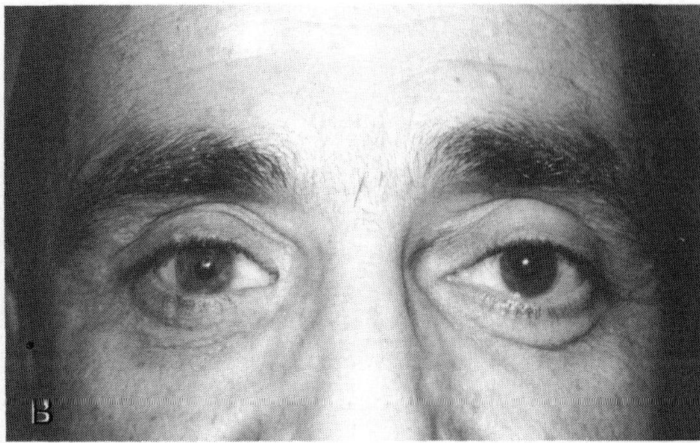

Figure 33–90. Anophthalmic orbit. *A,* A middle-aged patient with right-sided anophthalmic orbit, enophthalmos, superior sulcus depression, and lower lid ptosis. *B,* Appearance four years after RTV silicone augmentation of the orbital contents and (in a separate procedure) elevation of the lower lid with a fascial sling. (From Vistnes, L. M.: Surgical Reconstruction in the Anophthalmic Orbit. Birmingham, AL, Aesculapius Publishing Company, 1987.)

MISCELLANEOUS ORBITAL PATHOLOGY

Fibrous Dysplasia

Fibrous dysplasia, first described by von Recklinghausen in 1891, is an abnormal proliferation of the bone-forming mesenchyme. It may be *monostotic* (involving a single bone) or *polyostotic* (see Chap. 69). A unique type of polyostotic fibrous dysplasia is Albright's syndrome, characterized by sexual precocity, café au lait cutaneous lesions, early epiphyseal fusion, and various endocrine abnormalities.

The main differential diagnosis lies with Paget's disease and the skeletal pathology associated with hematopoietic diseases and meningioma. Meningioma occurs mainly in later life.

Orbital dystopia, proptosis, and diplopia can result from fibrous dysplasia, especially if the frontoethmoidal and maxillary regions are involved (Fig. 33–91).

In a series of patients with fibrous dysplasia reported by Georgiade and associates (1955), 10 per cent demonstrated ethmoidal and orbital involvement. Of the 46 patients with fibrous dysplasia in another series (Leeds and Seaman, 1962), the frontal bone was involved in 29, the sphenoid in 19, and the ethmoid in 13. In the same series of 46 patients the presenting symptoms were ophthalmologic in nine (decrease in visual acuity, proptosis, scotoma, and epiphora).

Fries (1957) classified the radiographic appearance into three types: (1) pagetoid (56 per cent) with alternate areas of radiolucency and density, (2) sclerotic (23 per cent) with a homogeneous density, and (3) cystic (21 per cent) with a single oval or round lesion having a dense border.

The preferred treatment of the orbital deformity is total or subtotal resection of the involved bone, and reconstruction with autogenous bone grafts (Munro and Chen, 1981). However, the bone resection may be limited when there is extensive involvement of the cranial base.

In the patient illustrated in Figure 33–92 there was extensive involvement of the frontal bone (with hyperpneumatization of the

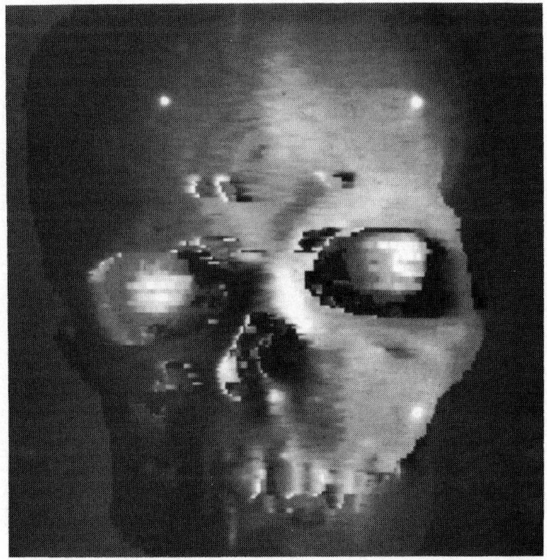

Figure 33–91. Three-dimensional CT scan showing massive involvement by fibrous dysplasia of the nasoethmoid and orbitomaxillary regions. Note the elevation and displacement of the globe.

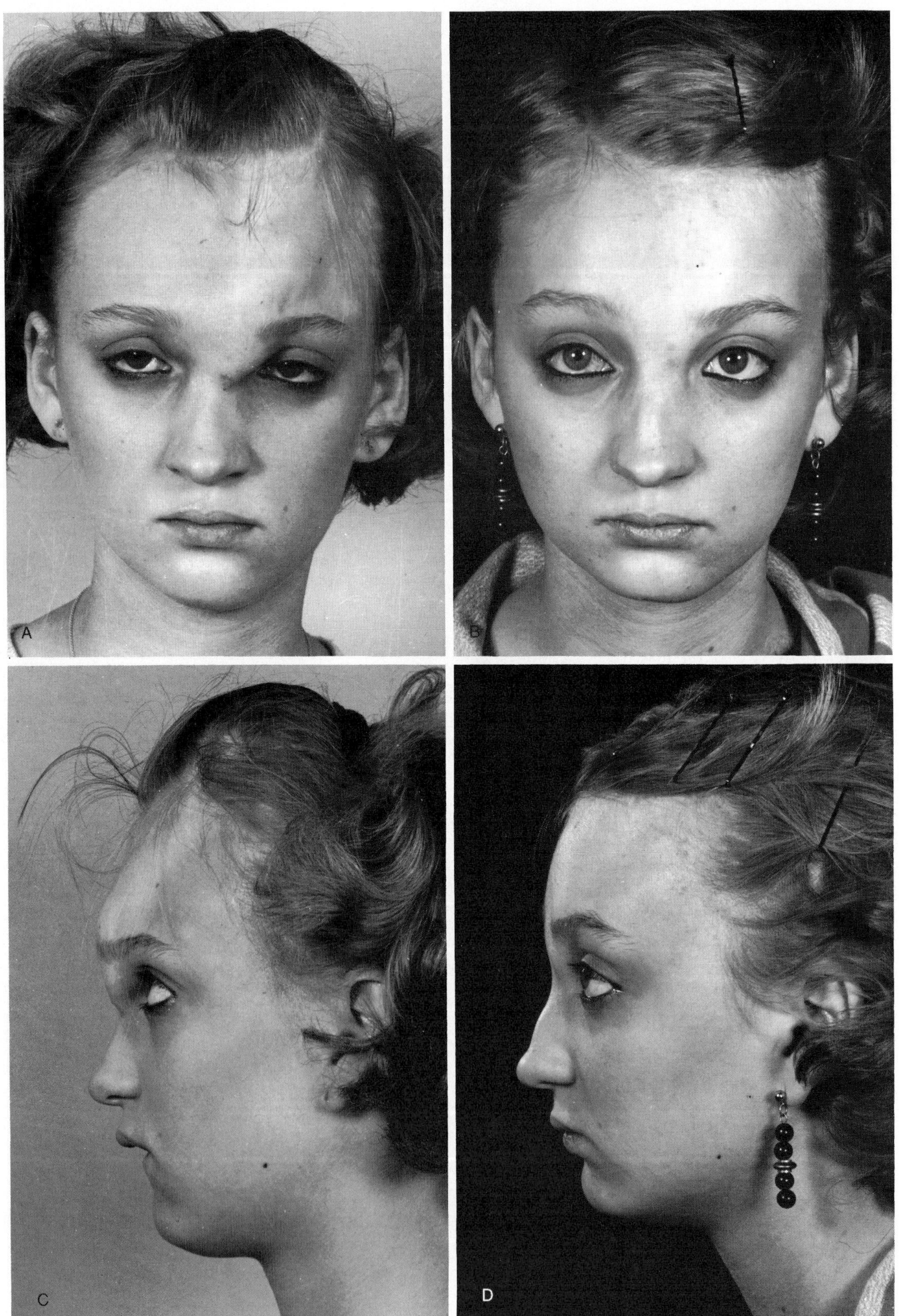

Figure 33–92. Fibrous dysplasia involving the left frontoethmoidal region. *A, C,* Preoperative views. Note the frontal bossing and displacement of the left globe. *B, D,* After resection of the involved bone and ablation of the frontal and ethmoid sinuses. The frontal bone and orbit were reconstructed with calvarial bone grafts.

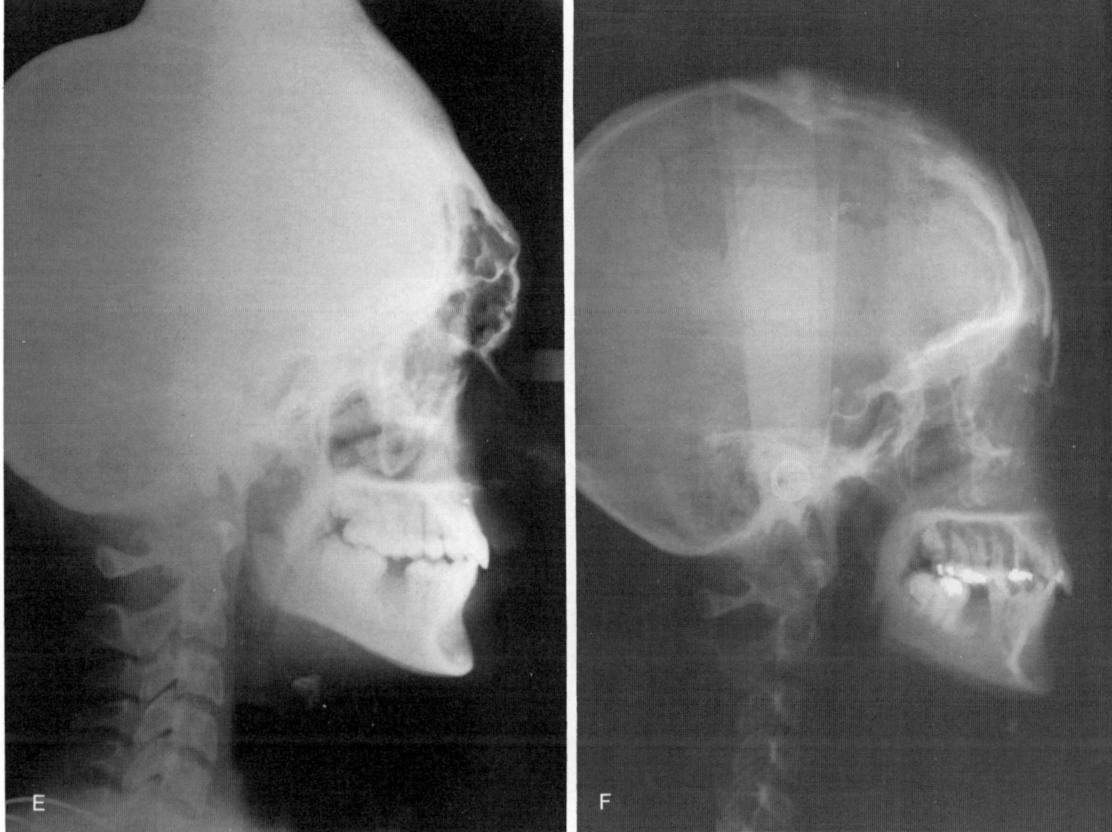

Figure 33–92 *Continued E,* Preoperative lateral cephalogram showing the hyperpneumatized sinus. *F,* Postoperative lateral cephalogram. Note the calvarial bone grafts.

frontal sinus) and ethmoid complex. In a single procedure the lesion was resected in a subtotal fashion (roof and medial wall of left orbit, frontal bone and sinus and part of nasal bone). The nasofrontal duct was obliterated with a bone graft, and the periorbita was radially incised to allow a repositioning of the globe and orbital contents. The resultant skeletal defect was reconstructed with a combination of calvarial and iliac autogenous bone grafts (Fig. 33–92*F*).

In another patient with more extensive involvement of the roof and cranial base (Fig. 33–93) the total lesion was resected through a combined craniofacial route and the resulting skeletal defect reconstructed with autogenous bone grafts.

Neurofibroma

Described by von Recklinghausen and Fastcher in 1882, neurofibromatosis is neuroectodermal in origin and can involve skin, subcutaneous tissue, and bone. Its mode of inheritance is autosomal dominant with variable penetrance.

Orbitopalpebral involvement is expressed in a variety of ways. It may be limited to the soft tissues of the eyelids and intraorbital contents. Craniofacial skeletal manifestations include enlargement of the middle cranial fossa, and widening of the superior orbital fissure and the optic foramen (van der Meulen and associates, 1982). In the typical case the patient presents with ptosis, hypertrophy of the eyelid, exophthalmos (occasionally pulsating), inferior displacement of the affected globe, and reduced visual acuity (Fig. 33–94) (Marchac, 1984).

The extent of the pathology is best defined by a three-dimensional CT scan. A bone defect is usually observed lateral to the optic foramen and involving the superior orbital fissure (Fig. 33–95). There is usually herniation of the brain through the bone defect into the orbit with displacement of the globe (pulsating exophthalmos).

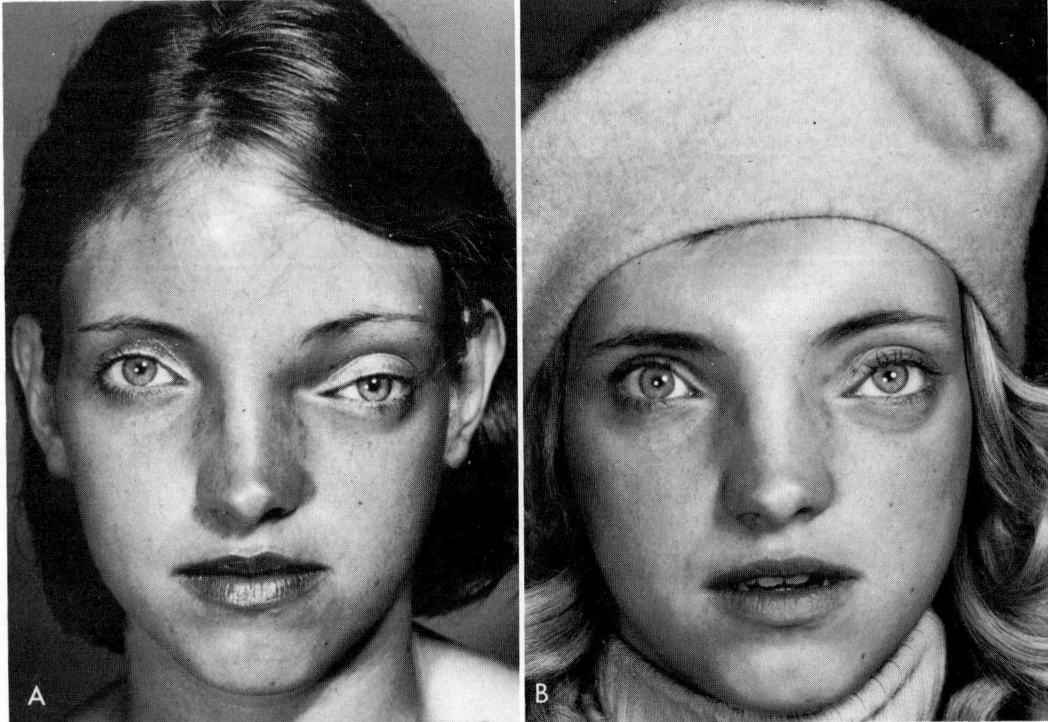

Figure 33–93. Orbital displacement associated with fibrous dysplasia of the frontoethmoid complex. *A,* Preoperative appearance. Note the inferolateral displacement of the orbit and frontal bossing. *B,* Postoperative appearance.

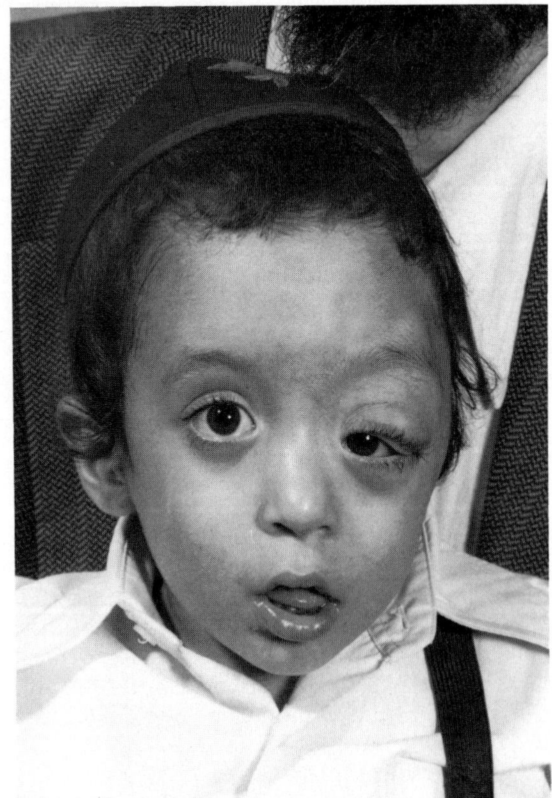

Figure 33–94. Neurofibromatosis of the orbit. Note the severe exophthalmos (pulsating), ptosis, esodeviation, and hypertrophy of the eyelid.

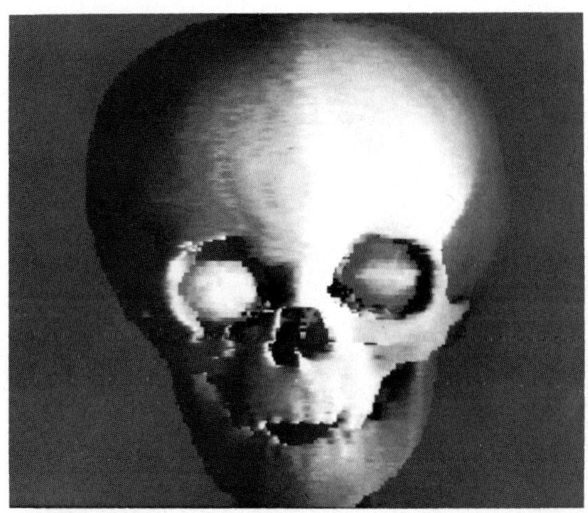

Figure 33–95. Three-dimensional CT scan of a patient with neurofibromatosis (see Fig. 33–97). Note the aplasia of the greater wing of the sphenoid with anteroinferior displacement of the right globe by the herniating brain.

Treatment of the skeletal deformity dictates an intracranial approach (Munro and Martin, 1979; Marchac, 1984; van der Meulen, 1987). Through a bicoronal incision a bilateral frontal bone flap is elevated and the anterior cranial fossa is exposed. The supraorbital rim and roof are osteotomized and temporarily removed (superior orbitotomy of Tessier). This maneuver provides excellent exposure of the herniating brain and allows its reduction into the cranial cavity after dissection separates the cranial and orbital components (Fig. 33–96).

The defect in the orbital roof is readily apparent and extends laterally from the area of the optic foramen. It is important to resect the periphery of the defect since this bone is usually too thin for adequate wire retention. The defect can be reconstructed by either a calvarial bone graft or an alloplastic material (Fig. 33–96). It is important that the periorbita be liberated circumferentially in order to elevate the globe into a normal position. This maneuver is also facilitated by scoring the periorbita and placing a calvarial bone graft in the floor of the orbit to maintain globe position (Fig. 33–96). The supraorbital bone segment is then wired into position and the canthopexies are performed if the respective ligament has been detached (Fig. 33–97).

If there is tumor involvement of the eyelid, a palpebral resection can be performed at this time, as discussed in Chapter 34.

Hemangioma

Vascular tumors of the orbit may present characteristic clinical and histopathologic findings (see Chap. 66). The simple benign hemangioendothelioma or capillary hemangioma (strawberry hemangioma, strawberry nevus) is the most common benign cutaneous tumor of infancy (Walsh and Tompkins, 1956; Bowes, Graham, and Tomlinson, 1970). The skin of the eyelid and the anterior orbital tissues are common locations for this lesion.

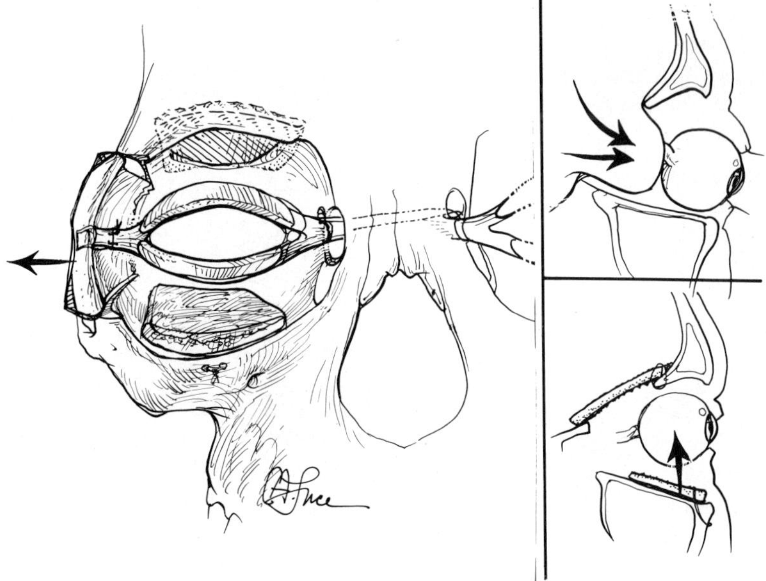

Figure 33–96. Neurofibroma and aplasia of the greater wing of the sphenoid. *Upper right panel,* Herniation of the brain into the orbit with displacement of the globe. *Lower right panel,* The brain has been returned to the cranial cavity and the defect repaired with a bone graft. Note also the bone graft on the floor to elevate the globe. *Left panel,* Frontal view showing the osteotomy of the lateral wall to increase orbital volume. Lateral and medial canthopexies complete the procedure (after Marchac).

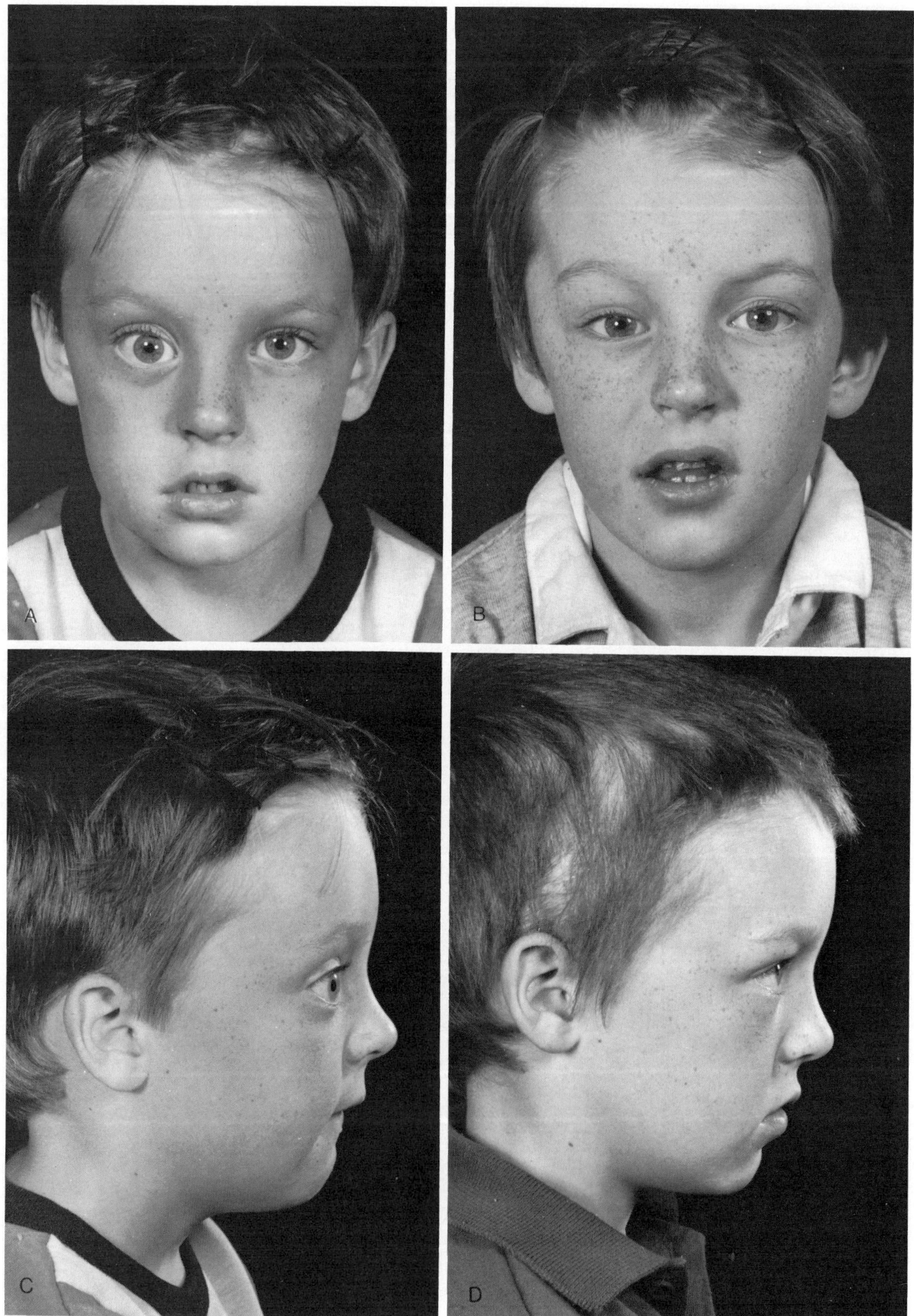

Figure 33–97. Young male with neurofibromatosis and a pulsating exophthalmos (right). *A, C,* Preoperative views. *B, D,* Appearance after correction by the technique illustrated in Figure 33–96.

The capillary hemangioma is more common in males than females, with a ratio of 3:2, and appears to be more common in low birth weight children. The lesion is usually apparent at birth or shortly thereafter. It is often unilateral with various degrees of red-purple or pinkish color.

When the deeper orbital tissues are involved, there may be ptosis and corneal exposure. Furthermore, if there is rapid expansion, complete occlusion of the eye may result (Fig. 33–98).

Refractive errors of myopia, astigmatism, or both are demonstrated in over 50 per cent of patients with large orbital hemangiomas. The refractive errors may remain after excision or regression of the hemangiomas (Robb, 1977).

A fortunate feature of capillary hemangiomas noted in early infancy is the capacity of these lesions to undergo spontaneous involution, often between 2 and 3 years of age (Fig. 33–98). Treatment of capillary hemangiomas with orbital involvement requires careful selection of noninterventive or invasive therapy. Most often, simple observation is all that is required. Early ophthalmologic evaluation with continued observation for astigmatic, defective, or occlusive amblyopia is mandatory when this approach is chosen.

Systemic corticosteroid therapy (de Venecia and Lobeck, 1970; Hiles and Pilchard, 1971) or direct injection with triamcinolone and betamethasone (Zak and Morin, 1981; Brown and Huffaker, 1982; Kusher, 1979, 1982) have been shown to produce satisfactory results.

Other forms of therapy include surgical excision, radiotherapy, and injections of embolization or sclerosing agents. The argon laser has proved helpful in obliterating the cutaneous manifestations of hemangiomas.

Cavernous hemangiomas are the most common vascular orbital tumor in adults. They usually present in the third to fourth decades of life as a painless, unilateral proptosis. The lesions are easily distinguished from other orbital tumors by ultrasonography and CT scans (see Fig. 33–16).

Lymphangioma

Orbital lymphangiomas may be present at birth but usually appear during the first decade of life as a slowly progressive mass with little propensity to regress (Hemmer, Marsh, and Milder, 1988). The orbital lymphangiomas characteristically cause cystic masses of the conjunctiva that periodically fill with blood (Fig. 33–99). Spontaneous bleeding into the cystic orbital structures can cause marked proptosis and ecchymosis (Dryden, Wak, and Day, 1985).

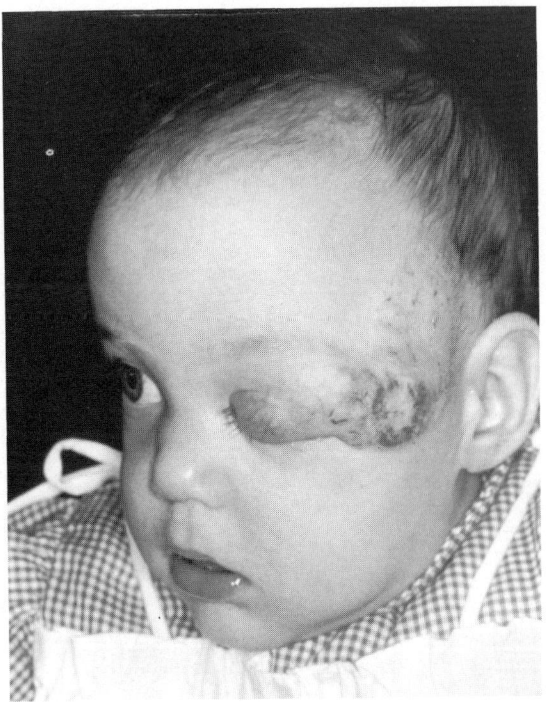

Figure 33–98. A 3 month old child with left orbital cutaneous capillary hemangioma. Note the complete occlusion of the left eye and evidence of partial involution of the lateral orbital mass (area of lighter color).

Like plexiform neurofibromas, lymphangiomas are difficult to manage surgically. The carbon dioxide laser has been shown to offer an alternative surgical tool for ablation with less blood loss (Kennerdell and associates, 1986).

RECONSTRUCTION OF THE ZYGOMA

The orbitozygomatic complex, located in the lateral portion of the midface skeleton, is formed by a skeletal framework consisting of the zygoma, the lateral wall of the orbit, and the zygomatic process of the maxilla. These bones are covered by the origins of the masseter, the zygomatic head of the quadratus

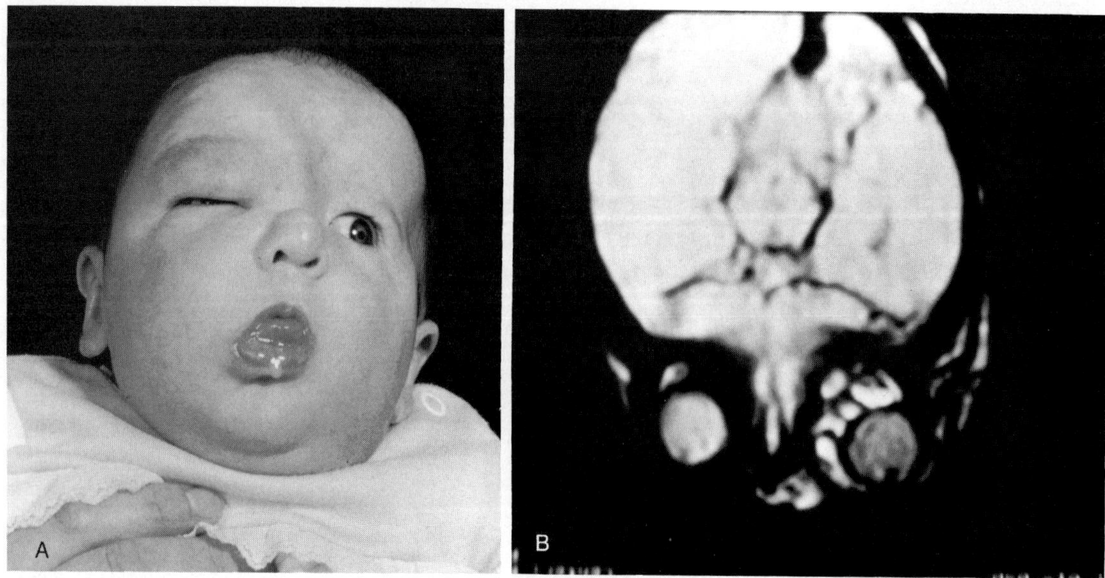

Figure 33–99. *A,* A 1 month old child with lymphangioma of the right orbit and periocular tissue. *B,* CT scan demonstrating apex involvement of the right orbit.

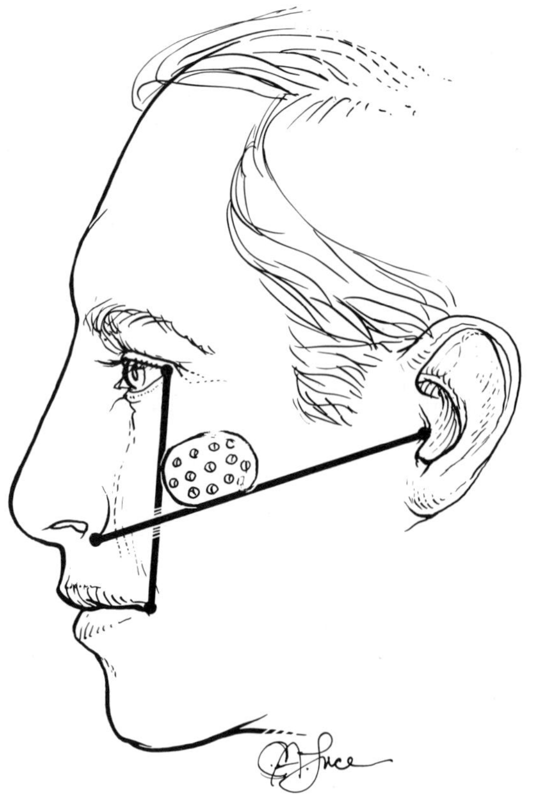

Figure 33–100. Placement of an alloplastic implant for zygomatic augmentation. The implant is placed in a subperiosteal position within an angle formed by a line drawn from the lateral canthus to the lateral commissure and a line from the tragus to the alar base (after Hinderer).

labii superioris and zygomaticus muscles, the lateral portion of the orbicularis oculi muscle, the subcutaneous tissues, and skin.

The prominence of the upper part of the cheek is formed by the zygoma; the most prominent point of the zygoma is sometimes referred to as the "tubercle" of the zygoma. Loss of the prominence due to malunited fracture of the zygoma results in a noticeable deformity.

Zygomatic deformities may be congenital or acquired. Congenital hypoplasia of the zygoma is a prominent feature of the Treacher Collins syndrome (Chap. 63) and the craniofacial synostosis syndromes (Chap. 61). There is also a group of patients with a mild form of zygomatic deficiency who seek augmentation for cosmetic reasons. Acquired zygomatic deformities are most commonly seen after zygomatic, orbitozygomatic, or panfacial fractures that have not been properly treated (Chap. 27).

Zygomatic deficiency can be treated by a variety of surgical techniques:

1. Onlay augmentation
   a. Alloplast.
   b. Cartilage : autograft, allograft, and xenograft.
   c. Bone : autograft (calvaria, rib, ilium) or calvarial bone flap.
2. Advancement osteotomy
   a. Zygomatic complex alone.
   b. Zygoma as part of the Le Fort III segment.

ALLOPLAST AUGMENTATION OF ZYGOMA

Patients request augmentation of the zygomatic complex to improve the appearance of the *facial oval* (Hinderer, 1975). Patients with elongated or excessively rounded faces (prominence of the cheek soft tissue) also benefit from this technique, since facial proportions are improved.

Hinderer (1975) described a procedure in which silicone rubber implants are placed over the zygomatic complexes. Two reference lines are helpful in establishing the implant position (Fig. 33–100): one drawn from the lateral canthus to the oral commissure, the other from the alar base to the tragus. The implant should be placed within the angle defined by the intersection of the lines.

A variety of incisions or approaches (eyelid and face lift) can be used, but the authors prefer an intraoral incision (4 cm) made above the labiobuccal sulcus. The dissection is extended to the zygomatic complex, and a subperiosteal pocket of a size slightly larger than the implant is made with an elevator. The pocket size and position are determined by the previously outlined skin markings. Implant position is further determined by guide sutures of catgut, which are passed through the implant and skin. After the intraoral incisions are closed, the catgut sutures are pulled and cut at the skin level (Fig. 33–101). Alternatively, the sutures can be temporarily tied over a cotton bolus dressing.

CARTILAGE/BONE GRAFT AUGMENTATION OF ZYGOMA

Cartilage has been used to augment the zygomatic complex as an autograft, allograft, or xenograft. There can be long-term distortion or warping after cartilage autograft (Dupertuis, 1950) reconstruction, and cartilage allografts are associated with a high rate of resorption (Gibson, 1977). Gillies and Millard (1957) augmented the malar prominences with cartilage allografts (preserved) or xenografts.

Bone grafts were used by Murphy to restore zygomatic contour as early as 1915. In like fashion, calvaria (Tessier, 1982b; McCarthy and Zide, 1984), rib (Longacre, de Stefano, and Holmstrand, 1961; Tessier, 1971), and ilium have also been transferred as nonvascularized grafts.

Extraoral Approach. Surgical access is gained by a transcutaneous or transconjunctival *eyelid* incision, which can be supplemented by a *bicoronal* scalp incision (see Fig. 33–24). In a subperiosteal plane, the soft tissues are elevated off the inferior and lateral orbital rims, the anterior wall of the maxilla, and the zygomatic complex. The masseter muscle is widely detached.

The grafts are properly positioned and wired to the exposed craniofacial skeleton, depending on the extent of the zygomatic deficiency (Fig. 33–102). It is usually necessary to perform a lateral canthopexy (see Chap. 34), since zygomatic deficiency is often associated with an inferior displacement of the lateral canthus (Fig. 33–103).

Intraoral Approach. The intraoral approach (Converse, 1950) is another way to expose the zygoma for the introduction of contour-restoring bone grafts. The approach is particularly indicated in malunited fractures of the zygoma. The procedure permits

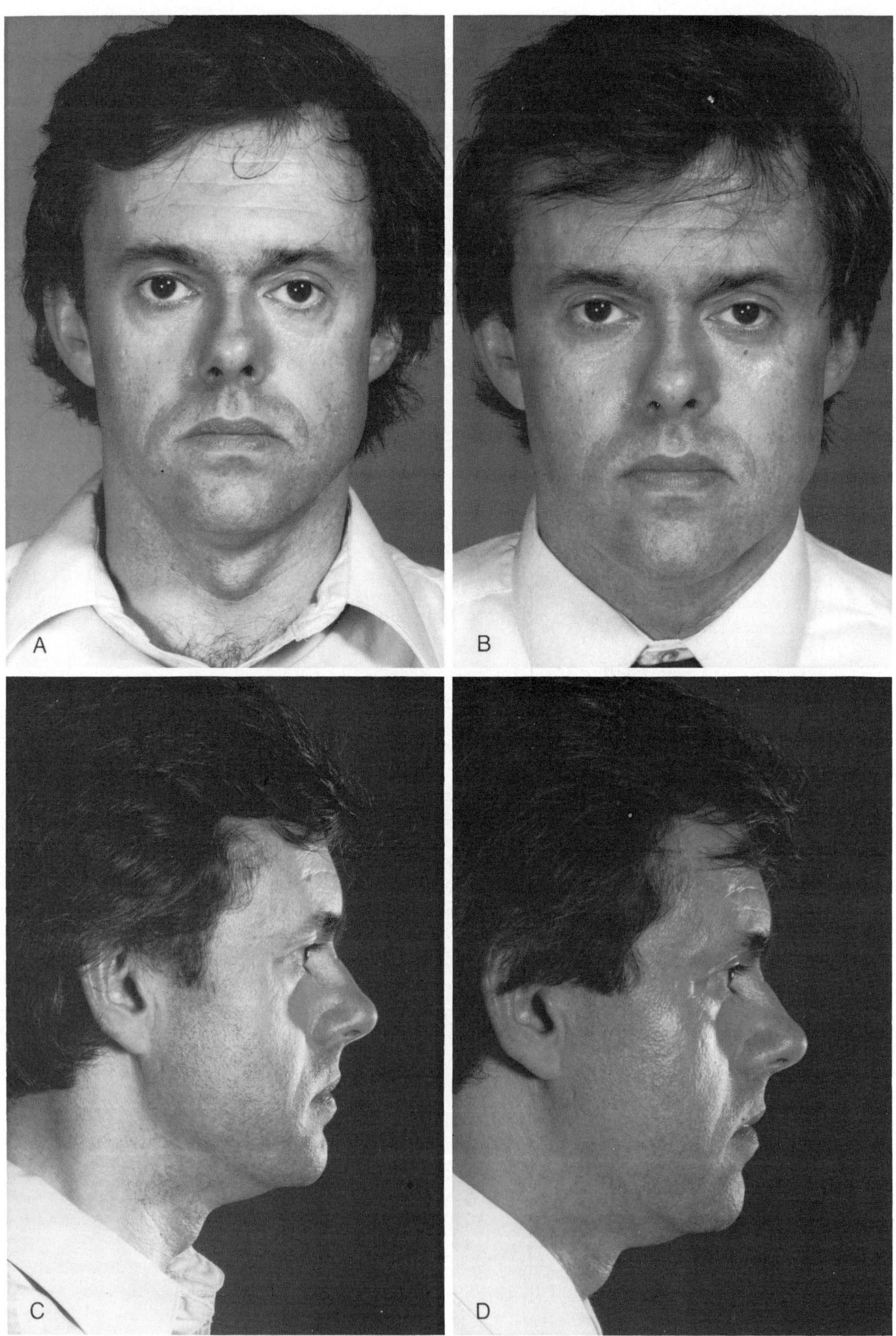

Figure 33–101. An adult male with zygomatic hypoplasia. *A, C,* Preoperative views. *B, D,* After zygomatic augmentation by the technique illustrated in Figure 33–100.

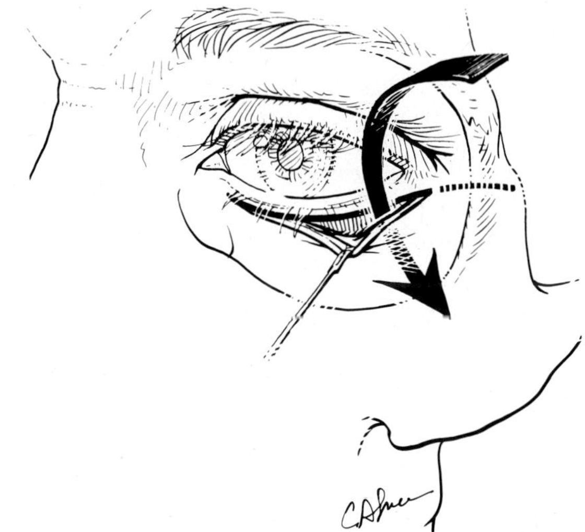

Figure 33–102. Onlay bone grafting of the zygomatic complex through an eyelid incision. The latter can be extended in a crow's foot line *(dots)* for additional exposure.

a direct view of the maxilla and zygoma from the piriform aperture medially to the infraorbital margin superiorly. The incision in the oral mucosa of the lip is placed lateral to the frenulum on the affected side above the vestibular sulcus (Fig. 33–104*A*). The periosteum is incised and elevated after the mucosa is dissected from the orbicularis oris muscle, thus exposing the defect (Fig. 33–104*B*). Wide exposure of the maxilla is obtained; the zygoma may be approached by extending the periosteal elevation laterally. The infraorbital nerve and vessels are avoided by carefully raising the periosteum around the neurovascular bundle and preserving its attachment to the elevated soft tissues. The bone defect may then be inspected under adequate lighting.

Bicoronal Approach (Tessier). When a major defect is present after severe trauma, a coronal scalp flap (see Fig. 33–24) is raised on the affected side; if sufficient exposure is not obtained, a full coronal flap is raised. The periosteum over the lateral orbital wall is incised. The periosteum over the zygomatic arch and zygoma is incised and elevated, exposing the area. This route provides satisfactory exposure for the introduction of contour-restoring bone grafts (calvaria or iliac bone). The placement of the grafts may be verified through a lower eyelid incision.

CALVARIAL BONE FLAP AUGMENTATION OF ZYGOMA

Calvarial bone flaps (see Chap. 18) are especially indicated for zygomatic augmentation in patients in whom there have been previous unsuccessful attempts at augmentation or who have unsatisfactory overlying soft tissue and skin, such as scars or irradiation-damaged skin (McCarthy and Zide, 1984; McCarthy, Cutting, and Shaw, 1987).

A bicoronal incision is made from ear to ear when bilateral flaps are elevated, but a more limited incision suffices for a unilateral flap (Fig. 33–105).

The scalp/skin is elevated in a subfollicular plane above the SMAS and galea. This is not a natural cleavage plane, but the dissection is facilitated by keeping the hair follicles in the elevated flap under direct vision. The scalp elevation must be extensive in order to expose the temporalis muscle, temporal crest, coronal suture, potential osseous donor sites, and vasculature of the superficial temporal system.

A metal template of the osseous defect is taken and transferred to the calvarial donor site. Care must be taken to ensure that the proposed flap pedicle provides sufficient length for transfer of the bone.

The overlying galea and periosteum are next incised with an excess 5 mm perimeter about the proposed bone donor site. A round, air-driven bur is then employed to create a trough about the bone component. Bleeding is observed as the diplopic space is entered. A curved osteotome is next driven by a mallet to elevate or separate the outer table of the calvaria (Fig. 33–106).

Drill holes are placed in the bone, and sutures are passed through the holes and overlying periosteum-galea to prevent disso-

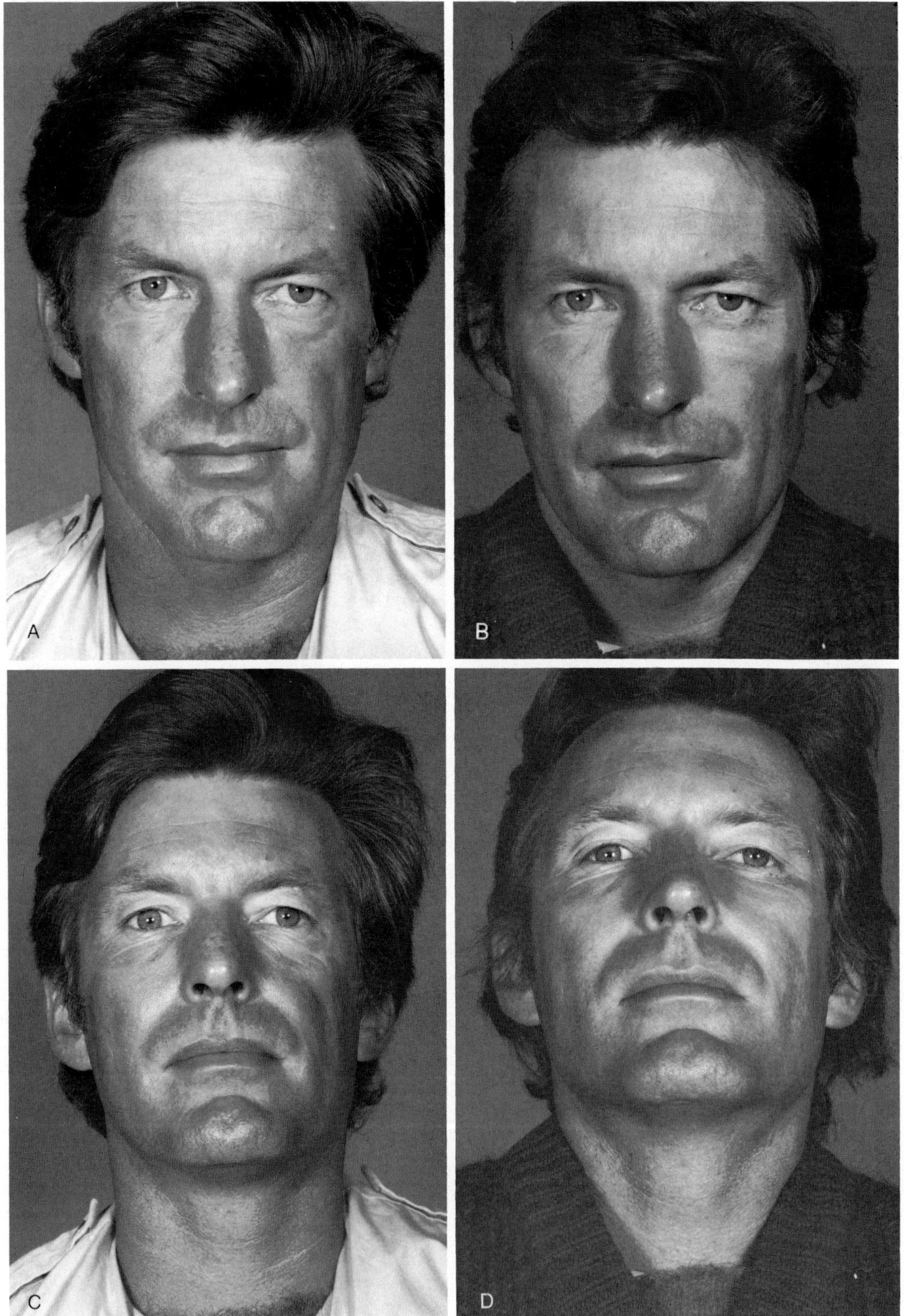

Figure 33–103. Onlay bone grafting of the left zygomatic complex (malunited fracture). The bone graft was inserted through an eyelid incision. *A, C, E,* Preoperative views. *B, D, F,* Postoperative views.

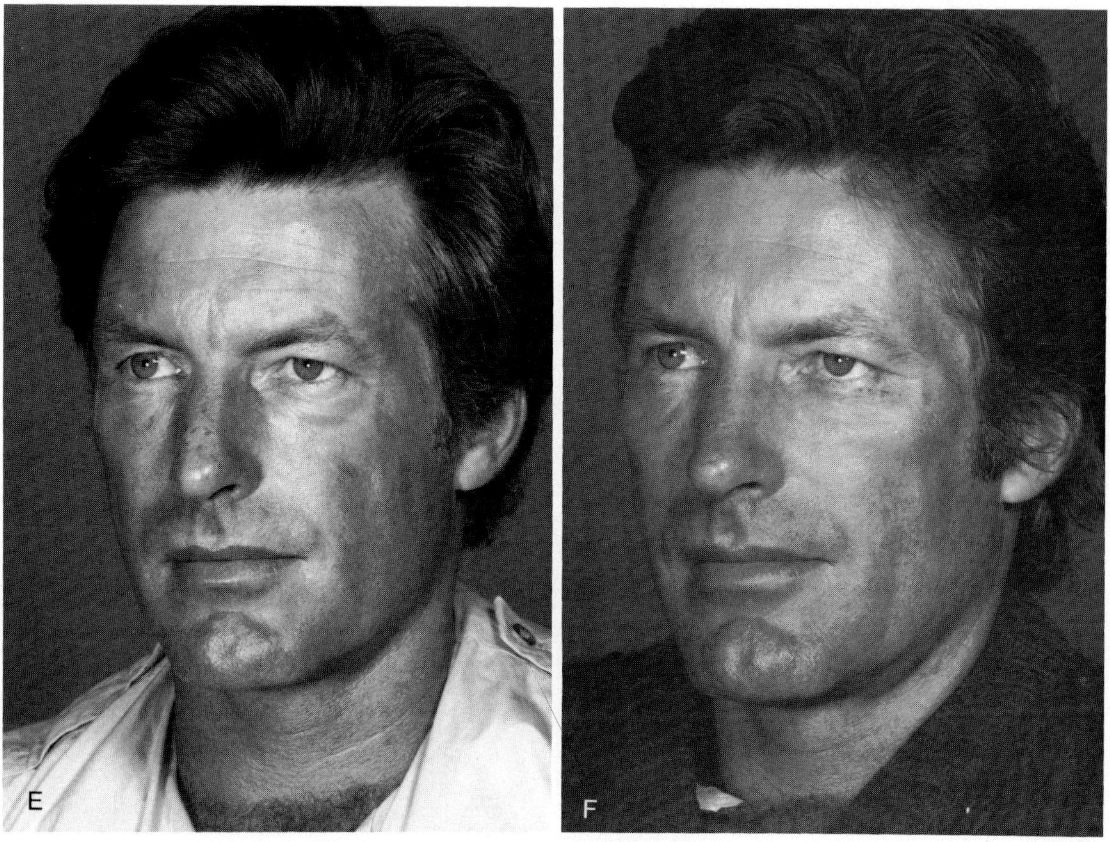

E

F

Figure 33–103 *Continued*

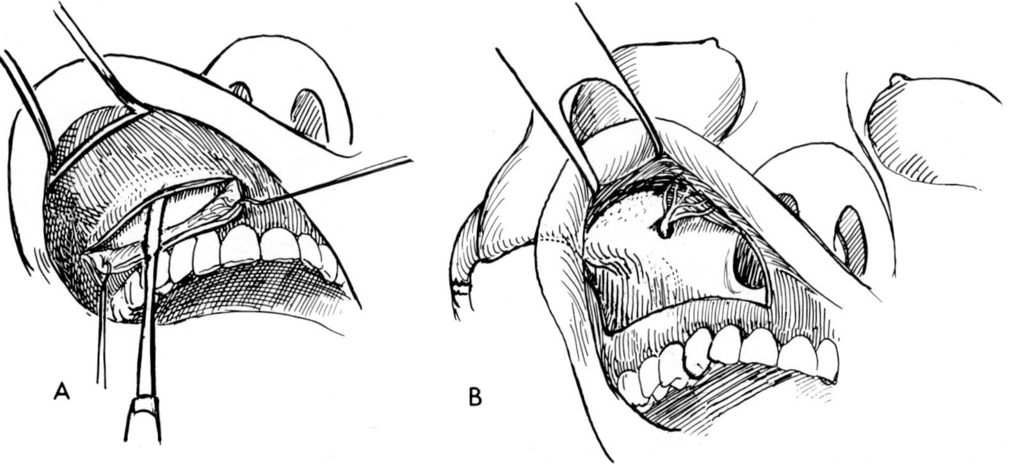

Figure 33–104. The intraoral approach to the maxilla and zygoma. *A,* The incision through the mucosa has been made on the labial aspect of the oral vestibule. *B,* The periosteum has been incised and elevated. The subperiosteal exposure has been extended to the infraorbital nerve, which is spared. The exposure is also extended to the edge of the piriform aperture and laterally over the zygoma.

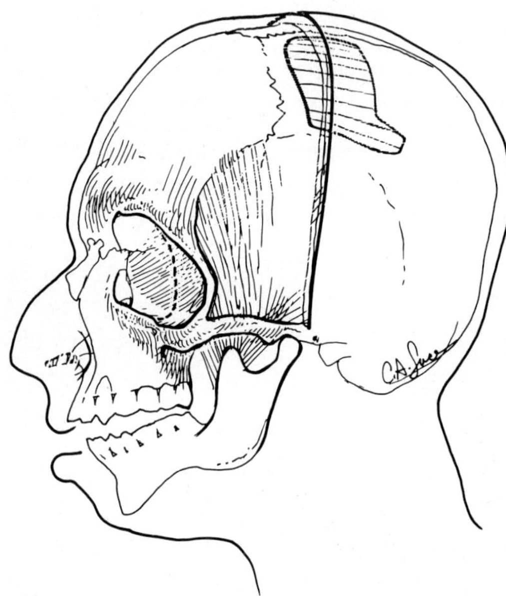

Figure 33–105. Temporoparietal flap. A coronal incision is made and the scalp is elevated in a subfollicular plane. The bone donor site is illustrated posterior to the coronal suture. (From McCarthy, J. G., Cutting, C. B., and Shaw, W. W.: Vascularized calvarial flaps. Clin. Plast. Surg., *14*:42, 1987.)

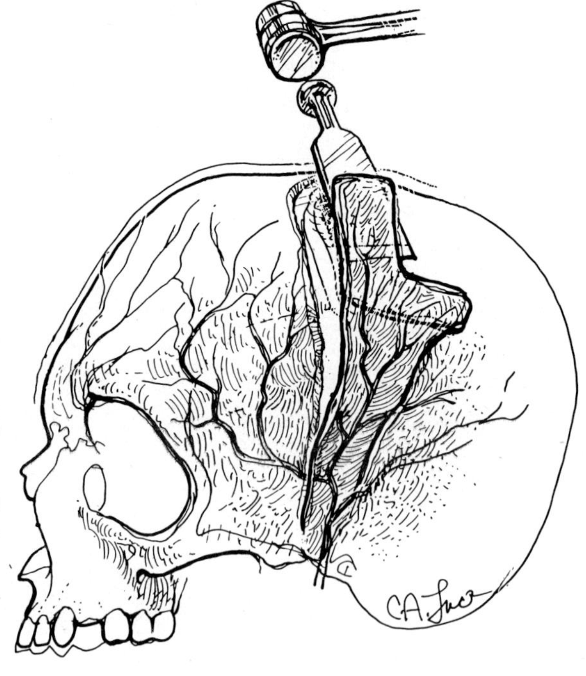

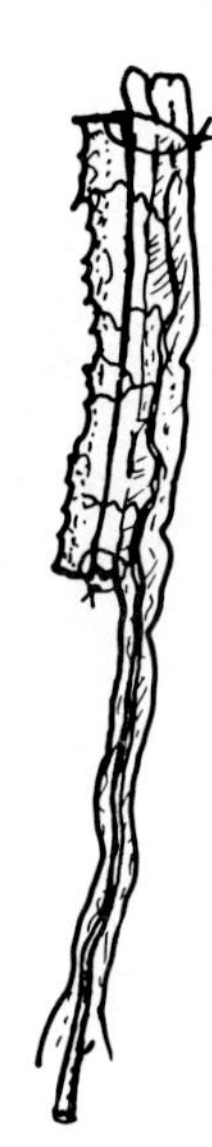

Figure 33–106. The superficial temporal arterial system is preserved along its main axis, and the outer table is harvested with a curved osteotome after a trough is created around the periphery with an air-driven bur. Inset shows the flap and pedicle. Note that sutures are passed between the overlying galea and the periosteum and calvaria in order to preserve the pedicle. The pedicle consists of the galea-SMAS as well as the deep temporal fascia (aponeurosis). (From McCarthy, J. G., Cutting, C. B., and Shaw, W. W.: Vascularized calvarial flaps. Clin. Plast. Surg., *14*:43, 1987.)

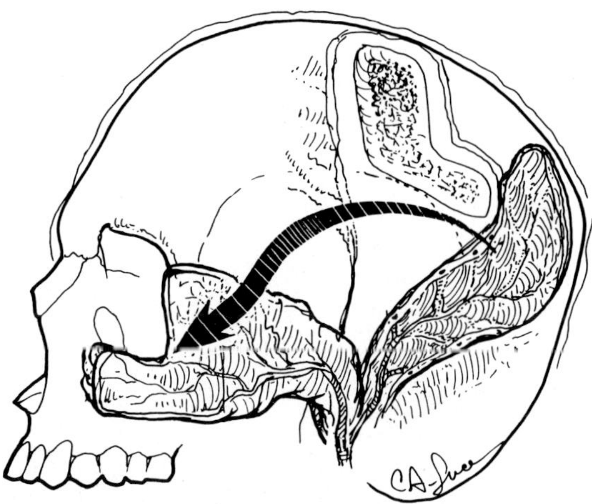

Figure 33–107. Composite flap in position to augment the zygomatic complex and lateral orbital wall. Note that a second flap can be taken from the same side when additional augmentation is required. (From McCarthy, J. G., Cutting, C. B., and Shaw, W. W.: Vascularized calvarial flaps. Clin. Plast. Surg., *14*:43, 1987.)

ciation of the pedicle from the bone component.

The flap pedicle is incised and elevated incorporating an axial component of the superficial temporal artery. The pedicle in the temporal region includes the galea-SMAS and the underlying aponeurosis (deep temporal fascia). The temporalis muscle is spared.

The skeletal donor site can usually be managed by burring the margins of the outer table defect. Methyl methacrylate can also be used to restore the contour in the adult, but

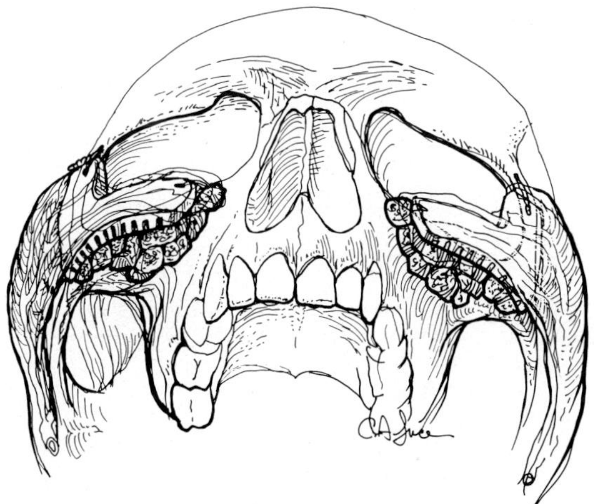

Figure 33–108. Nonvascularized calvarial bone grafts can be placed under the osseous component of the flap. (From McCarthy, J. G., Cutting, C. B., and Shaw, W. W.: Vascularized calvarial flaps. Clin. Plast. Surg., *14*:43, 1987.)

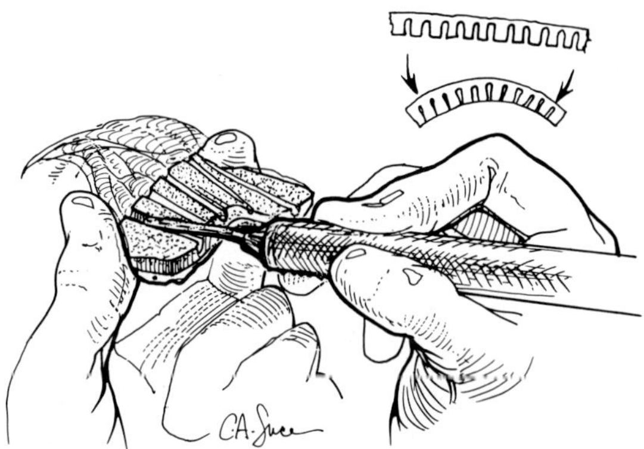

Figure 33–109. Recontouring the bone component with an air-driven bur. (From McCarthy, J. G., Cutting, C. B., and Shaw, W. W.: Vascularized calvarial flaps. Clin. Plast. Surg., *14*:43, 1987.)

is contraindicated if the operation also involves entry into the nose or paranasal sinuses.

If the outer and inner tables are harvested, split-thickness calvarial grafts can be removed from another site and placed in the defect.

Additional modifications include the simultaneous application of two flaps from the same side (Fig. 33–107) and the placement of nonvascularized calvarial bone grafts below the vascularized transfer (Fig. 33–108). The bone component of the flap can also be contoured with the aid of an air-driven bur (Fig. 33–109).

ADVANCEMENT OSTEOTOMY AUGMENTATION OF ZYGOMA

In cases of zygomatic hypoplasia of congenital origin a tripartite advancement osteotomy of the zygomatic complex may be indicated, especially if the maxilla is of normal proportions and occlusal relationships are satisfactory.

The craniofacial skeleton is exposed by a bicoronal and eyelid incision. The osteotomy is started in the region of the frontozygomatic suture and is extended in a full-thickness fashion through the lateral orbital wall and the inferior orbital rim (Fig. 33–110). This portion of the osteotomy is stopped in the region of the maxillozygomatic suture. The zygomatic arch is divided and the osteotomy is carried through the body of the zygoma. The segment is liberated, advanced, and secured by a combination of interosseous wires and/or miniplates. Onlay bone grafts can be

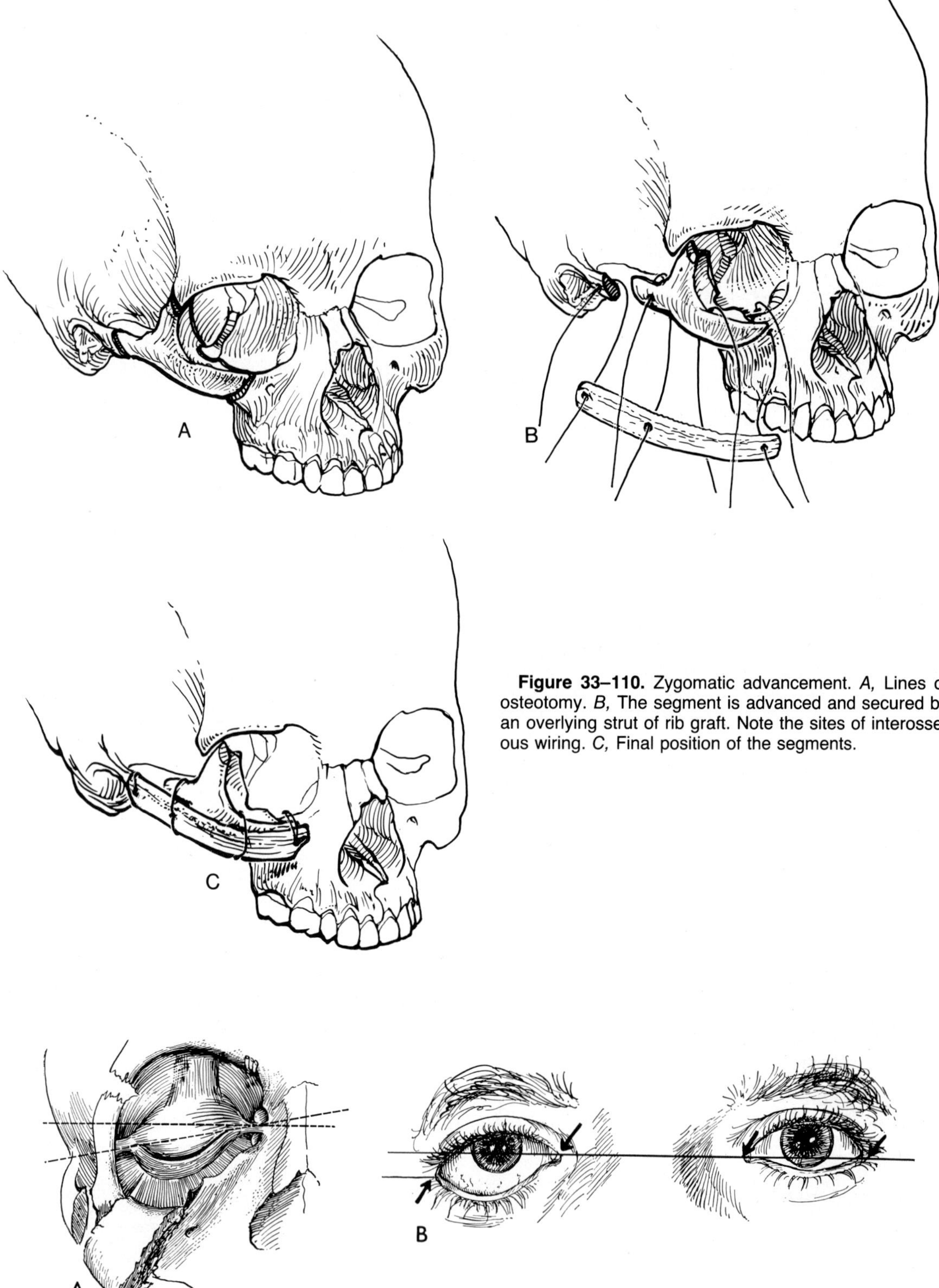

Figure 33–110. Zygomatic advancement. *A,* Lines of osteotomy. *B,* The segment is advanced and secured by an overlying strut of rib graft. Note the sites of interosseous wiring. *C,* Final position of the segments.

Figure 33–111. Deformity resulting from malunited fracture of the zygoma with frontozygomatic separation. *A,* Malunited fracture of the zygoma, frontozygomatic separation, and downward displacement of the lateral canthus. *B,* Downward displacement of the lateral canthus and vertical shortening of the lower lid.

secured to the advanced skeletal segment to obtain additional zygomatic prominence. The resulting defects are also filled with bone grafts.

Malunited Fractures of Zygoma and Lateral Orbital Wall

Deformity and functional disturbances resulting from a malunited fracture vary according to whether there is a fracture-dislocation or a comminuted fracture, and in particular whether there is a downward displacement with loss of continuity of the lateral orbital wall and lateral portion of the orbital floor. The latter is associated with a downward cant of the palpebral fissure.

Other functional disturbances also occur in fractures of the body of the zygoma and of the zygomatic arch. The displaced bone may press against the coronoid process of the mandible and interfere with mandibular function. This complication is particularly common after depressed fractures of the zygomatic arch.

In malunited fractures with downward displacement, the orbitozygomatic complex is detached from the frontal bone, and there is a gap in the continuity of the lateral wall of the orbit. The lateral canthal mechanism and its attachment are displaced downward (Fig. 33–111). Inasmuch as the lateral position of the floor of the orbit is formed by the zygoma, the comminution in fractures of considerable severity may extend to the entire orbital floor, with prolapse of the orbital contents into the maxillary sinus and enlargement of the bone volume of the orbit. Enophthalmos can be a prominent finding. An antimongoloid slant of the palpebral fissure and lateral canthus and vertical shortening of the lower lid with ectropion are characteristic deformities (Fig. 33–112), in addition to the flatness of the zygomatic prominence resulting from the malunited fractured zygoma.

TREATMENT

Osteotomy and Reduction. This method of treatment is indicated when the zygoma is displaced laterally and inferiorly with clinical evidence of enophthalmos.

As mentioned previously, the optimal treatment is osteotomy and open reduction of the malunited orbitozygomatic segment (see Fig. 33–40) (Kawamoto, 1982). This technique permits reestablishment of the cheek prominence and the position of the lateral canthal mechanism. In addition, bony orbital volume is reduced and the enophthalmos is corrected.

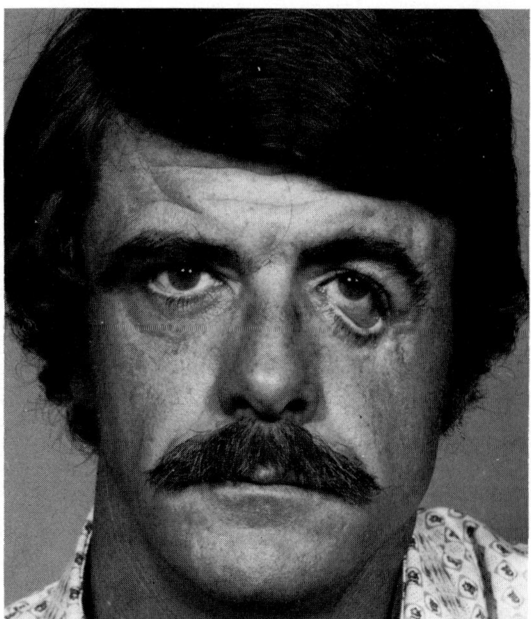

Figure 33–112. Comminuted malunited fracture of the left zygoma. Typical deformity: antimongoloid slant, vertical shortening, and ectropion of the lower lid.

Onlay Bone Grafting. If the zygoma and lateral orbital wall have been comminuted, the resultant bone loss or malposition will require bone grafts. In such cases, when there is no evidence of enophthalmos or displacement of the orbitozygomatic complex, onlay bone grafting of the complex should be considered.

There are two types of depression deformities of the zygoma. In Type I, the maxillary process of the zygoma and the zygomatic process of the maxilla are dislocated into the maxillary sinus, and the fractured bone is displaced laterally; the resultant deformity is seen as a depression in the infraorbital region of the cheek (Fig. 33–113). In Type II, the zygoma is depressed, causing loss of the cheek bone prominence and a generalized appearance of flatness (Fig. 33–114). Because of the relaxation of the musculature caused by the downward displacement of the bony origins of these structures, additional effects are

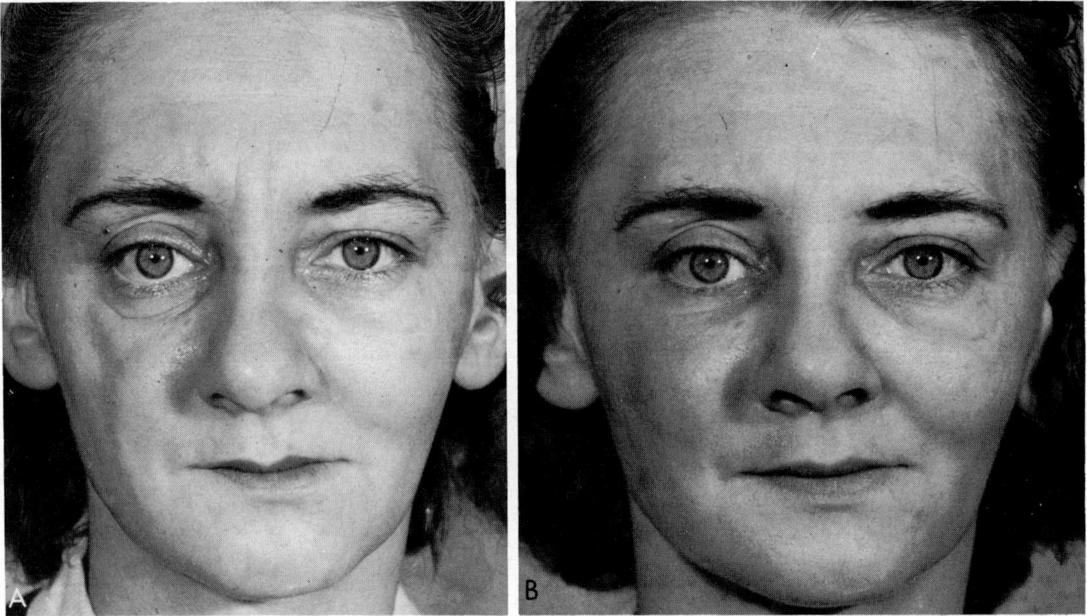

Figure 33–113. Malunited fracture of the zygoma: contour restoration by bone grafting through the intraoral approach. *A,* Type of deformity obtained when the fracture results in a rotation of the zygoma, with a backward displacement of the maxillary process of the zygoma and a lateral displacement of the frontal process of the zygoma. The displacement produces a depression in the infraorbital region. *B,* Result obtained by contour-restoring bone grafting through the intraoral approach. (From Converse, J. M.: Restoration of facial contour by bone grafts introduced through the oral cavity. Plast. Reconstr. Surg., *6*:295, 1950.)

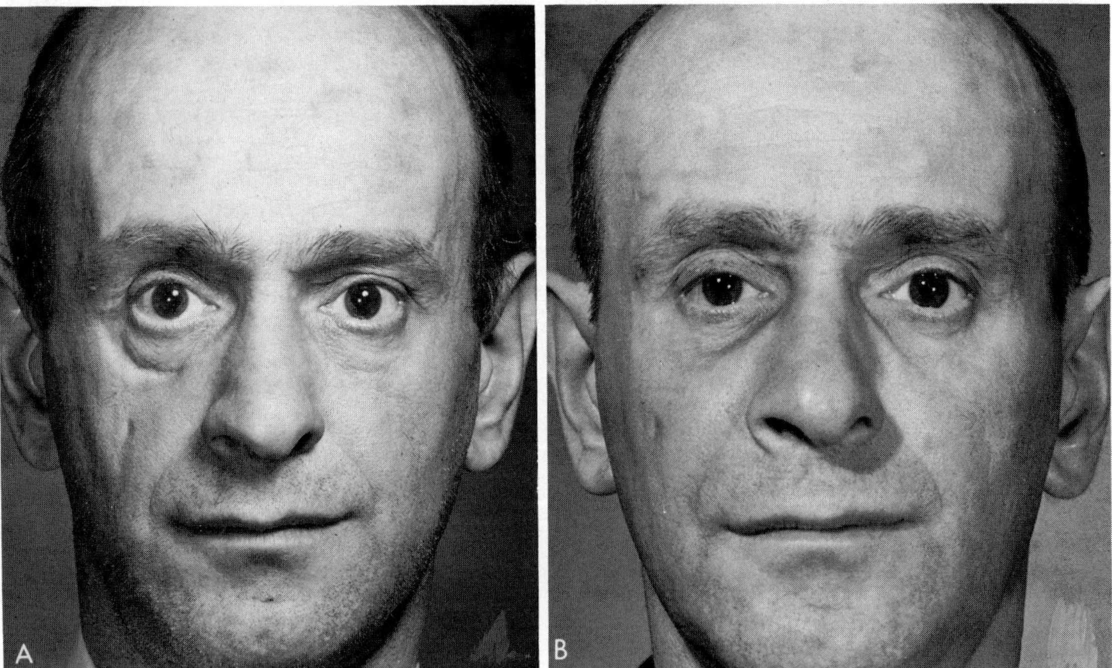

Figure 33–114. Malunited fracture of the zygoma: contour restoration by bone grafting through the intraoral approach. *A,* Depression over the right zygomaticomaxillary area resulting from a malunited fracture. *B,* Restoration of contour obtained by bone grafts placed over the right maxilla and zygoma after elevation of the periosteum. (From Converse, J. M.: Restoration of facial contour by bone grafts introduced through the oral cavity. Plast. Reconstr. Surg., *6*:295, 1950.)

noted, such as accentuation of the nasolabial fold, drooping of the upper lip, and deviation of the lip to the unaffected side.

Most defects are repaired by a single-piece bone graft, which is placed over the defect. Additional fragments of cancellous bone are packed beneath and around the bone onlay to improve the body contour.

One disadvantage of onlay bone grafting of the orbitozygomatic complex is resorption or eventual loss of the graft. Some situations are unfavorable for the nonvascularized bone transfer, e.g., overlying soft tissue deficiency and scarring. Calvarial bone grafts or flaps (McCarthy and Zide, 1984) are preferred in this situation.

REFERENCES

Adams, D. D.: Bioassay of long-acting thyroid stimulator (L.A.T.S.). The dose response relationship. J. Clin. Endocrinol. Metab., *21*:737, 1961.

Albert, A.: The experimental production of exophthalmos in Fundulus by means of anterior pituitary extracts. Endocrinology, *37*:389, 1945.

Alterman, K.: Exophthalmos: its reaction to adrenocortical function. I. Experimental exophthalmos. II. Clinical exophthalmos. Acta Endocrinol. (Suppl), *20*:59, 1954.

Andersson, E.: Ein Fall von schwerem Exophthalmus auf Grund von Morbus Basedowi bei einem 69-jährigen Manne operiert nach Dollinger. Acta Ophthalmol., *10*:396, 1932.

Ask, F.: Cited in Andersson (1932).

Basedow, C. von: Exophthalmos durch Hypertrophie des Zellgewebes in der Augenhöhle. Wochenschr. Ges. Heilk., *6*:197, 220, 1840.

Berke, R. N.: A modified Krönlein operation. Arch. Ophthalmol., *51*:609, 1954.

Berke, R. N.: Complications in ptosis surgery. *In* Fasanella, R. M. (Ed.): Complications in Eye Surgery. 2nd Ed. Philadelphia. W. B. Saunders Company, 1965.

Böhm, F.: Der Exophthalmus, seine Diagnose und Behandlung in der Chirurgie. Munch. Med. Wochenschr., *76*:51, 1929.

Bowes, R. E., Graham, E. A., and Tomlinson, K. M.: The natural history of strawberry nevus. Arch. Dermatol., *82*:667, 1970.

Boyden, G. L.: An otolaryngologic approach to malignant exophthalmos. Trans. Am. Laryngol. Rhinol. Otol. Soc., *66*:227, 1956.

Brant-Zawadski, M., Davis, P. L., Crooks, L. E., Mills, C. M., Norman, D., et al.: Nuclear magnetic resonance demonstration of cerebral abnormalities: comparison with CT. A.J.R., *140*:847, 1983.

Brown, B. Z., and Huffaker, G.: Local injection of steroids for juvenile hemangiomas which disturb the visual axis. Ophthalmic Surg., *13*:630, 1982.

Canadell, J. M.: Exophtalmie et Thyrostimuline. Extrait de la 5ème Réunion des Endocrinologistes de Langue Française, 1959, p. 178.

Chopra, I. J., and Solomon, D. H.: Graves' disease with delayed hyperthyroidism; onset after several years of euthyroid ophthalmopathy, dermopathy and high serum LATS. Ann. Intern. Med., *73*:985, 1970.

Converse, J. M.: Restoration of facial contour by bone grafts introduced through the oral cavity. Plast. Reconstr. Surg., *6*:205, 1950.

Converse, J. M.: Introduction to plastic surgery. *In* Converse, J. M. (Ed.): Reconstructive Plastic Surgery. 2nd Ed. Philadelphia, W. B. Saunders Company, 1977, p. 3.

Converse, J. M., Cole, G., and Smith, B.: Late treatment of blowout fracture of the floor of the orbit. A case report. Plast. Reconstr. Surg., *28*:183, 1961.

Converse, J. M., Firmin, F., Wood-Smith, D., and Friedland, J. A.: The conjunctival approach in orbital fractures. Plast. Reconstr. Surg., *39*:20, 1967.

Converse, J. M., Firmin, F., Wood-Smith, D., and Friedland, J. A.: The conjunctival approach in orbital fractures. Plast. Reconstr. Surg., *52*:656, 1973.

Converse, J. M., Ransohoff, J., Mathews, E. S., Smith, B., and Molenaar, A.: Ocular hypertelorism and pseudohypertelorism. Plast. Reconstr. Surg., *45*:1, 1970.

Converse, J. M., and Smith, B.: Enophthalmos and diplopia in fractures of the orbital floor. Br. J. Plast. Surg., *9*:265, 1957.

Converse, J. M., and Smith, B.: Naso-orbital fractures and traumatic deformities of the medial canthus. Plast. Reconstr. Surg., *38*:147, 1966.

Converse, J. M., and Smith, B.: Naso-orbital fractures and traumatic deformities of the medial canthus. Plast. Reconstr. Surg., *38*:147, 1966.

Converse, J. M., Smith, B., and Wood-Smith, D.: Orbital and Naso-orbital Fractures. *In* Converse, J. M. (Ed.): Reconstructive Plastic Surgery. 2nd Ed. Philadelphia, W. B. Saunders Company, 1977, p. 748.

Converse, J. M., Wood-Smith, D., McCarthy, J. G., and Coccaro, P. J.: Craniofacial Surgery. Clin. Plast. Surg., *1*:499, 1974.

Craig, W. M., and Dodge, H. W., Jr.: Surgical treatment of progressive exophthalmos. Trans. Am. Surg. Assoc., *70*:70, 1952a.

Craig, W., and Dodge, H. W., Jr.: The surgical treatment of malignant exophthalmos. Surg. Clin. North Am., *32*:991, 1952b.

Dallow, R. L.: Ultrasonography of the eye and orbit. *In* Gonzalez, C. F., Becker, M. H., and Flanagan, J. C. (Eds.): Diagnostic Imaging in Ophthalmology. New York, Springer, 1986.

de Venecia, G., and Lobeck, C. C.: Successful treatment of eyelid hemangioma with prednisone. Arch Ophthalmol., *84*:98, 1970.

Dingman, R. O., and Grabb, W. C.: Personal communication, 1974.

Dobyns, B. M., and Steelman, S. L.: The thyroid stimulating hormone of the anterior pituitary as distinct from the exophthalmos producing substance. Endocrinology, *52*:705, 1953.

Dollinger, J.: Die Druckentlastung der Augemhöhl durch Entfernung der äusseren Orbitalwand bei hochgrädigem Exophthalmus (Morbus Basedowii) und konsekutive Hosnhauterkrankung. Dtsch. Med. Wochenschr., *37*:1888, 1911.

Dryden, R. M., Wak, A. E., and Day, D.: Eyelid ecchymosis and proptosis in lymphangioma. Am. J. Ophthalmol., *100*:486, 1985.

Dupertuis, S. M.: Growth of young human autogenous cartilage grafts. Plast. Reconstr. Surg., *5*:486, 1950.

Edgerton, M. T., and Jane, J. A.: Vertical orbital dystopia—surgical correction. Plast. Reconstr. Surg., *67*:121, 1981.

Enzmann, D. R., Donaldson, S. S., and Kriss, J. P.: Appearance of Graves' disease on orbital computed tomography. J. Comput. Assist. Tomogr., *3*:815, 1979.

Eversman, J. J., Skillern, P. G., and Senhauser, D. A.: Hashimoto's thyroiditis and Graves' disease with exophthalmos with hyperthyroidism. Cleve. Clin. Q., *33*:179, 1966.

Fries, J. W.: The roentgen features of fibrous dysplasia of the skull and facial bones: a critical analysis of thirty-nine pathologically proved cases. Am. J. Roentgenol., *77*:71, 1957.

Fuchs, E.: Textbook of Ophthalmology. Philadelphia, J. B. Lippincott Company, 1924.

Furnas, D. W., and Achauer, B. M.: Two cases of orbital dystopia: Tessier III cleft and craniofacial osteomas. Ann. Plast. Surg., *6*:66, 1981.

Georgiade, N., Masters, F., Horton, C., and Pickrell, K.: Ossifying fibromas (fibrous dysplasia) of the facial bones in children and adolescents. J. Pediatr., *46*:36, 1955.

Gibson, T.: Transplantation of cartilage. *In* Converse, J. M. (Ed.): Reconstructive Plastic Surgery. 2nd Ed. Philadelphia, W. B. Saunders Company, 1977, p. 301.

Gillies, H., and Millard, D. R.: The Principles and Art of Plastic Surgery. Boston, Little, Brown Company, 1957.

Graefe, A. von: Ophthalmologische Miheilungen. Berl. Klin. Wochenschr., *4*:319, 1867.

Graefe, C. F. von: De Rhinoplastice. Berlin. Reimer. 1818. p. 13.

Graves, R.: Clinical lectures. Med. Classics. *5*:22, 1840.

Gruss, J. S.: Naso-ethmoid-orbital fractures: classification and role of primary bone grafting. Plast. Reconstr. Surg., *75*:303, 1985.

Guyton, J. S.: Decompression of orbit. Surgery, *19*:790, 1946.

Haid, B. G., Jakobiak, F. A., Ellsworth, R. M., et al.: Capillary hemangiomas of the lids and orbit: an analysis of the clinical features and therapeutic results in 101. Ophthalmology, *86*:760, 1979.

Haik, B. G., Saint-Louis, L., and Smith, M. E.: Nuclear magnetic resonance imaging in orbital disease. Ophthalmic Forum, *3*:31, 1985.

Hammerschlag, S., Hesselink, J. R., and Weber, A. L.: Computed Tomography of the Eye and Orbit. Norwalk, CT, Appleton-Century-Crofts, 1983, p. 25.

Handel, S. F., Stargardter, F. L., Glickman, M. G., and Newton, T. H.: Frequency of the ocular choroid blush during arteriography. Neuroradiology, *6*:50, 1973.

Hartman, D. C.: Anophthalmos and microphthalmos. *In* Troutman, R. C., Converse, J. M., and Smith, B. (Eds.): Plastic and Reconstructive Surgery of the Eye and Adnexa. Washington, DC, Butterworth, 1962.

Hemmer, K. M., Marsh, J. L., and Milder, B.: Orbital lymphangioma. Plast. Reconstr. Surg., *82*:340, 1988.

Henderson, J. W.: Relief of eyelid retraction; a surgical procedure. Arch. Ophthalmol., *74*:205, 1965.

Henderson, J. W.: Corrective surgery for endocrine lid retraction. *In* Proceedings of the Second International Symposium on Plastic and Reconstructive Surgery of the Eye and Adnexa. St. Louis, MO, C. V. Mosby Company, 1967, p. 490.

Heydenreich, A., Morczek, A., and Kurrals, U.: Behandlung des malignen Exophthalmus. Dtsch. Gesundheitsw. Wesen., *21*:1236, 1966.

Hildreth, H. R., and Silver, B.: Sensory block of the upper eyelid. Arch. Ophthalmol., *77*:230, 1967.

Hiles, D. A., and Pilchard, W. A.: Corticosteroid control of neonatal hemangiomas of the orbit and ocular adnexa. Am. J. Ophthalmol., *71*:1003, 1971.

Hinderer, U. T.: Malar implants for improvement of the facial appearance. Plast. Reconstr. Surg., *56*:157, 1975.

Hippel, E. von: Embryologischen Untersuchungen über die Entstehungweise der typischen augeborenen Spaltbildung (Colobome) des Augapfels. Arch. Ophthalmol., *55*:507, 1903.

Hirsch, O., and Urbanek, K.: Behandlung eines exzessiven exophthalmus (Basedow) durch Entfernung von Orbitalfett von der Kieferhohle aus. Monatsschr. Ohrenheilk., *64*:212, 1930.

Iverson, R. I.: Vistnes, L. M., and Siegel, R. J.: Correction of enophthalmos in the anophthalmic orbit. Plast. Reconstr. Surg., *51*:545, 1973.

Kawamoto, H. K.: Late posttraumatic enophthalmos: a correctable deformity? Plast. Reconstr. Surg., *69*:423, 1982.

Kennerdell, J. S., Maroon, J. C., Garrity, J. A., and Abla, A. A.: Surgical management of orbital lymphangioma with the carbon dioxide laser. Am. J. Ophthalmol, *102*:308, 1986.

Kistner, F. B.: Decompression of exophthalmos. Report of three cases. J.A.M.A., *112*:37, 1939.

Koornneef, L.: Current concepts on the management of orbital blow-out fractures. Ann. Plast. Surg., *9*:185, 1982.

Koyanagi, Y.: Embryologische Untersuchungen über die Genese der Augen—Kolobome und des Mikrophthalmus mit Orbitacyste. Graefes Arch. Ophthalmol., *104*:1, 1921.

Kroll, A. J., and Casten, V. G.: Dysthyroid exophthalmos. Palliation by lateral orbital decompression. Arch. Ophthalmol., *76*:205, 1966.

Krönlein, R.: Zur pathologie und Behandlung der Dermoidcysten der orbita. Beitr. Klin. Chir., *4*:149, 1888.

Kuehn, P. G., Newell, R. C., and Reed, J. F.: Exophthalmos in a woman with lingual, subhyoid and lateral-lobe thyroid glands. N. Engl. J. Med., *274*:652, 1966.

Kuhnt, H.: Zur Behandlung der Hornhautulzeration bei hochgradigem Basedow-Exophthalmos. Z. Augenheilk., *27*:1912.

Kusher, B. J.: Local steroid therapy in adnexal hemangioma. Ann. Ophthalmol., *11*:1005, 1979.

Kusher, B. J.: Intralesional corticosteroid injection for infantile adnexal hemangioma. Am. J. Ophthalmol, *93*:496, 1982.

Lagouros, P. A., Langer, B. G., Peyman, G. A., Matee, M. P., and Grisolano, J.: Magnetic resonance imaging and intraocular foreign bodies. Arch. Ophthalmol., *105*:551, 1987.

LaGrange, F.: De l'anaplerose orbitaire. Bull. Acad. Med. Paris, *80*:641, 1918.

Leeds, N., and Seaman, W. B.: Fibrous dysplasia of the skull and its differential diagnosis. A clinical and roentgenographic study of 46 cases. Radiology, *78*:570, 1962.

Ljungren, H., and Walander, A.: Transantral dekompression vid malign exophthalmus. Nord. Med., *61*:436, 1959.

Long, J. C.: Lateral decompression of the orbit for thyroid exophthalmos. *In* Proceedings of the Second International Symposium on Plastic and Reconstructive Surgery of the Eye and Adnexa. St. Louis, MO, C. V. Mosby Company, 1967, p. 463.

Long, J. C., and Ellis, G. D.: Temporal decompression of the orbit for thyroid exophthalmos. Am. J. Ophthalmol., *62*:1089, 1966.

Longacre, J. J., de Stefano, G. A., and Holmstrand, K.: The early versus the late reconstruction of hypoplasias of the facial skeleton and skull. Plast. Reconstr. Surg., *27*:489, 1961.

Low, J. G.: Transcranial decompression for relief of exophthalmos. *In* Proceedings of the Second International Symposium on Plastic and Reconstructive Surgery of the Eye and Adnexa. St. Louis, MO, C. V. Mosby Company, 1967, p. 478.

Manson, P. N., Clifford, C. M., Su, C. T., Iliff, N. T., and Morgan, R.: Mechanisms of global support and posttraumatic enophthalmos. I. The anatomy of the ligament sling and its relation to intramuscular cone orbital fat. Plast. Reconstr. Surg., *77*:193, 1986a.

Manson, P. N., Grivas, A., Rosenbaum, A., Vannier, M., Zinreich, J., and Iliff, N.: Studies on enophthalmos. II. The measurement of orbital injuries and their treatment by quantitative computed tomography. Plast. Reconstr. Surg., *77*:203, 1986b.

Marchac, D.: Intracranial enlargement of the orbital cavity and palpebral remodelling for orbitopalpebral neurofibromatosis. Plast. Reconstr. Surg., *73*:534, 1984.

Marchac, D., Cophignon, J., Achard, E., and Dufourmentel, C.: Orbital expansion for anophthalmia and microorbitism. Plast. Reconstr. Surg., *59*:486, 1977.

Maroon, J. C., and Kennerdell, J. S.: Radical orbital decompression for severe dysthyroid exophthalmos. J. Neurosurg., *56*:260, 1982.

Mayo, C. H.: The surgical treatment of exophthalmos. J.A.M.A., *63*:1147, 1914.

McCarthy, J. G., Cutting, C. B., and Shaw, W. W.: Vascularized calvarial flaps. Clin. Plast. Surg., *14*:37, 1987.

McCarthy, J. G., and Zide, B. M.: Spectrum of calvarial bone grafting. Introduction of the vascularized calvarial bone flap. Plast. Reconstr. Surg., *74*:10, 1984.

McCord, C. D., Jr.: Orbital decompression for Graves' disease. Exposure through lateral canthal and inferior fornix incision. Ophthalmology, *88*:533, 1981.

McCord, C. D., Jr.: Current trends in orbital decompression. Ophthalmology, *92*:21, 1985.

McCord, C. D., Jr., and Moses, J. L.: Exposure of the inferior orbit with fornix incision and lateral cantotomy. Ophthalmic Surg., *10*:53, 1979.

McKenzie, J. M.: An evaluation of the thyroid activator of hyperthyroidism. *In* Pett-Rivers, R. (Ed.): Transactions of the Fourth International Goiter Conference. Vol. 11. New York, Pergamon Press, 1961, p. 210.

Means, J. H.: The eye problems in Graves' disease. Illinois Med. J., *80*:135, 1941.

Merrill, H. G., and Oaks, L. W.: Extreme bilateral exophthalmos. Report of two cases with autopsy with findings in one. Am. J. Ophthalmol., *16*:231, 1933.

Merville, L. C., Derome, P., and de Saint-Jorre, G.: Fronto-orbito-nasal dislocations. J. Maxillofac. Surg., *11*:71, 1983.

Moran, R. E.: Surgical decompressions for enophthalmos and exophthalmos. Sect. on Ophthalmol., A.M.A., *109*:1622, 1937.

Moran, R. E.: The correction of exophthalmos and levator spasm. Plast. Reconstr. Surg., *18*:411, 1956.

Moran, R. E., Letterman, G. S., and Schurter, M. A.: The surgical correction of exophthalmos. History, technique, and long-term follow-up. Plast. Reconstr. Surg., *49*:595, 1972.

Mueller, W., Schemmel, K., Uthgenannt, H., and Weissbecker, L.: Die Behandlung des malignen Exophthalmos durch totale Thyroidektomie. Dtsch. Med. Wochenschr., *92*:2103, 1967.

Munro, I. R., and Chen, Y.-R.: Radical treatment for fronto-orbital fibrous dysplasia: the chain-link fence. Plast. Reconstr. Surg., *67*:719, 1981.

Munro, I. R., and Martin, R.: One stage correction of giant neurofibromas and arterio-venous hemangiomas by craniofacial techniques. *In* Transactions of the International Congress of Plastic Surgery, Rio de Janeiro, 1979, p. 256.

Mustardé, J. C.: The treatment of ptosis and epicanthal folds. Br. J. Plast. Surg., *12*:252, 1959.

Mustardé, J. C.: Personal communication, 1975.

Naffziger, H. C.: Progressive exophthalmos following thyroidectomy: its pathology and treatment. Ann. Surg., *94*:582, 1931.

Naffziger, H. C.: Pathologic changes in the orbit in progressive exophthalmos with special reference to alterations in the extraocular muscles and the optic discs. Arch. Ophthalmol., *9*:1, 1933.

Naffziger, H. C.: Exophthalmos, some surgical principles of surgical management from the neurosurgical aspect. Am. J. Surg., *75*:25, 1948.

Naffziger, H. C.: Progressive exophthalmos. Ann. R. Coll. Surg. Engl., *17*:25, 1954.

Neuhaus, R. W., and Shorr, N.: The use of room temperature vulcanizing silicone in anophthalmic enophthalmos. Am. J. Ophthalmol., *94*:408, 1982.

Nolan, W. B., and Vistnes, L. M.: Correction of lower eyelid ptosis in the anophthalmic orbit: a long-term follow-up. Plast. Reconstr. Surg., *72*:289, 1983.

Obwegeser, H. L.: Late reconstruction of large maxillary defects after tumor resection. J. Maxillofac. Surg., *1*:19, 1973.

Odell, W. D., Fisher, D. A., Korenman, S. G., et al.: Symposium on hyperthyroidism. Calif. Med., *113*:35, 1970.

Ogura, J. H.: Transantral orbital decompression for progressive exophthalmos. A follow-up of 54 cases. Med. Clin. North Am., *52*:399, 1968.

Ogura, J. H., and Walsh, T. E.: The transantral orbital decompression operation for progressive exophthalmos. Laryngoscope, *72*:1078, 1962.

Pavlicek, W., Modic, M., and Weinstein, M.: Pulse sequence and significance. Radiographics, *4*:49, 1984.

Pochin, E. E.: Exophthalmos in guinea pigs injected with pituitary extracts. Clin. Sci., *3*:75, 1944.

Poppen, J. L.: Exophthalmos. Diagnosis and surgical treatment of intractable cases. Am. J. Surg., *64*:64, 1944.

Poppen, J. L.: The surgical treatment of progressive exophthalmos. J. Clin. Endocrinol., *10*:1231, 1950.

Putterman, A. M., and Urist, M.: Surgical treatment of upper eyelid retraction. Arch. Ophthalmol., *87*:401, 1972.

Rao, V. M., and Gonzalez, C. F.: Plain film radiography and polytomography of the orbit. *In* Gonzalez, C. F., Becker, M. H., and Flanagan, J. C. (Eds.): Diagnostic Imaging in Ophthalmology. New York, Springer, 1986, p. 1.

Riley, F. C.: Orbital pathology in Graves' disease. Mayo Clin. Proc., *47*:973, 1972.

Rintoul, A. J.: Unilateral proptosis. Proc. R. Soc. Med., *61*:545, 1968.

Robb, R. M.: Refractive errors associated with hemangiomas of the eyelids and orbit in infancy. Am. J. Ophthalmol., *83*:52, 1977.

Rogers, B. O.: Embryology of the face and introduction to craniofacial anomalies. *In* Converse, J. M. (Ed.): Reconstructive Plastic Surgery. 2nd Ed. Philadelphia, W. B. Saunders Company. 1977, p. 2296.

Schall, L. A., and Regan, D. J.: Malignant exophthalmos. Ann. Otol. Rhinol. Laryngol., *54*:37, 1945.

Schimek, R. A.: Surgical management of ocular complications of Graves' disease. Arch. Ophthalmol., *87*:655, 1972.

Sedan, R., and Harter, M.: Irradiation interstitielle hypophysaire dans l'exophtalmologie oedemateuse maligne. Neurochirurgie, *12*:226, 1966.

Sewall, E. C.: Operative control of progressive exophthalmos. Arch. Otolaryngol., *24*:621, 1936.

Slansky, H. H., Kolbeit, G., and Gartner, S.: Exophthalmos induced by steroids. Arch. Ophthalmol., *77*:579, 1967.

Smelser, G. K.: Water and fat content of orbital tissues in guinea pigs with experimental exophthalmos produced by extracts of anterior pituitary gland. Am. J. Physiol., *140*:308, 1943.

Smelser, G. K.: Experimental studies on exophthalmos. Am. J. Ophthalmol., *54*:929, 1961.

Smelser, G. K., Ozanics, V., and Zugibe, F. T.: The production of exophthalmos in the absence of adrenal and ovarian hormones. Am. Rec., *131*:701, 1958.

Smith, B., and Lisman, R. D.: Use of sclera and liquid collagen in the camouflage of superior sulcus deformities. Ophthalmology, *90*:230, 1983.

Smith, B., Obear, M., and Leone, C. R.: The correction of enophthalmos associated with anophthalmos by glass bead implantation. Am. J. Ophthalmol., *64*:1088, 1967.

Sonnenberg, M., and Money, W. L.: Chemical derivatives of thyroid stimulating hormone preparations. *In* Modern Concepts of Thyroid Physiology. Ann. N.Y. Acad. Sci., *86*:625, 1960.

Spira, M., Gerow, F. J., and Hardy, S. B.: Correction of post-traumatic enophthalmos. Acta Chir. Plast., *16*:107, 1974.

Swift, G. W.: Malignant exophthalmos and operative approach. West. J. Surg., *43*:119, 1935.

Szily, A. von: Weitere Beitrage zu den embryologischen Grundlagen der Missbildungen des Auges. Erklaung der angerborenen umschrieben Loch- oder Grubenbildungen an der Papille. Berl. Ophthalmol. Ges. Heidelberg, *39*:344, 1913.

Tenzel, R. R., and Miller, G. R.: Orbital fracture repair, conjunctival approach. Am. J. Ophthalmol., *71*:1141, 1971.

Tessier, P.: Expansion chirurgicale de l'orbite. Ann. Chir. Plast., *14*:207, 1969.

Tessier, P.: Vertical and oblique facial clefts (orbito-facial fissures). *In* Mustardé, J. C. (Ed.): Plastic Surgery in Infancy and Childhood. Philadelphia, W. B. Saunders Company, 1971, p. 94.

Tessier, P.: The conjunctival approach to the orbital floor and maxilla in congenital malformation and trauma. J. Maxillofac. Surg., *1*:3, 1973.

Tessier, P. A. (Ed.): Plastic Surgery of the Orbit and Eyelids. Translated by Wolfe, S. A. New York, Masson Publishers, 1981.

Tessier, P.: Inferior orbitotomy. A new approach to the orbital floor. Clin. Plast. Surg., *9*:569, 1982a.

Tessier, P.: Autogenous bone grafts taken from the calvarium for facial and cranial applications. Clin. Plast. Surg., *9*:531, 1982b.

Tessier, P., Guiot, G., and Derome, P.: Orbital hypertelorism. II. Definitive treatment of orbital hypertelorism by craniofacial or by extracranial osteotomies. Scand. J. Plast. Reconstr. Surg., *7*:39, 1973.

Tessier, P., Guiot, G., Rougerie, J., Delbet, J. P., and Pastoriza, J.: Ostéotomies cranio-naso-orbital-faciales. Hypertélorisme. Ann. Chir. Plast., *12*:103, 1967.

Tinker, M. B.: The surgical treatment of exophthalmos. Sect. on Ophthalmol., J.A.M.A., *58*:353, 1912.

Valenti, G., and Cordella, M.: Sugli affetti di un betabloccante adrenergico sullo esoftalmo spetimentale da triiodotironin. Ann. Ottal., *93*:1037, 1967a.

Valenti, G., and Cordella, M.: Esoftalmo sperimentale de triiodotironina, da STHC e da proprietiouracile dopo timectomia. Ann. Ottal., *93*:1025, 1967b.

van der Meulen, J. C.: Orbital neurofibromatosis. Clin. Plast. Surg., *14*:123, 1987.

van der Meulen, J. C., Moscona, A. R., Vaandrachen, M., and Hirshowitz, B.: The management of orbitofacial neurofibromatosis. Ann. Plast. Surg., *8*:213, 1982.

Walsh, T. E., and Ogura, J. H.: Transantral orbital decompression for malignant exophthalmos. Laryngoscope. *65*:544, 1957.

Walsh, T. S., and Tompkins, V. N.: Some observations in the strawberry nevus of infancy. Cancer, *9*:869, 1956.

Weinstein, M. A., Modic, M. T., Risius, B., Duchesneau, P. M., and Berlin, A. J.: Visualization of the arteries, veins and nerves of the orbit by sector computed tomography. Radiography, *138*:83, 1981.

Welti, H., and Offret, G.: A propos des exophthalmies malignes basedowiennes. Ann. Endocrinol. (Paris), *3*:186, 1942.

Werner, S. C.: Management of the active severe eye changes of Graves' disease. Trans. Am. Acad. Ophthalmol. Otolaryngol., *71*:631, 1967.

Whitaker, L. A.: Aesthetic augmentation of the malar-midface structure. Plast. Reconstr. Surg., *80*:337, 1987.

Whitnall, E.: The structure and muscle of the eyelids. *In* Anatomy of the Human Orbit. London, W. H. Milford, 1932, p. 129.

Wolfe, J. R.: A new method of performing plastic operation. Med. Times Gaz., *1*:608, 1876.

Wolfe, S. A.: Modified three-wall orbital expansion to correct persistent exophthalmos or exorbitism. Plast. Reconstr. Surg., *64*:448, 1979.

Wood, A. C.: The ocular changes of primary diffuse toxic goitre. Rev. Med., *25*:113, 1936.

Worst, J. G. F.: Method of reconstructing torn lacrimal canaliculus. Am. J. Ophthalmol., *53*:520, 1962.

Würdemann, H. V., and Becker, W.: A typical exophthalmic goiter from endothelioma of the pituitary and thyroid bodies. Death from general sepsis. Autopsy. Ophthalmology, *2*:411, 1906.

Wybar, K. C.: The nature of endocrine exophthalmos. Ophthalmology, *49*:119, 1957.

Zak, T. A., and Morin, D. J.: Early local steroid therapy of infantile eyelid hemangiomas. J. Pediatr. Ophthalmol. Strabismus, *8*:25, 1981.

Zheutlin, J. D., Thompson, J. T., and Shofner, R. S.: The safety of magnetic resonance imaging with intraorbital metallic objects after retinal detachment or trauma. Am. J. Ophthalmol., *103*:831, 1987.

Zide, B. M., and Jelks, G. W.: Surgical Anatomy of the Orbit. New York, Raven Press, 1985.

Zide, B. M., and McCarthy, J. G.: The medial canthus revisited: anatomic basis of medial canthopexy. Ann. Plast. Surg., *11*:1, 1983.

Zimmerman, R. D., and Russell, E. J.: Angiography in the evaluation of visual disturbances. Int. Ophthalmol. Clin., *26*:187, 1986.

34

Glenn W. Jelks
Byron C. Smith

Reconstruction of the Eyelids and Associated Structures

ANATOMY
UNIQUE OPERATIVE CONSIDERATIONS
LACERATIONS OF THE EYELIDS
RECONSTRUCTION OF THE EYELID
Partial-Thickness Defects
Full-Thickness Defects
MEDIAL CANTHOPLASTY
LATERAL CANTHOPLASTY
RECONSTRUCTION OF THE LACRIMAL SYSTEM
Excretory Deformities and Developmental Defects
Diagnostic Tests
Repair of Lacrimal Apparatus
EYELID MALPOSITIONS
Entropion
Symblepharon
Ectropion
PTOSIS OF UPPER EYELID
Fasanella-Servat Operation and its Modifications
Aponeurosis Surgery
Levator Resection
Frontalis Muscle Suspension
EPICANTHUS
EPIBLEPHARON
BLEPHAROPHIMOSIS

The eyelids contain specialized structures that protect the eyes from excessive light, exposure to extremes of the elements, and airborne debris. During blinking, they distribute a protective and optically important tear film over the anterior surface of the eye. The upper eyelid is particularly suited for optimal protection of the cornea. Lacerations or deformities of the upper eyelid are, therefore, more emergent in terms of repair.

The lacrimal apparatus consists of those structures involved with the production, distribution, and drainage of tears. Proper tear film maintenance protects the eyes and provides a refractive surface. The lacrimal apparatus may be obstructed or destroyed by lacerations, bony disruptions, or disease processes involving the medial orbit and nasal cavity. The flow of tears through the nasolacrimal duct, although not essential in all cases, must often be restored by creating an alternative route for tear flow into the nose.

The extraocular muscles allow ocular movement and are essential to single binocular vision. A fascial system within the orbit supports the globe, limits ocular movements, and provides an interconnected scaffolding from one structure to another. In the reconstruction of orbital dislocations, the architecture of the orbit (see Chap. 33) must be restored if functional disturbances of the ocular globe are to be minimized.

For surgery in the orbital region, the primary consideration should always be the protection of the eye and the maintenance of vision.

ANATOMY

Extraocular Muscles and Associated Fascial Structures

The ocular globe occupies the anterior half of the orbital cavity, and its movements are controlled by the extraocular muscles. The posterior half of the orbital cavity contains the optic nerve, orbital fat, vessels, muscles,

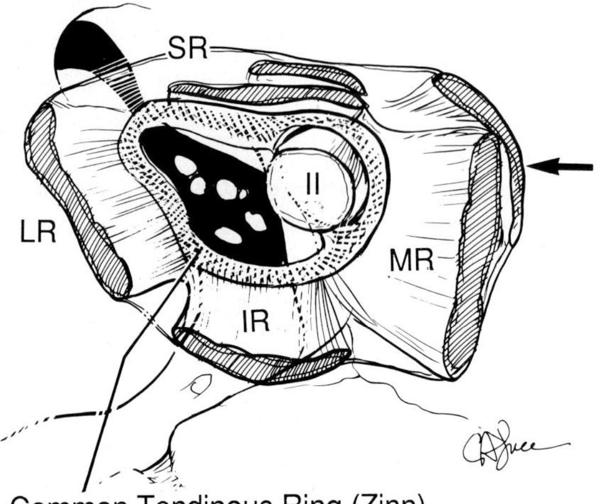

Figure 34–1. The annulus of Zinn or common tendinous ring. The superior origin of the lateral rectus (LR) muscle separates the superior orbital fissure into two compartments. The portion of the orbital apex enclosed by the annulus is called the oculomotor foramen, through which pass both divisions of the oculomotor nerve, the abducens nerve, and the nasociliary nerve. Those structures passing into the orbit laterally and outside the muscle cone or ring are the lacrimal, frontal, and trochlear nerves; the superior ophthalmic vein; and a communicating branch of the middle meningeal artery. The optic nerve (II) passes through the optic foramen lateral to the origin of the medial rectus muscle (MR). The ophthalmic artery enters the orbit with the optic nerve on its inferior aspect. The inferior rectus (IR) and superior rectus (SR) muscle origins complete the common tendinous ring. The superior oblique muscle *(arrow)* originates outside and superomedial to the annulus.

and motor and sensory nerves. All the extraocular muscles except the inferior oblique originate from a fibrous thickening of the periosteum at the apex of the orbit known as the Annulus of Zinn (Fig. 34–1). The superior origin of the lateral rectus muscle separates the superior orbital fissure into two compartments. The lowermost compartment, completely encompassed by the tendinous origins of the muscles, is termed the oculomotor foramen, through which pass both divisions of the oculomotor nerve, the abducens, and the nasociliary nerve. These nerves enter the inner surgical space of the orbit, and derangements in their function can be clinically correlated to a pathologic condition within the muscle cone and the inferior aspect of the superior orbital fissure. Those structures passing through the uppermost portion of the superior orbital fissure include the lacrimal, frontal, and trochlear nerves; the superior ophthalmic vein; and a communicating branch from the middle meningeal artery.

The optic nerve passes with its accompanying ophthalmic artery through the optic canal in the lesser wing of the sphenoid to enter the muscle cone. Knowledge of this specific orbital anatomy (see also Chap. 33) is invaluable in the clinical correlation of orbital pathology such as the localization of a superior oblique palsy (cranial nerve IV) associated with ipsilateral numbness of the forehead and lateral orbital skin (cranial nerve V) to the superior aspect of the superior orbital fissure. When ptosis, external ophthalmoplegia (cranial nerves III and VI), and anesthesia of the cornea (nasociliary nerve) are manifest, the pathology involves the structures within the oculomotor foramen of the superior orbital fissure *(superior orbital fissure syndrome)*. When visual loss is added to the above findings, the orbital apex, particularly the optic foramen, is involved *(orbital apex syndrome)*.

The extraocular muscles course forward from the orbital apex to insert on the ocular globe in such a way that balanced and complex movements can be achieved. The inferior oblique muscle originates from the anterior orbit just lateral to the nasolacrimal canal (Fig. 34–2).

The vascular supply to the extraocular muscles originates principally from the ophthalmic artery, with some contributions from the lacrimal and infraorbital arteries. Each rectus muscle is supplied by two anterior ciliary arteries, except the lateral rectus,

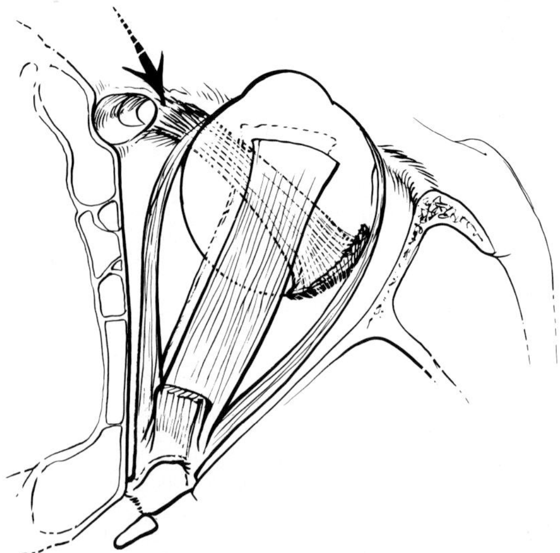

Figure 34–2. The course and relative positions of the extraocular muscles (superior orbital view). Note that the inferior oblique muscle originates from the periosteum lateral to the nasolacrimal canal *(arrow)*.

which has only one. The anterior ciliary arteries continue forward to penetrate the sclera at the muscle insertion and nourish the anterior segment of the eye. This explains how ocular anterior segment ischemia can occur if more than two extraocular muscles are detached from the globe.

The fascial framework of the orbit has classically been described as comprising (1) the bulbar fascia (Tenon's capsule), (2) the fascial sheaths surrounding the extraocular muscles, (3) the intermuscular fascial septa, and (4) the check ligaments of the medial and lateral recti. More recently, Koornneef (1977a, b, 1979, 1986) has classified the orbital and ocular fascial connections as being tripartite: (1) Tenon's capsule and the fascia around the extraocular muscles, (2) the connective tissue network connecting the posterior periorbita, and (3) the diffuse fascial connections between the extraocular muscles and the posterior periorbita. Koornneef has shown that the orbital connective tissue system allows the eye, eyelids, muscles, nerves, vessels, lacrimal gland, and orbital fat to move and be moved in concert. Tenon's capsule, or the fascia bulbi, is a dense fibroelastic layer that surrounds the globe. The extraocular muscles penetrate this fascia to insert on the globe. The intervening fascial network between the muscles is called the intermuscular septa. The anterior portion of the intermuscular septa is thick, providing an anatomic barrier to the escape of orbital fat. Tenon's capsule is tightly adherent to the globe just posterior to the muscle insertions and weakly adherent in the intervening quadrants. Posterior to the globe the orbit has been classically divided into an inner and outer space correlated to the space within or outside the area circumscribed by the extraocular muscles. Motais (1887) originally described a distinct common muscle sheath between the rectus muscles in the posterior orbit; however, Koornneef has virtually proved that no such structure exists. More posteriorly, the intervening intermuscular septa actually become thinner and discontinuous, thus allowing orbital fat to insinuate itself among the orbital structures and creating a less distinct muscle cone. Tenon's capsule continues posteriorly to encircle the optic nerve, which penetrates it as it enters the eye. More anteriorly, as the intermuscular septa thicken, the connective tissue mass between the inferior oblique and inferior rectus muscles forms the inferior suspensory ligament of Lockwood.

A thickening or condensation of fascia overlies and surrounds the levator muscle near the superior orbital margin, i.e., Whitnall's ligament. Extensions from the sleeves of fascia surrounding the medial and lateral recti muscles form condensations, called the check ligaments, that serve to secure them to the periorbita (Fig. 34–3).

Eyelids

The eyelids are composed of thin skin, areolar tissue, orbicularis oculi muscle, tarsus, levator palpebrae superioris muscle, Müller's muscle, septum orbitale, fat and conjunctiva.

The skin of the eyelids is thin and elastic. It is moderately adherent to the orbicularis muscle over the tarsus, and becomes more loose and mobile in the preseptal and orbital regions. The eyelid skin becomes thicker at the junction with the skin of the cheek and the other areas surrounding the orbit. The area of transition corresponds roughly to the bony orbital margins.

The tarsal plates are thin, elongated plates of connective tissue (Fig. 34–4) that contribute to the form and support of the eyelids. They are closely related to the levator palpebrae superioris muscle and the medial and lateral canthal structures. The superior tarsus is approximately 10 mm in height at its center and tapers gradually medially and laterally. The inferior tarsus varies from 3.8 to 4.5 mm in vertical height. The oil-secreting meibomian glands, approximately 20 in each lid, are within the substance of the tarsal plates, and their openings form a row of tiny dots on the central zone of the lid margin that corresponds to the mucocutaneous junction (gray line).

Orbicularis Oculi Muscle

The orbicularis muscle surrounding the palpebral fissure is responsible for lid closure. Although in appearance it is one continuous muscle, it has been divided arbitrarily into three subdivisions (Fig. 34–5): (1) the *pretarsal* muscle overlying the tarsus, (2) the *preseptal* muscle overlying the septum orbitale, and (3) the *orbital* muscle, which forms a ring extending over the orbital margin.

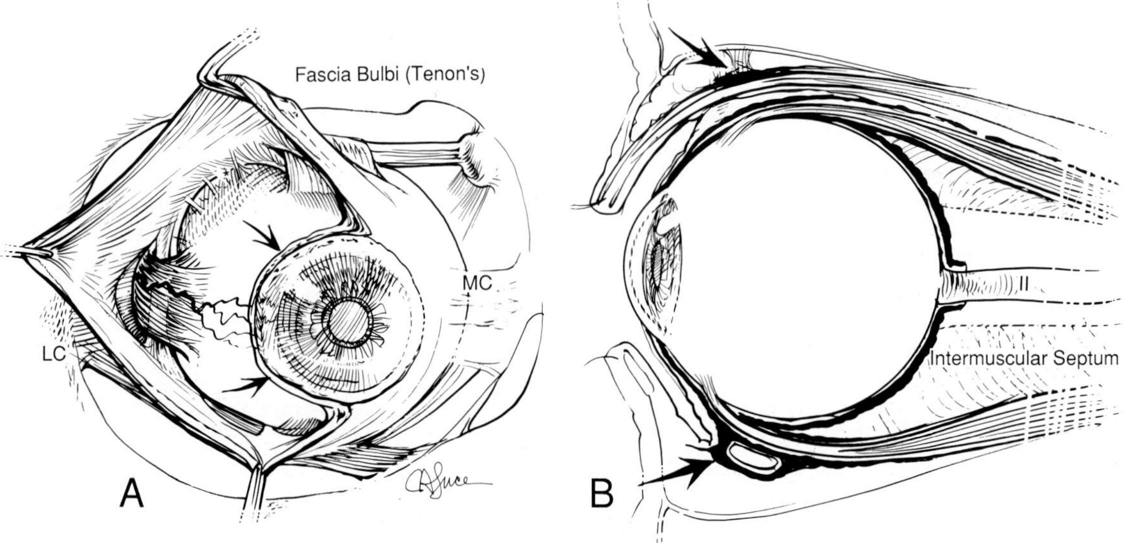

Figure 34–3. *A,* Tenon's capsule is elevated and retracted. The cut margin *(arrows)* is noted at the limbus. The extraocular muscles must penetrate this fascia to insert on the globe. The intervening fascial network between the muscles (better seen in *B*) is called the intermuscular septum. The anterior portion of the intermuscular septum is thick, providing an anatomic barrier in the front of the orbit. Tenon's capsule is tightly adherent to the globe just posterior to the muscle insertions and weakly adherent in the intervening quadrants. The medial check (MC) and lateral check (LC) ligaments are fascial extensions of the medial and lateral recti muscle sheaths that extend to the periorbita. Similarly, fascial extensions from the inferior oblique muscle extend onto the periorbita of the orbital floor. *B,* More posteriorly, the intervening intramuscular septa are thinner and may become discontinuous, thus opening the muscle cone. Tenon's capsule continues posteriorly, eventually to encircle the optic nerve (II), which penetrates it. More anteriorly, as the intermuscular septum thickens, the connective tissue mass between the inferior oblique and inferior rectus muscles forms the inferior suspensory ligament of Lockwood *(lower arrow).* Whitnall's ligament is a thickening or condensation of fascia located superiorly overlying the levator muscle *(upper arrow).*

The *orbital* portion of the orbicularis muscle extends in a wide circular fashion around the orbit, interdigitating with other muscles of facial expression (Figs. 34–5, 34–6). This portion of the muscle originates medially from the superomedial orbital margin, the maxillary process of the frontal bone, the medial canthal tendon, the frontal process of the maxilla, and the inferomedial orbital margin. The peripheral fibers sweep across the eyelid over the orbital margin in a series of concentric loops, the more central ones forming almost complete rings. In the upper eyelid, the orbital portion spreads upward

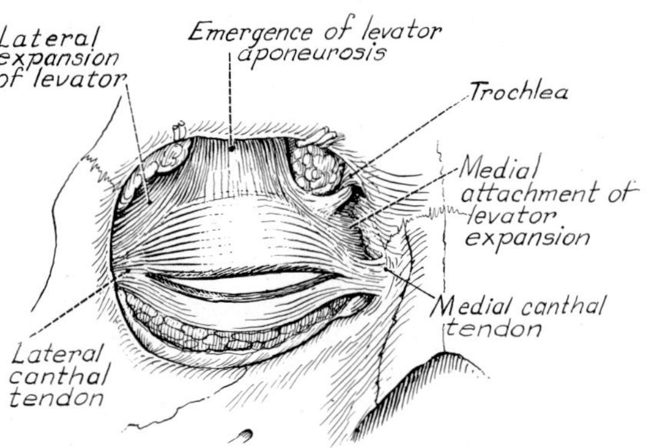

Figure 34–4. The tarsal plates, the levator palpebrae superioris, and their relationships to the medial canthal and lateral canthal tendons.

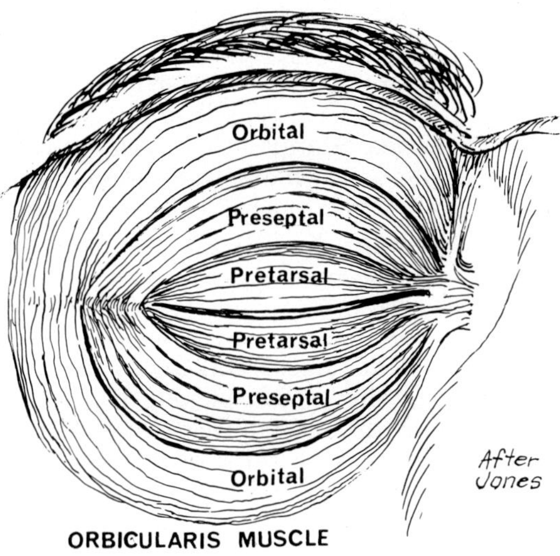

Figure 34–5. The three subdivisions of the orbicularis oculi muscle.

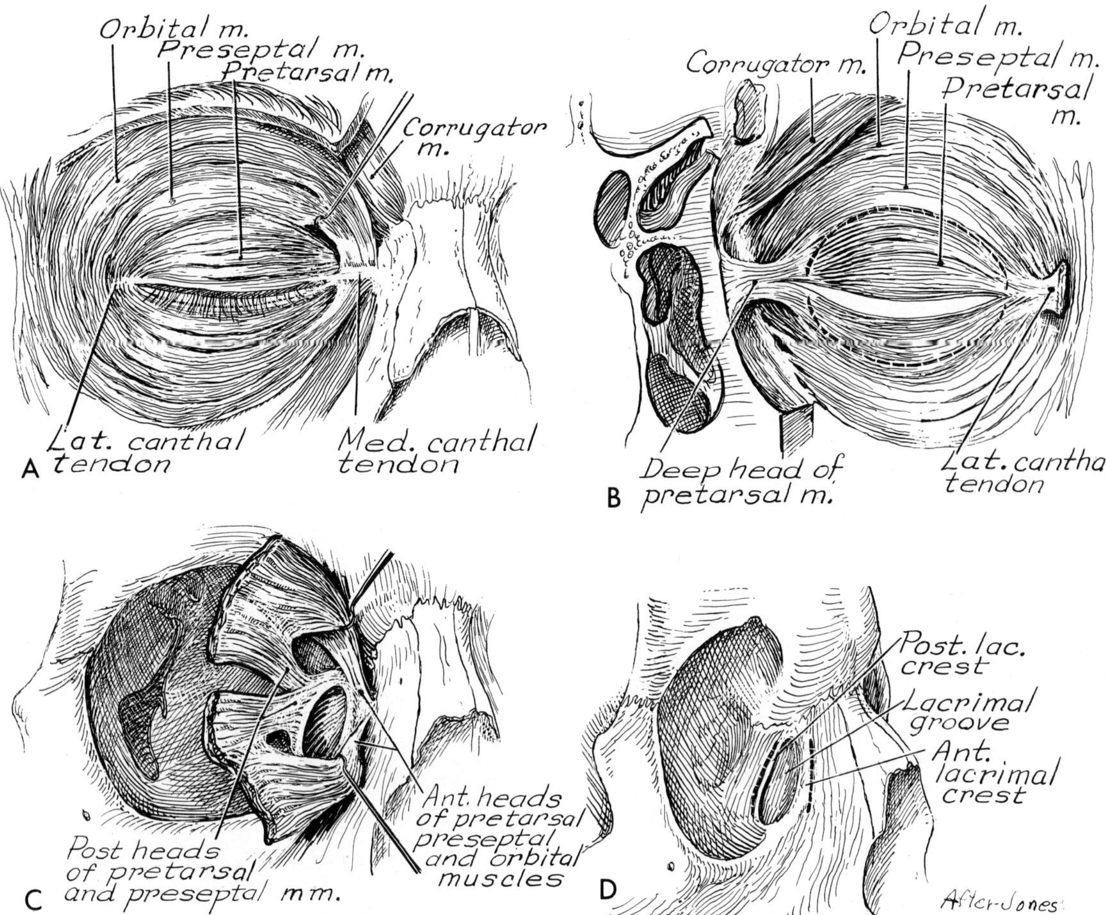

Figure 34–6. The orbicularis oculi muscle. *A,* The medial and lateral canthal tendons showing the superficial head of the pretarsal muscle, which joins its counterpart from the opposing lid to form the medial canthal tendon. The hook raises the preseptal muscle whose fibers insert on the orbital margin below the medial canthal tendon. *B,* The orbicularis oculi muscle seen from behind. The deep head of the pretarsal muscle after joining its counterpart extends posterior to the lacrimal sac, blending with the lacrimal sac diaphragm to insert behind the posterior lacrimal crest (Horner's muscle). *C,* Anterior view illustrating the anterior heads of the pretarsal and preseptal muscles, as well as the posterior heads. *D,* The skeletal anatomy of the medial canthus.

onto the forehead, covers the frontalis and corrugator supercilii muscles, and continues laterally over the temporalis fascia. In the lower eyelid, the orbital portion covers the origins of the elevator muscles of the upper lip and nasal ala, and continues in a temporal direction to cover part of the origin of the masseter muscle. Occasionally, the lower orbital portion may actually continue downward into the cheek.

The *pretarsal* muscle is divided medially into a superficial head and a deep head (Fig. 34–6, *A* to *C*). The superficial head joins its counterpart from the opposing lid to form the medial canthal tendon, which originates above and anterior to the anterior lacrimal crest. The deep head, after joining its counterpart, extends posteriorly to the lacrimal sac, blending with the lacrimal sac diaphragm to originate immediately behind the posterior lacrimal crest (Figs. 34–6*C, D,* 34–7). The deep head of the tarsal portions of the orbicularis is also known as Horner's muscle or the tensor tarsi muscle.

The *preseptal* muscle also has superficial and deep fibers (Figs. 34–6*A, B,* 34–7). The superficial fibers of each preseptal muscle (upper and lower) originate on the orbital margin below the medial canthal tendon (Fig. 34–8*A*). Deeper fibers originate from the lacrimal diaphragm. The deepest fibers originate from the posterior lacrimal crest just above the deep heads of the pretarsal muscles (see Fig. 34–6*C*). The lacrimal pump mechanism

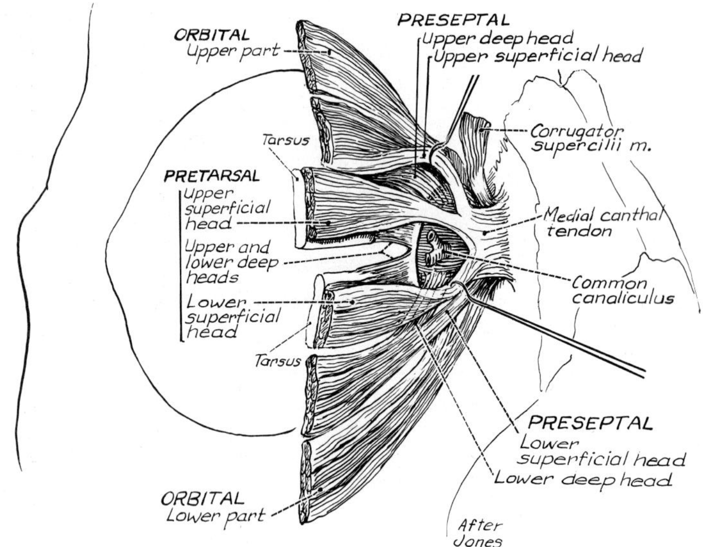

Figure 34–7. Details of the anatomy in the right medial canthal area (front view).

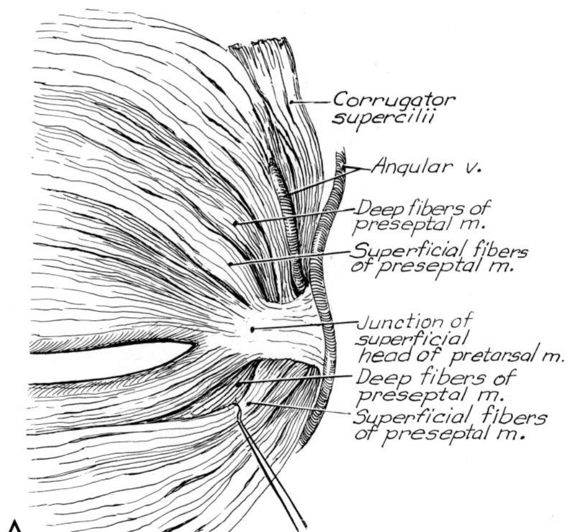

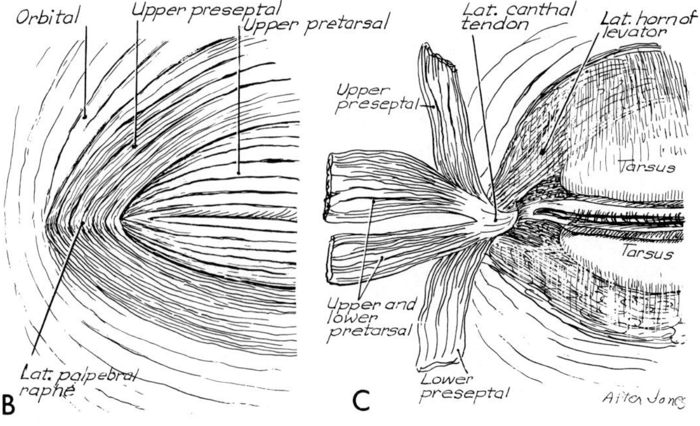

Figure 34–8. *A,* The anatomy of the orbicularis oculi muscle at the right medial canthus. *B,* The lateral palpebral raphé. *C,* The lateral canthal tendon and the anatomy of the structures of the lateral canthus.

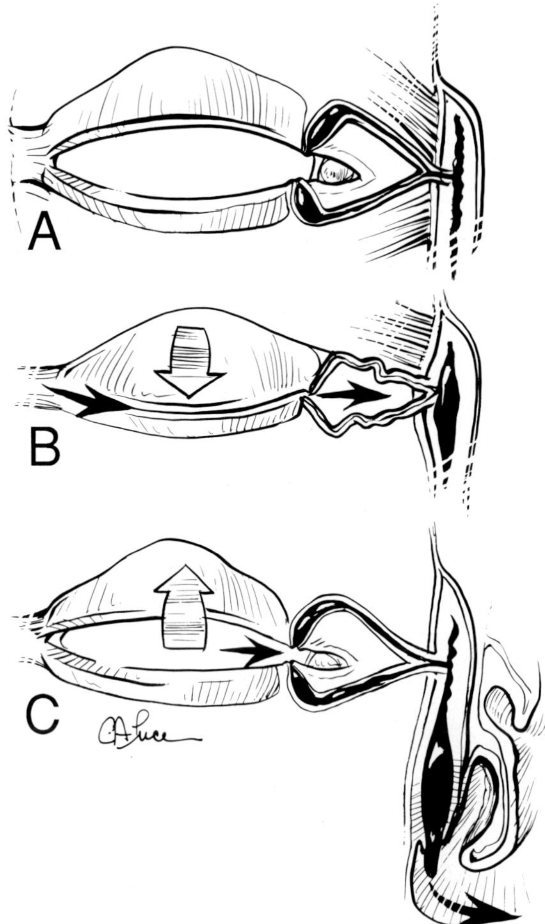

Figure 34–9. The lacrimal pump mechanism functions with the eyelids open; the puncta lie in contact with the lacrimal lake where the tears collect medially. The canaliculi remain patent as the lacrimal sac tends to collapse *(A)*. Upon eyelid closure, tears are milked laterally to medially. The deep heads of the pretarsal muscles contract, shortening the canaliculi and closing their ampullae. Simultaneously, the deep heads of the preseptal muscles, attached to the fascia of the sac (lacrimal diaphragm), contract and pull the fascia laterally to create a negative pressure within the sac *(B)*. As the lids reopen, the lacrimal diaphragm returns to its relaxed position, creating sufficient pressure to propel the tears into the nasolacrimal duct. The canaliculi reopen at this phase to allow collection of more tears *(C)*.

is explained by the medial movements of the lids during eyelid closure, emptying the ampullae, shortening the canaliculi, and thus forcing fluid into the lacrimal sac (Fig. 34–9). In addition, the preseptal muscles through their intimate connection with the lacrimal fascial diaphragm produce a negative pressure in the lacrimal sac, further drawing tears into the fundus. With eyelid opening, the elasticity of the lacrimal diaphragm returns the sac to a position of rest, forcing tears into the nasolacrimal duct. The heads of the pretarsal and preseptal muscles originating from the posterior lacrimal crest have a particular surgical importance. These structures not only aid active tear drainage but also maintain the eyelids against the ocular globe to create the depth of the naso-orbital valley. When anatomic disorganization of the medial canthal structures occurs, as in nasoethmoido-orbital fractures, flattening of the naso-orbital valley is due to disruption of the soft tissue attachments to the medial bony orbit. During reconstruction it is important to reattach the medial canthal structures sufficiently posterior and superior to the lacrimal groove to reestablish the depth of the naso-orbital valley (see Fig. 34–58).

In the lateral canthus, both preseptal muscles form a "raphé" (see Fig. 34–8*B*), a convenient term to designate the loops of muscle bundles that are firmly attached to the skin of the lateral canthus (Jones, 1974a). The pretarsal muscles of the upper and lower eyelids are inserted into the orbital tubercle, situated behind the orbital rim on the lateral orbital wall, through the intermediary of the lateral canthal tendon (see Fig. 34–8*C*). There is space between the tendon and the raphé, which deepens laterally. The lateral palpebral artery, a branch of the lacrimal artery, passes through this space to supply both eyelids.

Orbital Septum

The orbital septum (septum orbitale) is a fascial membrane that separates the eyelid structures from the deeper orbital structures. It is a barrier that helps prevent the spread of hemorrhage, infection, inflammation, and other disease processes. The orbital septum attaches to the orbital margin at a thickening of periosteum called the arcus marginalis (Fig. 34–10). The arcus marginalis is also the point of confluence for the facial bone periosteum and the periorbita. The orbital septum is usually thicker laterally in both lids. It lies anterior to the lateral canthal tendon, although this has not been proved to the satisfaction of all orbital anatomists (Doxanas and Anderson, 1984; Zide and Jelks, 1985). Superomedially, the arcus marginalis usually forms the inferior portion of the supraorbital groove. Therefore, the supraorbital neurovascular structures frequently exit from

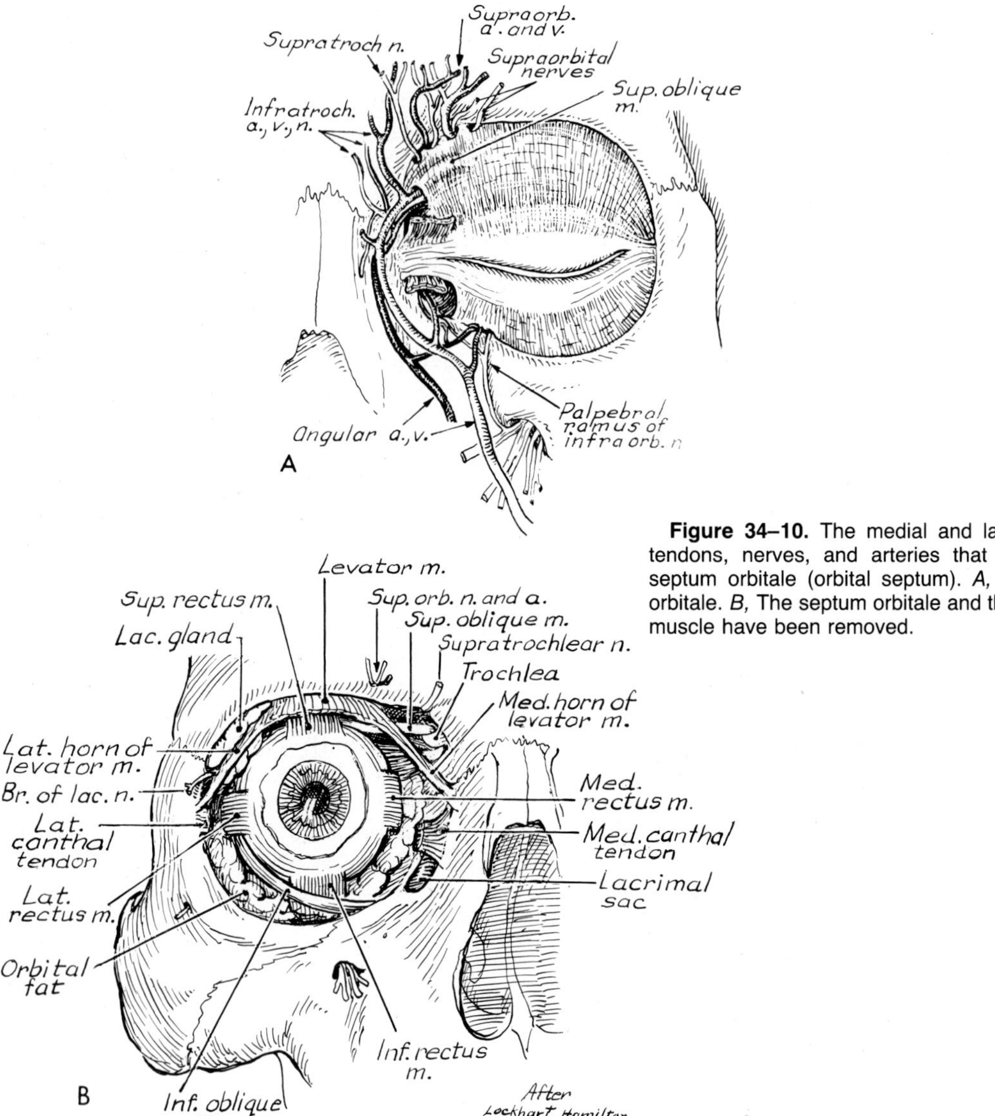

Figure 34–10. The medial and lateral canthal tendons, nerves, and arteries that traverse the septum orbitale (orbital septum). *A,* The septum orbitale. *B,* The septum orbitale and the orbicularis muscle have been removed.

a groove or notch closed by the arcus marginalis. Medially, the orbital septum passes anterior to the superior oblique trochlear pulley and is then directed posterior to the posterior lacrimal crest, and therefore posterior to the deep heads of the orbicularis oculi muscle. The orbital septum follows the orbital rim along the inferior portion of the anterior lacrimal crest and inferior orbital rim. In the lateral half of the inferior orbital rim, the orbital septum may originate a few millimeters inferior to the temporal orbital margin, forming a potential space on the facial aspect of the zygoma known as the recess of Eisler.

Levator Palpebrae Superioris and Müller's Muscle

The levator palpebrae superioris is a thin, flat, striated triangular muscle arising from the undersurface of the lesser wing of the sphenoid anterior and superior to the optic foramen (see Fig 34–1). At its origin it is narrow and tenuous; however, at a level corresponding to the equator of the globe it broadens into a wide aponeurosis that inserts onto the anterior lower third of the tarsus. The levator aponeurosis fans out medially and laterally into two extensions, termed

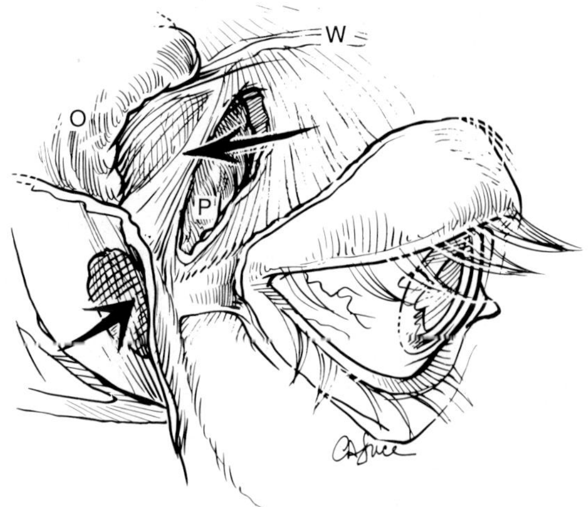

Figure 34–11. The lateral extension or horn of the levator aponeurosis *(upper arrow)* splits the lacrimal gland into its orbital (O) and palpebral (P) lobes and extends inferolaterally to join the lateral retinaculum. The lateral portion of Whitnall's ligament (W) inserts into the orbital lobe of the gland by way of the interglandular fascial septa. The inferolateral pole of the palpebral lobe of the lacrimal gland usually rests at the level of the lateral retinaculum *(lower arrow).* The lateral retinaculum is a confluence of the lateral horn of the levator, the lateral canthal tendon, Lockwood's suspensory ligament of the globe, and check ligaments from the lateral rectus muscle.

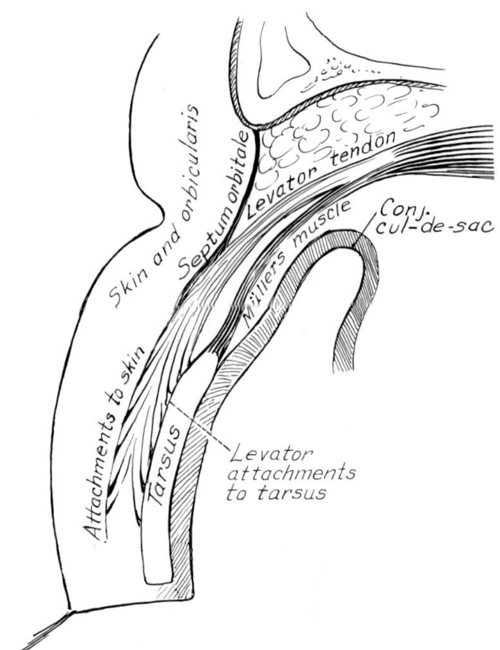

Figure 34–12. Sagittal section through the upper eyelid showing the relationship of the orbicularis oculi muscle, septum orbitale, levator palpebrae superioris, and Müller's muscle.

horns. The lateral extension is strong and divides the lacrimal gland into its orbital and palpebral lobes before attaching to the lateral retinaculum at the orbital tubercle of Whitnall (Fig. 34–11). The medial extension attaches to the posterior lacrimal crest (see Fig. 34–4). The levator aponeurosis has a firm attachment to the anterior surface of the tarsus and the skin of the eyelid via orbicularis muscle fascial fibers forming the superior tarsal fold of the upper eyelid. The levator aponeurosis is attached to and blends with the orbital septum for a distance of approximately 3 to 5 mm above the upper border of the tarsus. Above this level, the levator aponeurosis is separated from the septum orbitale by preaponeurotic fat. Thus, the preaponeurotic fat lies between the orbital septum and the levator aponeurosis and is a key surgical anatomic structure (Fig. 34–12). The preaponeurotic fat is characteristically looser in consistency and more easily separated and dissected than the deeper orbital fat. Müller's muscle (Fig. 34–13) extends from the junction of the muscular portion of the levator muscle and its aponeurosis to the superior border of the tarsus, and overlies the underlying conjunctiva. Whereas the levator muscle is a striated muscle innervated by the third cranial nerve, Müller's muscle is smooth and receives its innervation from the sympathetic nervous system. Manson and associates (1986) reported fluorescent staining and fluorescent microscopy studies documenting that the principal pathways for the sympa-

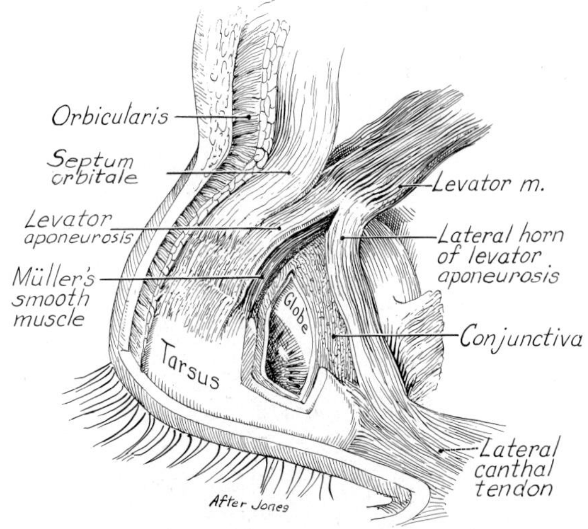

Figure 34–13. Sagittal section illustrating the structures of the upper eyelid, including the levator muscle, its aponeurosis, and its relationship with Müller's muscle and the septum orbitale.

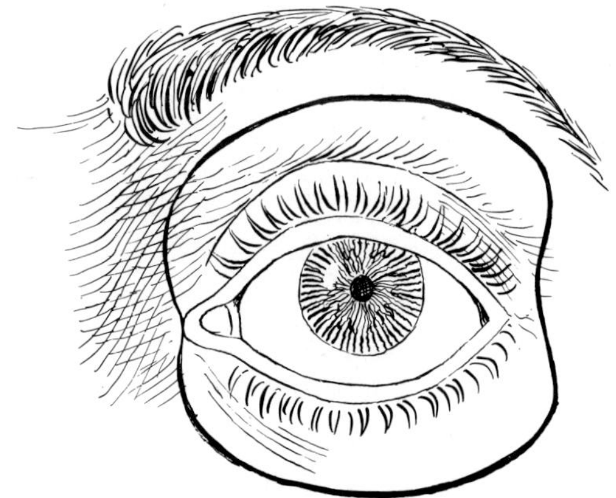

Figure 34–14. The depth of the conjunctival fornix.

thetic nerves to the eyelids are via the sensory (first division of the trigeminal) and the motor nerves (oculomotor, trochlear, and abducens) within the orbit.

Conjunctiva

The palpebral conjunctiva lines the inner aspect of the eyelid and is reflected onto the globe as the bulbar conjunctiva. The tarsal conjunctiva is densely adherent to the tarsal plates. The remainder of the conjunctiva is loosely bound to the underlying epibulbar and fornix tissues. The depth of the conjunctival cul-de-sacs varies (Fig. 34–14).

Sensory Innervation of Orbital Structures

Since local anesthesia is frequently employed for operations in the orbital region, an awareness of the sensory innervation is important. The eyelids are innervated by the ophthalmic and maxillary nerves, major branches of the trigeminal nerve.

The ophthalmic nerve, the first division of the trigeminal, enters the orbital cavity through the superior orbital fissure, distributing lacrimal, frontal, and nasociliary branches (Figs. 34–15 to 34–18). The lacrimal nerve contributes afferent filaments to the lacrimal gland and to the upper eyelid and skin in the region of the lateral orbital border. The frontal nerve (Figs. 34–15 to 34–18), bifurcating in the orbital cavity into supraorbital and supratrochlear branches, transmits sensation from the skin of the forehead and scalp, the frontal sinus, and the major portion of the upper eyelid. The nasociliary nerve is distributed mainly to the internal nose via posterior and anterior ethmoidal branches. The external nasal branch from the anterior ethmoidal nerve provides sensation to a small portion of the lateral aspect of the nose (Fig. 34–18).

The maxillary nerve, the second division of the trigeminal, leaves the cranium through the foramen rotundum, traverses the pterygopalatine fossa, supplies short sphenopalatine nerves to the sphenopalatine ganglion, and gives off zygomatic and alveolar branches as it traverses the floor of the orbit in a groove or canal as the infraorbital nerve (Fig. 34–18).

The zygomatic nerve is one of the orbital divisions of the maxillary nerve, branching from the latter in the pterygopalatine fossa and extending through the inferior orbital fossa into the orbit, where it bifurcates into the zygomaticofacial and zygomaticotemporal

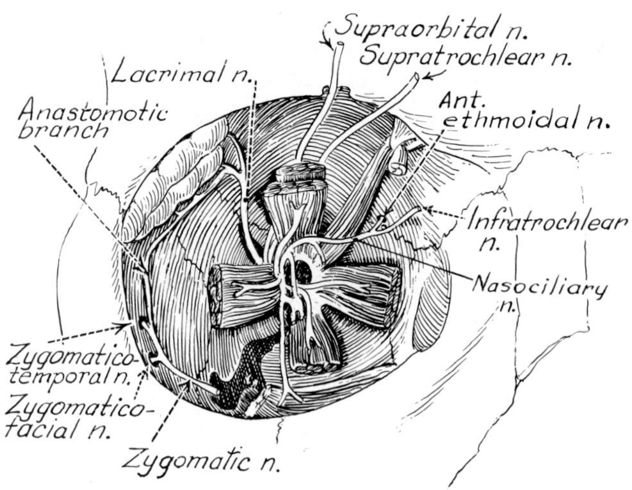

Figure 34–15. The sensory nerves of the orbit.

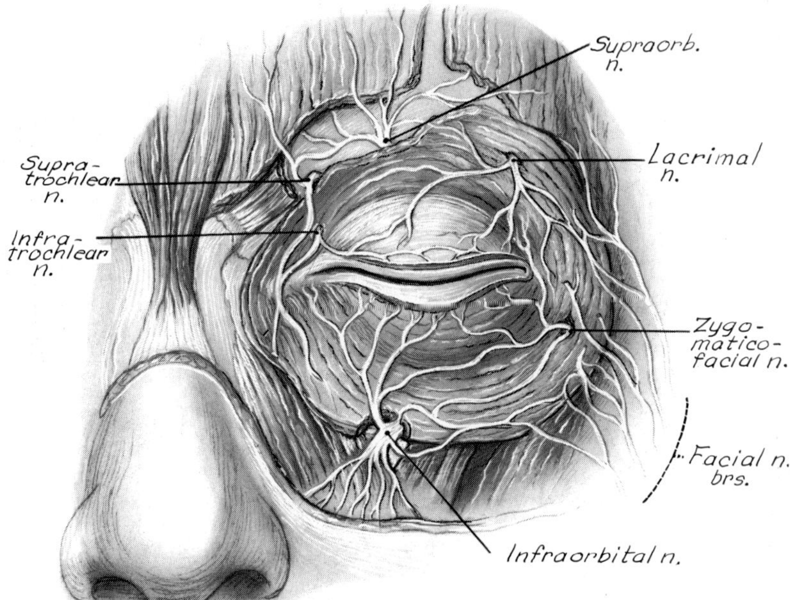

Figure 34–16. The peripheral distribution of the sensory nerves of the orbit.

branches. The zygomaticotemporal nerve joins the lacrimal nerve in the orbit, where it gives off parasympathetic secretomotor branches and then reaches the temporal fossa by way of the zygomaticotemporal foramen in the zygoma. It penetrates the temporal fascia to transmit sensation from the skin of the anterior temporal region. The zygomaticofacial nerve passes through its named foramen more inferiorly on the zygoma, and transmits sensation from the inferior lateral orbit and cheek (Fig. 34–15 to 34–18).

The infraorbital nerve (Figs. 34–16 to 34–18), after giving off middle and anterior superior alveolar branches from the floor of the orbit, emerges on the face through the infraorbital foramen and subdivides into terminal branches. The branches include the inferior palpebral, external nasal, and superior labial nerves, which transmit sensation from the remainder of the cheek, lid, lip, and adjacent nasal areas.

UNIQUE OPERATIVE CONSIDERATIONS

Surgical procedures for the eyelids and adnexal structures require careful attention to anatomy as well as gentle tissue handling. The introduction of more delicate surgical instruments and sutures with proper needles has made it more possible to attain optimal cosmetic and functional results.

Many surgical procedures may be performed with regional and infiltration local anesthesia. However, even with general anesthesia, local infiltration with a dilute anesthetic and epinephrine-containing solution is helpful. Regional block anesthesia of the eyelids may be achieved by injecting at various points along the superior rim of the orbit to produce block anesthesia of the lacrimal, frontal, supraorbital, and supratrochlear nerves. Additional injections into or near the infraorbital foramen and in the region of the zygomaticofacial foramen on the lateral as-

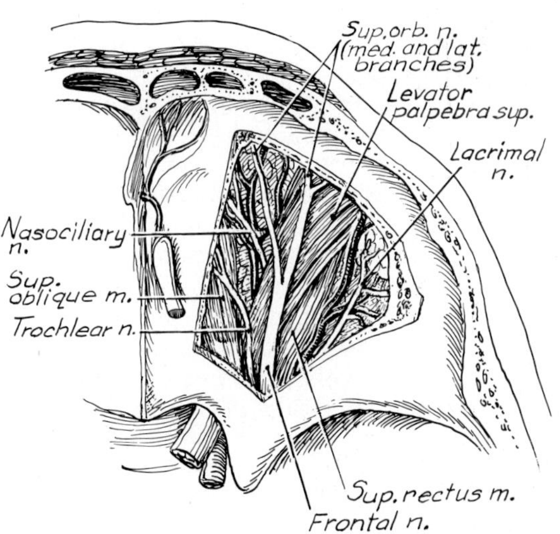

Figure 34–17. Transverse section after removal of the roof of the orbit, illustrating the position of the frontal nerve and the other nerves of the orbit.

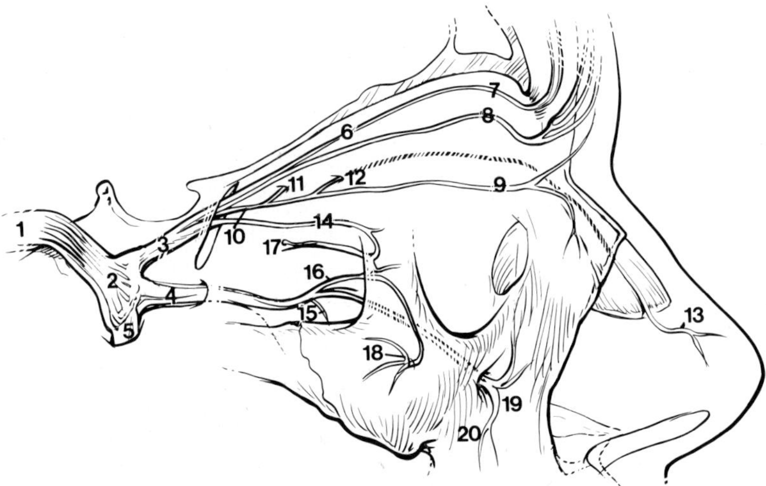

Figure 34–18. Sensory innervation of orbitonasal structures. (1) Cranial nerve V; (2) trigeminal ganglion; (3) ophthalmic division of trigeminal nerve (V_1); (4) maxillary division of trigeminal nerve (V_2); (5) mandibular division of trigeminal nerve (V_3); (6) frontal nerve; (7) supraorbital nerve; (8) supratrochlear nerve; (9) infratrochlear nerve; (10) nasociliary nerve; (11) posterior ethmoidal nerve; (12) anterior ethmoidal nerve; (13) external or dorsal nasal nerve; (14) lacrimal nerve; (15) posterior superior alveolar nerve; (16) zygomatic nerve; (17) zygomaticotemporal nerve; (18) zygomaticofacial nerve; (19) and (20) infraorbital nerve.

pect of the zygoma result in block anesthesia of the upper and lower lids.

An infratrochlear nerve block can effectively produce anesthesia of the medial orbit and proximal lacrimal drainage system. This block can be augmented with local infiltration of the lids to allow lacrimal probing, irrigation, intubation, and manipulation. With the addition of intranasal topical or infiltration anesthesia, lacrimal drainage procedures such as a dacryocystorhinostomy may be performed.

A convenient technique for obtaining regional anesthesia of the upper lid is to insert a 4 cm fine gauge needle beneath the midportion of the superior orbital rim, carefully staying on the orbital roof and injecting 1 to 2 ml of anesthetic solution. This maneuver effectively blocks the frontal nerve, which anatomically is the most superior structure within the orbit, just beneath the periorbita (Figs. 34–17, 34–18). The frontal nerve block is useful in operations for correction of upper lid ptosis or retraction, because it less frequently disturbs the motor innervation to the lid, permitting the patient to open and close the lids during the surgical procedure.

Protection of the cornea from desiccation, irritation, and trauma during and after the procedure is an essential consideration in all surgery for the eyelids and orbital region. Desiccation can be prevented by the administration of a few drops of balanced saline solution in the conjunctival cul-de-sac or directly onto the cornea periodically during an operation when the lids cannot be closed. During surgical procedures in the orbital areas, specially designed protective plastic contact corneal lenses should be routine. The contact shell prevents desiccation and inadvertent corneal injury by an instrument or gauze during the surgical procedure (Fig. 34–19).

A carefully applied dressing is essential to avoid corneal irritation during the postoperative period. It is distressing for the surgeon to be obliged to remove a pressure dressing

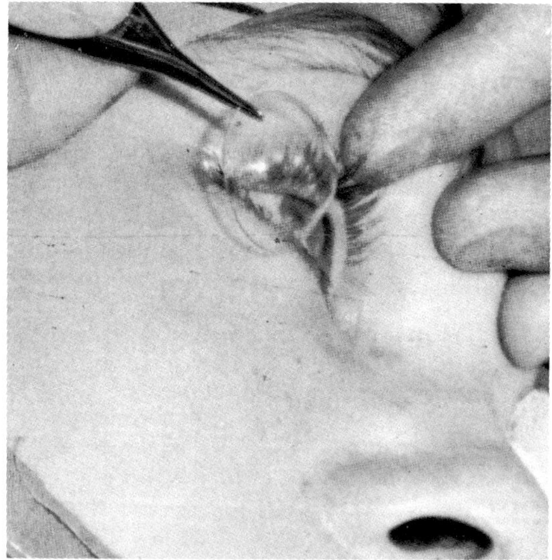

Figure 34–19. Protective lens being inserted into the conjunctival sacs. A transparent lens is shown in the photograph in order to allow the sclera and cornea to be seen through the lens. Colored lenses are preferable because they assist in filtering the bright operating room light from the patient during operations performed under local anesthesia. Colored lenses are also less often inadvertently left on the cornea postoperatively.

over a reconstructed lid, particularly if a skin graft has been used, because the patient complains of symptoms of corneal irritation (a grating sensation with recurring, shooting pains). At the end of the operation, the conjunctival sac should be washed carefully with balanced normal saline to free any loose particles of gauze, eyelash, cotton, or other foreign material. An occlusive suture should always be used if a pressure dressing is applied over the eye in order to avoid opening of the eyelids and exposure of the cornea to the dressing (Fig. 34–20). The dressing itself should be applied carefully so that it is not displaced during the postoperative period. A proper eyelid occlusion dressing is best applied in layers. The first layer is soft, fine-meshed gauze impregnated with a liberal amount of an ophthalmic ointment. This is followed by an eye pad placed over the orbital region and maintained in place with strips of paper adhesive tape. Further bulk may be added to these dressings in the form of fluff gauze or cotton. A figure-of-eight bandage with roll gauze can be employed to reinforce this dressing.

In order to avoid postoperative corneal abrasions, deep sutures should be placed in such a manner that the knots are buried in the tissue or placed externally when the lid is being reconstructed. A continuous buried suture that may be pulled out after healing is particularly useful in the approximation of tissue over the cornea. Skin grafts should not be placed in the conjunctival sac if they are to be in contact with the cornea; only conjunctiva or other mucosal tissue is tolerated by the cornea.

Temporary lid closure may be achieved by inserting one or two horizontal mattress sutures (see Fig. 34–20). A double-armed 4-0 silk suture is used for this procedure. One arm of the suture is passed through the lower lid tarsus 3 mm inferior to the lid margin (the marginal palpebral artery is usually 4 mm inferior to the lid margin) and exits from one of the meibomian gland orifices. The suture then enters the upper lid margin at a corresponding meibomian orifice and exits the lid 3 to 4 mm superiorly. This technique is repeated with the other arm of the suture in order that the knot may be tied in the upper lid, which facilitates removal of the suture.

Another method of occlusive suture is the continuous to-and-fro passage of a nonabsorbable monofilament suture (5-0 prolene) between the upper and lower eyelid margins (see Chap. 33). This type of suture may be left in position for many weeks with less risk of corneal or skin irritation.

Tarsorrhaphy, the formation of a lid adhesion, has been extensively used in the past to provide occlusion of the eyelids in order to protect the eye. The most common use of tarsorrhaphy is for protection of the cornea when there is a combined facial and trigeminal nerve palsy producing a neuroparalytic keratopathy. The two-pillar tarsorrhaphy technique is also useful in managing exposure keratopathy and other ocular pathology requiring only several months of lid occlusion. The lid adhesions may be divided with minimal residual deformity of the lid margin. However, lid margin abnormalities, trichiasis, or entropion may occasionally result if division is not performed precisely.

After local anesthesia has been obtained by infiltration, two fixation forceps are placed 1 cm apart on the lid (Fig. 34–21*A*). The lid is punctured and counterpunctured along its free margin with the tip of a sharp knife. A 1.5 × 4 mm strip of lid margin tissue is undermined with the knife and removed (Fig. 34–21*C*). The incision splits the lid (Fig. 34–

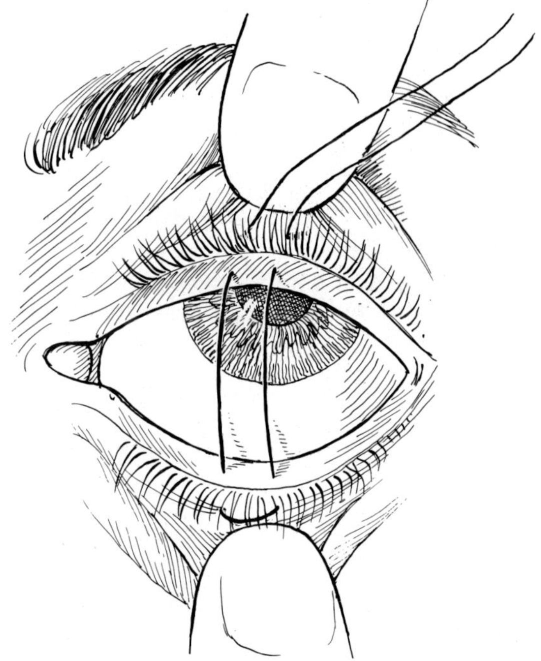

Figure 34–20. Occlusive suture used to prevent opening of the palpebral fissure and corneal abrasion when a pressure dressing is placed over the eye.

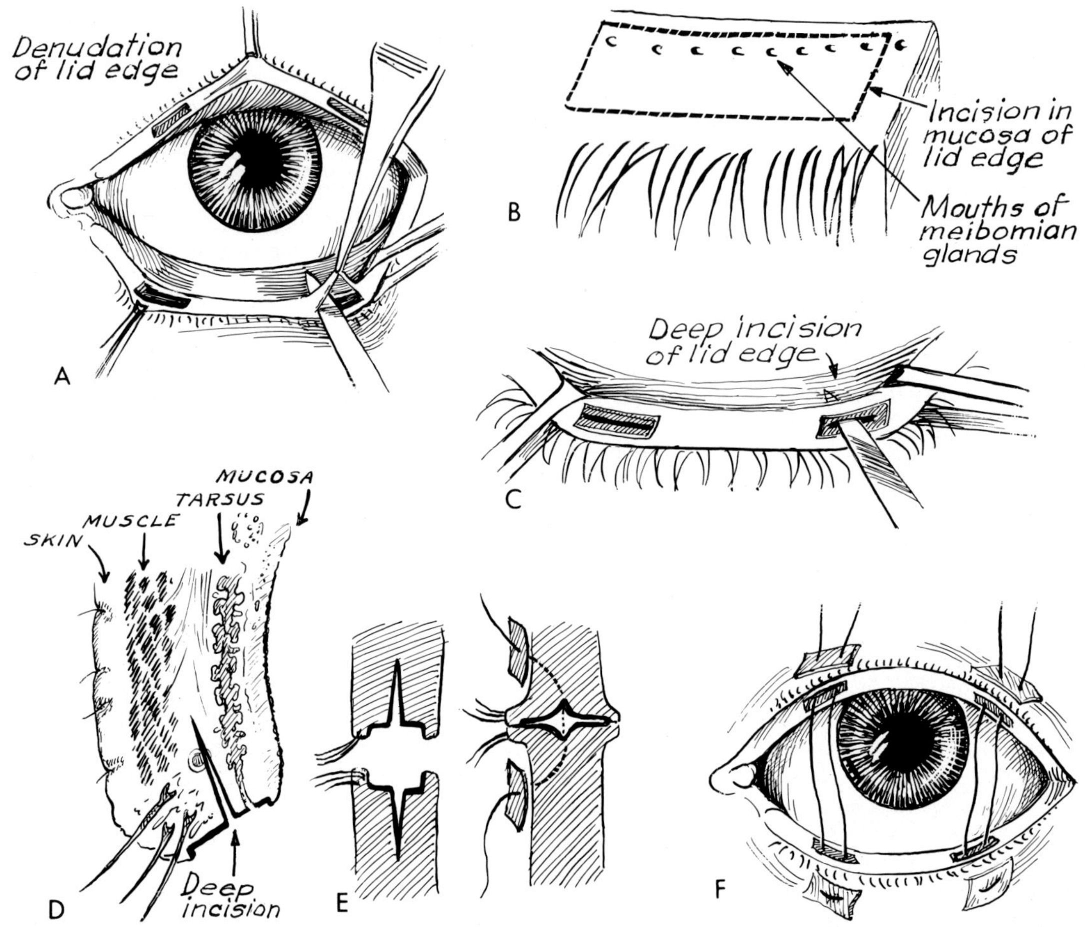

Figure 34–21. Technique of partial tarsorrhaphy. *A,* Excision of two small rectangles along the margin of each eyelid. *B,* Outline of the excised area. *C,* An incision 3 mm in depth is made into the tarsal plate. *D,* Sagittal section showing the depth of the incision in the denuded portion of the lid margin. *E,* The incision allows spreading of the denuded areas and a wider surface of contact. *F,* Sutures are placed through the denuded areas and through small pieces of rubber dam.

21*D*), thus increasing the surface contact between the raw areas of the lid, and improves the chance of successful adhesion (Fig. 34–21*E*). The procedure is repeated in another portion of the eyelid and also in two areas of the opposing eyelid. Mattress sutures of double-armed 4-0 silk or 5-0 nylon are placed through protective soft rubber dam plates, silicone sponges, or cotton to prevent undue pressure on the underlying skin. The sutures penetrate the skin 5 mm from the lid margin, entering the wound first through the lower lid and exiting through the upper lid, where they are tied (Fig. 34–21*F*).

Tarsorrhaphies of the lateral aspects of the lids were developed to reduce ocular exposure and avoid complete occlusion. The lateral tarsorrhaphy is used today for patients with mild degrees of orbicularis oculi palsy and lagophthalmos. In these patients, decreasing the horizontal lid aperture usually allows effective blink and eye coverage during sleep. In addition, the precorneal tear film may be more effectively supported. The McLaughlin (1952) lateral tarsorrhaphy is preferred because it preserves the lashes for camouflage of the lateral lid adhesion. The procedure consists of halving the lateral quarter of the two opposing lids at the mucocutaneous junction. A wedge of tarsus from the lower lid is developed and drawn into a recipient bed in the upper lid, prepared by excision of a triangular area of tarsus and conjunctiva (Fig. 34–22).

In certain ophthalmologic conditions, it may be necessary to perform a complete tarsorrhaphy, which requires denuding the entire length of both eyelid margins. This procedure should be used only when permanent and definitive tarsorrhaphy is required, since

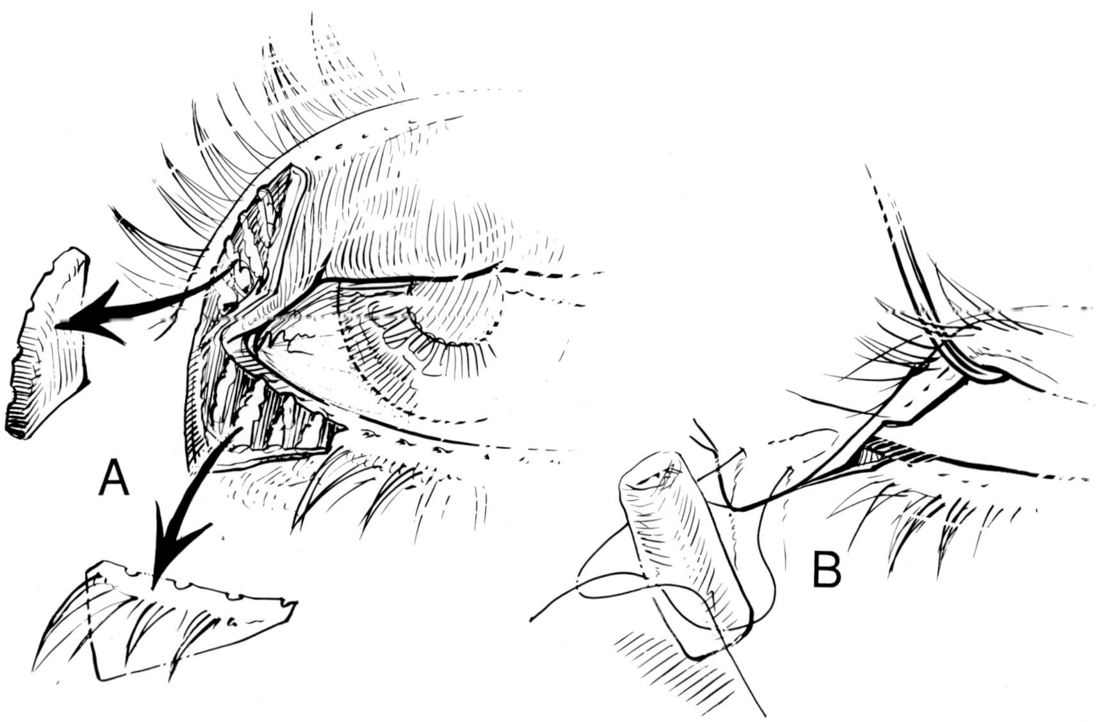

Figure 34–22. The McLaughlin lateral tarsorrhaphy consists of halving the outer quarter of the two opposing lids and removing a wedge of skin, cilia, and orbicularis oculi muscle from the edge of the lower lid, and a corresponding area of conjunctiva and tarsus from the deep surface of the upper lid. The raw surfaces are approximated by a horizontal mattress suture. The maneuver effectively narrows the palpebral fissure and elevates the lower lid for ocular protection.

it markedly damages the lid margins, and subsequent division is difficult.

LACERATIONS OF THE EYELIDS

Lacerations of the eyelids often present a challenge to reconstructive efforts. A distinction must be made between lacerations that extend through the eyelid skin only and those that extend through the tarsus and eyelid margin.

Superficial eyelid lacerations involving the skin and perhaps the orbicularis muscle require careful approximation of the wound edges, and usually leave an inconspicuous scar. Sutures are removed in 48 to 72 hours, otherwise epithelization along the suture tract may result in cystlike nests of sebaceous material that require subsequent removal.

A careful search for embedded foreign material and documentation of the integrity of the orbital septum and levator muscle should be carried out before repairing deeper eyelid lacerations. If a lacerated levator muscle or a detached levator aponeurosis is not anatomically repaired, postoperative ptosis may result. Furthermore, if the orbital septum is inadvertently incorporated in the repair, lid retraction or tethering of the upper lid may occur. Minimal debridement is usually necessary since the blood supply to the area is abundant. If there is a loss of tissue that cannot be replaced as a composite graft, primary split- or full-thickness skin grafting should be considered.

Lacerations involving the eyelid margin require precise suture placement and critical suture tension to avoid notches or irregularities of the lid margin. Various forms of overlapping dissections and complicated repairs have been described, including Wheeler's halving (1936) and Hughes' (1955) tongue and groove techniques. The Mustardé (1966) technique of direct approximation of the lacerated edges is currently recommended; however, the methods of Lekieffre and François (1976) and Tessier (1972) provide innovative approaches in difficult cases. It is often necessary to trim the lid tissues conservatively in order to freshen the wound edges. To ensure precise alignment of the lid margin, a 6-0 silk suture on an atraumatic ophthalmic needle is passed into the substance of the tarsus through one of the orifices of the meibomian tarsal glands, across the wound, and into the substance of the opposite tarsus to exit the lid margin at the meibomian gland orifice (Fig. 34–23*A* to *C*). The needle puncture should be approximately 1.5 mm from the edge of the laceration. Traction on this suture approximates the wound edges and aligns the anterior and posterior lid margins. Additional sutures are placed at the posterior and anterior lid margins and tied, leaving the suture ends long (Fig. 34–23*D* to *F*). After the three marginal sutures have been tied, moderate upward traction assists in positioning of the wound edges. Pretarsal and muscle sutures are placed, care being taken to avoid penetration of the conjunctiva (Fig. 34–23*F*). The skin is sutured with a continuous or interrupted suture technique. The skin sutures 2 mm inferior to the lashes are tied

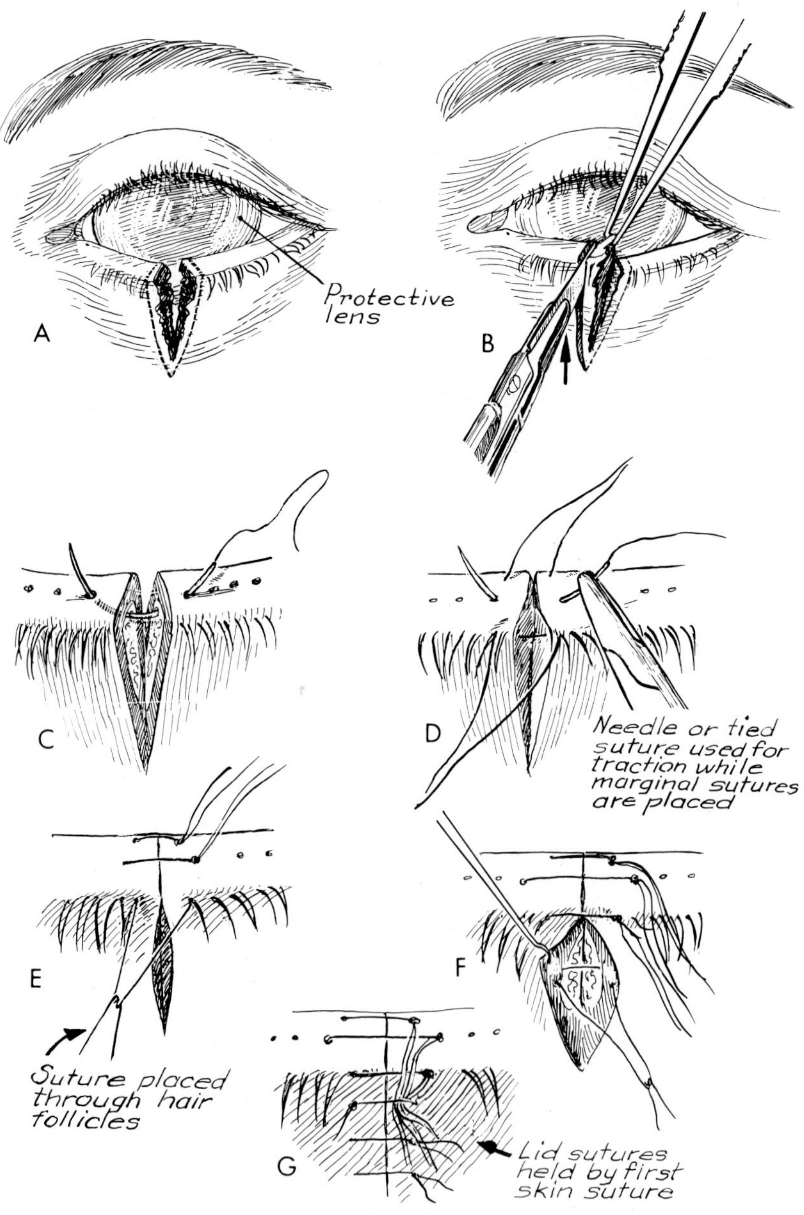

Figure 34–23. Repair of lacerations through the lid. *A,* A scleral lens has been placed in the conjunctival sac. *B,* The wound edges are freshened with a razor-blade knife. *C,* The first suture placed through the line of the ducts of the tarsal glands aligns the margins. *D, E,* Additional sutures are placed through the posterior and anterior edges of the lid margin and tied. *F,* The pretarsal and muscle sutures are placed and tied. *G,* Wound suture completed.

over the ends of the three marginal sutures (Fig. 34–23*G*). This prevents the sutures from irritating the cornea during the postoperative period. An eye patch is usually placed over the eye, but is not essential. The wound is examined after 24 hours and the skin sutures are removed after three or four days. The marginal sutures should be left in position for a week or longer, depending on the amount of tension in the wound. After the skin sutures have been removed, it is advisable to support the lid horizontally with a strip of surgical tape for three more days. The precision in approximation of lid margin lacerations depends on visual magnification. It is highly recommended to use loupes or the operating microscope to approximate the transected layers.

If there is tissue loss in the middle section of either the upper or lower lid, direct closure may exert undue tension on the horizontal dimensions of the lid. The release of the structures at the lateral canthus of the respective lid provides additional relaxation for a less tense closure. A lateral canthotomy is performed with scissors (Fig. 34–24*A*), and the skin and conjunctiva are dissected from the lateral canthal tendon to expose its substance. A lateral cantholysis or vertical incision of the respective limb of the lateral canthal tendon is made producing a noticeable release in horizontal tension (Fig. 34–24*B*, *C*). If the release is not achieved, further lysis of the structures between the skin and the conjunctiva is necessary. Ordinarily, 5 to 10 mm in the horizontal dimension of the lid may be gained by this method (Fig. 34–24*D*). The technique is applicable to the upper and lower lids.

Lacerations extending through the levator muscle or its aponeurosis must be repaired. The diagnosis and repair of the resulting traumatic ptosis is discussed later in this chapter.

Dog bites, human bites, and accidents of varying types have been the cause of partial or total avulsions of the eyelids. Silverman and Obear (1970) described a method of delayed primary repair of totally avulsed upper and lower eyelids 28 hours after the initial injury. If the eyelid is partially avulsed, the excellent blood supply of the area allows reattachment. Careful suture approximation of the corresponding recipient and donor structures is usually rewarded with anatomic and functional restoration.

A review of human bites of the eyelid (Spinelli and associates, 1986) reported five

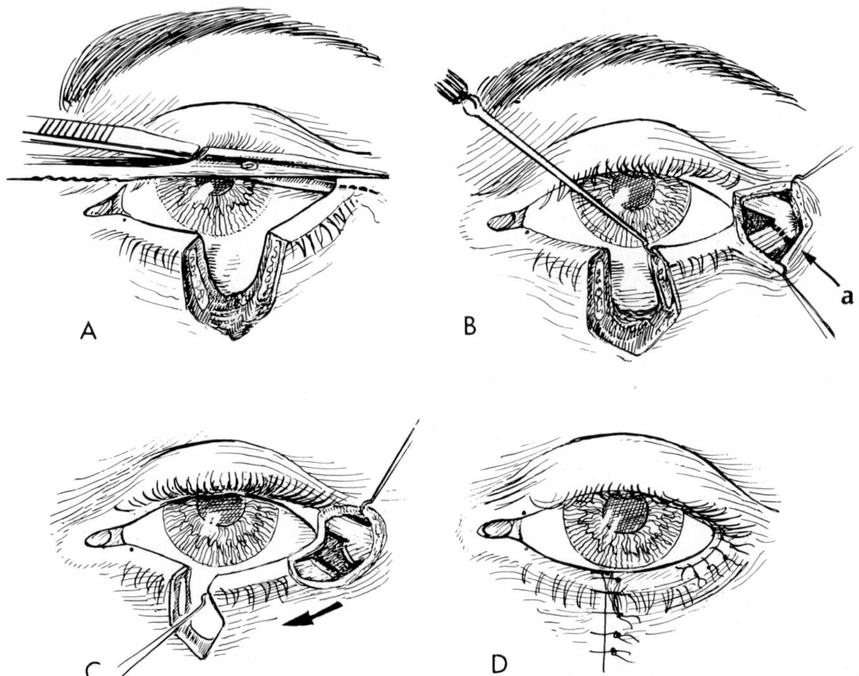

Figure 34–24. Lateral cantholysis to facilitate the closure of a moderate-sized defect. *A*, Lateral canthotomy. *B*, The conjunctiva is dissected from the lateral canthal tendon, and the lower crus of the tendon is severed (a). *C*, *D*, Closure of the defect is thus facilitated.

cases of full-thickness, lamellar, or total eyelid avulsion without associated lacrimal damage. The abundant vascular supply of the eyelid allowed successful composite grafting as late as 26 hours after trauma. Complications of replantation included loss of cilia and lid retraction. High dose antibiotic coverage with penicillin and oxacillin or cephalothin, combined with early replantation and careful debridement of recipient and donor tissue, were the factors associated with successful composite grafting (Fig. 34–25).

When replantation of the eyelid tissue is not possible because of loss or complete destruction, the eyeball remains exposed. When the upper eyelid is lost, desiccation of the cornea due to lack of corneal protection initiates a keratolytic process that terminates in destruction of the eye. Protection of the eye is therefore imperative if the avulsed tissues cannot be replaced. When the lower eyelid is destroyed, closure of the upper lid continues to protect the cornea and the destructive corneal changes are less likely to occur. Frequent observation and lubrication of the exposed surfaces of the eye are still required. It may be necessary to separate an intact lower eyelid into cutaneous, muscular, and tarsoconjunctival layers to mobilize and cover the eye when there is loss of the upper eyelid. The inner tarsoconjunctival layer is advanced as far as possible to unite with superior bulbar conjunctiva. The remaining raw areas are skin grafted.

The eye is in serious danger when both upper and lower eyelids are avulsed. Sectioning of the inferior rectus muscle permits upper rotation of the eyeball and some degree of protection of the cornea until later reconstructive procedures can be considered. The use of soft lenses and moisture chambers can also provide protection until adequate surgical measures can be undertaken. Destruction of both eyelids from trauma or extirpation for tumor fortunately is extremely rare. The goal in reconstruction should be preservation of a seeing eye behind protective conjunctival-lined and skin-covered surfaces. If sight in the opposite eye becomes defective, attempts to form an opening for functional vision can then be considered.

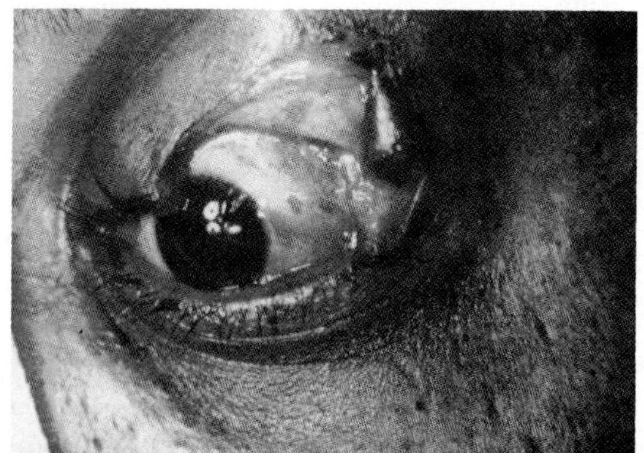
A

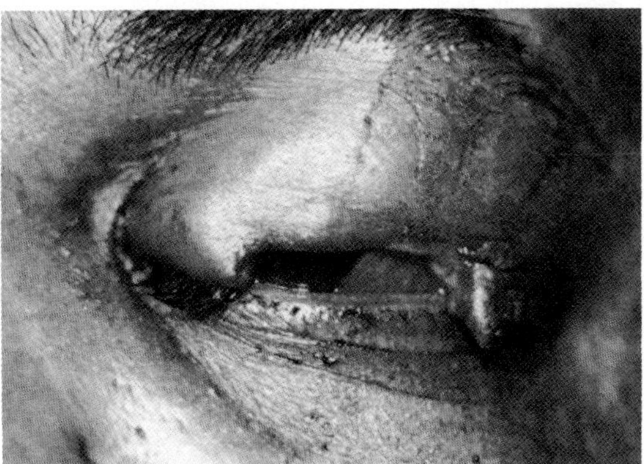
B

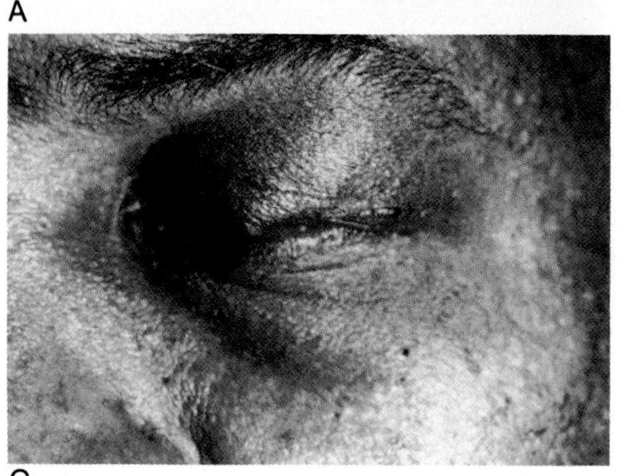
C

Figure 34–25. *A,* Large central and lateral defect of the upper eyelid resulting from a human bite. *B,* Appearance after further debridement. *C,* One year after replantation of the segment, with mild alopecia and minimal lid retraction. (*From* Spinelli, H. M., Sherman, J. E., Lisman, R. D., and Smith, B. C.: Human bites of the eyelids. Plast. Reconstr. Surg., *78*:610, 1986.)

RECONSTRUCTION OF THE EYELID

Eyelid tissue defects may be congenital (colobomas) or may result from neoplasm excision, trauma, irradiation, burns, or inflammatory conditions. In general, upper eyelid defects should be reconstructed early in order to prevent corneal damage (Paufique and Tessier, 1962). Eyelid defects that encroach on the medial canthal, lacrimal excretory, or lateral retinacular structures require more complex reconstructions (McCord, 1980a; Leone and Hand, 1979; Lekieffre and associates, 1970). The basic principles of successful eyelid reconstruction involve replacement of the outer layer of skin and muscle, an inner layer of mucosa, and a semirigid supporting structure interposed between them. These principles apply to all defects irrespective of their cause.

Rogers (1988) has detailed the history of the development of ophthalmic plastic surgery. Von Graefe (1818) constructed a lower lid with a cheek flap. His method was modified by Fricke (1829), who introduced a procedure for both upper and lower lid reconstruction using zygomatic and temporal skin flaps. The use of an arm flap to reconstruct the eyelid was a common practice among surgeons of the nineteenth century. Such large flaps, although generally successful, had several disadvantages: (1) considerable discomfort for the patient; (2) poorly matched transplanted skin in color, texture, and thickness; (3) scars and deformity at the donor site; and (4) compromised lid function.

After Reverdin (1869) introduced the concept of the skin graft, many attempts were made by the surgeons of the period to use this new technique in eyelid reconstruction. Lawson (1871) was the first to be credited with the use of a skin graft to correct ectropion. Le Fort (1872) in France and Wolfe (1876) in England also succeeded in transplanting full-thickness skin grafts. It was not until the principles of grafting full-thickness skin were well understood and widely employed that the number of satisfactory results with skin grafts exceeded those obtained with flaps.

Teale (1860) reported the correction of symblepharon by the use of a conjunctival flap. In 1884 Bock used mucous membrane as a graft repair to replace a conjunctival defect. Stellwag von Carion (1889) reported the use of vaginal mucosa for such a purpose.

The poor cosmetic results of eyelids reconstructed with skin grafts from arm or leg donor sites inspired Gradenigo (1904) to reconstruct an eyelid skin defect with a graft of eyelid skin. He was the first to introduce one of the basic principles in eyelid reconstruction: the use of similar available eyelid tissue to replace the deficient tissue.

Landolt (1881) was the first to employ the tarsoconjunctival flap in the reconstruction of lower eyelid defects. This concept was further expanded and developed by Cirincione (1901). In 1912 Ischreyt reversed the procedure and reconstructed an upper lid defect. This marked the beginning of full-thickness eyelid reconstruction with composite vascularized tissue. Esser (1919) first reported a full-thickness lower eyelid rotation flap to repair a defect of the upper eyelid. Cutler and Beard (1955) used a full-thickness flap from the lower lid for the same purpose, and Mustardé (1980) outlined a system for upper eyelid reconstruction with lower eyelid pedicled switch flaps. Since then, tarsoconjunctival advancement flaps for subtotal or total upper eyelid reconstruction have been described by Leone (1983).

In addition to the use of skin and mucosal grafts for eyelid reconstruction, Blaskovics (1918) reported the use of tarsal grafts. The use of mucosa-lined flaps in upper and lower eyelid defects has been reviewed by van der Meulen (1982). Youens and associates (1967) and Putterman (1978) reported composite full-thickness eyelid grafts for upper eyelid reconstruction.

The description of an advancement of an island of eyelid tissue by Kazanjian in 1949 (Fig. 34–26) was probably one of the first reports of an island flap with a subcutaneous pedicle for eyelid reconstruction. Stephenson (1983) reported the use of this island flap in the successful reconstruction of 91 eyelid defects.

The tarsoconjunctival flap, first described by Landolt (1881) and modified by Köllner (1911) and Hughes (1937), has proved useful in the reconstruction of lower eyelid defects. The Mustardé (1959, 1981) technique of lower eyelid reconstruction with a composite chondromucosal graft from the nasal septum covered with a cheek rotation flap has been helpful in the repair of extensive defects without obstructing vision. Paufique and Tessier

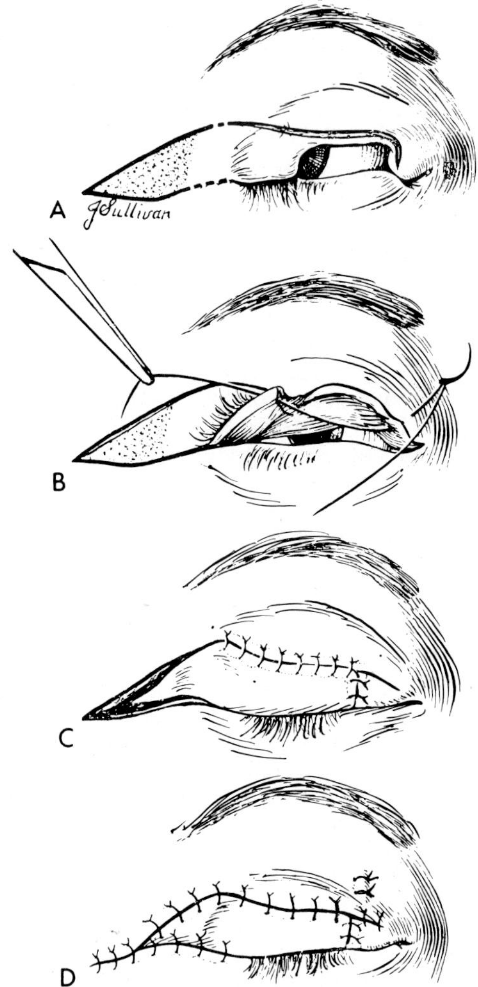

Figure 34–26. Full-thickness loss of eyelid tissue. Kazanjian's (1949) repair by an island flap. *A,* Incision of the flap, permitting advancement of the lateral portion of the upper lid. *B,* The edges of the defect are approximated by sutures. *C,* Lid reconstructed after advancement of the lateral portion. *D,* Operation completed.

(1962) advocated a composite graft consisting of the nasal upper lateral cartilage and overlying mucoperichondrium instead of the septal composite graft favored by Mustardé. A single-stage full-thickness upper eyelid bipedicle flap for total lower eyelid reconstruction, described by Anderson and Weinstein (1987), also allows maintenance of an open palpebral fissure. In this procedure, the levator aponeurosis and Müller's muscle are recessed to avoid upper eyelid retraction. Other advantages of this technique are (1) excellent tissue match, (2) minimal donor site deformity, (3) a posterior lamella of tarsus and conjunctiva, (4) an anterior lamella of skin and functional orbicularis, (5) simultaneous reconstruction of canthal defects, and (6) less lower eyelid retraction, ectropion, or laxity.

Further contributions of ophthalmic reconstructive surgeons such as Dupuy-Dutemps (1921), Wheeler (1939), Hughes (1937), Smith and associates (1987), Mustardé (1981), van der Meulen (1982), and Anderson and Weinstein (1987) have served to refine the techniques of eyelid reconstruction to the current level of predictability and effectiveness.

Partial-Thickness Defects

Repair of traumatic periorbital lacerations, avulsions, and contusions requires knowledge of the complex anatomy of the eyelids. The principles in the management of eyelid injuries have evolved from the reconstructions following tumor removal. Resection of tumors of the eyelids involves removal of an adequate amount of normal tissue around the apparent limit of the tumor. The amount of surrounding healthy tissue varies from 3 mm in a cystic basal cell carcinoma to 5 to 6 mm around a sclerosing basal cell carcinoma. When the lesion does not involve the lid margin and is confined to the subcutaneous tissue or the orbicularis muscle, the resection leaves a defect that can be covered with a local flap or skin graft. Retroauricular full-thickness skin is excellent for lower lid, medial and lateral canthal skin defects. However, upper eyelid skin, if available, is an excellent replacement for deficient lower (Fig. 34–27) and upper (Fig. 34–28) eyelid skin. When the lid and adjacent tissue defects are larger, local flaps can be designed to repair the deficient tissue (Figs. 34–29, 34–30). Small medial canthal tissue defects can be allowed to heal by secondary intention with satisfactory results (Fig. 34–31). If this method is chosen, careful attention to lid position during healing is necessary. A glabellar flap is also a versatile treatment alternative for larger medial canthal defects (Fig. 34–32).

Full-Thickness Defects

When a tumor extends to the lid margin and is fixed to the tarsus, a full-thickness resection of all layers of the lid, with an additional minimum of 4 mm of tissue sur-

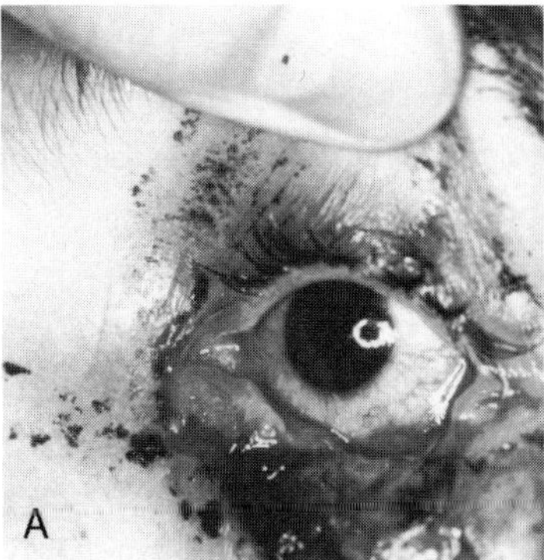

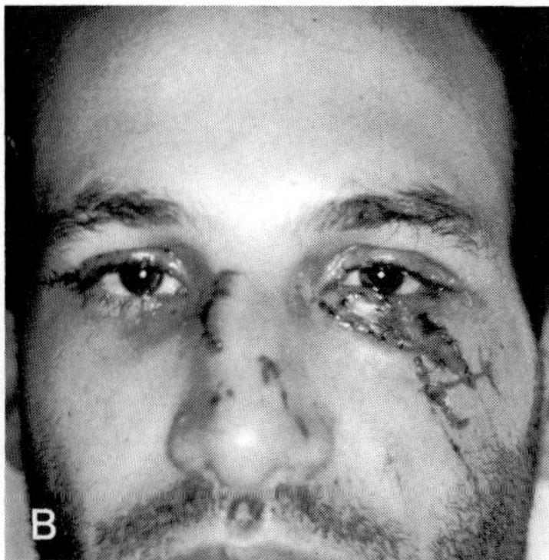

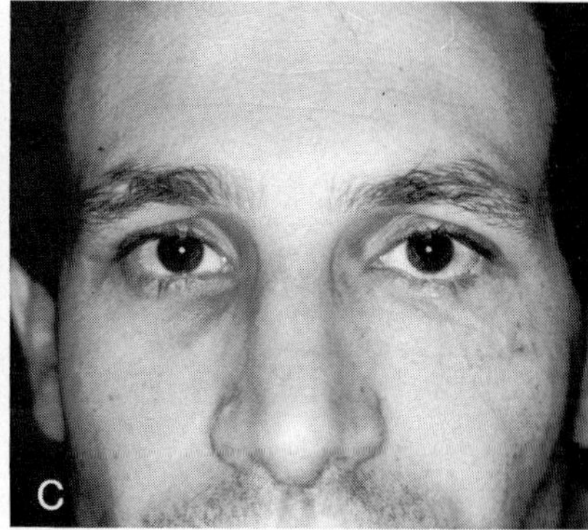

Figure 34–27. *A,* Traumatic injury to the left lower eyelid with avulsion of skin and marked derangement of anatomy. *B,* Patient four days postoperatively. Repair of eyelid structures (conjunctiva to the orbicularis muscle) resulted in a large full-thickness skin defect, which was reconstructed with a full-thickness skin graft from the right upper eyelid. *C,* The patient at one year.

rounding the apparent lesion, is needed. Reconstruction of the eyelid defect requires three elements: an outer layer of skin, an inner layer of mucosa, and a semi rigid supporting "skeleton" interposed between them. Equally important is the need to provide a stable margin that does not turn inward or outward. In addition, when the lateral or medial canthal structures require concomitant reconstruction, a varied repertoire of techniques must be employed. Mustardé (1981) promoted the basic principle that the lower lid should be used to reconstruct the upper lid, and other sources used to reconstruct the lower lid. Furthermore, he stated that only three-quarters of the width of either lid needs to be reconstructed. However, Smith (1959) and Smith and associates (1987) believed that lid sharing techniques, specifically the tarsoconjunctival flap, provide an excellent means of lower eyelid reconstruction, and rarely used a chondromucosal graft. Excellent eyelid reconstructions may be obtained with either the Mustardé or Smith techniques. Often the experience and expertise of the surgeon dictate the technique utilized. The modern reconstructive surgeon must be familiar with all techniques of eyelid reconstruction and incorporate them as required.

LOWER EYELID RECONSTRUCTION

Figure 34–33 depicts a summary of the most useful techniques for the subtotal or total reconstruction of lower eyelid defects. In all these procedures the lid margin is approximated by the method of Mustardé (1966). When the lower lid defect extends for less than 25 per cent of the horizontal dimension of the lid, the reconstruction can usually

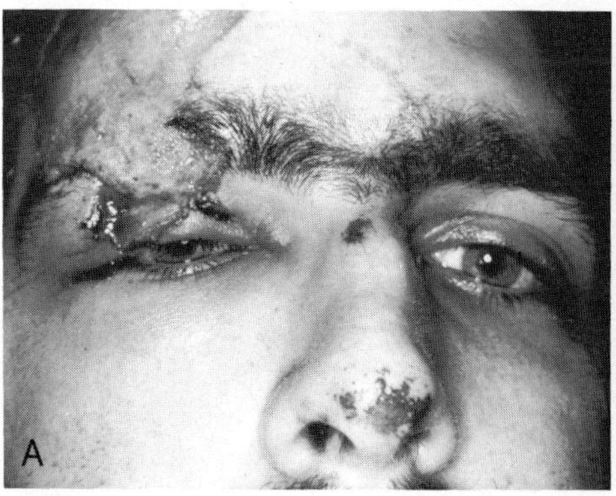

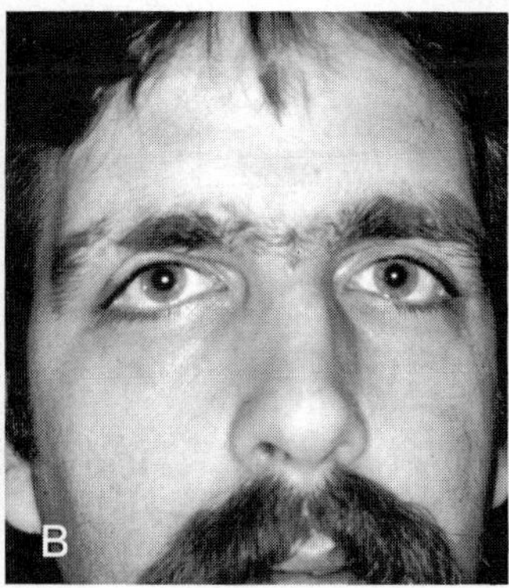

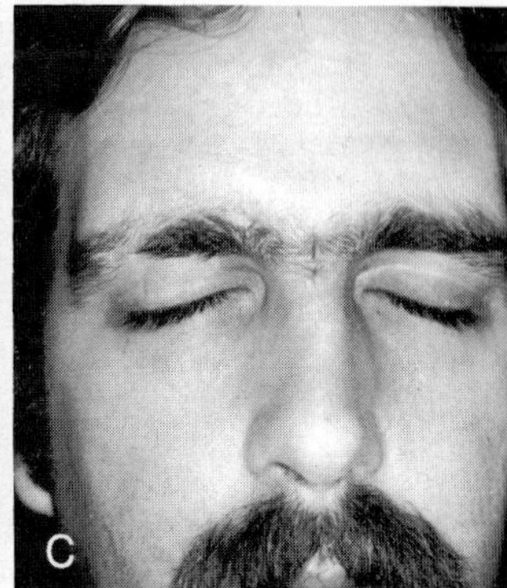

Figure 34–28. *A,* Post-traumatic full-thickness loss of the central and lateral aspect of the right upper eyelid, and partial-thickness loss of forehead and eyebrow skin. *B,* Four months after reconstruction of the right upper eyelid defect with a full-thickness skin graft from the left upper eyelid. The forehead and brow skin healed primarily. *C,* One year postoperatively, complete eyelid closure is possible and the color and texture match of the grafted tissue is satisfactory.

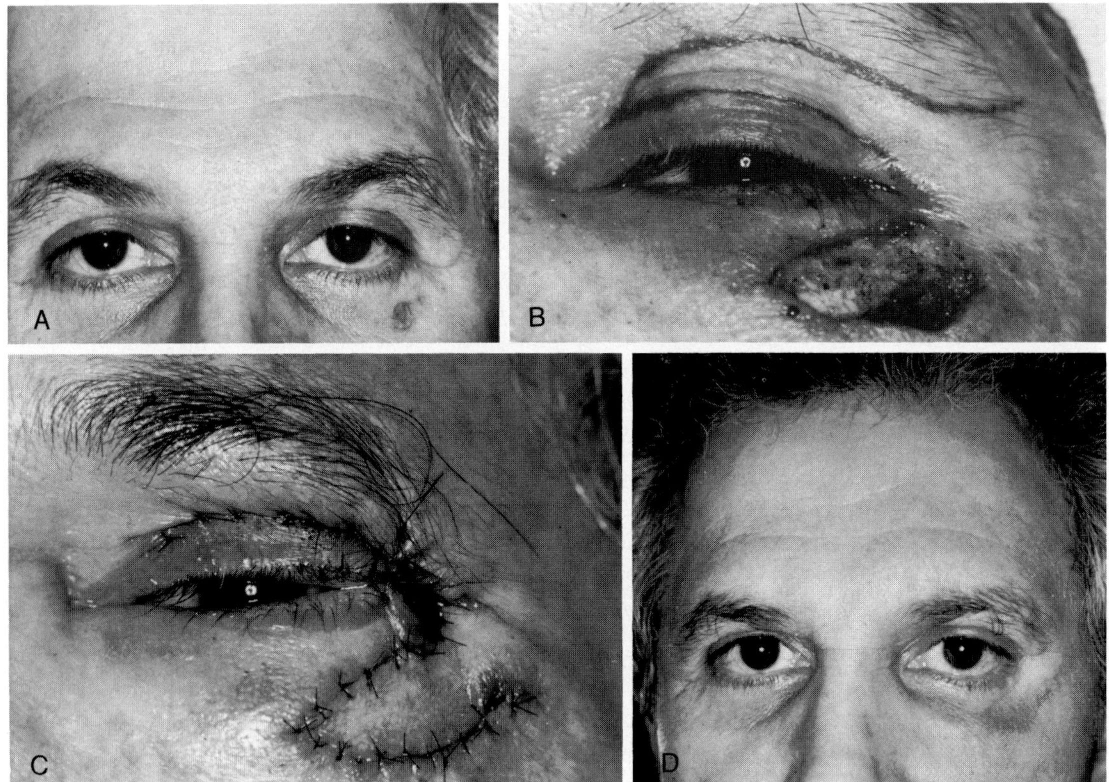

Figure 34–29. *A,* A patient, who had prevously undergone upper and lower blepharoplasty, with a basal cell carcinoma of the left lower eyelid. *B,* Resection of the lesion with frozen section controlled technique resulted in a full-thickness defect to the septum orbitale and periosteum of the superolateral maxilla. A laterally based upper eyelid musculocutaneous flap is outlined. *C,* The musculocutaneous flap has been transposed into the lower lid and cheek defect. A lateral canthal tendon plication to the lateral orbital rim periosteum has been performed and the donor site closed primarily. *D,* The patient six months after the one-stage reconstruction with acceptable lid position.

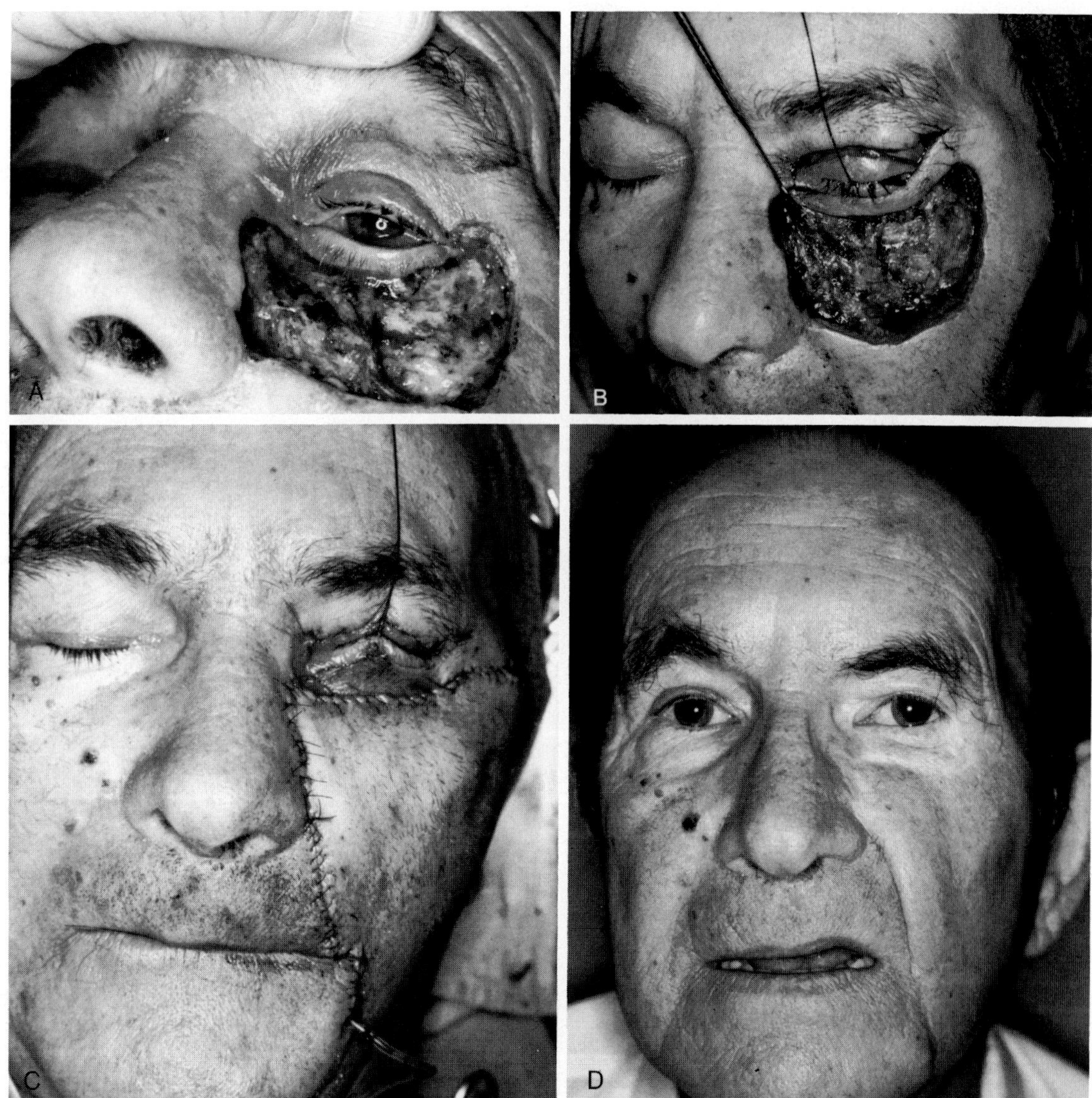

Figure 34–30. *A,* Defect of skin and muscle extending from the pretarsal level of the left lower eyelid to the nasal ala, with medial and lateral extensions, after frozen section controlled excision of a basal cell carcinoma. *B,* A laterally based left upper eyelid musculocutaneous flap has been transposed to reconstruct the deficient skin and muscle of the lower eyelid. A lateral canthal tightening procedure was also performed. *C,* The cheek defect has been reconstructed with an inferiorly based cervicofacial flap with attachment to the left medial canthus. *D,* The patient one year postoperatively.

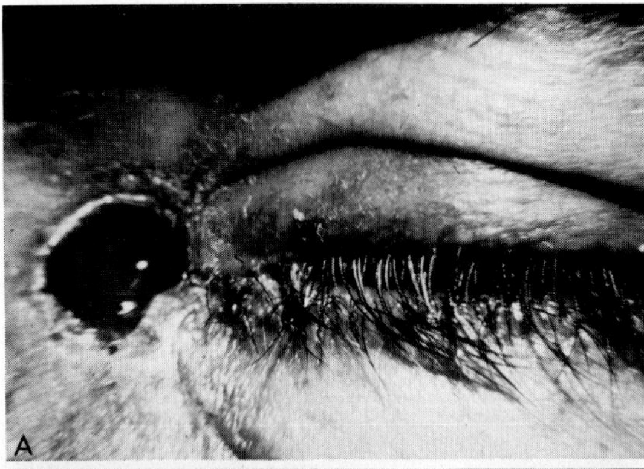

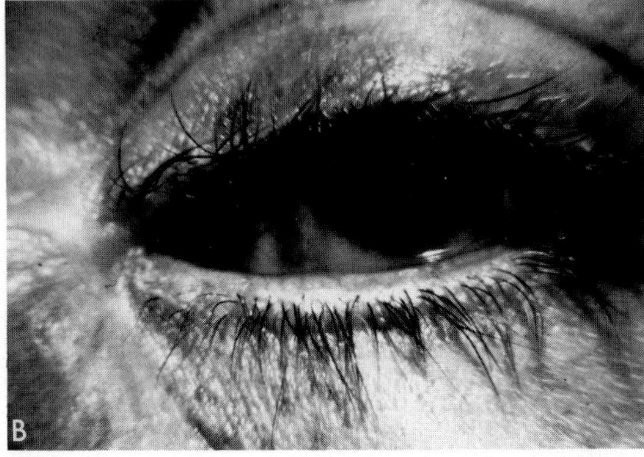

Figure 34–31. Excision of a canthal defect and healing by secondary intention. *A,* Defect resulting from resection of a malignancy of the medial canthus. *B,* After healing by secondary intention, the canthus is maintained in the depth of the naso-orbital valley.

be accomplished by direct approximation (Fig. 34–33*A, B*).

A lid defect of between 25 and 66 per cent is usually too large for primary approximation. Defects in this size range may require a selective lateral cantholysis of the inferior crus of the lateral canthal tendon with medial transposition of the lid elements alone (Figs. 34–33*C, D,* 34–34; see Fig. 34–43), or in combination with a local periorbital skin and muscle flap lined with conjunctiva (Figs. 34–33*E,* 34–35).

Defects of 75 to 100 per cent of the lower eyelid may be reconstructed with a two-stage tarsoconjunctival flap procedure (Figs. 34–33*F, G,* 34–36, 34–37; see Figs. 34–42, 34–43) or a Mustardé cheek advancement flap over a chondromucosal graft (Figs. 34–33*H,* 34–38 to 34–40).

In large defects in the central section of the

Text continued on page 1700

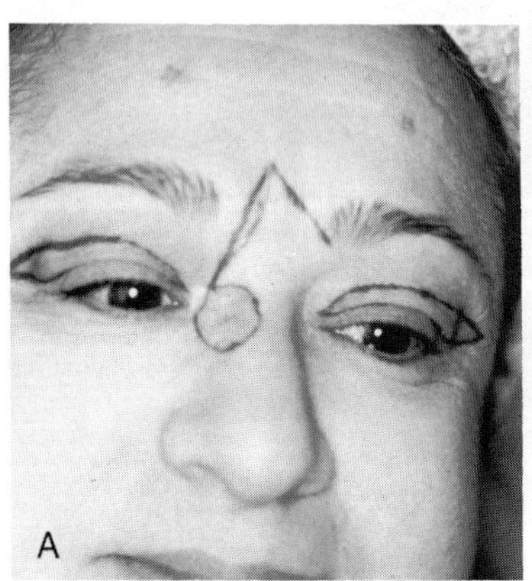

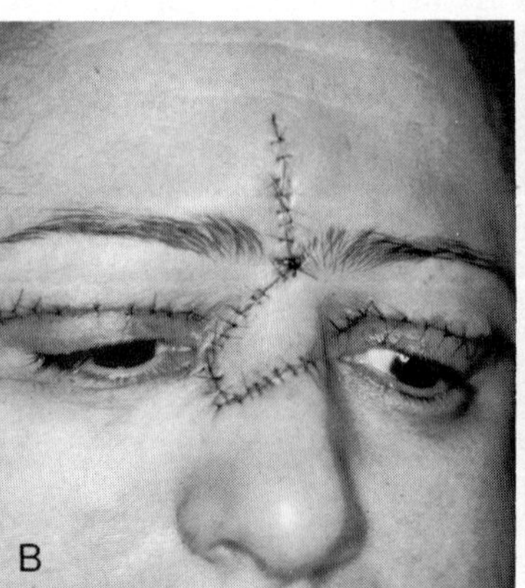

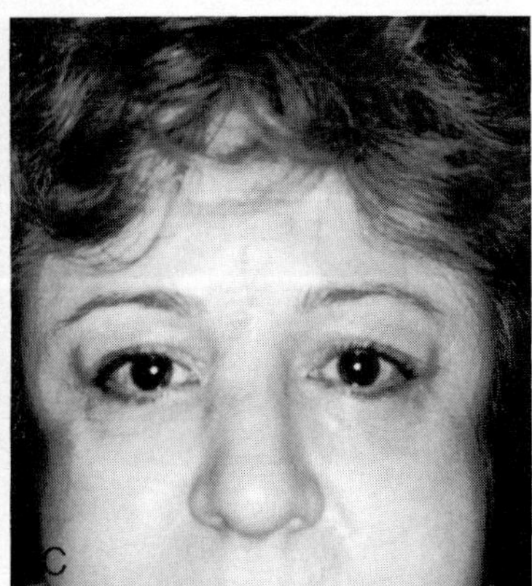

Figure 34–32. *A,* A patient before excision of a right medial canthal basal cell carcinoma and reconstruction with the glabellar flap outlined. *B,* After resection with frozen section control and flap transposition. The excess upper eyelid skin was also excised. *C,* The patient eight months postoperatively.

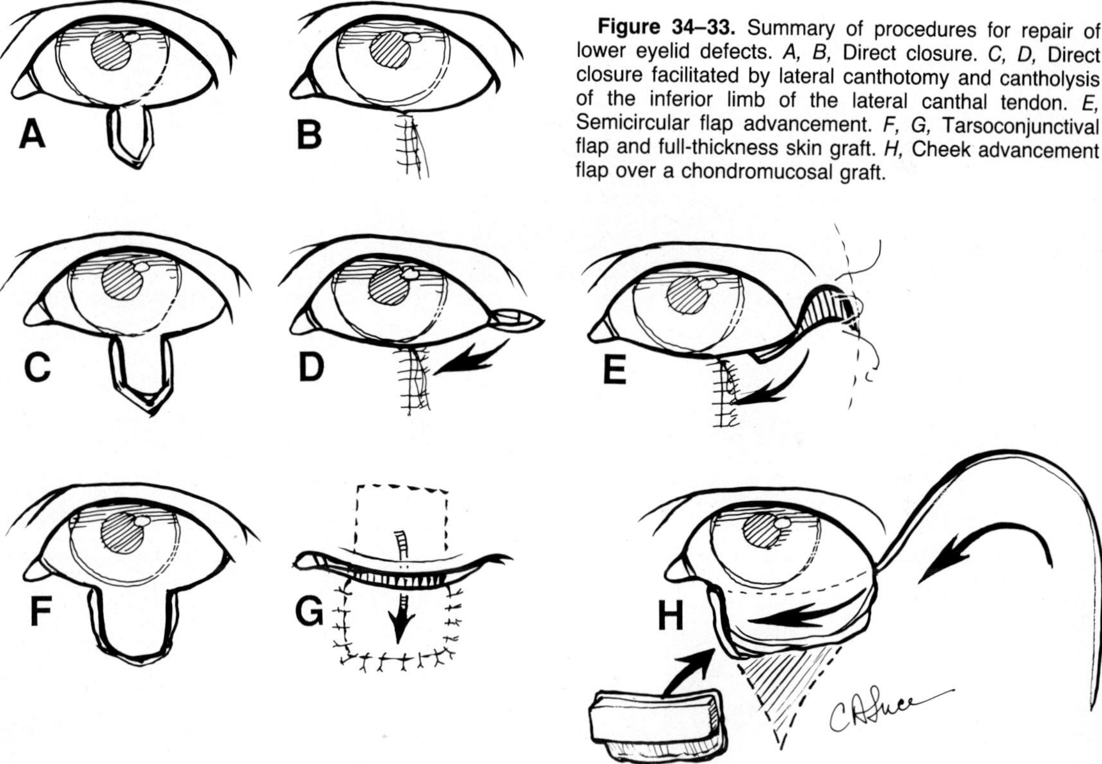

Figure 34–33. Summary of procedures for repair of lower eyelid defects. *A, B,* Direct closure. *C, D,* Direct closure facilitated by lateral canthotomy and cantholysis of the inferior limb of the lateral canthal tendon. *E,* Semicircular flap advancement. *F, G,* Tarsoconjunctival flap and full-thickness skin graft. *H,* Cheek advancement flap over a chondromucosal graft.

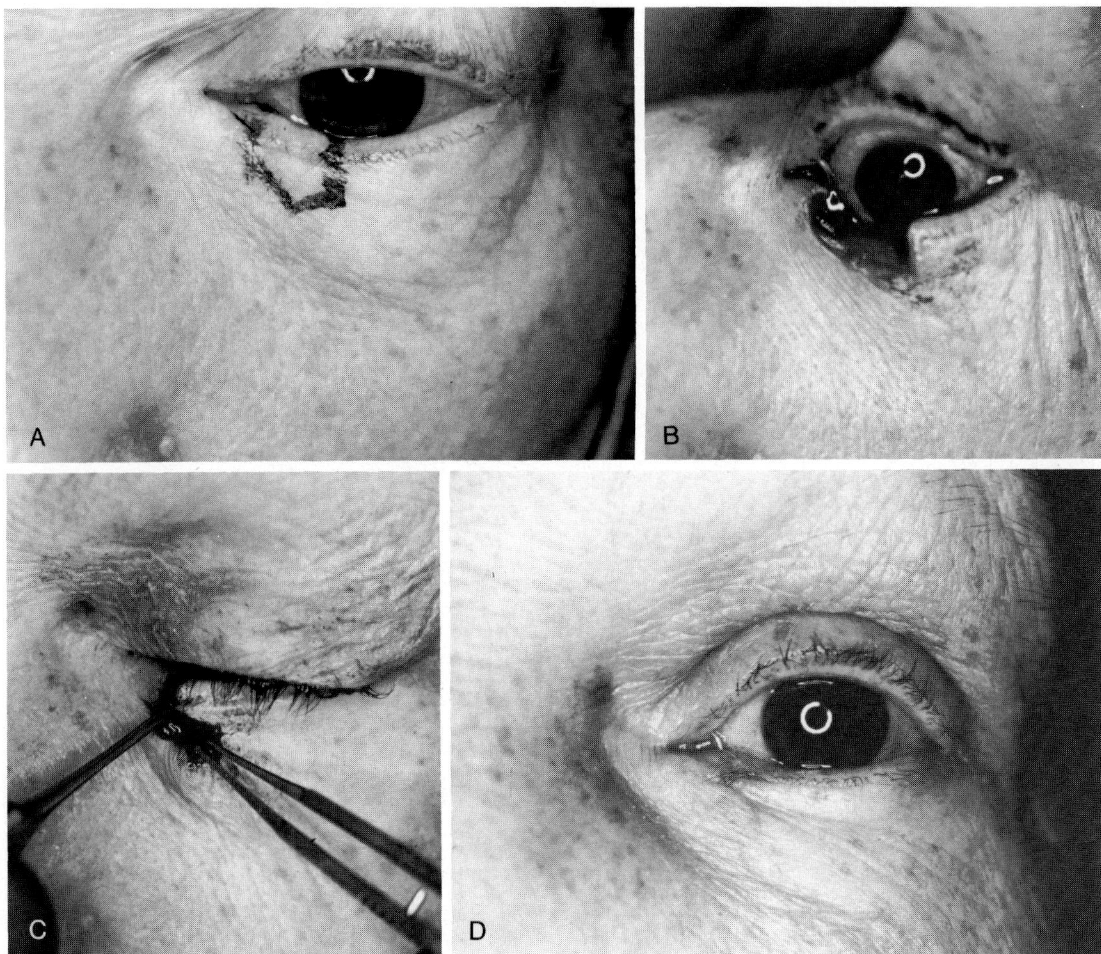

Figure 34–34. *A,* Basal cell carcinoma outlined with a 3 mm margin for pentagonal wedge resection. *B,* After resection of 33 per cent of the horizontal dimension of the lower lid. An encircling microsilicone tube canalicular intubation has already been performed. *C,* Direct approximation with appropriate lid tension was possible only after lateral canthotomy and cantholysis of the inferior limb of the lateral canthal tendon. *D,* Six months postoperatively with satisfactory lid contour and position. The microsilicone tube is visualized between the upper and lower canaliculi.

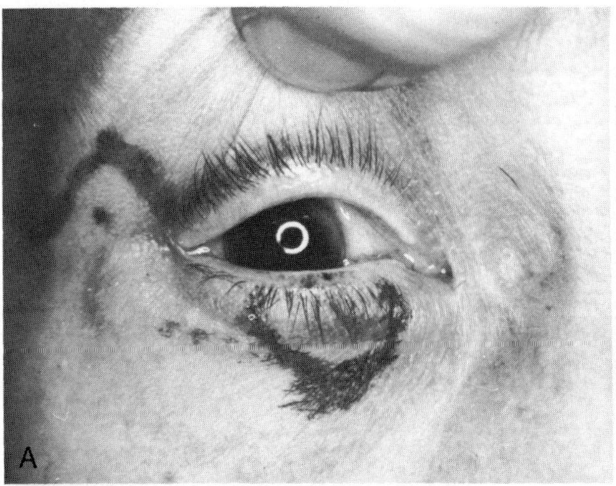

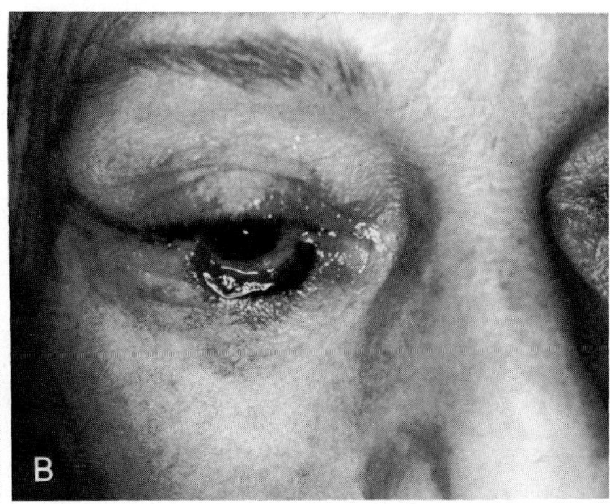

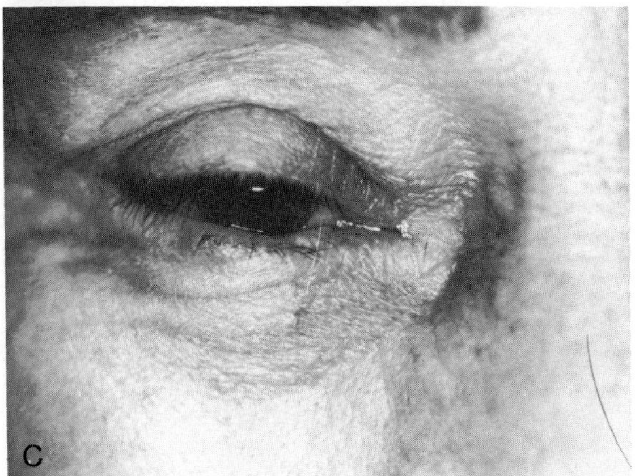

Figure 34–35. *A,* A melanocytic lesion of the right lower eyelid outlined for pentagonal wedge resection. A semicircular flap from the superolateral periorbital tissues is also outlined. *B,* After resection a 50 per cent defect of the lower lid is present. *C,* Patient one year after lateral canthal release and advancement of the semicircular flap to reconstruct the lid defect.

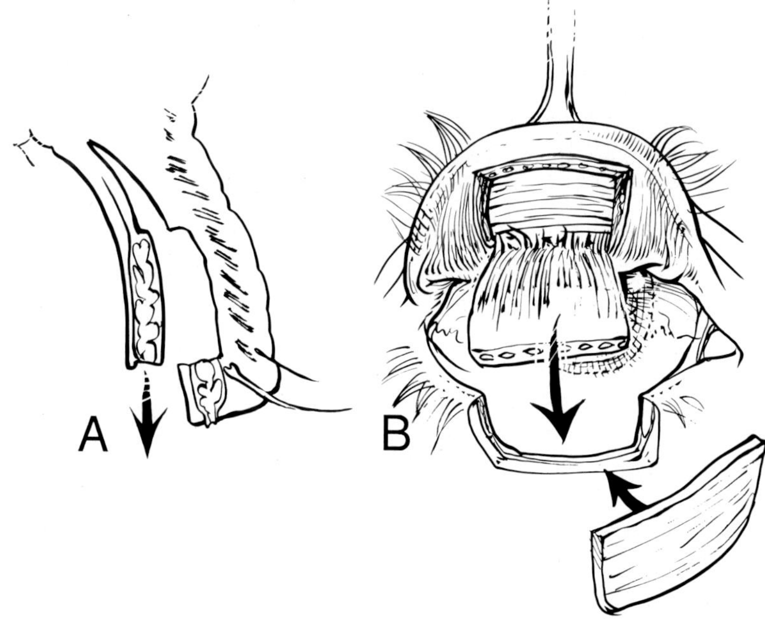

Figure 34–36. *A, B,* The Hughes tarsoconjunctival flap reconstruction of lower eyelid defects by replacement of the posterior lamella of the lid with vascularized upper eyelid tarsus and conjunctiva, and the anterior lamella with a skin graft.

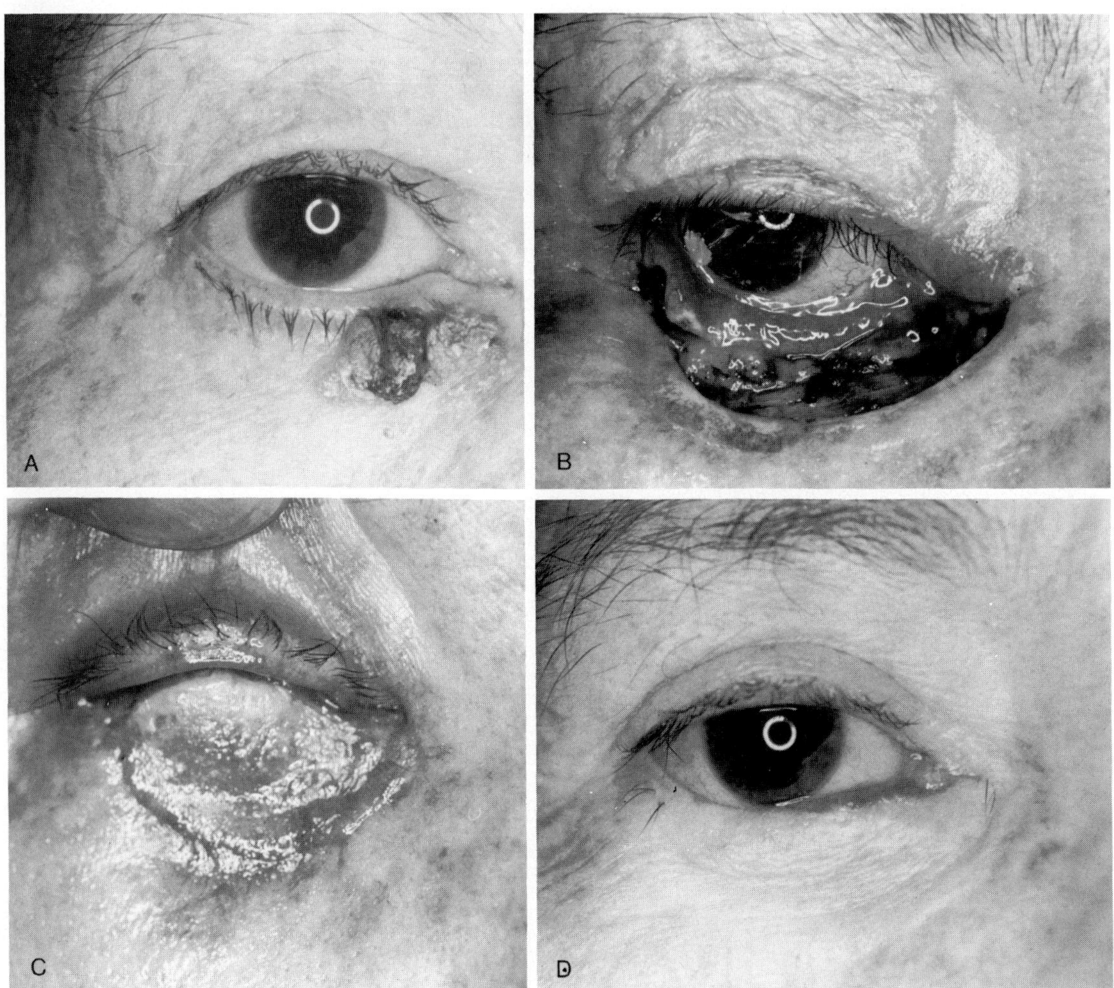

Figure 34–37. *A,* Basal cell carcinoma infiltrating the medial aspect of the right lower eyelid. *B,* 95 per cent defect of the lid and inner canthus after resection with frozen section control. *C,* Six weeks postoperatively showing a skin graft overlying the tarsoconjunctival flap. *D,* One year after division of the flap.

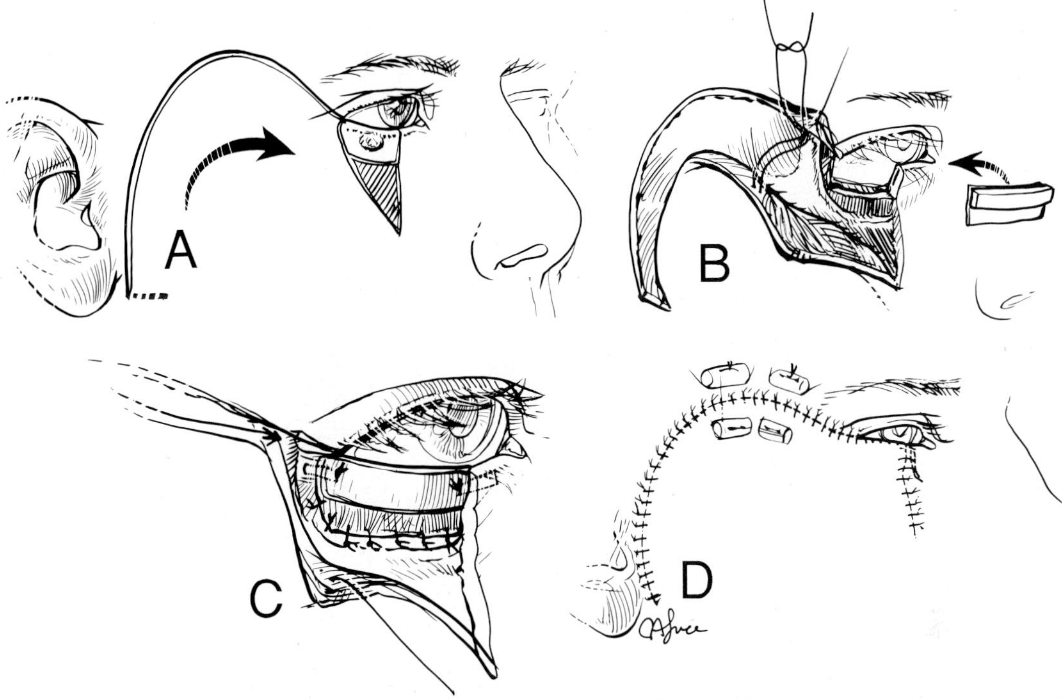

Figure 34–38. The Mustardé lower eyelid reconstruction. *A,* The area of excision and the rotation flap are outlined. Note the high arch of the cheek flap. *B,* The flap is elevated, rotated, and sutured to the periosteum of the zygoma, the lateral canthus, and the temporalis fascia with nonabsorbable "hitching" sutures. Note the chondromucosal graft *(arrow). C,* A septal chondromucosal graft of sufficient vertical and horizontal dimensions to fill the lid defect is sutured to the edges. *D,* The rotation flap in position.

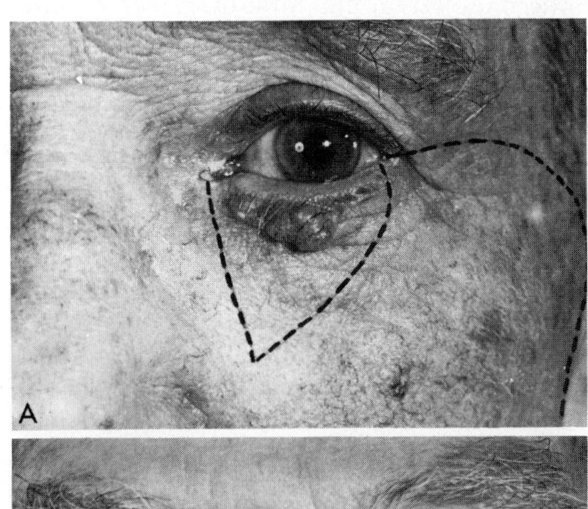

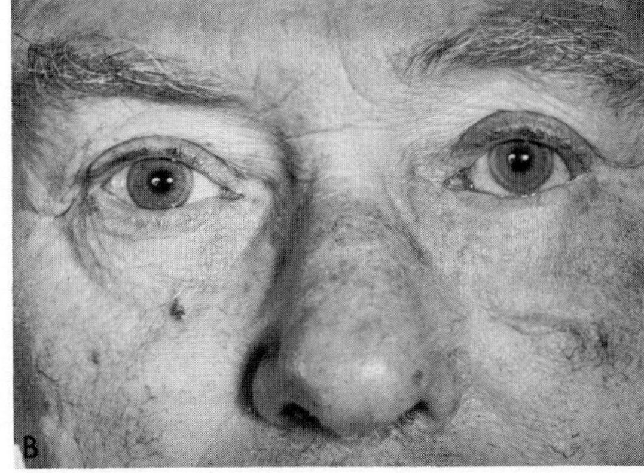

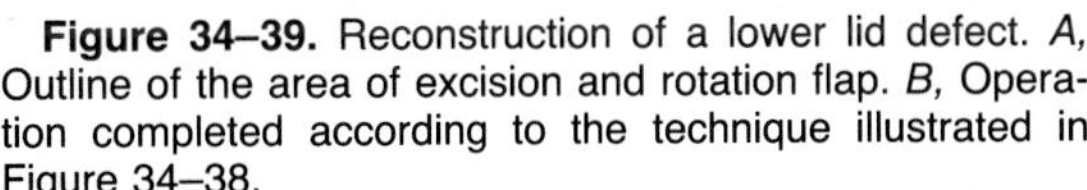

Figure 34–39. Reconstruction of a lower lid defect. *A,* Outline of the area of excision and rotation flap. *B,* Operation completed according to the technique illustrated in Figure 34–38.

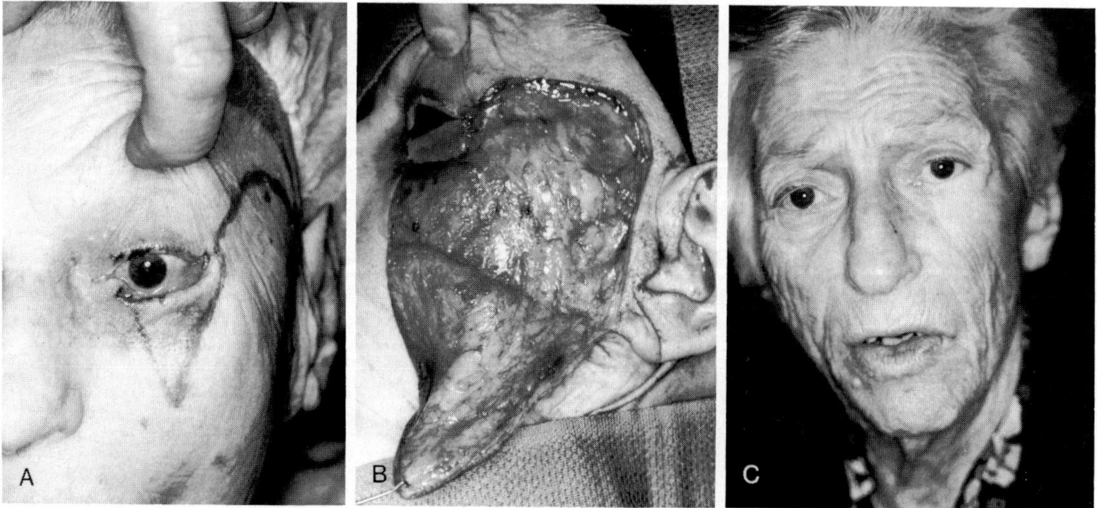

Figure 34–40. Reconstruction of a lower lid defect. *A,* A 95 per cent defect of the left lower lid after resection of a basal cell carcinoma. The rotation flap and tissue to be excised are outlined. *B,* A septal chondromucosal graft has been sutured to the edges of the lid defect. The amount of wide undermining of the cheek flap is illustrated. *C,* The patient one year postoperatively.

lower lid, replacement of the lid tissue by like tissue is usually possible. If borrowing techniques from the same, opposing, or contralateral lids are utilized, there should be only minimal structural, functional, and cosmetic consequences. The popularity of the tarsoconjunctival flap, first described by Landolt (1881) and advocated by Hughes (1937), waned when entropion and trichiasis occurred, complications that were attributed to the incision in the white line of the lid margin. Since that time the technique has been modified to correspond to the method of Köllner (1911), which places the horizontal incision parallel to the lid margin at least 4 mm from the edge of the lid margin. The addition of this modification, as well as the routine use of visual magnification, improved suture material, and specially designed needles, allows this procedure to be performed with ease and confidence. The tarsoconjunctival flap is an excellent choice when the lid defect is only 4 to 5 mm in vertical height, since the transposed tarsus and conjunctiva can be directly approximated to the remaining tarsal "skeleton" of the lower lid for a more stable type of reconstruction (Fig. 34–41).

Tarsoconjunctival Flap—First Stage. Inspection of the lower lid defect is made to determine the horizontal and vertical dimensions (Fig. 34–42*A*). Involvement of the lateral or medial canthal structures, including the lacrimal drainage structures, must also be documented. If the defect is irregular, it may be trimmed to make the lid margins perpendicular. The base of the defect should be inspected in terms of the conjunctiva, lid retractors, and residual orbicularis oculi. It is essential to maintain a well-supported upper lid margin, despite the fact that some of the upper lid tarsus is transposed. The horizontal incision parallel to the lid margin, which establishes the advancing edge of the tarsoconjunctival flap, *should be at least 4 to 5 mm above the internal surface of the upper lid margin* (Fig. 34–42*B, C*. With the scissors hugging the tarsus, the flap should be dissected high beneath the surface of the levator muscle (Fig. 34–42*C*). If the dissection is not carried sufficiently posteriorly and superiorly, residual upper eyelid retraction and increased arching of the upper lid may be the consequence of this error in technique.

The portion of the tarsoconjunctival flap used for the repair should be approximately 25 per cent narrower than the defect, especially in older patients with lax eyelids. A wider tarsoconjunctival flap would result in a reconstructed lower lid with laxity and ectropion due to excessive horizontal length.

After the tarsoconjunctival flap has been dissected and advanced into the defect, the leading margin of the advanced tarsus is attached to the recipient site conjunctival base by interrupted 6-0 absorbable sutures (Fig. 34–42*E*). The knots are tied externally so that they do not irritate the ocular globe. The margins of the tarsal flap are securely

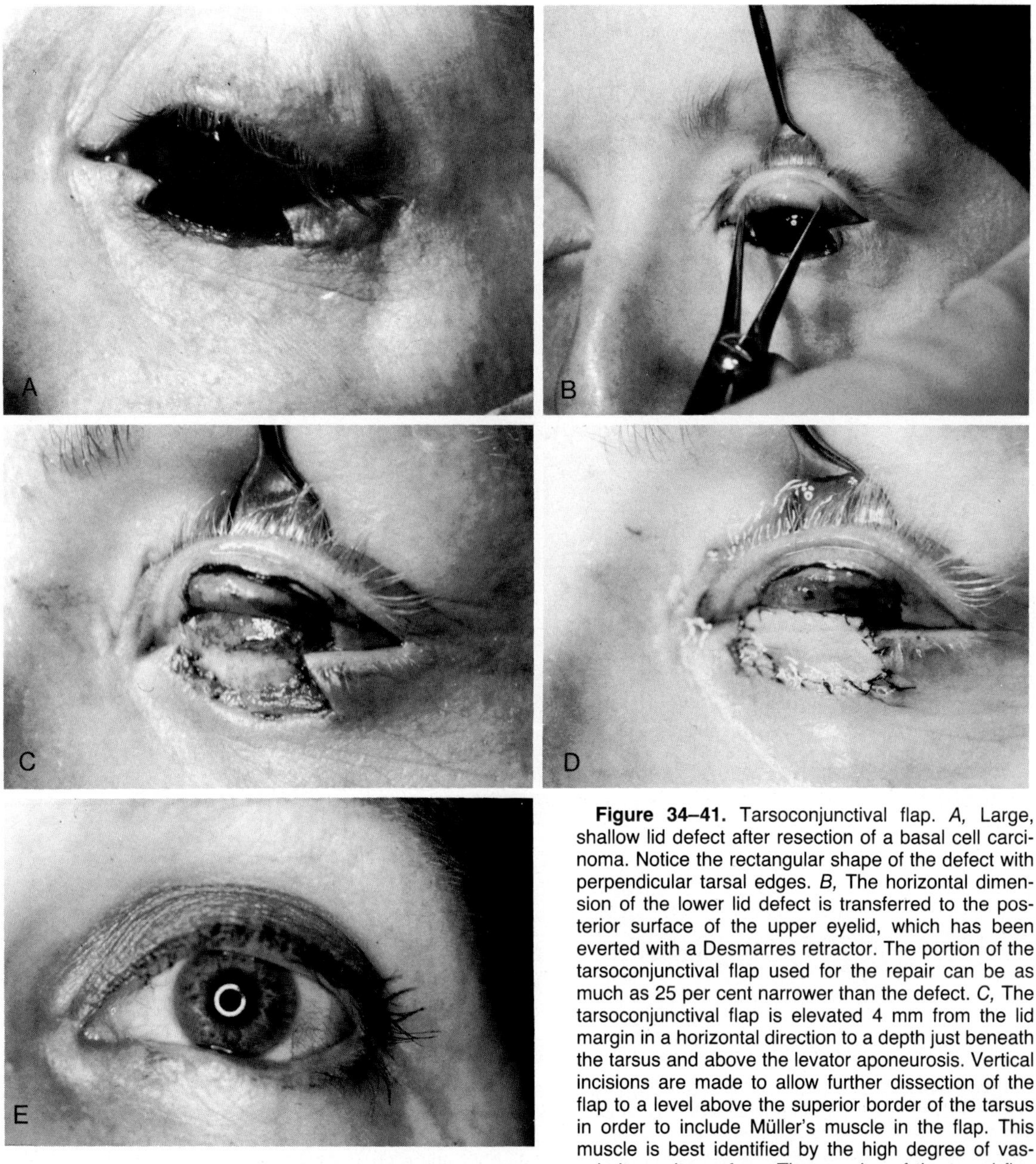

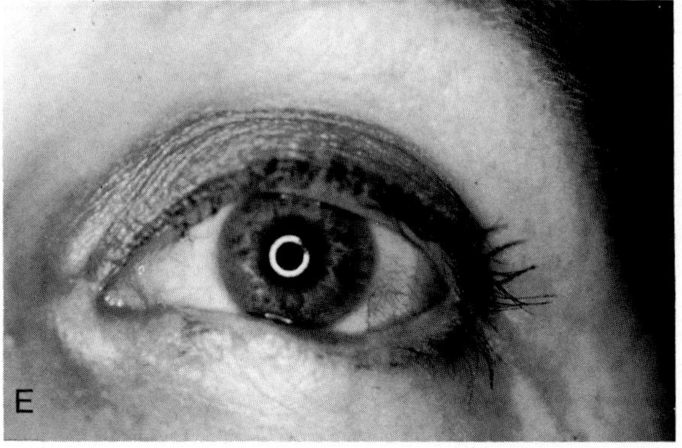

Figure 34–41. Tarsoconjunctival flap. *A,* Large, shallow lid defect after resection of a basal cell carcinoma. Notice the rectangular shape of the defect with perpendicular tarsal edges. *B,* The horizontal dimension of the lower lid defect is transferred to the posterior surface of the upper eyelid, which has been everted with a Desmarres retractor. The portion of the tarsoconjunctival flap used for the repair can be as much as 25 per cent narrower than the defect. *C,* The tarsoconjunctival flap is elevated 4 mm from the lid margin in a horizontal direction to a depth just beneath the tarsus and above the levator aponeurosis. Vertical incisions are made to allow further dissection of the flap to a level above the superior border of the tarsus in order to include Müller's muscle in the flap. This muscle is best identified by the high degree of vascularity on its surface. The margins of the tarsal flap are securely attached to the adjacent tarsal margins of the defect. *D,* A full-thickness retroauricular skin graft is sutured to the raw surface of the tarsoconjunctival flap with 6-0 silk sutures. *E,* The final result 18 months after division of the tarsoconjunctival flap.

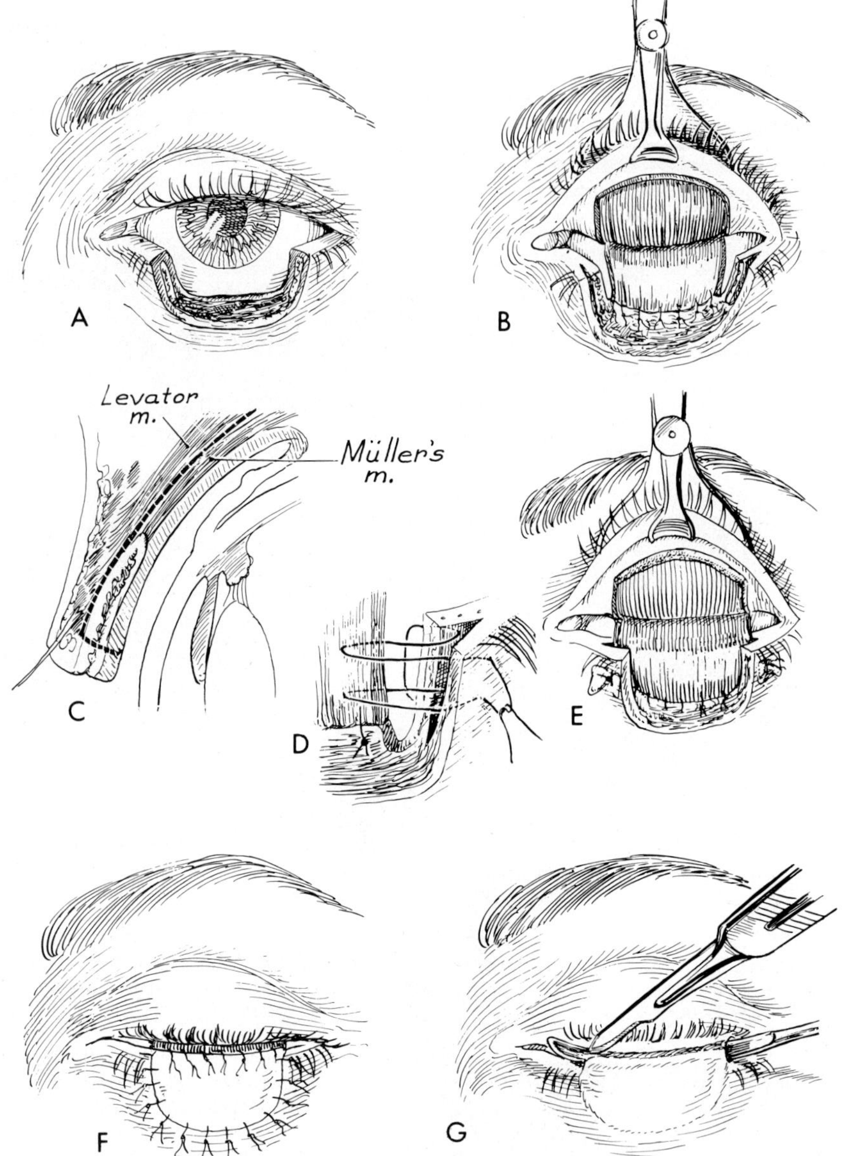

Figure 34–42. Reconstruction of a large central defect of the lower eyelid. *A,* Large lower eyelid defect. *B,* A tarsoconjunctival flap from the upper eyelid is sutured into the lower lid defect. An Erhardt clamp was used to evert the upper lid. Note that the incision through the tarsus is made parallel to the lid margin and no closer than 4 mm. The remaining tarsal border ensures stability of the lid margin and avoids entropion. *C,* In sagittal section, the incision through the conjunctiva and tarsus and the plane of dissection extending upward between the levator and Müller's muscles are outlined. Note the margin of tarsus left undisturbed, an essential precaution to prevent postoperative entropion of the upper lid. *D,* Technique of imbricating the tarsoconjunctival flap into the edge of the defect. *E,* The tarsoconjunctival flap is in position, each edge being imbricated into the wound edges of the defect. *F,* A full-thickness retroauricular or supraclavicular graft has been sutured over the tarsoconjunctival flap. *G,* Several weeks later a grooved probe is passed under the tarsoconjunctival flap, which is sectioned. (After Smith, B., and Cherubini, T. D., 1970.)

attached to adjacent margins of the lower lid defect by a tongue and groove technique (Fig. 34–42*D, E*).

Once in place, the tarsoconjunctival flap furnishes the posterior layers of the lid. This leaves a rectangular raw area over the tarsus (Fig. 34–42*E*), which is resurfaced with a full-thickness preauricular, retroauricular, or supraclavicular skin graft (Fig. 34–42*F*) or an advancement flap from the cheek. The choice of a graft or an advancement flap is determined by the laxity of the surrounding skin. The skin graft is sutured on all sides with 6-0 silk. The eyelids are covered with an antibiotic ophthalmic ointment and a moderately compressive dressing, which is removed after 48 hours. The sutures are removed after seven days. A protective bandage is kept in place for ten days. The patient is advised to avoid forceful opening of the eyelids until the second stage of the reconstructive procedure.

Tarsoconjunctival Flap—Second Stage. Six to nine weeks after the first stage, the palpebral fissure is opened by dividing the tarsoconjunctival flap and creating a stable, conjunctiva-lined lid margin. Under local anesthesia, the flap is divided with a knife over a grooved director (Fig. 34–42*G*). Care is taken to protect the cornea during this maneuver. The upper lid is everted on a Desmarres retractor, and the donor bed of the tarsoconjunctival flap is dissected of adhesions, scar tissue, and foreshortened Müller's muscle fibers. This maneuver helps to prevent residual upper eyelid retraction, secondary to Müller's muscle advancement. After the upper lid is released and is in proper position, a 0.5 to 1 mm horizontal strip of grafted skin is removed from the superior edge, preserving the underlying conjunctival layer. The conjunctiva is advanced inferiorly and sutured to the new superior edge of the skin grafted lower lid. This ensures that conjunctiva covers the new lower lid margin and is essential in preventing marginal entropion and corneal irritation. Any excess conjunctiva tends to keratinize and appear normal with the passage of time (see Figs. 34–37*D*, 34–41*E*). Attempts to reconstruct the eyelashes with eyebrow hair grafting is a technical possibility; however, it is not recommended.

Another method for reconstruction of large marginal defects of the lower lid is the use of a bipedicle skin muscle flap from the area of redundant tissue of the upper eyelid (Fig. 34–43*A*). The bipedicle, or Tripier (1889), flap should be elevated with the underlying preseptal orbicularis muscle, in order to provide adequate vascularity to the skin (Fig. 34–43*C, D*). The bipedicle is used to cover a septal chondromucosal composite graft (Fig. 34–43*C* to *E*). The two pedicles are divided after two to six weeks and returned to the upper lid (Fig. 34–43*F*). It is considered unnecessary, and indeed unwise, to insert a layer of lashes into a reconstructed lid because of the risk of distortion of the hairs and possible trichiasis at a later date. From a purely cosmetic point of view, an intact upper lash line disguises the lack of lashes in the reconstructed lid (Fig. 34–43*F, G*). Anderson and Weinstein (1987) eliminated the need to obtain a septal chondromucosal composite graft in total lower eyelid reconstruction by incorporating tarsus and conjunctiva within a bipedicle full-thickness upper lid flap.

UPPER EYELID RECONSTRUCTION

As in reconstruction of the lower lid, full-thickness upper lid reconstruction necessitates a skin-covering layer, a mucus-secreting lining layer, and a stable lid margin. Figure 34–44 depicts a summary of the most useful techniques for subtotal to total upper eyelid reconstruction. As with lower lid reconstruction, defects of up to 25 per cent of the horizontal dimension of the lid are usually closed by direct approximation (Figs. 34–44*A, B*, 34–45). Larger defects are reconstructed with selective lateral cantholysis of the superior crus of the lateral canthal tendon and medial transposition of the lid elements alone (Fig. 34–44*C, D*), or in combination with a Tenzel semicircular flap (Figs. 34–44*E*, 34–46).

When the upper lid has a defect of sufficient magnitude to require the addition of borrowed tissue from the lower lid, the Mustardé lid-switch (1981) provides excellent donor tissue (Figs. 34–44*F*, 34–47). For total upper eyelid reconstruction, the Cutler-Beard technique (1955) (Figs. 34–44*G, H*, 34–48, 34–49) or the Mustardé (1981) total upper lid reconstruction method (Figs. 34–44*I, J*, 34–47, 34–50 to 34–52) is appropriate. Marginal defects in the upper lid may be treated in the same way as in the lower lid by using a bipedicle Tripier flap from the loose peripheral skin of the upper lid with its subadjacent orbicularis muscle (see Fig. 34–43). The lining of the Tripier flap may consist of nasal chondro-

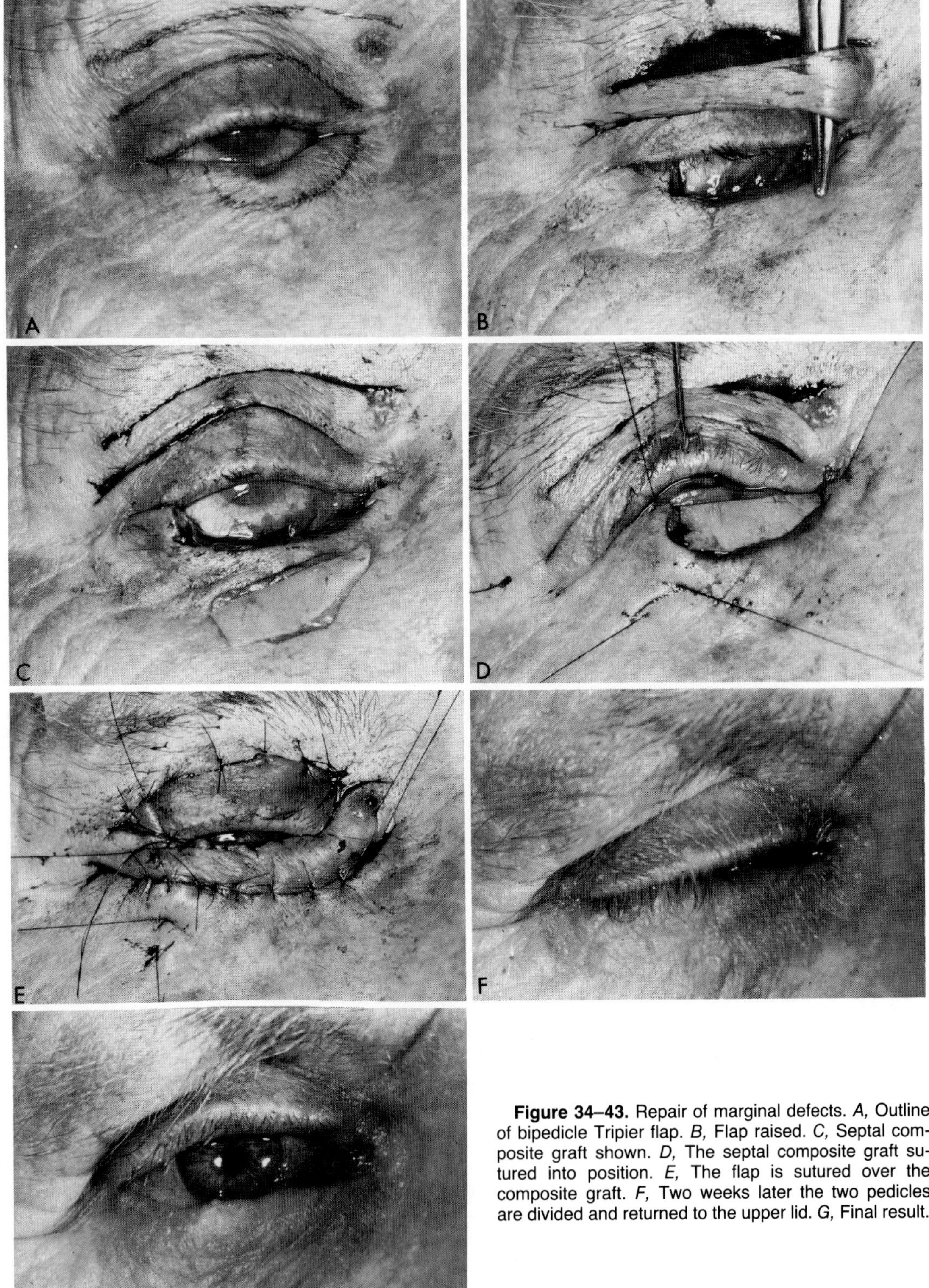

Figure 34–43. Repair of marginal defects. *A,* Outline of bipedicle Tripier flap. *B,* Flap raised. *C,* Septal composite graft shown. *D,* The septal composite graft sutured into position. *E,* The flap is sutured over the composite graft. *F,* Two weeks later the two pedicles are divided and returned to the upper lid. *G,* Final result.

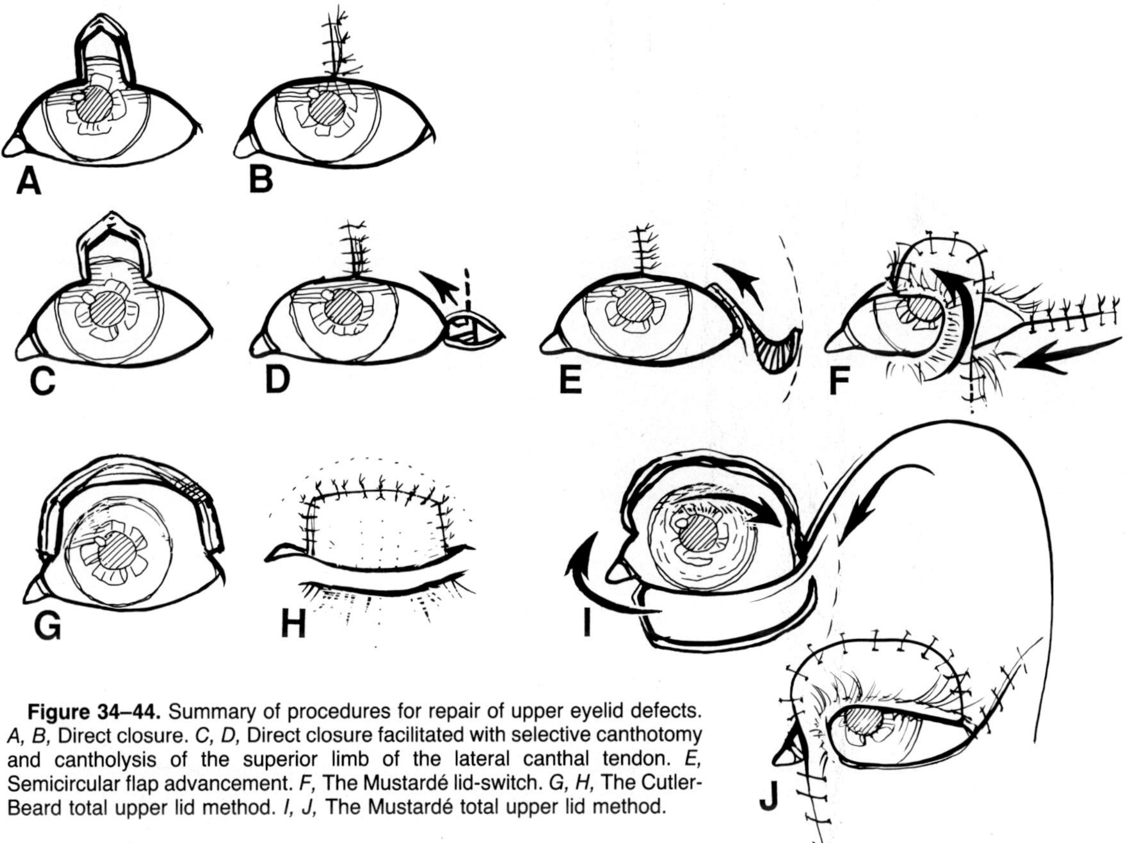

Figure 34–44. Summary of procedures for repair of upper eyelid defects. *A, B,* Direct closure. *C, D,* Direct closure facilitated with selective canthotomy and cantholysis of the superior limb of the lateral canthal tendon. *E,* Semicircular flap advancement. *F,* The Mustardé lid-switch. *G, H,* The Cutler-Beard total upper lid method. *I, J,* The Mustardé total upper lid method.

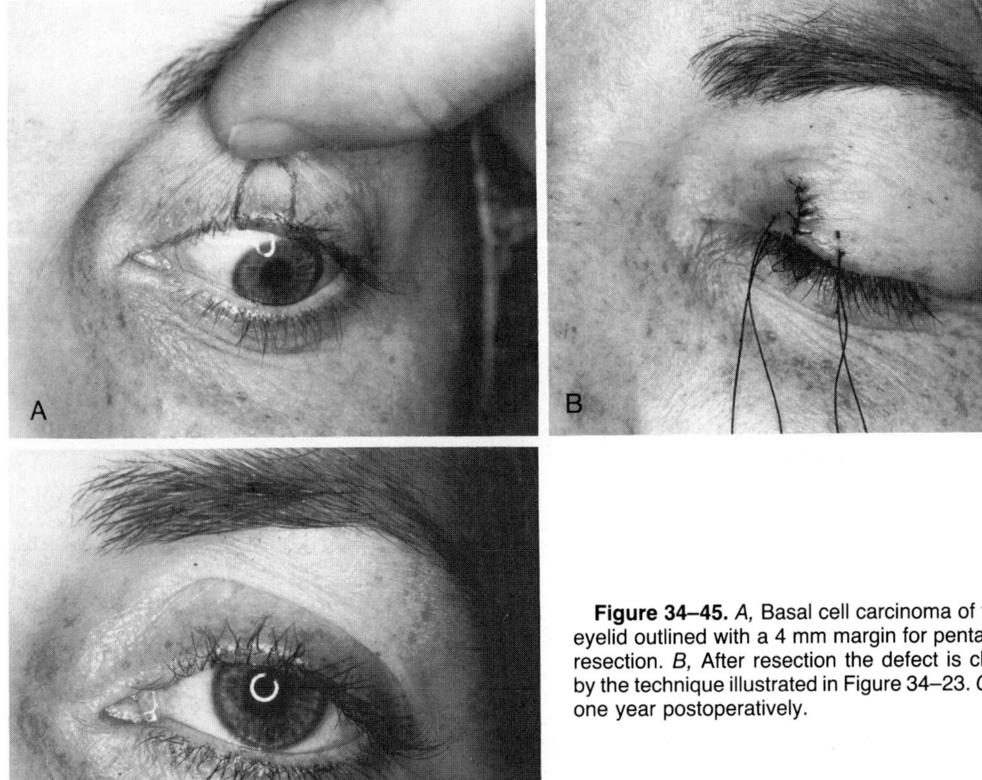

Figure 34–45. *A,* Basal cell carcinoma of the left upper eyelid outlined with a 4 mm margin for pentagonal wedge resection. *B,* After resection the defect is closed directly by the technique illustrated in Figure 34–23. *C,* The patient one year postoperatively.

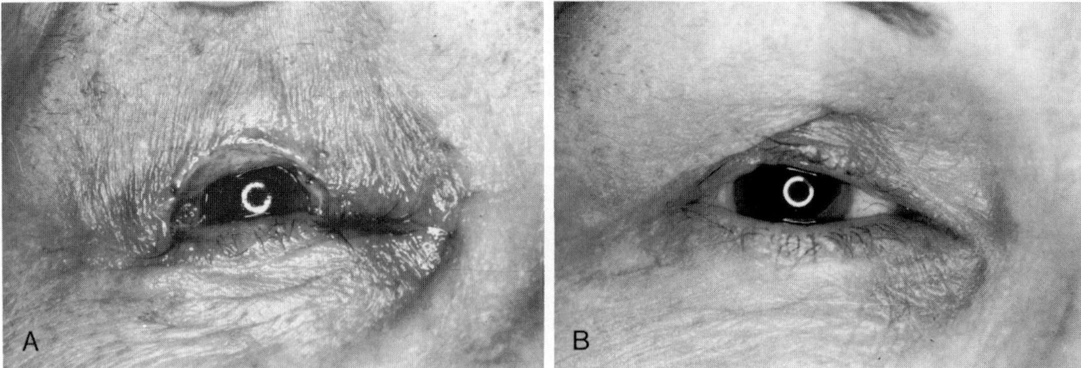

Figure 34–46. *A,* After resection of a squamous cell carcinoma of the right upper eyelid, a defect of approximately 50 per cent results. *B,* The eyelid eight months after reconstruction with a Tenzel semicircular flap as shown in Figure 34–44*E.*

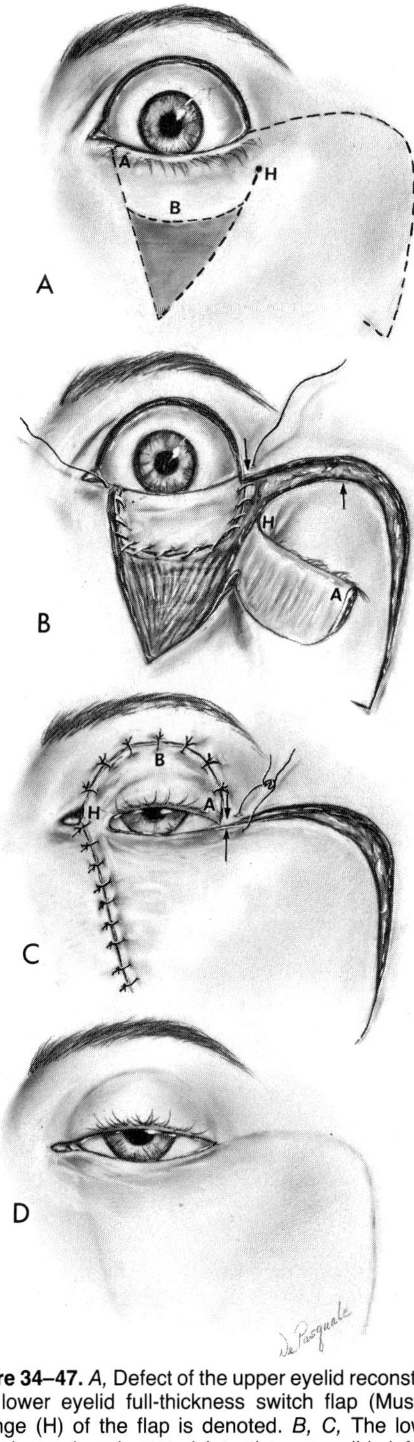

mucosa, palatal mucosa, or a tarsal graft from the opposite upper lid.

Most moderate-sized defects of the upper lid can be reconstructed with a lateral canthotomy and the Tenzel semicircular flap; however, defects of up to 60 per cent of the lid may also be reconstructed by rotating a

Figure 34–47. *A,* Defect of the upper eyelid reconstructed with a lower eyelid full-thickness switch flap (Mustardé). The hinge (H) of the flap is denoted. *B, C,* The lower lid flap is elevated and rotated into the upper lid defect. *D,* The lower lid defect is reconstructed with a lateral canthotomy, cantholysis, composite graft, and advancement of a cheek flap. The flap is divided and inset in three to four weeks.

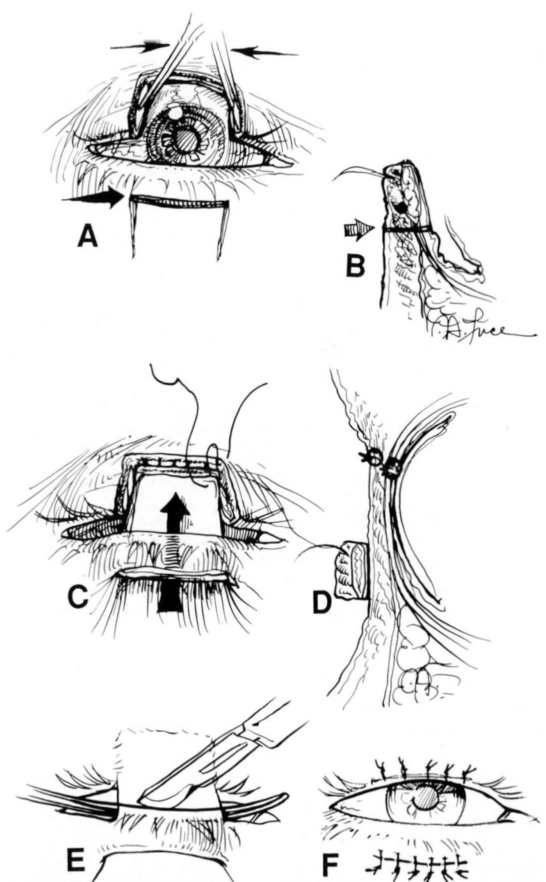

Figure 34–48. Reconstruction of a large central segment of the upper eyelid by the Cutler-Beard bridge flap technique. *A,* Defect of the upper eyelid and outline of the flap from the lower eyelid, designed 4 to 5 mm below the lid margin. *B, C,* The flap is incised and advanced beneath the bridge of tissue consisting of intact full-thickness lower lid margin. Interrupted sutures are used to approximate the conjunctiva of the flap and the edges of the tarsus. Autogenous cartilage or preserved sclera can be inserted between the conjunctiva and muscle to help prevent entropion of the reconstructed upper eyelid. *D,* In sagittal section, the relationship of the bridge flap to the upper lid structures is shown. *E,* The flap is divided after six to eight weeks, rotating the conjunctiva over the reconstructed upper lid to prevent skin from coming into contact with the ocular globe. *F,* The unused flap is resutured to the donor area after the edges are freshened.

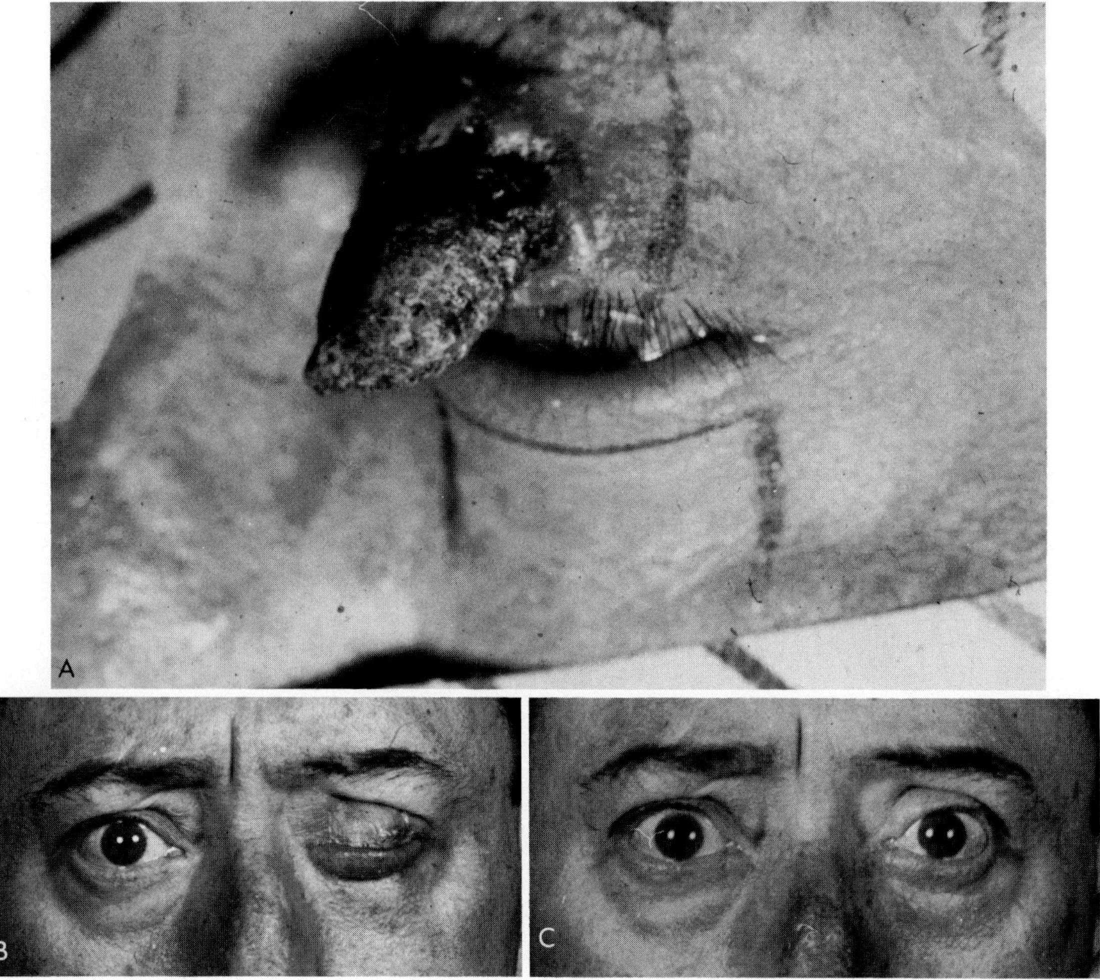

Figure 34–49. Reconstruction of a defect of the upper eyelid by the Cutler-Beard bridge flap technique. *A,* Large malignant lesion of the upper lid. Note the outline of the bridge flap from the lower eyelid. *B,* Appearance of the patient during the intermediate period when the bridge flap from the lower lid has been advanced into the upper lid defect. *C,* The patient one year postoperatively.

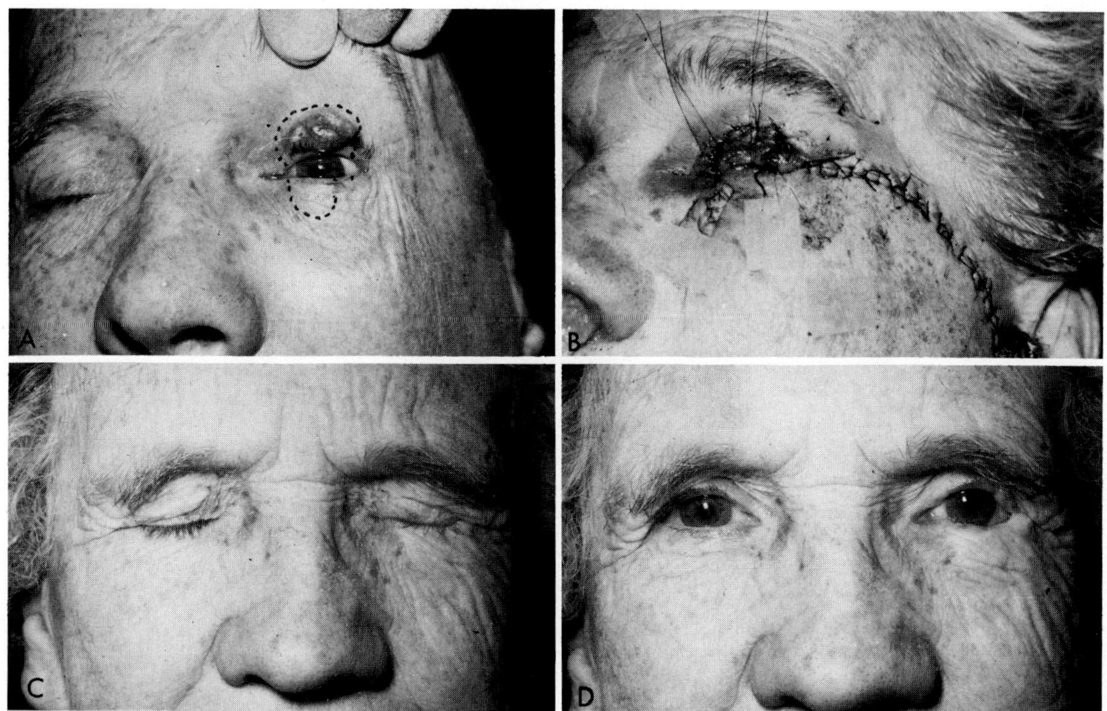

Figure 34–50. Reconstruction of a large defect of the upper lid by the technique of the lower lid "switch" flap. *A,* Outline of the upper lid lesion and of the portion of the lower lid to serve as the "switch" flap. *B,* After completion of the operative procedure outlined in Figure 34–47. *C,* Closure of the palpebral fissure after completion of the reconstruction. *D,* Appearance in the forward gaze position. (From Converse, J. M.: Reconstructive Plastic Surgery. 2nd ed. Philadelphia, W. B. Saunders Company, 1977, p. 890. Courtesy of Mustardé, J. C.)

small full-thickness flap of the lower lid based on the marginal artery (see Figs. 34–44*F*, 34–47). The marginal artery is 3 to 4 mm inferior to the lid margin, and therefore the pedicle should be at least 5 to 6 mm in vertical height. The horizontal dimension of the upper lid defect is measured and transferred to the lower lid. The central point of this transferred dimension marks the site for the lower lid hinge. The horizontal dimension of the lower lid flap can be reduced by up to one-quarter of the length of the lid; however, it is recommended that the full-thickness flap from the lower lid not be made smaller than one-quarter of the lower lid length, since it then becomes too small to manipulate adequately.

The flap can be designed on either the lateral or medial side of the hinge, and the defect in the lower lid is closed to within a few millimeters of the margin, care being

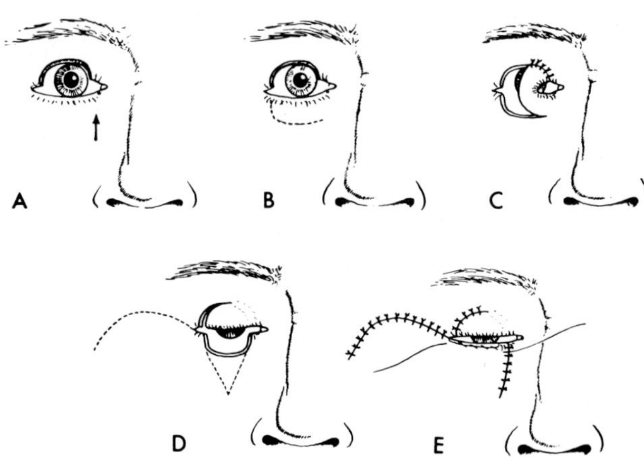

Figure 34–51. Reconstruction of a large defect of the upper eyelid with a broad-based flap of the full thickness of the lower lid. *A,* Large defect of the right upper lid. Arrow points to the broad, medially based flap hinge. Note that the hinge should be placed on the same side as the largest remnant of the upper lid (when this is present). If there is no upper lid remnant, the base should be placed on the lateral side. *B, C,* The flap consisting of the full thickness of the lower lid is outlined, incised, and sutured into the upper eyelid defect. *D, E,* Reconstruction of the lower lid is carried out by removing a triangle of tissue beneath the lower lid defect and rotating a large cheek flap over a chondromucosal composite graft. (From Mustardé, J. C.: Repair and Reconstruction of the Orbital Region. 2nd ed. New York, Churchill Livingstone, 1980.)

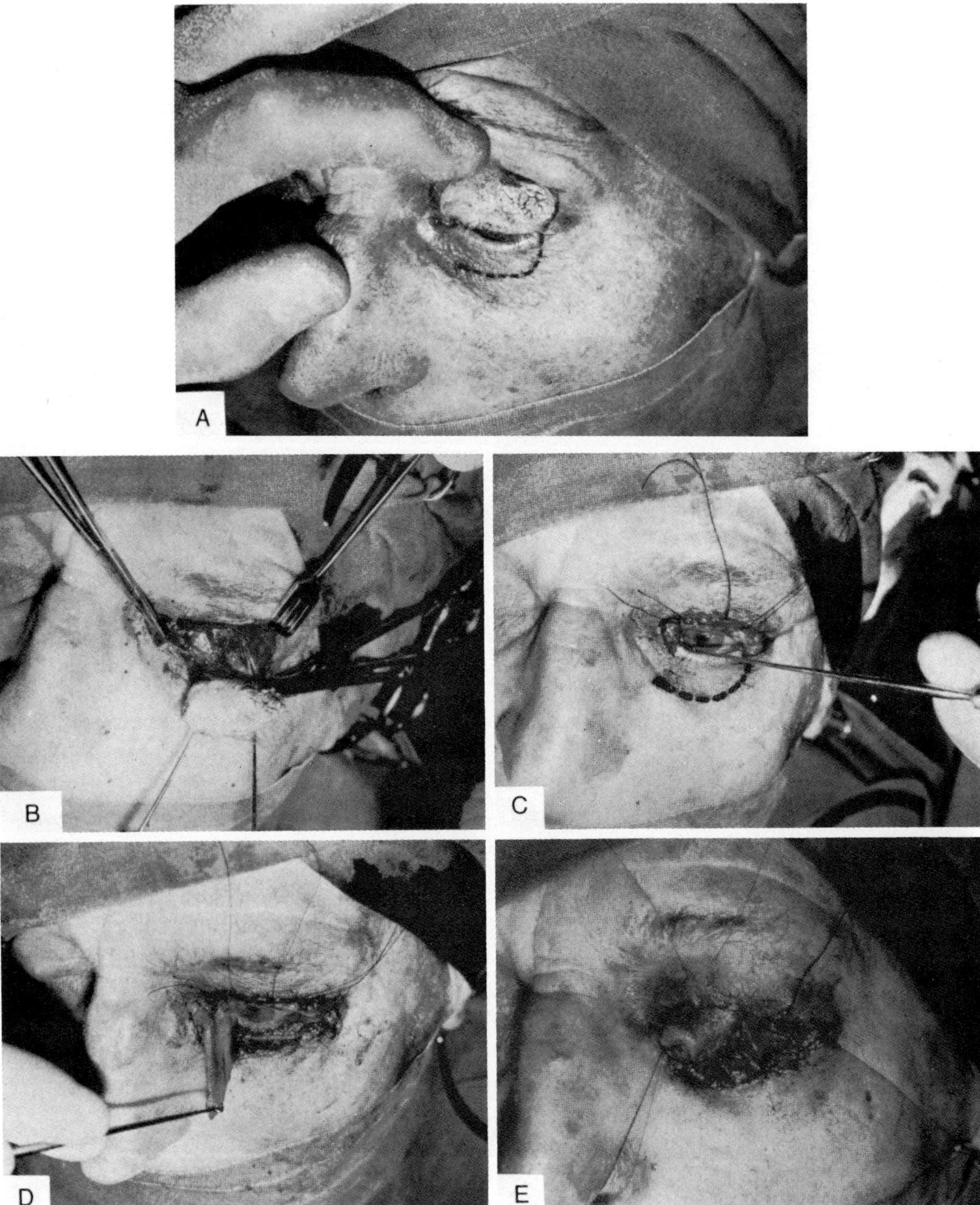

Figure 34–52. Reconstruction of the upper eyelid by the Mustardé technique. *A,* Large keratitic lesion involving the lid margin before excision. The broad lower lid flap is based medially, corresponding to the position where a remnant of upper lid will remain after resection of the lesion. *B, C,* Resection of the tumor and identification of the levator muscle. *D,* The tumor has been resected and silk sutures have been inserted to mark the levator muscle. The lower lid full-thickness flap has been developed and is shown transferred on its pedicle. *E,* The lower lid flap has been rotated upward on its base and is being inserted into the upper lid defect. Note that the suture marking the levator on the lateral side will not be removed until complete reconstruction of the lid in two weeks' time. The conjunctiva has been sutured to provide additional cover to the cornea.

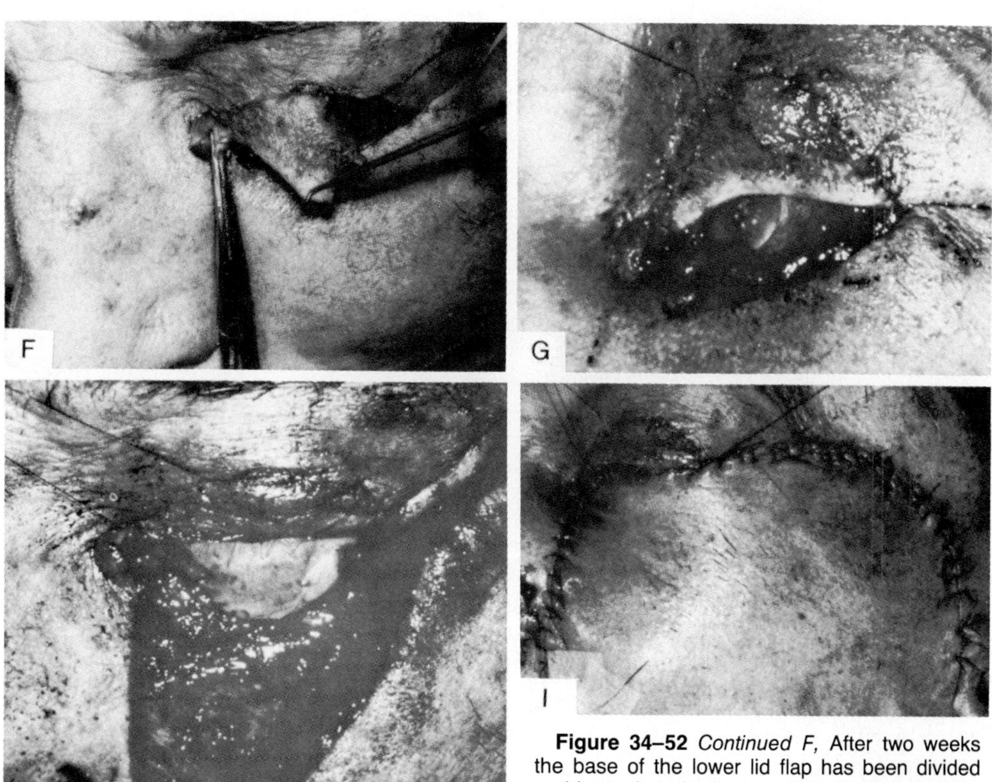

Figure 34–52 *Continued F,* After two weeks the base of the lower lid flap has been divided and is ready to be inserted into the defect of the upper eyelid. *G,* After insertion of the lower lid flap into the upper lid. *H, I,* Reconstruction of the lower lid is provided by a septal composite graft covered by a cheek flap.

Illustration continued on following page

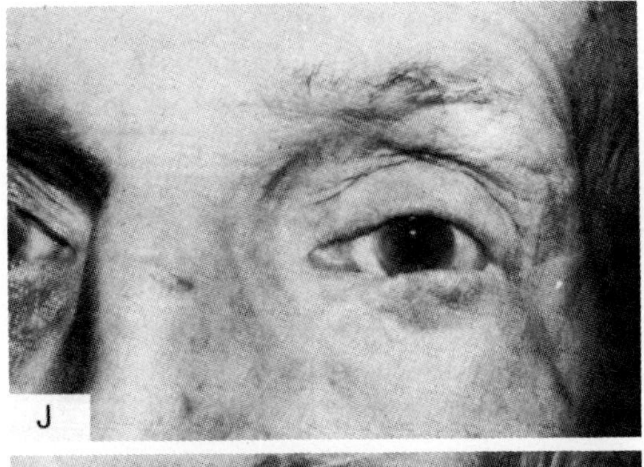

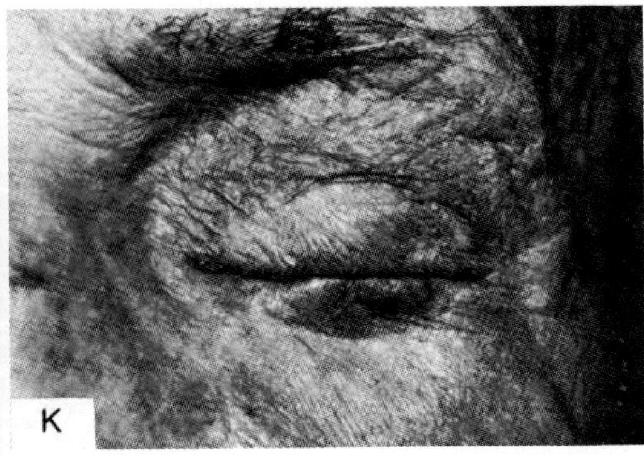

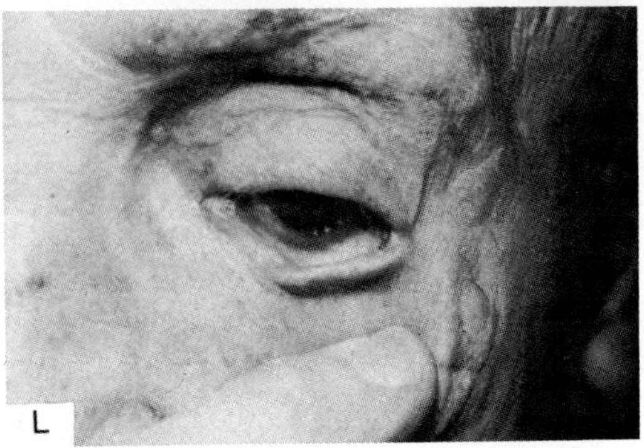

Figure 34–52 *Continued J,* Postoperative appearance after 18 months. Note the range of function of the upper lid on closure *(K),* and the adequate support of the reconstructed lower lid *(L).* (From Mustardé, J. C.: Repair and Reconstruction of the Orbital Region. 2nd ed. New York, Churchill Livingstone, 1980.)

taken to avoid damaging the small vessels in the pedicle. The conjunctiva and the tarsal plate are sutured with one or more continuous, pull-out 6-0 nylon sutures, which are removed after ten days. The cut ends of the levator muscle should be identified and sutured to the connective tissue in the center of the lower lid flap next to the tarsal plate. This maneuver provides satisfactory levator function, and the orbital portion of the orbicularis muscle with the assistance of gravity should produce adequate closure of the lid. The orbicularis muscle is approximated with 6-0 catgut, and the skin with 6-0 silk sutures.

The vascular pedicle is divided in two to four weeks and the lid margins revised. This usually requires splitting the edges of the lower marginal wound to a depth of several millimeters in order to equalize the edges. If the lower lid is too tight, a selective lateral cantholysis of the inferior crus of the lateral canthal tendon can be performed.

Larger defects of the upper lid may require the combination of a lower lid switch flap with a cheek rotation flap (see Figs. 34–47, 34–50). Because a larger secondary defect is produced in the lower lid, it is usually necessary to perform a rather extensive lower lid reconstruction. When a total upper eyelid reconstruction is required, Mustardé (1981) outlined a method consisting of first rotating a full-thickness flap of as much lower lid as necessary to fill the upper lid defect (see Figs. 34–44*I, J,* 34–51, 34–52). It is rotated and carried on a 7 to 8 mm pedicle. The pedicle is designed on the same side as the largest remnant of the upper lid (if any is present) so as to obtain a satisfactory scar line in the pupillary or near-pupillary area. After two weeks the base is divided and the rest of the full-thickness flap is inserted into the upper lid defect (see Figs. 34–51*D,* 34–52*F, G*). During the second operation, the donor defect in the lower lid is repaired with a cheek rotation flap, in combination with a composite septal chondromucosal graft (Fig. 34–52*H, I*). The upper lid remains somewhat edematous for several weeks. The reconstructed lid has adequate function and a lid margin that is free of any tendency toward instability. This result is assisted by the adhesion between the internal structures of the lid: the orbital septum, and the interfascicular tissue between the orbicularis muscle and the dermis of the skin.

The Cutler-Beard technique may also be used to reconstruct large to total defects of the upper lid (see Figs. 34–44*G, H,* 34–48,

34–49). This method uses a full-thickness flap from the opposing lower eyelid, preserving the margin of the donor lower eyelid.

In the first stage, the defect in the upper lid should be trimmed so that the edges are smooth and straight. The horizontal dimension of the defect in the upper lid is measured and the donor flap designed on the external surface of the lower lid (see Fig. 34–48*A*). In this technique, the margin of the lower lid is retained (see Fig. 34–48*C*). Within this small bridge, the marginal artery traverses the substance of the lid and provides its blood supply. It is essential to avoid injuring the bridge flap or its marginal artery. In order to include the marginal artery within the bridge flap, the horizontal incision delineating the advancing upper margin of the lower lid flap shoud be 5 mm below and parallel to the lid margin. Wesley and McCord (1980a) demonstrated that the vertical height of the bridge flap also includes all the lower lid vertical height of the tarsus. Therefore, the reconstructed upper lid may suffer from inadequate structural support, leading to shrinkage of the posterior lamella and cicatricial entropion with resultant ocular irritation. Because of this anatomic deficiency of the Cutler-Beard flap, Wesley and McCord (1980b), Carroll (1983), and McCord and Tanenbaum (1987) described methods of bolstering the transposed lower lid flap with eye bank sclera or autogenous septal or auricular cartilage.

After elevation of the lower lid flap, it is sutured to the remnants of the upper eyelid with a layered closure. Efforts should be made to attach any remnants of the levator muscle to the substance of the superior edge of the advanced flap. Six weeks after the first stage, the flap may be released, restoring the margin of the upper lid. As recommended by Reeh (1967), it is advisable to leave approximately 1 mm of excess on the upper lid to allow for ultimate contraction during healing. The flap from the lower lid is then freshened and replaced into its original position. The fact that the advancement flap is elongated during the early postoperative period is an element in avoiding ultimate retraction of the lower lid margin (see Fig. 34–49).

DEFECTS OF LATERAL SEGMENT OF EYELID

Small defects in the lateral canthus may be closed by direct approximation. If the tissues heal with a defective angle or shortened palpebral fissure, subsequent lateral canthoplasty may correct the residual defect.

If the defect in the lateral canthus is of significant dimensions, involving the upper lid, the lower lid, and the lateral canthus, a more involved technique becomes necessary. Carcinomas of the canthal regions are potentially dangerous and have a propensity toward recurrence unless widely excised. In addition, with the more widely available fresh tissue microscopically controlled excisions (see Chap. 74), a carcinoma resection of the lateral canthus ordinarily leaves a complex defect. Of the various means of closure of a lateral canthal defect, the tarsoconjunctival flap from the upper lid is the preferred technique (Fig. 34–53). The flap is prepared according to the technique employed in the large central lower lid defects (see Fig. 34–33*F, G*). After the flap has been sufficiently dissected and released, it is displaced downward and outward into the canthal defect. The advanced margin of the tarsoconjunctival flap is sutured to the recipient bed with 7-0 Vicryl sutures (Fig. 34–53*C*). The nasal extremity of the flap is interdigitated into the recipient lower lid margin. The temporal (lateral) edge of the flap is fixed to the orbital margin or tissues adjacent to the lateral retinaculum (Fig. 34–53*B, C*). An additional lateral canthal support can be designed using a turnover flap from the periosteum and superificial tissues of the lateral orbital margin. The fabricated tendon is sutured to the anterior surface of the tarsoconjunctival flap (Fig. 34–53*B, C*).

After the tendon has been sutured into position, the external raw surface is exposed. In older patients the defect may be covered by undermining and advancing skin from the adjacent area, or by rotating a flap, as advocated by Mustardé (1966) and McGregor (1973). If the skin in the area is scarred or is under tension or deficient, as in younger patients, a full-thickness skin graft can be employed (Fig. 34–53*D*). The flap is divided after six to eight weeks with occasional minor revisions required to produce a satisfactory functional and esthetic result (Fig. 34–53*E*).

DEFECTS OF MEDIAL SEGMENT OF EYELID

Cancers involving the medial canthus frequently are insidious, recognized late, and inadequately treated. They are particularly resistant to any type of treatment other than

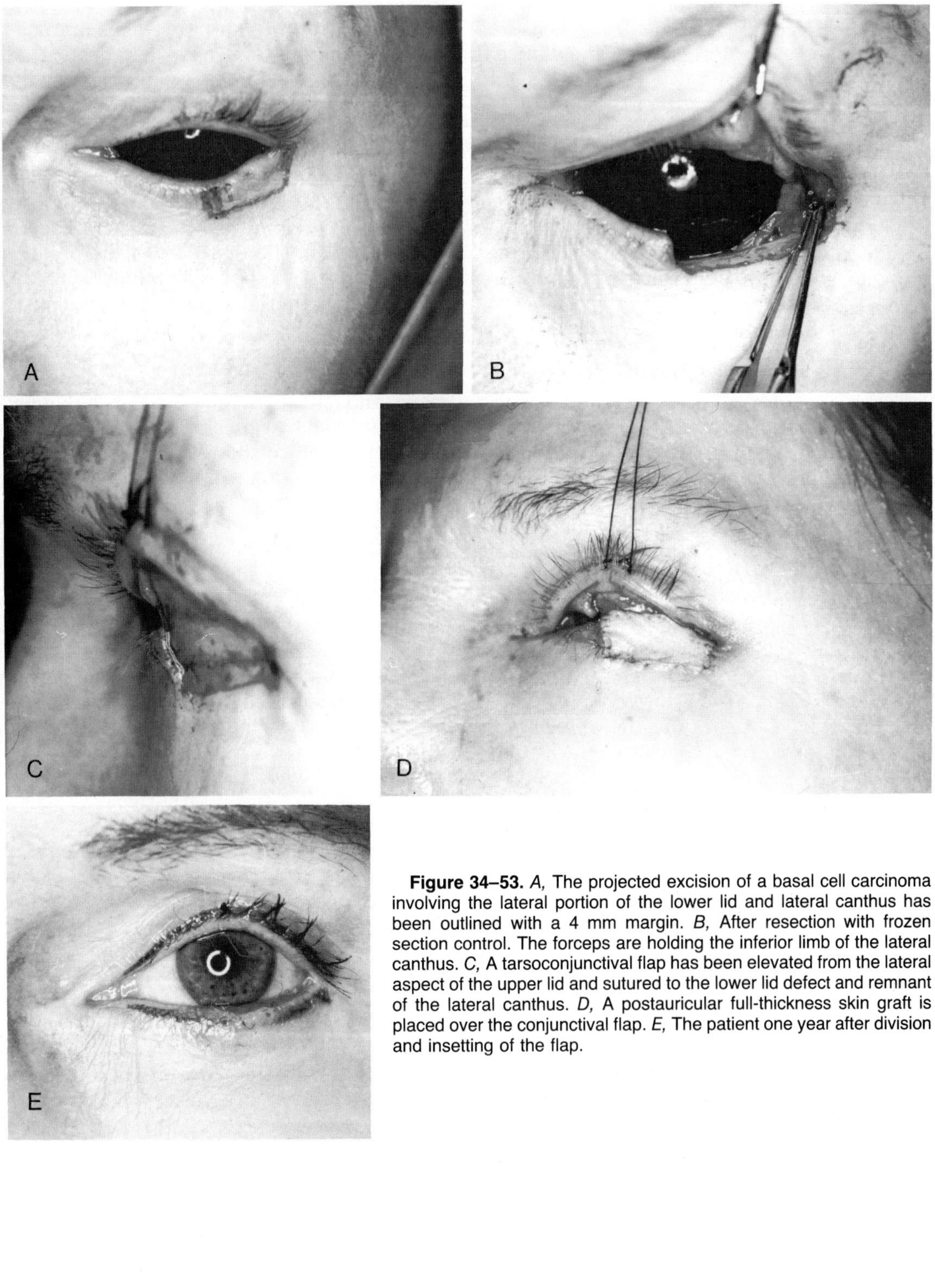

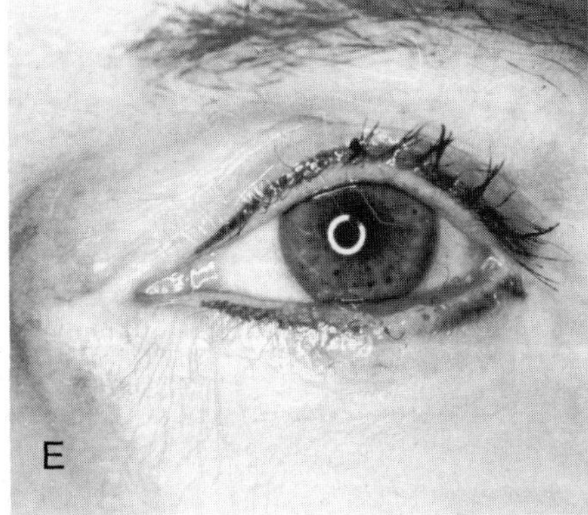

Figure 34–53. *A,* The projected excision of a basal cell carcinoma involving the lateral portion of the lower lid and lateral canthus has been outlined with a 4 mm margin. *B,* After resection with frozen section control. The forceps are holding the inferior limb of the lateral canthus. *C,* A tarsoconjunctival flap has been elevated from the lateral aspect of the upper lid and sutured to the lower lid defect and remnant of the lateral canthus. *D,* A postauricular full-thickness skin graft is placed over the conjunctival flap. *E,* The patient one year after division and insetting of the flap.

early radical surgical resection. Since the anatomy of the medial canthus is more complicated than that of the lateral canthus, surgical excision and restoration are more involved than similar surgery in the lateral canthal area. The lacrimal excretory ducts, the medial canthal tendon, and the caruncle are in close proximity. The resection may include all of these structures, including the lacrimal sac, if necessary. During resection of the entire medial canthal area, the tissues should be dissected down to the periosteum. If the conjunctiva in the caruncular area is involved, the dissection is extended toward the medial rectus muscle in order to include all the diseased tissue (Fig. 34–54*A*). Closure is started by outlining and elevating a tarsoconjunctival flap from the upper lid, as described for reconstruction of lateral canthal defects (Fig. 34–54*B*). The flap is advanced into the defect (Fig. 34–54*C*) and attached directly by transnasal wires to the stump of the medial canthal tendon (Fig. 34–54*C, D*). Since the skin overlying the medial aspect of the nose is difficult to advance, the resulting defect is best closed by a full-thickness skin graft taken from the preauricular, postauricular, or supraclavicular areas. The graft is sutured into position with a tie-over bolster, which is left in place for three to five days.

When the canalicular structures are removed with the tumor, they can be reconstructed by encircling silicone intubation, which acts as a stenting mechanism during the healing phase (see Fig. 34–34). When the lacrimal excretory system has been removed, postoperative epiphora is not unusual and can be bothersome to the patient. Successful conjunctivorhinostomy or conjunctivonasal drainage procedures are difficult to obtain in these situations.

The surgeon should study the pathology of the tumor. After the initial healing, the scarred area should be observed every three months for the first 18 months, and then every six months for three years. From that time on the patient should be examined carefully on a yearly basis.

COMPOSITE GRAFTS

Horizontal defects of the lids may be closed by composite grafts from one of the other unaffected lids, provided that the tissues can be made available without causing a permanent defect in the donor lid (Jones 1966; Putterman, 1978). The composite graft is taken full-thickness fashion from the donor lid and transplanted into the recipient bed in the defective lid (Fig. 34–55). The technique is more difficult and requires more skill than the procedures previously described. Since the composite graft consists of several layers of tissue, sutures must be placed in such a fashion as to avoid obliteration of the vasculature that will sustain the graft.

MEDIAL CANTHOPLASTY

The anatomy of the medial canthal region is complex and involves an intricate interweaving of the skin of the eyelids, the orbicularis oculi muscle, and the lacrimal drainage system with the medial canthal tendon structures. It has been documented that the medial canthal tendon inserts onto the medial orbit in a tripartite manner (Anderson, 1977; Zide and McCarthy, 1983; Zide and Jelks; 1985; Rodriquez and Zide, 1988) with a more anteriorly placed horizontal and vertical component and a deeper horizontal element (Fig. 34–56). The medial canthal tendon is formed from extensions from the nasal aspects of the tarsi blending with the superficial and deep portions of the pretarsal, preseptal, and orbital orbicularis oculi muscle (see Figs. 34–6, 34–7). The lacrimal drainage system is intimately related to this region (Fig. 34–57). Reconstructions of the medial canthus after cancer resection, traumatic displacements, or congenital deformities must incorporate knowledge of these anatomic relationships.

The medial canthoplasty may simply require repositioning the displaced soft tissue structures to their anatomic relationships, with or without lacrimal system silicone intubation. When the entire medial canthal complex is involved as in nasoethmoido-orbital fractures, orbital hypertelorism, or cancer invasion, the medial canthoplasty requires repositioning of the canthal structures according to the anatomic vector forces (Fig. 34–58). In order to perform a proper medial canthoplasty, transnasal wiring through a large bony opening after a 360 degree release of the periorbita must be performed. Extensive release of the periorbita involves incising at the arcus marginalis and subperiosteally disinserting the inferior oblique muscle origin and the trochlea of the superior oblique muscle. The technique of medial canthoplasty is also discussed in Chapters 33 and 60.

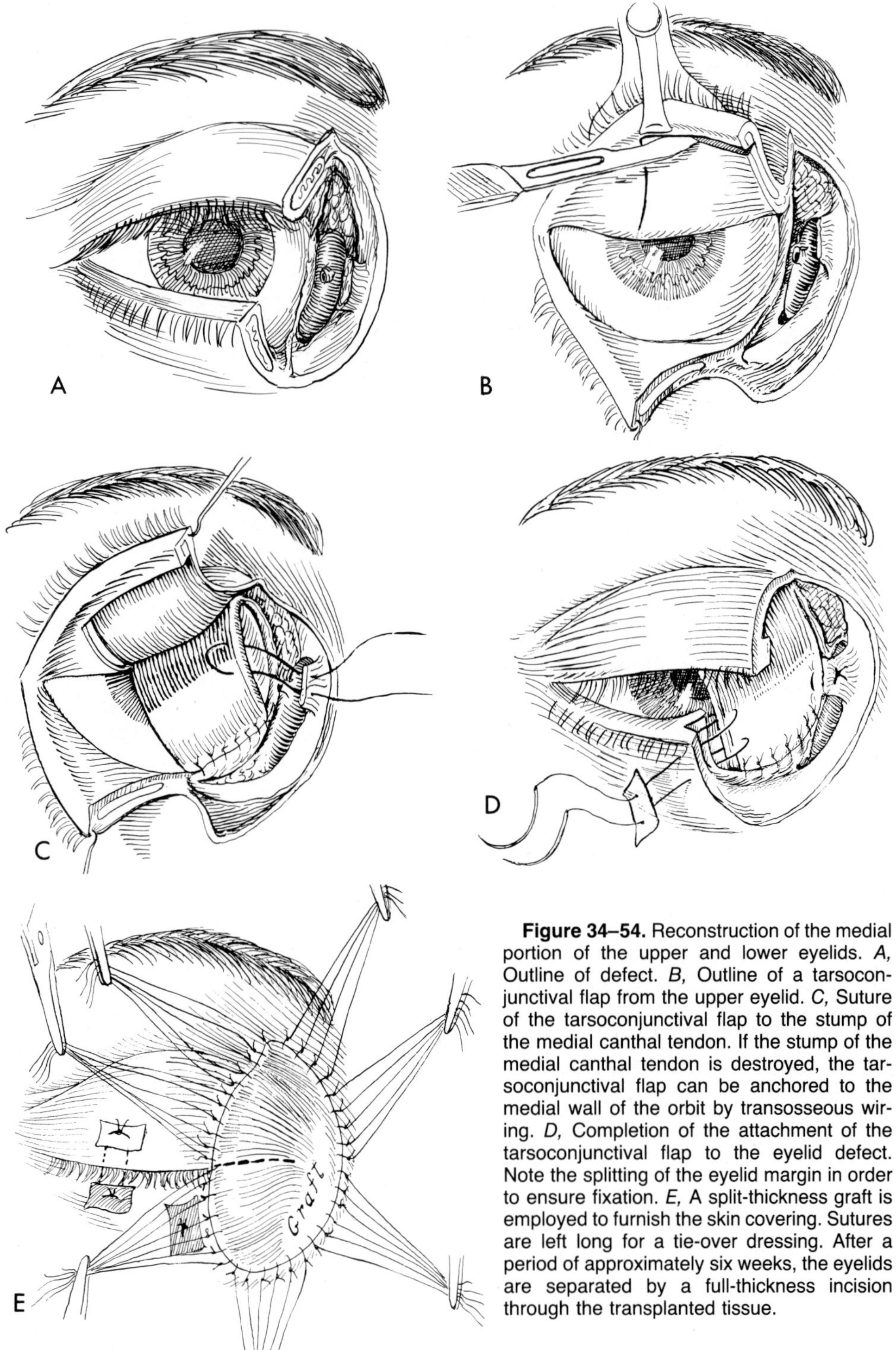

Figure 34–54. Reconstruction of the medial portion of the upper and lower eyelids. *A,* Outline of defect. *B,* Outline of a tarsoconjunctival flap from the upper eyelid. *C,* Suture of the tarsoconjunctival flap to the stump of the medial canthal tendon. If the stump of the medial canthal tendon is destroyed, the tarsoconjunctival flap can be anchored to the medial wall of the orbit by transosseous wiring. *D,* Completion of the attachment of the tarsoconjunctival flap to the eyelid defect. Note the splitting of the eyelid margin in order to ensure fixation. *E,* A split-thickness graft is employed to furnish the skin covering. Sutures are left long for a tie-over dressing. After a period of approximately six weeks, the eyelids are separated by a full-thickness incision through the transplanted tissue.

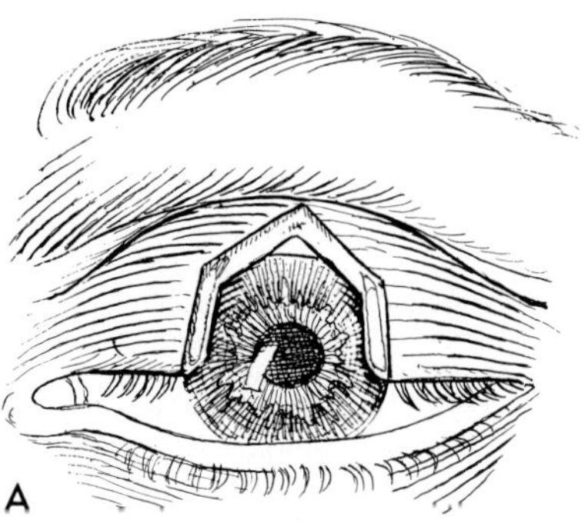

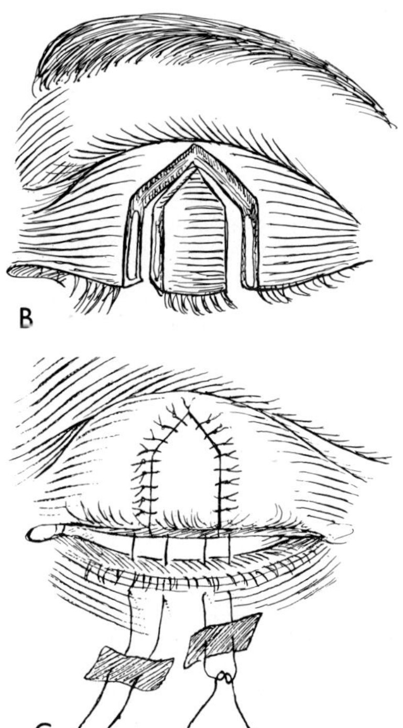

Figure 34–55. Composite graft reconstruction of eyelid defects. *A,* Moderate defect of the upper eyelid. *B,* Composite graft, smaller in width than the defect, has been removed from the donor eyelid and is placed in the defect. *C,* Sutures have been placed in the pretarsal fascia to approximate the edges of the tarsus to orient the graft. Suturing of the graft has been completed by interrupted sutures approximating the skin margins. Two occlusive mattress sutures are placed to join the eyelids and immobilize the area during the healing phase.

LATERAL CANTHOPLASTY

The lateral canthus is an integral anatomic unit defining the geometric pattern of the temporal or lateral aspect of the eyelids. The lateral canthus is more correctly termed a lateral retinaculum (see Figs. 34–8, 34–11) consisting of (1) the lateral horn of the levator superioris, (2) the continuation of the preseptal and pretarsal orbicularis oculi muscle (the lateral canthal tendon), (3) the inferior suspensory ligament of the globe (Lockwood's ligament), and (4) the check ligament of the lateral rectus muscle. Gioia, Linberg, and McCormick (1987) reported gross and histologic anatomic information that clearly demonstrates fibrous attachments from the lateral canthal tendon and the check ligament of the lateral rectus muscle. They also confirmed that the lateral retinacular structures attach to a confluent region of the lateral orbital wall that incorporates Whitnall's tubercle, a small promontory just within the lateral orbital rim.

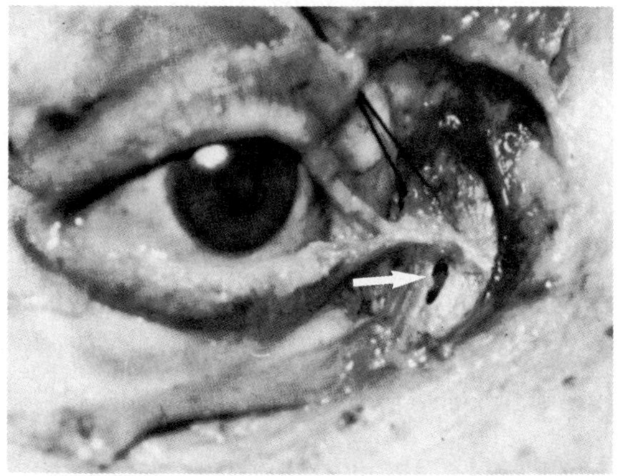

Figure 34–56. A suture is passed around the vertical component of the medial canthal complex. The horizontal component extends medially onto the nasal bones. The arrow denotes an opening into the lacrimal sac. (From Zide, B. M., and McCarthy, J. G.: The medial canthus revisited. An anatomical basis for canthopexy. Ann. Plast. Surg., *11*:1, 1983.)

Consideration of the anatomic complexities of the lateral canthal region must be incorporated into lateral canthal and contiguous eyelid reconstructions. Numerous surgical procedures directed to the lateral canthus have been developed to correct: (1) cicatricial, atonic, or paralytic lower eyelid ectropion; (2) lateral canthal dystopia; and (3) epiphora and corneal exposure. More recently, the lateral canthoplasty has found wide acceptance in esthetic surgery of the lower eyelid (see Chap. 43).

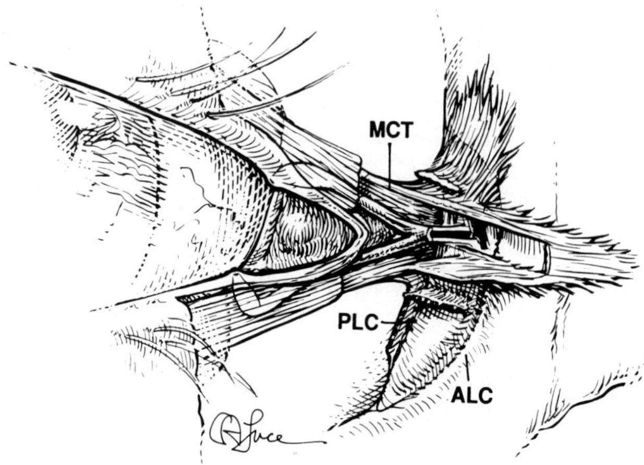

Figure 34–57. The lacrimal canaliculi pass between the superficial and deeper muscle heads to empty into the lacrimal sac. MCT = medical canthal tendon; PLC = posterior lacrimal crest; ALC = anterior lacrimal crest. (From Rodriquez, R.L., and Zide, B. M.: Reconstruction of the medial canthus. Clin. Plast. Surg., *15*:255, 1988.)

In 1826 Von Walther designed the simple lateral tarsorrhaphy procedure, which had the disadvantage of distorting the lid margins and decreasing the functional fields of vision. In 1950 and 1952 McLaughlin described a lateral tarsorrhaphy procedure that produces a more esthetic result in noncicatricial ectropion and paralytic lagophthalmos. The technique (see Fig. 34–22) retains the upper eyelashes to camouflage the lid adhesion. The lateral quarter of the upper and lower eyelids are split at the gray line, and a wedge of skin, cilia, and orbicularis oculi muscle is excised from the lower eyelid. A corresponding area of tarsus and conjunctiva is excised from the upper eyelid, so that the lower lid tarsoconjunctival wedge and upper lid recipient bed may be approximated. Although the retained upper lid cilia produce a satisfactory cosmetic effect, the lateral canthus may be displaced downward and the lateral peripheral visual field is diminished owing to the horizontal shortening of the lid aperture. If the tarsorrhaphy is released, there may be entropion and trichiasis due to the previous resection of tissue from both lids.

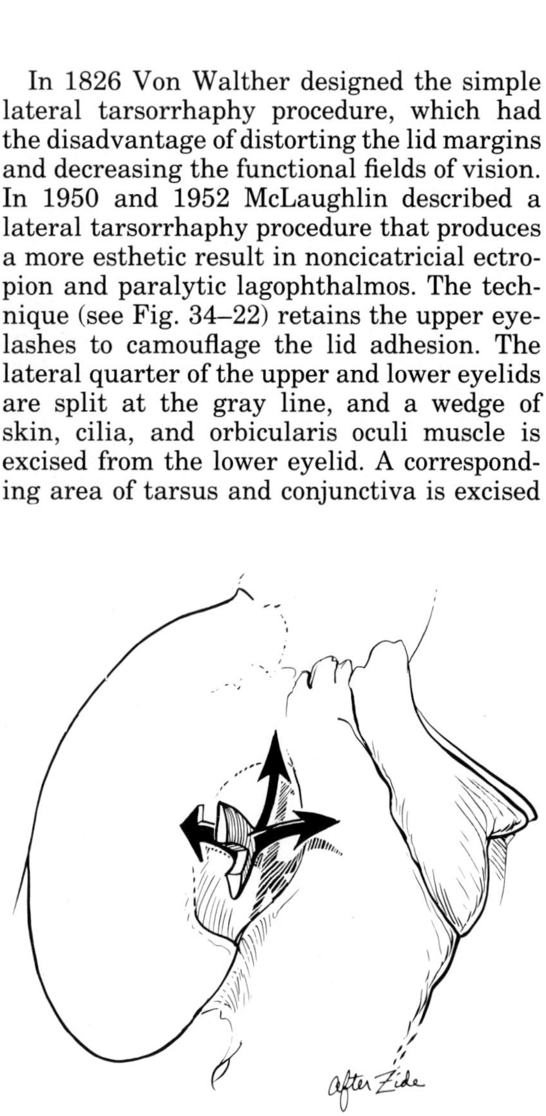

Lateral canthorrhaphies were developed to avoid the limitations and associated deformities of the tarsorrhaphy. These procedures utilized various methods of flap transpositions and removal of skin laxity to support the lower eyelid. Procedures described by Denonvilliers (1856, 1863) and Meller (1953) were widely employed. The Kuhnt-Szymanowski procedure for the correction of senile ectropion (Szymanowski, 1870; Kuhnt, 1912, 1916) required splitting the lateral two-thirds of the lower eyelid at the gray line into a deep tarsoconjunctival and a superficial skin–orbicularis oculi muscle layer. The lid was shortened by excising a wedge of the tarsoconjunctival layer large enough to bring the lid into contact with the globe. The tarsoconjunctival layer was reapproximated and the excess skin and muscle trimmed. The procedure caused occasional entropion and trichiasis due to the lid splitting. Modifications of the procedure were developed by Smith (1959) with an incision below the lashes, and by Kazanjian and Converse (1959) with excision of a tarsoconjunctival wedge medially.

Bick (1966) reported a technique for removal of the full-thickness temporal aspect

Figure 34–58. Each of the skeletal attachments of the medial canthal complex are represented by an arrow.

of the eyelid to correct laxity. This procedure became popular for the correction of senile ectropion of the lower eyelid, although it tended to blunt the lateral canthal angle.

Edgerton and Wolfert (1969) described a deepithelized dermal pennant flap of lateral canthal tissue that was passed through a drill hole in the lateral orbital rim to correct lower eyelid paralytic ectropion (Fig. 34–59). This procedure tightens the lateral lid elements and allows better apposition of the lids to the globe. A later modification of this procedure by Montandon (1978) included a lateral lid tarsorrhaphy (0.5 to 1.0 cm) of the lateral lid elements in association with the dermal flap. This procedure has the advantage of reducing the amount of exposure of the globe while tightening the lids (Fig. 34–59*C*). Internal lateral canthal suspensions have also been performed by Whitaker (1984) via the face lift incision (Fig. 34–60*A*), Whitaker (1984) and Ortiz-Monastario and Rodriguez (1985) from the bicoronal (Fig. 34–60*B*), and Paterson, Munro, and Farkas (1987) from the conjunctival approach (Fig. 34–60*C*).

Many surgeons developed their own methods of recreating the lateral canthal angle by various lateral canthal tendon suture techniques. The more effective methods involved isolating the lower lid contribution to the lateral canthus by a lateral canthotomy, followed by a cantholysis of the inferior limb of the lateral canthus at the orbital rim. The lower eyelid was thus isolated from the upper lid and lateral retinacular structures to allow more selective repositioning (Fig. 34–61*A*).

Tenzel (1969) described a technique of correcting lower eyelid lagophthalmos in patients wearing an ocular prosthesis. The procedure mobilizes the lower limb of the lateral canthal tendon to be passed through the attached superior limb and fixed with a periosteal suture. The procedure corrects the blunting of the lateral canthus, and suspends and horizontally shortens the lower eyelid (Fig. 34–61*B*).

Marsh and Edgerton (1979) reported the use of a pennant of orbital periosteum as a method of fixation for the lateral canthoplasty (Fig. 34–61*C*). A more recent variation of this

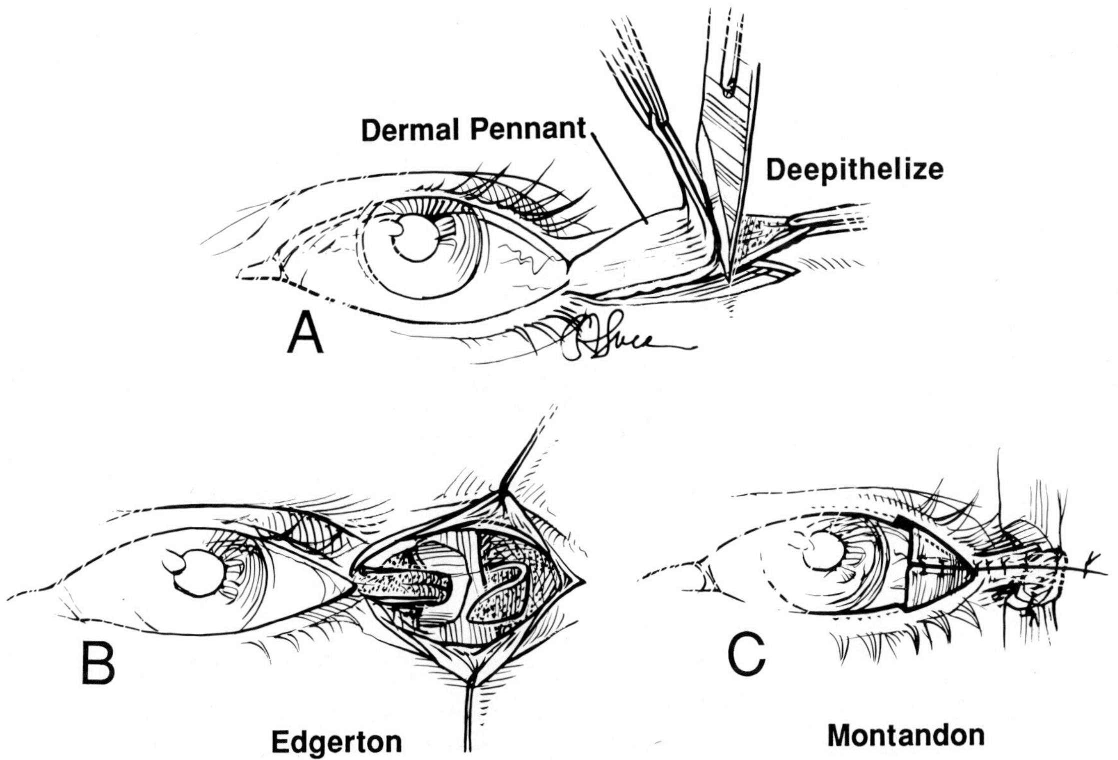

Figure 34–59. Lateral canthoplasty (pennant techniques). *A*, Technique of deepithelization of a pennant of lateral canthal tissue in continuity with the lateral canthus. *B*, Passage of the deepithelized pennant through a large drill hole in the lateral orbital rim for correction of a paralytic ectropion (Edgerton and Wolfert, 1969). *C*, Combining the same procedure as in *B* with a lateral lid tarsorrhaphy (Montandon, 1978).

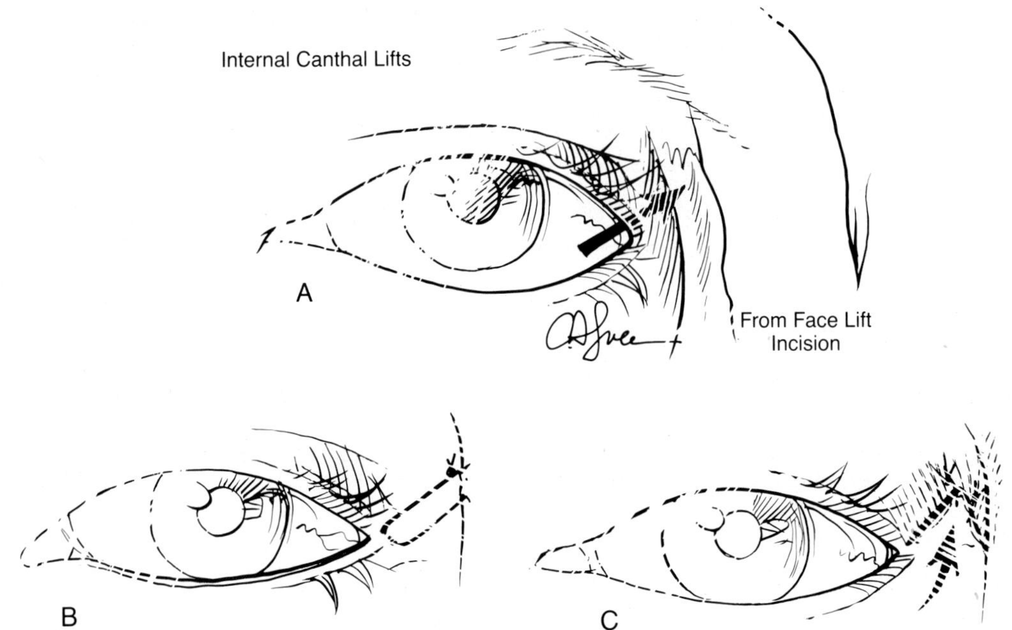

Figure 34–60. Lateral canthal suspension procedures performed via the *(A)* face lift, *(B)* bicoronal, or *(C)* conjunctival approach.

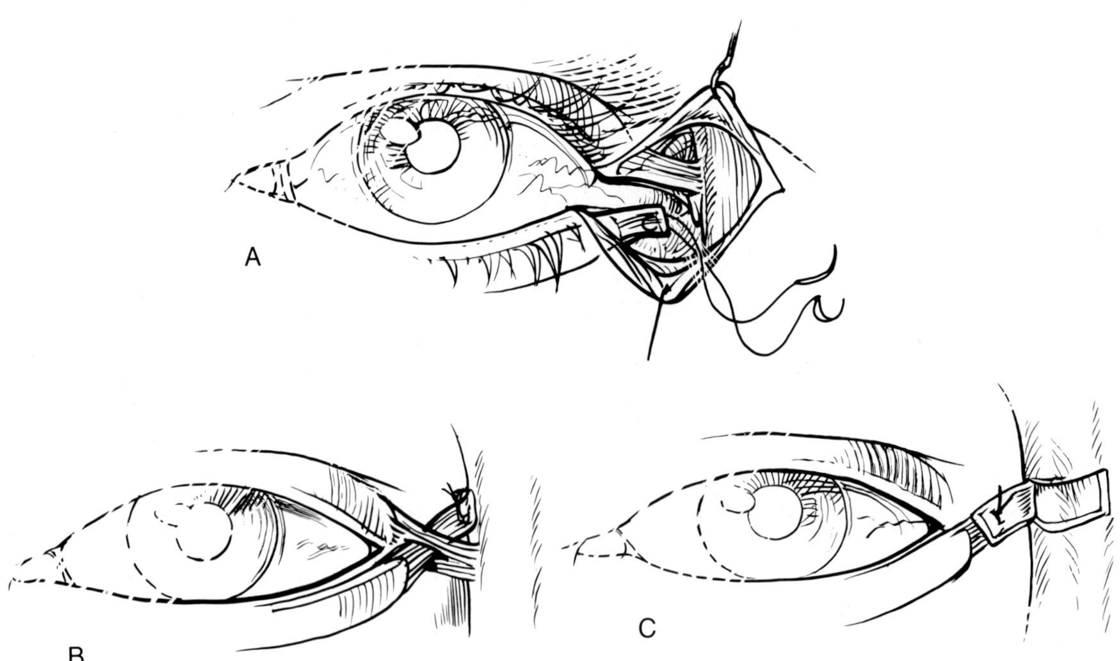

Figure 34–61. Lateral canthoplasty by isolation of the lower limb of the lateral canthal tendon. *A,* Lateral canthal suture technique. *B,* Tenzel (1969) lateral canthoplasty. *C,* Marsh and Edgerton (1979) periosteal pennant lateral canthoplasty.

innovation was described by Leone (1987). Bachelor and Jobe (1980) reported replacement of the absent lateral canthal tendon with a Y-graft of palmaris longus tendon, and Holt, Holt, and van Kirk (1984) used temporalis fascia for lower eyelid and lateral canthal reconstructions.

The basic principle in selective lower eyelid reconstruction with a lateral canthoplasty has evolved into various methods of tarsal fixation to the lateral orbital tissues (Fig. 34–62*A*). Anderson and Gordy (1979b) described the tarsal strip procedure for correction of senile or paralytic ectropion. The advantage of this technique is that the upper and lower lids can be individually sutured to the lateral orbital periosteum to vary the amount of correction. The amount of horizontal lid shortening and suspension can be varied with the suture placement. Furthermore, the vertical placement of the suture on the tarsal strip can assist in correction of entropion or ectropion (Fig. 34–62*B;* see also Figs. 34–92, 34–109, and 34–110). The lateral canthoplasty is also useful as an adjunct in full-thickness skin graft reconstruction of the lower eyelid for burn scar deformities and reconstruction after excessive skin removal during blepharoplasty (see Fig. 34–111).

Hamako and Baylis (1980) described a combined tarsal strip and periosteal pennant flap fixation type of lateral canthoplasty. The tarsal strip is sutured under a superiorly based lateral orbital periosteal flap to enhance fixation. To promote the suspension effect, a suture from the tarsal strip was passed through the base of the periosteal flap, brought out to the skin surface, and tied over a silicone bolster (Fig. 34–62*C*). More important, these authors described the lower lid deformity of lid retraction and its correction when the lateral canthoplasty is combined with surgical release of the retraction. Lower eyelid retraction is usually associated with a cicatricial fixation of the orbital septum to the lower lid retractors and orbital rim. Lower lid retraction is observed after (1) orbital floor explorations via an inadequately stepped skin-muscle eyelid approach (see Fig. 34–112*A*), (2) abnormal wound healing after lower lid blepharoplasty (Fig. 34–63), and (3) marked soft tissue trauma associated with orbital fractures (see Fig. 34–68). Lower eyelid retraction also occurs in thyroid ophthalmopathy due to lymphocytic infiltration of the lower eyelid tissues. Correction of lower lid retraction may only require incising the internal lid cicatricial component and lateral canthal fixation. However, if the vertical lid defect created is excessive, an interpositional autogenous auricular or septal cartilage graft (Figs. 34–64 to 34–66) or a vascularized,

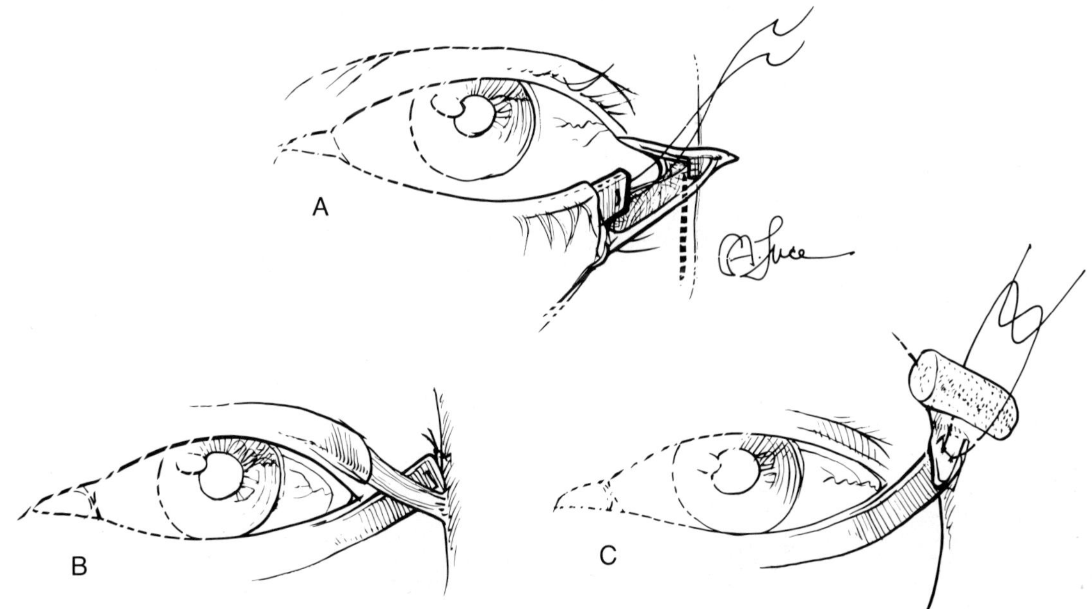

Figure 34–62. Lateral canthoplasty by development of a tarsal element for fixation. *A,* Tarsal fixation to the lateral orbital periosteum. *B,* The tarsal strip lateral canthoplasty (Anderson and Gordy, 1979). *C,* The Baylis and Hamako (1981) lateral canthoplasty for correction of ectropion and lid retraction.

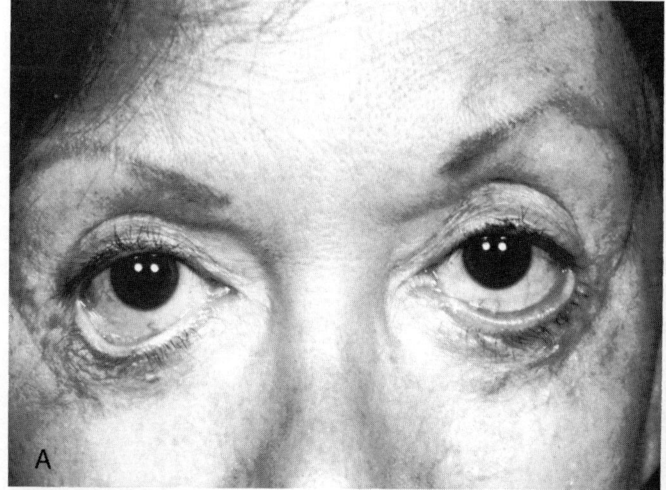

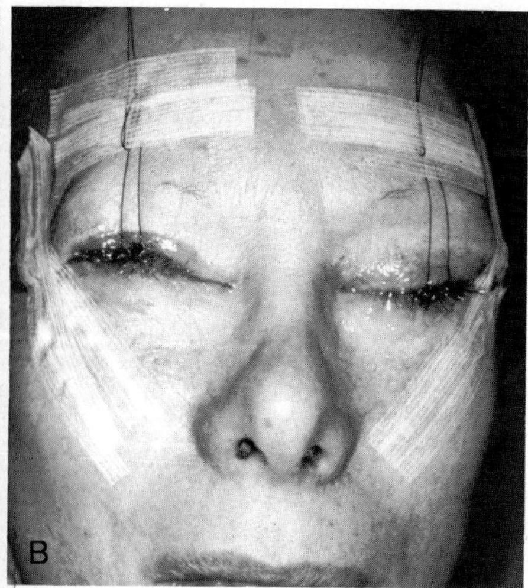

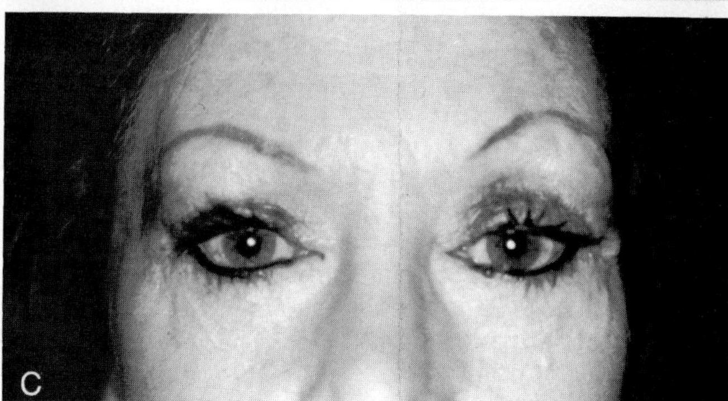

Figure 34–63. *A,* Patient 3½ weeks after evacuation of bilateral lower eyelid hematomas following blepharoplasty. There is marked eversion and ectropion of both lower eyelids and inferior corneal punctate stain, suggesting corneal desiccation. In addition there was marked cicatricial retraction of both lower lids, more evident on the right side. *B,* The patient immediately after extensive release of the cicatricial retraction, cheek suspension, and lateral canthoplasty similar to that illustrated in Figure 34–62*C*. Note the sutures from the lower eyelids taped to the forehead to assist in lid elevation during the early healing period. *C,* The patient one year postoperatively. Skin grafting was not necessary.

deepithelized lateral canthal dermal flap may be required (Figs. 34–67, 34–68).

The tarsal strip procedure and its many variations (Webster and associates, 1979; Wesley and Collins 1983; Lisman and associates, 1987) is also useful for primary (Fig. 34–69) or secondary (Fig. 34–70) reconstructions of the lax lower eyelid with lower eyelid blepharoplasty.

The key surgical points to achieve symmetric lateral canthal repositioning are summarized in Figure 34–71. The lateral canthal and lower eyelid incision should be horizontal (Fig. 34–71*A*). After selective release of the lower eyelid with its portion of the lateral canthal tendon, the lid is elevated to cover 1 to 2 mm of the inferior limbus (Fig. 34–71*B*). The tarsal strip is fashioned, the horizontal

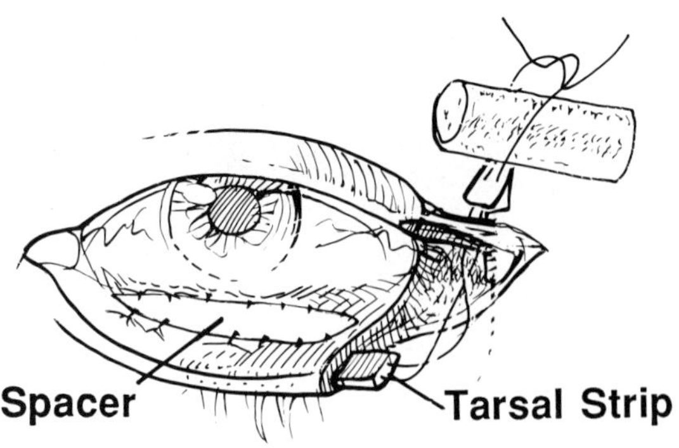

Figure 34–64. An autogenous cartilage graft to increase the vertical height of the retracted or deficient lower lid may be combined with the lateral canthoplasty to enhance the results in difficult cases (see Figs. 34–65 and 34–66).

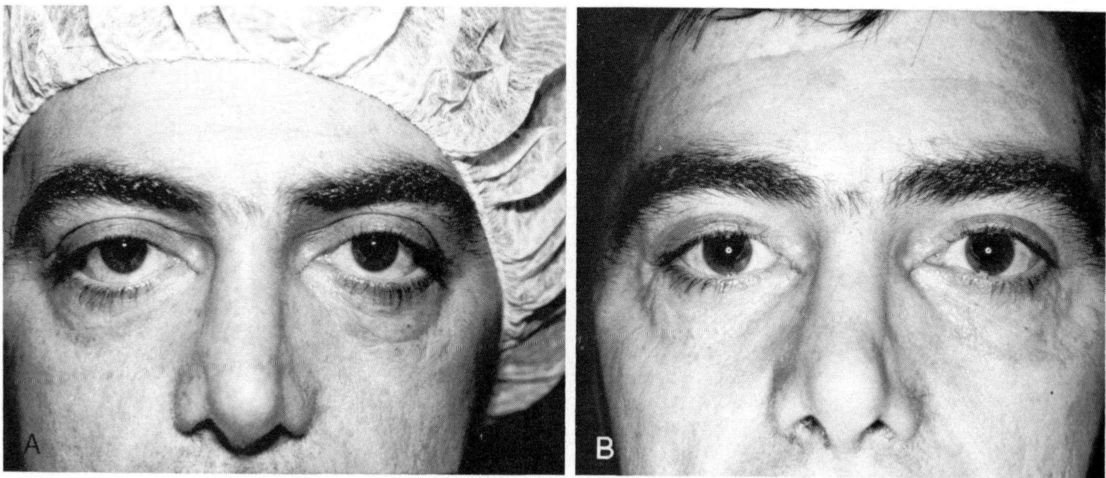

Figure 34–65. *A,* Patient with severe lid retraction of both lower eyelids after blepharoplasty. There is vertical shortening and temporal bowing of the lower lids with scleral show and inadequate support from the malar region. *B,* One year after autogenous auricular cartilage grafting and lateral canthoplasties of both lower lids as illustrated in Figure 34–64. Note that there is unavoidable narrowing of the horizontal dimension of the palpebral aperture with this procedure.

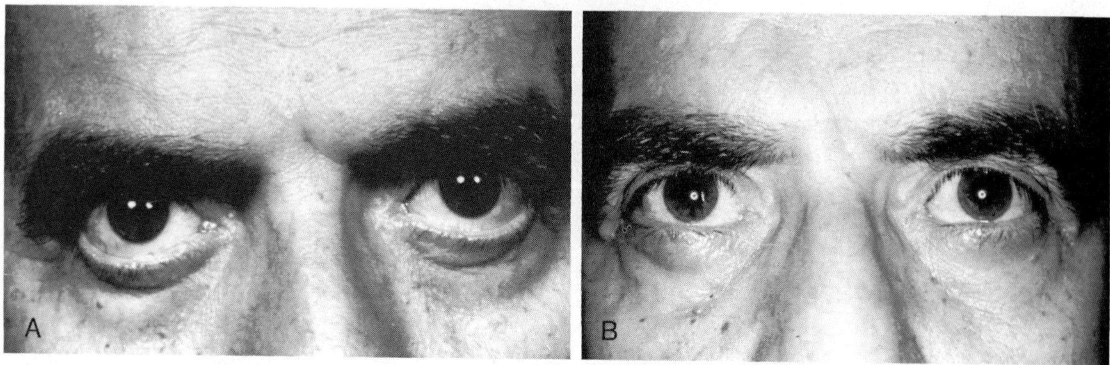

Figure 34–66. *A,* Patient with thyroid ophthalmopathy and lower eyelid retraction due to contraction of the vertical elements of the lower eyelids. *B,* One year after autogenous auricular cartilage grafting and lateral canthoplasties as illustrated in Figure 34–64.

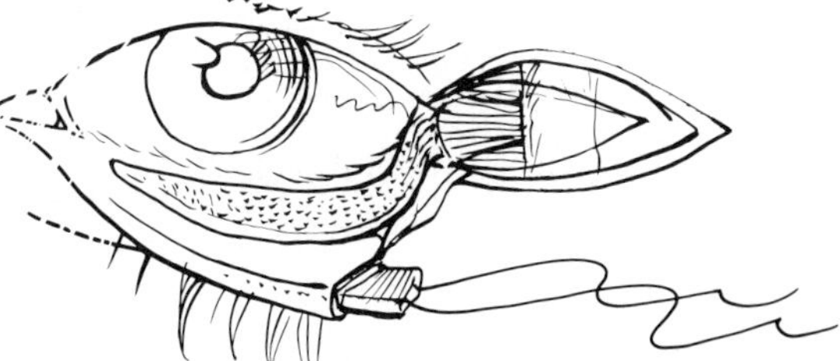

Figure 34–67. A vascularized deepithelized pennant of lateral canthal tissues may be incorporated with the lateral canthoplasty to provide vertical height and bulk to the lower eyelid.

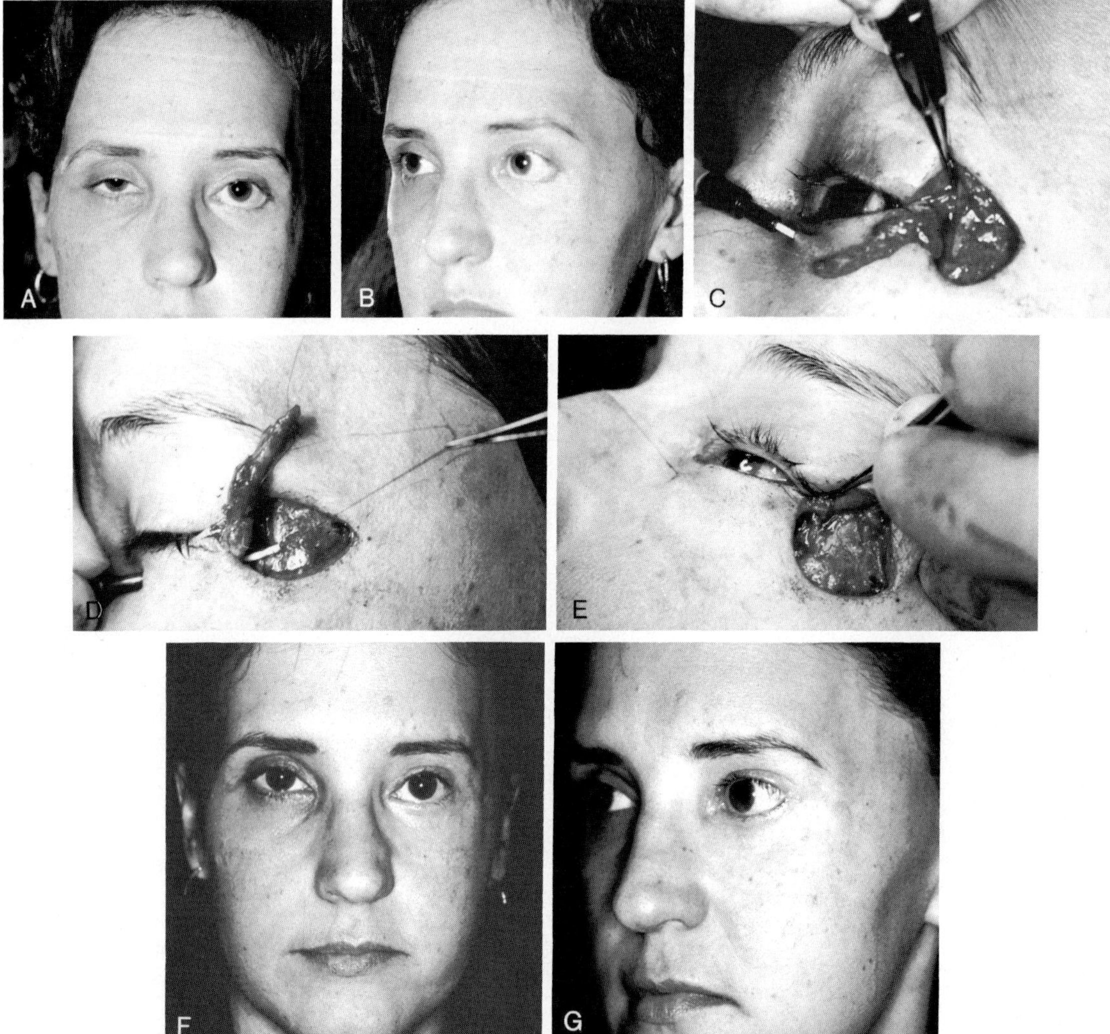

Figure 34–68. *A, B,* A patient eight months after left comminuted orbitozygomatic fracture requiring several surgical procedures to establish acceptable bone alignment. Persistent left lower eyelid retraction, soft tissue deficiency, and lateral canthal deformity are evident. *C,* A large deepithelized pennant of lateral canthal tissue has been elevated with a wide lateral canthal pedicle. There has been extensive dissection of the lower eyelid and lateral cheek area to allow the lateral canthus, which is held with the forceps, to be repositioned more superiorly. *D,* A catheter has been inserted into the medial eyelid skin to emerge at the lateral canthal area. The tip of the deepithelized flap is sutured to the catheter. When the catheter is withdrawn *(E),* the soft tissue deficiency of the lower lid is augmented. Elevation of the lateral canthus is also performed in an overcorrected position. *F, G,* The patient six months postoperatively with improvement in lid contour, position, and bulk.

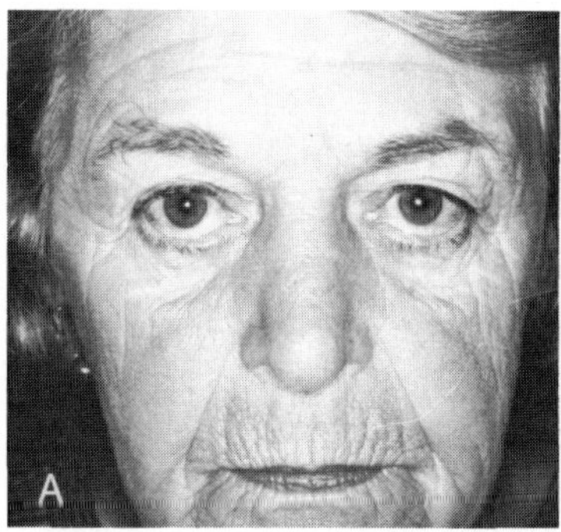
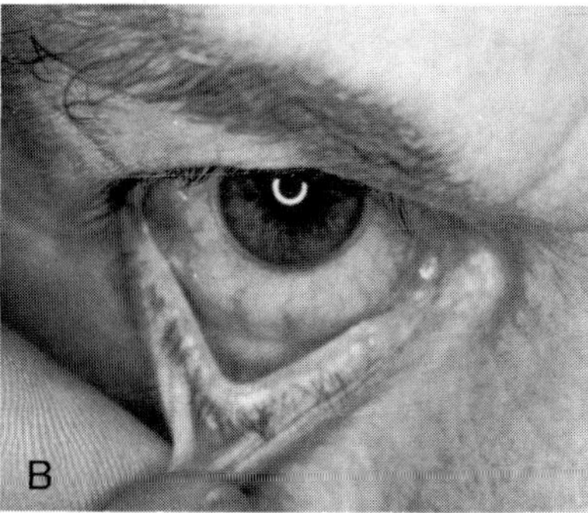
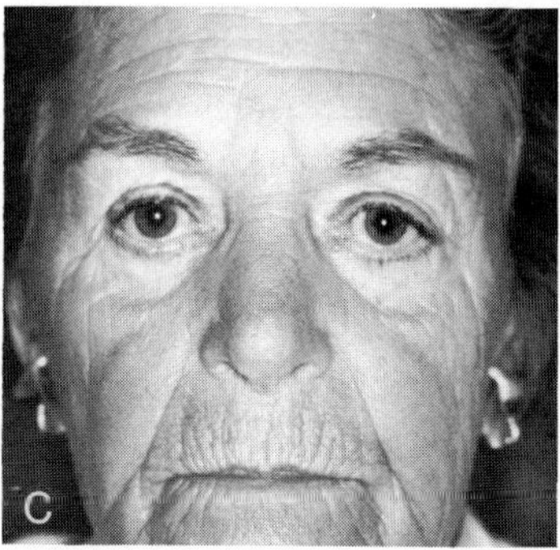

Figure 34–69. *A,* A patient with lower eyelid laxity and scleral show. *B,* The lower lid laxity is demonstrated by gentle anterior traction of the lower eyelid, which produces 8 to 10 mm of distraction from the globe. On release of the lid, there often is poor repositioning to the globe. *C,* The patient one year after four-lid cosmetic blepharoplasty combined with horizontal lid shortening and lateral canthoplasty as illustrated in Figure 34–62*A*. Note that the horizontal lid shortening is performed at the lateral canthus, and therefore no lid margin scar is produced.

lid shortening is performed, and fixation to the lateral orbital periosteum is accomplished at the inner aspect of the lateral orbital rim, at a vertical level corresponding to the superior aspect of the pupil in primary position (Fig. 34–71*C*). Upon closure of the lateral canthal skin incisions, the angle of divergence from the original horizontal orientation must be equal and symmetric to ensure lateral canthal and lower eyelid symmetry (Fig. 34–71*D*).

RECONSTRUCTION OF THE LACRIMAL SYSTEM

Anatomic Considerations. The lacrimal system (Figs. 34–72, 34–73) is a tripartite system consisting of those structures involved in the *secretion, distribution,* and *drainage* of tears. Proper tear film maintenance protects the eye and provides a refractive optical surface.

The precorneal tear film, produced by the lacrimal secretory system, is composed of three distinct layers (Fig. 34–74): the superficial lipid, the aqueous, and the mucin layers.

The lacrimal secretory system controls the amount of tears and is divided into basic and reflex secretors. (Viers, 1955; Jones, 1974b).

Basic Secretors. The mucin-secreting goblet cells of the conjunctival tarsus and limbal area contribute most of the lubrication of the lids, and form the innermost fixed polysaccharide layer of the precorneal tear film. This portion of the tear film interacts with the aqueous layer to help stabilize the tear film and prevent rapid desiccation of the cornea. Approximately 50 accessory lacrimal exocrine glands of Krause and Wolfring are located in the subconjunctival space of each upper lid. These form the intermediate aqueous layer, which is 98 per cent water and accounts for 90 per cent of the precorneal tear film. The third and last group of basic tear secretors consists of the oil-producing

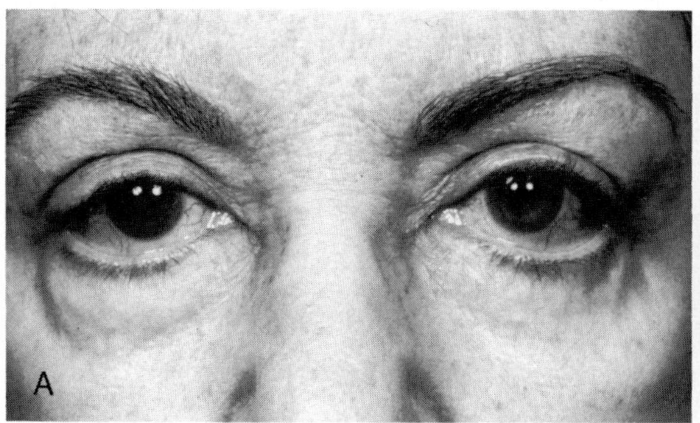
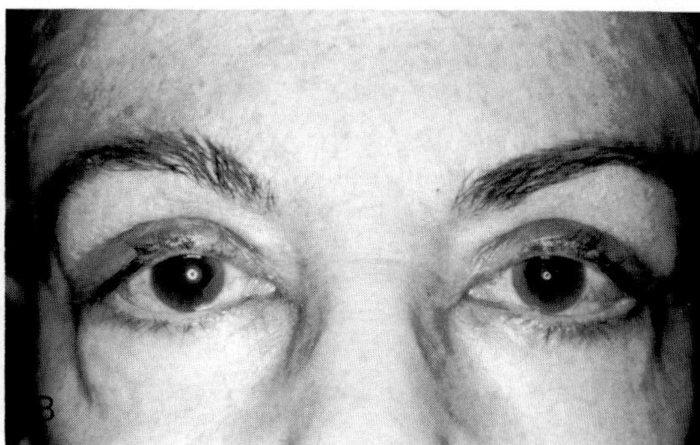

Figure 34–70. *A,* A patient with lower eyelid laxity, lid margin eversion, and scleral show after lower lid blepharoplasty. *B,* After horizontal lid shortening and lateral canthoplasties.

Lateral Canthoplasty

Key Points

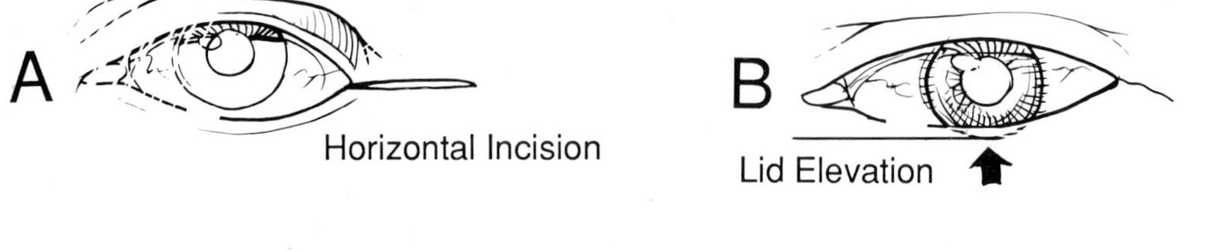

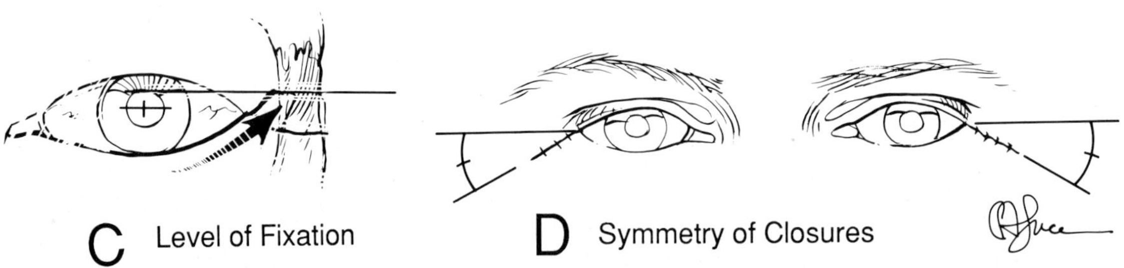

Figure 34–71. The key points to achieve symmetric lateral canthal repositioning. *A,* The lateral canthal and lower eyelid incision should be horizontal. *B,* The lid is elevated to cover 1 to 2 mm of the inferior limbus. *C,* The level of fixation to the lateral orbital periosteum is at a level corresponding to the superior aspect of the pupil in primary position. *D,* On closure of the lateral canthal skin incisions, the angle of divergence from the original horizontal orientation must be equal and symmetric to ensure lateral canthal and lower eyelid symmetry.

meibomian glands (approximately 20 in each lid) and the palpebral glands of Zeis and Moll. These glands produce the outermost lipid layer of the precorneal tear film, a very thin layer composed of cholesterol and cholesterol esters. The superficial lipid layer helps stabilize the tear film and retards evaporation of the underlying aqueous layer.

Figure 34–72. The lacrimal drainage system.

Basic tear secretion is the fundamental, indispensable function of the lacrimal secretory system. The basic secretors can produce all three layers of the precorneal tear film without the assistance of the reflex secretors. There is no known efferent nerve supply to the basic secretors; however, it is believed that mucin secretion increases in response to inflammation.

Reflex Secretors. These consist of the exocrine, parasympathetically innervated lacrimal glands. The main lacrimal gland connects to the palpebral portion of the gland by two to six excretory ducts. The palpebral portion of the gland empties into the upper lateral conjunctival cul-de-sac through 15 to 40 small excretory ducts (see Fig. 34–73). When basic lacrimal secretion is inadequate, corneal and conjunctival desiccation and its sensory awareness stimulate an increase in

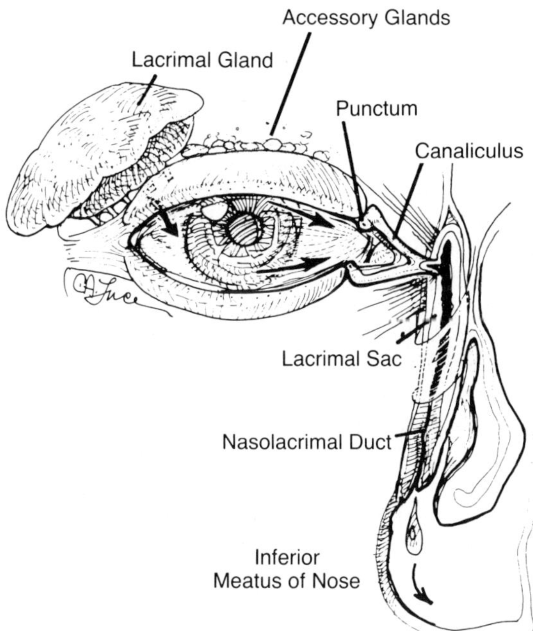

Figure 34–73. The lacrimal production, distribution, and drainage systems.

lacrimal gland output. This phenomenon explains the paradoxical situation of increased tearing in a dry eye state. When basic secretion is normal, further sensory stimulation of the cornea or conjunctiva causes increased lacrimal gland output. This response helps protect against damage from trauma, inflammation, foreign bodies, chemicals, noxious gases, heat, and wind.

Holly and Lemp (1971, 1973), Holly (1973), and Holly, Lamberts, and Price (1980) showed that the three-layered tear film is formed between blinks. When the eyelids close, each lid is stretched as it moves medially. During closure, the posterior lid margins are held tightly against the globe, squeezing the outer two layers off and rubbing mucus onto the corneal surface. Because the layer of mucus is hydrophilic, it aids in rapidly reforming the remainder of the precorneal tear film upon eyelid opening.

Thinning of the precorneal tear film occurs as a result of fluid movement into the fornices and evaporation between blinks. If blinking is prevented, observable areas of desiccation appear on the corneal surface. These dry spots represent focal areas of disruption of the tear film composition that become hydrophobic, causing the aqueous layer to retract. If blinking is further prevented, larger areas of tear film discontinuity develop, predisposing to more corneal desiccation and eventual epithelial damage. It is obvious that the precorneal tear film exhibits a dynamic role in the functional physiology of the eye.

The passage of tears into the nose occurs via the lacrimal drainage system. The tears collect along the border of each lid, and during blinking the fluid moves medially toward the upper and lower puncta and the lacrimal lake, assisted by the pressure of the lids against the globe. The orbicularis muscles also furnish the motor power for the lacrimal pump mechanism (see Fig. 34–9). The canaliculi are approximately 10 mm long, and consist of a vertical part 2 mm long and a horizontal component 8 mm long (see Fig. 34–73). The vertical part of each canaliculus

Figure 34–74. The composition of the precorneal tear film. (Modified from Holly, F. J., and Lemp, M. A.: Tear physiology and dry eyes. Surv. Ophthalmol., *22*:70, 1977.)

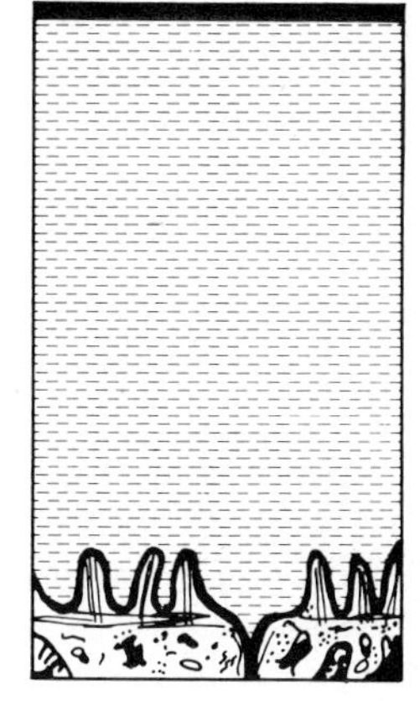

Superficial Lipid Layer

Source: Meibomian, Zeiss, Moll glands

Composition: Cholesterol (esters)

Function: Retard evaporation
Tear film stability

Aqueous Layer

Source: Main and accessory lacrimal glands

Composition: Inorganic salts, glucose, oxygen, proteins in aqueous solution

Function: Protective lubrication

Mucin Layer

Source: Conjunctival goblet cells

Composition: Mucous

Function: Interacts with aqueous layer to stabilize tear film begins with the punctum and lies in the apex of the lacrimal papilla. It is about 0.3 mm in diameter and is surrounded by a ring of elastic connective tissue. The lumen widens to form the ampulla, which is 2 to 3 mm in its greatest diameter. The horizontal part with the ampulla is 8 mm long and 0.5 mm in diameter. In 90 per cent of patients, both canaliculi join to form a single common duct that opens into the lacrimal sac just posterior and superior to the center of the lateral wall of the sac. The canaliculi and sac are lined with stratified squamous epithelium (see Figs. 34–57, 34–72, 34–73).

The lacrimal sac lodged in the lacrimal groove and the nasolacrimal duct are anatomically a single structure, with a wide fundus that extends 3 to 5 mm above the level of the medial canthal tendon. The isthmus is a narrowing of the sac just before it becomes the interosseous nasolacrimal duct. The combined length of the lacrimal sac and nasolacrimal duct is approximately 30 mm. The general direction is slightly lateral and backward as the nasolacrimal duct descends into the nasal cavity under the inferior turbinate to open via the valve of Hasner (see Figs. 34–72, 34–73).

Epiphora is the accumulation of tears that are not evacuated from the lacrimal lake and spill over the lower eyelid onto the cheek. The causes are varied and include obstruction of any portion of the lacrimal excretory system, paralysis of the orbicularis muscles and subsequent loss of the lacrimal pumping mechanism, and inflammatory conditions of the conjunctiva. It is noteworthy, however, that epiphora may be absent even when the lacrimal sac has been destroyed or removed.

Excretory Deformities and Developmental Defects

The excretory lacrimal passages are formed from a thickening of ectoderm in the naso-optic fissure. This cord buries itself in the mesenchyme, separating from the surface ectoderm as the lateral nasal and maxillary processes fuse. The cord thickens as it develops, and divides to form the duct and canaliculi extending through the mesenchyme from the medial canthus to the nasal fossa. The passages canalize just before birth.

The puncta may be absent or may appear only as a surface dimple separated slightly from the canaliculus. In adults it may be difficult to distinguish between congenital absence of the puncta and acquired stenosis. Membranous closure of the puncta may be treated by establishing an opening using the dissecting microscope. It is often clinically impossible to determine whether the canaliculi are absent or have failed to reach the surface. If an opening cannot be found, retrograde probing becomes necessary. A skin incision is made down to the lacrimal sac, and a probe is passed through the common canaliculus. If a duct is located, the probe is passed toward the punctum, and a small incision is made over the probe. A small silicone tube is inserted and left in place for approximately eight weeks. If both puncta are located, one can use a single piece of silicone tubing that bridges between the two puncta in an encircling fashion so that the ends lie in the lacrimal sac (Fig. 34–75). The silicone tubing is usually well tolerated and may be removed when desired. The silicone tube functions as a stent to maintain the patency of the canaliculi. If no canaliculi are found, a conjunctivodacryocystostomy, or direct connection of the lacrimal sac to the conjunctival sac, is required.

A membrane at the lower end of the nasolacrimal duct is the most common developmental defect encountered in the pediatric age group. Relief is usually achieved by passing a small probe down the passage and perforating the membrane (Fig. 34–76). If this fails, it may be concluded that a more extensive defect is present. The use of silicone tube placements in 150 patients with congenital nasolacrimal obstruction, canalicular lac-

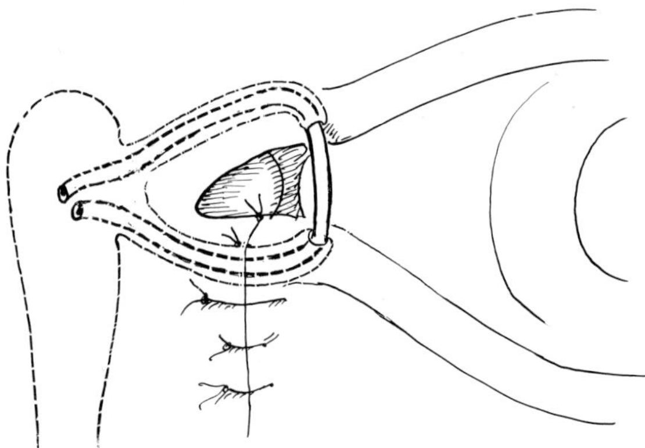

Figure 34–75. Technique of maintaining the patency of the canaliculus after repair consists of placing a silicone tube in a circular fashion into the upper and lower canaliculi.

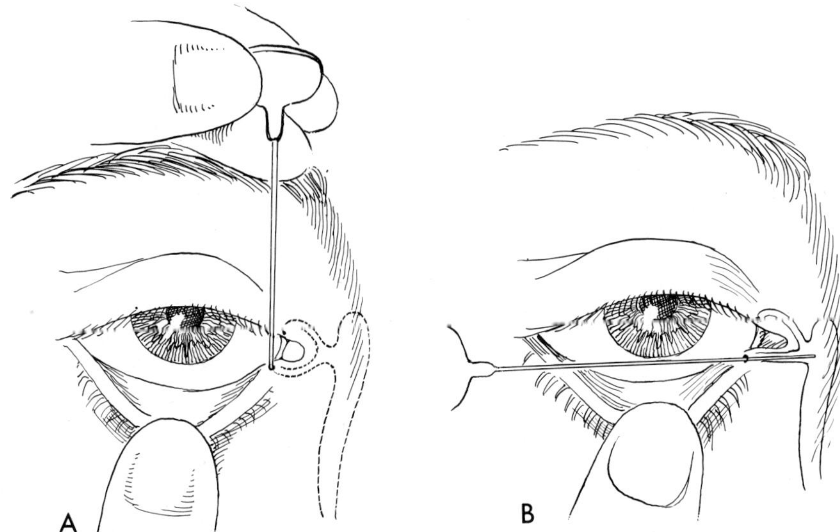

Figure 34–76. Probing the canaliculus. Successive positions assumed by the probe: first vertically *(A),* then horizontally *(B).* The probe is then directed vertically and advanced through the nasolacrimal system.

erations, primary canalicular disease, or complicated dacryocystorhinostomies was shown by Pashby and Rathbun (1979) to be helpful. Abnormalities of the lacrimal system in craniofacial malformations were studied by Whitaker, Katowitz, and Randall (1974).

Diagnostic Tests

The plastic surgeon dealing with nasoethmoido-orbital fractures or penetrating lacerations that have injured or obstructed the excretory lacrimal system should be familiar with tests to evaluate the patency of this system. Before specific testing, an objective and subjective evaluation of the tear quality and quantity should be performed. In addition, lid position and evidence of trichiasis, punctal stenosis, lagophthalmos, or lid retraction are determined. Palpation of the medial orbital region and pressure on the lacrimal sac may express mucous or purulent material into the conjunctival sac—strong evidence of nasolacrimal duct obstruction. Placing lateral traction on the eyelids while palpating the medial canthal tendon helps determine whether the medial canthal tissues are intact (Furnas and Bircoll, 1973). There is a high association of lacrimal disruption with medial canthal tendon disruption.

Dye Disappearance Test. A drop of 2 per cent fluorescein solution is placed in each conjunctival sac, and the clearance time is recorded. The dye should disappear within five minutes. Asymmetric or delayed clearance is diagnostic of a functional or anatomic obstruction of the nasolacrimal system.

Primary Dye Test (Jones I Test). This is helpful in determining the passive functional outflow of the lacrimal system. A cotton-tipped applicator, or a thin copper wire applicator with a small amount of cotton moistened with 4 per cent cocaine, is carefully introduced under the inferior turbinate at the opening of the nasolacrimal duct (valve of Hasner), which is situated approximately 4 cm from the nostril, anteriorly to the highest point of the cavity of the inferior turbinate. A solution of 2 per cent fluorescein dye is instilled into both conjunctival fornices and recovered after five minutes from the inferior turbinate cotton if the system is patent. If no dye is recovered, the test is considered negative and is indicative of a functional block. However, it does not exclude an anatomic block of the lacrimal outflow system.

Secondary Dye Test (Jones II Test). This test determines the anatomic patency of the lacrimal system. It is performed immediately after a negative Jones I test, and requires dilation and irrigation of the superior or inferior canaliculus via a lacrimal cannula and syringe with clear saline solution. Observation of the amount of fluid injected, the amount of reflux via the opposite canaliculus, and the time lapse until the patient tastes the fluid assist in the diagnosis of partial or complete obstruction of the lacrimal outflow system. If fluid without fluorescein dye is recovered, the dye could not have reached the lacrimal sac, and therefore a functional obstruction of the punctocanalicular system is present. This condition is usually observed in orbicularis oculi paralysis when the lacrimal pump mechanism is malfunctioning. Canalicular bypass by means of a conjunctivodacryocystorhinostomy is necessary to correct this situation.

Schirmer I or Schirmer II Test. These tests provide objective evidence of the lacrimal secretory capacity and are used in combination with tear break-up time, fluorescein disappearance, lysozyme assay, and rose bengal staining to evaluate tear deficiency states (Jelks and McCord, 1981).

Repair of Lacrimal Apparatus

The plastic surgeon is frequently involved in treating disturbances of the lacrimal system caused by trauma. In all acute trauma involving the nasoethmoido-orbital area, injury to the lacrimal system must be considered a possibility and verification of the integrity of the lacrimal system should be routine (see Chap. 27). Injuries to the lacrimal system occur most frequently in nasoethmoido-orbital fractures; in glass fragment, razor, or knife lacerations; in sports injuries; and through fragments impelled by high explosives. Direct trauma to the nasoethmoido-orbital region may fragment and fracture the bony nasolacrimal apparatus, which often leads to a chronic dacryocystitis requiring secondary reconstruction. Immediate diagnosis and treatment may be rendered impossible when hemorrhage, ecchymosis, and local tissue swelling are severe. In such cases, management may be deferred for several hours. However, with modern techniques of reconstruction, late treatment of lacrimal obstruction is usually successful.

Injury to the secretory portion of the lacrimal system is rare because the lacrimal gland is protected by the bony orbital rim. Lacrimal gland involvement in zygomaticofrontal fractures was described by Briggs and Heckler (1987), who recommended careful dissection and repositioning of the gland in the orbital cavity while the fracture is reduced.

Avulsion of the medial canthus is often complicated by transection of the upper or lower canaliculus (Fig. 34–77). Transection of the lid margin between the punctum and the medial canthus, disrupting the continuity of the canaliculus, also occurs in direct blunt trauma to the periocular tissues (Fig. 34–78). The orbicularis oculi muscle tends to enlarge the area of laceration and produce ectropion. Cicatricial coloboma with epiphora is frequent when the wound is not treated primarily. Canalicular injuries should be treated acutely with the assistance of loupe or operating microscope magnification. The punctum can usually be located and dilated to allow passage of a probe to identify the lumen of the canaliculus. The medial end of the lacerated canaliculus may be difficult to identify even with magnification, because it tends to retract deeply into the medial canthal tissues. After the tissues have become more edematous and hemorrhagic, identification of the

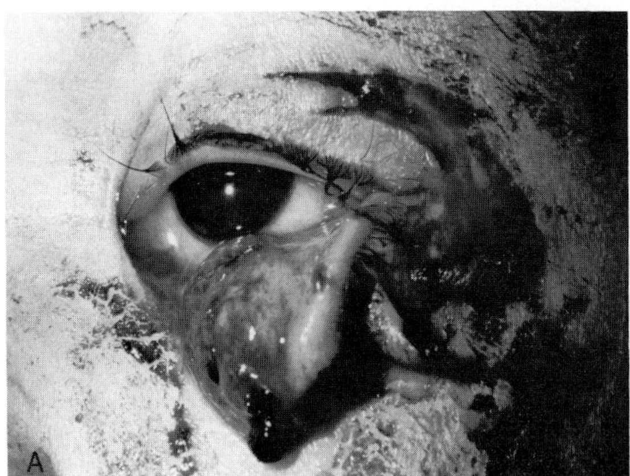

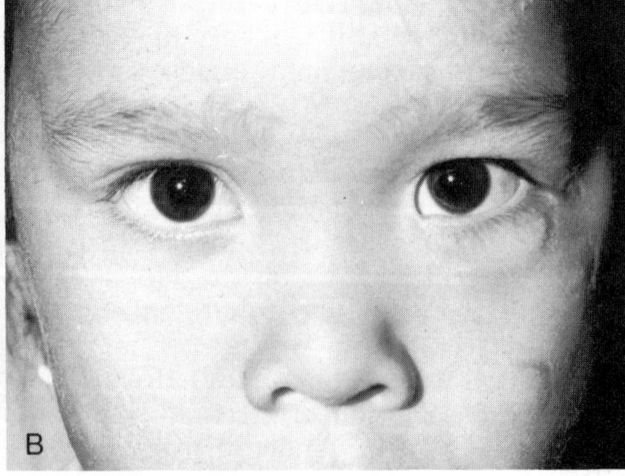

Figure 34–77. *A,* A 3 year old child attacked by a dog, sustaining laceration and avulsion of the left lower eyelid from the medial canthus. The canaliculus was also avulsed from its junction with the common internal punctum. *B,* Six months after repair of the injury by the technique illustrated in Figure 34–79. Microscopic controlled canalicular repair and encircling microsilicone intubation was also performed (see Figs. 34–78, 34–80, and 34–84).

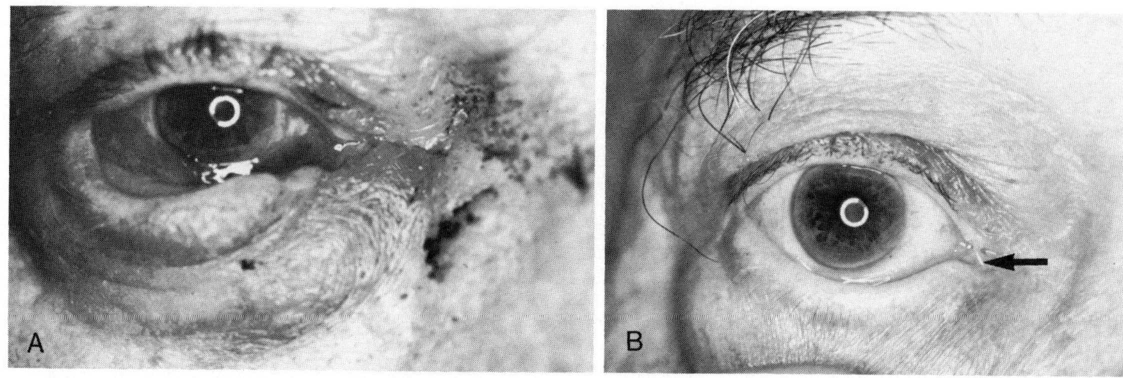

Figure 34–78. *A,* A patient with avulsion-laceration of the right lower lid and lower canaliculus. *B,* After repair of the avulsed canthal tissues and canalicular repair over an encircling microsilicone tube. The arrow points to the silicone tube exiting the upper canaliculus to enter a horizontally enlarged punctum of the lower canaliculus.

retracted canalicular stump is usually not possible. Therefore, canalicular lacerations should be repaired within a few hours. Irrigation of fluid or air through the intact upper canaliculus may assist in identifying the divided medial stump.

The most popular method of canalicular laceration repair requires passage of silicone tubing swedged onto a metal stent (Crawford tubes) in an encircling fashion through the canalicular-lacrimal system. The intact canaliculus is intubated and the metal probe is passed through the nasolacrimal duct to exit under the inferior meatus. The opposite end of the tubing is then passed through the punctum of the lacerated canaliculus and subsequently out of the temporal cut end. It is next passed into the lumen of the medial cut end of the canaliculus, lacrimal sac, and nasolacrimal duct to exit the inferior meatus, thus creating an encircling element. Appropriate tension placed on the tubing often approximates the cut ends of the canaliculus so that 9-0 nylon sutures can be placed. It is also recommended to suture the deep tissues of the lid and the cut ends of the medial canthal tendon to reduce tension on the canalicular repair. If the medial canthal tendon is difficult to locate, an additional incision is made over the frontal process of the maxilla. The proximal portion of the tendon is exposed and dissected as shown in Figure 34–79. If there is excessive tension on the canalicular repair, a selective cantholysis of the inferior crus of the lateral canthal tendon is performed (see Fig. 34–24).

When the canalicular system is surgically removed during the extirpation of medial canthal tumors, immediate reconstruction is mandatory with the use of the silicone encircling method (Fig. 34–80).

The Worst (1962) pigtail probe is a sharply

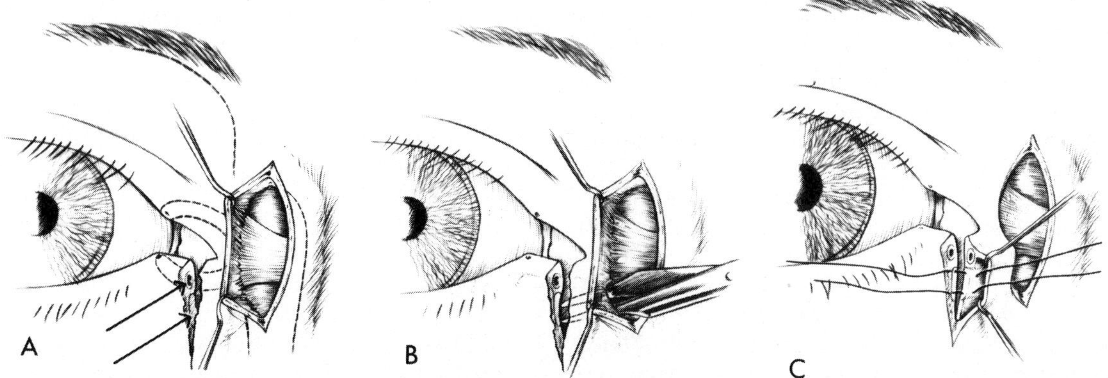

Figure 34–79. Treatment of a sectioned lower eyelid canaliculus and medial canthal tendon. *A,* The upper arrow indicates the sectioned canaliculus; the lower arrow indicates the sectioned portion of the medial canthal tendon. An incision has been made medially to expose the uninjured portion of the tendon. *B,* The dissection, extended laterally, facilitates exposure of the severed tendon. *C,* The severed tendon is sutured in an overcorrected position to the medial canthal tissues. The canaliculus is repaired with microscopic magnification over a microsilicone tube.

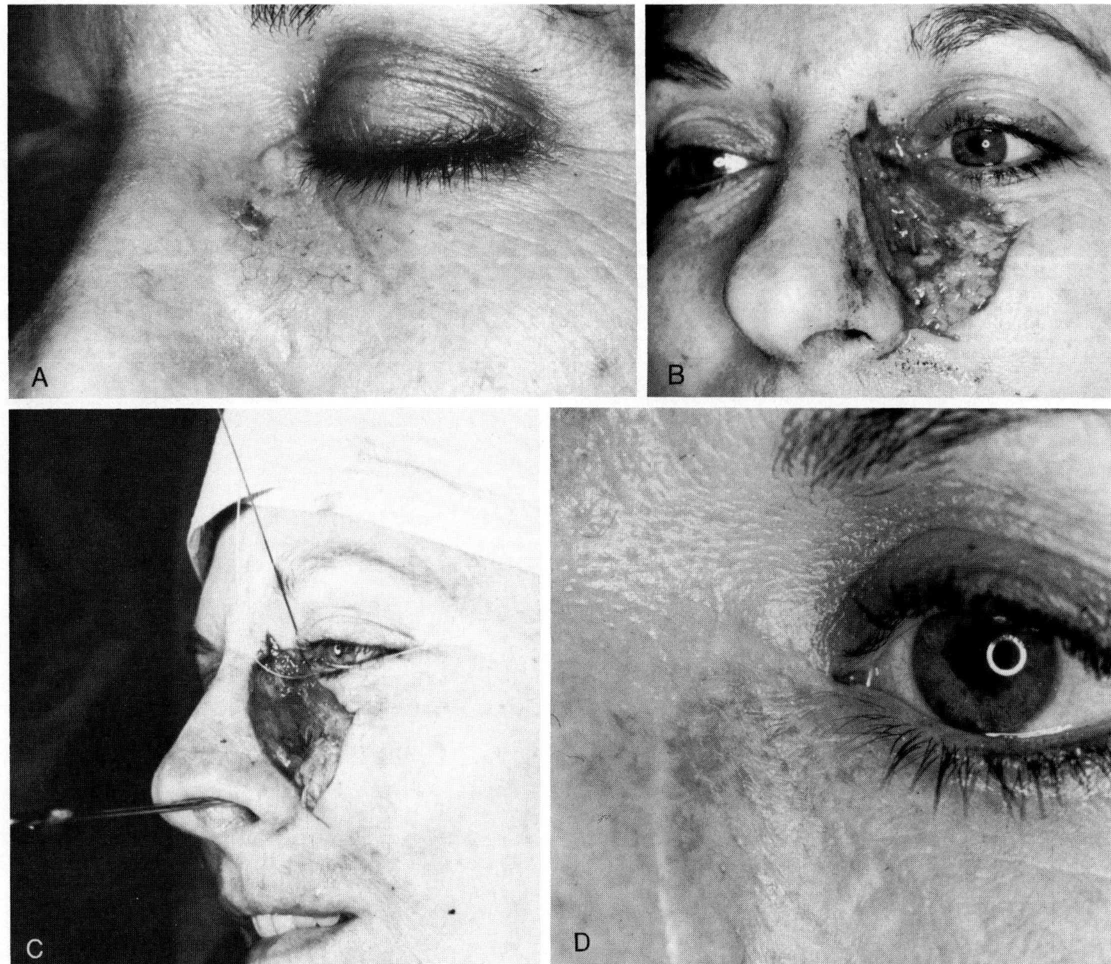

Figure 34–80. *A,* A patient with a recurrent medial canthal, cheek, and nasal basal cell carcinoma. *B,* After resection of the tumor with frozen section control. The inferior canaliculus has been sacrificed. *C,* A microsilicone tube swedged onto stainless steel probes is being passed through the canalicular system in an encircling fashion to stent the repair of the lower canaliculus. Note that retrieval of the probe from below the inferior turbinate is facilitated with the use of a grooved director. *D,* Seven months after reconstruction, before removal of the silicone tube. The skin defect was covered with a full-thickness skin graft. Note the silicone tubes passing from the upper to the lower canaliculus.

curved instrument that is inserted into the punctum of the unaffected canaliculus, into the common canaliculus, and back through the severed canaliculus, where it emerges into the area of the laceration. Silicone tubing is then passed through the punctum of the cut canaliculus and exits next to the pigtail probe to which it is affixed. Upon withdrawal of the pigtail probe, the canalicular system, including the laceration, is stented. The externalized silicone tubes are sutured together and are removed after several weeks. Beard (1967) confirmed excellent results from the use of this probe. In expert hands the instrument is useful, but considerable damage may be caused by inexpert use. Other methods of canalicular stenting include a Viers or Johnson metal rod (Anderson and Edwards, 1979b). Placement of an encircling silicone tube is the preferred technique.

Cicatricial stenosis of the punctum may result from lacerations of the medial lid. Isolated closure or stenosis of the punctum may be alleviated by a vertical stab in the papilla lacrimalis, but retrograde probing may be required for accurate location. Jones (1962) advocated the "end-snip" operation, in which a vertical 2 mm cut is made in the conjunctival wall of the canaliculus. He believed this technique superior to the "three-snip" procedure (Stallard, 1940), since it preserves the capillary attraction valve of the vertical canaliculus and the pumping action of the ampulla.

Dacryocystitis occurs when the lacrimal sac contents become infected. Acute dacryocystitis associated with redness, swelling, and pain occur with associated edema of the entire orbital area and occasional closure of the eyelids (Fig. 34–81). Warm compresses and antibiotics appropriate to culture and sensitivity are indicated. Incision and drainage should be performed only when the purulent collection cannot be controlled with local wound care and systemic antibiotics. Incision and drainage of the lacrimal sac via a skin approach may cause the development of a cutaneolacrimal fistula. A suppurating lacrimal sac is a source of constant danger because even a slight abrasion of the cornea may become infected and ulcerated by the contaminated lacrimal fluid.

The lacrimal sac becomes dilated when the nasolacrimal duct is obstructed, and part of its contents flows back through the lacrimal puncta into the palpebral fissure. Fluid injected into the lower canaliculus should pass through the lacrimal system and appear when the patient blows his nose. If pressure over the sac causes a backflow of this fluid through the canaliculi, there may be an obstruction without infection. If the sac is very dilated and difficult to evacuate, the mucoid contents indicate chronic obstruction. This condition is designated a lacrimal sac mucocele or dacryomucocele. The enlarged sac forms a visible and palpable mass in the medial canthal region (Fig. 34–82). A viscous fluid characteristic of the presence of a mucocele may be expressed by digital pressure over the swollen sac; this will help prevent an acute infection.

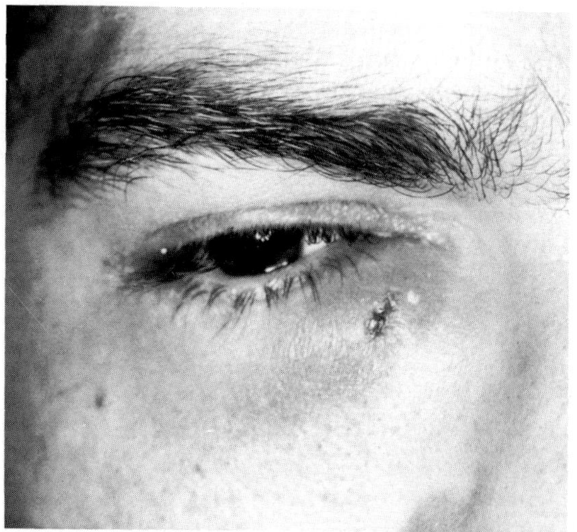

Figure 34–81. A patient with acute dacryocystitis. Note the swelling, induration, and inflammatory reaction overlying the lacrimal sac.

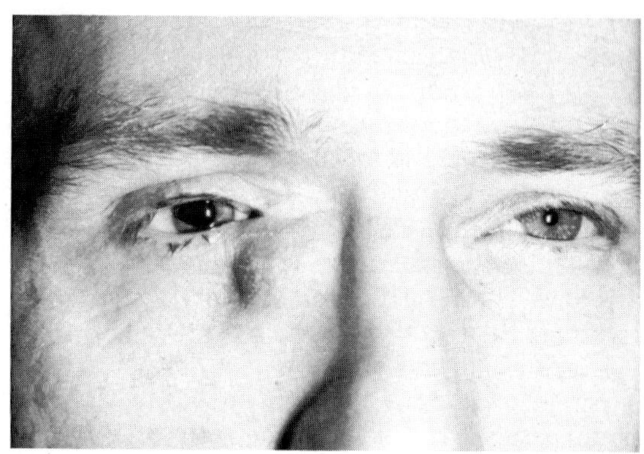

Figure 34–82. A patient with a chronic lacrimal sac mucocele. Note the relative lack of inflammatory reaction of the periorbital region.

The treatment of dacryocystitis must include dilation of the puncta with probing and irrigation of the lacrimal system. This can be performed under topical or infiltration anesthesia with appropriate sedation. The puncta is first dilated until a thin Bowman's probe can be introduced into the canaliculus. The probe is directed vertically, rotated 90 degrees, and advanced medially while the lower lid and canaliculus are stretched laterally. The probe is pressed forward until it reaches the sac. Penetration into the sac is evidenced by contact of the tip of the probe with the bony medial wall of the orbit. At this point the probe is elevated to the vertical position and inclined slightly forward to enter the nasolacrimal duct, which inclines posteriorly and laterally (see Fig. 34–76). The probing must be done carefully to avoid perforation of the canaliculus, lacrimal sac, or thin medial orbital wall. After the probe has reached the junction of the lacrimal sac and nasolacrimal duct, it is removed, and saline or an anesthetic agent is injected through the canaliculus with a lacrimal cannula. If the fluid passes into the nose, elimination of the obstacle in the nasolacrimal duct has occurred and further probing should be discontinued.

The appropriate treatment of chronic dacryocystitis is surgery, replacing the former method of periodic probing to relieve obstruction. However, extirpation of the sac may be necessary when it is irretrievably damaged by multiple lacerations and scarring, or by prolonged suppuration and necrosis.

Dacryocystorhinostomy is an operation often required in patients with nasolacrimal obstruction. The indications, according to Jones (1974b), are (1) primarily for lacerations of the common canaliculus; (2) for acute and chronic dacryocystitis; (3) for complete obstruction of either the lacrimal sac or the nasolacrimal duct; (4) for paralysis of the lacrimal pump, such as occurs in facial paralysis; and (5) for nasoethmoido-orbital fractures in which the continuity of the nasolacrimal duct may be interrupted.

Toti (1904) introduced dacryocystorhinostomy, allowing the tears to enter the nose by perforating the lacrimal groove. Mosher (1915, 1923) improved on the procedure by a technique in which the anterior margin of the opening in the sac was approximated with catgut sutures to the anterior margin of the bony opening. Further modification of this operation by Dupuy-Dutemps and Bourguet (1921) produced a higher percentage of successes and involved careful anastomosis of the nasal mucous membrane to the edges of the lacrimal sac. This technique (Fig. 34–83) is preferred because it ensures an epithelia-lined passage between the lacrimal sac and the nasal cavity.

Dacryocystorhinostomy may be performed under local or general anesthesia. The nasal cavity is inspected with a nasal speculum and headlight illumination to determine whether middle turbinate hypertrophy or septal deviation is present. These conditions must be remedied before dacryocystorhinostomy is performed. Nasal packing soaked in 4 per cent cocaine is inserted into the involved side. The lacrimal punctum is dilated and the patency of the proximal canalicular system confirmed before a dilute solution of methylene blue is instilled into the lacrimal sac under moderate pressure. A skin incision is made slightly below the medial canthal tendon and extended downward and slightly outward for approximately 25 mm. The incision is extended by sharp and blunt dissection to the underlying periosteum of the frontal process of the maxilla and the anterior lacrimal crest. The angular vessels are retracted or ligated as required. A subperiosteal dissection is performed posteriorly over the lacrimal groove as far as the posterior lacrimal crest and inferiorly into the nasolacrimal canal.

The nasal cavity is again inspected with the aid of a nasal speculum and headlight illumination. A local anesthetic solution containing 1:100,000 epinephrine is injected beneath the mucoperiosteum lining the frontal process of the maxilla. An incision is made intranasally near the base of the frontal process, and the mucoperiosteum is elevated upward and backward to the area of the lacrimal groove. A small epinephrine-soaked gauze pack is placed into this tunnel and left in position until the nasal mucosa is incised.

The bone forming the anterior lacrimal crest and the wall of the lacrimal groove is removed with an air drill and trephine or bur, exposing the gauze protecting the nasal mucosa (Fig. 34–83*B*). The most important area of bone to remove is that situated in front of the posterior lacrimal crest. Bone beneath the medial canthal tendon is removed without detaching the tendon by means of bone-biting instruments. Bone is also removed from the nasolacrimal canal for a distance of at least 5 mm below the opening of the common canaliculus into the lacrimal sac. This point is determined by passing a Bowman's probe through one canaliculus and tenting the medial wall of the sac. An opening is made into the lacrimal sac with a pointed knife blade immediately lateral to the tip of the probe. Scissors are used to extend the incision to the top of the fundus and the bottom of the nasolacrimal duct to create anterior and posterior lacrimal sac flaps. At this time the Bowman's probe should be visualized entering the lacrimal sac in direct line with the rhinostomy. Silicone tubes can now be placed within the punctocanalicular system if any possible common canalicular stenosis exists (see the discussion of canaliculodacryocystorhinostomy below). A parallel incision with H extensions is made through the nasal mucoperiosteum, creating posterior and anterior flaps that are anastomosed to the corresponding posterior and anterior lacrimal flaps with fine catgut sutures (Fig. 34–83*E*). The subcutaneous tissue and skin are closed separately.

When the medial orbital wall has been disrupted or disorganized as the result of previous nasoethmoido-orbital fractures, the bone landmarks are lost and the lacrimal sac may be abnormally scarred. In these situations, the ideal dacryocystorhinostomy with a completely epithelially lined continuity from the lacrimal sac to the nasal cavity may not be possible to obtain. In some cases, only posterior flaps can be joined with a single flap from the nasal mucosa; in others only an anterior lacrimal sac flap may be sutured to the nasal mucosa.

Failures of the dacryocystorhinostomy can

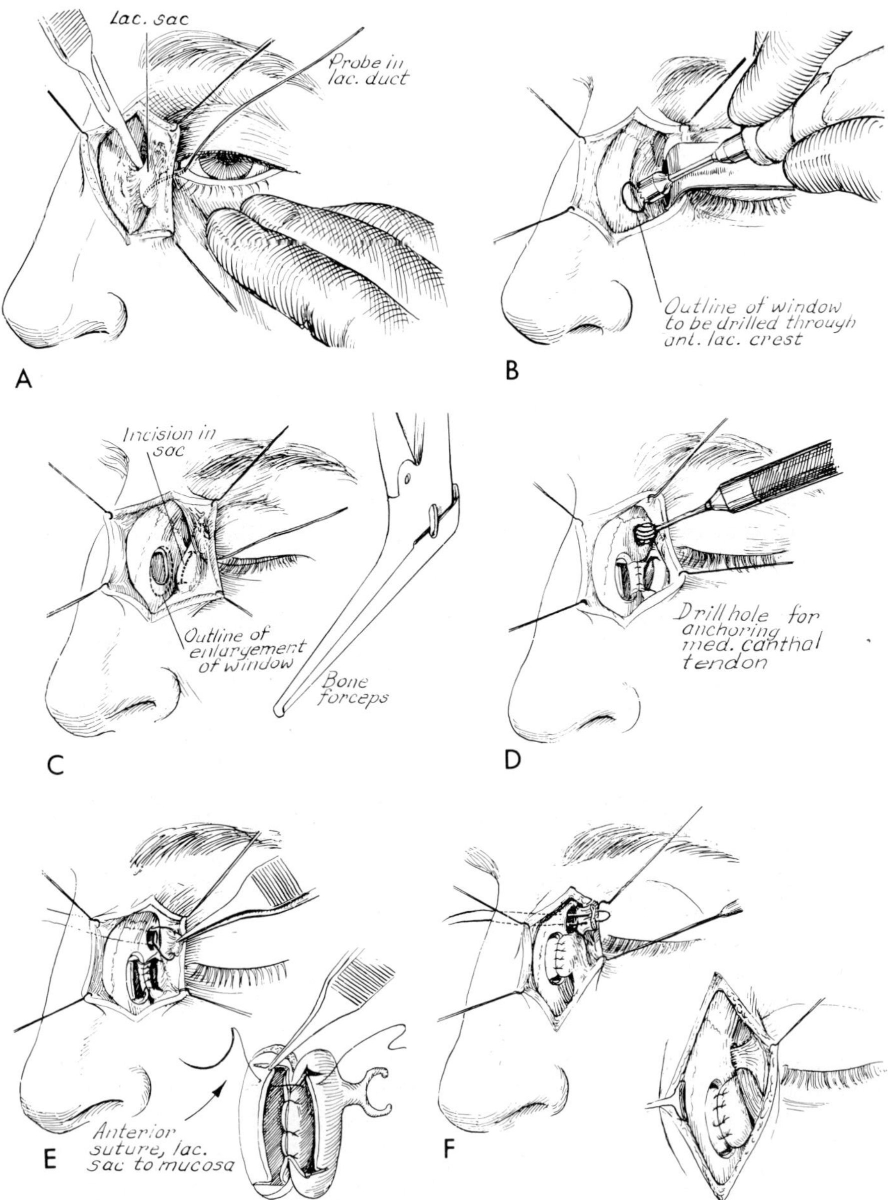

Figure 34–83. Technique of dacryocystorhinostomy combined with medial canthoplasty and canthopexy. *A,* Exposure of the medial orbital wall. The lacrimal probe placed into the lower lacrimal punctum (or an injection of methylene blue into the sac) helps to identify the lacrimal sac. The sac is dissected and raised from the lacrimal groove. *B,* A circular section of bone approximately 10 mm in diameter is removed from an area situated slightly below and anterior to the lacrimal groove without perforating the nasal mucoperiosteum. *C,* The bony opening is enlarged to a diameter of 15 to 20 mm, the diameter of the sac, which is usually dilated by the accumulation of secretion as a result of the obstruction of the nasolacrimal duct (mucocele). A vertical I-shaped incision is made through the sac and through the nasal mucoperiosteum. *D,* The posterior nasal flap is sutured to the posterior flap of the lacrimal sac. A drill hole is prepared for the attachment of the medial canthal tendon. *E,* The suture of the anterior flaps is begun. The transosseous wires have been passed through the medial canthal tendon. *F,* Suture is completed. The wires are twisted, and traction is exerted from the contralateral medial wall to maintain the fixation of the medial canthal tendon and canthus.

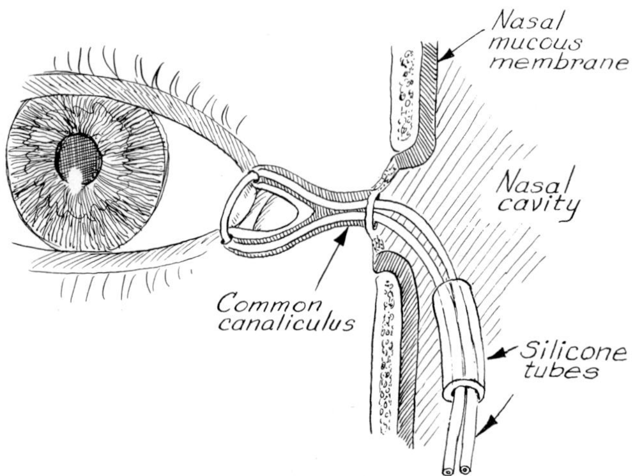

Figure 34–84. A silicone catheter placed through the upper and lower puncta into the canaliculi, maintaining continuity between the common canaliculus and the nasal opening.

be attributed to (1) faulty technique in the establishment of a lacrimal sac–nasal cavity fistula; (2) variations in intranasal anatomy resulting in the lacrimal fistula emptying into an anteriorly positioned ethmoid air cell, or obstructed by an enlarged middle turbinate or deviated nasal septum; (3) an improperly performed fenestration into the nasal cavity that is too small or inappropriately positioned; or (4) concomitant punctocanalicular functional or anatomic blockage.

A *canaliculodacryocystorhinostomy* is performed when a stricture is present at the junction of the common canaliculus and the lacrimal sac. A dacryocystorhinostomy is performed first. After the posterior flaps of the lacrimal sac and the nasal mucosa have been sutured, a metal probe to which a silicone tube has been attached (Crawford tube) is passed through each canaliculus. The end of the probes can be seen tenting the obstruction in the common canaliculus within the lacrimal sac. The obstructing mucosa around the common canaliculus is excised, thus exposing the probes. The probes are pulled through the respective canaliculi to form an encircling loop, which is subsequently passed intranasally and fixed to the mucosa (Fig. 34–84). The anterior flaps are sutured to form the epithelia-lined tract. The silicone tubes are removed after three to six months. The alternative techniques of Werb (1971) and Quickert and Dryden (1970) consist of placing a probe into either canaliculus through the site of obstruction, and subsequently placing a stent of silicone tubes to maintain the patency of the system.

A *conjunctivodacryocystorhinostomy with the insertion of a Pyrex tube* (Jones, 1962) is indicated when both canaliculi are obliterated. It may also be used in patients with facial paralysis and dysfunction of the lacrimal pump mechanism. A dacryocystorhinostomy is performed to the point of suturing the posterior flaps. The caruncle is then excised and a 22 gauge, 30 mm long needle is inserted 2.5 mm posterior to the cutaneous margin of the medial canthus. The needle is pushed in a direction that causes its point to penetrate the nose immediately anterior to the sutured posterior flaps. A knife is used to penetrate the conjunctival sac and enter the lacrimal sac, following the direction of the 22 gauge needle. The knife should incise a passageway above and below just large enough to allow insertion of a Pyrex tube. The distance between the medial canthus and the nasal septum is measured, and a Jones Pyrex tube is chosen to bridge this area. The Pyrex tube is threaded over a Bowman's probe, which is passed through the new opening into the nose via the dacryocystorhinostomy (Fig. 34–85). A 6-0 silk suture is tied around the collar of the Pyrex tube and anchored to the skin of the canthus. After one to three weeks, the Pyrex tube may be replaced with a smaller, shorter, collared version. Jones (1974b) stated that the Pyrex tube is well suited to its role of draining tears into the nose because it (1) has a natural capillary attraction effect on tears, (2) does not collapse or obstruct easily, and (3) causes minimal tissue irritation. The intranasal negative pressure during inspiration is an important factor in assisting the lacrimal flow through the Pyrex tube.

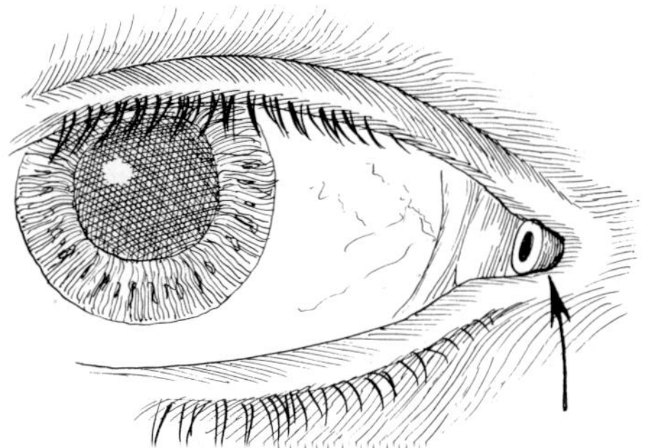

Figure 34–85. Pyrex tube for maintenance of a conjunctivodacryocystorhinostomy (Jones, 1962). The technique is employed when the canaliculi and lacrimal sac are destroyed; it establishes a direct communication between the conjunctival sac and the nasal cavity.

Postoperative care is the most important factor in successful conjunctivodacryocystorhinostomies. The length of the tube should be carefully determined so that it does not make contact with internal structures such as the middle turbinate or nasal septum. The tube should be replaced in one to three weeks with one with a smaller collar (3.5 mm) and just enough length to enter the nasal cavity by 1 to 2 mm. The patient must be instructed not to blow the nose. If the patient is obliged to blow the nose or sneeze, the eyelids must be closed tightly and digital pressure applied over the Pyrex tube to prevent its dislodgement. If the tube becomes obstructed, it can be irrigated with saline solution, or a fine wire can be passed through it.

If the tube becomes extruded, the patient should be seen within 24 hours. The conjunctivorhinostomy opening should be dilated with a probe and the tube reinserted.

Conjunctivitis may occur and is usually due to the formation of granulation tissue around the tube. The tube should be removed and granulation tissue excised before reinsertion of a new tube.

The Pyrex tube technique requires an intact medial (nasal) margin of the lower eyelid. Reconstruction of a defective eyelid should precede any attempt at placing a Pyrex tube.

The patient shown in Figure 34–86 suffered a nasoethmoido-orbital fracture with comminution of the right medial orbital wall and an avulsion-laceration of the medial canthal tendon, with disruption of the lacrimal apparatus. The lacrimal sac mucocele can be seen as a swelling below the medial canthus (Fig. 34–86*A*). During reconstruction of the right medial orbital wall, the lacrimal sac and distal canaliculi at the level of the common canaliculus were resected. The medial canthal tendon was reattached to the medial orbital wall by transosseous wiring (Fig. 34–86*B*). A silicone tube was threaded through both remnants of the canaliculi and passed into the nose. The ends of the tubes were brought out through the right nostril and taped to the cheek (Fig. 34–86*B*; see Fig. 34–84). This procedure was not successful and three months later a conjunctivorhinostomy with a Pyrex tube insertion was performed. The appearance of the patient five years later is shown (Fig. 34–86*C*). This case illustrates the difficulty of late correction of severe anatomic disruption of the medial orbital region by nasoethmoido-orbital fractures with lacrimal and medial canthal involvement. A one-stage, immediate surgical correction gives the best results. This case also shows the contrast between management with a conjunctivorhinostomy in the severely disrupted medial canthal region and that of a conjunctivodacryocystorhinostomy in less damaged or virginal tissues.

EYELID MALPOSITIONS

Disorders or conditions that affect the anatomic position of the eyelid margin and lashes are broadly categorized into eyelid malpositions. Entropion, ectropion, trichiasis, symblepharon, and lid changes associated with orbicularis oculi paralysis are the most commonly encountered eyelid malpositions. The management of these conditions requires a thorough understanding of their associated pathophysiology.

Entropion

Entropion is an inward turning of the eyelid margin and contact of the lashes against the cornea. The friction of the lashes or epidermized lid margin causes ocular irritation and corneal epithelial abrasions. In contrast, *trichiasis* is a condition in which only lashes are turned against the globe and the lid margin remains in a normal position. In *epiblepharon,* an abnormal fold of skin retracts over the lower lid, pushing the lashes onto the cornea. This can be observed in young children and Orientals (Fig. 34–87). *Distichiasis* is a condition in which extra rows of

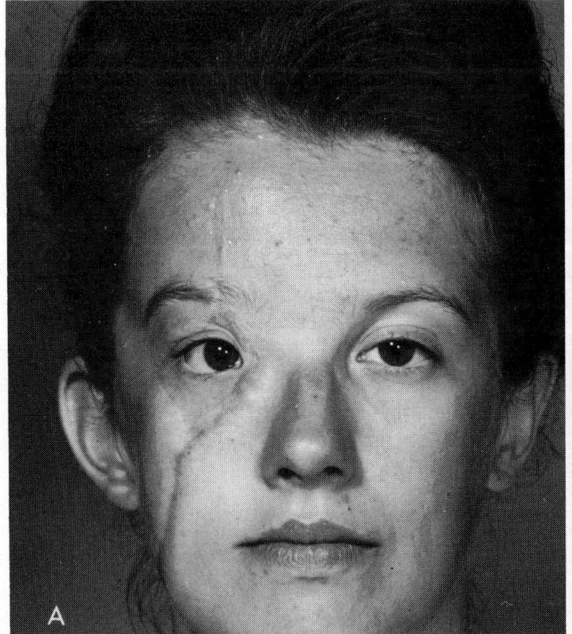

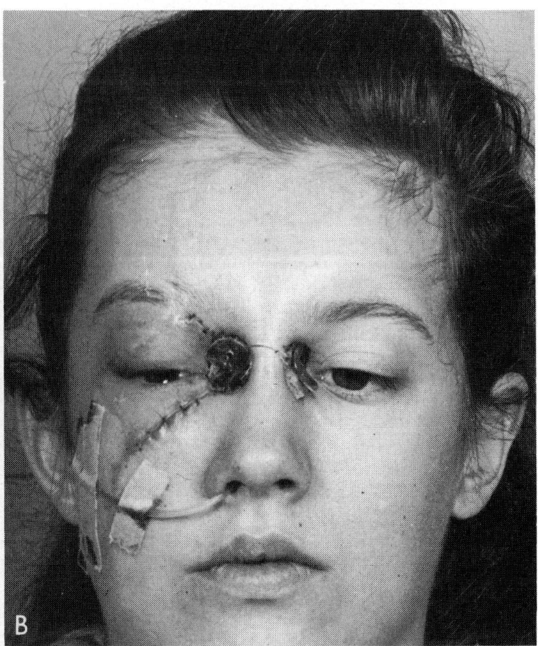

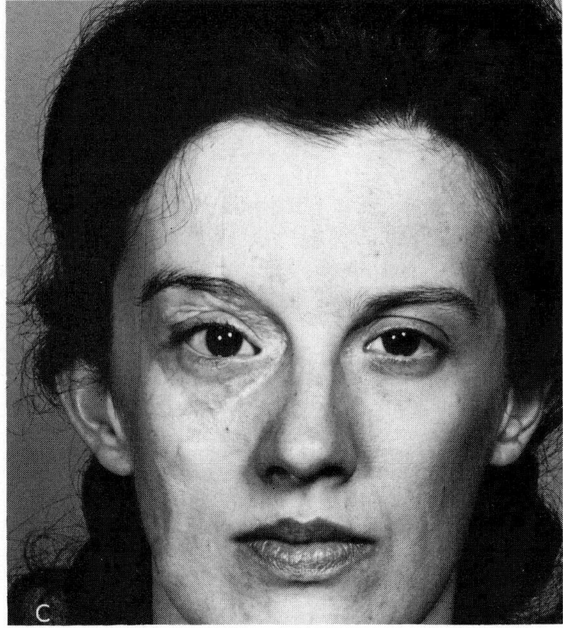

Figure 34–86. *A,* The patient, a 17 year old adolescent female, was a victim of an automobile accident in which she was projected through the windshield after striking the dashboard. She suffered a nasoethmoido-orbital fracture involving the medial wall of the right orbit, severe lacerations of the forehead and cheek, and a penetrating laceration through the medial canthus. Obstruction of the right lacrimal system resulted in a mucocele, which can be seen as a swelling immediately below the medial canthus. Note also the telecanthus on the right side. *B,* After reduction of the fracture and reestablishment of the position of the medial orbital wall, the mucocele was resected. A conjunctivorhinostomy was then performed, placing silicone tubing as illustrated in Figure 34–84. The patient is shown with the tubing taped to the cheek. The cheek laceration has been repaired, and the canthal plates maintained by transosseous wiring are in position. *C,* Reestablished medial canthal region after medial canthoplasty five years after surgery. A Jones Pyrex tube has been placed and maintained in position for a period of two years. The patient no longer needs the Jones tube, as the conjunctivorhinostomy remains patent. (From Converse, J. M., and Smith, B.: Naso-orbital fractures and traumatic deformities of the medial canthus. Plast. Recontr. Surg., *38*:147, 1966.)

eyelashes point inwardly from a normally positioned lid margin (Fig. 34–88).

Entropion is classified into congenital or acquired varieties and may be of the involutional (aging) or cicatricial etiologies (Fig. 34–89). *Congenital entropion* of the lower lid is rare and is due either to lack of a normal tarsal plate or to hypertrophy of the marginal fibers of the orbicularis oculi muscle. The condition is progressive and involves the whole of the lower lid margin. Spasm of the orbicularis oculi is a common clinical finding in this condition. Surgical correction is accomplished by excision of the infratarsal skin and hypertrophied pretarsal orbicularis muscle, with or without a lateral canthoplasty (Fox, 1956). A similar surgical procedure is used to correct *secondary entropion* caused by lack of lid support due to a small or absent globe, or the backward pressure on the ciliary

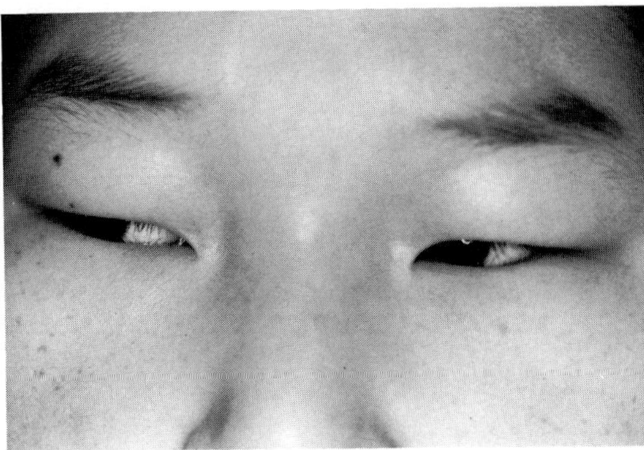

Figure 34–87. A young Oriental patient with epiblepharon of the lower eyelids, causing the lashes to contact the cornea.

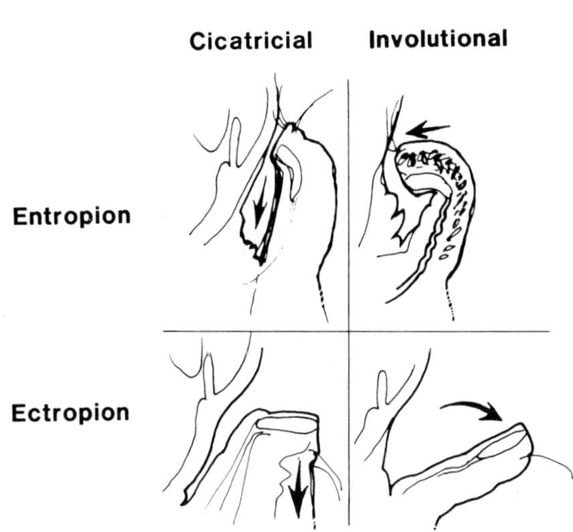

Figure 34–89. Classification of eyelid malpositions: entropion, cicatricial or involutional; ectropion, cicatricial or involutional (see text).

margin by a fold of excess skin with epiblepharon (Fig. 34–90).

Involutional entropion is caused by horizontal lid laxity that develops with advancing age. However, a similar condition known as spastic entropion may occur transiently in younger individuals and signal the eventual development of involutional entropion. The pathophysiologic mechanism of spastic and involutional entropion is the mechanical overriding of the preseptal orbicularis oculi onto the pretarsal orbicularis, causing inward rotation of the lid margin. When the lower eyelid margin rolls inward, the lower border of the tarsus rotates outward. This allows the preseptal orbicularis fibers to migrate further onto the pretarsal area, often forming a tight band that pushes the lid margin against the eye (see Fig. 34–89). Most patients present with a constant entropion and a red, irritated eye (Figs. 34–91, 34–92). Entropion can be intermittent and is usually elicited by having the patient tightly close the eyes. This allows the preseptal orbicularis to ride onto the pretarsal zone, precipitating the entropion (Fig. 34–91).

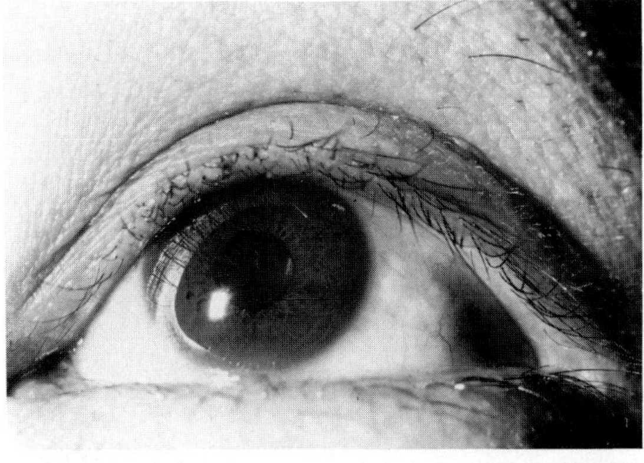

Figure 34–88. A patient with left upper eyelid distichiasis or an abnormal (extra) row of lashes on a normally positioned lid. The lashes may contact the cornea, causing irritation and serious damage.

Cicatricial entropion is caused by scarring of the conjunctiva or the subconjunctiva, which shortens the posterior lamella of the lid and pulls on the lid margin, causing a bowing of the tarsus toward the globe (see Fig. 34–89). The most common causes are trauma, chemical injuries, and inflammatory conditions such as the Stevens-Johnson syndrome, ocular pemphigoid, and ocular rosacea. In these conditions, trichiasis is common. Cicatricial entropion with trichiasis may also result from unsuccessful reconstructive procedures on the eyelids that produce scar tissue retraction of the posterior elements of the lid. Cicatricial entropion may also be caused by symblepharon or an abnormal adhesion of the palpebral and bulbar conjunctival surfaces. Correction of this condition requires release of the conjunctival adhesions and resurfacing of the bare surfaces with mobilized conjunctival flaps or buccal mucosal grafts.

The management of lower lid entropion first requires the determination of whether conjunctival scarring or symblepharon is present. If not, the methods of correction employed depend on the severity of ocular irritation and the degree of horizontal lid laxity.

A nonsurgical eyelid suture method of cor-

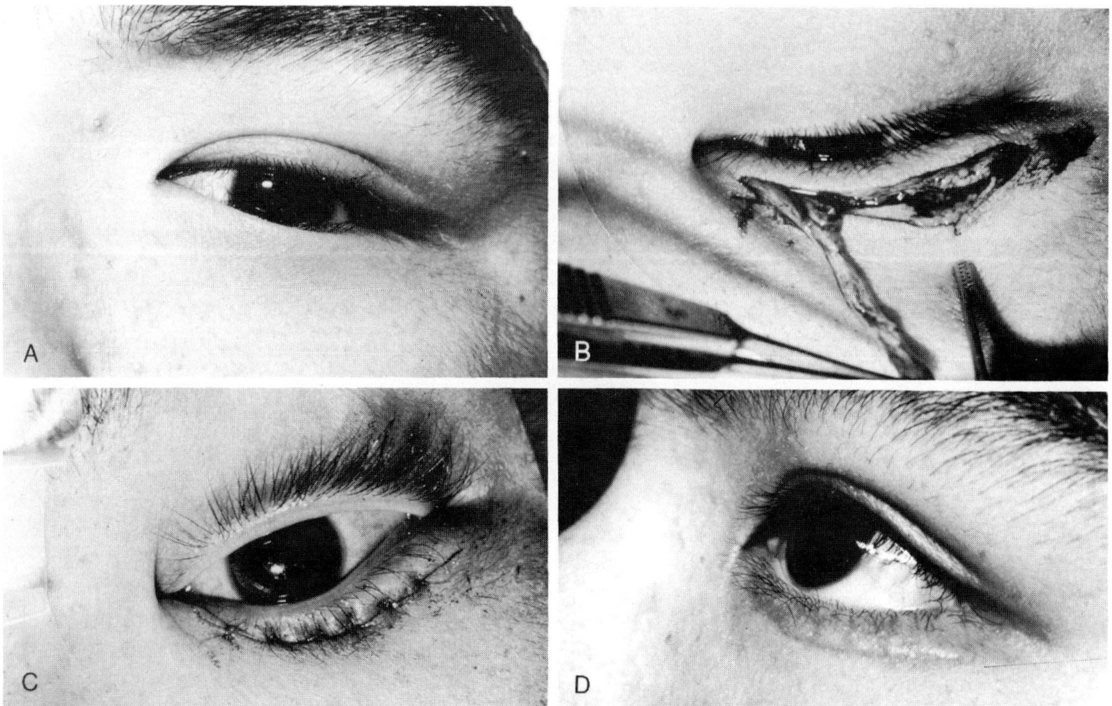

Figure 34–90. *A,* Secondary entropion of the left lower eyelid caused by epiblepharon (see Fig. 34–87). *B,* A strip of infraciliary skin and underlying pretarsal muscle is excised to expose the inferior border of the tarsus and the insertion of the lower eyelid retractors (capsulopalpebral fascia). *C,* Correction of the entropion is accomplished by suturing the infraciliary skin-muscle edge to the inferior border of the tarsus, incorporating the lower lid retractors, as well as the lower skin-muscle edge. *D,* Six months postoperatively, the lash eversion and the relative thinning of the pretarsal area secondary to orbicularis muscle resection are noted.

recting lower eyelid involutional entropion (Quickert and Rathbun, 1971), epiblepharon, and congenital entropion (Quickert, Wilkes, and Dryden, 1983) has proved to be a helpful and simple procedure (Fig. 34–93).

The surgical correction of congenital or secondary entropion associated with epiblepharon is performed by careful excision of the abnormal skin fold and underlying hypertrophied orbicularis muscle in the pretarsal and infratarsal region. Plication of the lower lid retractors (the capsulopalpebral fascia) to the lower border of the tarsus, and separate skin closure, complete the operation (see Fig. 34–90).

When involutional entropion is associated

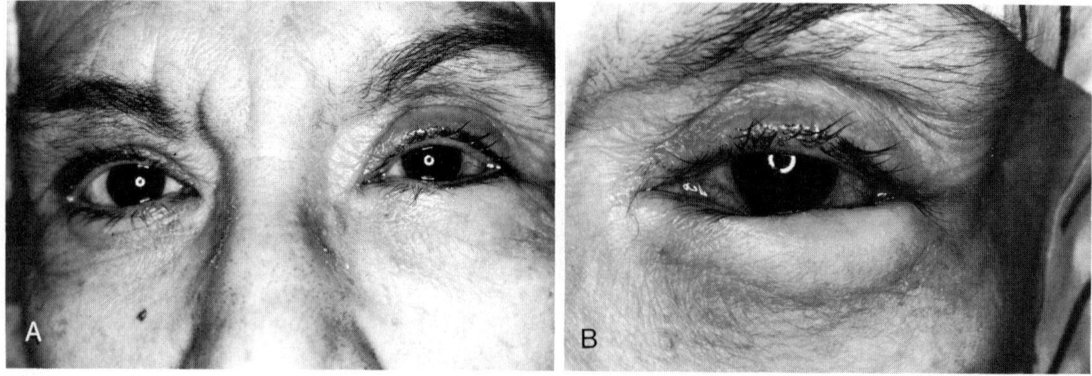

Figure 34–91. *A,* A patient with intermittent left lower eyelid spastic entropion in the relaxed posture position. *B,* Upon forced eyelid closure, the entropion and lash contact with the globe are elicited. This is caused by the preseptal orbicularis oculi migrating upward into the pretarsal area during contraction. This movement pushes the lid margin toward the globe.

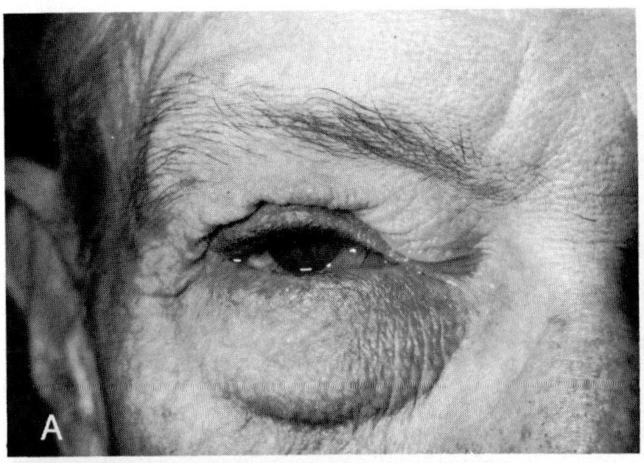

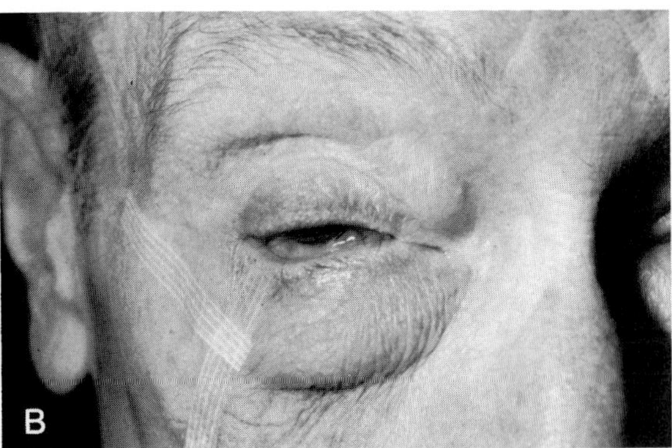

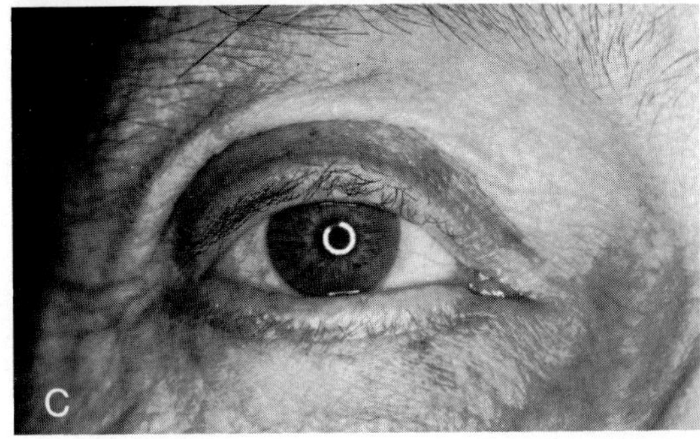

Figure 34–92. *A,* A patient with spastic, involutional entropion with a red, inflamed right eye. *B,* Temporary relief is afforded by taping to give lateral support and inferior distraction of the lid. *C,* One year after horizontal lid shortening, tarsal strip lateral canthoplasty (see Fig. 34–62*B*), tarsal rotation, and capsulopalpebral fascia tightening (see Fig. 34–90). Excess skin and fat from the eyelids were also removed.

with laxity of the horizontal dimension of the eyelid, correction must incorporate a horizontal lid-shortening procedure. This may be performed by excision of a triangular segment of full-thickness tarsus and lid retractors from the midportion of the lower lid. Closure of the defect produces lid shortening and a noticeable lid margin bulge (Fig. 34–94*A*). When the horizontal lid shortening is performed at the lateral canthus, a lower lid suspension, tarsal rotation, and capsulopalpebral fascia tightening can be added (Fig. 34–94*B*). If the involutional entropion occurs with little or no horizontal lid laxity, the

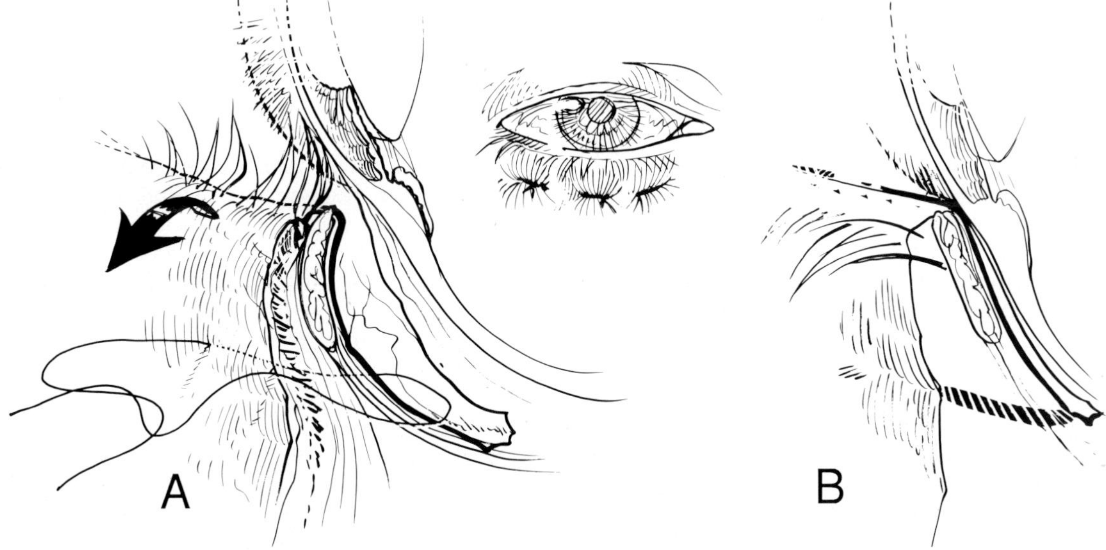

Figure 34–93. Nonsurgical eyelid suture method for the correction of entropion. *A,* Three double-armed 4-0 silk mattress sutures are passed from the conjunctival surface, below the inferior border of the tarsus, and tied anteriorly in the pretarsal region. *B,* The sutures are removed after two weeks. The scar produced by the horizontal mattress sutures usually maintains the lid in proper position.

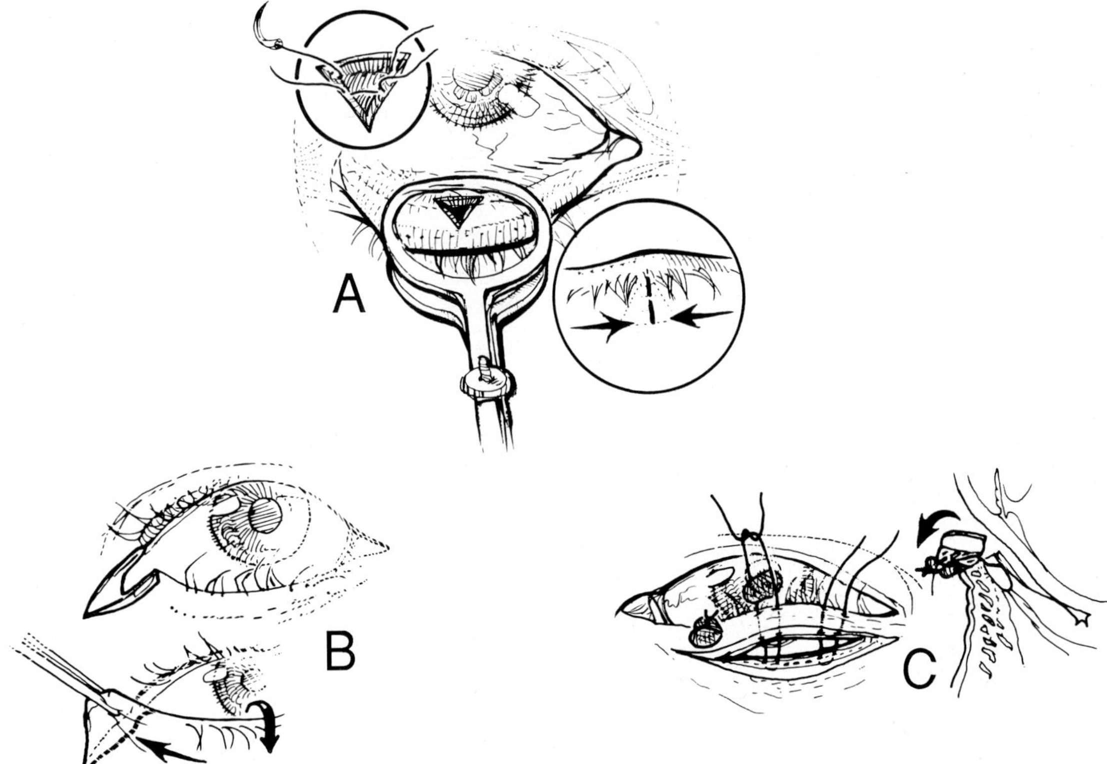

Figure 34–94. *A,* Correction of involutional entropion due to lid laxity with the resection of a base-down triangular segment of full-thickness tarsus and lid retractors. *B,* Correction with lid suspension, horizontal lid shortening, and tarsal rotation performed at the lateral canthus. *C,* The transverse infratarsal lid splitting and rotation technique (Weis) is indicated for difficult or recurrent situations.

method of correction should create a fibrous tissue (scar) barrier to the upward migration of the preseptal orbicularis muscle. The procedure demonstrated in Figure 34–90 is most commonly used; however, the Weis transverse lid split and marginal rotation technique is indicated for more difficult cases (Fig. 34–94*C*).

Cicatricial entropion is most appropriately treated by replacing the tissue deficiency. The sources for replacement tissue include eye bank sclera, autogenous tarsoconjunctiva, buccal mucous membrane, nasal chondromucosa, palatal mucosa, or conchal cartilage. In general, the graft tissue should have a smooth surface; however, some lower lid defects have been reconstructed with nonmucosa-lined tissue such as conchal cartilage.

Trichiasis, as mentioned previously, is the misalignment of the eyelashes with an inward direction toward the eye. This creates a foreign body sensation, pain, corneal erosion, or even corneal ulcer with perforation. Isolated eyelashes in contact with the cornea often resist standard entropion repairs and require individual electrolysis, cryoablation, or excision.

Symblepharon

Chemical burns are a frequent cause of symblepharon. Lacerations extending through the lid, conjunctival cul-de-sac, and sclera may result in symblepharon. The raw areas of the globe and inner surface of the lid fuse in a cicatricial band. The entire inner surface of the lid may adhere to the globe in extensive trauma. Localized areas of symblepharon may be corrected with a conjunctival Z-plasty (Fig. 34–95); however, the best method of correction is wide release of the adhesions and conjunctival grafting (Fig. 34–96).

Conjunctival Flap from Opposing Eyelid. The conjunctiva of the upper lid is a source for replacing the lower lid defect after release of an extensive symblepharon. The technique consists of freeing the lower lid

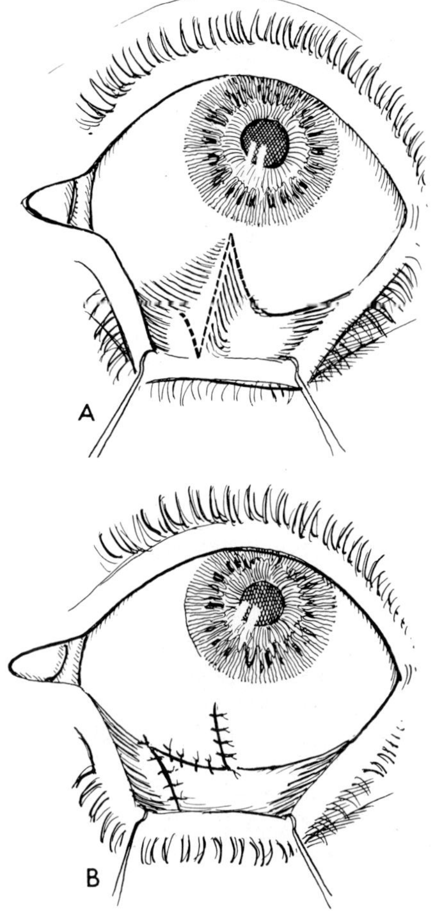

Figure 34–95. Z-plasty procedure for correction of symblepharon.

from the globe (Fig. 34–97*A*) and developing a conjunctival flap 4 mm from the upper lid. After undermining and advancing of the conjunctival flap into the lower lid defect, several fornix mattress sutures are passed to the skin (Fig. 34–97*B*). The lids are sutured together for four to six weeks, after which the lids and flap are separated and inset (Fig. 34–97*C*).

Conjunctival or Mucosal Grafts. A small conjunctival defect can be repaired by a conjunctival graft from the other eyelids (Fig. 34–98). Buccal wall or lower lip mucosa is used when larger surfaces must be covered. Sections of mucosa as large as 1.5 × 5.0 cm may be removed from the buccal wall (Fig. 34–99). The mucosa should be taken inferior to the parotid duct opening. The donor area may be left as a raw surface, which normally heals within a few weeks. A split-thickness mucosal graft may be removed with a Castroviejo electric mucotome. In extensive symblepharon, when wide areas of palpebral and bulbar conjunctival defects must be covered, the conjunctival cul-de-sac should be reconstructed. This is performed by anchoring the mucosal graft to the periosteum of the infraorbital rim before suturing to the lid and globe defect. To maintain the depth of the conjunctival fornix, the lower margin of the graft is anchored with through and through bolster sutures (Fig. 34–100). If more positive fixation is required, silicone tubing may be used to maintain the graft in the depth of the fornix (Fig. 34–100*A*). A doughnut scleral lens (symblepharon ring) can also be placed in the cul-de-sac to maintain fornical depth (Fig. 34–100*B*).

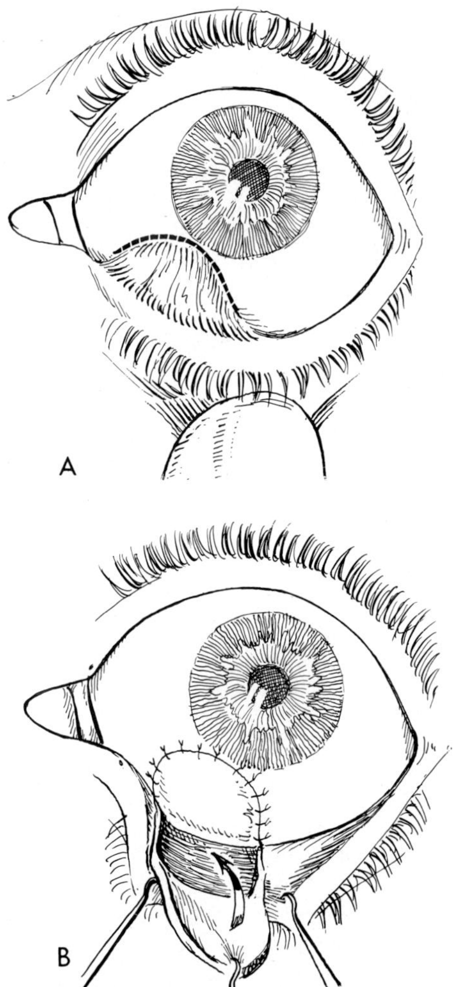

Figure 34–96. Correction of symblepharon. *A*, Freeing of an adhesion between the eyelid and the ocular globe. The scarred tissue over the sclera is employed to provide lining for the lower lid. *B*, The scleral defect is covered by a conjunctival graft.

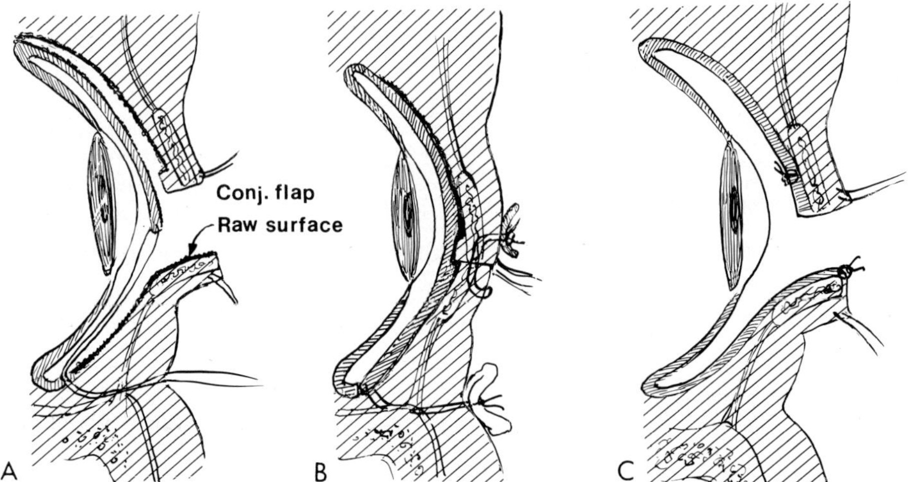

Figure 34–97. Conjunctival flap for the correction of symblepharon. *A,* The conjunctiva is outlined in sagittal section of the upper lid; the defect in the lower lid is also outlined. *B,* The upper lid flap has been advanced into the lid defect, and the lids are held together by occlusive sutures. *C,* After healing, the occlusive sutures are removed, the flap is divided, and the palpebral fissure is opened.

Transplantation of a split- or full-thickness skin graft to the mucosal surfaces of the eyelids or globe should not be performed. There is a high incidence of serious ocular damage from friction of the dermoepidermal graft on the globe.

Ectropion

The term ectropion denotes an outward turning or eversion of the eyelid. It may vary in degree from the mild eversion of a portion of the lid to a total eversion of the entire lid (Figs. 34–101, 34–102). The latter occurrence is more frequent in the lower lid because of the relatively greater effect of gravity, mechanical forces, and the laxity of the tarsocanthal structures on the smaller vertical height of the tarsus. Ectropion is classified into congenital and acquired forms that may have cicatricial, involutional (aging), or paralytic etiologies (see Fig. 34–89). Congenital ectropion is a rare condition usually associated with a deficiency of eyelid skin, and therefore can be considered a form of cicatricial ectropion (Fig. 34–101). The acquired forms of ectropion are most conveniently clas-

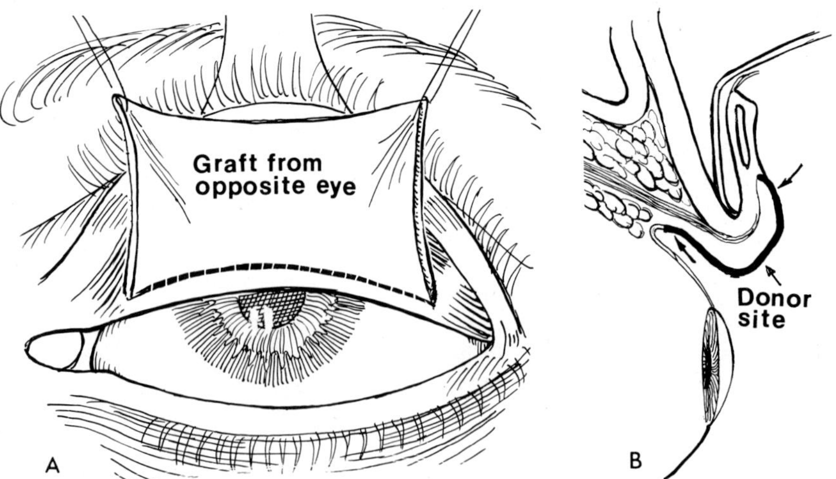

Figure 34–98. A conjunctival graft for the correction of symblepharon. *A,* Outline of graft from the upper lid. *B,* Sagittal view illustrating the position of the donor site on the upper lid.

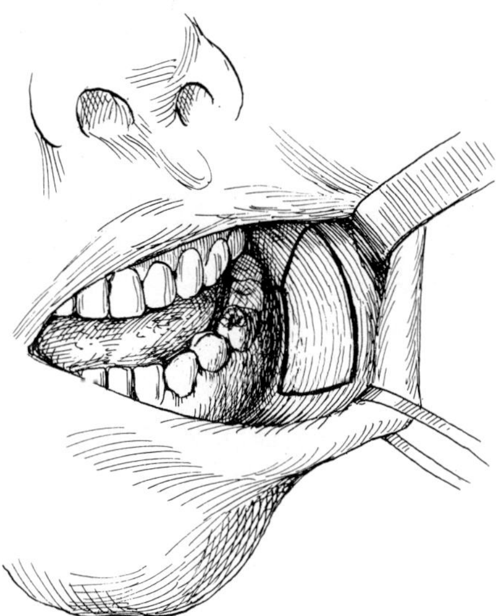

Figure 34–99. Area of the buccal mucosa from which a full-thickness mucous membrane graft may be removed. The graft is usually made thinner by trimming the undersurface with scissors.

sified as (1) involutional (Fig. 34–103), (2) cicatricial (Fig. 34–104), (3) complex, and (4) paralytic. A common factor in all forms of ectropion is conjunctival hyperemia or keratinization, punctal occlusion, and inflammatory changes as the ectropion becomes progressively worse. Involutional ectropion, also known as senile ectropion, is caused by laxity of the eyelid supportive structures, especially the lid retractors, the tarsus, and the canthal tissues. The condition usually begins with sagging of the lower lid to produce "scleral show." The lid margin may then evert, usually exposing the punctum medially and progressing to keratinization and possible occlusion (see Fig. 34–103). As the laxity progresses, the ectropion progresses to involve the whole lid with considerable exposure of the globe.

Correction of *involutional ectropion* is best performed early and usually involves correction of the medial lid ectropion. Several methods are available to correct ectropion of the medial half of the lower lid; however, the degree of the deformity and the experience of the surgeon dictate the most desirable means of management.

Minimal ectropion of the punctum of the lower lid may be tolerated when symptoms are insufficient to justify surgical correction. Cauterization of the internal layers of the lower lid is an uncontrolled method that has been employed for decades (Fig. 34–105). It

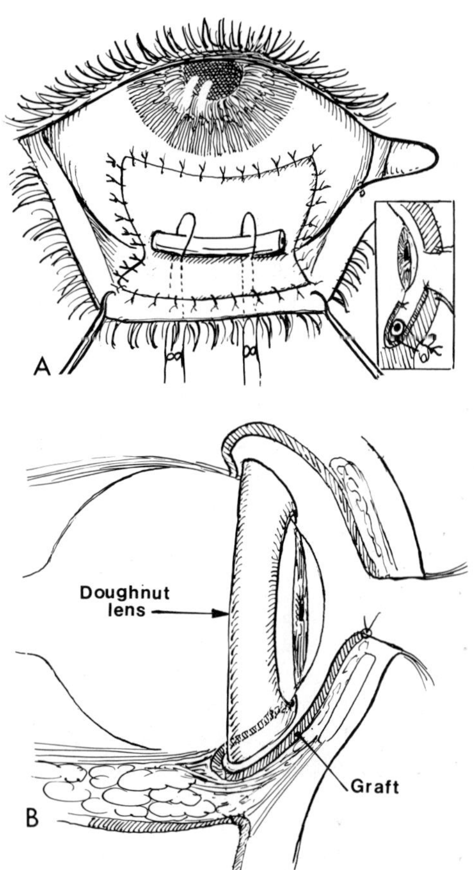

Figure 34–100. Relief of symblepharon by a mucosal graft. *A,* The graft has been sutured over the raw surface of the sclera and lower eyelid. The position of the mucosal graft and polyethylene tubing maintains the depth of the cul-de-sac (sagittal section). *B,* The cul-de-sac can also be maintained by a fenestrated scleral lens.

has met with some success, although the actual excision of a diamond-shaped portion of the retrocanalicular tarsus and conjunctiva, and suture placement to shorten the lid vertically, tends to provide more predictable

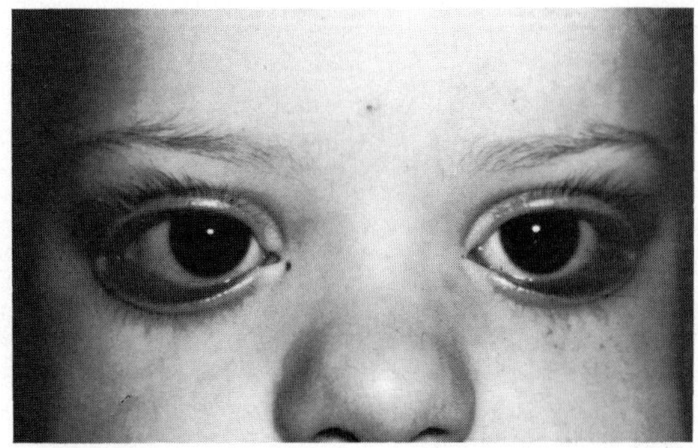

Figure 34–101. A 3 year old child with congenital ectropion of all four eyelids due to relative deficiency of skin.

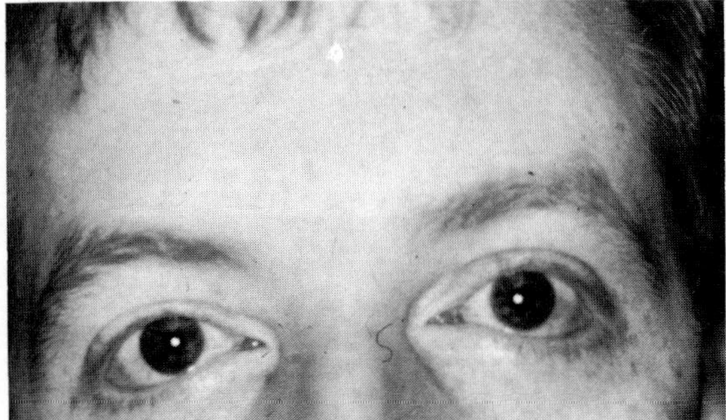

Figure 34–102. An adult with a mild form of congenital ectropion of the lower eyelids. Note the scleral show, lateral lid margin eversion, and bowing of the lower lids.

results (Fig. 34–106). The apex of the diamond should be approximately 0.5 to 1 mm inferior to the canaliculus. A Bowman's probe should be passed to protect the canaliculus during suture placement, which approximates the cut edges of the tarsus and conjunctiva.

In more severe deformities in which there is a need for both horizontal and vertical shortening of the lid, neither of the above methods provides sufficient means to produce the desired result. Therefore, the "lazy-T" method of treatment may be employed to effect a simultaneous vertical and horizontal shortening of the lid in order to correct moderately severe ectropion. As the term "lazy-T" implies, the incision for this procedure takes the shape of a "T," with the horizontal bar lying inside the lower lid (Fig. 34–107). The procedure may be done under local or general anesthesia. If local anesthesia is employed, the tissues should be distorted as little as possible by the injection. A lapse of 15 to 20 minutes between the injection and the start of surgery also allows time for some of the distortion from the anesthetic solution to dissipate. If general anesthesia is used, the amount of anesthetic infiltration can be reduced.

As indicated in Figure 34–108*A*, fixation of the lid margin is maintained with forceps, and gentle traction pulls the lid into an ac-

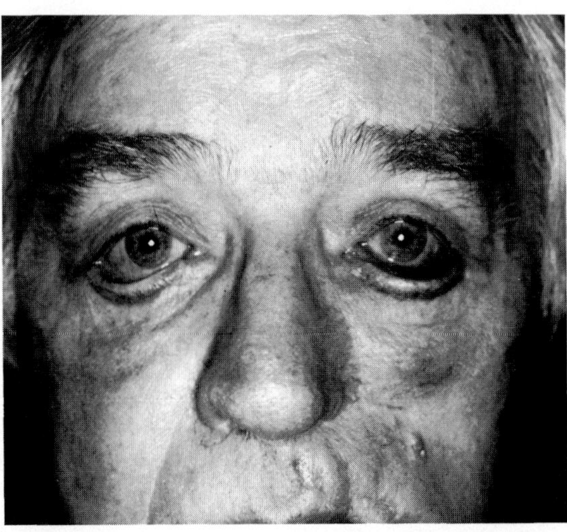

Figure 34–104. Bilateral lower eyelid cicatricial ectropion due to excessive skin removal during blepharoplasty.

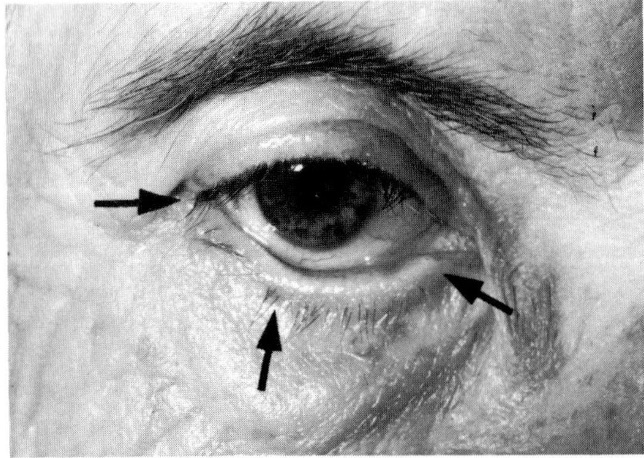

Figure 34–103. Involutional ectropion of the right lower eyelid. Note the progressive lid laxity and lid margin eversion from laterally to medially. The medial arrow points to the punctal eversion resulting from medial canthal laxity.

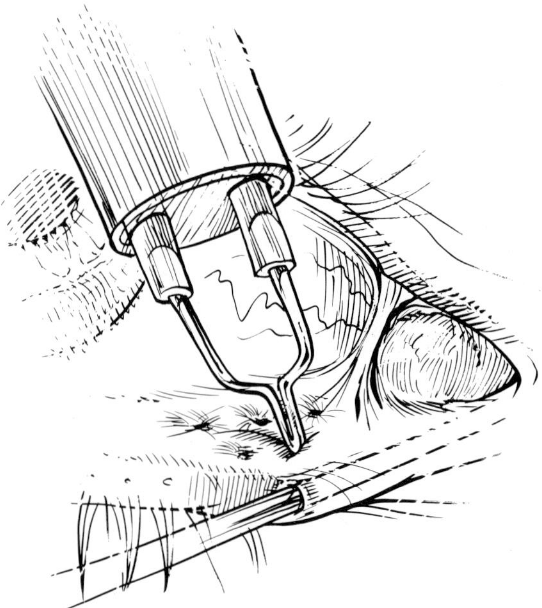

Figure 34–105. Technique of punctate cauterization of the inner layers of the medial portion of the lower lid for the correction of senile ectropion. Note the lacrimal probe in place.

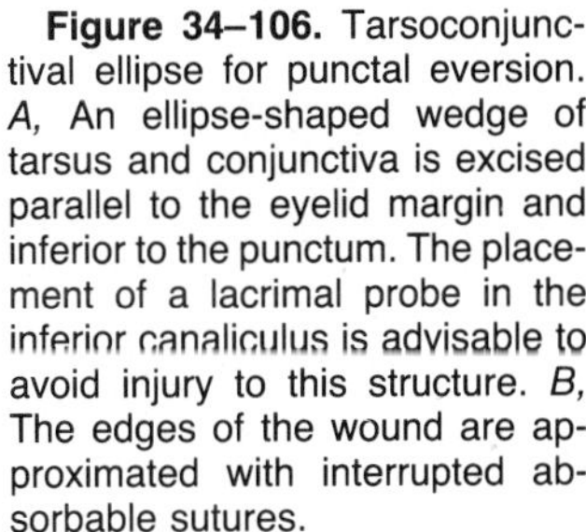

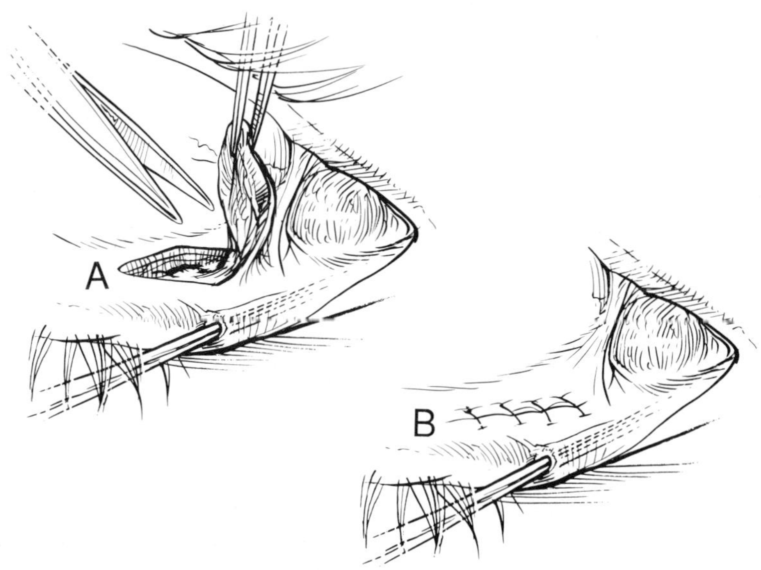

Figure 34–106. Tarsoconjunctival ellipse for punctal eversion. *A,* An ellipse-shaped wedge of tarsus and conjunctiva is excised parallel to the eyelid margin and inferior to the punctum. The placement of a lacrimal probe in the inferior canaliculus is advisable to avoid injury to this structure. *B,* The edges of the wound are approximated with interrupted absorbable sutures.

centuated position of ectropion. Using a razor knife, a horizontal incision is made below the level of the lower canaliculus. A lacrimal probe may be inserted into the lower canaliculus to identify the level of its location. The incision is made sufficiently deep to section the tarsoconjunctival layer of the lower lid, and long enough to allow for correction of the ectropion. The inferior margin of the incision is undermined (Fig. 34–108*B, C*) sufficiently to allow for adequate excess of tissue when the margins are overlapped by manipulation with two forceps (Fig. 34–108*D, E*). The amount of tissue to be resected is undermined, as the lower, undetached tissues help to maintain the corrected lid position. When the resection of tissue has been achieved (Fig. 34–108*F*), apposition of the wound edges corrects the vertical component of the deformity. In order to correct the horizontal component contributing to the ectropion, a vertical incision lateral to the punctum is extended inferiorly through all layers of the lower lid from the lid margin into the depth of the lower fornix. As shown in Figure 34–108*H*, the two sections of the lower lid are overlapped with forceps. Sufficient horizontal traction is applied to provide an estimate of the dimensions of the lid resection necessary to correct the horizontal component of the deformity. After resection of the wedge of lower lid tissue, apposition of the wound margins should restore the lower lid contact with the globe. Figure 34–108*I, J* shows the closure of the initial horizontal tarsoconjunctival incision with fine caliber, interrupted, absorbable sutures, such as plain catgut. The vertical transmarginal incision is then closed as a lid laceration or wound (Fig. 34–108*K*). This is usually done with 6-0 silk sutures. The initial suture is placed through the orifice of the meibomian glands on either side of the defect. Traction upon this suture aligns the lid margin in the correct position to allow accurate placement of an anterior and a posterior marginal suture (Fig. 34–108*L*). The anterior marginal suture is placed through ciliary exits. Two buried muscle sutures are placed and tied (Fig. 34–108*M*). The long ends of the middle and posterior marginal sutures are brought forward and held beneath the mar-

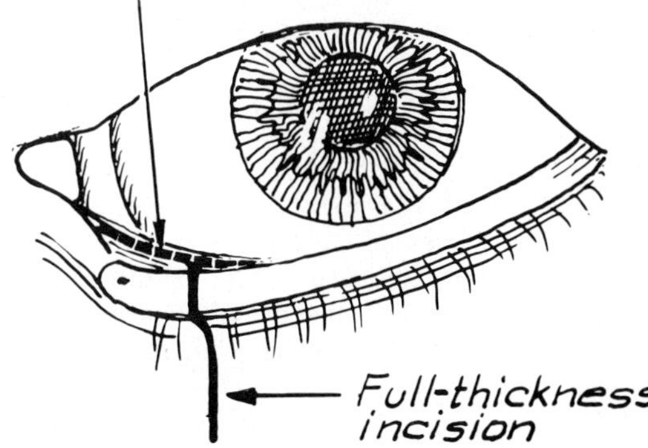

Figure 34–107. The "lazy-T" method. The incision is made in the form of a "T" with the horizontal bar inside the lower lid.

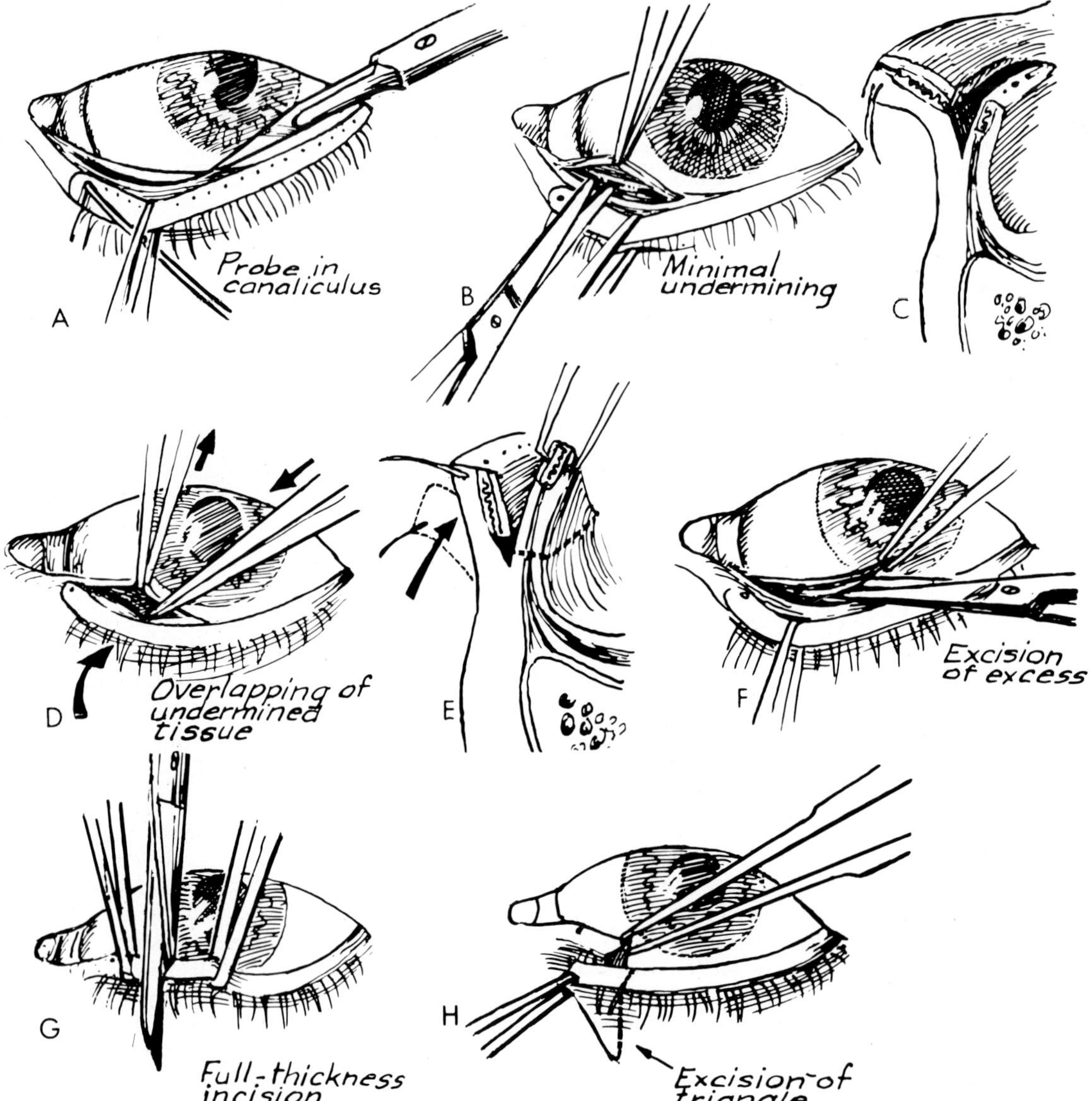

Figure 34–108. The technique of the "lazy-T" method. *A,* A forceps everts the lower lid. A razor knife incises horizontally below the canaliculus. *B,* The inferior margin of the incision is undermined. *C,* Sagittal section demonstrating the depth of the undermining. *D,* The lower margin of the incision is overlapped over the anterior margin. *E,* Sagittal section illustrating the overlap. The dotted line indicates the line of resection. *F,* The excess tissue is resected. *G,* A vertical incision lateral to the punctum extends through all layers of the lid down to the lower fornix. *H,* The two sections of the lid are crisscrossed and overlapped. As indicated by the dotted line, a triangle of excess tissue is resected.

ginal suture at the eyelash (Fig. 34–108*M, N*), to prevent the suture ends from floating into the palpebral fissure. The remainder of the skin incision is closed with interrupted silk sutures (Fig. 34–108*N*). Ointment is not applied, because it may seep into the wound and delay healing. A moderately compressive Telfa dressing is applied. The silk sutures may be removed in one week. After wound reaction subsides, the lid margin usually assumes a more normal position, enabling the punctum to make contact with the lacrimal lake.

Severe cases of medial ectropion cannot be corrected with the "lazy-T" operation, but combining a second horizontal lid shortening at the lateral canthus can produce the desired results (Fig. 34–109). When the "lazy-T" medial ectropion procedure is combined with lateral canthal tightening and lid shortening,

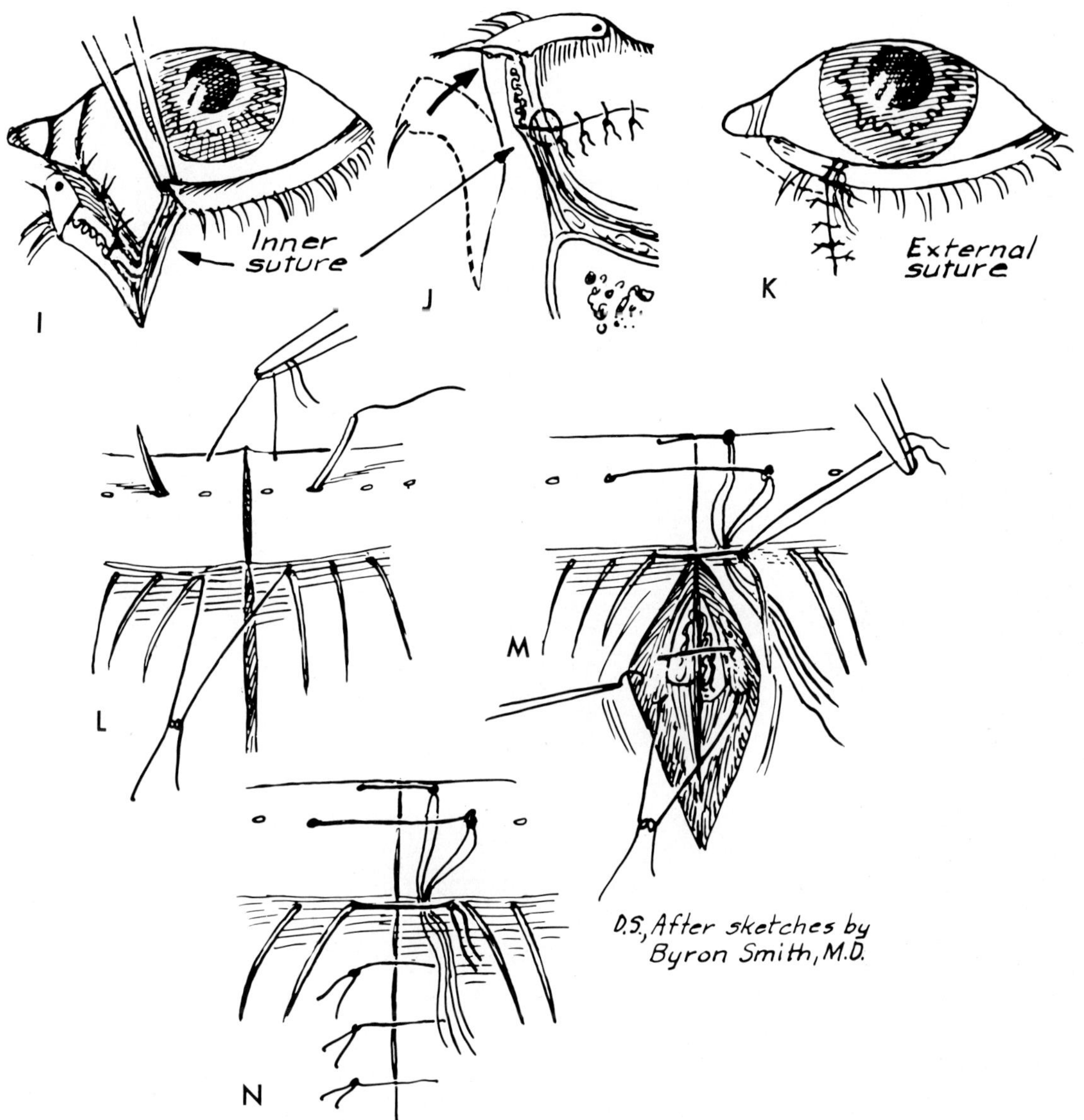

Figure 34–108 *Continued I, J,* Closure of the horizontal tarsoconjunctival incision. *K* to *N,* Closure of the vertical transmarginal incision in the same fashion as a full-thickness transmarginal laceration (see Fig. 34–23).

the surgery on the medial lid structures should be performed first.

If the medial ectropion is associated with marked medial canthal tendon laxity or disinsertion, the reconstruction may require sacrifice of a portion of the canaliculus and punctum with the lower lid resection. The canaliculus is then reconstructed with an encircling canalicular silicone intubation and stenting of the repair. Further lid malposition correction should be delayed several months to allow sufficient healing of the canalicular reconstruction (Fig. 34–110).

Cicatricial ectropion is caused by a deficiency of the skin or skin and muscle of the lid from a variety of causes, e.g., congenital conditions, trauma, thermal injuries, inflammatory conditions, cicatrizing skin tumors, or irradiation. This condition can also result from excess skin removal after blepharoplasty (Fig. 34–111) or resection of benign or malignant skin lesions. It may also result from a secondary cicatricial force in the periorbital area such as occurs after (1) inadequate skin grafting to the eyelids following burns, (2) retraction and contraction of cheek

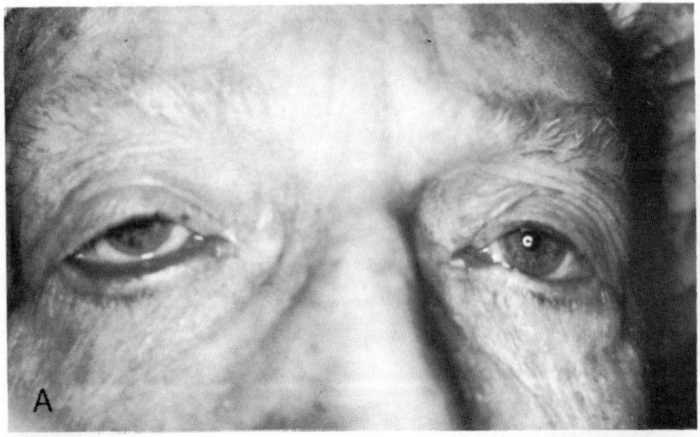

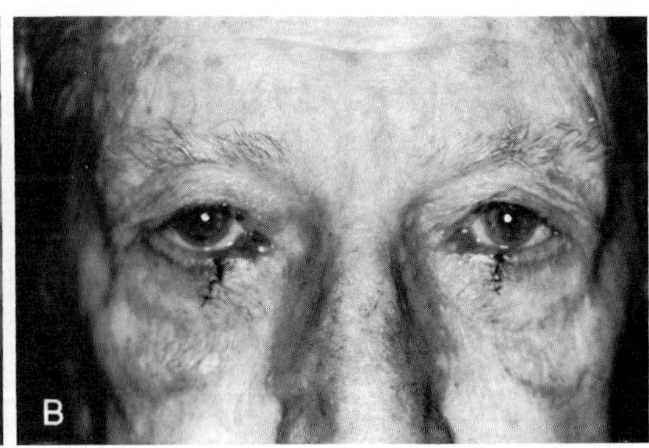

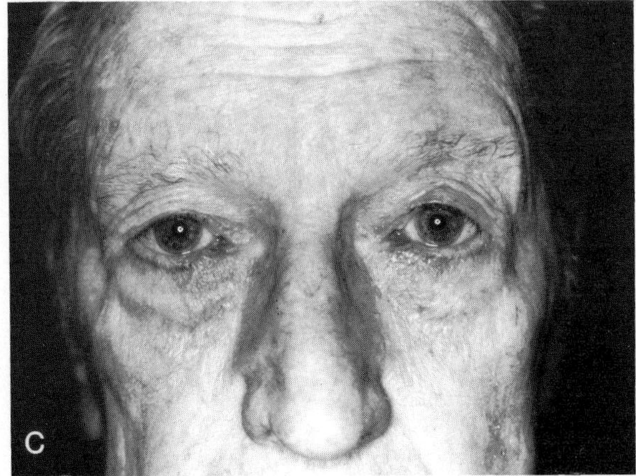

Figure 34–109. *A,* A patient with severe medial ectropion of the right lower eyelid, moderately severe ectropion of the left lower eyelid, and bilateral lower eyelid lateral canthal laxity. *B,* Ten days after bilateral "lazy-T" procedures (see Fig. 34–108) and lateral canthoplasties. *C,* Eight months postoperatively.

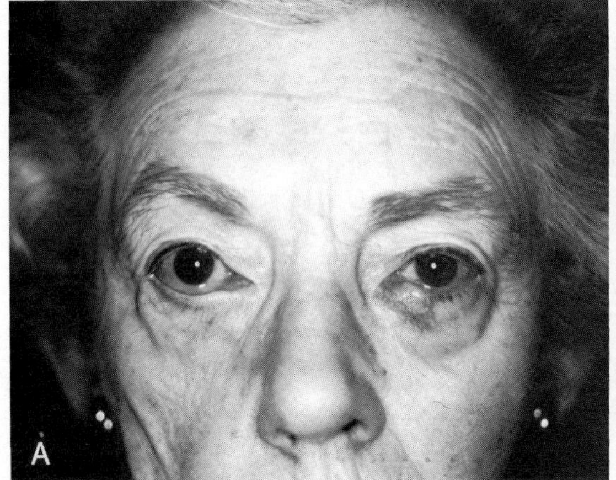

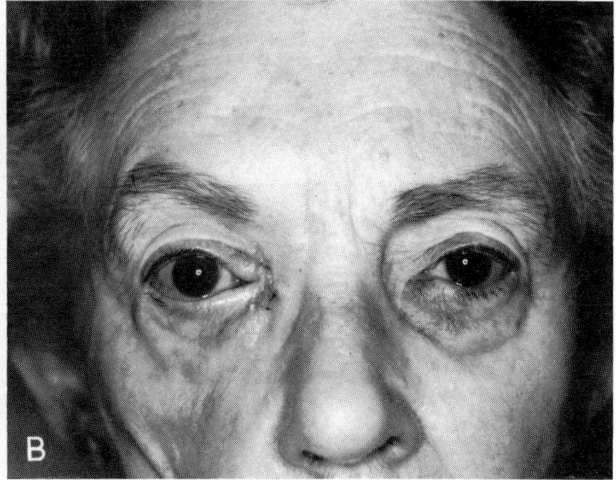

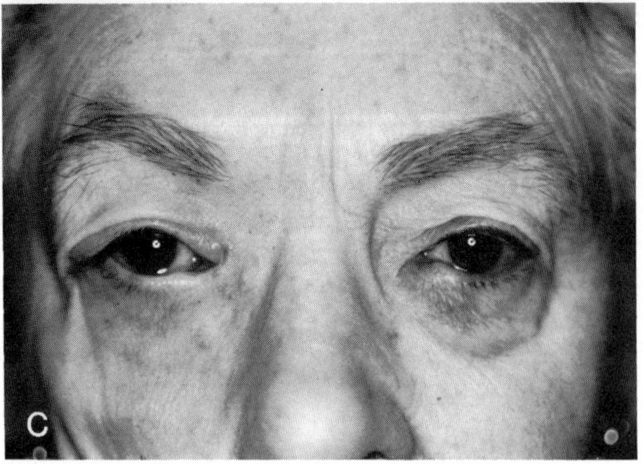

Figure 34–110. *A,* A patient with paralytic ectropion and severe medial canthal laxity of the right lower eyelid. *B,* After right inferior canalicular horizontal resection and reconstruction over a silicone stent. A medial canthal plication of the lower limb of the medial canthal tendon was also performed. *C,* Six months after procedure described in *B* and three months after a right lateral canthoplasty, tarsal suspension, and horizontal lid shortening.

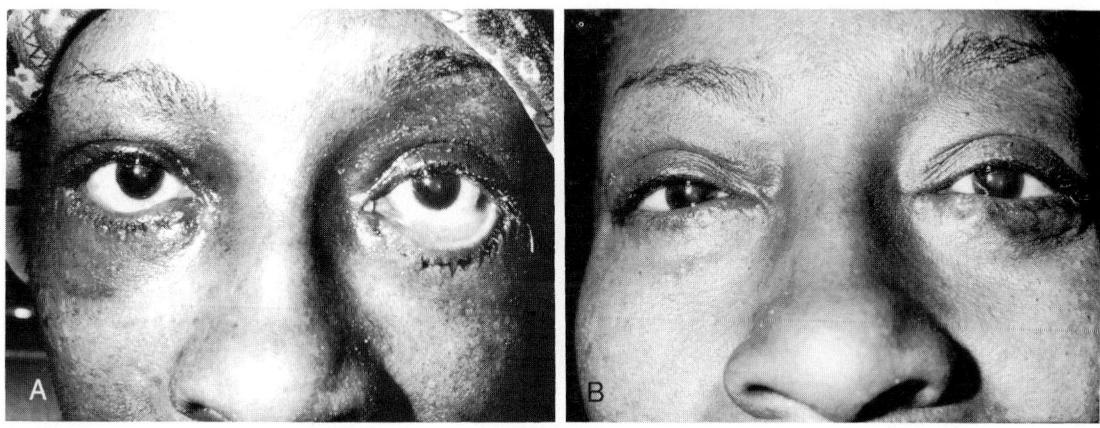

Figure 34–111. *A,* A patient with cicatricial and mechanical ectropion after excessive lower eyelid skin removal during blepharoplasty. *B,* Six months after left lateral canthoplasty and lid suspension with a full-thickness retroauricular skin graft to the left lower eyelid. The right lower eyelid responded to massage and lateral canthoplasty alone.

flaps placed in close proximity to the lids, or (3) the secondary contraction after the healing of medial canthal and lower lid wounds by primary intention.

Complex ectropion is closely associated with lid margin eversion and lid retraction, and results from a marked derangement in the anatomy of the lower lid after reaction to an organizing hematoma, severe lid lacerations, and multiple incisions in and around the lid for exploration of combined orbital fractures with open lid wounds. The common denominator in the formation of complex ectropion is a marked edematous and inflammatory phase during healing. It is proposed that the cause of complex ectropion is a fusion of the lid structures at the level of the orbital septum. This explains the fact that the condition is most often observed after multiple surgical explorations for orbital fractures (Fig. 34–112*A*) and after an organized hematoma (Fig. 34–112*B*).

Paralytic ectropion is caused by facial nerve palsy (see Chap. 42), resulting in a denervation of the orbicularis oculi muscle, the protractor muscles of the eyelids. A marked laxity of the tarsocanthal structures eventually results, which is more noticeable in older people (Fig. 34–113).

In younger individuals, the eversion of the lid may not be so obvious because of sufficient firmness of the tarsocanthal tissues. However, lid retraction of the upper eyelid may be so marked that the ocular globe is at risk of exposure keratopathy and potential ulceration. This finding is explained on the basis that the normal levator superioris, innervated by the third cranial nerve, is the retractor muscle of the eyelid and pulls against the paralyzed protractor orbicularis muscle. This results in lagophthalmos, or inability to close the eye (Fig. 34–114*A*). Surgical correction requires a levator exploration (Fig. 34–114*B*) and recession to allow the upper lid to

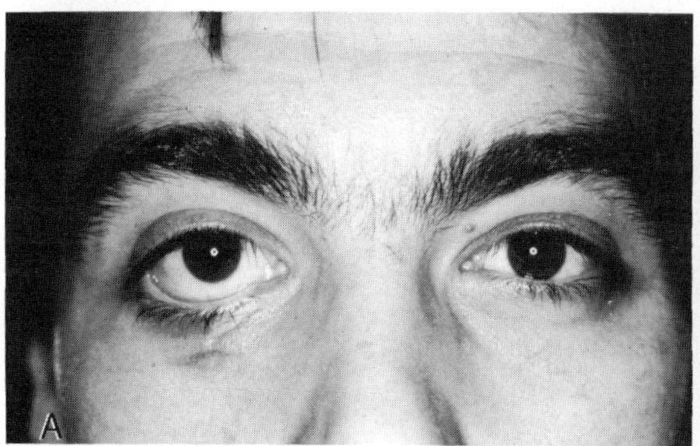

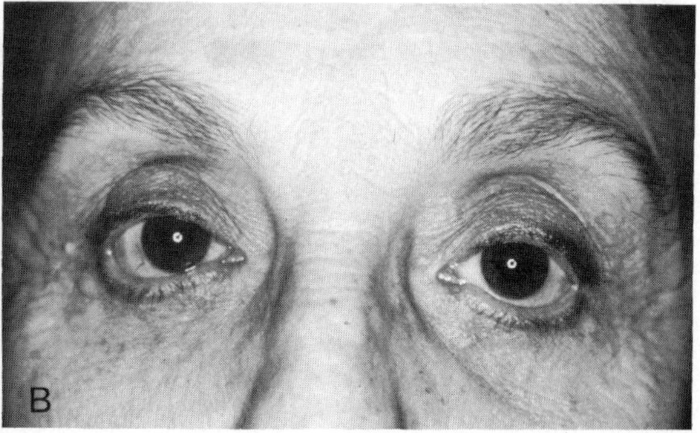

Figure 34–112. *A,* Complex ectropion of the right lower eyelid with associated lid retraction following orbital fracture and multiple surgical explorations via an infraciliary skin-muscle approach. *B,* Another patient with bilateral lower eyelid retraction six months after prolonged edema, and hematoma formation after blepharoplasty.

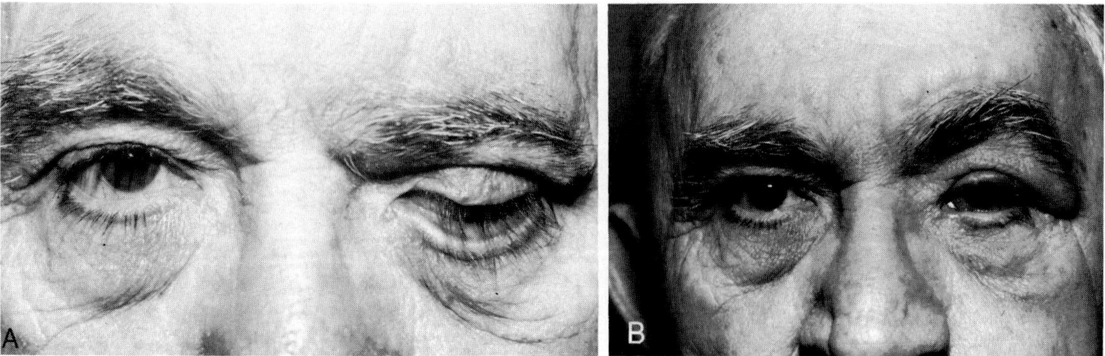

Figure 34–113. *A,* Severe left lower paralytic ectropion in an elderly patient. *B,* Six months after left lower eyelid (horizontal) shortening, tarsal suspension, and lateral canthoplasty.

be free from the relative overaction of the levator muscle and provide protective eyelid closure. A lateral canthoplasty and horizontal lid shortening (Hamako and Baylis, 1980, see Fig. 34–62*C*) of the affected lower lid may be performed at the same time (Figure 34–114*C*). Another method of correcting the upper eyelid retraction, paralytic ectropion and associated lagophthalmos is to insert a silicone elastic rod into the upper lid to simulate the counterbalancing effect of the protractor orbicularis oculi muscle. At the same time, a horizontal lid shortening and lateral canthal suspension to the lateral orbital periosteum can be performed (Fig. 34–115). This combined technique provides excellent ocular protection with less surgical intervention.

The details of skin grafting of the eyelids for the correction of ectropion are presented in Chapter 41.

PTOSIS OF UPPER EYELID

Ptosis of the upper eyelid, or blepharoptosis, refers to an abnormally low level of the upper eyelid during straight-ahead gaze. This finding suggests that in the relaxed position the upper lid is lower than normal and interferes with the visual field. The classification of ptosis can best be described by the time of onset and the mechanism producing the lowered lid level. Congenital ptosis, by definition, is present at birth and usually represents an isolated dystrophy of the involved levator muscle. However, birth injuries causing in-

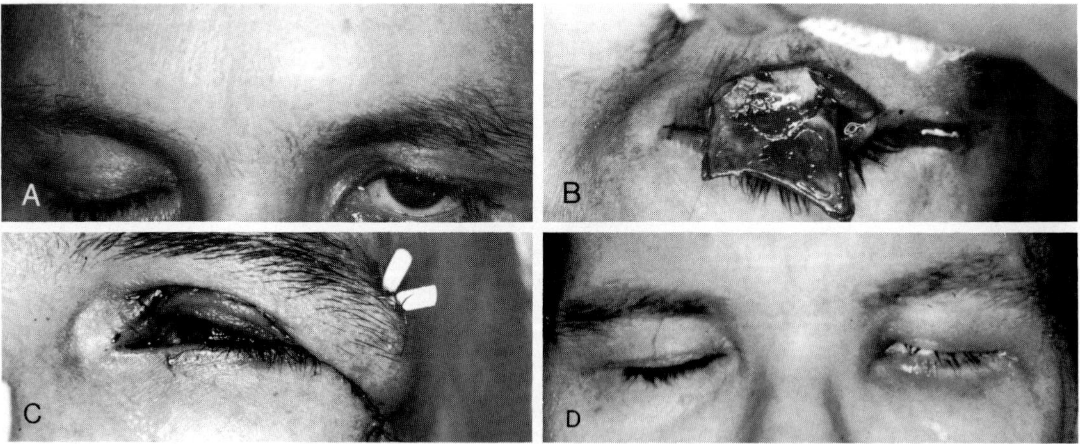

Figure 34–114. *A,* A 40 year old male 48 hours after resection of a left cerebellopontine angle acoustic neuroma with sacrifice of the facial nerve. Note the left upper eyelid retraction, poor Bell's phenomenon, and lagophthalmos on attempted lid closure. Frank lower lid ectropion has not yet developed. *B,* The left levator muscle has been dissected and freed from its attachments to allow a 15 mm recession to correct the lid retraction. *C,* Immediately after left upper eyelid levator recession and left lateral canthoplasty, tarsal suspension, and lower lid shortening as described in Figure 34–62*C*. *D,* The patient one month postoperative with improved lid function, decreased lagophthalmos, and corneal protection.

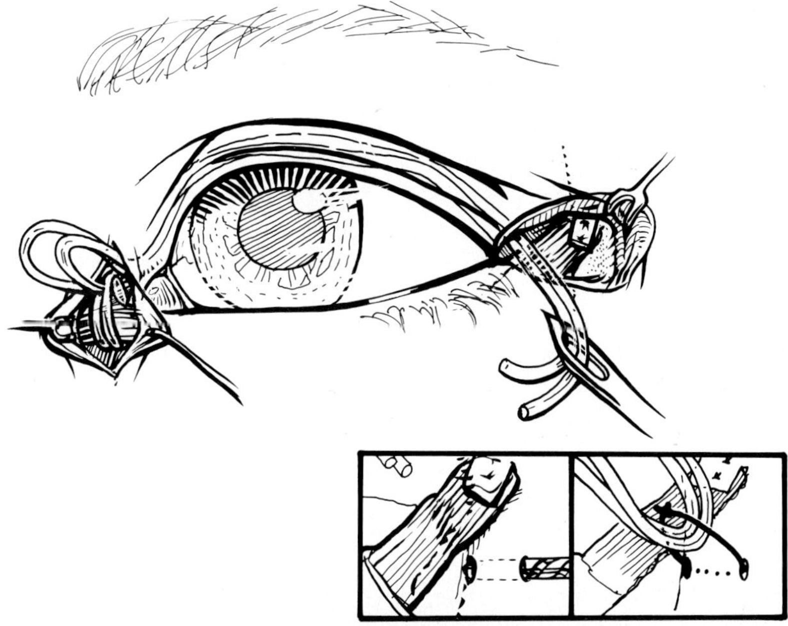

Figure 34–115. Correction of paralytic ectropion and lagophthalmos with placement of an upper eyelid silicone rod 0.5 mm in diameter from the medial canthus to the lateral canthal periosteum, in combination with a lateral canthoplasty, tarsal suspension, and lid shortening as described in Figure 34–62*C*. The insets show the suturing of the ends of the silicone rod to the lateral orbital rim.

jury to the levator muscle or the third nerve technically produce an acquired form of ptosis. Acquired ptosis may have (1) neurogenic, (2) myogenic, (3) aponeurotic, or (4) mechanical causes (Frueh, 1980).

Pseudoptosis may result from a myriad of conditions that simulate an asymmetry of the upper lid levels. Foremost in this group is the dysthyroid ophthalmopathic condition, which produces complex eyelid and ocular globe positional abnormalities (Fig. 34–116). Ocular globe hypertropia and a weakness of the superior rectus muscle, causing a downward oriented eye, also produce pseudoptosis. Conversely, ocular hypotropia and associated fullness of the upper lid and orbit can cause pseudoptosis (Fig. 34–117). Enophthalmos can also simulate a condition of ptosis (Fig. 34–118), and exophthalmos of the opposite side can produce a relative appearance of ptosis on the normal side (Fig. 34–119).

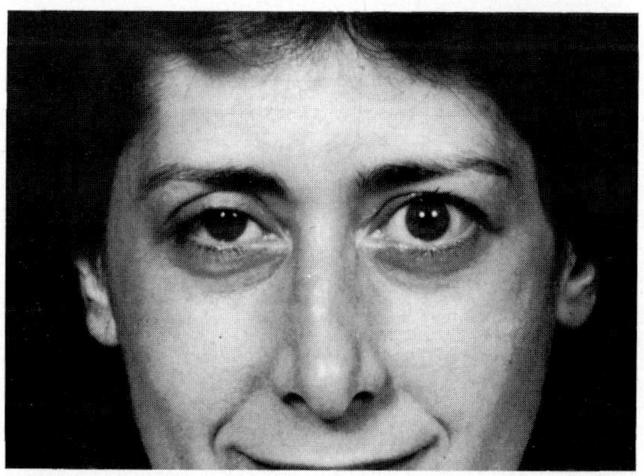

Figure 34–116. A patient with thyroid ophthalmopathy and left upper eyelid retraction, which accentuates the minimal ptosis of the right upper eyelid.

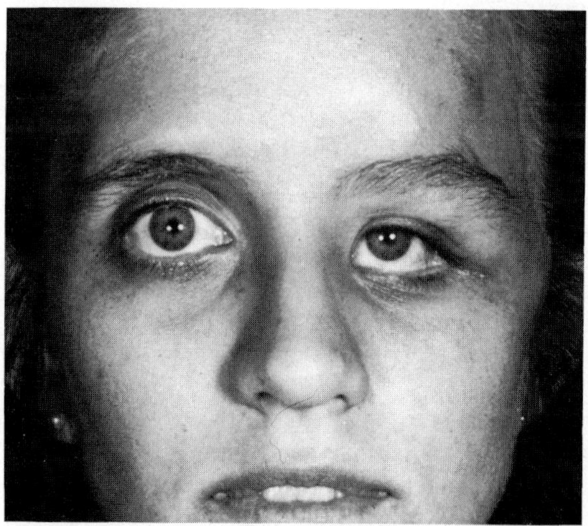

Figure 34–117. A patient with left ocular hypotropia and fullness of the upper eyelid due to neurofibroma accentuating the minimal left upper lid ptosis.

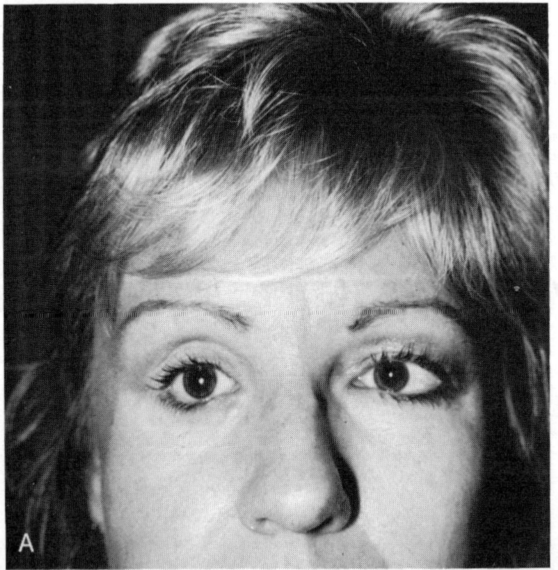

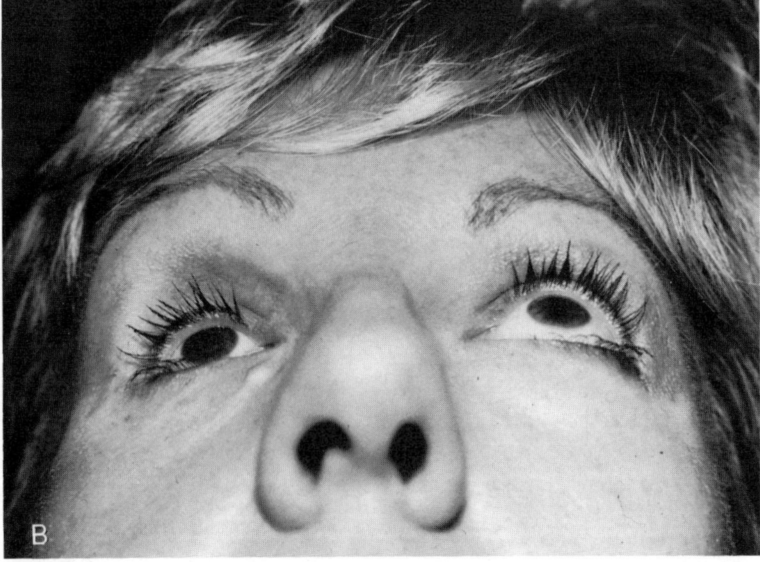

Figure 34–118. *A, B,* A patient with an artificial right eye, and enophthalmos/upper eyelid sulcus accentuation causing pseudoptosis.

Asymmetric upper eyelid folds can also simulate ptosis (Fig. 34–120*A*) or make minimal ptosis appear greater than it actually is (Fig. 34–120*B*).

Neurogenic causes of ptosis relate to conditions affecting the third cranial nerve anywhere along its course from the brain stem to the posterior third of the muscular portion of the levator muscle. Conditions that alter the function of the sympathetic nervous innervation to the eye, such as Horner's syndrome, also produce a neurogenic ptosis. The rare aberrant regeneration or synkinetic jaw winking forms of ptosis are also neurogenic in origin (Fig. 34–121).

Myogenic ptosis results from a dystrophy or myopathy of the levator muscle and is usually due to myasthenia gravis or chronic external ophthalmoplegia. Since the condition is often progressive and associated with poor ocular protective mechanisms, the correction should be conservative and easily reversible if the eyes become compromised (Fig. 34–122). Occasionally, the levator muscle may be infiltrated with fat, and correction may require an internal suspension to Whitnall's ligament to bypass the nonfunctioning levator muscle (Fig. 34–123).

Aponeurotic ptosis results from a dehiscence, stretching, attenuation, or complete

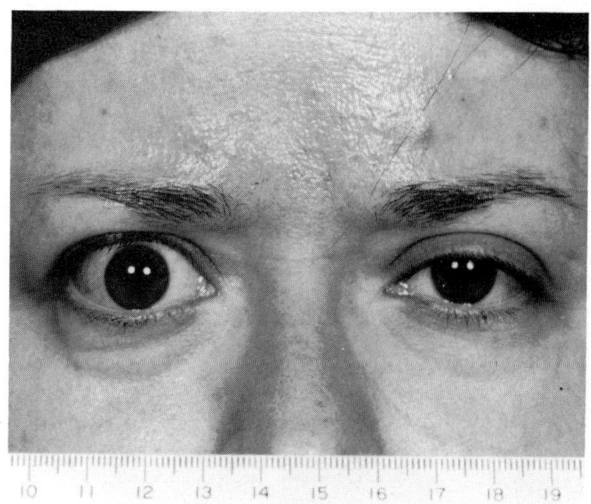

Figure 34–119. A patient with thyroid ophthalmopathy, 4 mm of proptosis of the right ocular globe, and upper lid retraction accentuating the minimal ptosis of the left upper eyelid.

detachment of the levator aponeurosis, with a resultant loss of levator power to the upper lid tarsus. This can result from congenital defects (Anderson and Gordy, 1979a) or from trauma (Fig. 34–124). However, the most common cause is a senile or involutional type resulting from aging changes. The patient presents with ptotic, extremely thin lids with high lid creases due to the aponeurosis pulling loose from its normal attachment or becoming extremely attenuated within the substance of the lid. There is often brow elevation in an attempt to elevate the ptotic lids (Fig. 34–125).

Mechanical ptosis results from excess weight of the eyelid, most commonly through aging or involutional changes. The excess upper eyelid skin can actually cause the eyelashes to be inferiorly directed, further impairing the visual fields. Correction of this type of ptosis is by blepharoplasty (see Chap. 43). Eyelid tumors or cicatricial foreshortening of the palpebral aperture may also cause mechanical ptosis.

The results of surgery for ptosis depend on (1) the nature of the ptosis, (2) the type of operation selected, and (3) the skill with which the operation is performed (Berke, 1949, 1952, 1957, 1959, 1962). The optimal esthetic and functional results in congenital or acquired ptosis are achieved by resection or advancement of the levator or its aponeurosis, provided that the levator muscle action is adequate. Before deciding what type of operation is indicated, one must measure the amount of levator function, note the position of the normal lid with respect to the cornea in primary position, and determine the position of the normal upper lid fold.

Measurement of the levator action of the ptotic lid is best made by placing a millimeter ruler over the lid with one hand and noting the amount of elevation of the lid, from a position of looking down to a position of looking up, while immobilizing the brow with the thumb of the other hand. This maneuver shoud be repeated several times until the excursion of the lid is the same on two or more tests while the head is held stationary. Smith (1974) used the retinoscope as a means of studying the relationship of the upper lid margin to the pupil. He also requested eating or gum chewing as part of the examination to detect the presence of the jaw winking phenomenon. The position of the cornea is examined during forced closure of the lids by opening the lids passively during voluntary

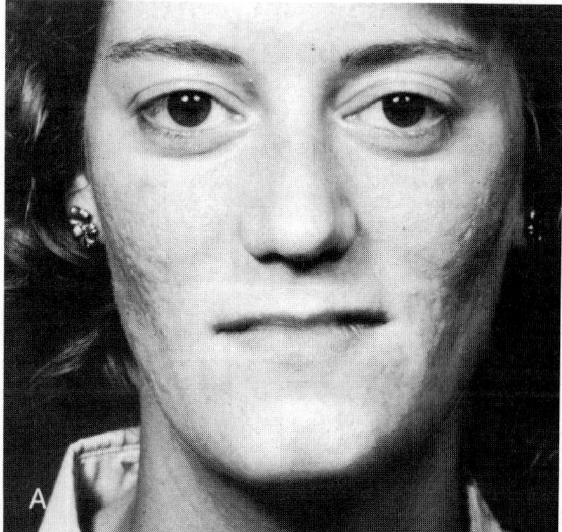

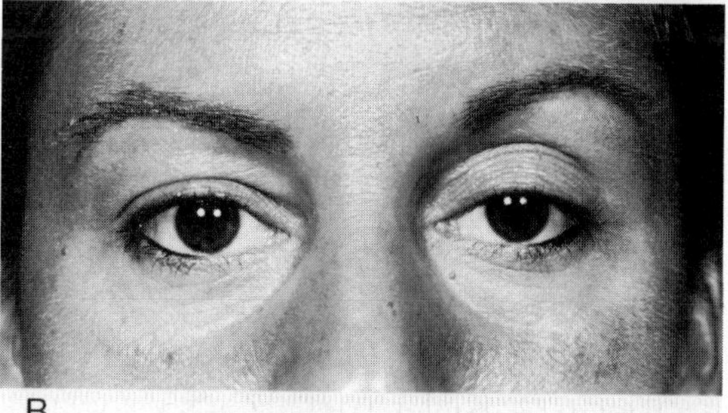

Figure 34–120. *A,* A patient with a single right upper eyelid fold and a double left upper eyelid fold causing left upper lid pseudoptosis. *B,* A patient with asymmetric upper eyelid folds accentuating the minimal ptosis of the left upper lid.

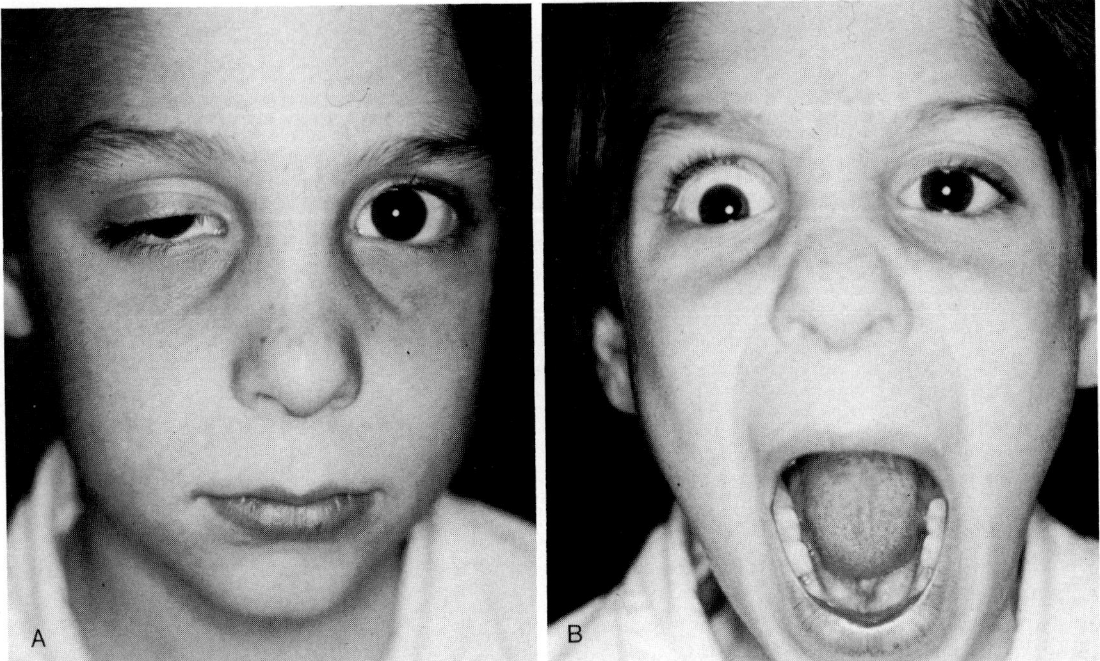

Figure 34–121. *A,* A 7 year old boy with severe ptosis of the right upper eyelid. *B,* With mouth opening, the ptosis is converted to lid retraction due to aberrant congenital nerve crossover between the trigeminal and oculomotor cranial nerves (the Marcus Gunn or synkinetic jaw winking syndrome).

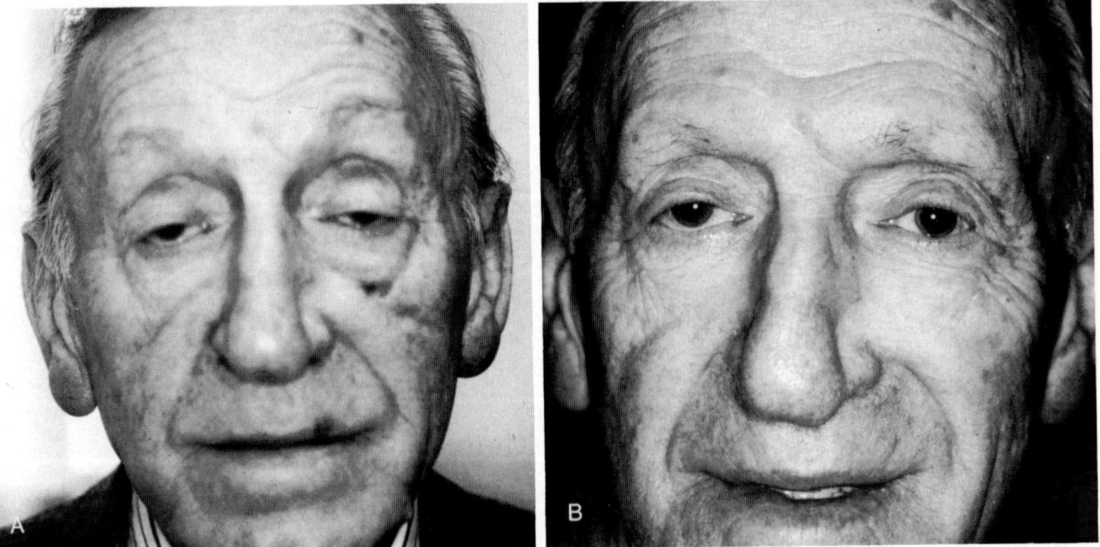

Figure 34–122. *A,* A patient with progressive external ophthalmoplegia causing severe myogenic ptosis and obstruction of the superior visual fields. *B,* After conservative upper eyelid ptosis correction by levator advancement.

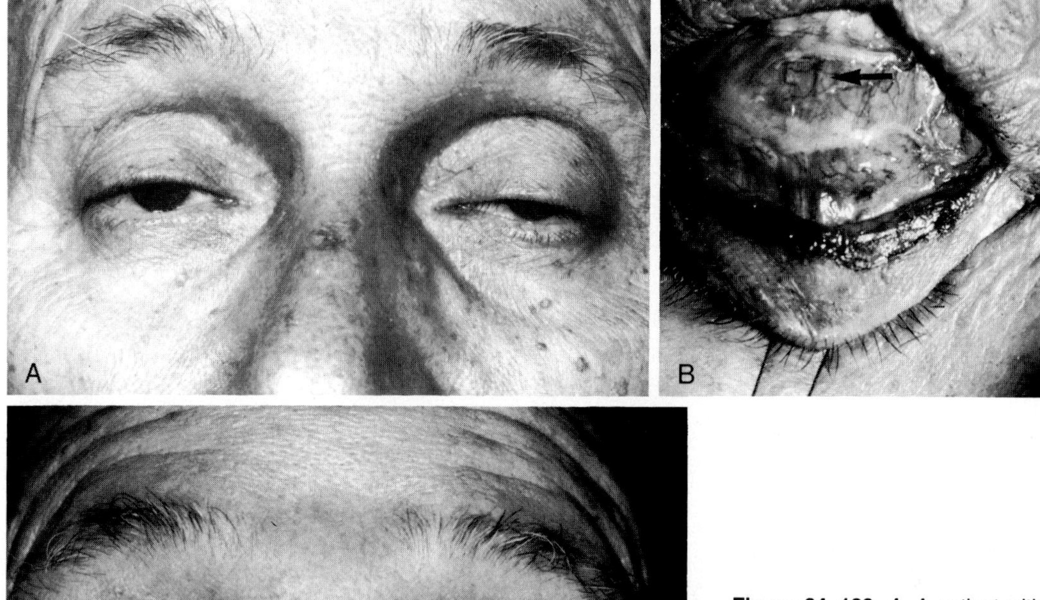

Figure 34–123. *A,* A patient with severe bilateral upper eyelid ptosis and obstruction of vision. *B,* During upper eyelid exploration the levator muscle *(arrow)* was replaced with fatty infiltration and did not contract. *C,* After internal suspension of the distal levator to Whitnall's ligament to provide adequate lid elevation.

forced closure of the eyelids. The position of the cornea during this act helps to disclose the position of the eye during sleep. It is encouraging to find that the eyes drift upward *(Bell's phenomenon)* to allow coverage of the cornea during sleep in the presence of various degrees of lagophthalmos commonly seen in the postoperative period after ptosis correction.

The position of the normal lid with respect to the cornea in primary position must be noted, because this position represents the point at which the ptotic lid should rest after surgical correction when healing is complete. Lid lag of the ptotic lid in relation to the normal lid on downward gaze strongly suggests that the ptosis is congenital in nature. The abnormal levator muscle in congenital ptosis neither contracts nor relaxes normally. In acquired ptosis the lid should have a normal excursion in downward gaze in relationship to the normal fellow eyelid. In general, it is difficult to overcorrect congenital ptosis and easy to overcorrect acquired ptosis by whatever surgical technique is chosen. However, the postoperative lid position should ideally be slightly overcorrected, since it is easier to remedy overcorrection than undercorrection. Overcorrection can be lessened by frequent lid massage, early postoperative suture release, a partial levator tenotomy, or levator recession. Undercorrection usually requires a second resection of the levator (provided that the levator action is adequate) under less favorable conditions, namely, obliterated tissue planes and scar tissue.

The position and contour of the normal upper lid fold are also important preoperative observations, because they indicate where the skin incision should be made in the ptotic lid in order to cause the ptotic upper lid fold to match that of the normal side after operation.

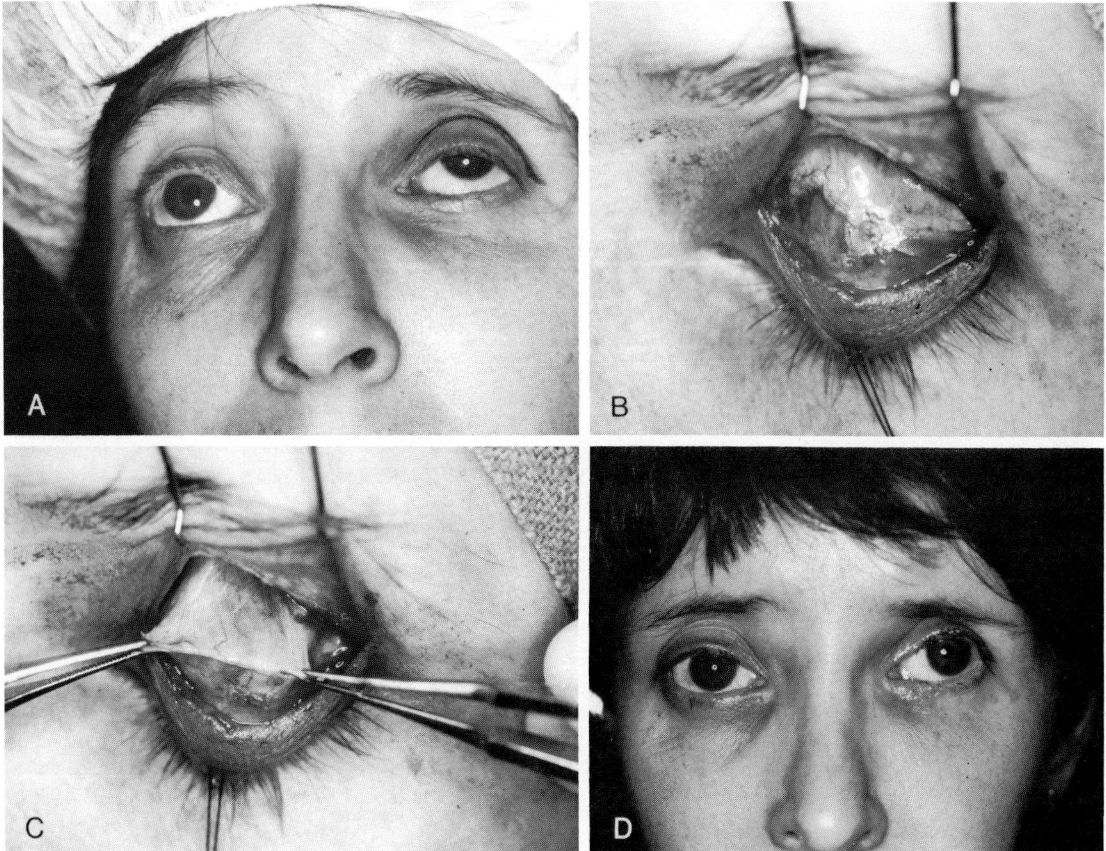

Figure 34–124. *A,* A patient with moderately severe ptosis of the left upper eyelid six months after trauma to the periorbital region. *B,* Exploration of the left upper lid demonstrates a levator dehiscence. *C,* The levator aponeurosis is freed and held with forceps before reinsertion onto the anterior surface of the tarsus. *D,* The patient six months postoperatively with adequate lid levels.

A high lid fold on the ptotic side suggests a levator defect. In most children the normal upper lid fold is 4 to 5 mm above the lashes in the midline, being 1 or 2 mm closer to the lashes in its temporal and nasal extremities. Therefore, the skin incision should be made to conform to this curve. In a few patients the normal lid fold may blend with the palpebro-orbital fold, which usually is 10 to 18 mm above the lashes, to create an unusually high upper fold. In bilateral ptosis correction the upper lid incision should be placed at the same distance above the lashes to result in symmetric lid folds.

Figure 34–125. A patient with the characteristic appearance of levator dehiscence. Note the ptosis, thin upper eyelid tissue, high lid creases, and brow elevation.

Figure 34–126 illustrates the surgical management of ptosis based on the logical application of the most effective procedures to correct ptosis in accordance with the amount of levator function and the degree of ptosis. According to Rycroft (1962), until 1811 ptosis of the upper eyelid was treated by the excision of skin alone, after the fashion of the ancient Arabian surgeons. Even Scarpa at that time used this time-honored technique. Von Graefe, however, no doubt influenced by the teachings of his father and Dieffenbach, recommended that a strip of orbicularis oculi muscle should also be excised. There is no doubt that von Graefe must have spoken of this technique on his trips to England and

Ireland. Bowman (1859), who was his friend, used the technique on several occasions, but clearly was not completely satisfied with it.

Numerous procedures are described for the correction of ptosis; however, the most useful are only those that address the anatomic defect producing the ptosis. The procedures to be described are (1) the Fasanella-Servat operation and its modifications, (2) aponeurosis surgery, (3) the levator resection, and (4) the brow suspension procedure.

When levator function is greater than 10 mm and the degree of ptosis is minimal or less than 2 mm, the *Fasanella-Servat operation* (Fasanella and Servat, 1961) or its various modifications may be used most effectively. When there is good levator function and the degree of ptosis is greater than 2 mm but less than 4 mm, exploration of the levator aponeurosis and advancement, plication, or reapproximation often produce the best result *(aponeurosis surgery)*. When the levator function is fair (4 to 10 mm) or poor (< 4 mm), the *levator resection operation* in the former and the *brow suspension procedure* in the latter are used (Fig. 34–126).

Fasanella-Servat Operation and its Modifications

This operation was first described in 1961. According to Fasanella (1973), the procedure is indicated in patients with mild ptosis (1.5 to 2 mm) in whom levator function and a satisfactory lid fold are present. The exceptions to this generalization are the ability to correct up to 3 mm of ptosis in the postenucleation situation, and 4 mm of ptosis in acquired myogenic ptosis. In all instances, levator function must be present or the operation will fail. The Fasanella-Servat operation has proved most helpful in (1) bilateral congenital ptosis, (2) unilateral congenital ptosis, (3) Horner's syndrome, (4) myogenic acquired senile ptosis, (5) postenucleation ptosis, (6) ptosis following incomplete ptosis correction, and (7) ptosis after cataract extraction. In most instances for aduts, and always for children, general anethesia is preferred. If local anesthesia is selected, the usual solutions of local anesthetic and epinephrine may be utilized. However, the epinephrine stimulates the sympathetically innervated Müller's muscle, and the local anesthetic paralyzes the orbicularis oculi muscle, causing an artificially elevated lid. These factors must be taken into consideration when adjusting the lid level during surgery and usually require placing the lid at a 1 to 2 mm overcorrected position.

The eyelid is everted with a Desmarres retractor or similar instrument, which pushes the skin and subcutaneous tissues inward, where they can be picked up in the bite of the hemostatic forceps. This maneuver avoids postoperative unwanted skin folds and "peaked" lids.

A selection of two thin, curved, hemostatic

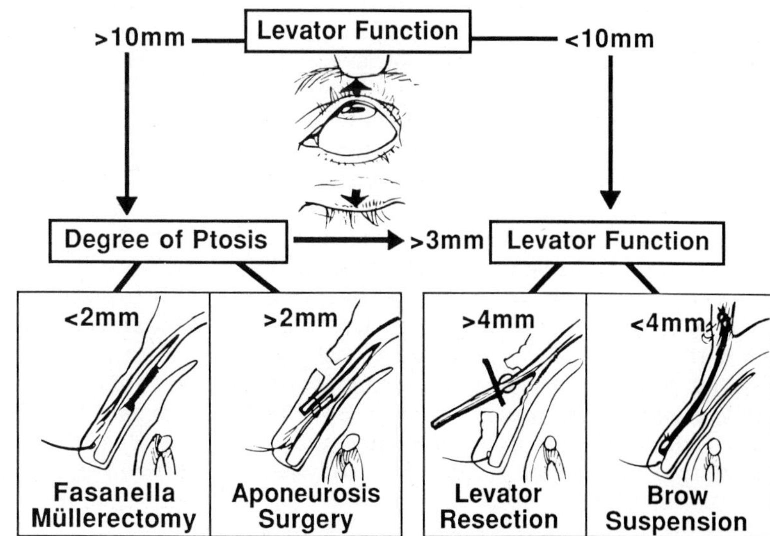

Figure 34–126. The surgical management of ptosis.

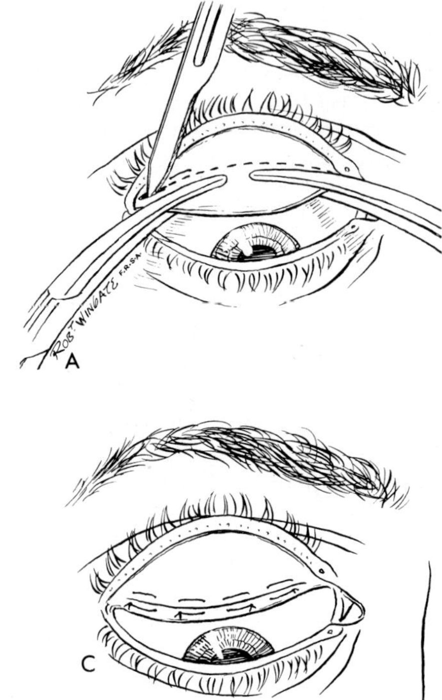

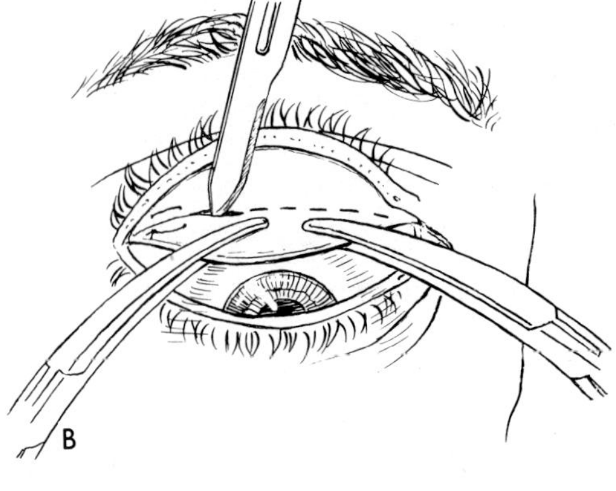

Figure 34–127. The Fasanella-Servat operation (1973). *A,* The eyelid is everted. *B,* Two thin, curved hemostatic forceps are placed on the lower edge of the everted lid 3 mm or less from the upper border of the tarsus. The first of the interrupted incisions is made. The interrupted incisions are extended in steps of 4 to 5 mm. A mattress suture is placed after each incision. *C,* The sutures are tied so as to hold the tissues firmly yet allow the lid to be returned to its normal position at the end of the procedure.

forceps and two straight forceps to match the variations of the tarsal plate should be available. Most tarsal plates have a "D" shape with an upward convexity, but a few are almost straight.

The height of the midportion of the adult tarsus is approximately 11 mm. The forceps are placed on the lower edge of the everted lid 3 mm or less from the everted upper border of the tarsus (Fig. 34–127*A*). The forceps grasp the conjunctiva, tarsus, levator (or some thin anterior fibers of the levator 4 or 5 mm below the superior edge of the tarsus), and Müller's muscle. A question arises as to whether any of the fibers of the levator are grasped by the clamp; in any event, all loose tissues are held taut by the clamps. The incisions are extended in steps of 4 to 5 mm, and a suture is placed after each incision (Fig. 34–127*B*). The interrupted incisions and subsequent sutures minimize bleeding and serve as a safety factor in preventing retraction of tissue. The sutures are tied tightly enough to hold the tissues firmly, yet allow the lid to be returned to its normal position at the end of the procedure (Fig. 34–127*C*). One should always avoid dog-ears and raggedness of the tarsal plate, which may cause corneal abrasion.

In the original Fasanella procedure, four or five interrupted 5-0 or 6-0 sutures were placed, but owing to reports of corneal abrasions Fasanella now recommends that such sutures be used exclusively for minimal ptosis after enucleations. In 1961 Fasanella and Servat pointed out that the danger of corneal damage could be averted by using a continuous suture to the point of origin (Fig. 34–128).

Beard's (1969) modification is a running serpentine suture of 5-0 to 6-0 plain catgut (Lukens double-armed, gas sterilized). The suture is placed from the temporal to the nasal aspect, passing back and forth between the tarsal and palpebral conjunctiva approximately 1 mm from the hemostatic forceps (Fig. 34–129*A*). The tissue included in the hemostats is excised and the suture is returned to its point of origin in a running fashion. Both ends of the suture are brought out through a small skin incision in the upper temporal eyelid fold, and tied in such a fashion that the knot retracts beneath the skin and cannot touch the cornea or sclera.

Tenzel (1970) suggested a modification of the Beard suture in that the return of the suture from medial to lateral is placed in the "subsubstance" tissue (Fig. 34–129*B*). In the

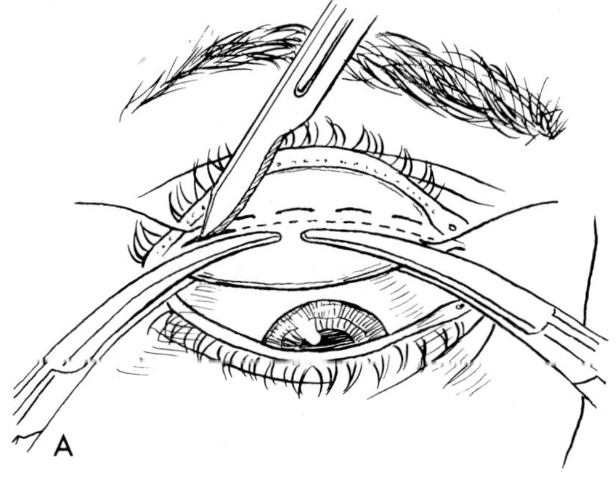

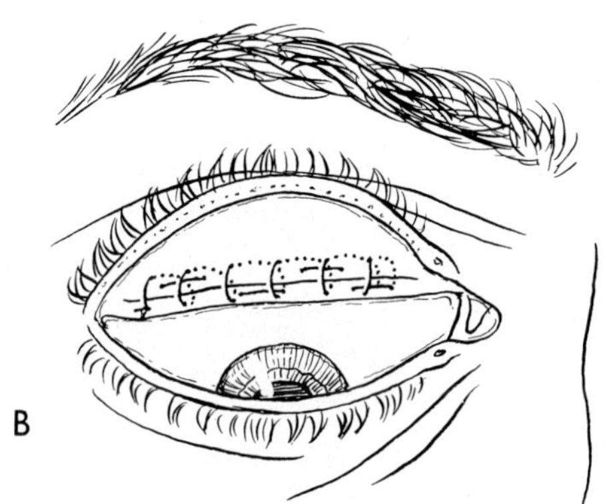

Figure 34–128. *A,* Fasanella's alternative method of suturing in a running continuous or "serpentine" fashion. *B,* The running continuous or "serpentine" suture is returned, and the suture is tied on the temporal side.

Smith modification, the lid is everted, and hemostats are placed 3 mm above the everted upper border of the tarsus (Fig. 34–130*A*). Figure 34–130*B* illustrates the anatomy of the eyelid. Note the position of the hemostat on the everted lid (Fig. 34–130*C*). A suture is inserted, entering above the lateral canthus and exiting just above the clamp on the palpebral conjunctival side (Fig. 34–130*A, D*). The anatomy of the lid before and after eversion is depicted in Figure 34–130*B, D*. The clamp grasps the conjunctiva, tarsus, the orbital septum, the levator aponeurosis, and Müller's muscle, avoiding the infolded skin and orbicularis muscle. The clamped portion of the lid is elevated, and the suture is brought from the palpebral-conjunctival side to the tarsal side, above the clamp (Fig. 34–130*E*). The suture is continued across the area held by the clamps (Fig. 34–130*F*). Each entrance of the needle is placed as close to the last exit of the suture as possible, and the suture is angled to form a "V" to the opposite side. In this way, abrasion of the cornea by a large amount of suture material is avoided. Figure 34–130*G* shows the minimal amount of suture material indented into the conjunctiva on the tarsal side. The clamp on the nasal side is removed and placed on the edge of the tarsus to act as a retractor. A through and through incision is made into the crushed tissue left after the removal of the hemostat (Fig. 34–130*H*). The suture is brought out into the wound through the subcuticular layer (Fig. 34–130*I*). The subcuticular suture

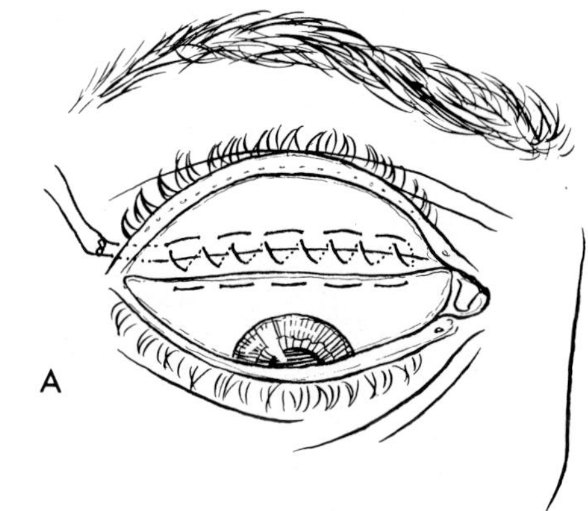

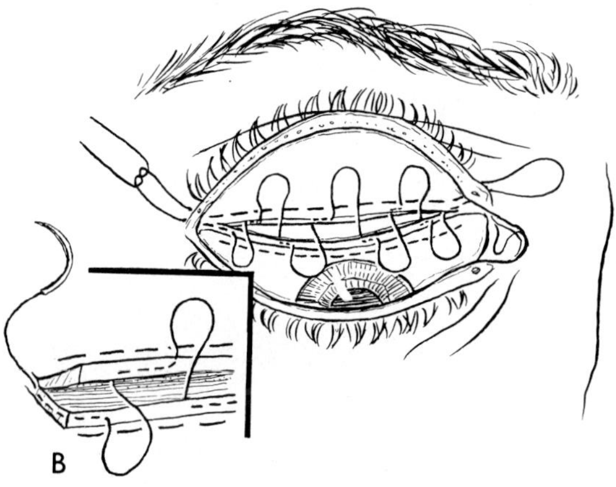

Figure 34–129. *A,* Beard's modification (1969). A running "serpentine" suture of 5-0 or 6-0 plain catgut is placed from the temporal to the nasal aspect approximately 1 mm from the hemostats; the suture passes back and forth between the tarsal conjunctiva and the palpebral conjunctiva. The tissue included in the hemostat is excised, and the suture is returned to its point of origin as a running continuous suture uniting the palpebral conjunctiva to the upper tarsal edge. The ends of the suture are brought out through the skin in the temporal portion of the supratarsal fold and tied. By this modification, no knots touch the cornea or the sclera. *B,* Tenzel's modification (1970) of the Beard suture. The return of the suture from medial to lateral is placed in the "subsubstance."

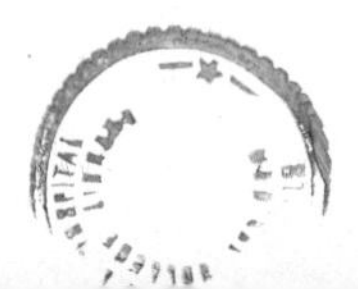

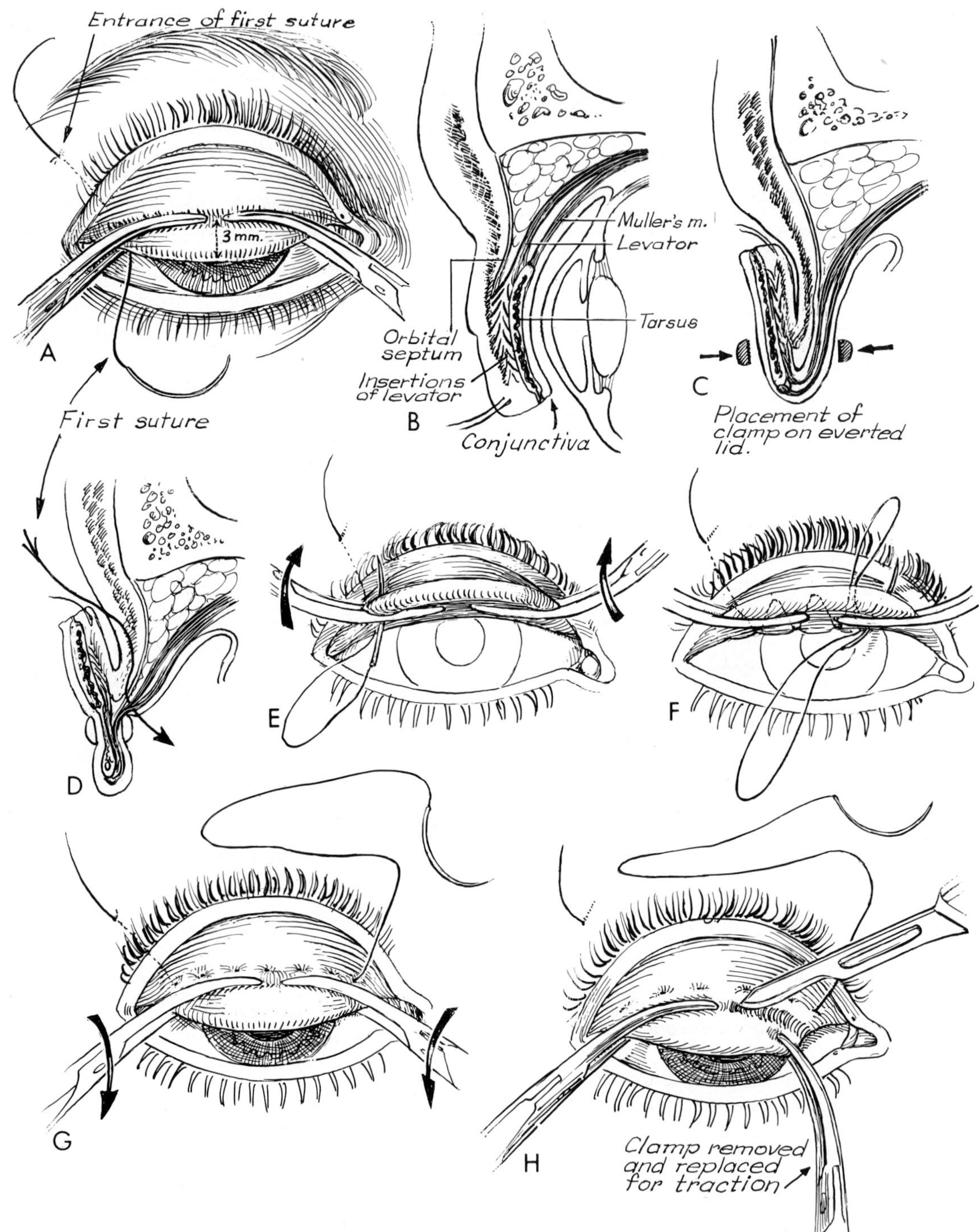

Figure 34–130. Smith's modification of the Fasanella-Servat operation. *A,* The lid is everted, and hemostats are placed 3 mm above the everted upper border of the tarsus. A suture is inserted, entering above the lateral canthus and exiting just about the clamp. *B,* Cross section illustrating the anatomy of the upper eyelid. *C,* The arrows indicate the position of the hemostat on the everted lid. *D,* Cross section illustrating the position of the lid after it has been everted and showing the tissues grasped by the hemostat: conjunctiva, tarsus, orbital septum, levator, Müller's muscle, and conjunctiva; the infolded skin and orbicularis muscle are avoided. *E,* The clamped portion of the lid is elevated, and suturing is begun. *F,* The suture is continued across the area held by the clamp. *G,* The suture is brought out through the conjunctiva beyond the clamped area. *H,* The clamp on the nasal side is removed and placed on the edge of the tarsus as a retractor. A scalpel makes a through and through incision into the crushed tissue left by the removed hemostat.

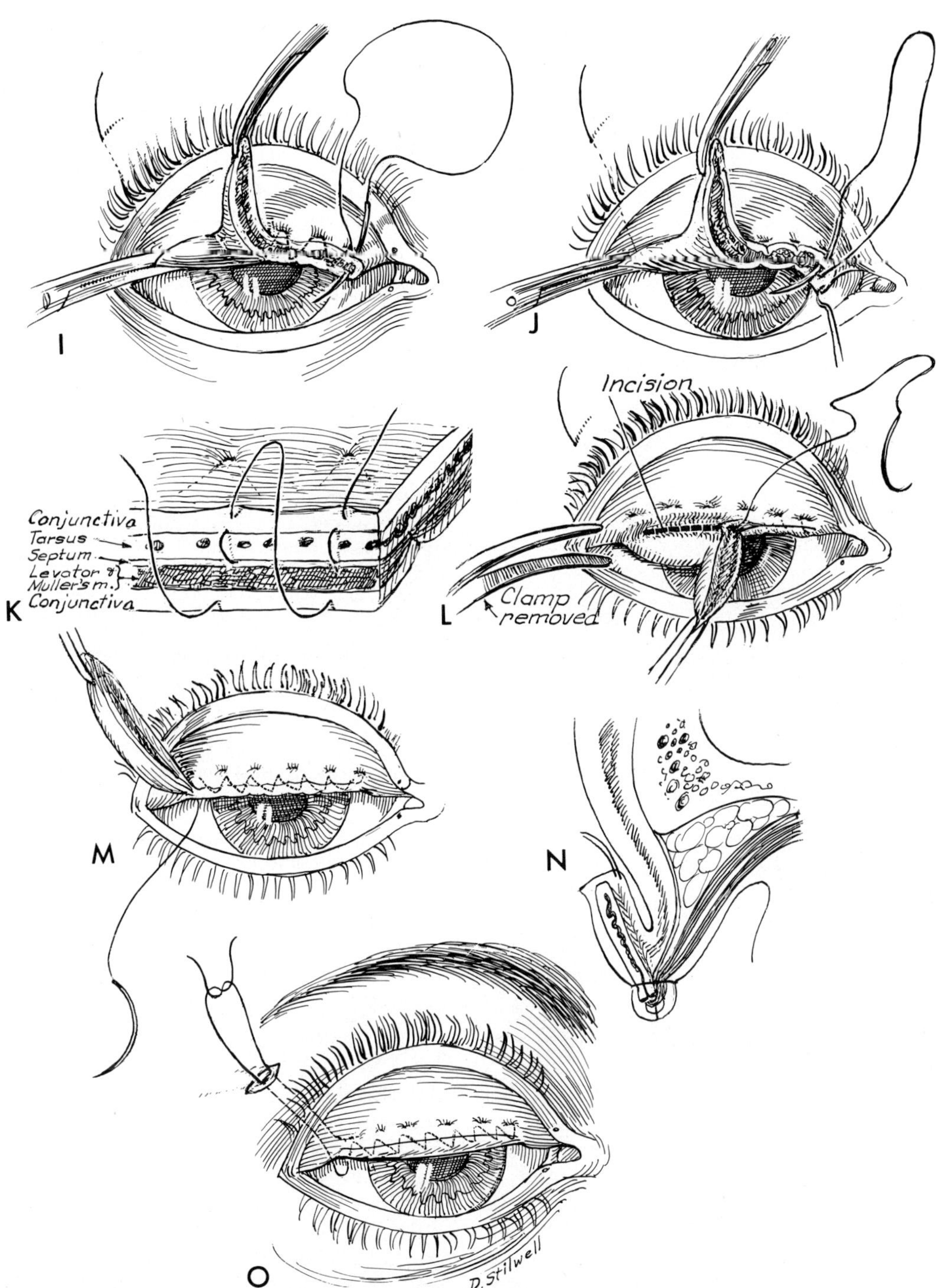

Figure 34–130 *Continued I,* The incised tissue is raised, and the suture enters the wound through the subsubstance layer. *J, K,* The subsubstance suture extends laterally, picking up the fibers of the levator, Müller's muscle, and the septum orbitale in the lower bites. *L,* The lateral clamp is removed, and the through and through incision and suture continued laterally. *M,* The suture is continued to the lateral edge. *N,* Cross section showing the position of the sutures. *O,* The suture is brought out through an incision at the lateral end of the supratarsal fold and tied beneath the skin.

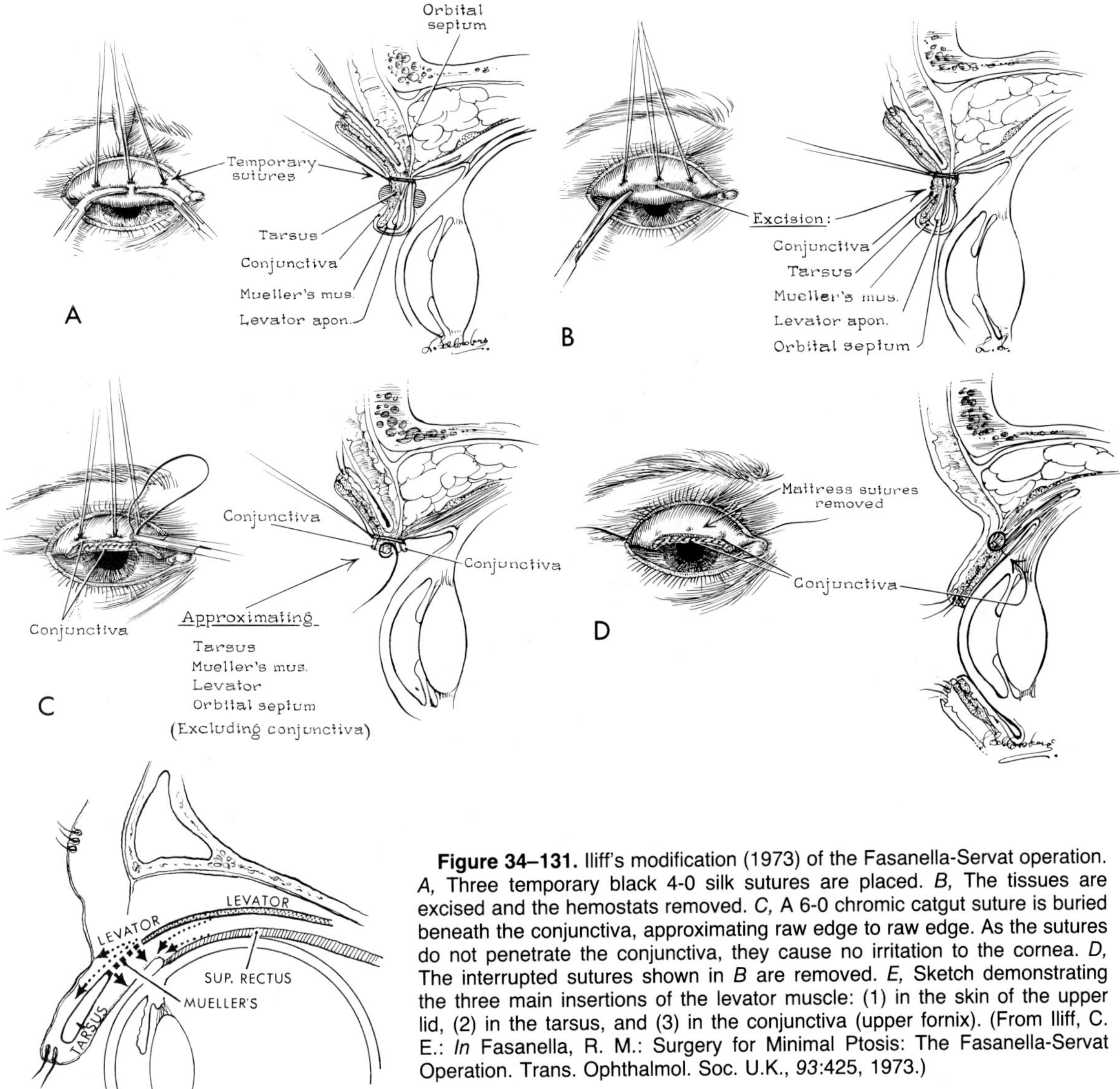

Figure 34–131. Iliff's modification (1973) of the Fasanella-Servat operation. *A,* Three temporary black 4-0 silk sutures are placed. *B,* The tissues are excised and the hemostats removed. *C,* A 6-0 chromic catgut suture is buried beneath the conjunctiva, approximating raw edge to raw edge. As the sutures do not penetrate the conjunctiva, they cause no irritation to the cornea. *D,* The interrupted sutures shown in *B* are removed. *E,* Sketch demonstrating the three main insertions of the levator muscle: (1) in the skin of the upper lid, (2) in the tarsus, and (3) in the conjunctiva (upper fornix). (From Iliff, C. E.: *In* Fasanella, R. M.: Surgery for Minimal Ptosis: The Fasanella-Servat Operation. Trans. Ophthalmol. Soc. U.K., *93*:425, 1973.)

is continued laterally, picking up the fibers of the levator, Müller's muscle, and the septum in the lower needle bites (Fig. 34–130*J*, *K*). The lateral clamp is removed and the through and through incision continued laterally along the bed of the clamp; a small area is left attached for traction purposes (Fig. 34–130*L, M*). The subcuticular suture is continued to the lateral edge (Fig. 34–130*M*). The sagittal section (Fig. 34–130*N*) shows the position of the suture. A stab incision is made at the site of the first entrance of the suture above the lateral canthus; the ends of the subcuticular suture are brought out through an incision at the lateral end of the supratarsal fold and tied beneath the skin (Fig. 34–130*O*).

The Fasanella operation modified by Iliff employs three interrupted 4–0 black silk stay sutures (Fig. 34–131*A*). These temporary sutures provide hemostasis and secure the tissue firmly. The hemostats are removed and the tissues excised (Fig. 34–131*B*). A modified, completely buried 6–0 chromic running suture is applied and knotted (Fig. 34–131*C*). The suture does not include the conjunctiva, and when the lid is returned to the normal position the suture tends to be covered by conjunctiva and causes little corneal irritation.

There are three insertions of the levator (Fig. 34–131*E*). The main insertion is in the skin through fibers that cross the antagonist, the orbicularis oculi, and its associated muscular fascia. This insertion is marked by the superior palpebral sulcus. The accentuation of the superior palpebral fold with the eyes looking up is an index of levator function. This is one of the main conditions looked for in selecting candidates for this operation. Part of the levator is inserted in the anterior face of the tarsus 4 to 5 mm below its superior edge, i.e., the superior third to half of the anterior aspect of the tarsus. The principal attachment to the tarsus is through the nonstriated Müller's muscle, which attaches to the superior edge of the tarsus. The third attachment of the levator is to the conjunctiva of the upper cul-de-sac via the fascial sheath of the muscle. There may be a similar attachment to the superior rectus muscle.

Other modifications of the Fasanella-Servat operation include (1) the Mustardé split-level resection (Mustardé, 1975), (2) the McCord external tarsoaponeurectomy (McCord, 1973), (3) the Putterman tarsal-müllerectomy (Putterman and Urist, 1975), and (4) the Lauring sutureless Fasanella-Servat procedure (Lauring, 1975). Beard (1969) was of the opinion that the Fasanella-Servat operation is successful because of the tarsectomy. Putterman (1973) believed that the results are due to resection and advancement of Müller's muscle. According to Fasanella (1973), a combination of both these factors may be responsible for the usually predictable and satisfactory results.

Another operation for the patient with minimal ptosis (1 to 2 mm) and levator function (>10 mm) is the levator shortening (plication) operation described by Jones (1974a). It has been used by Smith (1975) and Callahan (1974) with satisfactory results. The operation is performed on the sedated patient under local anesthesia. An incision is made 6 mm above the lash line through the skin and orbicularis muscle. An Erhardt clamp is attached near the lid margin and the skin-muscle layer is retracted upward, exposing the underlying orbital septum. The skin-muscle flap is elevated for 10 to 12 mm upward to visualize the preaponeurotic fat beneath the orbital septum. The patient is asked to look upward to assist in identification of the levator. The orbital septum is opened and a muscle hook is inserted to separate the attachment of the septum to the levator aponeurosis (Fig. 34–132*A*). A plication suture is passed into the central portion of the levator aponeurosis and into the midline anterior tarsus, incorporating approximately 7 to 10 mm of tissue (Fig. 34–132*B*). The Erhardt clamp is removed and a loose temporary knot is tied to assess lid level and contour. Removal and replacement of the suture is performed until the lid is lifted to a satisfactory level. After this is achieved, additional sutures are placed on each side of the central suture to elevate the medial and lateral thirds of the eyelid.

Aponeurosis Surgery

A more recent trend in the correction of minimal ptosis with levator function is to proceed to direct identification of the levator aponeurosis in order to repair, advance, or resect it instead of plicating it. The trend for more levator aponeurosis exploration and surgical manipulation developed from the realization that most acquired, late ptosis is caused by an abnormality in the distal aponeurosis. It has also been shown that a small but significant number of patients with congenital ptosis may have levator aponeurotic defects amenable to aponeurotic surgery (Anderson and Gordy, 1979a). The surgical technique includes simple repair of the levator aponeurosis dehiscence or some form of levator aponeurosis advancement (Anderson and Dixon, 1979a; McCord and Tanenbaum, 1987). Whether or not an advancement of the freed levator aponeurosis is required is determined at the time of surgery. The accuracy of this determination is directly proportional to the surgeon's experience in aponeurosis surgery.

The clinical findings that suggest a levator aponeurotic defect as the cause of ptosis are satisfactory (>10 mm) levator function, a high lid fold, and thinning of the upper eyelid tissues (see Figs. 34–124, 34–125). These findings are consistent with the anatomic defect of aponeurotic dehiscence or disinsertion. Figure 34–133 shows a sagittal section of the anatomic findings in a normal upper lid compared with the patient with involutional ptosis. Note that the lid crease attachments remain intact, and with levator dehis-

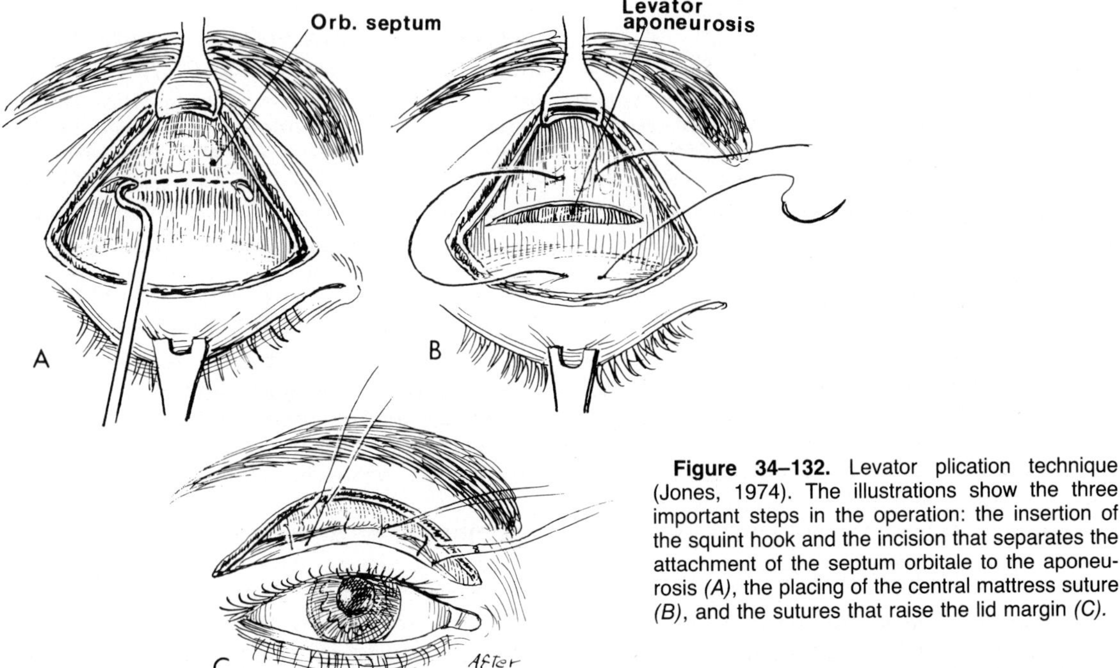

Figure 34–132. Levator plication technique (Jones, 1974). The illustrations show the three important steps in the operation: the insertion of the squint hook and the incision that separates the attachment of the septum orbitale to the aponeurosis *(A)*, the placing of the central mattress suture *(B)*, and the sutures that raise the lid margin *(C)*.

cence the lid fold is elevated. Fig. 34–124*A* shows a patient with 3 mm of left upper eyelid ptosis, satisfactory levator function, a lid crease, and thinning of the lid tissues. Upon exploration of the levator aponeurosis, a complete dehiscence with ragged edges was found (see Fig. 34–124*B*). Advancement of the aponeurosis (see Fig. 34–124*C*) and reapproximation to the superoanterior tarsus resulted in adequate ptosis correction (see Fig. 34–124*D*).

Levator Resection

The Conjunctival Approach. In 1859 Bowman described the first resection of the levator through the conjunctiva. He everted the lid, excised the upper edge of the tarsus with slightly more than 10 mm of the levator, and sutured the two edges together. Blaskovics (1923) described another method for conjunctival resection of the levator that could correct 4 to 8 mm of ptosis. Berke (1952)

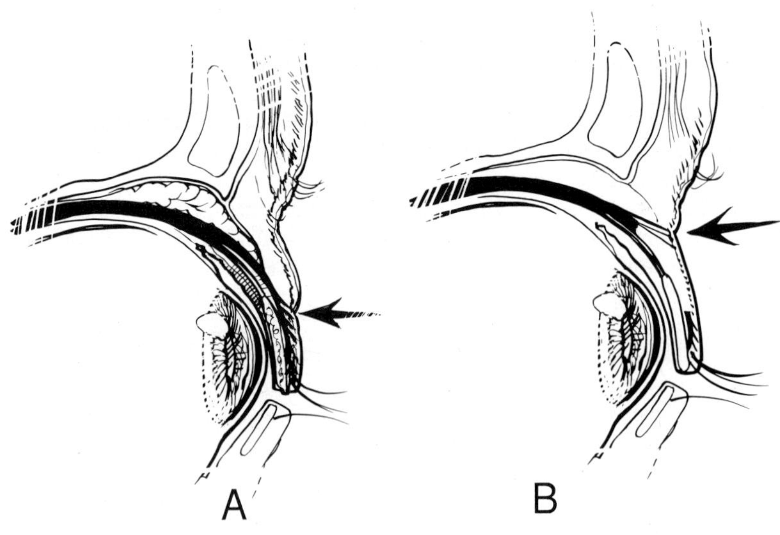

Figure 34–133. *A,* Diagram of the normal upper eyelid anatomy in sagittal section. *B,* The anatomic situation with levator aponeurosis dehiscence. The high lid fold is created because the lid crease (dermal) attachments from the levator aponeurosis remain intact *(arrow)*.

modified the Blaskovics procedure by completely freeing the levator attachments to gain additional correction. Iliff (1954) simplified the operation by excising the conjunctiva of the upper fornix with the levator. In general the conjunctival approach to levator resection gives excellent results when the levator function is adequate.

The Cutaneous Approach. The first operation for resection of the levator through a skin incision was described by Eversbusch (1883). Many modifications of this procedure have been made. In general, more levator can be excised through the external route and better results achieved when the levator function is poor. Berke (1959) attributed the superior results to better exposure and a firmer anchorage of the transplanted levator to the upper lid tissues. Thus, he concluded that the external approach is the method of choice when the levator action is fair or poor; either the cutaneous or conjunctival approach may be used if the levator action is good.

External Levator Resection. When the levator function is less than 10 mm and the ptosis greater than 4 mm, the levator resection operation through a cutaneous approach gives excellent results. Even when the levator function is poor (<4 mm), this procedure frequently produces an acceptable result. The operation is best suited for patients with moderate or severe congenital ptosis. It has also proved helpful in mild congenital and acquired ptosis; however, alternative forms of correction for these conditions, such as the Fasanella-Servat procedure, tarsal-müllerectomy, or aponeurosis advancement should be considered.

Surgical Technique. A scleral contact lens is inserted to protect the globe (Fig. 34–134*A*). The upper border of the tarsus is identified by slightly elevating the upper lid margin, causing the skin to form a crease at the supratarsal fold. This line is marked with ink and incised after subcutaneous injection of a solution of local anesthetic combined with 1:100,000 epinephrine (Fig. 34–134*B, C*). The skin is separated from the underlying orbicularis muscle superiorly about 3 to 4 mm and inferiorly to the lower margin of the tarsus deep to the roots of the eyelashes (Fig. 34–134*D*). At the lateral end of the incision, scissors undermine the pretarsal portion of the orbicularis muscle, separating it from the pretarsal fascia (Fig. 34–134*E*). The pretarsal portion of the orbicularis muscle is raised as a flap and excised (Fig. 34–134*F*). A puncture incision is made at the superolateral edge of the tarsus, lateral to the levator aponeurosis (Fig. 34–134*G*), and a straight hemostat is passed through the conjunctival cul-de-sac just above the tarsus; the other rests over the levator aponeurosis, Müller's muscle, and a few preseptal orbicularis fibers (Fig. 34–134*H, I*). The tissues incorporated within the blades of the hemostat are freed from the tarsus by an incision (Fig. 34–134*J*). The conjunctiva is separated from Müller's muscle and the levator. Saline solution injected between the layers (Fig. 34–134*K*) facilitates the dissection, which is extended upward (Fig. 34–134*L*), separating the conjunctiva from Müller's muscle; care is taken to avoid injuring the superior rectus muscle. The conjunctiva is approximated to the superior border of the tarsus with absorbable suture; Müller's muscle, the levator aponeurosis, and the orbital septum are contained within the clamp (Fig. 34–134*M*). The skin and orbicularis muscle are retracted upward while downward traction is exerted with the hemostat. The septum orbitale is incised laterally and medially (Fig. 34–134*N*), which allows the orbital fat to prolapse. The levator is freed medially and laterally from the levator expansions, upward toward the trochlea and along the lateral orbital wall (Fig. 34–134*O*). A double-armed suture is passed through the central portion of the tarsus but not through to the conjunctiva. It is passed through the structures held within the hemostat at a level 1 to 2 cm above the level of the hemostat, and tied (Fig. 34–134*P* to *R*). The level at which the suture is placed depends on the amount of shortening desired and is directly related to the amount of ptosis. The best guideline for setting the central portion of the upper eyelid at the proper level is to place it just below the upper limbus (after removal of the contact lens) (Fig. 34–134*S*). Additional mattress sutures are placed medially and temporally, and the tissue below the hemostat is excised (Fig. 34–134*T*). Three additional vertical mattress sutures are placed through the upper portion of the tarsus, incorporating all layers of the lid, to reinforce the attachment of the levator aponeurosis and ensure the position and depth of the supratarsal fold (Fig. 34–134*U, V*). A temporary lid occlusion suture is placed (Fig. 34–134*W*) to protect the cornea. This suture may be removed in 24 hours. Artificial tears

Text continued on page 1772

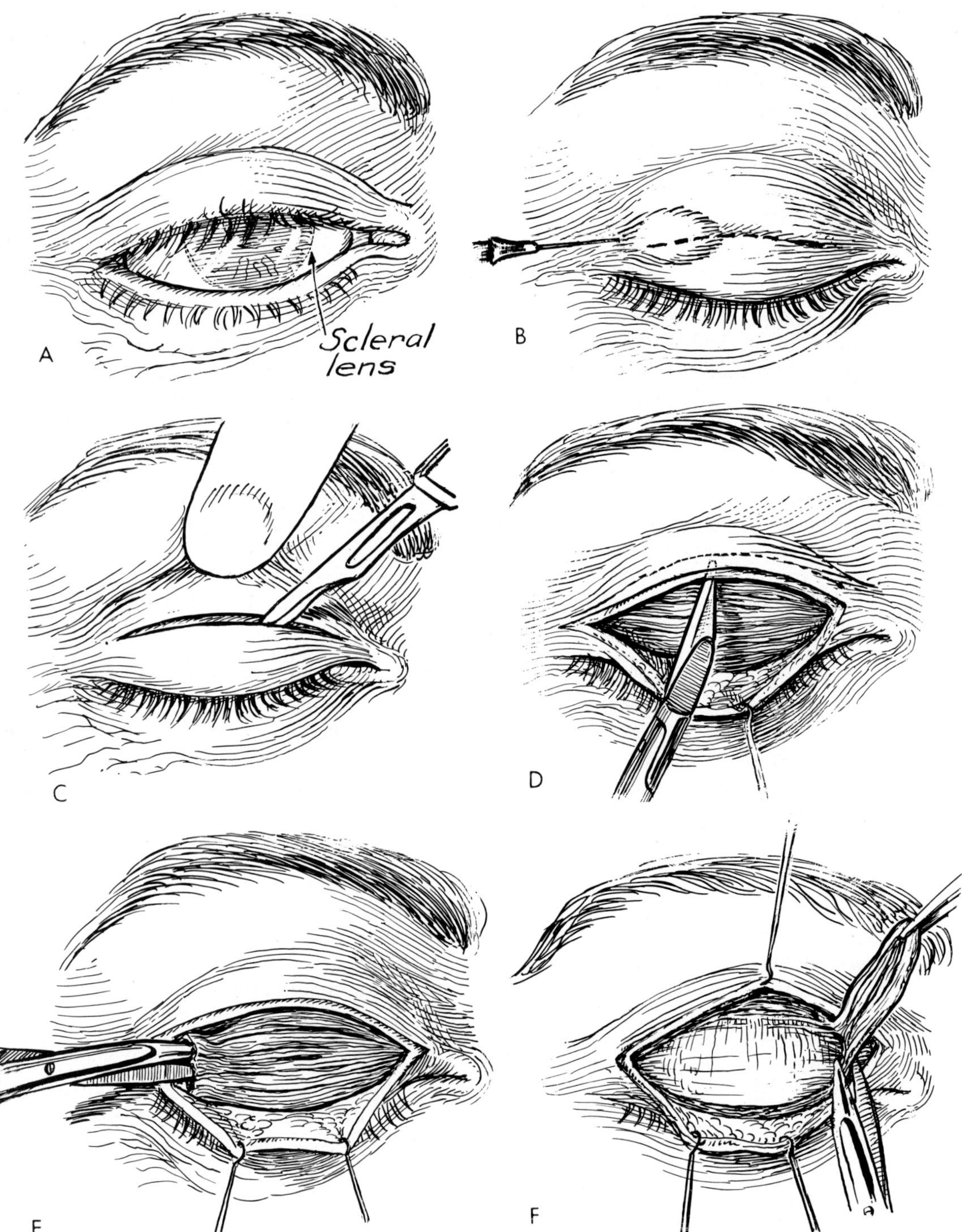

Figure 34–134. External levator resection: modified Blaskovics operation. *A,* The protective lens has been inserted. *B,* The upper border of the tarsus has been indicated by an ink line. Injection of a solution of lidocaine-epinephrine separates the skin from the underlying orbicularis muscle. *C,* An incision is made following the ink line. *D,* The skin is separated from the oribicularis muscle by sharp dissection. *E,* Scissors incise and undermine the pretarsal portion of the orbicularis muscle, separating it from the pretarsal fascia. *F,* The pretarsal portion of the orbicularis muscle is raised as a flap and excised.

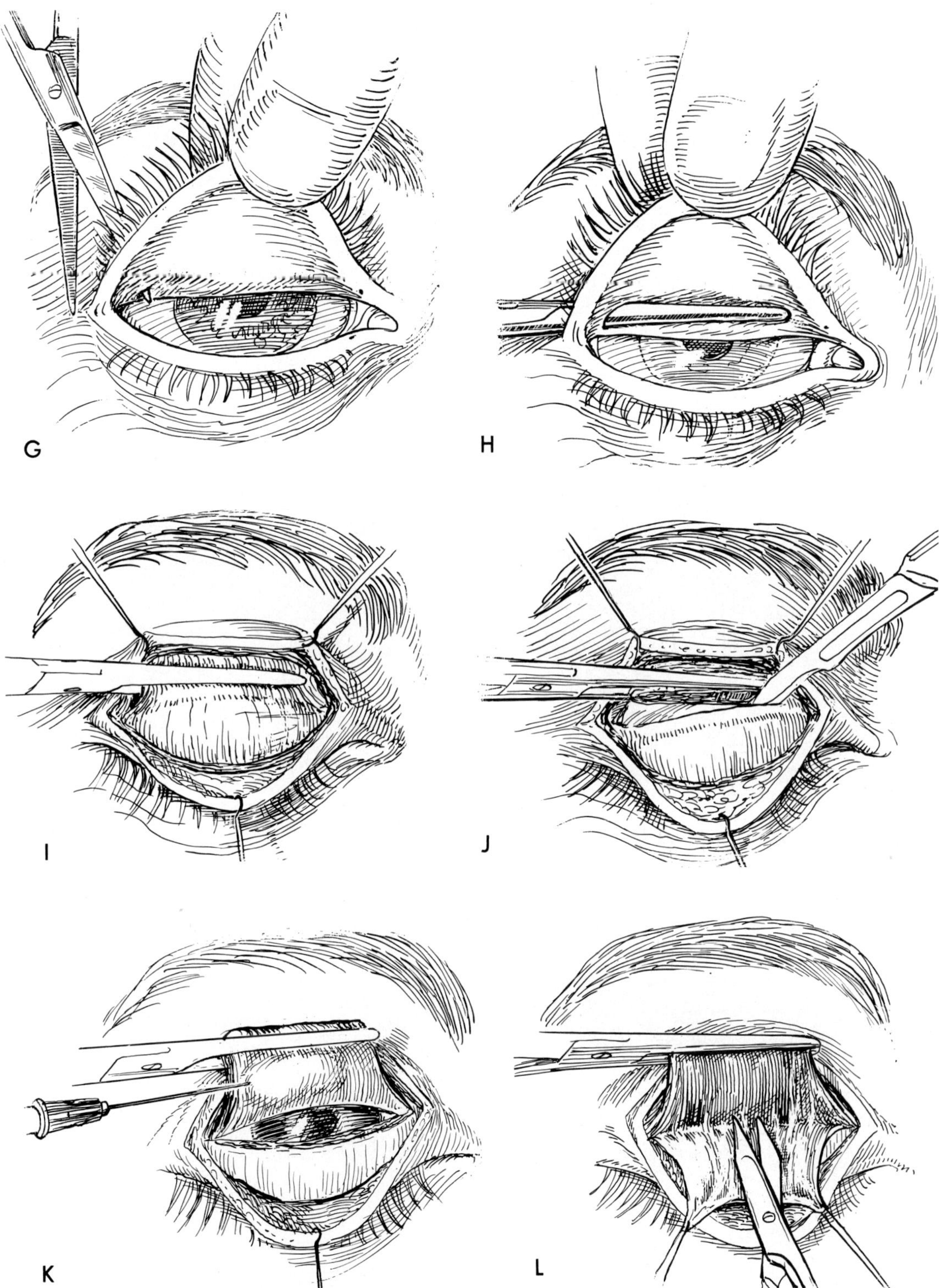

Figure 34–134 *Continued G,* A puncture incision is made at the superolateral edge of the tarsus, lateral to the levator aponeurosis. *H,* A straight hemostat is passed through the conjunctiva. *I,* One blade of the hemostat extends across the conjunctiva just about the tarsus. The other blade rests over the levator aponeurosis, Müller's muscle, and a few preseptal orbicularis fibers. *J,* The tissues incorporated within the blades of the hemostat are freed from the tarsus by an incision. *K,* Injection of saline solution separates the conjunctiva from Müller's muscle and the levator. *L,* The plane of dissection is found between Müller's muscle and the conjunctiva.

Illustration continued on following page

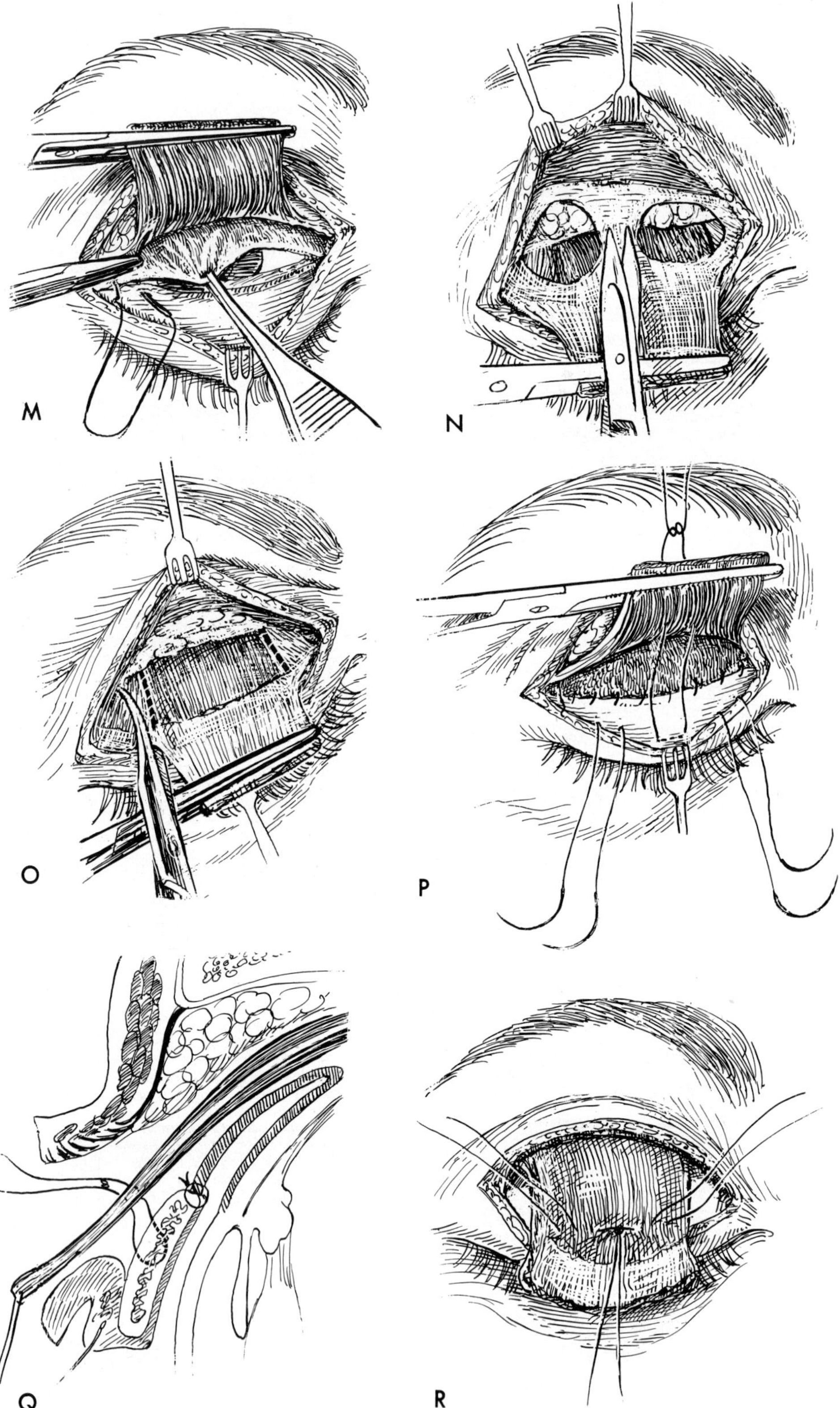

Figure 34–134 *Continued M,* Müller's muscle is sutured with catgut to the upper margin of the tarsus. *N,* The skin and orbicularis muscle are retracted upward, and the septum orbitale is incised laterally and medially. *O,* The levator is freed medially and laterally from the levator expansion. *P,* A double-armed suture of 6-0 silk is passed through the central portion of the tarsus but not through the conjunctiva; a suture is then placed through the structures held by the hemostat at a level situated between 1 and 2 cm above the level of the hemostat. *Q,* Sagittal section showing the position of the suture illustrated in *P. R,* A mattress suture is tied; additional sutures have been placed medially and laterally.

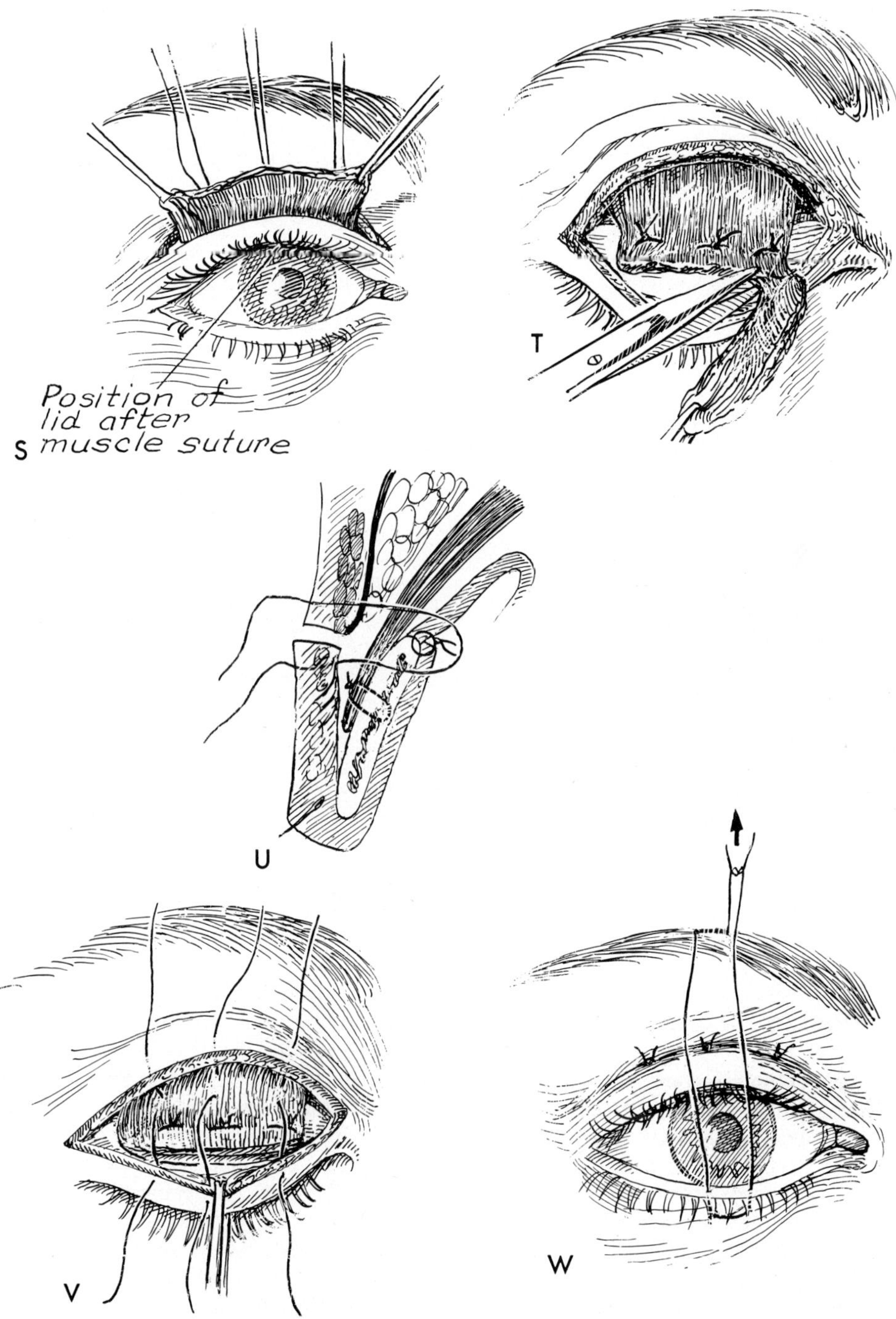

Figure 34–134 *Continued S,* The contact lens has been removed, and the operator is guided by the level of the eyelid margin in relation to the upper limbus when the suture is tightened. *T,* Additional mattress sutures have been tied, and tissue below the hemostat is excised. *U,* Sagittal section illustrating the position of a mattress suture of 6-0 chromic catgut placed through the upper portion of the tarsus, traversing the levator and the supratarsal fold. *V,* Position of three catgut sutures placed according to the technique shown in *U. W,* At the completion of the operation, an occlusive suture protects the cornea and relieves tension on the sutures, ensuring fixation of the levator aponeurosis to the tarsus.

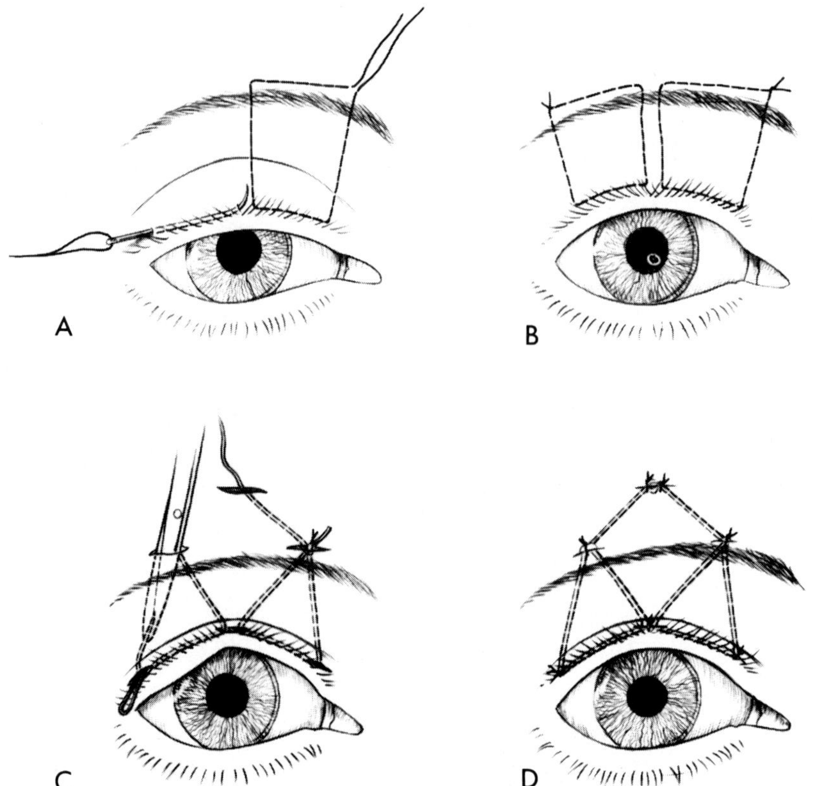

Figure 34–135. Frontalis fixation for ptosis when levator function is absent. Before location of the incisions above the eyebrow, the frontalis muscle is tested. If the frontalis is paralyzed, the suspension technique cannot be used. One part of the frontalis muscle may contract more than others, and the incisions should be placed to utilize that part. *A, B,* Double rhomboid frontalis fixation technique. Suspension material is threaded from the lid margin upward to emerge from the incision above the brow (see text for details). Note the special needle for introducing the suspension material. *C, D,* Double triangular suture.

and ointment are liberally applied to the eyes during the early postoperative phase.

Frontalis Muscle Suspension

Frontalis suspension is best indicated for the correction of bilateral severe congenital ptosis with very poor or absent levator function (see Fig. 34–126). Children with the blepharophimosis syndrome and the Marcus Gunn synkinetic ptosis syndrome often require bilateral frontalis suspension techniques to obtain the best results. According to Burian (1962), Hess in 1893 conceived a method of provoking the formation of fibrous bands between the frontalis muscle and the skin on the margin of the lid so that they would work as tendons. He made a long incision in the eyebrow and separated the skin of the lid from the orbicularis muscle down to the tarsus. Two or three mattress sutures were inserted from the brow to the lid and tied over glass bolsters under considerable tension. The sutures remained for two weeks, during which time fibrous bands developed between the brow and eyelids. Apparently some success was achieved in the ability to elevate the lids with the fibrous band connection to the brow; however, the results were unpredictable and not long-lasting. This led to the use of permanent suspension of the lid by sutures inserted subcutaneously to connect the tarsus with the frontalis muscle. The type of suture material ranged from silk to more physiologically inert substances such as silver and stainless steel wire, and finally to alloplastic materials.

As mentioned in König's (1928) monograph, it was Payr who originated the use of fascia (1928). Payr made incisions in the upper border of the tarsus, the eyebrow, and the forehead. He then undermined the skin between the incisions to introduce a large strip of fascia lata. Lexer (1923) introduced two narrow tapes of fascia through small incisions on the internal and external parts of the brow and on corresponding parts of the tarsus. Elschnig (1913) performed an operation similar to that of Payr but sutured the lower end of the strip transcutaneously. Many surgeons have used strips of fascia in different ways. Risdon (1945) made a small incision above the eyebrow and tunneled triangular tracts along the tarsal area to attach fascia strips to the frontalis muscle. The most popular suture technique is a modification of the Friedenwald-Guyton (1948) method, which employs a double rhomboid or triangular suture (Fig. 34–135). The suture material may be autogenous fascia lata, temporalis fascia, or strips of palmaris longis or plantaris tendon. Callahan (1974) reported success with the technique of Tillett and Tillett (1966), using a Silastic band for the frontalis suspension of the upper lids in the blepharophimosis syndrome (Fig. 34–136). A silicone rod frontalis suspension was recommended by McCord and Shore (1982) for patients with poor eye-protective mechanism because the procedure is easy to reverse or adjust in an office setting.

For the double rhomboid suspension (see Fig. 34–135*A*, *B*), three incisions are made above the eyebrow extending through the frontalis muscle. Two separate rhomboid suspensions are performed, the knots being tied laterally and medially. In performing the double triangular frontalis fixation (see Fig. 34–135*C*, *D*), two small incisions are made above the eyebrow to the frontalis muscle, one medially and the other laterally. Three incisions are made through the skin and orbicularis oculi muscle immediately above the eyelashes. Another incision is made 6 cm above the central portion of the eyebrow and extended through the frontalis muscle (see Fig. 34–135*C*). Two strips of fascia, tendon, Supramid, silicone rod, or other inorganic material are threaded upward through the

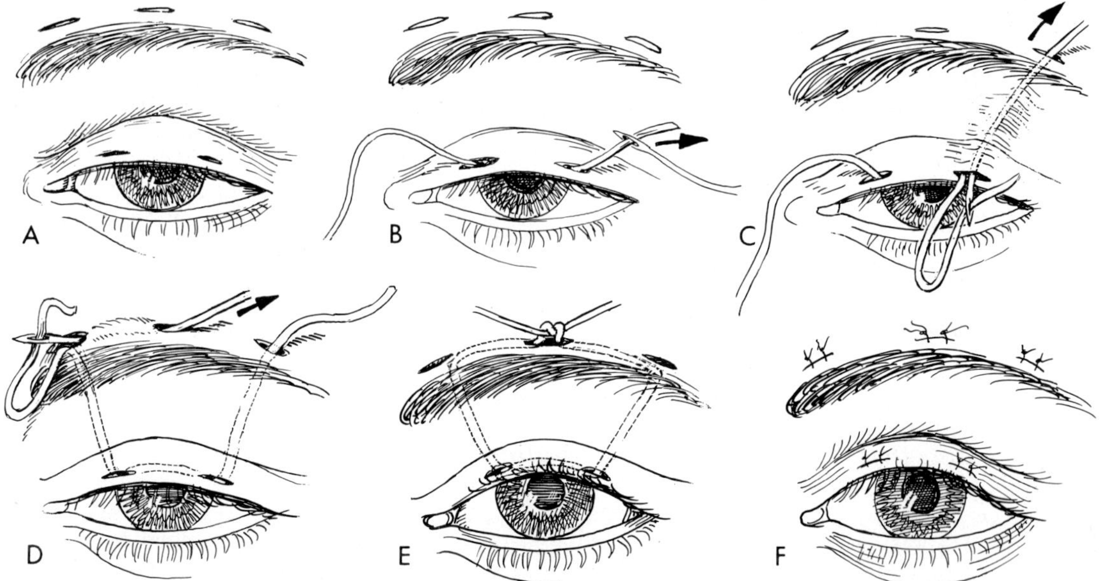

Figure 34–136. Frontalis suspension technique of Tillett and Tillett (1966). Modified placement of a Silastic strip. *A,* At the juncture of the horizontal thirds of the lid, two linear incisions are made 3 mm from and parallel to the lid margin. Each incision is 4 mm long. The skin, subcutaneous tissues, and orbicularis muscle are opened to expose the anterior tarsal surface. Three linear incisions are made just above the eyebrow. The first is placed in the midline of the brow directly over the lid. The medial incision is placed medially to a vertical line extending from the medial margin of the incision, and the lateral incision is made lateral to the lateral marginal incision. These incisions above the brow are opened to the frontalis muscle aponeurosis, but not to the periosteum. *B,* Insertion of the Silastic strip (No. 40). The Wright needle has been inserted from the lateral to the medial incision, the needle point having been pushed behind the orbicularis muscle, picking up some fibers of the epitarsus. When the point emerges through the medial incision, one end of the strip is inserted in the needle's eye. As the needle is withdrawn through the lateral incision, the strip is left in place in the lid near the margin. *C,* The needle has been directed down through the upper lateral incision and brought posterior to the orbicularis muscle in the plane of the orbital septum along the anterior surface of the tarsus to emerge in the lateral lid incision. One end of the strip has been inserted in the needle's eye. *D,* Both ends of the strip have been drawn through the respective brow incisions. The needle has not yet been detached from the strip at the medial end. The needle has been inserted in the midbrow incision and out through the medial incision. One end of the Silastic strip has been inserted through the eye of the needle so that it can be drawn out through the medial incision. *E,* Both ends have now been drawn up through the midbrow incision and through the Watzke sleeve. If desired, a suture may be tied around the ends of the sleeve to prevent slipping. *F,* The skin incisions have been closed. (After Callahan, 1974.)

incisions above the eyebrow, where they are fixed with sutures under sufficient tension to form a supratarsal fold and elevation of the lid. Occasionally, a separate upper eyelid incision with lid crease sutures may be required to ensure lid crease formation. The longer ends of the suspension material are passed subcutaneously to emerge through the central wound above the eyebrow, where they are tied together. The incisions are closed by interrupted sutures (see Fig. 34–135*D*). The lower eyelids may be sutured to the eyebrows with suspension sutures for 24 to 48 hours. Copious amounts of ophthalmic solution are instilled into the palpebral fissure every hour during the day, and ointment is applied during sleep. Stippling of the cornea may appear during the early postoperative phase, but usually within a few days the cornea becomes tolerant of the new lid position.

The main disadvantage of the frontalis suspension operation is that ptosis in upward gaze and lagophthalmos on downward gaze usually occur. The lid can be raised only by lifting the brow, and the pull exerted by the fascia for elevating the lid tends to pull the lid away from the globe.

EPICANTHUS

Congenital Epicanthus

Congenital epicanthus is often bilateral and is transmitted as a dominant trait. It is characterized by a fold of skin that extends from the bridge of the nose, overhanging and partially hiding the medial canthus. The fold may arise from the eyebrow, the tarsal fold, or the skin of the upper lid above the tarsal fold. It occurs with varying frequency in all races but is most common among Orientals. Variations include *epicanthus inversus,* characterized by a fold of skin that originates in the lower lid and swings upward into the upper lid. This is differentiated from the more common (1) *epicanthus palpebralis,* in which the fold arises from the upper lid above the tarsal region; (2) *epicanthus tarsalis,* in which the fold arises from the skin over the tarsus; and (3) *epicanthus superciliaris,* in which the fold runs from the eyebrows toward the normal lower lid.

Congenital epicanthal folds are corrected surgically; this can be performed at an early age. Various techniques have been proposed for the correction of congenital epicanthal folds (Blair, Brown, and Hamm, 1932); however, the Mustardé four-flap technique has proved capable of correcting the deformity in predictable fashion (Mustardé, 1963, 1980).

Rectangular (Four-Flap) Technique. The Mustardé method involves relieving the vertical shortness of the fold by transfer of the apparently excessive skin from the horizontal component of the fold. The final scar passes vertically through the medial canthus and does not lie in the nasal skin. Epicanthal folds, with or without telecanthus may be treated by the four-flap technique, irrespective of the position of the folds or their severity.

A point is marked on the skin of the nose (Fig. 34–137*A*) at the site of the proposed new canthus (halfway between the center of the nose and the center of the pupil). The nasal skin is pulled medially to obliterate the fold, and another mark is made at the actual canthus (Fig. 34–137*A*). The two points are joined, and from the midpoint lines are drawn at 60 degrees and only slightly shorter in length than the distance between the two points (Fig. 34–137*B*). From the top of the vertical lines, back cuts of 45 degrees are drawn, and again the length of these should be the same as that of the vertical lines (Fig. 34–137*B*). Finally paramarginal lines of the same length are drawn along each lid margin (Fig. 34–137*B*). The skin flaps so outlined are incised down to the orbicularis muscle and elevated (Fig. 34–138). If mild telecanthus is present, the excessive amount of medial canthal tendon is excised, and the medial canthus is sutured to the periosteum of the medial orbital wall with a nonabsorbable suture. In patients with wide telecanthus, medial orbital osteotomies are performed and the medial canthal tendons are medially displaced by transnasal wiring with stainless steel wire. The skin-muscle flaps are then transposed and sutured, trimming any excess tissue from the rectangular portions of the flaps (Fig. 37–138*C*). Epicanthal folds of mild to moderate severity may be corrected with minimal scarring by means of this technique (Fig. 34–139). Ethnic epicanthus may be corrected concomitantly with removal of upper lid fat and creation of an upper lid fold (Fig. 34–140).

It is essential that the final scar run through the medial canthus in order to avoid secondary cicatricial folds.

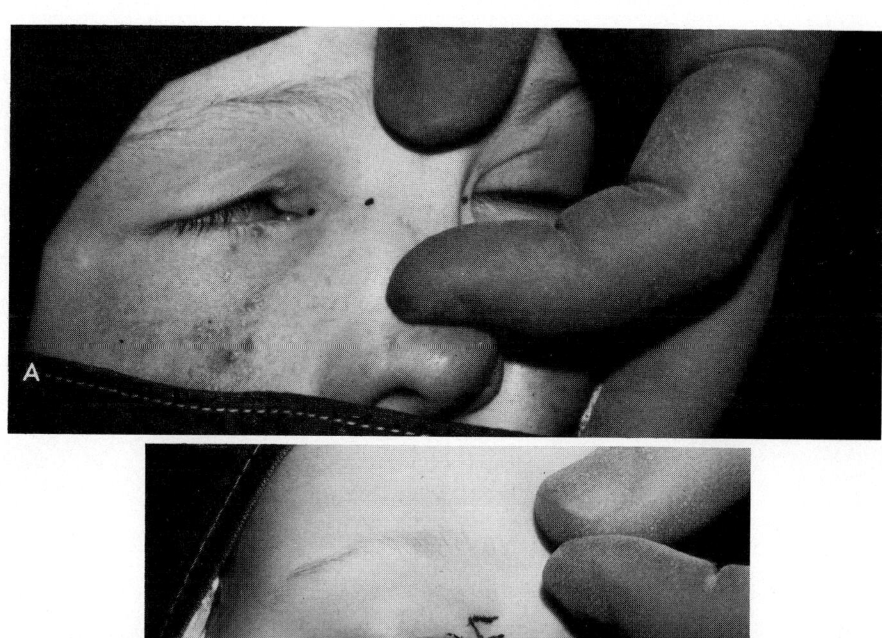

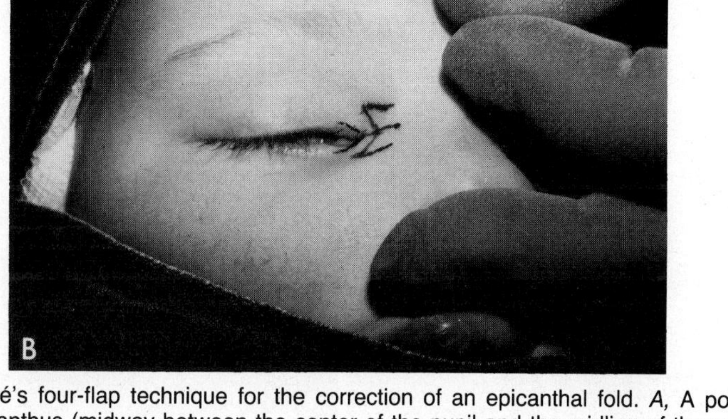

Figure 34–137. Mustardé's four-flap technique for the correction of an epicanthal fold. *A,* A point is marked at the proposed site of the new canthus (midway between the center of the pupil and the midline of the nose). The skin of the nose is pulled medially to obliterate any fold present, and a second point is marked at the site of the actual canthus. *B,* A line is drawn between the two points, and from the center two diverging lines are drawn at an angle of 60 degrees and slightly shorter in length (1 to 2 mm) than the original horizontal line. Back cuts of a similar length are now drawn at a 45 degree angle. Paramarginal incisions also of the same length are drawn on the upper and lower eyelids. (From Converse, J. M.: Reconstructive Plastic Surgery. 2nd ed. Philadelphia, W. B. Saunders Company, 1977, p. 940. Courtesy of Mustardé, J. C.)

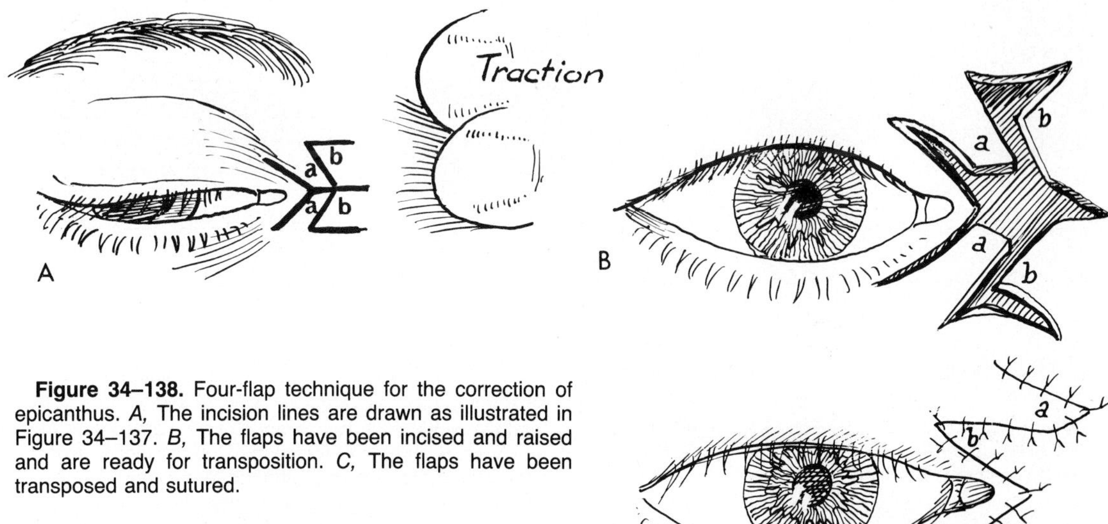

Figure 34–138. Four-flap technique for the correction of epicanthus. *A,* The incision lines are drawn as illustrated in Figure 34–137. *B,* The flaps have been incised and raised and are ready for transposition. *C,* The flaps have been transposed and sutured.

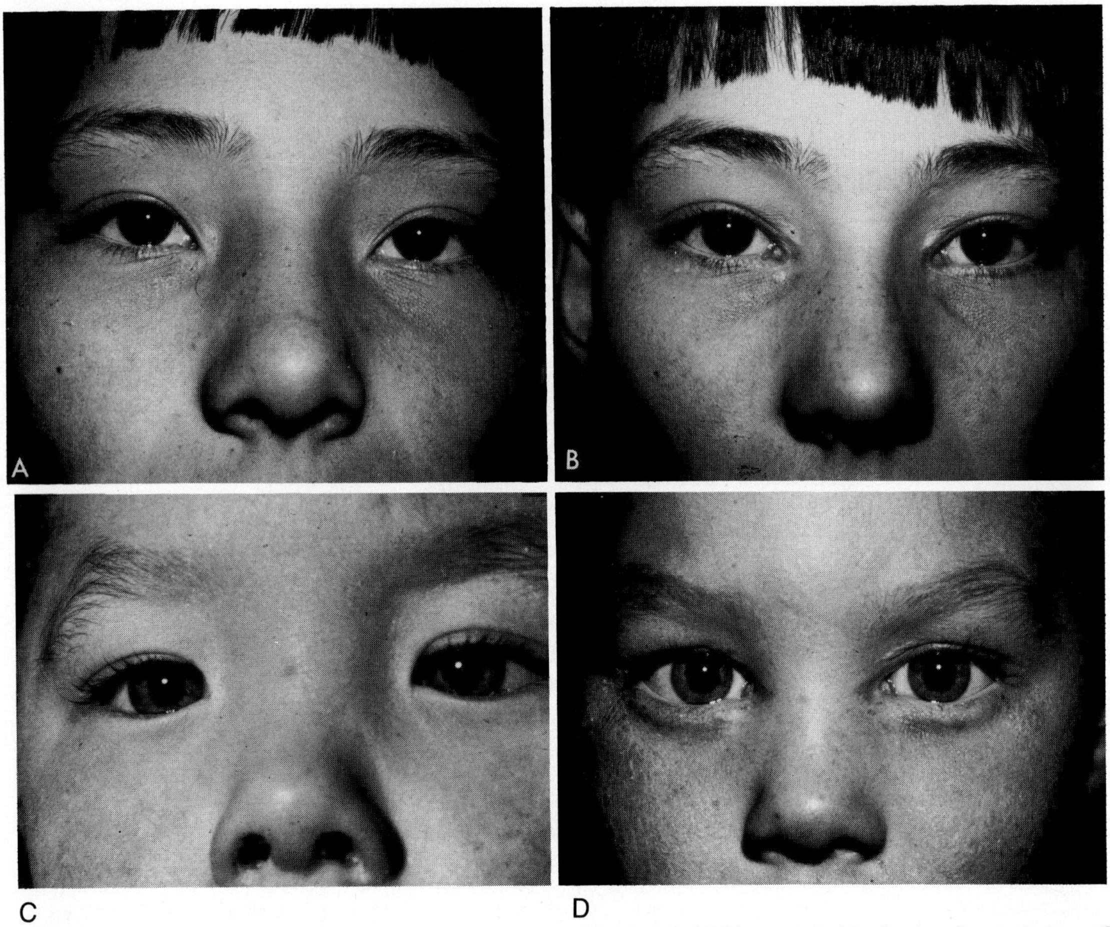

Figure 34–139. *A,* Preoperative and *B,* postoperative views of epicanthal folds corrected by the four-flap technique. *C,* Preoperative and *D,* postoperative views of more accentuated epicanthal folds corrected by the four-flap technique. (From Converse, J. M.: Reconstructive Plastic Surgery. 2nd ed. Philadelphia, W. B. Saunders Company, 1977, p. 942. Courtesy of Mustardé, J. C.)

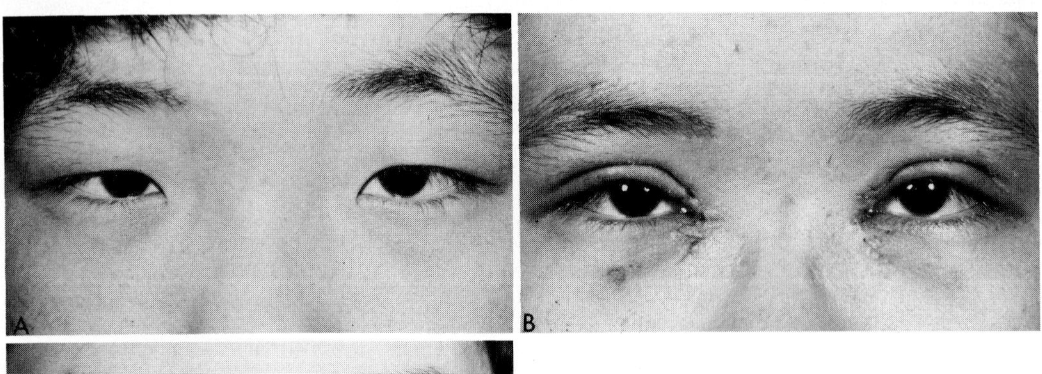

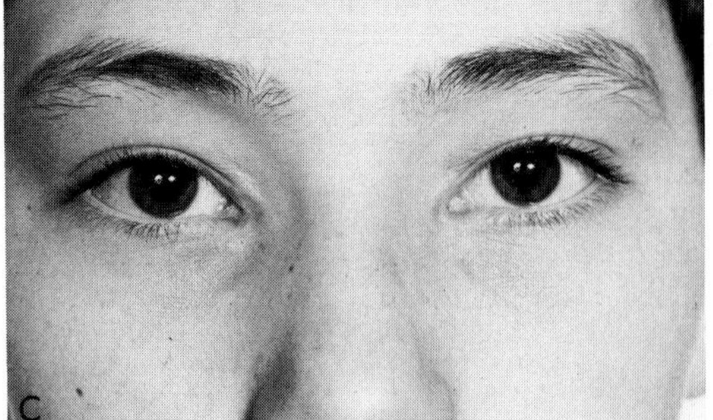

Figure 34–140. Example of more severe (ethnic) epicanthus with absence of superior palpebral folds and telecanthus. *A,* Appearance of the patient preoperatively. *B,* After the correction of the epicanthal folds by the four-flap technique and the formation of supratarsal folds. *C,* Appearance after healing of the wounds. (From Converse, J. M.: Reconstructive Plastic Surgery. 2nd ed. Philadelphia, W. B. Saunders Company, 1977, p. 943. Courtesy of Mustardé, J. C.)

Traumatic Epicanthus

Double-opposing Z-plasties have been used exclusively in the treatment of traumatic epicanthus (Converse and Smith, 1966). They may be preferable in cicatricial epicanthus, particularly in the repair of nasoethmoido-orbital fractures. The incisions made through the skin for double-opposing Z-plasties also serve as the point of surgical entry to the medial orbital wall and nasal dorsum. The usual cause of the traumatic epicanthal fold is disruption of the skeletal anatomy of the medial canthal area, or underlying scar tissue resulting in linear contractile bands. Whereas the epicanthal fold itself can be disregarded in the Mustardé technique, the incision for the traumatic epicanthal fold must extend through the scar itself (Fig. 34–141). If the scar is wide, it may have to be excised; however, in most cases the Z-plasty redistributes the scar and results in its progressive softening.

EPIBLEPHARON

Epiblepharon is a deformity characterized by a fold of skin and conjunctiva that covers the caruncle and a variable portion of the sclera. The deformity is frequently associated with congenital epicanthus and blepharophimosis. Epiblepharon also occurs in traumatic epicanthus, orbital hypertelorism, and postthermal deformities involving the medial canthal area (the nasoorbital valley). Treatment consists of replacing the medial canthus against the medial orbital wall and restoring its angular shape. The Mustardé four-flap technique, combined with shortening of the elongated medial canthal tendons as illustrated in Figure 34–142, may be sufficient to correct the deformity.

More complicated examples follow burns or facial fractures and usually require more extensive reconstruction. Resection of subcutaneous scar tissue, extensively raising the periorbita and sectioning the inferior portion of the lateral canthal tendon to release tension, may be required before transnasal medial canthoplasty (Fig. 34–142*C*).

BLEPHAROPHIMOSIS

Blepharophimosis is a congenital malformation involving the orbital region, usually associated with ptosis of the upper eyelids

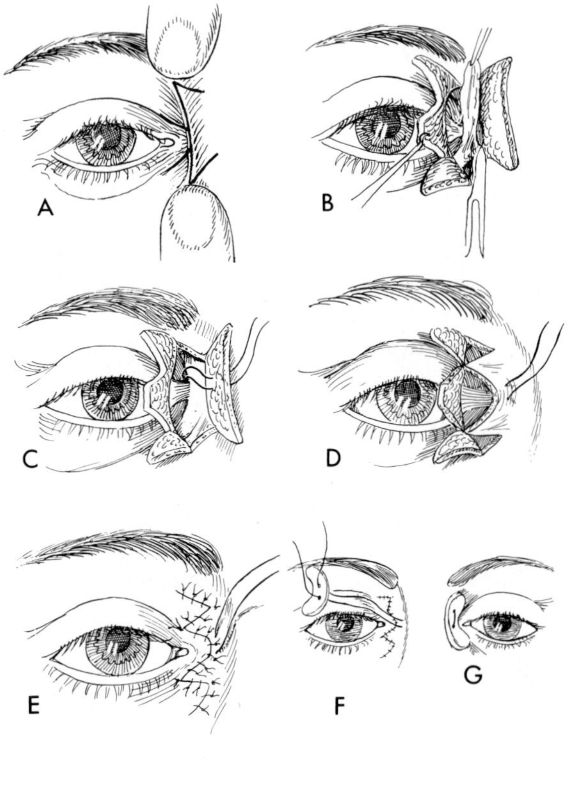

Figure 34–141. Double-opposing Z-plasties. Two Z-plasties done in opposing directions constitute an excellent technique for relaxing tension and releasing contracture of a linear scar. A limited amount of tissue in the confined naso-orbital valley limits the size of the Z-flaps. *A,* Design of the opposing Z-plasties. *B,* Flaps are raised, and deep scar tissue is excised. *C,* Transosseous wires have been placed through the bony skeleton of the nose for fixation of the canthal buttons (see *F* and *G*). *D,* The flaps have been transposed. *E,* Double-opposing Z-plasties completed. *F, G,* The canthal buttons are maintained by through and through wiring, ensuring the coaptation of the flaps to the underlying skeleton. (Converse, 1964.)

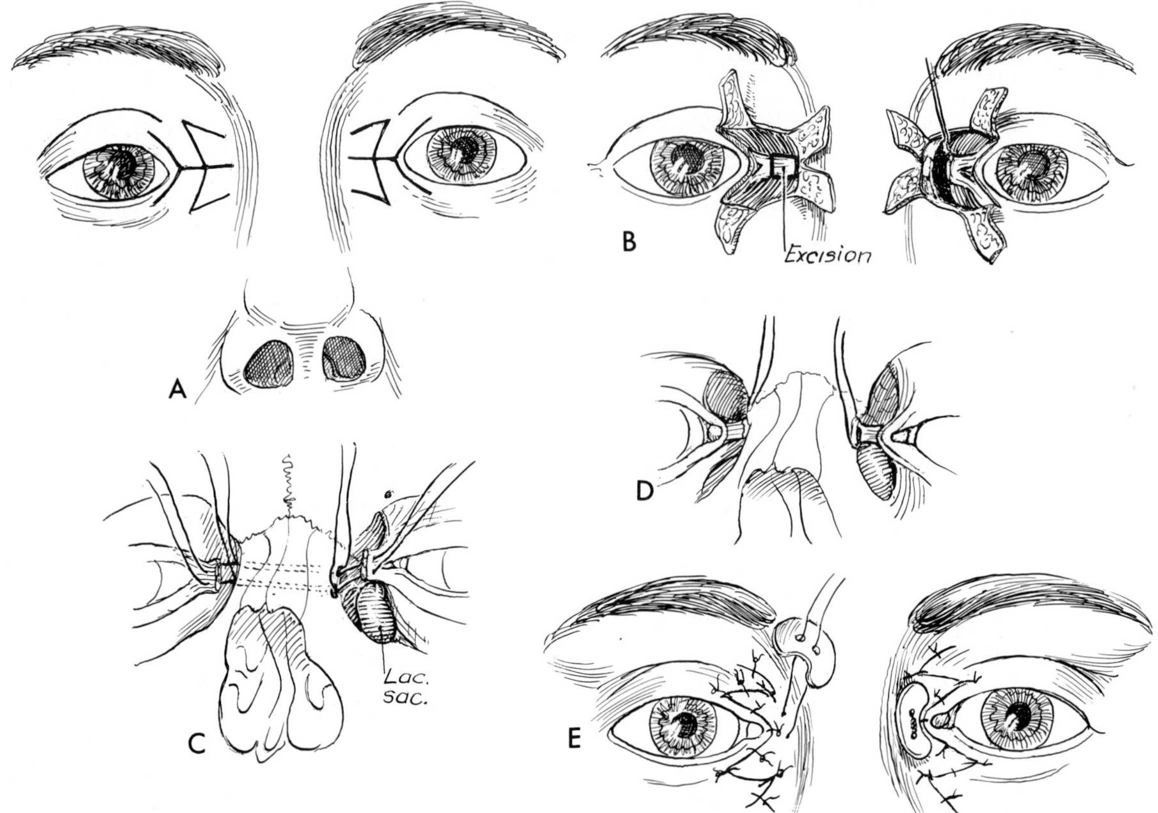

Figure 34–142. Correction of epiblepharon. *A,* Design of Mustardé's "jumping man" incisions. *B,* The flaps are raised. The medial canthal tendon is shortened. *C, D,* Transnasal wires are passed through the stump of the medial canthal tendons. *E,* Operation completed. The buttons are placed to prevent hematoma formation.

and epicanthal folds. The tissues of the medial canthal region encroach upon the ocular globe, covering the caruncle and a portion of the sclera (epiblepharon). The bridge of the nose appears flattened and widened, which makes the eyes appear far apart. Often the intercanthal distance is increased (telecanthus) and epicanthal folds are prominent. In severe cases of blepharophimosis, there may be minor degrees of orbital hypertelorism. The diminution of the transverse dimension of the palpebral fissure is accompanied by a diminution in the vertical dimension of the palpebral fissure caused by the eyelid ptosis. There is almost always an absence of the supratarsal fold in the upper eyelid, and the eyebrows are highly arched because of the severe ptosis.

Because of the lateral displacement of the medial canthi, the lacrimal puncta are also laterally displaced. Shortage of lower lid skin is frequent. Epicanthal folds may be present, but there is nearly always an excess of skin and also of subcutaneous tissue between the skin and the underlying skeletal structures of the nose.

As in many congenital syndromes, the malformation is rarely an isolated developmental anomaly. Auricular deformities and anomalies of the forehead are common. Patients have a characteristic posture, maintaining the neck extended backward in order to be able to see below the ptotic eyelids. They may appear mentally retarded, although in many cases their intellectual development may be higher than normal.

Genetic Aspects. According to Callahan (1974), Dimitry (1921) studied five generations of patients with blepharophimosis and coined the term from two Greek words—*blepharon* (eyelids) and *phimosis* (stricture). Dimitry's studies suggested that the malformation occurs more frequently in males, although it is not sex linked. Owens, Hadley, and Kloepfer (1960) confirmed Dimitry's observation that the hereditary pattern is usu-

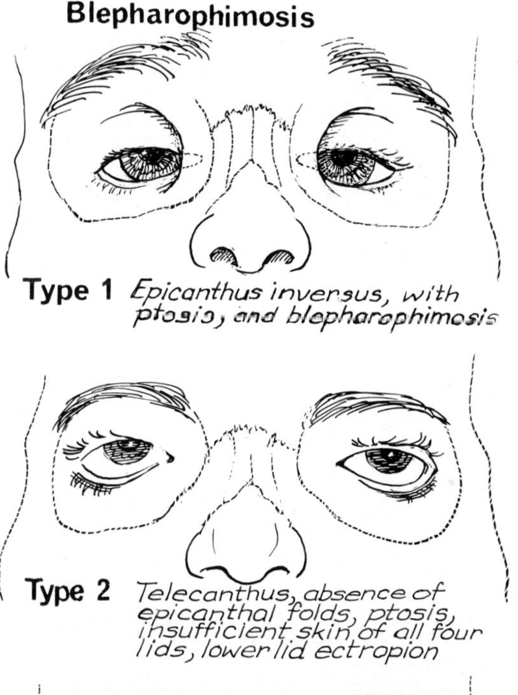

Figure 34–143. Types of blepharophimosis. (After Callahan, 1974.)

ally transmitted as an autosomal dominant with varying degrees of penetrance. Chromosome studies have been negative.

In the American and British literature, the treatment of patients with blepharophimosis has been reported by Berke (1953), Hughes (1955), Johnson (1956, 1964), Lewis and associates (1967), Fox (1963), and Mustardé (1963).

Classification and Treatment. Callahan (1974) recognized the characteristic features and the required treatment of three types of blepharophimosis (Fig. 34–143).

Blepharophimosis Type I. Type I blepharophimosis is characterized by large epicanthal folds extending upward from the lower lid with epicanthus inversus, a downward slant of the medial canthi. The eyelids are shortened in their horizontal dimension, and the upper eyelids are ptotic.

Three essential operative procedures are advocated to correct this deformity:

1. Elimination of the epicanthal folds by the quadrilateral flap technique of Mustardé (see Fig. 34–138) or by the double-opposing Z-plasty technique (see Fig. 34–141). McCord (1980b) advocated a crescent-shaped skin excision of the epicanthal fold, which had satisfactory results.
2. Resection of bone through the superoposterior portion of the lacrimal groove. The medial canthal tendons and the adjacent periorbita are advanced into the bony window by means of transnasal wiring.
3. Correction of the severe ptosis, usually by the frontalis suspension technique.

Blepharophimosis Type II. Type II blepharophimosis is characterized by telecanthus and the absence of epicanthal folds. Because there are no skeletal deformities, there is no increased distance between the medial orbital walls (hypertelorism). Type II patients have severe bilateral upper lid ptosis with absent levator function and marked shortage of the skin of all four lids. Correction of this type of blepharophimosis requires three procedures:

1. Skin grafting to the deficient eyelid skin.
2. Fixation of the medial canthal tissues into the bony openings of the medial orbital walls and fixation by transnasal wiring (Callahan, 1974). Alternatively, the medial orbital walls may be translocated medially after appropriate osteotomies and exenteration of the ethmoid air cells. The medial canthi are reattached by the transnasal wiring technique, which also maintains the medial displacement of the medial orbital walls.
3. The frontalis suspension technique to correct the ptosis. Figure 34–144 shows a patient in whom bilateral double-opposing Z-plasties and medial displacement of the medial orbital walls after resection of a central segment from the midline of the nose corrected the Type II deformity. In this case there was sufficient levator activity to permit levator resection procedures to correct the asymmetric ptosis.

Blepharophimosis Type III. This type is characterized by the lack of epicanthal folds, but the presence of telecanthus, antimongoloid slanting of the palpebral fissures, severe ptosis, mild orbital hypertelorism, and insufficient skin of all four lids. Correction requires skin grafting of the eyelids, followed

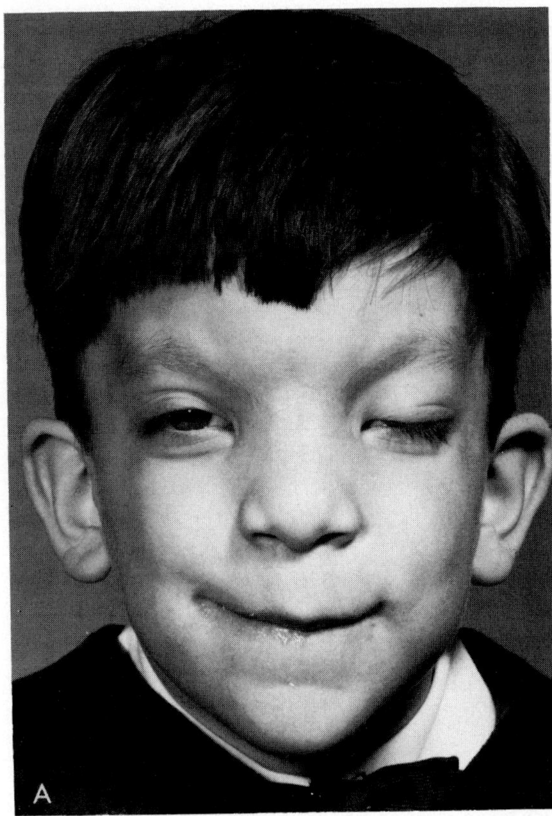

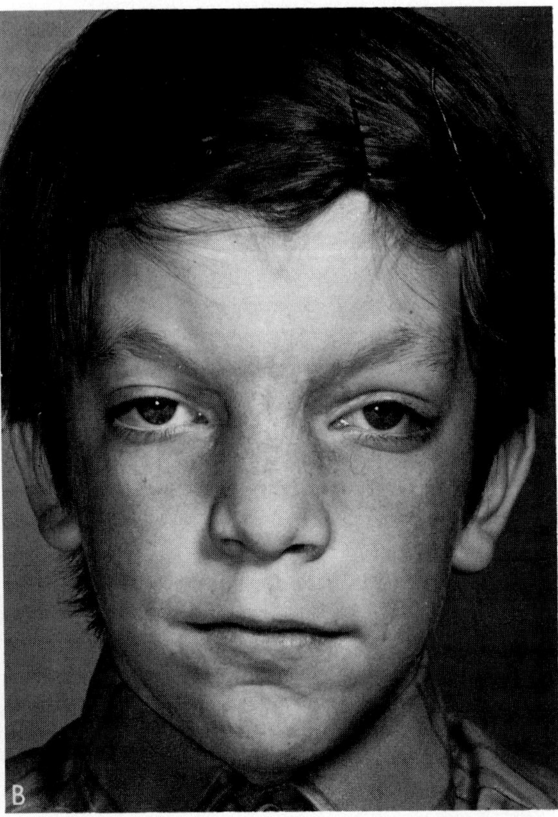

Figure 34–144. Corrective surgery for blepharophimosis. *A,* A patient aged 5 years with the typical characteristics of blepharophimosis. *B,* Appearance of the patient six years later following bilateral double-opposing Z-plasties, medial displacement of the medial orbital walls after osteotomy, and resection of a central segment of bone. Sufficient levator muscle activity was present to correct the ptosis by levator resection. The patient has a slight degree of orbital hypertelorism. (From Converse, J. M., Ransohoff, J., Mathews, E. S., Smith, B., and Molenaar, A.: Ocular hypertelorism and pseudohypertelorism. Plast. Reconstr. Surg., *45*:2. Copyright 1970. The Williams & Wilkins Company, Baltimore.)

by correction of orbital hypertelorism in which the entire orbital contents with their contiguous orbital walls are moved medially via an intracranial or subcranial approach (see Chap. 60). Medial canthoplasty by transnasal and interosseous fixation is performed at the same time. Ptosis correction by the frontalis suspension technique is usually performed as the final procedure.

REFERENCES

Anderson, R. L.: Medial canthal tendon branches out. Arch. Ophthalmol., *95*:2051, 1977.

Anderson, R. L.: The aponeurotic approach to ptosis surgery. *In* Bosniak, S. L., and Smith, B. C. (Eds.): Advances in Ophthalmic Plastic and Reconstructive Surgery. New York, Pergamon Press, 1982, p. 183.

Anderson, R. L., and Beard, C.: The levator aponeurosis. Attachments and their clinical significance. Arch. Ophthalmol., *95*:1437, 1977.

Anderson, R. L., and Dixon, R. S.: Aponeurotic ptosis surgery. Arch. Ophthalmol., *97*:1123, 1979a.

Anderson, R. L., and Dixon, R. S.: The role of Whitnall's ligament in ptosis surgery. Arch. Ophthalmol., *97*:705, 1979b.

Anderson, R. L., and Edwards, J. J.: Reconstruction by myocutaneous eyelid flaps. Arch. Ophthalmol., *97*:2358, 1979a.

Anderson, R. L., and Edwards, J. J.: Indications, complications and results with silicone stents. Ophthalmology, *86*:1474, 1979b.

Anderson, R. L., and Gordy, D. D.: Aponeurotic defects in congenital ptosis. Ophthalmology, *86*:1493, 1979a.

Anderson, R. L., and Gordy, D. D.: The tarsal strip procedure. Arch. Ophthalmol., *97*:2192, 1979b.

Anderson, R. L., and Weinstein, G. S.: Full-thickness bipedicle flap for total lower eyelid reconstruction. Arch. Ophthalmol., *105*:507, 1987.

Aurora, A. L., and Blodi, F. C.: Lesions of the eyelids: a clinicopathological study. Surv. Ophthalmol., *15*:94, 1970.

Bachelor, E. P., and Jobe, R. P.: The absent lateral canthal tendon: reconstruction using a Y graft of palmaris longus tendon. Ann. Plast. Surg., *5*:362, 1980.

Baylis, H. I., Cies, W. A., and Kamin, D. F.: Correction of upper eyelid retraction. Am. J. Ophthalmol., *82*:790, 1976.

Beard, C.: Repair of traumatic defects of the lacrimal system (acute). *In* Proceedings of the Second International Symposium on Plastic and Reconstructive Surgery of the Eye and Adnexa. St. Louis, MO, C. V. Mosby Company, 1967, p. 171.

Beard, C.: Ptosis. St. Louis, MO, C. V. Mosby Company, 1969; 2nd Ed., 1976; 3rd Ed., 1981.

Berke, R. N.: An operation for ptosis utilizing the superior rectus muscle. Trans. Am. Acad. Ophthalmol., *53*:499, 1949.

Berke, R. N.: A simplified Blaskovics operation for blepharoptosis. Arch Ophthalmol., *45*:460, 1952.

Berke, R. N.: A modified Krönlein operation. Trans. Am. Acad. Ophthalmol., *51*:193, 1953.

Berke, R. N.: Complications in ptosis surgery. *In* Fasanella, R. M. (Ed.): Management of Complications in Eye Surgery. Philadelphia, W. B. Saunders Company, 1957, p. 71.

Berke, R. N.: Results of resection of the levator muscle through a skin incision in congenital ptosis. A.M.A. Arch. Opthalmol., *61*:177, 1959.

Berke, R. N.: Types of operation indicated for congenital and acquired ptosis. *In* Troutman, R. C., Converse, J. M., and Smith, B. (Eds.): Plastic and Reconstructive Surgery of the Eye and Adnexa. Washington, DC, Butterworth, 1962.

Bick, W.: Surgical management of orbital tarsal disparity. Arch. Ophthalmol., *75*:386, 1966.

Blair, V. P., Brown, J. B., and Hamm, W. G.: Correction of ptosis and of epicanthus. Arch. Ophthalmol., *7*:831, 1932.

Blaskovics, L. de: Über Totalplastik des untern Lides. Bildung einer hinteren Lidplatte durch Transplantation eines Tarsus-und. Bindehautstriefeus aus dem Oberlide. Z. Augenheilk., *40*:222, 1918.

Blaskovics, L. de: New operation for ptosis with shortening of the levator and tarsus. Arch. Ophthalmol., *52*:563, 1923.

Bock, E.: Die Propfung von Haut and Schleimhaut auf ocultistischen Gebiete. Vienna, W. Braumuller, 1884.

Bowman, W.: Cited by Bader: Report of a chief operation performed at the Royal London Ophthalmic Hospital for the quarter ending 25th of September 1857, II. Eyelid. 51 Operations. Royal London Ophthal. Hosp. Rep., *1*:34, 1859.

Briggs, P. C., and Heckler, F. R.: Lacrimal gland involvement in zygomaticofrontal fracture sites. Plast. Reconstr. Surg., *80*:682, 1987.

Burian, F.: Operations in blepharoptosis: fascial and synthetic slings and dermomuscular suspension. *In* Troutman, R. C., Converse, J. M., and Smith, B. (Eds.): Plastic and Reconstructive Surgery of the Eye and Adnexa. Washington, DC, Butterworth, 1962.

Callahan, A.: Ptosis associated with congenital defects; blepharophimosis, epicanthus and other syndromes. *In* Symposium on Surgery of the Orbit and Adnexa. Transactions New Orleans Academy of Ophthalmology. St. Louis, MO, C. V. Mosby Company, 1974.

Carrol, R. P.: Entropion following the Cutler-Beard procedure. Ophthalmology, *90*:1052, 1983.

Cirincione, G.: Sulla blefaro plastica. Clin. Ocul., Palermo, *2*:449, 1901.

Converse, J. M., and Smith, B.: Naso-orbital fractures and traumatic deformities of the medial canthus. Plast. Reconstr. Surg., *38*:147, 1966.

Cutler, W. L., and Beard, C.: A method for partial and total upper lid reconstruction. Am. J. Ophthalmol., *39*:1, 1955.

Denonvilliers: Blepharoplastie. Bull. Soc. Chir. Paris, 1st series, *7*:243, 1856.

Denonvilliers: De la methode autoplastique par pivotment, appliqueé à la restauration des paupières. Bull. Gen. Ther. Med. Chir., *65*:110, 1863.

Dimitry, T. J.: Hereditary ptosis. Am. J. Ophthalmol., *45*:4656, 1921.

Doxanas, M. T., and Anderson, R. L.: Oriental eyelids. An anatomic study. Arch. Ophthalmol., *102*:1232, 1984.

Dupuy-Dutemps, L.: Autoplastie palpébro-palpébrale intégrale. Réflection d'une paupière détruite dans toute son épaisseur par greffe cutanée et tarso-conjonctivale prise à l'autre paupière. Ann. Ocul., *164*:915, 1921.

Dupuy-Dutemps, L., and Bourguet, J.: Plastic operation for chronic dacryocystitis. Bull. Acad. Natl. Med., *86*:293, 1921.

Edgerton, M. T., and Wolfert, F. G.: The dermal-flap canthal lift for lower eyelid support. Plast. Reconstr. Surg., *43*:42, 1969.

Elschnig, A.: Ueber Ptosisoperationen (Ptosisoperation mit Freier Fascientransplantation). Med. Klin., Berlin, *9*:1536, 1913.

Esser, J. F. S.: Ueber eine gestielte Ueber-Pfanzung eines senkcrechtangelegten Keils aus dem oberen Augenlid in das gleichseitige Unterlid oder Umgekehrt. Klin. Monatsbl. Augerheilk., *63*:379, 1919.

Eversbusch, O.: Zur operation der congenitalen Blepharoptosis. Klin. Monatsbl. Augenheilk., *21*:100, 1883.

Fasanella, R. M.: Personal communication, 1973.

Fasanella, R. M., and Servat, J.: Levator resection for minimal ptosis: another simplified operation. Arch. Ophthalmol., *65*:493, 1961.

Fox, S. A.: Primary congenital entropion. Arch. Ophthalmol. *56*:839, 1956.

Fox, S.: Blepharophimosis. Am. J. Ophthalmol., *55*:469, 1963.

Fricke, J. C. G.: Die Bildung neuer Augenlider (Blepharoplastik) nach Zerstoerungen and dadurch hervogebrachten Auswaertswendungen derselben. Hamburg, Perthes & Besser, 1829.

Friedenwald, J. S., and Guyton, J. S.: Simple ptosis operation: Utilization of the frontalis by means of a single rhomboid shaped suture. Am. J. Ophthalmol., *31*:411, 1948.

Frueh, B. R.: The mechanistic classification of ptosis. Ophthalmology, *87*:1019, 1980.

Furnas, D. W., and Bircoll, M. H.: Eyelid traction test to determine if the medial canthal ligament is detached. Plast. Reconstr. Surg., *52*:315, 1973.

Gioia, V. M., Linberg, J. V., and McCormick, S. A.: The anatomy of the lateral canthal tendon. Arch. Ophthalmol., *105*:529, 1987.

Gradenigo, P.: Scritti oftalmologici del conte Pietro Gradenigo. Padua Stabilimento della Societa Cooperativa Tipografica, 1904, pp. 115, 157, 158.

Hamako, C., and Baylis, H. I.: Lower lid retraction following blepharoplasty. Am. J. Ophthalmol., *89*:517, 1980.

Hess, H.: Eine Operationsmethode gegen Ptosis. Arch. Augenheilk., 1893.

Holly, F. J.: Formation and rupture of the tear film. Exp. Eye Res., *15*:515, 1973.

Holly, F. J., Lamberts, D. W., and Price, J. Scientific and clinical significance of tear film break up time. *In* Proceedings of the Annual Meeting of the American Academy of Ophthalmology, Chicago, 1980.

Holly, F. J., and Lemp, M. A.: Wettability and wetting of corneal epithelium. Exp. Eye Res., *11*:239, 1971.

Holly, F. J., and Lemp, M. A. (Eds.): The preocular tear

film and dry eye syndromes. Int. Ophthalmol. Clin., 13, 1973.

Holly, F. J., and Lemp, M. A.: Tear physiology and dry eyes. Surv. Ophthalmol., *22*:69, 1977.

Holt, J. E., Holt G. R., and van Kirk, M.: Use of temporalis fascia in eyelid reconstruction. Ophthalmology, *91*:89, 1984.

Hughes, W. L.: New method for rebuilding lower lid. Arch. Ophthalmol., *17*:1008, 1937.

Hughes, W. L.: Reconstructive Surgery of the Eyelids, 2nd Ed. St. Louis, MO, C. V. Mosby Company, 1943, 1954.

Hughes, W. L.: Surgical treatment of congenital palpebral phimosis. The V-Y operation. Arch. Ophthalmol., *54*:586, 1955.

Iliff, C. E.: A simplified ptosis operation. Am. J. Ophthalmol., *37*:529, 1954.

Ischreyt, G.: Verfahren für der plastichen Ersatz des Unterlides. Munch. Med. Wochenschr., *59*:479, 1912.

Jelks, G. W., and McCord, C. D., Jr.: Dry eye syndrome and other tear film abnormalities. Clin. Plast. Surg., *8*:803, 1981.

Johnson, C. C.: Operations for epicanthus and blepharophimosis. Evaluation and method for shortening medial canthal ligament. Am. J. Ophthalmol., *41*:71, 1956.

Johnson, C. C.: Surgical repair of the syndrome of epicanthus inversus, blepharophimosis, and ptosis. Arch. Ophthalmol., *71*:510, 1964.

Jones, L. T.: The cure of epiphora due to canalicular disorders, trauma, and surgical failures on the lacrimal passages. Trans. Am. Acad. Ophthalmol., *66*:506, 1962.

Jones, L. T.: The lacrimal secretory system and its treatment. Am. J. Ophthalmol., *62*:47, 1966.

Jones, L. T.: Levator resection. *In* Callahan, A.: Ptosis associated with congenital defects: blepharophimosis, epicanthus and other syndromes. Symposium on Surgery of the Orbit and Adnexa. Transactions of the New Orleans Academy of Ophthalmology. St. Louis, MO, C. V. Mosby Company, 1974a.

Jones, L. T.: Lacrimal surgery. *In* Symposium on Surgery of the Orbit and Adnexa. Transactions of the New Orleans Academy of Ophthalmology. St. Louis, MO, C. V. Mosby Company, 1974b.

Kazanjian, V. H.: Deformities of the eyelids, orbital and zygomatic regions. *In* Kazanjian, V. H., and Converse, J. M. (Eds.): The Surgical Treatment of Facial Injuries. Baltimore, Williams & Wilkins Company, 1949, p. 548.

Kazanjian, V. H., and Converse, J. M.: The Surgical Treatment of Facial Injuries. Baltimore, Williams & Wilkins Company, 1959.

Köllner, P.: Verfahren für den plastischen. Ersatz des Unterlids. Munch. Med. Wochenschr., *58*:2166, 1911.

König, E.: Die Körpereignee frei Fascienverpflanzung. Vienna, Urban & Schwarzenberg, 1928.

Koornneef, L.: New insights in the human orbital connective tissue: results of a new anatomic approach. Arch. Ophthalmol., *95*:1269, 1977a.

Koornneef, L.: Details of the orbital connective tissue system in the adult. Acta Morphol. Neerl. Scand., *15*:1, 1977b.

Koornneef, L.: Orbital septa: anatomy and function. Ophthalmology, *86*:876, 1979.

Koornneef, L.: Orbital connective tissue. *In* Duane, T. D., and Jaeger, E. A. (Eds.): Biomedical Foundations of Ophthalmology. Vol. 1. Philadelphia, Harper & Row, 1986, Chap. 32.

Kuhnt, H.: Zur Behandlung der Hornhautulzeration bei hochgradigem Basedow—Exophthalmos. Z. Augenheilk., *27*:1912.

Kuhnt, H.: Ueber plastische Operationen am Augeapfel, an den Lidern und der Orbita. Z. Augenheilk., *36*:1, 1916.

Kuhnt, H.: Plastische Operationen an Lidern und Bidhaut bei Krigsverletzen. Handb. d. arztl. Erfahr. im Weltkr., *5*:449, 1922.

Landolt, M.: Un nouveau cas de blépharoplastie suivant notre procédé. Arch. Ophthalmol., *1*:111, 1881.

Landolt, M.: De quelques operations pratiquées sur les paupières. Arch. Ophthalmol., *5*:481, 1885.

Lauring, L.: Sutureless Fasanella-Servat blepharoptosis correction (correspondence). Am. J. Ophthalmol., *80*:778, 1975.

Lawson, G.: On the transposition of portions of skin for the closure of large granulating surface. Trans. Clin. Soc. Lond. *4*:49, 1871.

Le Fort, L. C.: Blépharoplastie par un lambeau complétement détaché du bras et reporté à la face. Bull. Mem. Soc. Chir., *1*:39, 1872.

Lekieffre, M., and François P.: Les arrachements des paupières. Extraits Bull. Mem. Soc. Fr. Ophthalmol., 1976.

Lekieffre, M., Tessier, P., Lagache, G., and François, P.: Les cancers de la paupière inférieure et de la commissure interne. Traitement chirurgical. Ann. Chir. Plast., *15*:318, 1970.

Leone, C. R., Jr.: Tarsal-conjunctival advancement flaps for eyelid reconstructions. Arch. Ophthalmol., *101*:945, 1983.

Leone, C. R., Jr.: Lateral canthal reconstruction. Ophthalmology, *94*:238, 1987.

Leone, C. R., Jr., and Hand, S. I., Jr.: Reconstruction of the medial eyelid. Am. J. Ophthalmol., *87*:797, 1979.

Lewis, S. R., Arons, M. S., Lynch, J. B., and Blocker, T. G.: The congenital eyelid syndrome. Plast. Reconstr. Surg., *39*:271, 1967.

Lexer, E.: Ptosisoperation, Herstellung der Oberlidfalte und Herstellung des Unterlides durch Faszienzügel. Klin. Mbl. Augenheilk., *70*:464, 1923.

Lisman, R. D., Rees, T., Baker, D., and Smith, B.: Experience with tarsal suspension as a factor in lower lid blepharoplasty. Plast. Reconstr. Surg., *79*:897, 1987.

Manson, P. N., Lazarus, R. B., Morgan, R., and Iliff, N.: Pathways of sympathetic innervation to the superior and inferior (Müller's) tarsal muscles. Plast. Reconstr. Surg., *78*:33, 1986.

Marsh, J. L., and Edgerton, M. T.: Periosteal pennant lateral canthoplasty. Plast. Reconstr. Surg., *64*:24, 1979.

McCord, C. D., Jr.: An external minimal ptosis procedure—external tarsoaponeurectomy. Trans. Am. Acad. Ophthalmol. Otolaryngol., *79*:683, 1973.

McCord, C. D., Jr.: Canalicular resection and reconstruction by canaliculoplasty. Ophthalmic Surg., *11*:440, 1980a.

McCord, C. D., Jr.: The correction of telecanthus and epicanthal folds. Ophthalmic Surg., *11*:446, 1980b.

McCord, C. D., and Shore, J. W.: Silicone rod frontalis suspension. Adv. Ophthalmol. Plast. Reconstr. Surg., *1*:213, 1982.

McCord, C. D., Jr., and Tanenbaum, M. (Eds.): Oculoplastic Surgery. New York, Raven Press, 1987.

McGregor, I. A.: Eyelid reconstruction following subtotal resection of upper or lower lid. Br. J. Plast. Surg., *26*:346, 1973.

McLaughlin, C. R.: Epiphora in facial paralysis. Br. J. Plast. Surg., *3*:87, 1950.

McLaughlin, C. R.: Permanent facial paralysis. Lancet, *2*:647, 1952.

Meller, J.: Ophthalmic Surgery. 6th Ed. Translated by Daily R.D., and Daily, L., Jr. New York, Blakiston Company, 1953.

Montandon, D. A.: A modification of the dermal-flap canthal lift for correction of the paralyzed lower lid. Plast. Reconstr. Surg., *61*:555, 1978.

Mosher, H. P.: An operation for draining the lacrimal sac and nasal duct into the unciform fossa. Laryngoscope, *25*:739, 1915.

Mosher, H. P.: The combined intranasal and external operation on the lacrimal sac. Ann. Otol. Rhinol. Laryngol., *32*:1, 1923.

Motais, M.: L'Appareil moteur de l'oeil de l'homme et des vertèbres. Paris, Doin, 1887.

Mustardé, J. C.: The treatment of ptosis and epicanthal folds. Br. J. Plast. Surg., *12*:252, 1959.

Mustardé, J. C.: Epicanthus and telecanthus. Br. J. Plast. Surg., *16*:346, 1963.

Mustardé, J. C.: Repair and Reconstruction in the Orbital Region. A. Practical Guide. Baltimore, Williams & Wilkins Company, 1966.

Mustardé, J. C.: Problems and possibilities in ptosis surgery. Plast. Reconstr. Surg., *56*:381, 1975.

Mustardé, J. C.: Repair and Reconstruction in the Orbital Region. 2nd Ed. Edinburgh, Churchill Livingstone, 1980, pp. 188–192.

Mustardé, J. C.: Major reconstruction of the eyelids—functional and aesthetic considerations. Clin. Plast. Surg., *8*:227, 1981.

Ortiz-Monasterio, F., and Rodriguez, A: Lateral canthoplasty to change the eye slant. Plast. Reconstr. Surg., *75*:1, 1985.

Owens, N., Hadley, R. C., and Kloepfer, H. W.: Hereditary blepharophimosis, ptosis, and epicanthus inversus. J. Int. Coll. Surg., *33*:558, 1960.

Pashby, R. C., and Rathbun, J. E.: Silicone tube intubation of the lacrimal drainage systems. Arch. Ophthalmol., *97*:1318, 1979.

Paterson, R. S., Munro, I. R., and Farkas, L. G.: Transconjunctival lateral canthopexy in Down's syndrome patients: a nonstigmatizing approach. Plast. Reconstr. Surg., *79*:714, 1987.

Paufique, L., and Tessier, P.: Reconstruction totale de la paupière supérieure. *In* Troutman, R. C., Converse, J., M., and Smith, B. (Eds.): Plastic and Reconstructive Surgery of the Eye and Adnexa. Washington, DC, Butterworth, 1962.

Payne, J. W., Duke, J. R., Butner, R., et al. Basal cell carcinoma of the eyelids. Arch. Ophthalmol., *81*:553, 1969.

Payr, E.: Plastischen erfolgreicher Ersatz aller 4 Augenlider (von 3 durch Fernplastik aus den Arm). Arch. Klin. Chir., *152*:532, 1928.

Putterman, A. M.: Treatment of epiphora with absent lacrimal puncta. Arch. Ophthalmol., *89*:125, 1973.

Putterman, A. M.: Viable composite grafting in eyelid reconstruction. Am. J. Ophthalmol., *85*:237, 1978.

Putterman, A. M., and Urist M. J.: Müller's muscle–conjunctival resection. Arch. Ophthalmol., *93*:619, 1975.

Quickert, M. H., and Dryden, R. M.: Probes for intubation in lacrimal drainage. Trans. Am. Acad. Ophthalmol. Otolaryngol., *74*:431, 1970.

Quickert, M. H., and Rathbun, E.: Suture repair of entropion. Arch. Opthalmol., *85*:304, 1971.

Quickert, M. H., Wilkes, T. D., and Dryden, R. M.: Nonincisional correction of epiblepharon and congenital entropion. Arch. Ophthalmol., *101*:778, 1983.

Reeh, M. J.: Discussion of paper by Smith, B., and Obear, M. F.: The bridge flap technique for reconstruction of upper lid defects. Trans. Am. Acad. Ophthalmol. Otolaryngol., *71*:897, 1967.

Reverdin, J. L., Greffe epidermique. Expérience faite dans le service de M. le docteur Guyon à l'hôpital Necker. Gas. L'Op., *43*:15 Disc. 35, 1870 (reported on Dec. 15, 1869).

Risdon, F.: Plastic operations about the orbit. Bull. Acad. Med. Toronto, *18*:139, 1945.

Rodriquez R.L., and Zide, B. M.: Reconstruction of the medial canthus. Clin. Plast. Surg., *15*:255, 1988.

Rogers, B. O.: History of oculoplastic surgery: the contributions of plastic surgery. Aesth. Plast. Surg., *12*:129, 1988.

Rycroft, B.: Tearing—Management with transantral vidianectomy. *In* Troutman. R. C., Converse J. M., and Smith, B. (Eds.): Plastic and Reconstructive Surgery of the Eye and Adnexa. Washington, DC, Butterworth, 1962.

Silverman J. P., and Obear, M. F.: Delayed primary repair of totally avulsed upper and lower eyelids. Am. J. Ophthalmol., *70*:230, 1970.

Smith, B.: Eyelid surgery. Surg. Clin. North Am., *38*:367, 1959.

Smith, B.: Personal communications, 1974, 1975.

Smith, B. C., Della Rocca, R., Nesi, F., and Lisman, R. D. (Eds.): Ophthalmic Plastic and Reconstructive Surgery. St. Louis, MO, C. V. Mosby Company, 1987.

Spinelli, H. M., Sherman, J. E., Lisman, R. D., and Smith, B.: Human bites of the eyelids. Plast. Reconstr. Surg., *78*:610, 1986.

Stallard, H. B.: Operations for epiphora. Lancet, *2*:743, 1940.

Stellwag von Carion, K.: Rückblicke auf die augenärzt lichen Pfropfungsvesuche und ein neuer Fall von Schleimhautübertragung. Allg. Wien. Med. Ztg., *34*:341, 1889.

Stephenson, C.: Reconstruction of the eyelids using a myocutaneous island flap. Ophthalmology, *90*:1065, 1983.

Szymanowski, J. von: Handbuch der operativen Chirurgie. Braunschweig, F. Vieweg. & Sohn, 1870.

Teale, T. P.: On relief of symblepharon by transplantation of the conjunctiva. Ophthal. Hosp. Rev., *3*:253, 1860.

Tenzel, R. R.: Treatment of lagophthalmos of the lower lid. Arch. Ophthalmol., *81*:366, 1969.

Tenzel, R. R.: Personal communication to Fasanella, 1970.

Tessier, P.: Les lacerations palpebrales. L'urgence en chirugie palpebrale. Extraits Bull. Mem. Soc. Fr. Ophthalmol., *85*:423, 1972.

Tillett, C. G., and Tillett, G. M.: Silicone sling in the correction of ptosis. Am. J. Ophthalmol., *62*:521, 1966.

Toti, A.: Nuovo metodo conservatore di cura radicale delle suppurazioni croniche del sacco lacrimal (dacriocistorhinostomia). Clin. Med., *10*:385, 1904.

Tripier, L.: Lambeau musculo-cutane enforme de pont, applique a la restauration des paupières. Gaz. Hop. (Paris), *62*:1124, 1889.

van der Meulen, J. C.: The use of mucosa-lined flaps in

eyelid reconstruction: a new approach. Plast. Reconstr. Surg., *70*:140, 1982.

Viers, E. R.: The Lacrimal System. New York, Grune & Stratton, 1955.

von Graefe, C. F.: De Rhinoplastice. Berlin, Reimer, 1818, p. 13.

Von Walther, P.: Ectropium anguli oculi externi, eine neue Augenkrankheit, und die Tarsorraphie, eine neue Augenoperation. J. Chir. Augenheilk., 1826, p. 986.

Webster, R. C., Davidson, T. M., Reardon, E. J., and Smith, R. C.: Suspending sutures in blepharoplasty. Arch. Otolaryngol., *105*:601, 1979.

Werb, A.: Personal communication to Jones, L. T., 1971.

Wesley, R. E., and Collins, J. W.: McCord procedure for ectropion repair. Arch. Otolaryngol., *109*:319, 1983.

Wesley, R. E., and McCord, C. D., Jr.: Height of the lower tarsus of the lower eyelid. Am. J. Ophthalmol., *90*:102, 1980a.

Wesley, R. E., and McCord, C. D., Jr.: Transplantation of eyebank sclera in the Cutler-Beard method of upper eyelid reconstruction. Ophthalmology, *87*:1022, 1980b.

Wheeler, J. M.: Halving wounds in facial plastic surgery. Proc. 2nd Congr. Pan-Pacific Surg. Assoc., 1936, p. 229.

Wheeler, J. M.: Collected Papers of John Martin Wheeler, M. D. New York, 1939.

Whitaker, L. A.: Selective alteration of palpebral form by lateral canthopexy. Plast. Reconstr. Surg., *74*:611, 1984.

Whitaker, L. A., Katowitz, J. A., and Randall, P.: The nasolacrimal apparatus in congenital facial anomalies. J. Maxillofac. Surg., *2*:59, 1974.

Wolfe, J. R.: A new method of performing plastic operation. Med. Times Gaz., *1*:608, 1876.

Worst, J. G. F.: Method of reconstructing torn lacrimal canaliculus. Am. J. Ophthalmol., *53*:520, 1962.

Youens, W. T., Westphal, C., Barfield, F. T., Jr., and Youens, H. T., Jr.: Full thickness lower lid transplant. Arch. Ophthalmol., *77*:226, 1967.

Zide, B. M., and Jelks, G. W.: Surgical Anatomy of the Orbit. New York, Raven Press, 1985.

Zide, B. M., and McCarthy, J. G.: The medial canthus revisited—an anatomical basis for canthopexy. Ann. Plast. Surg., *11*:1, 1983.

Index

Index

Note: Page numbers in *italics* refer to illustrations; page number followed by *t* refer to tables.

Abbé flap
  for lower lip reconstruction, 2016, 2018, *2019*
  for repair of deficient lip tissue, 2779–2780, 2782–2783, 2785, *2782–2785*
  for tight lip or horizontal deficiency, 2844, 2849, 2851, *2850*
  for upper lip reconstruction, 553
Abdomen reconstruction
  for spina bifida, 3780–3781, *3781–3783, 3785–3787*
  muscle and musculocutaneous flaps for, 397
Abdominal wall
  anatomy of
    of fascia, 3762
    of layers, 3759
    of ligaments, 3762
    of muscles, 3759, 3761–3762
  circulation of, 3762–3763
  nerves of, 3763
  reconstruction of
    anatomic considerations for, 3755, 3759, 3761–3763
    closure for, 3763–3764
    fascial support for, 3768–3770, *3769, 3770*
    for gas gangrene, 3772–3774, *3773*
    for gastroschisis, 3774, 3775–3777, 3779–3780, *3776, 3778*
    for hernias, *3761*, 3770–3772
    for omphalocele, 3774, 3775–3777, 3779–3780, *3775, 3777, 3779*
    general approach to, 3764–3765
    incisions for, 3763–3764
    musculofascial flaps for, 3766–3768
    skin flaps for, 3765–3766, *3766, 3767*
    skin grafts for, 3765
Abdominoplasty
  autologous blood for, 3935
  combined with other procedures, 3953, *3958–3961*, 4021
  complications of, 3933
    prevention of, 3935–3936
  equipment for, 3933, *3933*
  full technique of
    closure in, 3939, 3949
    drains and dressings in, 3951, *3953*
    elevation of panniculus in, 3939, *3945, 3946*
    plication of diastasis recti in, 3939, *3946–3948*
    selection of incision for, 3937, 3939, *3942–3945*
    suctioning of adjacent deformities in, 3951
Abdominoplasty *(Continued)*
  full technique of, suctioning of dog-ears in, 3951, *3952*
    suctioning upper abdomen in, 3951
    tailoring umbilicus in, 3948, *3949–3951*, 3951
    trimming of flaps in, 3951, *3952*
  historical aspects of, 3929–3930, 3933
  incisions for, *3930*
  inpatient vs. outpatient setting for, 3934–3935
  mini technique for, 3951, 3953, *3954, 3955*
  patient selection for, 3933–3935, *3934, 3935*
  postoperative management of, 3961
  preoperative planning for, 3933–3935, *3934, 3935*
  results of, *3931, 3932*
  reverse technique for, 3953, *3956, 3957*
  secondary/revision procedures for, 3961
  suctioning of abdomen for
    results of, *3940–3942*
    technique of, 3936–3937, *3938, 3939*
Abductor digiti minimi muscle flap
  for foot reconstruction, 401
  for heel defect coverage, 4082
Abductor hallucis muscle flap
  for foot reconstruction, 401
  for heel defects, 4082
Abductor pollicis longus tendon, transfer of, *4944*, 4944–4945
Ablation, for lymphedema, of upper extremity, 5027–5028, *5028, 5029*
Abscess
  of hand, 5538, *5538*
  of web space, 5542–5543, *5542, 5543*
  subeponychial, 5539
  subungual, 5539
Accutane
  nerve cell death and, 2475, 2491
  teratogenicity of, 2464–2465
Acetylsalicylic acid, platelet function and, 458
Achondroplasia, 104
Acid burns, 5436–5438, *5437, 5438*
Acinic cell carcinoma, of salivary gland, 3308
Acne scarring
  chemical peeling for, 758
  dermabrasion for, 773, *774*
Acrocephaly
  clinical presentation of, 3018, *3018*

Acrocephaly *(Continued)*
radiographic findings in, 3018, *3018*
visual abnormalities in, 3025–3026
Acrochordon, 3579, *3580*, 3581
Acromiocervical flap, for complete cervical contractures, 2068, 2073, *2071, 2072*
Acrosyndactyly
clinical presentation of, 5246, 5248, 5252, 5255, *5249–5251, 5253–5254*, 5303, 5305
treatment of, 5248, 5255, 5305, *5306, 5307*, 5308
by metacarpal distraction lengthening, 5252, 5255, *5353–5354*
by metacarpal transfer, 5248
by phalangeal transfer, 5248, 5252, *5250–5251*
web deepening for, 5248
Acrylic splints, 1216, *1216*
Actinic keratosis
clinical presentation of, 3595–3596, *3596, 3597*
of hand, 5485, *5485*
Actin-myosin meshwork, 2462
Actinomycosis, 5552
Acuminate warts
of anogenital area, treatment of, 3565–3566, *3565*
pathology of, 3562–3563, *3563*
Acupuncture, for reflex sympathetic dystrophy, 4912
Adamantinoma, of jaw, *3341*, 3341–3342
Adenitis, tuberculous cervical, 3177
Adenocarcinoma, of salivary gland, 3309
Adenoid cystic carcinoma, of salivary glands, *3306*, 3306–3308
Adenoid pad, in velopharyngeal closure, 2729
Adenoidectomy
for obstructive sleep apnea, 3150
velopharyngeal incompetence from, 2729, 2906
Adenoma sebaceum, dermabrasion of, 777
Adenomatoid odontogenic tumor, of jaw, 3342
Adipose tissue, aging and, 3965–3967, *3966–3968*
Adnexal structures, operative considerations for, 1681–1685, *1681–1685*
"Adoption phenomenon," 667
Adson maneuver, 5000, *5000*
Advancement flap
for hand surgery, 4448–4449, *4448, 4449*
for coverage of digital amputation stumps, 4487–4489, *4488, 4489*
for lower lip and commissure reconstruction, *2230*, 2231
for neck resurfacing, 2194, 2196, *2196*
general description of, 276–277, *277*
of cheek, for nasal reconstruction, 1943, *1948, 1949*
random cutaneous types of, *288*, 288–289, *289*
Advancement-rotation flap, cervicofacial, for removal of cheek scars, 2167, 2169, *2168, 2170–2171*
Aerodigestive tract
anatomy of, 3416–3417, *3416, 3417*
cancers of. *See* Aerodigestive tract cancers.
Aerodigestive tract cancers
anatomic sites of, 3416*t*
clinical evaluation of, 3419–3425, *3421–3425*
erythroplakia and, 3419
etiologic factors for, 3417–3419, 3418*t*
flap reconstruction for, 3436, 3438, 3444, 3447–3449, *3436, 3437, 3439–3449*
historical aspects of treatment for, 3413–3415
incidence of, 3413
Aerodigestive tract cancers *(Continued)*
leukoplakia and, 3419
management of neck in, 3427–3435, *3429, 3430–3436*
primary, of unknown origin, 3469–3470
primary tumor management for, 3450–3452, *3451, 3453–3455*, 3455
staging of, 3425–3427, 3426*t*, 3427, 3427*t*
Afferent impulses, 4978
Age of patient
effect on patient selection, 119
for replantation surgery, 4358–4359
influence on skin, 44–45
peripheral nerve regeneration and, 662–663
Aging process
morphologic changes of, 2361, 2363, *2363*
of skin, 2360–2361
histologic features of, *2362*, 2362*t*
Agromegaly, facial hyperplasia of, *1300*, 1301
Air flow, nasal, *1806*, 1806–1807
Airway
complications of, in mandibular fracture treatment, 975–976
maintenance of, after cleft palate surgery, 2747
obstruction of
from lymphatic malformations, 3247
from orthognathic surgery, 1411–1412
in Down syndrome, surgery for, 3166, 3168
Alar base, resection of, *1836*, 1836–1837
Alar cartilage
anatomy of, *1794*, 1794–1795
ventilation and, 1807–1808
lateral crus of, relationship to alar rim, 1924, *1925*
Alar groove, 1788
Alar margin, sculpturing of, 1837, *1837*
Alar rim reconstruction, by local nasal flaps, 1936, *1938, 1939*, 1940
Albinism, basal cell carcinoma and, 3617
Alcohol consumption
cold injury and, 850–851
oral cancer risk and, 3418, 3418*t*
prenatal, pathogenesis of cleft lip/palate and, 2533, 2535
Alcoholism, Dupuytren's disease and, 5055–5056
Algal infections, 5553–5554
Alkali burns, 5438–5439, *5439*
Alkylating agents, craniofacial cleft formation and, 2929
Allen's test, 4276–4277, *4276–4277*
Allograft(s)
definition of, 54, 225
for bone transplants, 4687
of skin, for thermal burns, 804
of tendon, experimental studies of, 541–542
reaction mechanism of, 187
rejection mechanism of, modification of, 193–196
storage of, 247
Alloplastic implants
biologic testing of, 701–703
ceramics for, 714–718, *716–718*
development of, 698–699
dressing materials for, 722–724, *723, 724*
efficacy of, 702–703
for facial paralysis, 2304–2305, *2305*
for forehead contouring, materials for, 1567
for zygoma reconstruction, 1657, *1656, 1658*

Alloplastic implants *(Continued)*
future of, 724–726, 729, *725, 726, 728*
materials for
for secondary rhinoplasty, 1897, *1897*
mechanical testing of, 699–701, *699–701*
metals in, 703–706, 704*t*, 705*t*
polymers for, 706–714, *707, 708, 710, 711, 713*
suture materials for, 718–722, 719*t*
vs. autogenous grafts, 47
Allopurinol, for postoperative skin flap treatment, 318
Alopecia
after facialplasty in male, 2398
after forehead-brow lift, 2406
androgenic, 1519
nonsurgical treatment of, 1520
surgical treatment of, 1520–1536, *1521–1523, 1525–1535*
tissue expansion for, 492–493, 496
cicatricial, of scalp, 1553–1554, *1554, 1555*
from burn injury, 2223–2226, *2227, 2228*
post-traumatic, correction by tissue expansion, 491–492, *492–494*
Alpert's syndrome, 2488
Alpha particles, 832
Alpha-methyltyrosine (AMT), 3804
Alveolar nerve block, 147–148, *149*
Alveolar process
fractures of, 1013, *1015*
in children, 1157*t*, 1158–1160, *1158, 1159*
treatment of, *1013*, 1019
reconstruction of, 1457, 1463, *1459–1463*
Alveolar ridge, increasing vertical height of, 1454–1456, *1455, 1456*
Alveolus, cancers of, 3452, 3455
cleft, surgical repair of, abnormal facial growth and, 2568–2569, *2570, 2571*
Ameloblastic fibroma, of jaw, 3342, 3345
Ameloblastic fibro-odontoma, 3345
Ameloblastic fibrosarcoma, 3346
Ameloblastic tumors, of jaw, 3341–3342, 3345, *3341, 3343–3344*
Ameloblastoma, of jaw, 3341–3342, 3345, 3346, *3341, 3343*
of maxilla, 3342, *3343–3344*
Ameloblastoma carcinoma, 3346
American Association of Cleft Palate Rehabilitation Classification (AACPR), of craniofacial clefts, 2932, *2932*
American Association of Oral and Plastic Surgeons, establishment of, 14–*15*
American Joint Committee on Cancer Classification, staging of paranasal sinus cancer, 3322, *3322*
American Society of Plastic and Reconstructive Surgery, 21
6-Aminonicotinamide (6-AN), 2532, 2540
β-Aminopropionitrile (BAPN)
for abnormal scars, 738, 740
for lathyrism, 180–181
Aminopterin, 195
Amitriptyline (Elavil), for reflex sympathetic dystrophy, 4911
Amnion, for thermal burns, 804–805
Amniotic rupture sequence, disruptions of, 78
Amputation
challenge of, 4350
cineplasty and, 4347

Amputation *(Continued)*
complications of, 4330–4332
definition of, 4329
for brachial plexus root avulsion, 4789–4790
historical aspects of, 4329
in mutilating injuries of hand, 4339–4340, *4339, 4340*
indications for, 4329–4330
metacarpal hand from, *4338*, 4338–4339
of arm
at above elbow level, 4343, *4344*
at around shoulder level, 4343, 4345
at below elbow level, *4241, 4342*, 4341–4342
elbow disarticulation for, 4343
Krukenberg operation for, 4342–4343
replantation surgery for, 4376–4377
of fingers, 4335–4338, *4336, 4337*
bilateral, 4361, *4361*
levels of, 4334–4335
operative technique for, 4337–4338
principles of, 4332–4334, *4333, 4334*
of fingertip
composite type of, 4485–4487, *4486–4488*
guillotine type of, 4479
of foot, at forefoot level, 4074
of hand, for burn injury, 5467, 5469, *5469–5471*
of leg
at above knee level, 4074
at below knee level, 4074
at hind fore-ankle level, 4074
of thumb, replantation of, 4373
of upper extremity
bilateral, 4347, 4350, *4347*
caused by electrical injury, 5428
forequarter type of, 4345–4347, *4345, 4346*
zone I replantations of, 4371–4372, *4372*
zone II replantations of, 4372–4373, *4373, 4374*
postoperative care for, 4074–4075
psychosocial aspects of, 132–134
salvage attempts in, *4348, 4349*, 4350
self, of upper extremities, 131–132
standard midthigh, 4074
stump of, neuromas of, *4847*, 4848, 4849, *4849–4852*, 4852
surgical goals for, 4330
through knee level or knee disc articulation, 4074
transcarpal, 4340
wrist disarticulation, 4340–4341, *4341*
AMT (alpha-methyltyrosine), 3804
Analgesia, 140–141
Anaphylatoxins, 192
Anastomosis, lymphovenous, 5029–5032, *5030, 5031*
Anatomic snuffbox, 4275
Anemia, for postoperative skin flap treatment, 317
Anencephaly, embryology of, 2460–2461, *2461*
Anesthesia. *See also* Nerve blocks.
for blepharoplasty, 2335
for dermabrasion, 778
for extensor tendon repair, 4568
for facialplasty, 2368–2369
for forehead-brow lift, 2402
for hand injury, 4595–4596
for hand surgery, 4290–4291
for neck contractures, 2058–2060
for rhinoplasty, 1812, 1814–1815, *1813, 1814*
for treatment of nasal bone fractures, 985

Anesthesia *(Continued)*
for upper extremity
for replantation or revascularization, 4362
patient evaluation for, 4302–4305
regional, 4302
for upper lip reconstruction, 2027, *2027*
general, 153–155
for cleft palate repair, 2739
for soft tissue wounds in face, 902
techniques for, 155
vs. local, for suction-assisted lipectomy, 3967–3968
ketamine, 157–158
legal aspects of, 139–140
local
allergic reactions to, 144
chemistry of, 143
for soft tissue wounds in face, 902
mechanism of action of, 143
toxicity of, 144, 144*t*
vs. general, for suction-assisted lipectomy, 3967–3968
neural complications of, 4304–4305
pediatric, 155–157, 156*t*
Aneuploidy, midline posterior cervical lymphatic cysts and, 3243–3245, *3245*
Aneurysms, arterial
local, abnormal blood flow and, 452
true, 5007
Angiofibromas, 3184
Angiogenesis
dependency, hemangiomas and, 3199
stages of, 281
Angiography
for arteriovenous malformations, 3256
for venous malformations, 3252
of orbit, 1586, *1587*, 1588
Angiokeratoma circumscriptum, *3234*, 3235–3236
Angiokeratoma corporis diffusum universale, 3236, *3236*
Angiokeratomas
fucosidosis, 3236
histopathologic criteria for, 3234
of Fordyce, 3235, *3236*
of Mibelli, 3235
Angioma cavernosum, 3192
Angioma simplex, 3192
Angiosarcoma
of head and neck, 3371
of jaw, 3359
Angiosomes
concept of, *343–350*, 347, 349, 351–352
definition of, 334–335, *341*
Angle-rotation flap, for removal of cheek scars, 2167, 2169, *2168, 2170–2171*
Animal bites
delayed primary wound closure and, 900–901
hand infections from, 5534–5535, *5534*, 5535*t*
Ankle
cutaneous arteries of, *371*, 373–374
suction-assisted lipectomy of, 4019, *4020, 4021, 4023*
Ankles, suction-assisted lipectomy of, complications of, 3978
Ankylosis, of temporomandibular joint, 1494–1496, *1495*
Anomalies, minor, 78–81, *79*, 80*t*
frequency of, *80*
Anomalies *(Continued)*
significance of, 81*t*
Anophthalmos
primary congenital, 1639–1640, *1641, 1642*, 1644–1646, *1644–1646*
secondary, 1640
Anoxia, skeletal muscle and, 550
Antacids, for prevention of ulceration, 809
Anterior interosseous nerve syndrome
characteristics of, 4831
etiology of, 4832
management summary for, 4832–4833
surgical indications for, 4832, *4832, 4833*
Anterior neural plate, embryological development of, 2517, *2517*
Anthelical fold, restoration of, 2116–2117, *2117*
Anthrax, 5550
Antibiotics, for suction-assisted lipectomy, 4026
Antibodies, production of, 190–191
Anticoagulants, 458
Anticoagulation, 458–459
Anticonvulsants, craniofacial cleft formation and, 2928–2929
Anti-inflammatory agents, for reflex sympathetic dystrophy, 4910–4911
Antilymphocyte globulin, immunosuppression by, 194–195
Antimetabolic agents, craniofacial cleft formation and, 2929
AO fracture healing, *591*, 591–592
Aortic bodies and sinuses, embryological development of, 2478, *2479*
Apertognathism. *See* Open bite deformity.
Apert's syndrome
clinical presentation of, 3021, *3022*, 5293, 5296, *5296*
hand configuration in, 5296, *5297, 5298*
craniofacial manifestations of, 2488
face proportions in, 30–32, *30, 32*
hydrocephalus in, 3025
inheritance of
dominant type of, *91*
sporadic occurrence of, 89, *90*, 104
maxillary deformities in, 1360
pathogenesis of, 97–98
radiologic findings in, 3021, *3022*
treatment of, 5298–5300, *5299*
visual abnormalities in, 3025–3026
Apical ectodermal ridge (AER), 2482, 5217, 5219, *5218*
Aplasia cutis congenita, 1540–1542, *1541–1544*
Aponeurosis, 630
Aponeurosis surgery, for ptosis, *1758*, 1759, 1765–1766
Apron flaps, for intraoral reconstruction, 3438, *3441*
Arch and band appliances, for mandibular fixation, 3500, *3500–3506*
Arch bars, 1035, *1037*, 1216, *1217*
for intermaxillary fixation, 922, *923–926*, 925–926
prefabricated, for intermaxillary fixation, 944, *945, 946*
Arch wires, cable, 944
Areola, reconstruction of, *3907, 3908*
Argon laser
characteristics of, 3666
lesions amenable to, 3667–3669, *3667–3669*
Arhinencephaly, orbital hypotelorism and, 3005, *3005*
Arion prosthesis, for eyelid paralysis, 2310

Arm
amputation of
prostheses for, 4405, *4406, 4407*
replantation surgery for, 4376–4377
congenital anomalies of. *See also* Hand anomalies.
incidence of, 5225, 5229, 5231, 5229*t*, 5230*t*
intercalated phocomelia, 5242–5243, 5245, *5243, 5244*
timetables and, 5223, 5225
ultrasound examination of, *5234–5235*
uncertain etiology of, 5236
cutaneous arteries of, 359, *360*
embryology of
experimental studies of, 5217, 5219–5220, *5218, 5219*
morphologic development in, 5216–5217, 5216*t*, *5217, 5218*
of muscles, 5220–5221, *5222–5229*
of nerves, 5221, 5223
of vascular system, 5220, *5221*
skeletal development in, 5220
replantation of, 20
suction-assisted lipectomy of, complications of, 3977, 3978
upper, transverse absences of, 5241–5242
Arm flaps
for nose resurfacing, 2202–2203
lateral
anatomy of, 4471, *4472*
for free flap transfer in upper extremity, 4471–4472, *4472*
for sensory reconstruction of hand, 4867–4868, *4868*
medial
anatomy of, 4470–4471, *4471*
for free flap transfer in upper extremity, 4469–4471, *4471*
upper distal, for nasal reconstruction, 1971, *1971–1973*
Armenoid nose, 1853
Arterial ligation
for lymphedema, 4112
selection, for control of facial wound hemorrhage, 877
Arterial malformations, of hand, 5324, *5325, 5326, 5327*
Arterial revascularization, for erectile dysfunction, 4219
Arteries. *See also specific arteries.*
cutaneous
classification of, 352–353
regional anatomy of, 355, 358–359, 362–363, 367–368, 371–374, *356, 357, 360, 361, 364–366, 369–371*
damage to, microscopic signs of, 4367–4368, *4368*
interconnections of, 346–347, *348–350*
musculocutaneous, 277, *278, 283*, 283–284
of lower extremity, 4033–4035, *4034*
Arteriography, for free flap transfer in upper extremity, 4460
Arterioles, microstructure of, 449, *450*
Arteriovenous fistulas
microsurgical concerns for, 452–453
of hand, 5502–5503, *5503*
Arteriovenous malformations
clinical findings in, 3255–3256
Arteriovenous malformations *(Continued)*
histology of, 3255
of hand, 5324, 5326, *5325*
of wrist, 5008, *5008*
physiology of, 3255
terminology for, 3254–3255
treatment of, 3256–3258, *3258*
Arthritis
correction of systemic abnormalities of, 4698
incidence of, 4695
of hand. *See* Hand, arthritis of.
of temporomandibular joint, 1498–1501, *1500, 1501*
patient education for, 4697–4698
treatment problems in, 4695–4696
Arthrodesis
for degenerative arthritis of hand, 4699, 4700, *4701*, 4701–4702
historical aspects of, 4686
of small joints
complications of, 4677–4678
fixation techniques for, 4673–4677, *4674–4677*
general considerations for, *4672*, 4672–4673
indications for, 4671–4672
of wrist
complications of, 4681–4682
for rheumatoid arthritis, 4715–4716
general considerations for, 4678
indications for, 4678
limited, 4682–4686, *4683–4685*
operative techniques for, 4678–4681, *4680, 4681*
Arthrography, of temporomandibular joint, 1503–1505, 1504*t*, *1505*
Arthrogryposis
clinical presentation of, 5378–5380, *5378–5379*
treatment of, 5380–5381
Arthroplasty
gap, for temporomandibular ankylosis, 1494–1495
interpositional with alloplastic or biologic materials, for temporomandibular ankylosis, *1495*, 1495–1496
resection implant
for degenerative arthritis of hand, 4702
for rheumatoid arthritis, 4716–4718, *4717, 4720*
Articulation tests, for evaluation of velopharyngeal incompetence, 2912–2913
Artificial synapse theory, 4898, *4899*
Asch forceps, 985, *987*
Asian patients
beauty standards for, 2416–2420, *2417–2419*
cleft lip/palate susceptibility and, 2529–2530
corrective rhinoplasty in, 1879–1880
esthetic surgery for
for double eyelids, 2423–2426, *2424–2426*
for upper double eyelids, 2420–2422, *2421*
historical perspective of, 2415–2416
of corrective profileplasty, 2426–2428, *2427, 2428*, 2431
of orthopedic profileplasty, *2429–2432*, 2431, 2433
patient selection for, 2420
preoperative considerations of, 2422–2423, *2423*
rhinoplasty for, 2433–2435, *2433–2435*
nose shape of, 1926, *1926*
nose size of, 1926, *1926*
Aspirin, craniofacial cleft formation and, 2929
Ataxia-telangiectasia, 3227, *3238*, 3239
Atheroma, 3569, 3572

Atresia, aural
  bilateral
    evaluation of hearing loss in, 2146–2147
    rehabilitation from otologic surgery for, 2147
  middle ear surgery for, timing of, 2149
    indications for, 2146
  otologic surgery for, results and complications of, 2148–2149
Audiometry
  for aural atresia, 2146–2147
  for microtia, 2146–2147
Auditory canal, external
  aural atresia of, indications for timing of middle ear surgery in, 2146
  stenosis of, *2127*, 2127–2128, 2148–2149
Aufricht retractor, 1822, *1822*
Auricle. *See also* Ear(s).
  acquired deformities of, 2119
    in lower third area, 2137
    in middle third area, 2136–2137, *2137–2141*
    in upper third area, *2133*, 2135–2136, *2136*
    of helical rim, 2131, 2135, *2133–2135*
    with loss of tissue, 2128–2129
    without loss of tissue, 2125, 2127–2128, *2127*
  amputation of, replantation for, 2119–2121, 2124–2125, *2121–2126*
  anatomy of, *2095*, 2095–2096
  cartilage grafts of, 568–569, *568–571*
  congenital deformities of
    cryptotia, 2111, *2116*
    deformities associated with, 2099, *2099*
    diagnosis of, 2099, 2099*t*
    in Treacher Collins syndrome, 3120
    prominence of, 2111, 2116–2117, *2116–2119*, 2119
  earlobe. *See* Earlobe.
  hypoplasia
    clinical characteristics of, 2099–2100
    general treatment considerations for, 2100
  injuries to, 912–913, *914*
  lateral cartilage surface, alteration of, 2117, 2119, *2120*
  medial cartilage surface, alteration of, 2117, *2118, 2119*
  partial loss of, 2129–2130
    composite grafts for, 2131, *2132, 2133*
    structural support of, by contralateral conchal cartilage, 2130, *2130, 2131*
      by ipsilateral conchal cartilage, 2130, *2136*
  reconstruction of
    detaching posterior auricular region in, 2106, *2107, 2108*
    for microtia, 2100–2101
    hairline management for, 2106, 2108
    obtaining rib cartilage for, 2101–2103, *2102*
    preoperative consultation for, 2101
    rotation of lobule for, 2105, *2105*
    secondary, 2108, *2109, 2110*
    total, with autogenous tissue, 204
    tragal construction and conchal definition for, 2105–2106, *2106*
  sensory innervation of, 2095–2096, *2096*
  tumors of
    malignant types of, 2142, 2146, *2146*
    nonmalignant types of, 2142
Auricular composite grafts, for nasal reconstruction, 1931, *1931*
Auricular prostheses, 2129, 3549, *3551*
Auricular reconstruction, for microtia, preoperative consultation for, 2101
Auriculo-branchiogenic dysplasia, 3054
Auriculotemporal syndrome, 1409, 3314, *3314*
Austad prosthesis, 476
Autogenous grafts, vs. alloplastic grafts, 47
Autografts
  autogenous, 225
  banking of, 247
  biochemical studies of, 251
  definition of, 54
Autoimmune diseases, correlation with HLA-DR3, 188
Autologous blood, for suction-assisted lipectomy, 3977, *3977*
Autologous fat injection, 4021, 4025, *4025–4027*
Automobile accidents. *See* Motor vehicle accidents.
Autoregulation, 445
Avascular necrosis, after treatment of mandibular fracture, 976
Avulsions, of facial area, 909, 912, *911, 912*
Axial flaps, local, for genital reconstructive surgery, 4126
Axillary artery, compression of, 4999
  diagnosis of, 5002–5003, *5002–5004*
  management of, *5002–5004*, 5002–5005
Axillary block
  extent of analgesia from, 4306
  performance of, 4320, *4321*
Axillary contractures, from burn injury, 5471, 5473, *5474, 5475*
Axillary nerve, injuries of, 4800–4802
Axolemma, 635–636
Axon(s)
  at node of Ranvier, 641–642
  depolarization of, 639
  morphology of, 635–636
  regeneration of, 657–660, *658, 659*
    facilitation of, 675–676
  reinnervation and, 668–669
Axon blockers, postoperative treatment of skin flaps, 314–315
Axon hillock, 635
Axonotmesis, 656, 2252
Axoplasmic transport, in peripheral nerves, 637–638, *639*
Azathioprine (Imuran), 195

Baggy eyelid syndrome, 2322
Baldness, male pattern. *See* Alopecia, androgenic.
Banded dental arch, for intermaxillary fixation, of mandibular fractures, 944, 946
Bannayan's syndrome, 3264
BAPN (β-aminopropionitrile), for abnormal scars, 738, 740
Barbiturates, 142, 4315
Barraquer-Simons disease, 3136
Barsky technique for bilateral cleft lip repair, 2690, *2691*
Barter principle, 46–47
Basal cell adenoma, of salivary gland, 3296, 3299
Basal cell carcinoma
  clinical features of, 3619, 3621, 3623, *3620, 3622*

Basal cell carcinoma *(Continued)*
  curettage and electrodesiccation for, 3599–3600, *3600, 3601*
    complications and disadvantages of, 3600, 3602, *3602*
  etiologic factors for, 3615–3617, 3619, *3616–3619*
  incidence of, 3614–3615
  of hand, 5489, *5489*
  of perionychium, 4512
  superficial radiation therapy for, 3602–3604
  treatment of
    by cryotherapy, 3627
    by curettage and electrodesiccation, 3623
    by 5-fluorouracil, 3627–3628
    by radiation therapy, 3623, *3624, 3625*
    by surgery, 3623, 3625–3626
    by surgical reconstruction, 3628
    for recurrent lesions, 3626–3627, *3627*
Basal cell epithelioma. *See* Basal cell carcinoma.
Basal cell nevus syndrome, basal cell carcinoma and, 3616, *3616*
Basal metabolic rate (BMR), 797
Basicranium
  growth of, 2502
  synchondroses of, 2506–2507, *2507*
Bathing trunk nevus, 3589, 3591
Beauty
  criteria for, 28–29
  facial, standards for Asian patients, 2416–2420, *2417–2419*
  spectrum of, 116–117
Beauty index, 2417–2418, *2418*
Beckwith-Wiedemann syndrome, 73, 92, 3234
Bedsores. *See* Pressure sores.
Bell's palsy, neurologic signs in, *2252*
Bell's phenomenon, 1757, 2307
Belt lipectomy, *4016, 4017*, 4017, 4019
Benadryl (diphenhydramine hydrochloride), 738
Bennet fracture, *4611*, 4611–4612
Benzodiazepines, 141, 4315
Benzopyrones, for lymphedema, 4107
Bernard modification, for lower lip reconstruction, 2018, 2020, *2020*
Beta particles, 832
Beta-aminopropionitrile. *See* β-Aminopropionitrile (BAPN).
Betadine, for thermal burn management, 802–803
Bicoronal incision, *1592*, 1593
Bifurcations, blood flow through, 444, *444*
Bimaxillary dentoalveolar protrusion
  correction of, 1347, 1351, *1348–1351*
  in Asian face, surgical correction of, *2429*, 2431
Binder's syndrome. *See also* Nasomaxillary hypoplasia.
  dish-face deformity of, 1362
  nasomaxillary hypoplasia in, 3008, *3009*
  orbital hypotelorism and, 3006, *3006*
  surgical correction of, 3008, *3009*
Biobrane, 805
Biochemical defect syndromes, 84, *88*
Biofeedback therapy, for reflex sympathetic dystrophy, 4913
Bipedicle flaps, of scalp, 1530, *1531*
Bite wounds
  from animals
    delayed primary wound closure and, 900–901
    hand infections and, 5534–5535, *5534*, 5535*t*
Bite wounds *(Continued)*
  from humans, hand infections and, 5534–5535, *5534*, 5535*t*
Biteblocks, for mandibular fixation, 3500, *3500–3506*
Black method, for bilateral cleft lip repair, 2693, *2695, 2696*
Blacks
  corrective rhinoplasty in, 1880
  nose shape and sizes of, 1926, *1926*
Bladder exstrophy. *See* Exstrophy of bladder.
Blair, Vilray Papin, 9, 10, *12*, 13
Blair-Brown triangular flap closure, correction of tight lip after, *2785*
Blepharochalasis, 2320, *2321*, 2326
Blepharophimosis
  characteristics of, 1777–1779
  classification of, 1779, *1779*
  genetic aspects of, 1778–1779
  illusion of hypertelorism in, 2982, *2982*
  treatment of, 1779–1780, *1779, 1780*
Blepharoplasty
  anatomic considerations for, 2322–2324, 2326, *2323–2326*
  complications of, 2348–2349
    of asymmetry, 2353–2354
    of blindness, 2354
    of corneal injury, 2349
    of dermatologic types, 2349–2350, *2350*
    of dry eye syndrome, 2354–2355
    of ectropion, 2355–2357, *2355–2357*
    of enophthalmos, 2351–2353, *2352, 2353*
    of hematoma, 2350–2351
  indications for, 2320, 2322
  postoperative care for, 2348
  preoperative evaluation for, 2327–2328, 2330–2331, 2333–2335, *2328–2330, 2332–2334*
  secondary, 2357–2358
  surgical technique for
    anesthesia for, 2335
    for lower eyelids, 2337, 2339, *2340–2347*, 2345, 2348
    for upper eyelids, 2335, 2337, *2338*
    skin marking for, 2335, *2336*
Blindness
  after orbital or nasoethmoido-orbital fractures, 1105
  as complication of Le Fort fracture, 1031
  from blepharoplasty, 2354
Block anesthesia, for rhinoplasty, 1814–1815
Blood
  circulation of, temperature changes and, 853–854
  constituents of, abnormalities in blood flow and, 457–459
  embryology of, 3223–3224
Blood flow
  abnormalities of, 449, 451–453, 453–457, *453, 454*
    external compression and, 453–454, *453, 454*
  control mechanisms for, 445–447, *445–447*
  cutaneous, local control of, 309
  in skin flap, changes in, 311–312, *311, 312*
  normal
    in microvascular surgery, 442–449, *442–449*
    through bifurcations, 444, *444*
  patterns, normal microvascular, 442–443, *442, 443*
Blood supply
  cutaneous system of, 283–284, *283*
  for fracture healing, 592, *592*

Blood supply *(Continued)*
internal system of, 281–282, *282*
muscular system of, 282–283, *283*
of dermal plexus, 286, *286*
of fascial plexus, 284–285, *285*
of scalp, 1517, *1517*
of subdermal plexus, 285–286, *286*
of subepidermal plexus, 286, *286*
to bone, 600–605, *601–604*
to muscles, 302
Blood vessels. *See also specific blood vessels.*
elastic properties of, 443
embryology of, 280–281, *281*
Blood viscosity
blood flow and, 447–448, *448*
factors affecting, 457–458
Blood volume, microvascular procedures and, 457
Blue nevus, 3591, *3591*
B-lymphocytes, 178, 189–190
BMP (bone morphogenetic protein), 592, 594–597
BMR (basal metabolic rate), 797
Body contouring
autologous fat injection
for glabellar frown lines, 4021, *4025*
instrumentation and technique for, 4026, *4026, 4027*
belt lipectomy, *4016, 4017*, 4017, 4019
by suction-assisted lipectomy
equipment for, 3973, 3975, *3974, 3975*
preoperative planning for, 3975–3977, *3976*
combined procedures for, 4021
medial thighplasty, *4018*, 4019
Body fat
aging and, 3965–3967, *3966–3968*
environmental effects of, 3964–3965
genetic predisposition of, 3964, *3965*
Body image, 27–28
Body proportions, 35–36, *36, 37*
Body temperature
as index of flap perfusion, 319*t*, 320
decreased. *See also* Cold injuries.
physiologic responses to, 860*t*-861*t*
Bonding, for child with facial deformity, 2731
Bone(s)
anatomy of, in great toe vs. thumb, 5159, 5161, *5160–5162*
blood supply to, 600–605, *601–604*
flat or membranous, blood supply to, 602–603, *603*
healing of
in lower extremity, 4057–4058, *4060*, 4061
mechanism of, 197–198
of fractures, 590–592, *591*
histochemistry of, 583–586
in electrical burn injuries, 5425–5426
long, blood supply to, 600–601, *601*
microanatomy of, 583–586, *584, 585*
mineral equilibrium in, 587, 590
necrosis of, from orthognathic surgery, 1405
osteoblastic apposition of, 725, *725*
reconstruction of defects of
allograft transplants for, 4687
autogenous bone grafts for, 4686–4687
illustrative cases of, 4688–4689, *4688–4692*, 4691–4692
vascularized bone grafts for, 4687
Bone(s) *(Continued)*
remodeling of, 597–598, *598, 599*
resorption of, from orthognathic surgery, 1411, *1412*
transplantation of bone-producing tissue, 592–593
turnover, cellular mechanisms of, 586–587, 590
types of tissue in, 583–584
vascularized transfers of, 598, 600–605, *601–605*
Bone cysts, aneurysmal, 3351
Bone deposition, 2499, *2500*
Bone graft(s). *See also specific bone grafts.*
allografts
for mandibular defects, 1414
immune response to, 595–597
immunologic consequences of, 197–198
vascularized, 200
autogenous
bone formation in, 4686–4687
history of, 593–594
calvarial, nonvascularized autografts, 617–619, *617–619*
clinical uses of, 605–606, 608, 610, 612–614, 617–622, 624–625, *605–611, 613–625*
cranial, for secondary rhinoplasty, *1903*, 1908
for alveolar and anterior cleft palate, 2758–2759
incorporation of, 2762, *2764*
for bilateral cleft lip repair, 2676
for cleft alveolar arch deformities, 2439
for cleft palate closure, timing of, 2737–2738
for congenital hand anomaly correction, 5255, *5256*
for contour restoration, in microgenia, 1323, 1329, *1330*
for hand reconstruction, *4296*, 4296–4297
for mandibular defects, 1413
prerequisites for success of, 1414–1415
for maxillary deformities, secondary to cleft palate
technique of, 2825–2829, *2827–2829*
timing of, 2823–2825
for reconstruction of orbital floor fracture, 1075, *1075, 1076*
for restoration of orbital and nasal bone, 1097, *1098*
for saddle nose deformity, 1882, *1884*, 1885–1886
for thumb reconstruction, 5190
for zygoma reconstruction of, 1657, *1659–1661*
from ilium
for nasal contour restoration, 1886–1887, 1889, 1892, *1886–1888, 1890, 1891*
vascularized types of, 612
in orbital hypertelorism correction, 2998–2999
nonvascularized, for acquired deformities of mandible, 1422, 1426, 1432–1433, 1437–1438, *1421–1437*
of mandibular defects, of small and medium size, 1422, 1426, *1426–1428, 1431*
onlay, for maxillary micrognathia-retrognathia correction, 1367, *1367, 1368*
primary
after mandibular tumor resection, 1422, *1423–1425*
for panfacial fractures, 1039–1040, 1043, *1043*
of mandibular post-traumatic defects, 1422
rib, 613–614, 617, *613–617*
secondary, for alveolar and anterior cleft palate, 2757–2758
sources of, for alveolar and anterior cleft palate, 2759
tibial, 605, *605*
ultrastructural organization of, 586, *587–589*
vascularized, 4687

Bone graft(s) *(Continued)*
with canthopexy and dacryocystorhinostomy, for epicanthal fold correction, 1617–1618, *1618–1620*
with elongation osteotomy, 1277
with osteotomy and septal framework resection, 1892–1893
xenografts, immune response to, 595–597
Bone marrow, microanatomy of, 585–586
Bone morphogenetic protein (BMP), 592, 594–597
Bone transfers
allograft transplants for, 4687
vascularized, for acquired defects of mandible, 1438–1440, 1443, 1445, 1447, 1451, *1440–1446, 1448–1450*
Bone tumor(s), of hand
adjuvant treatment for, 5517
reconstructive surgery for, 5521–5522, 5524–5528, *5523–5527*
staging of, 5515, 5517, 5515*t*, *5517*
surgical excision of, 5517–5518, 5520–5521, 5517*t*, *5518–5521*
Bonnevie-Ullrich syndrome, correction of congenital neck webbing in, 2077–2078, *2079–2084*
Boutonnière deformity
after burn injury, 5465–5467, *5466*
clinical presentation of, 4579, *4584*
immobilization period for, 4586
splinting technique for, 4585–4586
treatment failures in, 4586–4587, *4587*
with closed injuries, 4580, *4581*
with established mobility, 4580–4582, *4582–4586*
with open injuries, 4579–4580
with passive motion, 4582–4583, *4585*
with proximal interphalangeal joint dislocation, 4580, *4582*
Boutons, 634
Bowenoid papulosis, 3594–3595, *3595*
Bowen's disease
of hand, 5487, *5488*
of vulva, *3604*, 3604–3605
Brachial plexus
anatomy of, 4313–4315, 4758
injuries of, 4788–4789
conservative treatment for, 4787, 4789
diagnosis of, 4781–4782
direct surgical treatment for, 4787–4788
etiology of, 4780–4781, 4781*t*
extraforaminal C5–C6 rupture and C7–T1 root avulsion, 4793–4794
extraforaminal rupture of C5 and root avulsion of C6–Th1, 4792–4793
historical aspects of, 4776–4780
preoperative considerations for, 4785–4786
severity of, 4781–4785, 4783*t*, 4784*t*
with C5–C6, possibly C7 paralysis, 4796–4797, 4799, *4797, 4798*
with C5–C6–C7 rupture and C8–T1 avulsion, 4794–4796, *4794, 4795*
with Klumpke-type lesions, 4799
with main nerve trunk lesions, 4799–4802, *4800, 4801*
with ruptures of trunks, cords, and individual terminal branches, 4799
Brachial plexus blocks
choice of, *4305*, 4305–4308
Brachial plexus blocks *(Continued)*
complications of, 4307*t*, 4307–4308
plasma levels of local anesthetic agents during, 4311*t*
Brachial plexus injuries
evaluation criteria for, 4808, 4809*t*-4810*t*, 4810
gunshot wounds of, 4810
irradiation therapy for, plexopathy following, 4811–4812
lacerations of, 4810
operative technique of
for exposure of plexus, 4802–4804
for grafting, 4805–4806
for nerve stump preparation, 4805
for osteotomy of clavicle, 4805
for suturing, 4805
for topographic orientation of grafts, 4806–4807
pain syndromes of, 4812–4813
surgical results for, 4807–4808
presentation of, 4810, 4811*t*, 4812*t*
treatment of
for root avulsion, C5–T1, 4789–4792, *4790, 4791*
problems of, 4813–4814
Brachioplasty
by suctioning alone, 3987–3988, *3989, 3990*
combined with other body contouring procedures, 4021
without suctioning, 3985, 3987, *3986, 3987*
Brachmann-de Lange syndrome, 3234
Brachycephaly, 1546
Brachycephaly-bilateral coronal synostosis, 3015, *3017*
Brachytherapy, 832
Bradycardia, 141
Brain injury, with nasoethmoido-orbital fractures, 1091–1092
Branchial arch syndrome, 2931
Branchial cleft anomalies, 3178–3180, *3179*
Branchio-otorenal syndrome, 2468–2469, 2491
Breast(s)
aberrant tissue, locations of, *3840*
anatomy of, 3840–3841, *3841*
asymmetry of, after augmentation mammoplasty, 3886
augmentation of. *See also* Mammoplasty, augmentation.
psychosocial aspects of, 125–126
with abdominoplasty, 3953, *3958, 3959*
blood supply of, 3843–3844, *3843, 3844*
embryology of, 3839–3840
loss of, emotional impact of, 3897
lymphatic supply of, 3844–3846, *3845*
nerve supply of, *3846*, 3846–3847
nipples of. *See* Nipple(s).
physiology of, 3841–3843, *3842*
proliferative disease of
risk of, 3873
subcutaneous mastectomy for, 3873, 3875, *3876–3878*, 3877
ptosis, surgical treatment of, 3861, 3864, *3864–3868*
reduction of. *See* Breast reduction.
suction-assisted lipectomy of
complications of, 3977, 3978
for axillary tissue removal, 3988, *3993, 3994*
for glandular resection, 3988, *3996*
for nonglandular resection, 3988, *3997*
symmetry of, breast reconstruction and, 3900, 3901

Breast cancer
breast reconstruction for. *See* Breast reconstruction.
chemotherapy for, 3900
incidence of, 3897
local management of, 3898–3899
prophylactic mastectomy for, 3922–3924, *3925*
risk factors for, 3897, 3897*t*
staging of, 3899, 3899*t*, 3900
survival from, 3898
Breast feeding, augmentation mammoplasty and, 3892
Breast flaps, for chest wall reconstruction, 3703, *3706*
Breast reconstruction
after mastectomy, psychosocial aspects of, 126–128
by tissue expansion, 482–491, *484–487, 489, 490*, 3906–3908, *3906–3910*, 3911
advantages of, 482
bilateral technique for, 485, *485*
disadvantages of, 482–483
for congenital breast abnormalities, 488–489, *489, 490*, 491
for tuberous breast, 489, 491
permanent expansion prostheses for, 486–487, *487*
reconstruction in conjunction with distant flaps, *487*, 487–488
surgical technique for, 483, *484*, 485
complications of, 3905–3906, 3916, 3922
immediate, by tissue expansion, 485–486, *486*
management of opposite breast in, 3924–3925
muscle and musculocutaneous flaps for, 387–393, *389, 390, 392, 393*
nipple-areola reconstruction for, 3926–3927, *3926, 3927*
preoperative planning for, 3900–3901, 3913–3914, 3919–3920
selection of method for, 3901–3902
suction-assisted lipectomy for, 3988, *3995*
timing of, 3901, *3902*
TRAM flap for, 3916–3920, *3917–3921*, 3922, 3925
with available tissue, 3902–3906, *3903–3905*
with gluteus maximus flap, 3922, *3923, 3924*
with latissimus dorsi flap, 3911–3914, 3916, *3912–3916*
Breast reduction
complications of, 3877, 3879
dermal pedicles for, 3847, *3848, 3849*
superior based, 3847, 3849, *3850–3854*, 3853
development of, 3847
for massively hypertrophied breasts, 3877, *3881*
for moderately hypertrophied and ptotic breasts, 3877, *3879, 3880*
free nipple graft for, 3854, 3856, *3858, 3859*
inferior pyramidal dermal flap technique for, 3856, *3860–3863*, 3861
psychosocial aspects of, 126
vertical bipedicle dermal flap technique for, 3853–3854, *3856, 3857*
with abdominoplasty, 3953, *3960–3961*
Breastfeeding, problems of, for cleft palate infant, 2731
Brephoplasty, 54
Bronchopleural fistula, chest wall reconstruction and, 3726, *3727–3730*
Brooke formula, 788, 792*t*, 793
modified, 792*t*, 793
Brow lift. *See* Forehead-brow lift.
Brow suspension, for eyebrow ptosis, 1759, *1759*
Brucellosis, 5550
Buccal fat pad excision, with facialplasty, 2384
Buccal mucosa, cancer of, 3452, *3453–3455*
Buccal sulcus
deficiency of, correction of, 2796–2797, *2797*
restoration of, 3508
by skin graft inlay technique, *1452, 1453*, 1457
secondary abnormalities of, from bilateral cleft lip repair, 2853, 2855, *2855*
Buccopharyngeal membrane, persistence of, 1998
Buffalo hump deformity, suction-assisted lipectomy for, 3981, *3983*
Bullet wound, nerve injury from, 678
Burkitt's lymphoma, 3359
Burn contractures
contraction process and, 167, *167*
history of treatment for, 787–788
of axilla, 5471, 5473, *5474, 5475*
of elbow, 5469, 5471, *5472*
of hand
dorsal, 5458, 5460–5461, *5460*
volar, 5464–5465, *5465*
of oral commissure, 2229, 2231
true vs. apparent defect of, *24*, 24–25, *25*
Burn injuries
causes of, 2153–2154
deaths from, 2153
of ear, 2204–2207, *2207–2209*, 2209–2210
of eyebrows, 2218–2222, *2219–2220*
of hand
amputations for, 5467, 5469, *5469–5471*
complications of, *5415*, 5415–5416
depth categories for, 5404*t*
historical aspects of, 5399–5402
inpatient treatment of, 5405–5414, *5411, 5412, 5414–5416*
outpatient treatment of, 5405
pathology of, 5402–5403
physical examination of, 5403–5405, *5404*
reconstruction for. *See* Hand reconstruction, after burn injury.
of male genitalia, *4234*, 4234–4235
of upper lip, 2183–2184
scalp alopecia from, 2223–2226, *2227, 2228*
to face. *See* Facial injuries, from burns.
Burn wound sepsis, *807*, 807–808
Buttock, cutaneous arteries of, 368, 371, *369*
Buttonhole incision, for cancellous chips, 610

Cable grafting, 4769
Calcaneal artery fasciocutaneous flap, lateral, 4085, *4087*
Calcitonin, for reflex sympathetic dystrophy, 4910–4911
Calcium channel blockers, in postoperative treatment of skin flaps, 316–317
Calcium gluconate injection, for acid burns, 5437–5438
Calculi, salivary, 3290, *3291, 3292*, 3312–3313
Caldwell projection
for plain films, 884–885, *885*
of orbit, 1584
Calf flap, posterior, for sensory reconstruction of hand, *4871*, 4871–4872
Caloric needs, of burn patients, 798–799, 799*t*

Calvarium
as bone graft donor site, 2759, 3111–3112
blood supply of, 603–605, *604, 605*
bone flaps of, 604–605, *605*
for maxillary and orbital deficiencies, 3112–3113, *3114–3115*
for zygoma reconstruction, 1659, *1662, 1663, 1663*
growth processes in, 2507, *2507*
nonvascularized autografts, 617–619, *617–619*
thickness measurement, *617*, 617–618, 618*t*
vascular anatomy of, 619–620, *620*, 620*t*
vascularized grafts, 619–622, *620–625*
Calves, suction-assisted lipectomy of
complications of, 3978
technique for, 4019, 4021, *4020, 4023*
Camouflage, vs. anatomic restoration, 46
Camptodactyly
anatomy of, 5332–5333, *5334*
clinical presentation of, 5328, 5330–5332, *5331, 5332*
treatment of, 5333, *5334–5337*, 5337
Canaliculi, 583
Canaliculodacryocystorhinostomy, 1736, *1736*
Cancellous bone, as bone graft source, 2759
Candidiasis
of hand, 5552
oral cancer and, 3418
Canines, eruption of, after alveolar bone grafting, 2765, *2765*, 2767
Canthopexy, for epicanthal fold correction, 1617–1618, *1618–1620*
Canthoplasty
for lagophthalmos, 2307, *2308–2310*, 2310
lateral, 1717–1719, *1719*–1726
medial, 2998, *2998*
Canthotomy, lateral, 1687, *1687*
Canthus deformity, lateral treatment of, 1609
Canthus inversus deformity
correction of, 1614, 1620, 1623, *1622*
illusion of hypertelorism in, 2982, *2982*
Cantilever bone graft, for nasal skeleton reconstruction, 1983, *1983*
Capillaries
blanching of, as index of flap perfusion, 319*t*, 320
microstructure of, 449, *450, 451*
temperature changes and, 853–854
vascular malformations of, in hand, 5316
Capillary hemangiomas
classification of, 3192
clinical presentation of, 3582–3583, *3583*
granular type of, 3204–3206, *3205*
of arm, 5502, *5502*
Capillary-cavernous hemangiomas
argon laser therapy for, 3668, *3668*
carbon dioxide laser therapy for, 3670
Capillary-lymphatic malformations, *3234*, 3234–3235, 3241
Capitate-lunate arthrodesis, 4684
Capsular contraction, after augmentation mammoplasty, 3886–3889, 3887*t*, *3889*
Capsular ligaments
loose or sprained, 1480
traumatized external, 1480–1481, *1481*
Capsulectomy, with flexor tendon tenolysis, 4550–4551
Capsulitis, posterior, 1479–1480, *1480, 1481*
Carbon dioxide laser
lesions amenable to, 3669–3670, *3670*
physiology and physics of, 3666
Carbon monoxide intoxication, diagnosis of, 795–796
Carbonic anhydrase histochemistry, of fascicle, 675
Carbons, for alloplastic implants, 718, *719*
Carcinogenesis, from radiation, 836–838, *837*
Carcinogenicity, of alloplastic implants, 702
Carcinoma ex pleomorphic adenoma, 3308
Cardiovascular anomalies, congenital, in Down syndrome, 3162
Cardiovascular malformations, congenital, embryology of, 2464
Carotid bodies, embryological development of, 2478, *2479*
Carotid cavernous sinus fistula, 1114, 1118–1119
Carotid sinuses, embryological development of, 2478, *2479*
Carpal bones. *See also specific carpal bones.*
dislocations of, 4605–4606, 4608–4609, 4605*t*, *4606–4608*, 4640–4641, *4641*, 4646–4650, *4647–4650*
fracture-dislocations of, 4605–4606, 4608–4609, 4605*t*, *4606–4608*
fractures of, 4596–4598, 4640–4646, *4642–4646, 4596, 4597*
transverse absence of, 5246, 5248, 5252, 5255, *5249–5251, 5253–5254*
Carpal tunnel
flexor tendon repair and, 4537
ulnar, 4281, *4281*
Carpal tunnel syndrome, 4742–4744, *4744*
anatomy of, 4823–4825, *4824, 4826–4828*
etiology of, 4825
management of, summary of, 4831
surgical correction technique for, 4825, *4829, 4830*, 4830–4831
Carpenter's syndrome
clinical and radiographic findings in, 3023, 3025
congenital heart defect in, 92
preaxial polydactyly in, 5123
Carpocarpal joint, in rheumatoid arthritis, 4714–4718, *4715–4717*
Carpometacarpal joint
degenerative arthritis of, 4701–4703, *4701, 4702*
dislocations of, 4609–4611, *4610*
fracture-dislocations of, *4611*, 4611–4612
subluxation of, 4611–4612
Carpue, Joseph, 5–6
Cartilage
antigenicity of, 564–566
banking and preservation of, 566–567
elastic, 563
fibrocartilage, 563
growth of, 2498–2499
hyaline, 563
hypertrophic, calcification of, 590
physical properties of, *560*, 561, 563–564, *563, 564*
warping of, 563–564, *564, 565*
Cartilage graft(s)
allografts, survival of, 565–566
autogenous, 559, 568–573, *568–572*
growth of, 560–561, *560–562*
of auricle, 568–569, *568–571*
of nose, 569, *572*
perichondrial, 573–576
physiology of, 560–561, *560–562*
conchal, for secondary rhinoplasty, 1904, *1906, 1907*, 1908
costal, for nasal contour restoration, *1892, 1892–1893, 1893*

Cartilage graft(s) *(Continued)*
for contour restoration, for microgenia, 1323, 1329, *1330*
for saddle nose deformity, 1882, *1884*, 1885–1886
for zygoma reconstruction, 1657, *1659–1661*
obtaining, for ear reconstruction, 2101–2103, *2102*
of nasal tip, 1838–1839, *1838–1840*
perichondrocutaneous graft, 576, *577–579*, 578
septal, for secondary rhinoplasty, 1902, 1904, *1904–1906*
Cartilaginous vaults, nasal, 1786, *1787*
Cast cap splints
disadvantages of, 1215–1216
for intermaxillary fixation, of mandibular fractures, 946, *947*
Castroviejo dermatome, *228*
Cataracts, from electrical injuries, 828
Catecholamines, vasoconstriction and, 5016
Catgut sutures, for alloplastic implants, 719, 719*t*
Catheters, for postoperative hypospadias repair, 4166
Caucasians, nose shape and sizes of, 1926, *1926*
"Cauliflower ear," 573, 2127
Causalgia, of reflex sympathetic dystrophy, 4892–4893
Cavernous hemangioma, 3583–3584, *3583*
Cebocephaly, orbital hypotelorism and, 3005, *3005*
Cecil-Culp technique, for hypospadia repair, 4158, *4159*
Cell dedifferentiation, 163
Cell mediated immunity, after thermal burn injury, 801–802
Cell mediated responses, 191
Cell survival theory, 516, *517, 518*
Cellulitis, of hand, 5537–5538
Celsus, 2, 7
Cement burns, 5439, *5439*
Cemental dysplasia, periapical, 3346
Cementifying fibroma, 3346
Cementoblastoma, 3345–3346
Central giant cell granuloma, of jaw, 3348, 3351
Central nervous system, complications of, in electrical injuries, 828
Central plasticity hypothesis, 669
Central venous pressure, monitoring of, in thermal burn injury, 793
Centralization, for longitudinal deficiencies of radius, 5262, 5264–5265, *5263, 5264*
Centrifugal sprouting theory, 3224
Cephalography
of maxillary deformity, *1378*
of open bite deformity, 1354, *1354*
Cephalometry
analysis techniques of, 1194
cephalostat for, 1195
control data for, 1198, 1199*t*, 1200
for preoperative evaluation, 1207–1209, *1208*, 1362
for cleft lip/palate, *2563, 2565*
for craniofacial microsomia, 3071–3076, 3077, *3071–3077*
for mandibular prognathism, *1230, 1231*
for obstructive sleep apnea, 3148–3149, *3149*
for short face deformity, 1384, 1386, *1385*
three-dimensional, for computer-aided surgical planning, 1209, *1211*, 1212, 1212*t*
tracings for, 1195, *1195*
of mandible after vertical osteotomy of ramus, *1246*
Cephalostat, 1195
Ceramics, for alloplastic implants, 714–718, *716–719*
Cerebral anomalies, in craniofacial microsomia, 3069
Cerebral injury, 870, *870*
Cervical cleft, congenital midline, with webbing, 2078, 2085, *2085*
Cervical contractures, complete, skin flaps for, 2068, *2069–2075*, 2073–2074, 2076
Cervical cord compression
anterior, 871
posterior, 871
Cervical metastases, management of, 3330–3331
Cervical region
anesthesia for, 2058–2060, *2060*
complete contractures of, 2057–2058
excision of scar in, 2060, *2061–2064*
limited contractures of, 2076, *2076, 2077*
Cervical ribs, vascular compression syndromes and, 4998
Cervical spine injuries, initial assessment of, 870–871
Cervicofacial advancement-rotation flap, for removal of cheek scars, 2167, 2169, *2168, 2170–2171*
Cervicofacial skin flap, for facialplasty, 2371, *2372*, 2373
Cervicohumeral flap, for cheek reconstruction, 2045–2046
Cervicomental angle
obtuse, 2378–2379, *2379, 2390, 2391*
pseudo-obtuse, *2389*
Cervicopectoral flap, for cheek reconstruction, 2043, 2045, *2045*
Chalone, 164
Charreterra flap, for complete cervical contractures, 2068, 2073, *2071, 2072*
Cheek flap
advancement type of, for nasal reconstruction, 1943, *1948, 1949*
nasolabial. *See* Nasolabial flap.
rotation type of, for eyelid reconstruction, *1707, 1709*, 1712
Cheek implant, with facialplasty, 2384
Cheek pouches, 2331, *2332*
Cheekbone, postnatal development of, 2497
Cheeks
anatomy of, 2037–2038, *2038*
for zone 1, 2038
bulk of, restoration of, 2053
reconstruction of
for buccomandibular defects (zone 3), 2048–2050, *2050–2052*, 2053
for perauricular defects (zone 2), 2042–2043, *2044–2048*, 2045–2048
for suborbital defects (zone 1), 2038–2040, *2039–2043*, 2042
regional entities of, 27
regional esthetic unit of, *2160*, 2161–2162, 2165
resurfacing of
esthetic considerations for, 2161
expanded skin flaps for, 2174–2178
for removal of large scars, 2160, 2169, *2172–2173*
for removal of moderate-sized scars, 2160, 2165, 2167, 2169, *2166, 2168, 2170–2171*
for removal of small scars, 2160, 2165
scar replacement and, 2160–2161
scar replacement with distant flaps or microvascular free flaps, 2183
scar replacement with regional tube pedicle skin flap, 2178–2179, *2180–2181*, 2182

Cheeks *(Continued)*
resurfacing of, scar replacement with skin graft, 2182–2183
single-sheet technique, *2163, 2164*
staged excision with sequential flap advancement, 2169, 2171
Chemabrasion, 781
Chemical carcinogenesis, squamous cell carcinoma and, 3629–3630
Chemical injuries
characteristics of, 5436
extravasation injuries from injections, surgical management of, 5442–5443, *5443*
first aid treatment for, 5436
from acids, 5436–5438, *5437, 5438*
from alkali, 5438–5439, *5439*
from injections, 5439–5443, *5441*
from phosphorus, 5439
Chemical peeling
chemical agents for, 754–757
complications of, 769–771, *770, 771*
description of, 748
for eyelid pigmentation after blepharoplasty, 2350, *2350*
histologic changes after, 751–754, *752–754*
histology of sun-damaged and aging skin and, 749–751, *750, 751*
historical background of, 748–749
indications for, 757–758, *758–761*
postoperative care for, 766–767, *768*, 769
preoperative evaluation for, 758–759, 761
technique of
for full face peeling, 761–764, *762–764*
for regional peeling, 764, 766, *767*
with dermabrasion, 781
Chemotherapeutic agents, topical, for thermal burn management, 802–804, 803*t*
Chemotherapy
adjuvant, for maxillary tumors, 3330
for hemangiomas, 3215–3216
Chemotrophic guidance, 675–676
Cherubism, 3348, *3350*
Chest wall reconstruction
anatomy of, 3676–3679, *3677, 3678*
clinical problems with, 3676*t*
historical aspects of, 3675–3676
muscle and musculocutaneous flaps for, 396–397, 3688–3691, *3689–3690, 3692–3693, 3694, 3695–3696, 3696–3697, 3698–3699*, 3700
breast flaps, unilateral or bilateral, 3703, *3706*
diaphragm mobilization for, 3703
external oblique muscle for, 3703
total arm flaps for, 3700, 3703, *3704*
omentum flaps for, 3700, *3701, 3702*
physiology of, 3676–3679, *3677*
principles of, 3679*t*
available flaps for, 3680, 3683, *3681–3683*, 3683*t*
for free flaps, 3703, 3705, 3707
fundamental goals of, 3679–3680
serratus anterior muscle flaps for, *3690*, 3697
skin flaps for, 3683, 3686, 3688, *3685, 3687*
tensor fasciae latae muscle flaps for, 3697, 3699–3700, *3698, 3699*
problems of, 3712–3713
bronchopleural fistula as, 3726, *3727–3730*
chronic empyema, 3726, *3728*
of chronic coverage, 3726
Chest wall reconstruction *(Continued)*
problems of, pressure necrosis, 3726
with benign neoplasms, 3713–3714, 3714*t*, *3715, 3716*
with chest wall injury, 3712–3713
with invasive chest wall tumors, 3716–3718, *3717*
with irradiated chest wall, 3718–3719, 3722, *3720–3723*
with malignant tumors, 3714–3716, 3715*t*, *3717*
with median sternotomy dehiscence, 3722, 3724, 3726, *3725*
with metastatic tumors, 3716
with pectus carinatum, 3742, 3745, *3744, 3746–3748*
with pectus excavatum, 3726, 3729, 3731–3733, 3737–3742, *3731, 3734–3736, 3738–3742*
with Poland's syndrome, 3749, 3752–3753, 3755, *3753, 3754, 3756–3761*
with sternal clefts, 3745, 3749, *3749–3752*
skeletal stabilization for
indictions for, 3707
method of, 3707–3708, *3707–3711*, 3712
Chilblain, 852, 5431
Child abuse, thermal burn injuries and, 789–790
Children
anesthesia for, 156*t*, 156–157, 4303
facial trauma of
aveolar fractures in, 1157*t*, 1158–1160, *1158, 1159*
clinical examination of, 1151–1152
complications of, 1183–1184
during birth, 1153–1154
during prenatal period, 1153–1154
emergency treatment for, 1153
etiology of fractures in, 1155–1156
frontal bone fractures in, 1174–1175, 1177, *1174, 1176–1177*
frontal sinus fractures in, 1175, 1177
in infant, 1153–1154
incidence of fractures in, 1156–1158, 1157*t*
mandible fractures in, 1160–1164, *1161, 1162, 1163*
radiologic evaluation of, 1152–1153, *1152*
fluid maintenance for, 156*t*, 156–157, 157*t*
growth in, of mandible, 1148–1150, *1149*
head and neck tumors of
benign types of, 3181–3184, *3183*
late sequelae of therapy for, 3188, *3188*
malignant, 3184–3188, *3188*
ilium autografts, nonvascularized, *609*, 610, 612, *610, 611*
malignancies of, incidence of, 3175
midfacial fractures in, 1164–1165, *1165*
compound, multiple and comminuted, 1179–1180, 1182–1183, *1179–1181*
nasal and nasoorbital fractures in, 1170–1171
nasoethmoido-orbital fractures in, 1171–1174, *1172, 1173*
orbital fractures in, 1167–1170, *1168, 1170*
postnatal growth of, nasomaxillary complex, 1150–1151
soft tissue injuries in, 1154–1155
supraorbital fractures in, 1177–1179, *1178, 1179*
thumb reconstruction in, by bone lengthening, 5205, 5209, 5211, *5208, 5209*
zygomatic fractures in, 1165, *1166–1167*, 1167
Chin
augmentation of, *1307*, 1307–1308
with autogenous rib cartilage graft, *574*

Chin *(Continued)*
burn injuries of, 2187–2188, *2189*
deformities of
anatomic considerations in, 1305, *1305, 1306*
macrogenia, 1332–1333, *1334, 1335*
microgenia. *See* Microgenia.
"double," suction-assisted lipectomy for, 3979, *3980,* 3981, *3981*
postnatal development of, 2497
surgery of, rhinoplasty and, 1802, *1802*
Chin implant, with facialplasty, 2383–2384
Chlorpromazine, in postoperative treatment of skin flaps, 316
Choanal atresia, congenital
anatomy of, 1999
diagnosis of, 1999–2000, *2000*
embryology of, 1998–1999
in Robin sequence, 3128–3129
incidence of, 1999
treatment of, 2001–2004, *2002–2004*
Choline acetylase activity, 675
Chondritis, suppurative, of ear, 2204–2205
Chondrocytes
functions of, 560–561, *560*, 563
neural crest cells and, 2462, 2464
storage of, 566–567
Chondrogladiolar deformity, surgical correction of, 3742, 3745, *3746, 3747*
Chondroma, chest wall reconstruction and, 3714, 3714*t*
Chondromatosis, in temporomandibular joint, 1490
Chondromucosal flap, from nasal septum, for nasal relining, 1981, *1981*
Chondrosarcomas
chest wall reconstruction and, 3714–3715
of jaw, 3356, *3357*
Chordee
correction of
in one-stage hypospadia repair, 4160
in two-stage hypospadia repair, 4157, *4158*
embryology of, 4154–4155
Chromium exposure, oral cancer and, 3418–3419
Chromomycoses, 5552
Chromosomal anomalies
cytogenetics of, 100, *101*
of syndromes, 84, *87*
midline posterior cervical lymphatic cysts and, 3243–3245, *3245*
of cleft lip/palate, 2539
of cleft palate, 2547
Chromosome banding, 100, 102*t*
Chronaxie, 2253
Chylous reflux, lymphedema and, 4117
Cigarette smoking
blood flow and, 5012
cleft palate and, 2546
oral cancer and, 3417–3418, 3418*t*
teratogenicity of, 2533
vasospasm form, 455
Cimetidine, 809
Cineplastic powered active prostheses, 4396
Cineplasty, 4347
Circulation, blood, temperature changes and, 853–854
Circumcision, complications of, 4236–4239, *4237, 4238*
Circumferential wiring techniques, for edentulous mandible fracture, 971, *972*
Clasped thumb deformities, 5116–5118, *5117*
Clavicle, osteotomy of, for brachial plexus injury repair, 4805
Claw hand, postburn deformity of, 5458, 5460–5461, *5460*
Clear cell adenoma, of salivary gland, 3299
Clear cell carcinoma, malignant, of salivary gland, 3309
Clearance tests, for flap perfusion assessment, 319*t*, 322
Cleavage lines
anatomy of, 216, *217*, 218
skin extensibility and, 218–220, *219*
tension lines and, 218, *218*
Cleft alveolus, abnormal facial growth and, surgical repair of, 2568–2569, *2570, 2571*
Cleft hand
clinical presentation of, 5267, 5269, *5268*
treatment of, 5269–5271, *5270, 5272, 5273*
types of, comparison of, 5267, 5269, 5269*t*, *5268*
Cleft lip
bilateral, 2653, *2654*
adaptation of Tennison unilateral cleft lip repair for, 2676, 2679, *2676–2679*
Barsky technique for, 2690, *2691*
Bauer, Trusler, and Tondra method for, 2679–2681, *2680–2682*
Black method for, 2693, *2695, 2696*
columella lengthening for, 2706, 2708, *2705–2708*
complications of repairs for, 2697–2698
development of, 2586–2587, *2586, 2587*
diagnosis of, 2653–2654, *2655, 2656*
gingivoperiosteoplasty for, 2702, *2703, 2704*
incidence of, 2653, 2654*t*
lip musculature in, 2603, 2608, 2612, *2603–2611*
Manchester method for, 2684, *2686, 2687*
Millard method for complete clefts of, 2683–2684, *2684, 2685*
Millard method for incomplete clefts of, 2681, *2682, 2683, 2683*
Mulliken method for, 2692–2693, *2693, 2694*
nasal deformity of. *See* Cleft lip nasal deformity.
Noordhoff technique for, 2696–2697, *2697, 2698*
postoperative care for, 2667
premaxilla in, 2581–2583, *2582*
presurgical orthodontic therapy for, 2702, *2702, 2703*
primary Abbé flap for, 2691–2692, *2692*
prolabium usage in repair of, 2656
repair of, 2698–2699
secondary lip deformities of, 2840–2843, 2849, 2851, 2853, 2855, *2841–2852, 2854*
secondary philtral abnormalities of, 2851, *2852,* 2853
secondary vermilion deficiency of, 2853, *2854*
Skoog method for, 2687, *2688, 2689*
straight line closure technique for, 2661, 2664, 2666–2667, 2673, 2675–2676, *2663–2666, 2668–2675*
timing of repair for, 2656
treatment principles and objectives for, 2654, 2656–2659, 2661, *2657–2660*
Wynn method for, 2687, 2689, *2690*
cephalometric tracings of, *2563, 2565*
classification of, 2442–2445, *2443–2445*
columella in, 2583
craniofacial development of, 2515, *2516*
dental anomalies in, 2882, 2885, *2884–2886*

Cleft lip *(Continued)*
embryogenesis of, 2526, 2528–2529, *2528*
epidemiology of, 2445–2446
parental age and, 2447
racial influences on, 2446–2447
sex ratio and, 2447
facial growth in, 2577–2578
intrinsic deficiencies of, 2553–2555
orthodontics and, 2575, 2577
orthopedics and, 2575, 2577
facial morphology in, 2553, *2554*
general growth and, 2557
genetics of, 2445–2446, 2447–2448
growth potential in, 2559–2561, *2560*
historical perspective of, 2437–2442
incidence of, 2446
lip anatomy in, 2583
mandible and, 2882, *2883*
maxillary retrusion from, Le Fort II osteotomy for, *2837, 2838*, 2838–2839
maxillary segment anatomy in, 2584, 2586, *2585, 2586*
multifactorial threshold model of, *2538*, 2538–2539
nasal septum anatomy in, *2582*, 2583–2584
nonsyndromic
environmental factors of, 2530, 2532–2533, 2535–2537, *2532, 2534–2537*
gene-environment interactions and, 2537–2539, *2538*
genetic factors of, 2529–2530, *2530*
premaxillary protrusion in, causes of, 2587–2588
prenatal environmental influences of, 2555–2557, *2555, 2556*
secondary deformities from, 2771
of buccal sulcus deficiency, 2796–2797, *2797*
of lip, 2647–2648, 2651, *2648, 2649*. *See also under* Lip deformities.
of lip landmarks, 2789–2790, *2789, 2790*
of orbicularis oris muscle, 2785–2787, 2789, *2786–2788*, 2851, *2851*
of vermilion deficiency or deformity, 2790–2791, *2791–2796*, 2793, 2796
surgery for, 2646–2647, *2647*
surgical repair of
abnormal facial growth and, 2565–2568, *2566–2568*
advancement in, 2636, *2638*
alar base cinch in, 2636, 2639, *2638*
early alar cartilage lift for, 2641–2643, *2642–2645*
evolution of method for, 2630, 2632, *2630–2633*
examples of rotation-advancement results, 2639, *2640*
facial growth after, 2561, 2564–2565, *2562, 2563*
goal of, 2632
measurements for, 2635–2636
modifications of rotation, 2639, 2641, *2641*
muscle dissection in, 2636, *2638*
rotation maneuver for, 2636, *2637, 2638*
suturing in, *2638*, 2639
syndromic, 2539–2540
unilateral
development of, 2591–2592, *2592*
lip adhesion for, 2632, 2635, *2634, 2635*
musculature in, 2600–2601, 2603, *2600–2603*
onset and rate of development of, 2592
secondary deformities of, evaluation of, 2771*t*, 2771–2772

Cleft lip *(Continued)*
unilateral, skeletal deformities in, 2588–2593, *2588–2594*
split appliance for, 2627–2628, *2627–2629*, 2630
treatment plan for, 2627–2628, *2627–2629*, 2630
Cleft lip nasal deformity, 2797–2798
bilateral
anatomy of, 2710
historical aspects of, 2714
pathologic anatomy of, 2855–2856, *2856*
surgical correction of, 2856–2857, *2857–2864*, 2859, 2863–2864
surgical repair of, 2714, 2716–2717, *2716–2718*
corrective rhinoplasty for, *2650*, 2651
dentoalveolar skeletal deformity in, 2879, *2880*
maxillary hypoplasia in, 2800–2801, *2801*
pathogenesis of, 2708–2709
primary nasal surgery for, 2643–2646, *2646*
secondary, pathologic anatomy of, 2798–2801, *2799–2801*
surgical correction of, 2801, 2803
alar cartilage mobilization and suspension, 2806–2810, *2808–2810*
ancillary procedures for, *2813*, 2813–2814
by graft augmentation, 2811–2813, *2812*
by incision and relocation of alar cartilage, 2810–2811, *2811*
rotation of cleft lip lobule and external incisions for, 2803, *2804–2807*, 2805–2806
timing of, 2801–2803
surgical repair of, 2643–2646, *2646*
unilateral
anatomy of, *2709*, 2709–2710
historical aspects of, 2710–2711
surgical repair of, 2711, 2713–2714, *2712, 2715*
Cleft lip/palate
embryogenesis of, 2526, 2528–2529, *2528*
nonsyndromic
environmental factors of, 2530, 2532–2533, 2535–2537, *2532, 2534–2537*
gene-environment interactions and, 2537–2539, *2538*
genetic factors of, 2529–2530, *2530*
orthodontic therapy for
during adult dentition period, 2897–2898, *2898, 2899*
during newborn period, 2885, 2887–2888, 2890, *2888–2891*
reasons for continuing care, 2898–2899, 2901, *2900*
Cleft nostril vestibular web, correction of, *2809, 2810*, 2813
Cleft palate
absence of midpalatal suture in, 2596
alveolar
closure of, 2753–2754
historical evolution of, 2754–2756
rationale for, 2754
secondary maxillary deformities from, 2822–2823
alveolar anterior
bone grafting for, 2758–2759
complications of surgical repair, *2766*, 2767
dental considerations for, 2753
flap design for, 2758
orthodontic considerations for, 2756–2757
secondary bone grafting for, 2757–2758
surgical results for, 2762, 2765, 2767, *2764–2766*
surgical technique for, 2760, 2762, *2760–2763*

Cleft palate *(Continued)*
anatomy of, 2726–2730, *2726–2728, 2730*
distortions in, 2729–2730, *2730*
bilateral, 2653, *2654*
development of, 2586–2587, *2586, 2587*
gingivoperiosteoplasty for, 2702, *2703, 2704*
incidence of, 2653, 2654*t*
premaxilla in, 2581–2583, *2582*
premaxillary protrusion in, causes of, 2587–2588
presurgical orthodontic therapy for, 2702, *2702, 2703*
secondary deformities of, 2864–2868
cephalometric tracings of, *2563, 2565*
classification of, 2442–2445, *2443–2445, 2730*, 2730–2731
craniofacial development of, 2515, *2516*
dental anomalies in, 2882, 2885, *2884–2886*
dental occlusion and, 2733–2734
embryogenesis of, 2543
epidemiology of, 2445–2446
parental age and, 2447
racial influences on, 2446–2447
sex ration and, 2447
facial growth in, 2577–2578
intrinsic deficiencies of, 2553–2555
orthodontics and, 2575, 2577
orthopedics and, 2575, 2577
feeding problems with, 2731
general considerations for, 2725–2726
general growth and, 2557
genetics of, 2445–2448
growth potential in, 2559–2561, *2560*
historical aspects of, 2437–2442, 2723–2725
in Robin sequence, 3127, 3133
incidence of, 2446
mandible and, 2882, *2883*
maxillary advancement in, 1373, *1375*
maxillary deformities in, bone grafts for, 2823
secondary, bone grafts for timing of, 2823–2825
secondary type of, 2821–2822
maxillary retrusion from, Le Fort II osteotomy for, 2838–2839, *2837, 2838*
maxillary segment anatomy in, 2584, 2586, *2585, 2586*
multifactorial threshold model of, *2538*, 2538–2539
musculature in, 2623–2625
nasal septum anatomy in, 2583–2584, *2582*
nonspecificity of, 72–73
nonsyndromic, embryogenesis of, 2545–2547
occult submucous, 2905
of secondary palate, 2593, *2595*, 2596
otology and, 2738–2739
palatoglossus in, 2619, *2622*
palatopharyngeus in, 2619, *2620, 2621*
postoperative care for, 2745–2746
premaxilla anatomy in, 2583–2584
prenatal environmental influences of, 2555–2557, *2555, 2556*
prostheses for, 3549, 3552–3553, *3552*
indications for, 3552
types of, 3553–3554, 3556, 3558, *3553–3557*
prosthetic obturation for, 2745
rare primary, 2540–2541, *2541*
repair of
Cronin technique for, 2699–2701, *2700, 2701*
double reverse Z-plasty for, 2701

Cleft palate *(Continued)*
secondary deformities of, fistula, 2814–2817, *2814–2821*, 2821
secondary deformities of, 2771
Simonart's band in, 2593, *2593, 2594*
speech problems of, 2731–2733
submucous, 2729–2730, 2905
surgical repair of, 2739
abnormal facial growth and, 2568–2569, *2570, 2571*
complications of, 2746–2747
double reversing Z-plasty for, *2740*, 2739–2742
effect on maxillary complex, 2569, 2572–2575, *2572–2577*
facial growth after, 2561, *2562, 2563*, 2564–2565
intravelar veloplasty for, 2742
velopharyngeal incompetence after, 2905
von Langenbeck operation for, 2742–2744, *2743*
Wardill-Kilner-Veau operation for, *2744*, 2744–2745
syndromic, 2539–2540, 2547
tensor veli palatini in, 2613–2614, *2614*
timing of treatment for, 2734–2735
early orthodontic therapy, 2736–2737
rationale for early soft palate closure, 2735–2736
unilateral
development of, 2591–2592, *2592*
onset and rate of development of, 2592
skeletal deformities in, 2588–2593, *2588–2594*
vomer anatomy in, 2583–2584, *2584*
with Klippel-Feil syndrome, 3145
Clicking, reciprocal, 1481–1482, *1482*, 1484–1485
Clinodactyly
clinical presentation of, 5337–5338, *5338*
treatment of, 5338, 5340, *5340*
Clostridial myonecrosis, abdominal wall reconstruction for, 3772–3774, *3773*
Clostridium, 5548
Clothing, protective, for cold injury prevention, 849–850
Clotting system, 192, *193*
Cloverleaf skull, 1546
Coagulopathy
for Kasabach-Merritt syndrome, 3219
localized intravascular, for venous malformations, 3252–3253
"Coated" vesicles, 637
Cobalt-chromium alloys, for alloplastic implants, 705, 705*t*
Coccidioidomycosis, 5552
Colchicine, for abnormal scars, 739–740
Cold
applications of, for extravasation injury, 5441–5442
vasoconstriction and, 5012–5013
Cold injuries
chilblain, 5431
frostbite, 5431–5436, *5433–5435*
generalized, 849, 858
historical aspects of, 859
late sequelae of, 864–865
pathophysiology of, 862
physiologic responses in, 860*t*–861*t*
treatment of, 862–864, *863*
with frostbite, 865
localized, 849
classification of, *851*, 851–852

Cold injuries *(Continued)*
localized, historical background for, 851–852
late sequelae of, 857–858
pathophysiology of, 852–854, 854*t*
treatment of, 854–857, *856*
with systemic hypothermia, 865
predisposing factors of, 849–851, *850*
Collagen
components of, 169, *170*
degradation of, in abnormal scars, 737
dermal, turnover in skin grafts, 244
epithelial migration and, 164
fibers of, structure of in dermis, 208, *208*, *209*, 210
in biologic dressings, for thermal burns, 805
in Dupuytren's contracture, 5057
in remodeling process, 4434
in scar tissue, 169
in tendon, 529
injectable, 781–782
complications of, 783–784
histopathology of, 782
indications for, 782–783
technique for, 783
metabolism of, 169–171
factors affecting, 175, 178–179
production of
hypoxia and, 735
in abnormal scars, 736–737
regenerated, in suture material for alloplastic implants, 719–720
remodeling of, 172, 175, *172–174, 176, 177*
synthesis, in tendon graft healing, 531
tensile strength of skin and, 161–162, *174*
types of, in abnormal scars, 737
Collagen-GAG membranes, 726, *728*, 729
Colles' fascia, 4190
Colles' fracture, 4635–4637, 4635*t*, *4636, 4637*
Colloid resuscitation, 793
Coloboma, correction of, in Treacher Collins syndrome, 3116, *3116*
Color transparencies, 37–38
Columella
anatomy of, 1788, 1797, *1797*
in cleft lip and palate, 2583
deformities of, in unilateral cleft lip and palate, 2590
growth of, relationship to bilateral cleft lip repair, 2856
hanging, correction of, 1857, *1858*
lengthening of, 2667, 2673, 2675–2676, *2674, 2675*
in bilateral cleft lip nasal deformity, 2856–2857, *2857–2867*, 2859, 2863–2864
reconstruction of, 1985–1987, *1986, 1987*
retracted, correction of, 1857–1858, *1859–1861*, 1860
wide base of, correction of, 1860–1861, *1861*
Columella-ala triangle, resection of, *1837*, 1837–1838
Columellar-lobar junction, 1788
Coma, 870
Commissure, reconstruction of, 2025, 2027, *2026*
Compartment syndromes
anatomic considerations of, 4032–4033, *4033*
treatment of, 4067–4068
Competence, embryological, 2454
Complement system, 191–192, *192*
Composite flaps
concept of, for facial reconstruction, 306, *307*
historical aspects of, 376–377
Composite grafts
for eyelid reconstruction, 1715, *1717*
of scalp, for alopecia treatment, 1520–1527, *1521–1523, 1525, 1526*
round punch types of, 1520–1523, *1521–1523*
square or hexahedral types of, 1523–1524
strip scalp types of, 1524, 1526–1527, *1525, 1526*
of skin and adipose tissue, for nasal reconstruction, 1932
of skin and cartilage, for nasal reconstruction, 1930–1932, *1931*
Compression arthrodesis, for small joints, 4675–4677, *4676, 4677*
Compression garments, as adjuncts for fat suctioning, 4026, *4027*
Compression syndromes
anterior interosseous nerve syndrome, 4831–4833, *4832*
costoclavicular, 4998–4999, *4999*
of hand, evaluation by wick catheter, 4287, *4287*
of median nerve, 4823. *See also* Carpal tunnel syndrome.
of upper extremity
anatomic structures associated with, 4998, *4998*
diagnosis of, 4999–5000, 5002–5005, *4999–5004*
pronator syndrome, 4833–4834, *4834*
Compression therapy, for hemangiomas, 3213
Computed tomography
in computer-aided surgical planning, 1212, 1214, *1214*
of facial injuries, 899
of nasoethmoido-orbital fractures, 1090–1091, *1090, 1091*
of optic nerve injury, 1118, *1119*
of orbit, 1584–1586
of temporomandibular joint, 1505
of velopharyngeal sphincter, 2914
of zygoma fractures, 998, *999, 1000*
Computer-aided surgical planning
three-dimensional, 1209
with three-dimensional cephalometrics, 1209, *1211*, 1212, 1212*t*, *1213*
Concha, alteration of, 2116, *2117*
Conchomastoid sutures, for reducing auricular prominence, 2116–2117, *2117*
Conduction test, evaluation of facial nerve function, 2253
Condylar growth, process of, 2505–2506
Condylar region, osteotomies of, 1235, *1236*
Condyle
dislocations of, 1487–1489, *1487–1489*
fractures of
classification of, *1490*, 1496
closed or conservative management of, 1497, *1497*
diagnosis of, 1496
open reduction for, 1497–1498, *1499*
roentgenography of, 1497
hyperplasia of
and unilateral mandibular macrognathia, 1294, *1294, 1295–1296, 1297*
with osteochondroma, 1490–1494, *1491–1493*
hypoplasia of, *1291*, 1292, *1293*, 1294. *See* Craniofacial microsomia.
idiopathic osteonecrosis of, 1502
movement of, 147–148

Condylectomy, for temporomandibular ankylosis, 1494
Congenital anomalies. *See also specific anomaly.*
  deformation sequence and, 5231, *5232*
  deformations and, 75
  distruption sequence and, 5231–5232, *5232*
  dysmorphologic approach to, 5231–5233, *5232*
  malformation sequence and, 5231, 5232, *5232*
  nonspecificity of, 5232
  pediatric tumors of, 3178–3181, *3179–3180*
  timing of repair for, 45–46
  with Robin sequence, 3129
Congestive heart failure
  multiple cutaneous and hepatic hemangiomas and, *3209*, 3209–3210
  with cutaneous-visceral hemangiomatosis, 3217–3219, *3218*
Coniotomy, 872, *872*, 873
Conjunctiva, anatomy of, 1680, *1680*
Conjunctival flap, for symblepharon correction, 1742–1743, *1744*
Conjunctival grafts, for symblepharon correction, 1743, *1744, 1745*
Conjunctivodacryocystorhinostomy, 1736–1737, *1737, 1738*
Connective tissue
  disorders of, differential diagnosis of, 4904
  peripheral nerves and, 642–644, *643*
Conotruncal outflow tract defects, 2464
Constriction ring syndrome, congenital
  clinical presentation of, 5373–5374, *5375*
  treatment of, 5374, 5376–5378, *5375–5377*
Contact inhibition, 163
Contour restorations. *See also specific restorations.*
  using autogenous rib cartilage grafts, *574, 575*
Contraction
  in wound healing, 165, 167–169, 4434–4435
  primary, 181, 243
  secondary, 181, 243
Contractures
  Dupuytren's. *See* Dupuytren's disease.
  flexion, from flexor tendon surgery, 4547
  from amputation, 4331
  from burn injury. *See* Burn contractures.
  importance of, 165, 167
  ischemic. *See* Ischemic contractures.
  of eyelid, 2213
Contralateral postauricular flaps, for nasal reconstruction, 1970–1971
Conversion disorders, differential diagnosis of, 4905
Core temperature, 858
Cornea
  injury of
    after blepharoplasty, 2349
    from maxillary surgery, 3333
  protection of
    after burn injury, 2212
    during surgery, 1682, *1682*
Coronary spasm, mechanisms of, 5015–5016
Coronoid process fractures, 968–969, *969*
Coronoid processes, impingement of, *1489*, 1489–1490
Corrugator supercilii muscles, 2400, 2404
Cortical osteotomy, 1223, *1224*, 1225
Corticosteroids
  for extravasation injury, 5442
  for reflex sympathetic dystrophy, 4910
  immunosuppression by, 194
  wound healing and, 179
Cortisone, for retardation of wound contracture, 168
Cosmetics, for port-wine stain, 3232
Costal cartilage grafts, for nasal contour restoration, 1892–1893, *1892, 1893*
Costoclavicular compression, 4998–4999, *4999*
Costoclavicular maneuver, 5000, 5002, *5001*
CPM, 2519
Crane principle, 2204
Cranial bones
  growth of, 1539–1540
  phylogeny of, 1539–1540, *1540*
Cranial fossa, anatomy of, 1579, *1580*
  of anterior, 2981, *2981*
  of middle, 2981–2982
Cranial nerve anomalies, in craniofacial microsomia, 3069–3070, *3070*
Cranial vault
  bone grafts of, for frontal bone repair, 1564–1565
  cranioplasty of, methylmethacrylate implants for, 1561–1562, *1563*
  defects of, reconstruction of—calvaria splitting, 1556–1558, *1557–1559*
  remodeling of, for craniosynostosis, 3035, *3035, 3036*
Craniectomies, strip, *3028*, 3028–3029
  with frontal bone advancement, *3028–3030*, 3029–3030
Craniocynostosis
  postoperative longitudinal studies of, 3051–3052
  surgical treatment of, New York University protocol for, 3045
Craniofacial anomalies. *See also specific anomalies.*
  analysis of, 92–94, 97–100, *92–96, 98–99*
Craniofacial clefts
  classification of, 2932–2937, *2932, 2936, 2937*, 2933*t*, 2934*t*, 2935*t*
    by American Association of Cleft Palate Rehabilitation Classification (AACPR), 2932, *2932*
    by Boo-Chai, *2932*, 2932–2934
    by Karfik, 2933*t*, 2934
    by Tessier, 2935–2937, *2936*
    by Van der Meulen and associates, 2934, 2934*t*
    of near-normal and excess tissue disorders, 2935
    of tissue deficiency malformations, 2934–2935, 2935*t*
  description of, 2937–2938
    for no. 6,7, and 8 combination type, *2956*, 2956–2957
    for no. 0 type, 2938–2941, *2938–2945*, 2943
    for no. 1 type, 2945, *2945, 2946*
    for no. 2 type, 2945–2946, *2947*
    for no. 3 type, 2947–2949, *2948, 2949*
    for no. 4 type, 2949–2951, *2950, 2951*
    for no. 5 type, 2951–2952, *2952*
    for no. 6 type, 2952, *2953*
    for no. 7 type, 2952–2955, *2954, 2955*
    for no. 8 type, 2955–2956, *2956*
    for no. 9 type, 2957, *2957*
    for no. 10 type, 2957, *2958*
    for no. 11 type, 2957
    for no. 12 type, 2957–2958, *2958*
    for no. 13 type, 2958–2959, *2959*
    for no. 14 type, 2959–2960, *2960, 2961*
  embryologic aspects of, 2923–2927, *2924–2926*
  etiology of, 2927–2930
  incidence of, 2922–2923
  morphopathogenesis of, 2930–2931
  numbering system for, *2936*, 2936–2937

Craniofacial clefts *(Continued)*
of mandibular process, 2927
of maxillary process, 2927
of midline craniofacial structures, *2926*, 2926–2927
severity of, 2937
treatment of, 2960, 2962–2963, 2966–2968, *2963–2964*
Craniofacial dysjunction, 1014, *1014*
Craniofacial microsomia
bilateral, 3089, *3094–3096*, 3096
bilateral microtia and, 2108
surgical reconstruction of mandible, 3096–3098, *3097*
vs. unilateral, 3055
contour restoration of skeletal deformity with onlay bone grafts in, 3089, *3091*
differential diagnosis of, 3054–3055
ear deformity in, 3056, *3057–3060*, 3067–3068, *3069*
embryology of, 3057–3061, 3061*t*
etiopathogenesis of, 3061, 3063, *3063*
jaw deformity in, 3056, *3062*
jaw reconstruction for, 3080, *3081*, 3082
after age 7 years, 3088–3089, *3090, 3091*
during adolescence, 3089, *3092, 3093*
muscles of mastication in, 3067
nervous system deformities in, 3068–3070, *3070*
pathogenesis of, reexamination of, *2490*, 2491–2492
pathology of, 3063–3064
of jaw deformity, 3064–3066, *3064–3066*
preoperative planning of
cephalometric analysis for, 3071–3076, *3071–3077*, 3077
for functional orthopedic appliance therapy, 3079–3080
for occlusal cant, 3074–3075, *3077*
for orthodontic therapy after combined surgical correction, 3079
for two-splint technique, 3077–3078
for unilateral vs. bilateral ramus osteotomies to reposition mandible, 3078–3079, *3087*
skeletal deformities in, 3066–3067, *3067, 3068*
soft tissue deformities of, 3070–3071
reconstruction for, after age 6 years, 3089
surgical treatment of
forehead deformity or orbital dystopia, under age 3 years, 3087, *3087*
New York University program for, 3086, *3085–3087*
reconstructive jaw surgery—functional appliance therapy, under age 6 years, 3087–3088, *3088, 3089*
restoration of soft tissue contour, 3082, *3083*
San Francisco program for, 3082–3084
Toronto program for, 3084, *3084*, 3086
terminology of, 3054
unilateral, 2471
auricular congenital deformities and, 2099, *2099*
classification of, 3057
historical aspects of, 3055
incidence of, 3055
surgical simulation for treatment of, 1212, *1213*
variations of, 3055–3057, *3056–3061*
vs. bilateral, 3055
Craniofacial skeleton
anatomy of, *2977–2981*, 2977–2982
in cleft lip and palate, 2581–2596
Craniofacial skeleton *(Continued)*
deformities of, psychosocial aspects of, 120
development of
early, of cleft lip and palate, 2515, *2516*
normal, 2451, 2453–2456, *2452–2455*
origins and migration of myoblasts of voluntary muscles, 2519, *2520*
origins of tissues in, 2517, 2519, *2518*
postnatal characteristics of, 2496–2498, *2497, 2498*
vertical growth of face and, 2508–2513, *2508–2513*
fractures of
dentition and, 916, *919*, 919–920
dentition as guide in reduction and fixation of, 921
dentoalveolar process and, 920–921, *921*
injuries of, from gunshot, 1127, 1130–1131
postnatal growth of, in horizontal direction, 2503–2505, *2503–2505*
tumors of
resection of, reconstruction after, *3405*, 3405–3406
surgical treatment for, 3371, 3373
Craniofacial surgery
complications of, 3008–3010
design of surgical procedure for, 2975
for fibrous dysplasia, 3008
for orbital hypertelorism
in children, *3000*, 3000–3001
postoperative treatment for, 2999–3000
for orbital hypotelorism, *3007*, 3007–3008
for tumors of frontoethmoid area, 3008
in Down syndrome, 3170–3171
intraoperative monitoring for, 2975–2976, *2976*
organization of team for, 2974–2977
postoperative period for, 2976–2977
preoperative planning for, 2974–2975
Craniofacial syndromes
Klippel-Feil syndrome. *See* Klippel-Feil syndrome.
mandibulofacial dysostosis. *See* Treacher Collins syndrome.
micrognathia and glossoptosis with airway obstruction. *See* Robin sequence.
obstructive sleep apnea, 3147–3152, *3149, 3151, 3152*
progressive hemifacial atrophy. *See* Romberg's disease.
Craniopagus, 1542–1543, *1544*, 1546
Cranioplasty
historical review of, 1554–1556, *1556*
split rib, 1558, *1559–1562*, 1560–1561
Craniosynostosis. *See also specific types of craniosynostosis.*
anatomic perspective of, 70*t*
clinical presentation of, 3015, 3018, 3020–3021, 3023, 3025, *3015–3024*
etiopathogenesis of, 3013–3015, *3014*
fronto-orbital remodeling for, *3028–3032*, 3029–3030, 3032
functional aspects of, 3025–3026
genetic perspective of, 70*t*
historical aspects of, 3013
inheritance of, *70*
monobloc advancement of orbits and midface for, 3043, 3045, *3045*
monobloc or craniofacial advancement for, 3035
pathogenesis of, 97–100, *98*
premature, 1546
radiographic findings in, 3015, 3018, 3020–3021, 3023, 3025, *3015–3024*

Craniosynostosis *(Continued)*
surgical treatment of, 3026*t*
by cranial vault remodeling, 3035, *3035*
by monobloc or craniofacial advancement, 3035
by shunt surgery, 3035, 3037
early performance of, 3026–3030, 3032, 3035, 3037, *3028–3036*
late performance of, 3037–3040, 3043, 3045, *3038–3045*
types of, 3013, 3014*t*
Cranium
as bone graft source, 2759
counterpart relationship with face, *2502*, 2502–2503
postnatal development of, 1147, 2497–2498
Creeping substitution, 602, 2758. *See also* Osteoconduction.
Crepitant infections, of hand, 5548
Crepitus, 1487
Cri du chat syndrome, 100
Cribriform plate, anatomy of, *2978*, 2978–2979
Cricothyroidotomy, 872
Critical closing pressure, 445
Cross arm flaps, 4454
Cross finger flap
arterialized side, for dorsal digital defects, *4495*, 4496
for coverage of fingertip amputations, 4489–4490, *4490, 4491*
for soft tissue injuries of thumb, *5098*, 5098–5099
radial innervated types for, 5100, 5103, *5103*
innervated, for soft tissue injuries of thumb, 5099, *5100, 5101*
side, for coverage of fingertip amputations, 4490, *4491–4493*, 4492–4493
upside-down, for dorsal digital defects, *4495*, 4495–4496
Cross leg flaps, 374
Crossbite
buccal, 1360
lingual, 1360
Croton oil, 756
Crouzon's disease
clinical presentation of, 84, *86*, 3018, 3020–3021, *3019–3021*
hydrocephalus in, 3025
involvement of cranial vault sutures in, 2488
maxillary deformities of, 1360
preoperative planning for, 1362, *1362*
radiological findings in, 3018, 3020–3021, *3019–3021*
treatment of, by strip craniotomy with frontal bone advancement, 3029–3030, *3028–3030*
visual abnormalities in, 3025–3026
Crura, lateral, malpositioned, correction of, 1856, *1857*
Cryoglobulinemia, 454
Cryotherapy, for basal cell carcinoma, 3627
Cryptotia, 2111, *2116*
Cubital tunnel syndrome, 4841–4842, 4844, *4842–4844*
Cupid's bow
deformity of, after cleft lip repair, surgical correction of, 2648, *2648*
reconstruction of, 2187, 2789–2790, *2789, 2790*
Curling's ulcer, 809
Cushing's disease, 214
Cutaneous tags, 3579, *3580*, 3581
Cutis hyperelastica. *See* Ehlers-Danlos syndrome.
Cutis laxa, characteristics of, 2364
Cutis marmorata telangiectatica congenita (CMTC), *3237*, 3237–3238
Cutler-Beard technique, for eyelid reconstruction, 1703, *1705, 1707, 1708*, 1712–1713
Cyclophosphamide, 195
Cyclopia, orbital hypotelorism and, *3005*, 3006
Cyclopia perfecta, 2458
Cyclosporine
immunosuppression by
in bone allografts, 197–198
in limb allografts, 198–200
in nerve allografts, 198
mechanism of action for, 195–196, *196*
wasting syndrome of, 200
Cylindroma, 3577, *3577*
Cystic hygroma, 3242
Cysts
aneurysmal bone, 3351
dermoid, 2986, 3181, *3182*
epidermal, 3569, 3572
gingival, 3337
myxoid, 3581
odontogenic, 3338–3340
of salivary gland, 3312–3313, *3313*
paradental, 3340
post-rhinoplasty, of mucous membranes, 1881
radicular, 3339
residual, 3340
Cytochalasin B, 638

Dacryocystitis
clinical presentation of, 1733, *1733*
treatment of, 1733–1734, *1735*, 1736
Dacryocystorhinostomy
canaliculodacryocystorhinostomy, 1736, *1736*
conjunctivodacryocystorhinostomy, 1736–1737, *1737, 1738*
with canthopexy and bone grafting, for epicanthal fold corection, 1617–1618, *1618–1620*
Dalmane (flurazepam), 140
Davis, John Staige, 10, *12*
DCIA (deep circumflex iliac artery), 4033
De Quervain's disease
anatomic features of, 4731, 4733–4735, *4733, 4734*
clinical features of, 4731, 4733–4735, *4733, 4734*
incision for, 4443, *4443*
treatment of, 4735, 4737–4739, *4735–4738*
triggering of finger and thumb and, 4729
Debridement, historical aspects of, 4029–4030
Decortication technique, 1990
Deep circumflex iliac artery (DCIA), 4033
Deep dorsal vein ligation, for erectile dysfunction, 4219–4220
Deep inferior epigastric artery (DIEA), 4033
Deep peroneal nerve, as source for free vascularized nerve graft, 4880, *4880, 4881*
Defects. *See also specific defects.*
shifting of, 47
true vs. apparent, 24–25, *24, 25*
Deformations. *See also specific deformations.*
interpretation of, 27
interrelationships of, with malformations and disruptions, 78, *78*
mechanical causes of, 74–75, 74*t*
time onset of, 76, 77
vs. malformations, 76, *76*
Degenerative arthritis, of hand, 4699–4703, *4701, 4702*

Degenerative joint disease, of temporomandibular joint, 1499–1502, *1500, 1501*
Degloving
 injuries, of lower extremity, 374
 of face, procedure for, *2833*, 2833–2834
 of mandible, procedure for, 1226–1227, *1226, 1227*
 of midface, procedure for, 1363, *1364*
Dehiscence, after cleft palate repair, 2747
Delay phenomenon
 description of, 314
 distant flaps and, 4451–4452
Delivery technique, 1845–1847, *1846*, 1851
Delta phalanx
 clinical presentation of, 5340–5341, *5342*
 treatment of of, 5341, *5342, 5343*, 5344
Deltopectoral flap
 anatomy of, 292, *292*
 development of, 275
 for cheek reconstruction, 2045, *2046*
 for chest wall reconstruction, 3686, *3687*
 for face reconstruction, 503
Dendrites, 634–635
Denis Browne technique, for hypospadia repair, 4158, *4159*
Dental anomalies, in cleft lip and palate, 2882, *2884–2886*, 2885
Dental casts, for preoperative planning, 1362
 for mandibular prognathism surgery, 1231–1232, *1232*
Dental examination, for open bite deformity, 1353–1354, *1354*
Dental measurements, 1198
Dental study models
 evaluation of, 1191, 1193
 for preoperative planning, 1205, *1206*, 1207
  for mandibular hypoplasia, *1265*
Dentigerous cysts, 3338
Dentition
 as guide in reduction and fixation of jaw fractures, 921
 maxillary, growth of, 2512–2513, *2513*
 maxillary and mandibular relationships of, *927*
 normal, 916, *919*, 919–920
 terminology for relationships of, *927*
Dentoalveolar arch deformities, in cleft lip or palate patients, 2439
Dentoalveolar complex, 1193
Dentoalveolar osteotomy, 1223, *1223*
Dentoalveolar processes, 920–921, *921*
 normal growth of, 2559
Dentoalveolar protrusion
 bimaxillary, 1347, *1348–1351*, 1351
 mandibular, 1347
Dentures
 retention methods for, 3524, 3528–3530, *3527–3534*
 temporary, 3523–3524, *3525, 3526*
Depressor labii inferioris muscle, 2247, *2248*
Dermabrasion
 by laser, 3666
 complications of, 780–781
 definition of, 771
 for scars on nose, 1929
 healing of abraded areas, 772–773
 historical background of, 771–772
 indications for, 773–774, *774–777*, 777
 limitations of, 777
 postoperative care for, 779–780
Dermabrasion *(Continued)*
 technique for, 778–779, *779, 780*
 with chemical peeling, 781
Dermal plexus, blood supply of, 286, *286*
Dermal transplants, for facial paralysis, 2304
Dermatofibroma, 3578–3579, *3579*
Dermatologic complications, of blepharoplasty, 2349–2350, *2350*
Dermatomes
 Castroviejo, *228*, 230
 development of, 13
 drum type, 230, *232–235*, 235–236
  selection of, 236–237
 power-driven, *229*, 229–230, *230*
Dermatosporaxis, 171
Dermis
 anatomy of, *222*, 222–223
 histologic changes of, after chemical peeling, 752–753, *753*
 rupture of, 214
 transplantation of
  complications of, 510, 515
  definition of, 508, *509*
  future of, 515
  graft fate in, 509–510, *511–514*
  historical aspects of, 508–509
  surgical technique for, 510, *514*
Dermis-fat grafting, 516, 520, *519, 520*
Dermochalasis, 2326–2327
Dermoepidermal junction, 223
Dermoid cysts, 2986, 3181, *3182*
Desensitization, for reflex sympathetic dystrophy, 4913
Desmoid tumor, chest wall reconstruction and, 3714, 3714*t*
Desmoplastic fibroma, of jaw, 3351
Desmoplastic melanoma, in head and neck, 3371, *3372*
Deviated nose
 septal deflection in, correction of, 1864–1865, *1865*
  anterior columnellar approach for, 1869, 1871, *1868, 1869*
  camouflage procedure for, 1871, 1873, *1872*
  internal splint for, 1869, *1871*
  morselization for, 1869
  mucoperichondrial splint for, 1866–1867, *1866, 1868*
  subcutaneous resection technique for, 1865–1866
  swinging door technique for, 1867, 1869, *1869–1871*
 types of, *1862*, 1862–1864
Dextran
 for fluid resuscitation, 793
 for treatment of cold injury, 856–857
 physiologic effects of, 458–459
Diabetes
 Dupuytren's disease and, 5055–5056
 hand infections and, 5533, *5533*
 morbid obesity and, 3968, *3972*
 postmaxillectomy management and, 3333
Diazepam (Valium)
 craniofacial cleft formation and, 2929
 for reflex sympathetic dystrophy, 4911
6–Diazo-5–oxo-L-nor-leucine (DON), 2540
Dibenzyline (phenoxybenzamine), 315, 4910, 5021
DIEA (deep inferior epigastric artery), 4033
Differential thermometry, for flap perfusion assessment, 319*t*, 321
Digastric muscle, 937

DiGeorge syndrome, 2471, 2478
Digital prostheses, 4399–4302, *4399–4302*
Digital sympathectomy, for chronic or recurring vasospasm, 5021
Digits. *See* Finger(s).
Dilantin (phenytoin), 2533
Dilated funduscopic examination, 1584
Dimethyl sulfoxide (DMSO), 316, 5442
Dioxin, cleft palate and, 2546
Diphenhydramine hydrochloride (Benadryl), 738
Diphenylmethane diisocyanate, 710
Diplopia
  binocular, 1599–1600
  from malunited orbital floor fracture, 1597, *1598*, 1599
  from orbital fractures, 1057*t*, 1058–1059
  monocular, 1599
  tests for, *1599*, 1599–1600
Dipyridamole (Persantine), platelet function and, 458
Direct flaps, 277, *277*
Disarticulation, of elbow, 4343
Disc dislocation, 1486
Dish-face deformity
  in Binder's syndrome, 1362
  nasomaxillary skin graft inlay for, 1975–1976, 1979, *1977, 1978*, 3543–3545, 3549, *3544–3548, 3550*
Displacement
  description of, 2498, *2499*
  of ethomaxillary complex, 2503–2504, *2504*
  of nasomaxillary complex, 2508, *2508*
Disruptions, 77–78, *78*
Distal interphalangeal joint
  deformities of, after burn injury, 5467
  dislocations of, *4624*, 4624–4625
  fracture-dislocations of, 4625–4627, *4626*
  subluxations of, 4624–4625
Distal radioulnar joint, in rheumatoid arthritis, 4712–4713, *4713, 4714*
Distant flap, delay phenomenon and, 4451–4452
Distichiasis, 1737–1738
Distoclusion, *1193*, 1193–1194
Distraction lengthening, of metacarpal, for congenital hand deformities, 5252, *5253, 5254*, 5255
Diuretics, contraindications for, in lymphedema, 4107
DMSO (dimethyl sulfoxide), 316, 5442
"Dog-ear," "depuckering" of, 52, *54*
Dopamine, in postoperative treatment of skin flaps, 314
Doppler ultrasound, for flap perfusion assessment, 320
Dorsal hand to thumb flap, for soft tissue injuries of thumb, 5099
Dorsal nasal rotation-advancement flap, 1936, *1936, 1937*
Dorsal thumb flap, noninnervated, for soft tissue injuries of thumb, *5103*, 5103–5104
Dorsal thumb island flap, innervated, for soft tissue injuries of thumb, 5104, *5104*
Dorsal web-plasty, for ulnar nerve palsy with median nerve palsy, 4958–4959, *4958–4960*, 4961
Dorsalis pedis artery, 4035, *4036*
Dorsalis pedis flap
  anatomy of, 4465, *4465*, 4862, *4863*
  for free transfer
    in lower extremity reconstruction, 4050–4051, *4051*
    in nasal reconstruction, 1971, 1974, *1974*
    in upper extremity, 4463, 4465, *4465, 4466*, 4467
  for sensory reconstruction of hand, 4861–4862
  operative technique for, *4466*, 4467
Double eyelid
  line from, 2421, *2421*
  surgery for
    incision method of, 2425–2426, *2426*
    operative technique of, 2423–2426, *2424–2426*
Down syndrome
  cardiovascular anomalies in, 3162
  chromosome abnormalities of, 103, 3161
  clinical features of, 3163–3164, *3163*
  corrective surgery in, 3163–3164, *3164*, 3164*t*
    complications of, 3171
    for esthetic improvements, 3168–3170, *3168–3170*
    for hypotonia of the tongue, 3164–3165, *3165*
    for macroglossia, 3165–3166, *3166, 3167*
    for strabismus, 3166
    longitudinal studies of, 3172–3173, *3172*, 3173*t*
    timing of, 3171–3172
  craniofacial surgery in, 3170–3171
  epidemiology of, 3161
  etiology of, 3161–3162
  hypotonia in, 3163
  immunologic defects in, 3161–3162
  karyotype for, *102*
  neuropathology of, 3162
  psychosocial aspects of, 121–122
  sensory deficits in, 3162–3163
Doxorubicin, extravasation injury from, 5440–5441, *5441*
Dressings
  biologic, for thermal burns, 804*t*, 804–805
  bolus tie-over or stent, 240–241, *241*
  circumferential compression, type of, 241
  external compression, for facial injuries, 877
  for burn injuries, 5400
  for eye, *1592*, 1593
  for eyelid surgery, 1682–1683, *1683*
  for facialplasty, 2384
  for hand surgery, *4297, 4297–4299, 4298*
  materials in, for alloplastic implants, 722–724, *723, 724*
  occlusive, for full face peeling, 764, *764–766*
  pressure, 52, 54–55
Droperidol, 141–142, 4315
Drug(s). *See also specific drugs.*
  extravasation injuries from, 5440
Drug abuse, hand infections and, *5533*, 5533–5534
Dry eye syndrome
  blepharoplasty and, 2331
  from blepharoplasty, 2354–2355
Duane's retraction syndrome, Klippel-Feil syndrome and, 3144
Dubreuilh, precancerous melanosis of, *3598*, 3598–3599
Duplay technique, for hypospadia repair, 4157–4158, *4158*
Dupuytren's disease
  anatomic considerations in, 5059, *5060–5064*, 5061–5062, 5064
  chromosomal changes in, 5055
  complications after surgery for, 5068–5069, 5069*t*
  diseases associated with, 5055–5056
  epidemiology of, 5053–5054, 5054*t*
  etiology of, 5054–5055
  historical aspects of, 5053
  mechanism of contraction in, 5058–5059, *5058, 5059*
  pathogenesis of, *5057*, 5057–5058
  pathology of, 5056–5059, *5057, 5058*
  postoperative management for, 5068

Dupuytren's disease *(Continued)*
  surgical results for, 5069–5070
  treatment of, 5083–5084
    by hyperextension at distal interphalangeal joint, 5076–5077, *5078*
    by subcutaneous fasciotomy, 5075–5076, *5077*
    for recurrent disease, 5077, *5079, 5079–5080, 5081–5083*, 5083
    goals for, 5065
    incisions for, 5067–5068, *5068*
    indications for, 5064
    types of surgery for, 5065, 5066*t*, 5067, 5067*t*
    when more than one finger is involved, 5072–5073, *5073, 5074*, 5075
    when single finger is involved, *5070–5071*, 5070–5072
    when thumb and thumb web are involved, 5075, *5076*
    wound closure methods for, 5067–5068, *5068*
  trigger finger and, 4731
Dura mater, injury of, from maxillary surgery, 3333
Dural cuffs, 4314
Dye disappearance test, 1729
Dynamic impedance, 443
Dysmorphophobia, 119–120
Dysmorphology
  disruptions of, 77–78, *78*
  malformations of, nonspecificity of, 72–75, *74, 75*
  principles of, 70–81
    malformations, *71*, 71*t*, 71–72, *72*
Dysostosis otomandibularis, 3054
Dysplastic nevus, 3593–3594, *3594*, 3636

Eagle syndrome, 1490
Ear(s). *See also* Auricle.
  anatomy of, 2095–2096, *2095, 2096*
  artificial, 3549, *3551*
  burn injuries of, 2204–2207, *2207–2209*, 2209–2210
  cartilage grafts of, for secondary rhinoplasty, 1904, *1906, 1907*, 1908
  cauliflower deformity of, 573, 2127
  congenital deformities of
    cryptotia, 2111, *2116*
    microtia. *See* Microtia.
  constricted, "cup" or "lop" deformity, 2110–2111, *2111–2115*
  deformity of, in craniofacial microsomia, 3056, *3057–3060*, 3067–3068, *3069*
  drawing of, 35, *35*
  embryology of, 2483, 2485, *2484, 2486, 2487*, 2487, 3058–3060
  external
    embryological development of, 2486, *2487*
    regional block of, 153, *154*
  full-thickness defects of, 2128
  inner, embryological development of, 2483, 2485
  microtia. *See* Microtia.
  middle
    complications from maxillary surgery, 3333–3334
    embryological development of, 2485, *2487*
    problem of, in microtia, 2096–2097, *2097*
  protrusion of
    in Down syndrome, 3170
    pathology of, 2111, 2116, *2116*
    treatment of, 2116–2117, *2117–2119*, 2119

Ear(s) *(Continued)*
  psychosocial aspects of disfigurement, 124
Ear reconstruction
  after burn injury, 2209–2210, *2211*
  for auricular hypoplasia, general treatment considerations for, 2100
  history of, 2094–2095
  tissue expansion for, 501–502
  total
    detaching posterior auricular region, 2106, *2107, 2108*
    fabrication of framework for, 2103, *2103*
    hairline management for, 2106, 2108
    implantation of framework for, 2103–2104, *2104*
    obtaining rib cartilage for, 2101–2103, *2102*
    planning and preparation for, 2101
    postoperative care for, 2104–2105
    preoperative consultation for, 2101
    secondary, 2108, *2109, 2110*
    tragal construction and conchal definition in, 2105–2106, *2106*
    using autogenous rib cartilage, 573, *573*
Earlobe
  acquired deformities of
    from burn injury, repair of, 2207, 2209, *2209*
    reconstruction for, 2141–2142, *2141–2145*
  transposition of, 2105, *2105*
Eccrine poroma, 3576–3577, *3577*
Ecthyma contagiosum, 5553
Ectoderm, differentiation of, 2456
Ectodermal dysplasia, hypohidrotic, pedigree for, 106–107, *107*
Ectodermal dysplasia-ectrodactyly-clefting, 2482–2483
Ectropion
  after orbital or nasoethmoido-orbital fractures, 1106
  cicatricial, 1749, 1751, *1751*
  complex, 1751, *1751*
  congenital, 1744–1745, *1745*
  correction of, 1745–1749, *1745–1753*
  from blepharoplasty, 2355–2357, *2355–2357*
  in hyperthyroidism, 2327, 2328, *2328, 2329*
  involutional or senile, 1745, *1746*
  of lower eyelid
    after chemical peeling, 770
    surgical correction of, 2215–2216, *2216–2218*
  of upper eyelid, surgical correction of, 2213–2215, *2214, 2215*
  paralytic, 1751, *1752, 1753*
  types of, 1744–1745
Edema
  hydrostatic, 4657, 4658
  inflammatory, 4657–4658
  lymphatic, 4657, 4658
Edgewise orthodontic and fixation appliance, 927, 929, *929*
Education in plastic surgery, development of, 13–14
EGF. *See* Epidermal growth factor.
Ehlers-Danlos syndrome
  characteristics of, 2363
  collagen metabolism in, 180
  hydroxylysine deficiency in, 171
Elastosis, 749–750, *750, 754*
Elavil (amitriptyline), for reflex sympathetic dystrophy, 4911
Elbow
  contractures of, from burn injury, 5469, 5471, *5472*
  disarticulation of, 4343

Elbow *(Continued)*
extension of, in tetraplegia, operative procedure for, 4986–4987, *4987*
longitudinal absence deformities of ulna, clinical presentations of, 5275
Elbow blocks, *4322*, 4323
Electrical injuries
classification of burns in, 815
complications of, 826, 828–829
diagnosis of, 5422–5423
fluid resuscitation for, 815–816, 816*t*
historical aspects of, 814
initial assessment of, 815–816
of lips and oral commissure, *2230*, 2231
of upper extremity, 5418, 5476, 5480, *5478, 5479*
assessment of, 5421
early management of, 5421–5423, *5424*, 5425–5426
later management of, 5426–5428, *5426–5428*
mechanism of, 5420–5421, *5421*
pathophysiology of, 823–824, 5419–5420
physiological considerations for, 5418–5419
wound management for
of extremities, 820–821, *821–827*, 823–824, 826
of scalp and skull, 817, *817, 818*, 819
of trunk and perineum, *819, 819–820, 820*
results of, 829
Electrocardiography, abnormalities of, in electrical injuries, 815
Electrodiagnosis
for facial paralysis, 2253, *2254*, 2255
intraoperative techniques of, 674
of peripheral nerves, 670–675. *See also specific techniques.*
Electrolysis, for hemangiomas, 3212–3123
Electromagnetic flowmetry, for flap perfusion assessment, 319*t*, 322–323
Electromagnetic spectrum
frequencies of, 3663*t*
position of lasers in, 3663–3664, *3664*
wavelengths of, 3663*t*
Electromyographic control, for active prostheses, *4397*, 4397–4398
Electromyography
evaluation of facial nerve function, 2253, *2254*
needle, 672–673
of nerve injuries, 4821, *4822*
of skeletal muscle, 549, *549*
Electroneurography. *See also* Electromyography; Nerve conduction velocity; Somatosensory evoked potentials.
evaluation of facial nerve function, 2255
information acquired from, 673
Electrostimulation, for brachial plexus injuries, 4787
Ellis–van Creveld syndrome, 106
Embolic therapy, for hemangiomas, 3218, *3218*
Embolism, in upper extremity, 5005
Embolization, for arteriovenous malformation, 3256–3258, *3258, 3259*
Embryo
normal development of, 2451, *2452–2455*, 2453–2456
skull of, 1539–1540, *1540*
Embryology
neural crest, normal and abnormal development of, 2461–2462, 2464–2465, 2466–2469, *2462–2464, 2466, 2468*
normal, of male genitalia, 4153–4154
Embryology *(Continued)*
of blood and vascular system, 3223–3224
of blood vessels, 280–281, *281*
of craniofacial clefts, 2923–2927, *2924–2926*
of craniofacial microsomia, 3057–3061, 3061*t*
of ear, 2096–2097, *2097*
of face, 1575, *1576*
of lymphatic system, 3224
of optic system, 1574–1575, *1574, 1575*
of orbital hypotelorism, *3006*, 3006–3007
tubulation process of (embryo folding), 2460–2461, *2461*
Emergency room, hand surgery in, general principles of, 4285–4289, *4286–4289*
Emotional or psychologic considerations, of facialplasty, 2364–2365
Empyema, chronic, chest wall reconstruction and, 3726, *3728–3730*
Encephalocele
frontal, with nasal cleft, surgical correction of, *2989*, 2990
frontoethmoidal, surgical correction of, 2989, *2989*
median frontal, with orbital hypertelorism, 2926
Enchondromas, *4510*, 4511
Endogenous opioid pain control system, in reflex sympathetic dystrophy, 4901–4902
Endoneurium, 642
Endoplasmic reticulum, 637
Endoscopy, of velopharyngeal sphincter, 2913–2914
Energy expenditure, balance of, in thermal burns, 798
Enophthalmos
after blepharoplasty, 2351–2353, *2352, 2353*
correction of, 1604–1606
in anophthalmic orbit, 1606, *1649*
with nonseeing eye, *1609*
etiopathogenesis of, 1600–1601
in nasoethmoido-orbital fractures, 1103
in orbital fractures, 1057*t*, 1059–1061, *1059, 1060*, 1068–1069, *1069*, 1103
late correction of, *1608*
measurement of, 1601
from orbital and naso-ethmoido-orbital fractures, 1103
with orbital fracture, *1060*, 1068–1069, *1069*
pseudoptosis of, 1753, *1754*
roentgenographic studies of, 1601, *1602–1604*
Enteral formulas, commercially available, 800*t*
Entropion
cicatricial, 1739, *1739*, 1742
clinical presentation of, 1737–1742, *1738–1742*
congenital, 1738–1739
from microphthalmos repair, 1645
involutional, 1739, *1739–1741*
surgical correction of, 1739–1742, *1740–1742*
Environmentally induced syndromes, 84, 87, 89, 92, *88–91*, 89*t*. *See also specific syndromes.*
Enzymes, for management of thermal burn wounds, 802
Eosinophilic granuloma, 3352, 3714, 3714*t*
Epaulette flap, for complete cervical contractures, 2068, 2073, *2071, 2072*
Ephelides, 3587
Epiblepharon, 1737, *1739*, 1777, *1778*
Epibolin, 164
Epicanthus
congenital, 1774, *1775, 1776*

Epicanthus *(Continued)*
folds in, *1612*, 1614
canthopexy, dacryocystorhinostomy and bone grafting for, 1617–1618, *1618–1620*
correction of, 1616, *1616*
surgical correction of, in Down syndrome, 3168, *3169*
traumatic, 1777, *1777*
Epicranius, anatomy of, 1516, *1517*
Epidermal appendage tumors, 3574–3576, *3574, 3575*
Epidermal cells, tissue culture of, for biologic dressings, 805
Epidermal cysts, 3569, 3572
Epidermal growth factor, 164
Epidermal nevus syndrome, *3262*, 3263–3264
Epidermis
anatomy of, 221–222, *222*
histologic changes after chemical peeling, 753–754, *755*
hyperplasia of, 165, 242–243
in sun-damaged skin, 750–751, *750, 751*
silastic, 805
Epidermodysplasia verruciformis, 3563
Epidermoid carcinoma, 165, *166*, 3606–3607, *3607*
Epidural space, extensions of, 4314
Epilepsy, Dupuytren's disease and, 5055–5056
Epinephrine
for prevention of local anesthetic systemic toxicity, 4310–4311, 4311*t*
humoral regulation and, 309
intraoperative administration of, for pediatric patient, 157
Epineurium
anatomy of, 642, 644
repair of, 676, *680*, 680–681
Epiphora, after blepharoplasty, 2349
Epiphyses, premature closure of, after frostbite, 858
Epispadias
embryology of, 4155
primary
characteristics of, 4167–4168
incidence of, 4167–4168
reconstruction for, 4168
secondary
characteristics of, *4170*, 4170–4171
reconstruction of, 4171–4175, *4171, 4172*
Epithelioid cell-spindle cell nevus, 3592–3593, *3592, 3593*
Epithelization, 162–165, *163, 164*
Epstein-Barr virus, nasopharyngeal carcinoma and, 3458–3459
Erb's palsy, 4796–4797, 4799, *4797, 4798*
Erectile dysfunction, pathophysiology of, 4213–4215, *4214, 4215*
Ergotamine, 5016
Erysipeloid, 550–551
Erythema
after chemical peeling, 769
after dermabrasion, 780
Erythroplakia, oral cancer and, 3419
Erythroplasia of Queyrat, 3605, *3605*
Esser, 14
Esthesioneuroblastoma, 3362–3364, *3363*
Esthetic surgery. *See also specific types of esthetic surgery.*
demand for, 20
Esthetic surgery *(Continued)*
for Asian patients
for upper double eyelids, 2420–2422, *2421*
patient selection for, 2420
historical aspects of, 23–24
incidence of, for males, 115*t*
vs. reconstructive surgery, 1–2
Estlander flap, for lower lip reconstruction, 2020–2021, *2022*
Ethmocephaly, orbital hypotelorism and, *3005*, 3006
Ethmoid bone, anatomy of, 1084, 2978, *2978*
Ethmoid carcinoma, surgical treatment of, 3390, *3390*
Ethmomaxillary complex, growth of, 2502
Ethnic variations, in nasal anatomy, 1803–1804, *1803–1805*
Etiology, relationship to pathogenesis and phenotype, 92, *92*
European Society of Structive Surgery, establishment of, 15, *18*
Evans formula, 792*t*
Eversion technique, for nasal tip exposure, 1844, *1845*
Ewing's sarcoma, 3356, 3359, 3716
Excision, surgical
for port-wine stain, *3232*, 3232–3233
of lymphatic malformations, 3247, *3248*, 3249
Exophthalmos. *See* Exorbitism.
Exorbitism, causes of, 1630
from orbital roof fracture-dislocation or loss, 1114
in Graves' disease, 1632, *1632*
orbital decompression for, 1632–1637, *1633, 1634, 1636–1638*, 1639
indications for, 1634–1635
with blepharoplasty, 2326
Expanders, for scalp reduction, *1535*, 1535–1536
Expression, lines of, 43–44
Exstrophy of bladder
embryology of, 4155
in female, 4211, *4211*
primary
characteristics of, 4167–4168, 4168–4169
complications of, 4170
incidence of, 4167
postoperative care for, 4169
reconstruction for, 4169
secondary
characteristics of, *4170*, 4170–4171
reconstruction of, 4171–4175, *4171, 4172*
Extensor digiti minimi tendon, as donor tendon for flexor tendon repair, 4552
Extensor digiti quinti minimus, 4570
Extensor digitorum communis tendon
anatomy of, *4571*, 4571–4572
extension of, 4569–4570, *4570*
function of, 4572
Extensor digitorum longus tendon
as donor tendon for flexor tendon repair, 4553
clinical transplantation of, 538–539, *538, 539*
Extensor digitorum muscles, function of, *4261*, 4261–4262
Extensor digitorum superficialis tendon, as donor tendon for flexor tendon repair, 4552
Extensor hypoplasia, secondary flexion deformity of digits in, 5328, *5329, 5330*
Extensor indicis muscles, function of, 4262, *4262*
Extensor indicis proprius, extension of, 4570, *4570*

Extensor pollicis brevis muscle, function of, 4262, *4264*
Extensor pollicis brevis tendon, in thumb extension, 4572–4573
Extensor pollicis longus muscle, function of, 4262, *4264*
Extensor pollicis longus tendon, in thumb extension, 4572–4573
Extensor sheath cyst, of wrist, 5496–5497, *5497*
Extensor tendons
anatomy of, 4569, *4570*, 4571–4572, *4571*
characteristics of, 4567–4568
closed avulsion of, 457
failures after surgery, 4578, *4578*
function of
in extrinsic finger extension, 4569–4570
in intrinsic finger extension, 4570–4571
in wrist extension, 4569
in rheumatoid arthritis, 4708–4711, *4709, 4710*
injuries of, 4565–4567, *4566*, 4573, 4591
at distal interphalangeal joint level, 4573–4578, *4573–4578*
at metacarpal level, 4589, *4589*
at metacarpophalangeal joint level, 4588–4589
at middle phalanx level, 4579
at proximal interphalangeal joint level, 4579–4583, *4579–4588*, 4585–4587
at proximal phalanx level, 4587–4588
at thumb joint levels, 4589–4590, *4590*
avulsion wounds of, 4566
by crush, 4566, *4566*
deep abrasion of, 4567
lacerations of, 4566, *4566*
paratenon of, 4567
repair of
active motion after, 4567
anesthesia for, 4568
exposure for, 4568
for replantation, 4365–4366, *4366*
golden period for, 4567
patient factors for, 4568
scar from, 4567
tendon retrieval for, 4568–4569
treatment conditions for, 4568
tenosynovectomy of, *4740–4741*, 4741
External oblique muscle flaps, for abdominal wall defects, 397
External pin fixation, of mandibular fractures, 946, *948–949*
External traction devices, 1288
Extraocular muscles
anatomy of, 1049, *1049*, 1671–1673, *1672*
dominant field action of, 1059, *1059*
evaluation of, in facial injuries, 881
function of, 1671
imbalance of, surgical correction of, 1606, 1609
injuries of, in nasoethmoido-orbital fractures, 1616
Extravasation injuries
from drugs, 5440–5442
from injections, surgical management of, 5442–5443, *5443*
Eye(s)
cyclopic, 2458–2459
embryological development of, 2478, *2480*, 2481
injuries of
after orbital fractures, 1103–1104
mobility of, 1583–1584
Eyeball, limitation of forced rotation of, 1062, 1065, *1065*
Eyebrow(s)
anatomy of, 2399–2400
burn injuries of, 2218–2222, *2219–2220*
lifts of, in facial paralysis, 2306–2307, *2306*
position of, 32–33, *33*
ptosis of, 2327, 2334–2335, *2334*
reconstruction of, 2219–2222, *2219–2220*
suspension procedure, for ptosis, 1759, *1759*
Eyelet method, of intermaxillary fixation, 921–922, *922*
Eyelid(s)
anatomy of, 1673, *1674*
burn injuries of, 2210, 2212–2218, *2214–2218*
Caucasian vs. Oriental, 2420–2422, 2422*t*
contractures of, 2213
deformities of
treatment of, in Treacher Collins syndrome, 3113, 3116–3117, *3116, 3117*
deformities of, classification of, 2326–2327
double, in Asian patients, anatomical considerations for surgery, 2420–2422, *2421*
functions of, 1671
hemangiomas of, intralesional steroids for, 3216, *3217*
hypertrophy of tissue, 2331, 2333
lacerations of, 1685–1688, *1686–1688*
lower
blepharoplasty technique for, 2337, 2339, 2345, 2348, *2340–2347*
contractures of, 2217–2218, *2217, 2218*
reconstruction of, 1691, 1694, 1700, 1703, *1694–1702, 1704*
in Treacher Collins syndrome, 3116–3117, *3117*
vertical shortening of, 1609
after orbital or nasoethmoido-orbital fractures, 1106
malpositions of
entropion, 1737–1742, *1738–1742*
symblepharon, 1742–1744, *1743–1745*
medial canthoplasty, 1715, *1717, 1718*
operative considerations for, 1681–1685, *1681–1685*
paralysis of, 2307, 2310, 2312, *2308–2313*
surgical methods for, 2307, 2310, 2312, *2308–2313*, 2312*t*
reconstruction of, 1689–1690, *1690*
for defects of lateral segment, 1713, *1714*
for defects of medial segment, 1713, 1715, *1716*
for full-thickness defects, *1690*, 1690–1691, 1694, 1700, 1703, *1694–1702, 1704*
for partial-thickness defects, 1690, *1691–1694*
for full-thickness defects, upper, 1703, *1705–1712*, 1707, 1709, 1712–1713
replantation of, 1687–1688, *1688*
"scleral show," 33, *33*
senile, ptosis of, 2327
skin of, 2323, *2323*
upper
blepharoplasty technique for, 2335, 2337, *2338*
block anesthesia of, 1639
loading of, for paralysis treatment, 2310, 2312, *2312*
ptosis of, 1752–1755, *1753–1759*
reconstruction of, 1703, 1707, 1709, 1712–1713, *1705–1712*
retraction of, 1639
surgical release of, 2213–2215, *2214*
wrinkling of, excessive, *2324*, 2333

Fabry's disease, 3236, *3236*
Face
abrasions of, 904
aging of, psychosocial aspects of, 124–125
anatomy of, 1671–1673, *1672*
anthropometric points of, 28, *28*
beauty standards of, for Asian patients, 2416–2420, *2417–2419*
bones of, blood supply of, 603–605, *604, 605*
clefts of. *See* Facial clefts.
color of, in burn injury, 2159
contours of, in burn injury, 2158
contusions of, 904, *904*
counterpart relationship with cranium, *2502*, 2502–2503
deformities of, correlation with correction of microtia, 2100
disfigurement of, psychosocial aspects of, 120–121
embryologic development of, 2923, *2924*
embryology of, 1575, *1576*
esthetic units of, *26*
forms of, 33, *34*, 35
growth centers in, 2455, 2481–2483, *2484*
growth of
abnormal, causes of, 2565
in cleft lip and palate, 2553–2578
lip reconstruction and, 2565–2568, *2566–2568*
normal, 2557–2559, *2558*
of nasomaxillary complex, 1150–1151
gunshot wounds of, 1124–1127, 1130–1131, *1126–1130*
measurements of
in horizontal lower area, 1198, *1197, 1198*
in horizontal midface area, 1196, *1197*, 1198
in vertical direction, 1195–1196, *1195*
midline structures of, duplication of, 2941, 2943, *2942–2944*
movement of, 2256
pain in, post-traumatic types of, 1131–1133
treatment of, 1133–1134
plain films of, lateral and profile view of, 886, *889*
postnatal development of, 1143, 1146–1148, *1143–1148*
characteristics of, 2496–2498
profile of, 1191, *1192*
proportions of, *30*, 30–36, 1190–1191, *1190, 1191*
regional entities of, *26*, 26–27, *27*
regional esthetic units of, 2159–2160, *2160*
skin cover of, in burn injury, 2158–2159
symmetry of, in burn injury treatment, 2159
texture of, in burn injury, 2159
vertical growth of, 2508–2513, *2508–2513*
Face lift. *See* Facialplasty.
Facial artery(ies), development of, 2470–2471, *2470*
Facial clefts. *See also* Craniofacial clefts.
classification of, 2442–2443, *2443*, 2934
epidemiology of, 2445–2446
formation of, theories of, *2924*, 2924–2926
genetics of, 2445–2446
historical aspects of, 2437–2442
oblique, 2540–2541
syndromic etiologic factors of, 2448
transverse, 3096, *3096*
with orbital hypertelorism, 2540, *2541*
Facial injuries
abrasions, management of, 904
clinical examination of, 879–882, *879–882*
computed tomographic scans of, 899
contusions, management of, 904, *904*
craniofacial skeleton fractures, dental wiring and intermaxillary fixation techniques for, 921–922, *922–930*, 925–930
emergency treatment
for hemorrhage, 876–877, *878*
for pulmonary aspiration, 877, 879
for respiratory obstruction, 871–873, *872, 873, 874, 875*, 875–876
evaluation of, in multiply injured patient, 869–871, *869t*
fractures of
complex or panfacial, *1032*, 1032–1033
treatment of, 1033, 1035, 1038–1040, 1043, *1034, 1036, 1037, 1041–1043*
Le Fort classification for, 1012–1015, *1013, 1014*
from burns
acute management of, 2154–2155
causes of, 2153–2154
cheek resurfacing in. *See* Cheeks, resurfacing of.
development of master plan for reconstruction of, 2157
esthetic considerations for reconstruction of, 2158–2160, *2160*
incidence of, 2154
of eyelids, 2210, 2212–2218, *2214–2218*
of forehead, 2222–2223, *2223*
of lower lip and chin, 2187–2188, *2189*
of nose, 2200, 2202–2204, *2203*
of oral commissure, 2226, 2228–2229, 2231, *2230*
of upper lip, 2183–2187, *2186*
patient-surgeon relationship in, 2156
timing of reconstruction for, 2156–2157
in children. *See* Children, facial trauma of.
incidence of, 867–868
initial assessment of, 868–869
lacerations, management of, 904, *905, 906*
roentgenographic diagnosis of, 882–887, 893–894, 897–899, *884–899*
soft tissue wounds
avulsed wounds of facial area, 909, 912, *911, 912*
lacerations of lips, 912, *913*
nonsuture closure technique, 916, *917, 918*
with loss of structure and tissue, 913, 916, *915*
treatment of
of soft tissue wounds. *See* Soft tissues, facial wounds of.
timing for, 869
Facial muscles
anatomy of, 2244, *2246*, 2246*t*, 2246–2247, *2247*
in facial paralysis, 2252–2253
Facial nerve
anatomy of, *2238, 2242, 2251*, 3277–3278, *3277, 3278*
branching of, 2241, *2241*
of extratemporal branch, 2239–2241, *2240*
of infratemporal branch, 2239
of mandibular branch, 2241, 2243, *2243*
of midfacial branches, 2243–2244, *2244*
evaluation of, 2250*t*, 2250–2251
injury of, 904, 906
after facialplasty in male, *2397*, 2397–2398
from salivary gland surgery, 3313–3314
vascular supply of, 2244

Facial paralysis
choice of corrective procedure for, 2312, 2314
crossface nerve grafting for, 2272–2274, *2274–2276*
diagnosis of, 2250*t*, 2250–2251
electrodiagnostic tests for, 2253, *2254*, 2255
etiology of, 2247, 2250
extratemporal nerve grafts for, 2259, 2262–2263, *2262–2264*, 2265, *2266–2270*, 2267, 2267*t*, 2270*t*, 2270–2271, 2271*t*
free muscle grafts for, 2294, 2298
historical perspective of, 2237, 2239
hypoglossal-facial nerve anastomoses for, 2277–2278, 2278*t*, *2278–2282*, 2281, 2283–2284
intracranial nerve grafting for, 2272
irradiation and facial nerve grafting for, 2272
limitations of reconstructions for, 2314–2315
location of lesion in, 2251, *2251*
microneurovascular muscle transfers for, 2298–2300, *2300–2303*
muscular changes in, 2252–2253
nerve-muscle pedicle techniques for, 2298
of eyelid, 2307, *2308–2313*, 2310, 2312
pathology of, 2251–2252
patterns of, 2237
phrenic-facial nerve anastomoses for, 2283
regional muscle transposition for, 2284
historical aspects of, 2284, 2286
of masseter muscle, 2286–2290, *2287–2291*
of temporalis muscle, 2291–2294, *2292–2297*
types of, *2285*
rehabilitation of, goals for, 2256
selective myectomy for, 2306
spinal accessory nerve-facial nerve anastomoses for, 2283–2284
spontaneous regeneration in, 2255, *2256, 2257*
static and ancillary techniques for, 2303–2307, *2304–2306*
surgical reconstruction for, 2255–2256, 2258
by direct nerve repair, 2258–2259, *2260–2261*
by extratemporal nerve grafting, 2259, 2262
treatment of, 2237
Facial reconstruction, for burn injuries
development of master plan for, 2157
timing of, 2156–2157
Facial skeleton, developmental malformations of, 1143, 1146–1148, *1143–1146*
Facial trauma, pediatric. *See* Children, facial trauma of.
Facialplasty
ancillary procedures for, 2383–2384
anesthesia for, 2368–2369
case studies of, *2385–2391*
cervicofacial, for males, 2392
chemical peeling and, 759
combined with other body contouring procedures, 4021
dressings for, 2384
emotional or psychologic considerations of, 2364–2365
historical aspects of, 2358–2360, *2358, 2359*
in facial paralysis, *2306*, 2306–2307
in male, 2392
complications of, 2393–2399, 2394*t*, *2397*
surgical incisions for, 2392–2393
laboratory evaluation for, 2367
limitations of, 2366–2367
Facialplasty *(Continued)*
patient instructions for, 2368
preoperative evaluation for, 2365–2366
preoperative orders for, 2368
preoperative photography for, 2367
psychosocial aspects of, 124–125
secondary, 2384, 2392
suction-assisted lipectomy with, 3981, *3981, 3984, 3985*
surgical techniques for
classical method for, 2369–2371, *2370–2372*, 2373
SMAS-platysma dissection and advancement, 2376, *2377, 2378*
Faciofacial anastomoses, for facial paralysis, 2272–2274, *2274–2276*
Factitious wounding, differential diagnosis of, 4905
Fahraeus-Lindqvist phenomenon, *448*, 448–449
Fasanella-Servat operation, technique for, 1759–1760, *1760*
Fascia, physical properties of, 522
Fascia transplantation
harvesting techniques for, 522, *523*
historical perspective of, 522
vascularized transfers for, 522, *524*, 525
Fascial grafts, for abdominal wall reconstruction, 3768, *3769*
Fascial infections, of hand, 5543–5544
Fascial or fascio-fat flap, 298, *298*
Fascial plexus, blood supply of, 284–285, *285*
Fascial transplants, for facial paralysis, 2304, *2304*
Fascicle
anatomy of, 4762
histochemical identification of, 675
intraoperative diagnosis and identification of, 674
Fascicular grafts, for facial nerve paralysis, 2315
Fasciectomy
extensive, for Dupuytren's disease, 5065, 5067
regional, for Dupuytren's disease, 5065
Fasciocutaneous flap
design of, 278
for chest wall reconstruction, 3688, *3688*
for lower leg reconstruction, 4044–4046, *4044–4049*, 4049
for soft tissue coverage, 4456–4457
historical aspects of, 376
Fasciotomy
for burn injuries, of upper extremity, 5423, 5425, *5423*
for Dupuytren's disease, 5065
subcutaneous, for Dupuytren's disease, 5075–5076, *5077*
Fat transplantation
clinical applications of, 516, 520–521, *519–521*
definition of, 515
fate of transplanted fat cells in, 516, *517, 518*
future of, 521–522
historical perspective of, 515–516
Fatigue curve, mechanical, 700–701, *701*
Felon, 5539–5540, *5540*
Festoons
clinical presentation of, 2324, *2326*
surgical removal of, 2339, *2342–2345*
Fetal alcohol syndrome
clinical presentation of, *88*
pathogenesis of, *2458, 2458–2459, 2459*
pathogenesis of cleft lip/palate and, 2533, 2535

Fibrillation potentials, 672–673
Fibrinolytic substances, 459
Fibroblasts
  collagen production by, 4434
  collagen production in abnormal scars, 736–737
  dermal, 243
  functions of, 169–170, 642
  in Dupuytren's contracture, 5056–5057
Fibroma, of hand, 5498–5499, *5499*
Fibroma durum, 3578–3579, *3579*
Fibroma simplex, 3578–3579, *3579*
Fibromatoses, Dupuytren's contracture and, 5056
Fibronectin
  functions of, 171–172
  in initial healing response, 4434
  neural crest cells and, 2461
Fibrosarcomas
  chest wall reconstruction and, 3716, *3717*
  of head and neck, 3368–3369
    in children, 3186
  of jaw, 3356
  of salivary glands, 3309–3310
Fibrous dysplasia
  chest wall reconstruction and, 3714, 3714*t*
  craniofacial surgery for, 3008
  in anterior skull base, surgical treatment for, 3377, *3378–3380*, 3381
  of jaw, 3347–3348, *3349*
  of orbit, 1649, *1649–1652*, 1651, 3396, *3396*
  resection of, primary reconstruction of mandible after, 1422, *1423–1425*
Fibrous histiocytoma
  of hand, 5500
  of head and neck, 3369
  of jaw, 3359
Fibula
  free flap of, for lower extremity reconstruction, 4055–4056, *4067*
  vascularized grafts, 624
Fillet flap
  for coverage of fingertip injury, 4482, *4482*
  of foot, for lower extremity reconstruction, 4052, *4053*
Finger(s). *See also* Hand.
  amputation of
    neurovascular pedicle method of digital transfer for, 5136, 5138, *5138–5141*
    of little finger, 4338
    operative technique for, 4337–4338
    principles in, 4332–4334, *4333, 4334*
    single, 4361
    through distal interphalangeal joint, 4334
    through middle phalanx, 4334
    through proximal interphalangeal joint, 4335
  anatomy of, of intrinsic muscles, 5332, *5334*
  collateral ligament avulsion fractures of, 4617
  congenital anomalies of
    clinodactyly of, 5337–5338, *5338–5340*, 5340
    delta phalanx, 5340–5341, *5342, 5343*, 5344
  cutaneous arteries of, *361*, 362
  derangements of, in spastic patient, 4982, *4983, 4984*
  dislocations of, *4610*, 4610–4611, 4614–4616
  duplication of
    in central locations, 5347–5348, 5351, *5348–5351*
    in small finger, 5352, 5356, *5353–5355*
  extension of, in radial palsy, tendon transfers for, 4945, *4946*, 4947
Finger(s) *(Continued)*
  extensor apparatus of, *4571*, 4571–4572
  flexion of
    in median nerve paralysis, 4957–4958
    secondary deformity of, from extensor hypoplasia, 5328, *5329, 5330*
  fractures of, *4598*, 4599–4601
  in Dupuytren's disease, *5060*, 5061–5062, *5061–5063*
  index
    amputations of, 4335–4336, *4336*
    transposition technique of, 5142, 5145, *5147–5151*, 5148–5149, 5151
  intrinsic muscles of, 4269–4271, *4270*
    examination of, 4271, *4271*
  ischemic contracture deformities of, 5044–5046, *5045*, 5045*t*
    surgical correction of, 5048–5051, *5049*
  joints of, in rheumatoid arthritis, 4718–4720, *4720*
  mallet deformity of, 4573–4576, *4573, 4574*, 4626–4627, *4626*
  metacarpophalangeal joints of, *4254*, 4254–4255
  mucous cysts of, 3581
  multidigit replantation surgery of, anesthesia for, 4304, 4305–4306
  proximal annular pulley of, surgical release of, 4730–4731, *4731, 4732*
  retinacular system of, anatomy of, 4572
  ring or long, amputations of, 4336–4337, *4337*
  spaces in, 4273, *4275*
  splinting techniques for, 4577, *4577*
    with boutonnière deformity, 4585–4586, *4587*
  swan-neck deformity of, 4576–4577
  synovial sheaths of, 4273, *4275*
  tip of. *See* Fingertip(s).
  transposition of
    for correction of transverse absence of carpals or metacarpals, 5248
    for index finger, 5142, 5145, 5148–5149, 5151, *5147–5151*
    for thumb reconstruction, 5138, 5142, *5143–5149*
  trigger
    anatomy of, 4727–4729, *4727, 4728*
    clinical features of, 4727–4729, *4727, 4728*
    treatment of, 4729–4731, *4730*
Finger pulleys, 4266, *4267*
Fingernail(s)
  anatomy of, 4478, *4478*
  bed of, anatomy of, 4499–4500, *4500*
  deformities of, after burn injury, 5467, *5468*
  growth of, physiology of, 4500–4502, *4500–4502*
Fingertip(s)
  amputation of, replantation of, 4371
  amputations of, composite types of, 4485–4487, *4486–4488*
  anatomy of, 4477–4479, *4478*
  injuries of
    general principles of, *4479*, 4479–4480
    local flap coverage for, 4487–4490, *4488–4494*, 4492–4493
    local tissue coverage for, 4481–4482, *4482*
    nonoperative treatment for, 4480–4481, *4481*
    on dorsal surface, 4493–4496, *4495*
    skin graft coverage for, 4482–4485, *4483–4485*
  nail bed injuries of, 4480
Finkelstein test, for de Quervain's disease, 4733, *4733*
First and second branchial arch syndrome, 3054

First branchial arch syndrome, 2931
First web space flap, for sensory reconstruction of hand, 4862, *4864, 4865–4867, 4866, 4867*
Fissural cysts, 3340
Fistula, palatal, closure of, 2814–2817, *2814–2821*, 2821
Fixation methods
  for acquired defects of mandible, 1415–1419, 1421–1422, *1416–1421*
    external types of, 1416–1419, 1421, *1417–1421*
    internal types of, 1421–1422, *1421, 1430*
    intraoral types of, 1415–1416, *1416*
  for jaw surgery, 1215–1216, *1216, 1217*
  rigid skeletal, for jaw, 1216, 1218, *1219–1222*
Flap(s). *See also specific types of flaps.*
  calvarial
    advantages of, 621
    anatomy of, 619–620, *620*, 620*t*
    design of, 620–621
    disadvantages of, 621
  combination types of, 383
  complications of, 306*t*, 306–308
  coverage by
    functional purpose of, 4443–4444
    historical aspects of, 4444–4445
  current surgical trends for, 276
  design of, for alveolar and anterior cleft palate repair, 2758
  distant, 4450–4451
    "delay" phenomenon and, 4451–4452
  for acquired defects of mandible, 1439–1440, *1440–1442*
  for aerodigestive tract reconstruction, 3436, 3438, 3444, 3447–3449 *3436, 3437, 3439–3449*
  for chest wall reconstruction, requirements for, 3679
  for soft tissue coverage, 279–280, 280*t*
  historical aspects of, *2*, 275–276
  microcirculation of, 308–309, *309*
  microvascular free scalp, 1531, *1532, 1533*
  microvascular osseous and osteocutaneous, for acquired defects of mandible, 1440, 1443, 1445, 1451, *1444–1446, 1448–1450*
  mucomuscular, for cleft palate closure, 2739–2742, *2741*
  multiple scalp, 1530–1531
  necrosis of, 506
  of lower extremity, 374
  of muscle, 301–304, *302, 303*
  specialized types of, 304–306, *305, 306*
  transposition types of, 4449–4450, *4450–4451*
  vascularized bone, 598, 600–605, *601–605*
Flexor carpi ulnaris tenosynovitis, 4742, *4742*
Flexor digitorum brevis muscle flaps
  for foot reconstruction, 401
  for heel and midplantar defects, 4082, *4085*
Flexor digitorum profundus muscle, examination of, 4269, *4269*
Flexor digitorum profundus tendon, 4262–4263, *4265*
Flexor digitorum superficialis tendon
  clinical transplantation of, 539–540
  examination of, 4269, *4269*
  in flexor tendon repair, 4534–4535
Flexor tendons
  avulsion of profundus, 4536
  blood supply of, 4516–4517, *4517, 4518*
  carpal tunnel and, 4537
Flexor tendons *(Continued)*
  complications of repair
    bowstringing of, 4547
    flexion contracture of, 4547
  exploration of, 4547–4551, *4549, 4550*
  fibrous flexor sheath of, 4518–4521, *4519–4520*
    reconstruction of, *4520*, 4521–4522, *4523*
  healing of, 4518
  importance of, 4516
  in rheumatoid arthritis, 4711–4712
  lacerations of
    at wrist, 4537–4538, *4538*
    oblique, 4539, *4539*
    proximal to fibrous flexor sheath, 4537
    with ragged or dammaged ends, 4539, *4540*
  musculotendinous junction of, 4538
  nutrition for, 4516–4517, *4517, 4518*
  of hand, 4264–4265
  one-stage tendon graft for
    complications of, *4558*, 4558–4559
    splintage for, 4558
    technique for, 4553–4559, *4555–4558*
  one-stage tendon graft of
    contraindications for, 4551
    donor tendon sites for, 4551–4553
  postoperative care for, 4560, *4560*
  primary repair of
    core suture for, 4531–4533, *4532*
    diagnosis for, 4524–4525, *4525*
    distal profundus laceration in, 4535–4536, *4536*
    for partial lacerations, 4535, *4535*
    intraoperative decisions in, 4529–4531
    peripheral running suture for, *4533*, 4533–4534
    technique for, 4525–4536, *4525–4533, 4535–4536*
    with FDS spiral, 4534–4535
    with flat superficialis, 4534
  repair of
    at double levels, 4539
    core suture for, 4526
    for replantation, 4366, *4367*
    incisions for, 4522–4524, 4526
    needles for, 4526–4528
  repairs of, postoperative management for, 4540–4544, *4541–4543*, 4542*t*
  secondary reconstruction of
    physical examination for, 4544–4547, *4546, 4547*
    preoperative considerations for, 4544
  sheath of, closure for, 4536–4537, *4537*
  staged reconstruction of, with silicone rod, 4559–4560, *4559, 4560*
  surgical results for, 4560–4561, *4561*
  tenolysis of, 4547–4551, *4549, 4550*
    with capsulectomy, 4550–4551
  tenosynovitis of, 4742, *4742*
  zones of, *4268*, 4268–4269
Fluids
  maintenance of, for pediatric patient, 156*t*, 156–157, 157*t*
  management of, for microsurgery, 457
  resuscitation with
    complications of, 794–795
    for electrical burn injuries, 815–816, 816*t*
    for thermal burn injuries, 791, 793–795, 794*t*, 5421–5422
5-Fluorouracil, 3627–3628
Flurazepam (Dalmane), 140

Foot
  anatomy of
    for midplantar aspect, 4035, *4036*
    of dorsal surface, 4035, *4036*
    vs. hand anatomy, 5156, *5156–5166*, 5159, 5161–5167
  closure of, for great toe to hand transfer, 5175–5176, *5176, 5177*
  cutaneous arteries of, *371*, 373
  dissection of
    for great toe to hand transfer, 5168–5173, *5168–5173*
    for thumb reconstruction, 5187–5190, *5187–5190*
  in great toe to hand transfer
    complications of, 5181, *5181*
    postoperative gait analysis for, 5178
  reconstruction of, muscle and musculocutaneous flaps for, 401–402, *402*
  soft tissue coverage of, 4080, 4082
    in distal plantar area, 4087
    in dorsal area, 4087–4088
    in weight-bearing heel and midplantar area, 4082, *4083–4087*, 4085, 4087
Foot flap
  fillet type of, for lower extremity reconstruction, 4052, *4053*
  from first web space, for sensory reconstruction of hand, 4862, 4865–4867, *4864, 4866, 4867*
"Football jersey" injury, 4536
Forced duction test, 1062, 1065, *1065*, 1601
Forceps
  Hayton-Williams, 1028, *1029*
  Row disimpaction, 1028, *1029*
Fordyce lesions, 3235, *3236*
Forearm
  cutaneous arteries of, 359, *360, 361*, 362
  longitudinal absence deformities of ulna, clinical presentations of, 5275
  muscles of, paralysis of
    in high median nerve injury, *4957*, 4957–4958
    in ulnar nerve paralysis, 4947, *4948*, 4949
  preparation of, for functioning muscle transfer, 4971
  transverse absence of, 5245–5246, *5247*
Forehead
  anatomy of, 2399–2400
  burn injuries of, 2222–2223, *2223*
  flaps of
    for intraoral wounds, 3436, *3437*, 3438
    for nasal lining, 1981
    midline, for nasal reconstruction, 1945, 1948, 1957–1958, *1950–1964*, 2202, *2203*
  parts of, *1566*, 1567
  reconstruction of, by tissue expansion, 496, *499, 500*
  regional nerve block of, *146*, 146–147
  resurfacing of, 2222–2223, *2223*
Forehead-brow lift
  alternative techniques for, 2410
  anatomical considerations for, 2399–2400
  bicoronal technique for, 2401–2402, 2404–2406, *2401–2405*
  case studies of, *2407–2409*
  complications of, 2406, 2410
  historical perspective of, 2399
  incision for, 2400, *2401*, 2402
  indications for, 2400
  patient evaluation for, 2400–2401
Foreign bodies, in male genitalia, 4236
Forequarter amputation, 4345–4347, *4345, 4346*
Foreskin, reconstruction of, 4238, *4238*
Forked wire extension, for class II mandible fracture, in edentulous posterior segment, *951*, 954, *955*
Forward traction test, 1604–1605, *1605*
Frank technique, of intermittent perineal pressure, 4206
Frankfort horizontal plane, 28, *28*, 1190
Freckles, 3587
Free flap. *See also specific types of free flaps.*
  design of, 277, *277*
  for cheek reconstruction, 2050, *2051*
  for chest wall reconstruction, 3703, 3705, 3707
  for lower extremity reconstruction, 4049–4052, 4054–4056, *4050–4053*
  in upper extremity reconstructions, 4459
    advantages of, 4460
    arteriography for, 4460
    composite tissue transfer technique for, 4461–4462
    disadvantages of, 4460
    dorsalis pedis flap as, 4463, 4465, 4467, *4465, 4466*
    gracilis flap as, 4474–4475
    groin flap for, 4462–4463, *4463, 4464*
    historical aspects of, 4459
    indications for, 4460
    lateral arm flaps as, 4471–4472, *4472*
    latissimus dorsi flap as, 4474
    medial arm flaps as, 4469–4471, *4471*
    parascapular flaps as, 4467–4468, *4468*
    posterior calf fasciocutaneous flap as, 4475
    primary vs. delayed coverage of, 4460–4461
    radial artery forearm flaps as, 4472–4474, *4473*
    scapular flaps as, 4467–4468, *4468*
    temporoparietal fascial flaps as, 4468–4469, *4469, 4470*
    types of, 4459–4460
  microvascular, for neck resurfacing, 2200, *2201*
  neurovascular, donor tissue for, 4861–4862, 4865–4868, 4870–4872, *4863, 4864, 4866–4871*
Free muscle transfer. *See* Functioning muscle transfer.
Free tissue transfers, innervated
  in restoration of sensation in hand, 4851
  of hand, 4859
Freeman modification, for lower lip reconstruction, 2018
Frey's syndrome, 1409, 3314, *3314*
Froment's paper sign, 4272, *4272*
Frontal area fractures, treatment of, 1119–1121, *1120, 1121*
Frontal bone
  contouring of, 1565
  fractures of, 1107–1108, *1108*
    in children, 1174–1175, 1177, *1174–1177*
  repair and contouring of
    for full-thickness defects, 1562–1564, *1564*
    iliac or cranial vault bone grafts for, 1564–1565, *1565*
    methylmethacrylate implants for, 1561–1562, *1563*
  repositioning of, 1565, 1567, 1570, *1564, 1568–1570*
Frontal lobe, injuries, signs and symptoms of, 1113, *1113*
Frontal nerve paralysis, after forehead-brow lift, 2406, 2410
Frontal sinus
  fractures of, 1107–1108, *1108*, 1121–1124, *1123–1125*
    in children, 1175, 1177
  postnatal development of, 1147

Frontal sinus *(Continued)*
size of, 1084, *1084*
Frontalis muscle
resection of, in forehead-brow lift, 2404–2405, *2405*
suspension of, for ptosis, 1772–1774, *1772–1774*
Frontobasilar region
anatomic characteristics of, 1109–1110, *1110*
fractures of, 1107–1108, *1108*
classification of, 1108–1109, *1108, 1109*
incidence of, 1111
signs and symptoms of, 1111–1115, *1112, 1113, 1115*
injury patterns of, 1110–1111, *1111*
Frontonasal dysplasia, 2540, *2541*, 2926
Fronto-occipital projection, for plain films, 885, *886*
Fronto-orbital remodeling, for craniosynostosis, 3029–3030, 3032, *3028–3032*
Frontoparietal flap, 622, 624, *624, 625*
Frontotemporal flaps
for nasal reconstruction, 1965
scalping flaps, 1965, *1966*
up-and-down flaps, 1965
for orbital and maxillary deficiencies, 3113, *3114–3115*
Fronto-temporo-orbital fracture, 1081
Frostbite
clinical presentation of, 5433–5434, *5433–5435*
environmental conditions for, 5431–5432
historical background for, 851–852
pathophysiology of, 852–854, 854*t*
physiology of, 5432–5433
treatment of, 854–857, *856*, 5434–5436
with systemic hypothermia, 865
Fry technique, 1426, *1431*, 1432
Fuchs position, for plain films, 886, *889*
Fucosidosis, 3227, 3236
Full-thickness defects, 55
Functional craniology, 3026
Functional matrix theory, 1294, 3026, 3067
Functioning muscle transfer. *See* Muscle transfer, functioning.
definition of, 4966
historical aspects of, 4966
indications for, 4970
muscle selection for, 4969–4970
operative technique of
for forearm preparation, 4971
for gracilis muscle preparation, 4971–4972
preoperative planning for, 4970–4971, *4971*
Funduscopic examination, 1118
Fungal infections, of hands, 5551–5553

Galeal frontalis myofascial flap, for fibrous dysplasia in anterior skull base, 3377, *3378–3380*, 3381
Galen, 2–3
Gamma rays, 832
Ganglion
of hand and wrist, 5494–5496, *5495, 5496*
of perionychium, 4511–4512, *4511–4513*
of wrist or hand, 4744–4746, *4746–4750*, 4749, 4752
Gangrene
of hand, 5548
vasospasm and, 5016
Gap arthroplasty, for temporomandibular ankylosis, 1494–1495
"Gap substance," 642
Gas gangrene, abdominal wall reconstruction for, 3772–3774, *3773*
Gastrocnemius muscle
applications of, 4043, *4043*
flaps of, for lower extremity reconstructions, 399
motor innervation of, 4043
origin and insertion of, 4043
vascular supply of, 4043
Gastrointestinal system complications, from burn injuries, 809, 828
Gastroschisis, abdominal wall reconstruction for, 3774, 3775–3777, 3779–3780, *3776, 3778*
Gastrulation, 2453, *2453*, 2456–2460, *2457–2460*
Generalized essential telangiectasia, 3239
Genetic conditions. *See also specific conditions.*
with collagen metabolism defects, 179–180
Genetics
chromosome studies, indications for, 104*t*
cytogenetic and chromosomal anomalies, 100, *100, 101, 102*, 103, *103*, 103*t*
monogenic inheritance patterns, 103–104, *105, 106*, 106–106, *107*
sporadicity, 109–111
vascular malformation pathogenesis and, 3227
Genioglossus muscle, 937
Geniohyoid muscle, 937
Genioplasty, 1312, *1313–1317*, 1318, *1318–1322*, 1323, *1324–1329*
Genital reconstruction
complication of, 4124
flaps for, 4126–4127
gracilis myocutaneous of, 4128, *4128–4137*, 4136–4137
of posterior thigh, 4141, 4143, *4144–4146*
of rectus femoris, 4149, *4149–4151*, 4152
of tensor fascia lata, 4148–4149
rectus abdominis of, 4137, 4139, *4140*, 4141
V-Y biceps femoris flap, 4147–4148
for male acquired defects
from traumatic injury, 4226–4239, *4229, 4232, 4234, 4235, 4237, 4238*
of lymphedema, 4180–4183, *4181, 4182*
of Peyronie's disease, 4183–4187, *4185, 4186*
of urethral strictures, 4187–4191, *4188, 4189, 4191, 4192, 4195–4201*
for male congenital defects. *See specific male congenital defect.*
embryology of, 4153–4155
free microvascular transfers for, 4152
in female
for congenital absence of vagina, 4203–4208, *4204–4207*
for exstrophy of bladder, 4211, *4211*
for lymphedema of vulva, 4211
for stenosis, 4210
for vaginal construction after ablative surgery, 4208–4210, *4209*
with vaginal fistulas, 4210
patient preparation for, 4123–4124
preoperative planning for, 4123–4124
principles of, 4121–4123
skin grafts for, 4125–4126
technical considerations for, 4124–4125
Genitalia, male
anatomy of, 4226–4227
avulsion injuries of, 4231, *4232*, 4233–4234

Genitalia, male *(Continued)*
burn injuries of, *4234*, 4234–4235
foreign bodies in, 4236
injuries of
anatomic considerations of, 4226–4228
nonpenetrating, 4228–4229, *4229*
normal anatomy of, 4156
normal embryology of, 4153–4154
penetrating injuries of, 4230–4231
radiation injuries of, 4235, *4235*
self-mutilation of, 131
Giant cell tumor
of hand, 5498, *5498*
of perionychium, 4512
Giant hairy nevus, malignant melanoma and, 3636–3637, *3637*
Giant pigmented nevus, 3589, 3591
Gigantism
hemihypertrophic type of, 5365, 5371, *5370–5371*
hyperostosis type of, 5365, *5368–5369*
neurofibromatosis type of, 5364–5365, *5366–5367*
of hand, 5362, 5364–5365, 5371, 5373, *5363, 5366–5372*
treatment of, 5371, 5373, *5372*
with nerve-oriented lipofibromatosis, 5362, 5364, *5363*
Gillies, Sir Harold Delf, 8–9, 10, *12*
Gillies fan flap, for lower lip reconstruction, 2021, *2022*
Gilmer technique of intermaxillary fixation, 921, *922*
Gingiva
attached, 2758
cysts of, 3337
of mandible, cancers of, 3451–3452
Gingivoperiosteoplasty, for bilateral cleft lip and palate, 2702, *2703, 2704*
Glabella, 1190
Glabrous skin receptors, 648–651, *648–650*
Glasgow Coma scale, 869, 869*t*, 870
Glass, for alloplastic implants, 717, *717*
Glass transition temperature, 707–708
Glial tumors, of root of nose, 2986
Glioma, neuromas of, 4852–4854, *4853*
Globulomaxillary cyst, 3340
Glomus tumor
of hand, 5504
of perionychium, 4510–4511
pathology of, 3586, *3586*
Glottal stop, 2734
Glottis
anatomy of, *3416*, 3416–3417
tumors of, 3466–3467
Glucose, total body stores, in thermal burns, 798
Gluteus maximus flap
applications for, 4038, *4039*
for groin and perineum reconstructions, 399
for pressure sore treatment, 402–403, *403*
motor innervation of, 4038
origin and insertion of, 4038
vascular supply of, 4038
Glycosaminoglycans
in Dupuytren's contracture, 5057
in wound healing, 740
Goldenhar's syndrome, 2469, 2491
Golgi tendon organ, 654
Golgi-Mazzoni receptors, 654, 655
Gonorrhea, 5551
Gorlin's cyst, 3338–3339
Gracilis flap
applications of, 4040, *4042*, 4043
for free flap transfer, in upper extremity, 4474–4475
for genital reconstructive surgery, 4128, *4128–4138*, 4136–4137
advantages of, 4136
disadvantages of, 4128, 4136
vs. regional flaps, 4136–4137
for groin and perineum reconstructions, 398, *398*
for lower extremity reconstruction, 4052, *4054*
for pressure sores, 404
for vaginal construction, after ablative surgery, 4208, *4209*, 4209–4210
motor innervation of, 4040
origin and insertion of, 4040
vascular supply of, 4040
Gracilis muscle
functioning muscle transfer of, operative technique for, 4972–4974, *4973, 4974*
microneurovascular transfers, for facial paralysis, 2299–2300, *2300–2303*
preparation of, for functioning muscle transfer, 4971–4972
Granular cell myoblastoma, 3586–3587, *3587*
Granuloma telangiectaticum, 3584–3585, *3585*
Graves' disease
orbital pathology in, 1630
scleral show of, 2327, 2328, 2330, *2328*
Great auricular nerve injury, after facialplasty, of male, 2396–2397
Great toe to hand transfer
failure of, 5181, *5181*
historical aspects of, 5153–5154
indications for, 5154–5156
operative steps of
for foot closure, 5175–5176, *5176, 5177*
for foot dissection, 5168–5173, *5168–5173*
for hand dissection, 5173–5174
for transfer and repair, 5174–5175, *5174, 5175*
in preoperative period, 5167–5168
postoperative gait analysis for, 5178
postoperative management for, 5176–5177
rehabilitation for, 5177–5178, *5177, 5178*
results from, optimization of, 5181, *5182*, 5183
secondary procedures for, 5179, *5180*, 5181
Great vessels, development of, 2470–2471
Greater trochanter autografts, 612–613
Greenstick fractures
nasal, 988
of mandible, 922, *931*
radiological evaluation of, 1152–1153, *1152*
Grenz radiation, for superficial basal cell epithelioma, 3600
"Grenz zone," 750, *750, 753*, 756
Groin flap
anatomy of, 4462, *4463*
design of, 292, 295, *293, 294*
disadvantages of, 4452–4453
for free flap transfer in upper extremity, 4462–4463, *4464*
for lower extremity reconstruction, 4049–4050, *4050*
for reconstruction of groin area, 397–399, *398*
for toe to hand transfer, 5156, 5159, *5157–5159*
Ground substance, 172, 210
Growth, skeletal, concepts of, 2498–2502, *2499–2502*
Growth factors, 179
Growth remodeling, 2499–2500, *2500*

Guanethidine
  for reflex sympathetic dystrophy, 4909–4910
  postoperative treatment of skin flaps, 314–315
Guérin fractures, 1013, *1014*
Gull-wing forehead flap, for nasal reconstruction, 1948, *1951, 1955–1956*, 1957–1958
Gunshot wounds, of face, 1124–1127, *1126–1130*, 1130–1131
Guyon's tunnel, *4281*, 4281–4282
Gynecomastia
  suction-assisted lipectomy for, 3988
  with ptosis, suction-assisted lipectomy for, 3988, *3988*

H_2blockers, 809
Hagedorn-LeMesurier technique, correction of short lip after, 2777, 2779, *2780*
Hair
  anatomy of, 1516
  growth cycle of, 1518–1519
  growth of, influencing factors for, 1519–1520
  sideburn, reconstruction of, 2226
  types of, 1519
Hair follicles
  anatomy of, 223
  hyperplasia of, in healing graft, 244–245
Hair replacement surgery, history of, 1514–1516, *1515*
Hairy skin receptors, 651–652, *652*
Halcion (triazolam), 140
Halo nevus, 3591–3592, *3592*
Hamartoma, 3192
Hamate, fractures of, *4597*, 4597–4598, 4645–4646
Hamstring muscle flaps, for pressure sores, 404
Hand. *See also* Finger(s); *specific structures of hand.*
  acute radiation injury of, 840–842, *840–843*
  adaptive elements of, *4253*, 4253–4254
  amputation of
    acquired vs. agenesis, 4385–4386, *4386*
    bilateral vs. unilateral loss, 4385
    patient's response to, 4387–4388, *4388*
  anatomy of
    historical aspects of, 4247–4248
    in Guyon's tunnel, *4281*, 4281–4282
    in opponens tunnel, *4281*, 4283
    in pisohamate tunnel, *4281*, 4282–4283
    mesotenon of, 4266, 4268
    synovial sheaths of, 4266
    vincula of, 4268, *4268*
    vs. foot anatomy, 5156, *5156–5166*, 5159, 5161–5167
  arthritis of
    analysis of kinesiologic problems in, 4697
    definition of patient problems in, 4696–4697
    degenerative, 4699–4703, *4701, 4702*
    maintenance of posttraumatic reconstruction, 4698–4699
    patient education for, 4697–4698
    treatment problems in, 4695–4696
  blood supply of, 4274–4275
    classical pattern of, 4275–4276
    examination of vascular system of, *4276*, 4276–4277
  bone tumors of
    adjuvant treatment for, 5517
    needle biopsy of, 5512

Hand *(Continued)*
  bone tumors of, open biopsy of, 5513, *5514*, 5515
    preoperative evaluation of, 5510–5512, *5511, 5512*
    staging of, 5515, 5517, 5515*t*, *5517*
    surgical excision of, 5517–5518, 5520–5521, 5517*t*, *5518–5521*
  bones of, 4252, *4252*
  burn injuries of
    amputations for, 5467, 5469, *5469–5471*
    complications of, *5415*, 5415–5416
    depth categories for, 5404*t*
    heterotopic ossification of, 5473, 5476, *5477*
    historical aspects of, 5399–5402
    inpatient treatment of, 5405–5414, *5406, 5407, 5411, 5412, 5414*
    outpatient treatment of, 5405
    pathology of, 5402–5403
    physical examination of, 5403–5405, *5404*
  circulation of
    adequacy of, 4994–4995
    ischemia and, 4995
  complete arches of, anatomic abnormalties of, 4993–4994, *4994*
  congenital anomalies of
    classification of, 5237, 5240, *5238–5239*
    dysmorphology approach to, 5231–5233, *5232*
    environmental causes for, 5233, 5236
    genetic causes for, 5233
    incidence of, 5225, 5229, 5231, 5229*t*, 5230*t*
    initial evaluation of, 5231
    of carpals, transverse absences of, 5246–5248, 5252, 5255, *5247, 5249–5251, 5253–5254*
    of metacarpals, transverse absences of, 5246–5248, 5252, 5255, *5247, 5249–5251, 5253–5254*
    of phalanges, transverse absences of, 5255, 5257, *5256*
    of upper arm, transverse absences of, 5241–5243, 5245–5246, *5243, 5244*
    syndromes of, 5236–5237
    timetables and, 5223, 5225
    timing of surgery for, 5240–5241, *5242*
    ultrasound examination of, *5234–5235*
    uncertain etiology of, 5236
  connective tissue tumors of
    benign types of, 5494–5500, *5495–5500*
    malignant types of, 5500–5501, *5501*
  cutaneous arteries of, *361*, 362
  dissection of
    for great toe to hand transfer, 5173–5174
    for thumb reconstruction, 5190
  dorsum of, incisions on, 4443
  electrical injuries of, 5476, *5478, 5479*, 5480
    assessment of, 5421
    early management of, 5421–5423, *5424*, 5425–5426
    mechanism of, 5420–5421, *5421*
    pathophysiology of, 5419–5420
  embryology of
    experimental studies of, 5217, *5218, 5219*, 5219–5220
    morphologic development in, 5216*t*, 5216–5217, *5217, 5218*
    of muscles, 5220–5221, *5222–5229*
    of nerves, 5221, 5223
    of skeletal development, 5220
    of vascular system, 4992–4994, *4993*, 5220, *5221*
  extrinsic flexors of, examination of, 4269, *4269*

Hand *(Continued)*
fingers of. *See* Finger(s).
fixed unit of, 4252–4253
flexor tendons of, 4264–4265
zones of, *4268*, 4268–4269
frozen, treatment of, 5434–5436
function of, dynamics of, 4272–4273, *4274*
gripping function of, surgical obtainment of, in tetraplegia, *4987, 4988*
hypothenar muscles of, 4271–4272, *4272, 4273*
infections of. *See* Hand infections.
injuries of
anesthesia for, 4595–4596
closed type of, evaluation for, 4286–4287, *4286*
dislocations of, 4607–4627, 4605*t*, 4605–4606, *4606–4608, 4610, 4611, 4613–4620, 4622, 4624, 4626*
equipment for, 4595, *4595*
fractures of, without joint injury, 4596–4602, *4596–4604*, 4604–4605
general patient evaluation for, 4593–4594
subluxations of, 4605*t*, 4605–4606, *4606–4608, 4607–4627, 4610, 4611, 4613–4620, 4622, 4624, 4626*
tetanus prophylaxis for, 4594, 4594*t*
treatment principles for, 4594–4596
intrinsic muscles of, ischemic contracture of. *See* Ischemic contractures, of intrinsic muscles of hand.
ischemia of, circulation and, 4995
joints of, 4252, *4252*. *See also Specific Joints.*
axes of, *4250*
lymphatic malformations of, 5503, *5504*
mirror, 5133
muscles of
extrinsic extensors of, 4261–4262, *4261–4264*
extrinsic flexors of, 4262–4264, *4265, 4266*
mutilating injuries of, *4339, 4339–4340, 4340*
nerve entrapment syndromes of, 4725–4726
neural tissue tumors of, *5505, 5505–5507, 5506*
open wound of, evaluation of, 4287–4288, *4288, 4289*
ossification centers of, *5215*
palmar fascia of, 4249–5252, *4251*
peripheral nerves of, 4277–4278, *4278, 4279*
anatomic considerations for repair of, 4758–4762, *4760, 4761*
dorsal branch of radial and ulnar nerves, 4280, *4280*
in crowded areas of, 4280–4281
internal anatomy of, 4762, *4763*
recovery potential for, 4757–4758
prosthesis for, fitting of, on children, 4386–4387, *4387*
replantation principles, 4289
restoration of sensation in, 4860–4861
retinacular system of, 4265–4266, *4267*
roentgenographic evaluation of, 4288–4289
sensory reconstruction of, 4872
skin of, 4248–4249, *4248, 4249*
soft tissue tumors of, 5483–5485
benign types of, 5485–5487, *5485, 5486*
distribution of, 5484*t*
incidence of, 5484*t*
malignant types of, 5487–5490, 5488, *5488, 5490t, 5491–5493*, 5492–5494
spaces in, 4273, *4275*
examination of infection of, 4274, *4274*

Hand *(Continued)*
splinting of, safe position for, 4433, *4433*
subcutaneous tissue of, 4248–4249
synovial sheaths of, 4273, *4275*
tendon and nerve entrapment of, associated disorders of, 4739, 4741–4746, 4749, 4752, *4740–4742, 4744, 4746–4751*
tendon entrapment syndromes of, 4725–4726
tendons of, nutrition for, 4268
thenar muscles of, 4271–4272, *4272, 4273*
therapy of
for joint stiffness, 4665–4666, *4666*
for reflex sympathetic dystrophy, 4912–4914
thumb of
first metacarpotrapezial joint and, *4256*, 4256–4257
skeleton of, *4255*, 4255–4256
trauma to, causing vascular injury, 4995–4997, *4996*
vascular conditions of, circulation and, 4995
vascular tissue tumors of, 5501–5505, 5502*t*, *5502–5504*
vasospastic disorders of, 5012
Hand anomalies
arthrogryposis, 5378–5381, *5378–5379*
cleft
clinical presentation of, 5267, 5269, *5268*
treatment of, 5269–5271, *5270, 5272, 5273*
types of, comparison of, 5267, 5269, 5269*t*, *5268*
combined venous-lymphatic malformations of, 5324
congenital constriction ring syndrome, 5373–5374, *5375–5377*, 5376–5378
delta phalanx, 5340–5341, *5342, 5343*, 5344
longitudinal ulnar deformities
clinical presentations of, 5274–5276, *5276*
lymphatic malformations of, 5319, *5323*, 5323–5324
mirror hand, 5356, *5357, 5358, 5359–5361*, 5361–5362
of duplication
classification of, 5344, *5345*, 5346
in small finger, 5352, 5356, *5353–5355*
incidence of, 5346
of central fingers, 5347–5348, *5348–5351*, 5351
of thumb, 5347
treatment of, 5346–5347
of failures of differentiation, 5279–5281, 5288–5293, *5280, 5282–5288, 5290–5292*
of flexion deformities, 5328, 5330–5333, 5337–5338, 5340–5341, 5344, *5329–5332, 5334–5343*
of high flow arterial malformations, 5324, 5326, *5325, 5327*
of hypoplasia, 5362
of longitudinal radial deficiencies, 5257–5258
classification of, 5258, 5260, *5259*
clinical presentation of, 5258, *5261*
defects associated with, 5258
treatment of, 5260, 5262, 5264–5265, 5267, *5263, 5264, 5266*
of overgrowth, 5362, *5363, 5364–5365, 5366–5372*, 5371, 5373
vascular malformations of
classification of, 5315, 5316*t*
hemangioma, 5315–5316, *5317*
of capillaries, 5316
of venous system, 5316, 5318–5319, *5318, 5320–5322*
Hand infections
antibiotics for, 5531–5532

Hand infections *(Continued)*
classification of, 5530–5531, 5531*t*
diagnostic studies for, 5536
high risk categories for, 5532–5535, *5533–5535*
historical aspects of, 5529–5530
of algal origin, 5553–5554
of bacterial origin, 5548–5551, 5549*t*
of deep space, 5539–5543, *5540–5543*
of fascia, 5543–5544
of fungal origin, 5551–5553
of parasitic origin, 5553–5554
of protozoan origin, 5553–5554
of viral origin, 5553, *5554*
organisms in, 5531–5532
osteomyelitis, 5546–5548
septic arthritis, 5545–5546, *5547*
subcutaneous, 5537–5539, *5537–5539*
tenosynovitis of, 5544–5545, *5545, 5546*
treatment of
by surgical techniques, 5536–5537, *5537*
principles of, 5535–5536
Hand prosthesis
esthetic considerations in, 4388–4389, *4390*
fitting of, vs. reconstruction for, 4389–4390, *4391–4392*
partial passive, 4402–4403, *4403*
passive, for total hand amputation, 4403, *4404*, 4405
Hand reconstruction
after burn injury
for dorsal contractures, 5458, 5460–5461, *5460*
for first web space adduction contractures, 5461, *5463, 5464*
for joint deformities, 5465–5467, *5466*
for postburn syndactyly, 5456, 5458, *5457–5460*
for volar contractures, 5464–5465, *5465*
general principles of, 5453, *5454, 5455*, 5456
historical aspects of, 5452–5453
web space contractures and, 5456, *5457, 5458*
by toe to hand transfer, 5178, *5179*
for bone tumors, 5521–5522, 5524–5528, *5523–5527*
for burn injuries, of complex deformities, 5469
of volar surface, 4366, *4367*
vs. prosthetic fitting, 4389–4390, *4391*
Hand surgery
anesthesia for, 4290–4291
draping for, 4292–4293, *4293*
dressings for, 4297–4299, *4297, 4298*
functioning muscle transfer. *See* Functioning muscle transfer.
general principles of
for operating room, 4289–4299, *4291–4298*
in emergency room, 4285–4289, *4286–4289*
harvesting of reconstructive tissues for, 4295–4297, *4296*
historical aspects of, 5213–5216, *5214*
instrumentation for, 4290
local anesthesia for, 4294
microvascular reconstructive toe to hand transfer
historical aspects of, 5153–5154
indications for, 5154–5156
operative procedure for, *4294*, 4294–4295
pneumatic tourniquet for, 4291
postoperative care for, 4299–4300, *4300*
preparation for, 4291–4294, *4291, 4292*
regional anesthesia for, choice of, *4305*, 4305–4308, 4306*t*, 4307*t*
Hand surgery *(Continued)*
tourniquet for, 4294
wound closure for, 4295, *4295*
Hand-Schüller-Christian disease, 3352
Hansen's disease, 5550
Hard palate
cancers of, 3452, 3455
reconstruction of, 1457, *1459–1463*, 1463
superoinferior occlusal views of, 887, *891, 892*
Harelip, 2438
Haversian canal, 583, *584*
HDPE (high density polyethylene), 711–712
Head
cancers of
interdisciplinary management of, 3412–3413
public education programs for, 3412
cutaneous arteries of, 355, *356, 357*, 358
embryology of, 2456–2460, *2457–2459*
of neural crest, 2461–2462, 2464–2465, 2466–2469, *2462–2464, 2466, 2468*
of peripheral nervous system, 2473–2475
of skeletal tissues, 2487–2489, 2491
of visceral arches and tongue, 2469*t*, 2469–2470, *2471*
origins of voluntary muscles, 2472–2473
pituitary gland development, 2475, *2477*, 2478
vascular development in, 2470, 2472, *2472*
injuries of, 870, *870*
pediatric tumors of
benign, 3181–3184, *3183*
developmental anomalies, 3178–3181, *3179–3181*
inflammatory masses of, 3176–3178
late sequelae of therapy for, 3188, *3188*
malignant, 3184–3188, *3188*
preoperative evaluation of, 3175–3176
radiographic imaging of, 3176, *3177*
proportions of, *29*, 29–30
soft tissue sarcomas of, 3366, 3368
Headaches, retro-orbital, in internal derangement of temporomandibular joint, 1482
Healing
by secondary intention, 1929
intrinsic vs. extrinsic, 531–532
of bone
in lower extremity, 4057–4058, *4060*, 4061
mechanism of, 197–198
of tendon graft, tendon, physiology of, 530–532, *531*
of wounds. *See* Wound healing.
Hearing problems
from hemangiomas, 3207
in microtia, 2096–2097, *2097*
Heat, applications of, for extravasation injury, 5442
Heel, soft tissue coverage of, 4082, *4083–4087*, 4085, 4087
Heister mouth prop, 1481, *1481*
Helical rim of auricle
deformities of, from burns, repair of, 2206–2207, *2207, 2208*
regional defects of, acquired, 2131, *2133–2135*, 2135
Hemangioendothelioma, of hand, 5504–5505
Hemangiomas
capillary
classification of, 3192
clinical presentation of, 3582–3583, *3583*
granular type of, 3204–3206, *3205*
of arm, 5502, *5502*

Hemangiomas *(Continued)*
capillary-cavernous
argon laser therapy for, 3668, *3668*
carbon dioxide laser therapy for, 3670
carbon dioxide laser therapy for, 3669–3670, *3670, 3671*
cavernous, 3583–3584, *3583*
classification of, 3193, 3193*t*
clinical presentation of, in hand, 5315–5316
complication of, in proliferation phase, *3206–3209*, 3206–3210
cutaneous-visceral, with congestive heart failure, 3217–3219, *3218*
differential diagnosis of
by clinical methods, 3201, 3203, *3202*
by radiographic methods, *3203, 3203–3204, 3204*
pyogenic granuloma and, 3204–3206, *3205*
differentiation from vascular malformations, 3193–3194
incidence of, 3199–3200
involution phase of, 3210–3212, *3210–3212*
multiple, 3200–3201, *3201*
of hand, 5501, 5502, 5502*t*
of jaw, 3352–3353, *3354–3355*
of orbit, 1653, 1655, *1655*
pathogenesis of, 3194–3199, *3195–3198*
angiogenesis dependency and, 3199
animal models of, 3194–3195
hormones and, 3199
involution, light and electron microscopy of, 3197, *3198*
proliferation
electron microscopy of, 3196–3197, *3197*
light microscopy of, 3195–3196, *3195–3196*
pathology of, 3584
port-wine. *See* Port-wine stains.
signs of, first, 3200, *3200*
treatment of
by laser therapy, 3219
by operative methods, 3219–3220, *3220–3224*, 3221–3222
chemotherapy for, 3215–3216
for emergent problems in proliferation phase, 3216–3219, *3217*
for Kasabach-Merritt syndrome, 3219
for local complications of bleeding and ulceration, 3214
historical aspects of, 3212–3213
in hand, 5316, *5317*
in salivary glands, 3299–3300, *3300*
in subglottic region, 3216–3217
primum non nocere, 3213–3214
steroid therapy for, 3214–3215, *3215*
with thrombocytopenia, 3584
Hemangiopericytoma
in children, 3187
of head and neck, 3369–3371, *3370*
Hemangiosarcomas, of hand, 5505
Hematocrit, blood flow and, 448, *448*
Hematologic disorders, craniosynostosis of, *99*, 99–100
Hematomas
after blepharoplasty, 2350–2351
after facialplasty, of male, 2393–2396
after forehead-brow lift, 2406
after orbital or nasoethmoido-orbital fractures, 1105–1106
from augmentation mammoplasty, 3885
Hematomas *(Continued)*
from orthognathic surgery, 1404
retrobulbar, after orbital and nasoethmoido-orbital fractures, 1103
Hemifacial hyperplasia, *1298–1299*, 1300–1301
Hemifacial microsomia, pathogenesis of, 2491, *2492*, 2493
Hemihypertrophy, gigantism of, 5365, 5371, *5370–5371*
Hemimandibular transplants, 201–203, *202*
Hemocoagulation, 178
Hemodynamic theories, of vascular malformation pathogenesis, 3226–3227
Hemodynamics, normal control of blood flow, 447–449, *448, 449*
Hemoglobin absorption curve, *3664*
Hemorrhage
in facial wounds, emergency treatment for, 876–877, *878*
in mandibular fracture treatment, 975
postoperative, 1881
Hemostasis, 48
Heparin
anticoagulation by, 458
for treatment of cold injury, 857
topical, 459
Hereditary hemorrhagic telangiectasia, 3227, 3238–3239, *3238*
Hereditary progressive arthro-ophthalmopathy, 73, 93, 3129
Heredity, in causation of craniofacial clefts, 2931
Hernias, abdominal, abdominal wall reconstruction for, *3761*, 3770–3772
Herpes simplex infections
of hand, 5553, *5554*
oral cancer and, 3418
Heterotopic ossification, in hand burns, 5473, 5476, *5477*
hGH. *See* Human growth hormone.
Hidden penis, 4177–4179, *4178, 4179*
Hidradenoma papilliferum, 3577
High density polyethylene (HDPE), 711–712
Hips
contour deformities of
classification of, *3999*, 4000
suctioning techniques for, 4004, 4015, 4017
type IV, 4002, *4009, 4010*
type V, suction-lipectomy of, 4002, 4004, *4013*
type VI, suction-assisted lipectomy for, 4004, *4014*
type VII, suction-assisted lipectomy for, 4004, *4015*
suction-assisted lipectomy of, complications of, 3978
Histiocytoma, 3578–3579, *3579*
Histiocytosis X, disorders of, 3351–3352
Histocompatibility antigens (HLA)
genetics of, 187, 187–188, *188*
keloid formation and, 735
testing of, 188–189
transplant rejection and, 190
transplantation and, 187
History of plastic surgery, 2–*22*
during early twentieth century, 8–18
during first half of nineteenth century, 7
during Renaissance, 3–*4*
during World War II and postwar era, 18–20
in ancient times, *2-3*
in seventeenth and eighteenth centuries, 4
rebirth of, 4–7, *7*
skin grafting, 7–8

HLA. *See* Histocompatibility antigens (HLA).
Hockeystick incision, 1843–1844
Hodgkin's lymphoma, staging classification for, 3185
Holocrine glands. *See* Sebaceous glands.
Holoprosencephaly
  dysmorphic facies associated with, *73*
  embryogenesis of, 2458, 2517, *2517*, 2926, *2926*
  fetal alcohol syndrome, pathogenesis of, 2458–2459, *2458, 2459*
  malformation sequence in, 72, 72*t*
  MNP deficiencies and, 2529
  types of, 2935, 2935*t*
Homans-Miller procedure, 5028, *5028, 5029*
Horizontal buttresses, 1021
Hormones
  breast development and, 3841–3842, *3842*
  for transsexualism therapy, 4240–4241
Horner's syndrome, 1754
  as nerve block complication, 4307
  development of, after brachial plexus block, 4313–4314
Hubbard tank immersion, for treatment of generalized cold injury, *863*, 863–864
Human growth hormone (hGH), 798
Human papillomavirus
  malignant transformation of, 3563
  types of, 3561*t*
Humby knife, 237, *237*
Hurler syndrome, 84, *88*, 98
Hyaluronidase (Wydase), 5442
Hydralazine, postoperative treatment of skin flaps, 316
Hydrocephalus, in craniosynostosis, 3025
Hydrodistention, for vasospasm, 456
Hydrofluoric acid burns, 5437, *5437, 5438*
  treatment of, 5437–5438
Hydrogel, 722–723, *723*, *724*
Hydron, 805
Hydroxyapatite, for alloplastic implants, 715–716, *716*, 725, *726*
Hydroxyzine, 4315
Hyperabduction maneuver, 5002, *5002*
Hyperalimentation, for thermal burn patients, 798–799, *799*, 800*t*, 800–801
Hyperbaric oxygen, for postoperative skin flap treatment, 318
Hyperhidrosis, from cold injury, 858
Hyperkalemia, from fluid resuscitation, 793, 795
Hypernasality, functional/hysterical, velopharyngeal incompetence and, 2906–2907
Hypernatremia, from fluid resuscitation, 793, 794–795
Hyperostosis, gigantism of, 5365, *5368–5369*
Hyperpigmentation
  after dermabrasion, 780–781
  after facialplasty in male, 2399
  blotchy, after chemical peeling, 770
  chemical peeling for, 758, *760, 761*
  familial, after blepharoplasty, 2349
Hyperplasia
  cellular, 242–243
  facial, *1300*, 1301
Hypersensitivity, delayed, from injectable collagen, 783
Hypertelorism, orbital, post-traumatic, 1088, 1625, 1628, *1628*
Hyperthyroidism
  orbital pathology in, 1630
  "scleral show" of, 2327, 2328, 2330, *2328*
  spasm of Müller's muscle in, 2327, 2328, *2328*, 2330
Hypertonic solutions
  extravasation injuries from, 5440
  of saline, for fluid resuscitation, 793
Hypertrophic scars
  after chemical peeling, 769, *770, 771*
  biochemical observations of, 735–738
  dermabrasion for, 773–774, *774–776*
  diagnosis of, 738
  formation of
    after dermabrasion, 781
    after thermal burn injury, 810
    causes of, 172, *173*
    in split-thickness donor site, 246–247
  from hand burns, 5458, 5460–5461, *5462*
  inhibition of, by mechanical pressure, 740–741
  microvasculature of, 735
  vs. keloids, 732, *733*, 737–738
Hypertrophy syndromes, with vascular malformations, 3258–3260, *3260–3263*, 3263–3264
Hypodermis, anatomy of, 224
Hypoglossal nerve
  anatomy of, 3280, *3280*
  injury of, from salivary gland surgery, 3314
Hypoglossal-facial nerve anastomoses, for facial paralysis, 2277–2278, 2278*t*, *2278–2282*, 2281, 2283–2284
Hyponatremia, from fluid resuscitation, 793, 794, 795
Hypopharynx
  anatomy of, 3416, *3416*
  cancers of, 3460–3462, *3461*
Hypoplasia
  condylar, *1291*, 1292, *1293*, 1294
  mandibular, 1260. *See also* Mandibular hypoplasia.
    variations of, functional disturbances associated with, 1262
  maxillary, 1360
    preoperative planning for, 1362, *1362*
Hypospadias
  anatomic description of, 4156, *4156*
  complications of, 4166–4167
  embryology of, 4154–4155
  incidence of, 4155
  one-stage repairs for, 4159–4161, *4160*
    by flip-flap method
      with distal flap chordee, 4162–4163, *4163*
      without chordee, 4161–4162, *4162*
    by meatal advancement glansplasty, 4161, *4161*
    by repair of proximal shaft, using full-thickness skin graft, 4163–4164, *4164*
    by vascularized preputial island flap, 4164–4165, *4165*
  postoperative care for, 4165–4166
  preoperative considerations for, 4157
  two-stage repairs of, techniques for, 4157–4159, *4158, 4159*
Hypothenar muscles, 4271–4272, *4272, 4273*
Hypothenar space infections, 5543
Hypothermia
  acute, 859
  chronic, 859
  subacute, 859
  systemic
    late sequelae of, 864–865
    pathophysiology of, 862
    physiologic responses in, 860*t*-861*t*
    predisposing diseases, 858
    treatment of, 862–864, *863*

Hypothermia *(Continued)*
with frostbite, 865
Hypotonia
in Down syndrome, 3163
Robin sequence and, 94
Hypovolemic shock, 4330
prevention of, after thermal burn injury, 791
Hypoxia
abnormal scar formation and, 735
and pathogenesis of cleft lip/palate, 2533
Hypoxia-selectivity hypothesis, of abnormal scar formation, 736–737

Ibuprofen, 317
Iliac bone grafts
for frontal bone repair and contouring, 1564–1565, *1565*
for mandibular defect, *1444–1446*
for secondary rhinoplasty, 1911
nonvascularized type of, 605
for children, 610, 612, *609–611*
technique of, 606, 608, 610, *606–608*
vascularized, 612
vs. split rib grafts, for mandibular defects, 1422, *1431*
Iliac crest free flap, 603
Imbibition, serum, 250–252
Imidazole, 317
Immunogenicity, of alloplastic implants, 702
Immunoglobulins, classes of, 191
Immunologic tolerance, 194
Immunology
defects of, in Down syndrome, 3161–3162
graft survival and, 193–194
in abnormal scar formation, 733, 735, 735*t*
of thermal burn injury, 801–802
Immunosuppressant drugs, 195–196
Immunosuppression
basal cell carcinoma and, 3617, 3619
modification of allograft rejection mechanism, 194–196
orthotopic composite tissue allografts with, 203*t*
squamous cell carcinoma and, 3629
transplantation and, 194–196
Immunotherapy, for malignant melanoma, 3651–3652
Implants. *See* Alloplastic implants; *specific implants.*
exposure of, 505–506
failure of, 505
for augmentation mammoplasty, 3884–3885
for reconstruction of orbital floor fracture, 1075–1077, *1077*
historical aspects of, 54–55
osteointegrated, for retention of denture, in reconstructed mandible, 1456
Impotence
nonsurgical treatment options for, 4219
pathophysiology of, 4213–4215, *4214, 4215*
surgical treatment options for, 4219–4220
Imuran (azathioprine), 195
Incisions
bicoronal, *1592*, 1593
bicoronal scalp, 1657, 1659
choice of site for, 44
conjunctival, 1594, *1595*
Converse subciliary, *1035*, 1072

Incisions *(Continued)*
coronal, 1098, 1100–1101, *1099–1101*
external, for rhinoplasty, 1847
eyelid
transconjunctival, 1593–1594, *1594*
transcutaneous, 1593, *1593, 1594*
for abdominal wall reconstruction, 3763–3764
for classical radical neck dissection, *3429*, 3429–3430
for face lift, 2369–2370, *2370*
for facialplasty, in male, 2392–2393
for flexor tendon repair, 4522–4524
for forehead-brow lift, 2400, *2401*, 2402
for full abdominoplasty, 3937, 3939, *3942 3945*
labiobuccal vestibular, 1226, *1226*, 1363
lateral brow, 1594, *1595*
local types of
general considerations for, 4443, *4443*
midlateral, *4442*, 4442–4443
on dorsum of hand, 4443
zigzag, 4441–4442, *4442*
medial canthal, 1594, *1595*
midlateral, *4442*, 4442–4443
mucogingival, 1226, *1226*, 1363
of lower extremity, 374
preauricular, 1227
submandibular, 1225, *1237*
technique for making, 48
to expose orbital floor, *1035*, 1072–1073, *1073*
transcartilaginous nasal tip, 1844, *1845*
vertical midline nasal, 1097–1098
Incisive foramen/papilla, 2726, *2726*
Inclusion cysts
of hand, 5485–5486, *5486*
of nail bed or distal phalanx, *4510*, 4511
Inderal (propranolol), 315, 4910
Indomethacin, 317
Induction, primary embryonic, *2453*, 2454
Inert buried appliances, for mandibular fixation, 3507–3508
Infant(s). *See also* Children.
feeding problems of
for cleft palate infant, 2731
in Robin sequence, 3128
orthostatic feeding of, 3130–3131
soft tissue injuries in, 1154–1155
Infection
after treatment of mandibular fractures, 976
craniofacial cleft formation and, 2928
effect on patency of microvascular anastomoses, 454
from orthognathic surgery, 1404–1405, *1408*
from radiation injury, 835–836, *836, 837*
postoperative, 1881. *See under specific surgical procedure.*
after tissue expansion, 505
from maxillary tumor surgery, 3332
potentiation of, by alloplastic implant, 703
Inflammatory lesions, of perionychium, 4512
Inflammatory mediators, 4897
Infraclavicular block, performance of, *4319*, 4320
Infraorbital nerve
anatomic relations of, 996, *996*
injury of, 1131
Infraorbital nerve block, 147–148, *147, 148*, 1609–1610, *1610*
after orbital or nasoethmoido-orbital fractures, 1106–1107

Infratemporal fossa tumors
low, 3397, 3401, *3398–3400*
superior, *3396*, 3397
Inguinal artery, anatomy of, 4033–4044, *4034*
Inhalation injury, from thermal burns, treatment of, *796*, 796–797
Inheritance
autosomal dominant, 104, *105*
sporadicity in, *110*
autosomal recessive, 104, 106, *106*
sporadicity in, *110*
multifactorial, 107–109
X-linked dominant, 107, *108, 109*
X-linked recessive, 106–107, *107*
Initial segment, 635
Injections, of chemicals or drugs, injuries from, 5439–5443, *5441*
Innervation, of skeletal muscle, 547–549, *547, 548*
Inspiratory muscles, anatomy of, 3677, *3677*
Insulin levels, in morbid obesity, *3971–3973*
Intercostobrachial nerve, anatomy of, 4314
Intercrural distance, 1802–1803, *1803*
Interdigital web space
anatomy of, *5280*
correction of, evolution of methods for, *5282–5287*
release of, 5289–5292
Interfragment wiring, chain-link fence technique, 1121, *1122*
Inter-island contraction phenomenon, 773
Interleukin 1, 190
Intermaxillary fixation
monomaxillary vs. bimaxillary, 930
splints in maintenance of, 929–930, *930*
Internal fixation, rigid, of mandible fractures
complications of, 965
intraoral approaches, 965, *966*
Internal nasal valve, 1786, *1788*, 1808, *1808*, 1925
Internervous planes concept, 4759–4760
Internuncial pool theory, of reflex sympathetic dystrophy, 4898–4900
Interorbital distance, measurement of, 2986, *2986*
Interorbital space, 1083, *1084*
Interosseous nerve syndrome, anterior. *See* Anterior interosseous nerve syndrome.
Interosseous wire fixation, for small joint arthrodesis, 4674–4675, *4675*
Interosseous wiring techniques, for edentulous mandible fracture, 971, *972*
Interphalangeal joint
anatomy of, 4255, 4258, 4655–4656, *4656, 4657*
arthrodesis of, indications for, of small joints, 4671. *See also* Arthrodesis
distal, degenerative arthritis of, 4699–4700
hyperextension of, 4261
pathophysiology of, 4655–4656, *4656, 4657*
proximal, degenerative arthritis of, 4700–4701
stiffness of
age and, 4661
anatomic restoration for, 4663, *4664*
from edema, 4657–4658
from immobility, 4656–4657
from mechanical obstruction, 4661, *4661*
from scar contracture, 4658–4661, *4659–4661*
hand therapy for, 4665–4666, *4666, 4667*
mobilization vs. immobilization for, 4663–4665, *4664, 4665*
motivational effects on, 4661–4663, *4662, 4663*
Interphalangeal joint *(Continued)*
stiffness of, surgical release for, 4667–4670, *4668*, 4669
Interpolation flaps, *29*, 277, *277*, 290, 292
Interscalene block
complications of, 4307*t*, 4307–4308
extent of analgesia from, 4306–4307
performance of, 4316, *4317*
Intersection syndrome, 4739
Intestinal flaps, for vaginal reconstruction, 4206–4207
Intra-arterial injections, of calcium gluconate, for acid burns, 5438
Intracapsular edema, 1479–1480, *1480, 1481*
Intracranial pressure
in head injury patients, 870, *870*
increased, in craniosynostosis, 3025
Intramedullary bone graft, for small joint arthrodesis, 4677
Intranasal block, 152–153, *152, 153*
Intranasal lining remnants, for restoration of nasal lining, 1979, *1980*
Intranasal prostheses, 3543–3545, 3549, *3543–3548, 3550*
Intraoperative monitoring, of craniofacial surgery, 2975–2976, *2976*
Intraoral appliances, for edentulous mandible fracture, 971, *971*
Intrauterine deformation, malformation sequence of, *75*
Intrinsic-plus test, for ischemic contracture evaluation, 5046, *5047*
Intubation, indications for, in inhalation injury, *796*, 796–797
Invagination procedure, for nasal tip, 1854, 1856, *1855*
Iron chelators, for prevention of abnormal scars, 740
Ischemia
secondary to vasospasm, 5018–5019
to peripheral digits, 5009
Ischemia-inducing agents, extravasation injuries from, 5440
Ischemic contractures
of intrinsic muscles of hand
clinical experience with, 5041–5042
etiology of, 5041–5042
finger deformities in, classification of, 5044–5046, *5045*, 5045*t*
historical aspects of, 5041
intrinsic-plus test for, 5046, *5047*
pathophysiology of, 5042, 5044, *5043*
surgical correction of, 5048–5051, *5049*
thumb deformities of, 5045*t*, 5046, *5048*
Volkmann's. *See* Volkmann's ischemic contracture.
Ischium, pressure sores of, 3823, 3823*t*, *3824–3826*, 3826
Island flaps
dorsal radial innervated, for soft tissue injuries of thumb, 5100, *5102*
midline forehead, for nasal reconstruction, 1958
neurovascular, 4860
for soft tissue injuries of thumb, 5095, 5097, *5096, 5097*
of innervated dorsal thumb, for soft tissue injuries of thumb, 5104, *5104*
of lower extremity, 374
of scalp, for eyebrow reconstruction, 2219–2222, *2220*
Isograft, 54
Isoxsuprine, postoperative treatment of skin flaps, 315–316

Jaw
acquired deformities of, 1189, 1412–1463
adenomatoid odontogenic tumor of, 3342
ameloblastic fibroma of, 3342, 3345
congenital deformities of, 1188
hemifacial hyperplasia, *1298–1299*, 1300–1301
in craniofacial microsomia, 3056, *3062*
cysts of
classification of, 3337
developmental odontogenic, 3337–3339
management of, 3340
developmental deformities of. *See under* Mandible, developmental deformities of; Maxilla, deformities of.
developmental malformations of, 1188–1189
fibrous dysplasia of, 3347–3348, *3349*
growth of, after surgical repair of cleft lip/palate, *2563*, 2564–2565
initial assessment of, 1189–1200
muscular incoordination of, 1478
nonodontogenic tumors of, 3346–3348, *3349–3350, 3351–3353, 3354, 3355, 3356, 3357, 3358*, 3359–3360
benign fibrous and fibro-osseous lesions of, 3347–3348, *3349, 3350*, 3351–3353
primary malignancies of, 3353, 3356, 3359–3360, *3354, 3355, 3357, 3358*
odontogenic cysts of, inflammatory, 3339–3340
odontogenic tumors of, 3340
epithelial, 3341–3342, *3343, 3344*, 3345
surgery of. *See* Orthognathic surgery.
tumors of, surgical treatment for, 3371, 3373
Jaw deformity, in craniofacial microsomia, 3064–3066, *3064–3066*
Joint(s). *See also specific types of joints.*
deformities of, after hand burn injury, 5465–5467, *5466*
in electrical burn injuries, 5425–5426
repair of, perichondrial grafts for, 574–575, *576*
salvaging of, for hand reconstruction, 4297
Joint effusion, 4658
Jones I test, 1729
Jones II test, 1729–1730
Joseph knife, 1818, *1819*
Joseph tip operation, 1844–1845, *1845*
Joule's law, 814–815
Juri flap, 1528–1529, *1529*

Kaposi's sarcoma, *5009*, 5009–5010
Karapandizic technique, for lower lip reconstruction, 2021, *2023*
Karfik facial cleft classification, 2933*t*, 2934
Karyotype, 100, *101–103*
Kasabach-Merritt syndrome, 3207–3209, *3208*, 3219, 3584
Kazanjian button, 927, *928*
Kazanjian technique, for nasal lining restoration, 1979, *1980*
Keloids
after blepharoplasty, 2350
biochemical observations of, 735–738
diagnosis of, 738
formation of, *733, 734*
causes of, 172, *172*, 175
immune system and, 735, 735*t*
Keloids *(Continued)*
from orthognathic surgery, 1411
microvasculature of, 735
on earlobe, 2141
recurrence of, 742
treatment modalities for, 738–741, *739*
vs. hypertrophic scars, 732, *733*, 737–738
Kent prosthesis, for temporomandibular ankylosis, *1495*, 1495–1496
Keratoacanthoma
clinical presentation of, 3607–3608, *3608*
of hand, 5486–5487, *5487*
Keratotic lesions, dermabrasion of, 774
Ketamine, 157–158, 4315
Kienböck's disease
description of, 4643–4644, *4644*
radiographic staging of, 4644*t*
treatment of, 4644–4645
Kinin system, role in rejection mechanism, 192
Kirschner wire fixation
for mandible fractures, 948, 958
for small joint arthrodesis, 4673, *4674*
for stabilization of proximal phalanx fractures, 4601–4602, *4602*
Kleeblattschädel anomaly, 3018, *3018*, 3025
Klippel-Feil syndrome
cleft palate and, 2547
clinical aspects of, 3144–3145
etiopathogenesis of, 3145–3146
treatment of, 3146
Klippel-Trenaunay syndrome, 3259–3260, *3260*, 5318–5319, *5318*
Knee
anatomy of, 4032
cutaneous arteries of, *371*, 372
suction-assisted lipectomy of, 4019, 4021, *4020, 4022, 4024*
complications of, 3978
Knuckle pads
clinical presentation of, 5486, *5486*
Dupuytren's disease and, 5055, 5061
Köle procedure, for closure of anterior open bite, 1356, *1357*
Krause end bulb, 652
Krönlein-Berke operation, *1634*, 1636
Krukenberg operation, for below elbow amputation, 4342–4343
Kufner procedure, for closure of anterior open bite, 1358, *1358, 1359*, 1360
Kutler lateral V-Y flaps, for coverage of digital amputation stumps, 4487–4488, *4488*

Labiobuccal sulcus, restoration of, by skin graft inlay technique, *1452, 1453*, 1457
Labyrinth, membranous, embryology of, 3058
Lacerations
facial, management of, 904, *905, 906*
of lips, 912, *913*
of nose, 909, *910*
of parotid duct, 906–907, *906–908*
Lacrimal apparatus
injury of, 1671
interruption of continuity of, after orbital or nasoethmoido-orbital fractures, 1105

Lacrimal apparatus *(Continued)*
malfunction of, in nasoethmoido-orbital fractures, 1614
repair of, 1730–1734, 1736–1737, *1730–1733, 1735–1738*
Lacrimal gland, prolapse of, *2333*, 2333–2334
Lacrimal pump mechanism, 1675, 1677, *1677*
Lacrimal system
diagnostic tests for, 1729–1730
excretory deformities and developmental defects of, 1728–1729, *1728, 1729*
injuries of, in nasoethmoido-orbital fractures, 1611, *1611*
injury to, reestablishment of continuity of, 1617
lacerations of, 907
reconstruction of, anatomic considerations for, 1725–1728, *1726, 1727*
Lactation fistula, after augmentation mammoplasty, 3889
Lactic dehydrogenase, in keloids, 735
Lag screw fixation, for mandible fractures, 961, *963–965*
Lagophthalmos, 1751–1752, *1752, 1753*
after forehead-brow lift, 2410
nonsurgical management of, 2307
Langer, Karl, *215*, 215–216
Langerhans' cells, 198
Langer's lines
anatomy of, 42, *42*, 216, *216, 217*
scar appearance and, 741–742, *742, 743*
Lanugo hair, 1519
Laryngocele, 3180
Larynx
anatomy of, 3416, *3416*
cancers of, management of, 3462, 3465–3467, *3463, 3464*
Laser Doppler, for flap perfusion assessment, 319*t*, 320–321
Laser light scanner, for preoperative planning, 1214–1215, *1215*
Laser therapy
argon, lesions amenable to, 3667–3669, *3667–3669*
carbon dioxide, lesions amenable to, 3669–3670, *3670*
components of optical system for, 3664–36676, *3665*
for hemangiomas, 3219
for lesions amenable to both carbon dioxide and argon lasers, 3670–3672, *3672*
lesions unresponsive to, 3672
physics principles of, 3663*t*, 3663–3667
Lateral brow incision, 1594, *1595*
Lateral calcaneal artery fasciocutaneous flap, for soft tissue coverage of heel and midplantar area, 4085, *4087*
Lateral canthoplasty, 1717–1719, *1719–1726*
Lateral canthotomy, for eyelid laceration correction, 1687, *1687*
Lateral canthus deformities, treatment of, 1609
Lateral femoral cutaneous nerve, 608, *608*
Lateral maxillary buttresses, 1021
Lateral nasal process
embryological development of, 2519, 2523, 2525–2526, *2522, 2525, 2527*
in embryogenesis of cleft lip, 2526, 2528, *2528*
Lateral nasal prominences, embryological development of, 2482
Lateral pharyngeal wall extrusion, maximal, level of, 2729
Lateral pterygoid muscle, 937
Lateral scalp flaps, 1529–1530, *1530*
Laterognathism, 1289–1290, 1292
Latham pin-retained appliance, for cleft palate, 2888, 2890, *2890*
Lathyrism, 180–181
Latissimus dorsi flap
anatomy of, 389–390, *390*
description of, 3448, *3449*
for abdominal wall defects, 397
for breast reconstruction, 3911–3914, 3916, *3912–3916*
for cheek reconstruction, 2047–2048
for chest wall reconstruction, 396, 3689–3691, *3689, 3690, 3692*
for mediastinal reconstruction, 396
for microneurovascular transfer, 2299
for soft tissue coverage, 4454–4456, *4455–4456*
for trunk coverage, 502–503
in head and neck reconstruction, 387
postoperative lumbar hernia and, 3771
Latissimus dorsi muscle, anatomy of, 3912–3913
Lazy-T procedure, for ectropion correction, 1746–1749, *1747–1750*
LDPE (low density polyethylene), 710–711
Le Fort fractures
Adams fixation of, 1019–1020, *1020*
classification of, 1012–1015, *1013, 1014*, 1022
complications of, 1030–1032
goals of treatment for, 1021–1022, *1021–1024*
in children, 1164–1165, *1165*, 1179–1180, 1182–1183, *1179–1181*
level I, stabilization of, 1024
level II, 1028
level II and III, stabilization of, 1026–1027, *1027*
simple level I, 1027–1028
Le Fort I advancement osteotomy, *1377, 1378*, 1379
Le Fort I osteotomy, 1369, 1371–1373, *1369–1372, 1374, 1375*, 3119
for correction of short face deformity, 1384, 1386–1387, *1385–1388*
for maxillary retrusion from cleft lip or palate, 2835, 2838, 2839, *2835, 2836, 2839*
to correct long face deformity, 1381, 1384, *1381–1383*
Le Fort II advancement, for craniosynostosis, 3045, *3046*
Le Fort II osteotomy
for maxillary retrusion from cleft lip or palate, *2837, 2838*, 2838–2839
for nasomaxillary hypoplasia, 1399, *1399–1401*, 1401
Le Fort III advancement osteotomy
for craniosynostosis, 3037
through subcranial route, for craniosynostosis, 3037–3039, *3038, 3039*
Le Fort III osteotomy
in growing child, for craniosynostosis treatment, 3039, *3041*
performed through a combined intracranial approach, for craniosynostosis treatment, 3039, *3042, 3043*
with Le Fort I osteotomy, for craniosynostosis, 3039, 3043, *3044*
Leg
anatomy of, compartments of, 4032–4033, *4033*
cutaneous arteries of, *369, 370*, 372–373
Leiomyosarcoma, in head and neck, 3371
Lentigines, 3587–3588
Lentigo maligna, *3598*, 3598–3599

Lentigo malignant melanoma, 3639, *3639*
Leprosy, 4964, 5550
Letterer-Siwe syndrome, 3352
Leukocyte typing, 188–189
Leukoderma acquistium centrifugum, 3591–3592, *3592*
Leukoplakia, 3596–3598, *3597*
  oral cancer and, 3419
Leukotrienes, 309
Levator aponeurosis, 1678–1679, *1679*
Levator eminence, 2619, 2623, 2727
Levator palatini muscles
  anatomy of, 2726, *2727*, 2728
  disorientation of, in cleft palate, 2729, *2730*
Levator palpebrae superioris, anatomy of, 1678–1680, *1679*
Levator resection, 1759, *1759*
  for ptosis, 1766–1767, *1768–1771*, 1772
Levator veli palatini
  in cleft palate, 2615, *2616–2618*
  normal, *2612, 2613*, 2614–2615
Lid magnets, for eyelid paralysis, 2310
Ligaments, of metacarpotrapezial joint, 4257, *4257*
Limb allografts
  primate, 201, *201*
  rejection of, 198–200
Limberg flap, modified, for cheek reconstruction, 2038–2040, *2039–2043*, 2042
Limberg operation, for anterior open bite correction, 1355, *1356*
Limbs, allografted, growth of, 200–201
Lines
  Langer's, 42, *42*, 216, *216, 217*, 741–742, *742, 743*
  of expression, 43–44, *43*
  of minimal tension, 43, *43*
  of skin relaxation, 43, *43*
  of skin tension
    cleavage lines and, 218, *218*
    hypertrophic scar formation and, 741
    scar appearance and, 741–742, *742, 743*
Lingual artery, injury of, from salivary gland surgery, 3314
Lingual flap
  anatomic considerations for, 3478–3480, *3479*
  from dorsum of tongue, 3480
    anteriorly based, 3481, 3483, 3488, *3483–3488*
    bipedicle transverse, 3488–3489, *3488, 3489*
    posteriorly based, 3480–3481, *3480–3482*
  from tip of tongue, 3489–3490, 3492–3493, *3490–3494*
  from ventral surface of tongue, *3494, 3494–3495, 3495*
Lingual nerve
  anatomy of, 3280, *3280*
  injury of, from salivary gland surgery, 3314
Lip(s)
  anatomy of, *2009–2011*, 2009–2012
    in cleft lip and palate, 2583
  closure techniques of, crossflap method of, 2438
  drawing of, *34, 35*
  electrical burns of, *2230*, 2231
  lacerations of, 912, *913*
  landmark abnormalities of, repair of, 2789–2790, *2789, 2790*
  lower
    burn injuries of, 2187–2188, *2189*
Lip(s) *(Continued)*
  lower, hypotonia of, surgical correction in Down syndrome, 3169–3170
    reconstruction of, 2011–2016, *2014–2026*, 2018, 2020–2021, 2023–2025, 2027
    staircase or stepladder reconstruction technique for, 2016, *2018*
  muscles of, 2598–2600, *2599*
  reconstruction of, abnormal facial growth and, 2565–2568, *2566–2568*
  scars on, from unilateral cleft repair, *2772*, 2773, *2774*, 2775
  upper
    burns of, 2183–2187, *2186*
    esthetic unit and subunits of, 2184
    reconstruction of, 2027–2028, *2027–2037*, 2030–2031, 2037
    resurfacing of, 2185–2187, *2186*
    skin grafting of, 2184–2185
Lip adhesion
  for bilateral cleft lip, 2704, *2704, 2705*, 2706
  for premaxilla deformity, in bilateral cleft lip, 2659, *2660*
  historical aspects of, 2632
  in treatment for cleft/lip palate in newborn, 2888, *2889*
  technical aspects of, *2634, 2635, 2635*
Lip deformities
  from bilateral cleft lip repair, 2840–2841
    of horizontal deficiency or tight lip, 2844, 2849, 2851, *2850*
    of vertical deficiency or short lip, 2844, *2844–2849*
    of vertical excess or long lip, 2841–2842, 2844, *2841–2843*
    scars from, 2841
  cleft repair
    of horizontal deficiency, *2781–2785*, 2779–2780, 2782–2783, 2785
    vertical deficiency, 2776–2777, *2776–2780*, 2779
    vertical excess, *2774*, 2775–2776
  unilateral cleft lip and palate, 2590
Lipectomy, submental, operative technique for, 2383
Lipoblastomatosis, infantile, 3183–3184
Lipodystrophy, 3136
Lipofibromatosis, nerve-oriented, gigantism of, 5362, 5364, *5363*
Lipoidal histiocytoma, 3578–3579, *3579*
Lipoma
  chest wall reconstruction and, 3714, 3714*t*, *3715*
  of hand, 5499, *5500*
  salivary gland, 3300–3301, *3301*
Lipomatosis, congenital infiltrating, *3183*, 3184
Lipomatous tumors, benign pediatric, *3183*, 3183–3184
Liposarcomas
  in children, 3187
  in head and neck, 3371
Lip-switch flap, 2031, *2035*, 2037, 2648, *2649*, 2651
Livedo reticularis, 3237
LNP, facial clefting and, 2540–2541
Load-deformation curve, 699–700, *700*
Lobule, nasal, anatomy of, 1924, *1925*
Local anesthetic agents
  choice of, 4311–4313
    concentration of, 4312
    volume of, 4311–4312

Local anesthetic agents *(Continued)*
mechanisms of action of, 4308–4309
pharmacokinetics for, 4309*t*, 4309–4310
systemic toxic reactions from, 4310
continuous infusion and, 4311
prevention by epinephrine of, 4310–4311
toxicity of, 4310
Long face deformity, 1381, *1381–1383*, 1384
L-osteotomy
description of, 1266, 1270, *1267*
Wassmund's inverted, of mandibular ramus, 1278–1279, *1279*
Louis-Bar syndrome, 3227, *3238*, 3239
Low density polyethylene (LDPE), 710–711
Lower extremity. *See also specific structure of lower extremity.*
anatomy of
arterial system, 4033–4035, *4034*
bones of, 4031–4032
compartments of, 4032–4033, *4033*
joints of, 4031–4032
nerves, 4035, 4038, *4037*
unique features of, 4031
bone healing in, 4057–4058, 4061, *4060*
cutaneous arteries of, 368, 371–374, *369–371*
lymphatics of, 4094, 4100, *4098, 4099*
nerve injuries of, 4064–4065
open fractures of, 4057–4058, 4061, *4059–4061*
open joint injuries of, 4063–4064
reconstruction of. *See* Lower extremity reconstruction.
soft tissue coverage of, after trauma, *4061*, 4061–4063
tissue expansion of, 503–504, *504*
trauma to, assessment of, 4056–4057
ulcer in, 4076–4077, *4078*, 4079, *4079*
vascular injuries of, 4063, *4063*
Lower extremity reconstruction
after tumor resection, 4079–4080, *4081*
amputation for
postoperative care for, 4074–4075
principles of, 4073–4074
chronic non-union and, 4065, *4066–4068*, 4067
fasciocutaneous flaps for, 4044–4046, *4044–4049*, 4049
for compartment syndromes, 4067–4068
historical aspects of, 4029–4030, *4030*
muscle and musculocutaneous flaps for, 399, *400*, 401
of bone gaps, 4065, *4066–4068*, 4067
osteomyelitis and, 4075–4076
principles of, 4030–4031, *4031*
replantation in, 4068–4069
indications for, 4070–4071
ischemia time and, 4069
nature of amputation injury and, 4070
operative technique for, 4071, 4073
postoperative management for, 4073
replacement of lost tissue in, 4070
salvage technique for, 4071, *4072*
surgical problems of, 4069
zone of injury in, 4069–4070
L-strut, for midline dorsal reconstruction of nose, 1982–1983, *1983*
Luhr plate method of fracture healing, *591*, 591–592
Luhr self-tapping system, 965, *966–967*, 968
Luhr system, 1218, *1219–1222*
Lumbrical muscles, function of, 4270–4271
Lunate
fractures, 4597, *4597*, 4643–4645, *4644, 4645*
load fractures, 4638, *4638*
volar dislocations, 4609
Lung, complications of, after thermal burn injury, 808
Lymph nodes, anatomy of, 3279, *3279*
Lymphadenectomy, for malignant melanoma, 5493–5494
Lymphadenitis, chronic cervical, in pediatric patients, 3177–3178
Lymphadenopathy, in pediatric patients, 3176–3177
Lymphangiectomy, for lymphedema of penis and scrotum, *4182*, 4182–4183
Lymphangiography, 5025–5026
Lymphangioma, 3300, 3585–3586
Lymphangioplasty, for lymphedema of penis and scrotum, 4182
Lymphangitis, of hand, 5538
Lymphatic cysts, midline posterior cervical, aneuploidy and, 3243–3245, *3245*
Lymphatic malformations
abnormalities associated with, 3243–3245, 3247, 3249, *3244–3246, 3248*
clinical findings in, 3241–3243, *3242, 3243*
diminution in size of, 3245, *3246*
histology of, 3241, *3241*
of hand, 5319, *5323*, 5323–5324, 5503, *5504*
combined with venous malformations, 5324
postoperative complications of, 3249
terminology for, 3240–3241
treatment of, 3245, 3247, *3248*, 3249
Lymphatic system
anatomy of, 4093–4094, *4094–4099*, 4100
augmentation of lymph flow to, 5028–5032, *5029–5031*
embryology of, 3224, 4992
insufficiency of flow through, 4101, 4101*t*, 4102*t*. *See also* Lymphedema.
physiology of, *4100*, 4100–4101
recreation of, for lymphedema treatment, 4112
transplantation of lymph collectors, for lymphedema therapy, 4115, *4116*, 4117
Lymphaticovenous malformation (LMV), 3241
Lymphatics, anatomy of, 3279, *3279*
Lymphatic-vein anastomoses, for lymphedema, 4113–4115
Lymphedema
chylous reflux and, 4117
classification of, 4105–4106, 5023–5024
historical aspects of, 4093
lymphatic system insufficiency and, 4101, 4101*t*, 4102*t*
of penis and scrotum
anatomic considerations for, 4181, *4181*
etiology of, 4180–4181
general considerations for, 4183
pathology of, 4181
therapy for, 4181–4183, *4182*
of upper extremity, 5023
diagnosis of, 5024–5026, *5024, 5025*
medical treatment of, 5026, *5026, 5027*
surgical treatment of, 5027–5032, *5027–5031*
of vulva, 4211
pathophysiology of, 4101–4105, *4103, 4104*, 5023
surgical problems with, 4102*t*

Lymphedema *(Continued)*
surgical techniques for, 4110*t*, 4110–4111
procedures to increase lymph drainage as, 4112–4115, *4114*
procedures to reduce load for lymphatic clearance as, 4111–4112
therapy for, 4106
complex decongestive physiotherapy as, 4107, *4108*, 4109*t*, 4109–4110
drugs as, 4107
heat and bandage treatment as, 4110
principles of, 4106–4107
surgical drainage procedures as, 4105
Lymphoid system, 189–190
Lymphokines, 191
Lymphomas
of head and neck, malignant, in children, 3185
of orbit, 3364
staging classification for, 3185
Lymphostasis, 4105
Lysine, hydroxylation of, 170–171
Lysine analogues, for abnormal scar prevention, 740
Lysozyme, 1806

Macrogenia, surgical correction of, 1332–1333, *1334, 1335*
Macroglossia, surgery for, in Down syndrome, 3165–3166, *3166*
Macrophage system, 190
Macrostomia, 3096, *3096*
Maddox rod test, 1599
Magnetic resonance imaging, of orbit, 1588–1590, *1589*
Magnification, for hand surgery, 4290
Magnifying loupes, 415
Major histocompatibility complex (MHC), 187
"Make a wish" maneuver, 4818, *4818*
Malar bone. *See* Zygoma.
Malar pouches, 2331, *2332*
Malar protuberance, growth of, 2509–2510
Male impotence, psychosocial aspects of, 128
Male pattern baldness. *See* Alopecia, androgenic.
Malformations. *See also specific deformity.*
interrelationships with deformations and disruptions of, 78, *78*
sequences of, 72, 72*t*
vs. malformation syndrome, 73–74, *74*
time onset of, 76–77, 77*t*
vs. deformations, 76, 76*t*
Malherbe, benign calcifying epithelioma of, 3576
Malignant hyperthermia, history of, anesthesia and, 4304
Malignant schwannoma, of hand, 5506–5507
Malingering, differential diagnosis of, 4904–4905
Mallet finger, 4573–4576, *4573, 4574*, 4626–4627, *4626*
Malocclusion, 919–920, *919, 920*, 1018
class II, preoperative orthodontic therapy for, 1201, 1203–1205, *1202*
classification of, 1193–1194, *1193, 1194*
myalgia from, 1478
Malunion, from orthognathic surgery, 1405
Mammoplasty, augmentation
approaches to, 3879
breast carcinoma and, 3889
complications of, 3885–3889, 3887*t*, *3889*
dissection of pocket for, 3883–3884

Mammoplasty *(Continued)*
implants for, 3884–3885
placement of, 3885
location of implant for, 3883, *3883*
operative technique for, 3881–3883, *3882*
postoperative management of, 3885
pregnancy and, 3892
preoperative evaluation of, 3879, 3881
results of, *3890–3892*
wound closure for, 3885
Manafo formula, 792*t*
Mandible
acquired defects of
historical review of, 1413–1415
methods of fixation for, 1415–1419, *1416–1421*, 1421–1422
nerve grafting and resection of body after bone graft reconstruction, 1438
nonvascularized bone grafting techniques for, *1421–1437*, 1422, 1426, 1432–1433, 1437–1438
procedure to increase area of labiobuccal sulcus and lingual sulcus in, 1454–1456, *1455, 1456*
restoration of buccal sulcus and functional alveolar ridge for, 1451–1452, 1454
vascularized bone transfers for, 1438–1440, 1443, *1440–1446, 1448–1450*, 1445, 1447, 1451
ameloblastomas of, 3341–3342, *3342*
basal bone of, normal growth of, 2557–2558
body of
elongation by retromolar step osteotomy, 1277, *1278*
elongation osteotomies of, 1277–1278
lengthening techniques for, 1270, 1272, *1273*
congenital deformities of, in craniofacial microsomia, 3064–3066, *3064–3066*
cysts of, classification of, 3336
deformation of, *74*
deformities of, maxillofacial prosthetics for, 3517, 3519, 3522–3523, *3518–3523*
developmental deformities of
combined extraoral and intraoral approach to, 1227
extraoral approach to, 1225, 1227, *1237*
intraoral approach to, 1225–1227, *1226, 1227, 1248*
prognathism as. *See* Prognathism, mandibular.
pseudoprognathism as, 1229
disarticulation of, 3373–3374
elongation of
by sagittal section of ramus, 1280–1282, 1285, *1282, 1284*
choice of technique for, 1287
osteotomy of ramus and body of mandible for, 1285–1286, *1286*
fractures of. *See* Mandible fractures.
fragments in, appliances for fixation of, 3500, *3500–3507*, 3504–3505, 3507–3508
growth of, after surgical repair of cleft lip/palate, 2561, *2562, 2563*, 2564
hypoplasia of, 1149–1150, *1150*, 1260
in cleft lip and palate children, 2882, *2883*
lateral deviation of, 1289–1290, 1292
resulting from bone loss, 1301
midline clefts of, 2482
muscles influencing movement of, 935, 937, *936, 938*
plain films of
oblique lateral views on, 894, *895, 896*
occlusal inferosuperior views on, 893, *893, 894*
postnatal development of, 2496

Mandible *(Continued)*
postnatal growth of, 1148–1150, *1149*
process clefts of, classification of, 2444
ramus of
condylar growth process of, 2505–2506
extraoral approach to, 1227, *1237*
hypomobility of, 1494–1496, *1495*
increasing of vertical dimension in, 1279–1280, *1279*
intraoral approach to, 1227, *1248*
operations on, to increase projection, 1278–1279, *1279*
osteotomies of, 1235–1239, *1236–1242*, 1241, 1243
for open bite deformity, 1357
reconstruction of, 1432–1433, 1437–1438, *1433–1437*
sagittal section of, 1285
surgical exposure of, 1237–1238, *1236, 1237*
vertical osteotomy of, 1280, *1281*
reconstruction of, 3374
bone grafting in, *1421*, 1426, *1429–1431*
vascularized bone transfers for, 600
resected, replacement of, 1414
severely comminuted, in panfacial fractures, 1038–1039, *1040*
skeletal relations of, 1194
tumors of
classification of, 3336
surgical treatment for, 3373–3374
Mandible fractures, 930
causes of, 933
class I type, treatment of, *943*, 943–944
class II
basal repositioning of, 959–961, *959, 960*
eccentric dynamic compression plate for, 961, *962*
external fixation of, 957–958, *959*
fixation when maxilla is edentulous, *953*, 968
Kirschner wire fixation of, 958
metal plates and screws for fixation of, 958–959
occlusal repositioning of, 959
open reduction and interosseous wiring for, 954, *955, 956*
titanium mesh tray for, 968, *968*
treatment of, 952, *952*
when horizontally and vertically favorable, 952–953, *953*
use of splint in edentulous posterior segment of, *953*, 953–954
classification of, 930, *931, 932*, 932–934
clinical examination of, 934
complications of, malunion of, 978–979
nonunion of, 977–978, *978*
treatment of, 975–979
compound comminuted, of anterior portion of, 946, 948, *950–951*
diagnosis of, 934–935
displacement of, factors influencing, 938, 940–941, *940, 941*
edentulous, management of, 969, 971, 973, *970, 972*
external fixation of, 975
horizontal interdental wiring of, 944, *944, 945*
in children, 1160–1164, *1161–1163*
intermaxillary fixation of
by banded dental arch, 944, 946
by cable arch wires, 944
by external pin fixation, 946, *948–949*
by prefabricated arch bars, 944, *945, 946*
Mandible fractures *(Continued)*
Luhr self-tapping system for, 965, *966–967*, 968
multiply fractured or comminuted edentulous, 973–975, *974*
roentgenographic examination of, 935
severity of, *931*, 932–933
soft tissues at site of, 940, *942*
Mandibular angle, development of, 598, *599*
Mandibular arch, growth of, 2510, *2511*
Mandibular cleft, 2941
Mandibular dentoalveolar protrusion, 1347
Mandibular hypoplasia
elongation osteotomies of body of mandible in, 1266, 1268, *1267, 1268*
elongation techniques for
age at operation, 1287
choice of, 1287
postoperative relapse and, 1287
interdental osteotomy for, 1272, 1274–1275
postoperative relapse, 1288–1289
preservation of soft tissue coverage and, 1268, *1269, 1270, 1271, 1272*
soft tissue deficiency in, 1288–1289
surgical correction of, suprahyoid musculature and, 1287–1288
treatment of, 1263
in Treacher Collins syndrome, *3118*, 3119
preoperative planning for, 1263–1264, *1264, 1265*, 1266
with maxillary dentoalveolar protrusion, *1274*, 1275, *1275, 1276*, 1277
Mandibular macrognathia, unilateral, with condylar hyperplasia, 1294, *1294–1297*
Mandibular nerve blocks, 149–150, *150*
Mandibular plane angle, 1196, *1196*
Mandibular process, clefts of, 2927
Mandibular prognathism, mandibular osteotomies for, 2840
Mandibular prostheses, for group I deformities, 3508, 3510–3512, 3514, 3516–3517, *3509–3511, 3513–3517*
Mandibular symphysis, oblique superoinferior submental projection of, 893–894, *894*
Mandibulofacial dysostosis. *See* Treacher Collins syndrome.
Mania operativa, 131, 132
Marcus Gunn pupil, 1583
Marcus Gunn pupillary test, 909, 1104, *1104, 1105*
Marcus Gunn syndrome, 1754, *1756*
Marffucci's syndrome, *3262*, 3263
Marjolin's ulcer, 165, 847
Maroon-Kennerdell four-wall orbital decompression, 1637, *1638*, 1639
Maryland bridges, 2738
Masseter muscle, 935
benign hypertrophy of, 1301, 1303, 1305, *1301–1304*
hypertrophy of, 1478–1479
neurovascular supply of, *2287*
pull of, 598, *599*
transposition of, for facial paralysis, 2286–2290, *2287–2291*, 2294
Masseteric hypertrophy, benign, 1301, 1303, 1305, *1301–1304*
Mastectomy
prophylactic, 3922–3924, *3925*
radical, breast reconstruction after, latissimus dorsi flap for, 3914, 3916, *3916*

Mastectomy *(Continued)*
subcutaneous, 3873, 3875, 3877, *3876–3878*
total, 3899
Masticatory muscles, intramuscular pathology of, causing TMJ dysfunction, 1479
Maternal impressions, 3191–3192
Maxilla
acquired defects of, 1456–1457
reconstruction of hard palate and alveolar process in, 1457, *1459–1463*, 1463
reconstruction of upper portion of, 1457, *1458*
ameloblastomas of, 3342, *3343–3344*
anatomy of, 1009, 1011, *1009, 1010*, 1579–1580, 2726, 2982
basal bone of, normal growth of, 2558–2559, *2558*
blood supply of, *1365*
classification of, 1360, 1362
cysts of, 3336
deficiencies of
in cleft lip and palate children, 2879, 2882, *2880, 2881*
treatment of, in Treacher Collins syndrome, 3111–3113
developmental deformities of, 1360
advancement procedures for, pharyngeal flaps and, 1379
correction for vertical excess in, 1381, 1384, *1381–1383*
dentoalveolar malocclusions in, 1360
from cleft palate correction, 2821–2840
nasomaxillary hypoplasia and, 1387, 1389, 1391, 1394, 1396, 1398–1399, 1401, *1389–1401*
preoperative planning for, *1362*, 1362–1363
prosthetics for, 3523–3524, 3528–3530, *3524–3532*
retromolar segmental advancement for, 1373, 1376, *1376*
short face, correction of, 1384, 1386–1387, *1385–1388*
surgical approach to midface, 1363–1364, 1366, *1365*
transverse, correction of, 1379–1381, *1380*
velopharyngeal incompetence after advancement for, 1376, 1379, *1379*
deformities secondary to cleft palate
onlay bone grafts for, 2829, 2832
osteotomies for, 2832–2835, *2833*
displacement of, 2503–2504, *2504*
fractures of, 1009
displacement of, 1015–1016, *1015–1017*
etiology of, 1015–1016, *1015–1017*
examination and diagnosis of, 1016, 1018, *1018*
Le Fort classification of, 1012–1015, *1013, 1014*
surgical anatomy of, 1011, *1011–1012*, 1012
without maxillary mobility, 1016
growth of, *2510*, 2510–2511
after surgical repair of cleft lip/palate, *2563*, 2564
surgical repair of cleft palate and, 2569, 2572–2575, *2572–2577*
micrognathia-retrognathia of onlay bone grafts for, 1367, *1367, 1368*
treatment for, 1366, *1366*
protrusion of, 1360
in Asian face, surgical correction of, *2429, 2430*, 2431
skeletal relations of, 1194
tumors of
adjuvant chemotherapy for, 3330
Maxilla *(Continued)*
tumors of, biopsy of, 3321
classification of, 3318, 3318*t*, 3336
complications of, 3331–3334, *3332*
diagnosis of, 3320–3321, *3321*
etiology of, 3318
examination of, 3320–3321, *3321*
from metastases, 3319
incidence of, 3317–3318
management of cervical metastases, 3330–3331
pathology of, 3318–3319, *3319*
postoperative management of, 3326–3328
radiation therapy for, 3330
signs and symptoms of, 3320
staging of, 3322, *3322*
surgical treatment of, 3375
treatment of, 3322–3330, *3324–3329*
Maxillary buttress, lateral, 1021
Maxillary dentoalveolar protrusion
treatment of, 1333, 1336, *1335*
with mandibular hypoplasia, *1274*, 1275, *1275, 1276*, 1277
Maxillary dentoalveolar retrusion, 1342, *1343–1346*, 1345–1347
Maxillary fractures
complications of, 1030–1032, *1031*
malunited or partially healed in malposition, 1028, 1030, *1029, 1030*
non-union of, 1031
of edentulous maxilla, 1028
of palate, 1024, 1026, *1025*
postoperative care of, 1030
Maxillary hypoplasia
in cleft lip nasal deformity, 2800–2801, *2801*
secondary to cleft lip or palate, segmental osteotomies for, *2839*, 2839–2840
Maxillary nerve, *1046*
Maxillary nerve block, 150–152, *151, 152*
Maxillary process, clefts of, 2927
Maxillary prominence, 2482, 2519, *2521*
Maxillary retrusion
from cleft lip or palate
Le Fort I osteotomy for, 2835, 2838, 2839, *2835, 2836, 2839*
Le Fort II osteotomy for, *2837, 2838*, 2838–2839
secondary to cleft deformity, 2829
Maxillary sinus
infections of, from orthognathic surgery, 1412
packing of, 1002, 1004
Maxillectomy
postoperative reconstruction following, 3334
total
historical aspects of, 3317
surgical procedure for, 3323–3326, *3324, 3325*
via midfacial degloving incision, 3328–3330, *3329–3331*
Maxillofacial injuries, treatment of, 871. *See also specific injuries.*
Maxillofacial prosthetics
auricular, 3549, *3551*
extraoral, 3530, 3534, 3536–3537, *3535, 3536*
for fixation of mandibular fragments, 3500, *3500–3507*, 3504–3505, 3507–3508
for mandibular deformities
of group 1 type, 3508, *3509–3511, 3510–3512, 3513–3517*, 3514, 3516–3517
of group 2 type, 3517, *3518–3523*, 3519, 3522–3523

Maxillofacial prosthetics *(Continued)*
for maxillary deformities, 3523–3524, *3524–3532*, 3528–3530
for nose deformities, 3541–3545, *3542–3548*, 3549
historical aspects of, 3497–3498
indications for, 3498–3499, *3499*
limitations of, 3549
orbital, 3537, *3537–3540*, 3540–3541
postoperative instructions for, 3549
Maxillofacial surgery, 21
Maxillomandibular disharmonies, *1402–1403*, 1403–1404, *1406–1407*
Maximal stimulation test, 2253
McGregor fan flap, for lower lip reconstruction, 2021, 2023–2024, *2024*
McIndoe technique
for hypospadias repair, 4158–4159
for split-thickness skin graft vaginal reconstruction, 4206
Meatal advancement glansplasty, for hypospadias, 4161, *4161*
Mechanical dilatation, for vasospasm, 455–456
Mechanical factors, in peripheral nerve regeneration, 661
Mechanical pressure, for inhibition of hypertrophic scar formation, 740–741
Meckel syndrome, 77, 92
Meckel's cartilage
anatomy of, 1540, *1540*
formation of, 1148, 1539, 2462
mandibular hypoplasia and, 2596
skeletal tissue development and, 2487, 3059, 3060–3061
Medial brachial cutaneous nerve, 4314
Medial canthopexy, transosseous wiring for, 1618, *1620*
Medial canthoplasty, 1617, 1715, *1717*, *1718*
Medial canthus deformities, 1609, 1614, *1614*
Medial gastrocnemius myocutaneous flap, *302*
Medial nasal process, embryological development of, 2519, 2523, 2525–2526, *2522, 2525, 2527*
Medial nasal prominences, embryological development of, 2482
Medial pterygoid muscle, 937
Median facial dysrhaphia, 2984
Median mandibular cyst, 3340
Median maxillary palatal cyst, 3340
Median nerve
anatomy of, 4278, *4278*, 4759
compression of, in carpal tunnel syndrome, 4742–4744, *4744*
entrapment syndrome of, in rheumatoid arthritis, 4704
injuries of
paralysis of forearm muscles in, *4957*, 4957–4958
with brachial plexus injuries, 4802
neuropathy of, 4823
regional block of, 4323
repair of, at wrist, 4767, *4770*
Median nerve palsy
distal muscle paralysis in, 4955, *4955–4957*, 4956
high, tendon transfer for, 4961–4963, *4962*
high and radial palsy, tendon transfer for, 4963
with ulnar nerve palsy, 4958–4959, *4958–4961*, 4961
Mediastinum reconstruction, muscle and musculocutaneous flaps for, 393–396, *394, 395*
Meissner's corpuscles
anatomy of, 648–649, *649*
reinnervation of, 668
Melanin, distribution in photo-damaged skin, 751, *751*
Melanoma
acral-lentiginous, 3640–3641, *3641*
in parotid gland, 3310
in situ, malignant, *3598*, 3598–3599
malignant
classification of, 3638–3642, *3639–3642*
clinical staging of, 5489–5490, 5492, 5490*t*, *5491*
diagnosis of, 3638
etiology of, 3636–3638, *3637*
immunotherapy for, 3651–3652
in hand, 5489, 5492, *5492–5494*
incidence of, 3635–3636, 5489
microscopic invasion as prognostic factor, 3642–3644, *3643*
Mohs micrographic surgery for, 3652–3653, 3655–3658, *3654–3656*
radiation therapy for, 3652
stage IA, IB, IIA and IIB, treatment for, 3644–3645, 3648–3650
stage III, treatment for, 3650
stage IV, treatment for, 3650–3651
staging of, 3644, *3646–3647*
nodular, 3640, *3641*
of nasal cavity and paranasal sinuses, 3361–3362, *3362*
of perionychium, 4514, *4514*
superficial spreading, 3639–3640, *3640*
unclassified type of, 3641–3642
Melanotic freckle of Hutchinson, *3598*, 3598–3599
Membranous bone, 1539
Meningitis, with frontobasilar region fracture, 1113–1114
Meningoencephalocele
classification of, 2984
nasoethmoidal type of, 2984, *2985*
nasofrontal type of, 2984, *2984*
nasoorbital type of, 2984, *2985*
Meningomyelocele, malformation sequence in, 72, 72*t*
Meniscus, anatomy of, 1477, *1477*
Mental protuberance, 1305, *1305*
Mental retardation
idiopathic, 79, 81
in craniosynostosis, 3025
Mental spines, 1305
Mental tubercles, 1305
Menton, 28, *28*, 1190
Meperidine, as premedication, 140*t*, 140–141
Merkel cell-neurite complex, 650, *650*
reinnervation of, 668
Mesenchyme, *2453*, 2454
Mesh grafts, cutting of, *237*, 237–238, *238*
Mesioclusion, *1193*, 1194
Mesoderm
deficiency of, theory of, 3063
organization of, 2456–2458, *2457*
otocephaly and, 2460, *2460*
Metabolic hypothesis, 445
Metabolic imbalance, maternal, craniofacial cleft formation and, 2928
Metacarpal arch
examination of, 4260
fracture of, 4260, *4260*

Metacarpal hand, *4338*, 4338–4339
Metacarpals
distraction lengthening of, for congenital hand deformities, 5252, *5253, 5254*, 5255
extension of, tendon tranfer for, in radial palsy, *4944*, 4944–4945
fractures of, without joint injury, 4598–4601, *4598–4601*
lengthening of, for thumb reconstruction. *See* Thumb reconstruction, by bone lengthening.
malunion or non-union of, 4601
transposition of, 5248
transverse absence of, 5246, 5248, *5249–5251*, *5252*, *5253–5254*, 5255
Metacarpophalangeal block, in flexor tendon repair, 4543, *4543*
Metacarpophalangeal joint
anatomy of, 4254–4255, *4254*, 4257–4258, *4258, 4259*, 4655–4656, *4656, 4657*
arthrodesis of, small joints, 4671. *See also* Arthrodesis.
indications for, small joints, 4671
deformities of, after burn injury, 5467
dislocations of, 4612–4616, *4613–4615*
fracture-dislocations of, 4616–4617, *4617*
locking of, 4728–4729
pathophysiology of, 4655–4656, *4656, 4657*
stiffness of
age and, 4661
from edema, 4657–4658
from immobility, 4656–4657
from mechanical obstruction, 4661, *4661*
from scar contracture, 4658–4661, *4659–4661*
hand therapy for, 4665–4666, *4666, 4667*
mobilization vs. immobilization for, 4663–4665, *4664, 4665*
subluxations of, 4612–4616, *4613–4616*, 4616–4617
Metacarpotrapezial joint
first, *4256*, 4256–4257
ligaments of, 4257, *4257*
Metal tray with bone chips, for mandibular defects, 1413–1414
Metals, in alloplastic implants, 703–706, 704*t*, 705*t*
Metatarsal artery, variability of course of, *1444*
Metatarsus, vascularized grafts of, 625
Methotrexate, 195
Methylmethacrylate implants, for craniofacial surgery, 1561–1562, *1563*
Metopic synostosis, 3032, 3035, *3034*
Meyer-Abul-Failat technique, for lower lip reconstruction, 2020, *2021*
MHC (major histocompatibility complex), 187
Mibelli lesions, 3235
Microcirculation, 449, *450, 451*
Microfilaments, 636
Microgenia
chin augmentation for, *1307*, 1307–1308
clinical presentation of, 1260, 1305–1306
contour restoration for
by alloplastic implant, 1308–1309, 1312, *1307, 1309–1311*
by cartilage or bone grafts, 1323, 1329, *1330*
by horizontal advancement osteotomy, 1312, 1318, *1313–1321*
by skin graft inlay and dental prosthesis, 1329, *1331, 1332, 1332*
Microgenia *(Continued)*
diagnosis and preoperative planning for, 1306–1307
surgical correction of, in Down syndrome, 3170, *3170, 3171*
with mandibular prognathism, 1258, *1259*
Micrognathia
definition of, 3123
mandibular, *1261*
contour restoration in, 1289, *1290*
etiology of, 1260–1262
maxillary, 1360
Micrognathia-retrognathia, maxillary
onlay bone grafts for, 1367, *1367, 1368*
treatment for, 1366, *1366*
Microneurovascular muscle transfers
for facial paralysis, 2298–2300, *2300–2303*
of skeletal muscle, 555–556, *556*
Microphthalmos, 1640–1642, *1643*
orbital expansion for, 1644–1646, *1646*
Microscope, operating, 412–414, *413, 414*
maintenance of, 415
preoperative preparation of, 414–415
Microsomia, craniofacial. *See* Craniofacial microsomia.
Microsurgery
development of, 20
for auricular replantation, 2125
interfascicular and perineural nerve repair, for facial paralysis, 2258–2259
of hand, operating room organization for, 4290
Microtia
auricular reconstruction method, 2100–2101
bilateral, 2108, 2110
complete
clinical characteristics of, 2099–2100
correlation of surgery with facial deficiency surgeries, 2100
general treatment considerations for, 2100
deformities associated with, 2099, *2099*
etiology of
hereditary factors in, 2098
specific factors in, 2098–2099
incidence of, 2097–2098
indications for timing of middle ear surgery, 2146
middle ear problem in, embryology and, 2096–2097, *2097*
middle ear surgery for, timing of, 2149
repair of, historical perspective of, 2094–2095
Microtubules, 636
Microvascular composite tissue transplantation, for breast reconstruction, 393
Microvascular free flaps, 3448–3449, *3449*
for Romberg's disease treatment, 3140, *3141*
Microvascular surgery
artery to vein repair ratio in, 4369
blood flow in, abnormal, 449, 451–453
continuous suturing in, 434–435
definition of, 4356
end-to-end anastomosis in
exposure for, 421
for normal or near-normal vessel tension, 423
for repair of normal vessels, 421–422, *422*
for similar diameter vessels, 423
operative technique for resection to normal vessels of, 423–427, *423–434*, 429–434
position and preparation for, 420–421
technique for, 421

Microvascular surgery *(Continued)*
end-to-side anastomosis, 435–437, *437*
for replantation and revascularization
nerve repair in, 4370
soft tissue coverage in, 4370–4371
vascular pedicles in, 4370
vein grafts in, *4369*, 4369–4370
for traumatic lesions, 449, 451
free flap transfers
advantages of, 461–462
complications of, 468–469
disadvantages of, 462–463
general aspects of, 459–461
indications for, 461
postoperative management of, 466
preoperative evaluation for, 463–465
results of, 466–468, 467*t*, 468*t*
secondary defects from, 469
technique for, 465–466
grafts for, 437–442, *439–441*
magnifying loupes for, 415
microinstrumentation for, 415–417, *416, 417*
bipolar coagulator in, 418
clamps in, 417–418, *417, 418*
Doppler monitors in, 418–419
suction in, 419
microsutures for, 419–420, *420*
normal blood flow in, 442–449, *442–449*
operating microscope for, 412–414, *413, 414*
maintenance of, 415
preoperative preparation of, 414–415
size discrepancy in, 435
sleeve anastomosis for, 435, *435*
vascular anastomosis for, *4368*, 4368–4369
venous anastomosis for, 434
zone of vascular injury for, 4367–4368
Microvascular transfers
for complete cervical contracture treatment, 2073–2074, *2074, 2075*
for foot reconstruction, 401–402, *402*
for genital reconstructive surgery, 4152
for lower leg reconstruction, 399, 401
Midazolam, 141
Middle ear surgery
for aural atresia, results and complications of, 2148–2149
timing of, 2149
Midface
advancement of, velopharyngeal incompetence from, 2906
degloving incision of, for maxillectomy, 3328–3330, *3329–3331*
fractures of, treatment of, 1019–1021, *1020, 1021. See also specific midfacial fractures.*
sarcomas of, surgical treatment of, 3390–3391
surgical approach to, 1363–1364, *1365*, 1366
tumors of, surgical treatment for, 3384, *3385–3389*, 3390
Midpalmar space infection, 5541–5542, *5542*
Migration, cellular, 163
Milia
after chemical peeling, 769
formation of, after dermabrasion, 780
treatment of, 3572
Milker's nodule, 5553
Millard operation, modification of, to prevent vermilion notching, 2793, 2795
Mini-abdominoplasty, technique for, 3951, 3953, *3954, 3955*
Minimal tension, lines of, 43
Minnesota Multi Personality Index (MMPI), 123, 125
Minoxidil, for androgenic alopecia, 1520
Mirror hand, 5133, 5356, 5358, 5361–5362, *5357, 5359–5361*
Mirror movements, 3144
Mitochondria, 636
Mitosis, 163
Mixed lymphocyte culture test, 189
MMPI (Minnesota Multi Personality Index), 123, 125
MNP, facial clefting and, 2540–2541
Möbius syndrome
Klippel-Feil syndrome and, 3144
temporalis muscle transposition of, 2289, *2297*
Mohs chemosurgery, for lower lip reconstruction, 2016, 2018, *2019*
Mohs micrographic surgery, for malignant melanoma, 3652–3653, 3655–3658, *3654–3656*
cure rate for, 3657–3658
indications for, 3653, 3655–3657, *3655, 3656*
procedure for, 3653, *3654*
Molluscum contagiosum, 3566, *3566*
Molluscum sebaceum, 3607–3608, *3608*
Monafo formula, 793
Mondor's disease, 3889
Mongolism. *See* Down syndrome.
Monocyte-macrophage cell system, 178
Morbid obesity. *See* Obesity, morbid.
Morel-Fatio Spring, for treatment of eyelid paralysis, 2310, *2310*
Morestin, 8
Morphine, 140, 140*t*
Morphogenesis, abnormal, resulting in malformations, 71, 71*t*
Morquio syndrome, 106
Morris appliance, 1038, *1040*
Morris external fixation splint, twin-screw appliance, *1417–1421*, 1418
Motor end organs, 655
Motor units, reinnervation of, 667
Motor vehicle accidents
multiple injuries in, 867, *868*
evaluation of, 869*t*, 869–870
pediatric facial trauma from, 1142
Mucocutaneous receptors, 652–653
Mucoepidermoid carcinoma, of salivary glands, 3304–3306, *3305*
Mucoperiosteal flap, palatal, for maxillary dentoalveolar retrusion correction, *1346*, 1346–1347
Mucoperiosteum, 2625
Mucosa, transposition or advancement of, for correction of misalignment of vermilion border of, 2791, *2791*, 2793
Mucosal graft inlay technique, for restoration of buccal sulcus and functional alveolar ridge, 1451–1452, 1454, *1452, 1453*
Mucosal grafts
for eyelid reconstruction, 1689
for symblepharon correction, 1743, *1744, 1745*
Mucous cysts
clinical presentation of, 3581, *3581*
of hand, *5497*, 5497–5498
of wrist or hand, *4750, 4751*, 4752
Müller's muscle
anatomy of, *1679*, 1679–1680

Müller's muscle *(Continued)*
  eyelid retraction and, 1639
  spasm of, 2327, 2328, *2328*, 2330
Mulliken method, for bilateral cleft lip repair, 2692–2693, *2693, 2694*
Multidisciplinary approach, 23
Multiple dysplasia syndromes, *3262*, 3263–3264
Multiple suture synostosis, hydrocephalus in, 3025
Muscle(s)
  applied physiology of, 4966–4968, *4967*
    length-tension relationships of, 4968–4969, *4968–4969*
  arc of rotation of, prediction of, 381, *383*
  blood supply of, 282–283, *283*
  embryology of, in hand and arm, 5220–5221, *5222–5229*
  evaluation of function of, in tetraplegia, spasticity and stroke patients, 4979–4980
  expiratory, anatomy of, 3677–3679, *3678*
  extraocular. *See* Extraocular muscles.
  fibers
    length-tension of, *4939*
  fibers of
    gross configuration of, 4967, *4967*
    isolated types of, 4926, *4926, 4927*
  length-tension curve of, 4926, *4926, 4927*
  mechanical qualities of, 4927–4931
  ocular, after orbital and nasoethmoido-orbital fractures, 1103
  of facial expression, evaluation of, in facial injuries, 881–882, *881–883*
  of lip, 2009–2012, *2009–2011*, 2598–2600, *2599*
    in bilateral cleft lip, 2603, 2608, 2612, *2603–2611*
    in unilateral cleft lip, 2600–2601, 2603, *2600–2603*
  of mandible, 935, *936, 937, 938*
  of mastication, in craniofacial microsomia, 3067
  of palate, 2612–2615, 2619, 2623–2625, *2612–2614, 2616–2618, 2620–2622*, 2726–2727, *2727*
  pH of, during ischemia, 5018–5019
  problems of, in rheumatoid arthritis, 4705–4707, *4706*
  voluntary, origins and migration of, 2471, *2472*, 2473, 2519, *2520*
Muscle flap. *See also specific flaps.*
  advantages of, 383–384
  arc of rotation of, prediction of, 381, *382*
  classification of, 380–381, *381*
  complications of, 405–406
  design of, 301–304, *302, 303*
  disadvantages of, 384
  distally based, design of, 382–383
  for abdominal wall defects, 397
  for breast reconstruction, 387, *389*, 389–393, *390, 392, 393*
  for chest wall and pulmonary cavity reconstructions, 396–397
  for foot reconstruction, 401–402, *402*
  for genitourinary reconstructive surgery, 4126–4127
  for groin and perineum reconstructions, 397–399, *398*
  for heel and midplantar defects, 4082, 4085, 4087, *4083–4087*
  for lower extremity, 399, *400*, 401, 4038–4040, *4039–4043*, 4043
  for mediastinal reconstruction, 393–396, *394, 395*
  for pressure sores, 402–404, *403*
  for soft tissue coverage, 4454–4456, *4455–4456*, 4457
Muscle flap *(Continued)*
  patient management for, 404–405
  refinements in, 383
  regional application of, to head and neck, 385–387, *386*
  selection of, 379–380, *380*, 384
  skin territory for, prediction of, 381–382
  SMAS-platysma, 2381–2382, *2381–2383*
Muscle grafts
  allografts
    vascularized, 200
  free
    for facial paralysis, 2294, 2298
    histology of, 553–555, *554*
    historical aspects of, 551–553, *552*
Muscle relaxants, in postoperative treatment of skin flaps, 316–317
Muscle spindle receptors, *653*, 653–654
Muscle transfer, functioning
  guidelines for, 4976*t*
  operative technique of, 4972–4974, *4973, 4974*
  postoperative care for, 4974–4975
  results of, *4975*, 4975–4976
Muscle transposition, regional, for facial paralysis, 2284
  historical perspective of, 2284, 2286
Muscular neurotization, 2255, *2256, 2257*
Musculocutaneous flaps. *See also specific flaps.*
  advantages of, 383–384
  complications of, 405–406
  disadvantages of, 384
  for foot reconstruction, 401–402, *402*
  for groin and perineum reconstructions, 397–399, *398*
  for heel and midplantar defects, 4082, 4085, 4087, *4083–4087*
  for lower extremity reconstructions, 399, *400*, 401, 4039–4040, 4043, *4038–4043*
  for pressure sores, 402–404, *403*
  for soft tissue coverage, 4454–4455, 4457, *4455–4456*
  historical aspects of, 376
  of latissmus dorsi, for breast reconstruction, 3911–3914, *3912–3916*, 3916
  patient management for, 404–405
  refinements in, 383
  regional application of, to chest wall and pulmonary cavity, 396–397
    to mediastinum, 393–396, *394, 395*
  selection of, 384
  skin territory for, prediction of, 381–382
Musculocutaneous nerve
  anatomy of, 4314, *4761*, 4761–4762
  injuries of, with brachial plexus injuries, 4802
  regional block of, 4323
Musculofascial flaps, for abdominal wall reconstruction, 3766–3768
Musculoskeletal problems, of amputation, 4331
Musculus uvulae, 2727, *2727*
Mustarde four-flap technique, for congenital epicanthus, 1774, *1775, 1776*
Mustarde lid switch, 1703, *1705, 1707*
Mustarde total upper lid method, 1703, 1712, *1705, 1707, 1709–1712*
Mycobacterial infections, of hand, 5548–5550, 5549*t*
Myectomy, selective, for facial paralysis, 2306
Myelin sheath, 640
Myeloma, chest wall reconstruction and, 3716

Mylohyoid muscle, 937
Myoblasts, origins and migration of, 2471, *2472*, 2473, 2519, *2520*
Myocutaneous flap, 277–278
Myofascial dysfunction
  differential diagnosis of, 4905
  reflex sympathetic dystrophy and, 4894–4896
  terminology for, 4895*t*
Myofascial pain dysfunction (MPD), 1483
Myofibroblasts, 167, *168*, 243
Myofibromatosis, infantile, 3184
Myogenic response, 445
Myoneurotization, 2255, *2256, 2257*
Myopia
  degenerative changes in, blepharoplasty for, 2345, *2346, 2347*
  preoperative evaluation for, 2328, *2329*
Myxoid cysts, 3581
Myxoma, 3301

Naevus maternus of infancy, 3192
Nager's acrofacial dysostosis, 3106, *3108*
Narcotics
  as premedication for regional nerve block, 4315
  premedication with, 140, 140*t*
  respiratory depression from, 141
Nares
  external, 1786, *1788*
  internal, 1786, *1788*, 1808, *1808*, 1925
Nasal area, weakness of, *1086*, 1086–1087
Nasal bone fractures, 979–980, *979, 980*
  comminuted, 990
  complications of, 990–991
  compound, 990
  in children, 1170–1171
  reduction of, instrumentation for, 985, 987, *986, 987*
  transnasal wiring with plastic or metal plates for, 990, *990*
  treatment of, *982*, 985
    anesthesia for, 985
  types and locations of, 980, *981–983*
Nasal bones
  plain films of
    axial projection of, 886–887, *890*
    lateral views of, 886, *890*
  short, 1847, *1848*
Nasal cartilage grafts, autogenous, 569, *572*
Nasal cavity
  metastatic tumors of, 3364
  tumors of, 3360–3364, *3362*
Nasal cycle, 1806
Nasal dorsum
  contour restoration of, in malunited nasoethmoido-orbital fractures, 1620, *1620–1622*, 1623
  depressed, bone and cartilage grafting for, 1882, 1885–1886, *1884*
  local nasal flaps, for reconstruction of, 1935–1936, *1935, 1936*
  recession of, 1843, *1844*, 1847
  straight, 1847, *1848*
Nasal escape speech distortion, 2733
Nasal flap, local, for nasal reconstruction, 1934–1936, *1935–1940*, 1940
Nasal index, 1879
Nasal packing, anteroposterior, technique for, 876–877, *878*
Nasal placodal porphogenesis, in normoxic vs. hypoxic embryos, *2536*
Nasal process, lateral. *See* Lateral nasal process.
Nasal prominence, lateral, embryological development of, 2482
Nasal prostheses, 3541–3545, 3549, *3542–3548*
Nasal reconstruction
  by tissue expansion, 496, 501, *501*
  cartilage warping in, 563–564, *564, 565*
  composite grafts for
    of skin and adipose tissue, 1932
    of skin and cartilage, 1930–1932, *1931, 1933–1934*
  distant flaps for, 1971, *1971–1974*, 1974
  for lining deformities, 1975–1976, 1979, 1981, *1976–1978, 1980, 1981*
  forehead flaps for, 1945
    frontotemporal, 1965
    midline, 1945, 1948, 1957–1958, *1950–1964*
  frontotemporal flaps for
    scalping, 1965, *1966*
    up-and-down, 1965
  of nasal skeleton, 1982–1984, *1982, 1983*
  planning for, 1926–1928, *1928*
  retroauricular flaps for
    and contralateral postauricular flaps, 1970–1971
    and Washio temporomastoid flap, 1966, 1970, *1970, 1971*
  scalping flaps for, 1965–1966, *1966–1969*
  skin closure for, 1928–1929
  skin flaps for, historical perspective on, 1932–1934
  skin grafts for, 1929–1930, *1930*
  tissue expansion for, 1974–1975
  total, 1984–1985, *1984–1985*
Nasal rim incisions, 1845–1847, *1846*
Nasal rotations, for nasal deformity in cleft lip, 2644–2646, *2646*
Nasal septum
  anatomy of, 1791, *1793*, 1793–1794
    sensory innervation of, *1813*
  deformities of, in unilateral cleft lip and palate, 2589–2590, *2589, 2590*
  fractures and dislocations of, 983–984, *983, 984*
    diagnosis of, 984, *984, 985*
    treatment of, 987–989, *988*
  hematoma of, *989*, 989–990
  in cleft lip and palate, 2583–2584, *2582*
  shortening of, 1822–1824, *1822–1824*
Nasal spine, resection of, 1837–1838, *1838*
Nasal splint, *988*
Nasal tip
  bifid, correction of, 1851, 1853, *1853*
  broad or bulbous, correction of, 1851, *1852*
  cartilage grafting of, 1838–1839, *1838–1840*
  corrective rhinoplasty for, 1824–1826, *1825–1827*
  definition/projection of, loss of, secondary rhinoplasty for, 1920–1921, *1920, 1921*
  deformities of, repairs for, *2811, 2812*
  deviated, 1853, *1854*
  drooping of, postoperative, 1881
  excessively pointed, correction of, 1849, *1851*
  exposure of, variations in technique for, 1843–1844, *1844, 1845*
  inadequate projection of, correction of, 1849, 1851
  landmarks of, 1802, *1802*

Nasal tip *(Continued)*
"plunging," correction of, 1853–1854, *1855*, 1856
projecting, 1847–1849, *1849–1851*
rhinoplasty for
Joseph operation for, 1844–1845, *1845*
Safian operation for, 1845, *1846*
"smiling" or mobile, 1856, *1856, 1857*
Nasal tip exposure, retrograde technique for, 1844, *1844*
Nasal valve, internal, 1786, *1788,* 1808, *1808,* 1925
Nasalis muscle, 2599, *2599*
Nasion, 28, *28*, 1190
Nasoethmoidal area, fractures of, 1107–1108, *1108*
Nasoethmoido-orbital fractures, 1043–1044, 1082, *1082*
clinical examination of, 1089–1090, *1088, 1089*
complications of, 1101–1107, *1102, 1104, 1105*
in children, 1171–1174, *1172, 1173*
malunited, 1610–1611, 1614, 1616, *1611–1616*
complications of, 1623, 1625, *1624–1627*
treatment of, 1616–1618, 1620, 1623, 1625, *1616–1627*
roentgenographic examination of, 1090–1091, *1090, 1091*
structural aspects of, 1082–1085, *1082–1084*
surgical pathology for, 1085–1086, *1085*
traumatic telecanthus and, 1087–1089, *1087, 1088*
treatment of, 1091–1092, *1092*
surgical approaches for, 1092, 1097–1098, 1100–1101 *1092–1096, 1099–1101*
weakness of nasal area and, *1086*, 1086–1087
Nasofrontal angle
anatomy of, 1788, *1788*
obtuse, 1847
deepening of, 1839, *1841*
Nasojugal transposition flap, 2217
Nasolabial angle
anatomy of, 1788
resection of, 1837–1838, *1838*
Nasolabial flap
for columellar reconstruction, 1986, *1986, 1987*
for intraoral reconstruction, 3438, *3439*
for nasal reconstruction, 1940, *1941–1949*, 1943
for nasal relining, 1979, *1980*
for total lower lip reconstruction, 2024–2025, *2025*
for upper lip reconstruction, 2031, *2032, 2033*
Nasolabial folds, 782, 1788, 2366
Nasolabial transposition flaps, for nasal reconstruction, 1943, *1945, 1946*
Nasolacrimal duct, obstruction of, in nasoethmoido-orbital fractures, 1614, *1615*, 1616
Nasolacrimal duct obstruction, from maxillary surgery, 3333
Nasomaxillary buttress, 1021
Nasomaxillary complex
displacement of, 2508, *2508*
postnatal growth of, 1150–1151
remodeling growth in, 2509
Nasomaxillary dysostosis. *See* Binder's syndrome.
Nasomaxillary hypoplasia, 1387, 1389, *1389–1401*, 1391, 1394, 1396, 1398–1399, 1401, 1800, *1800*. *See also* Binder's syndrome.
correction by naso-orbitomaxillary osteotomy, 1394, 1396, *1396–1398*, 1398
dish-face deformity of, 1362
in Binder's syndrome, 3008, *3009*
Nasomaxillary hypoplasia *(Continued)*
Le Fort II osteotomy for, 1399, *1399–1401*, 1401
surgical techniques for, 1389*t*
Nasomaxillary skin graft inlay, 3543–3545, 3549, *3544–3548, 3550*
for dish-face deformity, 1975–1976, *1977, 1978*, 1979
Naso-ocular clefts, 2444
Nasoorbital fractures, in children, 1170–1171
Naso-orbitomaxillary osteotomy, 1394, 1396, *1396–1398*, 1398
Nasopalatine duct cyst, 3340
Nasopharynx
anatomy of, 3416, *3416*
cancers of, 3458–3460
squamous cell carcinoma of, in children, 3187
Navicular bone, tubercle of, 4260, *4260*
Naviculocapitate syndrome, 4646, *4646*
Neck
burn injuries of, 2189–2190, *2191*, 2192–2194, *2194–2199*, 2196–2197, 2200
cancers of
interdisciplinary management of, 3412–3413
public education programs for, 3412
congenital webbing of, surgical correction of, 2076–2078, *2079–2085*, 2085
contracture of, excision of scar in, 2060, *2061–2064*
cutaneous arteries of, *356, 357*, 358–359
embryological development of, 2456–2460, *2457–2459*
lymph nodes of, management of, in aerodigestive tract cancer, 3427–3435, *3429, 3430, 3432–3436*
pediatric tumors of
benign, 3181–3184, *3183*
developmental anomalies and, 3178–3181, *3179–3181*
inflammatory masses of, 3176–3178
late sequelae of therapy for, 3188, *3188*
malignant, 3184–3188, *3188*
preoperative evaluation of, 3175–3176
radiographic imaging of, 3176, *3177*
radical dissection of
as prophylaxis for aerodigestive tract cancer, 3427–3429
classical technique for, 3429–3433, *3429, 3430, 3432*
functional technique for, 3433–3434, *3433–3436*
resurfacing of
after burn injury
ascending neck-chest advancement flaps for, 2197, *2199*
bilobed flaps for, 2194, *2195*
by vertical to transverse flap transposition, 2193–2194, *2194*
expanded skin flaps for, 2197, 2200
local and regional skin flaps for, 2193
microvascular free flaps for, 2200, *2201*
by combination of local flaps and skin grafts, 2196–2197, *2197*
laterally based advancement flaps for, 2194, 2196, *2196*
shoulder flaps for, 2197, *2198*
tube flaps for, 2200
scar contractures of, 2057–2058
soft tissue sarcomas of, 3366, 3368
torticollis of, congenital muscular, 2085, 2087–2090, *2086, 2089*

Neck mold, construction of, for splint, 2065–2068, *2065–2068*
Neck node biopsy, for aerodigestive tract cancer evaluation, 3422, *3422*
Neck webbing, correction of, 3146
Neck-chest advancement flaps, ascending, for neck resurfacing, 2197, *2199*
Neck-shoulder flaps, bilobed, for neck resurfacing, 2194, *2195*
Necrotizing fasciitis, 5543–5544
Needle electromyography, 672–673
Needles, for microsutures, 420, *420*
Neonate, cleavages lines in, *217*
Nerve(s)
  anatomy of
    in great toe vs. thumb, 5163–5164
    in lower extremity, 4035, *4037*, 4038
  control of blood flow by, 446–447, *446, 447*
  embryology of, in hand and arm, 5221, 5223
  in electrical burn injuries, 5425–5426
  local irritation of, differential diagnosis of, 4906
  of orbitonasal structures, 1680–1681, *1680–1682*
  of scalp, 1517–1518, *1518*
  problems of, in rheumatoid arthritis, 4704–4705
  recovery of, 4925
  repair of
    awake stimulation technique for, 4766
    delayed primary type of, with nerve retraction, 4768, *4770*
    with epineural splint, 4767–4768, *4767–4769*
Nerve allografts, cyclosporine immunosuppression in, 198
Nerve blocks
  alveolar, 147–148, *149*
  for increasing muscle function in tetraplegia, spasticity and stroke, 4979–4980, *4980*
  for post-traumatic facial pain, 1133–1134
  in head and neck surgery, 144–153, *146–152*, 153*t*
  infraorbital, 147–148, *147, 148*
  interscalene. *See* Interscalene block.
  lower incisor, 148–149
  mandibular, 149–150, *150*
  mental, 148–149, *149*
  neural complications of, avoidance and management of, 4324–4325
  of brachial plexus
    choice of, *4305*, 4305–4308
    complications of, 4307*t*, 4307–4308
    extent of analgesia from, 4306, 4306*t*
    plasma levels of local anesthetic agents during, 4311*t*
  of elbow, *4322*, 4323
  of external ear, 153, *154*
  of eyelids, 1639, 1681–1682, *1681, 1682*
  of forehead, *146*, 146–147
  of maxilla, 150–152, *151, 152*
  of nose, 152–153, *152, 153*
  of phrenic nerve, 4307
  of radial nerve, 4323
  of scalp, 145–146, *146*
  patient management of, 4315
  patient preparation for, 144–145
  patterns of onset and recovery of, 4314–4315
  performance of
    for axillary block, 4320, *4321*
    for digital block, 4323, *4325*
Nerve blocks *(Continued)*
  performance of, for elbow, *4322*, 4323
    for infraclavicular block, *4319*, 4320
    for interscalene block, 4316, *4317*
    for intravenous regional anesthesia, 4320, 4322
    for subclavian perivascular block, 4316, 4318, *4318*, 4320
    for wrist blocks, 4323, *4324*
    general aspects of, 4315–4316
  performed above clavicle, complications of, 4307–4308
  performed below clavicle, complications of, 4308
  premedication for, 4315
  recurrent laryngeal, 4307–4308
  subclavian perivascular, 4306, 4307
Nerve conduction velocity (NCV), 671–672
Nerve damage, from orthognathic surgery, 1409–1411, *1410, 1411*
Nerve excitability test (NET), evaluation of facial nerve function in, 2253
Nerve fibers, classification of, 4309*t*
Nerve grafts
  advantages of, 4771
  after resection of mandibular body and bone graft reconstruction, 1438
  autologous, for brachial plexus injury repair, 4805–4807
  choice of nerve for, 2262–2263, *2262, 2263*
  crossface, for facial paralysis, 2272–2274, *2274–2276*
  disadvantages of, 4771
  donor sites for, 4772
  extratemporal, for facial paralysis, 2259, 2262–2263, *2262–2264*, 2265, *2266–2270*, 2267, 2267*t*, 2270*t*, 2270–2271, 2271*t*
  facial, with irradiation, for facial paralysis, 2272
  for hand reconstruction, 4297
  for peripheral nerve reconstruction, *682*, 682–683
  free vascularized
    blood supply of, *4873*, 4873–4874
    donor sources for, 4875–4876, *4877–4881*, 4880
    experimental studies of, 4874–4875
    for upper extremity reconstruction, 4872–4873
    indications for, 4875
  historical aspects of, 4768–4769, 4771
  indications for, 4771–4772
  intracranial, for facial paralysis, 2272
  principles of, 4771
  technique of, 4772–4775, *4774*
  vascularized, for peripheral nerve reconstruction, 683–684
Nerve growth factor (NGF), 665–666, 2475
Nerve injuries
  after facioplasty, of male, 2396–2398, *2397*
  causing facial pain, 1131–1133
  classification of, 2252, 4819–4821, *4819–4821*
  clinical examination of, *4818,* 4818–4819, *4819*
  compression syndromes. *See specific compression syndromes.*
  electrodiagnostic evaluation of, 4821, *4822*, 4823
  from maxillary surgery, 3333
  historical aspects of, 4817–4818
Nerve territory oriented macrodactyly (NTOM), 5362, 5364, *5363*
Nerve-muscle pedicle techniques, for facial paralysis, 2298

Nervous system
deformities of, in craniofacial microsomia, 3068–3070, *3070*
vascular malformation pathogenesis and, 3227
Neural crest, 2517, 2519, *2518*
development of, 2461–2462, *2462–2464*, 2464–2465, *2466–2467*, 2467–2468
Neural crest cells, 2465, 2925, *2925*
Neural neurotization, 2255, *2257*
Neural plate, anterior, embryological development of, 2517, *2517*
Neural tissue tumors
granular cell myoblastoma, 3586–3587, *3587*
of hand, 5505–5507, *5505, 5506*
Neural tube
closure failure of, 2460–2461, *2461*
formation of, 2460
Neurapraxia, 656, 2252
Neurectomy, selective, for facial paralysis, 2305–2306
Neurilemomas, 3301–3304
of hand, *5505*, 5505–5506
Neuroblastoma, of head and neck, 3369, *3369*
Neurofibromas
benign pediatric, 3181–3183
of hand, 5506, *5506*
of orbit, 1651, 1653, *1652, 1653*, 3391, *3392–3395*, 3395–3396
Neurofibromatosis
chest wall reconstruction and, 3714, 3714*t*, *3716*
dermabrasion of, 777
gigantism and, 5364–5365, *5366–5367*
in children, 3181–3183, *3183*
Neurofibrosarcoma, of head and neck, 3369
Neurofilaments, 636
Neurogenic conditions, causing velopharyngeal incompetence, 2906
Neurogenic tumor, chest wall reconstruction and, 3714, 3714*t*
Neurologic sequelae, from amputation, 4331
Neurolysis procedures, 679–680
Neuromas
at amputation stump, *4847*, 4848, 4849, 4852, *4849–4852*
evaluation of, 4847–4848, *4847, 4848*
formation of, 669–670
historical aspects of, 4846–4847
in-continuity, 670, 674
and timing of repair, 678
of glioma, 4852–4854, *4853*
of hand, 5505
resection of, 4912
terminal bulb, 670
Neurons
morphology of, 634, 635, *635*
pathfinder type, 2475
regeneration of, 657–660, *658, 659*
Neuropathology, of Down syndrome, 3162
Neurotization, for brachial plexus root avulsion, 4790–4792, *4790, 4791*
Neurotmesis, 656, 2252
Neurotomy, for post-traumatic facial pain, 1134
Neurovascular free flaps, 304–305, *305*
Neurovegetative theory, 3227
Neutroclusion, 1193, *1193*
Nevus. *See also specific types of.*
of nail bed, 4509, *4509*
preexisting, malignant melanoma and, 3636
Nevus araneus, 3585, *3586*
Nevus cell nevus, 3588–3589, *3589, 3590*
Nevus flammeus. *See* Port-wine stains.
Nevus flammeus neonatorum, *3233*, 3233–3234
Nevus sebaceus, 3574–3576, *3575*
basal cell carcinoma and, 3617, *3617, 3618*
Nevus unius lateris, 3574, *3575*
Nevus verrucosus, 3574, *3575*
Nickel exposure, oral cancer and, 3418–3419
Nickel-titanium alloy (Nitinol), for alloplastic implants, 706
Nicotine, vasospasm from, 455. *See also* Cigarette smoking.
Nifedipine, for reflex sympathetic dystrophy, 4910
Nipple(s)
hypertrophy of, correction of, 3864, *3869, 3870*
inversion of, correction of, 3864, 3873, *3870–3872, 3874, 3875*
reconstruction of, *3907, 3908*
Nipple-areola reconstruction, *3926, 3926–3927, 3927*
Nissl bodies, 635
Nitroglycerin, postoperative treatment of skin flaps with, 316
Noack's syndrome, 5123
Node of Ranvier, 640, 641–642, *641*
Nodular fasciitis, 3184
Nodular synovitis, 4512
Nodulus cutaneus, 3578–3579, *3579*
Nonepidermoid carcinomas, of nasal cavity and paranasal sinuses, 3361
Non-Hodgkin's lymphoma
of bone, 3359
staging classification for, 3185
Nonunion, from orthognathic surgery, 1405
No-reflow phenomenon, 460, 5018–5019
Norepinephrine, 309, 310
Nose
anatomy of, 1786–1798, 1924–1926, *1925, 1926*. *See also specific structures of.*
ethnic variations in, 1803–1804, *1803–1805*, 1879
of accessory cartilages, 1795, *1795, 1796*
of alar cartilages, *1794*, 1794–1795
of bony structures, *1787*, 1788–1789, *1789*
of cartilaginous structures, *1787*, 1789, 1791, *1790*
of external landmarks, 1786, 1788, *1788*
of muscles, 1791, *1792*
of sensory innervation, *1813*
of soft triangle, 1795–1796, *1796*
of weak triangle, 1796, *1796*
artificial
coloring and camouflage for, 3543
materials for construction of, 3541–3542
modeling of, 3541
preliminary surgical procedures for, 3543
retention methods for, *3542*, 3542–3543
bifid, 2998–2999
bony hump of
double, rhinoplasty procedure for, 1839, 1841
resection of, 1827–1828, *1827–1829*
single, rhinoplasty procedure for, 1839
burn injuries of, 2200, 2202–2204, *2203*
contour restoration of
costal cartilage grafts for, 1892, *1892–1893*, 1893
iliac bone grafting for, 1886–1887, *1886–1888, 1889, 1890, 1891*
deformity of, in cleft lip. *See* Cleft lip nasal deformity.

Nose *(Continued)*
deviated, rhinoplasty for, 1862–1867, *1862–1872, 1869, 1871, 1873–1876*, 1876
dorsal hump of, recession of, 1843, *1844*, 1847
esthetics of, 1798–1800, *1799–1803*, 1802–1803
subunits for, 1927, *1927*
foreshortened
diagnosis of, 1990–1991, *1991, 1992*
etiology of, 1991, *1993, 1994*
surgical management of, 1991, 1994, *1995–1997*, 1997–1998
lacerations of, 909, *910*
lengthening procedure for, 1387, 1389, *1390, 1391*
middle vault problems of, secondary rhinoplasty for, 1917–1918, *1918, 1919*
physiology of, 1804, *1806*, 1806–1807
anatomic factors influencing ventilation and, *1807, 1807–1809, 1808*
postnatal development of, 2497
postoperative shortening of, 1998
psychosocial aspects of disfigurement of, 122–124, 123*t*
reconstruction of. *See* Nasal reconstruction.
regional block of, *152*, 152–153, *153*
regional entities of, 27
shape and size of, 1926, *1926*
skeleton of, reconstruction of, 1982–1984, *1982, 1983*
skin grafts within, 3543, *3543*
soft tissues of, 1786
surface measurements of, *1926*
tip of, 1788, *1788*
Nose-chin relationship, in preoperative planning for rhinoplasty, 1809–1810, *1810, 1811*, 1812
Nostrils
anatomy of, 1924–1925, *1925*
ventilation and, *1807*, 1807–1808
border of, 1795
outer angle of, and relationship to age, 2856, *2856*
problems with, correction of, 1856–1857, *1857*
shapes of, 1926, *1926*
soft triangle of, 1924, 1925, *1925*
Nové-Josserand technique, for hypospadias repair, 4158–4159
Nutrient artery, 600–601
Nutritional status, postmaxillectomy management and, 3333
Nylon fabric–silicone rubber composite dressing, *723*, 723–724

Obesity
definition of, 3965
hyperplastic, 3965
hypertrophic, 3965
morbid
diabetes and, 3968, *3972*
insulin levels and, *3971–3973*
SAL results and, *3969–3971*
surgical problems associated with, 3967–3968
type V hip/thigh contour deformity, suction-lipectomy of, 4002, 4004, *4013*
Oblique line, 1305
Oblique muscle flap, external, for abdominal wall defects, 397
Obstructive sleep apnea
clinical aspects of, 3147–3148
diagnosis of, 3148–3149
historical aspects of, 3147
nonsurgical treatment of, 3149–3150
surgical treatment of, 3150–3152, *3151, 3152*
Obturators, for cleft palate, 3553–3554, *3553–3557*, 3556, 3558
Occipital cerebral cortex, injury of, 1118
Occipitofrontalis muscles, 1538–1539
Occlusal cant, in craniofacial microsomia, preoperative planning for, 3074–3075, *3077*
Occlusion, dental
classification of, 916, 919, *919*
in cleft palate, 2733–2734
Occlusion test, 1599, *1599*
Occlusive suture, 1590, *1591*
Ocular globe, 1049, *1050*
Ocular prostheses, 3537, *3540*, 3540–3541
Oculoauriculovertebral syndrome malformation, 2469
Odontoameloblastoma, 3345
Odontogenic carcinomas, 3346
Odontogenic cysts
calcifying, 3338–3339
of jaw
developmental types of, 3337–3339
inflammatory types of, 3339–3340
Odontogenic fibroma, 3345
Odontogenic keratocysts, 3338, *3339*
Odontogenic myxoma, 3345
Odontogenic tumors
calcifying epithelial, 3342
of jaw
ectomesenchymal, 3345–3346
epithelial, 3341–3342, 3345, *3341, 3343, 3344*
malignant, 3346
squamous, 3342
Odontoma, 3345
Ohm's law, 814
Öhngren's line, 3417, *3417*
Olecranon autografts, 612–613
Olfactory nasal placodes, embryological development of, 2517, *2517, 2524*
Olfactory nerves, anatomy of, 2978–2979, *2979*
Oligohydramnios, *76*, 94
Omental flap
drainage of lymphedema through, 4112–4113
for chest wall reconstruction, 3700, *3701, 3702*
for mediastinal reconstruction, 395–396
for Romberg's disease, treatment of, 3140, *3142–3143*
vascularized transfer, 521, *521*
Omphalocele, abdominal wall reconstruction for, 3774, 3775–3777, 3779–3780, *3775, 3777, 3779*
Oncocytoma, of salivary glands, 3298–3299, 3309
Onlay bone grafts
for malunited zygoma fractures, 1665, *1666*, 1667
for maxillary deformities secondary to cleft palate, 2829, 2832
Open bite deformity
anterior, 1351, *1352*
classification of, 1352
clinical evaluation of, 1353–1354, *1353, 1354*
correction of, by Kufner procedure, *1361*
etiology of, 1352
incidence of, 1352

Open bite deformity *(Continued)*
treatment of, *1354*, 1354–1355
by anterior segmental dentoalveolar osteotomy of mandible, 1356–1357, *1357*
by anterior segmental dentoalveolar osteotomy of maxilla, *1357*, 1358
by mandibular ramus osteotomy, 1357
by orthodontic therapy, 1356
by posterior segmental dentoalveolar osteotomy of maxilla, 1358, *1358, 1359*, 1360
by tongue reduction, 1360
by total maxillary osteotomy, 1360, *1370*
by transverse posterior palatal osteotomy, 1360, *1376*
classification of modalities in, 1355–1356
surgical-orthodontic, historical background for, 1355, *1355, 1356*
with mandibular prognathism, 1258
Open reduction
extended
for Le Fort fracture treatment, 1022
of panfacial fractures, 1033, 1035, 1038, *1033–1037*
extraoral, of mandibular fracture, 971, *973*
for class II mandible fractures, 954, *955*
intraoral approach to, 956–957, *956–958*
intraoral, of mandibular fracture, 971, 973, *974*
of edentulous mandible, 969, 971, *971–974*
of mandibular parasymphyseal fracture, 948, *950*
with interfragment wiring or plate and screw fixation, of zygoma fracture, 1004–1005, *1005, 1006*
Open-sky technique, for nasoethmoido-orbital fractures, 1092, 1097, *1094–1097*
Operating room, organization of, for hand surgery, 4289–4290
Ophthalmic complications, from total maxillectomy, 3334
Ophthalmic prostheses, 3537
Opponens tunnel, anatomy of, *4281*, 4283
Optic atrophy, in craniosynostosis, 3026
Optic canal, *1048*, 1050
Optic chiasm injury, 1118
Optic cup, 1574
Optic foramen, 1050, 1110
Optic foramen–oblique orbital position, for plain films, 885, *888*
Optic nerve
anatomy of, 1115–1117, *1116*
injury of
computed tomography in, 1118, *1119*
treatment of, 1119
types of, 1117
visual examination techniques for, 1117–1118
Optic placode, 1574
Optic stalk, 1574
Optic sulcus, 1557
Oral cancers
of buccal mucosa, 3452, *3453–3455*
of hard palate and superior alveolus, 3452, 3455
of lower alveolar gingiva, 3451–3452
Oral cavity
anatomy of, 3416, *3416*
squamous cell carcinoma of
sites of, 3450
survival of, 3450*t*
Oral commissure
burn injuries of, 2226, 2228–2229, *2230*, 2231
electrical burns of, *2230*, 2231
Oral-facial-digital syndrome, Type I, 107
Orbicularis oculi muscle
anatomy of, 1673–1675, *1674–1676*, 1677
festoons of, 2324, *2326*
festoons of, surgical removal of, 2339, *2342–2345*
in blepharoplasty, 2324
Orbicularis oculi palsy. *See* Eyelid(s), paralysis of.
Orbicularis oculis muscle, hypertrophy of, 2327
Orbicularis oris muscle, 2246–2247, 2598, 2599, *2599*
abnormalities of, from unilateral cleft repair, correction of, 2785–2787, *2786–2788*, 2789
deformity of, after cleft lip repair, surgery for, 2646–2647, *2647*
secondary deformities of, from cleft lip repair, 2851, *2851*
Orbit
anatomy of, 1575, *1576–1580*, 1577–1580, 1671–1673, *1672*
anophthalmic syndrome of, reconstruction for, 1646–1647, *1647, 1648*
anophthalmos and, 1639–1640, *1641, 1642*
bony
anatomy of, 2979–2981, *2979–2981*
lateral wall of, total mobilization of, 2994–2995, *2994, 2995*
clinical evaluation of, 1580–1581, 1581*t*
by dilated funduscopic examination, 1584
by slit lamp examination, 1584
equipment for, 1580, *1581*
history for, 1580–1581
inspection and palpation in, 1582
motility and, 1583–1584
pupils in, 1582–1583
visual acuity for, 1581, *1582*
decompression of, 1630
four-wall approach to, 1634, 1635
indications for, 1634–1635
Krönlein-Berke approach (one-wall), 1635
lateral canthal or three-wall, 1637
lateral or one-wall, *1634*, 1636
Maroon-Kennerdell four-wall, 1637, *1638*, 1639
medial
through external incision (Sewal operation), 1635
two-wall or Walsh-Ogura operation, *1636, 1636–1637, 1637*
Naffziger-Poppen-Craig intracranial approach to, 1635
one-wall (Krönlein-type) approach to, 1632–1633, *1634*
Tessier-Wolfe three-wall, 1637, *1638*
three-wall approach, 1634, 1635
transantral (two-wall) approach to, 1635
two-wall approach to, 1633–1634, *1635*
upper lid retraction and, 1639
deformities of
in von Recklinghausen's disease, 3183
with microphthalmos, 1640–1642, *1643*
dislocation of, 1625, 1628, *1628*
dystopia of, vertical, 1628–1629
preoperative evaluation of, 1629, *1629*
surgical treatment of, 1629–1630, *1631*
embryology of, 1574–1575, *1574, 1575*
emphysema of, with frontobasilar region fracture, 1114
exenteration of, 3326, *3327*
fascial framework of, 1673, *1674*
fibrous dysplasia of, 1649, *1649–1652*, 1651

Orbit *(Continued)*
floor of, osteotomy for, 2995, *2997*
fractures of. *See* Orbital fractures.
functional, mobilization of, 2995, *2995–2997*
growth of, 2509, *2509*
hemangioma of, 1653, 1655, *1655*
injuries of, from gunshot, 1127
lymphangioma of, 1655, *1656*
neurofibroma of, 1651, *1652,* 1653, *1653,* 3391, *3392–3395*, 3395–3396
osteotomy-mobilization of, *1629*, 1629–1630
radiographic techniques for, 1584–1590, *1585, 1587, 1589*
reconstruction of, for Treacher Collins syndrome, 3111–3113, *3112*
roof of
fracture-dislocation or loss of, 1114
malunited fractures of, 1596–1597
soft tissues of, injury to, 909
structures of, innervation of, 1680–1681, *1680–1682*
surgical approaches to, *1592*, 1593–1594, *1593–1596*, 1596
surgical principles for, 1590, *1591, 1592*, 1593
surgical treatment of, 3381–3384, *3382–3384*
tumors of, 3364, 3366
Orbital apex, 1178
Orbital apex syndrome, 1115, *1115*, 1672
Orbital fat
anatomy of, 1049, *1049*
herniated, 2327
blepharoplasty for, 2320
Orbital fractures, 1043–1044
anatomic considerations for, 1044–1049, *1045–1048*
blow-out type of, 1046, 1050–1053, *1052*, *1062–1063*
classification of, 1052*t*
etiology of, 1052*t*, *1053*
impure, 1057
in children, 1057–1058, 1169–1170, *1170*
limitation of oculorotatory movements in, *1064, 1065*
mechanism of production of, 1053–1055, *1054–1056*
complications of, 1057, 1057*t*, 1101–1107, *1102, 1104, 1105*
diplopia in, 1057*t*, 1058–1059
enophthalmos in, 1057*t*, 1059–1061, *1059, 1060*, 1068–1069, *1069*
examination and diagnosis of, 1061–1062, *1062*
limitation of forced rotation of eyeball in, 1062, 1065, *1065*
impure, 1073, 1075
in children, 1167–1170, *1168, 1170*
linear, without blow-out, 1077–1082
comminuted, of orbital floor, 1078–1079
of lateral orbital wall, 1080–1081, *1081*
of medial orbital wall, 1079–1080, *1079, 1080*
of orbital roof, 1081–1082
malunion of
correction of extraocular muscle imbalance in, 1606, 1609
enophthalmos from, 1600–1601, *1602–1605*, 1604–1606
in nasoethmoido-orbital fractures, 1610–1611, *1611–1616*, 1614, 1616
infraorbital nerve anesthesia for, 1609–1610, *1610*
medial and lateral canthal deformity treatment of, 1609
Orbital fractures *(Continued)*
malunion of, superior sulcus deformity treatment of, 1609
surgical treatment for, 1601, 1604–1605, *1604, 1605, 1607–1610*
vertical shortening of lower eyelid, 1609
with zygoma fractures, *1664*, 1665, *1665*
of floor and medial and lateral walls, 1597, *1598*
of roof, 1107–1108, *1108*
radiographic evidence of, 1065, *1066–1069*, 1067–1069
secondary orbital expansion/contraction in, 1057
sensory nerve conduction loss with, 1069
surgical pathology of, 1057–1061, *1059, 1060*
surgical treatment of, 1069–1077
exposure of orbital floor in, 1071–1073, 1075, *1072–1074*
operative technique for, 1070–1071, *1071*
restoration of continuity of orbital floor for, 1075–1077, *1075–1077*
timing of, 1070
Orbital hypertelorism
classification of, 2988
clinical findings in, 2982, 2984, *2984–2986*, 2986
craniofacial surgery for
complications of, 3008–3010
in children, *3000*, 3000–3001
subcranial approach to, technique for, 3001, *3001*
design of surgical procedure for, 2975, *2975*
etiology of, 2926
operative procedures for, 2988
combined intra- and extracranial approach to, 2991–2995, *2991–3001*, 2998–3001
development of extracranial approach to, 2989
development of intracranial approach to, 2988–2989
in correction of associated deformities, 2989, *2989, 2990*, 2991
pathologic anatomy of, 2986, *2987*, 2988
postoperative extraocular muscle function and, 3002
postoperative period for, 2976–2977
preoperative planning for, 3001, *3002*
surgical correction of, longitudinal studies of, 3001, *3003, 3004*
terminology for, 2982, *2982, 2983*
with medial facial clefts, 2540, *2541*
Orbital hypotelorism
anomalies associated with, 3002, *3005*, 3005–3006
clinical findings in, 3002, 3005
differential diagnosis of, 3005*t*
embryological aspects of, *3006*, 3006–3007
surgical correction of, *3007*, 3007–3008
Orbital prostheses, 3537, *3537–3540*, 3540–3541
Orbital septum
anatomy of, 1677–1678, *1678*
in blepharoplasty, 2324
Orbitale, 28, *28*, 1190
Orbitotomy, marginal, 1601, *1604*, 1606
Orbitozygomatic complex, displaced, *1605*, 1605–1606, *1607*
Orf, 5553
Oriental people. *See* Asian patients.
Oro-aural clefts, 2444
Orofacial-digital syndromes, 2483
Oromandibular cancer, treatment of, 45–46
Oronasal fistula
after cleft palate surgery, 2747
closure of, 2754

Oro-ocular clefts, 2444
Oropharynx
anatomy of, 3416, *3416*
cancers of
management of, 3455–3458, *3456, 3458*
survival rates for, 3457*t*
squamous cell carcinoma of, in children, 3187
Orthodontic therapy
appliances of, for jaw fixation, 1216, *1217*
for cleft lip/palate
during adult dentition period, 2897–2898, *2898, 2899*
during deciduous dentition period, 2890–2891, *2892–2895*
during mixed dentition period, 2891, *2896*, 2897
during newborn period, 2885, 2887–2888, *2888–2891*, 2890
reasons for continuing care in, 2898–2899, *2900*, 2901
for cleft palate
bonded appliances for, 2738
timing of, 2736–2737
for open bite deformities, 1356
Orthodontics
and effect on facial growth in cleft lip/palate, 2575, 2577
for alveolar and anterior cleft palate, 2756–2757
historical aspects of, 2439
in alveolar cleft palate repair, 2823
in cleft lip and palate children, historical aspects of, 2878–2879
Orthodontist, and relationship with surgeon, 1189
Orthognathic surgery
complications of, 1404–1405, *1408*, 1409–1412, *1410–1412*
fixation techniques for, 1215–1216, 1217, *1216, 1217*
rigid skeletal types of, 1216, 1218, *1219–1222*
for craniofacial microsomia, 3080, *3081*, 3082
jaw reconstructive
for children under age 6 years, 3087–3088, *3088, 3089*
osteotomies for, 1222–1223, 1225, *1223, 1224, 1237, 1248, 1370*
postoperative care in, 1218, 1222
postoperative orthodontic therapy and retention for, 1222
preoperative orthodontic therapy for, 1200–1201, 1203, 1205, *1201–1205*
preoperative planning for, 1205, 1207–1209, 1212, 1214–1215, *1206–1208, 1210–1215*
reconstructive
after age 7 years, 3088–3089, *3090, 3091*
in adolescence, 3089, *3092, 3093*
Orthopedic appliance therapy, functional, for craniofacial microsomia, preoperative planning, 3079–3080
Orthopedic complications, of thermal burn injury, *809*, 809–810
Orthopedics
and effect on facial growth in cleft lip/palate, 2575, 2577
presurgical, 2736
Orthovoltage, 832
Osseocutaneous flap, 305–306, *306*
Ossification
centers of, in hand, *5215*
heterotropic, after thermal burn injury, 810
Osteitis, after treatment of mandibular fracture, 976
Osteoarthritis, 4699
Osteoblastoma, 3347
Osteoblasts, 584–585
Osteochondritis, of temporomandibular joint, 1502
Osteochondroma
chest wall reconstruction and, 3714, 3714*t*
with condylar hyperplasia, 1490–1494, *1491–1493*
Osteoclasts, 584, 585, 590
Osteoconduction, 593, 598
Osteocytes, 584, 585
Osteoid osteoma, of jaw, 3347
Osteoinduction, 594–595
Osteomas, of jaw, 3346–3347
Osteomusculocutaneous flaps, 384
Osteomyelitis
after lower extremity trauma, 4075–4076
after treatment of mandibular fracture, 976–977
diabetes mellitus and, 5533, *5533*
diagnosis of, 5547
etiology of, 5546–5547
treatment of, 5547–5548
Osteons, 583, *584*, 725, *725*
Osteoprogenitor cells, in alloplastic implants, *725*, 725–726, *728*
Osteoradionecrosis, 838, 838*t*, *839*
Osteosarcoma
chest wall reconstruction and, 3716
of jaw, 3353, *3355*, 3356
radiation exposure and, 838
Osteotomy
advancement augmentation for zygoma reconstruction, 1663, *1664*, 1665
and reduction, for malunited zygoma fractures, 1665
anterior segmental dentoalveolar, of mandible, for open bite deformity, 1356–1357, *1357*
C-shaped, of mandibular ramus, 1285–1286, *1286*
for bony hump of nose resection, 1827, *1827*
for elongation of mandibular body, 1277–1278
for malunited nasoethmoido-orbital fracture, 1616–1617, *1617*
for orthognathic surgery, 1222–1223, *1223, 1224*, 1225
horizontal recession in, *1313, 1320*, 1333, *1335*
in bilateral cleft lip and palate patients, 2868
infraorbital, 2995, *2996*
interdental, 1272, 1274–1275
Le Fort I technique for, 1401
Le Fort II technique for, for nasomaxillary hypoplasia, 1399, *1399–1401*, 1401
Le Fort III advancement
for craniosynostosis, 3037
through subcranial route, for craniosynostosis, 3037–3039, *3038, 3039*
naso-orbitomaxillary, 1394, 1396, *1396–1398*, 1398
Obwegeser-Dal Pont sagittal-splitting, 1247, *1248–1249, 1250*, 1250–1252, *1251*, 1253, 1255
Dautrey modification of, *1252*, 1252–1253, *1253, 1254*, 1255
of anterior cranial fossa and medial and lateral orbital walls, 2995, *2996, 2997*
of condylar region, 1235, *1236*
of jaw, 3080, *3081*, 3082
of lateral walls of nose, *1828–1832*, 1828–1833
of mandibular body, 1266, *1267, 1268*
of mandibular ramus, for open bite deformity, 1357

Osteotomy *(Continued)*
of maxilla
anterior segmental dentoalveolar, for open bite deformity, *1357*, 1358
for correction of skeletal deformities, 1367, 1369, *1369–1372*
for deformities secondary to cleft palate, 2832–2835, *2833*
of orbital floor, 2995, *2997*
perinasal, 1391, 1394, *1394, 1395*, 1994, *1997*
posterior segmental dentoalveolar, of maxilla, for open bite deformity, 1358, *1358, 1359*, 1360
premolar advancement, 1342, *1344–1346*, 1345–1347
premolar segmental, 1401
retromolar step, 1277, *1278*
segmental, for maxillary hypoplasia, secondary to cleft lip or palate, *2839*, 2839–2840
segmental dentoalveolar, 1333, *1336*, 1336–1337, *1338–1342*, 1342
advantages and disadvantages of, 1337, 1342
premolar recession or set-back type, 1336–1337, *1338–1341, 1360*
subnasal, 1337, *1342*
supraorbital, *2993*, 2993–2994, *2994*
technique of, for radioulnar synostosis, *5314*, 5314–5315
total maxillary, for open bite deformity, 1360, *1370*
transverse posterior palatal, 1360, *1376*
Otocephaly, 2460, *2460*
Otocraniocephalic syndrome, 3054
Otohematoma, 2127
Otology, cleft palate and, 2738–2739
Otorrhea, cerebrospinal, 1018
Outflow tract defects, 2470
Overexertion, cold injury and, 850
Oxide ceramics, for alloplastic implants, 717–718, *718*
Oxycephaly
correction of, *1566*, 1567, *1569*
definition of, 1546
visual abnormalities in, 3025–3026
Oxycephaly-multiple suture synostoses, clinical and radiographic findings in, 3018

Pacinian corpuscles, 649–650, *649*, 654–655
reinnervation of, 668
Padgett dermatome, 236, *236*
Paget's disease
extramammary, 3605, *3606*
of nipple, 3605, *3606*
Pain, after facialplasty in male, 2399
Palatal dimples, significance of, 2615
Palatal lengthening procedures, for cleft of secondary palate, *2907*, 2908, *2909*
Palatal process, deformities of, in unilateral cleft lip and palate, 2590–2591
Palate
anatomy of, 2726, *2726*
anterior, repair of, with bilateral cleft lip repair, 2664, *2665, 2666*, 2666–2667
congenital insufficiency of, 2905
fractures of, 1024, *1025*, 1026
growth of, 2509, *2509, 2510*, 2512–2513
muscles of, 2612–2615, 2619, 2623–2625, *2612–2614, 2616–2618, 2620–2622*
anatomy of, 2726–2729, *2727, 2728*

Palate *(Continued)*
primary, 2726
embryologic development of, 2519, *2521–2525, 2523, 2525–2526, 2527*
secondary, 2726
normal development of, 2541, *2542, 2543, 2544*
soft, functional movement of, 2729
Palatine foramina, anatomy of, 2726
Palatoglossus muscles, 2623–2624, 2728
Palatopharyngeus muscles, 2727, 2728, *2728*
anatomy of, *2612*, 2615, 2619, *2620, 2621*
in cleft palate, 2623–2624
Palmar bursae, 527, *528*
Palmar fascia, in Dupuytren's disease, 5059, *5060*, 5061
Palmar intercalate instability, 4647–4650, *4647–4650*
Palmar interossei muscle
examination of, 4271, *4271*
function of, 4270, *4270*
Palmaris longus muscle graft, 552, *552*
Palmaris longus tendon
anatomy of, 535–536
as donor tendon for flexor tendon repair, 4551–4552
clinical transplantation of, 535–536
transfer of, for radial palsy of thumb, 4944
transplantation of, 536
Palpebral aperture, slanting, surgical correction of, in Down syndrome, 3168–3169, *3169, 3170*
Palpebral spring, for treatment of eyelid paralysis, 2310, *2310*
Palpebral sulcus, creation of, 2425, *2425*
Panfacial fractures, involving anterior cranial fossa, 1039, *1042*
primary bone grafting for, 1039–1040, 1043, *1043*
treatment of, 1033, 1035, 1038–1040, 1043, *1034, 1036, 1037, 1041–1043*
when mandible is severely comminuted, 1038–1039, *1040*
when maxillary alveolus and palate are severely mutilated, 1039, *1041, 1042*
Panniculus, elevation of, for full abdominoplasty, 3939, *3945, 3946*
Papilledema, in craniosynostosis, 3025
Papillomas, schneiderian, 3360
Paradental cysts, 3340
Paranasal sinuses
anatomy of, 3417
cancers of
classification of, 3467*t*
management of, 3467–3469, *3468, 3469*
staging of, 3322, *3322*
surgical treatment complications of, 3331–3334, *3332*
metastatic tumors of, 3364
tumors of, 3360–3364, *3362*
Paraplegia, pressure sore development and, 3801
Parascapular flap, anatomy of, 4467–4468, *4468*
Parasitic infections, 5553–5554
Parasympathetic nervous system, control of blood flow by, 447, *447*
Paratenon, 527, *527*
Paré, Ambroise, 3–4
Parkes Weber syndrome, 3260, *3262*, 3263
Parkland formula, 792*t*
Parona's space, infection of, 5543
Paronychia, 5538–5539, *5539*
Parotid duct, 906–907, *907*
ascending, infection of, 3288–3290

Parotid duct *(Continued)*
fistulization of, 3312
lacerations of, *906,* 906–907, *907, 908*
perforations of, 3311–3312
transposition of, 3311, *3312*
Parotid duct (Stensen's), anatomy of, 2239–2240
Parotid fistula, from orthognathic surgery, 1405
Parotid gland. *See also* Salivary glands.
abscesses of, drainage of, 3312
accessory, 3303
anatomy of, 2239, *2240*, 3276–3279, *3277, 3278*
malignant lesions of, in deep segment of, 3310
masses of, 3282, *3282*, *3283*, *3286*
masseter hypertrophy and, 1478–1479
metastatic disease of, 3310
tumors of, biopsy specimen from, 3287, *3287*
Parotidectomy, incisions for, 3293–3294, *3294*
Parotitis, 3178, 3290, *3290*
Passavant's ridge or pad, 2623, 2625, 2727, 2729, 2746
Pasteurellosis, 5551
PDGF (platelet-derived growth factor), 178, 179
Pectoralis major flaps, 3438, 3444, *3444–3446*
anatomy of, 386, *386*, *388*, *389*
for acquired defects of mandible, 1439–1440, *1440, 1441*
for cheek reconstruction, 2047, *2048*, 2049, *2050*
for chest wall reconstruction, 396, 3691, *3693*, 3694
for head and neck reconstruction, 303, *303*, 503
for mediastinal reconstruction, 394–395, *394, 395*
Pectoralis minor muscle, microneurovascular transfer of, 2299
Pectus carinatum deformity
etiology of, 3742
surgical correction of, 3742, 3745, *3746–3748*
types of, 3742, *3744*
Pectus excavatum
cardiopulmonary function in, 3731–3732
chest wall reconstruction and, 3726, 3729, 3731–3733, 3737–3742, *3731, 3734–3736*
etiology of, 3729, 3731
indications for surgical correction of, 3732–3733
operative procedures for, 3733
roentgenographic studies of, 3732
severity of, 3729, *3731*
surgical techniques for
costoplasty as, 3739, *3739*
internal and external fixation as, 3739–3741, *3740, 3741*
Ravitch's technique for, 3733, 3737–3738, *3734–3736*
silicone implant reconstruction as, 3741–3742, *3741, 3743*
sternum turnover as, *3738*, 3738–3739
symptoms of, 3731
Pediatrics. *See* Children; Infant(s).
Pedicle flaps, subcutaneous, of cheek, for nasal reconstruction, 1940, *1941–1944*, 1943
Pedigree, *105*
Pedigree syndromes, 84, *86*
Penetrance, 104, *105*
Penile agenesis, 128–129
Penis
anatomy of
of arterial system, 4214, *4214, 4215*
of venous system, 4214, *4214*
artificial erection of, 4160, *4160*, 4176, *4176*, 4239
Penis *(Continued)*
avulsion injuries of, 4231, *4232*, 4233–4234
burn injuries of, *4234*, 4234–4235
constriction of, 4236
construction of, 4242
curvatures of
adjunctive diagnostic techniques for, 4177
differential diagnosis of, 4176, *4176*
etiology of, 4175–4176
surgical correction of, 4176–4177
erectile dysfunction of
evaluation of, 4215–4218, 4216*t*, 4217*t*
nonsurgical treatment options for, 4219
penile prosthesis for, 4220–4226, *4221–4224*, 4225*t*
surgical treatment options for, 4219–4220
erection of, normal physiology of, 4214–4215
foreign bodies in, 4236
fracture of, 4228–4229, *4229*
hidden, 4177–4179, *4178, 4179*
prosthesis for
complications of, 4224–4226, 4225*t*
for erectile dysfunction, 4220–4226, *4221–4224*, 4225*t*
surgical technique for, 4220–4224, *4221–4224*
reconstruction of, 4239–4240
psychosocial aspects of, 128–129
replantation of, psychosocial aspects of, 129
zipper injuries of, 4235
Pentoxifylline, for postoperative skin flap treatment, 317
PERCI, 2912
Perichondrial grafts, for joint repair, 574–575, *576*
Perichondrium, cartilage grafting and, 561
Perichondrocutaneous graft, 576, *577, 578, 579*
Pericranium, 1539
anatomy of, 1516–1518, *1517, 1518*
Perilunate
dislocations of, 4606, *4607, 4608, 4608*
dorsal transscaphoid fracture-dislocations of, 4608–4609
instability of, 4647–4650, *4647–4650*
volar dislocations of, 4609
Perinasal osteotomy, 1391, 1394, *1394, 1395*
Perineal pressure, intermittent, 4206
Perineum reconstruction, muscle and musculocutaneous flaps for, 397–399, *398*
Perineurium, 642, 643–644, 4762
Perinodal space, 642
Periodontal cysts, lateral, 3337–3338, 3340
Perionychium
anatomy of, 4499–4500, *4500*
embryology of, 4499
injury of
avulsion of, 4505–4507, *4506, 4507*
crushing, 4504–4505, *4506*
infection of, 4507–4509, *4508*
management of, 4502–4503
mechanisms of, 4502, *4503*
simple lacerations as, 4504, *4504*
stellate lacerations as, 4504, *4505*
subungual hematoma, 4503–4504
physiology of fingernail production, *4500–4502*
tumors of
benign, 4509–4512, *4509–4513*
malignant, 4512, 4514, *4514*
Periorbita, 1050, 2981, *2981*

Periorbital fat, compartmentalization of, 2323, *2325*
Periosteoplasty, 2756
Periosteum, blood vessels of, 600–602, *601, 602*
Peripheral nerve end organs, sensory receptors of, 646–655
Peripheral nerve grafting, historical background of, 630–632
Peripheral nerves
  central plasticity of, 669
  classification of fibers of, 634, 634*t*
  composition of, *632*, 632–634, *633*
    axoplasmic transport in, 637–638, *639*
    cellular morphology in, 634–637, *635*
    connective tissue elements in, 642–644, *643*
    intraneural architecture patterns in, *643*, 644
    Schwann cell in, 640–642
  conduction in, 638–640
  electrodiagnosis of, 670–675
  injury of, 655–657, *656*
    cause of, 664
    classification of, *656*, 656–657
    level of, 663–664
    timing of repair and, 676–680
  motor end organs and, 655
  neuroma formation and, 669–670
  of hand, physiology of, 4762–4764
  reconstruction of, 675–685, *680, 682*
    by nerve grafting, *682*, 682–683
    epineurium, *680*, 680–681
    nerve bed and, 683
    perineurium or fascicular repair as, *680*, 681
    postoperative care for, 684–685
    tension and, 681–682, *682*
    timing of, 676
    vascularized nerve grafts for, 683–684
  regeneration of
    in distal axon, 660
    in neuron, 657–660, *658, 659*
    in proximal axon, 657–660, *658, 659*
    influencing factors for, 661–666
    relationship to degree of injury in, 660–661
  reinnervation of, 666–669
  repair of
    delay in, 662
    techniques for, *4764–4768*
  structure of, 4314–4315
  vascular supply of, 644–646, *645*
Peripheral nervous system, embryologic development of, in head, 2473–2475, *2474, 2476–2477,* 2477
Persantine, platelet function and, 458
Pes anserinus, 2240
PET (polyethylene terephthalate)
  for alloplastic implants, 708*t*, 712, *713*
  in suture materials, for alloplastic implants, 719*t*, 721
Petit's triangle, 3771
Petrosectomy
  partial, 3401, *3402*
  total, 3401, *3403–3404*, 3404
Peyronie's disease
  Dupuytren's disease and, 5055
  etiology of, 4183–4184
  evaluation of, 4184
  general considerations for, 4185–4187
  penile curvatures in, 4175–4176
  surgical procedure for, 4185, *4185, 4186*
  treatment options for, 4184
Pfeiffer's syndrome, clinical and radiographic findings in, 3023, *3023, 3024*
PGA (polyglycolic acid), in suture materials, for alloplastic implants, 719*t*, 720–721
pH, tissue, as index of flap perfusion, 319*t*, 320
Phalanx
  distal, fractures of, *4604*, 4604–4605
  middle, fractures of, 4602, *4603*, 4604
  proximal, fractures of, 4601–4602, *4602*
  transverse absence of, 5255, 5257
Phalloplasty, 4242–4243
Phallus, reconstruction of, 4237–4239, *4238*
Phantom limbs, 127, 133, 4331
Pharyngeal abscesses, lateral, in pediatric patients, 3178
Pharyngeal constrictor muscles, superior, 2727–2729
Pharyngeal flap
  for velopharyngeal incompetence, operative technique for, 2915, 2917, *2917*
  for velopharyngeal incompetence correction, 2908
  postoperative velopharyngeal incompetence and, 2905–2906
Pharyngeal glands, embryologic development of, 2478, *2479*
Pharyngoplasty
  Hynes procedure for, 2910, *2911, 2912*
  postoperative velopharyngeal incompetence and, 2905–2906
Pharynx
  anatomy of, 3416, *3416*
  cancers of, management of, 3455–3462, *3456, 3458, 3461, 3462*
  walls of
    cancers of, 3457–3458, *3458*
    posterior, augmentation of, for correction of velopharyngeal incompetence, 2908, 2910, *2910–2912*
PHEMA (polyhydroxyethylmethacrylate), 723, *723*
Phenol
  application to skin. *See* Chemical peeling.
  for chemical peeling, 756–757
  full face technique of, 761–764, *762–766*
Phenoxybenzamine (Dibenzyline), 315, 4910, 5021
Phentolamine (Regitine), 315, 5019–5020, 5442
Phenytoin (Dilantin), 2533
Philtrum
  abnormalities of, from bilateral cleft lip repair, correction of, 2851, *2852*, 2853
  reconstruction of, 2185–2186, *2186*, 2789–2790, *2789, 2790*
Phocomelia, intercalated, 5242–5243, *5243, 5244,* 5245
Phosphorus burns, 5439
Photoelectric tests, for flap perfusion assessment, 319*t*, 320–321
Photographer, medical, role of, 37–38
Photographic records, mock surgery on, 1209, *1210*
Photography
  camera for, 38
  color transparencies, vs. black and white print, 38
  lighting for, 38
  of soft tissue wounds in face, 901
  patient positioning for, 38
  preoperative
    for corrective rhinoplasty, 1809–1810, *1810, 1811*
    for facialplasty, 2367
  standards for comparison of, 36–37
  studio for, 38

Photography *(Continued)*
through operating microscope, preoperative preparation of, 415
views for, 38, *39, 40, 41*
Photoplethysmography, for flap perfusion assessment, 319*t*, 321
Phrenic nerve
anatomy of, 4313
block of, complications of, 4307
paralysis of, after interscalene block, 4308
Phrenic-facial nerve anastomoses, for facial paralysis, 2283
Physical attractiveness, 113–116
Pickwickian syndrome, 3147
Pierre Robin sequence
cleft palate in, 2596
mandible in, 2554
mandibular hypoplasia or micrognathia in, 2882
pathogenesis of, 2547
Pierre Robin syndrome. *See* Robin sequence.
Piezoelectric effect, 597–598, *598, 599*
Pigmentation, dermabrasion of, 774
Pilar cysts, 3569, 3572, *3573*
Pilomatrixoma, 3576
Pin fixation, external, of mandibular fractures, 946, *948–949*
of zygoma fracture, 1004, *1004*
Pinched tip deformity, *1799*
Pindborg's tumor, 3342
Piriform aperture fractures, 980, *981*
Pisohamate tunnel
anatomy of, *4281*, 4282
syndrome of, 4282–4283
Pituitary gland, embryologic development of, 2477–2478, *2477*
Pivot flap, 277, 289–290, *290*
PLA (polylactic acid), in suture materials, for alloplastic implants, 720–721
Placodes, ectodermal, *2518*, 2519
Plagiocephaly, 1546, 3025–3026
Plagiocephaly–unilateral coronal synostosis, *3033*
clinical and radiographic findings in, 3015, *3017*, 3018
Plantar fibromatosis, Dupuytren's disease and, 5055
Plantar warts, treatment of, 3563, *3564*, 3565
Plantaris tendon
anatomy of, 536, *537, 538*
as donor tendon for flexor tendon repair, 4552–4553
clinical transplantation of, 536–538, *536–538*
Plasmacytoma, chest wall reconstruction and, 3716
"Plasmatic circulation" of skin graft, 250–252
Plaster of Paris, burns from, 5439
Plastic surgeon
integument and, 38, 42–45, *42–44*
qualities of, 1
training and education of, 23
Plastic surgery
future of, 22–24
incidence of procedures performed in, 113, 114*t*
patient selection for, psychosocial aspects of, 117–120
psychosocial aspects of. *See* Psychosocial aspects of plastic surgery.
scope of, 20–22
techniques of. *See specific techniques.*
Plate and screw fixation, for mandibular fractures by open reduction, 958–959, *962*
Platelet-derived growth factor (PDGF), 178, 179
Platelets, factors affecting function of, 458
Platysma muscle
anatomy of, 2247, 2373–2376, *2374, 2375*
microneurovascular transfer of, 2299
musculocutaneous island flap of, 385–386
Pleomorphic adenoma
of salivary gland, malignant, 3308
treatment of, *3296*, 3296–3297
Pleotropism, 5232
Plexuses
arterial, 281, *282*
nervous, topographic anatomy of, 633–634
Plummer-Vinson syndrome, 3418
PMMA (polymethylmethacrylate), for alloplastic implants, 708*t*, 713–714
Pneumatic tourniquet, for hand surgery, 4291
Pneumocephalus, with frontobasilar region fracture, 1114, *1114*
Pneumonia, as thermal burn injury complication, 808
Pneumothorax, from brachial plexus block, 4308
Pogonion, 28, *28*
Poland's syndrome
chest wall reconstruction and, 3749, 3752–3753, 3755, *3753, 3754, 3756–3761*
clinical presentation of, 5300, *5301, 5302*
tissue expansion for, 488–489, *489, 490*
treatment of, 5300, *5302–5305*, 5303
Polio, loss of function in, 4978*t*
Pollicization
for longitudinal deficiences of radius, 5262
of index finger, 5154–5155
Polyamide, in suture materials for alloplastic implants, 719*t*, 721
Polydactyly
central, 5347–5348, 5351, *5348–5351*
classification of, 5344, 5346, *5345*
high degrees of, 5133
incidence of, 5346
of thumb
classification of, 5123, *5123*
incidence of, 5121–5123
operative management principles for, 5123–5124, *5124*
secondary surgery for, 5129–5130, *5130*, 5133
types 1 and 2, surgical procedures for, *5123–5125*, 5124–5125
type 3, surgical procedures for, 5125, *5127*
type 4, surgical procedures for, 5125, *5127–5130*, 5129
types 5 and 6, surgical procedures for, 5129
type 7, surgical procedures for, 5129, *5131, 5132*, 5133
postaxial, 5352, *5353–5355*, 5356
preaxial, 5347
treatment of, 5346–5347
Polydimethylsiloxane, for alloplastic implants, 708*t*, 708–709, *710*
Polyethylene, for alloplastic implants, 710–712
Polyethylene terephthalate (PET)
for alloplastic implants, 708*t*, 712, *713*
in suture materials, for alloplastic implants, 719*t*, 721
Polyglycolic acid (PGA), in suture materials, for alloplastic implants, 719*t*, 720–721
Polyhydroxyethylmethacrylate (PHEMA), 723, *723*

Polylactic acid (PLA), in suture materials, for alloplastic implants, 720–721
Polymers
  for alloplastic implants, 706–714, *707, 708, 710, 711, 713*
  in suture materials, for alloplastic implants, 719*t*, 720–721
Polymethylmethacrylate (PMMA), for alloplastic implants, 708*t*, 713–714
Polymorphonuclear cells, migration of, 178
Polyolefin, in suture materials, for alloplastic implants, 721–722
Polypropylene, in suture materials, for alloplastic implants, 719*t*, 721–722, *722*
Polysomnography, 3148
Polytetrafluoroethylene (PTFE), for alloplastic implants, 708*t*, 712–713, *713*
Polyurethane, for alloplastic implants, 708*t*, 709–710, *711*
Popliteal artery
  anatomy of, 4034
  occlusion of, 4063, *4063*
Porcine xenograft, for thermal burns, 805
Porion, 1190
Port-wine stains
  argon laser therapy for, *3667*, 3667–3668
  clinical presentation of, 3227, 3229, *3228, 3230*, 3581–3582, *3582*
  in newborn, *3233*, 3233–3234
  treatment of, 3231–3233, *3232*
Postburn claw deformity, 5458, 5460–5461, *5460*
Posterior calf fasciocutaneous flap, for upper extremity skin coverage, 4475
Posterior interosseous nerve syndrome, 4834–4836, *4835–4837*
Posterior thigh flap, for genital reconstructive surgery, 4141, 4143, *4144–4146*
Postponement of surgery, 47–48
Postural deformities, mechanical origin of, 75
Potter sequence, 75, *76*
Pouce floutant, *5107*, 5107–5108, 5258
Povidone-iodine, 802–803
Preaxial polydactyly, 5121–5125, *5122–5132*, 5129–5130, 5133, 5347
Preaxial polydactyly-triphalangeal thumb, *5131, 5132*, 5133
Precancerous lesions, chemical peeling for, 758
Precorneal film tears, composition of, 1727, *1727*
Pregnancy
  anesthesia during, 4303
  augmentation mammoplasty and, 3892
Premaxilla
  anatomy of, 2726
  deformity of
    in bilateral cleft lip
      closure of clefts one side at a time and, 2658
      intraoral traction for, 2659, *2660*
      lip adhesion for, 2659, *2660*
      repair of, 2656–2657, *2657*
    with bilateral clefts, 2653, *2654*
  in cleft lip and palate, 2583–2584
  malformation of, in bilateral cleft lip and palate, 2581–2583, *2582*
  protrusion deformity of, in bilateral cleft lip, surgical setback of, 2659, 2661, *2662*
Premaxilla *(Continued)*
  protrusion of
    elastic traction for, 2658, *2659*
    in cleft lip and palate, causes of, 2587–2588
    surgical control of, 2657–2658
  retropositioning of, 2887
  tilting or retrusion of, 2697
Premaxillary segment, deformities of, in unilateral cleft lip and palate, *2589*, 2589–2590
Premedication
  dosages of, 140, 140*t*
  for pediatric patient, 156, 156*t*
  for regional nerve blocks, 4315
Premolar advancement osteotomy, 1342, *1344–1346*, 1345–1347
Premolar recession osteotomy, 1336–1337, *1338–1341, 1360*
Preoperative interview, psychologic preparation of patient during, 140
Preoperative medication, for rhinoplasty, 1812
Pressure dressings, 52, 54–55
Pressure sores
  clinical aspects of, 3806*t*, 3806–3807
  clinical studies of, 3803–3804
  conservative local treatment of, 3812–3813
  etiology of, 3798–3801, *3799*
  historical aspects of, 3797
  initial treatment of, 3801–3802
  pathology of, 3804–3806, *3804, 3805*
  spasticity and, 3803
  surgical treatment of
    complications of, 3834–3835
    general principles of, 3814, 3818
    in multiple sites, 3827, *3830–3834*, 3834
    procedure for, *3815–3817*, 3818–3821, 3819*t*, *3820–3826, 3823, 3826–3827, 3828–3834*, 3834–3835
    timing for, 3813–3814
    ulcer excision as, *3817*, 3819
  systemic treatment of, 3807–3812
    for relief of pressure, 3809
    for relief of spasm, 3808–3809
    in cooperation with other services, 3808
  treatment of, 3807
  type and level of lesion in, 3801–3803, *3802*
Prickle cell epithelioma, 3606–3607, *3607*
Primary Abbé flap, for bilateral cleft lip repair, 2691–2692, *2692*
Primary dye test (Jones I test), 1729
Procerus muscles, 2400
Procollagen, 171
Procollagen peptidase, 180
Prodromal phase, of radiation sickness, 833
Profileplasty, orthopedic, for Asian patients, *2429–2432*, 2431, 2433
Progeria, characteristics of, 2364
Prognathism
  mandibular
    children and adolescents with, *1257*, 1257–1258
    classification of, 1228–1229, *1230, 1231*
    clinical presentation of, 1228, *1228*
    correction in edentulous patients, 1255–1257, *1255–1257*
    etiology of, 1228
    intraoral vertical-oblique osteotomy of ramus for, *1244–1245*

Prognathism *(Continued)*
mandibular, osteotomy of ramus for, sagittal-split technique, 1247, *1248–1254,* 1250–1253, 1255
postoperative condylar changes, 1243, 1247
shape of mandible, after osteotomy of ramus, 1243
surgical correction procedures for, choice of, 1258, 1260
treatment of, 1229
evolution of techniques for, 1232–1235, *1234, 1235*
orthodontic vs. surgical, 1229, 1231
preoperative planning for, 1231–1232, *1232*
with microgenia, 1258, *1259*
with open bite, 1258
maxillary, 1362
in Asian face, surgical correction of, *2429*, 2431, *2432*, 2433
Prolabium, usage of, bilateral cleft lip repair and, 2656
Proline, hydroxylation of, 170
Proline analogues, for abnormal scar prevention, 740
Prolyl hydroxylase, in keloids, 735–736
Pronator quadratus, *4274*
Pronator syndrome, 4833–4834, *4834*
Pronator teres, *4274*, 4942–4943, *4944*
Propranolol (Inderal), 315, 4910
Proprioception, evaluation of, by two-point discrimination test, 4978–4979, *4979*
Prostacyclins, 309, 317
Prostaglandins, 309, 317
Prostanoids, in blister fluid, from frostbite patients, 854, 854*t*
Prosthetic material grafts, for abdominal wall reconstruction, 3769–3770, *3770*
Prosthetics
auricular, 2129, 3549, *3551*
cineplastic powered active, 4396
for amputations, with electrical injuries to upper extremity, 5428
for cleft palate, 3549, 3552–3553, *3552*
indications for, 3552
types of, 3553–3554, 3556, 3558, *3553–3557*
for hand. *See* Hand prosthesis.
for microphthalmos treatment, 1642, *1643*
for phocomelia, 5243, 5245
for temporomandibular ankylosis, 1495–1496, *1495*
for transverse absence of forearm, 5245–5246, *5247*
maxillofacial. *See* Maxillofacial prosthetics.
nasal, 3541–3545, 3549, *3542–3548*
ocular, 3537, 3540–3541, *3540*
penile. *See* Penis, prosthesis for.
shoulder cable powered active types of, 4394–4395, *4395*
Protein
in suture materials, for alloplastic implants, 719*t*, 719–720
needs of burn patients, 798–799, 799*t*
total body stores of, in thermal burns, 798
Proteus syndrome, *3263*, 3264
Protozoan infections, 5553–5554
Proximal interphalangeal joint
deformities of, after burn injury, 5465–5467, *5466*
dislocations of, 4617–4621, *4618–4620*
fractures of, 4621–4624, *4624*
Proximal ligation, for treatment of arteriovenous malformation, 3256
Pseudoenophthalmos, 2324
Pseudohypernasality, 2907
Pseudoprognathism, of mandible, 1229
Pseudoptosis
after orbital or nasoethmoido-orbital fractures, 1106
causes of, 1753–1754, *1754, 1755*
Pseudoxanthoma elasticum, characteristics of, 2364
Psychologic problems
from amputation, 4332
in reflex sympathetic dystrophy, 4900–4901, 4901*t*
Psychologic state of patient, tendon transfers and, 4924–4925
Psychosocial aspects of plastic surgery
facial disfigurement and, 120–124
of aging face, 124–125
of amputation, 132–134
of breast surgery, 125–128
of genitalia surgeries, 128–131
of otoplasty, 124
of replantation, 132–134
of self-mutilation, 131–132
patient selection and, 117–120
physical attractiveness and, 113–116, 114*t*, 115*t*
religion and, 117
spectrum of beauty and, 116–117
Psychotherapy, for reflex sympathetic dystrophy, 4914
Psychotropic drugs, for reflex sympathetic dystrophy, 4911
Pterygium colli, surgical correction of, in torticollis, 2076–2078, 2085, *2079–2085*
Pterygoid hamulus, 2726
Pterygoid muscle, 937
PTFE (polytetrafluoroethylene), for alloplastic implants, 708*t*, 712–713, *713*
Ptosis, eyelid
after orbital or nasoethmoido-orbital fractures, 1106
aponeurosis surgery for, *1758*, 1759, 1765–1766
Fasanella-Servat operation for
Beard's modification of, 1760, *1761*
Iliff's modification of, *1764*, 1764–1765
other modification of, 1765
Smith's modification of, 1761, *1762–1763*, 1764
technique for, 1759–1760, *1760, 1761*
frontalis muscle suspension for, 1772–1774, *1772–1774*
levator resection for, 1766–1767, 1772, *1768–1771*
upper, 1752–1755, *1753–1759*
Pulmonary aspiration, emergency treatment for, in facial injuries, 877, 879
Pulmonary cavity reconstruction, muscle and musculocutaneous flaps for, 396–397
Pulmonary fat embolism syndrome, in abdominoplasty, prevention of, 3936
Pulmonary thrombosis, in abdominoplasty, prevention of, 3936
Puncta adherentia, 641
Punctum, 2331
Pupillary reactivity, 1117–1118
Pupils, clinical evaluation of, 1582–1583
Pyogenic granuloma
clinical presentation of, 3584, *3585*
differential diagnosis of, hemangiomas and, 3204–3206, *3205*
of hand, 5499, *5499*
of paronychium, 5539, *5540*
pathogenesis of, 3584
treatment for, 3585–3586
Pyramidal fractures, 1013–1014, *1013, 1014*

Quadriga syndrome, 4331, *4332*, 4558, *4558*
Quadriplegia. *See* Tetraplegia.

Racial differences, in facial morphology, cleft lip/palate susceptibility and, 2529–2530
Rad, 832
Radial artery forearm flap
  anatomy of, *4473*, 4473–4474
  for free flap transfer, in upper extremity, 4472–4474, *4473*
  for sensory reconstruction of hand, 4868, *4869*, 4870
Radial bursae, infection of, 5543, *5543*
Radial forearm flap
  fasciocutaneous type of, *297*, 297–298
  for soft tissue coverage, 4457
Radial innervated dorsal skin flap, for soft tissue injuries of thumb, 5100, *5102*
Radial nerve
  anatomy of, 4758–4759
  dorsal branch of, 4280, *4280*
  injuries of, with brachial plexus injuries, 4802
  regional block of, 4323
Radial nerve paralysis, tendon transfers for, 4941–4947, *4942, 4944, 4946*, 4963
Radial styloid fractures, 4637–4638, *4638*
Radialization, for longitudinal deficiencies of radius, 5265
Radiation
  biologic effects of, 832–833
    diagnosis of, 833
    systemic, 833
  chronic, squamous cell carcinoma and, 3630, *3630*
  craniofacial cleft formation and, 2928
  exposure to, basal cell carcinoma and, 3615, *3616*
  historical background of, 831
  immunosuppression by, 195
  ionizing, 831–832
    irradiation injuries and, 5444–5445
Radiation dermatitis, 831
Radiation injuries
  acute, 834, 5445–5446
  chronic, 834, 5446, 5449, *5447, 5448*
  development of, 5443–5444, *5444*
  etiology of, 831–832
  infections in, 835–386, *836, 837*
  ionizing radiation and, 5444–5445
  local effects of, 833–834
  malignant transformation of, 836–838, *837*, 846–847, *847*
  of male genitalia, 4235, *4235*
  osteoradionecrosis and, 838
  subacute, 834
  treatment principles for, 838–842, *839–842*
  ulcers from, 844–846, *845, 846*
Radiation sickness
  latent phase of, 833
  main phase of, 833
  prodromal phase of, 833
Radiation therapy
  for breast cancer, 3899
  for hemangiomas, 3213
  for keloids, 741
  for malignant melanoma, 3652
  for maxillary tumors, 3330
    complications of, 3332–3333
Radiation therapy *(Continued)*
  injury from. *See* Radiation injuries.
  squamous cell carcinoma and, 3629, *3629*
  surgery after, 842–844, *843*
Radicular cysts, 3339
Radioactive microspheres, for flap perfusion assessment, 319*t*, 322
Radiocarpal joint, in rheumatoid arthritis, 4714–4718, *4715–4717*
Radiography
  cephalometric, 1194
  diagnosis of facial injuries by, 882–887, *884–889*, 893–894, 897–899
  for reconstruction planning, 25–26
  of aerodigestive tract cancers, 3423, 3425, *3423–3425*
  of facial injuries, 882–887, 893–894, 897–899, *884–889*
  of hand and wrist, 4288–4289
  of maxillary fracture, 1018, *1018*
  of nasoethmoido-orbital fractures, 1090–1091, *1090, 1091*
  of orbit, 1584–1590, *1585, 1587, 1589*
    for fractures of, 1065, 1067–1069, *1066–1068*
  of zygoma fractures, 997–998, *998*
  panoramic roentgenograms, of mandibular fracture, 897, 899, *899*
  plain films of
    Caldwell position of, 884–885, *885*
    for axial projection of nasal bones, 886–887, *890*
    for facial injuries, 883–884
    for lateral and profile views of face, 886, *889*
    for nasal bones, 886, *890*
    for occlusal inferosuperior views of mandible, 893, *893, 894*
    fronto-occipital projection of, 885, *886*
    Fuchs position of, 886, *889*
    lateroanterior projection of, 886, *889*
    of mandible, 894, *895, 896*
    of orbit, 1584, *1585*
    of temporomandibular joints, 894, 897, *897, 898*
    optic foramen-oblique orbital position in, 885, *888*
    reverse Waters position in, 885, *887*
    semiaxial projection for, 886, *888*
    submentovertex and verticosubmental positions for base of skull, 887, 893, *893*
    superoinferior occlusal views of hard palate, 887, *891, 892*
    Titterington position in, 886, *888*
    Waters position in, 884, *885*
Radionuclide bone scan, 590
  for diagnosis of reflex sympathetic dystrophy, 4904
Radioulnar synostosis
  clinical presentation of, 5309–5310, 5313, *5313*
  treatment of, 5313–5315, *5314*
Radius
  longitudinal absence deformities of, vs. ulnar longitudinal absence deformities, 5273*t*
  longitudinal deficiencies of
    classification of, 5258, 5260, *5259*
    clinical presentation of, 5258, *5261*
    complications of surgical procedures in, 5265, *5266*, 5267
    treatment of, 5260, 5262, *5263*, 5264–5265, *5264, 5266*, 5267
Ranvier, node of, 640
    ultrastructure of, *641*, 641–642

Rasp technique
for corrective rhinoplasty, 1841–1842, *1841, 1842*
for resection of bony hump of nose, 1827–1828, *1828, 1829*
Rathke's pouch, 2477–2478, *2477*
Ravitch's technique
for chondrogladiolar deformity, 3742, 3745, *3746, 3747*
for chondromanubrial deformity, 3745, *3747, 3748*
for pectus excavatum deformity, 3733, *3734–3736*, 3737–3738
Raynaud's phenomenon, initiation of, 5013–5014, *5014*. *See also* Vasospastic disorders.
Receptor blockers
and prostaglandins, for postoperative treatment of skin flaps, 317
for postoperative treatment of skin flaps, 315–316
Reciprocal clicking, 1481–1482, *1482*
Reconstructive surgery. *See also specific types of reconstruction.*
planning of, 24–26
vs. esthetic surgery, 1–2
Rectus abdominis flap
anatomy of, 390–391, 393, *393*
for abdominal wall defects, 397
for abdominal wall reconstruction, 3768
for chest wall and pulmonary cavity reconstruction, 396–397
for chest wall reconstruction, 3694, 3696–3697, *3695*
for genital reconstructive surgery, 4137, *4139–4141*
advantages of, 4139, 4141
disadvantages of, 4139
regional flap comparisons of, 4141, *4142, 4143*
for groin and perineum reconstructions, 399
myocutaneous type of, anatomy of, 299–300, *300*
Rectus abdominis muscle, microneurovascular transfer of, 2299
Rectus femoris flap
applications of, 4039–4040, *4041*
for abdominal wall defects, 397
for genital reconstructive surgery, 4149, 4152, *4149–4151*
for groin and perineum reconstructions, 398–399
motor innervation of, 4039
origin and insertion of, 4039
vascular supply of, 4039
Recurrent laryngeal nerve, anatomy of, 4314
Recurrent laryngeal nerve block, complications of, 4307–4308
Recurrent-pattern syndromes, 82, *83*, 84*t*
Red glass test, 1599
Reduction methods, for zygoma fractures, 1000–1001, *1001*
Reese dermatome, 230, *232–235*, 235–236
Reflex sympathetic dystrophy
clinical forms of, 4891–4894, *4893, 4895*
definition of, 4884–4886, 4885*t*
diagnosis of, 4885–4886, 4886*t*
diagnostic techniques for, 4903–4904
differential diagnosis of, 4904–4906, *4906*
endogenous opioid pain control system in, 4901–4902
etiology of
peripheral anatomic basis of, 4898–4903, *4899*
psychophysiologic basis of, 4902–4903
historical aspects of, 4886–4887
incidence of, 4887
Reflex sympathetic dystrophy *(Continued)*
mechanism of onset for, 4903
myofascial dysfunction and, 4894–4896
pain of, 4888–4889
precipitating causes of, 4888
prevention of, 4914–4916
prognosis for, 4887–4888
psychologic findings in, 4900–4901, 4901*t*
stages of, physical findings in, 4889–4891, 4890*t*, *4890–4892*
sympathetic nervous system and, 4897–4898
treatment of, 4907
by acupuncture, 4912
by hand therapy, 4912–4914
by pharmacologic agents, 4909–4911
by psychotherapy, 4914
by surgical control of peripheral nerve irritants, 4912
by sympathectomy, 4908–4909
by sympathetic block, 4907–4908
by transcutaneous electrical nerve stimulation, 4911–4912
trophic changes in, biologic mechanisms of, 4896–4898
"Registration peptide," 171
Regitine (phentolamine), 5019–5020, 5442
Reichert's cartilage, 2487–2488, 3059
Reinnervation, in muscle transfer, 4973, *4973*
Rejection, of limb allografts, 198–200
Relative afferent pupillary defect (Marcus Gunn pupil), 1583
Religion, plastic surgery and, 117
Relocation, of bone, 2500, 2502
Remodeling, 531
of mandible, 2502, 2504
of maxilla, 2508–2509, *2508*
Remodeling growth, 2499
Remodeling process, 4434
Rendu-Osler-Weber syndrome, 3227, 3238–3239, *3238*
Repair. *See also specific types of repair.*
choice of method of, 46–48
timing of, 45–46
Replantation
centers for, 4356–4357
definition of, 54, 4356, *4356*
for arm amputations, 4376–4377
for degloving or ring avulsion, 4374–4375
of forearm, 4375–4376, *4375, 4376*
of hand, 4289, 4375–4376, *4375, 4376*
of lower extremity, 4068–4069
indications for, 4070–4071
ischemia time and, 4069
nature of amputation injury and, 4070
operative technique for, 4071, 4073
postoperative management for, 4073
replacement of lost tissue in, 4070
salvage technique for, 4071, *4072*
surgical problems in, 4069
zone of injury in, 4069–4070
postoperative care for, 4377
psychosocial aspects of, 132–134
secondary procedures for, 4377–4378
techniques of, *4362*
with absent venous drainage, 4374
Research, in plastic surgery, 19

Reserpine
for postoperative treatment of skin flaps, 314
for vasospastic disorders, 5019
intra-arterial, for treatment of cold injury, 857
Residency programs, establishment of, 13–14
Residual cysts, 3340
Resorcinol, for chemical peeling, 756
Respiratory depression, narcotic-induced, 141
Respiratory obstruction
emergency treatment for, 871–873, *872, 873, 874, 875*, 875–876
from hemangiomas, 3207, *3207*
in Robin sequence, 3127–3129, *3128*, 3134
Restoration, anatomic, vs. camouflage, 46
Resuscitation
following electrical burn injuries, 815–816, 816*t*
formulas for, 792*t*
Retiform plexus, 3224
Retinacular system, of hand, 4265–4266, *4267*
Retinoic acid, 2491
13-cis-Retinoic acid, teratogenicity of, 2465, 2467–2468
Retinoic acid syndrome
craniofacial alterations in, 2465, *2466*, 2467
development of, 2468, 2469, 2473, 2478
Retroauricular flaps
for nasal reconstruction, contralateral postauricular flaps as, 1970–1971
Washio flaps as, 1966, 1970, *1970, 1971*
Retrobulbar hematoma, after blepharoplasty, 2351
Retrodiscitis, 1479–1480, *1480, 1481*
Retrognathia
definition of, 1260, 3123–3125
diagnosis of, 3127–3129, *3128*
etiology of, 3125–3127
of maxilla, 1360
treatment of, 3129–3131, *3132*, 3133
Retrograde lateral plantar artery flap, for foot reconstruction, 401
Retromolar step osteotomy, 1277, *1278*
Retrusion, maxillary, 1360
Revascularization
definition of, 4356
in muscle transfer, 4972
of skin grafts, 1931–1932
of tendon graft, 532
Reverse Waters position, for plain films, 885, *887*
Revue de Chirurgica Structive, 15, *16–17*
Rhabdomyosarcoma
of hand, 5500
of head and neck, 3368
in children, 3186
of orbit, 3364, 3366, *3367*
Rheology of blood, alteration of, to improve skin flap blood flow, 317
Rheumatoid arthritis
anesthesia for, 4303–4304
of temporomandibular joint, 1502–1503, *1503*
soft tissue problems of, 4704–4712, *4706, 4708–4710*
systemic effects of, 4703–4704
tendon and nerve entrapment of hand and wrist and, 4739
Rhinophyma
historical aspects of, 1987
nonsurgical treatment of, 1988
pathology of, 1987–1988, *1988*

Rhinophyma *(Continued)*
surgical treatment of, 3568–3569, *3569–3571*
extirpation of, 1988, *1989*, 1990
Rhinoplasty. *See also* Nose.
adoption of, 6–7
anesthesia for, 1812, 1814–1815, *1813, 1814*
complications of, 1881–1882
corrective, preoperative considerations for, 1809–1810, 1812, *1810, 1811*
cultural aspects of, 123*t*
deferral of, 1896
esthetic
for Asian patients, 2433–2435, *2433–2435*
in non-caucasians, 1876, 1879–1880
external, for foreshortened nose, 1994, 1997–1998, *1995–1997*
for asymmetric or deviated noses, camouflage technique for, 1896, *1896*
for augmentation, in Asian patients, 2426–2428, 2431, *2427, 2428, 2427, 2428*
for cleft lip nasal deformity, 2802
for deviated nose, 1862–1867, 1869, 1871, 1873–1874, 1876, *1862–1872, 1874–1876*
historical origin of, *2*, 5–6
history of, 1785–1786
open, 1845–1847, *1846*, 1851.
patient expectations and, 1896
postoperative care for, 1880–1881, *1881*
preoperative medication for, 1812
problem noses and, 1847–1849, *1848–1861,* 1851, 1853–1854, 1856–1858, 1860–1861,
psychosocial aspects of, 122–124, 123*t*
secondary
autogenous materials for, 1897, *1897*
consultation for, 1895–1896
diagnosis for, 1898–1899, *1899–1903*, 1901–1902
dissection in, limiting of, 1897–1898
esthetic goals for, 1898, *1898*
for loss of tip definition/projection, *1920,* 1920–1921, *1921*
for middle vault problems, 1917–1918, *1918, 1919*
for supratip deformity, 1911–1913, *1911–1917*, 1915
graft materials for, 1902, *1903–1911*, 1904, 1908–1909, 1911
technique of
evolution of, 1817
for adjunctive methods, 1836–1839, *1836–1839*
illumination for, 1815–1816, *1815, 1816*
patient positioning for, 1815, *1815*
stage 1, 1817–1818, *1818–1821*, 1821
stage 2, 1822–1826, *1822–1827*
stage 3, 1827–1828, *1827, 1828*
stage 4, 1828–1833
stage 5, 1833–1834, *1833–1835*
stage 6, 1834, *1835*
surface landmarks for, 1815–1817, *1816*
variations in, 1839, 1841–1847, *1841–1847*
with genioplasty, 1802, *1802*
Rhinorrhea, 1018
cerebrospinal, after orbital or nasoethmoido-orbital fractures, 1107
with frontobasilar region fracture, 1113–1114
Rhinoscope, *1816*
Rhytidectomy. *See* Facialplasty.

Rhytides, facial, injectable collagen for, 782
Rib grafts, 569, 572–573, *572–575*
for secondary rhinoplasty, 1909, *1909, 1910*
nonvascularized autografts of, 613–614, *613–616*
split, technique for obtaining, 614, *616, 617*
vascularized, 614, 617
Rickets
craniosynostosis of, 98–99
vitamin D resistant, 107
Riding breeches deformity of hip and thigh, suction-assisted lipectomy for, 4002, *4005, 4006*
Rigid intermaxillary fixation, 959
Riley-Smith syndrome, 3264
Risdon approach, 1227, *1237*
Robin sequence, *94*
cephalometric studies of, *3124*
complications of, 3133–3134
conditions associated with, 93*t*
congenital defects associated with, 3129
definition of, 3123–3125, *3124*
diagnosis of, 3127–3129, *3128*
etiology of, 75, 78, 3125–3127
growth and development with, 3133
historical aspects of, 3125, *3126*
malformation sequence of, 72, 72*t*
pathogenesis of, 92–94, *93*
treatment of, 3129–3131, *3132*, 3133
by modified Routledge procedure, 3131, *3132*, 3133
Roentgenography. *See* Radiography.
Roentgens, 832
Rolando fracture, 4611–4612
Romberg's disease
clinical aspects of, *3135*, 3135–3136
differential diagnosis of, 3136
pathophysiology of, 3136
treatment of, 3137, 3140, *3137–3143*
skeletal reconstruction for, 3137
soft tissue reconstruction for, 3137, 3140, *3137–3143*
Rotation flap
anatomy of, 277, *277*, 290, *290, 291*
design of, 4449
for radiation ulcer in sacral region, 846, *846*
of scalp, 1527
Rotation-advancement flaps
dorsal nasal type of, 1936, *1936, 1937*
for secondary long lip correction, *2774*, 2775–2776
for secondary short lip correction, 2776–2777, *2776–2780*, 2779
Rubber band flexion, for flexor tendon repair, *4541–4542*, 4541–4544
Rubinstein-Taybi syndrome, 73, 3234
Ruffini end organ, *650*, 650–651, 654
"Rugby jersey" injury, 4536

Sacrum, pressure sores of, 3819*t*, 3819–3821, *3820–3822*, 3823
Saddle nose deformity
bone and cartilage grafting for, 1882, *1884*, 1885–1886
clinical presentation of, 1881–1882
iliac bone grafts for contour restoration in, 1886–1887, 1889, *1886–1888, 1890, 1891*
surgical correction of, in Down syndrome, 3168, *3168*
Saddlebag deformity of hip and thigh, suction-assisted lipectomy for, 4002, *4005, 4006*
Saethre-Chotzen syndrome, clinical and radiographic findings in, 3023, *3024*
Safian tip operation, 1845, *1846*
Salivary glands
anatomy of, 3276–3281, *3277–3280*
cysts of, 3312–3313, *3313*
diseases of
diagnosis of, 3281–3284, *3282–3286*
historical aspects of, 3275–3276
with nonsalivary origin, 3309–3310
inflammatory masses of, 3288–3290, *3289*
minor
anatomy of, 3281
malignant lesions of, 3310–3311
surgery of, complications of, 3311–3315, *3313*
tumors of, 3187, 3187*t*
benign types of, surgical treatment of, 3295–3304, *3296, 3298, 3300–3302*
biopsy specimens from, 3287, *3287*
incidence of, 3284–3286
malignant types of, 3304–3309, *3305, 3306*
needle aspiration biopsy of, 3287–3288
primary types of, 3359–3360
surgical planning considerations for, 3290–3295, *3293, 3294*
Salivation, excessive, transposition of Stensen's duct for, 3311, *3312*
Saltatory conduction, 640
Saphenous flap, for sensory reconstruction of hand, *4870*, 4870–4871
Saphenous nerve, as source for free vascularized nerve graft, 4876, *4879*, 4880
Sarcomas. *See also specific types of sarcoma.*
of hand, 5500–5501, *5501*
of head and neck, 3366, 3368
of midface, surgical treatment of, 3390–3391
pediatric malignant, of head and neck, 3185–3187
Sartorius muscle, flap of, for groin and perineum reconstructions, 398
Scalp
alopecia of. *See* Alopecia.
anatomy of, 1516–1518, *1516–1518*, 1538–1539, *1539*
congenital defects of, 1540–1546, *1541–1545*
expansion technique for, *1544, 1545*, 1548, 1552–1553, *1553*
reconstruction of, by tissue expansion, 491–496, *492–495*
reduction of, 1533–1536, *1534, 1535*
regional nerve blocks of, 145–146, *146*
traumatic defects of, 1546–1554, *1547–1554*
avulsion, total as, 1546–1547, *1547*
partial, 1547–1548, *1548–1552*
Scalp flap
for alopecia, 1527–1533, *1527–1533*
for nasal reconstruction, 1965–1966, *1966–1969*
for partial scalp defects, 1547–1548, *1548–1552*
lateral, 1529–1530
Scalp grafts, strip, for eyebrow reconstruction, *2219*, 2219–2222
Scaphocephaly, 1546
Scaphocephaly-sagittal synostosis, clinical and radiographic findings in, 3015, *3015, 3016*
Scaphoid bone, 4260
fractures of, *4596*, 4596–4597, 4641–4642, *4642, 4643*

Scaphoid bone *(Continued)*
nonunions of, 4642–4643, *4643*
rotatory subluxation of, 4608
Scapho-trapezial-trapezoid fusion, 4683–4684, *4683–4685*
Scapula
flaps of, 294–295, *294*
anatomy of, 4467–4468, *4468*
vascularized grafts of, 624–625
Scarification, for port-wine stains, 3231
Scars
acne, dermabrasion for, 773, *774*
after facialplasty in male, 2398–2399
appearance of, mechanical factors of surgical wound closure and, 741–742, 745, *742–745*
collagen remodeling of, 172, 175, *173, 174*
contractures of
interphalangeal joint stiffness and, 4658–4661, *4659–4661*
metacarpophalangeal joint stiffness and, 4658–4661, *4659–4661*
depressed, injectable collagen for, 782–783
dermabrasion for, 773–774, *774, 775, 776*
formation of, 161
abnormal etiologies of, 732–733, 735, 735*t*
location of, 745
of lip, from cleft lip repair, removal of, 2646
of nose, 1928–1929
partial excision of, 52, *53*
replacement of, in cheeks
with distant flaps or microvascular free flaps, 2183
with regional tube pedicle skin flap, 2178–2179, *2180–2181*, 2182
with skin graft, 2182–2183
shape of, 742, *744*
tissue of, collagen content in, 169
Schirmer test, 1730, 2251
Schuchardt flap, for lower lip reconstruction, 2015–2016, *2017*
Schuchardt procedure, for anterior open bite correction, 1358, *1358*
Schwann cell, 198, 640–642
Schwannoma, of head and neck, 3369
Scleral show. *See* Ectropion.
"Scleroderma en coup de sabre," 3135, *3135*
Sclerosing angioma, 3578–3579, *3579*
Sclerotherapy
for hemangiomas, 3213
for venous malformations, 3253, *3253*
SC-pseudothalidomide-Roberts syndrome, 3235
Scrotum
avulsion injuries of, 4231, *4232*, 4233–4234
construction of, 4242
contusions of, 4229
Sebaceous cell lesions, 3299
Sebaceous cysts, 3569, 3572
Sebaceous glands
anatomy of, 223–224
in skin graft, 245
Sebaceous hyperplasia, 3574, *3574*
Seborrheic keratosis, 774, 3566–3568, *3567–3569*
Second branchial arch syndrome, 2931
Second toe autotransplantation
complications of, 4429
donor area of, 4409, *4410–4416*
foot dissection for, 4421–4425
Second toe autotransplantation *(Continued)*
for congenital autoamputations, *4424–4425, 4427*
for multiple digit reconstruction, 4409, *4411, 4415, 4419, 4423–4426*
for single digit reconstruction, 4409, *4420–4422*
for thumb reconstruction, 4409, *4416–4419*
hand dissection for, 4420–4421
historical aspects of, 4409–4410
indications for, 4410–4412
operative plan for, 4418, 4420
postoperative management for, 4425–4429
preoperative evaluation for, 4412–4414, *4414*, 4416, 4418
toe transfer for, 4425
Secondary dye test, 1729–1730
Secrétan's syndrome, 5024, *5025*
Sedation, 141–142
Seikeibigin, 2418–2420, *2419*
Self-mutilation, 131–132
Senile angioma, 3581, *3582*
Senile keratosis, 3595–3596, *3596, 3597*
dermabrasion of, 774
Senile lentigo, 751, *751*
Sensate flap, 304–305, *305*
Sensibility testing, in extremity, 4979–4980
Sensory changes, after forehead-brow lift, 2410
Sensory deficits, in Down syndrome, 3162–3163
Sensory evoked response, for evaluation of nerve injury, 4821, *4822*, 4823
Sensory mechanoreceptors, reinnervation of, 667–669
Sensory perception, basis for, 4859–4860, *4860*
Sensory receptors
adaptation of, 646–648, *647*
glabrous skin, 648–651, *648–650*
hairy skin, 651–652, *652*
mucocutaneous types of, 652–653
muscular and skeletal types of, 653–655, *653, 655*
of peripheral nerve end organs, 646–655, *647*
responses from, types of, 654, *655*
SEP (somatosensory evoked potentials), 673
Sepsis, from lymphatic malformations, treatment of, 3247
Septal cartilage
anatomy of, 1791, 1793–1794, *1793, 1794*
for secondary rhinoplasty, 1902, 1904, *1904–1906*
trimming of, in rhinoplasty, 1833–1834, *1833–1835*
Septal flap technique, for nasal relining, 1981, *1981*
Septal-turbinate synechiae, post-rhinoplasty, 1882
Septic arthritis, of hand, 5545–5546, *5547*
Septocutaneous arteries, 277, *278*, 283–284, *283, 284*, 292, 294
Septum, nasal
deviations of, ventilation and, 1808–1809
perforation of, 1882, *1883*
Septum orbitale, 1049–1050
Serotonin, 309, 2482
Serratus anterior flaps, for chest wall and pulmonary cavity reconstruction, 396
for chest wall reconstruction, *3690*, 3697
Sewal operation, 1635
Sex chromosome aneuploidy, 100
Sex reassignment surgery, 130
SHAFT syndrome, 132, 4332
Sheen technique, for corrective rhinoplasty, *1841*, 1841–1842, *1842*

Short face deformity, 1384, *1385–1388*, 1386–1387
Shoulder, cutaneous arteries of, 359, *360*
Shoulder cable powered active prostheses, 4394–4395, *4395*
Shoulder flap, for neck resurfacing, 2197, *2198–2199*
Shoulder-hand syndrome, *4893*, 4893–4894
Sialadenitis, 3178
Sialadenoma papilliferum, 3299
Side cross finger flap
  for coverage of fingertip amputations, 4490, *4491–4493*, 4492–4493
  for dorsal digital defects, *4495*, 4496
Silastic epidermis, 805
Silastic wrap, 670
Silicone, for alloplastic implants, 708–709, 708*t*, *710*
Silicone sling, for eyelid paralysis, 2310, *2311*
Silk sutures, for alloplastic implants, 719*t*, 719–720
Silvadene, 802, 803*t*, 803–804
Silver nitrate, 803, 803*t*
Silver sulfadiazine, 802, 803*t*, 803–804
Simianism, 1347, *1348–1351*, 1351
Simonart's band, 2557, 2593, *2593, 2594*
Sjögren's syndrome, 3282
Skeletal distortions, secondary to hemangiomas, 3210
Skeletal hypertrophy, in lymphatic malformations, 3243, *3244*
Skeletal maxillary protrusion, 1333, *1335*
Skeletal muscle
  blood supply to, 550
  fibers of, 546–547, *547*
  grafting of, 547, 551–555, *552, 554*
  injury to, 551
  innervation of, 547–549, *547, 548*
  microneurovascular transfers, 555–556, *556*
  tenotomy and, 547–548
Skeletal osteotomy, 1233, *1237, 1248, 1370*
Skeletal system, complication of, from electrical injuries, 828–829
Skeletal tissues, development of 2487–2488, *2487, 2489*, 2491
Skin
  aging process of, 44–45, 2360–2361
    histology of, 749–751, *750, 751, 2362*, 2362*t*
  anatomy of
    in foot vs. in hand, 5156, 5159, *5156–5159*
    skin grafts and, 221–224, *222*
  biologic functions of, 207–208
  blanching of, 214
  blood supply of, regional patterns of, 286, *287*, 288
  circulation of, 335, *336–344*, 344
  collagen fiber structure in, 208, *208, 209*, 210
  color and texture matching of, 46
  color of
    after cold injury, 858
    as index of flap perfusion, 319*t*, 320
  condition of, after chemical peeling, 770–771
  conductance of, for diagnosis of reflex sympathetic dystrophy, 4903
  crease lines in, 213
  cutaneous receptors in, 4859–4860, *4860*
  depigmentation of, after chemical peeling, 769
  disorders of. *See specific disorders.*
  extensibility of, 215
    cleavage lines and, 218–220, *219*
  functions of, 221
  mechanical studies of, *212*
  microcirculation of, 308–309, *309*
Skin *(Continued)*
  nonliving, storage of, 247
  of scalp, 1516, 1538
  physical properties of, 210
    directional variations in, 215–220, *216–219*
  problems of
    from amputation, 4332
    in rheumatoid arthritis, 4704
  stress-strain curve of, 210, *210*
  stretching or expansion of, 214
  striae formation in, 214
  structural studies of, *211*
  sun-damaged, histology of, 749–751, *750, 751*
  tattoos of, 3608–3610, *3609*
  tension properties of, 213–214
  thickness of, 224
  types of, 45
  venous drainage of, 353, 355, *354, 355*
  viscoelastic properties of, 210, 213, *213*
Skin closure, Steri-tape technique of, 49, *49*
Skin flap, 2348. *See also specific types of flaps.*
  alteration of rheology and, 317
  arterial cutaneous, *292*, 292–295, *293, 294*
  axes of, 374–375, *375*
  classification of
    by blood supply, 277–278, *278*
    by composition, *278*, 278–279
    by method of movement, 276–277, 277*t*
  dimensions of, *375*, 375–376
  drainage of lymphedema through, 4113, *4114*
  expanded, for neck, after burn injury, 2197, 2200
  expansion of, for cheek resurfacing, 2174–2178
  fasciocutaneous types of, 295–299, *296, 297, 298*
  folded, for nasal lining restoration, 1979, *1980*
  for abdominal wall reconstruction, 3765–3766, *3766, 3767*
  for cervical contractures, complete, 2068, *2069–2075*, 2073–2074, 2076
  for cheek reconstruction, 2049–2050, *2050, 2051*
    in zone 2, 2042–2043, *2044–2048*, 2045–2048
  for chest wall reconstruction, 3683, *3685, 3686, 3687*, 3688
  for correction of Cupid's bow, 2648, *2648*
  for lymphedema therapy, 4111
  for nasal reconstruction
    historical perspective on, 1932–1934
    local nasal flaps, 1934–1936, *1935–1940*, 1940
    nasolabial cheek flaps, 1940, *1941–1949*, 1943
  free, for nasal reconstruction, 1971, 1974, *1974*
  hypervascular planes of, 377
  hypovascular planes of, 377
  Limberg flap, modified, for cheek reconstruction, 2038–2040, *2039–2043*, 2042
  local vs. distant, 275, 277
  myocutaneous, *299*, 299–301, *300, 301*
  nasal turn-in, for nasal lining restoration, 1979, *1980*
  pathophysiologic changes in, 309–313, *310, 311, 312, 313*
    anatomic, 310, *310*
    hemodynamic, 311–312, *311, 312*
    metabolic, 312–313, *313*
  perfusion, monitoring of, 318–323, 319*t*
  pharmacologic studies of, 314–318
    increasing tolerance to ischemia and, 317–318
  radial innervated dorsal type of, for soft tissue injuries of thumb, 5100, *5102*
  random cutaneous, *288–291*, 288–292

Skin flap *(Continued)*
reconstruction of upper lip, 2186–2187
remote, for nasal reconstruction, 1971, *1971–1973*
tube pedicle, regional, for scar replacement in cheeks, 2178–2179, *2180–2181*, 2182
Skin graft(s)
acceptance of, 4437, *4438*
allografts
rejection of, 198
revascularization of, 252–259
autografts, revascularization of, 252–259
biologic behavior of, 249–267
choice of donor site for, 226, *227*, 228–229
contraction of, 243–244
dermal overgrafting technique of, 247–249, *248*, *249*
dermal/epidermal specificity of, 244
donor site for, healing of, 246–247
durability and growth of, 245
epithelial appendages in, 244–245
experimental studies of
biochemical studies and, 251
color changes in skin grafts and, 252
experimental orthotopic grafts and, 251
intravenous colloidal carbon suspension studies and, 251–252
microangiographic studies and, 251
failure of, causes for, 242, 242*t*
for abdominal wall reconstruction, 3765
for coverage of electrical burn injuries, 5426–5428, *5426–5428*
for eyelid reconstruction, 1689
for genital reconstructive surgery, 4125–4126
for hand reconstruction, 4295–4296
for lower eyelid, 2216–2217
for lymphedema therapy, 4111–4112
for scar replacement, in cheeks, 2182–2183
full-thickness, 226
choice of donor site for, 228–229
contraction of, 243–244
cutting of, *238*, 238–239, *239*
for complete cervical contractures, 2074, 2076
for coverage of fingertip injuries, *4483*, 4483–4485
for genital reconstructive surgery, 4125–4126
for nasal reconstruction, 1929–1930, *1930*
for vaginal reconstruction, 4204–4206, *4205*
for wound closure, 4439–4440, *4440*
healing of donor site for, 246
healing of
during initial stage, 242–243
maturation and, 243–246
historical origins of, 7–8
immobilization of, 240–241, *241, 242*
inlay method for, 241, *242*
innervation of, 245–246
maturation of, dermal collagen turnover in, 244
of upper lip, 2184–2185
outlay method for, 241, *242*
pigment changes in, 244
postoperative care for, 240–242, *241*, *242*
open technique for, 242
preliminary of reconstructive flap for nasal lining, 1981, *1981*
preparation of wound bed for, 239–240
rejection of, 187
relative thickness of, 243
Skin graft(s) *(Continued)*
selection of, 181–182, 225–226
skin anatomy and, 221–224, *222*
split-thickness, 225–226
choice of donor site for, 226, *227*
contraction of, 243
cutting of, *227*, 229–230, 235–238, *229–236*
development of, 12–13
for cheek reconstruction, 2038
for complete cervical contractures, 2057–2058
for coverage of fingertip injuries, *4484*, 4484–4485, *4485*
for genital reconstructive surgery, 4125
for muscle transfer coverage, 4973–4974
for nasal reconstruction, 1929
for neck contracture, 2063, 2065–2068, *2065–2068*
for neck resurfacing, 2190, 2192–2193
for radiation ulcer in sacral region, *845*, 845–846
for vaginal reconstruction, 4206
for wound closure, *4438*, 4438–4439, *4439*
freehand cutting method for, 237, *237*
healing of donor site for, 246–247
mesh grafts, cutting of, *237*, 237–238, *238*
storage of, 247
survival phases of, serum imbibition, 250–252
"taking" of, 242
thickness of, 225, *225*
types of, 225
with muscle flaps, 301–304
within nose, 1975, *1976*, 3543, *3543*
wound contraction and, 168–169
xenografts, revascularization of, 259–262
Skin graft inlay
for microgenia contour restoration, 1329, 1332, *1331, 1332*
for restoration of buccal sulcus and functional alveolar ridge, 1451–1452, 1454, *1452, 1453*
nasomaxillary, 1389, 1391, *1392, 1393*
Skin lines
dynamic, 2361, 2363, *2363*
gravitational, 2363, *2363*
orthostatic, 2361, *2363*
Skin marking, for blepharoplasty, 2335, *2336*
Skin slough, after facialplasty, of male, 2396
Skin surface temperature, for flap perfusion assessment, 319*t*, 321
Skin suture marks, 742, *744*, 745, *745*
Skin tags, 3579, *3580*, 3581
Skin tension, lines of, *42*, 42–43
Skin tumors
malignant. *See* Basal cell carcinoma; Melanoma, malignant; Squamous cell carcinoma.
of viral origin, 3560–3563, 3565–3566, 3561*t*, *3562–3566*
Skull
buttresses of, 1108–1109, *1108, 1109*
calvaria of. *See* Calvarium.
congenital defects of, 1540–1546, *1541–1545*
facial, postnatal growth of, 1143, 1146–1148, *1143–1148*
fractures of, during childbirth, 1154
plain films of, 887, 893, *893*
"tower" deformity of, 3018, *3018*
Skull base
anatomy of, 3376–3377, *3377*

Skull base *(Continued)*
tumors of
in central segment of posterior area, 3401, *3402, 3403*, 3404
in posterior area, 3391, 3395–3397, 3401, 3404–3406, *3392–3396, 3402–3405*, 3398–3400
in posterior segment, 3404–3405
malignant, in anterior area of, 3381
nonmalignant, in anterior area of, 3377, 3381, *3378–3380*
preoperative examination of, 3375–3376, *3376*
Sleep apnea
central, 3147
mixed, 3147
obstructive, 3147–3152, *3149, 3151, 3152*
Sliding (advancement) flap technique, historical origin of, *2*, 7
Slit lamp examination, 1584
SMAS, anatomy of, 619, 620, 2243–2244, *2244, 2245, 2374*, 2376
SMAS-platysma cervicofacialplasty
advancement of lateral SMAS-platysma and, *2378*, 2381
midline approximation of platysma and, *2378*, 2381
operative technique for, 2381–2382, *2381–2383*
partial-width platysma flaps for, *2377*, 2380–2381
platysma anatomy and, 2373–2376, *2374, 2375*
platysma techniques for, 2376, *2377, 2378*
full-width transection of, *2377*, 2378
SMAS anatomy and, *2374*, 2376
with submental lipectomy, 2383
SMAS-platysma flap, 2381–2382, *2381–2383*
Smile, anatomy of, 2247, *2249*
Smoke inhalation injury
diagnosis of, 795–796
treatment of, *796*, 796–797
Smoking. *See* Cigarette smoking.
"Snap-back" test, 2330, *2330*, 2345
Sodium thiosulfate, 5442
Soft fibroma (skin tags), 3579, *3580*, 3581
Soft palate, cancers of, 3457
Soft tissues
at mandibular fracture site, 940, *942*
coverage of, by skin flaps, 279–280, 280*t*
facial wounds of
anesthesia for, 902
cleaning of, 901
debridement and care of, 902, *903*
delayed primary wound closure for, 900–901
lacerations of nose, 909, *910*
photography of, 901
preoperative considerations for, 901
tetanus prophylaxis for, 899–900
hypertrophy of, in lymphatic malformations, 3243, *3244*
length-tension curves of, 4938, *4938*
reconstruction of, for Romberg's disease, 3137, 3140, *3137–3143*
Solar keratosis, 3595–3596, *3596, 3597*
Solar lentigo, 751, *751*
Soleus flap
applications of, 4043–4044
for lower extremity reconstructions, 399, *400*
motor innervation of, 4043
origin and insertion of, 4043
vascular supply of, 4043
Solid-state carcinogenesis, 702
Somatosensory evoked potentials (SEP), 673
Spasm, relief of, during microvascular surgery, 422
Spasticity
hand surgery for, 4977
finger derangements in, 4982, *4983, 4984*
for release abducted thumb, 4982, *4983*
indications for, 4980–4981
patient cooperation in, 4980
results of, 4982–4984, 4984*t*
wrist in, 4981–4982
in tetraplegia, 4985
kinesthesia and sensibility of, 4978–4979
loss of function in, 4978*t*
postoperative learning in, 4978–4979
pressure sores and, 3803
Speech
changes in, from orthognathic surgery, 1411
hypernasal quality of, 2732
hyponasal quality of, 2732
misarticulation of, 2732, 2733
patterns of substitution and omission in, 2734
problems with cleft palate and, 2731–2733
Speech pathologist, 2733
Sphenoid bone, anatomy of, 2977–2978, *2977*
Sphenomandibular ligament, mandibular hypoplasia relapse and, 1289
Sphenopterygoid bone, 2726
Spherical gliding principle, 960, *960*
Spider nevus, 3240, *3240*, 3585, *3586*
Spider telangiectasis, 3585, *3586*
Spina bifida, 75
deformations in, 75
parental counseling for, 3783–3784
surgical management of, 3784–3785, *3785–3787*, 3787–3788
timing of closure for, 3784
types of, 3780–3783, *3781–3783*
urologic evaluation of, 3783
Spinal accessory nerve–facial nerve anastomoses, for facial paralysis, 2283–2284
Spitz nevus, 3592–3593, *3592, 3593*
S-plasty, 58, *60*, 61
Splints
dynamic, for hand joint stiffness, 4665–4666, *4666*
for brachial plexus injuries, 4789
for class II mandible fractures, in edentulous posterior segment, *953*, 953–954
for dentures with circumferential wiring, in class II mandible fracture, *951, 953*, 954, *955*
for flexor tendon repair, *4541–4543*, 4541–4544, 4542*t*
for mandibular fixation, 3500, *3500–3506*
for nose, 1834, *1835*
for skin grafting of neck contracture, 2065–2068, *2065–2068*
in maintenance of intermaxillary fixation, 929–930, *931*
of wrist, for de Quervain's disease, 4735, *4735*
techniques of, for finger, 4577, *4577*
Split appliance, for unilateral cleft lip, 2627–2628, *2627–2629*, 2630
Split rib grafts, vs. iliac bone grafts, for mandibular defects, 1422, *1431*
Split-thickness excision, use of scar tissue after, 52, *53*
Sporadicity, 109–111

Sporotrichosis, 5552–5553
Spreader graft, 1904, *1906*, 1918, *1919*
Squamous cell carcinoma
  clinical presentation of, 3606–3607, *3607*
  differential diagnosis of, 3630
  etiologic factors for, 3628–3630, *3628–3630*
  of hand, 5488–5489, *5488*
  of nasal cavity and paranasal sinuses, 3360–3361
  of oropharynx and nasopharynx, in children, 3187
  of perionychium, 4512, 4514, *4514*
  of salivary gland, 3308–3309
  of tongue, management of, 3450–3451, *3451*
  treatment of, 3631, 3634–3635, *3631–3634*
Stab wound bleeding, as index of flap perfusion, 319*t*, 320
Stack splint, 4595, *4595*
Staige Davis, John, 10, *12*
Stainless steel, for alloplastic implants, 704–705, 705*t*
Steatoma, 3569, 3572
Stenosis, female genital reconstruction for, 4210
Stensen's duct. *See* Parotid duct.
Sternal clefts, chest wall reconstruction and, 3745, 3749, *3749–3752*
Sternocleidomastoid muscle
  anatomy of, 3433, *3433*
  flaps of, 3436, *3436*, 3438, *3442, 3443*
    anatomy of, 385
    for cheek reconstruction, 2049–2050
Sternotomy, infected, flap surgery for, 393–396, *394, 395*
Steroids
  cleft palate and, 2545–2546
  craniofacial cleft formation and, 2929
  for de Quervain's disease, 4735, 4737
  for hemangiomas, 3214–3216, *3215, 3217*
  for keloid therapy, 739
  for postoperative skin flaps, 317–318
  for trigger finger or thumb, 4730, *4730*
Stickler's syndrome, 73, 93, 3129
Stomion, 1190
Stout method, of intermaxillary fixation, 926–927, *928*
Strabismus, corrective surgery for, in Down syndrome, 3166
Straight line, 55
Strawberry marks. *See* Capillary hemangiomas.
Streeter's dysplasia, 2931
Strength-duration curves, for evaluation of facial nerve function, 2253
Streptokinase, 459
Stress-strain curve, 699–700, *700*
Stroke patient
  hand surgery for, 4977
    finger derangements in, 4982, *4983, 4984*
    for release of abducted thumb, 4982, *4983*
    indications for, 4980–4981
    patient cooperation in, 4980
    wrist in, 4981–4982
  kinesthesia and sensibility of, 4978–4979
  loss of function in, 4978*t*
  postoperative learning in, 4978–4979
Sturge-Weber syndrome, capillary malformations in, 3229–3231, *3231*
Stylomastoid artery, 2244
Subclavian artery, compression of, 4998
Subclavian perivascular block
  extent of analgesia from, 4306, 4307
  performance of, 4316, 4318, *4318*, 4320
Subcutaneous fasciotomy, for Dupuytren's disease, 5075–5076, *5077*
Subcutaneous pedicle flaps, for cheek reconstruction, 2049
Subcutaneous plexus, blood supply of, 285, *286*
Subcutaneous tissue, of scalp, 1538
Subcutaneous-assisted lipectomy, adjuncts for, 4026, *4027*, 4028
Subdermal plexus, blood supply of, 285–286, *286*
Subepicranial space, 1516, 1539
Subepidermal plexus, blood supply of, 286, *286*
Subeponychial abscess, 5539
Subglottic tumors, 3467
Subglottis, anatomy of, 3417
Sublingual gland. *See also* Salivary glands.
  anatomy of, 3281
  benign and malignant neoplasms of, surgical planning considerations for, 3294–3295
  malignant lesions of, 3310–3311
  mucoepidermoid carcinomas of, 3306
Submandibular gland. *See also* Salivary glands.
  anatomy of, 3279–3281, *3280*
  malignant lesions of, 3310–3311
  mucoepidermoid carcinoma of, 3306
Submaxillary duct, injuries of, 907
Submental fat collection, surgical correction of, in Down syndrome, 3170
Submucous approach for nasal profile resection, 1843, *1843*
Subnasal segmental dentoalveolar osteotomy, 1337, *1342*
Subnasale, 28, *28*, 1190
Subpial space, 4314
Substance P, inflammation and, 4897
Subungual abscess, 5539
Suction-assisted lipectomy
  complications of, 3977, 3979, *3978*
    prevention of, 3979
  equipment for, 3973, 3975, *3974, 3975*
  historical aspects of, 3930, 3933
  of abdomen, 3936–3937, *3938–3942*
  of arms and thorax, 3981, 3985, 3987–3988, *3986, 3987, 3989–3991*
  of breasts
    for axillary reduction, 3988, *3993, 3994*
    for breast reconstruction, 3988, *3995*
    for gynecomastia, 3988
  of face, chin and neck, 3979, 3980, *3979–3983*
  of hips and upper thighs, 3988, 4000, 4002, 4004, 4015, 4017
  of knees, calves, and ankles, 4019, 4021, *4020*
  patient selection for, 3975–3977, *3976*
  preoperative planning for, 3975–3977, *3976*
  secondary/revision procedures of, 4028
Sudeck's osteoporosis, 4894, *4895*
Sulfamylon (mafenide acetate), for thermal burn management, 802, 803, 803*t*
Sunlight, chemically peeled skin and, 769
Super voltage, 832
Superficial circumflex iliac artery (SCIA), 4033
Superficial femoral artery (SFA), 4034
Superficial inferior epigastric artery (SIEA), 4033
Superficial musculoaponeurotic system (SMAS), anatomy of, 619, 620, 2243–2244, *2244, 2245, 2374*, 2376
Superficial radial nerve, as source for free vascularized nerve graft, 4876, *4877*

Superficialis flexor digitorum tendon, clinical transplantation of, 539–540
Superior mesenteric artery syndrome, 809
Superior orbital fissure, 1110, *1110*
Superior orbital fissure syndrome, 1081–1082, *1114*, 1114–1115, 1178, *1179*, 1672
Superior palpebral fold, 2420–2421
Superior pharyngeal constrictor, *2612, 2613*, 2623
  in cleft palate, 2624–2625
Superior sulcus deformity, correction of, 1609
Superoinferior projection (Titterington position), for plain films, 886, *888*
Superoxide dismutase, 313, 318
Superoxide radical scavengers or blockers, for postoperative skin flap treatment, 318
Supraglottic tumors, treatment of, 3465–3466
Supraglottis, 3416
Suprahyoid musculature, in correction of mandibular hypoplasia, 1287–1288
Supraorbital foramen, anatomic palpation of, 147, *147*
Supraorbital fractures, in children, 1177–1179, *1178, 1179*
Supraorbital nerve, injury of, 1131
Supraorbital ridge, nasal profile and, *1800*
Suprascapular nerve
  anatomy of, 4313
  injuries of, with brachial plexus injuries, 4800
Supratip
  deformity of
    diagnosis of, 1899, *1899–1901*, 1901
    secondary rhinoplasty for, 1911–1913, 1915, *1911–1917*
  postoperative protrusion of, 1881
  protrusion in, 1833
Supratrochlear nerve injuries, 1131
Sural nerve, as source for free vascularized nerve graft, 4876, *4878*
Surgeon, and relationship with orthodontist, 1189
Suture(s)
  continuous running, 51, *52*
  everting interrupted, 49, *50*
  "figure-of-eight," 48, *48*
  for genital reconstructive surgery, 4124
  historical aspects of, *48*, 48–49
  horizontal mattress, 50–51, *51*
  inverting, 49–50, *50*
  materials for, in alloplastic implants, 718–722, 719*t*
  microsutures, 419–420, *421*
  midpalatal, absence of, 2596
  of nerve, for brachial plexus injury repair, 4805
    techniques for, *4764*, 4764–4765, 4766–4767
  proper placement of, *4435*, 4435–4436
  reinforcement of, 48–49, *49*
  removable continuous intradermal, 51, *52*
  subdermal buried, 50, *50*
  variations in technique for, 52, *53*
  vertical mattress, 50, *51*
Swallowing
  muscles involved in, 2727
  tongue thrust type of, 1352
Swan-neck deformity, correction of, in spastic patient, 4982, *4983*
Sweat glands
  anatomy of, 224
  in skin graft, 245
  of hand, carcinoma of, 5494
  tumors of, 3576–3578, *3576–3578*
Symblepharon, 1742–1744, *1743–1745*
Sympathectomy
  for reflex sympathetic dystrophy, 4908–4909
  for treatment of cold injury, 857
Sympathetic block
  for reflex sympathetic dystrophy, 4907–4908
  for treatment of cold injury, 857
Sympathetic chain, anatomy of, 4313–4314
Sympathetic nervous system
  control of blood flow by, 446–447, *446*
  in reflex dystrophy, 4897–4898
Sympatholytic agents, for reflex sympathetic dystrophy, 4909–4910
Symphalangism
  clinical presentation of, 5308–5309, *5308, 5310*
  treatment of, 5309, *5310–5312*
Synchondroses, 2506–2507, *2507*
Syndactyly
  after burn injury, 5456, 5458, *5457–5460*
  anatomy of, 5280–5281, *5280*
  classification of, 5279, *5280*
  incidence of, 5279
  syndromes related to
    acrosyndactyly and, 5303, 5305, *5306, 5307*, 5308
    Apert's syndrome and. *See* Apert's syndrome.
    Poland's syndrome and. *See* Poland's syndrome.
    radioulnar synostosis and, 5309–5310, *5313*, 5313–5315, *5314*
    symphalangism and, 5308–5309, *5308, 5310–5312*
  treatment of
    complications of, 5293, *5295*
    evolution of methods for, *5282–5287*
    for interdigital web space release, 5289–5292
    for thumb-index web space release, 5292–5293, *5294–5295*
    immobilization for, 5292, *5292*
    principles of, 5281, 5288–5289, *5288–5289*
    timing of, 5289, *5290–5291*
Syndrome delineation
  pace of, 89, 89*t*
  process of, 84, 89, *89*
  significance of, 89, 92
Syndromology
  definition of, 70
  known-genesis syndromes of, 84, 87, 89, 92, *86–91*
  unknown-genesis syndromes
    provisionally unique-pattern, 81–82
    recurrent-pattern syndromes, 82, *83*, 84*t*
  vs. classical medicine, 89, 89*t*, *91*
Syngenesiotransplantation, 54
Synkinesis, 2258–2259
Synkinetic jaw winking syndrome, 1754, *1756*
Synostosis, sagittal, 98
Synovial cell sarcoma, in head and neck region, 3371
Synovial sheaths, of hand, 4266
Synovioma, malignant, of hand, 5500–5501, *5501*
Syphilis, oral cancer and, 3418
Syringomas
  clinical presentation of, 3576, *3576*
  dermabrasion of, 777

T lymphocytes, 178, 189, 190
Tagliacozzi, Gaspare, *4*, 6
Tagliacozzi method, 1971, *1971–1973*
Tantalum, for alloplastic implants, 706

Tarsal strip procedures, for eyelid reconstruction, 1722, *1725, 1726*
Tarsoconjunctival flap, for eyelid reconstruction, 1689–1690, *1690*, 1700, 1703, *1702, 1704*
Tarsorrhaphy
  clinical presentation of, 1590
  disadvantages of, 2212
  for lagophthalmos, 2307
  McLaughlin's lateral, 1684–1685, *1685*
  partial, 1683–1684, *1684*
Tattoos
  dermabrasion of, 774, *777*
  for port-wine stain correction, 3231–3232
  removal of, 3608–3610, *3609*
    by laser, 3671–3672, *3672*
Teeth
  buccolingual relationships of, 1194, *1194*
  congenital absence of, in cleft lip and palate, 2882, *2884*
  development of, 3336–3337
  embryologic development of, 2488, *2489–2490*, 2491
  fused, in cleft lip and palate, 2885, *2886*
  grinding of, myalgia from, 1478
  in mandibular fractured segment, presence or absence of, 940–941, *941*
  incisal edges of, relationship of, *1194*
  relations of, after surgical repair of cleft lip/palate, *2563*, 2564–2565
  sensibility and vitality of, loss of, from orthognathic surgery, 1405, 1409
  supernumerary, in cleft lip and palate, 2882, 2885, *2885*
  terminology for
    description of maxillary and mandibular relationships, *927*
    relationships of, *927*
  variations in size of, in cleft lip and palate, 2885, *2886*
Telangiectasias
  argon laser therapy for, 3668, *3669*
  clinical presentation of, 3237–3240, *3237, 3238*
  generalized essential types of, 3239
Telangiectasis
  after blepharoplasty, 2349
  spider, 3240, *3240*
Telecanthus
  post-traumatic, *1610*, 1611, *1615*
  traumatic, 1087–1089, *1087, 1088*
Television, through operating microscope, preoperative preparation of, 415
Temperature tests, for flap perfusion assessment, 319*t*, 321
Temporal arterial system, 619–622, *620, 622*
Temporal fascia, for secondary rhinoplasty, 1909, *1911*
Temporal vertical flap, 1530
Temporalis fascial flap, 298, *298*
Temporalis muscle
  anatomy of, 935
  flaps of, 385
    for reconstruction after craniofacial tumor resection, 3405–3406, *3405*
  neurovascular supply of, *2287*
  transfers of
    for eyelid paralysis, 2312, *2313*
    for facial paralysis, 2291–2294, *2292–2297*
Temporomandibular joint (TMJ)
  anatomy of, 937–938, *939*, 1475–1477, *1476*
    abnormal, 1481–1487, *1482–1486*
  ankylosis of
    after treatment of mandibular fracture, 977
    with mandibular hypoplasia, 1262
  arthritis of, 1498
  capsular and ligamentous problems of, 1479–1481, *1480, 1481*
  condylar action and, 1477–1478
  developmental abnormalities of, 1489–1496, *1489, 1491–1493, 1495*
  dysfunction of, 1478
    evaluation and examination of, 1482–1487, 1483*t*, *1483, 1485, 1486*
    muscular problems and, 1478–1479
  dysfunctions of, from condylar dislocations, 1487–1489, *1487–1489*
  function of, 937–938, *939*
  internal derangement of, 1481–1487, *1482, 1483, 1485, 1486*
  osteochondritis of, 1502
  plain films of, 894, 897, *897, 898*
  radiographic study of, 1503–1505, *1504, 1504t, 1505*
  rheumatoid arthritis of, 1502–1503, *1503*
  surgical approach to, 1505–1506, *1506*
    procedure during exposure in, 1508–1510, *1509*
    subfascial technique for, 1506–1507, *1507*
    suprafascial technique for, 1507–1508, *1508*
Temporoparietal fascial flap
  anatomy of, 621–622, *621–624*, 4468–4469, *4469*
  for free flap transfer, in upper extremity, 4468–4469, *4469, 4470*
Temporo-parieto-occipital flap, 1528–1529, *1529*
Tendon(s). *See also specific tendons.*
  anatomy of, 527–529, *528, 529*
    in great toe vs. thumb, 5161–5163, *5162, 5163*
  biochemistry of, 549–550
  blood supply to, 528
  clinical transplantation of. *See* Tendon transfer.
  experimental transplantation of, 541–542
  gliding of, 532
  graft healing of, physiology of, 530–532, *531*
  grafts of, for hand reconstruction, 4297, *4297*
  histology of, 550
  in electrical burn injuries, 5425–5426
  in functioning muscle transfer, 4973
  nutrition of, physiology of, 530
  problems of, in rheumatoid arthritis, 4707–4712, *4708–4710*
  wound healing in, 182
Tendon sheath
  anatomy of, 527–529, *529*
  reconstruction of, *540*, 540–541
Tendon transfer, 532–533, 535–536
  balance of muscle strength from, 4925–4927, *4926, 4927*
  changes after, 4927, 4936
  donor sites for, 534
  drag in, 4937–4939, *4938–4940*
    reduction of by surgical techniques, 4939–4941, *4940*
  for high median and radial palsy, 4963
  for longitudinal deficiencies of radius, 5262
  for radial and ulnar palsy, 4963

Tendon transfer *(Continued)*
for radial nerve paralysis, 4941–4947, *4942, 4944, 4946*
for thumb reconstruction, 5179, 5181
for ulnar nerve paralysis, 4947, *4948, 4949, 4949–4955, 4952–4954*
of extensor digitorum longus, 538–539, *538, 539*
passive soft tissue resistance in, management of, 4937–4939, *4938–4940*
psychologic state of patient and, 4924–4925
recovery of nerves and, 4925
technique of, 533–534, *533–535*
tendon excursions after, changing of, 4935–4936
tendon excursions in
matching of, 4932
terminology for, 4932–4935
timing of, 4923
tissue adaptation and, 4923–4924
Tenolysis, of flexor tendon, 4547–4551, *4549, 4550*
Tenon's capsule, 1049, 1673, *1674*
Tenosynovitis
de Quervain's. *See* De Quervain's disease.
of extensor digiti minimi, 4739
of hand, 5544–5545, *5545, 5546*
Tenotomy, 547–548
Tensor fasciae latae, strips of, for drainage of lymphedema, 4112
Tensor fasciae latae flap
applications of, 4038–4039, *4040*
for abdominal wall defects, 397
for chest wall reconstruction, 3697, *3698, 3699*, 3699–3700
for genital reconstructive surgery, 4148–4149
for groin and perineum reconstructions, 398
for groin coverage, 4136–4137
for lower extremity reconstruction, *4054*, 4054–4055
for pressure sores, 403–404
motor innervation of, 4038
origin and insertion of, 4038
vascular supply of, 4038
Tensor palatini muscles, 2727, 2728, *2728*
Tensor veli palatini, 2612–2614, *2612–2614*
Tenzel semicircular flap, *1705, 1706*, 1707, 1709
Teratogens
associated with cleft lip/palate, 2530, *2532, 2532–2533, 2534–2537*, 2535–2539
inhibition of electron transport, 2532, *2532*
Teratomas
malignant, of nasal cavity or paranasal sinuses, 3364, *3365*
of head and neck, in pediatric patients, 3181, *3182*
Terminal hair, 1519
Terminology, 1
Tessier-Wolfe three-wall orbital decompression, 1637, *1638*
Testicle, fracture of, 4229
Tetanus prophylaxis
description of, 899–900
for hand injuries, 4594, 4594*t*
Tetraplegia
classification of, 4985, *4985*
evaluation of patient in, 4985–4986
future of surgery for, 4988, 4990
hand surgery for, 4977
patient cooperation in, 4980
Tetraplegia *(Continued)*
hand-gripping function of, surgical obtainment of, *4987, 4988*
kinesthesia and sensibility in, 4978–4979, *4979*
operative procedures of, for elbow extension, 4986–4987, *4987*
postoperative learning in, 4978–4979
surgical results in, *4989*
treatment of, 4984–4985
TGF-beta, 179
Thalidomide
craniofacial cleft formation and, 2929
teratogenicity of, 2465, 2468, 2491
Thenar flap, for fingertip amputations, 4492–4493, *4493, 4494*
Thenar muscles, 4271–4272, *4272, 4273*
Thenar space, infection of, 5540–5541, *5541, 5542*
Thermal biofeedback, for chronic or recurring vasospasm, 5021
Thermal burns
biologic dressings for, 804*t*, 804–805
complications of, *807–809*, 807–810
epidemiology of, 789–790
history of treament for, 787–789
hyperalimentation for, 798–799, *799*, 800*t*, 800–801
immunology of, 801–802
inhalation injury of
diagnosis of, 795–796
treatment of, *796*, 796–797
metabolism of, 797–799, 801
pathology of, 790–791
rehabilitation for, 810–811, 811*t*
resuscitation for, 791, 793–795, 794*t*
second degree or partial thickness, 790–791
supplemental feeding for, 801*t*
third degree or full-thickness, 791
treatment of, protocol for, 790
wound management for, 802–807, 803*t*, 804*t*, *806, 807*
excision of burn eschar in, 805–807, *806*
Thermal shock, 853
Thermocautery, for hemangiomas, 3212–3213
Thermography, for diagnosis of reflex sympathetic dystrophy, 4903
Thiersch-Duplay technique, for hypospadias repair, 4157–4158, *4158*
Thigh(s)
contour deformities of
classification of, *3999*, 4000
complications of suction-assisted lipectomy, 4000, 4002, *4004*
medial thighplasty for, *4018*, 4019
reduction of anterior thighs, 4019, *4019*
type I, suction-assisted lipectomy for, 4000, *4001–4004*, 4002
type III, 4002, *4007, 4008*
type IV, 4002, *4009, 4010*
type V, suction-lipectomy of, 4002, 4004, *4013*
type VI, suction-assisted lipectomy for, 4004, *4014*
type VII, suction-assisted lipectomy for, 4004, *4015*
cutaneous arteries of, *369–370*, 371–372
flaps of, *294*, 294–295
suction-assisted lipectomy of, complications of, 3978
type II contour deformity, saddlebag deformity of, suction-assisted lipectomy for, 4002, *4005, 4006*

Thighplasty, combined with other body contouring procedures, 4021
Thiphenamil hydrochloride (Trocinate), 168
Thompson buried dermal flap procedure, for lymphedema, 5028, *5029*
Thoracic flap, for upper extremity reconstructions, *4452*, 4453, *4454*
Thoracic outlet syndrome, 4836, *4838–4840*, 4839–4841
Thoracic rib, rudimentary first, vascular compression syndromes and, 4998
Thoracobrachiobreastplasty
  with suctioning, 3988, *3991, 3992*
  without suctioning, *3986*, 3988, *3989, 3991*
Thoracobrachioplasty
  with suctioning, 3988, *3991, 3992*
  without suctioning, *3986*, 3988, *3989, 3991*
Thoracodorsal artery, 3913, *3913*
Thorax, suction-assisted lipectomy of, complications of, 3977, 3978
Thrombophlebitis, suppurative, secondary to thermal burn injury, 808–809, *809*
Thrombosis, arterial
  in upper extremity, 5005–5006
  local, abnormal blood flow and, 452
Thromboxanes, 309
Thumb
  abduction of, 5119
    release of, 4982, *4983*
  adduction of, 5118, *5118*
  amputated, replantation of, 4373
  amputation of, 5135
    historical aspects of, 5135–5136, *5137*
    neurovascular pedicle method of digital transfer for, 5136, 5138, *5138–5140*
    reconstruction of by finger transfer, 5138, 5142, *5143–5149*
    subtotal level of, 5138
    surgical technique for, choice of, 5155
    total level of, 5138, *5140–5141*
    treatment of. *See* Toe(s), microvascular transfer to hand.
  aplasia or hypoplasia of, 5106–5108, *5107*
    principles of operative management for, 5108–5110, *5108–5110*
  carpometacarpal joint of, arthrodesis of, of small joints, 4671–4672. *See also* Arthrodesis.
  collateral ligament tears of, differentiation of complete and incomplete, *4613*, 4613–4614
  congenital anomalies of, 5106, 5106*t*
    aplasia or hypoplasia of, operative steps for, 5110–5115, *5110–5115*
    differentiation failures of, 5115–5121, *5115–5118, 5120*, 5119*t*
    duplication of parts of, 5121–5125, 5129–5130, 5133, *5122–5132*
  dislocations of, 4609–4610, 4613–4614, *4614*
  extension of, 4572–4573
    with radial palsy, 4943–4944
  first metacarpotrapezial joint and, *4256*, 4256–4257
  flexion of, in median nerve paralysis, 4957–4958
  fracture-dislocations of, 4616–4617, *4617*
  fractures of, 4598–4599, *4598*
  function of, 5186
  hypoplastic or absent, 5119–5121, 5119*t*, *5120*
  in Dupuytren's disease, 5062, 5064
  in ulnar nerve paralysis, 4953–4955, *4954*
Thumb *(Continued)*
  ischemic contracture deformities of, 5045*t*, 5046, *5048*
    surgical correction of, 5051
  pulley system of, *4519–4520*, 4519–4521
    reconstruction of, *4520*, 4521–4522
    surgical release of, 4730–4731, *4731, 4732*
  reconstruction. *See* Thumb reconstruction.
  skeleton of, *4255*, 4255–4256
  soft tissue injuries of
    dorsal skin transfers for, *5098, 5098–5099, 5100–5104*, 5103–5104
    minor types of, 5087, *5088, 5089*, 5090
    volar skin transfers for, 5090–5093, *5090–5094, 5095, 5096–5098*, 5098
  tendon injuries of, 4589–4590, *4590*
  thenar and hypothenar muscles and, 4271–4272, *4272, 4273*
  trigger
    anatomy of, 4727, 4727–4729, *4728*
    clinical features of, 4727–4729, *4727, 4728*
    treatment of, 4729–4731, *4730*
Thumb pulleys, 4266, *4267*
Thumb reconstruction
  by bone lengthening
    bone grafting of gap in, 5202, *5204*
    complications of, 5205, *5208*
    distraction device for, 5197, *5198*
    distraction period for, 5198, 5200
    historical aspects of, 5195–5196, *5196*
    immobilization period for, 5200
    in children, 5205, 5209, 5211, *5208, 5209*
    indications for, 5196, *5196*
    limits of distraction in, 5196, *5197*
    long-term results of, *5210, 5211*
    operative technique for, 5197–5198, *5199*
    removal of distraction device, 5205
    secondary operations for, 5205, *5206–5208*
    spontaneous osteogenesis in, 5200, *5201–5204*, 5202
    tissue response to stretching in, 5200
  by wrap-around technique
    bone graft for, 5190
    foot closure for, 5192, 5194, *5193*
    foot dissection for, 5188–5190, *5188–5190*
    hand dissection for, 5190
    modifications of, 5194
    operative technique for, 5190–5192, *5191, 5192*
  considerations for thumb function in, 5186
  preoperative evaluation for, 5186–5188, *5187*
    skin marking for, 5187–5188, *5187, 5188*
  second toe autotransplantation for, 4409, *4416–4419*
  secondary soft tissue pulp plasty for, 5179, *5180*
Thumb web, in Dupuytren's disease, 5062, 5064
Thumb-index web space
  deepening of, 5248
  release of, 5292–5293, *5294–5295*
Thymus, cellular immunity and, 189
Thyroglossal duct remnants, 3180, *3180, 3181*
Thyroid gland carcinoma, 847, 3187–3188
Thyrotropin (TSH), 798
Thyroxine, 98, *98, 99*, 798, 2928
Tibia
  blood supply of, *4057*, 4057–4058
  open fractures of, 4057–4058, *4059–4061*, 4061
    classification of, 4058, *4059*
Tibia-fibula synostosis, for bone defects, 4065, *4067*

Tibial grafts, 605, *605*
Tip-columellar angle, 1788, *1788*, *1797*
Tissue expansion
  biology of, 477–478, *477–479*
  complications of, 504–506
  for breast reconstruction, 482–491, *484–490*
  for ear reconstruction, 501–502
  for extremities, 503–504, *504*
  for face reconstruction, 496, *497–500*, 501
  for nasal reconstruction, 1974–1975
  for scalp alopecia, 2224–2226, *2227, 2228*
  for scalp reconstruction, 491–496, *492, 493, 494, 495*
  for trunk, *502*, 502–503
  historical aspects of, 181, 475–476, *476*
  implant choice and placement in, 481
  inflation of implant in, 481–482
  patient selection for, 480–481
  source of increased tissue surface, 479–480, *480*
  types of implants for, 476–477
Titanium, for alloplastic implants, 705*t*, 705–706
Titterington position, for plain films, 886, *888*
Tobacco
  risks of, 3412
  smokeless, oral cancer and, 3418
Toe(s)
  microvascular transfer to hand, 5178, *5179*
    historical aspects of, 5153–5154
    indications for, 5154–5156
  mucous cysts of, 3581
  second, autotransplantation of. *See* Second toe autotransplantation.
  transposition of, for correction of transverse absence of carpals or metacarpals, 5248, *5250–5251*, 5252
TONAR, 2912
Tongue
  anatomy of, 3478–3480, *3479*
  displacement of, in Robin sequence, 3128
  embryologic development of, 2468, *2469*, 2470
  flaps of. *See* Lingual flap.
  hypotonia of, corrective surgery for, in Down syndrome, 3164–3165, *3165*
  posterior, cancers of, 3457, *3458*
  squamous cell carcinoma of, management of, 3450–3451, *3451*
Tongue flap
  for cheek reconstruction, 2049
  for intraoral reconstruction, 3438, *3440*
Tongue reduction, for open bite correction, 1360
Tongue-to-lip adhesion, 3134
  modified Routledge procedure, 3131, *3132*, 3133
Tonsillectomy
  for obstructive sleep apnea, 3150
  velopharyngeal closure and, 2729
Tonsils
  cancers of, 3455–3457, *3456*
  enlarged, velopharyngeal incompetence from, 2906
Torticollis, congenital muscular, 2085, 2087–2090, *2086, 2089*
Toxicity, of alloplastic implants, 701–702
Toxoplasmosis, craniofacial cleft formation and, 2928
Tracheal intubation, of retrognathia infant, 3130, 3131
Tracheostomy, for obstructive sleep apnea, 3150
Tracheotomy
  complications of, 876
  elective, 872–873, *873, 874, 875*, 875–876
  emergency low, 872, 873, *873*
Tracheotomy *(Continued)*
  indications for, 873
  techniques of, 873, 875–876, *873–875*
Traction devices, external, 1288
Tragion, 28, *28*
TRAM flap, 3908
  anatomy of, 3918–3919, *3918, 3920*
  for breast reconstruction, 3916–3920, 3922, *3917–3921*, 3925
  for genital reconstructive surgery, 4139, *4139, 4141, 4142, 4143*
  limitations to usage of, 3917–3918
  postoperative abdominal hernia and, 3771–3772
Tranquilizers, craniofacial cleft formation and, 2929
Transcarpal amputation, 4340
Transcutaneous electrical nerve stimulation (TENS), for reflex sympathetic dystrophy, 4911–4912
Transcutaneous pO_2, as index of flap perfusion, 319*t*, 320
Transfixion incision
  for rhinoplasty, 1818, *1820, 1821, 1821*
  transseptal, 1853
  variations in, 1842–1843, *1843*
Transforming growth factor (TGF-beta), 179
Translation, 2498, *2499*. *See also* Displacement.
Transplantation
  allograft reaction and, 187
  allograft rejection mechanism, modification of, 193–196
  general aspects of, 54–55
  histocompatibility antigens and, 187
  histocompatibility genetics of, 187
  historical background of, 186–187
  immediate, 55
  lymphoid system and, 189–190
  macrophage system and, 190
  mediate, 55
  of composite tissue, 196–203, *197*
  of craniofacial modules, 201–203, *202*
  rejection mechanism of
    afferent limb of, 190–191, *191*
    efferent limb of, 191–192, *192*
  success of, 196
Transposition flap
  design of, 289–290, *290*
  for coverage of soft tissues of hand, 4449–4450, *4450–4451*
  of scalp, 1527–1528
  Z-plasties, 4445, 4447–4448, *4446, 4447*
Transsexualism
  etiology of, 4239–4241
  hormonal therapy for, 4240–4241
  psychosocial aspects of, 129–131
  vaginoplasty for, *4241, 4241–4243, 4242*
Transverse rectus abdominis musculocutaneous flap. *See* TRAM flap.
Trapdoor effect, on scars, 742, *743, 744*
Trapezius flap
  for acquired mandibular defect, 1440, *1442*
  for cheek reconstruction, 2046–2047, *2047*, 2049
  for head and neck reconstructions, 386–387
  for intraoral and external reconstructions, 3444, 3447–3448, *3447, 3448*
Trauma
  basal cell carcinoma and, 3619
  Dupuytren's disease and, 5055–5056

Trauma *(Continued)*
  malignant melanoma and, 3637
Traumatic segmental arterial spasm (TSAS), 5016–5017
Treacher Collins syndrome
  auricular deformities in, 3120
  bilateral microtia and, 2108
  causation of, heredity and, 2931
  classification of, 3105–3106
  clinical features of, 3105*t*, 3105–3106
  congenital aural atresia and, 2148
  craniofacial skeletal features of, 3111, *3111*
  description of, *2956*, 2956–2957
  differential diagnosis of, 3054
  ear deformities and, 2098
  embryologic development of, 2475, *2476–2477*, 2491–2492
  embryology of, 2455
  genetic considerations in, 3106, 3109
  historical aspects of, 3101, *3104*, 3104–3105
  incomplete form of, 2952, *2953*
  pathogenesis of, 2547, 3109–3110, *3110*
  phenotypic expression of, variations in, 3101, *3102, 3103*
  racial groups and, 3106, *3109*
  radiographic features of, 3105–3106, 3106*t*, *3107*
  sideburns, anterior placed in, 3119, 3123
  treatment of, 3110–3111
    for eyelid deformities, 3113, 3116–3117, *3116, 3117*
    for mandibular hypoplasia, *3118*, 3119
    for maxillary and orbital deficiencies, 3111–3113, *3111, 3112, 3314–3315*
    using multiple operations, *3120–3122*, 3123
Trefoil flap technique, for columella lengthening, 2856–2857, *2858*
Trench foot (immersion foot), 852
Triamcinolone, intralesional injection of
  for abnormal scars, 738
  for keloids, 739, *739*
Triangular fibrocartilage complex (TFCC), rupture of, in rheumatoid arthritis, 4713, *4713*
Triazene, craniofacial cleft formation and, 2929
Triazolam (Halcion), 140
Tricalcium phosphate, for alloplastic implants, 716–717
Trichiasis, 1737, 1742
Trichion, 28, *28*, 1190
Trichloroacetic acid, for chemical peeling, 754–756
Trichoepitheliomas
  clinical presentation of, 3577–3578, *3578*
  dermabrasion of, 777
  laser therapy for, 3671
Trigeminal nerve, injury of, 906
Trigger points, in myofascial dysfunction, 4894–4896
Trigger thumb, congenital, 5116, *5116*
Trigonocephaly
  description of, 1546
  orbital hypotelorism and, 3005
  visual abnormalities in, 3025–3026
Trigonocephaly-metopic synostosis, clinical and radiographic findings in, 3015, *3016*
Triiodothyronine, 798
Tripier flap, 1703, *1704*, 1707
  modified, 2217
Triquetrum, fractures of, 4597
Trismus
  from maxillary surgery, 3333
  intramuscular pathology of, 1479
Trisomy 13 syndrome, 84, *87*
Trisomy 13–15 syndrome, 3234
Trisomy 18 syndrome, 79
Trisomy 21 syndrome, 79
Trochanter, pressure sores of, 3826–3827, *3826, 3828*, 3827*t*
Trocinate (thiphenamil hydrochloride), 168
Trophic influences, in peripheral nerve regeneration, 664–666
Tropocollagen, 171
Trunk
  cutaneous arteries of, 362–363, 367–368, *364–366*
  tissue expansion for, *502*, 502–503
TSAS (traumatic segmental arterial spasm), 5016–5017
Tube flap, 277, *277*
  development of, 20
  for neck resurfacing, 2200
Tularemia, 5551
Turban tumor, 3577, *3577*
Turbinates, 1798, 1809
Turner's syndrome, 79
  congenital neck webbing in, 2076–2077
    surgical correction of, 2077–2078, *2079–2084*
Turnover flaps, for cheek reconstruction, 2049
Turricephaly–multiple suture synostosis, clinical and radiographic findings in, 3018, *3018*
Twin-screw Morris biphase appliance, for mandibular fixation, 3500, *3503–3507*, 3504–3505, 3507
Two-point discrimination test, 4818, *4818*, 4859, *4860*, 4862, 4978–4979, *4979*

UHMWPE (ultra high molecular weight polyethylene), 711–712
Ulcers
  in hemangiomas, 3206, *3206*
  in lower extremity, 4076–4077, *4078, 4079*
  radiation injury, 844–846, *845, 846*
Ullrich-Noonan syndrome. *See* Turner's syndrome.
Ulna
  distal
    dislocations of, 4639–4640, *4640*
    fractures of, 4638–4639, *4639*
    subluxations of, 4639–4640
  duplication of, 5133
  longitudinal absence deformities of, 5271, 5273
    classification of, 5273–5274, *5274*
    clinical presentations of, 5274–5276, *5276*
    treatment of, 5276–5277, 5279, *5276–5278*
    vs. radial longitudinal absence deformities, 5273*t*
Ulnar artery, thrombosis of, 452, 5006
Ulnar bursae, infection of, 5543, *5543*
Ulnar carpal tunnel, 4281, *4281*
Ulnar dimelia, 5133, 5356, 5358, 5361–5362, *5357, 5359–5361*
Ulnar nerve
  anatomy of, 4278, 4280, *4279*, 4759
  dorsal branch of, 4280, *4280*
  entrapment of, 679
  entrapment syndrome of, in rheumatoid arthritis, 4704–4705
  injuries of, with brachial plexus injuries, 4802
  regional block of, *4322*, 4323
Ulnar nerve palsy
  distal effects of, 4949, *4949*
  high, tendon transfer for, 4961–4963, *4962*

Ulnar nerve palsy *(Continued)*
of forearm muscles, 4947, *4948*, 4949
tendon transfer for, 4947, 4949–4955, *4948, 4949, 4952–4954*, 4963
choice of methods for, 4949–4953, *4952, 4953*
timing of, 4947
thumb involvement in, 4953–4955, *4954*
with median nerve palsy, 4958–4959, *4958–4961*, 4961
Ulnar tunnel syndrome, 4844–4846, *4845, 4846*
Ultra high molecular weight polyethylene (UHMWPE), 711–712
Ultrasonography
for reflex sympathetic dystrophy, 4913
in suction-assisted lipectomy, 4026, 4028
of orbit, 1586, *1587*
Ultraviolet radiation
basal cell carcinoma and, 3615
malignant melanoma and, 3637–3638
squamous cell carcinoma and, 3628
Umbilicus
anatomy of, 3755, 3759
tailoring of, in full abdominoplasty, 3948, *3949–3951*, 3951
Undifferentiated carcinoma, of salivary gland, 3309
Unknown-genesis syndromes
provisionally unique-pattern, 81–82, *82*
recurrent-pattern, 82, *83*, 84*t*
U-osteotomy, for orbital hypertelorism correction, 3001
Upper extremity. *See also specific structures of upper extremity.*
anesthesia for
evaluation of patient for, 4302–4305
regional, 4302
cutaneous arteries of, 359, *360, 361*, 362
dislocations of, with burn injuries, 5422
electrical injuries of, 5476, *5478, 5479*, 5480
assessment of, 5421
early management of, 5421–5423, *5424*, 5425–5426
mechanism of, 5420–5421, *5421*
pathophysiology of, 5419–5420
embryology of, of vascular system, 4992–4995, *4993*
fractures of, with burn injuries, 5422
free flap transfer in, 4459–4475
advantages of, 4460
arteriography for, 4460
composite tissue transfer technique for, 4461–4462
disadvantages of, 4460
dorsalis pedis flap for, 4463, 4465, 4467, *4465, 4466*
gracilis flap for, 4474–4475
groin flap for, 4462–4463, *4463, 4464*
historical aspects of, 4459
indications for, 4460
lateral arm flaps for, 4471–4472, *4472*
latissimus dorsi flap for, 4474
parascapular flaps for, 4467–4468, *4468*
posterior calf fasciocutaneous flap for, 4475
primary vs. delayed coverage of, 4460–4461
radial artery forearm flaps for, 4472–4474, *4473*
scapular flaps for, 4467–4468, *4468*
temporoparietal fascial flaps for, 4468–4469, *4469, 4470*
types of, 4459–4460
ischemia of, onset of, 4997
ischemic conditions of, historical aspects of, 4991–4992
lymphatics of, 4094, *4096–4097*
Upper extremity *(Continued)*
microvascular surgery of, zone of vascular injury for, 4367–4368
nerves of, anatomy of, 4758–4762, *4760, 4761*
occlusive disease of, 5005–5007
replantation and revascularization of
anesthesia for, 4362
mechanics of operation from emergency room to operating room, 4361–4362
replantation of
age of patient for, 4358–4359
by level of amputation, *4371–4376*, 4371–4377
centers for, 4356–4357
definition of, 4356, *4356*
goals of, 4358
historical aspects of, 4355–4356
indications for, 4358, 4358*t*, 4359*t*
ischemic time and, 4359
level of amputation and, 4360–4361
mechanism of injury and, 4360, *4360*
patient care for, *4357*, 4357–4358
patient motivation for, 4359
perfusion of parts for, 4359
replantation surgery for
bone shortening and fixation in, 4364–4365, *4365*
cold ischemia in operating room and, 4363
debridement and structure dissection for, *4363*, 4363–4364
sequence of structure repair for, 4364, 4364*t*
tendon repairs for, 4365, *4366, 4367*
revascularization of
definition of, 4356
goals of, 4358
historical aspects of, 4355–4356
patient care for, *4357*, 4357–4358
tissue expansion of, 503–504, *504*
traumatic injuries of, 4995–4997, *4996*
incidence of, 4477
vascular tumors of, 5007
diagnosis of, 5007–5010, *5007–5009*
Upper limb prostheses
active, 4390–4392, *4393*
externally powered types of, 4396–4398, *4397*
powered by body, 4394–4396, *4395*
fitting of, 4405, 4408
for children, 4386–4387, *4387*
vs. reconstruction for, 4389–4390, *4391–4392*
for hand amputee, esthetic considerations in, 4388–4389, *4390*
passive, 4392, *4393*, 4394, 4398, *4398*
color matching for, 4398–4399
for fingers or thumb, *4399–4402*, 4399–4402
for major upper arm amputations, 4405, *4406, 4407*
for partial hand amputation, 4402–4403, *4403*
for total hand amputation, 4403, *4404*, 4405
planning for, 4384–4385, *4385*
Urethral fistula, from circumcision, 4237
Urethral stricture
anatomic considerations for, 4188–4191, *4189*
classification of, 4187–4188, *4188*
etiology of, 4187
from trauma, 4236
surgical procedure for, 4191, *4191, 4192, 4193–4197, 4195–4201*, 4204
treatment options for, 4187–4188
Urethroplasty, for urethral strictures, 4191, *4191, 4192, 4193–4197, 4195–4201*, 4204

Urinary anomalies, congenital, Klippel-Feil syndrome and, 3144
Urine output, monitoring of, for fluid resuscitation evaluation, 793–794
Urokinase, 459
Uvulae, *2612*, 2619, 2623
bifid, *2730*, 2730–2731
Uvulopalatopharyngoplasty (UPPP), for obstructive sleep apnea, 3150–3152, *3151, 3152*
Uvulus muscle, in cleft palate, 2624

Vacuum, physics of, 3973, *3974*, 3975
Vagina
congenital absence of
correction of, 4239
diagnosis of, 4204, *4204*
historical aspects of, 4203–4204
surgical techniques for, 4204–4207, *4205, 4206*
construction of, after ablative surgery, 4208–4210, *4209*
fistulas of, 4210
reconstruction of, 129
comparison of techniques for, 4207–4208, *4208*
complications of, 4207–4208, *4208*
Vaginoplasty, for transsexualism, 4241–4243, *4241, 4242*
Valium (diazepam), 2929, 4911
Van der Woude's syndrome
cleft lip/palate and, 2539–2540
pathogenesis of, 2547
Variant additive patterns, 109–111, *111*
Vascular anomalies, cutaneous pediatric
classification of, 3191–3194
terminology for, 3191
Vascular changes, after tissue injury, 178
Vascular malformations
capillary
associated morphogenetic deformities in, 3229, *3230*
nevus flammeus neonatorum as, 3233, *3233*
port-wine stains as, 3227, 3229, *3228*
classification of, 3193, 3193*t*
differentiation from hemangiomas, 3193–3194
high flow, 3254–3258, *3258*
hyperkeratotic stains, 3234–3236, *3234, 3236*
of hand, 5501–5505, *5502–5504*, 5502*t*
pathogenesis of, 3222–3227, *3225, 3226*
telangiectasias, 3237–3240, *3237, 3238*
with hypertrophy syndromes, 3258–3260, 3263–3264, *3260–3263*
Vascular problems, from amputation, 4331–4332
Vascular resistance, normal, in microvascular surgery, 443, *444*
Vascular spiders, 3240, *3240*
Vascular status, monitoring of, in replantation and revascularization surgery, 4377
Vascular supply, of facial nerve, 2244
Vascular territories
historical background of, 329–334, *330–333*
research on, 334–335
Vascular tumors, 3581–3586, *3582, 3583, 3585, 3586. See also specific tumors.*
malignant, of hand, 5504–5505
Vasculature
embryology of, 3223–3224
in hand and arm, 5220, *5221*
in upper extremity, 4992–4995, *4993*
in head, embryologic development of, 2470, 2472, *2472*
intrinsic and extrinsic, of peripheral nerves, 644–646, *645*
of skin and deeper tissues, 329
basic research on, 334–335
historical aspects of, 329–330, *330–333*, 332–334
interconnections of, 346–347, *348–350*
of vessels following connective tissue framework of body, 335, *336–344*, 344
of vessels' size and orientation as products of tissue growth and differentiation, 344, *345*
response to cold temperatures, 5432
response to thawing of, 5432–5433
Vasoconstriction, 5012, *5013*
Vasospasm
chronic or recurring, treatment for, 5020–5021, *5021*
definition of, 5012
management of, 455–457
mechanisms of, 5015–5018, *5017*
microsurgery and, 454–457
no-reflow phenomenon and, 5018–5019
pharmacologic, 455
physiologic, 454–455
post-traumatic, 454
Vasospastic disorders
anatomic considerations in, 5012–5015, *5013–5015*
localized, 5017
pharmacologic agents for, 5016
traumatic segmental arterial spasm, 5016–5017
treatment of
by pharmacologic agents, 5019–5020
by surgical methods, 5020
Vastus lateralis flap
applications of, 4040
motor innervation of, 4040
origin and insertion of, 4040
vascular supply of, 4040
Veau III operation, for bilateral cleft lip, 2661, 2664, 2666–2667, 2673, 2675–2676, *2663–2666, 2668–2675*
Veau-Wardill-Kilner operation, for cleft of secondary palate, *2907*, 2908
Vein grafts, in replantation and revascularization surgery, *4369*, 4369–4370
Velar elevation, 2903–2904, *2904*
Vellus hair, 1519
Velocardiofacial syndrome, 2471
Velopharyngeal closure, 2726
adenoid pad in, 2729
for normal speech, 2732
incompetence of, in cleft palate patients, 2732–2733
Velopharyngeal incompetence
after maxillary advancement, 1376, 1379, *1379*
after osteotomy for maxillary advancement in cleft patients, 2840
anatomic and functional considerations of, 2903–2904
causes of, 2904–2907
evaluation and measurement of, 2910–2914
long-term surgical results for, 2918–2919

Velopharyngeal incompetence *(Continued)*
management of, 2910–2914
choice of surgery for, 2914–2915
operative technique for, 2915, *2916*, 2917
postoperative speech therapy, 2917–2918
surgical correction of, historical aspects of, 2907–2908, 2910, *2907, 2909–2911*
Velopharyngeal sphincter
in speech production, 2903–2904
inability to close. *See* Velopharyngeal incompetence.
lace of movement for speech, velopharyngeal incompetence and, 2906
Veloplasty, intravelar, 2742
Venae comitantes, 353, *354, 355, 355*
Venae communicantes, 353
Venous anatomy, in great toe vs. thumb, 5165–5167, *5166*
Venous malformations
clinical findings in, 3250, *3251*, 3252
histology of, 3249–3250
of hand, 5316, *5318, 5318–5319, 5320–5322*
combined with lymphatic malformations of, 5324
terminology for, 3249
treatment of, 3252–3254, *3253*
Venules, microstructure of, 449, *451*
Venus, necklace of, 29, *29*
Veratrum californicum, craniofacial cleft formation and, 2930
Vermilion. *See also* Lip(s), upper.
adjustments of, 2187
anatomy of, 2184
deficiency or deformity of, 2790–2791, *2791–2796*, 2793, 2796
of upper lip, reconstruction of, 2027–2028, *2028–2031*, 2030–2031
reconstruction of, 2013–2105, *2014–2016*
repair of, perimeter flaps from lingual tip for, 3490, *3490–3492*, 3492
secondary deficiency of, from bilateral cleft lip repair, 2853, *2854*
Vermilionectomy, 2014–2015, *2015*
Verruca vulgaris
clinical description of, 3561–3562, *3562*
epidemiology of, 3561
etiology of, 3560
incidence of, 3560–3561
malignant transformation of, 3563
of perionychium, 4509–4510
pathology of, 3562–3563
treatment of, 3563, 3565, *3564, 3565*
Vertebrobasilar insufficiency, transient, 5007
Vessel wall tension, microvascular surgery and, 444–445
Vestibule, nasal
anatomy of, 1797–1798, *1797*, 1925
ventilation and, *1807*, 1807–1808
atresia of, 1882
Vestibules, nasal, 1804
V-excision, for lower lip reconstruction, 2015
Vibrio hand infections, 5551
Vincula, 4268, *4268*
Viral infections
craniofacial cleft formation and, 2928
of hand, 5553, *5554*
squamous cell carcinoma and, 3630
Viral warts, of perionychium, 4509–4510
Visceral arches
embryologic development of, 2468, 2468*t, 2469*, 2470
growth centers in, 2455, 2481–2483, *2484*
in development of voluntary muscles, 2471, *2472*, 2743
of head and neck, 2519, *2520*
Vision
abnormalities of, in craniosynostosis, 3025–3026
decreased, after orbital or nasoethmoido-orbital fractures, 1105
obstruction of, by hemangiomas, 3206–3207
Visual acuity, 1117, 1581, *1582*
Visual evoked response (VER), 1118
Visual examination techniques, for optic nerve injury, 1117–1118
Visual field testing, 1118
Visual loss, with frontobasilar region fractures, 1115
Vital dye tests, for flap perfusion assessment, 319*t*, 321–322
Vitamin A, corticosteroids and, 179
Vitamin deficiencies, cleft palate and, 2546
Vitamin supplements, cleft lip/palate prevention and, 2535–2537
Volar advancement flap, for soft tissue injuries of thumb, 5092–5093, *5092–5094*
Volkmann's canals, 583
Volkmann's ischemic contracture
development of, 4286–4287
differential diagnosis of, 4905–4906, *4906*
historical aspects of, 5033
management of
in evolutionary stage, 5036
in final stage
with clawhand, *5037*, 5037–5038
without clawhand, 5036, *5037*
in initial stage, *5034*, 5034–5036
pathophysiology of, 5033–5038
surgical treatment of
for correction of type I deformity, 5038–5039, *5039*
for correction of type II deformity, 5039–5040, *5040*
for correction of type III deformity, 5040
to restore sensation, 5040
treatment of, for initial stage, 5034–5036, *5035*
Volume loading, for abdominoplasty, 3935–3936
Vomer
anatomic distortion of, in cleft palate, 2730
deformities of, in unilateral cleft lip and palate, 2590–2591, *2591*
in cleft lip and palate, 2583–2584, *2584*
Von Langenbeck operation, for cleft palate repair, 2742–2744, *2743*
Von Recklinghausen's disease. *See also* Neurofibromatosis.
in children, 3181–3183, *3183*
V-Y advancement
double, for vermilion deformities, 2793, *2795*, 2796
flap design for, 289, *289*
for soft tissue injuries of thumb, 5090–5092, *5090, 5091*
for vermilion border misalignment, 2791, *2791*
V-Y advancement flaps
design of, 65–66
V-Y biceps femoris flap, for genital reconstructive surgery, 4147–4148
V-Y volar flaps, for coverage of digital tip amputation stumps, 4488, *4489*

Waardenburg's syndrome
cleft lip/palate and, 2539
illusion of hypertelorism in, 2982, *2982*
Wallerian degeneration, 662, 4762–4763
Walsham forceps, 985, *987*
Walsh-Ogura operation, *1636*, 1636–1637
Wardill-Kilner-Veau operation, for cleft palate repair, *2744*, 2744–2745
Warping, in craniofacial skeleton, 3073, *3074*
Wartenberg's syndrome, 4733
Warthin's tumor, 3297–3298, *3298*
Warts. *See also* Verruca vulgaris.
on hand, 5485, *5485*, 5553
plantar, 3562, *3562*
Washio temporomastoid flap, for nasal reconstruction, 1966, 1970, *1970, 1971*
Water, free replacement therapy of, for thermal burns in infants, 793
Waterproof mask, application after full face peeling, *763*, *763–764*, *764*, *765*, *766*
Web space
abscess of, 5542–5543, *5542, 5543*
burn contractures of, 5456, 5458, *5457–5460*
first, adduction contractures of, 5461, 5464, *5463, 5464*
Webster modification, for lower lip reconstruction, 2018, 2020
Webster-Bernard technique, for total lower lip reconstruction, 2024, *2025*
Wen, 3569, 3572
Werner's syndrome, 2364
Whistle deformity, 2697–2698, 2791, *2791*, 2793, *2794*
Williston's law, 1539
Wind-chill index, 849, *850*
Witch's chin deformity, 2383
Wolff's crest, 5216, *5217*
Work simulation therapy, for reflex sympathetic dystrophy, 4914
Wound healing, 4433
abnormal, 161
biologic principles, clinical application of, 181–182
collagen and, physical property changes in, 179–181
collagen remodeling in, 172, *172*, *173*, *174*, 175
contraction and, 162, 165, 167–169
corticosteroids and, 179
epithelization and, 162–165, *163*, *164*
in tendon, 182
initial response to injury and, 4433–4434
of dermabraded areas, 772–773
of skin graft, initial events of, 242–243
structure and synthesis of fibrous protein and matrix in, 169–172, *170*
tendon graft in, physiology of, 530–532, *531*
tensile strength and, 161–162
Wounds
closure of
acceptance of graft and, 4437, *4438*
mechanical factors affecting scar appearance in, 741–742, 745, *742–745*
mechanism of, for nasal reconstruction, 1927
nonsuture technique of, 916, *917*, *918*
primary type of, *4435*, 4435–4436
soft tissue coverage using skin flaps, 279–280, 280*t*, *280*
tertiary type of, 4436, *4436*, *4437*
types of grafts for, 4437–4440, *4439*, *4440*
Wounds *(Continued)*
contraction process of, 4434–4435
coverage of
quality of, for nasal reconstruction, 1927
quantity of, for nasal reconstruction, 1927–1928, *1928*
drainage of, 4436–4437
environment of, 179
initial care for, 4430–4431, *4431–4433*
management of, for thermal burns, 802–807, 803*t*, 804*t*, *806*, *807*
W-plasty
and Z-plasty, in depressed scars of partially avulsed trapdoor flaps, 64–65, *65*
contraindications for, 64
for abdominoplasty, *3943*, *3944*
for lower lip reconstruction, 2015, *2016*
indications for, 64
technique of, 63–64, *63*, *64*
Wright's maneuver, 5000, 5002, *5001*
Wrinkles
dermabrasion of, 774, 777, *778*
facial, chemical peeling for, 758, *758*, *759*
Wrist
anatomy of, 4725–4726, *4726*
dorsal compartments of, 4725, *4725*
of bones in, 4630, *4630–4632*
of ligaments in, 4630–4633, *4632–4634*
of triangular fibrocartilage complex, 4629, *4630*, *4631*
arthrodesis of
complications of, 4681–4682
general considerations for, 4678
indications for, 4678
limited, 4682–4686, *4683–4685*
operative techniques for, 4678–4681, *4680*, *4681*
de Quervain's disease of, 4731, 4733–4738, *4733–4738*
disarticulation of, 4340–4341, *4341*
distal radioulnar joint problems of, in rheumatoid arthritis, 4712–4713, *4713*, *4714*
extension of, 4569
in radial palsy, 4942
flexor tendon laceration of, 4537–4538
in hand surgery for spastic or stroke patient, 4981–4982
injuries of, 4635
dislocations of carpal bones in, 4640–4641, *4641*
fractures of carpal bones in, 4640–4646, *4642–4646*
to distal radius, 4635*t*, 4635–4638, *4636–4638*
to distal ulna, 4638–4640, *4639*, *4640*
intersection syndrome of, 4739
kinetics of, 4634–4635
longitudinal absence deformities of ulna, clinical presentations of, 5275
motion of, 4258
nerve entrapment syndromes of, 4725–4726
roentgenographic evaluation of, 4288–4289
skeletal system of, 4258–4261, *4260*
tendon and nerve entrapement of, associated disorders of, 4739, *4740–4742*, *4741–4746*, *4744*, *4746–4751*, 4749, 4752
tendon entrapment syndromes of, 4725–4726
Wrist blocks, 4323, *4324*
Wrist disarticulation, vs. below the elbow amputation, 4342

Wrist powered active prostheses, 4395–4396
Wrist pulley, 4265–4266, *4267*
Wynn method for bilateral cleft lip repair, 2687, 2689, *2690*

Xenografts, 54, 225, 542
Xeroderma pigmentosum
  basal cell carcinoma and, 3616–3617
  squamous cell carcinoma and, 3629
X-rays, 832

Y-V advancement flap, 289, *289*

Zigzag incisions, 4441–4442, *4442*
Zinn, annulus of, 1672, *1672*
Zisser-Madden method, for upper lip reconstruction, 2030, *2031*
Zona pellucida, 2730
Z-plasty
  and W-plasty, in depressed scars of partially avulsed trapdoor flaps, 64–65, *65*
  compound right angle in, 63, *63*
  contraindications for, 64
  design of, 57–58, *58*
  development of, 55–56
  double reverse, for cleft palate repair, 2701, 2739–2742, *2740*
  double-opposing, 61, *61*
    for correction of epicanthal fold, 1616
    for epicanthus correction, 1777, *1777*
  elongation, degree of, 57
  for Apert's syndrome treatment, 5298–5300, *5299*
  for correction of misalignment of vermilion border, 2791, *2791*
  for limited cervical contracture, 2076, *2076*
  for linear scar contracture in nasal stenosis, 1975, *1976*
  for neck scarring, 2190, 2192
Z-plasty *(Continued)*
  for realignment of scar in lines of minimal tension, 57–58, *58*
  for symblepharon correction, 1742, *1743*
  four-flap, 61, *61, 62*
  "half-Z" procedure for, 58, *59*
  indications for, 64
  of alar rim, 1936, *1938*, 1940
  purposes of, 55
  scar appearance and, 742, *742, 743*
  technical aspects of, 4445, 4447–4448, *4446, 4447*
  technique of, *56, 56–57, 57*
  variations in technique, 58–62, *59, 60, 61*
Zyderm collagen, 781–784
Zygoma
  anatomy of, 991–992, *992, 1577*, 1580
  deformities of, 1655, 1657
  depression deformities of, 1665, 1667, *1666*
  fractures of
    classification of, 996
    comminuted, 1001–1002, *1003*
    complications of, 1007–1009, *1007, 1008*
    compound comminuted, 1006–1007, *1007*
    computed tomography of, 998, *999, 1000*
    delayed treatment of, 1006–1007, *1007*
    diagnosis of, *995*, 997–998, *997, 998*
    in children, 1165, 1167, *1166–1167*
    intraoral approach, *1003*, 1004
    pin fixation of, 1004, *1004*
    surgical pathology of, 992–993, 996, *993, 994, 996*
    treatment of, 998, 1000–1001, *1000–1002*
  hypoplasia of, surgical correction of, in Down syndrome, 3169, *3170*
  malunited fractures of, *1664*, 1665, *1665*
    treatment of, 1665, 1667, *1666*
  reconstruction of
    by advancement osteotomy augmentation, 1663, 1665, *1664*
    by alloplast augmentation, *1656*, 1657, *1658*
    by calvarial bone flap augmentation, 1659, 1663, *1662, 1663*
    by cartilage/bone graft, 1657, *1659–1661*
Zygomatic maxillary-mandibular osteotomies, for craniosynostosis, 3045, *3048–3050*
Zygomaticomaxillary buttress, 1021
Zyplast collagen, 781–784

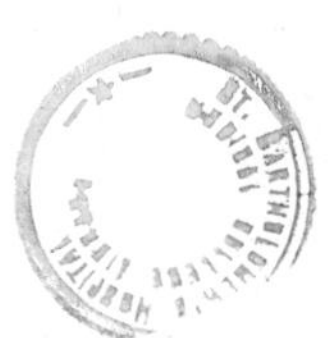